DENTAL ASSISTING

A COMPREHENSIVE APPROACH

Fifth Edition

DENTAL ASSISTING
A COMPREHENSIVE APPROACH

Fifth Edition

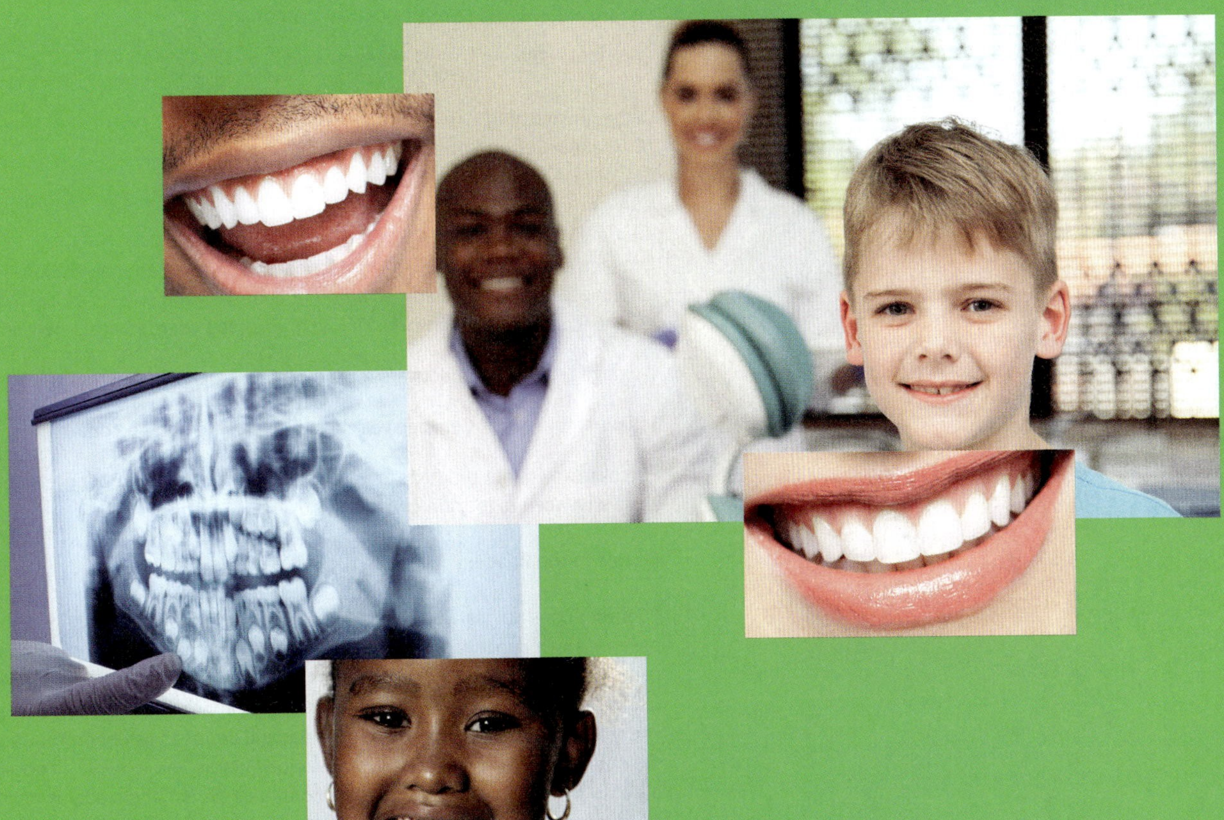

DONNA J. PHINNEY, CDA, FADAA, BA, MED

Professor Spokane Community College

JUDY H. HALSTEAD, CDA, BA

Professor Emeritus Spokane Community College

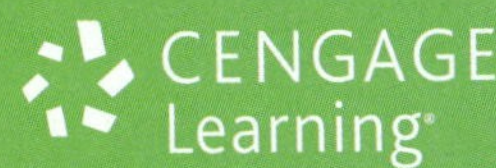

CENGAGE Learning®

Australia • Brazil • Mexico • Singapore • United Kingdom • United States

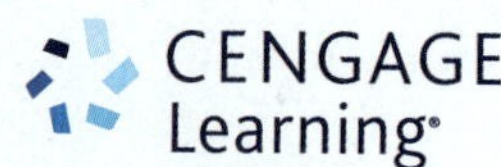

Dental Assisting: A Comprehensive Approach, Fifth Edition
Donna Phinney and Judy Halstead

SVP, GM Skills & Global Product Management: Jonathan Lau

Product Team Manager: Matthew Seeley

Associate Product Manager: Lauren Whalen

Senior Director, Development: Marah Bellegarde

Senior Product Development Manager: Juliet Steiner

Senior Content Developer: Darcy M. Scelsi

Product Assistant: Mark Turner

Vice President, Marketing Services: Jennifer Ann Baker

Marketing Manager: Jonathan Sheehan

Senior Production Director: Wendy Troeger

Production Director: Andrew Crouth

Senior Content Project Manager: Kenneth McGrath

Senior Art Director: Jack Pendleton

Cover images: kurhan/Shutterstock.com; karelnoppe/Shutterstock.com; michaeljung/Shutterstock.com; wavebreakmedia/Shutterstock.com

For product information and technology assistance, contact us at
Cengage Learning Customer & Sales Support, 1-800-354-9706
For permission to use material from this text or product,
submit all requests online at **www.cengage.com/permissions**.
Further permissions questions can be e-mailed to
permissionrequest@cengage.com

Library of Congress Control Number: 2016961828

Book Only ISBN: 978-1-305-96763-2

Cengage Learning
20 Channel Center Street
Boston, MA 02210
USA

Cengage Learning is a leading provider of customized learning solutions with employees residing in nearly 40 different countries and sales in more than 125 countries around the world. Find your local representative at **www.cengage.com**.

Cengage Learning products are represented in Canada by Nelson Education, Ltd.

To learn more about Cengage Learning, visit **www.cengage.com**

Purchase any of our products at your local college store or at our preferred online store **www.cengagebrain.com**

Notice to the Reader

Publisher does not warrant or guarantee any of the products described herein or perform any independent analysis in connection with any of the product information contained herein. Publisher does not assume, and expressly disclaims, any obligation to obtain and include information other than that provided to it by the manufacturer. The reader is expressly warned to consider and adopt all safety precautions that might be indicated by the activities described herein and to avoid all potential hazards. By following the instructions contained herein, the reader willingly assumes all risks in connection with such instructions. The publisher makes no representations or warranties of any kind, including but not limited to, the warranties of fitness for particular purpose or merchantability, nor are any such representations implied with respect to the material set forth herein, and the publisher takes no responsibility with respect to such material. The publisher shall not be liable for any special, consequential, or exemplary damages resulting, in whole or part, from the readers' use of, or reliance upon, this material.

Printed in the United States of America

Print Number: 01 Print Year: 2017

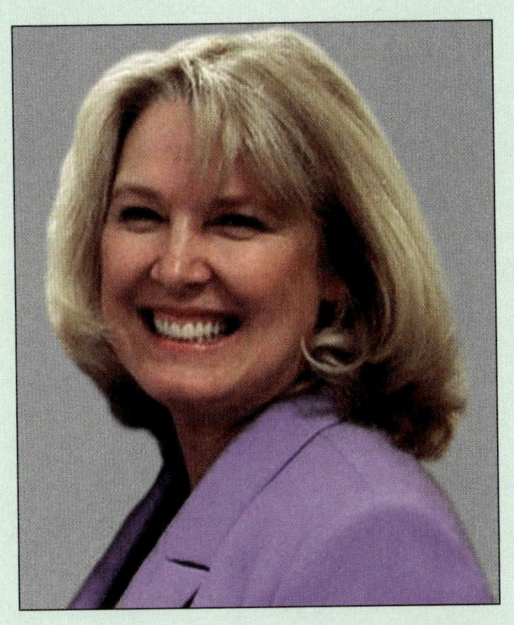

In Memory

This fifth edition was completed and is dedicated to Donna's memory. Never did I ever think I would be writing this dedication. There really are not words or maybe there are just too many. I have been so blessed to have had Donna in my life as a coworker, team mate, coauthor, friend and "sister." Donna and I took a journey together that took us in many amazing directions. We shared a love of dental assisting, the dental profession and especially of teaching dental assisting students. The biggest and best opportunity and adventure was authoring this textbook for dental assistants together. Through this experience we kept our love for dental assisting education and yet entered a whole new world of publishing. We have worked together for many years on the original textbook and then on each new edition. I am so grateful to have had this opportunity to work with my best friend-sister. She was dedicated, positive, supportive, forward thinking, and just plain fun. Now as I look back I can clearly see the wonderful journey Donna and I had. I miss her greatly and this textbook will be our bond forever. Many thanks to Darcy and all from Cengage Learning for their patience and assistance in completing this fifth edition, it has been difficult to say the least, but I know Donna would be proud of the results. Thank you.

Judy

I met and began working with Donna over 11 years ago when we began the revision of the third edition of the book. We developed a great relationship both professionally and personally. We would often exchange book suggestions, comparisons of the weather here in the east versus out west, and exchange stories about what was happening in our lives. I especially loved hearing about the wildlife that would end up in her yard—most particularly the moose. Trips out to Spokane for photo shoots were always a treat due to her hospitality. She enjoyed sharing the history and sites of a very lovely city. She tried many a time to get me out on a jet ski and I am sorry to say that never happened. To say it has been very difficult to complete the fifth edition of the book would be an understatement.

Donna touched the lives of so many people. She treated her students like family. When working with all of them at the school their respect and admiration of her was always quite apparent. She cared and went above and beyond in providing the support and assistance they needed. She had a quiet, soft-spoken manner and a smile that brightened a room. She will be missed as an author, an educator, a mother, and a wife. Donna, thank you for enriching my life and for sharing your knowledge, skills, and compassion with so many of us.

Darcy and all of us at Cengage Learning

BRIEF CONTENTS

LIST OF PROCEDURES

CONTENTS

NEW TO THIS EDITION

Chapter 1

- Added discussion of:
  - Dr. Samuel D. Harris
  - Expanded Function Dental Assistant
  - Sterilization Assistant

Chapter 2

- Added discussion of:
  - Dental phobias and patient concerns
  - Generation "Z"
  - Stress in the dental office
  - Conflict resolution

Chapter 3

- Added discussion of emotional abuse, domestic violence, and elder abuse
- Some additional minor updates and points of clarification

Chapter 4

- Added discussion of:
  - Updates related to the latest advances in mechanical toothbrushes
  - Fluoride varnish, including the procedure for application
- Revised content on age characteristics into tabular form for ease of comprehension

Chapter 5

- Added discussion of:
  - Technology-related health and fitness devices, such as the FitBit, as well as a variety of fitness and weight loss apps.
  - Trend of consumption of energy drinks and shots
  - Add more on diet and culture and how it relates to oral health

Chapter 10

- Added discussion of:
  - MRSA
  - Swine Influenza
  - Ebola
  - Pandemic

Chapter 11

- Added discussion of:
  - National Institute of Health
  - National Institute of Occupational Safety and Health
  - Recommendations for environmental infection control
  - Greener infection control
  - Surface disinfectants
  - Sanitation and disinfection wipes
  - Mechanical sterilization monitoring
  - Updated CDC regulations/recommendations throughout
  - Expanded content on dental unit waterlines
  - Procedure for treatment of dental unit waterlines

Chapter 12

- Includes updates to the Hazardous Materials Standard including
  - Switch from MSDS to SDS
  - Hazard communication pictograms
  - Globally Harmonized System of Classification and Labeling of Chemicals (GHS)

Chapter 15

- Includes an added discussion of pharmacokinetics

Chapter 16

- Added the following procedures:
  - Treating the patient with asthma
  - Treating the hyperventilating patient
  - Treating patients experiencing a seizure
  - Treating a hypoglycemic patient
  - Treating the patient with angina

Chapter 17

- Minor updates throughout, particularly of updates to equipment

Chapter 18

- Added three procedures: identification of cutting, non-cutting, and rotary instruments.
- Added discussion on the ultrasonic and laser handpiece.

Chapter 19

- Content on the dental dam, formerly covered in Chapter 34, has been moved to this chapter.

Chapter 21

- Updates throughout the chapter

Chapter 22

- Added procedure for the assembly of film positioning devices
- Added discussion of care for visually and hearing impaired patients
- Added discussion on the communication of radiation risks

Chapter 23

- Updated to include more content and discussion related to digital radiography

Chapter 24

- Added more information on the endodontic microscope

Chapter 25

- Added discussion of surgical rotary instruments
- Content on dental implants has been moved to its own chapter (see Chapter 26).
- Added discussion of paresthesia as a complication of dental surgery

Chapter 26

- Content on dental implants has been moved to its own chapter; this was formerly covered in Chapter 25.

Chapter 27

- Formerly Chapter 26
- Added discussion of thrush, cellulitis, oral cancer, and leukemia

Chapter 28

- Formerly Chapter 27
- Added discussion of short-term orthodontic treatment for cosmetic reasons

Chapter 29

- Formerly Chapter 28
- Added discussion of patients with special needs
- Added discussion of diet and its relationship to pediatric dentition
- Content on dental sealants has been moved to its own chapter (see Chapter 30)

Chapter 30

- Content on dental sealants has been moved to its own chapter; this was formerly covered in Chapter 28.
- Content has been expanded to cover more detail in types of materials and techniques.

Chapter 31

- Formerly Chapter 29
- Expanded discussion of the use of lasers
- Added discussion of additional types of graft surgeries
- Added discussion of periodontal plastic surgery
- Content on coronal polish has been moved to its own chapter (see Chapter 32).

Chapter 32

- Content on coronal polish, formerly covered in Chapter 29, has been moved to its own chapter, this was formerly covered in Chapter 29.

Chapter 33

- Formerly Chapter 30
- Added information on digital shade guides
- Added discussion of the steps for fixed prosthesis procedures

Chapter 34

- New chapter covering CAD/CAM systems
- Expanded on information and added a procedure

Chapter 35

- Formerly Chapter 31
- Added content on in office whitening with the laser
- More information on patient preparation and maintenance.

Chapter 36

- Formerly Chapter 32
- Added discussion of home care instructions

Chapter 37

- Formerly Chapter 33
- Added discussion of fluoride varnish
- Added procedure for placement of desensitizing agents
- More content on the types of glass ionomer cements

Chapter 38

- Formerly Chapter 34
- Dental dam content moved to its own chapter (see Chapter 19)

Chapter 39

- Formerly Chapter 35
- Updates to materials where appropriate
- Content on CAD/CAM moved to Chapter 34

Chapter 40

- Formerly Chapter 36
- Added discussion of online marketing, websites, and social media, as well as paperless practices
- Eliminated content on paging systems
- Minimized content on pegboard systems and expanded content on computerized billing systems

Chapter 41

- Formerly Chapter 37
- Added discussion of state requirements

PREFACE

The world of health care changes rapidly. The twenty-first century presents health care professionals with more challenges than ever before—but with challenge comes opportunity. Job prospects for dental assistants have never been better. The Bureau of Labor Statistics expects employment in our field to grow much faster than the average for all occupations through the year 2024. Population growth and greater retention of natural teeth will fuel demands for dental services. As the health care industry requires more services to be completed by dentists, the dental assistant will be more valuable and needed than ever before. Many states are passing legislation allowing for an expansion in the skills that dental assistants can provide—with additional training. Placing restorations, obtaining virtual impressions, and monitoring general sedation are a few examples.

As dental assistants, you'll be expected to take on an increasing number of clinical and administrative responsibilities to stay competitive. Now is the time to equip yourselves with the range of skills and competencies you'll need to excel in the field. Now is the time to maximize your potential, to expand your base of knowledge, and to dedicate yourself to become the multi-faceted dental assistant required in the twenty-first century.

This text and complete learning system, *Dental Assisting: A Comprehensive Approach*, fifth edition, will guide you as a dental assisting student on this journey. The result of years of research, writing, and testing, this system is designed to prepare the dental assisting student for the Dental Assisting National Board (DANB) certification examination, some state credentialing and the workplace. It presents information in a unique manner, using a variety of formats that account for the many ways in which today's students learn.

To receive the full value of *Dental Assisting: A Comprehensive Approach*, fifth edition, it's important to understand the structure of the text, chapters, and supplements and how they are all integrated into a complete learning system. Together, these materials will make your dental assisting education comprehensive and meaningful, providing you with the skills, knowledge, principles, values, and understanding needed to excel in your chosen profession.

The Learning System

The components of the learning system were developed with today's learner in mind. The authors and Cengage Learning recognize that students learn in different ways—they read, write, listen, watch, interact, and practice. For this reason, we've created a variety of products learners can use to fully comprehend and retain what they are taught. An instructor's manual ties the components together, making classroom integration easy and fun.

The Text

This text delivers comprehensive coverage of dental assisting theory and practice, supported by full-color illustrations and photographs throughout with 169 step-by-step procedures in nine sections. Section I—*Introduction*—introduces learners to the profession and its history as well as communication and legal issues. Section II—*Prevention and Nutrition*—covers general techniques to maintain health and wellness of the oral cavity and the dentition. Section III—*Basic Dental Sciences*—covers the basics of general anatomy, head and neck anatomy, embryology, histology, tooth morphology, charting, and microbiology, creating a foundation on which learners can move forward in skills training. Section IV—*Preclinical Dental Skills*—prepares students in the areas of infection control, hazardous materials management, patient care, pharmacology, and emergency management, which are critical elements to the profession. Section V—*Clinical Dental Procedures*—the introduction to the dental office and equipment, covers chairside assisting, instruments, and the management of pain and anxiety. Section VI—*Dental Radiography*—provides updated information on radiographic techniques and procedures, including the latest on digital and 3-D radiography. Section VII—*Dental Specialties*—introduces learners to the specialized areas of endodontics, oral maxillofacial surgery, dental implants, oral pathology, cosmetic dentistry, orthodontics, pediatric dentistry, periodontics, fixed prosthodontics, computerized impression and restorative systems, and removable prosthodontics. This section also includes information on advanced functions, such as coronal polish, dental sealants, and tooth whitening and retraction cord placement. Section VIII—*Restorative and Laboratory Materials and Techniques*—covers chairside restorative materials and techniques, and laboratory and impression materials and techniques. Section IX—*Dental Practice Management*—contains coverage of dental office management, dental computer software, dental insurance, employment portfolios, and legal and ethical considerations, which are important components for managing a dental practice properly.

HANDWASHING

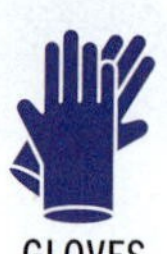
GLOVES

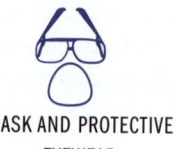

MASK AND PROTECTIVE EYEWEAR

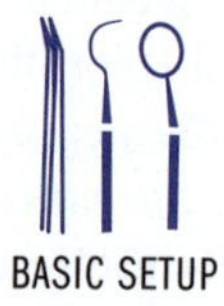
BASIC SETUP

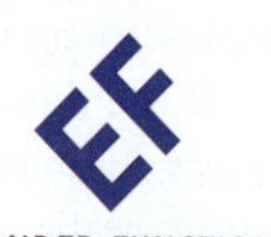
EXPANDED FUNCTIONS

LEGAL

SAFETY

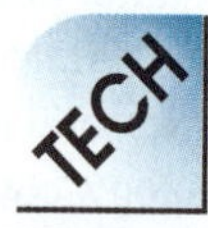

TECHNOLOGY

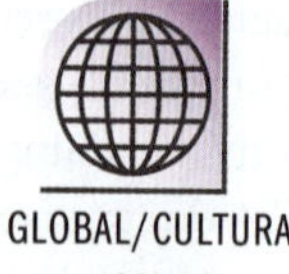
GLOBAL/CULTURAL ISSUES

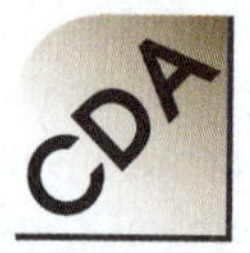

DANB EXAM COMPONENT

Each chapter includes the following pedagogical features:

- Specific Instructional Objectives
- Key Terms (key terms also appear in color in the text)
- Pronunciation of difficult terms the first time they appear in the text
- Introduction
- Step-by-step procedures with icons indicating handwashing, gloves, mask and protective eyewear, basic setup, and expanded functions
- In-text icons identifying legal, safety, technology, and global/cultural issues, as well as DANB exam components
- Boxed information containing tips and summaries
- Summary
- Case Studies
- Web Activity boxes
- Review questions, including critical thinking

MindTap

It's 1 AM, there are 20 tabs open on your computer, you lost your flashcards for the test, and you're so tired you can't even read. It'd be nice if someone came up with a more efficient way of studying. Luckily, someone did. With a single login for MindTap® Dental Assisting for *Dental Assisting: A Comprehensive Approach*, fifth edition you can connect with your instructor, organize coursework, and have access to a range of study tools, including the ebook and apps all in one place!

- **Manage your time and workload without the hassle of heavy books!** The MindTap Reader keeps all your notes together, lets you print the material, and will even read text out loud.
- **Need extra practice?** Find pre-populated flashcards and the entire e-book in the MindTap Mobile App, as well as quizzes and important course alerts.
- **Want to know where you stand?** Use the Progress app to track your performance in relation to other students.
- **Engage with the material.** Videos and animations help your understanding of key concepts while simulations and quizzing helps you bridge the gap from learning to real-world application.
- The **MindTap eReader** takes the textbook experience to a whole new level with the ability to have the material read to you with **Readspeaker**, print the material and take it with you for on the go preparation, and take notes or highlights within the eReader, which feeds to the StudyHub App for easy study guide creation.
- The **New MindTap Mobile App** not only includes access to the ebook both online and off, but keeps you connected to your instructor and your course with alerts and notifications. It also arms you with on-the-go study tools like flashcards and quizzing, helping you to manage your limited time efficiently.
- **Flashcards** are pre-populated to provide a jump-start on your course preparation and studying. You can also create your own customized cards as you move through the course material.

Instructor Companion Web Site

An Instructor Companion Web Site is available to facilitate classroom preparation, presentation, and testing. This content can be accessed through your Instructor SSO account. To set up your account:

- Go to www.cengagebrain.com/login.
- Choose **Create a New Faculty Account**.
- Next you will need to select your **Institution**.
- Complete your personal **Account Information**.
- Accept the **License Agreement**.
- Choose **Register**.
- Your account will be pending validation—you will receive an email notification when the validation process is complete.
- If you are unable to find your Institution, complete an **Account Request Form**.

Once your account is set up, or if you already have an account:

- Go to www.cengagebrain.com/login.
- Enter your email address and password and select **Sign In**.
- Search for your book by author, title, or ISBN.
- Select the book and click **Continue**.
- You will receive a list of available resources for the title you selected.
- Choose the resources you would like and click **Add to My Bookshelf**.

Components available on the Instructor Companion Web Site include a(n):

- Computerized test bank, a 2,300-question bank with questions geared to text chapters and the DANB exam; available for download in many different LMS options

- Instructor presentations on PowerPoint™ with talking points, designed to support and facilitate classroom instruction
- An electronic version of the *Instructor's Manual*, so that notes and ideas can be customized
- Dental assisting curriculum cross referencing all of Cengage Learning's dental assisting materials to create a dynamic learning system
- Correlation guide to help make a smooth transition from the third edition to the fourth edition
- Additional handouts on Key Terms Review and additional activities such as crossword puzzles, word searches, matching, and labeling exercises
- Skill checklists to use for student evaluation.

- **Student Workbook (Order #978-1-3059-6764-9)**
  The workbook, which corresponds to the text, contains chapter objectives, summaries, exercises in a variety of formats, and skill sheets to test competencies. The workbook contains a section with activities that allow you to practice with the Dentrix software.

- **Other Supporting Materials Include:**
  - Dental Terminology, 3rd Edition (Charline Dofka) (Order #978-1-13301-9718)
  - Dental Assisting Coloring Book (Donna Phinney and Judy Halstead) (Order #978-1-4390-5931-9)
  - Dental Assisting Instrument Guide (Donna Phinney and Judy Halstead) (Order #978-1-1336-9159-4)
  - Dental Assisting Materials Guide (Donna Phinney and Judy Halstead) (Order #978-1-4180-5199-0)
  - Dental Assisting Video Series (Order #978-1-4180-2963-0)

  When you use all these components together, you'll discover an innovative, comprehensive system of teaching and learning that prepares students for success in the twenty-first century.

About the Authors

Donna J. Phinney is the Program Director for Spokane Community College's Dental Assisting Program. She has spent more than 25 years in the dental field as a dental assistant, a dental office consultant, an office manager, and an educator. Donna holds a bachelor of arts from Eastern Washington University, a master in education from Whitworth College, and an associate of science and certificate in dental assisting from Spokane Community College. A certified dental assistant, she is active in the Washington State Dental Assisting Association, where she served as president from 1992 to 1993. She obtained her fellowship from the American Dental Assisting Association in 2002. Donna was a consultant for the American Dental Association, Commissioner on Dental Accreditation for 17 years and was on the Dental Assisting Review Committee, and she was a Commissioner for the American Dental Association, appointed by the American Dental Assistants Association.

Judy H. Halstead is Professor Emeritis at Spokane Community College. She has more than 25 years' experience teaching and more than 10 years' experience as a dental assistant. She was a program director for dental assisting in a private college and for a high school skills center. Judy holds a bachelor of arts from Eastern Washington University, is a certified dental assistant, and has an expanded functions certificate. She has been a member of local, state, and national Dental Assistants Associations for the past 25 years. She served as president of the Washington State Dental Assisting Association from 1994 to 1995. Judy has presented lectures and workshops at local, state, and regional dental conferences.

Acknowledgments

The authors would like to thank Cengage Learning and its staff, whose assistance and encouragement in this pursuit are greatly appreciated.

We would also like to thank the many dentists with whom we have had the opportunity to work and who made dental assisting a career to be proud of.

We would like to thank our peers across the nation, especially the Allied Health Department and staff and friends at Spokane Community College, who encouraged us throughout this endeavor. The students, who in the end make everything worthwhile, are to be thanked for their desire to learn and the ongoing challenge they present to their instructors.

We would like to thank our daughters, Heidi and Traci, who continue to love and support us and who took part in this revision.

Last, but never least, we would like to thank our husbands, Dwayne and Chuck, and our families, who supported and encouraged us throughout this project. Their understanding, patience, and love allowed us to stay on track and to complete the task at hand. Thank you!

We also want to thank the following individuals and facilities for providing valuable assistance in the development and production of this project:

- Pat Norman, CDA, who continues to give so much; we appreciate all her help in revising the chapters on radiography and orthodontics.
- Helen Fairchild, RDA, for revising chapters on Management of Hazardous Materials and Laboratory Materials and Techniques.
- Cynthia Lamkin, RDA, RDH, for revising the chapter on Dental Office Management.
- Julie Davitt, CDA, who supported and encouraged us throughout this project.
- Peg Jacobs Bloy, CDA, RDH, MS, and Middlesex Community College, for their coordination and assistance while allowing us to photograph in their facility.

- Rita Johnson, CDA, COA, RDH, MA, and Dr. Vincent DeAngelis, who provided assistance and many pictures for the text.
- Dr. Clifton Caldwell, who continues to help us with our endeavors both in student education and in publishing.
- Dr. Dale Ruemping, Dr. Steven Crump, Dr. Ola England, Dr. George Velis, Dr. Gary Shellerud, Dr. Dwight Damon, Dr. Earl Ness, Drs. Rodney Braun and Chris Chaffin, and Dr. Steven Gregg, who continue to help us with student education, and provided pictures for the text.
- The reviewers who spent their time and energy to make this a better text.
- Anderson's Dental Laboratory, for continuing to help us with student education, and providing pictures and models for the text.
- Dr. Joseph Konzelman, who provided many pictures for the text.
- Dr. Steven Bates, Dr. Greg Miller, and their staff for assisting us with numerous photos of their office.
- Nici Roberts, CDA, who assisted with photos and time.
- Kathy Thurber, Dental Assistant, who assisted with photos and time.
- Dr. Jay Enzler, pediatric dentist, who allowed us to take numerous photos of his entire pediatric office, including photos of his staff and patients during routine procedures.
- Dr. Duane Grummons, orthodontist, who allowed us to take photos of his office and provided us with additional photos of advanced technology for use in the textbook.
- Dr. Charles Rigalotto, general and cosmetic dentist, and his assistant Judy Miner, for assisting us with numerous photos of his office, equipment, and tray setups.
- Students in the Dental Assisting Class of 2011–2012. With special thanks to Stephanie Alcock, Ivan Chavdar, Rebekah Ehlers, Aimee Nimri, Heather Layson and Alysia Cross and her children. Johnson, Stephanie Mueller, Laura Potts, Kristine Smasel, Hong-Van tran, and Amorette Verduin for going the extra mile.
- Dr. Dale Ruemping, pediatric dentist; Dr. Kenji Higuchi, oral maxillofacial surgeon; and Dr. Steven Crump, general dentist, for providing pictures of various procedures and techniques.
- Troy Schmidt, sales representative for KaVo Technologies/ Gendex Imaging.

Reviewers of the Fifth Edition

Terri Bannor
Northwest Technical College

Miriam Chacon
Passaic County Technical Institute

Cindy Cronick, BS, CDA
Metro Community College in Omaha

Cynthia Gasparik, CDA
Institute of Medical Careers

Robin Givens, CDA
Westwood College

Yolanda Johnson Gray
Fortis College

Carol Hall-Pace
Martin Luther King Jr. Career Center

Tija Hunter, CDA, EFDA, CDIA, FADAA
Dental Careers Institute

Shauna Phillips
Fortis College

Judith Shannon, CDA, RDH
Massasoit Community College

Donna Zagame, AS
Milwaukee Career College

Reviewers of the Fourth Edition

Annette Scranton, EFDA
Remington College/West Campus
North Olmsted, Ohio

Bobby A. Sconyers, BA, CDA, CPFDA
Professor
South Florida State College
Avon Park, Florida

Connie Myers Kracher, PhD, MSD
Chair, Department of Dental Education
Indiana University-Purdue University Fort Wayne
Fort Wayne, Indiana

Deborah K. LeBeau, AACOM, CDA
Fortis College
Stow, Ohio

Diana M. Sullivan, CDA, LDA, M.Ed
Program Director
Dakota County Technical College
Rosemount, Minnesota

Jan DeBell, CDA, EFDA, BS
Front Range Community College
Fort Collins, Colorado

Jennifer Dumdei, LDARF, CDA
South Central College
North Mankato, Minnesota

Jill Brunson, CDA, RDA
Dental Assisting Instructor
Texas State Technical College Harlingen
Harlingen, Texas

Joyce T. Uyeda Yamada, CDA, RDH, MS
Program Coordinator and Instructor
University of Hawaii Maui College
Maui, Hawaii

Judith A. McCauley, RDH, MA
Associate Professor
Chair, Dental Hygiene Department
Palm Beach State College
Lake Worth, Florida

Kerri H. Friel, RDH, COA, CDA, MA
Dental Health Programs, Assistant Professor
Community College of Rhode Island
Lincoln, Rhode Island

Lea Anna Harding, CDA, B.S.Ed
Gwinnett Technical College
Lawrenceville, Georgia

Michelle Bissonette, CDA, EFDA, BS
Indiana University School of Dentistry
Bloomington, Indiana

Professor Teresa A. Macauley, CDA, EFDA, MS
Ivy Tech Community College of Indiana
Kokomo, Indiana

Stephanie Joyce Schmidt, CDA, CPFDA, CDT, RDAEF2, MS
Pasadena City College
Pasadena, California

Stephanie Olson, BA, CDA
Coordinator, Dental Assisting Program
University of Alaska Anchorage
Anchorage, Alaska

Terry R. Dean, DMD
Associate Professor
Western Kentucky University
Bowling Green, Kentucky

Tracie E. West
Dental Assistant
Remington College-Cleveland West
North Olmsted, Ohio

Reviewers of the First, Second, and Third Editions

Betty Ladley Finkbeiner, CDA, RDA, BS, MS
Washtenaw Community College
Ann Arbor, Michigan

Cynthia S. Cronick, CDA, AAS, BS
Dental Assisting Instructor
Southeast Community College
Lincoln, Nebraska

Denis Campopiano, CDA, RDH, BS
Dental Assisting Program Director
Ogeechee Technical College
Statesboro, Georgia

Dennis Garcia, DMD, RDA
Curriculum Manager, Health Sciences
Corinthian Colleges, Inc.

Diana M. Sullivan
Director Dental Assisting Program/Instructor
Dakota County Technical College
Rosemount, Minnesota

Heidi Denson
Instructor
Ogden Weber Applied Technology
Ogden, Utah

Janet Wilburn, BS, CDA
Director Dental Assisting Program
Phoenix College
Phoenix, Arizona

Jenny Schuler, CDA, BS
Dental Assistant Instructor/Program Coordinator
Bellingham Technical College
Bellingham, Washington

Karen F. Sperry, CDA, RDA, BVE
Professor Emeritus Dental Assisting
College of the Redwoods
Eureka, California

Kathy Foust, CDA, MS
Western Wisconsin Technical College
LaCrosse, Wisconsin

Kelly Svanda, CDA
Southeast Community College
Lincoln, Nebraska

Krista M. Rodriguez, RDH, CDA, BA, NYCDA, FADAA
Assistant Professor
Monroe Community College
Rochester, New York

Le Ann Schoelne, CDA, RDA, RF, BS
Director, Dental Assisting Program
Central Lakes College
Brainerd, Minnesota

Linda Kay Hughes, RDA, NRDA
Owner/Educator
PDE/Excelle College
San Diego, California

Lynette Sickelbaugh, CDA
Dental Assisting Instructor
Washington Local Adult Education
Toledo, Ohio

Lynn Tyler
Director, Dental Assisting Program
The American Institute of Medical-Dental Technology
Provo Utah

Marie Desmarais Cecil, CDA, MA
Central Community College
Hastings, Nebraska

Pamela G. Zarb, CDA, RDA, RDH, MA
Dental Assisting Program Discipline Chair
Wayne County Community College
Detroit, Michigan

Paulette Kehm-Yelton, CDA, EFDA, MPA
Assistant Professor
Northeast State Community College
Elizabethton, Tennessee

Rebecca Mattney, CDA, RDA
Vatterott College
Springfield, Missouri

Robert Bennett, DMD
Texas State Technical College
Harlingen, Texas

Robin Caplan, CDA
Medsafe, Inc.
Waltham, Massachusetts

Sandra Lo, DDS
Sacramento City College
Sacramento, California

Sharon K. Dickinson, CDA, CDPMA, RDA
Professor
Dental Assisting Program Director

El Paso Community College
El Paso, Texas

Sheila Semler, CDA, RDH, MS, PhD
San Juan College
Farmington, New Mexico

Stephanie J. Schmidt, CDA, RDAEF, CDI, CDT, BA, MS
Faculty
Pasadena City College
Pasadena, California

Susan Thaemert, CDA, RDA, BS
Hennepin Technical College
Minneapolis, Minnesota

Valerie Blackenship, CDA, RDA
Program Director
Simi Valley Adult School and Career Institute
Simi Valley, California

Vivian Koistinen, ASDA
Corporate Dental Assistant Program Manager
High Tech Institute, Inc.
Phoenix, Arizona

HOW TO USE THIS TEXT

Dental assisting is an ever-evolving profession full of opportunity and challenge. *Dental Assisting: A Comprehensive Approach*, fifth edition, is designed to help you acquire the knowledge, skills, and values necessary to become a successful dental assistant. The text is organized into nine main sections that reflect the broad areas of dental assisting responsibility. These sections are then divided into a total of 41 chapters of related information. The text has many unique features that will make it easier for you to learn and integrate theory and practice, including:

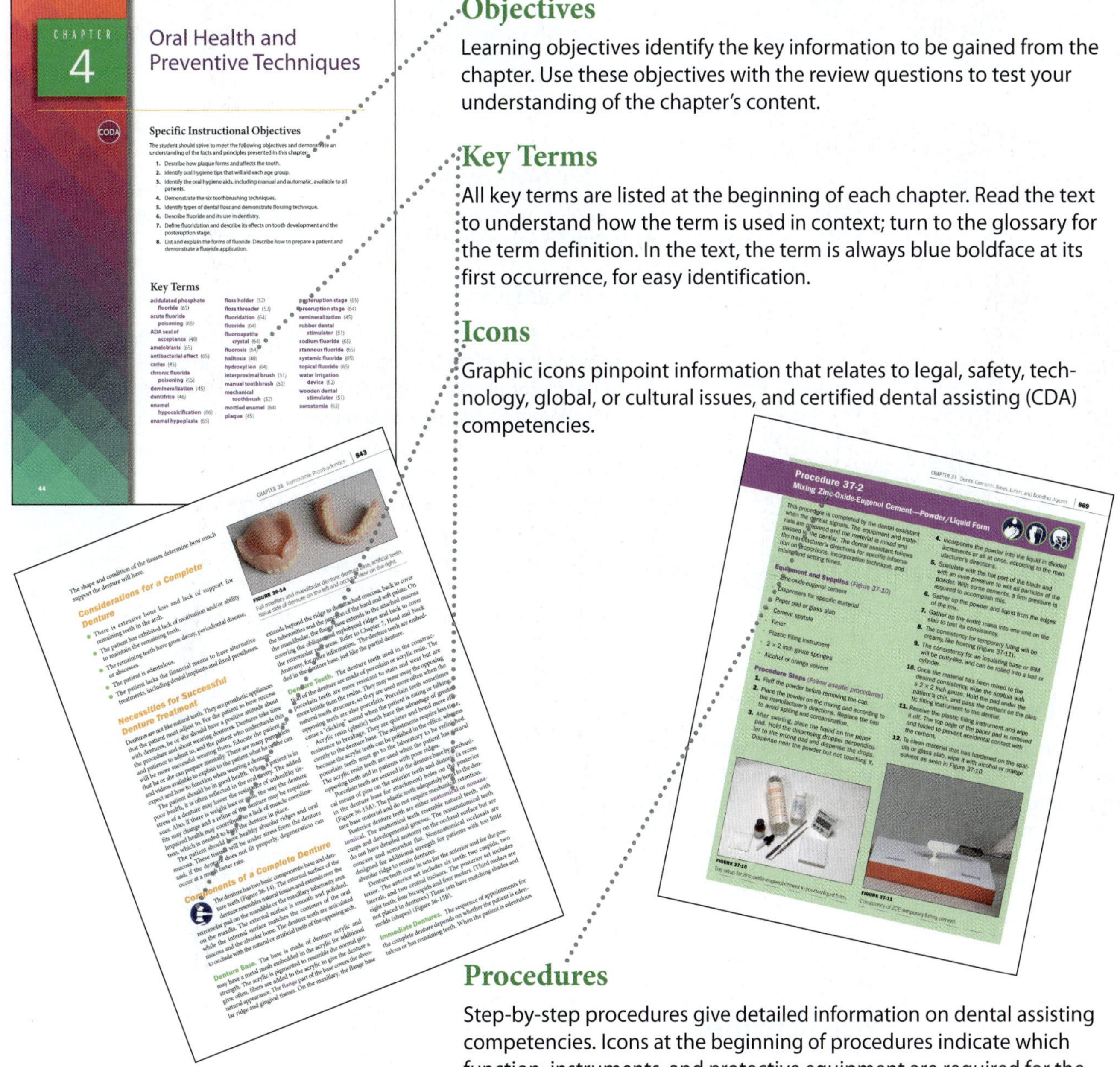

Objectives

Learning objectives identify the key information to be gained from the chapter. Use these objectives with the review questions to test your understanding of the chapter's content.

Key Terms

All key terms are listed at the beginning of each chapter. Read the text to understand how the term is used in context; turn to the glossary for the term definition. In the text, the term is always blue boldface at its first occurrence, for easy identification.

Icons

Graphic icons pinpoint information that relates to legal, safety, technology, global, or cultural issues, and certified dental assisting (CDA) competencies.

Procedures

Step-by-step procedures give detailed information on dental assisting competencies. Icons at the beginning of procedures indicate which function, instruments, and protective equipment are required for the procedure.

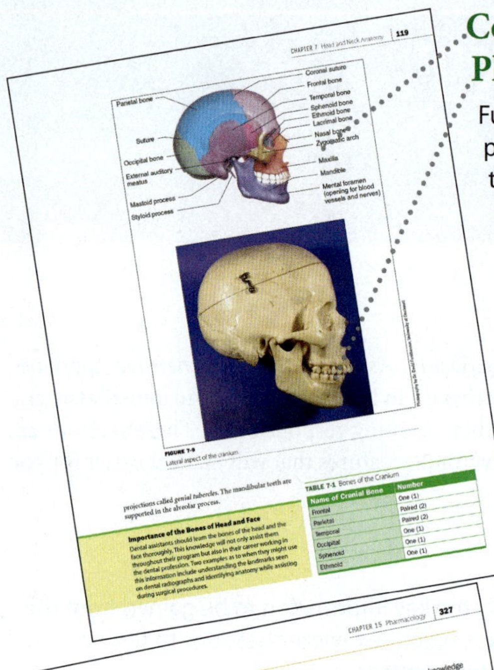

FIGURE 7-9
Lateral aspect of the cranium.

projections called genial tubercles. The mandibular teeth are supported in the alveolar process.

Importance of the Bones of Head and Face

TABLE 7-1 Bones of the Cranium

Name of Cranial Bone	Number
Frontal	One (1)
Parietal	Paired (2)
Temporal	Paired (2)
Occipital	One (1)
Sphenoid	One (1)
Ethmoid	One (1)

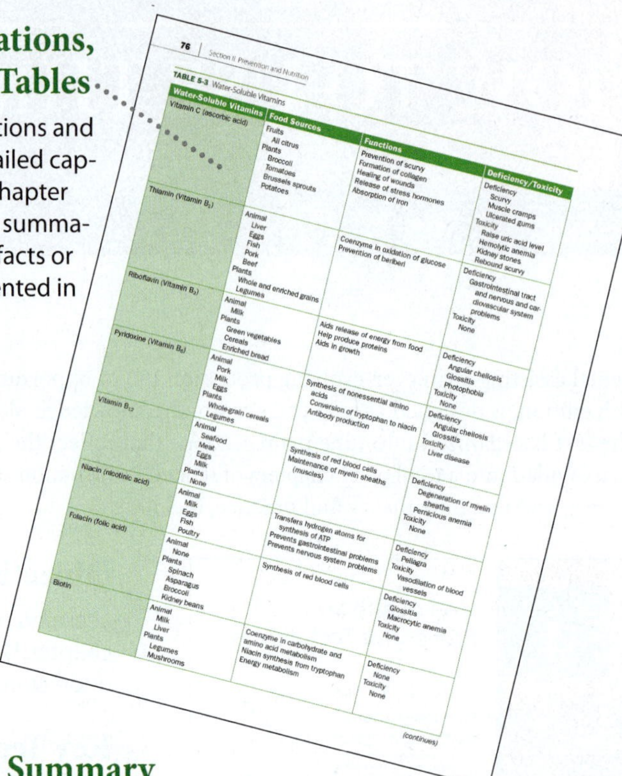
76 | Section II Prevention and Nutrition

TABLE 5-3 Water-Soluble Vitamins

Water-Soluble Vitamins	Food Sources	Functions	Deficiency/Toxicity
Vitamin C (ascorbic acid)	Fruits All citrus Plants Broccoli Tomatoes Brussels sprouts Potatoes	Prevention of scurvy Formation of collagen Healing of wounds Release of stress hormones Absorption of iron	Deficiency Scurvy Muscle cramps Ulcerated gums Toxicity Raise uric acid level Hemolytic anemia Kidney stones Rebound scurvy
Thiamin (Vitamin B_1)	Animal Liver Eggs Fish Pork Beef Plants Whole and enriched grains Legumes	Coenzyme in oxidation of glucose Prevention of beriberi	Deficiency Gastrointestinal tract and nervous and cardiovascular system problems Toxicity None
Riboflavin (Vitamin B_2)	Animal Milk Plants Green vegetables Cereals Enriched bread	Aids release of energy from food Help produce proteins Aids in growth	Deficiency Angular cheilosis Glossitis Photophobia Toxicity None
Pyridoxine (Vitamin B_6)	Animal Pork Milk Eggs Plants Whole-grain cereals Legumes	Synthesis of nonessential amino acids Conversion of tryptophan to niacin Antibody production	Deficiency Angular cheilosis Glossitis Toxicity Liver disease
Vitamin B_{12}	Animal Seafood Meat Eggs Milk Plants None	Synthesis of red blood cells Maintenance of myelin sheaths (muscles)	Deficiency Degeneration of myelin sheaths Pernicious anemia Toxicity None
Niacin (nicotinic acid)	Animal Milk Eggs Fish Poultry	Transfers hydrogen atoms for synthesis of ATP Prevents gastrointestinal problems Prevents nervous system problems	Deficiency Pellagra Toxicity Vasodilation of blood vessels
Folacin (folic acid)	Animal None Plants Spinach Asparagus Broccoli Kidney beans	Synthesis of red blood cells	Deficiency Glossitis Macrocytic anemia Toxicity None
Biotin	Animal Milk Liver Plants Legumes Mushrooms	Coenzyme in carbohydrate and amino acid metabolism Niacin synthesis from tryptophan Energy metabolism	Deficiency None Toxicity None

(continues)

Color Illustrations, Photos, and Tables

Full-color illustrations and photos with detailed captions reinforce chapter material. Tables summarize important facts or concepts presented in the text.

CHAPTER 15 Pharmacology | 327

Chapter Summary

At no other time have drugs been as widely used and misused as they are today. The dental assistant will need to pay attention to the patient's medical and dental history and carefully document the drugs used by the patient. The dental assistant will have to become knowledgeable about pharmacology, the side effects of drugs, and drug interactions. Dental assistants are concerned with prescribed drugs, but they must also have knowledge about the illegal drugs that patients may be using, and what will happen if the two types of drugs interact. It is also important to know the signs and symptoms that individuals may experience if under the influence of drugs. Background knowledge about drugs and their effects aids the dental assistant in providing better patient care.

CASE STUDY

Jordan Taylor, a 20-year-old male, comes in because an upper anterior tooth is abscessed. He is a smoker and has just had four shots of espresso (coffee) in a drink. He seems nervous about the upcoming treatment. Further information obtained from Jordan is that he has also had two regular soft drinks and a candy bar in the past two hours.

Case Study Review

1. What reaction should the dental team expect from Jordan due to the drugs he has ingested recently?
2. Are these drugs stimulants or depressants?
3. Would giving other drugs to Jordan be a problem?

Review Questions

Multiple Choice

1. The most commonly used resource to obtain information about drugs in the dental office is (the)
   a. *United States Pharmacopoeia.*
   b. *National Formulary.*
   c. *Dental Therapeutics.*
   d. *Physician's Desk Reference.*
2. Dental ointment that is placed on the mucosal surface is administered by which route?
   a. Sublingual
   b. Oral
   c. Topical
   d. Intravenous
3. Addictive depressants used to relieve pain are
   a. narcotics.
   b. amphetamines.
   c. hallucinogens.
   d. barbiturates.
4. The legislation that was established to identify drugs according to five schedules of abuse potential is the
   a. Pure Food, Drug, and Cosmetic Act.
   b. Comprehensive Drug Abuse Prevention and Control Act of 1970.
   c. Occupational Safety and Health Act.
   d. Controlled Substances Act.
5. If an antibiotic is said to be broad spectrum, it means that
   a. a culture can be taken to identify the type of microorganism.
   b. many microorganisms resist it.
   c. it causes side effects, such as nausea or an allergic rash.
   d. it is effective against a wide range of bacteria.
6. The drug schedule number that has the highest abuse potential, and is more dangerous is
   a. Schedule I.
   b. Schedule II.
   c. Schedule III.
   d. Schedule IV.
7. The route of administration of a drug that is delivered right under the skin level is
   a. intravenous.
   b. intramuscular.
   c. subcutaneous.
   d. intradermal.
8. Tylenol with codeine is under which schedule number of controlled substances?
   a. Schedule I
   b. Schedule II
   c. Schedule III
   d. Schedule IV

Chapter Summary

The chapter summary emphasizes key concepts from the chapter to help you focus on your study.

Case Studies

The case studies and review questions present real-life scenarios requiring a problem/solution approach. Use the case studies to put your knowledge into practice and to arrive at a deeper understanding of the dental assisting profession.

CHAPTER 12 Management of Hazardous Materials | 269

Review Questions

Multiple Choice

1. The Bloodborne and Hazardous Materials Standard covers all the following except
   a. housekeeping.
   b. laundry.
   c. hours of employment.
   d. safety data sheets.
2. An example(s) of engineering or work practice controls is (are)
   a. personal protective equipment.
   b. splash guards on model trimmers.
   c. gloves, masks, and glasses.
   d. dental uniforms.
3. After an exposure incident, the employer provides a copy of the health care professional's written opinion within ____ days of a completed evaluation.
   a. 5
   b. 10
   c. 15
   d. 30
4. The color and number method often used to label various chemicals was developed by the
   a. Occupational Safety and Health Administration.
   b. American Dental Association.
   c. Environmental Protection Agency.
   d. National Fire Protection Association.
5. A skull and crossbone pictogram indicates
   a. a health hazard.
   b. acute toxicity or fatal.
   c. corrosion.
   d. PPE is needed.
6. Broken glass must be cleaned up and placed in ____
   a. a plastic bag
   b. a leak-proof sharps container
   c. a cardboard container
   d. a garbage container
7. Yellow on the chemical warning label determination identifies a
   a. fire hazard.
   b. health hazard.
   c. PPE is needed.
   d. reactivity or stability of a chemical.
8. The OSHA hazard communication standard is set up so that the ____ receives training about the risks of using hazardous chemicals and the safety precautions.
   a. employee
   b. employer
   c. patient
   d. both a and b
9. The following are accepted work practice controls except
   a. no two-handed recapping.
   b. no bending of needles.
   c. mouth pipetting.
   d. handwashing following glove removal.
10. The housekeeping area of the OSHA Bloodborne and Hazardous Materials Standard shows that all of the following must be done except
    a. following a written schedule for cleaning and disinfection.
    b. protective covering may be used over equipment.
    c. carpets in all operatories.
    d. If no contamination has occurred, the equipment and surfaces must be cleaned at the end of the work shift.

Critical Thinking

1. Would the scope of the OSHA Bloodborne and Hazardous Materials Standard cover the employee while traveling to the place of employment?
2. Employees have a lunchroom that becomes untidy and disorderly. The dentist never uses the lunchroom. If one of the employees has an accident in the room, who is responsible?
3. Standard precautions are issued by whom? To protect whom?

Web Activities

1. Go to http://www.osha.gov and find information on SDSs and print the two pages of requirements for the OSHA 174 document.
2. Go to http://www.osha.gov and find information about biohazardous waste. Have there been any changes in this area since the publication of this textbook? If so, note these changes and bring information to class for discussion.
3. Go to the Web and identify a source with a list of SDSs. Find two chemicals that are used in the school clinic. Were they on the list you found? What information did you find on the SDSs for the two identified chemicals?

Review Questions

Test your comprehension of the chapter with structured multiple-choice questions and open-ended critical thinking questions that require you to combine an understanding of chapter material with your personal insight and judgment.

Web Activities

Internet exercises in each chapter encourage Web searches to locate information.

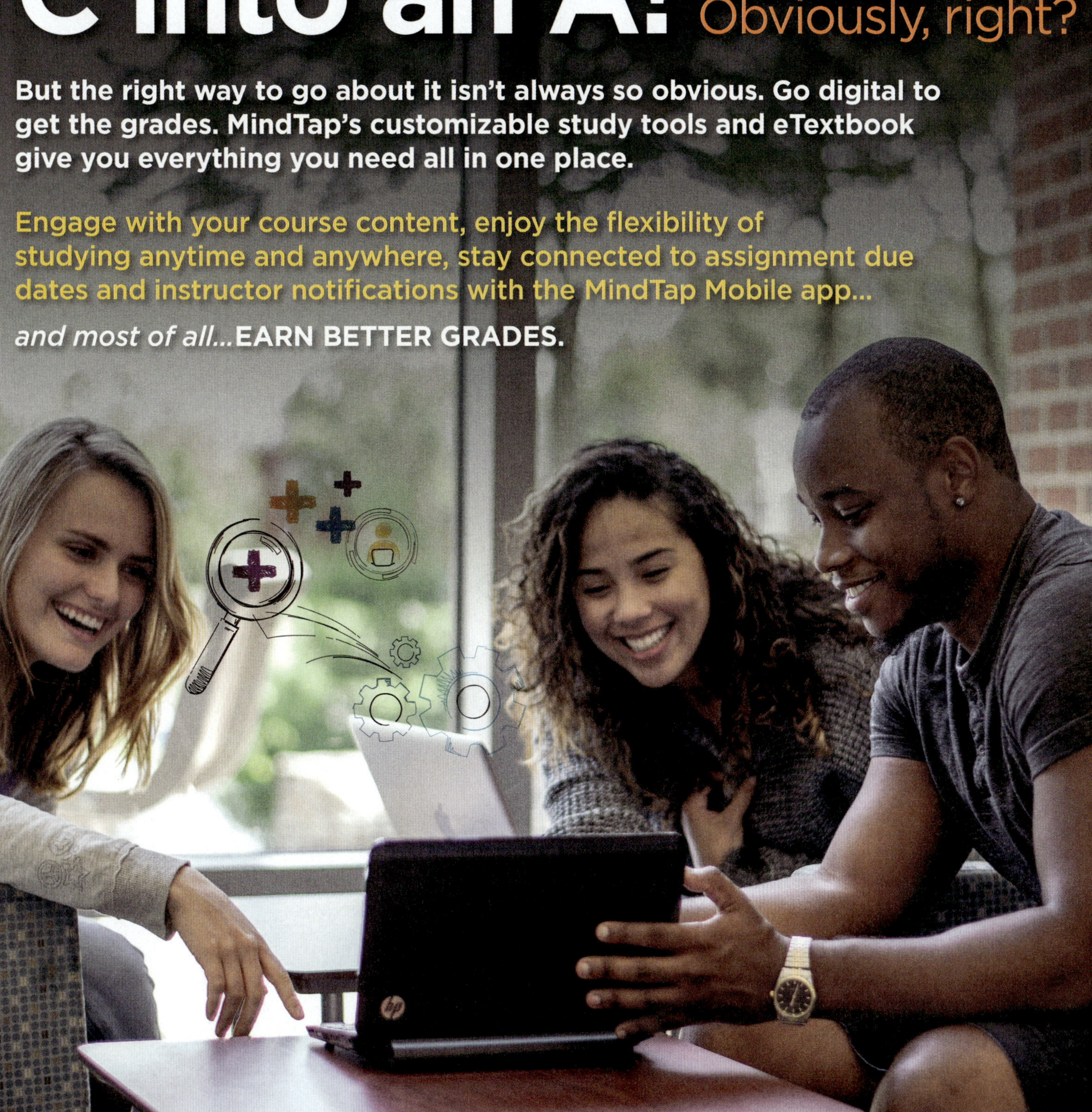
Want to turn your
C into an A? Obviously, right?
But the right way to go about it isn't always so obvious. Go digital to get the grades. MindTap's customizable study tools and eTextbook give you everything you need all in one place.
Engage with your course content, enjoy the flexibility of studying anytime and anywhere, stay connected to assignment due dates and instructor notifications with the MindTap Mobile app...
and most of all...EARN BETTER GRADES.
TO GET STARTED VISIT
WWW.CENGAGE.COM/STUDENTS/MINDTAP
CENGAGE Learning
MindTap®

Section I

Introduction

CHAPTER

1

Introduction to the Dental Profession

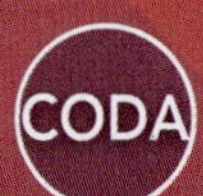

Specific Instructional Objectives

The student should strive to meet the following objectives and demonstrate an understanding of the facts and principles presented in this chapter:

1. Review dental disease and dentistry from the "beginning of time."
2. Identify the items on the timeline of dental history.
3. Name the individuals who had a great impact on the profession of dentistry.
4. Identify the people who promoted education and organized dentistry.
5. Explain what DDS and DMD stand for.
6. Identify the nine specialties of dentistry.
7. Describe, generally, the career skills performed by dental assistants, dental hygienists, and dental laboratory technicians.
8. List the education required for, and the professional organizations that represent, each dental career path.

Key Terms

American Dental Assistants Association (ADAA) (10)
American Dental Association (ADA) (7)
American Dental Hygienists' Association (ADHA) (12)
American Dental Laboratory Technician Association (ADLTA) (12)
certified dental assistant (CDA) (10)
Chapin A. Harris (6)
Dental Assisting National Board, Inc. (DANB) (10)
Dental public health (9)
Dr. C. Edmund Kells (10)
Dr. Greene Vardiman Black (7)
Dr. Samuel D. Harris (6)
Endodontics (9)
Expanded Function Dental Assistant (10)
forensic dentistry (9)
Guy de Chauliac (4)
Hippocrates (4)
Horace H. Hayden (6)
James B. Morrison (6)
John Greenwood (5)
Josiah Flagg (5)
Juliette Southard (10)
Lucy Beaman Hobbs Taylor (7)
Oral and maxillofacial pathology (9)
Oral and maxillofacial radiology (9)
Oral and maxillofacial surgery (9)
Orthodontics and dentofacial orthopedics (9)
Paul Revere (5)
Pediatric dentistry (9)
Periodontics (9)
Pierre Fauchard (4)
Prosthodontics (9)
Robert Woofendale (5)
sterilization assistant (10)
Wilhelm Conrad Roentgen (5)

Introduction

Humans have been plagued with dental problems from the very beginning of time. Over the years, a number of different dental treatments were tried and perfected. Tools of various types were developed and used to repair and clean teeth.

It is important to be familiar with the historic struggles that took place and contributions that were made to advance the dentistry profession into what it is today (Table 1-1).

History of Dentistry

Beginning in ancient times, dental work was done by physicians. Often, each physician specialized in only one area of care for one part of the body. In fact, during the fifth century BC, a Greek historian named Herodotus wrote that medicine had become so fragmented that each physician was a specialist in a particular disease. "All the country is full of physicians, some of the eyes, some of the teeth, some of what pertains to the belly, and some of the hidden diseases." One Egyptian doctor of teeth named Hesi-Re, the first dentist whose name was recorded, practiced in 3000 BC.

TABLE 1-1 Timeline of Dental History

Era	Events
Beginning of time	Tooth decay is noted.
3000 BC	First dentist, Hesi-Re, is recorded.
460–322 BC	Written information about tooth decay is recorded by Aristotle and Hippocrates.
460–377 BC	Oath of Hippocrates (Hippocrates).
384–322 BC	Attention to oral hygiene (Diocles of Carystus).
1300–1368	Hygienic rules (Guy de Chauliac).
1452–1519	Tooth morphology identified (Leonardo da Vinci).
1678–1761	Founder of modern dentistry (Pierre Fauchard).
1760–1819	Josiah Flagg develops the dental chair.
1768–1770	Paul Revere places advertisements in a Boston newspaper offering his services as a dentist.
1790	James B. Morrison constructs the first known dental foot engine, which he adapted from his mother's spinning-wheel foot treadle.
1832	James Snell invents the first reclining dental chair.
1840	Horace Hayden and Chapin Harris establish the Baltimore College of Dental Surgery.
1840	American Society of Dental Surgeons established.
1841	Alabama enacts the first dental practice act to regulate dentistry.
1844	Horace Wells, a Connecticut dentist, discovers that nitrous oxide can be used for dental pain relief.
1859	American Dental Association (ADA) created.
1866	Lucy Beaman Hobbs Taylor, the first woman to earn a dental degree, graduates from Ohio College of Dental Surgery.
1869	Dr. Robert Tanner Freeman, the first African-American to earn a dental degree, graduates from Harvard University Dental School.
1871	First commercially manufactured foot-treadle dental engine is patented by James B. Morrison.
1885	First "lady in attendance" employed by Dr. C. Edmund Kells.
1890	Dr. Ida Gray, the first African-American woman to earn a dental degree, graduates from University of Michigan School of Dentistry.
1895	X-rays discovered (Wilhelm Conrad Roentgen).
1907	"Lost wax" casting machine is invented by William Taggart.
1913	Fones School of Dental Hygiene established.
1923	American Dental Hygienists' Association (ADHA) created.
1924	American Dental Assistants Association (ADAA) established; first president was Juliette Southard.
1930	First dental specialty board is founded, the American Board of Orthodontics.
1938	First synthetic bristle (nylon) toothbrush appears on the market.

(continues)

TABLE 1-1 Timeline of Dental History (continued)

Era	Events
1945	Water fluoridation era begins in the cities of Newburgh, New York and Grand Rapids, Michigan.
1947	Dental Assisting National Board, Inc. (DANB) is established.
1950	First fluoride toothpastes are marketed.
1960	Four-handed, sit-down dentistry is utilized.
1970	The Occupational Safety and Health Administration is created by the U.S. Congress.
1982	Hepatitis B vaccine becomes available.
1989	Tooth-whitening commercial products are marketed.
1992	Occupational Safety and Health Administration's Bloodborne Pathogens Standard becomes effective.
1997	The laser, approved by the Food and Drug Administration, is used to treat tooth decay.

Dentistry during these early times primarily consisted of removing teeth when pain occurred. Some evidence has been found on human skulls that holes were drilled near the roots to allow infection to drain so that pressure in an abscessed tooth could be relieved. Other dental problems that date from ancient times derived from food preparation techniques. Grains were ground in stone bowls with stone pestles. During this process, particles of stone mixed with the grain. This grit in the food caused severe wear of the biting (occlusal) surfaces of the teeth and possible pulp exposure.

Hippocrates (460–377 BC), the father of medicine, attempted to explain health and disease. He suggested that four main fluids in the body, namely blood, black bile, yellow bile, and phlegm, along with heat, cold, dry air, and wet air, must remain in balance. Disruption of these four fluids and four elements would result in disease. Among Hippocrates' numerous writings is a book titled *On Affections*. In this book he wrote, "Teeth are eroded and become decayed partly by the mucus, and partly by food, when they are by nature weak and badly fixed in the mouth." Even though much of what Hippocrates thought about health and teeth was inaccurate, his writings provided much-needed information for the progress of medicine. Even today, the Oath of Hippocrates is used as a basis for the code of ethics used by the medical and dental professions in regard to the solemn obligation these professionals undertake when caring for patients.

During Aristotle's time (384–322 BC), some attention was given to oral hygiene and this was reflected in his writings. An Athenian physician, Diocles of Carystus, stated that oral hygiene should get proper attention, and he even gave instructions to this end. During the next couple of centuries, more importance was placed on good oral hygiene. A number of cleaning powders were made from crushed bones, oysters, and egg shells. At times, these substances were mixed with honey to make a paste to clean with. Guests in the homes of the wealthy who were invited to dinner were given silver- and even gold-decorated toothpicks with which to clean their teeth after the meal. At the time, picking one's teeth was considered proper etiquette.

Later Progress of Dentistry

In France, a surgeon named **Guy de Chauliac** (1300–1368) became one of the fourteenth century's most influential authors on surgery. He also wrote the "Hygienic Rules for Oral Hygiene."

Hygienic Rules for Oral Hygiene,
Written by Guy de Chauliac

1. Avoid food that putrefies readily.
2. Avoid food or drink that is too hot or too cold, and especially avoid swallowing extremely cold food after extremely hot food, and vice versa.
3. Do not bite into things that are too hard.
4. Avoid foods that stick to the teeth, such as figs and confections made with honey.
5. Avoid certain foods known to be bad for the teeth (his example was leeks).
6. Clean the teeth gently with a mixture of honey and burnt salt to which some vinegar has been added.

It is now known that the information given by de Chauliac was not entirely accurate. However, because it was based on sound logic, much of it is used today. For example, it is well known that sticky, sweet foods increase dental decay. In his writings, de Chauliac noted that surgery on the teeth should be performed under the supervision of doctors but could be done by "barbers or dentatores." This notation was the first to refer to "dentatores," the specific group of practitioners caring for the oral cavity and the teeth.

During the fifteenth and sixteenth centuries, artists became more interested in human anatomy to enhance the accuracy of their artwork. Leonardo da Vinci (1452–1519) painstakingly dissected the human skull and then drew his discoveries. He was the first to make a distinction between premolars and molars. His writings further define the morphology of teeth.

Pierre Fauchard (1678–1761), a French dentist, organized all known information about dentistry in a manuscript titled

"Le Chirurgien Dentiste," relating to a title he used to refer to himself as a surgical dentist. It was clearly written and had step-by-step pictures that depicted easy-to-follow procedures. In those times, dentistry was about removing teeth and he was one of the few who restored teeth. He rejected the idea that a tooth worm caused decay and noted that "caries" (his term for decay) were a result of a "hormonal imbalance." Fauchard wrote of his perceived causes of decay and prevention techniques and was an early advocate of treating diseased gingival tissue. He combined early information and operative methods for replacing or transplanting teeth. He even noticed that he could straighten teeth by using gold braces that were fastened by waxed linen or silk threads and allowed the teeth to follow a pattern of wires. He went to jewelers, barbers, and watchmakers to gather ideas for instruments that could be used on teeth. Pierre Fauchard developed a manual drill for use in dentistry that was powered by a catgut twisted around a cylinder. Fauchard perfected a number of dental treatments and instruments that are still used today, almost three centuries later. Many refer to Pierre Fauchard as the "Founder of Modern Dentistry."

Wilhelm Conrad Roentgen (1845–1923), a German physicist, discovered X-rays in 1895. This discovery allowed dentists to further their knowledge of the diseases and structures of the mouth.

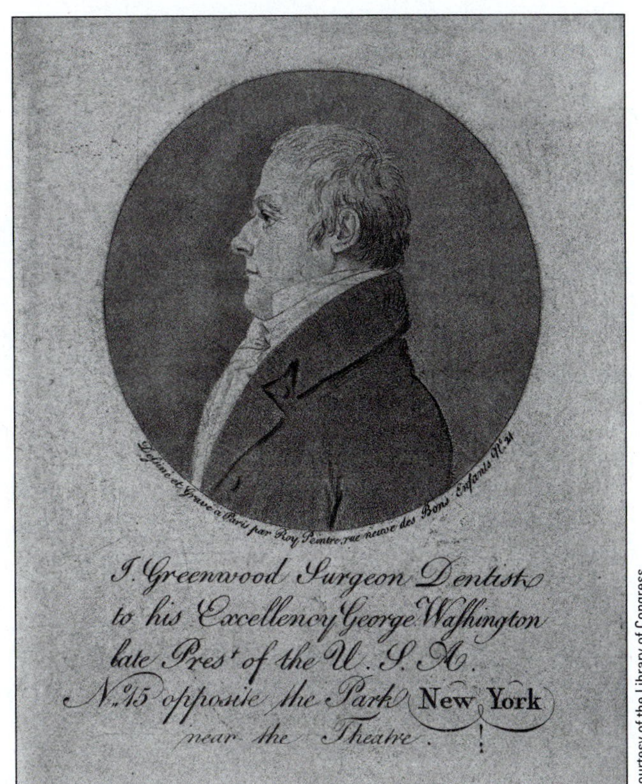
I. Greenwood Surgeon Dentist
to his Excellency George Washington
late Pres^t of the U.S.A.
N°15 opposite the Park New York
near the Theatre

Courtesy of the Library of Congress

FIGURE 1-1
John Greenwood

Progress of Dentistry in the United States

One of the first dentists to arrive in the United States from England was **Robert Woofendale**. Woofendale placed an advertisement in the *New York Mercury* on November 17, 1766, stating that he "performs all operations upon the teeth, sockets, gums, and palate, likewise fixes artificial teeth, so as to escape discernment." Soon after Woofendale arrived, John Baker came and started advertising in the Boston area. He spoke and wrote about fillings and artificial teeth. Baker was well known and was one of the dentists who treated George Washington. **John Greenwood** (1760–1819) was said to be the first president's favorite dentist (Figure 1-1). Greenwood had very little formal education but was a proficient practitioner in the eighteenth century. He thought children should care for their teeth and offered parents reduced rates for children's dental care. He also thought that tartar came from bad breath and was adamant about the regular removal of it for good oral health.

At one time or another, George Washington was probably treated by every notable dentist of the time. A number of references in his diary note continual pain and discomfort from his teeth. At the time the picture that is currently on the one-dollar bill was painted, the president had only one tooth left, a lower left bicuspid (premolar). In fact, the artist had to pad out the cheeks and lips with cotton to give the president's sunken face a more normal appearance. Washington's last set of dentures, made by Greenwood, were comprised of ivory and gold and had two springs holding them together (Figure 1-2). A number of dentures were made for the president; however, contrary to popular belief, they were not made of wood.

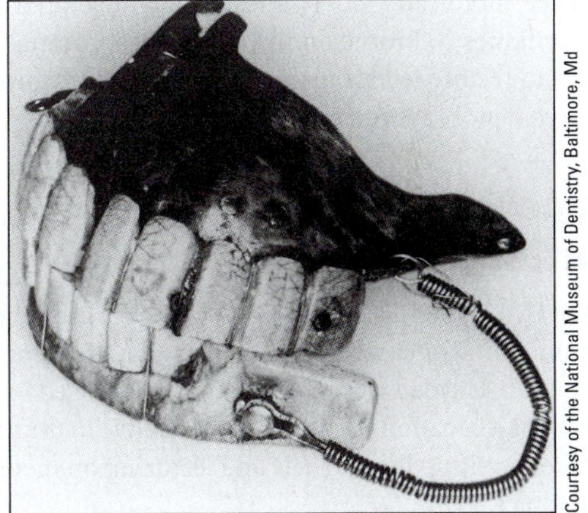

Courtesy of the National Museum of Dentistry, Baltimore, Md

FIGURE 1-2
The last dental prosthesis worn by George Washington was made for him by John Greenwood. It is made of gold and ivory and is held together with springs.

Paul Revere (1735–1818), a silversmith (Figure 1-3), was a dentist for several years, but his greatest contribution to dentistry was in his making surgical instruments and artificial teeth. He may have had a part in training a notable dentist of the late 1700s, **Josiah Flagg**. Flagg's father was a partner to Revere. Flagg, a skilled surgeon, was accomplished in corrective procedures on cleft lips, orthodontics, endodontics, and operative dentistry. However, one of his major contributions to dentistry

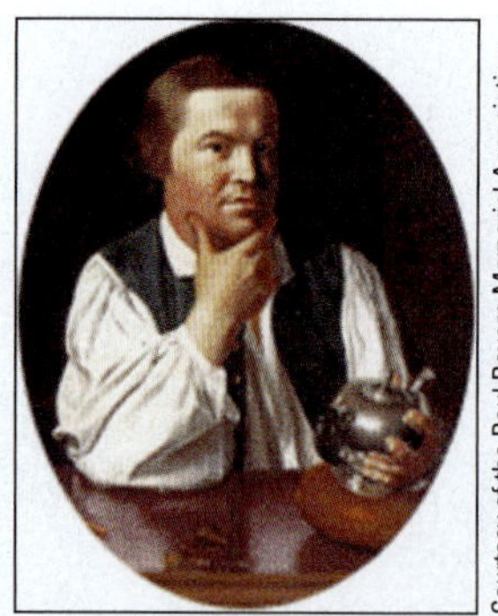

FIGURE 1-3

Paul Revere, shown as a silversmith.

was the construction of a dental chair. It had an extension on the arm to hold dental instruments and an adjustable head rest.

In the early 1800s, U.S. dentistry took a giant leap forward. The establishment of a popular democracy—with the opportunity for personal financial gain, free public school education, and population growth—prompted some of the most notable dentists in the world to relocate to America. The literature and knowledge base expanded a great deal during this time. Most large cities now had resident dentists rather than traveling barbers who extracted teeth and sold tooth powders. The dentists of the time were better educated and involved in the communities they served. The profession was progressing far beyond massive tooth removals and occasional cleanings. Additionally, as dental techniques improved and developed, so did dental materials. The first dental engine with a functioning handpiece, motor, and foot treadle was manufactured and patented by **James B. Morrison** in 1871. This apparatus allowed dentists to restore teeth much more quickly. Organized dentistry was rapidly approaching.

Education and Organized Dentistry

Horace H. Hayden (1769–1844) (Figure 1-4) sought dental care from John Greenwood, the dentist who cared for George Washington. Hayden was inspired and encouraged to take up dentistry as a vocation. He became very active in the dentistry profession, writing for journals and lecturing on medical and dental topics.

One of the students who studied with Hayden was **Chapin A. Harris** (1806–1860) (Figure 1-5). Harris believed in education and built an extensive library of dental literature, including his own work, *The Dental Art: A Practical Treatise on Dental Surgery*. Due to the efforts of Hayden and Harris, the first dental college in the world, the Baltimore College of Dental Surgery, was founded on March 6, 1840. It is now called the School of Dentistry at the University of Maryland, and is the home of the Dr. Samuel Harris National Museum of Dentistry.

Dr. Samuel D. Harris, whom the museum was named after, was instrumental in founding the museum. It is the largest and most complete museum of dental artifacts and history (Figure 1-6). Visitors can learn about the heritage of dentistry

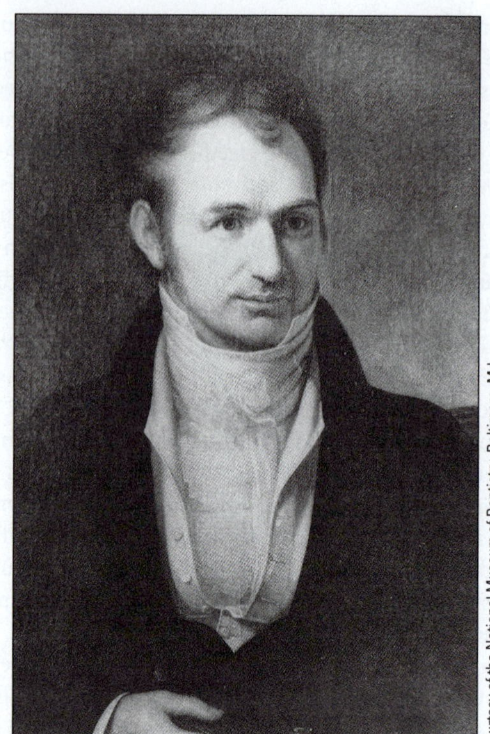

FIGURE 1-4

Horace Hayden, one of the founders of professional dentistry in the United States, helped establish the world's first dental college.

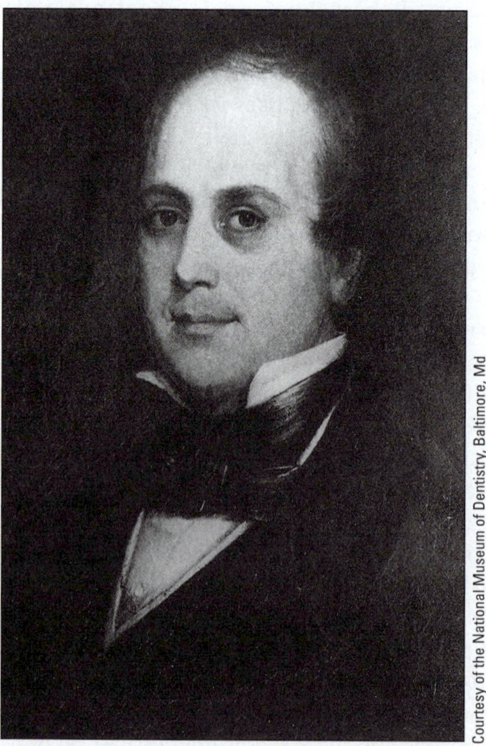

FIGURE 1-5

Chapin Harris, one of the founders of professional dentistry in America, helped establish the first dental college in the world and the first national association representing dentistry.

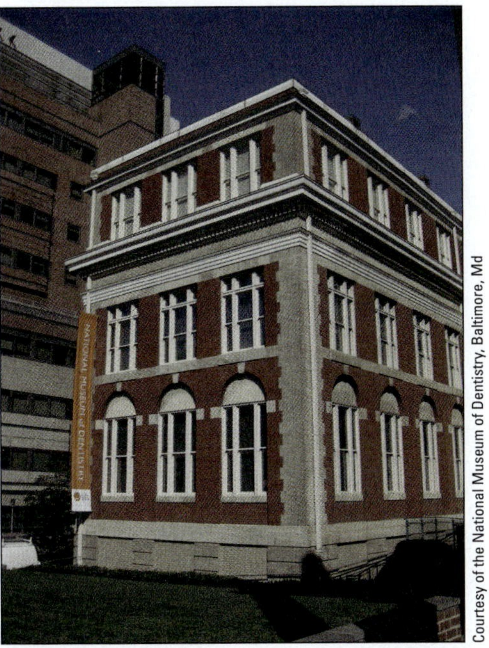

Courtesy of the National Museum of Dentistry, Baltimore, Md

FIGURE 1-6
National Museum of Dentistry

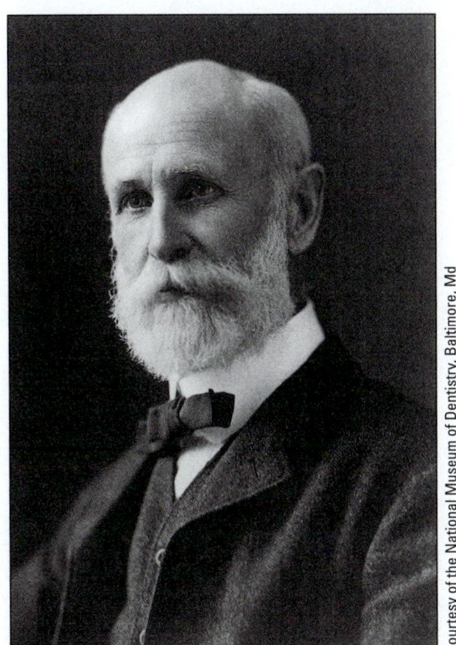

Courtesy of the National Museum of Dentistry, Baltimore, Md

FIGURE 1-7
Dr. Greene Vardiman Black (1836–1915), known as the "grand old man of dentistry" or as one of the "founders of modern dentistry in the United States."

and how to maintain their oral health. They can learn if President George Washington's teeth were really made of wood, engage in interactive exhibits, and partake in educational programs.

Dr. Greene Vardiman Black (1836–1915), known as G.V. Black (Figure 1-7), taught in dental schools such as the University of Iowa and the Northwestern University Dental School in Chicago. As the dean, he increased the library holdings and authored more than 500 articles and several books. He invented numerous machines for testing alloys and instruments to refine cavity preparations. Black later enlarged these instruments for demonstrations to students in the classroom. Many refer to him as the "grand old man of dentistry" or as one of the "founders of Modern Dentistry in the United States." His son, Arthur D. Black, followed in his footsteps, becoming dean of the Northwestern University Dental School in Chicago. In 1921 he developed the *Index to Dental Periodical Literature in the English Language*. Not only did this allow researchers to access the literature, but also it provided access to general practicing dentists who wanted to improve their knowledge and skills.

Lucy Beaman Hobbs Taylor, the first woman to graduate from a recognized dental college, earned her dental degree in 1866 (Figure 1-8). She was a teacher who became interested in medicine and then pursued further education. She met with resistance, but after the Iowa State Dental Society amended its constitution and bylaws, she was admitted into the dental college.

Dr. Robert Tanner Freeman (Figure 1-9), the first African-American to earn a dental degree, graduated from Harvard University Dental School in 1869. Eleven years later in 1890, Ida Gray became the first African-American woman to earn a dental degree upon graduation from the University of Michigan, School of Dentistry. George Franklin Grant (Figure 1-10), an African American, graduated from the second class in dentistry in 1870 at Harvard University. He is credited as an authority on the cleft palate, but many golfers may consider his contribution to the game of golf as his most important achievement. He invented and owned the first patent on the golf tee. Prior to his invention, the method of teeing up a ball came from bending over and pinching enough sand to make a raised area for the ball. It was both a messy and an inaccurate way of launching a ball.

American Dental Association

At a time when dentistry education and literature were developing, it was thought that organizing dentists would promote sharing of information concerned with excellence in dentistry. Horace Hayden and Chapin Harris collaborated on endeavors such as forming the first nationwide association of dentists. The American Society of Dental Surgeons was formed in 1840, but was dissolved in 1856. Harris had long believed in the need for an informative dental periodical and was instrumental in its founding in 1839. This journal was called the *American Journal of Dental Science (AJDS)*. Later, in 1859, twenty-five delegates gathered in Niagara Falls, New York, and organized the **American Dental Association (ADA)** (Figure 1-11). The association was small at first, but after grouping all local associations according to states, and

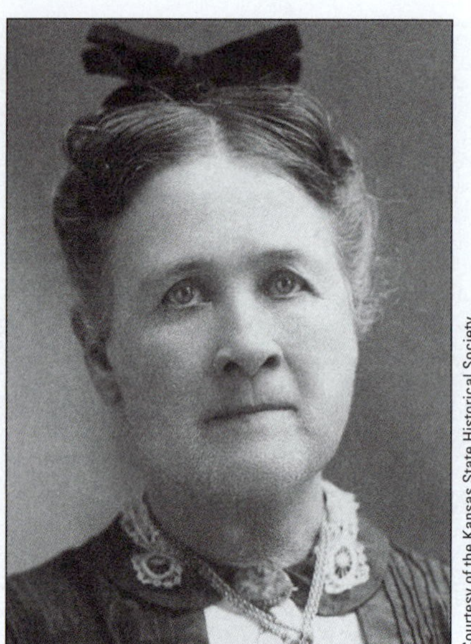

FIGURE 1-8
Lucy Beaman Hobbs Taylor

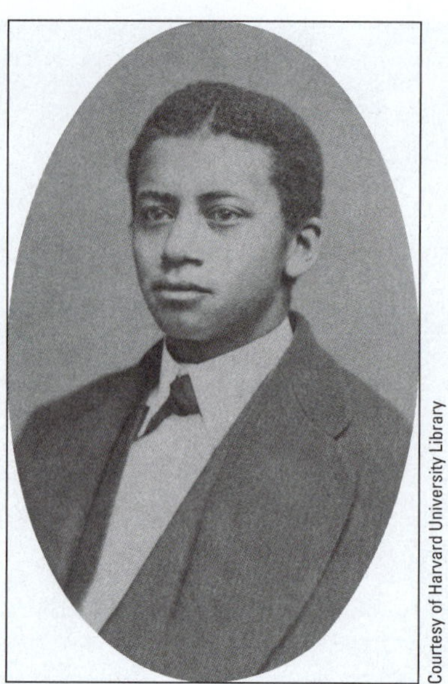

FIGURE 1-10
Dr. George Franklin Grant graduated from the second class of Harvard School of Dental Medicine.

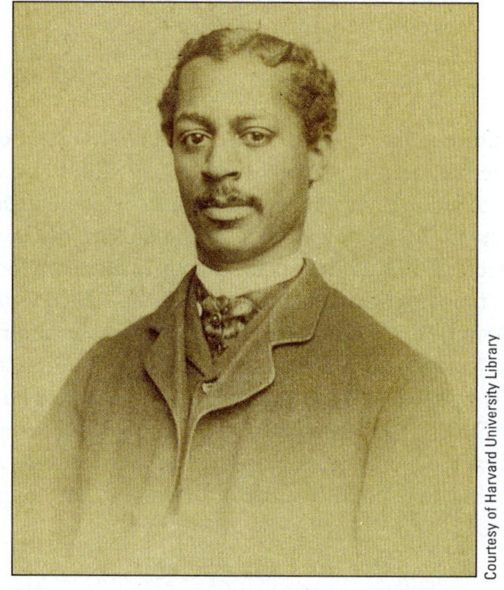

FIGURE 1-9
The first African American to earn a DMD, Dr. Robert Tanner Freeman graduated from the Harvard School of Dental Medicine in 1869.

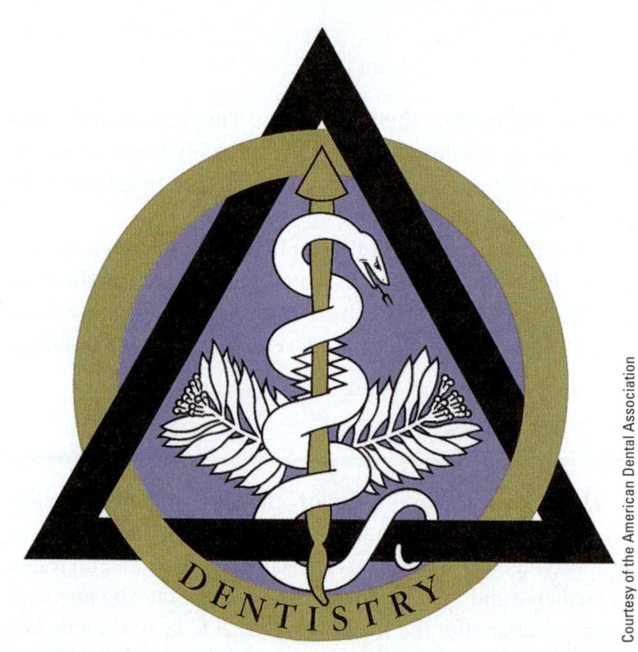

FIGURE 1-11
Logo for dentistry.

then giving all states representation in the national organization, membership began to increase. Today each state has its own organization with bylaws approved by the ADA, and each local (regional) organization has ADA-approved bylaws that are sent to each state organization. For example, Texas is represented to the ADA by the Texas State Dental Association, and the Texas State Dental Association comprises individual local dental associations. The official publication of the ADA is the *Journal of the American Dental Association (JADA)*. The ADA also has a Web site, http://www.ada.org, which provides a link to the ADA for dental professionals and dental consumers.

The Dental Team

Many people working together make up the dental health team: dentists, dental assistants, dental hygienists, dental lab technicians, and other members of the dental team (Figure 1-12). Each member of the team has specific skills, roles, and responsibilities. This team approach to dentistry improves efficiency and the overall patient experience. Dental team members often attend continued education together. All members of the dental team need to keep current on the knowledge and skills required for dentistry. Each member of the team must commit to being a lifelong learner within the ever-changing field of dentistry.

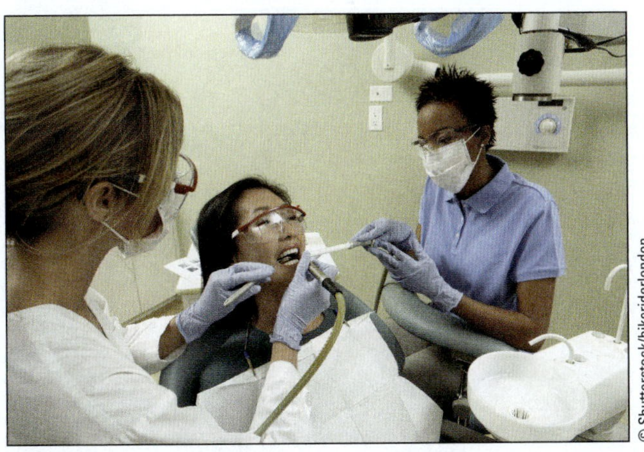

© Shutterstock/bikeriderlondon

FIGURE 1-12
Dental team.

Dentists

Once dentistry was established as a profession, the need for formal education became apparent. Only half the dentists practicing during the nineteenth century had formal educations. The requirements for state regulations began in Alabama in 1841, and by 1899 every state had enacted laws regulating the practice of dentistry. The requirements set forth for dentistry include an undergraduate education and graduation from a dental school approved by the ADA Commission on Dental Accreditation. Currently, 3 to 4 years of undergraduate work and 4 years of dental school (5 years at Harvard) are required to achieve a dental degree. Depending on program emphasis, a doctor of dental surgery (DDS) or a doctor of medical dentistry (DMD) degree is granted. Specialist training includes two or more additional years of postgraduate education in an approved, specialized training area. All dentists must take and pass both written and clinical examinations in the states in which they practice. All dental team members are responsible for following the regulations in their states. These regulations are defined in each state's dental practice act. The dental practice acts are defined to protect the public. Each state's act specifies what can be performed legally by the dental professionals in that state. Dentists supervise the dental team members in their offices.

Dental Specialists. A dentist who practices all phases of dentistry is called a general dentist. General dentists may encounter cases for which treatment is required that goes beyond the scope of their training. The general dentist would refer these cases to a dental specialist. The ADA recognizes the following nine specialties:

1. **Dental public health** is the specialty concerned with the prevention of dental disease (Chapter 4). The public health dentist works with the community to promote dental health. (www.aaphd.org)
2. **Endodontics** is concerned with the pathology and morphology of the dental pulp and surrounding tissues due to injury and disease (Chapter 24). Patients referred for root canals would see an endodontist. (www.aae.org)
3. **Oral and maxillofacial pathology** is the specialty concerned with the diagnosis and nature of the diseases affecting the oral cavity (Chapter 27). A patient who has a lesion unknown to the general dentist may be referred to the oral pathologist for further treatment and diagnosis. (www.aaomp.org)
4. **Oral and maxillofacial radiology** is the specialty of dentistry and the discipline of radiology concerned with the production and interpretation of images and data produced by all modalities of radiant energy that are used for the diagnosis and management of diseases, disorders, and conditions of the oral and maxillofacial region (Chapters 21 through 23). (www.aaomr.org)
5. **Oral and maxillofacial surgery** is concerned with the diagnosis and surgical treatment of the oral and maxillofacial region due to injury, disease, or defects (Chapter 25). A patient having third molars (wisdom teeth) removed may be referred to an oral and maxillofacial surgeon. (www.aaomos.org)
6. **Orthodontics and dentofacial orthopedics** is concerned with the diagnosis, supervision, guidance, and correction of malocclusion in the dentofacial structures (Chapter 28). Braces for straightening teeth are placed by the orthodontist. (www.aaortho.org)
7. **Pediatric dentistry** is concerned with the prevention of oral disease and the diagnosis and treatment of oral disease in children, from birth through adolescence (Chapters 29 and 30). Other patients requiring special care due to emotional, mental, or physical problems are referred to the pediatric dentist. (www.aapd.org)
8. **Periodontics** is the specialty concerned with the diagnosis and treatment of the diseases of the supporting and surrounding tissues of the tooth (Chapters 31 and 32). The periodontist is also concerned with the prevention of disease in this area. Patients who have plaque and calculus buildup and patients who have lost some of the bone around the tooth due to periodontal disease would be referred to the periodontist for further evaluation and treatment. (www.perio.org)
9. **Prosthodontics** is concerned with the diagnosis, restoration, and maintenance of oral functions (Chapters 33 and 36). This specialty is also concerned with the replacement of missing teeth through artificial means.

Another area that requires additional training but is not regarded as a specialty of dentistry is **forensic dentistry**. This is a relatively new area that deals with a wide range of services, such as the identification of bite marks on the body and/or the identification of an individual through tooth restorations and morphology using dental records.

The specialist works with the general dentist to provide the optimum oral health and patient care. During and once the specialty treatment is completed, the patient continues regular visits with the general dentist.

Dental Assistants

Before the early twentieth century, dentists hired men and boys to assist them in their dental practices. **Dr. C. Edmund Kells**, who practiced in New Orleans, hired a female to replace a male assistant in 1885. He wanted this "lady assistant" to be "quick, quiet, gentle, and attentive." A number of dentists were unsure about a female in the dental office, but the public accepted it quickly. This change allowed a woman to go to a dental office without being accompanied by her husband or maiden aunt. Due to the popularity of "ladies in attendance," dentists advertised the fact that they had hired female dental assistants by displaying signs in their windows.

Today, the educationally qualified dental assistant normally graduates from an institution accredited by the ADA Commission on Dental Accreditation. Training is approximately one academic year in length, and includes didactic, laboratory, and clinical content. Each state has a dental practice act that governs which duties dental assistants can perform. This varies from performing intraoral procedures, such as placing retraction cord and dental dams, to extraoral procedures, such as patient education. Dental assistants enable dentists to care for many more patients and to produce more dentistry than they could alone. Almost all dental offices employ one or more dental assistants. In the office, the person working directly with the dentist during patient procedures is the dental assistant.

Certified Dental Assistants. A 104-hour course was developed in 1947, along with a certifying board, to give credentials to assistants who passed the written and clinical examinations. That test is currently replaced by a written test that can be taken at designated sites. See Chapter 41, Employment Strategies, for pathways to sit for the examination. The **Dental Assisting National Board, Inc. (DANB)** provides a means for competent, qualified dental assistants to obtain credentials. By passing a comprehensive written examination from DANB, the dental assistant can use the title of **certified dental assistant (CDA)**. Other specialized certification can be obtained in areas such as certified dental preventive assistant (CDPA) and certified orthodontic assistant (COA). Some state dental practice acts allow assistants to obtain the credential of registered dental assistant (RDA).

Expanded Function Dental Assistant. Some states require registration and or licensure in expanded functions (i.e., functions and skills considered to be above the normal scope of dental assisting). Additional education and training may be required to allow dental assistants to perform a coronal polish, place a dental dam, or place dental restorations for example (Figure 1-13). Each state or providence will define the scope of practice and requirements. Dental Assistants can earn the title of Registered Expanded Functions Dental Assistant (REFDA) or **Expanded Function Dental Assistant** (EFDA) (see Chapter 41, Employment Strategies).

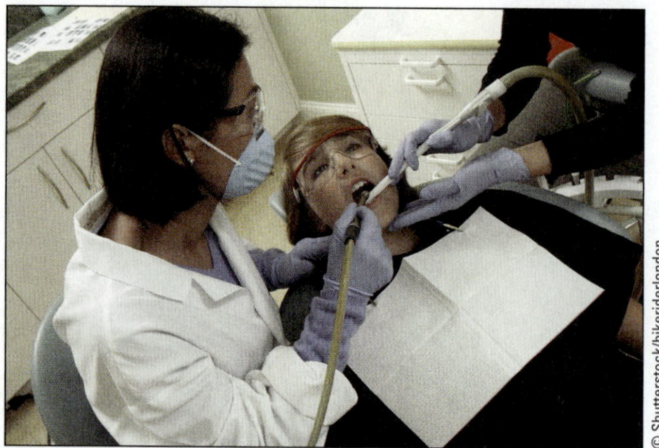

FIGURE 1-13
Expanded Function Dental Assistant with patient.

Dental Receptionists/Dental Practice Management Assistants. The dental receptionist position is becoming a more specialized area of dental assisting with the use of computers and computerized insurance claims. The dental receptionist or practice management assistant attends seminars to upgrade skills in front office management, computer technology, marketing, and accounting. The dental receptionist is most likely the first contact for the patient. It is critical that this person greet the patient and start the experience off in a positive manner. Scheduling the patients to allow for greater efficiency for the office and not requiring the patient to spend additional time in the dental office is important. The business office administrator may be responsible for additional responsibilities such as accounts payable and receivable, staff evaluations, staff meetings, and so on. In larger offices, several individuals may fill these positions.

Sterilization Assistant. Some office/clinics are hiring a dental assistant to do all the disinfecting/sterilizing of treatment rooms and instruments, called a **sterilization assistant**. This individual is responsible for monitoring all sterilizers, water lines, ultrasonic, cold chemical solutions, and biohazard materials. They stay informed on updates on chemicals and the personal protective equipment required when using them.

American Dental Assistants Association. The **American Dental Assistants Association (ADAA)** was founded in 1924 by **Juliette Southard**, its first president (Figures 1-14 and 1-15). It was founded on four principles: education, efficiency, service, and loyalty. Membership offers a voice in national affairs regarding the career of dental assisting, opportunities in continuing education, professional liability insurance, and interaction with other professionals in the field. ADAA members can remain current in their knowledge through the ADAA publication *The Dental Assistant, Journal of the American Dental Assistants Association,* or by accessing the ADAA Web site (http://www.dentalassistant.org).

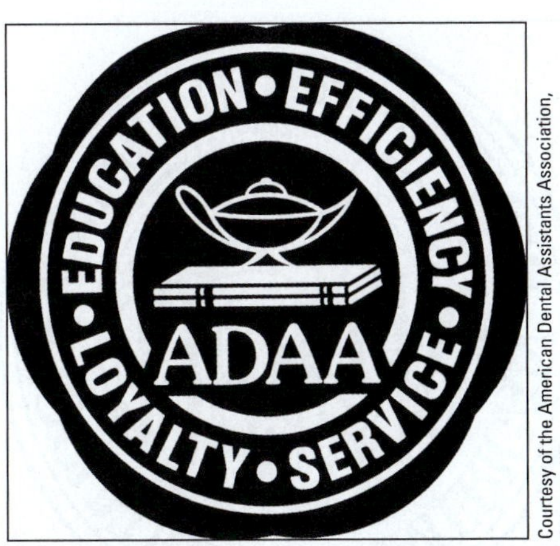

Courtesy of the American Dental Assistants Association, Chicago, Ill

FIGURE 1-14

Logo for the American Dental Assistants Association.

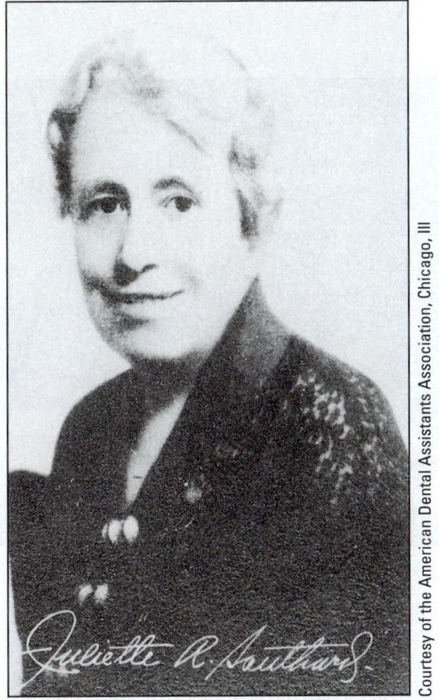

Courtesy of the American Dental Assistants Association, Chicago, Ill

FIGURE 1-15

Juliette Southard, founder and first president of the American Dental Assistants Association.

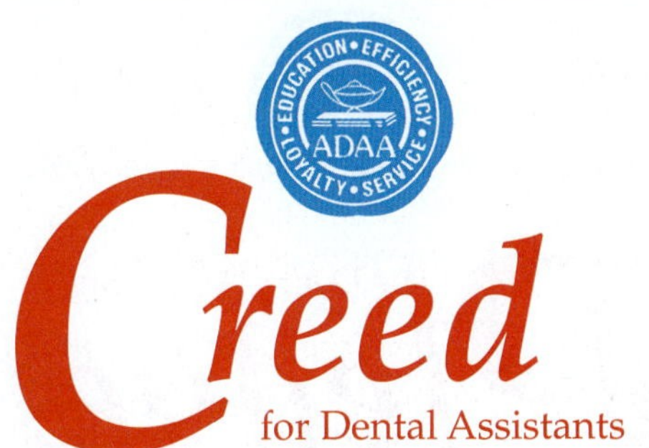

"To be loyal to my employer, my calling, and myself.

To develop initiative–having the courage to assume responsibility and the imagination to create ideas and develop them.

To be prepared to visualize, take advantage of, and fulfill the opportunities of my calling.

To be a co-worker–creating a spirit of co-operation and friendliness rather than one of fault-finding and criticism.

To be enthusiastic–for therein lies the easiest way to accomplishment.

To be generous, not alone of my name but of my praise and my time.

To be tolerant with my associates, for at times I too make mistakes.

To be friendly, realizing that friendship bestows and receives happiness.

To be respectful of the other person's viewpoint and condition.

To be systematic, believing that system makes for efficiency.

To know the value of time for both my employer and myself.

To safeguard my health, for good health is necessary for the achievement of a successful career.

To be tactful–always doing the right thing at the right time.

To be courteous–for this is the badge of good breeding.

To walk on the sunny side of the street, seeing the beautiful things in life rather than fearing the shadows.

To keep smiling always."

– *Juliette A. Southard*

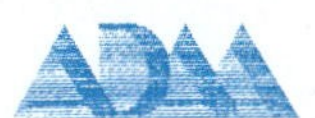

American Dental Assistants Association

Courtesy of the American Dental Assistants Association, Chicago, Ill

FIGURE 1-16

The "Creed for Dental Assistants" by Juliette A. Southard.

When pursuing a career in dental assisting, it is beneficial to use the "Creed for Dental Assistants" (Figure 1-16) and the "Dental Assistants Pledge" (Figure 1-17) as guidelines for professional behavior.

Dental Hygienists

Early in the 1900s in Bridgeport, Connecticut, several dentists, along with a leader named Dr. Alfred Civilon Fones, stated that the dentists would not be able to both be surgeons and give preventive treatments. It was suggested that women be trained to clean teeth because "they have smaller and gentler hands." At that time, it was uncommon for women to work outside the home. A dental assistant, Irene Morgan, was the first to be trained by Dr. Fones in dental hygiene. Dr. Fones established a school in 1913, and it survives today as the Fones School of Dental Hygiene, University of Bridgeport. Graduates of 2- or 4-year dental hygiene schools receive the title Registered Dental Hygienist (RDH) after passing written and clinical tests in the states in which they practice, and they are granted licenses. Dental hygienists specialize in providing dental prophylaxis, including the removal of plaque, stains, and calculus from the teeth. They also specialize in patient education. Many state practice acts allow licensed hygienists to apply tooth sealants; to expose, process, and mount dental radiographs; and to chart conditions in the oral cavity. Some of the states allow hygienists to place restorative materials and to administer local anesthetics.

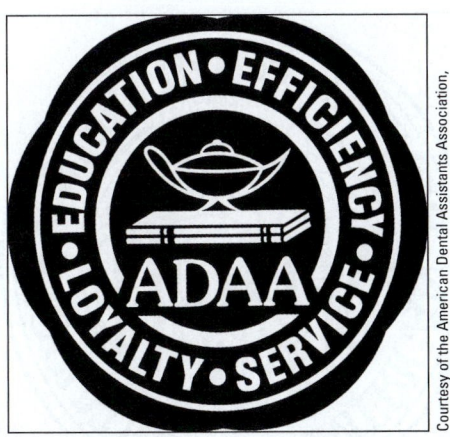

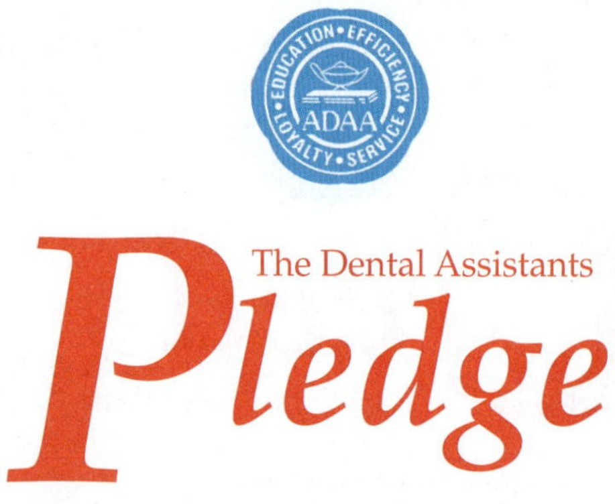

"I solemnly pledge that,
in the practice of my profession, I will always be loyal
to the welfare of the patients who come under my care,
and to the interest of the practitioner whom I serve.

I will be just and generous to the members of my profession,
aiding them and lending them encouragement to be loyal,
to be just, to be studious.

I hereby pledge to devote my best energies to the service
of humanity in that relationship of Life to which I consecrated
myself when I elected to become a Dental Assistant."

- Dr. C.N. Johnson

Printed and Distributed through the American Dental Assistants Association

Courtesy of the American Dental Assistants Association, Chicago, Ill

FIGURE 1-17

"The Dental Assistants Pledge" by Dr. C. N. Johnson.

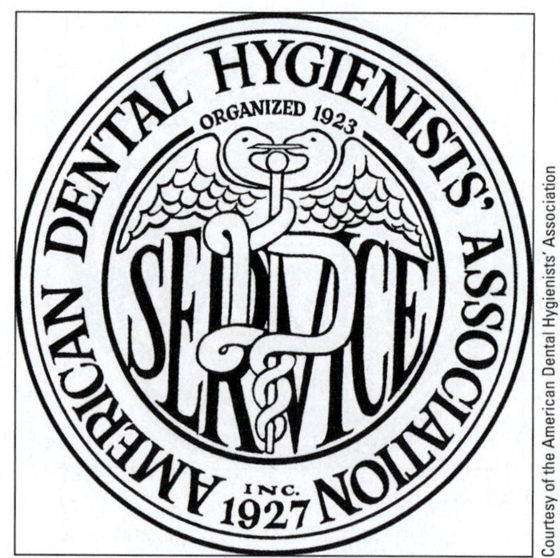

Courtesy of the American Dental Hygienists' Association

FIGURE 1-18

Logo for the American Dental Hygienists' Association.

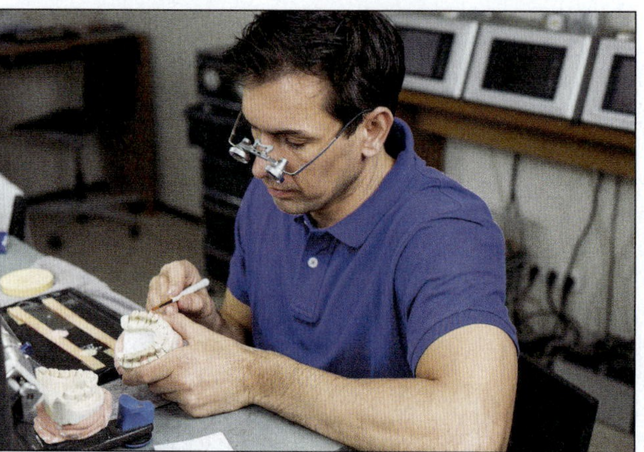

© Shutterstock/Ikonoklast Fotografie

FIGURE 1-19

Dental lab technicians.

American Dental Hygienists' Association. The **American Dental Hygienists' Association (ADHA)** was formed in 1923 in Cleveland in conjunction with the ADA annual meeting (Figure 1-18). In 1927, the *Journal of the American Dental Hygienists' Association* was founded and continues to be the official publication of the organization. This organization, like the ADA, has the leadership of national, state, and local societies working together to promote oral health.

Dental Laboratory Technicians

Dental laboratory technicians may not work in the dental office with the other members of the team, but they are essential team members (Figure 1-19). Some dental laboratory technicians are employed by the dentist; others work in privately owned dental laboratories.

Originally, dentists performed their own laboratory procedures; however, they eventually became too busy to complete the laboratory work and hired trained technicians to perform these tasks. The first commercial dental laboratory was opened in Boston in 1883 by Dr. William H. Stowe, a dentist, and Frank F. Eddy, a toolmaker. By the turn of the century, dental laboratories were firmly established. Today, whether the technicians are in the dental office or in a commercial dental laboratory, they provide such extraoral services as fabricating gold and porcelain restorations and partial and full dentures.

In most states, a dental laboratory technician is not required to have formal training and may be trained on the job. Many technicians have graduated from 2-year, ADA-accredited dental laboratory technician programs. These programs require extensive knowledge of dental anatomy and dental materials and the development of detailed mechanical skills. Individuals seeking credentials must pass an examination to become certified dental technicians (CDTs). Membership in the **American Dental Laboratory Technician Association (ADLTA)** is also offered to dental technicians.

Other Members of the Dental Team

Additional members of the dental team are dental service technicians, dental representatives, and dental supply companies and representatives. The dental service technicians maintain dental equipment. The dental assistant works with the technicians and identifies equipment problems. The technicians may be required to make service calls, or they will direct the assistant to rectify a problem. Dental representatives demonstrate how to use new materials. Normally, they are trained in the materials they represent. Dental supply companies and representatives also give information on new materials and help the dental assistant order supplies for the dental office. They normally make weekly calls to the dental office. Dental supply companies could be mail order companies through which the assistant can order office supplies.

Chapter Summary

It is important to know the historic struggles that took place and contributions that were made to advance the dentistry profession into what it is today. Organized dentistry was formed with the intent to promote the sharing of information concerned with excellence in dentistry. To provide excellence in dentistry, additional dental team members (such as dental assistants, dental receptionists, dental hygienists, and dental laboratory technicians) would become recognized and add contributing roles to the field. Therefore, the dental assistant will need to be able to identify and define those who contribute to the dental profession and look forward to the future of dentistry.

CASE STUDY

Lori Ann Smith was 18 years old in 1880 and was seeking a position in a dental office. The opinion of the dentists was to not allow women access to the profession. Lori's career dreams were denied. Over 100 years later, her great-great-granddaughter, Traci Lynd, was seeking a position in a dental office and found a very different environment. What changes and advancements took place for dental assistants during that time frame to allow Traci to reach her goal?

Case Study Review

1. When were gender barriers eliminated for dental assistants?
2. What career changes for dental assistants took place over four generations?
3. With the current educational advancements in the profession, what credentials are available to dental assistants today?

Review Questions

Multiple Choice

1. The basic code of ethics used by the medical and dental professions originated with
   a. Aristotle.
   b. Leonardo da Vinci.
   c. Pierre Fauchard.
   d. Hippocrates.
2. Who is the teacher and inventor recognized as the "grand old man" of dentistry?
   a. Chapin A. Harris
   b. G.V. Black
   c. John Greenwood
   d. Josiah Flagg
3. Which of the following is not an ADA-recognized dental specialty?
   a. Endodontics
   b. Oral and maxillofacial pathology
   c. Forensic dentistry
   d. Pediatric dentistry
4. The first president of the ADAA was
   a. Juliette Southard.
   b. Dr. Lucy Hobbs Taylor.
   c. Dr. C. Edmund Kells.
   d. Dr. Alfred Fones.
5. Whose greatest contribution to early dentistry was the creation of artificial teeth and surgical dental instruments?
   a. George Washington
   b. Robert Woofendale
   c. Paul Revere
   d. John Greenwood

6. Who was the first African-American woman to earn a dental degree?
   a. Ida Gray Nelson
   b. Juliette Southard
   c. Lucy Beaman Hobbs Taylor
   d. Loretta Fones
7. Which dental specialty deals with the diagnosis and nature of diseases affecting the oral cavity?
   a. Endodontics
   b. Periodontics
   c. Oral and maxillofacial pathology
   d. Oral and maxillofacial surgery
8. Where was the first commercial dental laboratory opened?
   a. Boston, Massachusetts
   b. Bridgeport, Connecticut
   c. Baltimore, Maryland
   d. Chicago, Illinois
9. Which dental specialty is concerned with the replacement of missing teeth through artificial means?
   a. Periodontics
   b. Prosthodontics
   c. Pediodontics
   d. Endodontics
10. Which dental team member allows the dentist to care for more patients and increase productivity?
    a. Dental assistant
    b. Dental laboratory technician
    c. Dental practice management assistant
    d. Dental hygienist

Critical Thinking

1. If a patient fell and fractured a front tooth, and it seemed to have pulpal involvement (nerve damage), what specialists could the general dentist refer the patient to?
2. Who would you contact for information about dental assisting organizations?
3. Which dental team member(s) besides the dentist requires a license?

Web Activities

1. Go to http://www.dentalmuseum.org and identify which exhibits are available for viewing at the Samuel Harris Museum of Dentistry.
2. Go to http://www.ada.org and identify how many people have ADA membership.
3. Go to http://www.dentalassistant.org and download and print a membership application for the ADAA.

CHAPTER 2

Psychology, Communication, and Multicultural Interaction

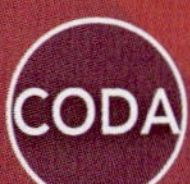

Specific Instructional Objectives

The student should strive to meet the following objectives and demonstrate an understanding of the facts and principles presented in this chapter:

1. Define psychology and paradigm.
2. Describe the components of the communication process.
3. List the skills used in listening.
4. Differentiate the terms used in verbal and nonverbal communication.
5. Demonstrate how the following body language is used in nonverbal communication behavior: spatial, posture, facial expression, gestures, and perception.
6. Discuss how Maslow's hierarchy of needs is used, and how it relates to communication in today's dental office.
7. Discuss how defense mechanisms can inhibit communication.
8. Identify and explain dental patient phobias and concerns.
9. Describe how the baby boomer generation may differ from generations X, Y, and Z.
10. Identify office stress, and demonstrate how to achieve conflict resolution.
11. Describe some general behaviors of multicultural patient populations.

Key Terms

Abraham Maslow (20)
baby boomer generation (22)
communication (16)
conflict (23)
culture (24)
dental phobia (22)
echo generation (23)
encoding (17)
ethnicity (24)
generation X (23)
generation Y (23)
generation Z (23)
Maslow's hierarchy of needs (20)
MTV Generation (23)
nonverbal communication (19)
paradigm (16)
psychology (16)
race (25)
resolution (24)
stress (23)
verbal communication (19)

Introduction

Communication is the foundation of dental care. The dental assistant must gain an understanding of the patients being treated, i.e., how and why they think and act as they do. In order to achieve this, the assistant must develop good communication skills. Communication is behind every action taken by the dental team. The message is to be transmitted as clearly as possible, and when the patient, or other staff member, sends the response, it is critical to listen before providing feedback. Watching for nonverbal communication is essential for obtaining the entire message. The dental assistant must develop the skills needed to overcome the patient's defense mechanisms and fears, as well as understand how people from other cultures and generations interact. Stress will be encountered in the dental office, and it is important to recognize it and be able to effectively achieve conflict resolution.

Psychology and Understanding Individual Paradigms

Every dental team member is responsible for communicating well, and treating each patient and coworker respectfully. Through these efforts, patients can overcome their fear of dental treatment. Employees can do many things to enhance the mental and physical comfort of patients; but employees must first have a positive attitude toward patients and their treatment. The dental assistant must understand patients, and how to meet patient needs during dental treatment.

The science of the mind and of the reasons people think and act as they do is **psychology**. Historically, individuals have associated dental treatment with discomfort. Patients may think and react using past reasoning. Today's dentistry works diligently to make treatment pain free, and does whatever is possible to make every patient comfortable. It is critical to understand patients' attitudes toward dentistry, and listen to their views about their dental experiences. With this information, the dental assistant can better help patients overcome any fears they may have.

A person's **paradigm**, or acquired belief system, may also be a factor. Individuals have different life experiences that have contributed to their personal belief systems or paradigms. For example, people may believe that a toothbrush with hard bristles gets their teeth cleaner. They may have always used hard-bristled brushes and have no cavities. Therefore, they believe hard brushes clean teeth better. Even though the evidence now shows that soft-bristled brushes do a better job, the dental assistant may have a difficult time changing these people's paradigm. Through good communication, the dental assistant can make an assessment. If the teeth are indeed clean in all areas, and it does not appear that damage is being done to the tooth or tissue, then the dental assistant can encourage the patient to continue existing practice. If the hard-bristled brush is damaging the teeth or gums, or failing to clean the entire tooth surface, then the dental assistant will have to begin educating the patient and changing the patient's paradigm. It may be difficult for the patient to associate clean teeth with a soft-bristled brush. Good communication skills, such as listening, are essential to understanding the patient's viewpoint and introducing new information that may challenge it. Listen first, and tell the patient what to expect when trying the new toothbrush. For instance, the brush is going to feel different in the mouth. Continue to listen to the patient's concerns, such as feeling the need to brush harder, or that the brush may wear more quickly. Acknowledge and address each of the patient's concerns. Watch the patient's nonverbal behavior and work with the patient to understand necessary changes in behavior. The patient's behavior may not change immediately. Share with the patient that it may take a while before the change feels comfortable, and that this is normal. Motivate the patient to continue the changed behavior.

Communication

Understanding how individuals think and feel is only part of interacting successfully with patients. A dental assistant must also have excellent communication skills. These skills, which can be learned and developed, are very important in patient care. The act of passing along information (the message), transmitting an idea (or receiving the message), or connecting with another individual (providing feedback) is **communication**. Transmitting thoughts, ideas, feelings, facts, and other information is done through verbal and nonverbal behavior. Every time a person communicates with another person, even if no verbal comments are taking place, information is being transmitted. In fact, people cannot avoid communicating with each other. In dental assisting, this communication is essential in establishing a relationship with the patient. This method of connecting with patients allows for patient comfort and safety so that the treatment can take place. The quality of the communication, and the way the patient feels connected to the dental assistant and dentist, directly relate to the patient's total experience while in the dental office. Listening is important. The adage, "You have two ears and one mouth so you can listen twice as much," is true. Often, people begin formulating their responses before they hear the entire question. In the dental office, pay special attention to what the person is saying, and then give the correct response (Figure 2-1).

In the dental office, when a staff member is going over the case presentation, a patient may say something like, "I just want to fix the front teeth." This may communicate a message to the dentist or auxiliary staff that appearance is important to this individual. Further communication with the patient will help determine why she or he wants the front teeth restored. If staff members listen carefully, they may find that this individual is applying for new employment, or that she or he is going to be in a daughter's wedding and wants to look good in the pictures. Once an understanding is reached as to where patients are coming from, and what their desires and needs are, then a treatment plan can be established to help meet these needs.

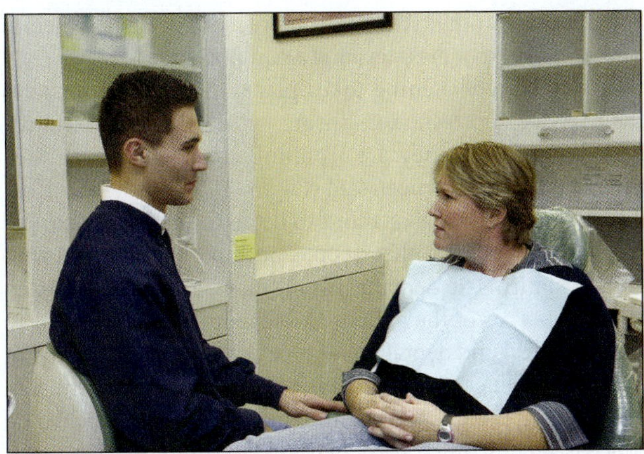

FIGURE 2-1
Communication with the patient is extremely important. Pay special attention to what the patient is saying. If the patient does not seem to understand, go over it again using another method until understanding occurs.

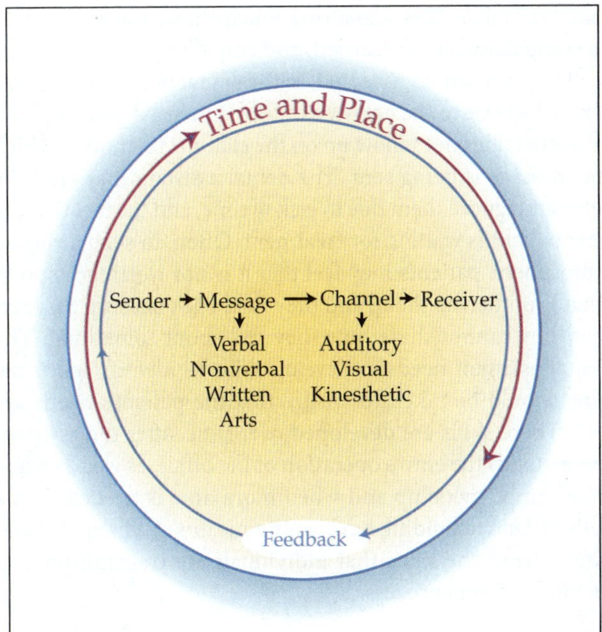

FIGURE 2-2
A communication model.

Components of the Communication Process

The communication process consists of five major components: sender, message, channel through which the message is delivered, receiver, and feedback (Figure 2-2).

Sender

The sender is the individual who begins the communication process by generating a message. The senses of taste, touch, smell, or other external stimuli may inspire the individual to begin communication. Other internal stimuli may include feelings of delight, hunger, fatigue, or anger; and thinking or fantasizing about a particular activity or scenario. Anything could be the source (or encoding) of the stimulus for communication. The use of specific signs, symbols, interpersonal communication, or language in sending a message is called **encoding**.

An example of a sender is a really good teacher who everyone talks about. Most people remember that the teacher could really get the message across. A good sender engages others when sending a message, and can transmit a message in a manner that is clear and concise. It may be beneficial to evaluate what an admired person in your life did to enhance their message. Use those qualities to become a better sender.

Message

An individual starts with an idea, and then formulates that idea and sends it through a message to another individual. The sender must shape the idea, which often starts as an image the sender visualizes, into a message by translating the image into words that others can understand. This complicated process happens so routinely during the day that most people are unaware of it.

The message is the stimuli—written, verbal, or nonverbal communication—produced by the sender to which the receiver will respond. Reception of the message could occur through visual, auditory, or kinesthetic channels. The message may be received by different individuals in different ways, depending on each individual's paradigm.

Channel

The channel is the communication medium through which a message is delivered. Three major communication channels are *auditory*, which is hearing or listening to the verbal message; *visual*, which is observing, perceiving, and seeing the visual message; and *kinesthetic*, which is a caring or procedural touch. Dental assistants use each of these channels during a clinical procedure. It is critical to be a good listener. Patients may feel comfortable because of the connection they have with the auxiliary; and may share more information with the auxiliary than they would with the dentist. In addition, when the dentist arrives, items are placed into the mouth, and it is more difficult for the patient to communicate verbally. Dental assistants also observe the patient during the procedure. Is the patient tightening his or her eyes? Are his or her knuckles white because his or her hands are tightly clutching the arms of the chair? The dentist is focusing on the procedure at hand, but the assistant can view the entire situation. Many dentists count on assistants to be their eyes, and to notify them if the patient is uncomfortable. Dental assistants normally possess the quality of empathy for patients. They also have the ability to communicate through the kinesthetic channel, by using the procedural touch, and by asking the patient, "How does that feel?" The dental assistant may also use the caring touch by touching a patient's arm during the anesthesia process, or any other procedure that appears to make the patient fearful or uncomfortable. This reassuring touch shows the auxiliary to be compassionate, concerned, and empathetic.

It is important to note that, in the dental office, the channel can be lost due to the pressure of time. Often a dental assistant or dentist does not follow up on the channel method in which the message is being sent. The dental assistant may read the signs and ignore them due to lack of time, and the fact that the next patient is waiting for treatment. Often, in such a rushed atmosphere, patients may feel that it is not worth going into what is bothering them, and they hold back because they feel that they cannot share how they feel about something. The dental assistant needs to develop skills to identify when the time should be taken to ensure that the patient's needs are met. These skills are developed over time, after the assistant understands the entire operation of the office, as well as when time can be made up and when more time is needed with a patient. Understanding how communication is channeled and how to read the signs that individuals are transmitting is a lifelong learning process.

Receiver

The receiver takes the message and must make some sense of it. This process uses feelings, intentions, and thoughts from a person's paradigm. Much of the message encoding comes from all the nonverbal clues the sender used to transmit the message. Much credence is given to the way in which the message was delivered.

Feedback

It is critical that the message is decoded correctly before providing feedback. Is the intent of the message clear? If not, state it back to the sender for correct interpretation. After making sure the message is clear, the individual formulates a response, much like the initial sender did. An idea is given shape and words are picked to mirror, or express, the idea to the other person. This interchange occurs until both people feel their ideas are expressed in the manner in which they intended, or they continue to another area of discussion.

Listening Skills

As noted, listening is an important element of communication. We spend more time listening than performing any other type of communication. Most college students spend about 50 percent of their time listening and 35 percent reading and writing. About 15 percent is spent talking. Some of the barriers to listening are preoccupation, message overload, external noise, and effort. People are often preoccupied with concerns that are more important to them, which, therefore, diminish their ability to listen. We experience overload because the quantity of messages we encounter each day is tremendous. Because we spend half our time listening, it is impossible to stay focused and listen actively. The mind wanders and listening stops. Often, there is additional external noise, which distracts us and makes it hard to listen. The external noise comes from others speaking, telephones ringing, music, or any number of other sources. Each person identifies when to actively listen to a message of great importance.

When active listening takes place, the receiver encodes the message and responds, during two-way communication. People can tell if they are listening actively, because they understand what has been said (Figure 2-3). In a dental office, it is critical to train your mind to listen to the patient so that you can understand other people, both more often, and with greater clarity. The dental assistant may be required to listen to the concerns of the patient and respond accordingly, or to chart medical and dental patient history correctly. The dental assistant may need to listen to the directions of the dentist in carrying out patient treatment. Often, listening in the dental office is accompanied with analyzing and interpreting information. It may help to repeat the content back to the patient. For example, "I understand that you said the discomfort started several days ago in the upper left side of your face, close to this tooth." The dental assistant should spend time developing and becoming more adept at active listening skills.

Telephone Listening Skills

Listening on the telephone is especially critical. It is often said that the telephone is where the patient derives his or her first impression of the office, and that the telephone is the office's lifeline. That being said, a telephone conversation is often like a conversation between two blindfolded individuals. The inflections in each auxiliary's voice, along with the verbal communication dialogue, give the message to the patient. Speaking in short sentences with a hard tone to the voice may not sound inviting to the patient. Patients may interpret this communication to mean that the auxiliary does not want them in the office. The message itself could say something like, "I am looking forward to seeing you in our office on May twenty-fifth," but the tone and perceived attitude may reflect a different message. The dental assistant will need to concentrate and obtain feedback from others on how the message is coming across. When listening on the telephone, sit in the correct posture and respond with

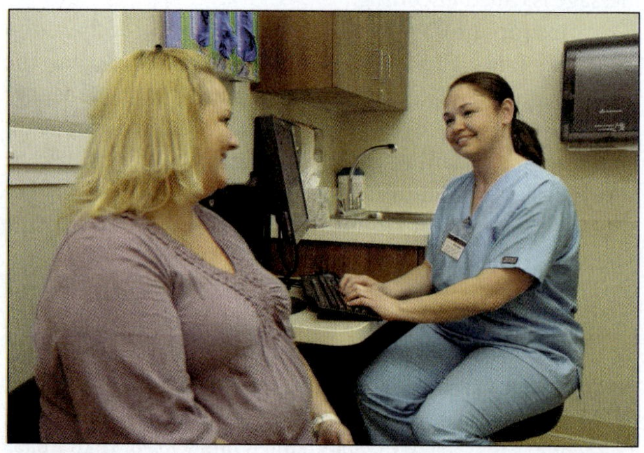

FIGURE 2-3
Good posture and position encourage positive communication with the patient. Shown here are open spatial seating, and an operator with a smile and a positive attitude.

the correct facial expression. These actions will have an effect on the message sent to the caller, and will convey the message that you want to listen. When talking on the telephone, listen with full attention to make certain that the messages sent and received are correct and accurate (Figure 2-4).

Verbal and Nonverbal Communication

It is often said that communication is less than 20 percent **verbal communication** (speaking words) and 80 percent nonverbal. Communication without using words is defined as **nonverbal communication**. It is the way in which we express ourselves by what we do, and not by what we say. Body language can communicate more than spoken words (Figure 2-5). Body language includes the unconscious way we move our bodies, the physical/spatial distance kept between individuals, posture and position, facial expressions, gestures, and perceptions.

Nonverbal communication is first learned when we are infants. The tone of a voice, and the presence, or absence, of a smile are picked up readily by an infant through nonverbal means. The infant adapts learned behaviors that bring positive responses from the caregiver.

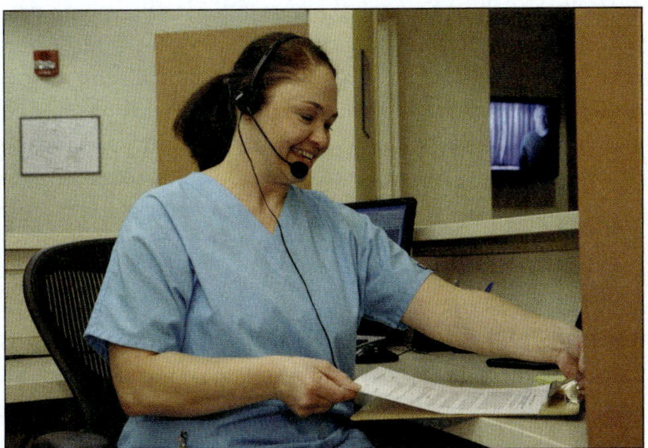

FIGURE 2-4
Give the patient on the telephone your full attention, and make certain the message is sent and received correctly.

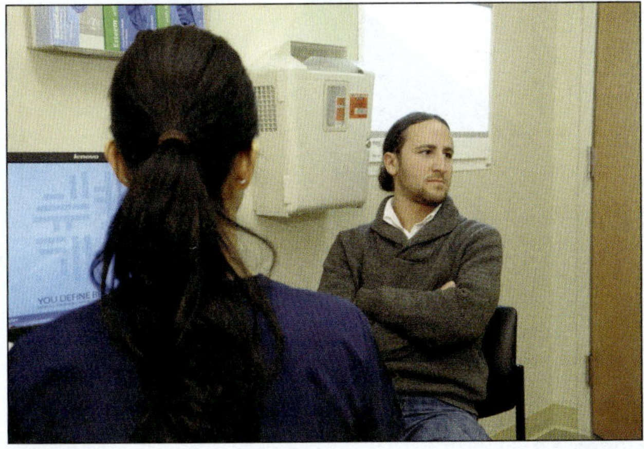

FIGURE 2-5
Body language and gestures often say more than the spoken word.

In the dental office, much of the communication with the patient is nonverbal. Sometimes, the patient cannot respond verbally due to the placement of the dental dam or other items in the oral cavity. The dental assistant should become aware of a patient's nonverbal communications, which could be a tightening of the hands on the chair arms, a look that indicates a need the patient may have, posture or movement in the chair, or just a muffled noise the patient makes. Watch for this nonverbal communication and try to identify, with the patient's help, which feelings and emotions are being communicated nonverbally.

Territoriality or Spatial Relation

Territoriality or spatial relation indicates the amount of space an individual needs to feel comfortable with others. This distance changes with the group we are in. Intimate touching, normally within six inches, is usually encountered with close family members or close friends. In the classroom, students often define their space on the first day of class with textbooks and papers. In the dental office, sometimes the procedures the dental assistants are doing require the assistants to invade the patient's space. It is best that the dental assistant tells the patient about the procedure so that it will not be perceived as threatening. The patient can then feel empowered by deciding to allow the treatment to proceed. This interaction helps to build a sense of trust with the patient. After informing the patient, sit and perform invasive procedures, if possible, from the side of the patient. When working straight toward a patient, the spatial distance required for comfort is much greater. Individuals are normally much more comfortable sharing the space to their side. People of various cultures handle territoriality and personal space differently.

Posture and Position

Posture indicates to dental assistants how patients are responding. If the patient is tight, it may indicate that the patient feels threatened. The patient may be seated with the arms and legs crossed, which is a message of closure or resistance. Slumped shoulders may indicate the patient is depressed or discouraged. The patient who sits with legs uncrossed, hands loose on the chair arms, and a slightly laid-back posture in the chair may appear to be open to suggestions. The manner in which dental assistants position themselves is also important. Standing over the patient may indicate superiority. Sitting close to the patient and leaning toward the patient expresses interest, warmth, acceptance, and caring (Figure 2-6). This arrangement allows the patient to feel valued, listened to, and cared for.

Facial Expression

Facial expression is considered one of the most observed and critical components of nonverbal communication. The sender's eyes give the message receiver great insight; emotions,

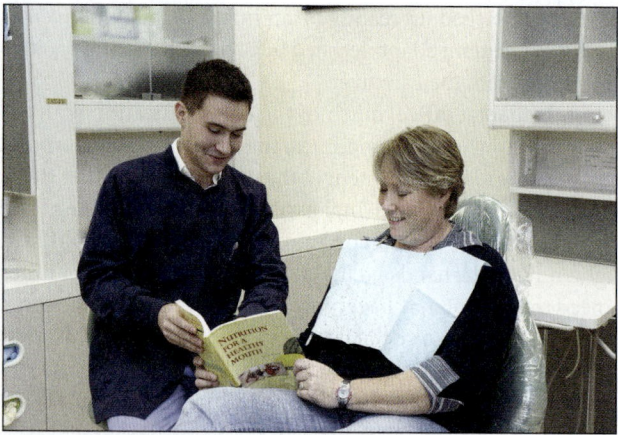

FIGURE 2-6
The operator's posture and correct positioning makes patients feel more comfortable, and that the dental assistant is interested in them.

such as happiness, sadness, and anger, are reflected in the eyes. The eyebrows also indicate such nonverbal clues as puzzlement, worry, questioning, and surprise. The dental assistant should check the patient's eyes during the procedure and watch for nonverbal communication. Practitioners, hygienists, and assistants should be mindful of the facial expressions (e.g., eye expressions) behind the treatment masks.

Gestures

Like facial expressions, gestures are a common form of nonverbal communication, and one of the most observed. Even while in a car at a stoplight, nonverbal communication can be observed inside the cars close to us. Gestures make it fairly easy to see if someone is angry, happy, or just trying to make a point to another individual. When we talk, we often use our hands to communicate. It enhances the spoken word by emphasizing the content, and holding the attention of the receiver.

Perception

It is critical that dental assistants develop good perception skills as they relate to patient communication. The dental assistant must be aware of the feelings of others and be able to sense patients' moods and their attitudes toward the dental treatment. Initially, the dental assistant can watch and observe other health care workers using good perception skills, and then emulate the others' examples. Soon, the dental assistant will master good perception skills.

Maslow's Hierarchy of Needs

Abraham Maslow (1908–1970), an American psychologist, is considered the founder of a movement called *humanistic psychology*. Maslow studied well-adjusted persons in society and identified several levels of human needs. His philosophy is that the most basic needs must be satisfied before the next levels of human needs can be fulfilled. The most basic needs are bodily drives, such as hunger, thirst, and sleep. The succeeding levels include the needs for safety, then belongingness and love. Above these are the needs for prestige and esteem. The highest need is the one for fulfillment of one's unique potential or, as Maslow termed it, *self-actualization*. **Maslow's hierarchy of needs** (Figure 2-7) aids in communication and patient treatment. When patients' most basic needs are not met, they cannot go forward and feel safe and cared for. Keeping this hierarchy in mind helps the dental assistant understand the patient's perceptions and needs, and it helps facilitate dental treatment and care.

Survival or Physiological Needs

In the context of Maslow's hierarchy of needs, an individual will seek to fulfill survival or physiological needs first. These needs include the need to breathe, regulate body temperature, quench thirst, sleep, eat, and dispose of bodily waste. In the dental office, most patients try to have their basic needs met prior to the dental appointment. However, during the treatment some patients may indicate that they are having difficulty breathing through the nose if fluid in the mouth prevents breathing through the mouth. The treatment must stop or the fluid must be removed so that the patient can swallow and breathe. Breathing through the nose may be obstructed in several other ways, such as by the rubber dam covering the patient's nose, or the nosepiece on the nitrous mask becoming dislodged. The dental assistant should recognize that this need must be taken care of immediately, before the patient becomes too anxious and panics. The need to dispose of bodily wastes is another area that cannot wait, and, often, in the dental office patients may need to excuse themselves to use the restroom. Survival or physiological needs cannot be ignored and they are immediate in nature. When a particular need is not being met, a person becomes entirely focused on that need, and it is the only thing that the individual can think about until it is fulfilled.

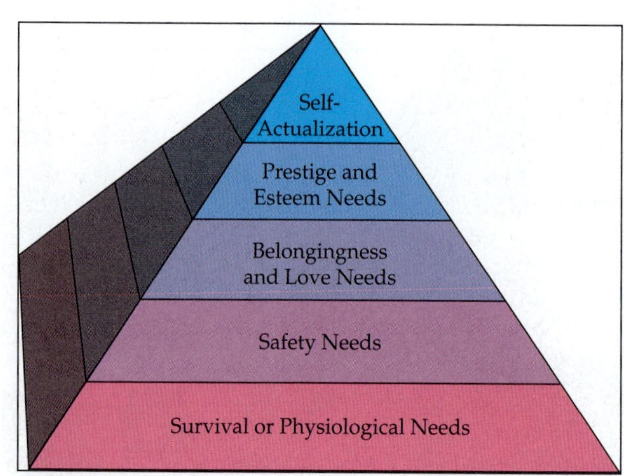

FIGURE 2-7
Maslow's hierarchy of needs.

Safety Needs

After survival or physiological needs are met, the most critical need is for safety. This need covers a variety of areas, such as safety from violence, family and health security, security in employment, and being able to pay the bills. In the dental office, this security most often comes into play under the area of insurance, and the individual's need to understand both the fee that will be charged for the service, and what portion will be paid by the individual's insurance. If patients lose a job, or otherwise have to contend with lower incomes or higher expenses, they may contact the office to discontinue services, make arrangements to pay for services over time, or both. They would seek out ways to meet financial obligations until their employment status changes. People often do not receive necessary services due to loss of insurance, or not being able to pay for the services rendered.

Dental office staff may also observe this need being met by parents who watch over their children during services to ensure their safety and security. Even auxiliaries seeking employment may prefer employment in one office to another because the former provides better insurance and, thus, fulfills their security needs. This benefit may be more important to the prospective employee than other benefits or a higher salary.

Belongingness and Love Needs

After physical and safety needs are fulfilled, the focus shifts to the desire to be accepted. Individuals want others to accept them, and they wish to be needed. This level of Maslow's hierarchy is focused on social needs, which encompass belonging to or having a family, feeling loved (sexually and non-sexually), and having interactions with friends. Patients may wish to belong to the dental office, and wish to be cared for (and thus they wish to be needed as a patient in that practice). It is also very important that all members of the dental team feel that they belong, and are accepted as part of the team as providing quality patient care. Because dental assistants work with individuals every day, those who feel fulfilled with their work (and that they belong in their workplace) will be more effective. The more that members share the feeling that everyone is part of a team and is needed, with each person contributing, the more harmonious the workplace will be. Successful office teams that experience friendship and acceptance in the workplace show greater satisfaction; and patients often notice this positive atmosphere in the office. Dental office staff often attend seminars in order to aid in positive interpersonal communications within the office.

Prestige and Esteem Needs

Humans have a need to gain recognition and self-esteem. This can only be realized after the previous needs have been fulfilled. At this level, individuals respect others and find a level of self-respect, whether it is in work or personal accomplishments. Emotional fulfillment at this level overcomes low self-esteem, and feeling inferior, or second rate in comparison to others, and is the opposite of pretentiousness, arrogance, and vanity. Ideally, a person needs to have confidence, and value others' successes. This is apparent with patients who are seeking cosmetic dentistry. A new smile, without missing teeth, spaces, and decay, gives an individual new self-esteem. On several television shows, people are brought in and given designer clothes, dentistry, and put through an exercise routine, and their personalities virtually change right before us. This happens in the dental office as well. After placing crowns and veneers, whitening teeth, and completing cosmetic dentistry, patients walk out with a new smile that positively affects their entire life.

Dental assistants work to feel the accomplishment of elevating their own skill level, as well as to feel confident in their own performance without walking over other individuals in the office who seek to obtain the same. Many dentists work to provide recognition and meet the employees' need for self-value within the workplace. A dental team that respects others and values each employee's accomplishments is primary for job satisfaction and enjoyment. When a dental assistant does not feel valued and has low self-esteem, it affects all office personnel. This problem either needs to be overcome, or the dental assistant will eventually seek employment in another office in search of the feeling of self-value.

Self-Actualization

Self-actualization is the highest level on Maslow's hierarchy of needs. This is where individuals seek to become the best that they can be. Maslow described self-actualization as follows: "Self-actualization is the intrinsic growth of what is already in the organism, or more accurately, of what the organism is" (*Psychological Review*, 1949).

Maslow wrote that self-actualizing people are spontaneous in their ideas and actions. He stated that they are creative, interested in solving problems, feel close to others, generally appreciate life, judge others without prejudice, and embrace the facts and realities of the world.

Maslow stated that the reason some individuals do not seek self-actualization is that obstacles have been placed in their way by society to hold them back. Education (or lack thereof) can become such an obstacle. Individuals should be taught to transcend their cultural conditioning, become world citizens, and understand that life is precious and that controls are good. They must be taught to make good choices. In short, Maslow's message was that each individual should seek to reach his or her fullest potential.

Defense Mechanisms

Individuals often use defense mechanisms to block communication. The individual may feel ashamed, guilty, or threatened and, therefore, respond with defense mechanisms. It becomes difficult to go forward when the patient may be unconsciously defensive in order to gain control. For instance, when talking to the patient about the course of treatment to care for an area of decay, the patient may say, "The last dentist didn't find decay there!" or "You said that if I brushed and flossed, I wouldn't get cavities!"

In order to go forward, the dental assistant must recognize common defense mechanisms, and work with patients so that communication can be more effective. Denial is a common defense mechanism in health care. When patients do not brush and floss, and believe they will never get decay because they have not had it in the past, they are in denial. Patients may respond with regression, moving back to a former time to escape the fear, a tactic that creates temporary amnesia and an inability to cope with a situation. Often in the dental office, the patient uses rationalization to justify a situation. For instance, a patient may say, "We live in Spokane, a city that does not have fluoride in the water. Therefore, of course my children have a great deal more decay."

Understanding and recognizing patients' defense mechanisms help the dental assistant get to the truth. This, in turn, helps patients improve communication and get beyond their defenses to achieve better outcomes. Dental assistants must constantly observe nonverbal behaviors and look for cues, as well as listen intently to verbal messages. Give patients your full attention so that communication has every opportunity to succeed.

Dental Phobias and Concerns

Some patients may have a fear of dentistry and of receiving dental care, this is called **dental phobia**. It may also be called dental anxiety. Patients with dental phobias have fear and severe anxiety that is excessive, unreasonable, and irrational; and they are often unable to overcome it without professional help. These patients often create a cycle that adds to their fear of dental treatment. The cycle begins with the patient being so fearful of dental treatment that they won't get care until the problem becomes an emergency. At this point, their treatment often requires invasive procedures, which only adds to their fear, so the phobia continues. The causes of dental phobias can be direct or indirect. Direct causes often begin with the patient experiencing difficult and/or painful treatment. The experience can be more traumatic if the dentist's behavior is not personable, understanding, and caring toward the patient. The indirect causes may be from several sources including the following:

- Hearing about another person's traumatic experience, or their negative views on dentistry and dental treatment.
- The media, which often portrays dentistry and dental treatment in a very negative way, such as portraying dental treatment as a means of torture, incompetent dentists, and painful procedures.
- Bad experiences with medical doctors or hospitals may lead people to fear any type of treatment.
- People who have experienced sexual, physical, or emotional abuse may also transfer their fear to dental treatment.
- Fear of needles/injections, or the side effects of the anesthetic; and questioning whether the anesthetic will work or if the needle will break.
- Embarrassment of the condition of their teeth and oral hygiene.
- Lack of control, feeling of helplessness, and loss of personal space.

Treatment of a patient with dental phobia often includes behavior and pharmacological techniques. Some patients are treated in the dental office, while others require specialized treatment where psychologists and dentists work together to help patients decrease and manage their fears. Behavior techniques include: taking more time to explain procedures using visual aids, such as models and photos that are not too graphic; use of the "look, see, then do" approach to relax the patient; listening to their concerns and making sure they understand; or by allowing the patient some control by giving them a sign when they want the dentist to stop. Pharmacological techniques include medicine in pill form, intravenously, or use of nitrous oxide. The dentist can also use slow, careful injection techniques with the anesthetic. The dentist and dental auxiliary can aid dental phobia patients by being understanding and using gentle dental techniques.

Understanding Different Generations

The dental assistant will encounter a wide variety of patients, often spanning all ages. Individuals of different ages can be grouped by generation. It helps to have a basic understanding of the primary concerns of each generation. This will help the dental office aid the patient in getting their needs and wants met. It should be stated that this discussion is only a general description of the generations, and, certainly, individuality abounds within each characterization.

Baby Boomers

Many have heard about the **baby boomer generation**. It is loosely defined as the set of individuals who were born in the United States between the years 1946 to 1964, and is often thought of as those born after World War II. Due to the high birth rate, in 1964 about one-third of the population was under 19 years of age. When the baby boomers came of age, there seemed to be a great deal of parental defiance that played out with the so-called flower children, and the impact of drugs on this generation. However, many great minds came from this generation, and currently many of the large corporations are run by baby boomers, who will be passing the torch on to the next generation within the next decade. The baby boomers were often two-income families and were often tagged as the me generation. Due to their parents, they grew up as one of the healthiest and wealthiest generations, but it was still expected that the world would improve for this generation. Most of the individuals in this generation saw a president assassinated, people walk on the moon, and the birth of personal computers. This generation is interested in cosmetic dentistry, teeth whitening, and keeping their teeth for a lifetime.

Generation X

Generation X (also called the **MTV generation**) is thought to be those born during the 1960s and 1970s, and some consider it to include the 1980s. According to the U.S. Census Bureau, this generation statistically holds the highest education level when looking at age groups. They are a very diverse group in aspects such as race, ethnicity, sexual orientation, politics, and religion. They were influenced by heavy metal and disco music, Desert Storm, the recession in the 1980s, and the oil and energy crisis. This generation is unsure about their future due to the savings and loan crisis, and the overall economy. This generation has grown up with video games, cable television, and the Internet. When working with this group of individuals in dentistry, note that they may search out offices on the Internet and may want to be contacted by texting versus phone interaction. They may be interested in deals that are offered in the dental office, such as half off for whitening if a dental examination is completed.

Generation Y

Most refer to **Generation Y** (those born between 1977 and 1994) as the generation following Generation X; they are also referred to as the **echo generation** (children of the baby boomers). This generation varies greatly in their social and economic conditions. It is known that this generation is delaying adulthood longer than prior generations, and staying in their parents' homes longer. This may be due to the housing crisis and high unemployment levels facing this generation. This generation communicates through texting and email, and follows Web sites, such as YouTube, and especially social networking sites, such as Facebook and Twitter (Figure 2-8). Most individuals in this group are fascinated with communication and the latest gadgets in technology. Knowing this helps us to communicate with them as patients in the dental office. This individual is going to check out Web sites, and choose an office that uses the latest in digital technology. They may also want to have digital images of their braces or teeth sent to their phones. All communication will be done through their phones.

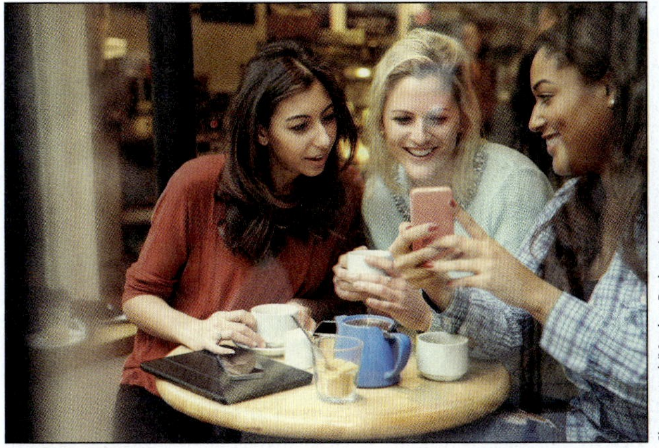

Shutterstock/Monkey Business Images

FIGURE 2-8
Many from the Y Generation communicate using their cell phone or email.

Generation Z

Generation Z was born in the mid-1990s to early 2000s. In American culture specifically this group is a more diverse mix of ethnicities than the generations before them. As a generation growing up at the peak of technology advancement they are technology proficient using, on average, five devices, and communicating across many devices. Technology has given them opportunities to engage with people all over the world, preparing them for global communication and interaction. As a group they are mature, fast learners, curious, driven, tolerant, and open-minded. They often feel they can't depend on the advice of older adults as they have watched the economy decline and seen the mistakes other generations have made. This generation wants to be heard and have input, which has led them to be active in their communities; and they care about the world and each other because they have always been connected through technology. They believe in investigating, experiencing, and creating things they love, which has led many to be mini entrepreneurs. Generation Z has taken hobbies and turned them into jobs, and then into businesses. These businesses become their own reality. To appeal to this generation, create communication that they relate to, using various technologies. Be authentic and appeal in a human sense, while listening to them and getting them involved.

Stress in the Dental Office

Working closely with other employees, waiting patients, and procedure change are all issues occurring in the dental office that cause **stress**. Stress is the body's method of reacting to specific conditions or stimuli. How each member of the dental team handles stress is an important aspect of how the dental office runs. Even with the best dental team members, it is a very stressful environment. The stress comes from the sources noted previously, along with overbooking appointments, being understaffed, equipment malfunctioning, and unavailable supplies, along with all of the skills that have to be done in a timely manner. Things that often cause the most problems with stress are employees unhappy with their jobs, lack of advancement, salary, and poor communication. Stress can cause conflicts with patients and team members. Learning to deal with stress and conflict will enable you to be able to make sound decisions at work and home. Maintaining a healthy lifestyle, eating properly, exercising regularly, setting realistic goals and expectations, and communicating well with others will aid in reducing stress.

Conflict

A disagreement or power struggle between individuals or groups is defined as **conflict**. This may result from being contradictory, or having a difference of opinion. Conflicts in the dental office with the employer or other colleagues create an atmosphere of stress. Conflicts continue to fester when ignored; they stay with us until we face them or resolve them. Conflicts trigger strong emotions. Gaining the conflict resolution skills that can turn conflicts into opportunities is a normal part of any healthy relationship.

Conflict Resolution

The act of finding an answer or a solution to a problem is defined as **resolution**. An individual must first understand that a response to a conflict is based on individual perceptions of the situation, and not always on the facts. Good communication will aid in finding a method to resolve the conflict. If the problem or conflict is too out of control for the parties to resolve on their own, use of a mediator should be considered. This could be the office manager or dentist. If involved in a conflict, it is important to understand that it is not all about you. For example, your perception may be that a coworker is angry with you when in fact something has happened in their life and they are having a bad day, and it has nothing to do with you. Try to depersonalize the conflict from "me versus you," and work on the situation. Be specific about the conflict and try to not bring in any other complaints. Be open and listen to the other person's point of view. Seeing it from an opposing side may help to understand the issue better. Try to resolve the dispute or conflict to allow for less stress in the working environment and, therefore, allow for better communication and patient care in the office.

Culture, Ethnicity, and Race

Understanding the concepts of culture, ethnicity, and race is necessary to gain insight into people of different backgrounds. The beliefs, behaviors, attitudes, customs, languages, symbols, ceremonies, rituals, knowledge, and practices that are distinctive to a specific group defines **culture** (Figure 2-9). Individuals in a particular cultural group may behave according to the strict traditional dictates of their culture; or their behavior may diverge from this pattern in minor to major ways. Diversity within a cultural group originates from long-term changes in the social environment (e.g., political or economic transformation and pressures) that cause cultural change, which in turn may affect group members unevenly.

Cultural traditions are transferred from one generation to the next by how grandparents and parents model behavior, or through discussions within the family or group. Many families have traditions that date from previous centuries. Often, traditions are shared through informal or formal activities such as mealtimes (Figure 2-10).

Defined as a subgroup's shared ancestry, history, linguistic characteristics, religion, and/or culture, **ethnicity** emerges, and is made relevant through ongoing social situations and encounters, as well as through people's ways of coping with the demands and challenges of life. Typically, members of an ethnic group share a sense of solidarity and a desire to preserve their culture, traditions, religion, or language, or some combination of these. An ethnic group is self-conscious with a strong sense of oneness. People usually do not become members of an ethnic

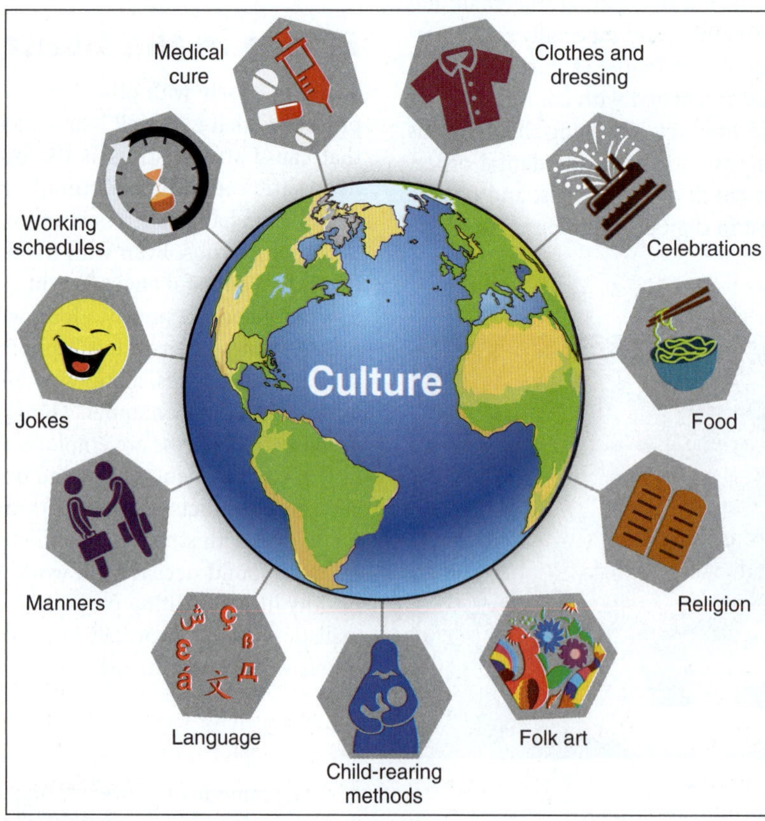

FIGURE 2-9

Things are done differently within each culture.

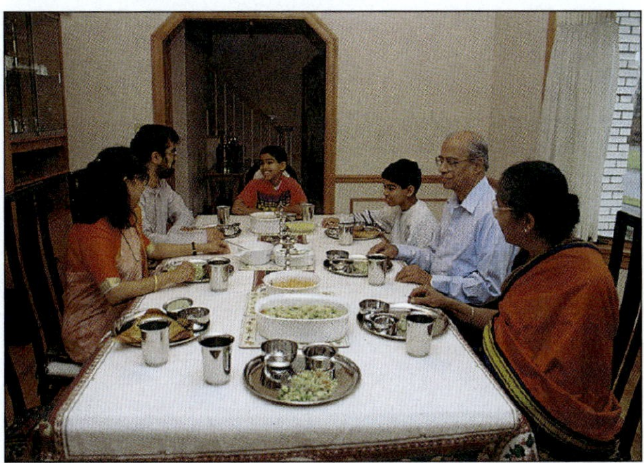

FIGURE 2-10

Mealtimes are often opportunities for families to share traditions and cultural customs.

group voluntarily; they are born into it. By choice or necessity, members of an ethnic group tend to marry within the group.

A **race** is a subgroup that is believed to be distinct in some way from other groups based on real or imagined *physical* differences (Figure 2-11). Racial classifications are rooted in the idea of biological classification of humans according to morphological features, such as skin color or facial characteristics. Individuals are usually externally classified (meaning someone else makes the classification) into a racial group, rather than choosing where they belong as part of their identity (as occurs with ethnic identity). Conceptions of race, as well as specific racial groupings, are often controversial due to their impact on social identity and how those identities influence an individual's position in social hierarchies.

Many social scientists believe that race is a social construct, meaning that it does not have a basis in the natural world, and, instead, is simply an artificial distinction created by humans. Others continue to believe that race is a valid measure when understood as genetic clusters or extended families.

In general, regardless of whether *race* is accepted as a useful descriptor, social and physical scientists agree that genetic variation *within* racial groups is much greater than genetic variation *between* them. In the face of the increasing rejection of race as a valid classification scheme, many have replaced the concept of *race* with *ethnicity*.

Cultural subgroups are also based on other individual differences such as gender, age, profession and occupation, political/ideological beliefs and attitudes, nationality, socioeconomic status, skills, education, residence, geographic location, and family structure. One or more of these (or other distinctions) may be more salient or important to an individual than ethnicity.

Multicultural Interaction

It is important that dental assistants avoid stereotyping individuals according to their cultures, customs, traditions, or beliefs. Each patient is to be treated with respect and care. Make no assumptions about the behaviors and paradigms of the multicultural patient populations you serve. According to the U.S. Census Bureau, vast numbers of immigrants have relocated to the United States and Canada in recent years; many speak English as their second language. It would benefit any dental assistant to study the geographical data, cultural beliefs, and practices that have shaped the paradigms for the patients in the region where employment is sought.

Treating everyone in the manner in which you would like to be treated may not work across cultures. Eye contact, for example, may be disrespectful in some cultures; a person may instead show respect by looking down and away. In western culture, because doing so may be viewed as disinterest, some communication difficulties may occur. When calling a patient back for treatment, it may be appropriate in western culture to use a patient's first name to put the patient at ease. In other cultures, it may be appropriate to use the formal name to address the patient. Right away, a person can see that mistakes can be made and, therefore, inappropriate messages can be inadvertently given to the patient. Speak with patients and discover how to give them the best care. Individuals may come to the dental office having used folk medicine in the past, or they may be using it currently. Find out what is working for the patient, and then inform the doctors so they can design treatments that will achieve the best results.

When addressing individuals who speak English as a second language, face the patient and speak slowly, not more loudly. Try to avoid unnecessary words. Lots of information may result in information overload. In western culture, the belief is that the caregiver is to tell us everything, and that the informed patient should be included in the health care decisions. Many other cultures rely on the caregiver to make decisions without consulting the patient. Summarize information in a simple manner, and obtain feedback from the patient by asking questions that require more than a yes or no answer.

If necessary, bring a translator to the dental office. When using an interpreter for your patient, make sure the interpreter understands the information. It may be appropriate to state it a couple of different ways for the interpreter to translate. Make sure that the information is accurate and unchanged in the translation.

Also, always try to avoid behavior or treatment that conflicts with the patient's belief system. Some cultures find it inappropriate to have the female patient alone with the dental team. The dental team should respond to this and allow someone to accompany the patient in the office, and in the treatment room during treatment. If both the doctor and dental assistant working on a female patient are males, having a female assistant in the room as well is advisable. Occasionally, an instrument is placed on the patient's chest. This is not appropriate, especially with a female patient, and is even more inappropriate if a male assistant is working with a female patient. Be conscious of gender boundaries to ensure that no patient feels uncomfortable with the treatment methods. When providing patient care, it is prudent to err on the conservative side in order to avoid conflict with the patient's cultural beliefs and preferences. Remember, do not assume that everything should be handled in one manner; listen without judgment and provide the optimal care for every patient.

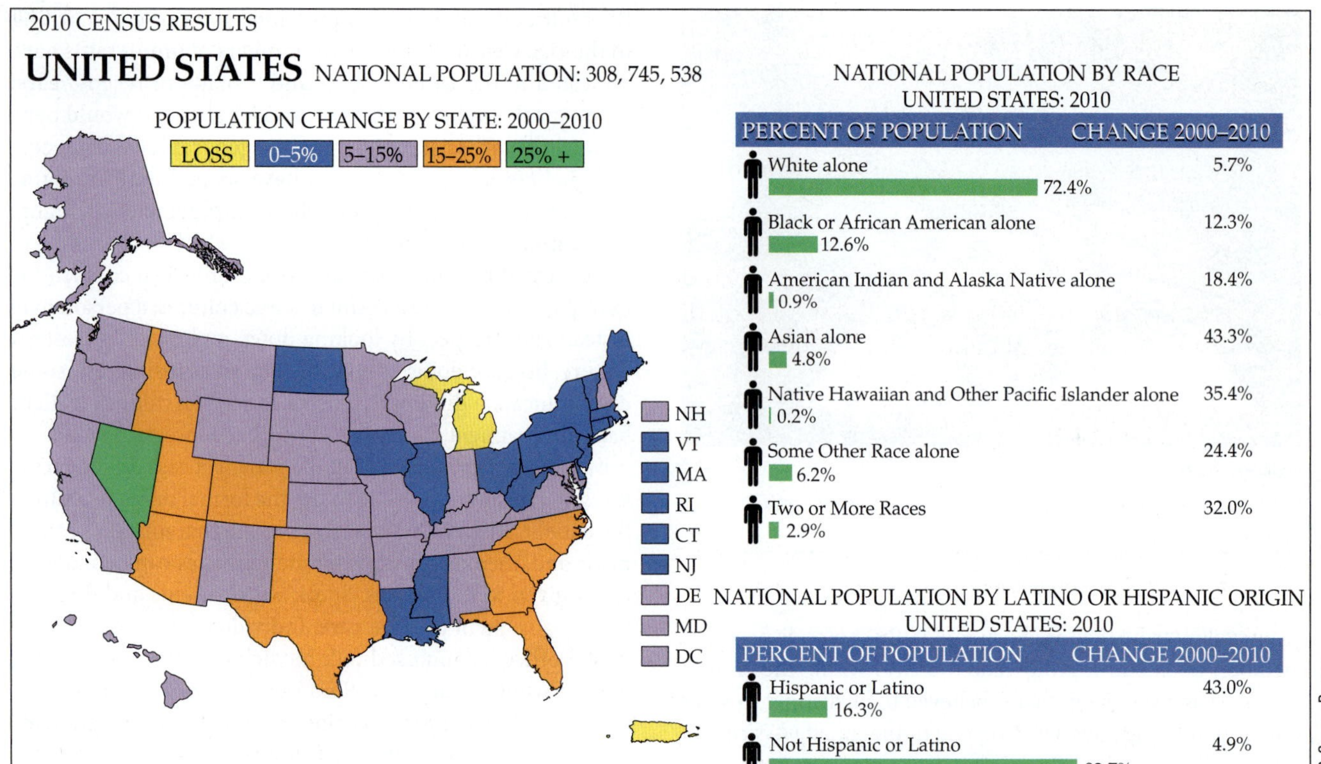

FIGURE 2-11

United States population of 308,745,538 divided into racial/ethic categories, with the population changes by state noted. (From U.S. Census Bureau, July 1, 2010).

Chapter Summary

The role of the dental assistant includes making dental treatment comfortable for patients of any culture or generation by understanding those patients' psychological backgrounds and their paradigms concerning dentistry. Appropriate communication is the key to successful interaction. A dental assistant should have skills in listening and in verbal and nonverbal communication, and should know how to overcome defense mechanisms to meet patient needs. Stress is a part of life in the dental office, however, recognizing its causes, and being able to acknowledge and resolve conflict, will aid in keeping the office running smoothly.

CASE STUDY

Maci Smith is a dental assistant in Dr. Jones' office. The office is currently working on dental teamwork and Maci cannot stay focused. In the past, Maci was involved and ready to accomplish the task at hand, but now everyone has noticed that Maci is no longer acting as part of the team. What the rest of the dental team members do not know is that Maci's husband has left her and she is about to have her home repossessed. Maci has not shared this with anyone at the office. According to Maslow's hierarchy of needs, what must happen in Maci's life before she can be emotionally present in the discussions and seek to become part of the team again at the office?

Case Study Review

1. What levels of Maslow's hierarchy of needs are addressed in this scenario?
2. According to Maslow, is it true that the basic levels of need must be met before seeking a higher level?
3. At what level in the hierarchy of needs does dental office teamwork belong?

Review Questions

Multiple Choice

1. Self-actualization is a term used by:
   a. Laurence Peter
   b. Carol Rogers
   c. Abraham Maslow
   d. Harry Levinson
2. The American psychologist that is considered the founder of a movement called humanistic psychology is named:
   a. Edmund Kells
   b. Horace Hayden
   c. Chapin Harris
   d. Abraham Maslow
3. Communication is said to be ________ percent verbal and ________ percent nonverbal.
   a. 50 50
   b. 30 70
   c. 70 30
   d. 20 80
4. Communication without words is said to be ________.
   a. gestures
   b. expressions
   c. nonverbal communication
   d. perceptions
5. When treating individuals from other cultures, it is best to treat the patient in the manner that you would like to be treated.
   a. True
   b. False
6. The science of the mind and the reasons people think and act as they do is ________.
   a. communication
   b. psychology
   c. paradigms
   d. encoding
7. A person's acquired belief system is their ________.
   a. communication
   b. psychology
   c. paradigm
   d. encoding
8. Most college students spend about ________ percent of their time listening.
   a. 25
   b. 35
   c. 50
   d. 70
9. The communication channels that are most often used are:
   a. auditory
   b. visual
   c. kinesthetic
   d. all of the above
10. Intimate spatial relationships with family members or close friends is normally within ________ inches.
    a. 3
    b. 6
    c. 10
    d. 24

Critical Thinking

1. Identify defense mechanisms that you may have used, and then identify what helped you to go forward and communicate.
2. What nonverbal communication might be seen in the dental office? What could be the intent of this behavior?
3. Define self-actualization.
4. Outline Maslow's hierarchy of needs.

Web Activities

1. Search for "cross-cultural communication" in *Wikipedia*, the free encyclopedia. Find the sections on "Interdisciplinary Orientation," "Global Rise," and "Incorporation into College Programs," and be prepared with questions and comments.
2. Go to *http://www.diversityhotwire.com*. Identify some common issues related to diversity in the workplace, as well as effective strategies for overcoming diversity issues.
3. Look up information on the Web about generations X, Y, and Z, and be prepared to discuss these generations in class. Do you think that the information you obtained is true? Why?

CHAPTER

3

Ethics, Jurisprudence, and the Health Information Portability and Accountability Act

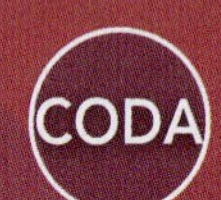

Specific Instructional Objectives

The student should strive to meet the following objectives and demonstrate an understanding of the facts and principles presented in this chapter:

1. Identify the difference between statutory, civil, and criminal law.
2. Define the Dental Practice Act and what it covers.
3. Identify who oversees the Dental Practice Act and how licenses for the dental field are obtained.
4. Define expanded functions.
5. Identify the components of a contract.
6. Identify due care and give examples of malpractice, doctrine of ***res ipsa loquitur***, and torts.
7. Define fraud and where it may be seen in the dental office.
8. Identify care that can be given under the Good Samaritan Law.
9. Describe emotional abuse, domestic violence and elder abuse.
10. Identify the four areas of the Americans with Disabilities Act.
11. Identify the responsibilities of the dental team in regard to dental records, implied and informed consent, subpoenas, and the statute of limitations.
12. Define ethics and give examples of the American Dental Association and American Dental Assistants Association's principles of ethics.
13. State how dentistry follows ethical principles in regard to advertising, professional fees and charges, and professional responsibilities and rights.
14. State how the HIPAA law has impacted the dental office and identify the parameters of the law.
15. Identify how patient health information can be used and disclosed, as well as the rights of patients.
16. Gain an understanding of the training that the staff must follow to be compliant with the HIPAA laws.
17. Identify the CDT transactions and code sets.

Key Terms

abandonment (32)
agent (31)
Americans with Disabilities Act (33)
assault (32)
battery (32)
breach of contract (31)
business associates (37)
civil law (29)
contract (31)
covered entities (37)
criminal law (29)
Current Dental Terminology (CDT) (36)
defamation of character (32)

(continues)

Key Terms (continued)

defendant (29)
dental jurisprudence (29)
Dental Practice Act (30)
direct providers (37)
direct supervision (31)
doctrine of respondeat superior (30)
domestic violence (33)
due care (32)
elder abuse (33)
emotional abuse (33)
ethics (35)
expanded functions (30)
expressed contract (31)
fraud (33)
general supervision (31)
Good Samaritan Law (33)
health information (HI) (37)
Health Insurance Portability and Accountability Act of 1996 (HIPAA) (36)
implied consent (34)
implied contract (31)
indirect providers (37)
informed consent (34)
libel (32)
malpractice (32)
negligence (32)
noncompliant (32)
plaintiff (29)
preemption (40)
privacy officer (36)
protected health information (PHI) (36)
reciprocity (30)
res gestae (31)
res ipsa loquitur (32)
security rule (39)
slander (32)
statutory law (29)
subpoena (34)
tort (32)

Introduction

Each dental team member is faced with daily decisions that require judgments regarding legal and ethical principles. Maintaining professional ethical standards at all times is essential. The area of **dental jurisprudence**, the law(s) that governs dentistry, is more clearly defined than dental ethics, or moral judgment(s). At a minimum, ethical behavior in the dental office must follow the letter of the law or dental jurisprudence. The consequences of not doing what should be legally done or doing what should not be done can be imposed on an individual in the form of fines or imprisonment.

The Law

The U.S. Constitution is the supreme law in the United States of America. If a question of how to read or interpret this law occurs, a decision is made in a court of law. The first case that relates to that particular question is referred to as the precedent. A precedent that is familiar to many is the *Roe vs. Wade* case, in which the U.S. Supreme Court established that most laws prohibiting abortion violate a constitutional right to privacy. Although this case remains very controversial, it is currently the precedent that all similar cases are evaluated against. After the precedent, all cases relating to that same situation are based on the primary decision, adhering to the principle of *stare decisis*, meaning "let the decision stand." All future cases are determined in the same manner. Following these guidelines, everyone is treated fairly under the same circumstances. These laws and rules are known as common laws and are to be followed by everyone. Law written and enacted by a legislative body is defined as **statutory law** (or statute law).

Civil and Criminal Law

Law (jurisprudence), the set of rules established and enforced by local, state, and federal governments, can be divided into two primary classifications: **civil law** and **criminal law**. The most frequent law exercised in the dental care setting is civil law, which can be divided into two subclassifications, contracts and torts, which are discussed later.

If a civil charge is brought against a dentist, he or she becomes the **defendant**. The **plaintiff**, the person who is bringing the charges against the defendant, must prove that a civil wrong was committed. If able to prove wrongdoing, restitution is awarded to the plaintiff in a monetary amount for any pain, suffering, and loss of wages that the dentist or dental treatment has caused.

Criminal law addresses wrongs committed against the welfare and safety of society as a whole. Criminal charges are brought against the defendant by the state to prevent any further harm to society and its members. If a case is proven against a defendant in criminal law, the defendant faces fines and/or imprisonment (Figure 3-1). A dentist would also face disciplinary action from the board of dentistry in his or her practicing state.

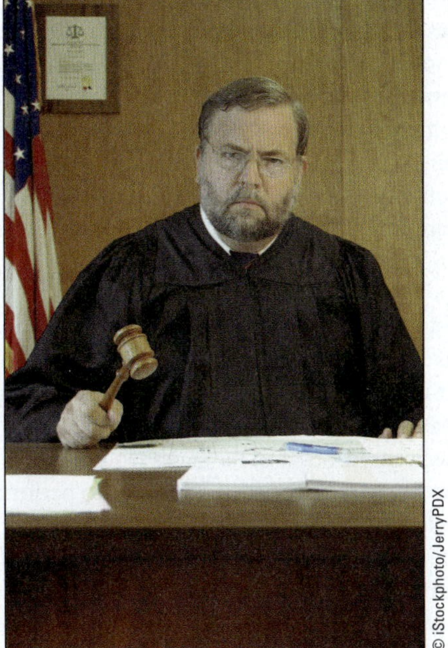

FIGURE 3-1
Judge handing down a verdict in the courtroom.

Dental Practice Act

In each state, statutes are enacted by each legislative body to make rules and regulations. The state board of dentistry is an administrative agency in each state that enforces these statutes and rules in regard to performance of specific functions. Each state has a **Dental Practice Act** that describes the legal restrictions and controls on the dentist, hygienist, and other dental assistants. The Dental Practice Act describes the dental team members as either licensed or non-licensed. It also lists the duties that are allowed or disallowed for each dental team member, including which **expanded functions** (i.e., delegated functions that require increased responsibility and skill) each dental team member may perform. Even if the job classification or title is unused in the state Dental Practice Act, any employee working in a dental office is covered in the law. The Dental Practice Act of each state gives guidelines for eligibility for licensing and identifies the grounds by which this license can be suspended or repealed. Dental assistants are advised to access the current Dental Practice Act when moving to another state to determine that state's guidelines for dental auxiliaries. Changing the content of the Dental Practice Act can be done by an amendment of the dental law, by enacting an entirely new law and new regulations to replace the old law, or by a combination of the two.

State Board of Dentistry

The dental practice act includes the name of the administrative board that supervises the act, such as the State Board of Dental Examiners or the state's Dental Quality Assurance Board. This board has the basic responsibility of enforcing adherence to the Dental Practice Act of that specific state. The members of this board are appointed by the state's governor, normally from a list of recommendations from the state dental association. The membership usually has one lay member from the state, and the rest of the board members are normally licensed dentists. In some states a dental assistant and/or a dental hygienist are appointed to the dental board. The dental assistant and dental hygienist are normally appointed to participate and bring their profession's viewpoints into discussions, but often are nonvoting members. Another function of this board is to examine applicants for dental licenses and grant licenses if the criteria are met.

License to Practice. A license is granted to a dentist if he or she has met all the minimum requirements. The license is to protect the public from unqualified individuals providing dental treatment. Each state also requires the dental hygienist to become licensed. Some of the states require dental assistants to become licensed or registered in order to perform specific dental tasks.

To obtain a license, an individual must meet educational and moral requirements and pass a written theory examination and a clinical practice examination as specified by the administrative board of that state or region. The requirements may vary from state to state, so if the individual wants to practice in another state, an additional license may be required. In some states, an individual who has passed the requirements for one state may apply for a **reciprocity** agreement in another state and be allowed to perform dental skills without taking a written or clinical examination again. Reciprocity is an agreement between two or more states that allows an individual licensed in one state to receive, without further examination and testing, a similar license in the other state(s) identified in the reciprocity agreement. The reciprocity agreement normally takes place in states with adjoining borders and similar testing requirements.

The factors for revoking, suspending, or denying renewal of a license vary from state to state. Most states take action if the licensed person has a felony conviction and/or misdemeanors of drug addiction, moral corruption, or incompetence, or a mental/physical disability that may cause harm to patients under his or her dental care.

Expanded Functions. Expanded functions are specific advanced tasks that require increased skill and responsibility (Figure 3-2). These functions are delegated by the dentist according to the Dental Practice Act within the state. Some states require additional education, certification, or registration to perform these functions. Like all functions the dental assistant performs, the expanded functions fall under the **doctrine of respondeat superior**. Translated, this means "Let the master answer." So, if wrongdoing took place, under the guidelines of employment the dentist is liable for the negligent act. However, this does not mean that the dental assistant is not held responsible and cannot be sued. It merely means that a suit can be filed against either the employee or the dentist, or both. Dental assistants who perform expanded functions are advised to carry their own malpractice/liability insurance. The dental assistant who is a current member of the American Dental Assistants Association (ADAA) has a $50,000 professional liability insurance policy that is included in ADAA dues. Other organizations and professional groups offer medical malpractice/professional liability insurance and risk management information. The Health Providers Service Organization and many others are available to provide this coverage. Often, the dentist is sued because the plaintiff

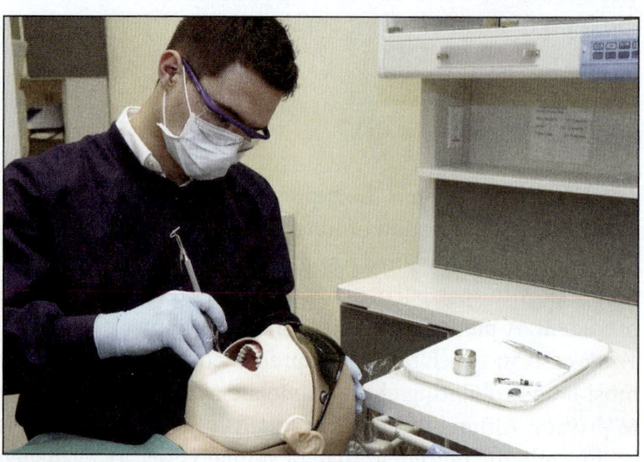

FIGURE 3-2
Student placing an amalgam restoration in a typodont, practicing for regional board examination.

anticipates greater recovery in financial damages from the dentist. The doctrine itself is based on the assumption that the dentist has the right to direct and control the employees; therefore, along with the right comes the responsibility for the consequences of their actions. In addition, if the patient is damaged, it is due to the employer exposing the patient to his or her employee. Therefore, the dentist is required to compensate the patient for any harm that was caused.

The expanded functions are most often specified in the dental practice acts according to how they are to be delegated. They may be stipulated for general supervision, which means that the procedure authorized in the dental practice act can be performed legally on a patient of record by the dental assistant under the **general supervision** of the dentist. Definitions vary from state to state, but most often general supervision means the dentist is to diagnose and authorize the work to be performed on the patient by the dental auxiliary, but the dentist is not required to be on the premises while the treatment is being completed.

If the expanded function is specified to be delegated under **direct supervision**, the dentist must be physically in the treatment facility to authorize this function, must be available within an immediate distance to respond to the patient's needs, and must evaluate the performance of the procedure.

Certification, Licensure, and Registration. Dental assistants can become nationally certified by the Dental Assisting National Board, Inc. (DANB) (see Chapter 37, Employment Strategies). Some states require dental assistants to be certified, licensed, or registered to perform specific functions in the dental office. The first state to grant licensure to dental assistants was Minnesota. Certification from DANB is granted after education or work requirements have been met and a written test covering general chair-side skills, radiology, and infection control has been passed. Continuing education is required to maintain current certification from DANB, and many states require continuing education to maintain registration or licensure.

The Dentist, the Dental Assistant, and the Law

The dental assistant must thoroughly understand the law in order to protect the patient, the dentist, and the profession. Dental health care continues to change, and the dental assistant must understand how these changes are impacted by the law.

Contracts

A **contract** is a binding agreement between two or more people. This agreement must be between two competent people, to do or not to do something lawful, in exchange for a payment. The term "competent" eliminates the mentally incompetent, individuals under the influence of drugs or alcohol, infants, and minors. The dentist has a legal obligation to care for a patient under the principles of contract law after a patient arrives for dental care and the dentist accepts him or her by providing dental care.

A contract can be expressed or implied. An **expressed contract** is written or verbally agreed upon. It describes specifically what each party in the contract will do. An **implied contract** is implemented by actions, not words. Most of the dentist/patient contracts are implied. If a patient comes to the dentist with a toothache and the dentist checks the area and requests that a radiograph be taken, this is an implied contract because it exists due to the circumstances. The law says that the dentist does what is necessary and what the patient would have requested had there been an expressed contract.

A dental assistant is an **agent** of the dentist. What a dental assistant says and does can be used in a court of law against the dentist. For instance, if a dental assistant said the dentist can cure a problem but the dentist does not cure it, the dentist—not the dental assistant—is at fault. This is considered an admission by an employee. Under the doctrine of respondeat superior, this would be the legal equivalent of the dentist himself or herself saying that this can be accomplished, even if it cannot be done. The dental assistant should be cautious because his or her actions and words at work may become binding on the employer, the dentist. Any statements either pro or con made spontaneously at the time of an alleged act can be admissible as evidence in a court of law. This is true because the principle of **res gestae**, which translates to "part of the action," is in effect at the time of the offense and therefore the statement becomes admissible evidence in a case.

Termination of a Contract. A contract can be terminated when one of the parties does not meet contractual obligation. Until the contract is broken, or a **breach of contract** occurs, the dentist is legally bound to treat the patient. The contract can be terminated if:

- The patient discharges the dentist or fails to return to the office.
- The patient fails to follow instructions given by the dentist.
- The dentist formally withdraws from patient care.
- The patient no longer needs treatment/all requirements agreed upon have been met.

Patient Discharges the Dentist. The patient often discharges the dentist by not continuing to return to the office to complete services or continued care appointments. Legally, the dentist should send a letter to the patient to confirm and document the termination of the contract. This is normally done with a recall notification, documentation on the chart, and follow-up notification. Ideally, it should be done through certified mail, requesting a return receipt, so that a copy is in the patient's chart.

Patient Fails to Follow Instructions from the Dentist. The patient may fail to follow the instructions of the dentist in regard to the dental treatment. For instance, a patient has dental implants and is told by the dentist that ongoing cleaning appointments are necessary in order to maintain the health of the area. The patient is warned that failing to undergo ongoing cleaning may cause the implants to fail. The dental office repeatedly contacts the patient to have the prophy (cleaning) appointments, yet the patient does not return. Further, the dentist writes a letter telling the patient again that the implants may fail without the ongoing cleaning appointments and asks the patient to schedule necessary appointments. If the patient chooses not to follow the instructions from the dentist and fails to schedule the needed appointments, the contract would be broken. Any time the patient fails to respond to or follow instructions of the dentist, the contract between the dentist and the patient is broken.

Dentist Formally Withdraws from the Case. To avoid any charges of **abandonment** (desertion), the dentist should send the patient a certified letter, with return receipt requested, to formally withdraw from a dental case. This would happen if the dentist feels that he or she can no longer provide service to the patient or if the patient becomes **noncompliant** (failure to follow instruction) and the dentist can no longer work with the patient.

Patient No Longer Needs Treatment. The dentist is responsible for providing treatment until the patient no longer needs treatment or the dentist has formally withdrawn from the case. For example, if an oral surgeon has seen a patient to remove four wisdom teeth and this service has been completed, and the patient has healed accordingly and therefore no longer needs this treatment, the contract would be terminated.

Standard of Care

The dentist and the dental team members have the responsibility and duty to perform **due care** (what any reasonable and prudent dental care professional in the same circumstances would do) in treating all patients. The dental professional must provide sufficient care, within his or her scope of training, in all dental procedures, not excluding prescribing, dispensing, or administering drugs.

Malpractice

The failure to use due care in dental treatment is **malpractice**, which is considered **negligence**. Negligence is the failure to exercise the standard of care that a reasonable person would exercise in similar circumstances. Negligence is the primary cause of malpractice suits. Negligence comes about when an individual suffers injury because of another person's failure to live up to the normal standard of care. Malpractice is professional negligence. There are normally four elements of negligence (sometimes called the four "Ds"): duty, derelict, direct cause, and damage. Dental professionals are held to a high standard of care by virtue of their knowledge, intelligence, and skills. It is their duty to provide high performance, and they are expected not to be derelict (careless) in their skills. If they directly cause injury due to deviation from the normal standard of care and damage or harm occurs, they are negligent. At times, in a court of law, expert witnesses will testify in regard to the standard of care that is to be expected. If a dentist does something such as removing the wrong tooth, an expert witness is not needed because of the doctrine of ***res ipsa loquitur*** ("the act speaks for itself"). The situation shows very clear evidence and there is no refuting that the wrong tooth was removed.

Torts

A **tort** is a wrongful act that results in injury to one person by another. For example, a dental assistant breaks the aseptic chain and causes the patient to be exposed to infection. If this infection causes the patient damage or harm, then the case may result in litigation. If the dental assistant broke the aseptic chain but the patient care did not result in infection, damage, or harm, then a tort did not result. A tort must have a wrongful act that is a breach in due care that causes injury because of this action. Some wrongful areas of negligence may result in torts when the standard of care is not followed. Practicing good risk management protects the dentist and dental assistant from litigation.

Assault and Battery

The threat of touching a person without consent is called **assault**, and **battery** is the actual touching. The basis of the tort of assault and battery is the threat of or unprivileged touching of one person by another without consent. For example, an assault would be to insinuate that a desired touch is indicated. If dental personnel touch any areas other than the oral cavity or perioral region (i.e., palpation of neck, TMJ, lymph nodes, and so on), this could be considered battery. An unwanted hug without consent is battery. If a child was refusing treatment and the dental assistant threatened and restrained him or her without parental consent, assault and battery charges could be brought against the dental assistant according to the tort law.

Defamation of Character

Another tort law protects against an individual(s) causing injury to another person's reputation, name, or character. This injury, called **defamation of character**, can come from written or spoken words. Defamation of character can come from either libel or slander. Comments made in writing that are false and malicious is defined as **libel**. In the dental office, untrue comments on the patient's chart may be libel. For instance, if the dental assistant wrote on the chart that he or she suspected the patient's grinding of the teeth was a result of a bad marriage, it would be libel if someone else read the chart and took it as truth. False or maliciously made comments that are spoken words is defined as **slander**. For example, a patient said, "Dr. Smith removes teeth even if they do not need to be removed." If the statement was overheard by another individual, it would be considered slander if untrue. A third party must hear or see it and understand what was said in order for defamation of character to exist.

Invasion of Privacy

Another kind of tort is the invasion of privacy. It includes unwanted publicity and exposure to public view and unauthorized publicity of patient information or anything in the patient's records. (See information on HIPAA later in the chapter.)

The dental office must take great care to protect against the disclosure of any patient information, spoken or written, on patient records. A dental assistant cannot use any medical or personal information about the patient that was obtained in the course of treatment without the person's approval or permission.

> ✱ In the dental office, unwanted exposure to public view is not a problem; however, this problem does occur in the medical field, where body parts are exposed for treatment.

Fraud

Deliberate deception that is practiced to secure unfair or unlawful gain is **fraud**. The most common area of fraud in the dental office is insurance fraud. Dental personnel who send information that they know to be incorrect to the insurance companies for payment are committing fraud.

Good Samaritan Law

The **Good Samaritan Law** is for individuals who do not seek payment but render medical assistance to the injured. This care is usually given because of an accident, and the law protects people or grants immunity for acts performed while providing emergency care. If this care is given without the intent to do bodily harm and without being compensated for this care, the Good Samaritan Law provides protection. Contents of the Good Samaritan Law vary from state to state, and each individual is responsible for understanding state laws.

Child Abuse and Neglect

Each of the 50 states has passed some form of a mandatory child abuse and neglect reporting law. This allows the state to qualify for funding and meet the criteria under the Child Abuse Prevention Treatment Act (CAPTA) of 1996. Every state requires certain professionals and institutions to report suspected abuse. Included are providers of medical, dental, and mental health care; teachers and other education personnel; social workers; and law enforcement personnel. In many states, individuals who work in film processing may also fall under this law. Some states require "any individual" to be responsible for reporting child abuse and neglect. Dental assistants in all states fall under this reporting law. Failure to report suspected child abuse and neglect can result in civil or criminal liability that may be punishable by a fine. False reports are unacceptable; cases must be made according to a standard under which a "reasonable person" would believe that the report is true.

Emotional Abuse, Domestic Violence, and Elder Abuse

Behaviors used by one person in a relationship to control the other person in the relationship are defined as **emotional abuse** or **domestic violence**. More and more individuals live in a situation where they are abused and controlled. Often they are afraid to tell anyone for fear of retaliation or losing the only security they have. In the dental office the staff may see signs of abuse and have conversations with the patient indicating abuse. The patient may appear withdrawn, have physical bruising, broken teeth, etc. Abuse of persons 65 and older is defined as **elder abuse** and may come from care takers or family. This presents a problem to those who cannot care for themselves. They find it difficult to speak up for themselves, especially if the abuse comes from their family. The dental office staff should be aware of the signs of abuse and violence and be prepared to refer or assist the patient in obtaining help with the situation.

Americans with Disabilities Act

The **Americans with Disabilities Act** (ADA) of 1990 and the ADA Amendments Act of 2008 (which revised the definition of "disability" to more broadly encompass impairments that substantially limit a major life activity) mandate nationally that individuals will not be discriminated against because of their disabilities. The four areas noted in the act refer to the following:

- Employment discrimination due to disabilities.
- The disabled are provided access to public services.
- Public accommodations and access to equal goods and services are open to the disabled.
- Telecommunication services to the hearing and speech impaired are extended.

In the dental offices, ramps must be provided to allow access for individuals with disabilities. The doorways and treatment rooms should allow for care to be provided for individuals with disabilities. One dental operatory needs to have access for patients confined to wheelchairs.

Dental Records

The dentist and the dental team members must be responsible to maintain accurate, up-to-date patient records. In litigation, the accuracy of the dental record directly relates to the credibility of the professionals. All actual care and charges must be reflected in the patient's dental records. Charts must be written in ink and be legible. All necessary corrections should be made by drawing a line through the initial content and then making the correction, initialing it, and dating the new data (Figure 3-3). Many offices are now utilizing software that allows for paperless charting. The dental record, radiographs,

Chart No. ______

Patient's Name Bradley Plummley

Date 4/9/16 #2 MOD Amal

#3 DO Amal dycal

#4 O Amal

2 anes. KJM

5/2/16 #15 Full cold Crown prep

acrylic temp cemented w/tempbond KJM

5/13/16 #15 Full Gold Crown

cemented with zinc phosphate KJM

R 250 mg V-cillin K ~~20 tabs~~ 10 tabs KJM 5/13/16

FIGURE 3-3

When changes are made on the dental chart, a red line must be drawn through the initial content; then the correction is made, with the person initiating the change notating it by initialing the chart and dating it.

medical and dental history, and all other aspects of the chart are maintained through a computer backup system. These electronic files constitute a legal record that must be securely maintained. All HIPAA documents should be copied and scanned into the electronic record. Any prescriptions used in patient care would also be saved as part of the record, and a copy printed for the patient.

Informed Consent

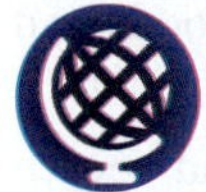

One important area of documentation is the **informed consent** form. Each patient has the right to know and understand any procedure that is to be performed. The patient is informed in words that can be understood. The patient should be told of the procedure, risks involved, expected outcome, other optional methods to treat the same problem, and the risk of denying the treatment. The health care worker must make certain that the patient understands the treatment. In today's society, a large number of patients speak English as a second language or do not speak it at all. An interpreter must be used to explain the procedure to the patient, if necessary. If the patient is a minor child, the parent or legal guardian must give consent. If the parents are separated and share custody, both parents must provide authorizing consent and ability to provide emergency treatment if needed. If the parents live separately, the custodial parent must provide authorizing consent. This should be noted on the child's record.

If surgical procedures are to be performed, it is advisable to receive a consent form. The dental assistant may sign as a witness on the consent form. One copy is kept in the patient's chart and one is given to the patient for his or her records.

There are situations when a written informed consent is required such as:

- Use of the patient's photo for marketing or on the Web page
- Use of new drugs or an experimental treatment
- When patient is put under general anesthesia
- When treatment is going to take longer than 1 year to complete
- When student dentists are providing treatment

Implied Consent

Implied consent may happen in a number of subtle ways. When a dentist sits down and the patient opens his or her mouth, the patient is implying consent for the dentist to begin treatment. Patients rolling up their sleeves prior to blood pressure being taken are implying that the actions for the blood pressure procedure can be taken. This suggestion of acceptance without voicing it is defined as **implied consent**.

Subpoenas

A court orders mandating that an individual show up at a specific time and date and with a specific reason to testify is called a **subpoena** (Figure 3-4). Dental records can also be subpoenaed by the court and must be released to the court. Any records that provide documentation about sensitive material, such as sexually transmitted diseases (including AIDS), substance abuse, and so forth, may require an additional court order.

Statute of Limitations

The statute of limitations is different in every jurisdiction (i.e., states and counties). The statute of limitations defines the period of time in which legal action can take place. Some time limits run from the beginning of treatment, some from the time the accused neglect took place, and others from the time the treatment was completed. Most timeframes run for 3 to 6 years. Given the confusion about the time limits, most dentists keep their records for indefinite time periods.

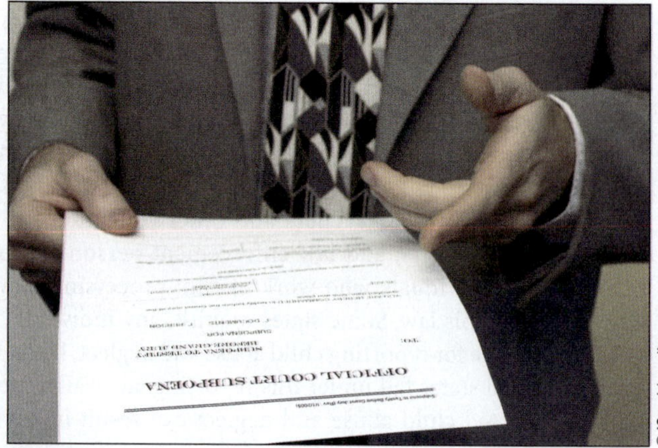

© iStock/tacojim

FIGURE 3-4

Serving a subpoena.

Ethics

Determination of what is right or wrong, or moral judgments regarding these two is referred to as **ethics**. Ethics in dentistry covers a broad range of activities, from not taking extra toothbrushes from the dentist without the dentist being aware of this act to treating patients with high standards of conduct. People learn ethical behavior throughout life. Examples of learning experiences in teaching ethics include schoolteachers talking about cheating, parents talking about treating others the way you would like to be treated, or simply that internal moral conduct message that tells you the difference between right and wrong. Ethics encompasses the concepts of good and evil. To be ethical would be to follow the "good" pathway. Unethical behavior can be legal or follow the jurisprudence of the law, but ethical behavior cannot be illegal. In dentistry, it is defined by a code such as the *American Dental Association Principles of Ethics*. Unlike the law, which rarely changes, ethics constantly changes and evolves just as personal values and morals change and evolve.

Advertising

Traditionally, dentists as professionals did not advertise. Advertising was not illegal if the advertising was truthful and not misleading, but many thought it to be unethical. Currently, it is not thought to be unethical, and there is a trend to advertise in a number of ways, such as telephone books, television, radio, media, Internet, and dental service coupons. Advertising is becoming more popular in the dental profession (Figure 3-5). Patients who are satisfied with their dental care are still the best advertising source.

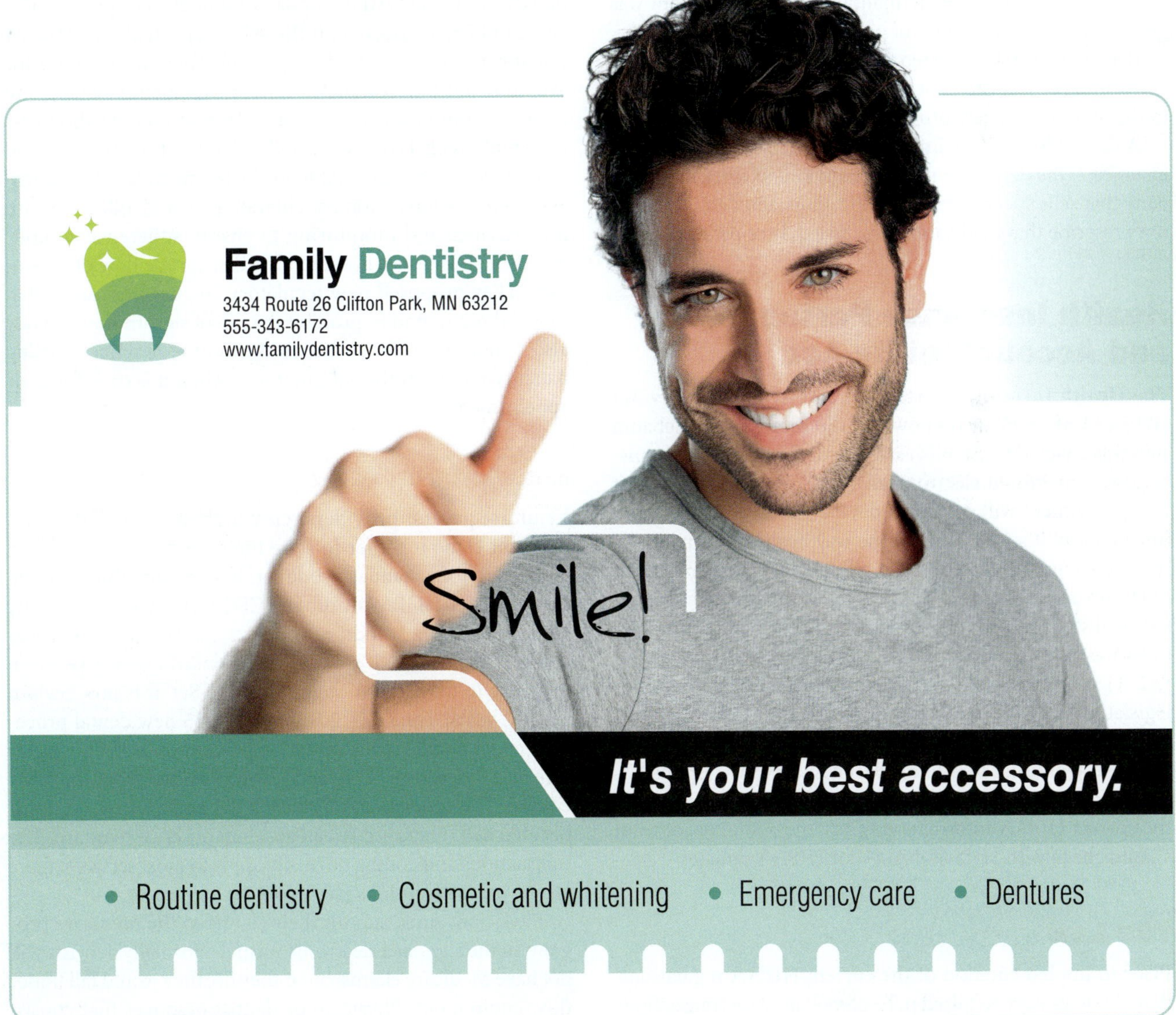

FIGURE 3-5
Advertising for dental care.

Professional Fees and Charges

Professional fees are based on what is customary to the locale and should represent the difficulty of the dental procedure and the quality of the services rendered. The services documented on the patient's chart are the ones that are charged. The office can also charge the patient for insurance processing and missed appointments if the patient has been reminded of the appointment (see Chapter 36, Dental Office Management, for further information).

Professional Responsibilities and Rights

The dentist has professional responsibilities and rights when treating patients. Dentists cannot refuse to serve a patient on the basis of race, color, religion, national origin, sexual preference, or because he or she is an HIV-infected individual. If the dentist takes a dental patient for treatment, the dentist must provide the care in a timely manner unless that patient was given official written notice of possible delays.

If a dentist is HIV infected, the dentist should refrain from performing procedures that may risk transmission of the virus to the other health care providers or patients.

A dentist is not to be influenced by financial interests. For instance, if the dentist owns a large amount of stock in a company that sells specific dental medications, the dentist should not prescribe that medication only to enhance personal gain.

Health Insurance Portability and Accountability Act

The **Health Insurance Portability and Accountability Act (HIPAA) of 1996**, also known as the Kennedy-Kassebaum Act, was enacted to establish safeguards for health care transactions transmitted electronically. This does not mean that the government will develop a database of everyone's health information; it speaks only to the way health information is transacted and protected in the office. The U.S. Department of Health and Human Services (HHS) was mandated to adopt national standards for electronic administrative and financial health care transactions. The American Dental Association (ADA) was named consultant to the secretary of HHS for this legislation. The HIPAA laws are designed to protect patient rights. Every dental office that chooses to transmit transactions electronically falls under HIPAA. It is the responsibility of providers to ensure that they are up to date and have the correct HIPAA information. Thus, the dental office team should check with HHS and ADA for HIPAA updates.

The Law

Prior to implementation of the current HIPAA regulations, dental offices were required to be compliant with transactions and code sets by April 14, 2003. The HHS released guidance on July 6, 2001, that provided further information and explanations about the initial HIPAA Privacy Rule. In March 2002, HHS released proposed modifications to the final rule. The principal modification was elimination of the need for written patient consent for uses and disclosures of **protected health information (PHI)**. It was noted that a dentist having a direct treatment relationship with an individual is required to make a good faith effort to obtain that person's written acknowledgment of Receipt of Notice of Privacy Practices. Form design, however, is left to the dentist, but must be written. The Centers for Medicare and Medicaid Services (CMS) is the enforcement authority for transactions, code sets, identifiers, and security. The Office for Civil Rights (OCR) is the enforcement authority for the privacy rule. It is critical that each dental professional know the HIPAA legislation and be familiar with the regulations and terms used in the HIPAA. It is the provider's responsibility to ensure that the office and personnel are up-to-date and have the correct HIPAA information. The HHS administrative website is http://www.hhs.gov/hipaa. It is advisable that the **privacy officer**, the person in the office responsible for keeping all office personnel updated on HIPAA, review HIPAA updates routinely. The privacy officer should also check with the ADA repeatedly for HIPAA updates to ensure compliance. Education and training for everyone must be completed initially upon employment and on an ongoing basis thereafter. It should include all efforts to comply with HIPAA through routine office policies and procedures. It is beneficial to evaluate the "areas of concern" and then develop an implementation plan and follow up with maintenance and monitoring to ensure adherence compliance. The HHS does not intend to disrupt the flow of patient care. They proposed new regulatory language to clarify that they did not intend to prohibit the use of sign-in sheets. They also noted that HIPAA did not forbid the practice of using patients' names in the waiting room when it is time for their appointments.

Transactions and Code Sets

Vendors, payers, providers, clearinghouses, and the government came together to state their needs and reached an agreement for a standard code set. In dentistry, this code set, **Current Dental Terminology (CDT)**, is revised biennially at the beginning of odd number years. The first CDT was completed in 1969. It was initially revised every 5 years; in response to the HIPAA Standard Code Set, it is now revised every 2 years. The CDT 2015 contains 15 new dental procedure codes and 52 revisions to the procedure code nomenclature and descriptors. Five codes were omitted from the prior edition. The codes currently have a "D" and a four-digit number attached. There are 12 categories in the code standard. The transactions and coding normally apply to most services; there are very few exceptions (see Table 3-1).

Physicians must submit their claims to the Medicare program in the standard electronic format. Normally dentists will not have Medicare claims, but if they do, they would fall under this requirement. Physician or dentist practices that consist of fewer than 10 full-time employees are not subject to this standard. Medicare contractors will not accept transactions that do not meet the new standards.

TABLE 3-1 CDT 2016—Current Dental Technology Standard Codes

Diagnostic	D0100–D0999
Preventive	D1000–D1999
Restorative	D2000–D2999
Endodontics	D3000–D3999
Periodontics	D4000–D4999
Prosthodontics, removable	D5000–D5899
Maxillofacial Prosthodontics	D5900–D5999
Implant Services	D6000–D6199
Prosthodontics, fixed	D6200–D6999
Oral and Maxillofacial Surgery	D7000–D7999
Orthodontics	D8000–D8999
Adjunctive General Services	D9000–D9999

What Does HIPAA Encompass?

The key element of HIPAA is the safeguarding of PHI. Dental personnel must understand how HIPAA defines **health information (HI)** as well as PHI. The privacy rule regulates how PHI may be used and disclosed. It also provides certain rights to patients and contains administrative requirements to protect the confidentiality of PHI. The Privacy Standard covers the following:

- Protected health information
- Rights of the individual
- New policies that cover the Privacy Standard for dental offices
- Disclosures that do not require authorization
- Uses and disclosures of PHI with patient authorization
- Minimum necessary use and disclosure
- Enforcement
- Preemption

Who Must Comply with HIPAA?

The HIPAA provisions, by statute, apply to all direct and indirect providers of health care services and supplies. HIPAA defines **direct providers**, also referred to as **covered entities**, as hospitals, clinics, nursing homes, assisted-living facilities, home health agencies, physicians, dentists, and alternative medicine. It defines **indirect providers**, or **business associates**, as laboratories, pharmacies, surgical centers, and any services that deal with any patient information. Health care services and supplies would include any medical and dental suppliers, information systems, record and data storage and destruction, maintenance services that may have access to patient information, and so on. The HIPAA provisions apply to any entity transmitting health information in an electronic form. Therefore, business associates that use or disclose the protected health information, or create, obtain, and use this information to perform a function or activity on behalf of the covered entity (in this case the dentist), are covered under the HIPAA provisions. Examples of business associates would include accounting firms, consultants, legal firms, management companies, data/record copying, storage and destruction companies, and suppliers.

Business Associates. It should be noted that both the covered entities and their business associates must comply with HIPAA. The dental office must have contracts with any business associates who will be able to access individuals' PHI. These parties may even include cleaning services and any other persons with patient file access. The covered entity (dentist) should make the business associates aware of HIPAA requirements and document that the information has been provided. The business associate contract must establish the required uses of patient information and outline safeguards against inappropriate disclosure. Contracts must prohibit other uses and disclosures of the patient information, and must provide for return and destruction of protected health information at the end of the contract, if possible, or require that the associates continue protection. Covered entities may be penalized for HIPAA infractions, and business associates may not. If the covered entity knows of a violation by a business partner and takes no action, that entity is violating the privacy standard. The dental office needs to exercise good judgment with business associates. For instance, if remodeling occurs when no office personnel are present, all PHI should be locked up. Charts for the following day should not be left out unprotected. This does not mean that dentists cannot discuss a patient's case with other dentists and fax information back and forth on the case. If the patient is made aware of how this information is to be used in his or her treatment and he or she signs a document that allows the dentists to discuss or fax information about the case with other dentists or specialists, such PHI distribution falls within the HIPAA guidelines.

Protected Health Information

Any information that identifies the individual or gives a reasonable basis toward identifying the individual is protected health information. PHI covers the individual's name (including nickname), telephone numbers, fax numbers, e-mail addresses, Social Security numbers, student identification numbers, photographs, oral health information, birth date, appointment date, and any geographic identifier more specific than state (e.g., zip code, county, region, or address). It also covers any individually identifiable health information such as the individual's past, present, or future physical or mental health condition as well as payments for any past, present, or future physical or mental health treatment. The privacy rule excludes any health information that a covered entity maintains in its capacity as an employer.

What this means to a dental office is that all patient records must be protected. Doors must be locked when patient records are left unattended. In an office's HIPAA policy manual, an individual should be identified as the person responsible for locking the doors. Records cannot be left out for others to see;

day sheets—sheets that show the daily schedule and patients' names with services required—cannot be left out for everyone to see in the operatories. Day sheets can be placed in a cabinet for the staff to view when necessary (Figure 3-6). Other offices have responded to this rule by taping the day sheet upside down and toward the wall (the sheet is flipped up for viewing when necessary). Screen savers could be set to come on within a few seconds of reviewing patient information and computer screens should be placed out of view of other patients. Charts cannot be left in potential view of other patients and individuals in the office. When the business office is confirming appointments for the following day or making an appointment for a patient, dental office employees should not repeat a patient's telephone number or any other PHI out loud if others could hear it. The last four numbers could be repeated but not the initial numbers that would identify a geographic area for the patient. If the office is located in an area where only one or a few telephone prefixes are used, then repeating out loud the last four numbers is also prohibited.

Location of the fax machine and copy machine is critical. It is important that any patient PHI that is copied or faxed is not visible or accessible to individuals passing by the machines. Spend the extra time to verify the number that any information is being sent to and remember that patient knowledge and consent for this transaction must have been obtained. If the dental office receives a facsimile that was sent in error, contact the sender and notify him or her immediately of the error.

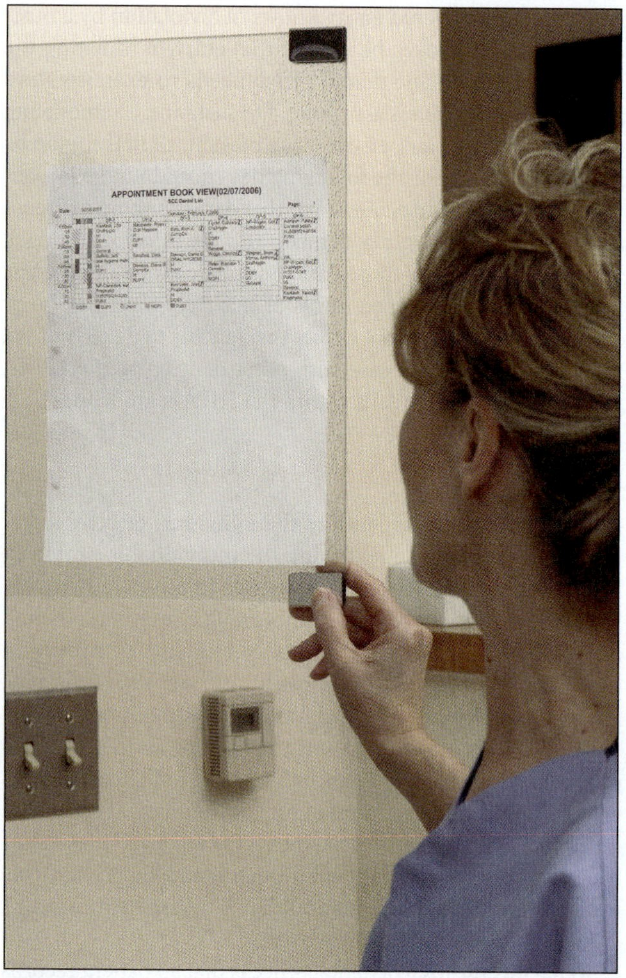

FIGURE 3-6

Due to the privacy rule, many offices are keeping the day sheet (daily schedule with patient names on it) inside a cabinet so that it is not available for viewing by other patients.

Rights of the Individuals. Individuals have the right to access, inspect, and get copies of their dental information. They have the right to request amendments or corrections of their dental information. HIPAA requires that they receive written notice of information practices and an accounting of disclosures.

Privacy Policies and Procedure Statements. Dental offices write their own health information privacy policies and procedure statements and must present this information to patients for their acknowledgment and signature. There are a number of template formats available for adoption by dental offices. The *HIPAA Privacy Kit*, available from the ADA, contains policies and procedures for dental offices along with forms, checklists, and other helpful information (Figure 3-7).

A dental office's privacy officer (PO) may be an auxiliary, or this responsibility may be shared by two or more dental auxiliaries. The PO(s) provides information to patients about their privacy rights and how their information may be used. This information must be written so that it is easily understood by the patient. The notice of privacy practices for the patient should describe how the health information about the patient may be used and disclosed and accessed by the patient. It should also cover how a patient should proceed if he or she feels that privacy rights have been violated. It should note that retaliation against the patient will not occur if a complaint is filed. The dentist and/or privacy officer(s) are responsible for ensuring that privacy procedures are adopted and followed. Employees must be trained to ensure that they understand privacy policies. This can be accomplished by giving the employees copies of the privacy policies and having each employee read the information and sign a document

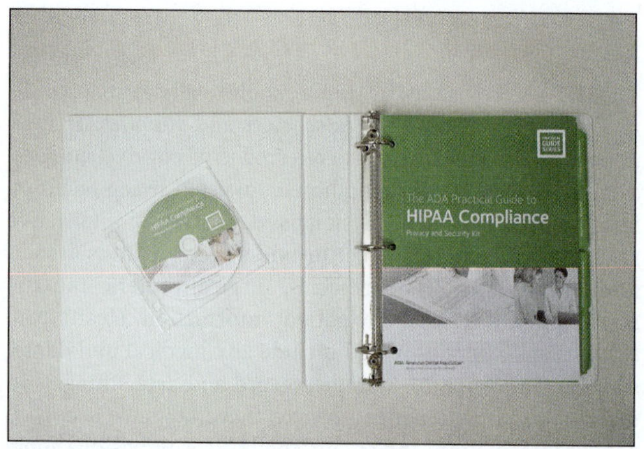

FIGURE 3-7

The American Dental Association developed the ***HIPAA Privacy Kit*** to aid members with HIPAA regulations.

that they have read the policies and understand them. These signed documents should be dated and kept as part of the office records. The office must also create and display a patient rights notice that states all rights that patients have regarding PHI. Staff training is to occur initially upon employment and annually thereafter.

HIPAA requires the following:

- Reasonable steps to protect PHI
- Identification of PO(s) by dental offices
- Employee privacy training
- Compliance with an individual's rights to a notice of dental policy, access to the individual's information, and the right to ask for an amendment and accounting of how information is used
- Administrative, technical, and physical safeguards of PHI
- A policy for handling grievances
- Business associate agreements

Patient Health Information Use and Disclosure. Patients have the right to an understandable written explanation of the use and disclosure of their health information. Patients have the right to know about all instances in which their health information has been disclosed for something other than treatment, payment, or health care operations. Patients also have the right to complain about privacy violations, without repercussion. Dental offices should develop a tracking system for all PHI and note each transaction so that they can ensure safety and protection for their patients.

Consent Requirements

1. Plain language.
2. Inform the individual of the notice of information practices.
3. Refer the individual to the notice of information practices.
4. Inform the individual of the right to review the notice before signing the consent.
5. State that the notice may change.
6. Inform the individual of the right to restrict use and disclosure of the information.
7. State that the individual may revoke consent.
8. Signature and date by patient.

A valid authorization must identify the nature of the information to be disclosed, must be in writing, and must be dated and signed by the patient. It must also identify the name, address, and institutional affiliation of the person to whom the information is being disclosed. The office may comply with this requirement by faxing a form containing all necessary information to the patient to sign and date; the patient's return fax containing signature and date is considered valid. It is a good idea to stamp any copies of PHI that leave the office so that if copies are made they can be traced to the source. Stamps for "patient copy," "insurance copy," and "copied for ___" cover most areas. Stamping in red may help determine if the information has been copied again.

Permitted Use and Disclosure. PHI should not be used or disclosed except as required or permitted by regulations and standards. It can be used for treatment and care coordination, to pay doctors and hospitals for health care, and to help run their businesses. It can be shared with family, relatives, and friends who are identified by the patient as involved in the patient's health care or health care billing. Patient PHI can be used for public health purposes, such as in reporting flu in the locale, and to make reports to the police as required. Dental offices should minimize information release. Only "reasonably needed" information should be released from the office. Patients have the right to determine how their information may be used. The dental office must honor a patient's authorization to disclose information.

Remember, release only required information, and minimize information releases. For instance, if patients ask for transfer of all records, what are they really asking for? Are the radiographs that were taken 20 years ago pertinent for the next provider? Dental offices can verify in the Office HIPAA Manual that office policy for transferring records states that the transfer can be limited to the past 5 years of information and the most recent radiographs. This would then be the standard for transferring information unless a specific request is made. The dental office does have the right to charge for copying and transferring this information for the patient. The goal is to protect the privacy and the security of PHI without hindering dental care.

Security Rule

The **security rule** mandates the safeguards required to control access to patient information and to protect it from both accidental and intentional disclosures to unauthorized persons and from alteration, destruction, or loss. This rule can be understood as implementation of the privacy rules. The dental office is not required to store all PHI in a safe, nor are locks necessary on all cabinets. Instead, office staff must be responsible in preventing the inadvertent or intentional exposure of PHI to unauthorized persons.

Office Manual

An office HIPAA manual must identify the PO and a contact person to receive complaints (who may be the same person). The manual must include job descriptions for all employees. When the dental office is creating a manual, it is a good time to evaluate how PHI is handled and what measures can be taken to ensure compliance to the HIPAA privacy standard. The manual must also include the HIPAA training plan and training dates for each employee. Training must include information about coding and electric claims submission, privacy, and security, as well as procedures and processes to be used in the office to protect the PHI. It is advisable to cover relationships with business associates during the training, as well as including a copy of business associate audits and forms in the manual. The manual should contain the privacy policy statement, HIPAA forms and supporting documentation, how compliance is maintained and ongoing, method of reporting violations, confidentiality agreements, notice about contents, notice that policies may change, and employee responsibilities for following up on change notices. Document everything to maintain a record of compliance.

The dental office staff manual must include but is not limited to the following:

- PO identified
- Job descriptions for all employees
- HIPAA training plan and dates
- Business associate audits and forms
- Privacy policy statement
- HIPAA forms and supporting documentation
- Documentation of HIPAA compliance and ongoing evaluation
- Method of reporting violations
- Confidentiality agreements
- Notice that policies may change, and employee responsibilities for following up on change notices

Staff Training and Review

Dental offices should provide training for all employees in safeguarding PHI and its usage and disclosure. Training for new employees should be organized by the PO within a reasonable time from the hire date. Retraining for employees should take place when duties change or privacy policies change. If an employee appears not to follow the office's privacy policies, then discussion should occur and additional training should be provided. Continued violation of office privacy policies can be grounds for dismissal. Dentists should encourage incident identification by employees so that ongoing evaluation and monitoring take place. Dentists must develop a policy for disciplining employees who violate and continue to violate the office privacy policy. This policy should be part of the office HIPAA manual.

Enforcement of HIPAA

The HHS Office of Civil Rights polices HIPAA. If requested, covered entities—dentists—must provide records and compliance reports. Anyone, including an employee, may file a complaint with the HHS. These complaints are covered under the whistleblower provision, and thus retaliation against the complainant is not acceptable. There are no HIPAA inspectors who will show up unannounced at the dental office to evaluate what is being done. Dental offices must self-monitor and self-evaluate their HIPAA practices and be responsible for rule compliance.

Preemption. The U.S. Congress enacted several sections of the HIPAA that are known as the Administrative Simplification provisions. Congress mandated that certain standards must be followed in protecting the privacy of individually identifiable health information. Under the **preemption** doctrine, wherever state laws are contrary to federal law, the federal law is to be followed. State law is therefore preempted by federal law. However, if state law provides greater privacy than the federal HIPAA, then the state law must be followed and not preempted. It should be noted that a request to make a state law provision exempt from preemption may be submitted in writing to the secretary of HHS.

Federal Civil and Criminal Penalties for Violations of a Patient's Right to Privacy

Civil, or noncriminal, violations of a patient's right to privacy result in prescribed monetary penalties. Penalties for disclosures made in error with no intent of violation are $100 per incident, and up to $25,000 per year per standard or individual. Criminal penalties for "knowingly" violating the patient's right to privacy upon obtaining or disclosing PHI are up to $50,000 and 1 year of imprisonment. Other criminal penalties for "knowingly" violating a patient's right to privacy are as follows: up to $100,000 and 5 years of imprisonment for obtaining or disclosing PHI under "false pretenses"; and up to $250,000 and 10 years of imprisonment for obtaining PHI with the intent to sell, transfer, or use it for commercial advantage, personal gain, or malicious harm.

HIPAA Challenge

The greatest HIPAA challenge is training and monitoring office personnel. Doing so requires that everyone be responsible for protecting patients' privacy. Ongoing training is necessary as rules and regulations change. A recommended strategy for dental offices is to "document, document, and document." A number of sources can be contacted for help. Many template training programs (on CD) contain sample forms that can be adapted to the dental office. Consultants are available for writing policies and procedures. Finally, many Web-based systems are available that can be adapted to the dental office.

The American Dental Assistants Association Principles of Ethics and Professional Conduct

Each individual involved in the practice of dentistry assumes the obligation of maintaining and enriching the profession. Each member shall choose to meet this obligation according to the dictates of personal conscience based on the needs of the general public that the dentistry profession is committed to serve.

The member shall refrain from performing any professional service that is prohibited by state law and has the obligation to constantly strive to upgrade and expand technical skills for the benefit of both the employer and the consumer public. The member should additionally seek to sustain and improve the local organization, state association, and the American Dental Assistants Association through active participation and personal commitment.

Code of Professional Conduct

As a member of the American Dental Assistants Association, I pledge to:

- Abide by the bylaws of the Association;
- Maintain loyalty to the Association;
- Pursue the objectives of the Association;
- Hold in confidence the information entrusted to me by the Association;
- Maintain respect for the members and employees of the Association;
- Serve all members of the Association in an impartial manner;
- Recognize and follow all laws and regulations relating to activities of the Association;
- Exercise and insist on sound business principles in the conduct of the affairs of the Association;
- Use legal and ethical means to influence legislation or regulation affecting members of the Association;
- Issue no false or misleading statements to fellow members or to the public;
- Refrain from disseminating malicious information concerning the Association or any; member or employee of the Association;
- Maintain high standards of personal conduct and integrity;
- Not imply Association endorsement of personal opinions or positions;
- Cooperate in a reasonable and proper manner with staff and members;
- Accept no personal compensation from fellow members, except as approved by the Association;
- Promote and maintain the highest standards of performance in service to the Association;
- Assure public confidence in the integrity and service of the Association.

(Source: ADAA, House of Delegates, (1980))

Dental Assistants Following Ethics and Jurisprudence

The profession of dentistry will continue to advance, and dental assistants will have more decisions to make in the arena of ethics and jurisprudence. It is necessary to stay abreast of the changes and it is essential to make decisions that are educated and apply specific principles. The dental assistant should always strive to stay within the law, handle patients in a professional manner, maintain a high standard of care, obtain patient consent, preserve confidentiality, maintain legible and accurate records, and avoid judging others who have belief systems that are different.

Chapter Summary

Each dental team member is faced with daily decisions that require judgments regarding legal and ethical principles. Maintaining professional ethical standards at all times is essential. The consequences for not doing what should be legally done or doing what should not be done can include fines or imprisonment. A license is granted to protect the public from unqualified individuals providing dental treatment. Some states require dental assistants to become licensed to perform specific dental tasks. The expanded functions are most often specified in the Dental Practice Act according to how they are to be delegated. They may be stipulated for general supervision, which means that the procedure authorized in the Dental Practice Act can be legally performed on a patient of record by the dental assistant under the general supervision of the dentist, or they may be specified to be delegated under direct supervision. The dental assistant must thoroughly understand the law in order to protect the patient, the dentist, and the profession. Dental health care continues to change, and the assistant must understand how the law affects these changes and must stay within the law. HIPAA regulations are required to protect patient information. It is the responsibility of the dental team members to stay informed and comply with the standards.

CASE STUDY

Desiree is a dental assistant for Dr. Wyatt. Jack, her best friend Kendra's boyfriend, came in as a patient. When he filled out the health history, she learned that he was HIV positive. He asked that she not share that with her best friend.

Case Study Review

1. Should Desiree discuss this with her best friend?
2. Can she discuss this with her friend legally?
3. How should she handle this information?
4. Should she discuss this with her dentist?

Review Questions

Multiple Choice

1. Occasionally, a dentist is sued for negligence committed by a dental assistant employee, even though the dentist himself or herself is not guilty of the negligent act. This is done on the basis of the doctrine of
   a. contract law.
   b. expressed law.
   c. respondeat superior.
   d. civil law.
2. The contract that most often exists between the dentist and the patient is:
   a. civil.
   b. implied.
   c. expressed.
   d. proximate.
3. The legal restrictions and controls that governs dentistry in each state are
   a. statutes.
   b. expanded functions.
   c. Dental Practice Acts.
   d. reciprocities.
4. A binding agreement between two or more people is a(n)
   a. agent.
   b. reciprocity.
   c. contract.
   d. breach.
5. A wrongful act that results in injury to one person by another is a(n)
   a. tort.
   b. contract.
   c. assault.
   d. libel.
6. Hospitals, clinics, physicians, dentists, and alternative medicine are described as ________ according to HIPAA provisions.
   a. indirect providers
   b. direct providers
   c. covered entities
   d. b and c
7. HIPAA was enacted in
   a. 1990.
   b. 1996.
   c. 2001.
   d. 2005.
8. In dentistry, the code set Current Dental Terminology is revised how often?
   a. every 2 years
   b. every 5 years
   c. every 10 years
   d. every 15 years
9. The office HIPAA manual must include
   a. job descriptions of all employees.
   b. PO identity.
   c. business associate audit and forms.
   d. all of the above.
10. The law that covers individuals who are not seeking payment but are rendering medical assistance to the injured is the
    a. Americans with Disabilities Act.
    b. Good Samaritan Law.
    c. ADAA Code of Ethics.
    d. HIPAA.

Critical Thinking

1. Explain the standard of care as it applies to dental assistants. Give an example.
2. What is the Good Samaritan Law? What must the dental assistant remember when giving first aid during an accident?
3. Differentiate between ethics and jurisprudence.
4. Does the HIPAA law allow patients to sign in for appointments, or is this in violation of the patient's right to privacy?
5. When calling a patient to enter the treatment room, is it allowable to use the patient's name spoken out loud in a room of other patients? Does this practice violate HIPAA guidelines?

Web Activities

1. Research the ADA Web site at http://www.ada.org and the U.S. Department of Health and Human Services Web site at http://www.hhs.gov/hipaa/ for any HIPAA updates.
2. Visit http://www.usdoj.gov and review the requirements for small businesses to aid in the treatment of individuals with disabilities.
3. Look up the state dental practice act for the state that you reside in and find the information that states what dental assistants can do legally in your state. Be prepared to discuss this in class.

Section II

Prevention and Nutrition

CHAPTER

4

Oral Health and Preventive Techniques

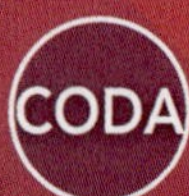

Specific Instructional Objectives

The student should strive to meet the following objectives and demonstrate an understanding of the facts and principles presented in this chapter:

1. Describe how plaque forms and affects the tooth.
2. Identify oral hygiene tips that will aid each age group.
3. Identify the oral hygiene aids, including manual and automatic, available to all patients.
4. Demonstrate the six toothbrushing techniques.
5. Identify types of dental floss and demonstrate flossing technique.
6. Describe fluoride and its use in dentistry.
7. Define fluoridation and describe its effects on tooth development and the posteruption stage.
8. List and explain the forms of fluoride. Describe how to prepare a patient and demonstrate a fluoride application.

Key Terms

acidulated phosphate fluoride (65)
acute fluoride poisoning (65)
ADA seal of acceptance (48)
ameloblasts (65)
antibacterial effect (65)
caries (45)
chronic fluoride poisoning (65)
demineralization (45)
dentifrice (46)
enamel hypocalcification (66)
enamel hypoplasia (65)
floss holder (51)
floss threader (52)
fluoridation (64)
fluoride (64)
fluoroapatite crystal (64)
fluorosis (64)
halitosis (48)
hydroxyl ion (64)
interproximal brush (51)
manual toothbrush (52)
mechanical toothbrush (52)
mottled enamel (64)
plaque (45)
posteruption stage (65)
preeruption stage (64)
remineralization (45)
rubber dental stimulator (51)
sodium fluoride (65)
stannous fluoride (65)
systemic fluoride (65)
topical fluoride (65)
water irrigation device (52)
wooden dental stimulator (51)
xerostomia (63)

Introduction

Dental assistants in the dental office have an important role in preventive dentistry. Dentistry is about preventing oral disease, such as dental decay, and preventing and caring for periodontal disease. It is important to educate the public on how to prevent disease. The dental assistant must be knowledgeable about the many products available that aid patients in maintaining their teeth and gums. The dental assistant must be a good listener and be able to evaluate the needs of patients. Dental assistants must also know how to motivate patients to be effective in their oral hygiene care. Fluoride has been proven to be effective in reducing dental caries. Therefore, the dental assistant will need to have background knowledge of fluoride to educate patients in its usage and benefits.

Preventive Dentistry

CDA The goal of preventive dentistry is that each individual maintains optimal oral health. Preventive concepts are woven in throughout each modern dental practice. To be effective in preventive dentistry, dental assistants must first care for their own teeth properly and practice good nutrition.

- Brush and floss daily to remove plaque and bacteria.
- Periodically disclose to evaluate the effectiveness of brushing and flossing.
- Follow a fluoride program while the teeth are developing to allow them to be strong and decay resistant. The fluoride program includes office applications and home treatments.
- See a dentist for routine care and, especially, when teeth newly erupt in order to have the dentist evaluate if enamel sealants need to be placed in areas where there are faulty unions in the enamel. (See Chapter 28, Pediatric Dentistry and Enamel Sealants.)
- Follow a good nutrition and exercise program to maintain overall health. Good nutrition over a lifetime allows strong teeth and bones to develop and be maintained (See Chapter 5, Nutrition).
- Schedule regular dental visits for a thorough examination, cleaning, and any necessary dental treatment.

Plaque Formation

Dental **plaque** is a sticky mass that contains bacteria, and grows in colonies on the teeth (Figure 4-1). Most people miss areas while brushing their teeth, and have noted that a soft, white, sticky mass has formed on their teeth. This consists of plaque and other soft deposits. The bacteria in plaque are fed by the sugar in food. The bacteria-rich plaque converts the sugar to acid. After a period of time, the acid attacks the tooth and eventually causes **demineralization**, in which minerals, calcium, and phosphate are lost from the enamel surface (Figure 4-2). People who have had orthodontic appliances may have demineralization on the tooth surfaces where the brackets were located. When the brackets are removed, demineralization appears as a whitish area on the tooth. It developed because plaque was not removed routinely around the brackets. In the field of dentistry, many dentists like to term decalcification as incipient (i.e., beginning to develop) decay. The dentist may decide to watch this area and hope that, with special care, remineralization may occur in the patient's tooth. When the minerals are replaced in the tooth **remineralization** occurs. Other dentists may decide to restore the tooth before the condition becomes more serious.

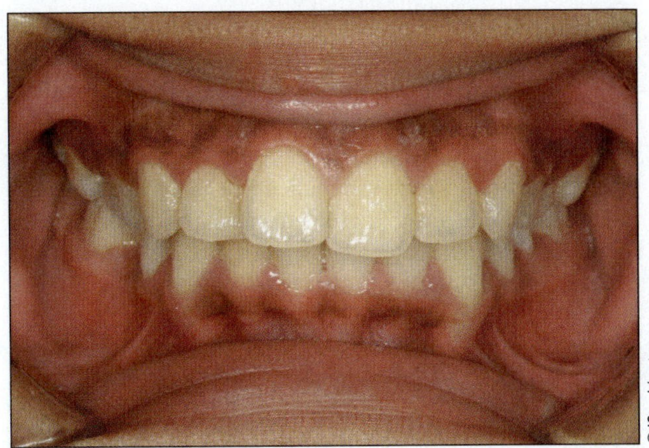

FIGURE 4-1
Plaque on the teeth has been stained with disclosing solution so it can be identified easier.

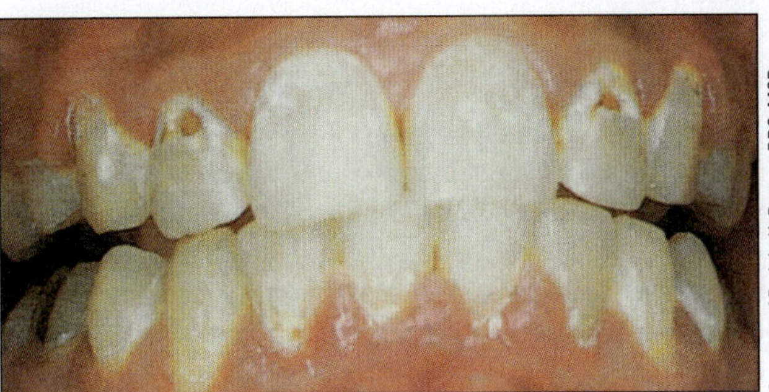

FIGURE 4-2
Demineralization of the tooth enamel appears as a white chalky area.

If plaque continues to attack the tooth, it will cause decay, or **caries**. Once dental decay has begun, a dentist should restore the area.

> **Dental Decay (Caries) Equation**
> Sugar + plaque = acid + tooth = decay

Patient Motivation

Preventing dental disease is ultimately the responsibility of the patient, but dental auxiliaries spend a great deal of time educating and motivating patients to care for their teeth and oral cavities. The first aspect of patient motivation is for the dental assistant to assess oral hygiene and to listen to the patient. Listening to the patient gives insight into the patient's attitude toward oral hygiene, and allows the assistant to get a better idea how to communicate with, and motivate, the patient. It is best to work with patients to help them recognize their dental problems and problem solve together to develop solutions, and then provide motivation and help them set oral hygiene goals.

Age Characteristics

Each patient should be treated as an individual, taking into consideration the patient's age, oral hygiene knowledge, skills, attitude, and any special considerations (Figure 4-3). Different age groups have characteristics that are normally identifiable; however, these characteristics are not absolute. A few general characteristics pertaining to each age group are discussed in Table 4-1.

Home Care

Patients are ultimately responsible for caring for their oral health at home. The dental assistant can suggest ideas that will make this task simpler while still having every section of every tooth cleaned every day. The dental assistant's goals should closely resemble the ideas that stimulated the patient's desire to meet these goals. These ideas, of course, will differ for each patient. If what patients have been doing is working, and they are not developing periodontal disease or dental decay, then acknowledge that they are doing a good job and encourage them to keep it up.

Patients should be made aware that the gingival tissue may be sore and may bleed when they first start a vigorous oral hygiene program. This means that the tissues are not healthy, but they will improve over time. It is much like the rest of the body. For instance, if a body is out of shape and an exercise program including sit-ups is started, the abdominal area will be sore for a week or so until the area is in shape. The same is true for gingival tissue. In about a week, the tissue will firm up and become healthier if the patient maintains the program. Patients should be told to expect soreness and bleeding for the first few days and not to stop because of it. They should be encouraged to continue the daily routine to maintain healthy gingival tissues and to prevent decay.

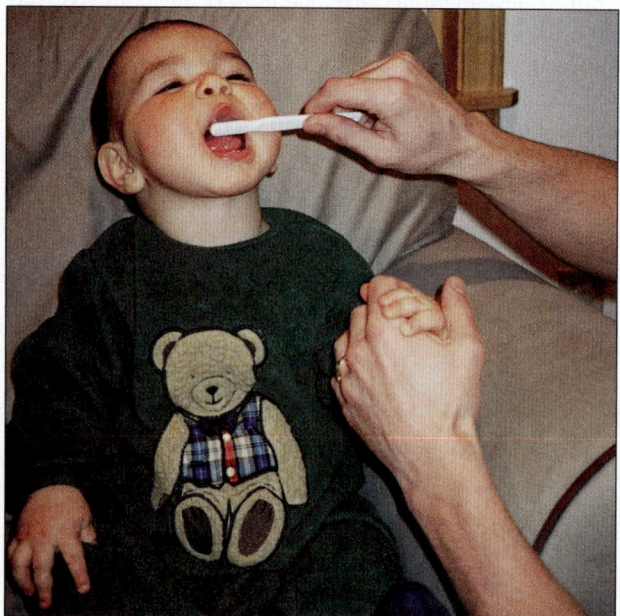

FIGURE 4-3
Parent brushing an infant's teeth.

Oral Hygiene Aids

A number of oral hygiene aids are on the market today for patient use. It is important to keep in mind that the simpler the task, the greater the chance of getting it accomplished. Adding a large number of steps will make it more difficult to accomplish the task daily. Dental team members will make suggestions for the best oral hygiene aids and the correct usage for each patient depending on their needs and abilities. The dental assistant should stay abreast of the dental aids on the market, and know how they can help specific patients.

Disclosing Agents

Most individuals are visual in their approach to life. Being able to see plaque makes it easier for the dental assistant to show what it is, and how and when it should be removed. Disclosing agents are used as a motivating factor in oral hygiene (Procedure 4-1). The agent is a temporary coloration (normally red, blue, or purple) that makes plaque visible. The disclosing agent comes in a tablet that can be chewed, a solution the dental assistant can paint on the teeth, a drop that can be placed on the tongue, or a "Snap-n-Go" swabs that highlights the older plaque with blue and the new plaque with red (Figures 4-5A to B). Also available is a fluorescent disclosing agent, which glows under a blue light. The color adheres to the plaque. Disclosing agents can be used in the dental office or at home to identify plaque. The patient should be warned that the oral cavity will change color due to the use of the disclosing agent. Before use, it is advisable to place petroleum jelly on the lips to prevent the color from sticking to the tissue. The color will go away within 30 minutes, but patients may not want it noticeable when they leave the office.

Dentifrice

The toothpaste used with brushing and flossing for patient oral hygiene self-care is called a **dentifrice** (DEN-ti-fris). All dentifrices have mild abrasives to help remove surface stains, and most contain fluoride to help reduce tooth decay. They can also contain other ingredients, such as those that help reduce gingivitis, sensitivity, or bad breath; ingredients to help prevent the buildup of tarter; and special mild abrasives that help whiten teeth by removing surface stains. As with all over-the-counter (OTC) products used

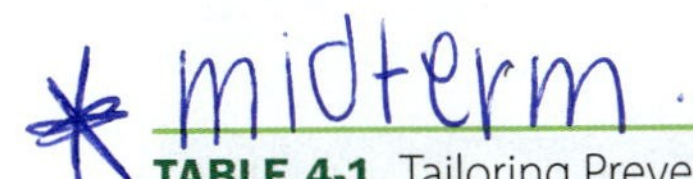

TABLE 4-1 Tailoring Preventive Care to Age

Age Range	Characteristics	Needs	Teaching
Infants (birth to one year)	• Unable to care for teeth on their own	• Must be accomplished by parent or guardian • Needs to be a positive experience • Make it fun	• Positioning child in arms or sitting in chair • How to hold hand and use washcloths or infant tooth brushes (Figure 4-3)
Preschool (one year to four years)	• Lacks highly developed motor skills • Attention span of about 5 minutes • Unable to read • Loves to imitate parents	• Use visual aids (fun toothbrush or puppet) • First appointment with dentist around the age of three • Should be positive and pleasant • Still need parental assistance	• Use "Mr. Air" to blow "wind" on the tooth • Use "Mr. Water" to give the child a drink • Count the "upstairs" and "downstairs" teeth • Demonstrate use of the toothbrush to "tickle" the teeth • At home, sit and watch TV or listen to a story while brushing teeth • Have parents role play • Must get a thorough monitored brushing at least once a day (at bedtime) but twice a day is best • Try to floss between molars once per day
Five through eight years	• Attention span increases to 10 to 15 minutes • Learning to read • Expanding vocabulary • Likes to please adults and enjoys learning • Loves facts • Requires constant guidance • Dexterity is improving	• Use positive reinforcement • Make it fun and entertaining	• Teach better brushing techniques • Teach how to floss • Use cartoon videos for demonstration and teaching • Coloring sheets, matching, and finding items in pictures make learning fun (Figure 4-4) • ADA has videos for use in teaching
Nine through twelve years	• Wants to fit in with peers • Very curious • Are able to brush and floss proficiently • Attention span around 30 minutes	• Mixed dentition may need special care	• Use realistic visual aids • Give rewards for good hygiene • Take pictures for an honor wall in the office or online with parental permission • ADA has videos for use in teaching
Thirteen through Fifteen years	• Motivated by peer pressure and personal appearance • May be uncoordinated	• Improved nutrition • More diligence with hygiene • Provide positive reinforcement	• May need practice flossing • Teach good nutrition
Sixteen through nineteen years	• Peer pressure continues to be a factor • Questioning of authority • Wants to avoid bad breath • Improved coordination	• Improve nutrition habits • Improve techniques	• Teach good nutrition • Allow them to take responsibility • Teach about the role of sugar in tooth health, plaque formation, and decay • Demonstrate improved brushing and flossing techniques
Twenty through sixty years	• May develop gingivitis or periodontal disease • Plaque may build up with lack of dental care	• Have more specialized needs and concerns that are individualized • Must be involved and motivated	• Teach how to unlearn bad habits • Assistance with identifying problems • Teach that bleeding indicates care or attention is required
Sixty plus years	• Motivated to keep teeth for lifetime • May develop physical impairments • May be taking medications	• Repair or replacement of restorations and appliances	• Teach value of routine appointments • Discuss age-related changes that impact oral health • Techniques to adapt to arthritis • Discuss impact of medications on oral health

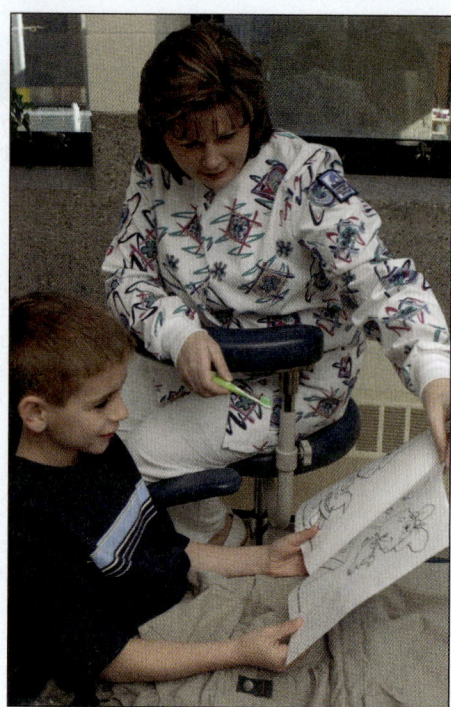

FIGURE 4-4

A 7-year-old patient is learning how to improve brushing technique.

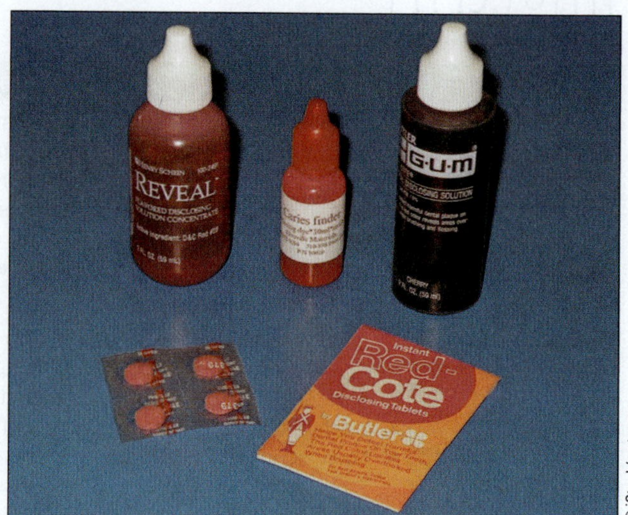

© iStock/watanyou

FIGURE 4-5A

Examples of disclosing solutions (tablets and liquids).

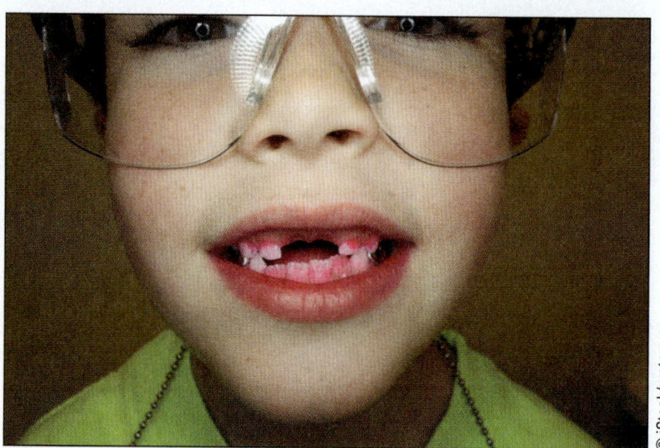

© iStock/watanyou

FIGURE 4-5B

Disclosing solution on the patient's teeth indicating where improved oral hygiene is needed.

in oral hygiene, use only those that have been reviewed and accepted by the ADA. In order to be awarded the **ADA seal of acceptance** (Figure 4-7), products are first subject to a rigorous scientific review by the ADA Council on Scientific Affairs (CSA) to determine if they meet ADA criteria for safety and effectiveness. Products that meet these criteria are awarded the ADA seal, which will appear on product packaging and labeling. Products are awarded the ADA seal for a period of five years; after that, products can be resubmitted for continued ADA acceptance for successive five-year periods.

Toothpaste is used by most individuals for dental care. Many types of toothpaste are available to patients, with numerous different flavors and consistencies (Figure 4-8). It should be chosen carefully based on the abrasives, as well as how well it controls caries. The dentifrice (toothpaste) most often recommended is one that contains fluoride, especially for children and adults who are prone to caries. A small, pea-sized amount should be expelled onto the toothbrush for use. Toothpaste should not be ingested (because of the possibility of excessive intake of fluoride), and the excess should be expectorated (spat) into the sink. Toothpaste with low abrasives is also recommended, because extremely high abrasives can permanently damage the patient's teeth with repeated use (they actually abrade the tooth structure). If a patient is prone to calculus (hard deposits mineralized on the teeth), there are toothpastes on the market with active ingredients that inhibit the growth of supragingival calculus. Other specialized toothpaste products whiten teeth or reduce gingival sensitivity when used routinely.

Mouth Rinses

Mouth rinses are used for cosmetic or therapeutic reasons (Figures 4-9A and B). Advertisements may lead patients to believe that mouthwashes do more than is possible. Vigorous rinsing with mouthwashes may loosen debris and give the patient a pleasant taste and feel, and will temporarily eliminate **halitosis** (bad breath). They can also reduce the total number of microorganisms in the mouth. However, mouth rinses should not be used to replace brushing and flossing. The ADA has approved oral rinses that contain fluoride, which helps reduce dental decay and supragingival plaque. Individuals using these rinses must follow manufacturer's directions.

Rinses with fluoride are often prescribed for patients who have a high incidence of decay. Rinses that can be purchased at the pharmacy or the grocery store generally contain 0.05 percent sodium fluoride and are for daily use. The fluoride that is prescribed generally contains 0.2 percent sodium fluoride or 0.63 percent stannous fluoride. The stannous

Procedure 4-1
Applying Disclosing Agent for Plaque Identification

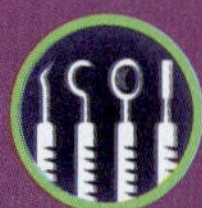

The dental assistant or dental hygienist performs this procedure. During the hygiene appointment, disclosing would be done to identify plaque and its location for the patient and operator. In some offices, a record of plaque location is charted and referred to during future appointments. Means of removing the plaque are then discussed and demonstrated.

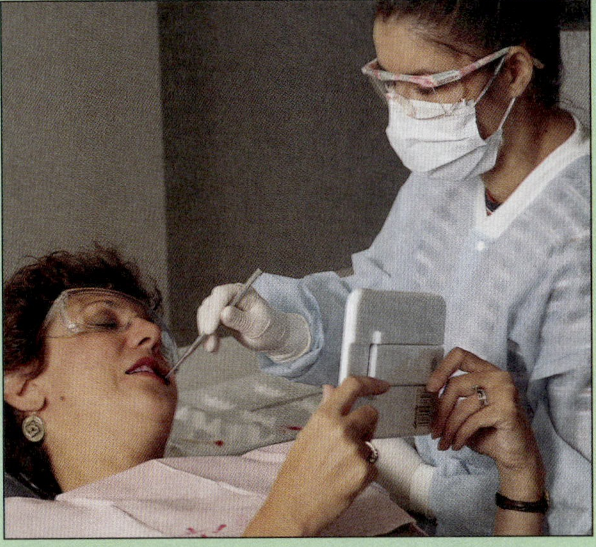

FIGURE 4-6

Dental assistant working with a patient to identify dental plaque. Disclosing agent on the patient's teeth identifies plaque.

Equipment and Supplies

- Basic setup: mouth mirror, explorer, and cotton pliers
- Saliva ejector, evacuator tip (HVE), and air–water syringe tip
- Cotton rolls, cotton-tip applicator, and gauze sponges
- Petroleum jelly (lubricant)
- Disclosing agent (liquid, tablet, or swab) and dappen dish
- Plaque chart and red pencil, or software program

Procedure Steps

1. While seating the patient, the operator reviews the medical and dental history with the patient.
2. After washing hands and donning personal protective equipment (PPE), such as a mask, gloves, and glasses, the operator examines the oral cavity.
3. The operator applies the lubricant to the patient's lips (some dentists may want lubricant applied on any tooth-colored restorations to prevent staining).
4. The operator applies the liquid using the dappen dish and cotton-tip applicator. All accessible surfaces of the teeth should be covered with the disclosing solution.
5. If using the tablet, the patient chews and swishes for 15 seconds.
6. The remaining solution is rinsed only once or twice, and then is evacuated from the area.
7. The patient uses a hand mirror to see the plaque, and the operator uses a mouth mirror and an air–water syringe to identify the plaque (Figure 4-6).
8. Overgloves are placed over treatment gloves to record the plaque in the chart or on the computer. It should be noted that some states do not allow overgloves to be used for any type of treatment, even in the case of placing them over treatment gloves to write on a chart. The dental assistant would then have someone else chart for him or her, or place a barrier on the computer or writing utensil to allow for charting to occur.
9. The operator removes the overgloves (treatment gloves remain in place), and then he or she demonstrates for the patient the methods of brushing and flossing for plaque removal.

fluoride can also be used for decreasing the sensitivity of the tooth to hot and cold (dental hypersensitivity). Fluoride rinses are used for their antiplaque properties. When using the fluoride rinse it is best to brush and floss thoroughly, and then dispense about 10 mL of solution, swish in the mouth for one minute, and then spit it out. Adults should not swallow the solution and children should be monitored so they do not swallow the rinse. It is not advisable to ingest excessive fluoride. After rinsing with the solution, the patient should not eat or drink for 30 minutes. This allows the rinse to have time

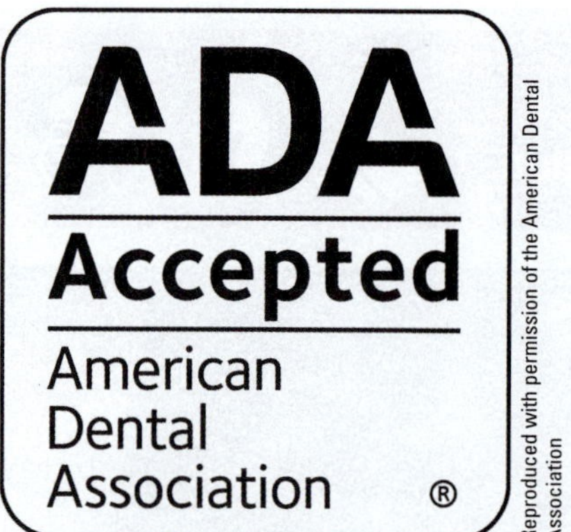

FIGURE 4-7

American Dental Association (ADA) Seal of Acceptance. The Program began in 1930 to promote the safety and effectiveness of dental products.

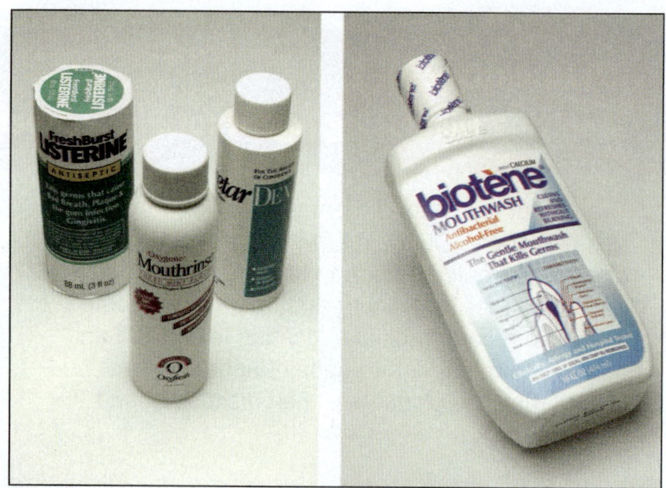

FIGURE 4-9A

Antimicrobial mouth rinses.

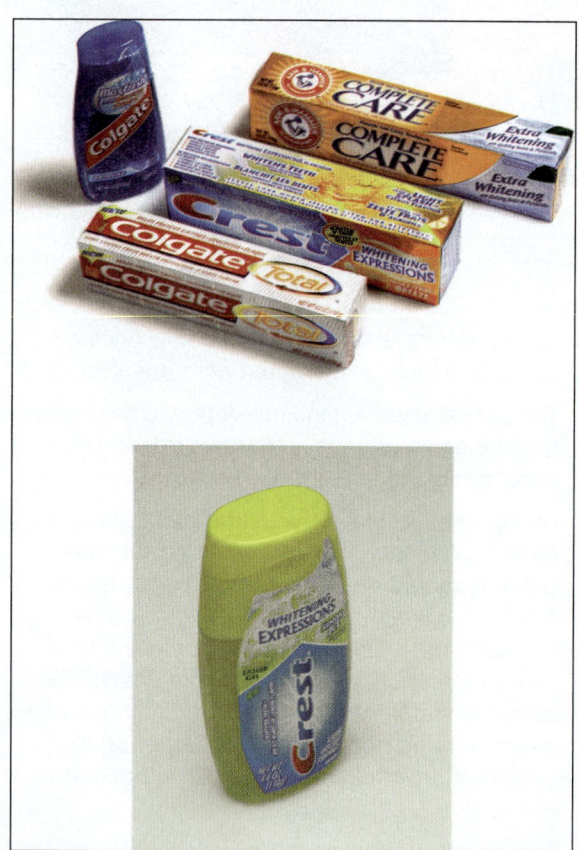

FIGURE 4-8

Examples of toothpastes used with brushing.

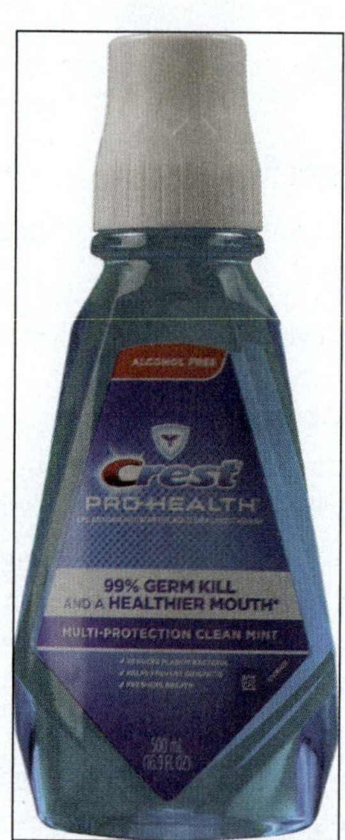

FIGURE 4-9B

Multi Protection Oral Rinse

to be effective. Other fluoride rinses contain antimicrobial properties that can be used for the prevention and control of periodontal disease.

Chewing Gum

Chewing gum designed specifically for oral hygiene purposes is a fairly new aid on the market (Figure 4-10). It is recommended for use after the intake of carbohydrates. Gum chewing stimulates saliva that buffers the plaque acid and is said to have carious-inhibition properties. The chewing action also helps dislodge particles from the teeth.

Interdental Aids

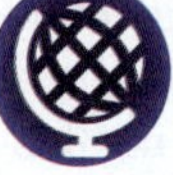

Interdental aids are used to aid in cleaning the area between the teeth and to stimulate the gingival tissue in that area. In ancient oriental cultures, women would put spices between the teeth to have good breath. These women did not develop periodontal disease at the

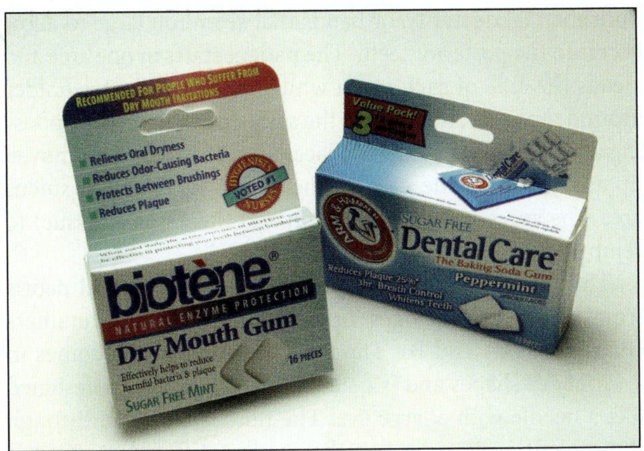

FIGURE 4-10
Xylitol-containing chewing gum used to prevent tooth decay.

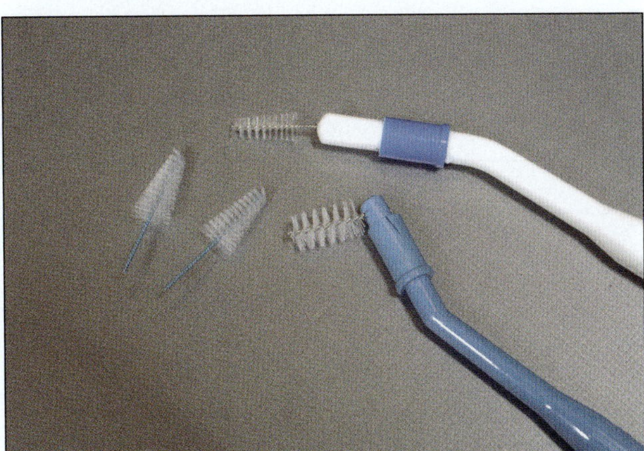

FIGURE 4-11A
Interproximal brushes.

same rate as other individuals, and it was found that the spices being placed and removed routinely cleaned the plaque in that area, therefore, eliminating periodontal disease. In other early cultures, it was said that a "chew stick" was used to clean the interproximal areas of the teeth. It resembled the toothpick and, after the end was chewed, the small fibers spread out slightly. As it was inserted into the areas between the teeth, it cleaned the opposing surfaces. Some individuals today use the toothpick in this manner, and it is quite effective at removing plaque between the teeth. A number of other products are on the market for use today.

The **interproximal brush** is a small hand-held brush with soft nylon bristles twisted in wire and adapted into a handle (Figures 4-11A and B). It comes in different shapes and sizes and can be disposable. The brush is placed in the interproximal area and rotated back and forth using light pressure. Patients who have open contact areas, or a substantial amount of bone loss due to periodontal disease, would benefit from the interproximal brush. This brush is also useful to individuals who have open bifurcation or trifurcation areas (where the roots of the teeth come together). It is also handy to use around orthodontic brackets to clean the difficult-to-access areas.

The devices called a **rubber dental stimulator** and a **wooden dental stimulator**, respectively, are placed in the interproximal area, angled toward the occlusal (biting) surface, and rotated in a circular pattern. This action stimulates the soft tissues and removes plaque in this area. Many toothbrushes have a rubber stimulator at one end that can be used for this purpose (Figure 4-12). Wooden stimulators often come in a pack, much like a book of matches. These elongated, softwood wedges are first moistened before use. The wood, normally balsam, has a little give as it stimulates the tissue. Another type of wooden dental stimulator has a plastic handle device that holds a moistened toothpick tip, and is used in the same manner as the rubber and wooden stimulators.

The **floss holder** is a Y-shaped device with a handle used by some individuals to hold floss tightly as it is placed into

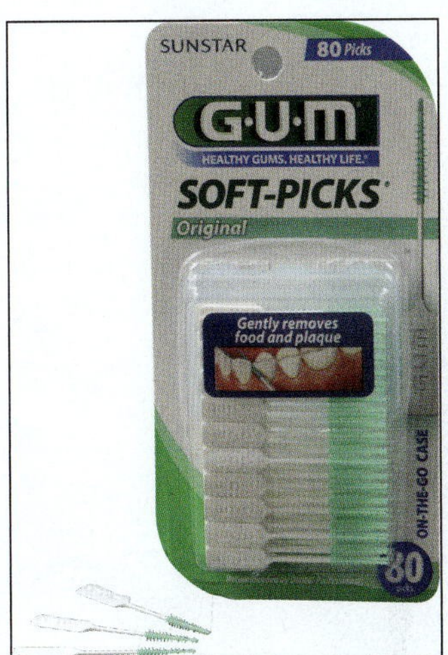

FIGURE 4-11B
Soft picks for easy on the go cleaning

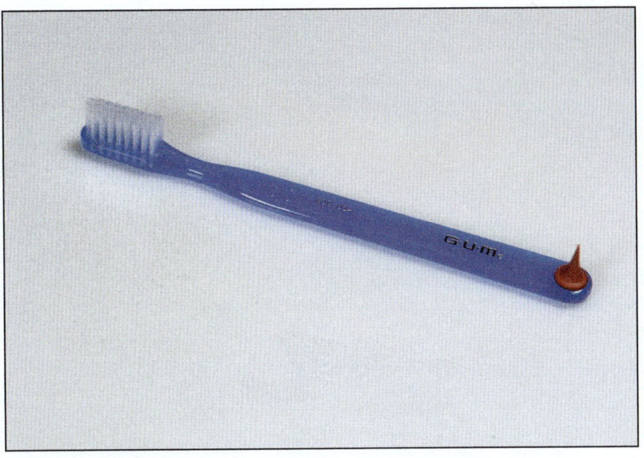

FIGURE 4-12
Rubber tip stimulator on the end of a toothbrush.

the interproximal area of the teeth and around the posterior end of the last tooth in each quadrant (Figure 4-13). The floss holder makes flossing easier for individuals who have arthritis, poor manual dexterity, or hands that seem too large to allow access to the posterior teeth. The patient starts in one area and cleans the side of each tooth while rotating the floss holder around the arch, and then, in the same manner, on the opposing arch. The floss holder is placed into each area and moved up and down on the sides of the tooth, and into the sulcus area (the space between the tooth and the gingival tissue) to remove plaque, and clean the area.

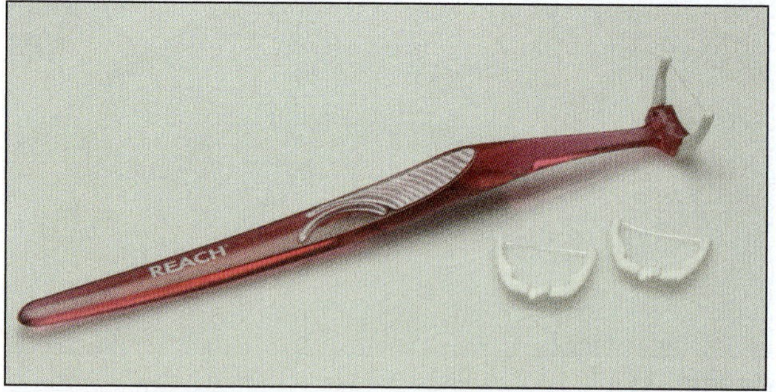

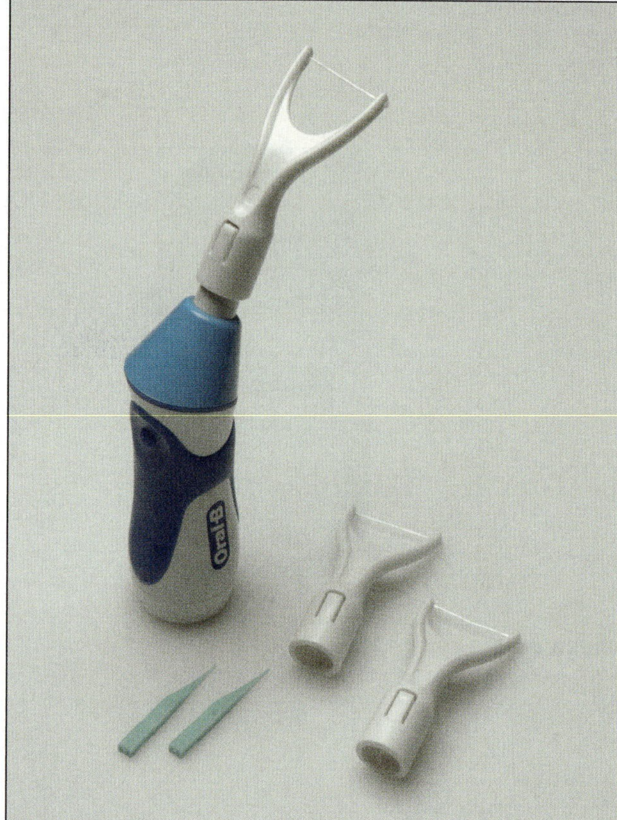

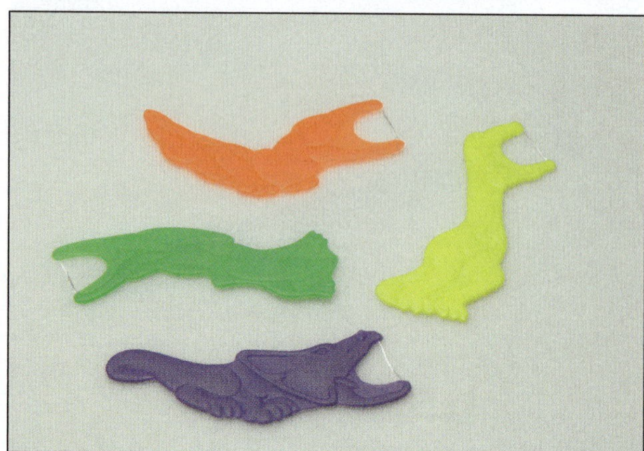

FIGURE 4-13

Floss holders and flossers.

The **floss threader** is used to remove plaque and debris from under fixed bridges, orthodontic wires, and retainers (Figures 4-14A and B). The floss threader, which comes in a variety of shapes and is made from stiff plastic, is designed like a needle with a large eye. The floss is threaded through the eye of the threader and the needle (stiff end) portion is then threaded through the intended area by the patient. When the floss reaches the opposite side, the floss threader can be removed, leaving the floss in place to clean this difficult-to-reach area. This allows the patient to direct the floss under the appliance and to clean away plaque and debris. After the entire area is cleaned, the floss can be removed. The area should be flossed daily using the threader to maintain proper oral hygiene.

A **water irrigation device** is used to flush away debris from orthodontic brackets and other prosthetic devices. It does not remove plaque and should not replace brushing

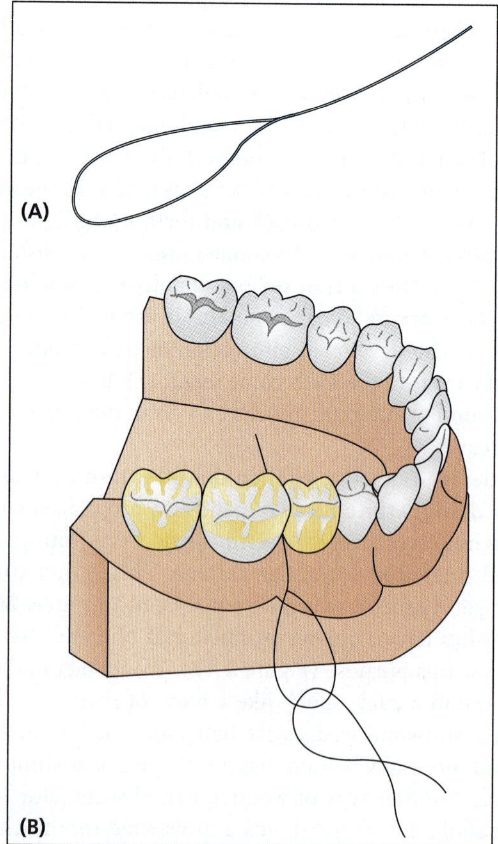

FIGURE 4-14

(A) Floss threader. (B) Floss threader threaded under the pontic area of a three-unit bridge.

and flossing. The pulsating water flow allows food debris to be removed easily; some patients place mouthwash in the fluid-holding container to gain fresh breath in the process. The patients should be instructed to use the water irrigation device carefully, because it can cause tissue damage when turned on high and directed toward the gingival sulcus (it could force debris into the tissue and damage the periodontium). It should be used at low speed and in a direction that forces debris to be pushed away from the gingival area.

Toothbrushes and Techniques

Most patients use toothbrushes, but many have never been shown proper techniques and the methods recommended today. Patients should be shown that the toothbrush only cleans three of the five tooth surfaces. The proximal (between-the-teeth) tooth surfaces normally are not accessible with a toothbrush.

Patients have a variety of toothbrushes to select from today. Dental assistants must stay informed of these choices so they can answer patients' questions appropriately. Various styles and designs of both the **manual toothbrush** (powered by the human hand) and the **mechanical toothbrush** (powered by electricity or batteries—the toothbrush moves while being held by the individual) are on the market today. Mechanical toothbrushes normally come with recharging units.

Correctly designed toothbrushes are sized and shaped to allow for efficient cleaning and easy management. The toothbrush should be durable and inexpensive, and have bristles that are flexible and soft (normally polished on the end), allowing for repeated use. The handle must be firm and strong as well as lightweight. The choice of a toothbrush should reflect individual needs. Some adult patients use children's toothbrushes to gain access to the teeth in the most posterior areas of their mouths.

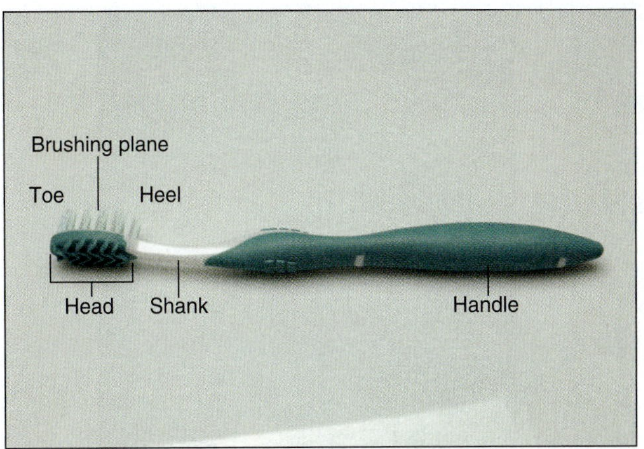

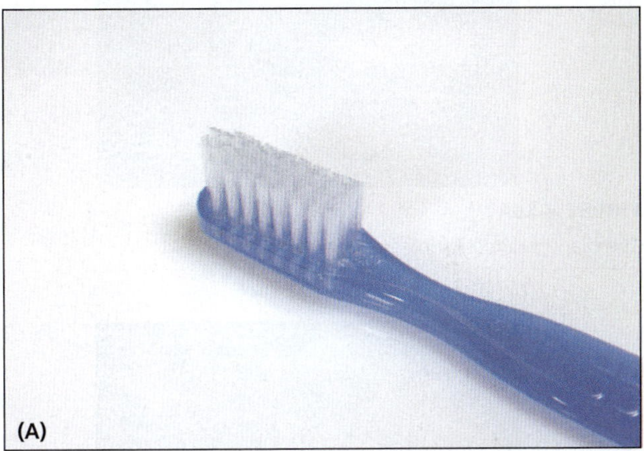

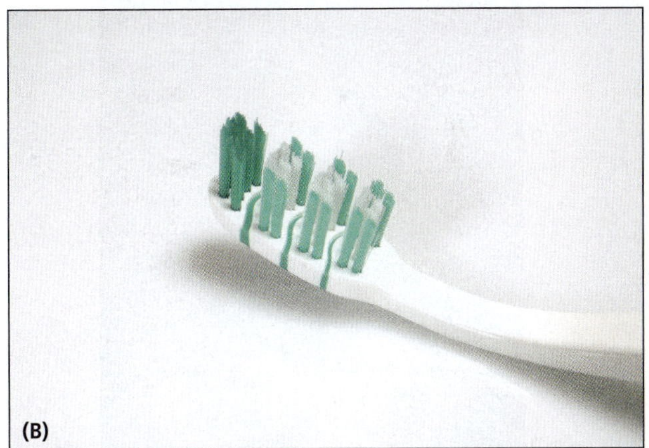

FIGURE 4-15

Manual toothbrush parts identified. (A) Spaced. (B) Multi-tufted.

Manual Toothbrushes

The parts of a manual toothbrush are the head, shank, and handle (Figures 4-15A and B). The bristles are placed on the head of the brush. They can be multitufted or spaced, and come in a number of patterns. Normally, the handle, shank, and head are in a relatively straight plane. Nylon bristles are recommended because they maintain their shape longer than natural bristles, and they dry quickly. The ends of the nylon bristles are often run over a flame to cause rounded ends that will not abrade the tooth. Soft bristles are recommended over medium and hard because they do not abrade the tooth or the gingival surface.

Mechanical Toothbrushes

Many patients use mechanical toothbrushes (Figures 4-16A and B). Like manual toothbrushes, there are many models of mechanical toothbrushes on the market today. They have larger handles and chargers (the handles have to be larger to hold the rechargeable battery and circuit board). The heads of the mechanical toothbrush can move in several different directions, and are available in different sizes and shapes for all oral health needs. Dental assistants must be familiar with each motion to be able to recommend the appropriate toothbrushing method for each motion. The motions can be reciprocating, orbital, vibratory, arched, elliptical, or a combination of two or more of these motions (Figure 4-17). Newer

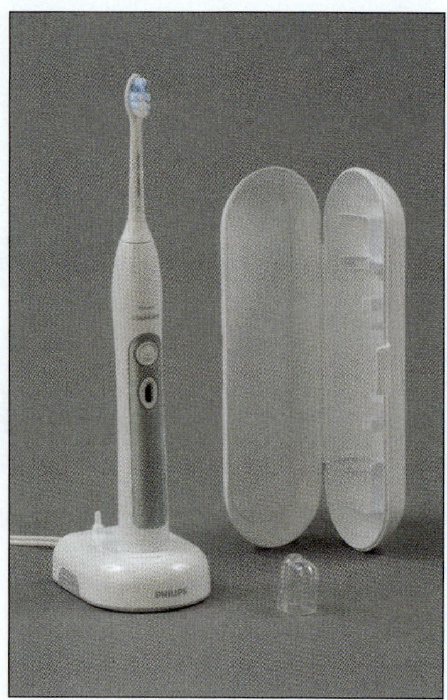

FIGURE 4-16A

The diamond head Sonicare toothbrush.

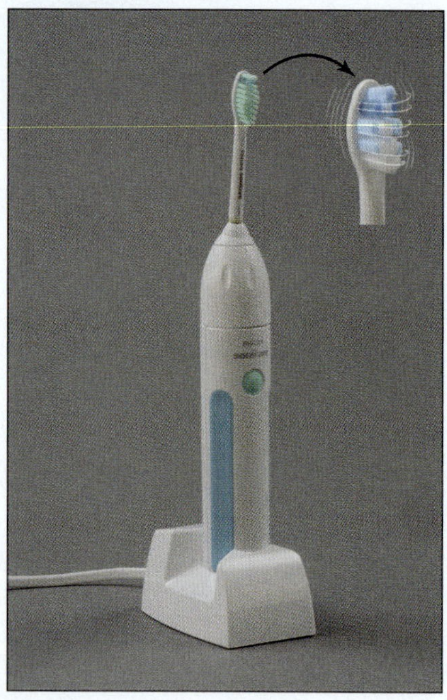

FIGURE 4-16B

Phillips Sonicare® dynamic action gently and effectively reaches deep between teeth and along gumlines.

Motion	Illustration
Reciprocating motion—moves back and forth in a line	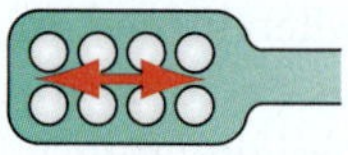
Orbital motion—moves in a circle	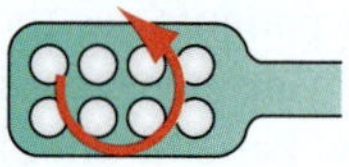
Vibratory motion—vibrates quickly back and forth	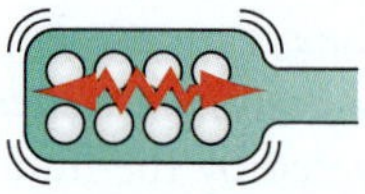
Semicircular motion—moves in an arc	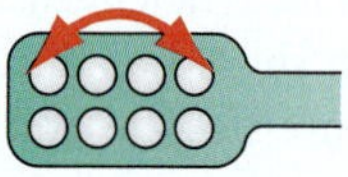
Elliptical motion—moves in an oval	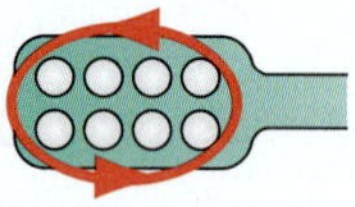

FIGURE 4-17

Motions of mechanical toothbrushes.

models also incorporate sonic action that seems to be particularly effective in removing plaque and extrinsic stains. Some of the automatic units have built-in timing devices that allow 30 seconds for each of the four quadrants and stop when 2 minutes have elapsed. An automatic toothbrush can be used in place of a manual toothbrush. Care should be taken to apply light pressure and to let the action of the bristles clean the teeth and gums.

Advanced mechanical toothbrushes incorporate the latest oral technology (Figures 4-18A and B). These toothbrushes connect with your smart phone through Bluetooth. It allows for personalized guidance, tracks your performance over time

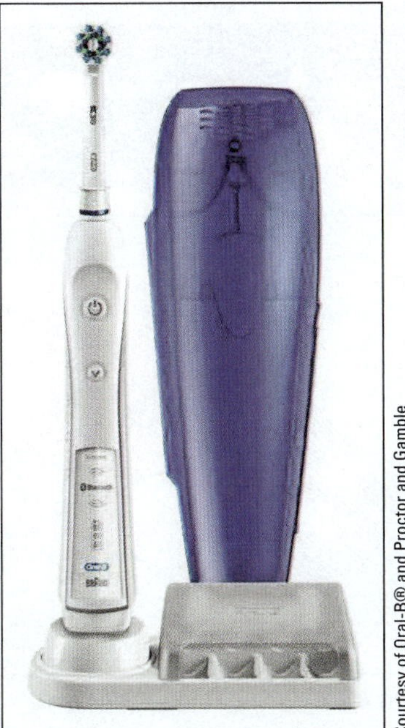
Courtesy of Oral-B® and Proctor and Gamble

FIGURE 4-18A

Oral B® pro 5000 automatic toothbrush with bluetooth communications.

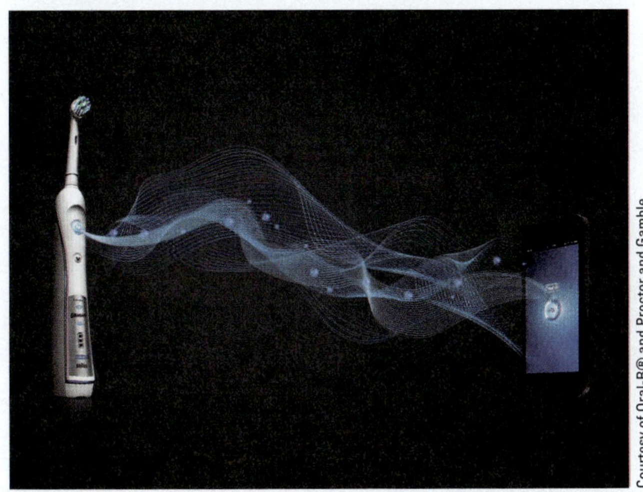
Courtesy of Oral-B® and Proctor and Gamble

FIGURE 4-18B

Action with the bluetooth communication.

with graphs and charts, and stores up to 6 months of brushing data. It senses when the patient is brushing too hard, has unique adjustable settings based on dental professional input, and motivates the patient to brush with news, reminders, recommendations, and rewards.

Brushing Techniques for the Manual Toothbrush

Several toothbrushing techniques can be used to obtain proper oral hygiene. Any technique should allow for all the surfaces of all the teeth to be cleaned. Brushing will not clean the interproximal areas. Some patients will be successful in noting the amount of time spent on brushing by using a timer. Normally, 2 to 3 minutes is recommended to clean the facial, lingual, occlusal, and incisal surfaces of all the teeth. A pattern should be developed by the patient to ensure that no area is missed. Some patients like the counting system in which five to ten strokes are made in each area. Starting at the same point each time when brushing is a good idea. For example, one could start at the maxillary (upper) right facial surface area (cheek and lip side), and then continue around the entire surface to the maxillary left. From this position, the lingual side (tongue side) of the arch can be cleaned from the left to the right. The mandibular (lower) teeth can then be cleaned in the same manner, starting from the right, continuing to the left, and then cleaning the lingual side from the left to the right. It does not matter what the pattern is; it only matters that no teeth are left uncleaned. The heel or the toe of the toothbrush can be used effectively on the narrower anterior areas. There are six commonly used brushing techniques: Bass or modified Bass, Charters, modified Stillman, rolling stroke, Fones, and modified scrub.

Bass or Modified Bass Brushing Technique. The Bass or modified Bass is the most popular in the dental community. The Bass technique is named for Dr. C. Bass, a dentist who was an early advocate of preventive dentistry. The Bass brushing technique is used to remove plaque next to, and directly beneath, the gingival margin (Procedure 4-2).

Charters Brushing Technique. This brushing technique is used to loosen plaque and debris and to stimulate both the marginal and interdental gingiva (Procedure 4-3). The primary difference from the Bass technique is the angle of toothbrush placement.

Modified Stillman Brushing Technique. The modified Stillman technique is designed to do a good overall cleaning, remove plaque, and stimulate and massage the gingiva (Procedure 4-4). Again, bristle placement distinguishes this technique from the Bass and Charters techniques. They are positioned so that the bristles point apically (toward the root of the tooth), with the toothbrush handle level with the biting surface of the tooth.

Rolling Stroke Brushing Technique. The rolling stroke is a method used to remove food debris and plaque from teeth and to stimulate the gingival tissue (Procedure 4-5). The brush is placed parallel to the tooth with the bristles pointed apically.

Fones Technique. The Fones technique is used as an initial brushing method to achieve a good overall cleaning. Most individuals can easily learn to make the small circles over the teeth as they are in the closed position. It is very easy to do on the outside surface of the teeth (see Procedure 4-6).

Procedure 4-2
Bass or Modified Bass Brushing Technique

This procedure is explained to an individual to teach a toothbrushing technique.

Equipment and Supplies

- Toothbrush

Procedure Steps

Bass

1. Grasp the brush and place it so that the bristles are at a 45-degree angle, with the tips of the bristles directed straight into the gingival sulcus (Figure 4-19).
2. Using the tips of the bristles, vibrate back and forth with short, light strokes for a count of 10, allowing the tips of the bristle to enter the sulcus and cover the gingival margin.
3. Lift the brush and continue into the next area or group of teeth until all areas have been cleaned.
4. The toe bristles of the brush can be used to clean the lingual (tongue) anterior area in the arch.

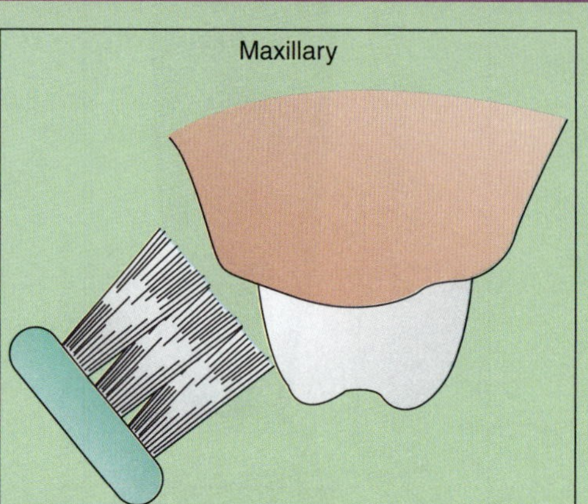

FIGURE 4-19
Initial position of the toothbrush when using the Bass technique.

Modified Bass

1. Follow all the steps of the Bass technique.
2. After the vibratory motion has been completed in each area, sweep the bristles over the crown of the tooth, toward the biting surface of the tooth.

Procedure 4-3
Charters Brushing Technique

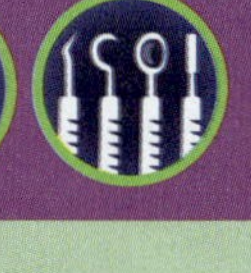

This procedure is explained to an individual to teach a toothbrushing technique.

Equipment and Supplies

- Toothbrush

Procedure Steps

1. Grasp the brush and place it so that the back of the head is directed apically (toward the end of the root), with the bristles placed downward on the maxillary and upward on the mandibular (Figure 4-20).
2. The bristles should be placed over the tissue, where the tooth and gingiva meet.
3. Press the bristles into the space between the teeth.
4. Vibrate gently back and forth while maintaining this position. Count to 10.
5. Reposition, and repeat the technique for each subsequent area.

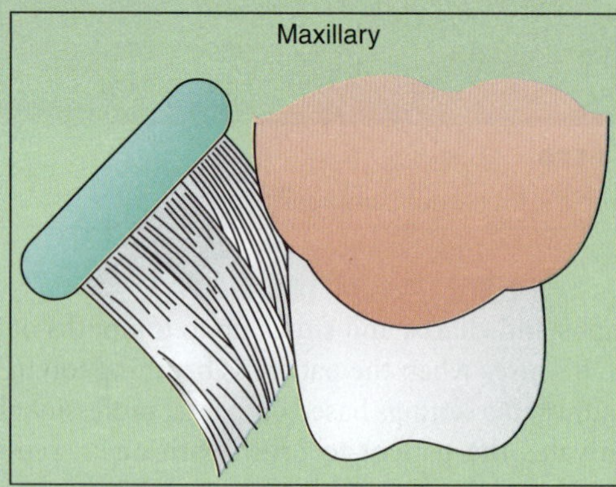

FIGURE 4-20
Initial position of the toothbrush when using the Charters technique.

6. For anterior areas, hold the brush parallel to the teeth and use the sides of the toe bristles to clean the area. Count to 10.

Procedure 4-4
Modified Stillman Brushing Technique

This procedure is explained to an individual to teach a toothbrushing technique.

Equipment and Supplies

- Toothbrush

Procedure Steps

1. Place the toothbrush so that the bristles are pointing apically and the handle of the brush is level with the biting surface of the tooth (Figure 4-21).

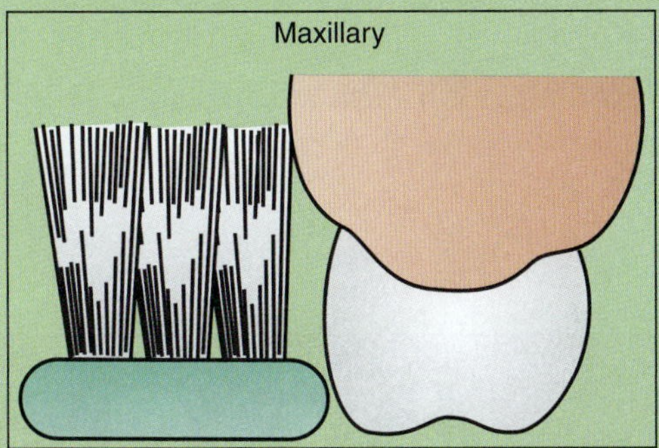

FIGURE 4-21
Initial position of the toothbrush when using the modified Stillman technique.

2. Rotate the bristles downward and vibrate back and forth until the brush has rotated over the entire surface of the tooth (Figure 4-22). Do this motion slowly and count to 10.

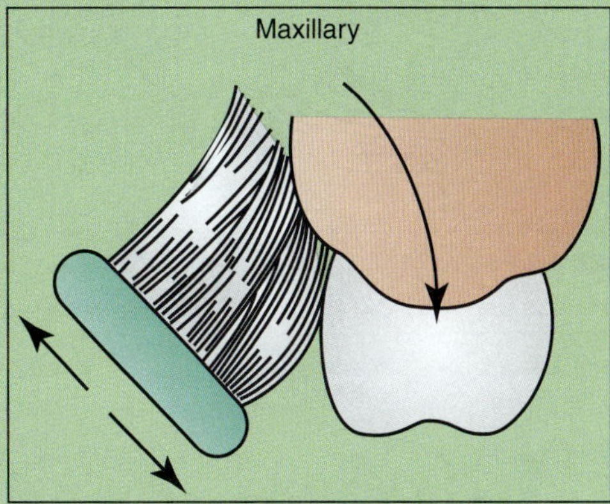

FIGURE 4-22
Brush stroke used with the modified Stillman technique.

3. Repeat this motion over the same area at least five times.
4. Continue until each area and every tooth have been cleaned in this manner.

Procedure 4-5
Rolling Stroke Brushing Technique

This procedure is explained to an individual in order to teach a toothbrushing technique.

Equipment and Supplies

- Toothbrush

Procedure Steps

1. Grasp the brush and place it parallel to the tooth so that the bristles are pointing apically, upward for the maxillary arch, and downward for the mandibular arch, as in the modified Stillman method (Figure 4-23).
2. Firmly but gently press the bristles against the gingiva and roll them slowly over the tissue and the teeth, toward the biting surface (Figure 4-24).

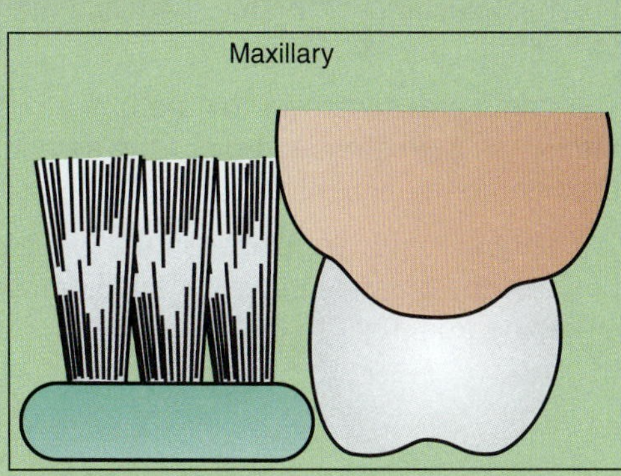

FIGURE 4-23
Initial position of the toothbrush when using the rolling stroke technique.

(continues)

Procedure 4-5 (continued)

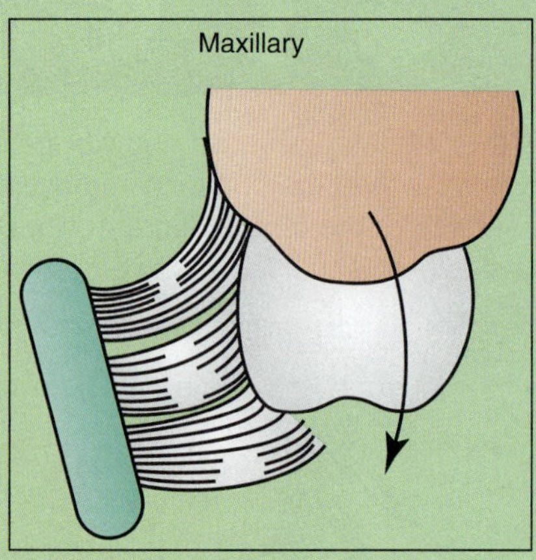

FIGURE 4-24

Brush stroke used with the rolling stroke technique.

3. Repeat this rolling stroke over the same surface a total of five times.
4. Move the brush to the next area and repeat the five rolling strokes.
5. Use the heel or the toe of the toothbrush to clean the lingual surfaces of the anterior teeth. The bristles will still need to be pressed gently into the area and rolled toward the biting surface.

Procedure 4-6

Fones Brushing Technique

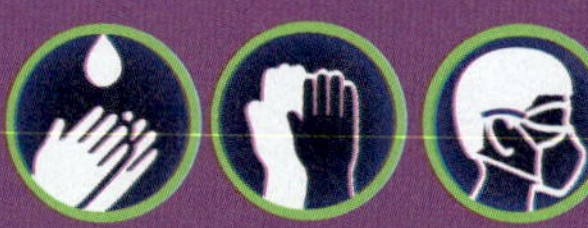

This procedure is explained to an individual in order to teach a toothbrushing technique.

Equipment and Supplies

- Toothbrush

Procedure Steps

1. Close the jaws and place the brush against the cheek. Starting with the posterior teeth, the brush is placed over the maxillary and mandibular teeth (Figure 4-25).
2. The brush proceeds over the teeth in a circular motion as it progresses toward the anterior teeth in a sweeping motion.
3. The anterior teeth are placed in the biting position and the brush is used in a circular motion sweeping from right to left.

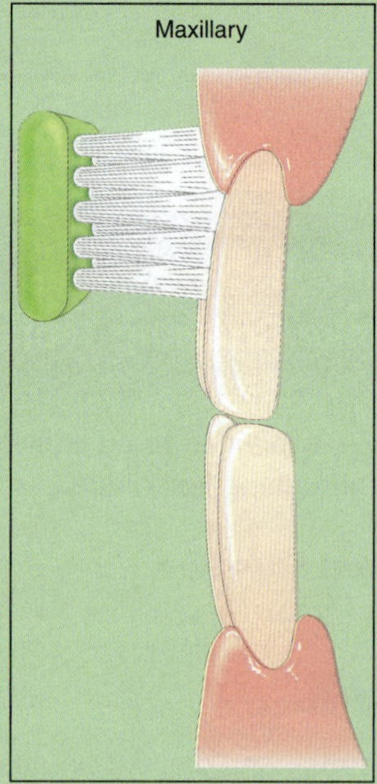

FIGURE 4-25

Brush stroke used with the Fones technique.

Procedure 4-7
Modified Scrub Brushing Technique

This procedure is explained to an individual to teach a toothbrushing technique.

Equipment and Supplies

- Toothbrush

Procedure Steps

1. Grasp the brush and place the bristles at a right angle to the tooth surface (Figure 4-26).
2. Use gentle but firm pressure and place the bristles over the area where the tooth and gingiva come together.
3. Activate the brush with back-and-forth scrubbing strokes.
4. Repeat this action throughout the mouth until all areas have been cleaned.

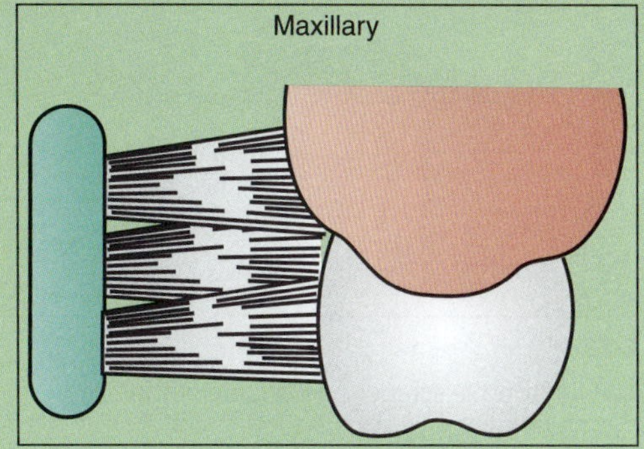

FIGURE 4-26
Initial position of the toothbrush when using the modified scrub technique.

Modified Scrub. The modified scrub brushing technique uses a scrubbing motion to remove plaque, and to stimulate the gingival tissue (Procedure 4-7).

Tongue Brushing

For centuries, individuals have known that it is important to clean the surface of the tongue. Bacteria can collect in the irregular dorsal (top) surface of the tongue. The daily ritual of oral hygiene historically included the scraping of the tongue with a tongue scraper (Figures 4-27 and 4-28). Several different tongue cleaners are on the market today.

A conventional toothbrush is most often used to ensure cleaning of the tongue surface. The size of the toothbrush head may limit access to the posterior area of the tongue because it may initiate gagging. To clean the tongue, the toothbrush should be placed as far back as is comfortable, and then be drawn forward to the tip, allowing the bristles to clean the debris that has accumulated. Repeat this process until the entire tongue has been cleaned.

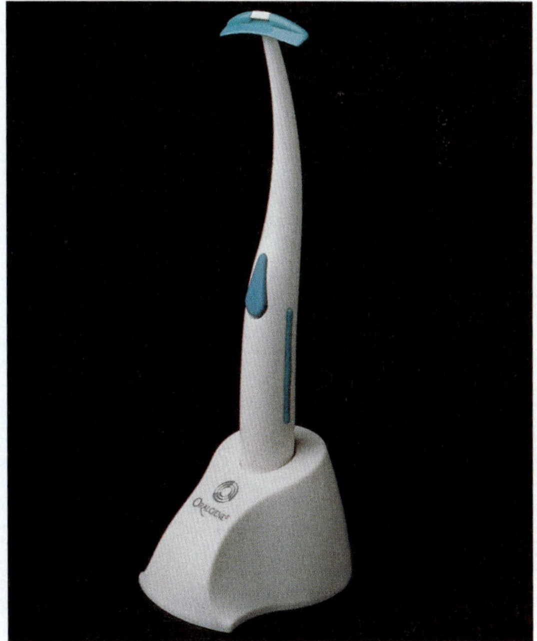

FIGURE 4-27
Automatic tongue scraper.

Dental Flossing

Dental flossing (Procedure 4-8), the second essential element of a good oral hygiene program, should be done daily. Dental floss has been shown to be the most effective way to remove bacterial plaque and other debris from otherwise inaccessible areas, that is, the interproximal surfaces of the teeth.

Types of Floss

Dental floss is available in several forms (Figure 4-29). Floss should be chosen according to patients' manual skills, dental restorations, and preferences. Following the office's

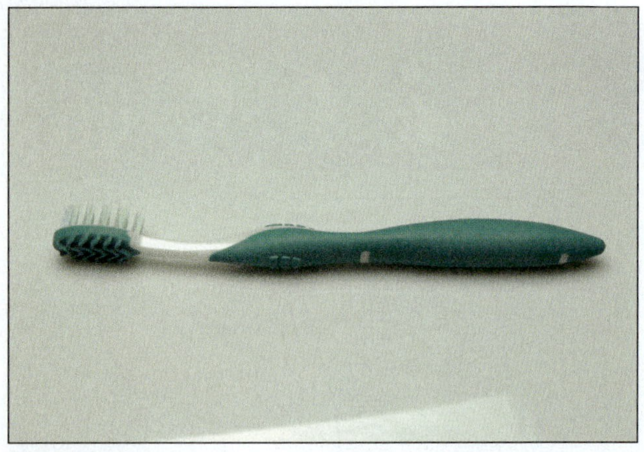

FIGURE 4-28
Toothbrush with tongue scraper on backside of the head.

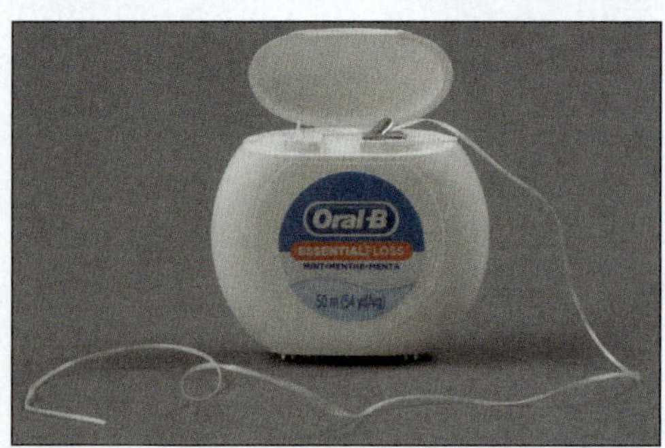

FIGURE 4-29
Dental Floss.

Procedure 4-8
Dental Flossing Technique

This procedure is explained to an individual to teach a dental flossing technique.

Equipment and Supplies

- Dental floss

Procedure Steps

1. Obtain the appropriate dental floss and dispense 18 inches of it.
2. Wrap the ends of the floss around the middle or ring finger as anchors (Figure 4-30).
3. Grasp the floss between the thumb and index finger of each hand, allowing ½ to 1 inch to remain between the two hands (Figure 4-31).

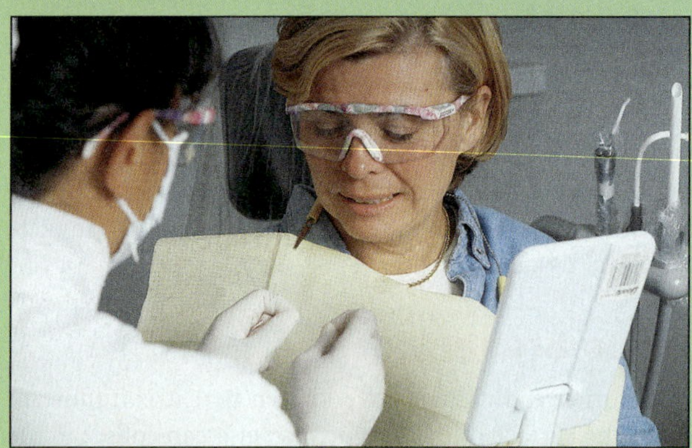

FIGURE 4-31
Floss adapted between fingers, prepared for use.

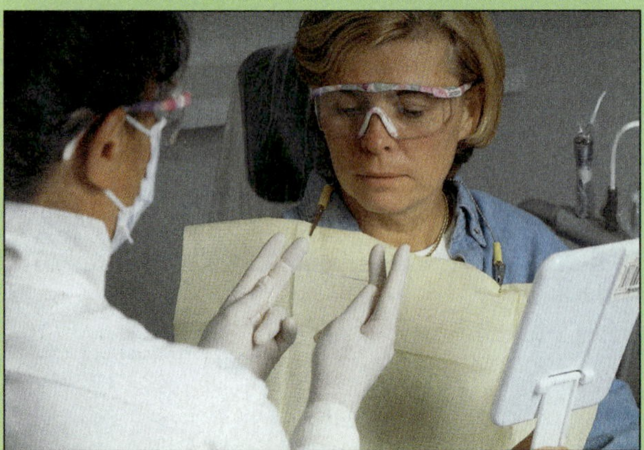

FIGURE 4-30
Adapting floss to the fingers for use.

4. For the maxillary teeth, pass the floss over the two thumbs or a thumb and finger, and direct the floss upward (Figure 4-32A). For the mandibular teeth, pass the floss over the two index fingers and guide it downward (Figure 4-32B).
5. Direct the floss to pass gently between the teeth, using a sawing motion. Try to avoid snapping the floss through the contacts because it may damage the interdental papilla (gingival point between teeth).
6. Curve the floss into a C-shape to wrap it around the tooth and allow access to the sulcus area (Figure 4-33). Resistance indicates that the bottom of the gingival sulcus has been reached.

(continues)

Procedure 4-8 (continued)

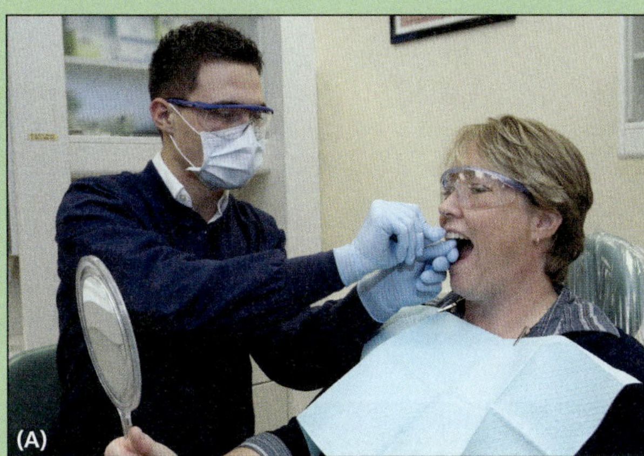

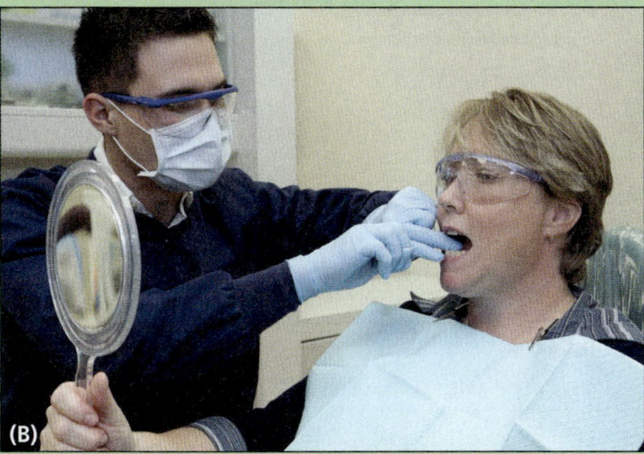

FIGURE 4-32
(A) Finger position on the floss for the maxillary arch. (B) Finger and thumb position on the floss for the mandibular arch.

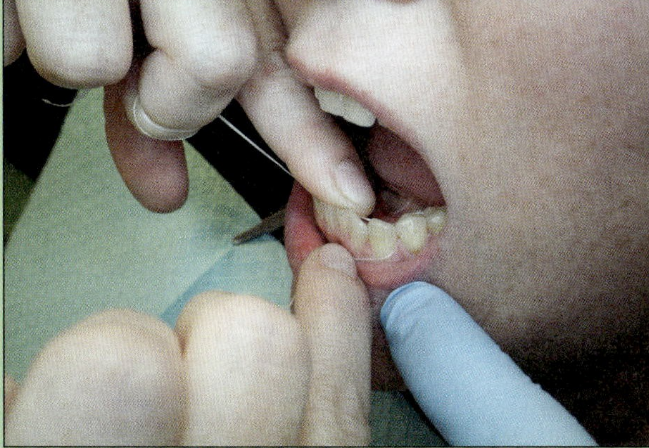

FIGURE 4-33
Patient placing the dental floss around the tooth, wrapped into the sulcus.

7. Move the floss gently up and down the surface of the tooth to remove the plaque.
8. Slightly lift the floss over the interdental papilla to the adjacent tooth.
9. Lift slightly and wrap the floss in the opposite direction in a C-shape over the adjacent tooth.
10. Move the floss gently up and down the surface of this tooth before removing it from the area.
11. Rotate the floss on the fingers to allow for a fresh section to be used each time, and continue to clean between every tooth. It does not matter where an individual begins, but it is best to proceed systematically to ensure that no area is missed.
12. Use the dental floss around the distal surface of the most posterior tooth by wrapping it into a tight C-shape and moving it gently up and down with a firm pressure (Figure 4-34). Floss the most posterior teeth in all four quadrants in the same manner.

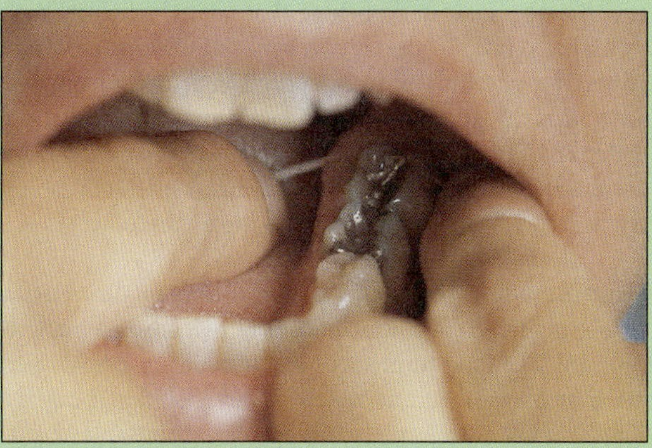

FIGURE 4-34
Patient placing the dental floss around the last molar.

philosophy, the dental assistant can make suggestions to the patient that will meet the patient's dental needs. Historically, patients have been advised to use unwaxed dental floss with small, individual filaments that aid in plaque removal as the floss is moved over the surface of each tooth. Some patients become frustrated while using unwaxed floss because it is thinner and more likely to shred or to catch on old dental restorations, making it difficult to remove from the inter-proximal areas. These patients should be encouraged to use waxed, lightly waxed, or nonshredding dental floss. Waxed floss will slide over the surface with greater ease for patients who have tight contacts and roughened surfaces.

Dental floss can also be purchased as extra fine, or as larger flat tape, or even with a tufted texture that, when tightened, changes sizes. Some patients will be attracted to the different colors and flavors of floss available on the market today. Colored and flavored floss does not perform any better than plain floss, but it may motivate patients to use it routinely. Flossing daily is more important than the type of floss that is used.

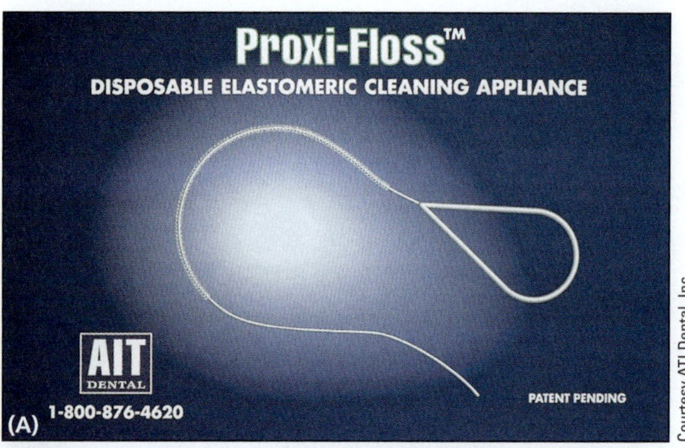

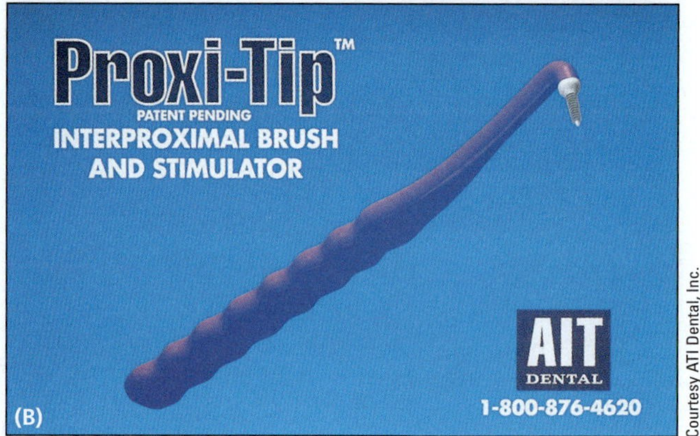

FIGURE 4-35

Dental hygiene aids for implants. (A) Proxi-Floss. (B) Proxi-Tip™.

Hygienic Care of Prosthetic Devices

An individual may have prosthetic devices that require special oral hygiene care for obtaining the desired plaque-free result each day. Professional knowledge and guidance will aid patients in the care of their prosthetic devices, such as fixed bridges, implants, orthodontic brackets, and full or partial dentures.

Fixed Bridges. A fixed bridge that is anchored on both sides with a pontic in the middle will not allow for normal flossing. The patient will need special instructions on how to use a floss threader (see previous information on the floss threader and Figure 4-13) to remove plaque and debris from under the bridge. The patient may also need special brushing instructions to clean the gingival area more carefully.

Implants. Many patients have dental implants to replace their missing teeth. The implants are a great advancement in dental care. The long-term success of implants is determined partially by the patients and how well they maintain the areas. Patients can use yarn in place of floss, or a disposable elastomeric cleaning appliance and interproximal brushes to clean around the implants (Figures 4-35A and B). A plastic scaler is used in the dental office to thoroughly clean the implant and remove any calculus.

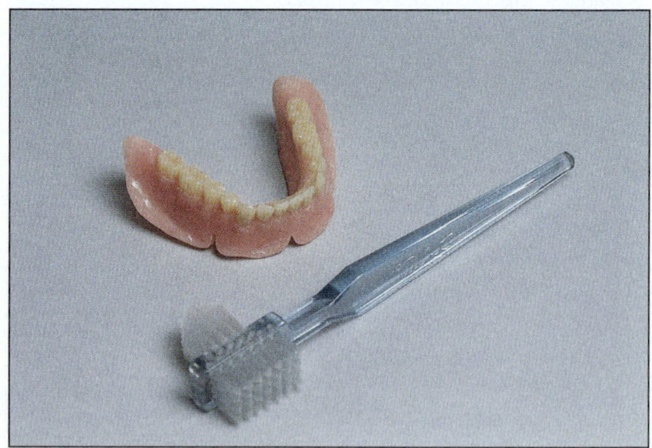

FIGURE 4-36

Denture and denture toothbrush.

Full and Partial Dentures. All removable dentures and appliances should be carefully cleaned daily and rinsed following a meal or as needed. A denture brush is used to brush the appliance (Figure 4-36). It is a larger brush that can be used with toothpaste or a mild soap. A soft brush should be used on the tissue under the appliance to clean and to stimulate circulation in that area.

Commercial cleaning agents can be used daily on a denture. These chemical agents remove stains and help freshen breath. The dentures normally are immersed in solutions according to the manufacturer's directions, and rinsed after the specified time has elapsed. The soaking solutions can be made at home with the following ingredients:

- Warm water (1 cup)
- Bleach (1 tsp.) (*Note:* The bleach should not be used with a partial denture as it may corrode the metal.)
- An anticorrosive agent (2 tsp.)

When calculus is heavy, a solution of 1 cup of warm water with a teaspoon of vinegar can be used. These home solutions should be used only once a week.

Orthodontic Appliances. As stated earlier in this chapter, special oral hygiene techniques must be practiced in order to maintain orthodontic appliances. The appliances must be kept plaque free. When care is improper, the tooth structure around the brackets may decay, and the gingival tissue will become irritated and virtually grow over the appliances. Special orthodontic toothbrushes and aids can be used (Figure 4-37). The bristles of the brush are designed to allow contact with the surface of the tooth. In special cases, an interproximal brush can be used to gain access to difficult areas. In addition to removing food and debris with a toothbrush and flossing, a water irrigation device can be used for overall cleaning.

Oral Hygiene for Patients with Special Needs

Dental assistants may be called on to be creative to meet the oral hygiene needs of patients with special needs (Figure 4-38). Patients who are mentally or physically compromised are often fed soft foods that lack the cleaning effects of normal foods. Devices can be developed to clean these patients' teeth. The dental assistants may need to show caregivers how to clean the patient's teeth routinely. For example, putty or a rubber ball can be wrapped over the handle of a toothbrush to allow the patient to grasp it more easily, or handles may be extended with tongue depressors or rulers so that patients can reach their oral cavities. Keep the focus on the desired outcomes, and establish methods to meet those goals. A moist washcloth can be used to wipe the surfaces of the teeth, if necessary. Be creative in meeting the needs of patients with special needs.

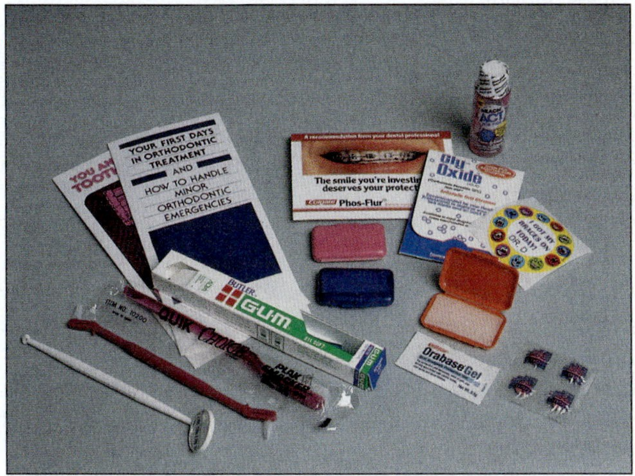

FIGURE 4-37
Orthodontic information and oral hygiene and comfort aids.

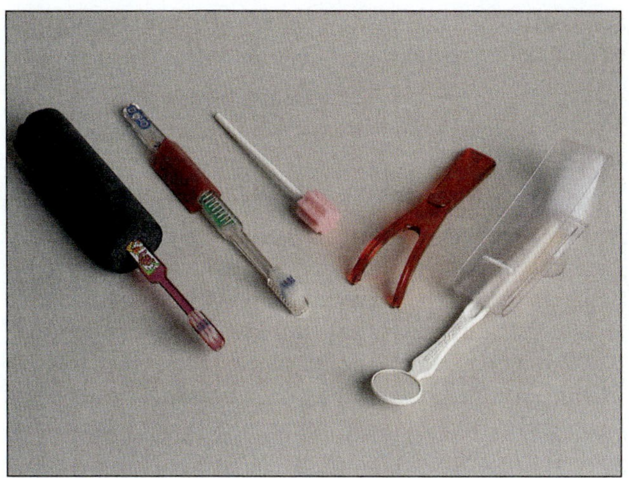

FIGURE 4-38
Aids for patients who have difficulty brushing and flossing.

Pregnant Patients

Pregnant patients may require special dental hygiene techniques because of the nausea that often accompanies pregnancy. Regurgitation will repeatedly bring acid from the stomach over the surface of the teeth (this will also be a concern for patients with bulimia). Patients should be educated on the possible destruction of the teeth from this acid repeatedly contacting the teeth. In addition, placing a toothbrush into the mouth may cause the patient to gag. Problem solve with the patient, and find a way to meet the goal of proper oral hygiene. Normally, eliminating toothpaste, and identifying specific times of the day when the pregnant patient is less nauseated, allows toothbrushing and flossing to be made more comfortable during pregnancy. The dental assistant should tell the obstetrical patient that increased gingival bleeding is normal and that routine prophylaxis (cleaning) is recommended during pregnancy. The patient's physician should approve any dental treatment.

Patients with Cancer

Patients with cancer may have a number of oral manifestations due to the cancer and the therapy. Loss of muscle function, gingival bleeding, rampant caries, and **xerostomia** (zee-roh-STOH-me-ah) may compromise the skills of good oral hygiene. Xerostomia is abnormal dryness of the mouth, and may be due to radiation or chemotherapy treatments. The patient may have a number of problems to overcome, such as root caries. Home topical fluoride treatments are often suggested to help eliminate these problems. Listen and problem solve with the patient. It will be important that infection does not perpetuate in the oral cavity and compound the patient's condition. The dental assistant may suggest that an extra-soft toothbrush, or a moistened foam toothbrush, be used on the tender tissues along with a nonabrasive fluoride toothpaste. Maintaining the teeth and tissues will allow the patient to eat properly and regain a healthier state. Use empathy, encouragement, and sincerity to motivate the patient.

Patients with Heart Disease

Patients with heart disease may express a number of the same problems that cancer patients have due to medication usage. Many have xerostomia, gingival bleeding, and rampant caries. Patients with congestive heart disease will be uncomfortable in the chair if the chair is reclined (this brings increased fluid around the heart and patients feel as if they are suffocating). Be aware of the patient's health status, address the problems that are identified, and aid the patient through education and being understanding when seeking a method to accomplish good oral hygiene.

Older Patients

For many older patients with arthritis, holding floss and a toothbrush is difficult. There are toothbrushes with large, soft handles that help these patients. A floss holder can be used to secure the floss tightly as it is placed between the teeth. Listen to these patients and keep in mind that they want to save their teeth to be able to eat properly. Many are afraid of having dentures. The wonderful thing about older patients is that they often have time to listen carefully to oral hygiene directions, and to ask questions to clarify what is required of them to meet their oral hygiene goals.

Additional Preventive Procedures Performed in the Dental Office

Other procedures that are performed in the dental office to aid patients in good oral hygiene are topical fluoride treatments, and pit and fissure sealants.

Fluoride Treatments

The use of **fluoride** (a natural mineral nutrient) in dentistry is based on the knowledge that, when the fluoride content of the teeth is increased to the optimum level, there is significant reduction in dental caries. Fluoride was once thought to be beneficial only during tooth development years, but, through further research, fluoride has been proven to be beneficial throughout the life span.

Fluoride is derived from fluorine, which comes from fluorspar, the thirteenth most abundant chemical element in the earth's crust. Fluoride is essential to the formation of healthy bones and teeth, just as calcium and phosphorus are. These minerals are obtained from water and certain foods.

Fluoride Content in the Bones and Teeth

- Normal bone contains 0.01 to 0.3 percent fluoride.
- Dental enamel contains 0.01 to 0.02 percent fluoride.
- Carious teeth contain as little as 0.0069 percent fluoride.

History of Fluoride in Dentistry. Early in the 1900s, Dr. G.V. Black and Dr. F. McKay of Colorado first revealed that people with **mottled enamel** (discolorations) did not have as much dental decay. In the 1930s, a chemist found a definite relationship between fluoride and mottled enamel. Eventually, an optimum level of fluoride was found. This level prevents dental caries without mottling the teeth. The optimum level was found to be 1 part per million (1 ppm). In some climates, this level may be adjusted slightly. For example, in hot climates where people are likely to drink more water, the level may be reduced.

Fluoridation. The process of adding fluoride to the water supply is called **fluoridation**. The first city to test the benefits of fluoride through fluoridation was Grand Rapids, Michigan. In 1945, 1 ppm fluoride was added to the water supply. Several other cities also fluoridated their water supplies when it was proven that dental caries in Michigan were reduced by approximately 60 percent. Since then, numerous cities have added fluoride to their water supplies.

Adding fluoride to community water supplies is a very controversial issue in many areas. It has been proven that adjusting the amount of fluoride to the optimum level does reduce dental caries, but some people oppose fluoridation. Much has been written about the fluoride controversy, and dental assistants need to stay up to date on what is going on in their communities. Knowing whether the water is fluoridated, the benefits of fluoridation, and the effects of too much fluoride will better prepare the assistant to answer patients' questions.

Effects of Fluoride. Fluoride is a natural substance needed for the development of healthy teeth and bones. It is absorbed almost entirely through the bloodstream from the gastrointestinal tract. Fluorides also are absorbed through the lungs in places like industrial settings, where people have occupational exposure to fluorine.

Once fluoride is absorbed by the body and deposited in the bones and teeth, the remaining fluoride is excreted. The developing child requires more fluoride than a 40-year-old person, and so the body adjusts the amount absorbed and excretes the excess fluoride.

Tooth Development. When the fluoride reaches the tooth, it replaces part of the tooth structure called the **hydroxyl ion**. The hydroxyl ion is on the surface of the apatite crystal in the enamel. The new tooth structure that is formed is called a **fluoroapatite crystal**.

Fluoride affects the tooth both before and after the tooth has erupted into the oral cavity. During the **preeruption stage**, the fluoride ion replaces the hydroxyl ion when the teeth are calcifying. Fluoride is supplied from drinking water, some foods, and fluoride tablets or drops. During this stage, excessive amounts of fluoride may disturb the normal pattern of development. This condition is known as **fluorosis**, or mottled enamel (Figures 4-39A and B).

Children who are given prescribed doses of fluoride at birth and continue receiving fluoride during the development of both the deciduous and permanent teeth benefit the most in reducing the number of dental caries.

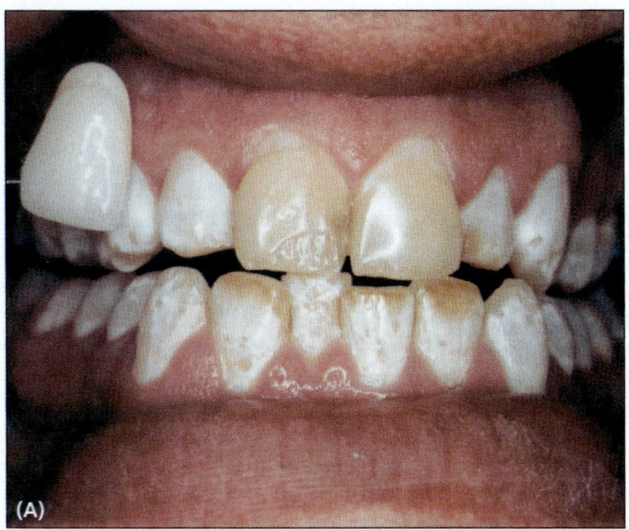

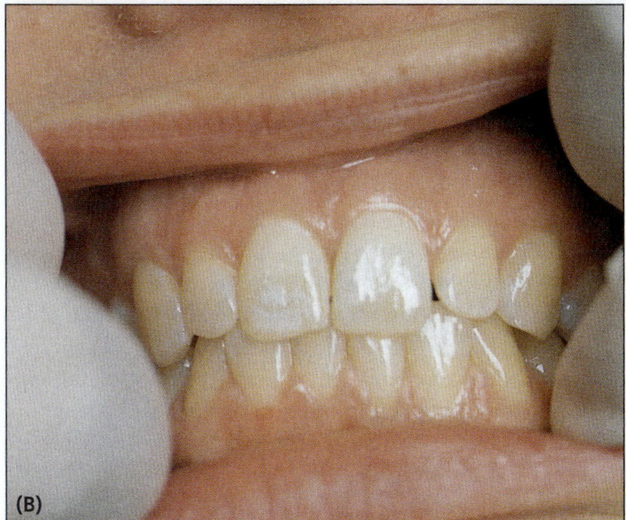

FIGURE 4-39

(A) Dental fluorosis on a new patient who was seeking cosmetic dentistry. Notice the shade guide to the side. (B) Mild dental fluorosis.

During the **posteruption stage**, the absorption rate of fluoride is the highest just after the tooth has erupted; it tapers off afterward, as the enamel matures. Absorption is also affected by the amount of fluoride exposure. Once the teeth have erupted, they receive fluoride through the bloodstream, and also through exposure in the oral cavity to fluoride in toothpastes, tablets, gels, and rinses.

Fluoride in Dental Plaque. Fluoride in dental plaque has been found to have a favorable effect. The amount of fluoride in plaque is relative to the amount of fluoride exposure. Fluoride in plaque is bound within bacteria. This condition causes an **antibacterial effect** that inhibits the production of acids responsible for dental decay.

Fluoride Toxicity. Fluoride, like many other substances, can be toxic when absorbed in excessive amounts. Today, fluorides are regulated carefully by occupational health legislation and governmental agencies. Over the years, it has been found that the toxicity of fluoride depends on the duration and dosage of ingestion. Fluoride used in dentistry presents little or no risk for acute toxicity. However, the dental assistant should be aware of the possibilities of fluoride poisoning, and when and where it has occurred, because patients may have questions.

Dangers Associated with Fluoride Ingestion. When large amounts of fluoride are ingested, inhaled, or absorbed into the body at one time **acute fluoride poisoning** occurs; it is extremely rare. The lethal dose varies from 2.5 to 10 grams in adults to as low as 0.25 grams in infants. A medical doctor should be contacted whenever excessive amounts of fluoride are ingested at one time. When there is suspected toxicity, the patient should drink milk, and then seek medical treatment immediately. Milk acts as a demulcent, a medicine that soothes irritated mucous membranes. It also helps with the mild nausea the patient may have.

Ingestion of high fluoride levels in water, or combinations of several fluoride sources over a period of time, results in **chronic fluoride poisoning**. Two effects of chronic fluoride overdose are crippling fluorosis (skeletal hypermineralization of ligaments) and mottled enamel. With today's health and safety controls in industry, crippling fluorosis can be avoided. Mottled enamel is caused by excess exposure to fluoride during the time of tooth development. When the fluoride level is from 1.8 to 2.0 ppm, the enamel shows varying degrees of white areas or brown lines, a condition called **enamel hypoplasia**. Because high levels of fluoride occur naturally in some areas, mottled enamel would be more common in those areas, unless the amount of fluoride in the water supply were adjusted to the optimum level.

Mottled enamel is pitted because of a deficiency in the number of **ameloblasts** (enamel-forming cells) and chalky because of a lack of mineral deposits. See Table 4-2 for the appearance of teeth with varying degrees of mottled enamel.

Benefits of Fluoride. The dental health benefits of fluoride have been shown in numerous studies. The benefits are in proportion to the length of time an individual received fluoride, and the amount of fluoride given. The primary benefit is the reduction of dental caries in both primary and permanent dentition, but there are also long-term benefits, such as the reduced need for extensive dental care, and the time and cost of such care. Through the use of fluoride, primary teeth are not lost prematurely to decay. This results in less malocclusion in permanent dentition; therefore, the need for orthodontic treatment is reduced. There is also less permanent tooth loss at early ages. Thus, adults require fewer bridges, partials, or dentures. Improved bone density can affect bone resorption, loss of bone, and resistance to local mastication or chewing. With stronger alveolar bone and less decay, the periodontal tissues stay healthier.

Forms of Fluoride. Fluorides are available for dental health care needs in two forms: **systemic fluoride** and **topical fluoride**. The fluoride compounds used in dentistry are **sodium fluoride**, **stannous fluoride**, and **acidulated phosphate fluoride**.

TABLE 4-2 Appearance of Teeth with Exposure to Different Levels of Fluoride

Amount of Fluoride Exposure	Appearance of the Teeth
Exposure between 0.7 and 1.2 ppm (the optimum level depending on average temperature of the area)	Teeth are white, opaque, and shiny without blemishes.
Exposure up to 1.8 ppm	The structure of the enamel is not affected, but chalky bands or flecks can be seen on the surface.
Exposure over 1.8 ppm	Chalky bands or flecks appear on the surface and the enamel structure is affected; this is known as **enamel hypocalcification**. The chalky bands and flecks discolor with time. With increased exposure to fluoride, the enamel may become cracked and pitted.

Systemic Fluoride. Systemic fluoride is ingested and then circulated through the body to the developing teeth. Sources of systemic fluoride include fluoridated water, foods with fluoride, fluoride tablets, and drops.

- Fluoride may be added to the community or school water supply. The level of natural fluoride is evaluated to adjust water supplies to the optimum level prescribed for dental health.
- Sodium fluoride is used in the community water supply.
- Foods such as meat, vegetables, cereals, and citrus fruits naturally contain small amounts of fluoride. Tea and fish have slightly higher amounts of fluoride.
- Tablets and drops require a prescription from a dentist or physician. They are prescribed from birth until the second permanent molar erupts. Vitamins with fluoride are also available.
- The ADA's Council on Dental Therapeutics recommends that specific amounts of fluoride be prescribed according to the child's age and weight.
- Studies have shown a 50 to 65 percent reduction in caries for patients who have received the optimum prescribed amount of fluoride during tooth development.
- Not all bottled water contains fluoride. Be sure to check the label if you want fluoride benefits, and you rely on bottled water for your water supply.

The amount of natural fluoride in a water supply can be determined by tests done by private laboratories, as well as by state and county agencies. In rural areas and cities without fluoridated water, children should receive topical fluoride. The dentist should assist the parents in determining the best methods and amount of fluoride the child should receive for maximum benefit. It is important that the fluoride supplement be taken continuously during tooth development to be most effective.

Topical Fluoride. Topical fluoride is another method that makes the tooth more resistant to demineralization, and also assists in the remineralization of decalcified areas. Because topical fluoride only penetrates the outer layer of the enamel, it is most effective if the tooth is cleaned before application. Cleaning can be accomplished by toothbrushing or a rubber-cup polish.

Topical fluoride is available for direct application in a variety of forms, such as gels, rinses, foams, and liquids. Polishing paste and dentifrice that are applied to the teeth also contain fluoride.

Dual Benefit of Chewing Fluoride Tablets

If fluoride tablets are chewed before being swallowed, the teeth benefit from both the topical and systemic fluoride applications.

Topical Fluoride Application in the Dental Office. In order for a child to achieve the optimal benefit, topical fluoride is applied to clean teeth once or twice a year in the dental office. By using this method, caries can be reduced by 40 to 50 percent.

In the dental office, fluoride gels, foams, and rinses are commonly applied (Procedure 4-9). The gel and foam solutions are convenient to use, and remain in the fluoride tray. Fluorides come in many flavors and, usually, the dental office will have several for the patients to choose from. The dental assistant should read and follow the directions for the type of fluoride being applied in order to determine the length of application, and helpful hints. The most common agents are 2 percent sodium fluoride, 8 percent stannous fluoride, and 1.23 percent acidulated phosphofluoride.

Advantages and Disadvantages of Fluoride Preparations.

- *Two Percent Neutral Sodium Fluoride:* Sodium fluoride solutions are relatively stable, have an agreeable taste, are nonirritating to soft tissue, and do not discolor the teeth or restorative materials. The disadvantage is that they must be used at one-week intervals for four weeks. Sodium fluoride solutions are applied after an initial prophylaxis of the crowns. The teeth are isolated and air-dried and fluoride is applied for three minutes. The complete series is performed at ages 3, 7, 11, and 13.
- *Eight Percent Stannous Fluoride:* The aqueous solution of eight percent stannous fluoride is not stable, and must be made up immediately before application. The eight percent solution has a disagreeable taste, is astringent, causes gingival blanching, and causes discoloration of the teeth. This discoloration is due to the tin, not the fluoride.
- *1.23 Percent Acidulated Phosphate Fluoride (APF):* APF solutions and gels are commonly preferred because of patient acceptability, and greater uptake of the fluoride by the surface enamel of the tooth. They are not irritating to soft tissue, do not discolor teeth or restorative material, and are slightly astringent. They are stored in plastic containers because they become more acidic when stored in glass. The application

Procedure 4-9
Fluoride Application

This procedure is performed by the dental assistant, after the rubber-cup polish has been completed. In some states, the application of fluoride may be an expanded function.

Equipment and Supplies

- Basic setup: mouth mirror, explorer, and cotton pliers
- Saliva ejector, evacuator tip (HVE), air–water syringe tip
- Cotton rolls, gauze sponges
- Fluoride solution
- Appropriately sized trays
- Timer (for 1 or 4 minutes)

Procedure Steps (*Follow aseptic procedures*)

1. Seat the patient in an upright position, review health history, and confirm that he or she has not had any allergic reactions to fluorides.
2. Explain the procedure to the patient. Inform the patient that they should try not to swallow the fluoride.
3. Explain that, in order for the fluoride to be most effective, he or she should not eat, drink, or rinse for 30 minutes after the fluoride treatment.
4. Place glasses and mask on, wash hands, and don treatment gloves.
5. Select the trays, and try them in the patient's mouth to ensure coverage of all the exposed teeth.
6. Place the fluoride gel or foam in the tray. The tray should be about one-third full. Show the patient how to use the saliva ejector.
7. Dry all the teeth with the air syringe. In order to keep the teeth dry while reaching for the tray, keep your finger in the patient's mouth and tell him or her to keep it open.
8. Place the tray over the dried teeth. The maxillary and mandibular arches can be done at the same time or individually (Figure 4-40).
9. Move the trays up and down to dispense the fluoride solution around the teeth.
10. Place the saliva ejector between the arches and have the patient close gently.
11. Set the timer for the designated amount of time.
12. When the timer goes off, remove the saliva ejector and the trays from the patient's mouth.
13. Quickly evacuate the mouth with the saliva ejector, or the evacuator (HVE), to completely remove any excess fluoride.
14. Remind the patient not to eat, drink, or rinse for 30 minutes.
15. Place on overgloves and make the chart entry, including the date, the fluoride solution applied, and any reactions.

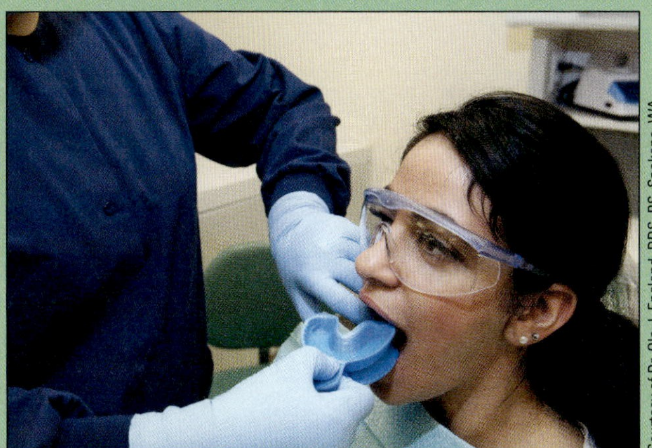

Courtesy of Dr. Ola J. England, DDS, PS, Spokane, WA.

FIGURE 4-40
Dental assistant placing a loaded fluoride tray into the patient's mouth.

procedure involves prophylaxis, isolation, and drying of teeth, which is then followed by an application of solution, gel, or foam for either one or four minutes (both solutions are available). The single application is repeated at 6- or 12-month intervals. The choice of solution is up to the practitioner, but foams appear to be more popular at this time.

The trays used with fluoride gels and foams come in a variety of materials and sizes (Figure 4-41). It is important to select a tray that covers all the erupted teeth, and does not extend beyond the most posterior tooth. Some trays come with the maxillary and mandibular arches connected, so they are placed at the same time. Others are individual for each arch, with the maxillary arch slightly larger. Often, the trays are color coded for different sizes.

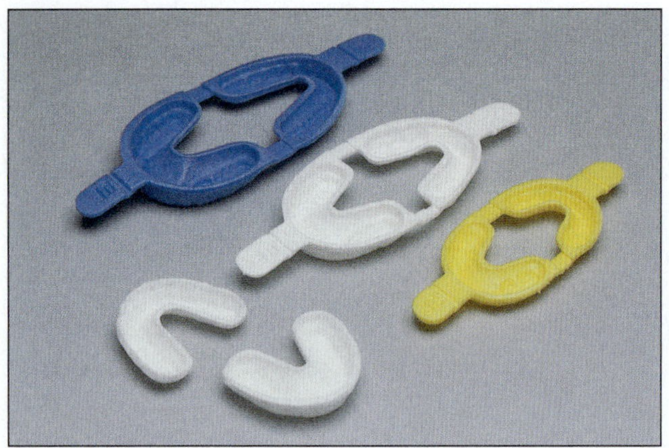

FIGURE 4-41
Various fluoride trays.

Contraindications. Note that fluoride should not be applied before placement of orthodontic bands, before placement of sealants, or before seating of cosmetic dentistry because it may inhibit adhesion.

Fluoride Varnish. **Fluoride varnishes** are often applied on the coronal surfaces of the teeth after a coronal polish, and pit and fissure sealants have been placed. They offer professional protection against dental caries and can be used on children, adolescents, and adults. Fluoride varnish contains five percent fluoride in an alcohol solution with natural resins. The resins are a sticky solution that adheres to the teeth, while the alcohol evaporates. It is painted on the teeth and sets when it contacts saliva. There is no mixing required, and the wait time is one minute after the varnish is applied. The varnish is barely visible, but can be felt on the teeth for a while until the varnish begins to wear off. Some other advantages include remineralization of incipient caries, inhibition of microleakage, and reduction of hypersensitivity for up to six months. (See Chapter 29, Pediatric Dentistry.)

Fluoride Rinses. Fluoride rinses are available as a means of fluoride treatment. The fluoride comes in a higher-concentration liquid and, because it is easy to swallow, the patient must be reminded not to swallow after rinsing.

After the patient's teeth have been cleaned with a toothbrush or a rubber-cup polish, apply the fluoride rinse. Follow the instructions for the individual rinse. Usually, the patient is directed to take half the dosage and then swish for a specific time (1 minute). The patient then empties this amount, and then repeats with the second portion for the same amount of time.

Procedure 4-10
Fluoride Varnish

This procedure is performed by the dentist, dental hygienist, or dental assistant, after the coronal polish and pit and fissure sealants have been applied. In some states, the application of fluoride varnish may be an expanded function.

Equipment and Supplies

- Basic set up: mouth mirror, explorer, and cotton pliers
- Saliva ejector, evacuator tip (HVE), air–water syringe tip
- Cotton rolls, gauze sponges
- Fluoride varnish (premeasured unit doses or individual applications with applicator brushes and tubes)

Procedure Steps (*Follow aseptic procedures*)

1. Thoroughly clean the coronal surfaces of the teeth and apply pit and fissure sealants.
2. Dry the tooth/teeth with air and isolate the area.
3. Depending on the application method, apply varnish (Figure 4-42) to the teeth using an applicator.
4. Dental floss can be used to apply the varnish to the proximal surfaces.
5. Evenly dispense and then air dry.
6. Keep the area isolated for one minute.
7. Ask the patient not to rinse, eat, or brush for 45 minutes after the placement of the fluoride varnish.

(continues)

■ Procedure 4-10 (continued)

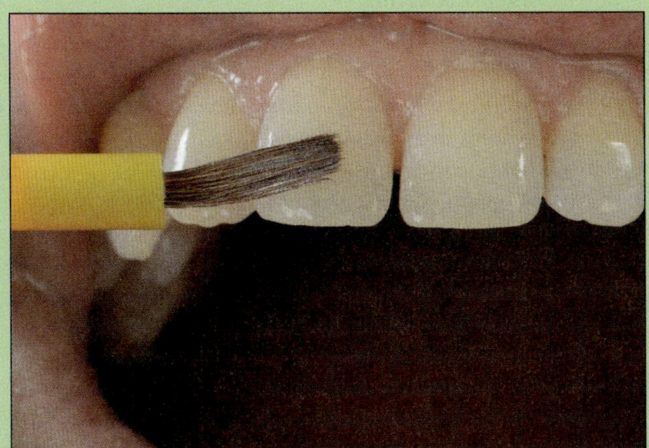

FIGURE 4-42
Applying fluoride varnish to the maxillary right central incisor.

Because of the taste of the fluoride, patients do not always look forward to fluoride treatments. The dental assistant can be the motivating factor and set the stage for the patient's attitude. Children under 6 years of age should not use fluoride rinses or mouthwashes because they may accidentally swallow them.

Pit and Fissure Sealants

Discussion and the procedures related to pit and fissure sealants are covered in more depth in Chapter 28, Pediatric Dentistry.

Chapter Summary

In order to be effective in preventive dentistry, dental assistants must first care for their own teeth properly. Becoming knowledgeable about the oral disease process will aid the dental assistant in educating patients on how to prevent it. The dental assistant must have the knowledge to solve oral hygiene concerns, know what preventive aids are available, and then aid patients in maintaining their teeth and gums.

CASE STUDY

Heidi Ann Jones, a 17-year-old, came into the dental office concerned with the discoloration of her teeth. After a thorough examination by the dentist, the findings showed that she had no caries, one restoration, and marginal gingivitis. What further questions would be important to ask Heidi? What preventive techniques would benefit Heidi?

Case Study Review

1. Was Heidi given fluoride drops or pills during the development of her permanent teeth?
2. Was she raised in an area that had fluoridated water?
3. What oral hygiene aids and habits did Heidi use in her daily routine?
4. Because Heidi is seeking information about her discolored teeth, and not about her gingivitis, the operator must first make sure that Heidi also wants help with the gingivitis before proceeding with home care instruction.
5. Home care instructions should include toothbrushing and flossing appropriate for a 17-year-old.

Review Questions

Multiple Choice

1. The most widely used brushing technique is the
   a. Stillman technique.
   b. Charters technique.
   c. Bass technique.
   d. Rolling stroke technique.
2. What is the most effective way to remove bacterial plaque from the proximal surfaces of the teeth?
   a. Use of a toothbrush
   b. Use of a tongue cleaner
   c. Use of an interproximal brush
   d. Use of dental floss
3. What is the optimal level of water fluoridation?
   a. 1 ppm
   b. 5 ppm
   c. 10 ppm
   d. 25 ppm
4. When dispensing dental floss, an appropriate length is about ________ inches.
   a. 4
   b. 10
   c. 18
   d. 25
5. The condition that causes an abnormally dry mouth is called
   a. fluorosis.
   b. demineralization.
   c. caries.
   d. xerostomia.
6. A sticky mass that contains bacteria and grows in colonies on the teeth is called
   a. caries.
   b. demineralization.
   c. plaque.
   d. acid.
7. The age group in which children are very concerned with fitting into a group and doing what others in that group are doing is
   a. 5 through 8.
   b. 9 through 12.
   c. 13 through 15.
   d. 16 through 19.
8. Dentifrice refers to
   a. toothpaste.
   b. disclosing agents.
   c. mouth rinses.
   d. dental floss.
9. A condition where the enamel shows varying degrees of white areas or brown lines could be
   a. demineralization.
   b. enamel hypoplasia.
   c. caries.
   d. xerostomia.
10. Which foods naturally contain small amounts of fluoride?
    a. Vegetables
    b. Cereals
    c. Citrus fruits
    d. All of the above

Critical Thinking

1. If you had a choice between hard candy and a candy bar, which would be more damaging to the teeth? Why?
2. Can dental fluorosis occur on a permanent tooth after eruption into the mouth?
3. Is it important to use one particular type of tooth brushing technique? Why?

Web Activities

1. Go to *http://www.ada.org* and read the article about the ADA seal of acceptance, and print the article.
2. Go to *http://www.sonicare.com* and identify the types of replacement brush heads available for the Sonicare toothbrush.
3. Go to *www.crest.com*, find "What's New." See if there are any samples available for trial usage. Fill out information to obtain the free sample.

CHAPTER 5

Nutrition

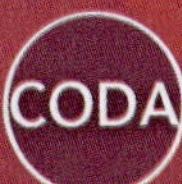

Specific Instructional Objectives

The student should strive to meet the following objectives and demonstrate an understanding of the facts and principles presented in this chapter:

1. Describe how an understanding of nutrition is used in the profession of dental assisting.
2. Define nutrients found in foods, including carbohydrates, fiber, fats, proteins, and amino acids. Explain how they affect oral hygiene.
3. Identify the food sources, functions, and implications of deficiencies of fat-soluble vitamins, water-soluble vitamins, and the seven major minerals.
4. Define a Calorie and the basal metabolic rate.
5. Identify and explain how vitamins, major minerals, and water function in the body.
6. Explain how to interpret food labeling.
7. Discuss the implications of eating disorders.
8. Discuss various technologies available to aid with nutrition and good health.
9. Explain how energy drinks and shots affect the body.
10. Discuss diet and culture and how it relates to oral health.

Key Terms

amenorrhea (81)
anorexia nervosa (81)
basal metabolic rate (BMR) (79)
binging (80)
biotin (75)
body mass index (BMI) (83)
bulimia (80)
calcium (77)
Calorie (78)
carbohydrates (72)
cariogenic (72)
carotene (74)
cheilosis (75)
chlorine (77)
chromium (77)
cobalt (77)
copper (77)
diet (72)
diuretic (77)
electrolytes (75)
emaciation (81)
essential amino acid (74)
fats (73)
fluorine (77)
folic acid (75)
glossitis (75)
iodine (77)
iron (77)
lanugo (81)
lipids (73)
magnesium (77)
malnutrition (72)
manganese (77)
metabolic rate (78)
metabolism (72)
molybdenum (77)
niacin (75)
nursing bottle syndrome (NBS) (73)
nutrient (72)
nutrition (72)
organic (80)
pantothenic acid (75)
phosphorus (77)
potassium (77)
preservatives (79)
prothrombin (74)
purging (80)
regurgitation (80)
retinol (74)
riboflavin (75)
selenium (77)
sodium (77)
sulfur (77)
thiamin (75)
triglycerides (73)
undernourished (72)
Vitamin B_{12} (75)
Vitamin B_6 (75)
vitamins (74)
zinc (77)

Introduction

Nutrition affects the entire body as well as the oral cavity. It directly impacts how an individual feels and functions throughout the day. Poor nutrition can affect the dental assistant in his or her career. It is critical that dental assistants maintain good health through proper food choices. This chapter covers an overall basic understanding of nutrients, including fats and lipids, proteins, vitamins, minerals, and water. Information on how to interpret food labeling is provided. Content on the implications of eating disorders is included in this chapter. Knowledge of nutrition provides the individual with the information to make sound decisions. The old saying "You are what you eat" is true.

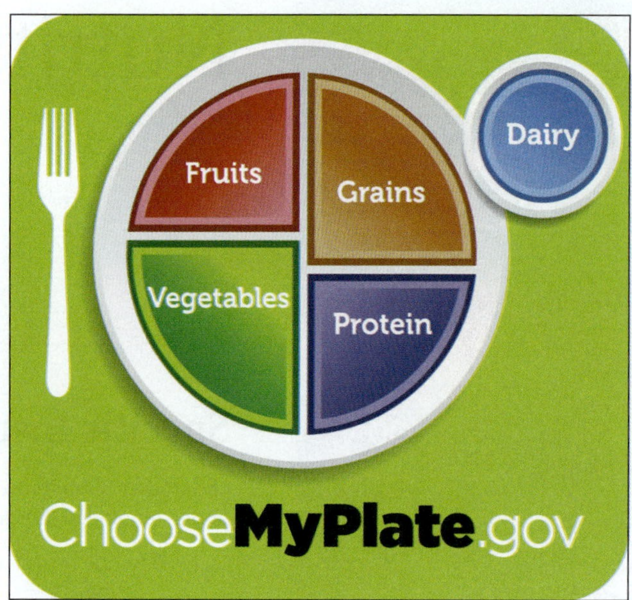

FIGURE 5-1
Myplate "new generation" food icon.

Nutrition

To remain healthy, dental assistants must first be knowledgeable about **nutrition** the manner in which foods are used to meet the body's needs. Dental assistants also need to be able to help patients with **diet** which is the food the individual eats. Dental assistants cannot sell health if they do not practice it themselves. Many patients may have the meaning of the word "diet" confused with weight loss. Everything that is taken into the mouth is the diet. An *adequate diet* meets all the individual's nutritional needs. People can eat large amounts of food and still be **undernourished** or lacking the correct nutrients for the body. A disorder resulting from being undernourished is **malnutrition**. This is often seen in individuals with alcoholism who may experience malnutrition due to the intake of alcohol (they feel full and do not eat the food necessary for an adequate diet).

The U.S. Department of Agriculture (USDA) first developed a guide to a balanced diet in 1992. This guide was presented in the shape of a pyramid with the items at the top to be used sparingly and the items at the bottom to be consumed in larger amounts. This food guide has undergone multiple revisions since it was originally developed. The latest revision of the USDA food guide is *MyPlate,* released in June 2011 (Figure 5-1). *MyPlate* uses a familiar visual, a place setting, to remind consumers to build a healthy meal. When making up your plate the USDA recommends:

- Make half your plate fruits and vegetables
- Make at least half your grains whole grains
- Switch to fat free or low fat (1%) milk

The USDA website, *ChooseMyPlate.gov*, offers tips and interactive tools to help educate and aid consumers in making smarter, healthier nutrition choices.

More than 60 percent of Americans are overnourished, leading to obesity and the diseases related to obesity. Americans are eating an abundance of fast foods that are high in fat content. Consistent with its lack of exercise, the overall population gains a minimum of a half pound a year.

Nutrients

Any chemical substance in food that provides the body tissues and structures with the elements necessary for growth, maintenance, and repair is a **nutrient**. Forty-plus essential nutrients are required by the human body. These can be obtained from a diet comprised of foods from all the food groups. Having a variety of foods daily helps ensure that essential nutrients are obtained and the body's **metabolism** is maintained. There are six broad classifications of nutrients: carbohydrates, fats, proteins, vitamins, minerals, and water.

Carbohydrates

The nutrients classified as **carbohydrates** primarily come from fruits, grains, legumes (peas, beans, and lentils), and some vegetable roots (Figure 5-2). This group encompasses sugars, starches, and fibers and provides quick energy. People in athletic events normally take in carbohydrates before the events to increase their energy levels.

Dental assistants will need to advise patients on carbohydrates because they are potentially **cariogenic**. Cariogenic foods break down into simple sugars in the mouth that can be used by bacteria to cause dental caries. Most patients will be aware that carbohydrates already broken down into simple sugars, such as candies, soft drinks, and sweet desserts, will cause decay. It will be the other carbohydrates that patients are unaware of that may cause decay, such as raisins, crackers, fruits, and a few vegetables. The intake of fruits and vegetables normally is not a problem because fruits and vegetables do not

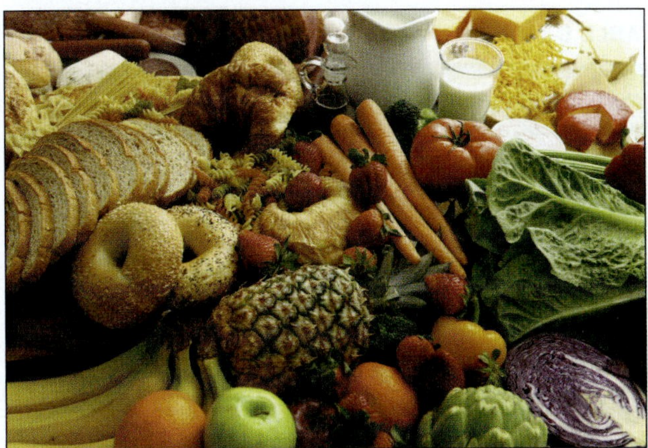

FIGURE 5-2

Fruits, vegetables, grains, and some dairy products are good sources of carbohydrates.

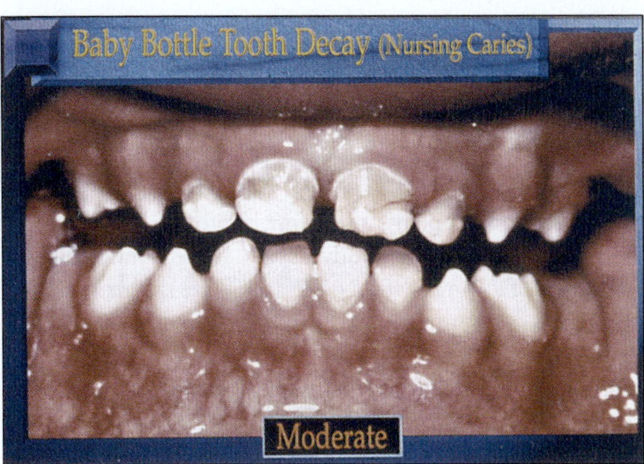

FIGURE 5-3

Moderate baby-bottle tooth decay.

stick to the teeth and are not converted to simple sugars until they reach the stomach.

Evaluating cariogenic foods in patients' diets is accomplished by having the patients record their diets over several days. The dental assistant can review the diet and identify cariogenic foods with the patient. The assistant can discuss the texture of the foods and whether they are retentive sugars, such as caramels, that remain in a concentrated sugar form on the tooth. Evaluation of each food in the patient's diet provides a better understanding of which types of foods are cariogenic.

Other pertinent information that the dental assistant can discuss with the patient is the number of times cariogenic foods are being eaten, whether they are eaten with other foods, and at what time of day they are eaten.

One other factor in the equation of decay is that the more often the teeth are exposed to cariogenic food, the greater the probability of decay. For instance, the person who drinks a soft drink very slowly and allows the sugar to soak on the teeth over and over will have a greater chance of decay.

Eating cariogenic foods with other foods may offer some neutralization of the acid that feeds the bacteria. Eating cariogenic foods at bedtime, when the flow of saliva decreases, increases the chance of decay. Saliva is a buffer to the acid and, if the flow rate of the saliva is inadequate, the cariogenic substances may not be washed away.

Infants who have erupted teeth and are given bottles of milk, fruit juice, or sweet substances for long periods may develop **nursing bottle syndrome (NBS)** or baby bottle tooth decay (BBTD) (Figure 5-3). This extensive decay of newly formed teeth is due to the sweetened liquid frequently bathing the teeth, often at bedtime. Parents should be informed and advised of the possibility of NBS so they can take preventive measures.

Suggest to patients that they choose carbohydrates that will not remain on the teeth for long periods. Caution patients about medicines and mouth fresheners that have sugars in them because they dissolve in the mouth, bathing the teeth with sugar for a long period. These may cause a large number of caries if used over time.

Fiber. Fiber is obtained from fruits, vegetables, and the grain food groups. It is suggested that 20 to 30 grams of fiber be eaten daily. Currently, an average of 15 grams or fewer are taken in by most Americans. Recent evidence has shown that consuming greater amounts of fiber can reduce the occurrence of colon cancer and reduce blood cholesterol levels. Increasing the levels of fiber should be done gradually to prevent unnecessary gastrointestinal problems, such as constipation.

Fats and Lipids

The nutrient classification of **fats** encompasses substances derived from a solid, and **lipids** are the oils from a liquid. Fat provides an alternate source of energy to carbohydrates. Fats and lipids share one commonality: They are insoluble in water. It is often called a backup source of energy. Fat also insulates the body from heat loss, protects vital organs, and aids in the transportation of the fat-soluble vitamins: A, D, E, and K.

The fats in normal diets derive from plant and animal foods, and are identified as **triglycerides** or neutral fats. Everyone needs fat in their diet, but there is widespread concern that Americans are consuming too much fat. The American Heart Association suggests that the diet contain 30 percent fat content, but currently most Americans' diets are 40 to 45 percent fat. The excess fat has a direct correlation to cholesterol levels and heart disease, which is the number one cause of death of Americans over the age of 40.

Even though people know fat consumption is a problem, they are drawn to foods that have fat in them. Food manufacturers are aware that fat enhances the taste and smell of food. People need to read food labels and reduce the intake of fast-food products to reduce the fat in their diets. Choosing foods that contain less fat is often difficult unless the individual has an understanding of comparative claims. For instance, if the label states *reduced fat,* then fat is normally reduced about 25 percent from the original; and if it states that it is *light,* then fat is typically about 50 percent less than in the original.

Proteins

Found naturally in plants and animals, protein is essential for the growth and repair of body tissues. Protein molecules are composed of a combination of 20 amino acids. The quality of a protein is determined by the distribution and kinds of amino acids in its structure. They are classified as "complete" if they have all 10 essential amino acids and "incomplete" if they do not have all 10. Most animal proteins such as eggs, milk, and meat are complete, and vegetable or grain proteins are incomplete (Figure 5-4). Incomplete proteins can be combined to make complete proteins if complementary foods are eaten at the same meal. For example, corn (an incomplete protein) can be eaten with beans (another incomplete protein) to make a complete protein. Macaroni with cheese, as well as cereal with milk, form complementary proteins.

Amino Acids. There are 10 **essential amino acids** that the body cannot synthesize or produce in the needed amounts, so they must come from the individual's diet (Table 5-1). Nonessential amino acids can be produced or synthesized by the body.

Vitamins

A class of nutrients that doesn't provide the body with energy, but instead, performs other necessary functions are **vitamins**. *Vita* comes from the Latin word meaning "life." The first vitamins were discovered by a group of scientists in 1913. They named the first vitamin "A" and the second vitamin "B," the third "C," and so on. Later, they found that Vitamin B was not a single vitamin but several, so they added numbers to the letter B (e.g., Vitamin B_1, B_2, and B_3). Some of the other vitamins were given names, rather than letters or numbers. In the 1940s, a committee of scientists named the vitamins A, B, C, D, E, and K with number subscripts where applicable. All vitamins fall in one of two groups: fat soluble or water soluble.

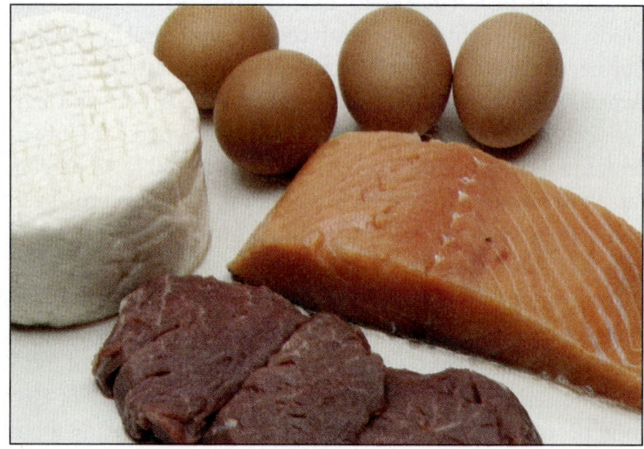

FIGURE 5-4
Animal sources of proteins.

TABLE 5-1 Essential and Nonessential Amino Acids

Essential Amino Acids	Nonessential Amino Acids
Arginine	Alanine
Histidine	Asparagine
Isoleucine	Aspartate
Leucine	Cysteine
Lysine	Glutamate
Methionine	Glutamine
Phenylalanine	Glycine
Threonine	Proline
Tryptophan	Serine
Valine	Tyrosine

Fat-Soluble Vitamins. The fat-soluble vitamins are Vitamins A, D, E, and K. These vitamins are stored in the fatty cells, especially the liver, and are not easily carried in the bloodstream.

Vitamin A. Vitamin A has two forms: the plant form **carotene** and the animal form **retinol**. Vitamin A is essential for healthy skin and maintenance of mucous membranes and gives strength to epithelial tissue (Table 5-2). It aids in the continual reshaping of bone but is best known for its contribution to vision.

Vitamin D. Vitamin D can be manufactured by the body if exposed to ultraviolet rays (Table 5-2). Dark-skinned people require additional sun exposure to manufacture the same amount of Vitamin D. Individuals need Vitamin D to ensure healthy bones and tooth development. Most milk is fortified with Vitamins A and D.

Vitamin E. Vitamin E has been related to childbearing and aging. It protects nutrients from destruction by oxidation. Scientific proof relating Vitamin E to slowing the aging process has not been demonstrated, but many feel the vitamin is effective in conditioning the skin.

Vitamin K. The last fat-soluble vitamin is Vitamin K. It promotes the formation of **prothrombin**. Prothrombin is responsible for blood clotting and coagulation. A small amount of Vitamin K is stored in the liver.

Water-Soluble Vitamins. Vitamin C, which is probably the most well-known vitamin of all, and the B-complex vitamins fall into the group of water-soluble vitamins. The body maintains the balance of water-soluble vitamins through the kidney; any excess is excreted through urine. Vitamin B_6 or

TABLE 5-2 Fat-Soluble Vitamins

Fat-Soluble Vitamins	Food Sources	Functions	Deficiency/Toxicity
Vitamin A (carotene or retinol)	Animal Liver Whole milk Butter Cream Cod liver oil Plants Dark green leafy vegetables Deep yellow or orange fruit Fortified margarine	Dim light vision Maintenance of mucous membranes Growth and development of bones Healthy skin	Deficiency Night blindness Xerophthalmia Respiratory infections Bone growth ceases Toxicity Cessation of menstruation Joint pain Stunted growth Enlargement of liver
Vitamin D (cholecalciferol)	Animal Eggs Liver Fortified milk Plants None	Bone growth Healthy tooth development	Deficiency Rickets Osteomalacia Poorly developed teeth Muscle spasms Toxicity Kidney stones Calcification of soft tissues
Vitamin E (alpha-tocopherol)	Animal None Plant Margarines Salad dressing	Antioxidant Skin conditioning	Deficiency Destruction of red blood cells Toxicity Hypertension
Vitamin K	Animal Egg yolk Liver Milk Plant Green leafy vegetables Cabbage	Blood clotting	Deficiency Prolonged blood clotting Toxicity Hemolytic anemia Jaundice

niacin can become toxic when intake is excessive because the kidneys cannot easily eliminate the surplus.

Vitamin C, Ascorbic Acid. A large number of people take Vitamin C for everything from toothaches to cancer (Table 5-3). Tragic stories of individuals who developed scurvy (a disease resulting from Vitamin C deficiency) during long sea voyages, wars, and famines are widely known. Vitamin C acts to hold cells together and is a component of connective tissue. Oral manifestations of Vitamin C deficiency include improper tooth development, ulcerated gums, and slow healing processes. It was discovered that citrus products prevented and treated this deficiency. Fruits and vegetables contain Vitamin C, especially citrus fruits and tomatoes.

Vitamin B Complex. Even though all vitamins in the B classification are grouped together, each has distinct functions (Table 5-3). Vitamin B_1 (**thiamin**), Vitamin B_2 (**riboflavin**), and **niacin** work together in the production of energy, but they also have separate functions. For example, thiamine prevents cardiovascular changes and a disease called beriberi, riboflavin helps produce proteins and is essential in growth, and niacin prevents gastrointestinal and nervous system disorders. Oral manifestations of Vitamin B deficiency include angular **cheilosis** (kee-**LOH**-sis), where the lips become red and fissures develop in the corners of the mouth; **glossitis** (glos-**EYE**-tis), which is inflammation of the tongue; and pellagra, where mucous membranes atrophy and ulcers develop (Figure 5-5).

Vitamin B_6 is essential in the synthesis and metabolism of protein, carbohydrates, and fat. **Vitamin B_{12}** and **folic acid** are important for the functioning of red blood cells and DNA. **Pantothenic acid** and **biotin** aid in energy metabolism.

Minerals

Minerals are classified as major or trace. A "major" classification indicates that the human body requires larger amounts. Minerals differ from vitamins in that they are elements rather than complex molecules. Some of the minerals that are positive or negatively charged are called **electrolytes**. When a person is healthy, the electrolytes are in balance.

TABLE 5-3 Water-Soluble Vitamins

Water-Soluble Vitamins	Food Sources	Functions	Deficiency/Toxicity
Vitamin C (ascorbic acid)	Fruits All citrus Plants Broccoli Tomatoes Brussels sprouts Potatoes	Prevention of scurvy Formation of collagen Healing of wounds Release of stress hormones Absorption of iron	Deficiency Scurvy Muscle cramps Ulcerated gums Toxicity Raise uric acid level Hemolytic anemia Kidney stones Rebound scurvy
Thiamin (Vitamin B_1)	Animal Liver Eggs Fish Pork Beef Plants Whole and enriched grains Legumes	Coenzyme in oxidation of glucose Prevention of beriberi	Deficiency Gastrointestinal tract and nervous and cardiovascular system problems Toxicity None
Riboflavin (Vitamin B_2)	Animal Milk Plants Green vegetables Cereals Enriched bread	Aids release of energy from food Help produce proteins Aids in growth	Deficiency Angular cheilosis Glossitis Photophobia Toxicity None
Pyridoxine (Vitamin B_6)	Animal Pork Milk Eggs Plants Whole-grain cereals Legumes	Synthesis of nonessential amino acids Conversion of tryptophan to niacin Antibody production	Deficiency Angular cheilosis Glossitis Toxicity Liver disease
Vitamin B_{12}	Animal Seafood Meat Eggs Milk Plants None	Synthesis of red blood cells Maintenance of myelin sheaths (muscles)	Deficiency Degeneration of myelin sheaths Pernicious anemia Toxicity None
Niacin (nicotinic acid)	Animal Milk Eggs Fish Poultry	Transfers hydrogen atoms for synthesis of ATP Prevents gastrointestinal problems Prevents nervous system problems	Deficiency Pellagra Toxicity Vasodilation of blood vessels
Folacin (folic acid)	Animal None Plants Spinach Asparagus Broccoli Kidney beans	Synthesis of red blood cells	Deficiency Glossitis Macrocytic anemia Toxicity None
Biotin	Animal Milk Liver Plants Legumes Mushrooms	Coenzyme in carbohydrate and amino acid metabolism Niacin synthesis from tryptophan Energy metabolism	Deficiency None Toxicity None

(continues)

TABLE 5-3 Water-Soluble Vitamins (continued)

Water-Soluble Vitamins	Food Sources	Functions	Deficiency/Toxicity
Pantothenic acid	Animal Eggs Liver Salmon Yeast Plants Mushrooms Cauliflower Peanuts	Metabolism of carbohydrates, lipids, and proteins Synthesis of acetylcholine Energy metabolism	Deficiency None Toxicity None

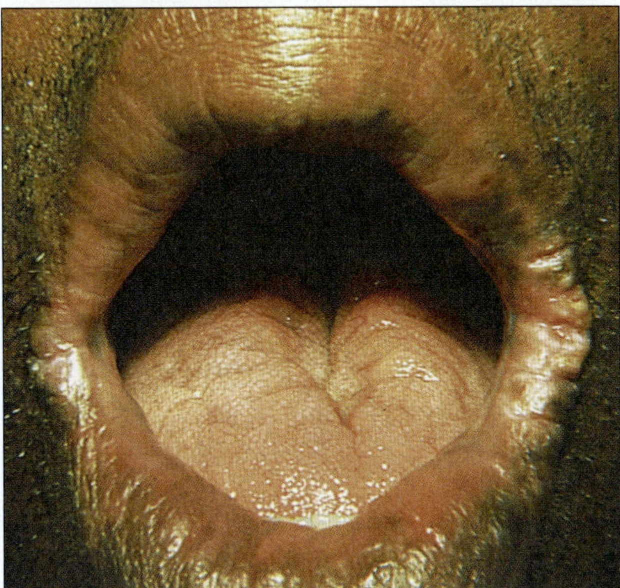

FIGURE 5-5

Cheilosis at the corners of the mouth is an indication of a riboflavin deficiency.

Major Minerals. Seven major minerals are in the body (see Table 5-4):

- **calcium** (Ca)—makes up the largest quantity and is found in bones and teeth; also functions in muscle contraction, the nervous system, and the blood (Figure 5-6).
- **phosphorus** (P)—found in bones and teeth and is involved in energy metabolism and maintenance of proper pH balance in the blood.
- **sodium** (Na)—works with potassium to regulate the electrolyte balance; maintains fluid balance in the blood.
- **potassium** (K)—works with sodium to regulate the electrolyte balance; helps to release energy and synthesize protein.
- **sulfur** (S)—found in protein and is involved in energy metabolism.
- **magnesium** (Mg)—involved in energy metabolism and in stabilizing components of bones and teeth once they are formed.
- **chlorine** (Cl)—maintains the correct pH balance in the blood.

Trace Minerals. Trace minerals are present in smaller quantities, yet are equally as important as the major minerals. The trace minerals **copper, chromium, molybdenum, selenium,** and **manganese** are important to our bodies in the process of metabolism. Found in the thyroid gland, **iodine** regulates metabolism of the body as well.

The primary function of **iron** is to carry oxygen is carried through the blood to the cells. People who are deficient in iron become anemic, which reduces their energy levels. Women tend to be more prone to this condition. The trace mineral **zinc** aids in tissue growth and maintenance of the immune system; **cobalt** helps in the functioning of red blood cells; and **fluorine** helps strengthen teeth, and research also indicates that it helps prevent osteoporosis, a condition in which calcium deficiency makes the bones weak and brittle.

Water

Water, by far, is the most abundant nutrient in the body. Water makes up 60 to 70 percent of total body weight. A turnover of 5 percent of total water each day is experienced by the average human adult. A person can go far longer without food than without water. In excessive heat, the body requires additional intake of water to prevent dehydration.

Water is used by the body in several ways, but the primary function is as a solvent for biochemical reactions. For instance, a large part of the blood is composed of water, and this allows for transport and necessary reactions to occur. This solvent action also serves to remove toxic waste from the body. Water acts as a lubricant, especially in the digestive system and the joints. It also helps control body temperature, releasing excessive heat through perspiration, and dispersing heat evenly throughout the body.

The body does not store water and it must be replenished daily. It is lost primarily through perspiration, urination, and fecal output. Some water is obtained from foods, but an additional eight glasses of water per day are recommended. Note that coffee and alcohol cannot be counted as water intake; in fact, they act as a **diuretic** and cause the body to lose water through increased urine output.

Balancing Energy

Ideally, people should take in enough nutrition to equal the amount of energy used daily. The amount of energy a substance can supply is measured in the form of Calories. One

TABLE 5-4 The Seven Major Minerals and Their Food Sources

Name	Food Sources	Function	Deficiency/Toxicity
Calcium (Ca)	Milk exchanges Milk, cheese Meat exchanges Sardines Salmon Vegetable exchanges Green vegetables	Development of bones and teeth Permeability of cell membranes Transmission of nerve impulses Blood clotting Muscle contraction	Deficiency Osteoporosis Osteomalacia Rickets
Phosphorus (P)	Milk exchanges Milk, cheese Meat exchanges Lean meat	Development of bones and teeth Transfer of energy Component of phospholipids Maintain pH balance in the blood	Same as calcium
Potassium (K)	Fruit exchanges Oranges, bananas Dried fruits	Contraction of muscles Maintaining water balance Transmission of nerve impulses Carbohydrate and protein metabolism	Deficiency Hypokalemia Toxicity Hyperkalemia
Sodium (Na)	Table salt Meat exchanges Beef, eggs Milk exchanges Milk, cheese	Maintaining fluid balance in blood Transmission of nerve impulses Works with potassium to regulate fluid balance in the blood	Toxicity Increase in blood pressure
Chlorine (Cl)	Table salt Meat exchanges Fish, pork	Gastric acidity Regulation of osmotic pressure Activation of salivary amylase Energy metabolism	Deficiency Imbalance in gastric acidity Imbalance in blood pH
Magnesium (Mg)	Vegetable exchanges Green vegetables Bread exchanges Whole grains	Energy metabolism Transmission of nerve impulses Activator of metabolic enzymes Relaxation of skeletal muscles	
Sulfur (S)	Meat exchanges Eggs, poultry, fish	Maintaining protein structure Formation of high-energy compounds	

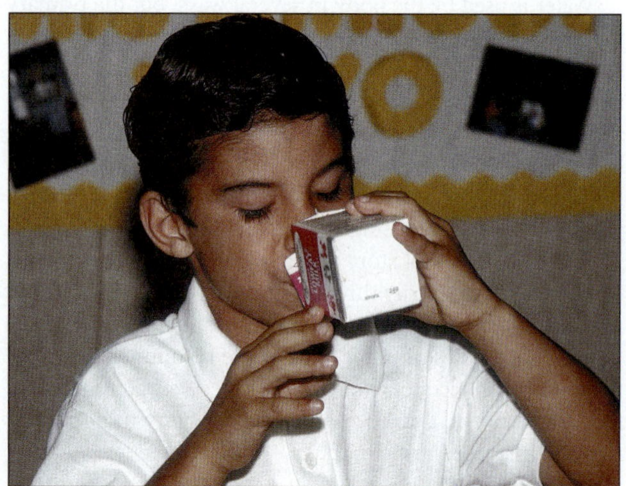

FIGURE 5-6

Milk is a good source of calcium and phosphorus, which aid in tooth development.

Calorie of food energy is understood to mean one kilocalorie (a kilocalorie is equivalent to one thousand true Calories). (When referring to a Calorie, always capitalize it or abbreviate it by using a capital C or Cal.) Carbohydrate and protein grams yield 4 Calories per gram; in contrast, 1 gram of fat yields 9 Calories. For example:

- 5 grams of carbohydrates × 4 Calories = 20 Calories of carbohydrates
- 5 grams of proteins × 4 Calories = 20 Calories of protein
- 5 grams of fat × 9 Calories = 45 Calories of fat

The total of all three categories would be 85 Calories. Fats are more energy rich than carbohydrates or proteins.

Calories are taken into the body to use as energy for everything from running to breathing. The body uses what it needs and stores the rest as fat. The physical and chemical changes that take place in relationship to the usage of energy are called the **metabolic rate**. If the rate of metabolism is less than the consumed Calories, then the person will store fat; if the rate of metabolism is greater, the stored fat will be used.

The energy that is used when a person is at rest is called the **basal metabolic rate (BMR)**. The BMR will be higher for pregnant women, children, and leaner individuals because it takes more energy to fuel muscle than it does to store fat in the body. Optimum energy balance would include the same amount of Calories taken into the body as are used. Ideally, most Calories would come from carbohydrates. Fats and protein should make up less than half the Calories taken in.

Nutrition Labels

For dental assistants to make good choices and be able to advise patients to do the same, they must be knowledgeable about nutrition labels on food products. Information is provided on the label according to government standards. Manufacturers of food products know that people are attracted to descriptive words on the product packages such as "lite" or "healthy." These terms may or may not describe the product, so it is important to read the details on the nutrition label. Consumers are paying more attention to the Calories and fat content when they compare two similar items. Information such as **preservatives** (the chemicals added to food to keep it fresh for a longer period) and artificial flavors and colors is also found on the food label.

Listed Items on Labels

Standard information is listed on nutrition labels. The government requires that the labels be easy for the consumer to read, so nutritional information is most often listed in a standard format. The 1990 Nutritional Labeling and Education Act was passed by Congress and enacted in 1994. This requires manufacturers to list all ingredients in the product. Individuals who have special dietary needs can readily identify ingredients, and all consumers can make comparisons from one product to another. The labels provide the serving size, percent of daily nutritional value, Calories, fat and cholesterol, sodium, carbohydrate, and other pertinent information on each label. In 2016 the Nutrition Label received an update making it more consumer-friendly (Figure 5-7). On the new label serving sizes

SIDE-BY-SIDE COMPARISON

Original Label

Nutrition Facts
Serving Size 2/3 cup (55g)
Servings Per Container About 8

Amount Per Serving	
Calories 230	Calories from Fat 72
	% Daily Value*
Total Fat 8g	**12%**
Saturated Fat 1g	**5%**
Trans Fat 0g	
Cholesterol 0mg	**0%**
Sodium 160mg	**7%**
Total Carbohydrate 37g	**12%**
Dietary Fiber 4g	**16%**
Sugars 1g	
Protein 3g	
Vitamin A	10%
Vitamin C	8%
Calcium	20%
Iron	45%

*Percent Daily Values are based on a 2,000 calorie diet. Your daily value may be higher or lower depending on your calorie needs.

	Calories:	2,000	2,500
Total Fat	Less than	65g	80g
Sat Fat	Less than	20g	25g
Cholesterol	Less than	300mg	300mg
Sodium	Less than	2,400mg	2,400mg
Total Carbohydrate		300g	375g
Dietary Fiber		25g	30g

New Label

Nutrition Facts
8 servings per container
Serving size 2/3 cup (55g)

Amount per serving	
Calories	**230**
	% Daily Value*
Total Fat 8g	**10%**
Saturated Fat 1g	**5%**
Trans Fat 0g	
Cholesterol 0mg	**0%**
Sodium 160mg	**7%**
Total Carbohydrate 37g	**13%**
Dietary Fiber 4g	**14%**
Total Sugars 12g	
Includes 10g Added Sugars	**20%**
Protein 3g	
Vitamin D 2mcg	10%
Calcium 260mg	20%
Iron 8mg	45%
Potassium 235mg	6%

*The % Daily Value (DV) tells you how much a nutrient in a serving of food contributes to a daily diet. 2,000 calories a day is used for general nutrition advice.

Courtesy of the FDA

FIGURE 5-7
Food label.

have been updated and the serving size and calories are now in bold and larger print. Daily values have been updated. There are new requirements to included added sugars. It includes nutrients required and the actual amounts present in the product. It also contains a new footnote relating daily values to a 2,000 calorie diet.

If the product packaging indicates that it is **organic** or organically grown, it must have been grown without the use of herbicides, chemical pesticides, or fertilizers. In addition, to qualify as organically grown, plant seeds must not have been prepared with the use of hormones or any other enhancement.

The *serving size* is listed on the label in a measurement or number of the product (for instance, ½ cup, or 2 cookies on a cookie package). It also gives the total number of servings per package. The rest of the information pertains to a single serving size.

The *ingredients* and *percent of daily value* are also listed. The daily value percent is based on a diet of 2,000 Calories per day for one adult. So, if the amount listed for total carbohydrate is 15 grams, this indicates that it is 5 percent of the daily value required according to calculations for the carbohydrate group.

Total *Calories* per serving are noted along with specific Calories derived from fat. The Calories from fat should total less than 30 percent of total Calories. Remember that this is the Calories in one serving and not the entire package.

Fat and *cholesterol* notations are valuable to the consumer because of various health concerns, including heart disease and weight control. The listing on the sample label in Figure 5-7 breaks out total fat as well as saturated fat. Saturated fat primarily comes from animal sources, while unsaturated fat primarily comes from vegetable sources. The total cholesterol content for one serving is also noted on the label.

Patients with heart disease or other diseases on sodium-restricted diets will want to watch the levels of *sodium* in foods. The total amount of sodium for one serving is listed on the nutritional label.

The total amount of *carbohydrate* is also listed, which may be broken down into dietary fiber (complex carbohydrates) or sugar (simple carbohydrates).

The nutritional labels show other information, such as the protein, vitamins, and minerals in the product.

Eating Disorders

It seems as if everyone is either overeating or doing everything possible to stay thin. The media and the fashion industry have brought forth the idea that all individuals should aspire to be thin. Advertisers repeatedly assert that taking this or that pill will allow for significant weight loss within a very short time. Eating disorders such as chronic dieting syndrome, compulsive overeating, bulimia, and anorexia nervosa are widespread and can be very serious and even life-threatening. They can have psychological, physical, and medical implications. The population most affected is females (at a ratio of 10 females to 1 male), aged 12 to 30, and often from white, affluent families.

Chronic dieting syndrome causes the individual to experience continuous weight loss and gain, and compulsive overeating can cause a number of psychological, physical, and medical implications that increase risk factors for diabetes and other diseases. Bulimia and anorexia can become life-threatening.

Chronic Dieting Syndrome

Chronic dieting syndrome is commonplace. A large percentage of people are ingesting pharmaceuticals and/or diet supplements to control their weight. This is important to dental assistants because the drugs may cause problems in dental treatment. The dieting may cause the heart to race or other chemical imbalances. Adding the anxiety of dental treatment may be enough to cause problems for the patient. Paying special attention to patients' medical and dental histories will be extremely beneficial.

Bulimia

A disorder that is characterized by secretive bouts of gross overeating followed by methods of weight control such as self-induced vomiting (**purging**), laxative abuse, excessive exercise, and overuse of diuretics (drugs that increase urine output) is **bulimia**, also called bulimia nervosa. Bulimia is attempted when other weight loss attempts do not work. Once tried, it quickly becomes obsessive, resulting in an out-of-control cycle of overeating and purging. An estimated 3 to 5 percent of women in the United States have been affected by bulimia at some time in their lives. Far fewer men are affected with this disorder. Bulimia and anorexia nervosa behaviors are very secretive and therefore difficult to diagnose. Individuals with bulimia may experience weight gains and losses, but normally do not show extreme weight loss such as in anorexia nervosa. The overeating (**binging**) is not caused by the desire for food but is a response to stress or depression. Eating brings about overwhelming happiness or a euphoric feeling that is quickly followed by the feeling of self-hatred and depression because of the binging. The individual experiences loss of control and then begins the purging or other behaviors that allow them to feel that they have regained control. Individuals may take laxatives, participate in excessive exercise, take diuretics, or use other weight loss methods to rid the body of the weight gained during the overeating.

There are a number of systemic complications that can result from bulimia. The vomiting can erode the tooth enamel, especially on the lingual surface of the teeth (Figure 5-8). Vomit is highly acidic. When the enamel has thinned or completely eroded, the teeth are more susceptible to decay and are more sensitive to hot or cold. The recurring **regurgitation** (vomiting) can cause the parotid glands and the saliva glands to become tender and swell, which can be very uncomfortable.

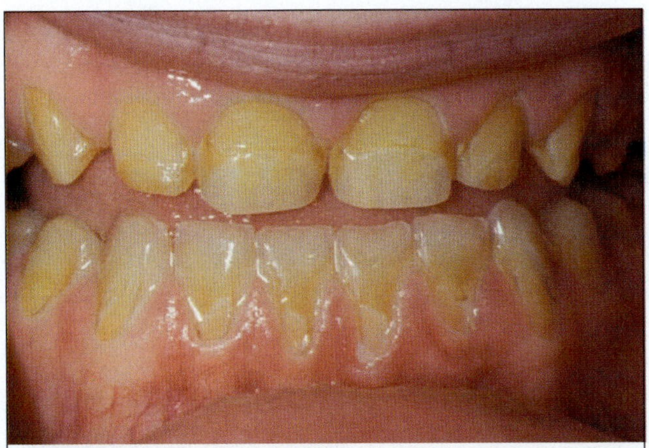

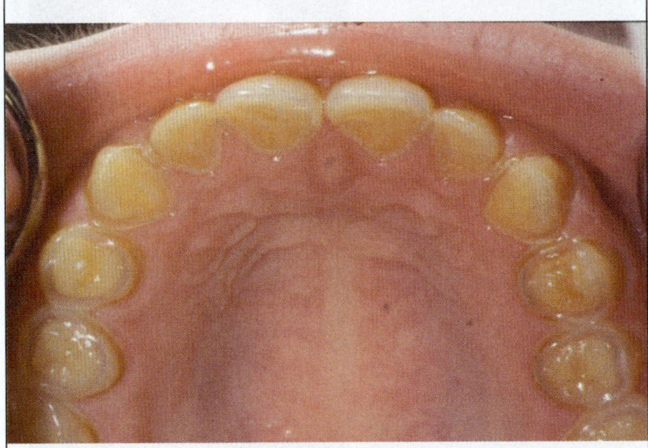

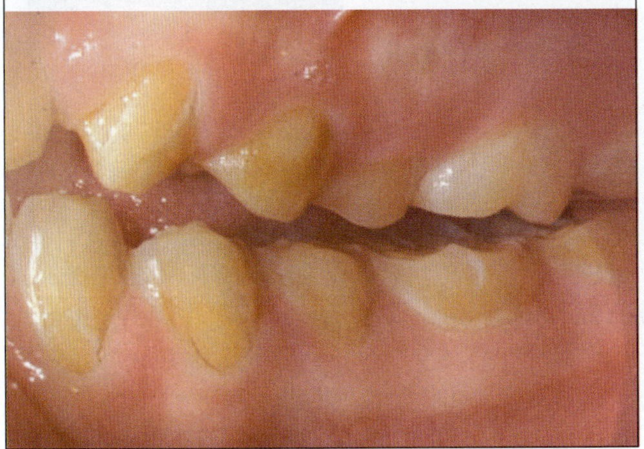

FIGURE 5-8

Eroded tooth structure shown on the facial, lingual, and buccal surfaces of the teeth due to bulimia.

Anorexia Nervosa

An eating disorder characterized by severe weight loss, an extreme aversion to food, and an extreme fear of being fat is **anorexia nervosa** (Table 5-5). Individuals with this disorder have a distorted body image, and see themselves as fat even though they may be overly thin. This psychological disorder centers on control, and behavioral symptoms focus on the fear of putting on weight or eating foods that contain fat or carbohydrates. Individuals with anorexia nervosa may have psychological, physical, and behavioral symptoms such as flaky skin, brittle nails, thinning of hair on the head, **amenorrhea** (absence of monthly menstrual periods), heart complications, kidney function issues, gastrointestinal complications, impaired organ function, **lanugo** (baby-like hair) on the body, food obsession, extreme use of laxatives, depression, social withdrawal, and obsessive exercising. The individual often feels intensely hungry but will deny fulfillment of this need. Individuals with anorexia nervosa are obsessed with food and thinking of food. They may find it difficult to go out to eat with others. They usually have eating rituals and may cut their food into small pieces and arrange and rearrange it on their plate; typically anorexics know every Calorie in each bite consumed. Individuals suffering from this disorder may prepare Calorie-laden foods for others but would feel extreme distress if they had to eat it themselves. The disorder is not focused on the weight loss or food intake but on control and/or other fears relating to the body.

Treating this disease is difficult. It is much easier to diagnose in the later stages because of **emaciation**, or extreme thinness. It is more complicated to diagnose in the early stages due to secrecy and attempts to hide the disorder from others. There are numerous types of therapies that can be helpful to people with anorexia nervosa, including psychological therapy, group therapy, family therapy, cognitive behavior therapy, and drug therapy, along with numerous hospital treatments that focus on correcting the malnutrition. Intravenous feeding may be recommended to treat the malnutrition. Working with a nutritionist during any of these therapies may enhance the outcome. The individual may require day treatment or longer inpatient care. Even if the treatment is successful, relapses can easily occur because the slightest stress triggers the disorder again. Of the individuals who have been hospitalized for anorexia nervosa, an estimated 8 to 10 percent later die from suicide or starvation. This condition is on the rise in the United States; an estimated 1 in every 100 adolescent females has anorexic symptoms.

The individuals that come to the dental office with this disorder have numerous physical problems, so special attention to the medical and dental history is crucial. They may also be very uncomfortable lying back in the dental chair if the dental treatment continues for any length of time. The oral cavity may show signs of the disorder, such as sore tissues resulting from poor periodontal health. The binging and purging may be reflected in the state of the teeth, as noted in the section on bulimia. Calcium intake may be limited; therefore, the teeth may not be as strong as normal and decay may progress more rapidly.

Nutrition, Health, and Technology

Today's health conscious individual has numerous devices to aid them in obtaining and maintaining good health and wellness. Most of the devices track food choices and exercise on tablets and smart phones. A popular health monitoring device is the Fitbit (Figure 5-9). It can track the steps taken, distance covered, calories burned, floors climbed, active minutes, and sleep habits.

TABLE 5-5 Stacia's Story

Stacia's parents have shared this story and the pictures with the hope that they will help someone else identify and overcome this disorder. They tried everything that they were aware of to help Stacia, but were unable to turn this eating disorder around. People with this disorder become quite skillful in their methods of weight loss and control.

Stacia was an outgoing, well-liked child. She was born into a family who cared about their children, and was loved and supported throughout her life. She was not pressured to be perfect but was allowed to seek her own desires. When she was 12 years old, an incident occurred that her parents did not know about. Other things occurred that seemed to perpetuate this disorder. This is a picture of Stacia at around 16 years old. She was a great athlete and gave it her all. She had been purging for 4 years at this time. Her parents were just becoming aware of what she was doing.	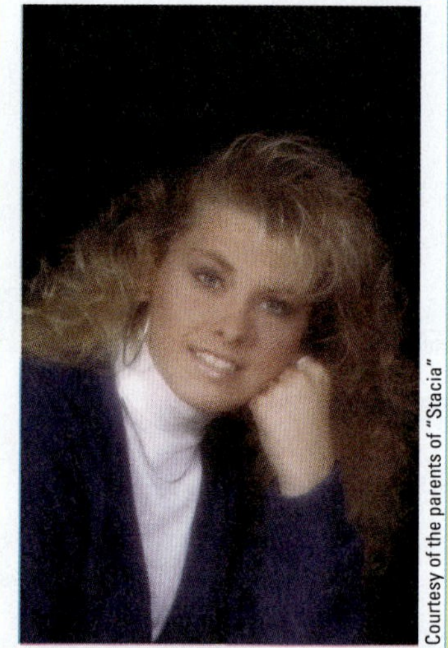 Courtesy of the parents of "Stacia"
Stacia spent part of her senior year in treatment facilities, and missed the senior picture opportunity. In this picture, she is about 21. She is 5 feet, 6 inches tall. In this picture she weighs about 100 pounds.	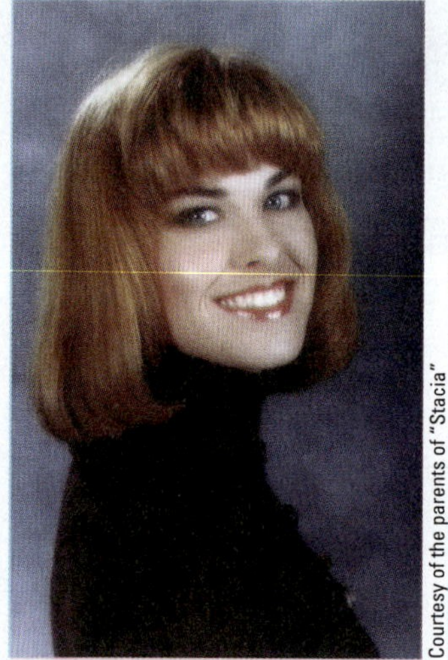 Courtesy of the parents of "Stacia"
Stacia weighs about 85 pounds in this picture, and the disorder has progressed. She now is taking many laxatives a day, and she focuses on food. In this photo she is about 22.	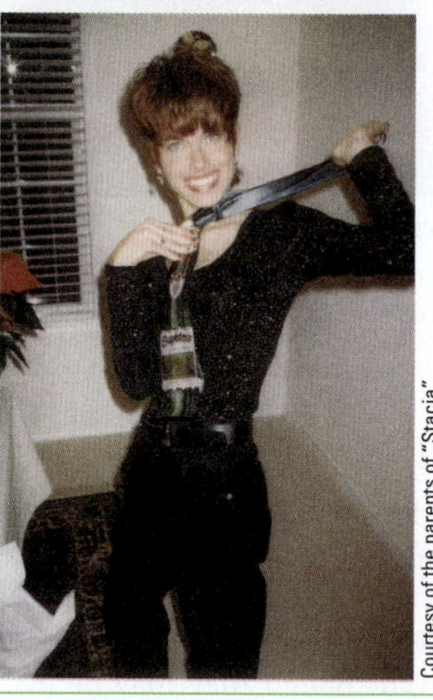 Courtesy of the parents of "Stacia"

(continues)

TABLE 5-5 Stacia's Story (continued)

Stacia continues to lose weight. She now is down to 82 pounds, and lacks the energy to work full time. She is about 24.	 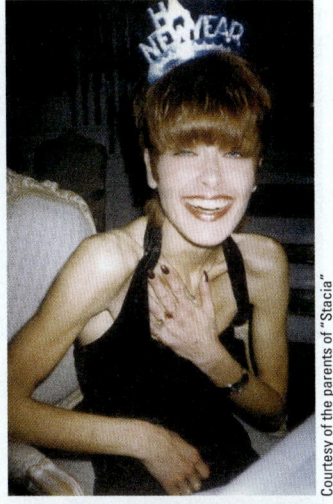 Courtesy of the parents of "Stacia"
The disorder becomes more apparent to everyone she comes in contact with. Stacia has a distorted view of her appearance. She does not see herself as thin and is still obsessed with controlling her food intake. Her weight has now dropped to about 78 pounds.	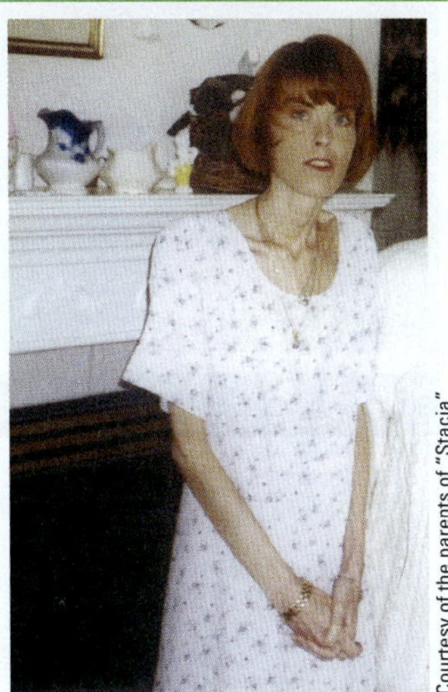 Courtesy of the parents of "Stacia"
This is one of the last pictures of Stacia. Her weight declined to around 62 pounds around the time that she passed away at age 27. At the time of her death, she was taking over 100 laxatives a day.	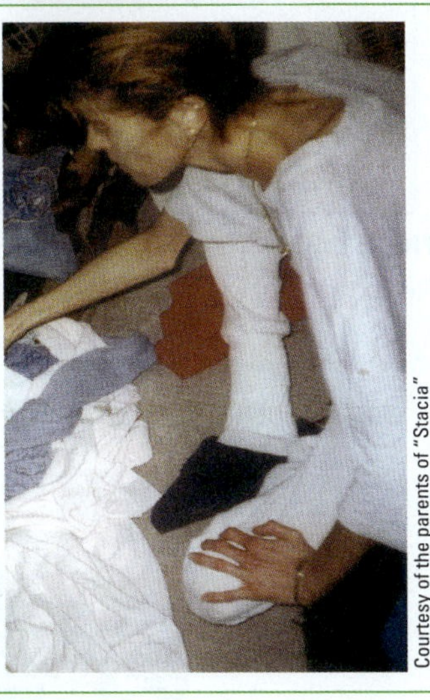 Courtesy of the parents of "Stacia"

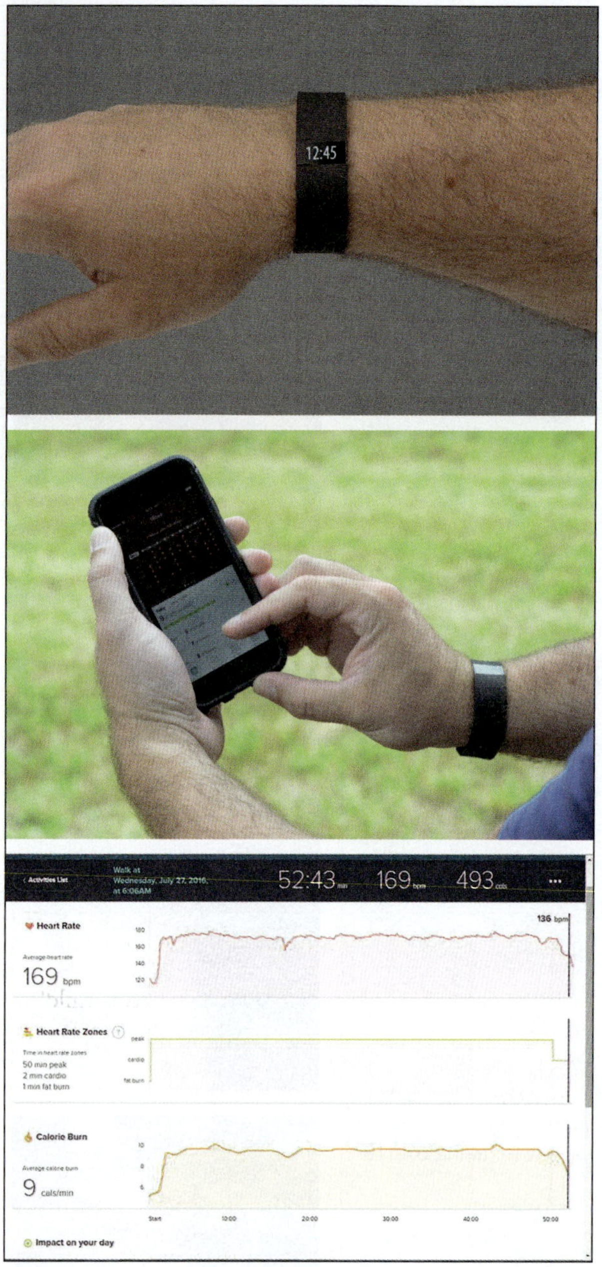

FIGURE 5-9

Fitbit, an example of a health monitoring system.

It also has a WiFi Smart Scale that measures weight, BMI, lean mass, and body fat percentage. The **body mass index (BMI)** is a value derived from the mass and height of an individual.

Numerous apps are available online that can be downloaded to aid in weight management, diet information, recipe suggestions, to improve health, and track your fitness stats. One example is *Fooducate* which serves as a dietary partner, health eating educator, and encourages you if you have health concerns. It has a barcode scanner which can be used for the foods you eat or to give you healthy alternatives to consider before choosing foods. Another example, *Lose It*, helps you set goals and track your progress to success. Its barcode scanning is used to track eating habits only. There are options to appeal to everyone's lifestyle and needs from *Weight Watchers*, *Cronometer*, *SparkPeople*, *Calorie King*, and *Techlife* just to name a few. Each individual should research the apps to identify the one that meets their needs. Almost all of them work with the iPhone or Android and many have a built in message center. Getting healthy is getting easier with the help of technology.

Energy Drinks and Shots

Energy drinks and shots have become extremely popular and it is recommended that an individual does not have more than two drinks each day to stay within a safe level (Figure 5-10). These drinks contain high levels of caffeine and sugar. People take these drinks to give them a boost, making them more alert. These drinks may cause dehydration, seizures, insomnia, heart problems, etc. The dental concerns come from repeated sugar over the teeth which may cause decay.

Diet and Culture

Dental assistants will come into contact with patients who come from a variety of cultural backgrounds. As stated in Chapter 1, each patient must be treated as an individual, and stereotyping must be avoided. Patients may eat foods that are unfamiliar to the dental assistant. Some examples include cultures that may drink specific teas that stain the teeth, or they may come into the United States and go from eating fruits and vegetables to a high-carbohydrate diet. Dental assistants should be informed of patients' diet choices so they can make suggestions that will aid them in achieving and maintaining good oral habits.

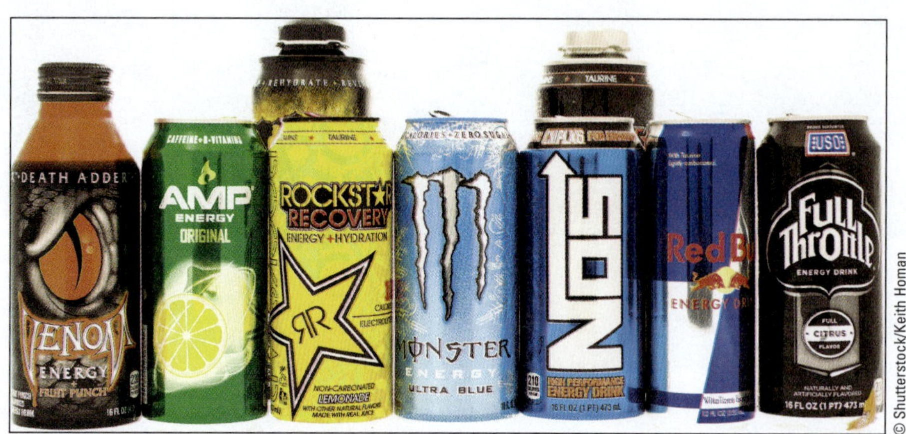

FIGURE 5-10

Energy drinks and shots.

Chapter Summary

Dental assistants need to have a background in nutrition to maintain good overall health as well as aid patients in decision making. Everyone can benefit from knowledge of how to read nutrition labels and what it means when a product is organic or organically grown. Having an understanding of eating disorders may prove beneficial in the work environment with other coworkers and patients.

CASE STUDY

Maci Smith was a beautiful 17-year-old who had been involved in chronic dieting to keep her weight down. Recently when she came into the dental office, staff members noticed that she had lost an extreme amount of weight. Signs of erosion on the lingual surface of her teeth were also noted. She told the dentist that her teeth were sensitive to heat and cold.

Case Study Review

1. What should the dental assistant do if he or she observes this condition?
2. What diagnosis may be indicated with these symptoms?
3. Should the dentist discuss with her the possibility that she has been purging?
4. What other areas in the oral cavity could be examined?

Review Questions

Multiple Choice

1. Water-soluble vitamins include
   a. B_1, B_2, D, and niacin.
   b. D, E, K, and C.
   c. D, E, B, and K.
   d. B_1, B_2, C, and niacin.
2. The major minerals are calcium, phosphorus, potassium, sodium, chlorine, magnesium, and
   a. copper.
   b. sulfur.
   c. chromium.
   d. manganese.
3. ________ primarily derive from fruits, grains, legumes, and some vegetable roots.
   a. Proteins
   b. Cariogenic foods
   c. Fats and lipids
   d. Carbohydrates
4. Fats in normal diets occur in plant and animal foods and are identified as
   a. amino acids.
   b. proteins.
   c. triglycerides.
   d. thiamin.
5. The "vita" in vitamin came from the Latin word
   a. Calorie.
   b. life.
   c. health.
   d. energy.
6. The fat-soluble vitamin that aids in the continual reshaping of bone, but is best known to help with vision is
   a. Vitamin A.
   b. Vitamin B.
   c. Vitamin C.
   d. Vitamin D.
7. The fat-soluble vitamin that has been related to childbearing and aging is
   a. Vitamin A.
   b. Vitamin E.
   c. Vitamin C.
   d. Vitamin D.
8. Water makes up ________ percent of total body weight.
   a. 40–50
   b. 50–60
   c. 60–70
   d. 70–80
9. The baby-like hair on the body that occurs with anorexia nervosa is called
   a. amenorrhea.
   b. lanugo.
   c. emaciation.
   d. regurgitation.
10. The eating disorder that is characterized by secretive bouts of gross overeating followed by purging is called
    a. anorexia nervosa.
    b. bulimia.
    c. chronic dieting syndrome.
    d. compulsive overeating.

Critical Thinking

1. How can knowledge of nutrition benefit the dental assistant?
2. If the dental assistant learns that a patient is bulimic, what should the dental assistant do? Should this information be disclosed to the dentist? What information should be offered to the patient about the effects on the oral cavity?
3. How should food labels be interpreted? What information is most helpful to the consumer? What should the dental assistant suggest that patients look at on food labels?

Web Activities

1. Go to http://www.nutrition.gov and find the Food and Drug Administration (FDA) page on food labels. Identify which foods are required to have FDA food labeling. Identify which foods only require voluntary food labeling.
2. Go to http://www.usda.gov/wps/portal/usdahome and find *Food and Nutrition*. Proceed to *Food Labeling and Packaging*. From there go to *Food Defense and Emergency Response* and learn what is new in this area.
3. Go to http://www.usda.gov/wps/portal/usdahome and find *Food and Nutrition*. From this point, go to *ChooseMyPlate.gov* and develop a customized food guide plan. This individual plan allows for tracking. Track food intake and physical activity for the following week.

Section III

Basic Dental Sciences

CHAPTER

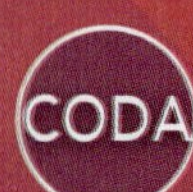

General Anatomy and Physiology

CODA

Specific Instructional Objectives

The student should strive to meet the following objectives and demonstrate an understanding of the facts and principles presented in this chapter:

1. List the body systems, body planes and directions, and cavities of the body, and describe the structure and function of the cell.
2. Explain the functions and structure of the skeletal system, list the composition of the bone, and identify the types of joints.
3. List the functions and structure of the muscular system.
4. List the functions and structure of the nervous system.
5. List the functions and structure of the endocrine system.
6. Explain dental concerns related to the reproductive system.
7. List the functions and structure of the circulatory system.
8. List the functions and structure of the digestive system.
9. List the functions and structure of the respiratory system.
10. List the functions and structure of the lymphatic system and the immune system.
11. List the functions and structure of the integumentary system.

Key Terms

alveolar sacs (105)
alveoli (105)
anatomy (89)
antagonistic pair (96)
aorta (101)
aponeurosis (96)
appendicular skeleton (91)
arteriole (101)
artery (101)
articulation (93)
autonomic nervous system (ANS) (97)
axial skeleton (91)
axons (97)
bile (105)
blood (101)
body cavity (91)
bronchi (105)
bronchioles (105)
cancellous bone (92)
capillary (101)
Cardiac muscle (95)
cartilage (93)
cell (91)
central nervous system (CNS) (97)
chyme (103)
compact bone (92)
cuticle (108)
deglutition (103)
dendrites (97)
digestion (103)
endocardium (101)
epiglottis (103)
esophagus (103)
excitability (96)
exhalation (105)
extensibility (96)
fascia (96)
gallbladder (105)
heart (101)
heart valves (101)
hemostasis (102)
homeostasis (91)
hormone (99)

(continues)

Key Terms (continued)

inhalation (105)
insertion point (96)
irritability (96)
large intestine (103)
laryngopharynx (105)
larynx (105)
ligaments (96)
liver (105)
lungs (105)
lymph (107)
lymph nodes (107)
myelin sheath (97)
nasopharynx (105)
neuron (97)
nonspecific immunity (107)
oral cavity (103)
organs (91)
origin (96)
oropharynx (105)
osseous tissue (92)
osteoblast (93)
osteoclasts (93)
pancreas (105)
pericardium (101)
peripheral nervous system (PNS) (97)
peristalsis (103)
pharynx (103)
physiology (89)
planes (90)
plasma (102)
pulmonary circulation (101)
reflex arc (97)
respiration (105)
Rh factor (102)
skin (108)
small intestine (103)
Smooth muscle (95)
specific immunity (107)
spinal canal (91)
spleen (107)
stomach (103)
Striated muscle (95)
synapse (97)
systemic circulation (101)
systems (91)
tendon (96)
thymus (107)
tissues (91)
tonsils (107)
trabeculae (92)
trachea (105)
vein (101)
vena cava (101)
vocal cords (105)

Introduction

To give the quality of care each patient deserves, the dental assistant needs to be familiar with the terminology of body systems and how each system functions. The study of the body structure is **anatomy** and **physiology** is the study of how the body functions. The anatomy and physiology of each body system will be briefly discussed.

Specific terms are used to establish a means for the health professional to communicate more effectively. Depending on the information and understanding needed, the human body can be studied on many different levels. The body is divided into systems, planes, cavities, and basic units. This chapter provides common references and terms for studying and communicating information about the human body.

As a dental assistant you should be able to use proper terminology to describe and locate various anatomical features and disease conditions. The key terms highlighted in the chapter focus on the foundations. Additional terms are placed in italic and should be learned as well.

Body Systems

The human body is comprised of many body systems. Each body system consists of specific organs and serves a specific purpose. Some of the body systems to be discussed relative to dentistry include: skeletal, muscular, nervous, endocrine, reproductive, circulatory, digestive, respiratory, lymphatic, immune, and integumentary. Information about each system is presented according to its relationship with dentistry. Refer to Table 6-1 for a list of the systems and their major functions.

TABLE 6-1 Body Systems

System	Function
Skeletal	Provides the basic framework of the body; protects, shapes, and gives support to the body; source of attachment for muscles; stores minerals and manufactures blood cells.
Muscular	Muscles contract and relax to allow external body movement and production of the body's heat; internal muscles work to move food along the digestive track and keep the heart beating.
Nervous	Provides a communication system for the body; response to both internal and external stimuli.
Endocrine	Controls growth; stimulates sexual development; regulates use of calcium; aids in regulating the body's water balance; produces insulin.
Reproductive	Produces new life.
Circulatory	Carries life-sustaining substances, such as nutrients and oxygen, throughout the body; carries away waste materials; maintains a balance between intracellular and extracellular fluids.
Digestive	Takes food in, breaks it down, and converts it to substances the body needs to sustain life; provides a means for the body to eliminate solid wastes.
Respiratory	Brings oxygen into the body that is transported to all cells; the waste product, carbon dioxide, is picked up and exhaled.
Lymphatic	Provides nutrients, drains body fluids, and absorbs fats.
Immune	Protects the body from disease and harmful substances.
Integumentary	Provides body protection; includes skin, hair, and nails.

Refer to Table 6-2 for terms commonly used to describe areas of the body. The dental assistant will use these terms in many circumstances. For example, when discussing radiographic images, an abscess that shows on the radiograph may be mesial and superior to the root, or an abnormal lesion may be found on the dorsal surface of the tongue.

Body Planes and Directions

The body is divided into three primary **planes** (an imaginary line used to define areas of the body and parts within those areas) (Figure 6-1). The *sagittal plane* divides the body into left and right halves. If the sagittal plane divided the body

TABLE 6-2 Terms to Describe Areas of the Body

Term	Definition	Example
Anterior	In front of; in the front of the body or body section.	The eye is anterior to the ear.
Ventral	On the front.	The belly or abdominal area of the body is on the ventral side of the body.
Posterior	In back or behind; in the back of the body or body section.	The ear is posterior to the nose.
Dorsal	On the back.	The dorsal surface is on the back of the body or organ.
Medial	Toward the middle of the body; the medial is closest to the midline.	The midline or median line divides the body into left and right halves.
Mesial	Toward the midline of the body (primarily used in dentistry).	The surface of a tooth that faces the median line is the mesial surface.
Lateral	Toward the outside or away from the midline that divides the body.	The ear is on the lateral surface of the head.
Distal	Away from the midline of the body or body section.	The hand is the distal portion of the arm. In dentistry, the surface of a tooth that faces away from the median line is the distal surface.
Proximal	Refers to the part of the body closest to the point of attachment.	The thigh is the proximal surface of the leg.
Inferior	Below or under.	The mouth is inferior to the nose.
Superior	Above or higher.	The eyes are superior to the mouth.

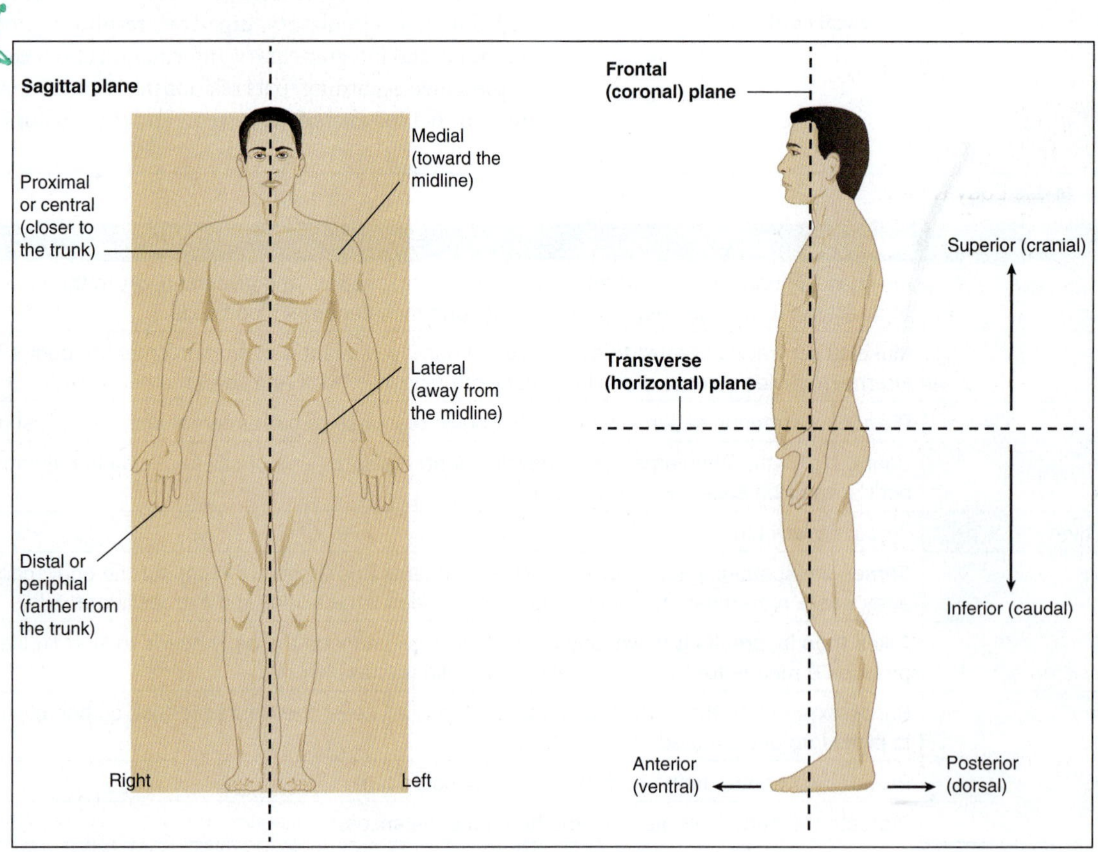

FIGURE 6-1
Body Planes and directions.

into equal left and right halves, it would be referred to as the *mid sagittal plane.* The plane that divides the body into upper and lower sections is known as the *transverse plane*, sometimes called the horizontal plane. The *frontal plane* divides the body into front and back sections. This vertical division divides the body into a front section, called the ventral or anterior, and a back section, referred to as the dorsal or posterior.

Body Cavities

A **body cavity** is a space or area in the body where various structures and organs are found. The body cavities are divided into two sections: the dorsal and the ventral.

The *dorsal cavity* is in the posterior portion of the body and contains two parts: the **spinal canal**, which contains the spinal cord, and the *cranial cavity*, which contains the brain. These two occupy one continuous space.

The *ventral cavity* is in the anterior portion of the body and contains three main parts: the *thoracic cavity*, the *abdominal cavity*, and the *pelvic cavity*. These cavities contain organs that maintain the basic life processes. The thoracic cavity or chest cavity contains the lungs, the heart, and all accessory parts needed for their functioning. The abdominal cavity is divided into upper and lower sections. The upper cavity is called the abdominal and includes most of the digestive tract and supporting organs needed for the process of digestion. The lower portion is called the pelvic cavity and contains the urinary bladder, the rectum, and the reproductive system (Figure 6-2).

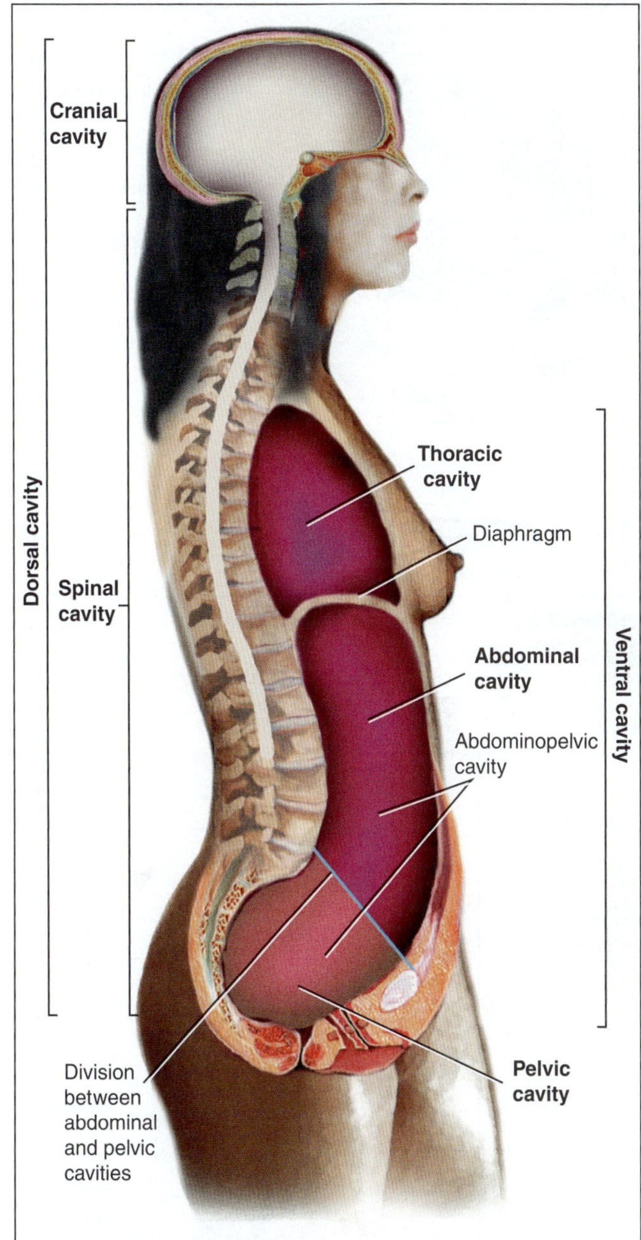

FIGURE 6-2
Body cavities.

Basic Structure and Functions of the Cell

The **cell** is the basic unit of all systems and the smallest functioning unit of the body (Figure 6-3). The basic components of a cell include the cell membrane, nucleus, cytoplasm, and chromosomes. The *cell membrane* is the outer wall of the cell. This thin wall is composed of proteins, lipids, and carbohydrates. This membrane controls the exchange of materials coming into and out of the cell. The *nucleus*, the controlling body of the cell, contains genetic codes. *Cytoplasm* comprises all the substance of a cell except the nucleus. *Chromosomes* are in the nucleus and contain DNA, which transmits genetic information.

Cells differ in appearance, function, and structure according to what they do. Specialized groups of cells form **tissues** and tissues group together to form **organs**. Tissues and organs unite to form **systems**. These cells, tissues, organs, and systems all function together to maintain harmony in the body, which is called **homeostasis** (hoh-me-o-STAY-sis).

Skeletal System

Functions of the Skeletal System

The functions of the skeletal system include support for the body's framework and overall body shape. The skeleton provides a surface for muscles to attach to and protects the fragile organs of the body. Also, the skeletal system manufactures blood cells and stores minerals for use when they are needed. An example is calcium.

Divisions of the Skeletal System

The skeleton is divided into two main divisions: the axial skeleton and the appendicular skeleton. The **axial skeleton** includes bones of the cranium, face, spinal column, ribs, and sternum. It is the framework of the head and the trunk of the body. The spinal column is divided into five sections including: cervical vertebrae, thoracic vertebrae, lumbar vertebrae, sacrum, and coccyx. Knowledge of the areas of the spinal cord is useful when learning the correct ergonomic positioning for the dental assistant. The **appendicular skeleton** is composed of the bones from the upper and lower extremities

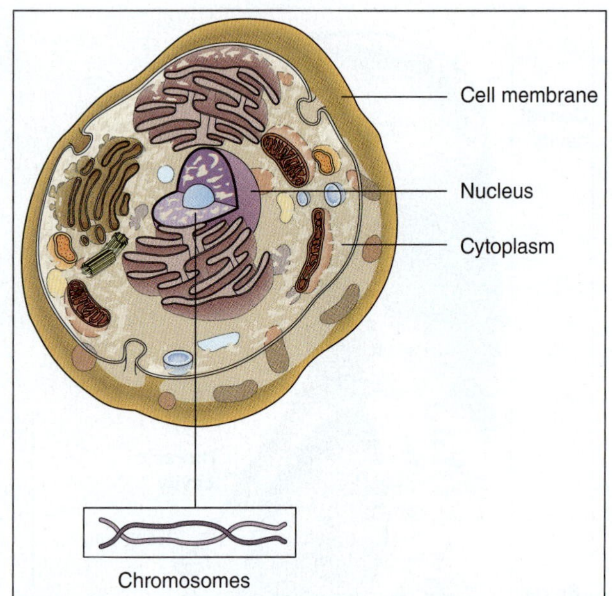

FIGURE 6-3
Basic cell structures.

and includes the arms, hands, legs, feet, shoulders, and hips. Together, the two divisions total 206 bones in an adult skeleton (Figure 6-4).

Bone Composition

The bone or **osseous tissue** is composed of connective tissue. This connective tissue is rendered hard by the deposits of mineral salts. The bone tissue is 20 percent water; of the remaining 80 percent, two thirds is composed of minerals and inorganic matter and one third is organic matter, including blood cells, lymphatic vessels, and nerves.

There are two types of bone tissue: cancellous or spongy bone, and compact or dense bone. The **cancellous bone** consists of a meshwork of interconnecting bone called **trabeculae** (trah-**BEK**-you-lay). The pattern of the trabeculae gives the bone a sponge-like appearance and strength without adding weight. Cancellous bone is found in the ends of long bones and in the middle of other bones. The **compact bone** is the strong and hard section of the bone. Compact bone is dense and forms the main shaft of long bones and the outer layer

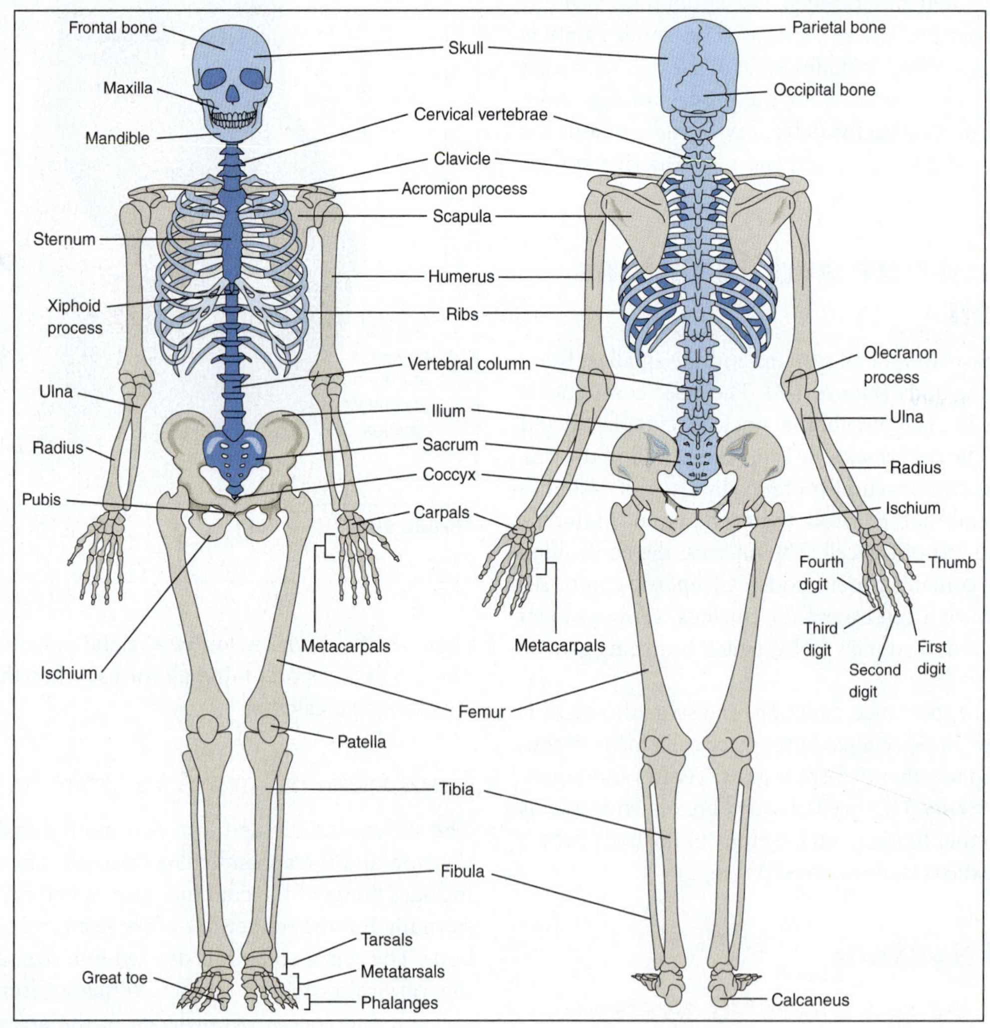

FIGURE 6-4
Axial (highlighted in blue) and appendicular (highlighted in grey) skeleton.

of other bones. **Osteoclast** cells are found in the compact bone. When bone is damaged or stressed, the osteoclasts dissolve and reabsorb the calcium salts of the bone matrix. The compact bone is covered with a layer of tough, fibrous tissue called the *periosteum*. The periosteum contains blood and lymph vessels, bone-building cells called **osteoblasts**, and nerve tissue.

Inside the spaces of the cancellous bone is *red bone marrow*. Red bone marrow is filled with blood vessels and small amounts of connective tissue. Red bone marrow manufactures red and white blood cells and platelets. It is found in the ends of long bones and the middle of other bones. *Yellow bone marrow* contains mainly fat cells and is found in the center shafts of long bones. As the body ages, the active red bone marrow is slowly replaced with yellow bone marrow (Figure 6-5).

Cartilage is found where bones join and forms part of such structures as the nose and ears. It is a tough, non-vascular, resilient connective tissue.

Types of Joints

A joint or **articulation** is an area where two or more bones meet or form a junction. A joint is usually composed of fibrous connective tissue and cartilage. Table 6-3 illustrates the three types of joints, explains how they are divided, and gives an example of each.

Synovial joints make movement possible and comprise most of the joints in the body (Figure 6-6).

Importance to the Dental Assistant

The skeletal system contains the cranium and facial bones, including the maxilla and the mandible. These bones support the teeth and surrounding tissues and are the primary focus of dentistry. Conditions of the skeletal system may alter patient treatment. Knowledge of this system aids dental assistants in correct patient positioning and movement at the dental unit, as well as providing sound ergonomic principles for themselves.

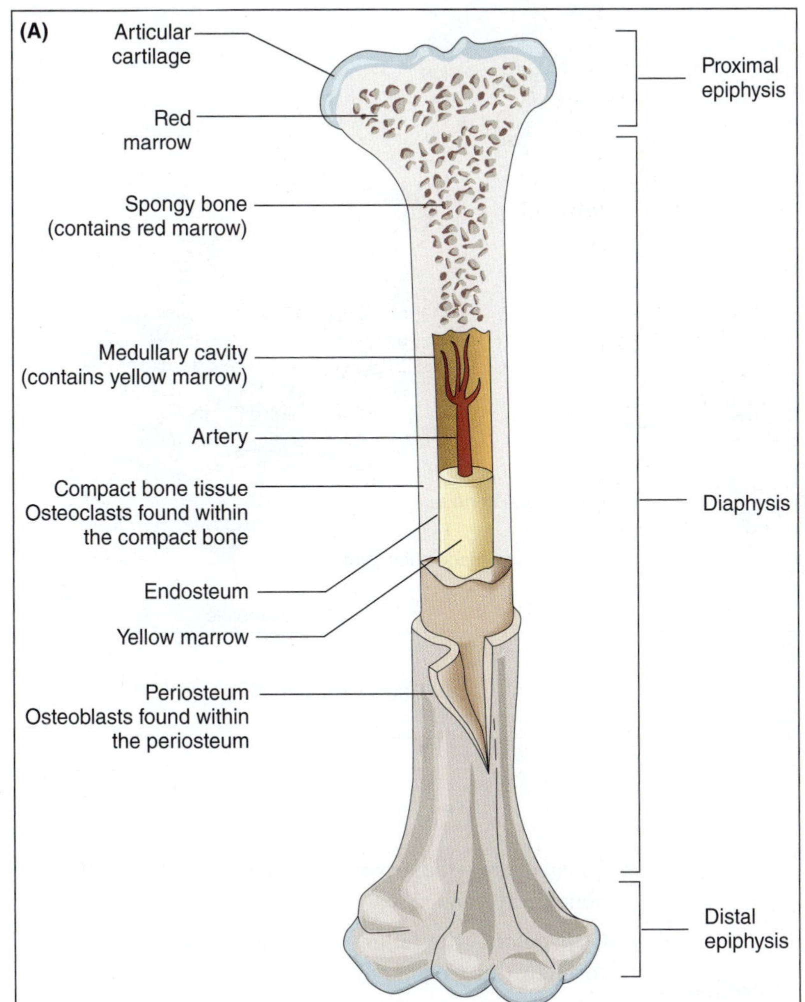

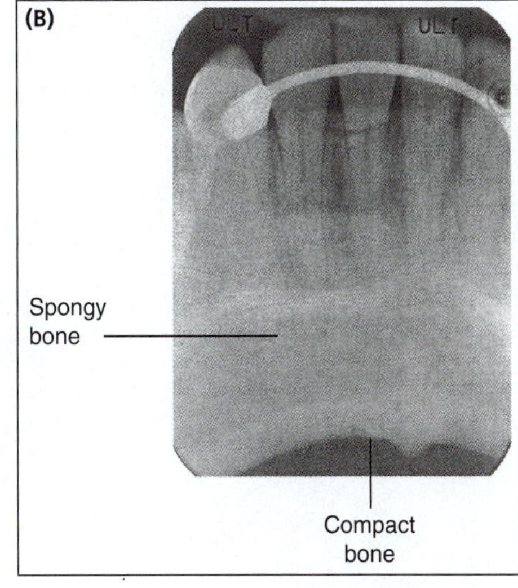

FIGURE 6-5
(A) Anatomic features of the bone. (B) Dental radiograph showing compact and spongy bone.

TABLE 6-3 Joints

Name of Joint	Description of Joint	Type of Movement	Example
Fibrous joint	Fibrous connective tissue	Immovable or fixed	Sutures found between the bones of the cranium.
Cartilaginous joint	Connective tissue, cartilage	Slightly movable	Joints found between bones of the vertebrae.
Synovial joint	Fluid within the joint (synovial fluid)	Considerable or free movement	There are six types of synovial joints: ball and socket, hinge, pivot, gliding, saddle, and condyloid. The temporomandibular joint is a synovial joint.

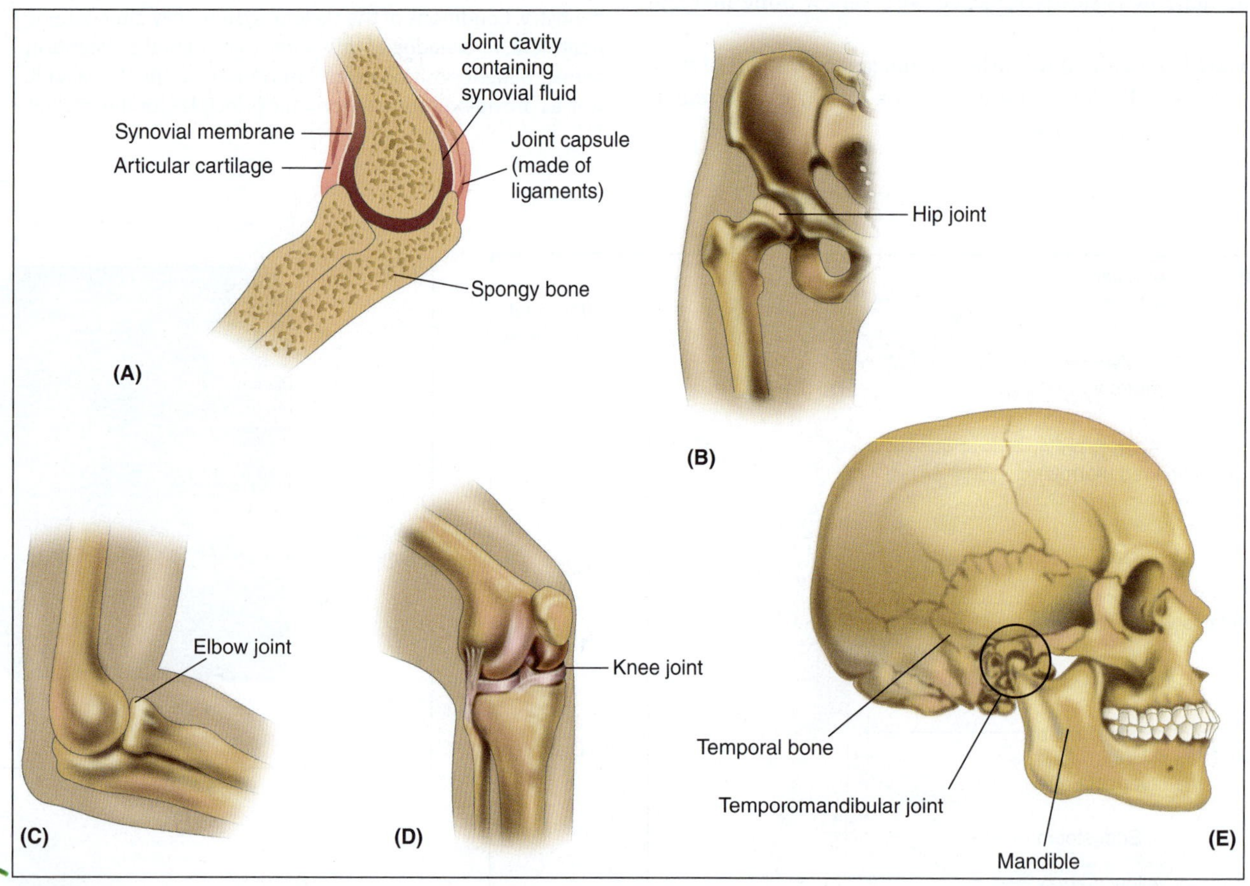

FIGURE 6-6

Skeletal joints: (A) Structures of a synovial joint and several examples of synovial joints. (B) Ball and socket joint of the hip. (C) Hinge joint of the elbow. (D) Hinge joint of the knee. (E) Temporomandibular joint.

Common Diseases and Conditions of the Skeletal System

Diseases of the bone include:

- *Osteomyelitis* (oss-tee-oh-my-eh-**LYE**-tis)—an infection of the bone-forming tissue. There is inflammation, edema, and circulatory congestion in the bone marrow. Pus may form and inflammatory pressure may cause small pieces of bone to fracture.
- *Osteoporosis*—the loss of bony material, thus leaving the bones brittle and soft.
- *Cleft palate*—the failure of the palate to form and join correctly (see Chapter 8).
- *Fractures*—breaks of the bone or cartilage.
- *Temporomandibular joint disease (TMJ)*—degeneration or disease of the joint where the mandible articulates with the temporal bone (see Chapter 25).

Muscular System

Functions of the Muscular System

The muscular system makes up 30 to 40 percent of total body weight. The muscles contract and relax to provide for all movements of the body, both internally and externally. Internal muscles move food along the digestive track and keep the heart beating. External muscles allow the body to walk, run, stand straight, and communicate. Muscles also produce body heat.

Types of Muscles

There are three types of muscle tissues: striated, cardiac, and smooth. Figure 6-7 shows these muscle tissues, locations, appearances, and functions.

Striated muscle is made of long, thin cells that have stripes or bands across them. Because these muscles are in bunches of fibers that attach to the skeleton, they are sometimes called skeletal muscles. This type has the largest amount of muscle tissue of the three types and its function is to provide for external body movement, from facial expression to bike riding. The skeletal muscles are under voluntary control. They are the only group of muscles an individual has conscious control over and are sometimes called voluntary muscles.

Cardiac muscle has the same striated or striped appearance as skeletal muscle but is involuntary in action. Cardiac muscles are found only in the heart, where they receive approximately 75 stimuli per minute. These muscle cells are specially designed in a chain-like arrangement and are able to receive an impulse, respond, and relax very rapidly, thereby keeping the heart beating in an even rhythm.

Smooth muscle is nonstriated tissue. The smooth muscles are also involuntary, which means they are controlled by the autonomic nervous system and are not consciously controlled. These muscles are found in internal organs (except the heart), blood vessels, skin, and ducts from glands.

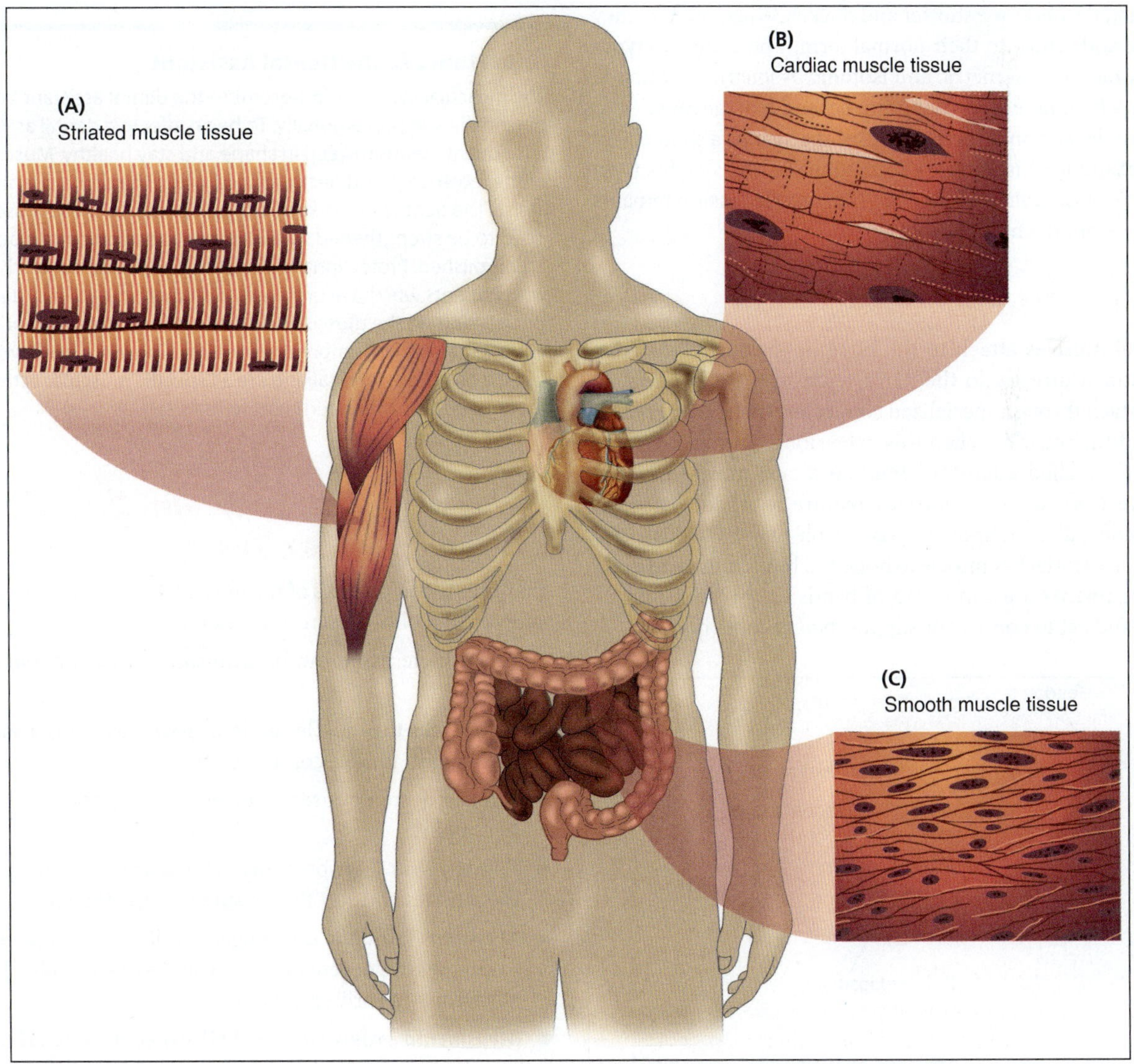

FIGURE 6-7

(A) Striated muscle. (B) Cardiac muscle. (C) Smooth muscle.

Muscle Characteristics

Each muscle is made of cells in various shapes and sizes depending on muscle function. Groups of muscle cells are often called fibers. Each fiber is about the size of a human hair and can support 1,000 times its own weight. Humans have over a trillion fibers in over 600 muscles in their bodies. Each fiber has nerves and a blood supply; it also has a fibrous sheet of connective tissue that covers, supports, and separates the muscle fibers. This sheet is called the **fascia**.

Muscle tissue has the capacity, called **excitability** or **irritability**, to respond to stimuli. This response puts the muscle into motion or activity. The ability of the muscle to stretch or spread in order to perform tasks is **extensibility**. Muscle tone is the tension of the muscular system. The brain and spinal cord continually send stimuli to the muscles on a subconscious level. The increase or decrease of the constant stimuli from the nervous system affects muscle tone. When the muscles are used, they stay toned and ready in a healthy state, while muscles that are not used become flabby and begin to deteriorate.

Muscles work by *contracting* and *relaxing*. When muscles contract, they become shorter and thicker. When relaxed, they release and return to their normal form. There are two types of contractions: isometric and isotonic. *Isometric contraction* occurs when there is no change in the length of the muscle but the muscle tension is increased. Pushing against a solid object is an example of isometric contraction. Lifting weights is an example of *isotonic contractions*—the muscle tension remains the same but the muscles shorten.

Muscle Attachments

Skeletal muscles attach to the bone in various ways. They may attach directly to the periosteum of the bone or they may attach through specialized connective tissue that extends beyond the muscle. When this extension is in the form of a cord, it is called a **tendon**. Tendons attach muscle to bone (Figure 6-8). Certain muscles require a broad, flattened extension called an **aponeurosis** (ap-oh-new-**ROH**-sis). The aponeurosis attaches muscle to bone and binds muscle to muscle. **Ligaments** are composed of bands or sheets of fibrous tissue and act to connect or support two or more bones.

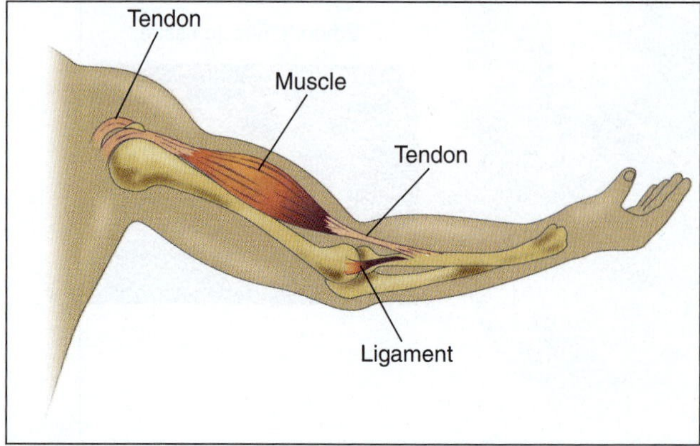

FIGURE 6-8
Muscle tissues and attachments of the arm.

The **origin** of the muscle is where the muscle attaches to the more stationary bone. The **insertion point** of the muscle is where the bone is moveable.

Muscle Function

Muscles contract and relax to provide movement. Most skeletal muscles function in **antagonistic pairs**. This means that while one set of muscles contract, another corresponding set relaxes. The body moves and functions through these coordinated efforts.

It takes energy for muscles to function. Energy is received in the form of oxygen and glucose. Oxygen comes to the muscle through the circulating blood and glucose is stored as a substance called *glycogen*. Muscles go through chemical changes to provide energy for body functions. Sometimes, when the activity is too rapid, there is not enough oxygen and an incomplete breakdown of glycogen occurs, resulting in a waste product called *lactic acid*. When the activity stops, the normal metabolic process readjusts and sufficient oxygen is restored.

Importance to the Dental Assistant

The muscular system is important to the dental assistant both personally and professionally. To be an effective dental assistant, it is advantageous to keep in shape and stay healthy. Muscles of the lower back and neck are used when the dental assistant assists the dentist or works directly on patients. These muscles need to be strengthened so that correct positioning can be accomplished. Professionally, the dental assistant will work with patients who have problems with their muscular systems. Understanding the muscular system can help the assistant make patients' dental visits more comfortable. Chewing, swallowing, facial expressions, and talking are all specific muscular activities that make this system pertinent to dentistry.

Common Conditions and Diseases of the Muscular System

Conditions and diseases of the muscular system are numerous and varied. Following are a few examples:

- The muscle tissue can be *strained, sprained, cramped*, or *inflamed*.
- Sometimes the muscles go into *spasm*, which is a sudden, involuntary muscle contraction.
- If muscles are not used, they begin to deteriorate, known as *atrophy*.
- *Fibromyalgia* (figh-broh-my-**AL**-jee-ah) is chronic pain in the muscles and soft tissues surrounding the joints.
- *Muscular dystrophy* is a congenital disorder characterized by progressive degeneration of the skeletal muscles. It usually strikes in early childhood.
- *Myasthenia gravis* (my-as-**THEE**-nee-ah **GRAH**-vis) is an autoimmune disorder that leaves the muscles weak and fatigued. One of the first symptoms is weakness in the facial or swallowing muscles.

Nervous System

Functions of the Nervous System

The nervous system transmits stimuli from outside and inside the body; it is the body's communication system. It has the ability to respond and transmit stimuli to maintain the body's unity and harmony.

Structure of the Nervous System

The nervous system consists of three sections: brain, spinal cord, and nerve cells. The brain and the spinal cord make up the **central nervous system (CNS)**. All the nerves outside the CNS make up the **peripheral nervous system (PNS)**. There is also a specialized group of peripheral nerves that function mainly automatically; this group is called the **autonomic nervous system (ANS)**.

The basic structural unit of the nervous system is a **neuron** or nerve cell. The neuron structure includes a nucleus surrounded by a cell membrane with thread-like projections called nerve fibers. The nerve fibers that conduct impulses toward the cell body are called **dendrites**. **Axons** are nerve fibers that conduct impulses away from the cell body. Some dendrites and axons can be up to 2 feet long. Nerve fibers move impulses from one cell body to another through a **synapse**. This is a junction where chemicals are released from the ends of axons to allow the stimuli to jump to the next dendrite. Some nerves in the PNS are covered with layers of Schwann cells. These layers insulate and protect nerves, and are known as the **myelin sheath** (Figure 6-9).

Sensory neurons work together to carry messages from all over the body to the spinal cord and the brain. Neurons that carry a message away from the spinal cord and brain are *motor neurons*. Motor neurons carry messages that direct the body to act. A third type of neuron, *interneurons or associate neurons*, transmits impulses from sensory neurons to motor neurons in the CNS.

The Spinal Cord and Spinal Nerves

The spinal cord is a major part of the nervous system. The activity of the spinal cord is twofold. First, it is a center for reflex or involuntary responses. When a stimulus is sent through the sensory neurons into the spinal cord and a response is automatically processed and sent back through motor neurons for an action a **reflex arc** occurs (Figure 6-10).

Second, the spinal cord transmits stimuli from the body to the brain, where the message is interpreted and then a response is sent back to an organ or a muscle.

Thirty-one pairs of spinal nerves originate in the spinal cord. The nerves are named and numbered according to the closest vertebrae.

The Brain and Cranial Nerves

The brain consists of many interlinked parts. The brain receives incoming stimuli and interprets and processes the information. Stimuli are directed to various parts of the brain, depending on which area of the body the stimuli is coming from.

Twelve pairs of cranial nerves mainly involve the head. They are numbered with Roman numerals beginning in the front of the brain and moving toward the back (Table 6-4).

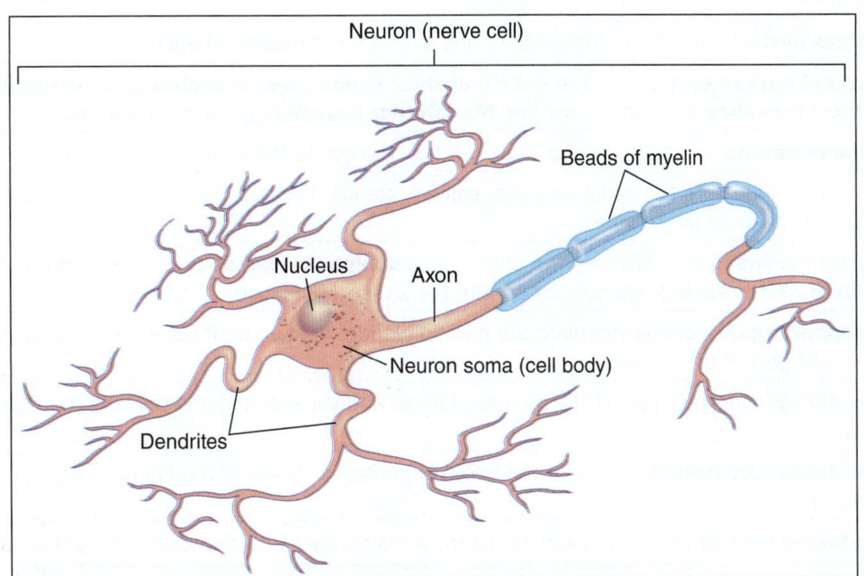

FIGURE 6-9
Structure of a neuron.

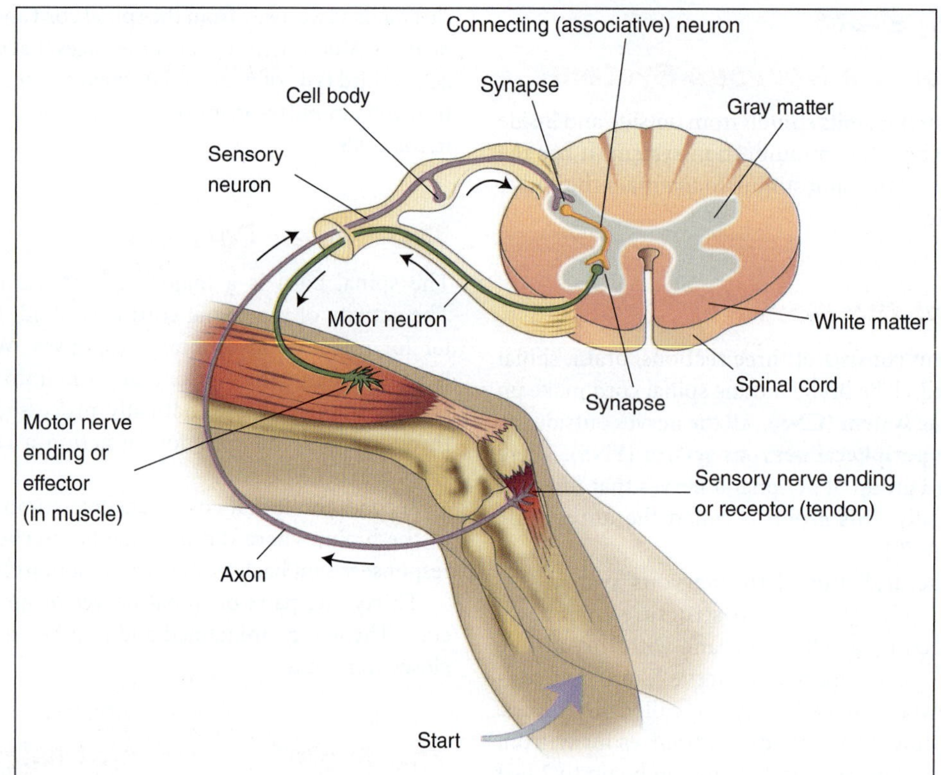

FIGURE 6-10

Simple reflex arc.

TABLE 6-4 Cranial Nerves and Their Functions

I.	**Olfactory nerves** conduct impulses from receptors in the nose to the brain and are sensory in function.
II.	**Optic nerves** conduct impulses from receptors in the eyes to the brain and are sensory in function.
III.	**Oculomotor nerves** send motor impulses to four of the external eye muscles, as well as to certain internal eye muscles.
IV.	**Trochlear nerves** send motor impulses to one external eye muscle of each eye.
V.	**Trigeminal nerves** each divide into three branches: **Ophthalmic branches** go to the eyes and forehead. **Maxillary branches** go to the upper jaw. **Mandibular branches** go to the lower jaw.
VI.	**Abducens nerves** innervate the muscles that turn the eye to the side.
VII.	Facial nerves innervate the facial muscles, salivary glands, lacrimal glands, and the sensation of taste on the anterior two-thirds of the tongue.
VIII.	**Acoustic nerves** each divide into two branches: **Cochlear branches** are concerned with the sense of hearing. **Vestibular branches** are concerned with the sense of balance.
IX.	**Glossopharyngeal nerves** innervate the parotid glands, the sense of taste on the posterior third of the tongue, and part of the pharynx.
X.	**Vagus nerves** innervate part of the pharynx, larynx, and vocal cords, and parts of the thoracic and abdominal viscera.
XI.	**Spinal accessory nerves** innervate the shoulder muscles. Some of the fibers of these nerves arise from the spinal cord.
XII.	**Hypoglossal nerves** primarily innervate the muscles concerned with movements of the tongue.

Importance to the Dental Assistant

Understanding its structure and how the nervous system works will help the dental assistant work with the dentist and the patient. Patients often fear going to the dentist because they assume it will be a physically painful experience. Anesthesia blocks patients' pain and makes dental procedures possible. Dental assistants must know the nerves in the face and oral cavity to effectively assist the dentist during the administration of anesthetic, as well as during many types of surgical procedures. Dental team members sometimes experience physical problems themselves, especially with the sciatic nerve located in the lower back and traveling down the back of the thigh. This is due to the positions they must hold for long periods of time.

Common Diseases of the Nervous System

- *Neuritis* is the inflammation of nerves. It may be the result of a fall or blow and can affect one or more nerves in the body. The term neuritis is also used when describing nerve tissue degeneration.
- *Multiple sclerosis (MS)* is a disease that usually appears in people aged 20 to 40. This disease destroys the myelin sheath of neurons in the CNS. When this happens, impulses cannot be transmitted to their destinations.
- *Parkinson's disease* is a chronic nervous disease characterized by slowly spreading tremors, muscular weakness, and a peculiar gait.
- *Bell's palsy* is a sudden onset of facial paralysis.

Endocrine System and Reproductive System

Functions of the Endocrine System

The endocrine system, like the nervous system, is a control and communication system. The nervous system acts rapidly to transmit stimuli, whereas the endocrine system is much slower and the results are longer lasting. The nervous system and the endocrine system are connected because the nervous system controls the pituitary gland and this gland controls the other glands. The endocrine system generally controls the body's growth; protects the body in stressful situations; controls development of sex characteristics; regulates utilization of calcium; aids in regulating the body's water balance; and produces insulin, which aids in the transport of glucose into cells (Table 6-5).

Parts of the Endocrine System

The endocrine system is made of glands spread throughout the body (Figure 6-11). They are grouped according to structures and interrelated functions. These glands produce secretions and are ductless—there is no tube for secretions from the glands to pass through, so the secretions empty directly into the bloodstream and circulate throughout the body. These secretions are called **hormones**. Hormones are released from the endocrine glands. Hormones control the internal environment of the body from the cellular to the organ level. They are analogous to the furnaces and thermostats in our homes. We set the thermostat to a particular temperature, and when the temperature falls below that temperature, the

TABLE 6-5 Major Glands of the Endocrine System

Gland	Main Function(s)	Examples of Hormones Produced
Pituitary	Master gland that releases hormones, which affect the workings of other glands.	Growth hormone and thyroid stimulation hormone
Thyroid	Increases metabolic rate, which affects both mental and physical activities. Needed for normal growth.	Thyroxin
Parathyroid	Increases the level of calcium in the blood. Regulates the calcium between bone and blood.	Parathyroid hormone
Adrenal	Releases the fight or flight hormone, which increases heart rate and blood pressure and aids in the metabolism of carbohydrates, proteins, and fats during stress.	Cortisol and adrenalin
Pancreas (Islets of Langerhans)	Produces hormones, including insulin and glucagon.	Insulin
Testes	Responsible for the development of male sex characteristics.	Testosterone
Ovaries	Responsible for the development of female sex characteristics.	Estrogen and progesterone

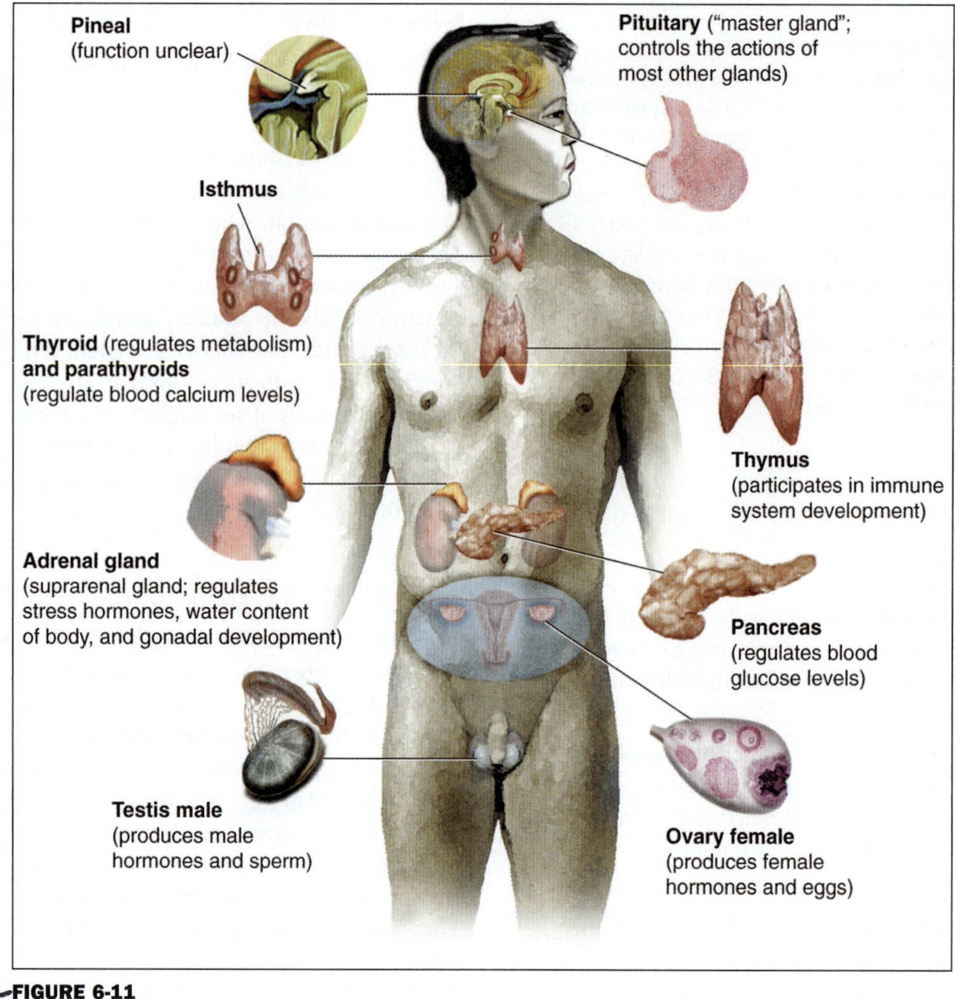

FIGURE 6-11
Structures of the endocrine system.

thermostat causes the furnace to turn on. Once the temperature reaches the set temperature on the thermostat, the furnace turns off. The hormonal system functions in a similar manner. When the concentration of a particular hormone reaches a certain level in the body, the endocrine gland that secretes that hormone is inhibited and secretion of the hormone ceases or decreases. Later when the concentration of that gland's hormone falls below normal levels, the inhibition of the gland stops and it begins to produce and secrete the hormone once again.

Importance to the Dental Assistant

There are diseases and conditions of the endocrine system, such as diabetes, that affect patients and how they respond to dental treatment. The dental assistant can prepare for possible emergencies with an understanding of the patient's needs. With young patients going through puberty and older patients going through menopause, better communication and understanding will be enhanced by knowledge of this system. The dental assistant is responsible for knowing and following all precautions and standards regarding radiation and the use of nitrous oxide in the dental examination room.

Reproductive System

The reproductive system includes male and female reproductive organs. The male and female reproductive systems' main function is the creation of life. In both sexes, primary and accessory organs must be protected in certain procedures used in dentistry. Two examples of procedures requiring protection are using a lead apron when exposing radiographs and providing adequate ventilation during nitrous oxide sedation. Safety guidelines are routinely followed in the dental office to protect the patient and the dental staff.

Common Diseases and Conditions of the Endocrine and Reproductive Systems

- *Diabetes mellitus* is a disease that occurs when the pancreas produces an insufficient amount of insulin.
- During *pregnancy*, dental treatments may need to be altered depending on the stage of pregnancy.

- *Hypothyroidism* is an underactive thyroid gland.
- *Hyperthyroidism* is an overactive thyroid gland with excessive secretion of hormones.

Circulatory System

Functions of the Circulatory System

The circulatory system is the body's means of transporting a continuous supply of oxygen, nutrients, hormones, and antibodies throughout the body while carbon dioxide and other cellular wastes are being removed from the body. This system maintains a balance between intracellular and extracellular fluids.

Parts of the Circulatory System

Circulation is divided into two pathways. The first pathway circulates blood through the heart to the lungs and back to the heart. This is **pulmonary circulation**. The second pathway, **systemic circulation**, carries the blood from the aorta to the smallest blood vessels and back to the heart (Figure 6-12). Main components of the circulatory system include the heart, blood vessels (arteries, veins, and capillaries), and blood.

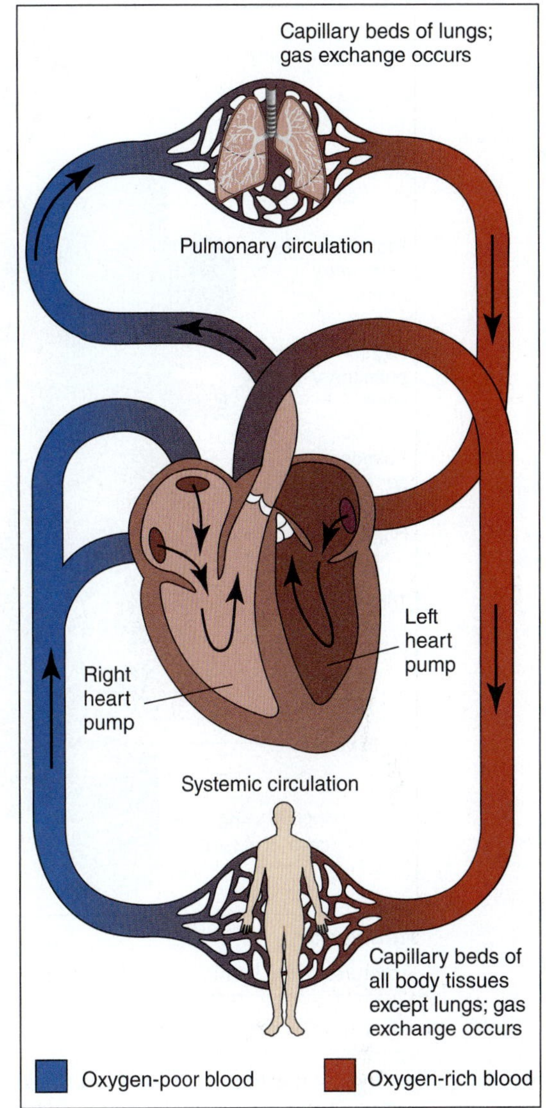

FIGURE 6-12
Systemic and pulmonary circulation.

Heart. The **heart** is a pump that circulates the blood throughout the body. It is a triangular-shaped muscular organ that is approximately the size of a closed fist (Figure 6-13). The heart is covered with three layers: the **pericardium**, the outer layer that is composed of a double-walled sac; the **myocardium**, a tough, muscular wall; and the **endocardium**, a thin lining on the inside of the heart. A wall divides the heart into right and left halves. Each half is divided again into upper chambers called the *atria* or *auricles* and lower chambers called *ventricles*. Four **heart valves** regulate the flow of blood in one direction. The blood comes into the heart through large vessels called the **vena cava**. From the superior and inferior vena cava, blood enters the right atrium, and then is pumped through the *tricuspid valve* into the right ventricle. It then goes through the *pulmonary valve* into the pulmonary artery, which carries the blood to the lungs to get rid of waste and gases, and picks up fresh oxygen. From the lungs, the blood is carried by the pulmonary vein to the left atrium, and then through the *mitral valve (bicuspid valve)* into the left ventricle and then through the *aortic valve* into the aorta to be distributed to all parts of the body. The *chordae tendineae* are found in the ventricular side of the heart (the lower chambers). They are strong, fibrous strings attached to the cusps of the heart. They originate from the papillary muscles which are small mounds of muscle tissue that project inward from the walls of the ventricle and connect to the tricuspid and mitral valves in the heart.

Blood Vessels, Arteries, Veins, and Capillaries. An **artery** carries oxygenated blood from the heart to the capillaries of the tissues. The walls of the arteries are tough and composed of three layers to withstand the pressure. The largest artery is the **aorta**, which receives blood directly from the heart; an **arteriole** is the smallest artery.

A **vein** carries blood that has drained from the capillaries back to the heart. The walls of the veins are composed of three layers like the arteries, but they are much thinner and less muscular. Within the inner layer are folds that form valves that keep the blood flowing toward the heart.

A **capillary** is the connection between the arteries and the veins. The exchange between the blood and body cells occurs in the capillaries. Here, oxygen and nutrients are delivered to the cells and carbon dioxide and wastes are removed. The walls of the capillaries are comprised of a single thin layer, which is an extension of the lining in arteries and veins. There are thousands of miles of connecting capillaries in the body.

Blood. The **blood** has three main functions: transportation of nutrients, gases, waste products, and hormones; regulation of the amount of body fluids, pH balance, and body temperature; and protection against pathogens and blood loss after

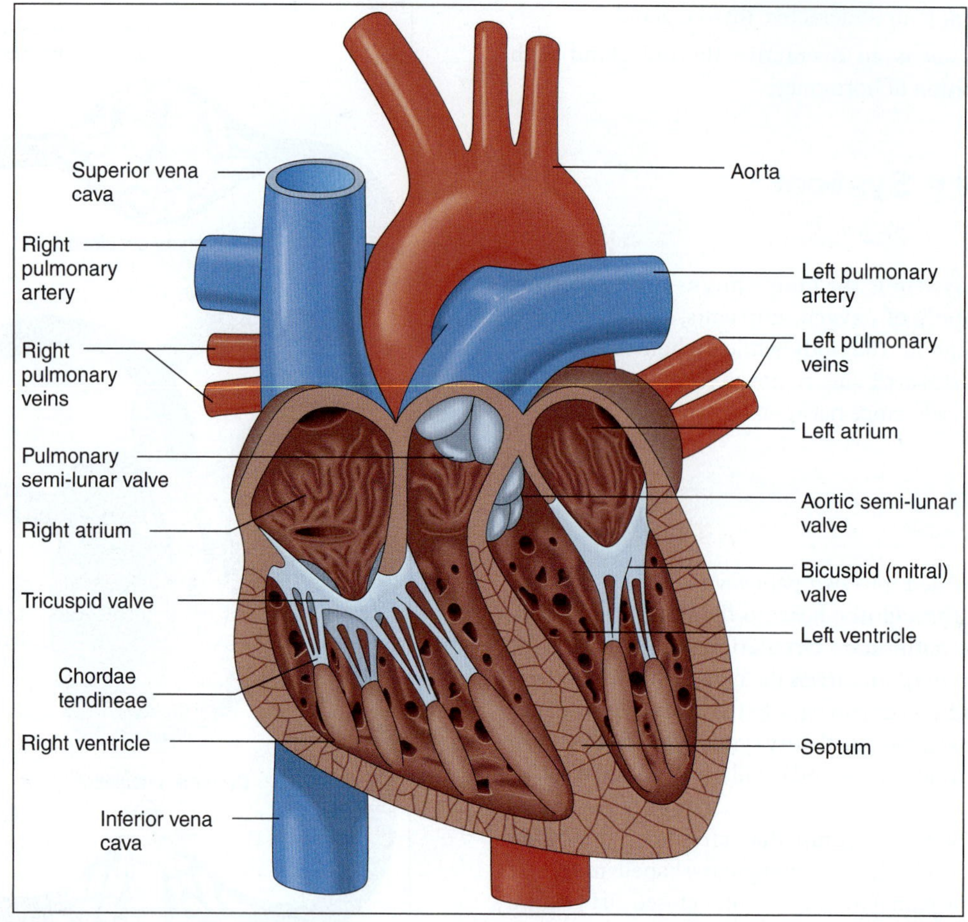

FIGURE 6-13
Structures of the heart.

injury through the clotting mechanism. Blood is a thick fluid that varies in color from bright red to a darker, brownish red. The average adult has four to six quarts of blood. The liquid portion of the blood, **plasma**, is 91 percent water and carries nutrients, hormones, and wastes. The cells or solid portion of the blood are called *corpuscles*. There are three types of corpuscles: erythrocytes, leukocytes, and platelets.

- *Erythrocytes*, or red blood cells, contain the protein *hemoglobin*, which gives the erythrocytes the ability to carry oxygen.
- *Leukocytes*, or white blood cells, protect the body from infection and disease. There are five types of leukocytes, all with specific tasks to defend the body against viruses, bacteria, and other foreign substances.

Thrombocytes, or platelets, are fragments or pieces of cells that are necessary for blood clotting (coagulation). The process by which the body controls bleeding is called ***hemostasis***.

Blood Groups. There are five main blood type categories: A, AB, B, O, and the ABO system. The ABO system is primarily used for blood transfusions. Refer to Table 6-6 for blood types, donors, and recipients. If patients were to receive blood that is not compatible with their blood type, the result could be fatal. Additionally, the **Rh factor** should be considered when treating patients who may require blood transfusions from a donor. Serious transfusion reactions could occur if the Rh factor is not matched. The Rh factor is also an important consideration during pregnancy; if the child is Rh positive and the mother is Rh negative, incompatibility between the mother and the fetus may result. People with the Rh antigen are Rh positive and those without are Rh negative. The mother may become sensitized by the blood of the Rh-positive fetus. To prevent problems in future pregnancies, if the fetus is Rh positive, during the second trimester of the first pregnancy the mother is given RhoGAM, an immunoglobulin.

Importance to the Dental Assistant

The circulatory system is important to the dental assistant as our population is aging and geriatric dentistry is growing. Understanding heart disease and frequently prescribed medications helps the assistant to be alert for possible complications. Heart disease is the leading cause of death for both men and women; therefore, another consideration is to be prepared for an emergency—dental treatment can present a stressful situation to an already compromised patient.

TABLE 6-6 Blood Types, Donors, and Recipients

Blood Group/Type	Percent of Population	Antigen/Agglutinogen on Red Blood Cells	Antibody/ Agglutinin in Plasma	Can Receive	Can Donate to
A	41	A	Anti-B	A or O only	A or AB only
B	12	B	Anti-A	B or O only	B or AB only
AB	3	A and B	None	A, B, AB, O (Universal recipient)	AB only
O	44	None	Anti-A and Anti-B	O only	A, B, AB, O (Universal donor)

Common Diseases and Conditions of the Circulatory System

- *Bacterial endocarditis* is an inflammation of the lining of the heart. Patients who have a history of rheumatic fever, congenital heart disease, open-heart surgery, joint replacement, organ transplants, or dental implants should always be treated with antibiotics before dental treatment.
- A disorder called *hemophilia* is the failure of the blood to clot.
- *Leukemia* is a malignant, progressive disease of the blood-forming organs that is marked by unrestrained growth of abnormal leukocytes. Leukemia cells infiltrate the bone marrow and lymph tissue. These cells then advance to the bloodstream and various body organs.

Digestive System

Functions of the Digestive System

The digestive system provides a means for consumed food to be prepared for use by the body, circulated to all cells, and eliminating wastes. This is done by **digestion**, breaking down food into small nutrient molecules the cells can use. After food has gone through digestion, it is transferred into the bloodstream; this is the absorption process. Here, the small nutrient molecules are circulated by the bloodstream to all cells of the body. Another function of the digestive system is the process of elimination, which provides a means for the body to eliminate solid wastes.

Parts of the Digestive System

The digestive system is divided into two groups: the *alimentary canal* and *accessory organs*. The alimentary canal forms a canal or tube from the mouth to the anus. The canal includes the mouth (oral cavity), pharynx, esophagus, stomach, small intestine, and large intestine. Accessory organs aid in the process of digestion. Included are the teeth, tongue, salivary glands and ducts, liver, gallbladder, and pancreas (Figure 6-14

Alimentary Canal. The mouth **(oral cavity)** receives food and begins breaking the food down. The teeth, tongue, lips, cheeks, and salivary glands all work together to mechanically break food into small pieces and then move the food to the throat area.

The **pharynx** connects the oral cavity to the esophagus, which is where food is swallowed. The pharynx also functions as part of the respiratory system. Therefore, sometimes during swallowing, food may go into the larynx instead of the esophagus. To prevent this from occurring, the **epiglottis** (a small, leaf-shaped cartilage) covers the larynx. Swallowing is a complex, multi-stepped process that is controlled by the medulla part of the brain. Swallowing, or **deglutition**, provides movement for the food to proceed from the mouth to the stomach.

The **esophagus** extends from the pharynx to the stomach. Muscles help to keep food moving toward the stomach, even when the body is reclined. The lower esophageal sphincter (**SFINK**-ter) muscle, at the end of the esophagus, relaxes to allow food into the stomach, and then contracts to prevent it from flowing backward.

The **stomach** is an organ that extends from the esophagus to the small intestine. It is located in the upper left area of the abdominal cavity, and can expand to hold a half gallon of food. The stomach acts as a storage area and a churn to mix the food with gastric juices. Two components of gastric juices are hydrochloric acid and pepsin. These gastric juices are secreted by glands in the stomach lining. Then the muscular movement of the walls, called **peristalsis**, mixes the food with gastric juices and breaks it down to a mixture called **chyme**. After about 3 hours, chyme leaves the stomach in spurts and enters the small intestine.

The **small intestine** connects the stomach to the large intestine and is approximately 20 feet long and 1 inch in diameter. The first section of the small intestine is called the *duodenum*. Here, other digestive juices enter and the breakdown process continues. In the walls of the small intestine are finger-like projections called *villi*. Here, the digested food is absorbed into the bloodstream.

The **large intestine** extends from the small intestine to the rectum. The large intestine is shorter, approximately 5 feet long, and 0.5 to 2.5 inches in diameter. The large intestine stores and excretes the waste products of digestion.

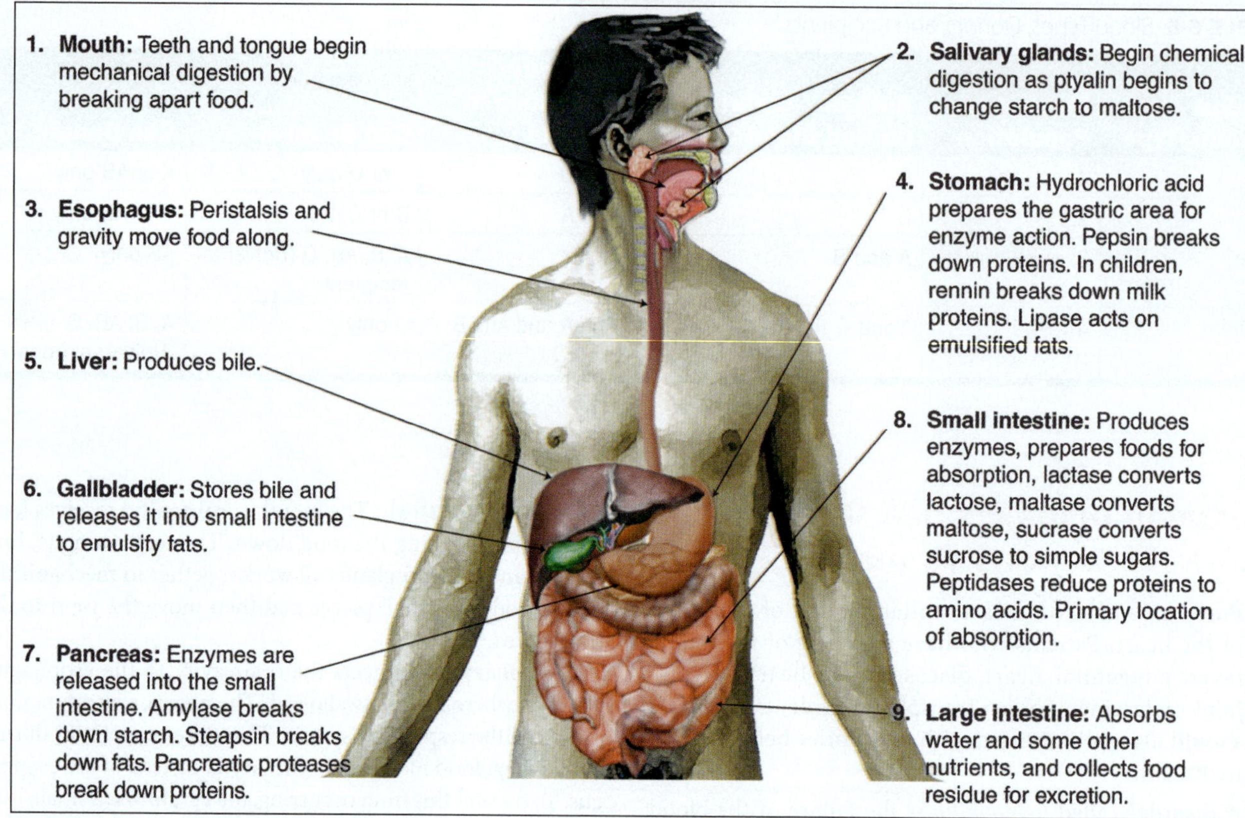
1. Mouth: Teeth and tongue begin mechanical digestion by breaking apart food.
2. Salivary glands: Begin chemical digestion as ptyalin begins to change starch to maltose.
3. Esophagus: Peristalsis and gravity move food along.
4. Stomach: Hydrochloric acid prepares the gastric area for enzyme action. Pepsin breaks down proteins. In children, rennin breaks down milk proteins. Lipase acts on emulsified fats.
5. Liver: Produces bile.
6. Gallbladder: Stores bile and releases it into small intestine to emulsify fats.
7. Pancreas: Enzymes are released into the small intestine. Amylase breaks down starch. Steapsin breaks down fats. Pancreatic proteases break down proteins.
8. Small intestine: Produces enzymes, prepares foods for absorption, lactase converts lactose, maltase converts maltose, sucrase converts sucrose to simple sugars. Peptidases reduce proteins to amino acids. Primary location of absorption.
9. Large intestine: Absorbs water and some other nutrients, and collects food residue for excretion.

FIGURE 6-14
Structures of the digestive system.

TABLE 6-7 Mechanism of Digestion

Organ	Process	Description of Process
Oral cavity (mouth, teeth, tongue, and saliva)	Taste Mastication Swallowing or deglutition	Receives the food, tastes Mechanical breakdown of food Saliva glands produce enzymes to start chemical digestion
Pharynx	Deglutition	Movement of food as a result of swallowing Passageway for food and air
Esophagus	Deglutition Peristalsis	Mucus is secreted as food is transported in waves toward the stomach
Stomach	Churning Peristalsis	Chemical breakdown continues as stomach enzymes are released and mechanical movements churn the contents
Small intestine	Absorption Peristalsis	Absorption of digested food Move contents along intestinal track
Large intestine	Peristalsis Defecation	Mechanical movements occur Emptying of the rectum

Accessory Organs. The accessory organs have specific functions, but each organ relies on the functions of the others in order to complete the digestive process.

- The *teeth* begin the digestive process by biting, tearing, and grinding the food.
- The *tongue* moves food from the anterior teeth to the posterior teeth and gathers the food before it is swallowed.
- The *salivary glands* produce saliva to dissolve food, facilitate the process of chewing (mastication), and coat food for ease in swallowing. The salivary glands excrete mucus to lubricate the food; amylase, an enzyme to begin the digestive process of starches; sodium bicarbonate to increase pH, which accelerates amylase function; and water to dilute and facilitate food mixing. Three salivary glands surround

the mouth, the parotid gland, the submandibular gland, and the sublingual gland. More information on the tongue and salivary glands is found in Chapter 7, Head and Neck Anatomy.

- The **liver**, the largest of the glandular organs, is on the right side of the body, just below the diaphragm. The liver has many functions that aid in the digestion process, but the main function is the production of **bile**. Bile contains salts that emulsify fats.
- The **gallbladder** is a muscular sac that stores bile from the liver. It is on the right side on the inferior surface of the liver.
- The **pancreas** produces juices that are emptied into the duodenum to aid digestion and produce insulin.

Even before food is ingested, the sight, smell, and thought of food stimulate the saliva glands to produce saliva and stomach secretions begin to flow. Then the process of digestion begins as outlined in Table 6-7.

Importance to the Dental Assistant

The digestive system begins with the oral cavity, which is the focus in dentistry. Knowing the components of this system and how each contributes to the processing of food enables the dental assistant to detect disease and communicate with the patient.

Common Diseases and Conditions of the Digestive System

Many diseases and conditions of the digestive system directly relate to dentistry.

- *Tooth decay* is destruction of the tooth surface.
- *Periodontal disease* is inflammation and deterioration of the periodontal tissues (see Chapter 29).
- *Bulimia* is a disease in which individuals "purge" or vomit after eating large quantities of food. With time, the hydrochloric acid from the stomach left in the oral cavity after vomiting can cause serious dental problems for bulimic patients. The acid eventually dissolves tooth structure.
- *Hepatitis* is inflammation of the liver caused by several viruses. There are three main hepatitis viruses: hepatitis A, hepatitis B, and hepatitis C. Hepatitis B is contracted by exposure to body fluids of infected individuals, and is of the most concern because of its serious prognosis. For more information, see Chapter 10, Microbiology.

Respiratory System

Functions of the Respiratory System

Breathing is the main function of the respiratory system. Air is inhaled through the nose into the lungs, where it is absorbed into the bloodstream and carried to all body cells. Once the oxygen reaches the cells, it is exchanged for the waste product carbon dioxide. Carbon dioxide is then transported by the blood back to the lungs and exhaled.

Parts of the Respiratory System

The respiratory system consists of the nose, pharynx, larynx, trachea, bronchi, and lungs (Figure 6-15).

The nose is the passage for outside air to enter the body. The nose contains two *nasal cavities*, which are divided by the *nasal septum*. The inner surface of the nose is lined with the *nasal mucosa*, which warms and humidifies the air as it passes through. The nose also contains the *olfactory receptors*, which facilitate the sense of smell.

The pharynx, or throat, serves as a passageway for two systems: respiratory and digestive. Air and food pass through the pharynx as they move downward. This tube is about 5 inches long and is divided into three sections. The first is the **nasopharynx**, the upper section behind the nasal cavity. The *eustachian* (you-**STAY**-shun) (auditory) *tubes* open into the pharynx. The **oropharynx** (o-ro-**FAIR**-inks), the middle section, is the portion behind the mouth. It is lined with the same mucosa as found in the oral cavity. The lower section, the **laryngopharynx** (lah-ring-goh-**FARE**-inks), divides and has an opening in the front to the larynx and in the back to the esophagus.

The **larynx**, or voice box, connects the pharynx and the trachea. The larynx is made up of cartilage and is supported by muscles. At the upper end of the larynx is the leaf-shaped epiglottis. Its function is to close off the larynx during swallowing to prevent food from entering. The thyroid cartilage, or Adam's apple, lies anterior to the larynx. In the interior of the larynx, the **vocal cords** stretch across the width of the larynx to produce sound.

The **trachea**, or windpipe, the next section for air passage, is 4 to 5 inches long and extends to the lungs. The trachea consists of C-shaped cartilage that allows for expansion of the esophagus during the process of swallowing. The trachea can become blocked by the inhalation of an object or from swelling.

The **bronchi** are the two branches that form at the end of the trachea and enter the lungs. The bronchi branches divide into smaller tubes called **bronchioles**. At the end of the bronchioles are **alveolar sacs**, which resemble clusters of grapes. These alveolar sacs consist of individual **alveoli**. Gaseous exchange takes place here in the alveoli. The thin walls of the alveoli make for easy passage of air entering and leaving the blood capillaries.

The **lungs** are two cone-shaped organs inside the rib cage. Each lung consists of a spongy mass that is pink at birth and then darkens to blue-gray or black, depending on air quality and personal habits. Each lung is surrounded by a sac called the *pleura*.

Respiration is the process of breathing and exchanging gases (oxygen and carbon dioxide) between the body and its environment. There are two phases to this process: inhalation and exhalation. During **inhalation**, muscles contract, the chest enlarges, and air flows into the lungs. **Exhalation** occurs when the muscles relax and the air is moved out of the lungs.

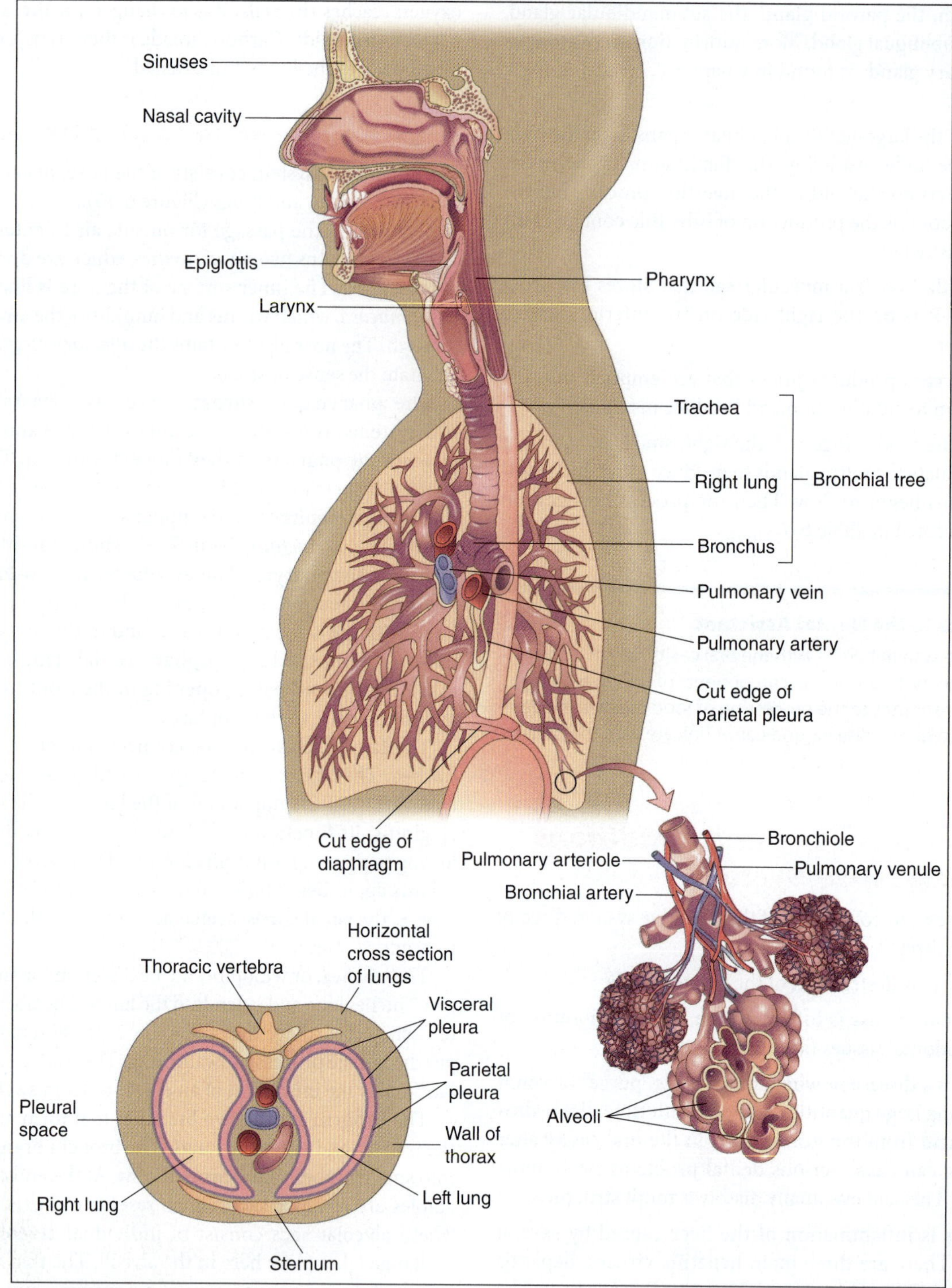

FIGURE 6-15

Structures of the respiratory system.

Importance to the Dental Assistant

The dental assistant should watch the patient for signs of discomfort or problems with breathing. The use of nitrous oxide may be contraindicated when a patient has respiratory disease. Allergic reactions can and do occur in the dental office. A patient could choke on materials that fall to the back of the throat, and respiratory diseases or conditions can make treatment difficult. Understanding the respiratory system could save a patient's life.

Common Diseases of the Respiratory System

- *Asthma* is the muscular spasm of the walls of the bronchi. The air passages are constricted so the person cannot easily exhale.
- *Tuberculosis* is a highly contagious disease of the respiratory system. Tuberculosis is transmitted by breathing or swallowing droplets contaminated by the TB bacillus.

- *Lung cancer* is a malignancy of the lung tissue. It is a very common form of cancer and is often caused by cigarette smoking.
- Other conditions include the common cold, pneumonia, and bronchitis. Following standard precautions protects the office staff and the patient when treatment is required during times of infection.

Lymphatic System and Immune System

Functions of the Lymphatic System

The lymphatic system is a network of vessels that drains and filters the tissue fluid surrounding cells.

Parts of the Lymphatic System

The parts of the lymphatic system include the lymph, lymph vessels, lymph nodes, spleen, and thymus gland.

Lymph, also called *tissue fluid*, is a clear liquid formed in tissue spaces. The lymph enters the lymphatic capillary system and drains away excess fluid and carries proteins back to the bloodstream.

Lymph is transported through a specialized network of vessels called *lymphatic capillaries*. These capillaries are very thin-walled and only allow lymph to travel in one direction on the way back to the general circulation system.

Lymph nodes are found in groups along the lymphatic vessels. They are small, round masses that vary in size and location. The lymph nodes most commonly known are the ones in the armpit, neck, and groin. The purpose of the lymph nodes is to filter the lymph as it journeys back to the bloodstream and to manufacture antibodies and other active materials of the immunity process.

The **spleen**, located behind the stomach, is protected by the rib cage. It is the largest lymphoid organ in the body and contains a very rich blood supply. If the spleen is damaged, it may have to be removed to stop blood loss. As the blood moves through the spleen, it removes bacteria and other foreign materials, filters out old red blood cells, produces red blood cells before birth, and acts as a storage area for blood in case of hemorrhage. Humans can live without the spleen because other lymphoid tissues take over its functions. However, without the spleen, the person may be more susceptible to certain bacterial infections.

The **thymus** is under the sternum, just below the thyroid. It is large and active from before birth through puberty, but then shrinks and almost disappears in adults. The thymus gland is important to immune system development.

Tonsils form a protective circle around the inside of the oral cavity. They consist of masses of lymphoid tissue that guard against bacteria that may enter the body through the digestive and respiratory systems. There are three groups of tonsils: the *palatine tonsils*, on each side of the throat; the *lingual tonsils*, on the base of the tongue; and the *pharyngeal tonsils* (adenoids), on the posterior wall of the nasopharynx area (Figure 6-16).

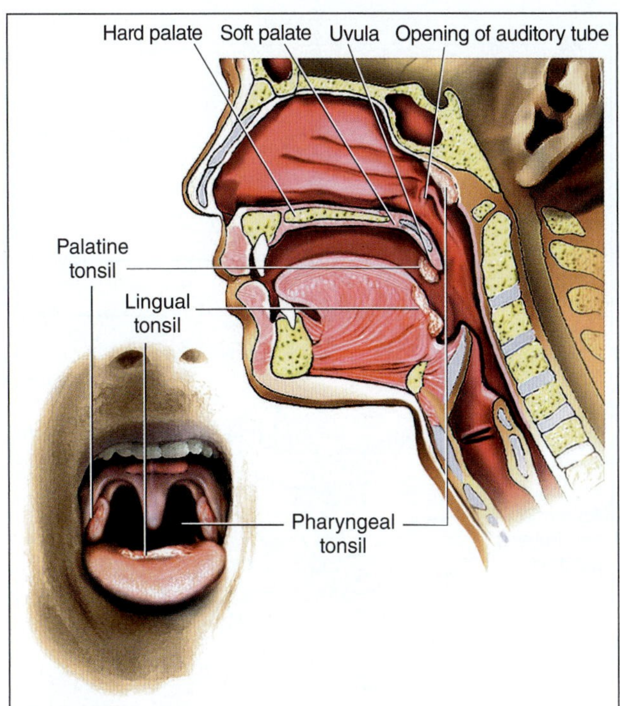

FIGURE 6-16
Tonsils.

Functions of the Immune System

The immune system is part of the body's defense against harmful organisms. It protects the body from pathogens, foreign materials, debris, and damaged cells by removing these elements. The immune system is composed of specialized cells (phagocytes and lymphocytes) and molecules (antibodies and antigens). The system is organized into nonspecific and specific defenses. **Nonspecific immunity** is the body's defense against any harmful agents, while **specific immunity** acts against selected agents. The immune system involves organs or vessels from several other systems (Figure 6-17).

Importance to the Dental Assistant

The dental assistant is constantly exposed to disease and infection. A major responsibility of each dental team member is to maintain a safe environment. Continuing education on prevention of and protection from health risks is necessary for all dental professionals.

Common Diseases and Conditions of the Lymphatic and Immune Systems

- *Tonsillitis* is a chronic infection of the tonsil tissue.
- *Hodgkin's disease* is a malignant disorder that causes enlargement of the lymph nodes.

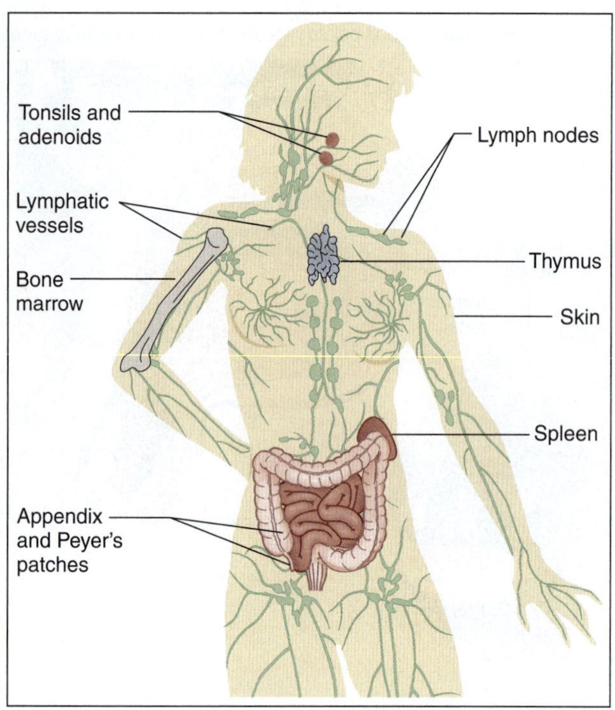

FIGURE 6-17

Organs and vessels from other body systems involved in the immune system.

- *Allergies* are a hypersensitivity to certain substances. These are often common substances such as pollen, pet dander, or cigarette smoke, which are referred to as allergens. The reaction to allergens can cause an inflammatory response or a severe allergic reaction.
- *Immune deficiency disease* is a failure in some part of the immune system.

Bacterial and viral infections, fungi, parasites, cancer cells, and foreign tissue implants are all conditions that the immune system protects and fights against.

Integumentary System

Functions of the Integumentary System

The integumentary (in-teg-u-men-tear-ee) system is a body system we don't always think about and yet it plays a very important role in relation to body functions. This system is composed of the largest organ of the body: the skin, hair, and nails. It comprises 16 percent of the body's weight and is composed of many types of cells and tissues. The integumentary system acts as a sensory receptor and informs the brain of external stimuli. Messages are sent to the brain to signal that the body is experiencing something that is hot or cold and also when something that the body is in contact with is hard or smooth. This system has many other important functions including:

- Protection—the skin is the body's first defense against foreign invaders, injury, and harmful sunrays
- Temperature regulation
- Metabolic regulation
- Prevention of water loss
- Synthesis of vitamin D
- Production of melatonin (skin color)
- Production of keratinocytes (fibrous protein)
- Storage of water, fat, and vitamin D
- Amazing wound-healing abilities that require extensive intercellular cooperation

Parts of the Integumentary System

The **skin** (cutaneous layer) is composed of several layers including the epidermis, dermis, and subcutaneous layers (Figure 6-18). The *epidermis* is the outer layer of the skin and is composed of epithelial tissue. This layer contains the skin pigment melanin. It is also coated with keratin, a tough, rough protein that is also the main component of hair and nails. The epithelial cells are shed from the skin's surface and replaced with new cells from the base of the epidermis every 10 to 30 days.

The *dermis* supports the epidermis and is comprised of connective tissue. In this layer the nerve endings of the skin, blood vessels, elastic fibers, sweat glands, and sebaceous glands are found. The sweat glands keep the body cool and sebaceous glands provide oil to keep the skin supple.

The *subcutaneous* layer (*hypodermis*) of the skin lies beneath the dermis and is rich in blood vessels and fat.

Abnormal skin colorations which may be seen in the dental office include:

- Albinism—a patient with pale skin, white hair, and pink coloration of the iris.
- Cyanosis—the skin appears bluish as a result of oxygen deficiency in the circulating blood.
- Erythema—skin appears reddish.
- Hematoma—bruising of the skin; skin color may appear reddish to purple.
- Jaundice—skin and sclera (white of the eyes) appear yellowish.
- Pallor—skin is ashen and pale due to white collagen fibers in the dermis.

Nails are a hard, scale-like modification of the epidermis that forms flat plates on the dorsal surface of the end of the fingers and toes. These fingernails and toenails are composed of two parts: the body and the root. Both portions lay on the nail bed, or matrix. The body is the exposed section and is made of keratin. The root is hidden under a fold of skin called the **cuticle**. The nails grow through activity of cells in the root; the average rate of growth in fingernails is about 1 mm per week, while toenails grow slower. Nail growth varies with age and is affected by disease and certain hormone conditions.

Hair grows on every part of the skin except the palms of the hand and the soles of the feet. Each hair consists of a root portion and a thin, flexible shaft. The hair shaft grows from hair follicles found in the dermis and sometimes the subcutaneous tissue. Hair color is due to the pigment (melanin) which is

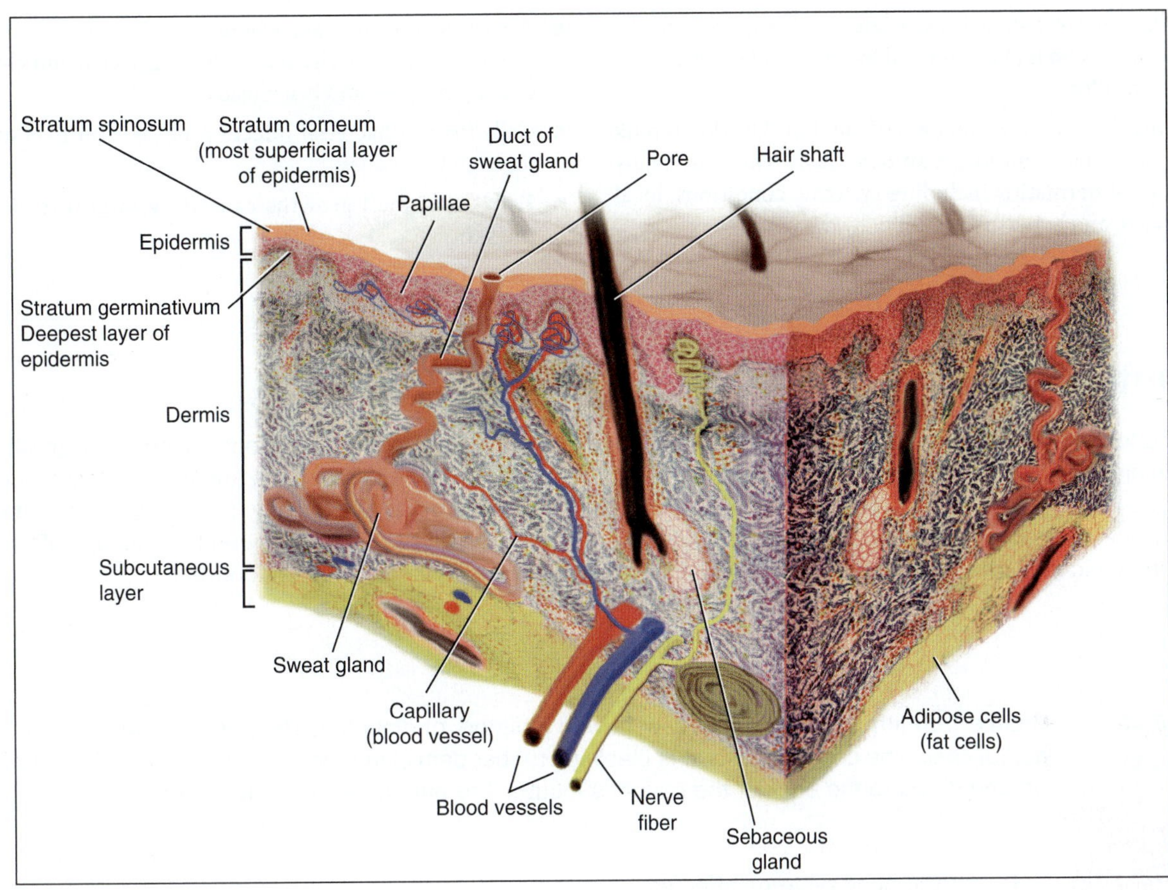

FIGURE 6-18

Parts of the integumentary system including the different sections of the skin and hair follicles.

found in the center of the shaft. There is constant growth and loss of hair for the adult human. Each part of the body has a specific growth pattern. For example, the hair of the eyebrows only lasts for three to five months, while hair of the scalp lasts for two to five years.

Importance to the Dental Assistant

The dental assistant works very closely with a patient and should always perform a quick visual exam of the patient's face and neck areas while the patient is seated. The assistant should take note of any discolorations, lesions, sores, and/or rashes found on the skin and inform the dentist. Many dental offices have discovered a suspicious lesion on a patient's face and referred the patient to another doctor for further examination. With the increase in skin cancer, early detection often contributes to successful treatment.

Diseases and Conditions of the Integumentary System

There are many diseases and conditions of the integumentary system that are related to dentistry. Here are just a few of the more common ones:

- *Carcinoma* is a cancerous tumor in the mucous membrane, skin, or similar body tissue. Basal cell carcinoma is the most common form of skin cancer. It begins as a small elevated area of the skin like a pimple, ulcer, or mole. It may be red, brown, black, or white in color and it may occur singly or in a group (Figure 6-19).

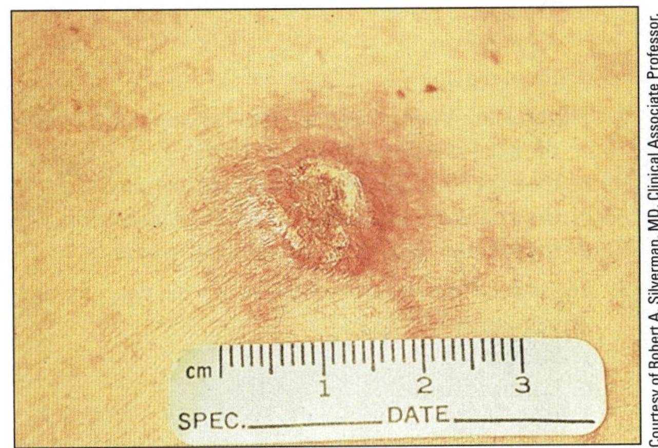

Courtesy of Robert A. Silverman, MD, Clinical Associate Professor, Department of Pediatrics, Georgetown University

FIGURE 6-19

Basal cell carcinoma.

- *Malignant melanoma* is associated with exposure to the sun. The lesion is characterized by an irregular border and uneven color.
- *Dermatitis* is an inflammation of the skin. The skin is pink to red in color and forms an itchy rash. There are many causes of dermatitis including systemic conditions, local irritants, and hypersusceptibility by the patient.
- *Acne* is a skin disorder where the sebaceous glands and the hair follicles of the skin become infected and clogged, causing pimples and blackheads.
- *Cellulitis* is a bacterial infection of the skin that spreads through the tissues.
- *Warts* are small growths caused by viral infections of the skin.

Chapter Summary

Specific terms are used to establish a means for health professionals to communicate more effectively. The body is divided into systems, planes, cavities, and basic units that provide common references and terms for studying and communicating information about the body.

The dental assistant needs to be familiar with the terminology of body systems and how each system functions to provide the quality of care that each patient deserves. Both the anatomy and physiology of all body systems will need to be understood.

CASE STUDY

Charlie T. Smith is a 23-year-old patient with a history of diabetes. The patient is reclined in the dental chair. The dental assistant is placing a rubber dam clamp on a tooth when the clamp pops off and drops to the back of the patient's mouth. The patient swallows the clamp.

Case Study Review

1. List the body systems affected.
2. List the specific structures of the primary system that could become involved.
3. Would the patient's age or medical condition impact the situation? If so, how?

Review Questions

Multiple Choice

1. Which of the following divides the body into left and right halves?
   a. Horizontal plane
   b. Transverse plane
   c. Sagittal plane
   d. Frontal plane
2. The skeletal system is divided into two main divisions:
   a. the axial skeleton and articulations.
   b. the appendicular skeleton and articulations.
   c. the axial skeleton and the appendicular skeleton.
   d. the pulmonary system and the axial system.
3. The skeletal muscles are comprised of what type of muscle tissue?
   a. Striated muscle
   b. Cardiac muscle
   c. Smooth muscle
   d. Involuntary muscle
4. The neurons that carry messages away from the spinal cord and brain are:
   a. sensory neurons
   b. motor neurons
   c. associated neurons
   d. inter neurons
5. The thyroid, adrenal glands, and the pancreas are all part of what system?
   a. Digestive system
   b. Lymphatic system
   c. Endocrine system
   d. Nervous system
6. All of the following are true statements about the reproductive system *except*:
   a. This system includes only the male and female reproductive organs.
   b. Primary and accessory organs must be protected in both sexes in certain dental procedures.
   c. Safety guidelines are followed in the dental office to protect the patient only.
   d. Placing a lead apron on the patient when exposing radiographs is an example of a safety guideline that is followed in the dental office.

7. All of the following are true statements about the blood *except*:
   a. Blood is a clear liquid formed in tissue spaces.
   b. Blood transports nutrients, gases, waste products and hormones.
   c. Blood is a thick fluid that varies in color from bright red to a darker, brownish red.
   d. Blood regulates body temperature.
8. The alimentary canal is part of what system?
   a. The circulatory system
   b. The digestive system
   c. The muscular system
   d. The skeletal system
9. All of the following are true statements about the respiratory system *except*:
   a. Breathing is the main function of the respiratory system.
   b. Respiration is the process of breathing and exchanging gases.
   c. The larynx, trachea, and alveoli are part of the respiratory system.
   d. During inhalation the muscles relax and air is moved out of the lungs.
10. The body system that drains and filters the fluid around cells is the:
   a. Respiratory system.
   b. Lymphatic system.
   c. Circulatory system.
   d. Immune system.

Critical Thinking

1. Name the synovial joint that has significance to the dental assistant.
2. Explain why the pulmonary arteries are called arteries even though they carry deoxygenated blood, and the pulmonary veins are called veins even though they carry oxygenated blood.
3. Why it is harder to replace lost blood in elderly patients?

Web Activities

1. Go to: http://www.heart.org and look for the warning signs of heart attack, stroke, and cardiac arrest.
2. Go to: http://www.lungusa.org and learn how to help your patients stop smoking.
3. Go to: http://www.ada.org and search related disorders discussed in this chapter such as oral cancer, diabetes, bulimia, and pregnancy. What is the significance of these disorders to dental health?

CHAPTER 7

Head and Neck Anatomy

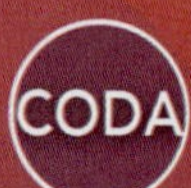

Specific Instructional Objectives

The student should strive to meet the following objectives and demonstrate an understanding of the facts and principles presented in this chapter:

1. List and identify the landmarks of the face and the oral cavity, including the tongue, floor of the mouth, and salivary glands.
2. List and identify the bones of the cranium and the face as well as the landmarks on the maxilla and the mandible.
3. Identify the parts of the temporomandibular joint (TMJ) and describe how the joint works.
4. List and identify the muscles of mastication, facial expression, the floor of the mouth, the tongue, the throat, the neck, and the shoulders. Explain their functions.
5. List and identify the nerves of the maxilla and the mandible.
6. List and identify the arteries and veins of the head and the neck.

Key Terms

articular disc (121)
bones of the cranium (118)
bones of the face (118)
common carotid (130)
facial nerve (127)
floor of the mouth (115)
glossopharyngeal nerve (127)
hyoid bone (123)
hypoglossal nerve (127)
landmarks of the face (113)
landmarks of the oral cavity (113)
mandible (118)
mastication (116)
maxilla (118)
muscles of facial expression (122)
muscles of mastication (122)
muscles of the floor of the mouth (123)
muscles of the neck (124)
muscles of the soft palate (124)
muscles of the tongue (122)
palate (114)
palatine bone (118)
papilla (115)
saliva (116)
salivary gland (116)
taste buds (115)
temporomandibular joint (TMJ) (120)
tongue (115)
torus (114)
trigeminal nerve (127)

Introduction

This chapter provides information on the anatomy of the head and neck. The dental assistant must be able to describe this anatomy, including the locations of structures and their functions. Patients often have questions, and knowing this anatomy will allow the assistant to answer these patient questions in a manner that will improve both patient understanding of different procedures and pre- and post-dental treatment care. Identifying parts of the head and neck anatomy will aid the assistant in many ways, including taking x-rays, taking study model impressions, and preparing for anesthetic application. Identifying the anatomy of the head, face, and neck in normal, healthy tissues enables the dental assistant to recognize the abnormal.

As a dental assistant you should be able to use proper terminology to describe and locate various anatomical features of the head and neck. The key terms highlighted in the chapter focus on the foundations. Additional terms are placed in italic and should be learned as well.

Landmarks of the Face and Oral Cavity

Landmarks of the anatomy are usually skeletal or soft tissue structures that are easily recognizable. They are used as reference points in describing the locations of anatomical structures or for taking measurements. It is important for the dental assistant to be familiar with the landmarks that make up the face and oral cavity.

Landmarks of the Face

The **landmarks of the face** include: ala of the nose, nasolabial groove, philtrum, vermilion border, vermilion zone, the tubercle of the lip, labial commissures, and the labio-mental grooves (Figure 7-1). As a dental assistant, you should be able to describe and locate each of these landmarks.

The *ala of the nose* is the wing of the nose or outer edge of the nostril. From the ala of the nose to the corners of the mouth is a groove called the *nasolabial groove*, or sulcus. Between the bottom of the nose and the middle of the upper lip is a shallow, V-shaped depression known as the *philtrum*. All these landmarks are covered with skin consistent with the skin in other parts of the face. These are areas to look at for scarring from accidents, surgeries, or physical conditions, such as cleft lip.

The lips are covered externally with skin and internally with mucous membrane. The reddish portion of the lips is called the *vermilion zone*. The vermilion zone is highly vascular and covered with a thin layer of epithelium. The *vermilion border* is where the skin meets the vermilion zone and forms a line around the lips. In the middle of the upper lip is a small projection that sometimes enlarges or thickens. It is called the *tubercle of the lip*. The corners of the mouth, where the upper lip meets the lower lip, are known as *labial commissures*. The commissures should be observed for cracks, color changes, and variations in form. Just below the lower lip is the *labio-mental groove*, which runs horizontally and separates the lip from the chin.

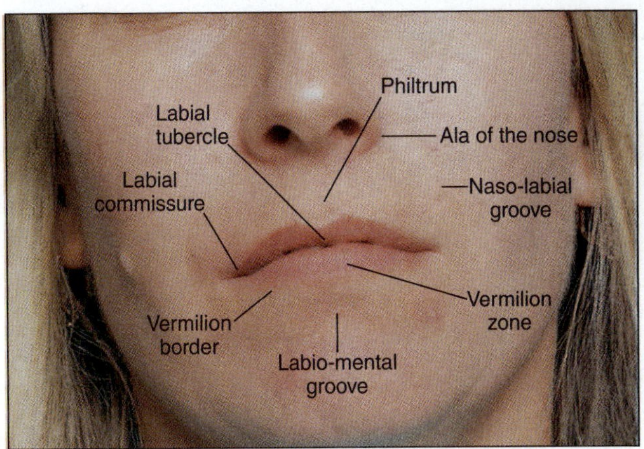

FIGURE 7-1
Landmarks of the face.

> **Importance to the Dental Assistant**
> The dental assistant may notice scars or sores around the nose, mouth, and chin areas. By knowing the normal landmarks of the face, the dental assistant can use correct terminology to describe any deviation and record the information on the health history. Sometimes facial scars can indicate the person has been in an accident and may have had many x-rays taken and possibly had surgery. He or she may have had seizures or had a cleft palate or lip. Knowing this information may assist in the details of the health history and treatment plan.

Landmarks of the Oral Cavity

Understanding the **landmarks of the oral cavity** aids the dental assistant when taking radiographs, placing topical anesthetic, recognizing healthy tissue, and recording information or medical history on a patient's chart.

The landmarks of the oral cavity include the following: vestibule, vestibule fornix, labial mucosa, buccal mucosa, parotid papilla, Stensen's duct, linea alba, Fordyce's spots, alveolar mucosa, gingiva, labial frenum, and buccal frenum (Figures 7-2A and B). As a dental assistant, you should be able to describe and locate each of these landmarks.

Inside the mouth, a pocket is formed by the soft tissue of the cheeks and the gingiva. This is the *oral vestibule* (mucobuccal fold). The deepest point of the vestibule is called the *vestibule fornix*. The fornix forms a U-shaped pocket that is continuous throughout the anterior and posterior areas.

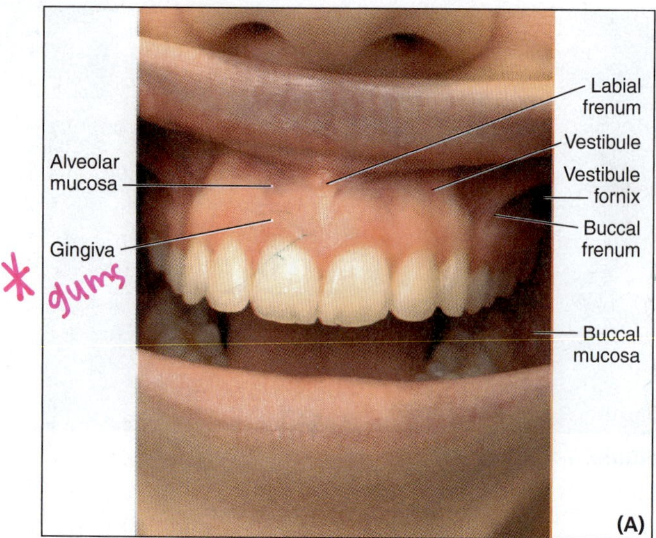

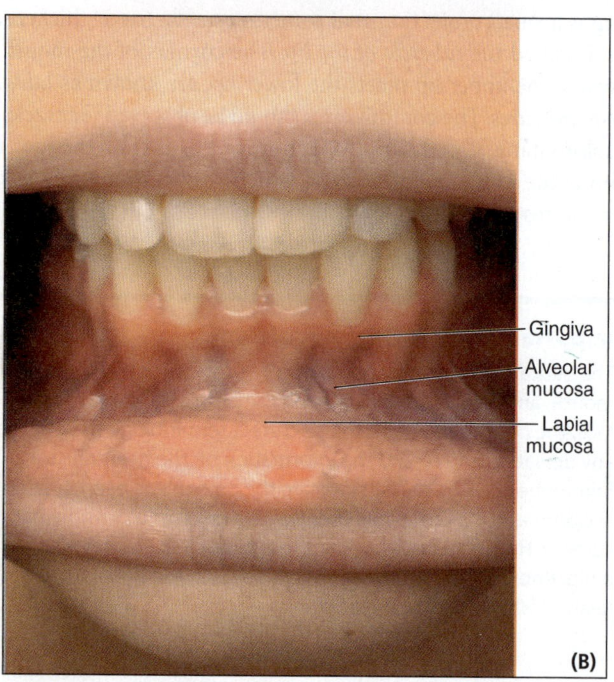

FIGURE 7-2
Landmarks of the oral cavity.

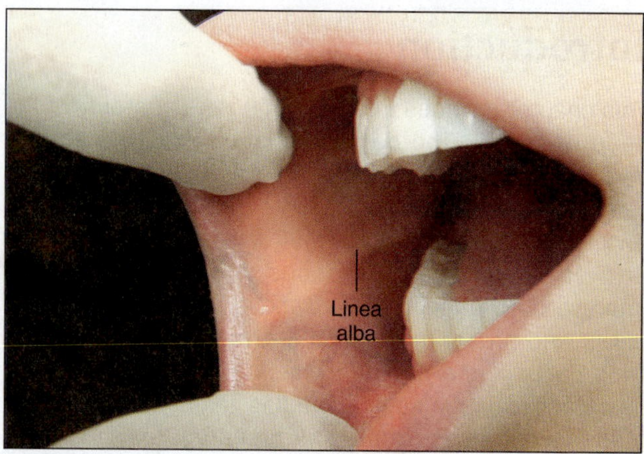

FIGURE 7-3
The oral vestibule with the linea alba on the buccal mucosa.

The tissue that lines the inner surface of the lips and cheeks is called *mucosa*. The mucosa is named according to location. The inner surface of the lips is called the *labial mucosa*, and the inner surface of the cheeks is the *buccal mucosa*. On the labial mucosa are small, yellowish glands near the commissures called *Fordyce's spots*, which become larger and more visible with age. On the buccal mucosa, opposite the maxillary second molar, is a flap of tissue called the *parotid papilla*, which is where the opening of the *Stensen's duct* is located. On the buccal mucosa is a raised white line that runs parallel to where the teeth meet, called the *linea alba* (Figure 7-3). Mucosa also covers the alveolar bone that supports the teeth. It is called the *alveolar mucosa*. The alveolar mucosa is loosely attached and is highly vascular, giving the mucosa a reddish color. Moving from the alveolar mucosa toward the teeth is the *gingiva*. The gingiva is firmly attached and usually pale pink or brownish pink, depending on pigmentation. This dense, fibrous tissue covered with mucous membrane can withstand pressure during chewing. The portion of the gingiva that meets the tooth is called the free gingiva or marginal gingiva.

When the lips are pulled out, frena become visible. Frena (plural form of *frenum*) are raised lines of mucosal tissue that extend from the alveolar mucosa through the vestibule to the labial and buccal mucosa. On the labial, the main frena are between the maxillary central incisors and the mandibular central incisors, with minor frena along the vestibule of both arches in the labial and buccal areas.

Palate Area of the Oral Cavity

On the inside of the maxillary teeth is the **palate**, or "roof of the mouth." The palate is divided into hard and soft sections. The hard palate, the anterior portion, is a bony plate covered with pink to brownish-pink keratinized tissue. The soft palate, the posterior portion, covers muscle tissue and is darker pink or yellowish. On the hard palate is the *incisive papilla*, which is a raised area of tissue lying behind the maxillary central incisors (Figure 7-4A). Extending from the back of the incisive papilla is a slightly raised line that extends down the middle of the hard palate, known as the *palatine raphe*. The ridges that run horizontally across the hard palate behind the incisive papilla are the *palatine rugae*. Occasionally, in the middle of the palate a lump or prominence of bone (exostosis) may be found. This excess bone is called a *torus* (plural is tori), or specifically a torus palatinus.

The following landmarks are on the soft palate and in the oropharynx areas: the uvula, anterior tonsillar pillars, posterior tonsillar pillars, palatine tonsils, and the fauces (Figure 7-4B). The *uvula* is a projection that extends off the back of the soft palate. Extending horizontally from the uvula to the base of the tongue are folds of tissue called

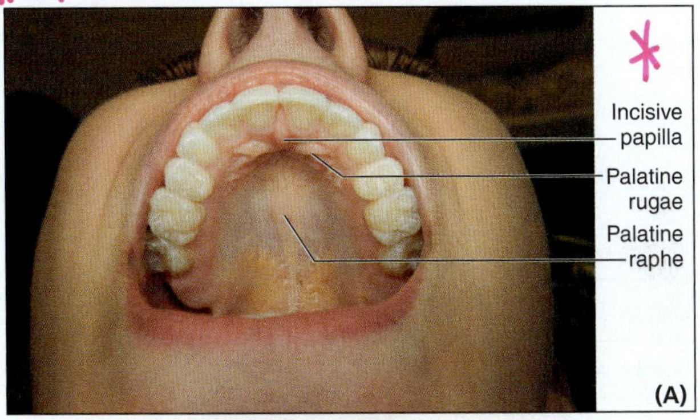

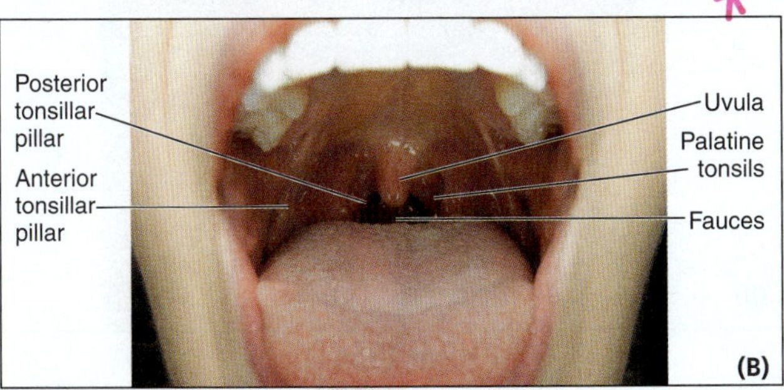

FIGURE 7-4

(A) Landmarks of the oral pharynx area. (B) Landmarks of the palate.

anterior tonsillar pillars or *palatoglossal arches*. Another set of arches is found farther back in the throat. This set is the *posterior tonsillar pillars* or *palatopharyngeal arches*. Between the two sets of pillars is a depressed area where the palatine tonsils are situated. The *palatine tonsils* are often marked with deep grooves and are red and inflamed when they are infected. The space in the back of the oral cavity where food passes into the pharynx is the *fauces*.

Tongue

The **tongue** is a significant region of the oval cavity with the following landmarks: sulcus terminalis, circumvallate papilla, filiform papillae, fungiform papillae, foliate papilla, and median sulcus on the dorsal or top surface of the tongue. On the ventral or underside of the tongue are the lingual frenum, the lingual veins, and the fimbriated folds. When the tongue is extended, a shallow, V-shaped groove is apparent on the posterior portion. This is the sulcus terminalis. This groove separates the anterior two-thirds, or body of the tongue, from the base of the tongue. Anterior to the sulcus, covering the dorsal side of the tongue (Figure 7-5A), are small, raised projections called **papilla**, where taste buds are located. The largest papilla, which are mushroom shaped, are anterior to the sulcus terminalis in a row of 8 to 10 and are called *circumvallate papillae*. Anterior to the circumvallate papillae and covering the dorsal side of the tongue are hair-like projections called *filiform papillae*. Papillae that give the tongue the "strawberry effect" are the *fungiform papillae*. On the lateral border of the tongue near the base are the *foliate papillae*, which are slightly raised, vertical folds of tissue. The tongue is divided in half by the *median sulcus*, which runs from the base to the tip of the tongue. The median sulcus is a groove that varies in depth from person to person.

In the middle of the ventral side of the tongue, a line of tissue extends from the tongue to the floor of the mouth, called the *lingual frenum* (Figure 7-5B). On either side of the lingual frenum are the *lingual veins*. They are bluish and run the length of the tongue. Lateral to the lingual veins are folds of tissue called *fimbriated folds*. Sometimes, under the tongue on the alveolar bone are excess bone formations called *torus mandibularis*.

Sensation of Taste. The **taste buds**, also known as taste receptors, are oval structures that are located on the dorsal surface of the tongue. When stimulated with different chemicals these receptors carry taste impulses to the brain. To stimulate the sense of taste, substances (food) must be mixed with liquid to form a solution. The solution stimulates these receptors to generate one or a combination of the four fundamental taste sensations. The four fundamental taste senses include: sweet, salty, sour, and bitter. These basic taste buds are located on different but overlapping areas of the tongue (Figure 7-6). Sweet tastes are located on the tip of the tongue, salty tastes are on the anterior sides of the tongue, sour tastes are on the posterior sides of the tongue, and the bitter tastes are located in the center posterior section of the tongue.

Importance to the Dental Assistant

The dental assistant should be aware that certain drugs cause patients to lose their sense of taste. Taste bud cells are continually being renewed because they have an average life span of only 10 to 10½ days. If a patient is receiving certain toxic agents, such as a cytotoxic agent used to treat cancer, the taste buds may be destroyed and the patient's sense of taste will take a minimum of 10 days, usually longer, to return.

Floor of the Mouth

The **floor of the mouth** includes the sublingual caruncles, sublingual folds, and sublingual sulcus (Figure 7-5B). There are two small, raised folds of tissue where the lingual frenum attaches to the floor of the mouth, one on either side of the frenum. These are the *sublingual caruncles*. On top of these folds of tissue lie the ducts of two salivary glands. The *sublingual folds* begin at the caruncles on either side of the frenum and run backward to the base of the tongue. Lateral to the sublingual fold is a horseshoe-shaped groove that follows the curve of the dental arch, called the *sublingual sulcus*. This sulcus marks the end of the alveolar ridge and the beginning of the floor of the mouth.

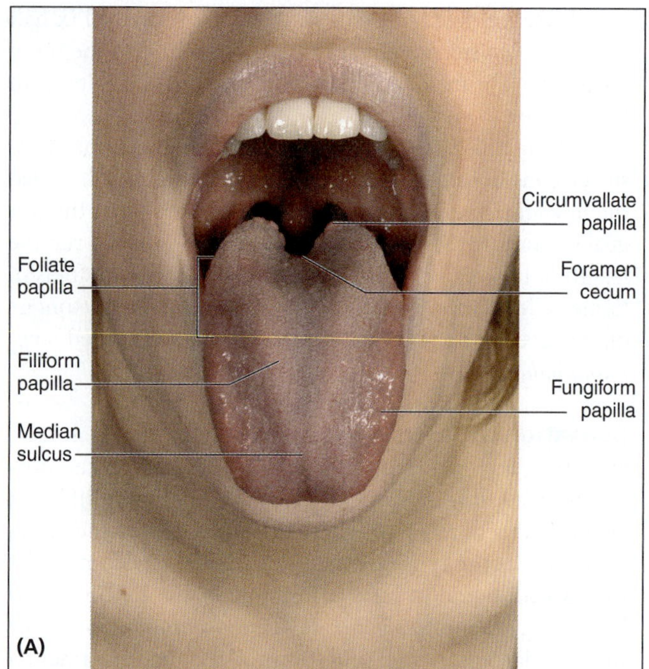

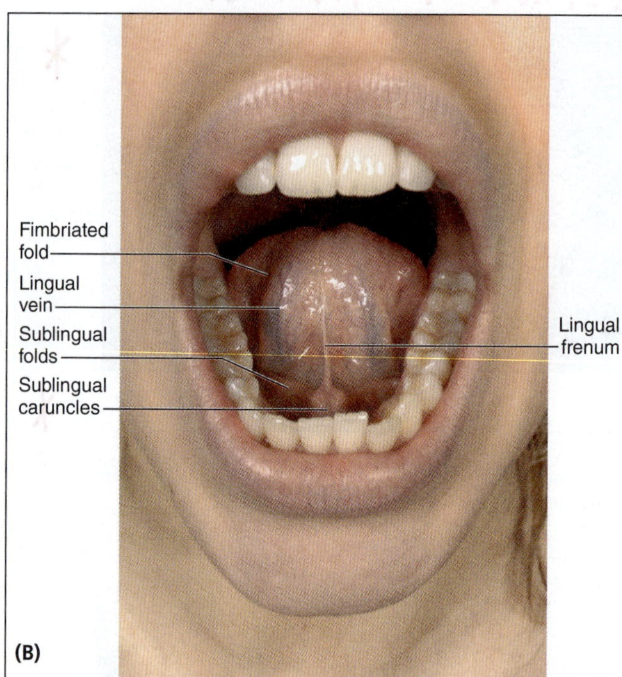

FIGURE 7-5

(A) Dorsal surface of the tongue. (B) Ventral surface of the tongue.

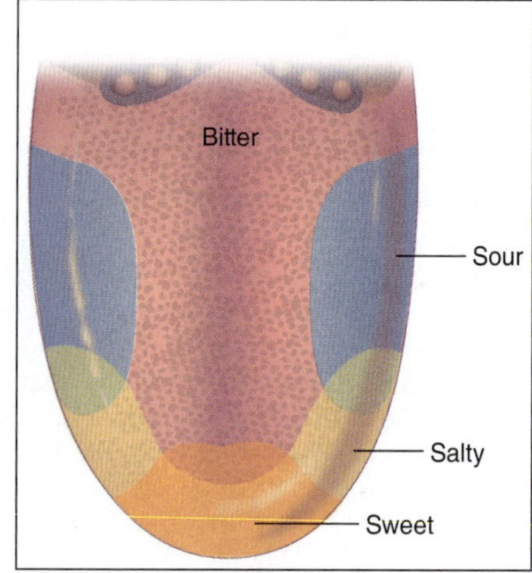

FIGURE 7-6

The location of the basic taste buds of the tongue.

Salivary Glands

Three major pairs of **salivary glands** supply the oral cavity with saliva: the parotid, submandibular, and sublingual (Figures 7-7 and 7-8). These glands secrete saliva to assist in the process of digestion. The largest of the salivary glands are the *parotid glands*, which lie just below and in front of the ear. The parotid glands empty into the mouth through the *parotid duct* (also known as Stensen's duct). The duct empties into the mouth through the parotid papilla, which is just opposite the maxillary second molar. The *submandibular glands* are about the size of a walnut and lie on the inside of the mandible in the posterior area. They empty saliva into the mouth through the *Wharton's duct*, which ends in the sublingual caruncles. The third set of glands and smallest are the *sublingual glands*, located on the floor of the mouth. These glands either empty directly into the mouth through the *ducts of Rivinus* or through the sublingual caruncles by means of the *ducts of Bartholin*. The ducts of the sublingual glands are similar in function to a "soaker hose."

There are also smaller minor salivary glands that are in the buccal, labial, and lingual mucosa; the floor of the mouth; the posterior portion of the dorsal surface of the tongue; the soft palate; and the lateral (side) portions of the hard palate. The saliva from these glands is mucous saliva.

Saliva. **Saliva** is a clear fluid secreted by the salivary and mucous glands throughout the mouth. This fluid varies in viscosity depending on an individual's chemical makeup, diet, and medications. Saliva contains water, mucin, organic salts, and the digestive enzyme ptyalin. It is normally odorless, tasteless, and slightly alkaline. Approximately 1,500 mL of saliva is produced daily.

The function of the saliva is to moisten and lubricate the oral cavity and to moisten food, aiding in the **mastication** (chewing) and swallowing of food. Saliva also initiates the digestion of starches and helps regulate water balance. Excess dryness of the mouth is called xerostomia (refer to Chapter 4). Dry mouth is caused by an abnormal reduction in the amount of saliva secretion. It can be related to certain diseases, such as diabetes, or result from radiation or chemotherapy. There are a number of products on the market to assist the patient with dry mouth symptoms.

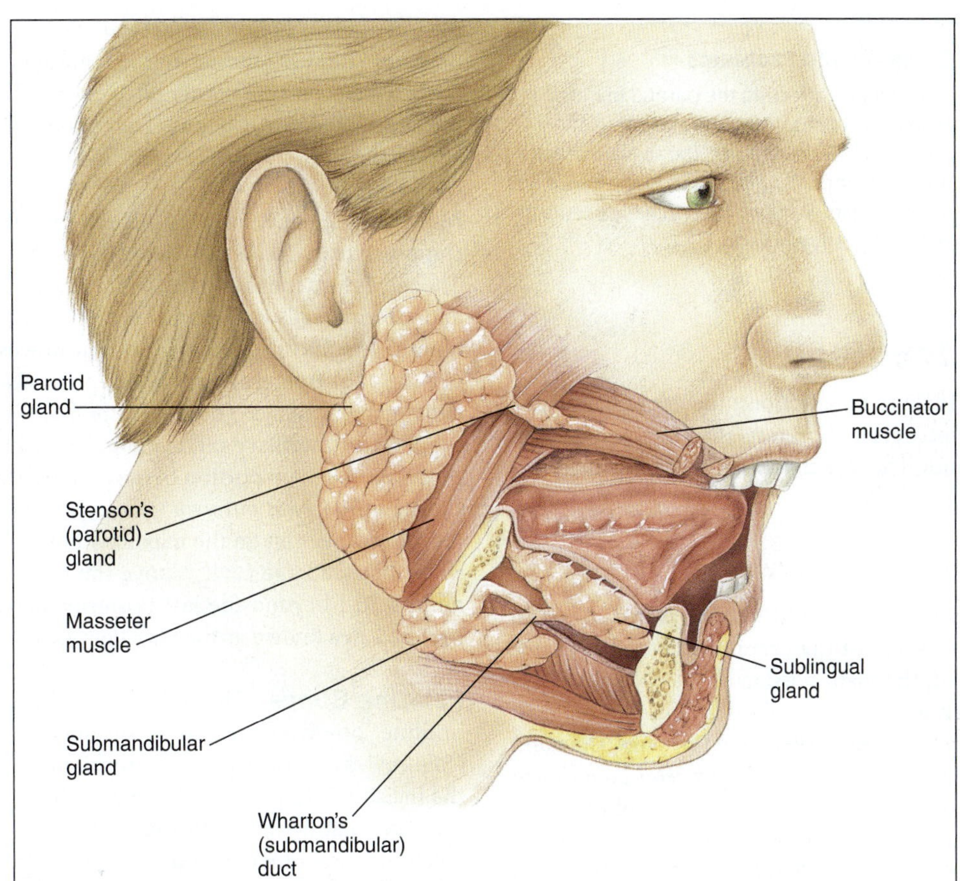

FIGURE 7-7

Salivary glands and ducts.

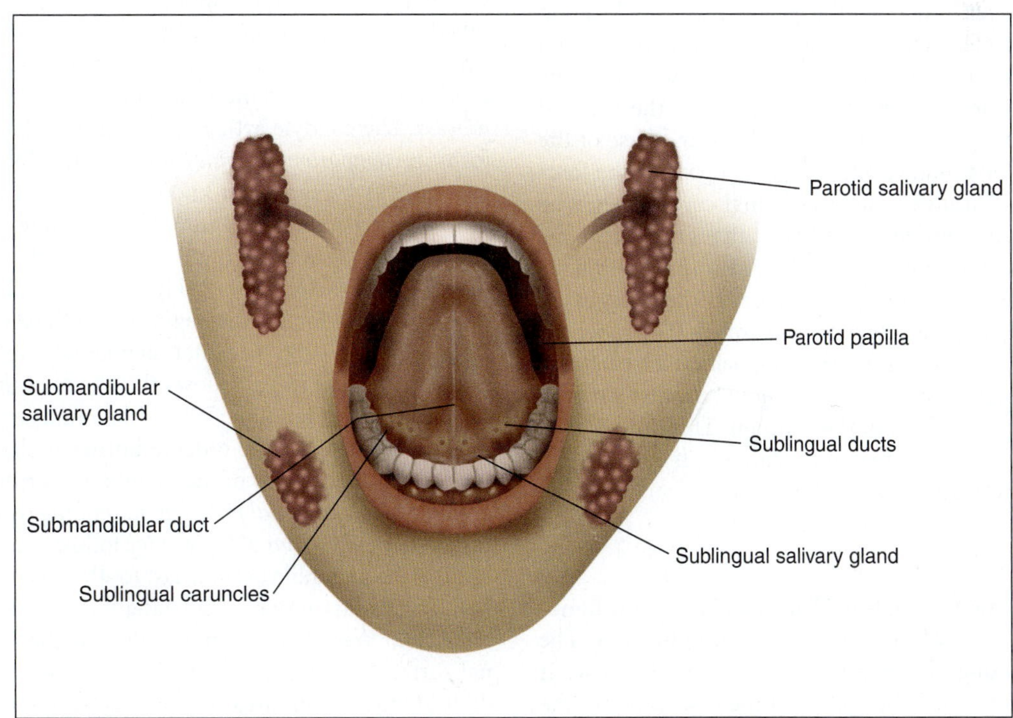

FIGURE 7-8

A frontal view of the major salivary glands and ducts.

Salivary Gland Diseases and Problems

The mumps are a viral infection affecting the parotid glands. Characterized by swelling and tenderness, mumps often affect children between ages 5 and 15. Sometimes, the salivary glands develop crystallizations or stones. When these stones try to leave the glands, they block the ducts. Swelling immediately occurs and the stones must be surgically removed.

Bones of the Head

The skull is divided into two sections: the cranium and the face. The cranium covers and protects the brain and is composed of eight bones. The face consists of 14 bones, including the maxilla and the mandible.

Bones of the Cranium

As a dental assistant you should be able to identify and describe the eight **bones of the cranium**. The *frontal bone* forms the forehead, the main portion of the roof of the eye socket (orbit), and part of the nasal cavity. On the skull just behind the frontal bone are the two parietal bones, right and left halves joining at the midline. The *parietal bones* form most of the roof of the skull and the upper half of the sides. Below each parietal bone, forming the lower sides and the base of the skull, are the *temporal bones*. Each temporal bone contains the following landmarks: external auditory meatus, mastoid process, glenoid fossa, and styloid process. The *external auditory meatus* is the opening for the ear. The *mastoid process* is the bony projection found on the bottom border of the temporal bone. A pit or depression found anterior to the mastoid process is the *glenoid fossa*, the location where the mandible articulates with the skull. The *styloid process* is a sharp projection on the under-surface of the temporal bone between the glenoid fossa and the mastoid process. The *occipital bone* forms the back and base of the skull. The occipital bone contains a large opening, the foramen magnum, through which the spinal cord passes. The *sphenoid bone* is a wedge-shaped bone that goes across the skull anterior to the temporal bones. It is a single continuous bone, shaped like a bat with its wings spread. The wings of the sphenoid bone are called the *pterygoid process*. The sphenoid bone forms the anterior base of the skull behind the orbit and contains the *sphenoid sinuses*. The *ethmoid bone* forms part of the nose, orbits, and floor of the cranium. This bone is thin and spongy or honeycombed in appearance. It contains the *ethmoid sinuses* (Figure 7-9 and Table 7-1).

Bones of the Face

It is also important to be able to identify and locate the **bones of the face.** The *nasal bones* form the bridge of the nose. The *vomer bone* is a single bone on the inside of the nasal cavity. It forms the posterior and the bottom of the nasal septum (the nasal septum is a cartilage structure that divides the nasal cavities). On the outside of the nasal cavities are scroll-like bones called *inferior nasal conchae*. Each concha consists of thin, cancellous bone. The *lacrimal bones* are small and very delicate. They are anterior to the ethmoid bone, comprising part of the orbit (the corner of the eye). The tear ducts pass through the lacrimal bones. The *zygomatic bones* form the cheeks (Figures 7-9 and 7-10 and Table 7-2).

Maxilla. The **maxilla** is the largest of the facial bones and is composed of two sections of bone joined at the *median suture*. The maxilla extends from the floor of each orbit and the floor and exterior walls of the nasal cavity to form the roof of the mouth. The maxilla is formed by four processes (outgrowths of bone). The frontal and zygomatic processes meet the frontal and zygomatic bones. The *alveolar process* forms the bone that supports the maxillary and mandibular teeth, and the palatine process is the main portion of the hard palate.

The *infraorbital foramen* (*foramen* means an opening) is just below the orbit on the maxillary bone, and the *maxillary sinus* forms a large cavity above the roots of the maxillary molars. Just beyond the last posterior maxillary tooth is a rounded area known as the *maxillary tuberosity*.

Palatine Bones. The **palatine bones** are joined at the midline, often referred to as the median *palatine suture* (Figure 7-11). Just behind the maxillary central incisors is the incisive (nasopalatine) foramen, which is an opening for the nasopalatine nerve. In the posterior region of the hard palate are three other openings on each side. The first of these three, the largest, is the *greater palatine foramen*. Behind the greater foramen are two smaller or *lesser palatine foramen*.

Mandible. The **mandible** is the only movable bone of the face (Figure 7-12A). The mandible consists of a horseshoe-shaped body that is horizontal, with two vertical extensions called *rami* (plural form of *ramus*). At the top of the rami are two projections. The posterior projection is the *condyle* or *condyloid process*, and the anterior projection is the *coronoid process*. The condyle articulates with the temporal bone to form the *temporomandibular joint (TMJ)*. Between the two processes is a depression known as the *mandibular notch* (also referred to as the sigmoid or coronoid notch). From the top of the rami moving downward is the body of each ramus. On the inside of the body of the ramus is the *mandibular foramen*, which is the beginning of the *internal oblique ridge* (Figure 7-12B). The internal oblique ridge, also known as the *mylohyoid ridge*, follows the inside of the ramus and the body of the mandible. Where the ramus meets the body of the mandible on the outside border is the *angle of the mandible*. On the body of the mandible near the apex of the premolars is the *mental foramen*. Extending from the mental foramen, the *external oblique ridge* follows the length of the body of the mandible past the last tooth and up to the ramus. Behind the last molar is a triangular area known as the *retromolar area*. In the center of the mandible on the external surface is a concave area where two bones of the mandible are fused. This area is known as the *symphysis*. The tip of the chin is called the *mental protuberance* Figure 7-12C. On the internal surface at the center of the mandible is the *lingual foramen*, which is surrounded by small, bony

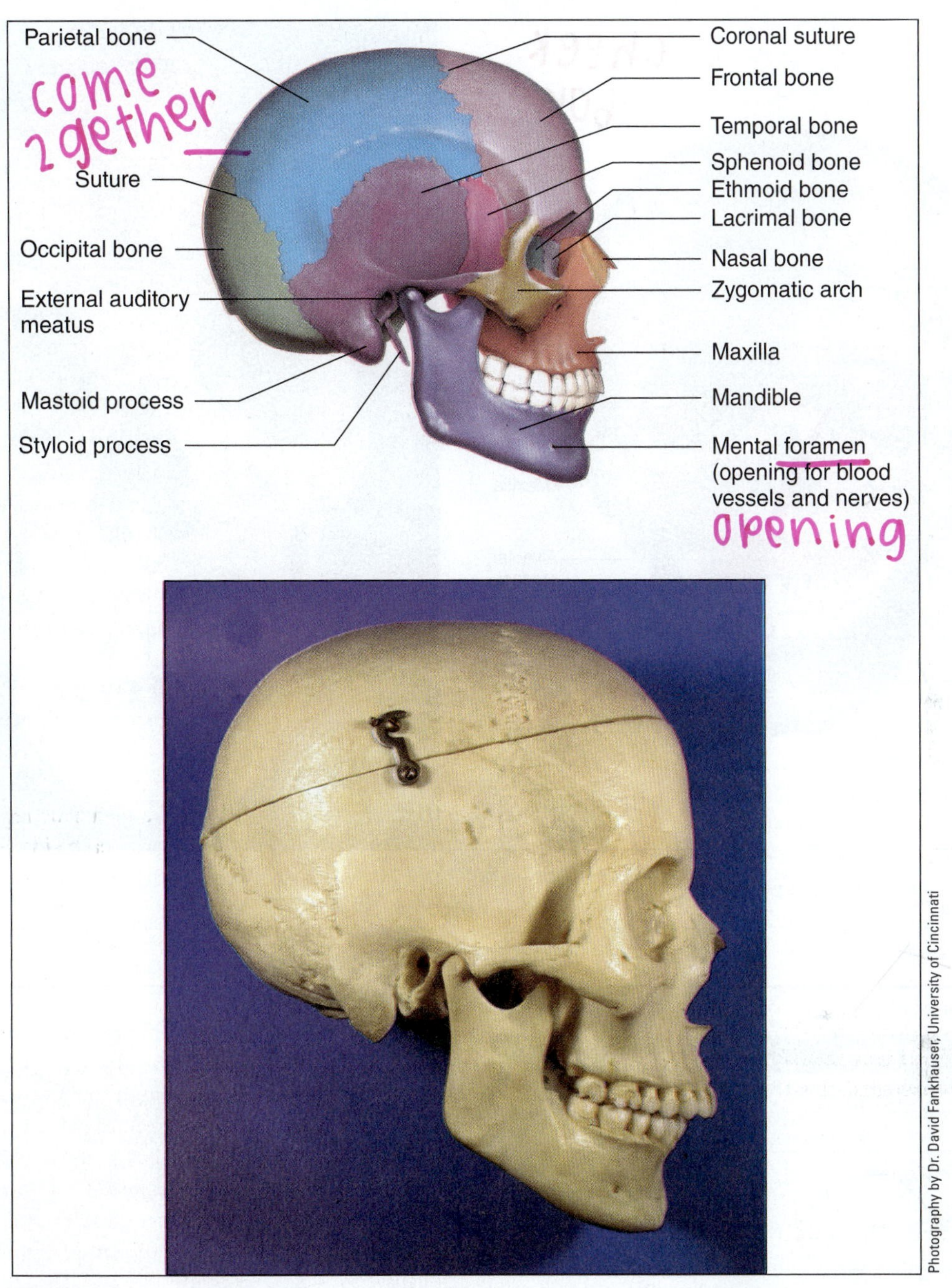

FIGURE 7-9

Lateral aspect of the cranium.

projections called *genial tubercles*. The mandibular teeth are supported in the alveolar process.

Importance of the Bones of Head and Face

Dental assistants should learn the bones of the head and the face thoroughly. This knowledge will not only assist them throughout their program but also in their career working in the dental profession. Two examples as to when they might use this information include understanding the landmarks seen on dental radiographs and identifying anatomy while assisting during surgical procedures.

TABLE 7-1 Bones of the Cranium

Name of Cranial Bone	Number
Frontal	One (1)
Parietal	Paired (2)
Temporal	Paired (2)
Occipital	One (1)
Sphenoid	One (1)
Ethmoid	One (1)

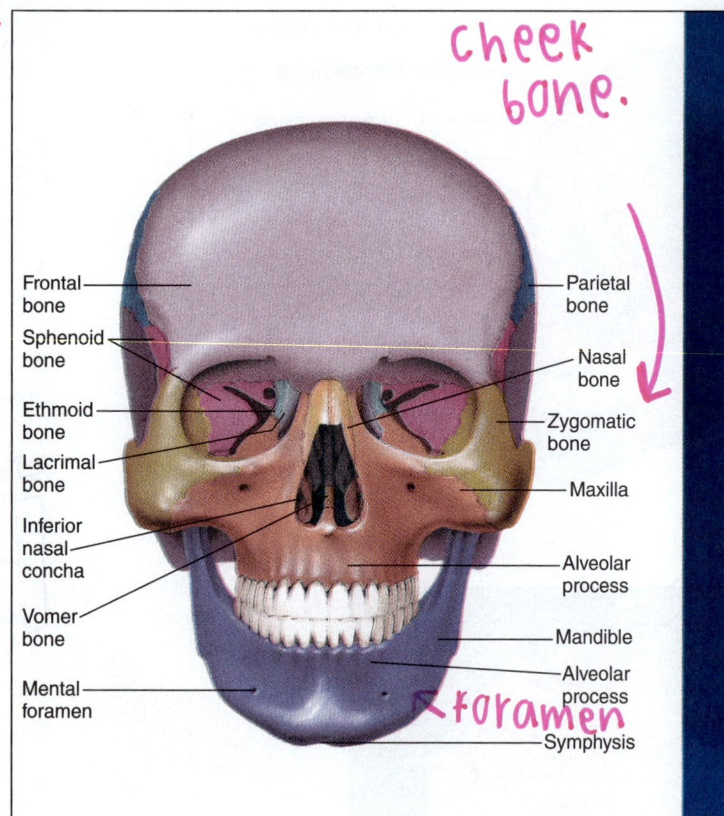

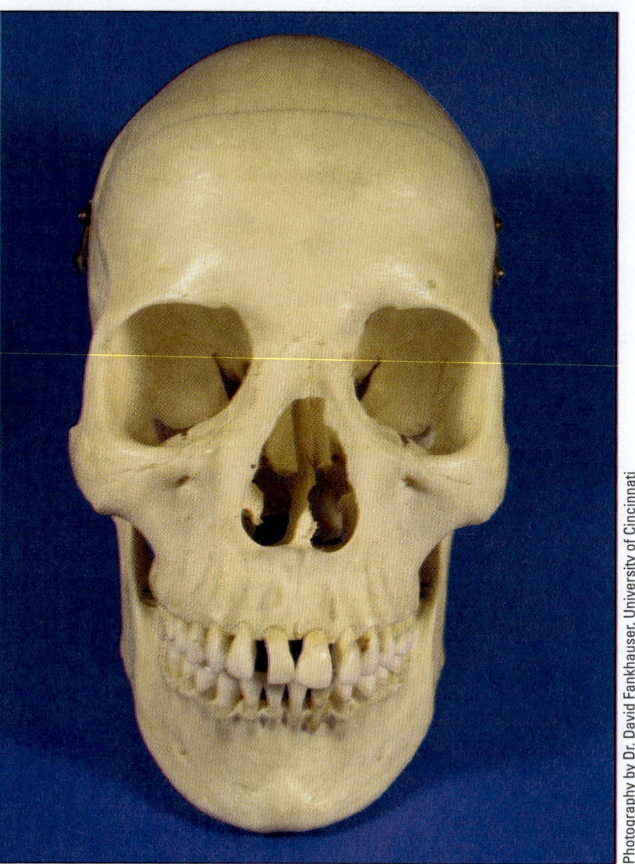

FIGURE 7-10

Bones of the face.

TABLE 7-2 Bones of the Face

Name of Facial Bone	Number
Nasal	Two (2)
Vomer	One (1)
Inferior nasal conchae	Two (2)
Lacrimal	Two (2)
Maxillae	Two (2)
Zygomatic	Two (2)
Palatine	Two (2)
Mandible	One (1)

Temporomandibular Joint

Once the bones of the cranium and the face have been identified, it is easy to locate the **temporomandibular joint (TMJ).** The joint is named for the two bones that form the union: the temporal and the mandible bones. The TMJ is composed of three parts:

1. Glenoid fossa of the temporal bone
2. Articular eminence of the temporal bone
3. Condyloid process of the mandible

These bones are covered with thick cartilage and are surrounded by several ligaments. There are no blood vessels or nerves in this connective tissue, but *synovial fluid* bathes these bone structures, providing nourishment and lubrication that enable the bones to glide over each other without friction. (*Synovial* means a thick, sticky fluid found in the joints of bones.)

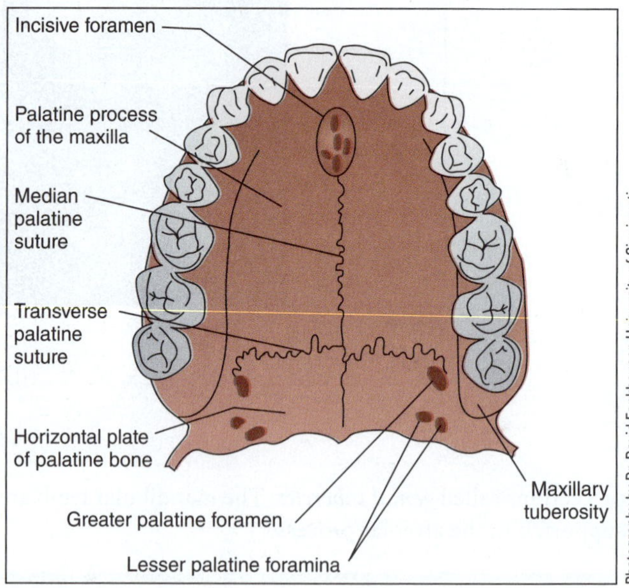

FIGURE 7-11

Landmarks of the palate.

The TMJ is formed by the condyle of the mandible articulating with the glenoid fossa and the articular eminence of

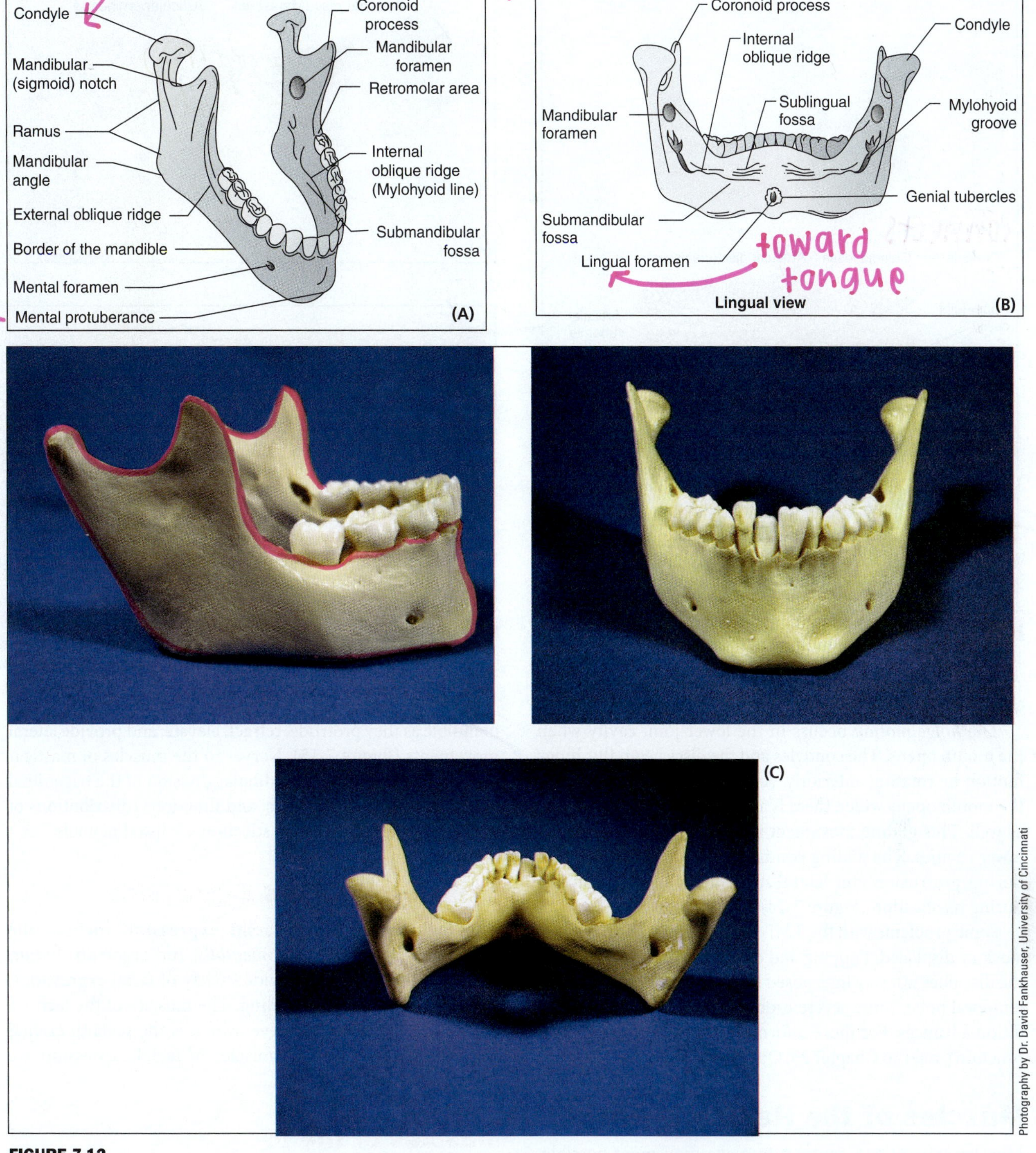

FIGURE 7-12

(A) Lateral view of the external surface of the mandible. (B) Internal (lingual) view of the mandible. (C) Frontal view of the external surface of the mandible.

the temporal bone (Figure 7-13). The condyle rests closer to the glenoid fossa, and then moves forward to the articular eminence when the mouth opens.

Between the condyle and temporal bone is the **articular disc** (meniscus). This disc is a dense, fibrous connective tissue that is thicker at the ends. The articular disc is attached to the condyle, so when the condyle glides forward and backward, the disc moves with it.

Surrounding the articular disc is a dense, fibrous *capsule* that encloses the entire joint. The capsule is divided into upper and lower cavities by the disc; these cavities are filled with synovial fluid.

The TMJ is supported by ligaments, and the muscles of mastication control the movements. The left and right TMJs function in unison and move in two ways: hinge (swinging) motion and gliding movement.

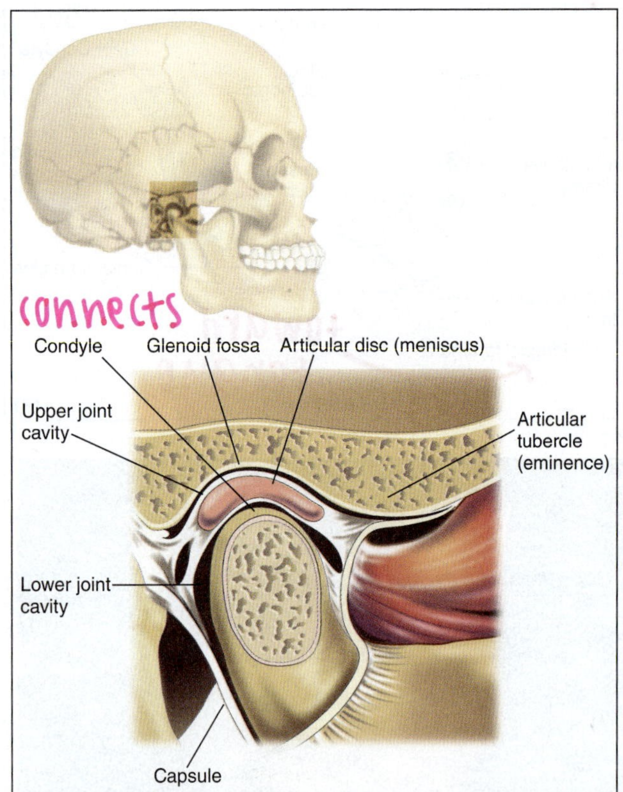

FIGURE 7-13
Temporomandibular joint (TMJ).

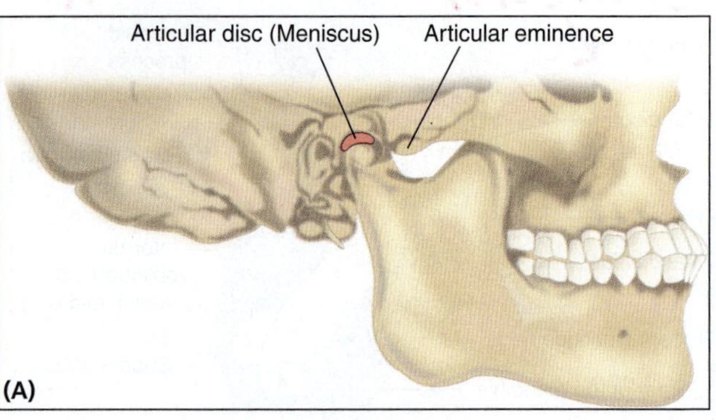

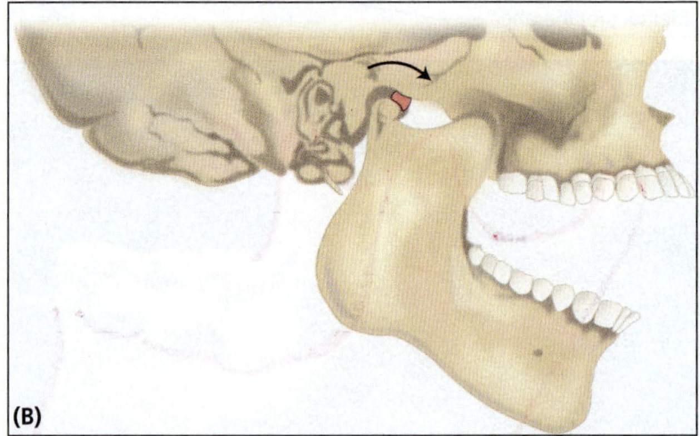

FIGURE 7-14
Movement of the TMJ. (A) Hinge joint. (B) Gliding joint movement.

The *hinge motion* occurs in the lower joint cavity when the mouth opens. The condyles and the discs begin this hinge motion by rotating anteriorly. As this motion continues and the mouth opens wider, there is an anterior *gliding movement* as well. This gliding movement involves both the upper and lower cavities. The gliding continues along the articular disc during protrusion and lateral movements of the mandible during mastication (Figure 7-14).

Some problems with the TMJ occur when the disc becomes stuck or displaced. Popping and clicking sounds may result if the disc does not stay interposed between the condyle and the temporal bone. More severe problems may occur as the condition advances. For more information on TMJ disease (dysfunction), refer to Chapter 25, Oral and Maxillofacial Surgery.

Muscles of the Head and Neck

Muscles expand and contract to make movement possible. Each muscle has an origin (fixed point) and insertion (movable point). Muscles of the head and neck include muscles of mastication, muscles of facial expression, muscles of the floor of the mouth, muscles of the tongue, muscles of the soft palate, the pharynx, and muscles of the neck.

Muscles of Mastication

There are four pairs of **muscles of mastication**: *temporal muscles, masseter muscles, internal pterygoid muscles,* and *external pterygoid muscles.* These muscles provide movement for the mandible as they protrude, retract, elevate, and provide lateral movements (Figure 7-15). Nerves to the muscles of mastication originate from the mandibular division of the trigeminal labor. The origins, insertions, and functions (distributions of nerves) of the muscles of mastication are listed in Table 7-3.

Muscles of Facial Expression

The major **muscles of facial expression** include the *orbicularis oris, buccinator, mentalis,* and *zygomatic major.* These muscles allow for a wide variety of facial expressions, including smiling and whistling. The muscles of the face are innervated by the facial nerve, which is the seventh cranial nerve (Figure 7-16). The muscles of facial expression are described in Table 7-4.

Muscles of the Tongue

The **muscles of the tongue** are divided into intrinsic and extrinsic groups. The *intrinsic muscles* are all within the tongue and are responsible for shaping the tongue during speech, mastication, and swallowing. There are four *extrinsic muscles* to assist in the movement and functioning of the tongue: *genioglossus, hyoglossus, styloglossus,* and *palatoglossus* (Figure 7-17). (The palatoglossus is discussed with the palate.) All the muscles of the tongue are innervated by the hypoglossal nerve except the palatoglossus muscle. See Table 7-5 for the origin, insertion, and function of each extrinsic muscle of the tongue.

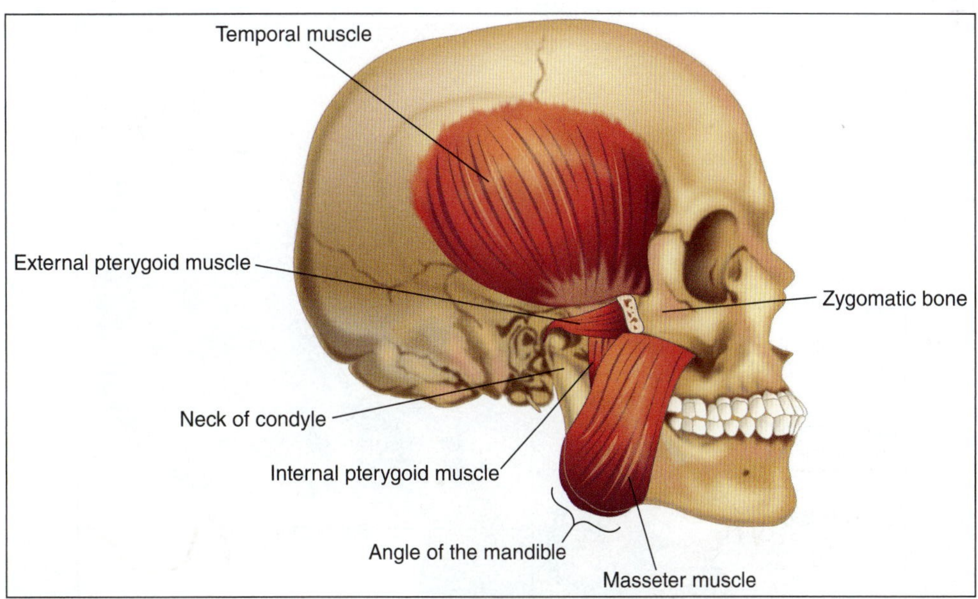

FIGURE 7-15

Muscles of mastication. Lateral view of the internal pterygoid muscle, the external pterygoid muscle, the temporal muscle, and the masseter muscle.

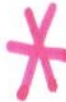

TABLE 7-3 Muscles of Mastication

Muscle	Origin	Insertion	Function
Temporal	Fan shaped across the temporal fossa of the temporal bone.	Inserts into the coronoid process of the mandible and down the anterior border of the ramus.	Elevates the mandible—closing the jaw. Contraction of the posterior fibers retracts the mandible.
Masseter	Two portions: superficial portion (strong, tendinous fibers from the zygomatic process of the maxilla and from the anterior two-thirds of the lower border of the zygomatic arch), and deep portion (muscular and smaller from the medial aspect and inferior border of the posterior one-third of the zygomatic arch).	The superficial portion inserts into the angle and lower border of the mandible; the deep portion is inserted into the upper section of the ramus and the lateral surface of the coronoid process.	Strong elevator of the jaw. This muscle is easily seen when the teeth are clenched.
Medial (internal) pterygoids	Medial surface of the lateral pterygoid plate of the sphenoid bone, the lateral portion of the palatine bone, and the maxillary tuberosity.	The medial pterygoids insert into the interior surface of the angle of the mandible (opposite the insertion of the masseter muscle).	Elevates the mandible.
Lateral (external) pterygoids	Superior portion from the lateral surface of the greater wing of the sphenoid bone; inferior portion from the lateral surface of the lateral pterygoid plate.	Superior portion inserts into the articular capsule of the temporomandibular joint; inferior portion inserts into the neck of the condyle of the mandible.	Opens jaw by depressing the mandible. If both lateral pterygoid muscles contract, the jaw protrudes; if only one contracts, the mandible shifts laterally.

Hyoid Bone. There is also a horseshoe-shaped bone lying at the base of the tongue called the **hyoid bone**. Muscles of the tongue and the floor of the mouth attach to this bone for support (Figure 7-18).

Muscles of the Floor of the Mouth

The **muscles of the floor of the mouth** are the *digastric*, *mylohyoid*, *stylohyoid*, and *geniohyoid*. These four muscles are located between the mandible and the hyoid bone. Unlike

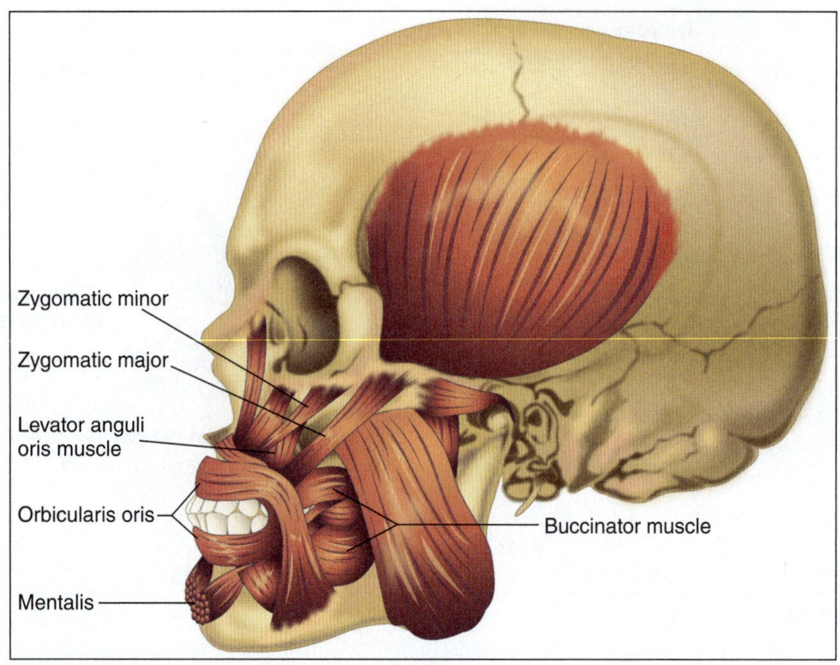

FIGURE 7-16
Muscles of facial expression.

TABLE 7-4 Muscles of Facial Expression

Muscle	Origin	Insertion	Function
Orbicularis oris	Complex origin—There is no skeletal attachment. The origin is from muscle fibers that surround the mouth.	Insertion is into itself and the surrounding skin.	Closing the lips or protruding them.
Buccinator	Alveolar processes of the maxilla and the mandible and the pterygomandibular raphe.	Inserts into the corners of the mouth, becoming part of the muscles that surround the mouth.	Compresses the cheeks against the teeth to assist during mastication. Assists in blowing air out of the mouth.
Mentalis	Incisive fossa of the mandible.	Inserts into the skin of the chin.	Wrinkles the skin of the chin and protrudes the lower lip.
Zygomatic major	Zygomatic bone.	Insertion into the corners of the mouth.	Lifts the corners of the mouth upward and backward, as in smiling.

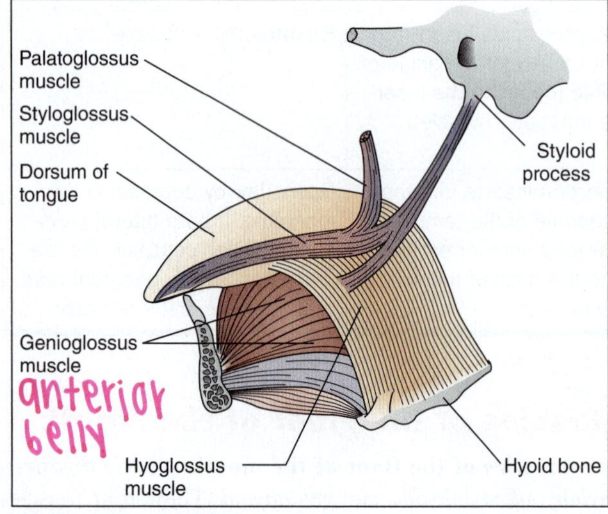

FIGURE 7-17
Extrinsic muscles of the tongue.

some other muscle groups, the muscles of the floor of the mouth are innervated by distinct nerve branches (Figure 7-18 and Table 7-6).

Muscles of the Soft Palate

There are two **muscles of the soft palate**, called the *palatoglossus muscle* and *palatopharyngeal muscle* (Table 7-7). These muscles raise the soft palate during the swallowing process (deglutition) and are both innervated by the pharyngeal plexus (Figure 7-19).

Muscles of the Neck

The three **muscles of the neck** are the *platysma*, *trapezius*, and *sternocleidomastoid* (Figure 7-20). Knowing the muscles of the neck helps the dental assistant to perform chairside functions in positions that are not tiring and will not cause injury (Table 7-8).

TABLE 7-5 Extrinsic Muscles of the Tongue

Muscle	Origin	Insertion	Function
Genioglossus	Genial tubercle in the center of the lingual of the mandible.	Fans out to insert in the inferior surface of the tongue and to the hyoid bone.	Most of the work of the tongue. Protrudes the tongue and retracts or depresses the tongue.
Hyoglossus	Hyoid bone.	Runs vertically to insert in the inferior sides of the tongue.	Mainly depresses the tongue.
Styloglossus	Anterior surface of the styloid process of the temporal bone.	Part of the styloglossus inserts into the sides of the tongue while the rest of the muscle continues forward to the tip of the tongue.	Retracts the tongue and raises the tip of the tongue.

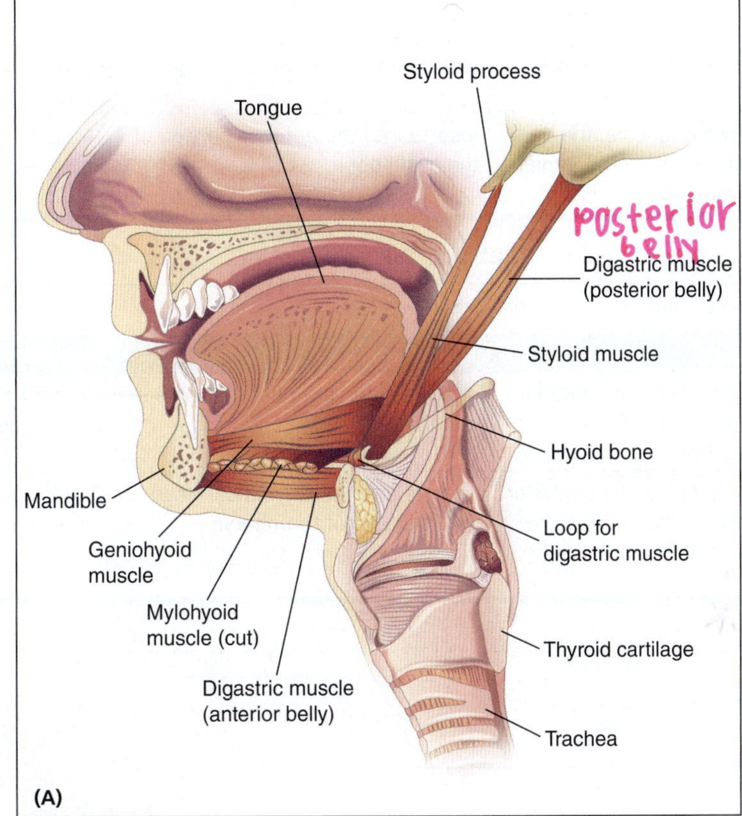

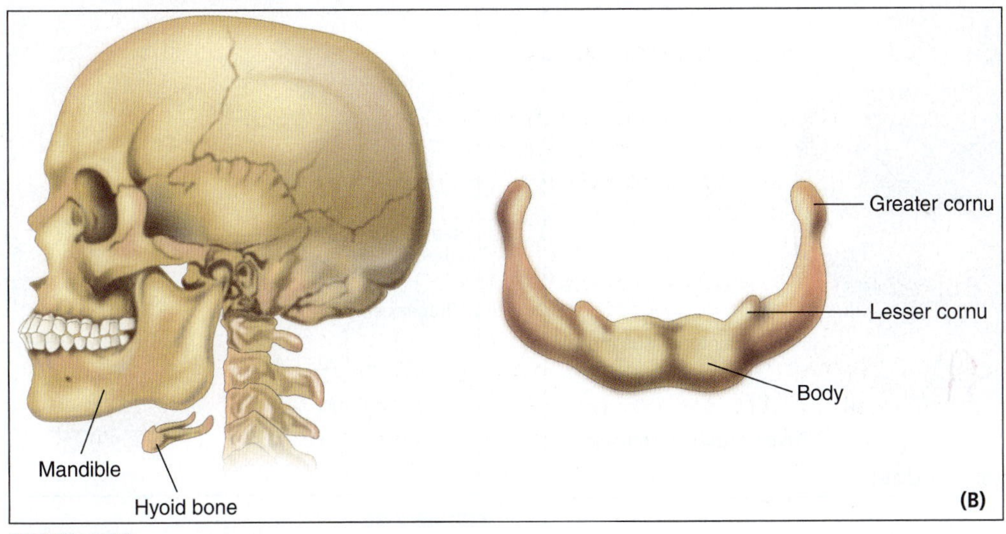

FIGURE 7-18

(A) Muscles of the floor of the mouth. (B) The hyoid bone.

TABLE 7-6 Muscles of the Floor of the Mouth

Muscle	Origin	Insertion	Function
Digastric	There are two portions, called bellies. The posterior belly originates from the mastoid process of the temporal bone; the anterior belly begins on the lingual surface of the mandible at the midline.	Both the posterior belly and the anterior belly insert into the intermediate tendon on the hyoid bone.	Together, the digastric muscles lift the hyoid bone and assist in opening the mouth; separately, the posterior belly draws the hyoid bone posteriorly and the anterior belly pulls the hyoid bone anteriorly.
Mylohyoid	This muscle is composed of left and right halves that join at the midline of the mandible. From the midline, each half attaches in a fan shape to the last molar area, thus following the mylohyoid line.	Inserts into the body of the hyoid bone.	Forms the floor of the mouth and assists in depressing the mandible and elevating the tongue.
Stylohyoid	The styloid process of the temporal bone.	Inserts into the body of the hyoid bone.	Draws the hyoid bone superiorly and posteriorly and stabilizes it.
Geniohyoid	Above the mylohyoid muscle, the geniohyoid originates from the genial tubercle of the mandible.	Inserts into the anterior portion of the hyoid bone.	Pulls the hyoid bone and the tongue anteriorly.

TABLE 7-7 Muscles of the Soft Palate

Muscle	Origin	Insertion	Function
Palatoglossus	This muscle forms the anterior arch on each side of the throat and arises from the soft palate.	Inserts along the posterior side of the tongue.	Elevates the posterior portion of the tongue and narrows the fauces.
Palatopharyngeal	This muscle forms the posterior arch on each side of the throat and also arises from the soft palate.	Inserts into the thyroid cartilage and the wall of the pharynx.	Constricts the nasopharyngeal passage and elevates the larynx.

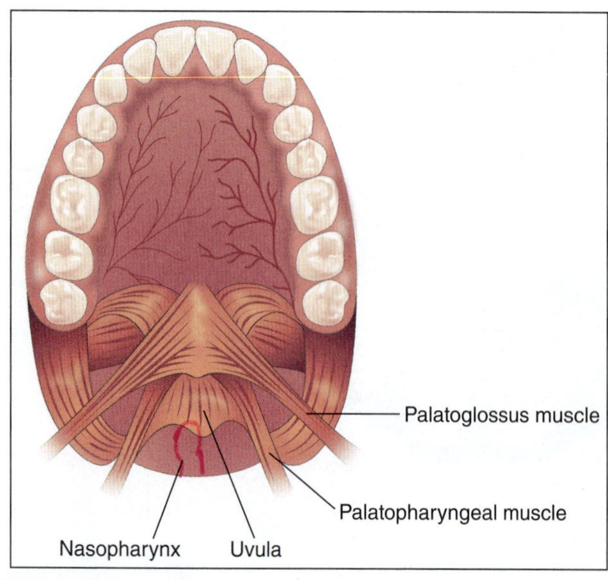

FIGURE 7-19
Muscles of the soft palate.

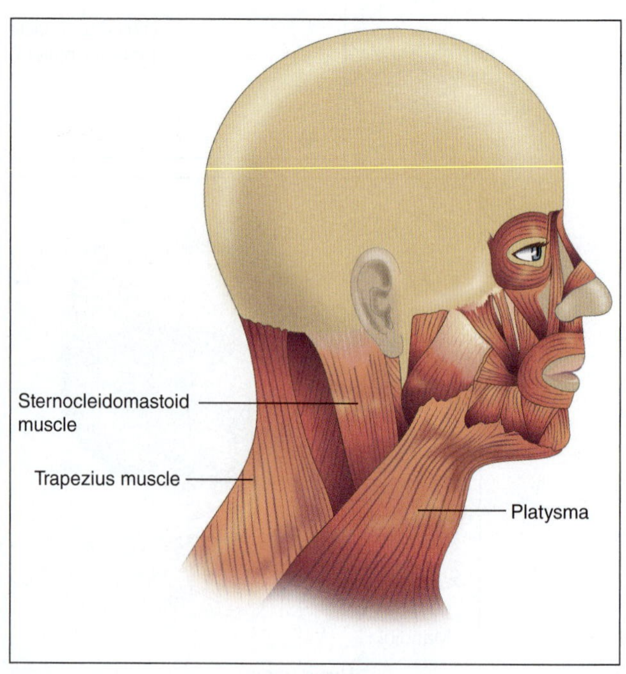

FIGURE 7-20
Muscles of the neck.

TABLE 7-8 Muscles of the Neck

Muscle	Origin	Insertion	Function
Platysma	Clavicle and the shoulder.	Inserts into the inferior border of the mandible.	This sheet of muscle draws down the mandible as well as the corners of the mouth and the lower lip.
Trapezius	Protuberance on the occipital bone.	Inserts into the clavicle and shoulders.	This large muscle moves the head backward and laterally.
Sternocleidomastoid	The top of the sternum and the clavicle.	Inserts into the mastoid process and the anterior of the occipital bone.	One on each side of the neck assists in elevating the chin.

Nerves of the Head and Neck

Four cranial nerves innervate the face and oral cavity: **trigeminal nerve**, **facial nerve**, **glossopharyngeal nerve**, and **hypoglossal nerve**. The largest cranial nerve and the most important to dental auxiliaries is the trigeminal nerve, because this cranial nerve innervates the maxilla and the mandible. The trigeminal nerve divides at the semi-lunar (gasserian) ganglion into three branches: the ophthalmic nerve, maxillary nerve, and mandibular nerve (Figure 7-21). (Refer to Chapter 20, Anesthetic and Sedation, for correlation to injection sites.)

Maxillary Branch of the Trigeminal Nerve

The *maxillary nerve branch* is a sensory nerve that innervates the nose, cheeks, palate, gingiva, maxillary teeth, maxillary sinus, tonsils, nasopharynx, and other facial structures. The maxillary nerve branch is divided into four branches: zygomatic, infraorbital, posterior superior alveolar, and pterygopalatine (Figure 7-22A).

Pterygopalatine Nerve Branch. After the maxillary nerve leaves the semilunar ganglion, one branch becomes the *pterygopalatine nerve branch*. This branch divides into the *greater palatine nerve*, the *lesser palatine nerve*, and the *nasopalatine nerve* (Figure 7-22B). The greater palatine nerve extends downward from the pterygopalatine nerve and reaches the palate through the greater palatine foramen. This nerve serves the soft palate, hard palate, medial gingiva, and mucous membrane as far forward as the anterior teeth. The lesser palatine nerve is a smaller branch that innervates the soft palate, uvula, and tonsils. The nasopalatine nerve extends anteriorly from the pterygopalatine nerve and exits through the incisive foramen. This nerve innervates the anterior hard

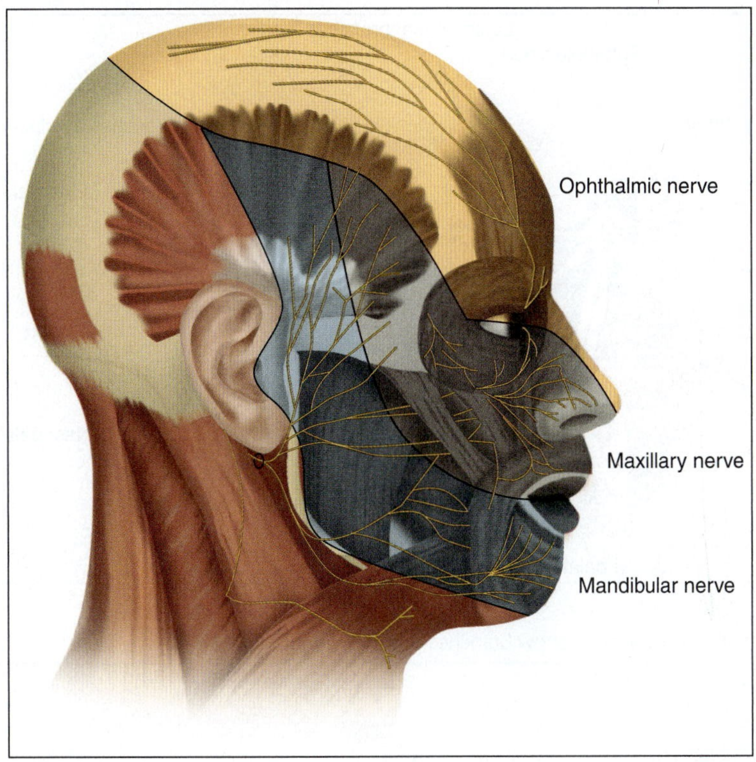

FIGURE 7-21
Area of distribution of the three divisions of the trigeminal nerve.

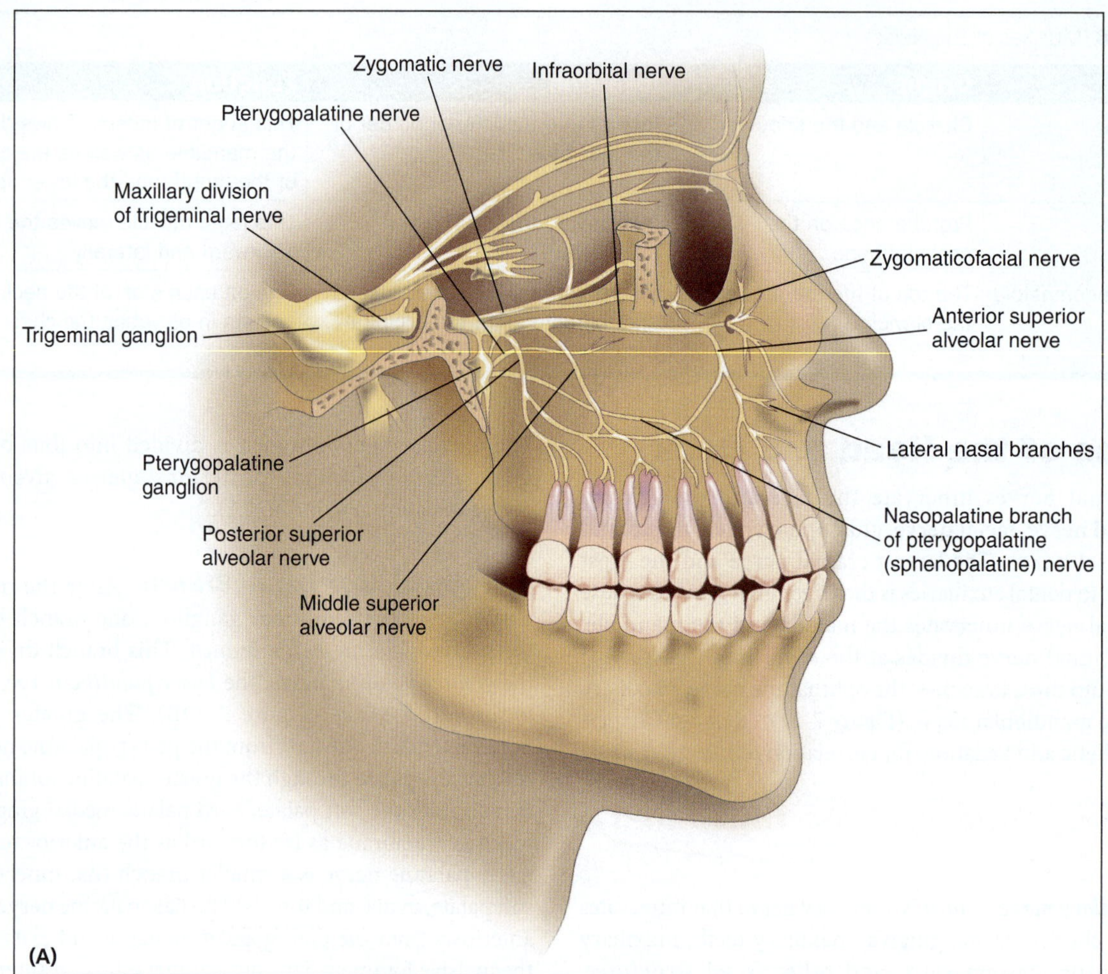

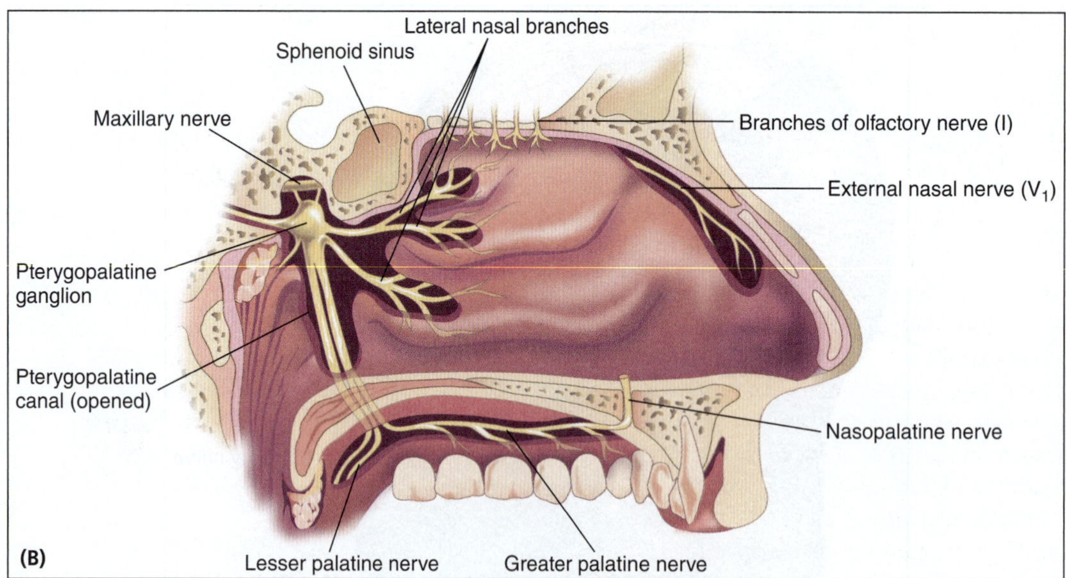

FIGURE 7-22

(A) Nerves of the maxillary arch. (B) Medial view to show branches of the pterygopalatine nerve.

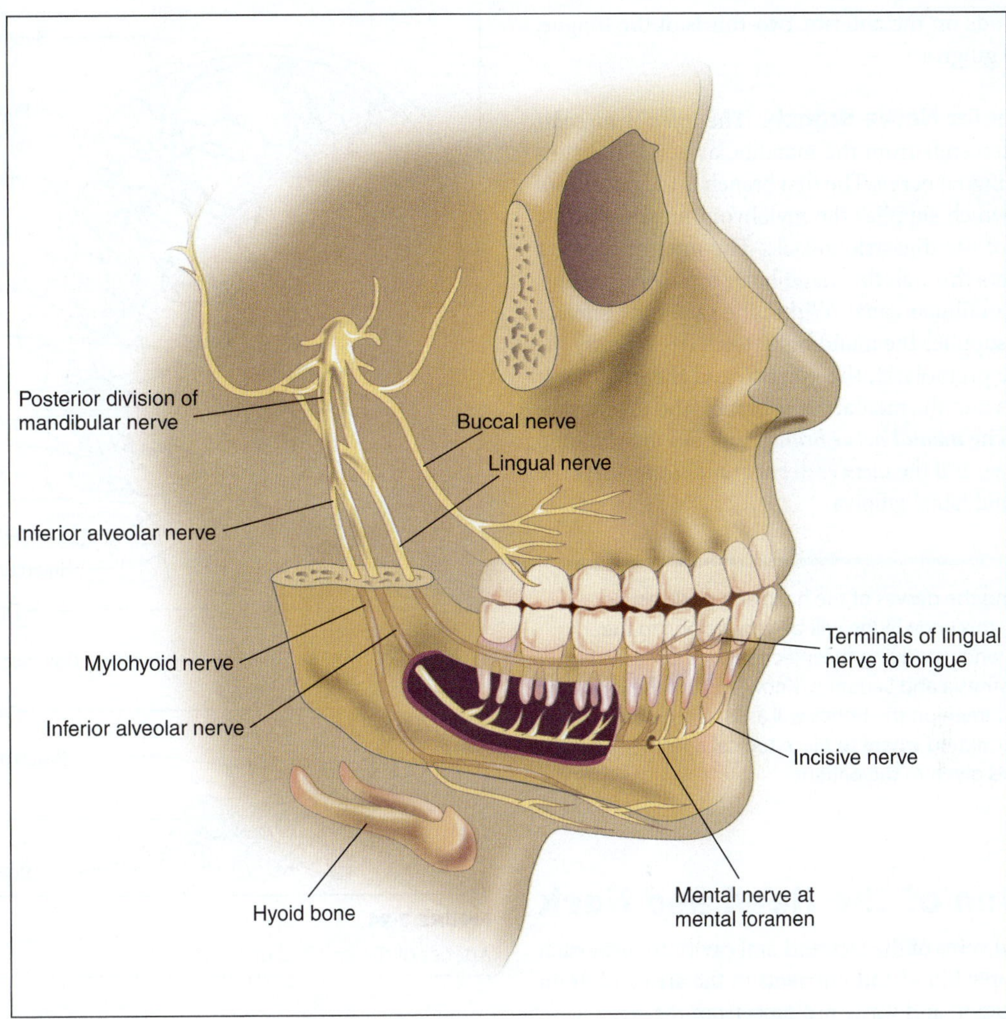

FIGURE 7-23
Mandibular nerves.

palate, gingiva, mucous membrane, and the anterior teeth from the cuspids forward.

Infraorbital Nerve. The *infraorbital nerve* is another branch of the maxillary nerve. Two nerves come from the infraorbital nerve before it exits through the infraorbital foramen. These are the *middle superior alveolar nerve* and the *anterior alveolar nerve*.

The middle superior alveolar nerve supplies the lateral wall of the maxillary sinus, gingiva, mesial buccal root of the first molar, and all the roots of the bicuspids (premolars). The anterior superior alveolar nerve is the next nerve to come from the infraorbital nerve. It innervates the anterior maxillary sinus, gingiva, cuspids, laterals, and central incisors.

Posterior Superior Alveolar Nerve. The *posterior superior alveolar nerve* branches downward from the maxillary nerve. It supplies the gingiva, maxillary sinus, cheeks, and maxillary molars with the exception of the mesial buccal root of the first molar, which is innervated by the middle superior alveolar nerve.

Zygomatic Nerve. The *zygomatic nerve* innervates the orbicularis oculi, the area around the eye, and the area around and behind the zygomatic arch.

Mandibular Branch of the Trigeminal Nerve

The *mandibular nerve branch* is composed of both sensory and motor neurons and is the largest division of the trigeminal nerve. There are three branches of the mandibular nerve: *buccal*, *lingual*, and *inferior alveolar* (Figure 7-23).

Buccal Nerve Branch. The *buccal nerve branch* passes through the buccinator muscle to the cheek, where it innervates the buccal mucosa and buccal gingiva, as well as the buccal of the mandibular molars.

Lingual Nerve Branch. The *lingual nerve branch* descends from the mandibular nerve to the underside of the tongue and extends from the posterior to the anterior of the mouth. This nerve innervates the floor of the mouth, the ventral side of the tongue, taste buds on the anterior two-thirds of the tongue, and the lingual gingiva.

Inferior Alveolar Nerve Branch. The *inferior alveolar nerve branch* descends from the mandibular nerve and runs parallel to the lingual nerve. The first branch is the *mylohyoid nerve branch*, which supplies the mylohyoid muscle and the anterior belly of the digastric muscle. The inferior alveolar nerve then enters through the mandibular foramen and runs through the mandibular canal. Within the canal, the inferior alveolar nerve supplies the mandibular teeth (specifically the molars and the premolars), the gingiva, and the mucosa. It then subdivides into the mental nerve branch and the incisive nerve branch. The *mental nerve branch* supplies the chin and the lower lip area, and the *incisive nerve branch* innervates the anterior teeth and labial gingiva.

Although learning the nerves of the head and neck can be difficult to learn, this knowledge will be very helpful to the dental assistant when studying the injection sites discussed in Chapter 20 Anesthesia and Sedation. Knowledge of the location of nerves and foramen on the bones will assist the dental assistant in determining where to place topical anesthetic before a local injection is given to the patient.

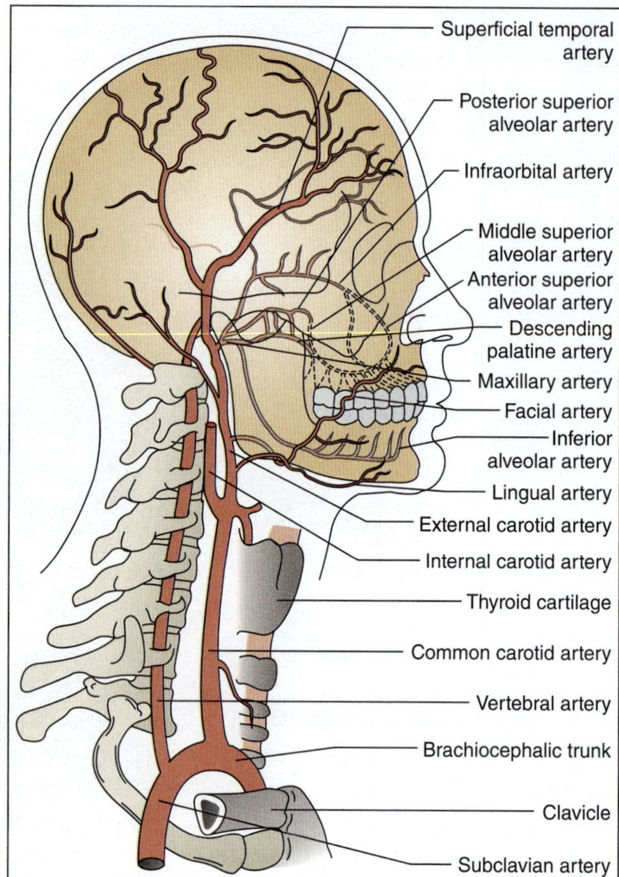

FIGURE 7-24
Arteries of the face and oral cavity.

Circulation of the Head and Neck

The arteries and veins of the face and oral cavity are near each other. They supply blood and nutrients to the area and drain unoxygenated blood and waste products from the area.

Arteries of the Face and Oral Cavity

The **common carotid** supplies blood to most of the head and neck. As the common carotid ascends up the neck, it divides into the internal and external carotid arteries. The *internal carotid artery* supplies blood to the brain and eyes, while the *external carotid artery* supplies blood to the face and oral cavity and has many branches (Figure 7-24). Information presented in this section is limited to the arteries that supply the teeth, tongue, and surrounding tissues.

External Carotid Artery

The external carotid artery branches go to the throat, tongue, face, and ears and also to the wall of the cranium. Branches are named according to the areas they supply and are nearer the surface (more superficial).

Lingual Artery. The lingual branch is about even with the hyoid bone and has several branches that supply the entire tongue, floor of the mouth, lingual gingiva, a portion of the soft palate, and the tonsils.

Facial Artery. The *facial artery* is above the lingual artery, near the angle of the mandible. It branches across the mandible to the corners of the mouth and then upward toward the eye. The facial artery has six branches that supply the pharynx muscles, soft palate, tonsils, posterior of the tongue, submandibular gland, muscles of the face, nasal septum, nose, and eyelids.

Maxillary Artery. The *maxillary artery* is the largest of the branches of the external carotid artery. It moves anteriorly across the ramus of the mandible, near the condyle, and supplies facial structures. The maxillary artery divides into three sections: mandibular, pterygoid, and pterygopalatine.

Mandibular Artery. The *mandibular artery* is behind the ramus of the mandible and branches into five arteries. The *inferior alveolar artery* descends into the ramus, enters the mandibular foramen, and bifurcates around the first premolar tooth to form the incisive and the mental arteries. The *mylohyoid artery* and the *dental arteries* are additional branches. The *mylohyoid artery* branches off the inferior alveolar artery before entering the mandibular canal. It supplies the mylohyoid muscle. As the inferior alveolar artery travels through the mandibular canal, the *dental arteries* supply the roots and periodontal ligaments of the molars and premolars. The *incisive arteries* continue anteriorly to supply blood to the roots and periodontal ligaments of the anterior teeth. The *mental artery* branches off the inferior alveolar artery, and then exits the mandibular canal at the mental foramen and supplies the chin and lower lip.

Pterygoid Artery. The *pterygoid artery* supplies blood to the temporal muscle, masseter muscle, pterygoid muscles, and buccinator muscles. The pterygopalatine artery divides into these branches: *posterior superior alveolar artery, infraorbital artery, middle superior alveolar artery, anterior superior alveolar artery,* and *greater palatine artery*. The posterior superior alveolar artery branches from the maxillary artery and descends along the maxillary tuberosity, where it enters the posterior superior alveolar foramen. This artery supplies the maxillary sinus, maxillary molar teeth, and surrounding gingiva with blood. The infraorbital artery ascends from the maxillary artery and travels anteriorly to the infraorbital foramen, where it supplies the face with blood. From the infraorbital artery, the middle superior alveolar artery branches to the maxillary premolar teeth, and the anterior superior alveolar artery branches to supply the anterior teeth. The greater palatine artery travels through the greater palatine foramen to supply the hard palate and the maxillary lingual gingiva.

Veins of the Face and Oral Cavity

Some of the veins of the face and oral cavity are located with corresponding arteries and have similar names. There are many variations of venous drainage, but ultimately the blood from the face and oral cavity drains into either the external jugular vein or internal jugular vein and then into the brachiocephalic vein, which flows into the superior vena cava. The veins are divided into the superficial veins and the deep veins. Only the primary veins of importance to the dental assistant are discussed in this section (Figure 7-25).

Superficial Veins. The *facial vein* drains the facial structures, beginning near the eye and descending toward the mandible. One of the tributaries is the *deep facial vein*, which connects the facial vein to the pterygoid plexus of veins. Near the border of the mandible, the facial vein heads posteriorly to the angle of the mandible, where it joins with the retromandibular vein. The *retromandibular vein* is frequently formed within the parotid gland. This vein drains the maxillary artery and the superficial temporal arteries. Below the facial vein is the *lingual vein*, which drains the floor of the mouth. The tongue empties into the internal jugular vein.

Deep Veins. The *maxillary vein* drains the pterygoid plexus of veins. It is a short vein that follows the maxillary artery. The *pterygoid plexus of veins* is a junction or center of veins that directly or indirectly drain a vast area, including the nasal cavity, eye, paranasal sinuses, muscles of mastication, buccinator muscle, palate, and teeth. The pterygoid plexus of veins is between the temporal and pterygoid muscles.

Jugular Vein. The *external jugular vein* drains the superficial veins of the face and neck into the subclavian vein. The *internal jugular vein receives* blood from the cranium, face, and neck, and drains into the brachiocephalic vein, and then into the superior vena cava, which drains into the heart.

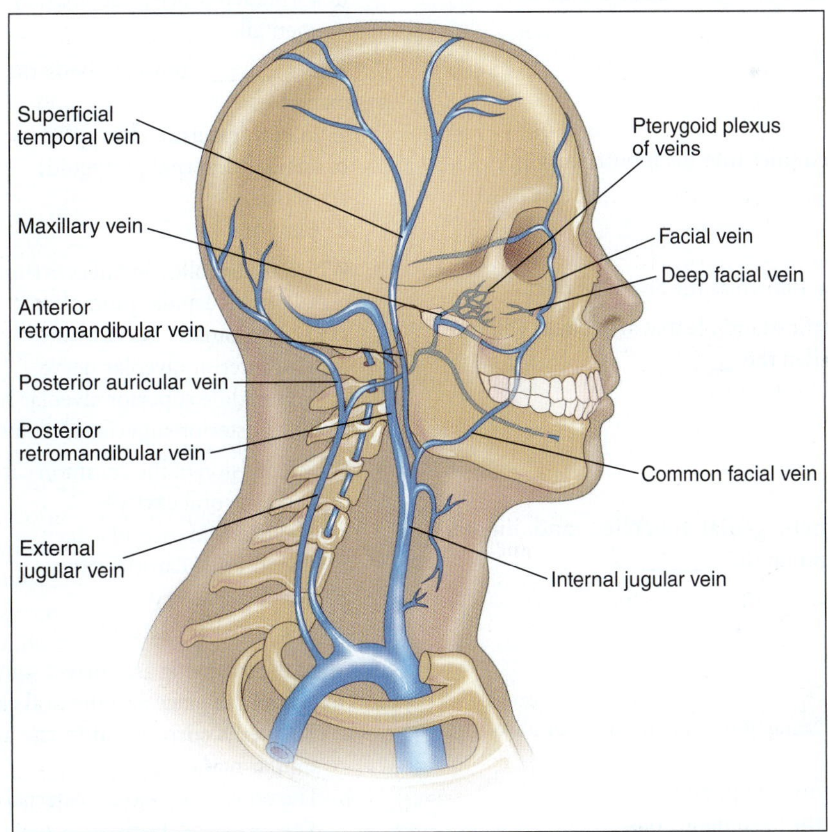

FIGURE 7-25
Veins of the face and oral cavity.

Chapter Summary

As a vital team member, the dental assistant needs to be able to recognize factors that may influence the general physical health of the patient. Understanding landmarks of the oral cavity, as well as being able to describe head and neck anatomy as it relates to location of structure and function, enables the dental assistant to recognize the abnormal. For this reason, accuracy is especially important when completing the patient's dental chart. This information provides a point of comparison for future visits.

CASE STUDY

Pat Boyer is a 35-year-old patient at Dr. Olson's office. Pat has had a series of headaches and pain during mastication (chewing). She also experiences clicking and popping when opening her mouth. These symptoms have continued for 6 months and seem to be worsening.

Case Study Review

1. List the components of the head and neck affected, identifying the specific anatomy.
2. Identify the possible conditions.
3. How might the dental assistant be involved in this patient's care?

Review Questions

Multiple Choice

1. What are the raised lines of mucosal tissue that extend from the alveolar mucosa to the vestibule called?
   a. Gingiva
   b. Alveolar mucosa
   c. Frenum
   d. Papilla
2. The parotid gland empties into the mouth through:
   a. Wharton's duct
   b. Sublingual duct
   c. Duct of Rivinus
   d. Parotid duct also known as the Stensen's duct
3. The vertical part of the mandible that articulates with the temporal bone is called the ________.
   a. oblique ridge
   b. ramus
   c. maxilla
   d. palatal
4. The mental foramen, genial tubercles, and lingual foramen are all found on the ________.
   a. maxilla
   b. mandible
   c. temporal bone
   d. nasal bone
5. The temporomandibular joint is composed of all of the following *except*:
   a. Glenoid fossa of the temporal bone
   b. Greater wing of the zygomatic bone
   c. Articular eminence of the temporal bone
   d. Condyloid process of the mandible
6. Which of the following are muscles of mastication?
   a. Temporal, masseter, buccinators, and internal pterygoid
   b. Temporal, masseter, internal pterygoid, and external pterygoid
   c. Masseter, mentalis, buccinators, and external pterygoid
   d. Orbicularis oris, buccinators, zygomatic major, and mentalis
7. The ________ muscle opens the jaw by depressing the mandible.
   a. lateral (external) pterygoid
   b. medial (internal pterygoid)
   c. masseter
   d. temporal
8. Which of the following nerves supplies all the roots of the maxillary bicuspids (premolars)?
   a. The zygomatic nerve branch
   b. The anterior alveolar nerve
   c. The middle superior alveolar nerve
   d. The posterior superior alveolar nerve
9. Which division of the common carotid artery supplies the face and the oral cavity?
   a. The external carotid artery
   b. The internal carotid artery
   c. The facial artery
   d. The maxillary artery
10. All of the following are correct statements about the veins that supply the face and the oral cavity *except*
    a. The veins correspond to the arteries and often have similar names.
    b. The veins drain into the external or internal jugular vein.
    c. The veins are classified as deep or superficial veins.
    d. The lingual vein drains the muscles of mastication, the sinuses, and the palate.

Critical Thinking

1. Which maxillary nerve is involved if a patient has a toothache on tooth 4?
2. Between the bottom of the nose and the middle of the upper lip is a shallow, V-shaped depression. Identify this landmark and any developmental disturbances that occur in this area.
3. Prominence of excess bone is sometimes found in the bones of the arches. What are these prominences called, and where are they located?

Web Activities

1. Go to http://www.tmjoints.org to find out who is affected, causes and symptoms of TMJ disease.
2. Go to http://www.mayoclinic.org, search for Bell's Palsy, and learn about facial paralysis and its causes.
3. Go to http://www.webmd.com and lookup salivary gland stones. Find what causes the stones to form and how this condition is treated. What is another name for the "stones"?

CHAPTER 8

Embryology and Histology

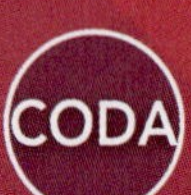

Specific Instructional Objectives

The student should strive to meet the following objectives and demonstrate an understanding of the facts and principles presented in this chapter:

1. Identify the terms and times of the three prenatal phases of pregnancy.
2. Describe how the human face develops and changes during the zygote and embryonic phases.
3. Describe the life cycle of a tooth and identify the stages.
4. Identify the four primary structures of the tooth and the location and function of each.
5. Identify the substances of enamel, dentin, cementum, and pulp and their identifying marks.
6. Identify the components of the periodontium and the considerations of the alveolar bone.
7. Describe the structures of the gingiva and the mucosa.

Key Terms

alveolar crest (149)
alveolar mucosa (151)
alveolar process (149)
alveolodental ligament fiber groups (149)
alveolus (149)
ameloblasts (146)
apposition (146)
attached gingiva (151)
attrition (146)
bell stage (146)
bud stage (143)
calcification (146)
cap stage (145)
cemental spur (148)
cementoblasts (146)
cementoclasts (148)
cementum (146)
cleft lip (142)
cleft palate (142)
cleft uvula (142)
contour lines of Owen (147)
cortical bone (149)
cytodifferentiation (135)
dental lamina (143)
dental sac (146)
dentin (146)
dentinal fluid (147)
dentinal hypersensitivity (148)
dentinal tubule (147)
embryo (135)
embryology (135)
embryonic layers (135)
embryonic phase (135)
enamel (146)
enamel dysplasia (147)
enamel lamellae (147)
enamel matrix (147)
enamel spindles (147)
enamel tufts (147)
epithelial attachment (152)
eruption (146)
evanesce (146)
fetal phase (138)
fibroblast (148)
free gingiva (152)
gestational period (138)
gingiva (151)
gingival fiber groups (150)
gingival groove (151)
gingival sulcus (152)
histodifferentiation (135)
histology (142)
hypercementosis (148)
imbrication lines (147)
Imbrication lines of Von Ebner (147)
initiation (143)
intercellular substances (148)
interdental gingiva (152)
interdental septum (149)

(continues)

Key Terms (continued)

interprismatic substance (147)
interradicular septum (149)
lanugo (141)
lamina dura (149)
lamina propria (150)
ligament fiber groups (149)
lines of Retzius (147)
mesenchyme tissue (146)
morphodifferentiation (135)
mucogingival junction (151)
Nasmyth's membrane (147)
nasolacrimal groove (135)
neonatal line (147)
odontoblast (146)
odontogenesis (143)
perikymata (147)
periodontium (148)
periodontal fiber groups (149)
periodontal ligament (149)
primary palate (136)
proliferation (145)
pulp (146)
pulp canal (146)
pulp chamber (146)
pulp horns (146)
pulp stones (148)
pulpitis (148)
rod core (147)
secondary palate (136)
Sharpey's fibers (148)
stippled (151)
stomodeum (135)
Tome's process (147)
zygote (135)

Introduction

Dental assistants should be familiar with the general embryological development of the face and the oral cavity and with general histology to understand the composition, formation, and eruption of the teeth. In addition to embryology and histology, this chapter covers the components of the periodontium and describes the structures of the gingiva.

As a dental assistant you should be able to use proper terminology to describe embryology and development. The key terms highlighted in the chapter focus on the foundations. Additional terms are placed in italic and should be learned as well.

Embryology

The study of prenatal growth and the developing process of an individual are called **embryology** (Figure 8-1). The **embryo** is the organism in the earliest stages of development. *Oral embryology* refers to the study of the development of the oral cavity. The following information provides the dental assistant with a basic understanding of embryology.

Human pregnancy is approximately 9 months (38 weeks [often counted 40 weeks from the first day of the pregnant woman's last menstrual period]) in duration. This period starts with conception, when the ovum is fertilized by the sperm. The following terms and times identify the three prenatal phases of the pregnancy:

1. Conception through the first two weeks—zygote
2. Two weeks through the eighth week—embryo
3. Nine weeks through birth—fetus

The **zygote** phase is when cells rapidly increase in number, or *proliferate*. During the **embryonic phase**, many critical changes are taking place. The cells are differentiating (developing individual characteristics) and integrating to form cell layers that develop into a human being. There are three stages of differentiation:

1. **Cytodifferentiation**—the development of different cells
2. **Histodifferentiation**—the development of different tissues
3. **Morphodifferentiation**—the development of different forms

Three primary **embryonic layers** are formed early in the embryo phase. The *ectoderm* layer differentiates into skin, hair, nails, brain, nervous system, lining of the oral cavity, and enamel of the teeth. The second layer, the *mesoderm*, differentiates into the lining of the abdominal cavity, bones, muscles, circulatory system, reproductive system, internal organs, dentin, cementum, and pulp of the teeth. The *endoderm*, the third layer, gives rise to the epithelial linings of the respiratory system, some glandular organs, and the digestive tract. To remember the layers, recall that *derm* refers to tissue and *ecto* refers to outside, *meso* refers to middle, and *endo* refers to inside (Figure 8-2). The first sign of a developing tooth is noted during the embryonic phase, in the area that will eventually become the lower mandibular anterior region (Figure 8-3).

Primitive Facial Development

The face begins to form during the fourth week of prenatal development (Figure 8-4A). This embryonic phase involves all three embryonic layers. At this time, the future face appears to be squeezed between the bulging brain and the large heart, with the eyes and nose spread out toward the sides. The face further develops from the three embryonic layers (Figures 8-4B and C). The first area, the frontonasal process, forms the upper portion of the face, the forehead, eyes, nose, and the *b* (vertical groove on the midline of the upper lip). The second area forms the middle of the face, called the maxillary (medial nasal) process. This area consists of the cheeks, sides of the upper lip, midface, secondary palate, zygomatic bones, a portion of the temporal bones, and the maxilla embryonic surface. The third area, called the mandibular process, forms the two mandibular arches (first branchial arches) and makes up the lower lip, lower face, temporal area, and the mandible. The **stomodeum** (stoh-mah-DE-um), or primitive mouth, appears between the maxillary and mandibular processes. It initially appears as a shallow depression in the embryonic surface.

The face continues developing until the twelfth week, changing shape considerably during this time. The eyes move forward, the nose comes together, and the face appears much narrower than during the first formation. The maxillary processes on each side of the face fuse at the *labial commissures*, or corners of the mouth, with the mandibular arch (Figure 8-4B). The frontonasal process fuses with the maxillary process along the line of the **nasolacrimal groove**. This groove

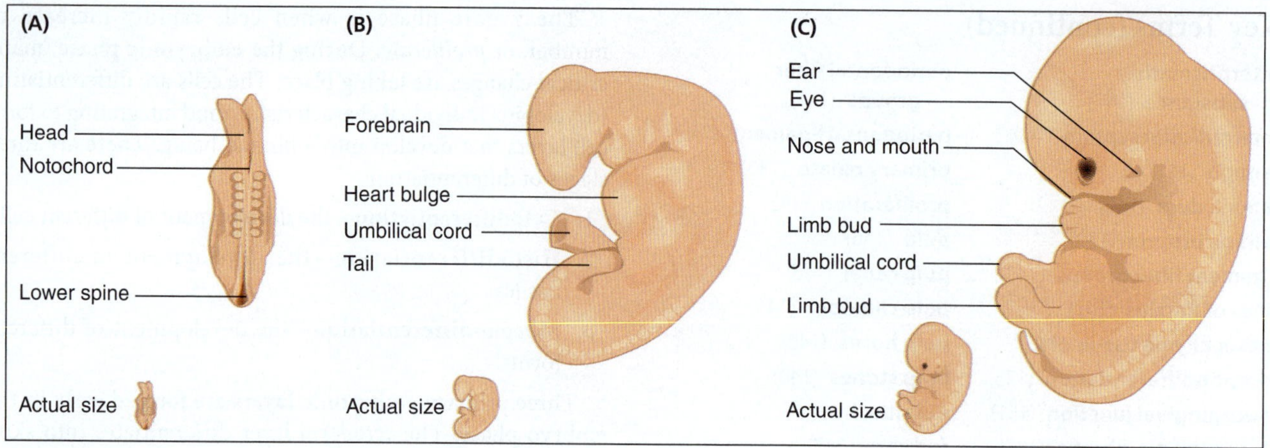

FIGURE 8-1

(a) at 3 weeks the embryo becomes pear shaped and has a rounded head and a rather pointed lower spine, and the **notochord** (a long flexible rod of cells that supports the body, referred to as a primitive backbone) runs along its back. (B) At 4 weeks the embryo becomes C-shaped and has a visible tail. The forebrain enlarges and an umbilical cord forms. There is also a bulge where the heart is located. (C) At 6 weeks the embryo has visible eyes, mouth, nose, and ears, and the arms and legs are growing from the limb buds. The umbilical cord has enlarged.

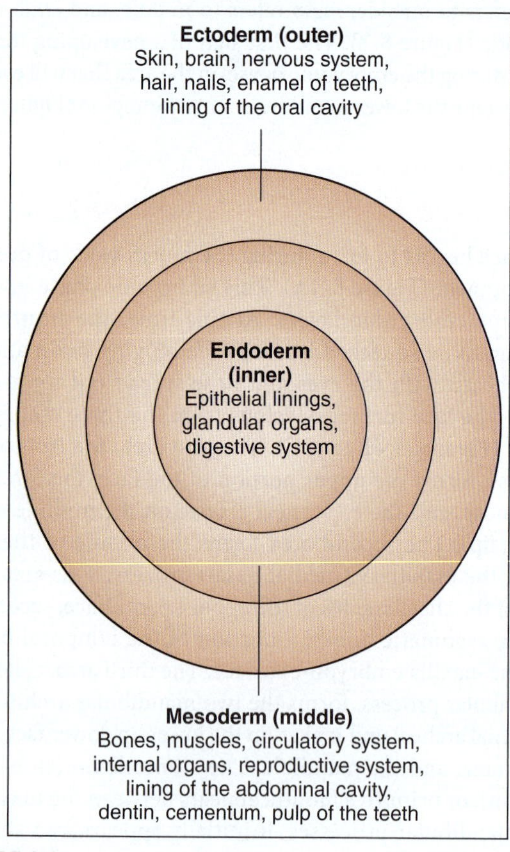

FIGURE 8-2

The three primary embryonic layers—ectoderm (outer), mesoderm (middle), and endoderm (inner)—and associated tissues.

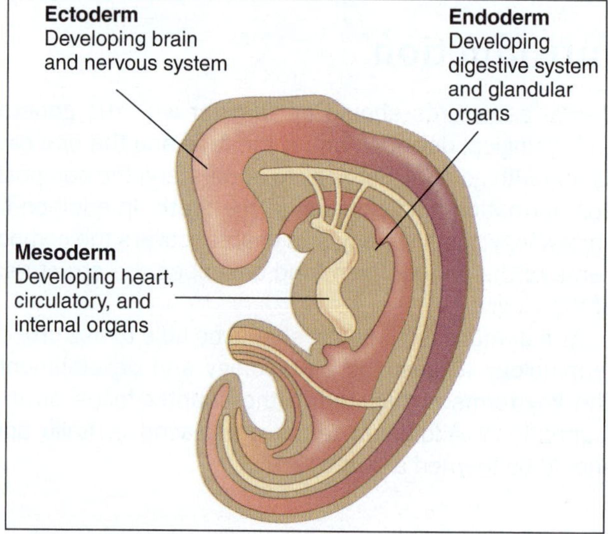

FIGURE 8-3

Developing embryo with primary embryonic layers identified.

extends from the medial corner of the eye to the nasal cavity along the maxillary process to the medial nasal process. This fusion normally is completed during the sixth week of prenatal development.

Inside the oral cavity, the **primary** (primitive) **palate** is developing. It appears as a triangular mass and contains the four maxillary incisor teeth. It serves to separate the developing oral cavities from the nasal cavities. The two palatal shelves develop and move medially toward each other, fusing to form the **secondary palate**, which will become two-thirds of the hard palate (Figure 8-5). The secondary palate contains the remaining teeth and forms the remaining two-thirds of the hard palate and the soft palate, including the uvula. During the twelfth week of prenatal development, the primary palate and the secondary palate meet and fuse, forming the final palate. Thus, the oral cavity and the nasal cavity are completely separated.

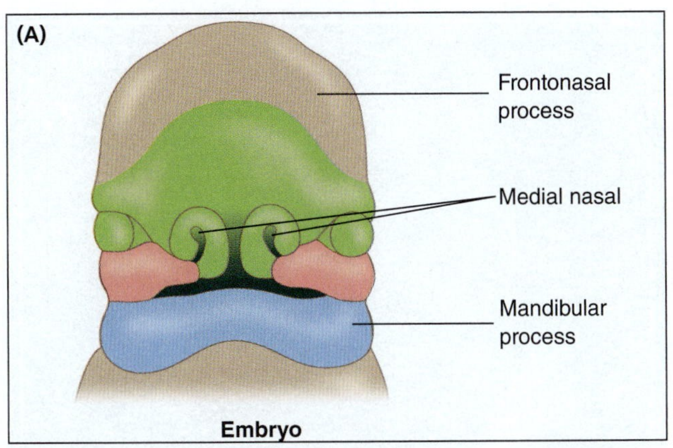

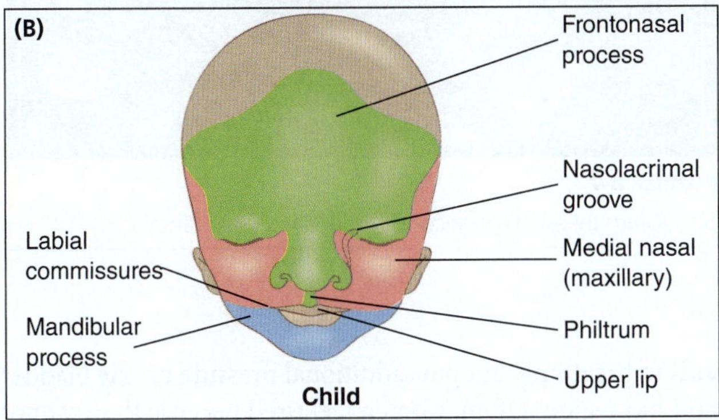

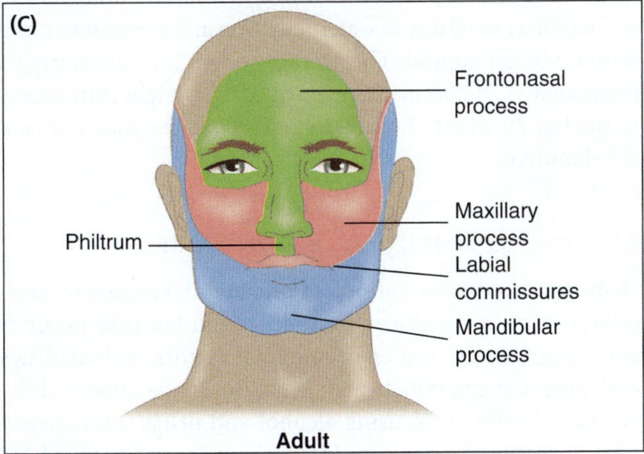

FIGURE 8-4

Embryonic facial processes shown on (A) embryo, (B) child, and (C) adult.

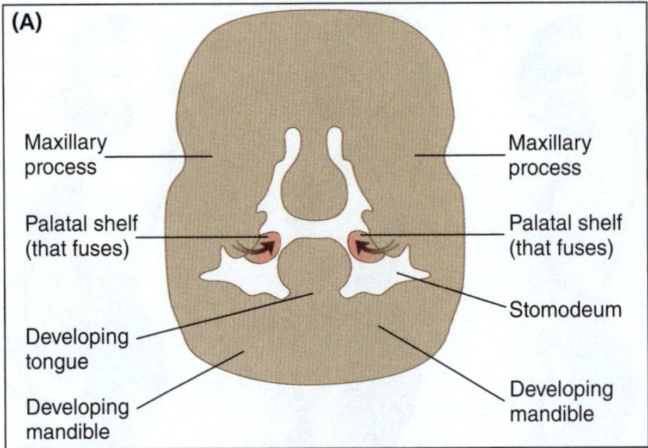

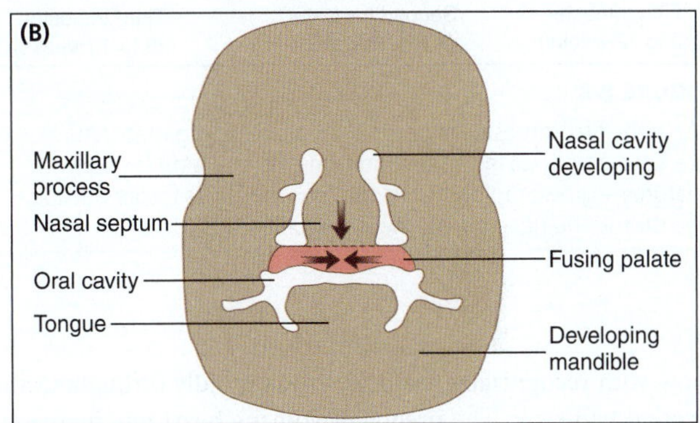

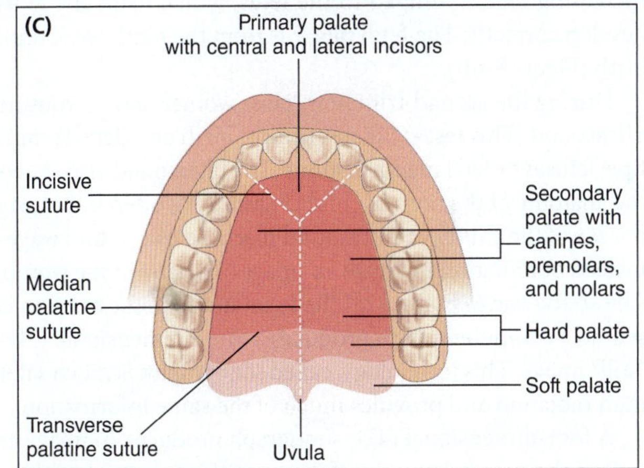

FIGURE 8-5

Development of the palate. (A) Palate forming from three sections. (B) Frontal view. (C) Palatal view of the three sections and where the secondary and primary palates fuse.

Stages and Features of Pregnancy

The first trimester is from week zero to week 12. The first sign of pregnancy is usually the absence of a menstrual period, although some women have breakthrough bleeding during their normal cycles. The breasts swell and may become tender. This is because the mammary glands develop to prepare for breastfeeding. The veins over the surface of the breasts become more prominent and the nipples begin to enlarge.

During the first 6 to 8 weeks, nausea and vomiting are common. Most women are tired and require more rest. Some women notice cravings for certain foods and may have a metallic taste in the mouth. After the vomiting decreases, weight begins to increase. All major organs in the embryo/fetus begin developing (Figure 8-6A).

The second trimester is from week 13 to week 28. The woman begins to look noticeably pregnant. Her weight increases, as does her appetite. The nausea is less and the woman may feel better and more energetic than during the first trimester. The woman's breasts and abdomen enlarge. The woman feels the baby moving between the eighteenth and the twentieth weeks. The fetus,

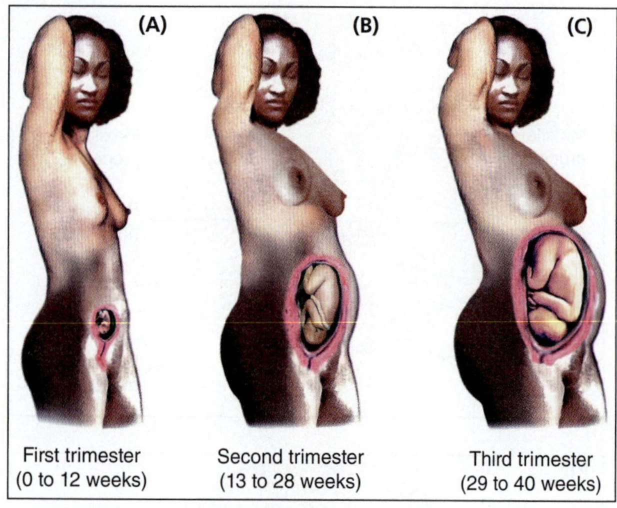

FIGURE 8-6

(A) In the first trimester of pregnancy, all major organ structures are developing. (B) In the second trimester, the fetus—now with features—grows rapidly. (C) As the fetus prepares for life outside the uterus, the head drops low in the pelvis.

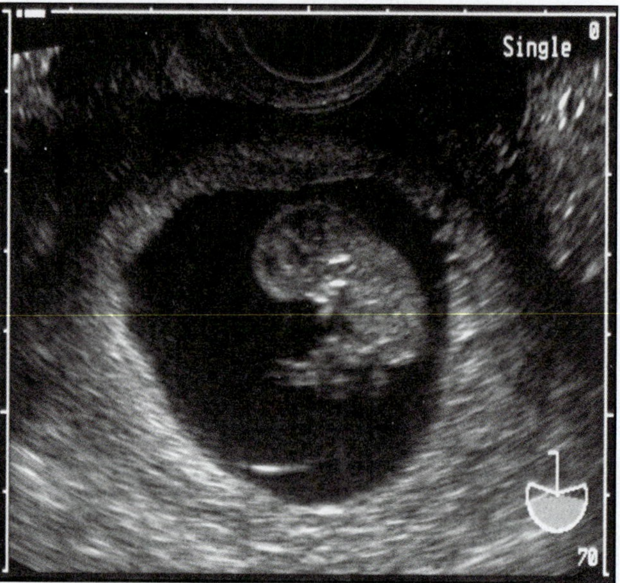

Courtesy of Nici Peterson

FIGURE 8-7

Sonogram taken in the second trimester of pregnancy.

now with recognizable features, grows rapidly throughout the second trimester. The pregnant woman's heart rate increases, increasing blood pumped to the fetus, which helps the fetus develop correctly. The **fetal phase** is from the ninth week until birth (Figure 8-6B).

During the second trimester, most women have a routine ultrasound. This test estimates time of birth and detects multiple fetuses or fetal malformations. The ultrasound also shows the anatomy of the normal child (Figure 8-7), often indicating the sex of the child. An ultrasound machine uses sound waves instead of radiation to create an image of a baby in the womb. The sound waves bounce off the fetus and that information is sent to a computer, which produces a three-dimensional (3D) "still" image. This technology, called sonography, is much safer than radiation and provides much of the same information.

A four-dimensional (4D) sonograph produces an image as well as showing movement of the fetus (Figures 8-8A and B). Both the 3D and the 4D tests can be considered safe as long as trained medical professionals are performing them. The number of nonmedical people offering ultrasound exams has increased. These individuals may not be trained and could give parents inaccurate information. The Food and Drug Administration (FDA) and professional medical organizations discourage the use of these nonmedical ultrasound examinations.

The third and final trimester is from week 29 to week 40. During the **gestational period** (the time span in the womb until offspring are born), the fetus can grow to a length (height) of 48 to 52 centimeters (19 to 21 inches) (Figure 8-9). The woman may experience stretch marks on the breasts, abdomen, and thighs due to the expansion and stretching of the skin. The woman may also experience hot flashes and perspire easily. The fetus matures and prepares for birth. During weeks 36 to 37 the baby's head drops low into the pelvis (Figure 8-6C). This relieves pressure in the woman's chest and aids in breathing, but puts additional pressure on the bladder and hip region. Often, women feel tired because they cannot find a comfortable position in which to rest. The woman's feet and legs may swell due to water retention and it becomes more difficult to get around. The average weight increase during a pregnancy is 28 pounds; 70 percent of this weight gain occurs in the last 20 weeks. Table 8-1 summarizes the stages of fetal development.

Developmental Disturbances

Disturbances during periods of prenatal development most often occur during the embryonic period but may occur at any time. Genetic and environmental factors such as drugs and infections can initiate malformations in the unborn child. Women should avoid using alcohol and drugs immediately after suspicion of pregnancy. Infants born to women who have persisted taking alcohol during pregnancy may exhibit fetal alcohol syndrome (FAS). Symptoms of FAS include, but are not limited to, small head circumference, low nasal bridge, indistinct philtrum, thin upper lip, and a small mandible.

Specific infections contracted by pregnant women may cause malformations and developmental disturbances in the unborn child. For example, German measles may cause heart, eye, or hearing defects in the unborn child. Syphilis, another infection, can cause paralysis, blindness, deafness, and defects in the incisors and molars.

Varying degrees of disfigurement may be caused by the failure of the tissues to fuse. Children born with disabilities of this kind should be seen by medical and dental specialists. Initially, the infant may face problems that limit nursing and feeding. Decisions need to be made to allow proper nutritional care for the child. Developmental disturbances that deal with the failure of tissues to fuse normally require long-term attention. If the palate has not fused, the teeth may not erupt in

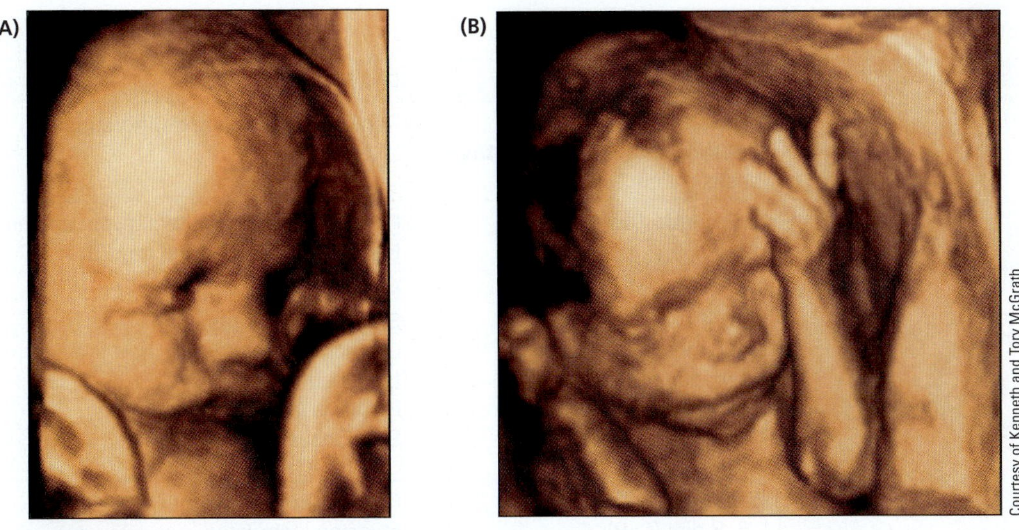

Courtesy of Kenneth and Tory McGrath

FIGURE 8-8

(A) 4D ultrasound at 37 weeks. (B) 4D ultrasound at 20 weeks.

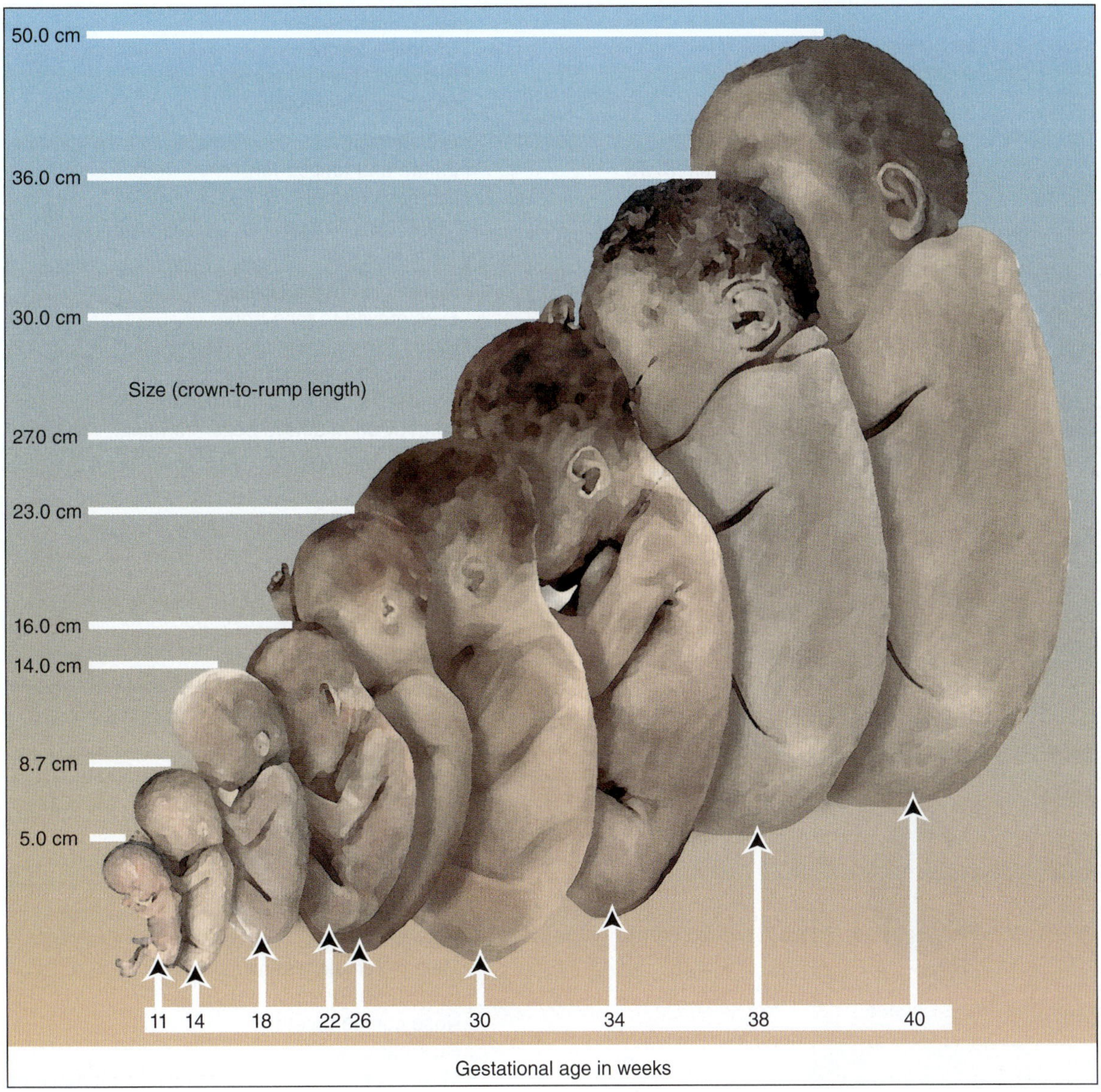

Size (crown-to-rump length): 50.0 cm, 36.0 cm, 30.0 cm, 27.0 cm, 23.0 cm, 16.0 cm, 14.0 cm, 8.7 cm, 5.0 cm

Gestational age in weeks: 11, 14, 18, 22, 26, 30, 34, 38, 40

FIGURE 8-9

Fetal size by gestational age.

TABLE 8-1 Stages of Fetal Development

Stage	Fetal Development
First Trimester **Embryonic or Germinal Stage** Weeks 1 and 2	Rapid cell division and differentiation.
Embryonic Stage Week 3	Primitive nervous system, eyes, and ears present. Heart begins to beat on day 21.
Week 4 Wt 0.4 g L 4–6 mm crown–rump (C–R)	Half the size of a pea. Brain differentiates. GI tract begins to form. Limb buds appear. Primitive face develops. Stomodeum appears.
Week 5 L 6–8 mm (C–R)	Cranial nerves present. Muscles innervated.
Week 6 L 10–14 mm (C–R)	Fetal circulation established. Central autonomic nervous system forms. Primitive kidneys form. Lung buds present. Cartilage forms. Primitive skeleton forms. Muscles differentiate.
Week 7 L 22–28 mm (C–R)	Eyelids form. Palate and tongue form. Stomach formed. Diaphragm formed. Arms and legs move.
Week 8 Wt 2 g L 3 cm (1.2 in) (C–R)	Resembles human being. Eyes moved to face front. Heart development complete. Hands and feet well formed. Bone cells begin replacing cartilage. All body organs have begun forming.
Fetal Stage Week 9	Fingers and toenails form. Eyelids fuse shut.
Week 10 Wt 14 g (¼ oz) L 5–6 cm (2 in) crown–heel (C–H)	Head growth slows. Bone marrow forms. Bladder sac forms. Kidneys make urine.
Week 11	Tooth buds appear. Liver secretes bile. Urinary system functions. Insulin forms in pancreas.
Week 12 Wt 45 g (1.5 oz) L 9 cm (3.5 in) (C–R) 11.5 cm (4.5 in) (C–H)	Oral cavity and nasal cavity are separated. Lungs take shape. Palate fuses. Heartbeat heard with Doppler ultrasound. Primary palate developing. Swallowing reflex present. External genitalia appear. Male or female distinguished. Eyes move forward. Nose comes together. Face narrows. Maxillary processes fuse at labial commissures. Frontonasal process fuses with maxillary process.

(continues)

TABLE 8-1 Stages of Fetal Development (continued)

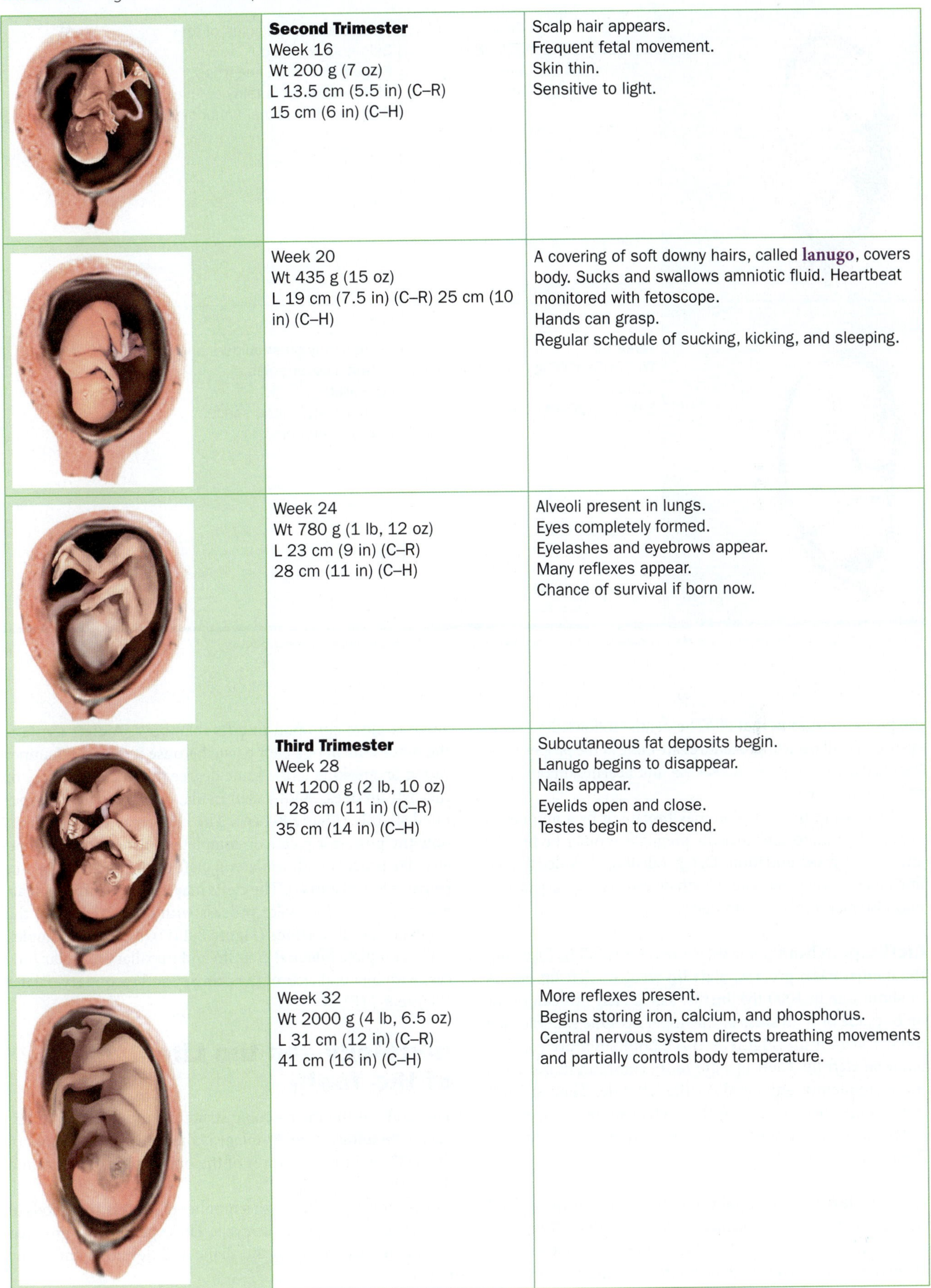

	Second Trimester Week 16 Wt 200 g (7 oz) L 13.5 cm (5.5 in) (C–R) 15 cm (6 in) (C–H)	Scalp hair appears. Frequent fetal movement. Skin thin. Sensitive to light.
	Week 20 Wt 435 g (15 oz) L 19 cm (7.5 in) (C–R) 25 cm (10 in) (C–H)	A covering of soft downy hairs, called **lanugo**, covers body. Sucks and swallows amniotic fluid. Heartbeat monitored with fetoscope. Hands can grasp. Regular schedule of sucking, kicking, and sleeping.
	Week 24 Wt 780 g (1 lb, 12 oz) L 23 cm (9 in) (C–R) 28 cm (11 in) (C–H)	Alveoli present in lungs. Eyes completely formed. Eyelashes and eyebrows appear. Many reflexes appear. Chance of survival if born now.
	Third Trimester Week 28 Wt 1200 g (2 lb, 10 oz) L 28 cm (11 in) (C–R) 35 cm (14 in) (C–H)	Subcutaneous fat deposits begin. Lanugo begins to disappear. Nails appear. Eyelids open and close. Testes begin to descend.
	Week 32 Wt 2000 g (4 lb, 6.5 oz) L 31 cm (12 in) (C–R) 41 cm (16 in) (C–H)	More reflexes present. Begins storing iron, calcium, and phosphorus. Central nervous system directs breathing movements and partially controls body temperature.

(continues)

TABLE 8-1 Stages of Fetal Development (continued)

	Week 36 Wt 2500–2750 g (5 lb, 8 oz) L 35 cm (14 in) (C–R) 48 cm (19 in) (C–H)	A few creases on soles of feet. Skin less wrinkled. Fingernails reach fingertips. Sleep–wake cycle fairly definite. Transfer of maternal antibodies.
	Week 38	L/S ratio 2:1
	Week 40 Wt 3000–3600 g (6 lb, 10 oz–7 lb, 15 oz) L 50 cm (20 in) (C–H)	Lanugo only on shoulders and upper back. Creases cover soles. Ear cartilage firm. Less active, limited space. Ready to be born.

Adapted from Littleton, L. and Engelbreson, J. (2005). *Maternal, Neonatal, and Women's Health Nursing* (2nd ed.). Clifton Park, NY: Delmar Cengage Learning.

the proper positions, if at all. The dentist follows the case to ensure that all needed procedures are done at the proper time. Reconstructive surgery and speech and hearing therapy may be recommended.

Disturbance in the fusion may be caused by a number of factors. It is important that the pregnant mother be healthy and enjoys good nutrition. Drugs (alcohol included) taken during pregnancy may cause birth defects. Hereditary factors may also play a role in birth defects.

Cleft Lip. When the maxillary processes fail to fuse with the medial nasal process, **cleft lip** results. Cleft lip occurs in about one in 1000 live births. These cleft lips can occur on one side or both sides of the upper lip. One side is called *unilateral cleft lip* (Figure 8-10A); both sides are called a *bilateral cleft lip*. Cleft lips are more common in boys and more frequently unilateral on the left side. They are also more severe in boys than girls. Clefts can be as small as a notch in the lip to more severe cases that extend into the floor of the nostril.

Cleft Palate. A **cleft palate** is the failure of the palatal shelves to fuse with the primary palate or with each other. A cleft palate may occur with or without a cleft lip. Cleft palate occurs in one of every 2500 births. Cleft palate occurring alone is more common in girls than boys. A **cleft uvula** is the mildest form of a cleft palate because it does not hamper eating or speaking to the same degree that the cleft palate or the cleft lip does. With a cleft uvula, only the uvula is separated slightly (Figure 8-11A). The clefts may be bilateral in only the posterior palate or complete unilateral cleft lip and alveolar process with unilateral cleft of the primary palates (Figures 8-11B and C). The clefts may also be complete bilateral cleft lip and alveolar process with bilateral cleft of the primary palatal portions (Figure 8-11D). The most complex is the complete bilateral cleft lip and maxillary alveolar process with bilateral cleft of the primary and secondary palates (Figure 8-11E).

Histology and the Life Cycle of the Tooth

The study of the microscopic structure and function of tissues is **histology**. *Oral histology* is the study of the tissues of the teeth and the structures of the oral cavity that surround the teeth.

Each tooth goes through a number of successive periods of development during its life cycle. These periods are grouped into stages according to the shape and development of the organ.

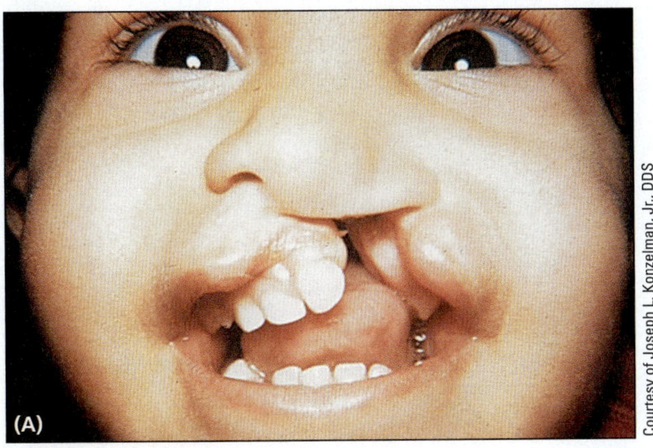

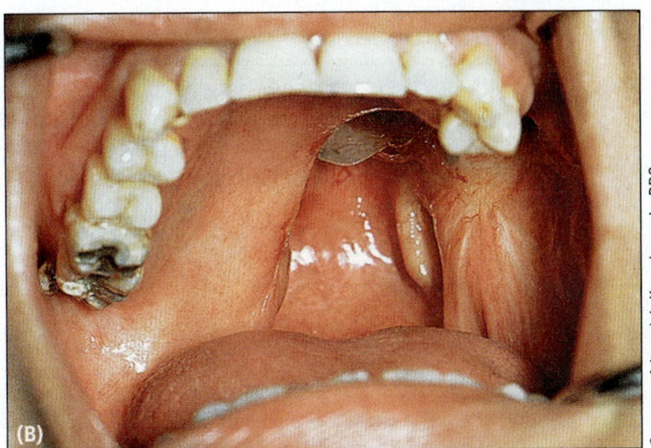

FIGURE 8-10
(A) Cleft lip. (B) Cleft palate.

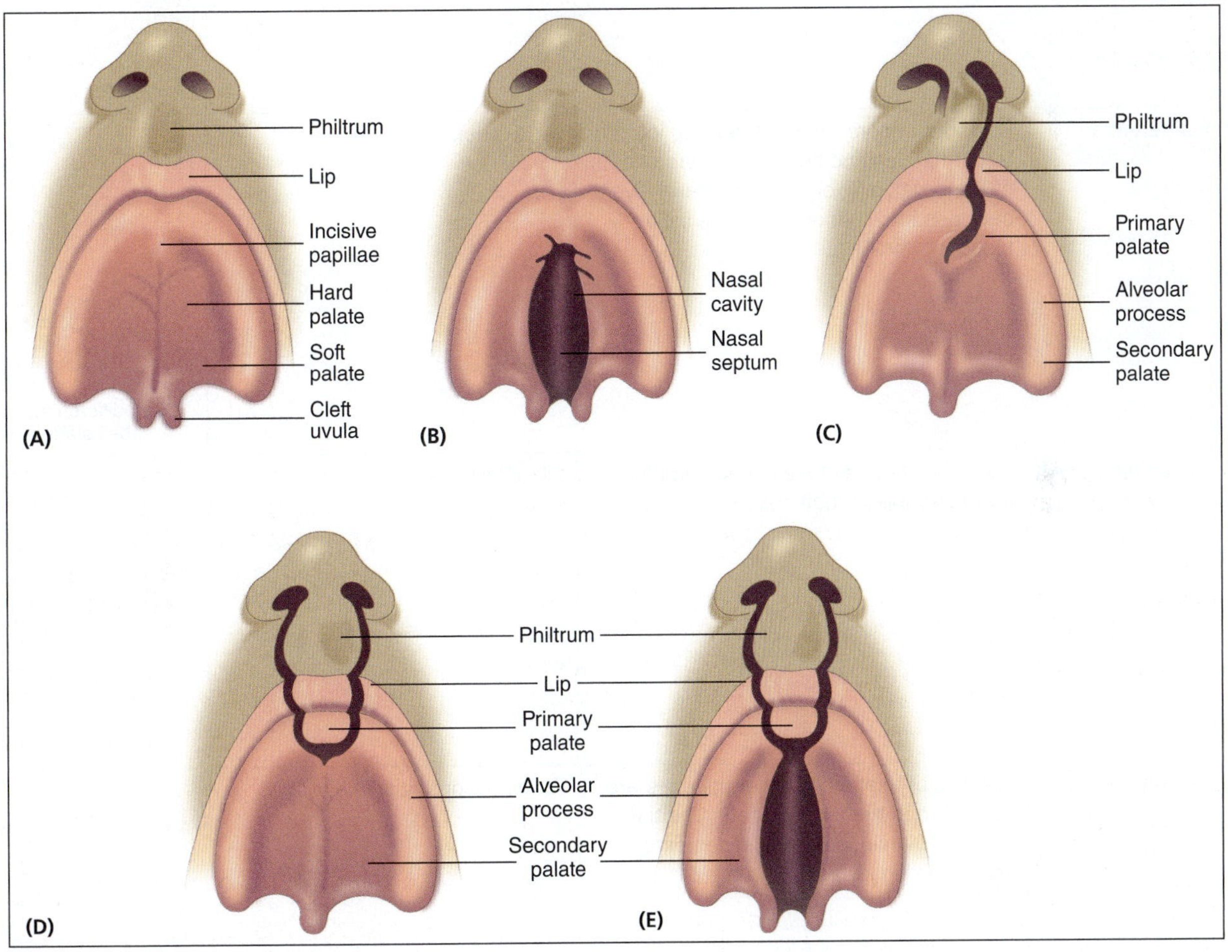

(A) Philtrum, Lip, Incisive papillae, Hard palate, Soft palate, Cleft uvula
(B) Nasal cavity, Nasal septum
(C) Philtrum, Lip, Primary palate, Alveolar process, Secondary palate
(D) (E) Philtrum, Lip, Primary palate, Alveolar process, Secondary palate

FIGURE 8-11
(A) Cleft uvula. (B) Bilateral cleft of the secondary palate. (C) Unilateral cleft lip, primary palate, and alveolar process. (D) Bilateral cleft of the lip, alveolar process, and primary palate. (E) Bilateral cleft of the lip, alveolar process, and primary and secondary palates.

Bud Stage

The first stage of **odontogenesis** (origin of the tooth) is called the **bud stage** (Table 8-2). During this stage, **initiation** takes place. Initiation is when the tooth begins formation from the **dental lamina**. The dental lamina is a growth from the oral epithelium that gives rise to the tooth buds. Therefore, on a deciduous dentition, 10 growths on each arch are apparent or 10 buds later become the primary teeth. The first sign of

TABLE 8-2 Life Cycle of the Tooth

Initiation	Odontogenesis (origin of the tooth) begins. The tooth begins formation from the dental lamina, which is a growth from the oral epithelium that gives rise to the tooth buds.	6–7 weeks	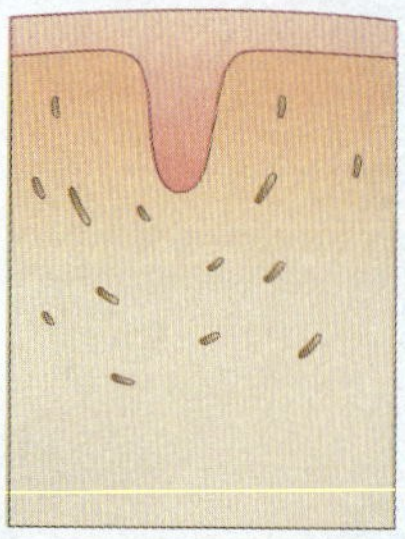 Initiation (bud stage)
Proliferation	Cap stage (begins proliferation, histodifferentiation, and morphodifferentiation) where the primary embryonic ectoderm layer matures into the enamel of the developing tooth.	8–9 weeks	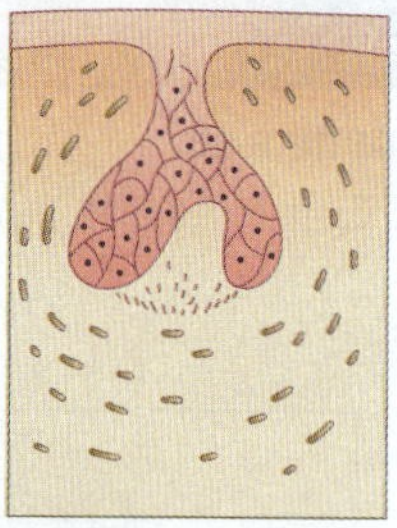 Proliferation (cap stage)
Histodifferentiation	Bell stage where the cells develop into different tissues and begin the future shape of the developing organ. Mesoderm layer develops into connective tissue called mesenchyme tissue.	9–11 weeks	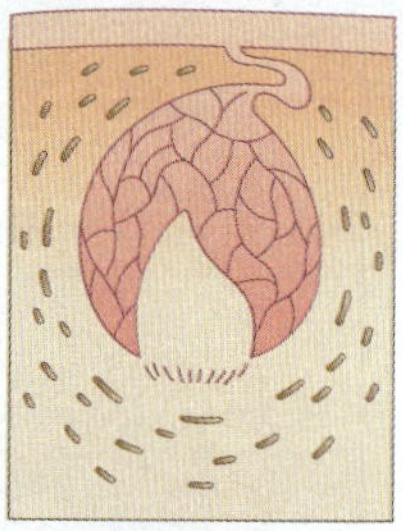 Histodifferentiation (bell stage)
Morphodifferentiation	The forming organ takes shape and further resembles a bell shape.	11–12 weeks	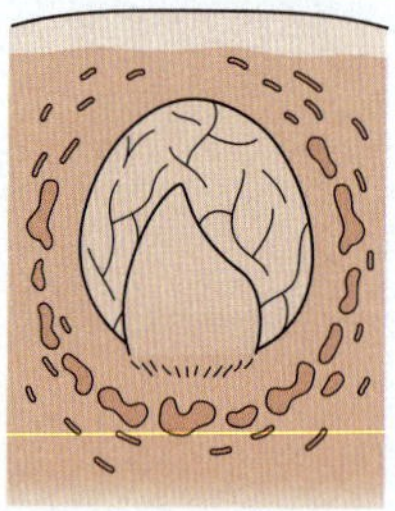 Morphodifferentiation
Apposition	The calcium salts and other minerals are deposited in the formed tooth. The tissues or enamel, dentin, and cementum are formed in layers.	Varies according to the tooth	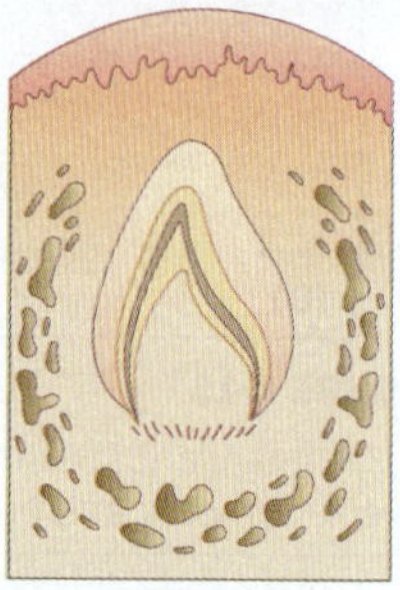 Apposition (maturation stage)

(continues)

TABLE 8-2 Life Cycle of the Tooth (continued)

Calcification	The layers of the tooth tissue become calcified.	Varies according to the tooth	Calcification
Eruption	The tooth emerges from the gum tissue and becomes visible.	Varies according to the tooth. "See 'Stages of Tooth Eruption' in Appendix B" or refer to the actual schedule in Chapter 9, Table 9-1.	Eruption
Attrition	The tooth wears away the incisal or occlusal surfaces during normal function and use.	Varies according to dentition, occlusion, stress, and lifestyle	Attrition

a developing tooth is noted during the embryonic phase in the area that will eventually be the lower mandibular anterior region of the child's oral cavity. The permanent teeth develop in a similar manner. Each arch has 16 buds developing into one tooth each. The last three molars in each quadrant develop behind the primary dentition. The 6-year molar begins developing at birth, the 12-year molar starts developing when the baby is about 6 months old, and the third molars (wisdom teeth) start when the child is approximately 5 years old.

Cap Stage

The bud of the tooth grows and changes shape during the cap stage. The organ is indented on the lower side and appears much like a cap, therefore the name **cap stage** (Table 8-2). The primary embryonic ectoderm layer that has developed into the oral epithelium matures into the enamel of the developing tooth. The processes of **proliferation**, when the cells multiply, and histodifferentiation, when the cells develop into different tissues, take place along with early morphodifferentiation, which is when the cells begin to outline the future shape of the developing organ. During this process, the primary embryonic mesoderm layer develops into connective tissue that is called the **mesenchyme tissue**. This connective tissue forms an enclosed area, called a **dental sac**, and further matures into the dentin, cementum, and the pulp of the tooth. A portion of the mesenchyme surrounds the outside of the enamel organ, the cementum, and the periodontal ligament of the tooth.

Bell Stage

Further specialization of the cells, or histodifferentiation, takes place in the **bell stage** (Table 8-2). The inner epithelium of the enamel organ becomes **ameloblasts**, enamel-forming cells. The peripheral cells of the dental papilla become **odontoblasts**, cells that form dentin. The **cementoblasts**, cementum-forming cells, form from the dental sac. Continued morphodifferentiation takes place, forming the organ into a shape that resembles a bell (Table 8-2).

Maturation Stage

The odontogenesis reaches completion in these final stages. The tissues of enamel, dentin, and cementum are formed in layers and fused in the appropriate manner. The process of depositing calcium salts and other minerals in the formed tooth takes place during the **apposition** stage (Table 8-2). This process, called **calcification**, is the last developmental stage before **eruption** of the tooth, when the growing tooth emerges from the gum (Table 8-2). The final stage of the life cycle of the tooth is **attrition**, or the wearing away of the incisal or occlusal surfaces of the tooth during normal function (Table 8-2 and Figure 8-12).

The root of the tooth does not develop fully before eruption. Eruption is the phase when the tooth passes through the bone and the oral mucosa and into its place in the oral cavity. An eruption schedule for the primary and permanent teeth appears in Chapter 9, Tooth Morphology. Twenty of the permanent teeth are below and distal to the primary teeth. As the permanent teeth erupt, they apply pressure to the apices of the roots of the primary teeth. During this force, *osteoclasts*, bone resorption cells, **evanesce** (ev-a-NES) (dissolve) the root of the primary tooth. This resorption first takes place at the apex and continues up toward the crown of the tooth. When very little of the root structure of the primary tooth is left, the tooth loosens due to lack of support. Children often assist in the final stages of loosening the tooth by moving it back and forth until they break the attaching fibers.

The primary teeth occupy and maintain space in the dental arches for the permanent teeth and act as guides during the eruption process. If the primary teeth are removed early, the spaces may be diminished, causing crowding when the permanent teeth erupt.

Tooth Structure

Each tooth is comprised of four primary structures (Figure 8-13). The **enamel** is the structure that covers the outside of the crown of the tooth. It is the hardest living tissue in the body. Enamel can be very brittle if not supported by dentin and a vital pulp. The bulk of the tooth structure is made up of **dentin** but is not normally visible. It surrounds the pulp cavity and lies under the enamel, within the anatomical crown and under the cementum within the root. The **cementum** is the third structure and is located around the root. It covers the dentin on the root portion of the tooth. The pulp tissue is at the center of the tooth, within the **pulp** cavity. It is made of the nerves and blood vessels that provide nutrients to the tooth. The pulp cavity is made of a pulp chamber with pulp horns and pulp canal(s). The **pulp canal**(s)/*radicular pulp* is (are) in the root(s) of the teeth. The **pulp chamber**/*coronal pulp* is a large portion of the pulp, which is in the crown of the tooth. The **pulp horns**, pointed elongations of the pulp, extend toward the incisal or occlusal portion of the tooth. The pulpal portion of the tooth is often larger in primary teeth and newly

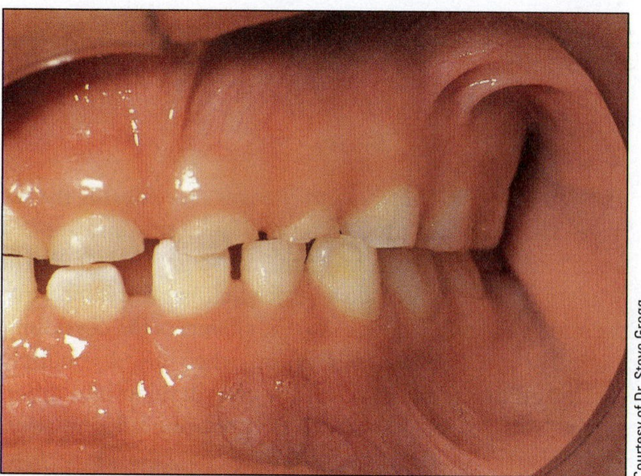

FIGURE 8-12

Attrition of the primary dentition.

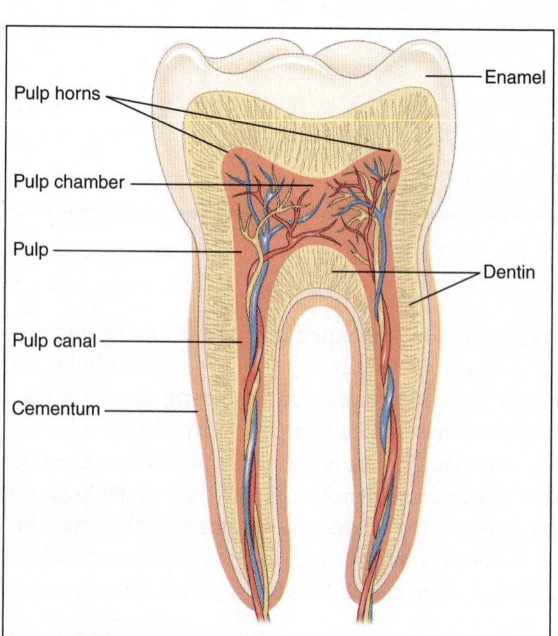

FIGURE 8-13

Tissues of the tooth.

formed permanent teeth. As a person ages, the pulpal portion may decrease in size. For example, adults over 70 years of age may have small pulp chambers or the pulpal portion may be totally calcified.

Enamel

Enamel is thicker on the biting surfaces, occlusal cusps, and the incisal edge than in other areas. Ameloblasts aid in developing enamel rods. These rods, which are not visible to the naked eye, are 4 micrometers in diameter, have variable lengths, and are shaped in the pattern of a fish (Figure 8-14). Their location in the enamel is such that the head is surrounded by the tails of two other enamel rods. The substance surrounding the inner portion, the **rod core**, of each enamel rod is the **interprismatic substance**. Of these substances, the enamel rods are hardest and the interprismatic substance is the weakest.

The **enamel matrix** is produced by the ameloblast cells. **Tome's process**, a secretory surface of the ameloblast, is responsible for laying down the enamel matrix. Tome's process guides the enamel matrix into place. As the second layer is laid down, the first becomes more mineralized and this process follows until the last layer is placed.

Enamel rods under a microscope show several developmental identification marks. The **lines of Retzius**- (**RET**zee-us) appear as incremental lines or bands around the layers, much like the growth rings on a tree. Very few lines are indicated prenatally, but one, known as the **neonatal line**, an accentuated incremental line, indicates the trauma of birth. It is found in all the primary teeth and several of the permanent teeth. Along with the lines of Retzius are the **imbrication lines**, slight ridges on the cervical third of certain teeth that extend mesiodistally, and the **perikymata** (pear-ee-**KIGH**-mah-tah), small grooves noted on some teeth.

Short, dentinal tubules that seem to have crossed over into the enamel and were trapped there during the process of enamel mineralization are called **enamel spindles**. Noted with bases near the dentinoenamel junction are the **enamel tufts**. They appear as small, dark brushes. Narrower and longer enamel tufts are called **enamel lamellae**. These thin structures extend from the dentinoenamel junction to the enamel surface.

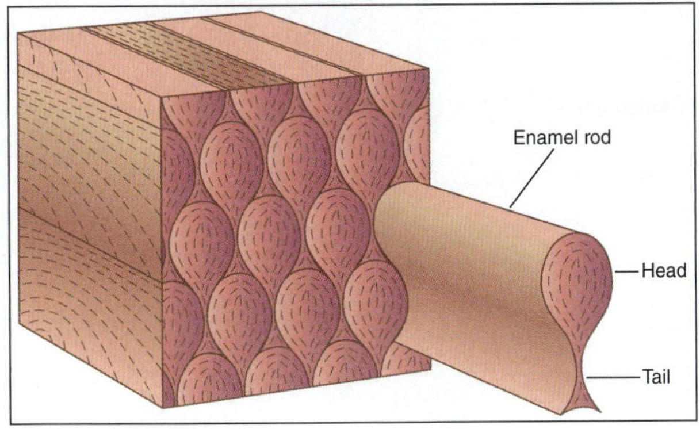

FIGURE 8-14

Drawing representing the enamel rods.

Clinical Considerations Regarding Enamel

- Primary teeth may erupt with a covering over the enamel that is left over from the epithelium and the ameloblasts, called the **Nasmyth's membrane**. Nasmyth's membrane may absorb stain easily. This membrane is easily removed by a thorough polishing. No lasting effects on the condition of the enamel are observed following removal of the membrane.
- Certain developmental disturbances can occur during the apposition stage. A loss of nutritional support may result in the surface of the teeth becoming grooved and pitted, called **enamel dysplasia**. The patient may be concerned with the appearance of the tooth, and the weakened surface is more susceptible to decay. With today's dental materials, the surface of the tooth can be restored.
- Fluoride can aid in strengthening the enamel to prevent demineralization. Fluoride can be ingested or applied topically.
- Dentists prepare the teeth for the placement of restorations in a manner in which isolated enamel rods are protected from fracture.

Dentin

Mature dentin is softer than enamel but harder than cementum and bone. If the dentin is exposed, it appears yellowish white. It is what gives the translucent enamel its underlying yellow hue. The cuspid is a bulky tooth with a greater amount of dentin; therefore, it appears more yellow than the teeth surrounding it. Dentin is less dense and appears rougher in surface texture than enamel. The odontoblasts form dentin, beginning at the dentinoenamel junction and continuing toward the pulp chamber. The long tubes that pass through the entire surface of the dentin are called **dentinal tubules** and contain the **dentinal fluid**, which is presumably tissue fluid surrounding the cell membrane of the odontoblast.

As with enamel, developmental marks are apparent in the dentin. **Imbrication lines of Von Ebner** are the stained growth rings or incremental lines in dentin. Contour lines that demonstrate a disturbance in the body metabolism are called **contour lines of Owen**. Again, the most pronounced stained contour line is the neonatal line that occurs due to the trauma of birth.

Types of Dentin. Dentin differs from area to area and is not uniform throughout. *Peritubular dentin* is the dentin that creates the wall of the dentinal tubule. Dentin found between the tubules is called *intertubular dentin*. The first predentin that is formed and matures within the tooth is called *mantle dentin*. The layer of dentin that surrounds the pulp is called *circumpulpal dentin*. Forming the bulk of the tooth is *primary dentin*, which is formed before the completion of the apical foramen (opening of the root's pulp canal). *Secondary dentin* forms after the completion of the apical foramen and slowly throughout the life of the tooth. Due to continued growth, the pulp chamber narrows and may become calcified later in life. *Tertiary dentin* repairs and is reactive to irritations. It forms quickly in response to localized injury. Injury may be caused by dental caries, cavity preparation, recession, attrition, or erosion. Tertiary dentin may be more irregular than primary or secondary dentin.

Clinical Considerations Regarding Dentin

- If the antibiotic tetracycline is taken during the formation of dentin, it binds chemically to the dentin and causes permanent yellow staining.
- Cavities that appear small on the outside of the tooth extend more rapidly through the dentin because its density is lower than enamel.
- Patients may experience **dentinal hypersensitivity** if the dentin is exposed. This may be very painful for the patient. In some individuals, the enamel and cementum do not come together at the cementoenamel junction (CEJ), leaving exposed dentin. Using the air-water syringe in an area that is not anesthetized causes discomfort.

Pulp

The pulp of the tooth evolves from cells similar to the dentin. Its function is to provide nourishment, support, and maintenance for the dentin. Also, when the dentin or pulp is injured, sensory nerves send the messages to the brain for interpretation. The pulp identifies the temperature and chemical changes, vibrations, and bacterial invasion of the tooth and transmits this information to the brain. It is a warning system that works as a defense system for the tooth.

The pulp is made partially from **fibroblasts** (cells from which connective tissue evolve), which synthesize protein fibers and **intercellular substances** (substances between the cells) to form pulp tissue. The pulp is fed continually through the opening at the apex of the root, the apical foramen.

Clinical Considerations Regarding Pulp

- If the pulp is damaged due to an injury, the tissue may become inflamed, causing **pulpitis.** The pressure increases and cannot escape. The structures of the tooth form a hard encasement and, when the tooth becomes inflamed, cause a great deal of pressure and discomfort. The patient may need to have root canal therapy, which opens the pulp and releases the pressure.
- If endodontic treatment (root canal therapy) is performed on a tooth, the pulp tissue is removed and the tooth becomes nonvital.
- The use of water-cooled handpieces prevents overheating of the pulp during dental treatment.
- **Pulp stones,** calcified masses of dentin, are sometimes found in the pulp tissue. They can be attached or unattached to the pulpal wall. They are quite common and normally cause a problem only if root canal therapy is necessary.

Components of the Periodontium

The **periodontium** consists of portions of the tooth structure that support hard and soft dental tissues and the alveolar bone. The cementum is part of the periodontium as well as the last tooth structure.

Cementum

Surrounding the root of the tooth, attaching it to the alveolar bone by anchoring the periodontal ligaments, is the cementum (Figure 8-15). It is a dull light yellow, lighter than dentin and darker than enamel. It is softer than both dentin and enamel and has a grainy feel. Cementum continues to develop throughout life, similar to dentin and pulp. Cementum is formed by cementoblasts and is thicker at the apex than elsewhere. Cementum does not resorb and regenerate like bone, which allows orthodontic treatment to move the teeth through the bone and not destroy the cementum. The cells that resorb cementum are called **cementoclasts.** Within the outer part of the cementum are collagen fibers from the periodontal ligament, called **Sharpey's fibers** (Figure 8-16). They act as anchors between the alveolar bone and the tooth.

Clinical Concerns Regarding Cementum

- In the case of gingival recession, the cementum may become exposed. The cementum is very thin at the cementoenamel junction (CEJ) and can quickly wear away. This exposes the dentin and causes pain.
- **Cemental spurs** are found near the CEJ. During dental cleaning (scaling and curettage), the operator may find it difficult to differentiate cemental spurs from calculus. One difference is that the calculus is much easier to remove.
- If the tooth is traumatized due to force from the occlusal or incisal surface, a condition known as **hypercementosis** may take place. This causes a thickening of cementum around the apex, which may show on the x-ray as a mass at the apex.

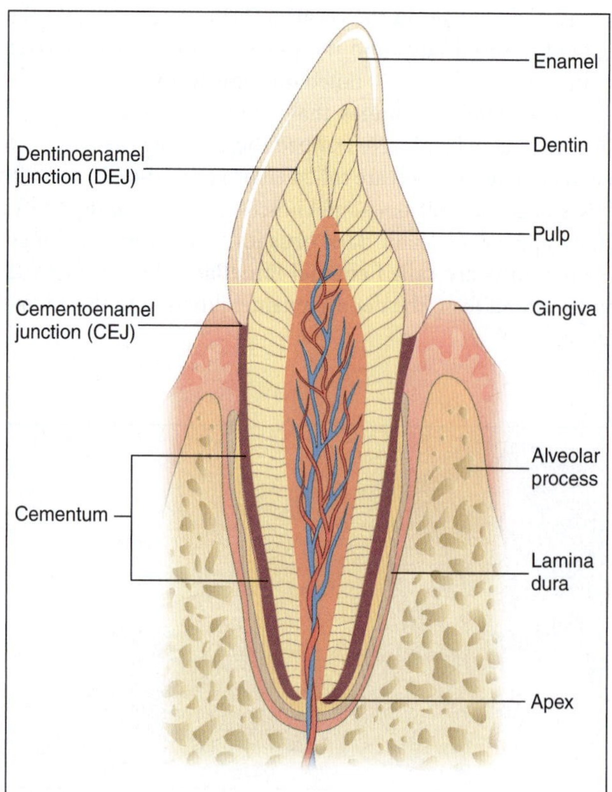

FIGURE 8-15
The tooth and surrounding tissues.

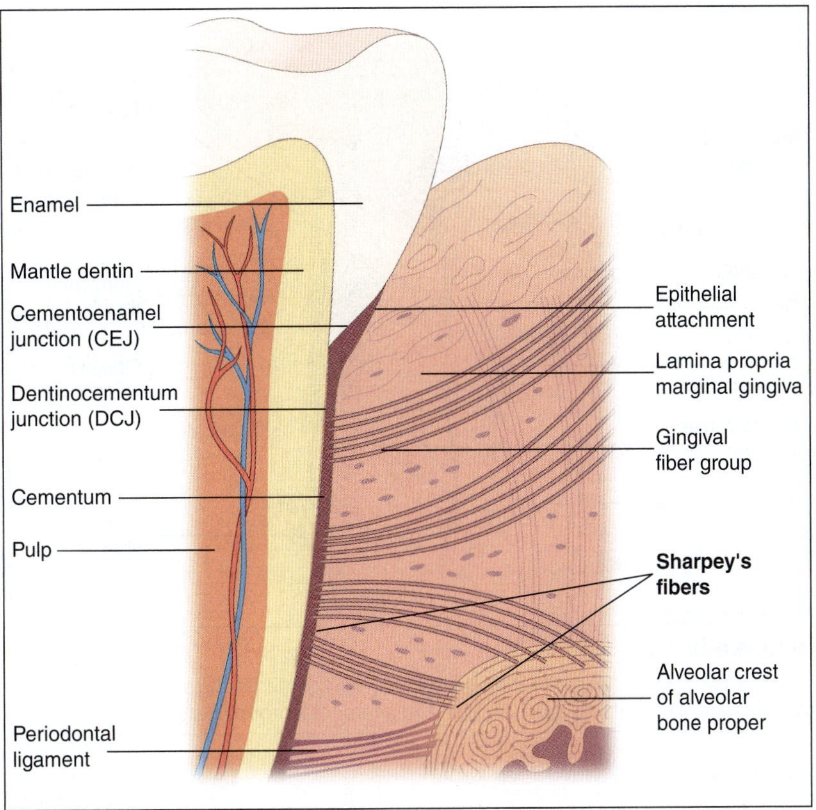

FIGURE 8-16

Section of tooth and tissue identifying Sharpey's fibers and cementum attachments.

Alveolar Bone

The bones of the mandible and maxilla are formed by *osteoblasts*, bone-forming cells. The cells that remodel and resorb bone are called *osteoclasts*. The extended areas of bone in each arch that are tooth bearing are called the **alveolar process**. The compact bone plates on the facial and lingual surfaces are called the **cortical bone**. The bone that surrounds the root of the tooth, the socket, is the **alveolus**. On a dental radiograph, the **lamina dura**, or radiopaque line, represents the thin, compact alveolus bone lining the socket. This alveolus does not actually contact the root because the periodontal ligament suspends it in place. The two cortical bone plates come together between each tooth. This is called the **alveolar crest** and should be slightly below the CEJ in a healthy mouth (Figure 8-17). If the tooth has multiple roots, the bone that separates the roots is identified as the **interradicular septum**. Each socket is separated by a bony projection called the **interdental** septum.

Periodontal Ligament

The **periodontal ligament**, like all connective tissue, is formed by the fibroblast cells and secures the tooth in the socket by a number of organized fiber groups. The Sharpey's fiber is attached in the cementum and to the alveolar bone. The periodontal ligament has two types of nerves: one sensory and one to regulate the blood vessels. This ligament is wider at the cervix (CEJ) and at the apex and narrow between these points.

Clinical Concerns Regarding the Alveolar Bone

- Periodontal disease can cause bone loss. The bone does not regenerate and the diseased tissue must be removed.
- The bone is stimulated from mastication and speech. If the teeth are removed, this stimulation is lost and the bone can resorb. The bone supports the teeth and the teeth support the bone.
- Modern implants placed in the bone are more successful if proper dental hygiene of the area is maintained. The implant has no movement in the bone; unlike teeth, it remains stable.

Periodontal Fiber Groups. Most of the fibers in the **periodontal fiber groups** are principal fibers, meaning they are organized into bundles or groups dependent on their functions. These fibers allow for some flexibility during mastication, speech, and other forces that would be exerted on the teeth. Six principal fiber groups consist of the five **alveolodental** (al-vee-oh-loh-**DENT**-al) **ligament fiber groups** and one interdental or transseptal ligament group

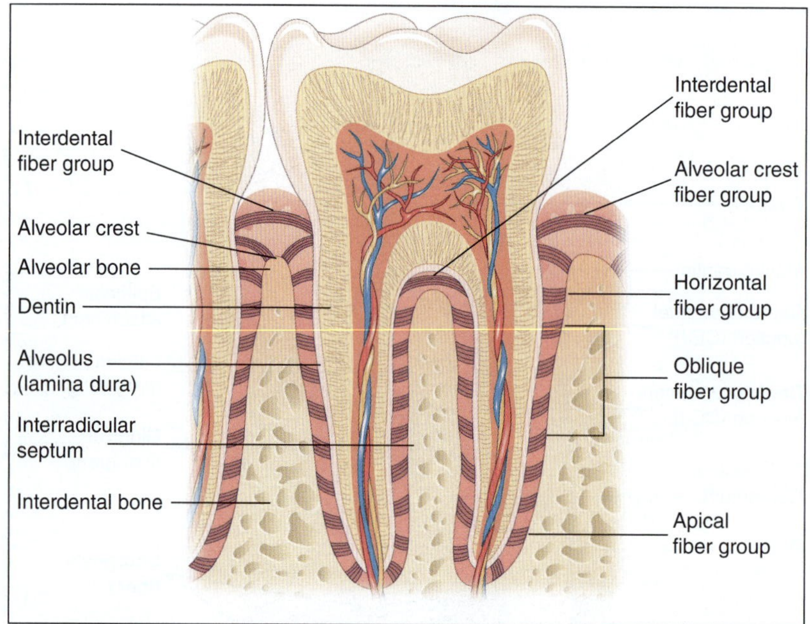

FIGURE 8-17

Section of a mandibular molar showing periodontal ligaments and alveolar crest, horizontal, oblique, apical, interradicular, and interdental group fibers.

(Figure 8-17). The alveolodental dental ligaments include the following:

- *Alveolar crest fiber groups* function to resist rotational forces and tilting. They originate in the alveolar crest of the alveolar bone and then insert into the cervical cementum at various angles.
- *Horizontal fiber groups* function in much the same manner as the alveolar crest fiber group. They are, however, in a different area. They originate in the alveolar bone, apical to the alveolar crest, and then insert into the cementum horizontally.
- *Oblique fiber groups* constitute the most abundant of the fiber groups. Their function is to resist intrusive forces that try to push the tooth inward. The oblique fiber group covers two-thirds of the root, attaching in the alveolar bone and extending in an oblique (diagonal) manner into the cementum.
- *Apical fiber groups* function to resist forces that try to pull the tooth outward, as well as rotational forces. They attach at the apex of the tooth and radiate outward to attach in the surrounding alveolar bone.
- *Interradicular fiber groups* are found only in multirooted teeth. Their function is to resist rotational forces and to hold the teeth in interproximal contact. They run from the cementum of one root to the cementum of the other root(s), over the interradicular septum.
- *Interdental (or transseptal) ligament groups* function to resist rotational forces and hold teeth in interproximal contact. They run above the crest of the alveolar bone interdentally, from the cervical cementum of one tooth to the cervical cementum of another tooth.

Clinical Considerations Regarding the Periodontal Ligaments

- Occlusal trauma does not cause periodontal disease but can accelerate an existing disease.
- Chronic periodontal disease causes the fiber groups to become disorganized and lose attachment due to resorption.
- The fiber group that is retained the longest during periodontal disease is the interdental ligament. As the disease progresses, this ligament reattaches itself in a more apical manner.

Gingival Fiber Groups. The **gingival fiber groups** are found in the **lamina propria**, the connective tissue of the marginal gingiva (Figure 8-18). They support the marginal gingival tissues in relationship to the tooth. They lie above the alveolar bone crest and below the epithelium.

- *Dentogingival fiber groups* act to maintain the gingival integrity of the marginal gingiva. They are attached to the cementum and extend into the lamina propria of the marginal gingiva.
- *Circular ligament fiber groups* circle and tighten the gingival margin around the neck of the tooth. This fiber group is in the lamina propria of the marginal gingival.
- *Alveologingival fiber groups* aid in attaching the gingiva to the alveolar bone. They extend from the alveolar bone and diffuse into the overlying lamina propria of the marginal gingiva.
- *Dentoperiosteal fiber groups* are supportive fibers that anchor the tooth to the bone. They originate from the cementum, near the CEJ, and extend across the alveolar crest.

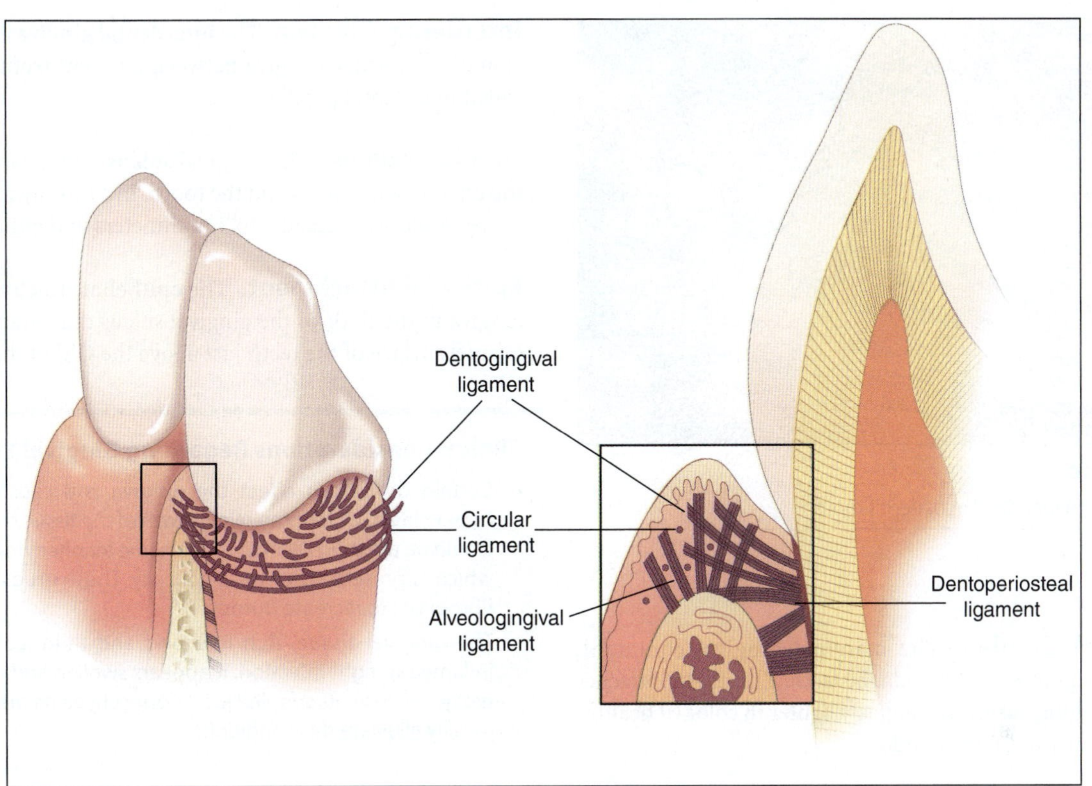

FIGURE 8-18

Gingival fiber groups: dentogingival, circular, alveologingival, and dentoperiosteal.

Gingiva

The **gingiva**, composed of a mucosa that surrounds the necks of the teeth and covers the alveolar processes, is commonly called the *gums*. It can be attached to the underlying bone or unattached (free) (Figures 8-19 and 8-20). (The plural of gingiva is *gingivae.*) The gingival tissue surrounds the teeth and, in a healthy state, is firm and tightly adapted to the tooth. The texture appears similar to the outside of an orange—**stippled**. The color of the gingiva may differ according to the pigmentation of the person.

Alveolar Mucosa. The **alveolar mucosa** appears thin and loosely attached, covering the alveolar bone. It flows into the tissue of the cheeks and lips and the inside floor of the mandible. It is found immediately apical to the mucogingival junction.

Mucogingival Junction. The **mucogingival junction** is the line of demarcation between the attached gingiva and the alveolar mucosa.

Attached Gingiva. The **attached gingiva** extends from the mucogingival junction to the gingival groove. The tissue is stippled and attached tightly to the alveolar bone.

Gingival Groove. The **gingival groove**, or free gingival groove, is the line of demarcation between the attached gingiva and the marginal gingiva.

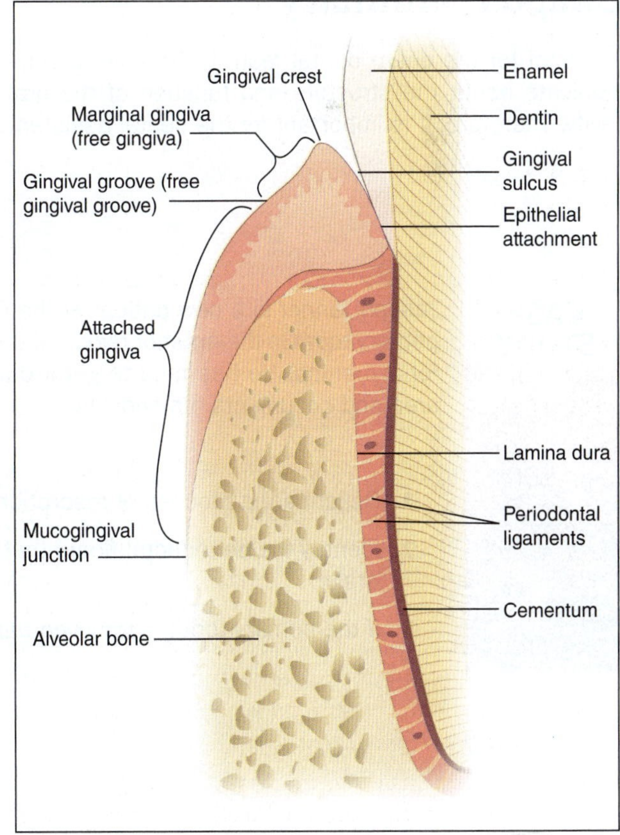

FIGURE 8-19

Periodontium.

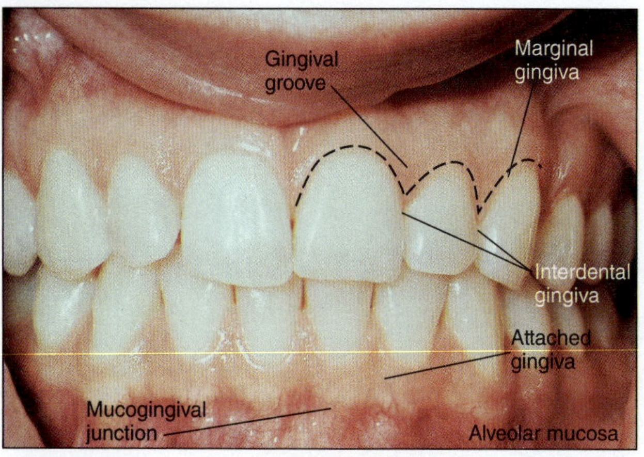

FIGURE 8-20
Periodontium identified in patient's mouth.

Marginal Gingiva. The marginal gingiva, commonly called **free gingiva**, surrounds the teeth. This tissue, attached only at the gingival groove, appears lighter in color (if healthy) and is about 1 millimeter wide.

Interdental Gingiva. The **interdental gingiva** is an extension of unattached gingiva between adjacent teeth. It is also called interdental papilla.

Gingival Sulcus. The **gingival sulcus** is the space between the unattached gingiva and the tooth. In a healthy mouth, this space would not exceed 2 to 3 millimeters in depth.

Epithelial Attachment. The **epithelial attachment** is the gingiva in the floor of the gingival sulcus that attaches to the enamel surface of the teeth just above the CEJ of the teeth.

Clinical Considerations Regarding Gingival Tissue

- Certain drugs can affect the gingiva and cause **gingival hyperplasia**, which is an overgrowth of the tissue. An example would be the drug Dilantin (trade name for phenytoin sodium), which is prescribed to treat epilepsy. These drugs cause the fibroblasts to increase output.
- The gingival tissue, rich in blood and fluid, can become inflamed to fight infection. It appears swollen and red, bleeds easily, and loses its stippled look. Correct hygiene measures can usually alleviate this condition.

Chapter Summary

It is vital for the entire dental team to be able to communicate about the structure and function of the oral cavity. Therefore, it is important for the dental assistant to understand the structure/function of tissue, the prenatal growth/development process of oral embryology, and the oral cavity that surrounds the teeth.

CASE STUDY

Joseph Tanner is a new patient at the Community Dental Clinic. He is a 6-year-old with a loose primary tooth in the anterior region of the mandible. He stated that the tooth has been "wiggling" for 2 months. He has tried to get it out but has been unsuccessful. The dentist examines the area and documents his findings.

Case Study Review

1. Describe the process of resorption of the root of the primary tooth.
2. Identify the periodontal fibers that may remain attached around the loose tooth at this stage.
3. If the primary tooth is removed early, what possible complications may occur?

Review Questions

Multiple Choice

1. The term used to identify the third prenatal phase of pregnancy from 9 weeks through birth is
   a. fetus.
   b. embryo.
   c. zygote.
   d. ovum.
2. The embryonic layer that differentiates into enamel and the lining of the oral cavity is the
   a. ectoderm.
   b. mesoderm.
   c. endoderm.
   d. stomodeum
3. Enamel-forming cells are called
   a. ameloblasts.
   b. odontoblasts.
   c. cementoblasts.
   d. fibroblasts.
4. An incremental line in the enamel indicating the trauma of birth, found in all primary teeth and several permanent teeth, is the
   a. line of Retzius.
   b. imbrication line.
   c. Tome's process.
   d. neonatal line.
5. The softest tooth structure is the
   a. alveolar bone.
   b. cementum.
   c. dentin.
   d. enamel.
6. The development of different tissues is
   a. cytodifferentiation.
   b. histodifferentiation.
   c. morphodifferentiation.
   d. proliferation.
7. The vertical groove on the midline of the upper lip is called the
   a. stomodeum.
   b. labial commissure.
   c. nasolacrimal groove.
   d. philtrum.
8. A tooth emerging from the gum is called
   a. eruption.
   b. attrition.
   c. apposition.
   d. proliferation.
9. The structure of the tooth that covers the outside of the crown is called the
   a. pulp.
   b. dentin.
   c. cementum.
   d. enamel.
10. Name the connective tissue that is formed by the fibroblast cells and secures the tooth into the socket by a number of organized fiber groups.
    a. Lamina dura
    b. Periodontal ligaments
    c. Gingiva
    d. Epithelial attachment

Critical Thinking

1. While in the hospital maternity ward, a dental assistant sees a newborn child with a severe unilateral cleft lip. Based on what the dental assistant knows about the probability of a child having this condition, what assumption would be made regarding the child's sex? What initial steps would be taken to help the baby and parents?
2. If a child has enamel dysplasia, a dental assistant would assume that a disturbance took place during which cycle of tooth development? Which stage?
3. If a calcified mass of dentin material is in the pulp chamber, what procedures can it inhibit? What are such masses called?

Web Activities

1. Go to http://www.operationsmile.org and read how many babies are born with cleft lips or cleft palates each year.
2. Search the Web to identify the dental specialty that would treat a child born with a cleft lip. Be prepared to discuss this in class.
3. Go to http://www.babycenter.com and compare fetal development at 4 weeks, 8 weeks, and 12 weeks.

CHAPTER 9

Tooth Morphology

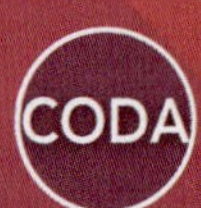

Specific Instructional Objectives

The student should strive to meet the following objectives and demonstrate an understanding of the facts and principles presented in this chapter:

1. Identify the dental arches and quadrants using the correct terminology.
2. List the primary and permanent teeth by name and location.
3. Explain the eruption schedule for the primary and permanent teeth.
4. Identify the different divisions of the tooth, including clinical and anatomical divisions.
5. Identify the surfaces of each tooth and their locations.
6. List the anatomical structures and their definitions.
7. Describe each permanent tooth according to location, anatomical features, morphology, function, position, and other identifying factors.
8. Describe each deciduous (primary) tooth according to its location, anatomical features, morphology, function, position, and other identifying factors.

Key Terms

agenesis (169)
anatomical crown (159)
anatomical root (160)
apex (162)
apical foramen (162)
apical third (161)
bicanineate (176)
bicuspids (157)
bifurcated (162)
buccal (161)
buccal groove (163)
canine (156)
canine eminence (169)
central incisor (156)
central groove (163)
cervical line (160)
cervical third (161)
cingulum (163)
clinical crown (159)
clinical root (160)
concave (161)
contact area (161)
convex (161)
crown (159)
cusp (163)
cusp of Carabelli (164)
deciduous (156)
dentition (155)
developmental groove (164)
diastema (161)
distal (160)
embrasure (161)
exfoliated (157)
facial (160)
fissure (164)
fossa (164)
furcation (164)
imbrication lines (168)
incisal edge (160)
incisal third (161)
interproximal (161)
labial (160)
lateral incisor (156)
lingual (160)
lobes (164)
mamelons (164)
mandibular arch (155)
marginal groove (165)
marginal ridges (165)
maxillary arch (155)
mesial (160)
middle third (161)
mixed dentition (157)
molars (156)
nonsuccedaneous (157)
oblique ridge (166)

(continues)

Key Terms (continued)

occlusal (161)
occlusal third (161)
peg lateral (169)
permanent teeth (156)
pit (166)
premolars (157)
primary teeth (156)
quadrants (155)
ridge (166)
root (159)
sextants (156)
succedaneous (157)
supplemental groove (166)
tooth morphology (155)
transverse ridge (166)
triangular ridge (166)
tricanineate (176)
trifurcated (166)

Introduction

Tooth morphology is the study of the structure and form of teeth. In this chapter, the morphology of the teeth is discussed, along with the location, eruption schedule, and function of each tooth in the primary and permanent dentition. The terms in this chapter are the building blocks of dental terminology used in the dental office.

Dental Arches

The **dentition** (natural teeth in position) are arranged in two arches. The upper arch is the **maxillary arch**, because the teeth are set in the maxilla bone. The lower teeth are located in the mandible bone, and therefore are located in the **mandibular arch** (Figure 9-1). The maxillary arch is fixed to the skull and the mandibular arch is movable, bringing the biting force toward the maxillary arch. Each arch has an identical number of teeth, and the teeth are designed so that proper function and positioning can be maintained. The teeth in the maxillary arch slightly overlap the mandibular teeth when in proper alignment. The teeth in each arch touch the teeth *adjacent* (next) to them, except for the last tooth in each arch. The teeth from the maxillary arch contact the teeth from the mandibular arch each time the mouth is closed. Each tooth supports the teeth beside it and the teeth in the opposing arch so that displacement does not occur.

Dental Quadrants

Each of the dental arches is divided in two halves by an imaginary line called the *midline* (median line), which creates two sections called **quadrants** (one-fourth of the dental arches). Thus, there are four quadrants, containing eight permanent teeth each, found in the dentition. The arrangement of the teeth is identical in each quadrant, and each quadrant is named according to its location in the dentition (Figure 9-2).

The quadrants are labeled according to the patient's right or left. Looking into the oral cavity from the front of the

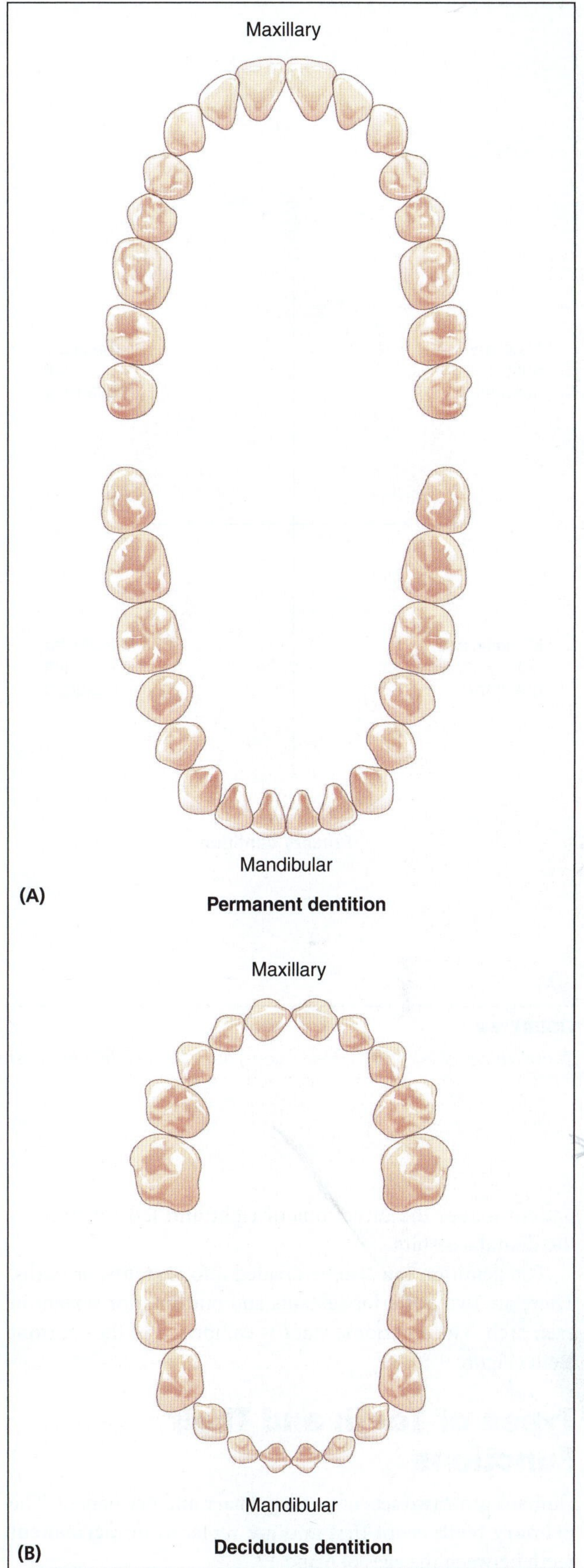

FIGURE 9-1
(A) Maxillary and mandibular dentition of an adult (permanent dentition). (B) Maxillary and mandibular dentition of a child (deciduous dentition).

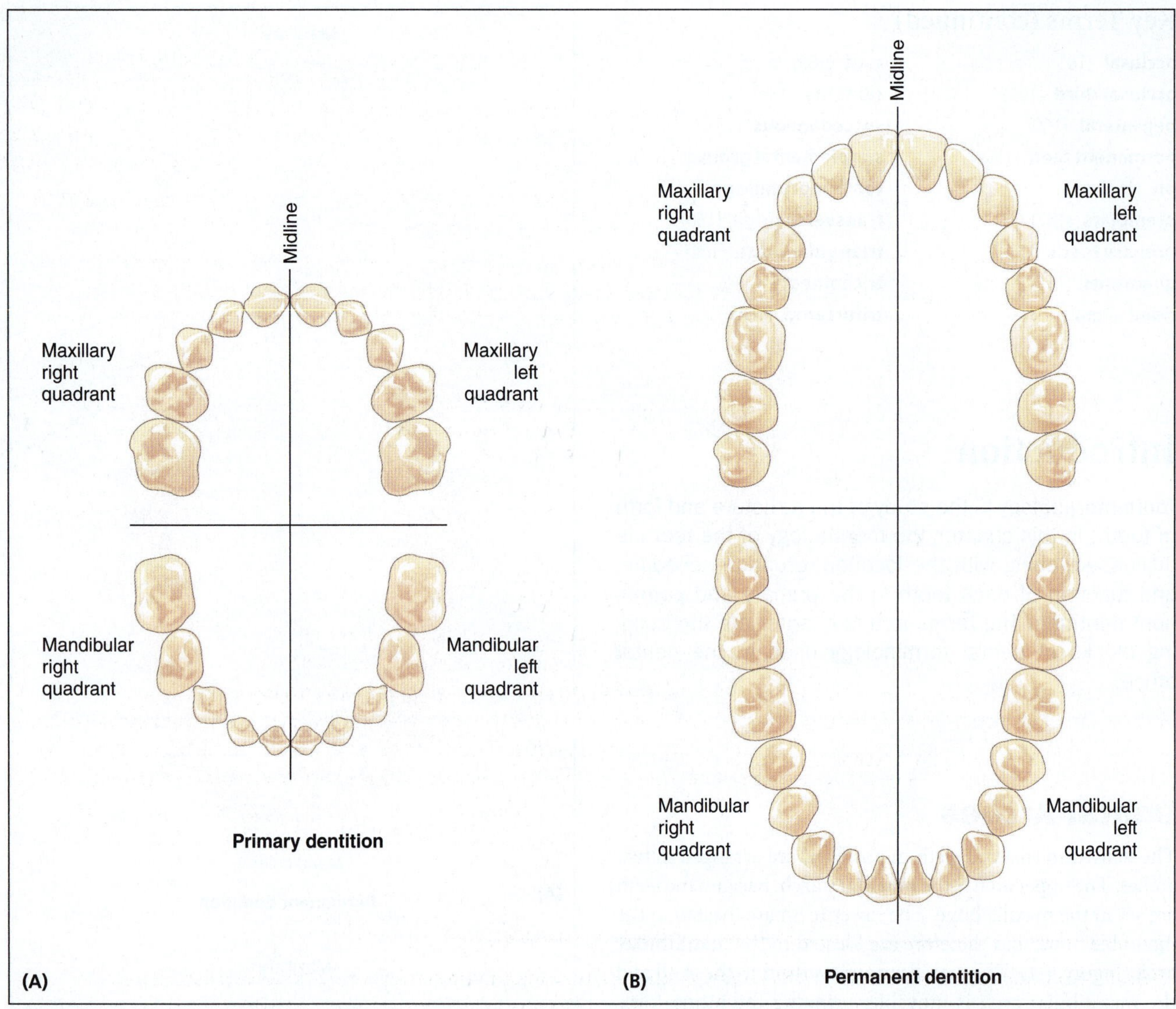

FIGURE 9-2
Dental arches of (A) primary (deciduous) dentition and (B) permanent dentition divided into quadrants with the midline identified.

patient makes the directions of right and left reversed to the dental assistant.

The dentition can also be divided into **sextants**, or sixths. There are two posterior sextants and one anterior sextant in each arch. The anterior sextant is comprised of the six front teeth (Figure 9-3).

Types of Teeth and Their Functions

Humans grow two sets of teeth: primary and permanent. The **primary teeth** erupt first and are replaced by **permanent teeth** between the ages of 6 and 17.

Primary Teeth

The primary (**deciduous** [di-**SI**-jeh-wus]) teeth in each quadrant are named similar to the permanent teeth. The deciduous (i.e., first) dentition consists of 20 teeth: 10 in each arch and 5 in each quadrant. The following teeth are found in each quadrant: Starting from the midline, the first tooth is called the **central incisor** and is used to cut or bite the food that is ingested. The second tooth from the midline, the **lateral incisor**, is also used for cutting. The third tooth from the midline is the **canine** (cuspid). This tooth is slightly bulkier in size and aids in tearing food. The next two teeth are **molars** and are named the first molar, which

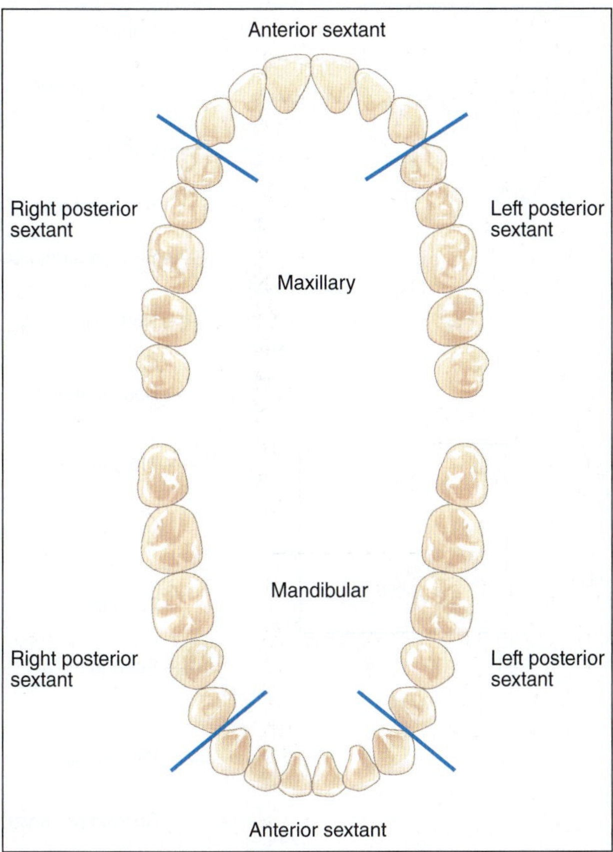

FIGURE 9-3

Permanent dentition divided into sextants. The maxillary and mandibular arches each have two posterior sextants and one anterior sextant.

is the one closest to the midline, and the second molar. Molars are used to chew food.

Both the first and the second primary teeth from the midline are incisors; to incise something is to cut it.

When compared to the permanent dentition, the deciduous dentition contains an identical number of central incisors, lateral incisors, and canines, but has no premolars and one less molar per quadrant (Figure 9-4).

Permanent Teeth

Permanent teeth are arranged similarly to the deciduous teeth. Adults have 32 permanent teeth: 16 in each arch and 8 in each quadrant. Each quadrant has the permanent central incisor, the lateral incisor, and the canine (cuspid), as did the deciduous quadrant. Directly after the canine (cuspid) in the permanent dentition are the first and second **premolars**.

The premolars are often called **bicuspids** because they usually have two (bi) *cusps* (pointed or rounded mounds on the crown of the tooth). However, two of the eight bicuspids may have three cusps; therefore, the term *bicuspid* is not technically correct. However, it is important to be aware of the names commonly used for the same teeth (for example, canines or cuspids and premolars or bicuspids).

The premolars are used to pulverize food. In other words, the premolars break the food down into smaller sizes to ready them for the chewing process, which is performed by the molars.

After the premolars, the permanent dentition has the first, second, and third molars. The first molars are closest to the midline, and the third molars—which are farthest from the midline—are commonly termed the "wisdom teeth."

The teeth in either arch that are toward the front of the mouth from cuspid to cuspid are the *anterior* teeth. The central incisors, lateral incisors, and canines (cuspids) are termed anterior teeth for both the deciduous and permanent dentition. Anterior teeth have single roots and a cutting or tearing edge called the *incisal edge.*

The teeth in either arch that are located in the back of the mouth are termed *posterior* teeth. The molars are posterior teeth in the deciduous dentition, and the premolars (bicuspids) and molars are posterior teeth in the permanent dentition. Posterior teeth normally have more than one root and multiple cusps for pulverizing and chewing.

Eruption Schedule

The primary dentition (deciduous teeth) begins eruption (emerges into the oral cavity) around 6 months of age. All 20 teeth are normally erupted by the age of 3 years (Table 9-1). The period when both primary teeth and permanent teeth are in the dentition is called the **mixed dentition** period (Figure 9-5). This period lasts from approximately 6 to 12 years of age. After the age of 12, most of the primary teeth have **exfoliated** (shed from the oral cavity). The permanent dentition begins to erupt from about 6 years of age until around 17 to 21 years of age (Table 9-2).

The permanent teeth that replace the primary teeth are called **succedaneous** teeth (Figure 9-6). The term refers to succeeding the deciduous teeth. Therefore, because there are 20 primary teeth, there are also 20 succedaneous teeth. **Nonsuccedaneous** teeth pertain to the teeth that do not replace primary teeth. This would reference the molars in each quadrant. Therefore, there could be up to 12 nonsuccedaneous teeth in the permanent dentition. The premolars would replace the primary molars; therefore, they are succedaneous teeth.

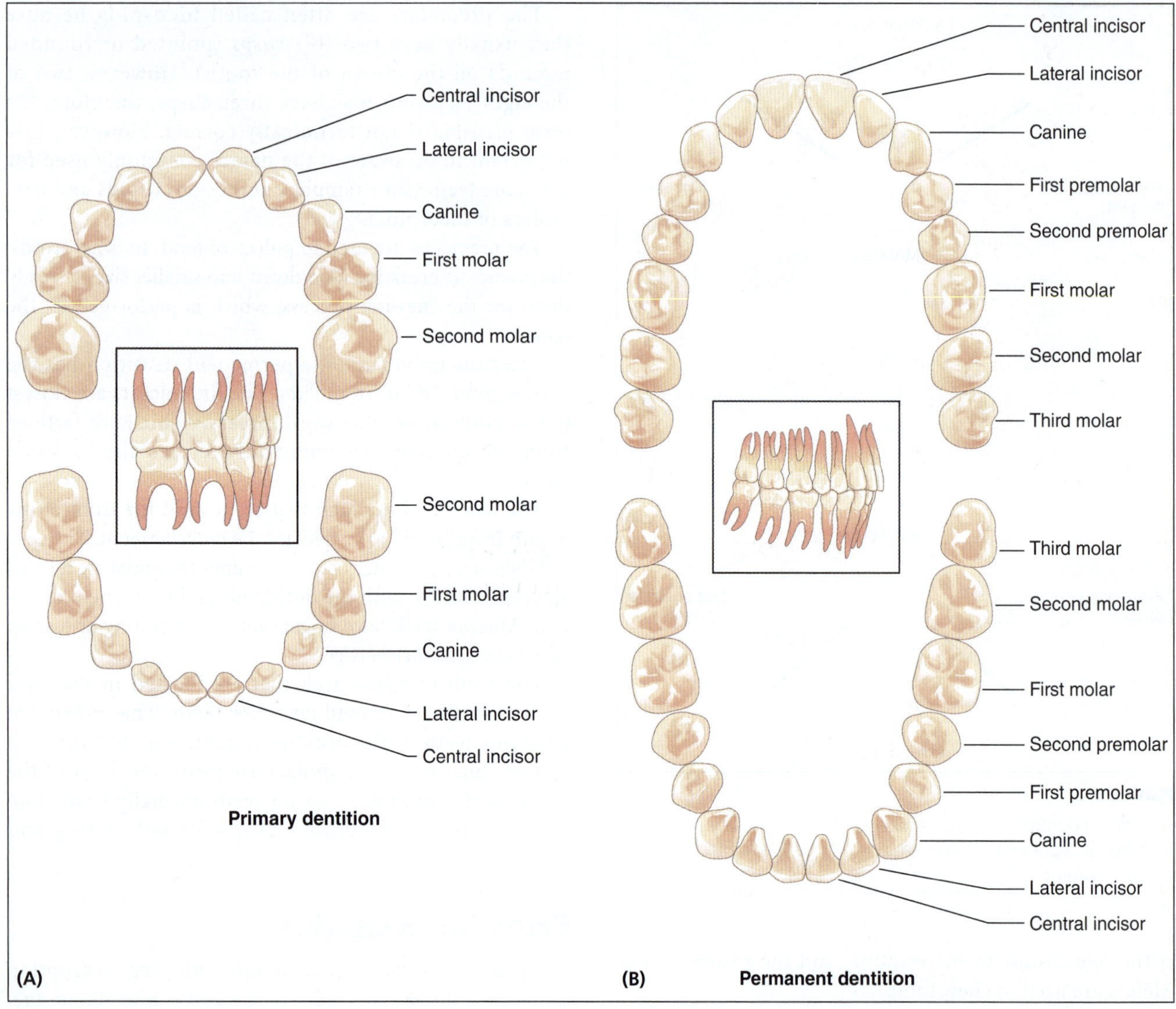

FIGURE 9-4
(A) Deciduous dentition, identifying each tooth by name. (B) Permanent dentition, identifying each tooth by name.

TABLE 9-1 Eruption and Exfoliation Dates for Primary Teeth

Tooth	Eruption Date (Months)	Exfoliation Date (Years)	Maxillary Order
Central incisor	6–10	6–7	#1
Lateral incisor	9–12	7–8	#2
Canine	16–22	10–12	#4
First molar	12–18	9–11	#3
Second molar	24–32	10–12	#5
Tooth	**Eruption Date (Months)**	**Exfoliation Date (Years)**	**Mandibular Order**
Central incisor	6–10	6–7	#1
Lateral incisor	7–10	7–8	#2
Canine	16–22	9–12	#4
First molar	12–18	9–11	#3
Second molar	20–32	10–12	#5

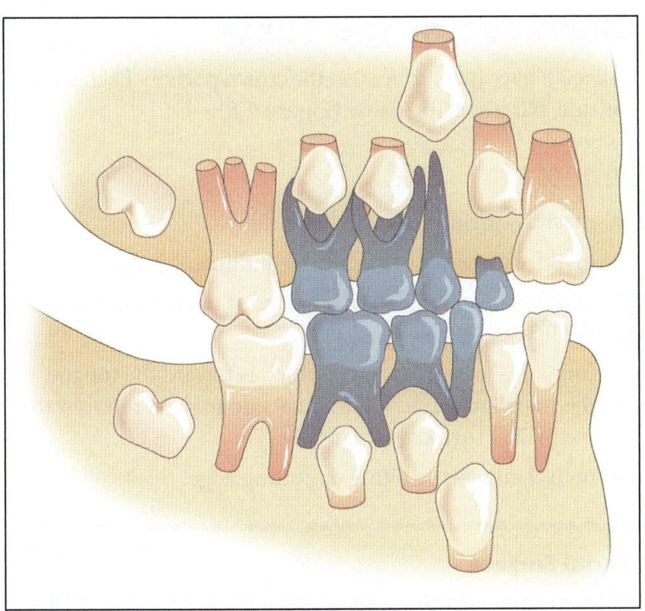

FIGURE 9-5

Mixed dentition of a 7- or 8-year-old.

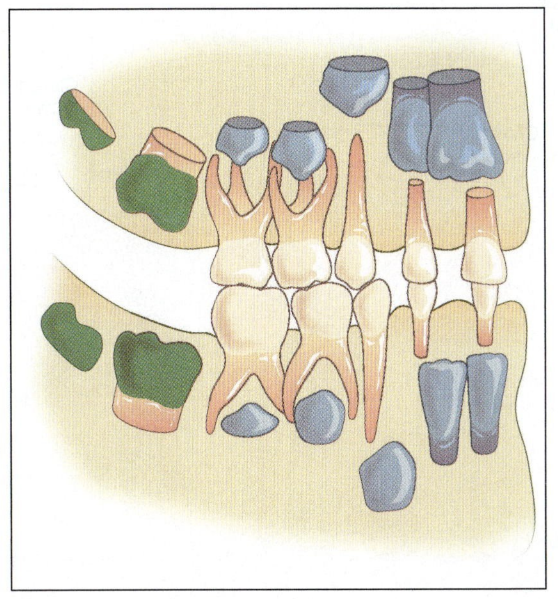

FIGURE 9-6

Mixed dentition of a 5-year-old. Unerupted succedaneous teeth are shaded in blue, nonsuccedaneous teeth are shaded in green.

TABLE 9-2 Eruption Dates for the Maxillary and Mandibular Permanent Teeth

Tooth	Eruption Date (Years)	Order of Eruption (Maxillary)
Central incisor	7–8	#2
Lateral incisor	8–9	#3
Canine	11–12	#6
First premolar	10–11	#4
Second premolar	11–12	#5
First molar	6–7	#1
Second molar	12–13	#7
Third molar	17–21	#8
Tooth	**Eruption Date (Years)**	**Order of Eruption (Mandibular)**
Central incisor	6–7	#2
Lateral incisor	7–8	#3
Cuspid	9–10	#4
First premolar	10–11	#5
Second premolar	11–12	#6
First molar	6–7	#1
Second molar	11–13	#7
Third molar	17–21	#8

Divisions of the Tooth

Each tooth has two basic parts: the **crown** and the **root**. The crown of the tooth is described as either anatomical or clinical (Figure 9-7). The **anatomical crown** is the portion of the tooth that is covered with enamel. The **clinical crown** is the portion of the crown that is visible in the mouth. The clinical crown may be smaller than the anatomical crown if the gingiva covers a portion of the crown (for example, during tooth

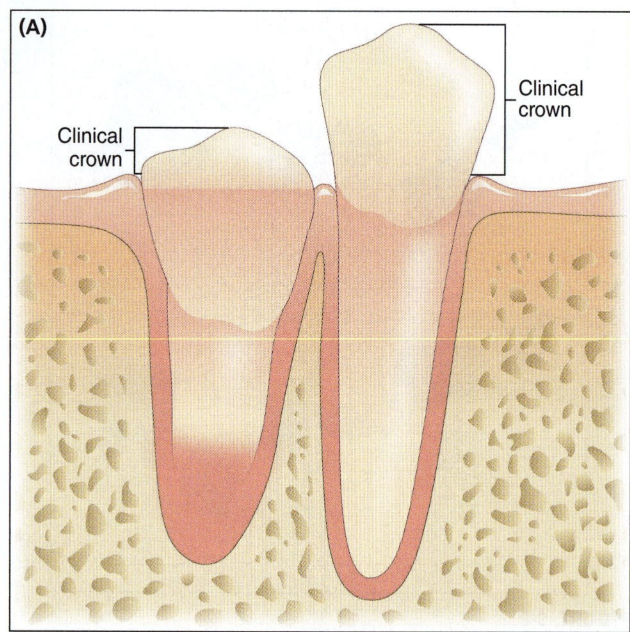

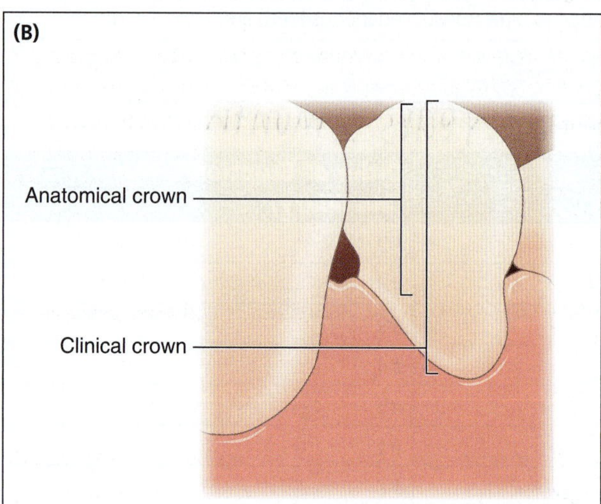

FIGURE 9-7

(A) Clinical crown shown on a partially erupted tooth and an erupted tooth. (B) Comparison of anatomical crown to clinical crown on mandibular left first bicuspid that has gingival recession.

eruption). The root of the tooth is also divided into anatomical and clinical portions. The **anatomical root** is the portion covered with cementum, and the **clinical root** is the portion of the root seen in the oral cavity (for example, where the gingiva has receded). It should be noted that often when referring to periodontics or coronal polishing the operator may refer to the clinical crown length as both the crown portion and the root portion exposed in the oral cavity. See Chapter 31, Periodontics. The **cervical line** divides the crown and the root; the anatomical crown and the root join together here as well. (Cervical comes from the word *cervix*, meaning "the neck of.") The cervical line is also termed the cementoenamel junction (CEJ).

Surfaces of the Teeth

All teeth have five surfaces on the crown portion. Each surface, or side, has a specific name (Figure 9-8).

Anterior Teeth

- **mesial**—surface toward the midline.
- **distal**—surface away from the midline.
- **labial**—"outside" surface on anterior teeth, which is toward the lips.
- **lingual**—"inside" surface, which is toward the tongue. On the maxillary arch, the lingual side may be referred to as the palatal surface.
- **incisal edge**—the biting or cutting edge.

Facial Surface

The term **facial** may be used for either the labial surface of the anterior teeth or the buccal surface of the posterior teeth.

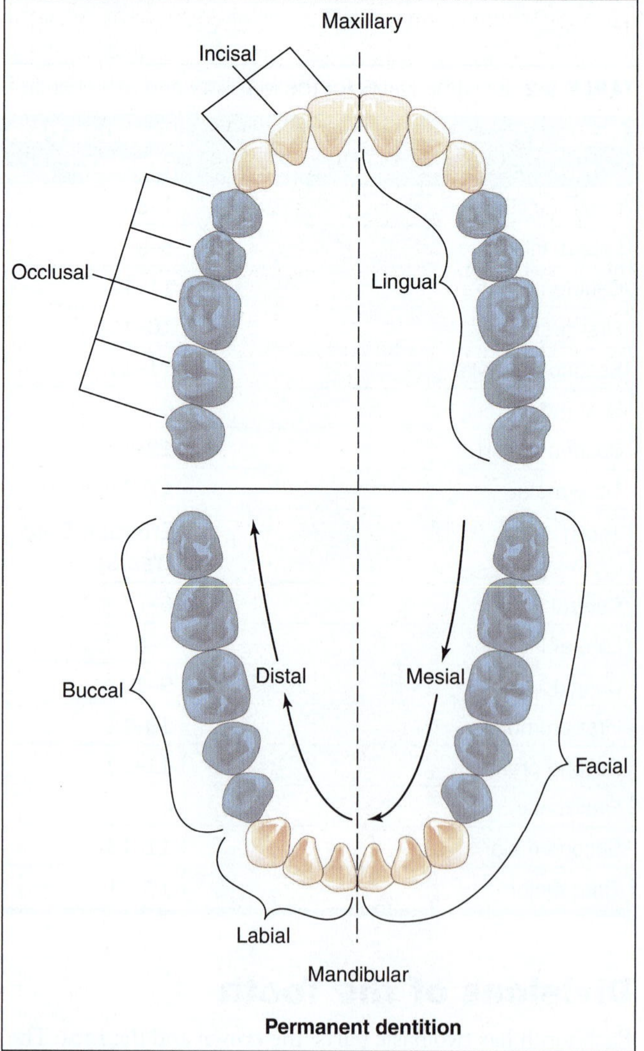

FIGURE 9-8

Surfaces of the teeth identified on the dental arches in a permanent dentition. Posterior teeth colored in blue.

Posterior Teeth

- mesial—surface toward the midline.
- distal—surface away from the midline.
- lingual—"inside" surface, which is toward the tongue.
- **buccal**—"outside" surface on posterior teeth, which is toward the cheek.
- **occlusal**—pulverizing or chewing surface.

All of the above tooth surfaces are flat, convex, or concave (Figure 9-9). **Convex** means to bulge or curve outward, and **concave** means recessed or indented. (A memory cue is to think of a "cave" in concave; a cave is hollow and not bulging outward.)

Tooth Surfaces Divided into Thirds

Tooth surfaces are further identified by dividing them into approximate thirds. This practice helps dental staff in identifying specific areas on each surface. Also identified are the spaces between the teeth and where the teeth are touching.

The crown of the tooth and the root of the tooth are divided in approximate thirds (Figure 9-10). The area on the crown of the tooth that is nearest the incisal edge on the anterior tooth is called the **incisal third** of the tooth, and the occlusal surface of the posterior tooth is called the **occlusal third** of the tooth. The area on the crown of the tooth that is closest to the cervical area (or to the gingiva) is called the **cervical third** of the tooth. The area between the incisal third and the cervical third is called the **middle third**. The root is also divided into imaginary thirds with the area nearest the apex as the **apical third** and the area nearest the crown of the tooth as the cervical third of the root. The area between the apical third of the root and the cervical third of the root is called the middle third of the root.

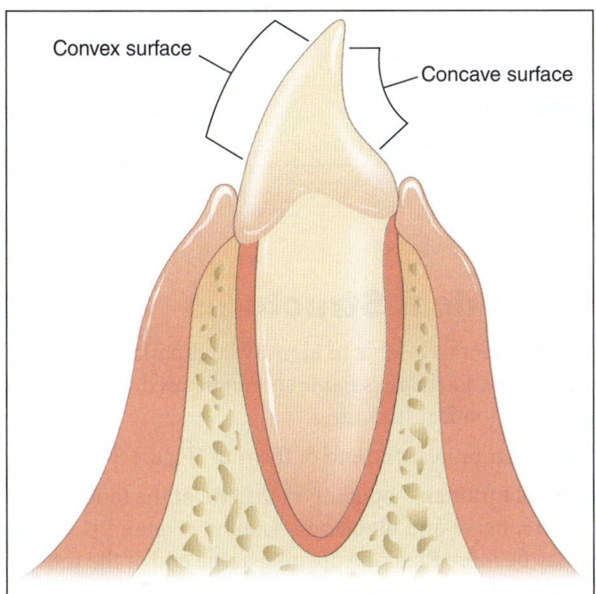

FIGURE 9-9
Concave and convex surfaces of the mandibular incisor.

Identifying these areas allows the dentist to give clearer information about a tooth. For instance, if the dentist is describing the shade of the tooth to the dental laboratory technician, the dentist can say that the incisal third is a lighter shade and the cervical third is a darker shade. This information enables better color matching, thereby preventing creation of a single-color tooth. Another example is when the dentist describes a lesion on the root of the tooth, noting that it is on the apical third of the root. These terms also facilitate better diagnosis through greater specificity in identifying the location on the root. All such terms are used frequently in the dental office to identify a specific area of the tooth.

Contact

Identifying the **contact area** on the tooth refers to where the proximal sides of two teeth come together and touch (Figure 9-11). This is normally the mesial of one tooth and the distal of another tooth, except where the two central incisors come together in each arch. This area is generally in the middle third of the tooth, and is also the area that dental floss tends to snap through. Such contact holds teeth in place so that they do not drift and shift around. Where the two proximal surfaces contact and the area where an individual flosses is called the **interproximal** (in between proximal surfaces). It should also be noted that food that remains caught in the teeth after eating is common in places where teeth do not contact. Good contact areas protect the gingiva from trauma during mastication (chewing food).

Embrasure

The **embrasure** (im-*bray*-zhur) is the triangular space in the gingival direction when two adjacent teeth are in contact (Figure 9-11). When discussing flossing with patients, the dental assistant will show the patient how to hold the floss and guide it through the contact area and make a half circle and wrap the floss tightly around the tooth as it goes down the embrasure toward the gingival sulcus of the tooth. The floss is then wrapped around the proximal tooth on the other side of the embrasure, and this area is cleaned with the dental floss as well. The embrasure allows the dental papilla to remain healthy.

Diastema

A **diastema** (plural *diastemata*) is a space or gap between teeth. Many animals, such as deer, have diastemata between incisors and the molars. In humans, the term *diastema* is most often used in reference to the "front teeth" maxillary central incisors (Figure 9-12). In some cases, the frenum attachment is removed at a young age or prior to orthodontics to allow this space to be closed. It can also be closed with cosmetic dentistry by veneers or composite restorations being done on the adjacent teeth. Treatment is at the desire of the patient. Many well known people have a diastema,

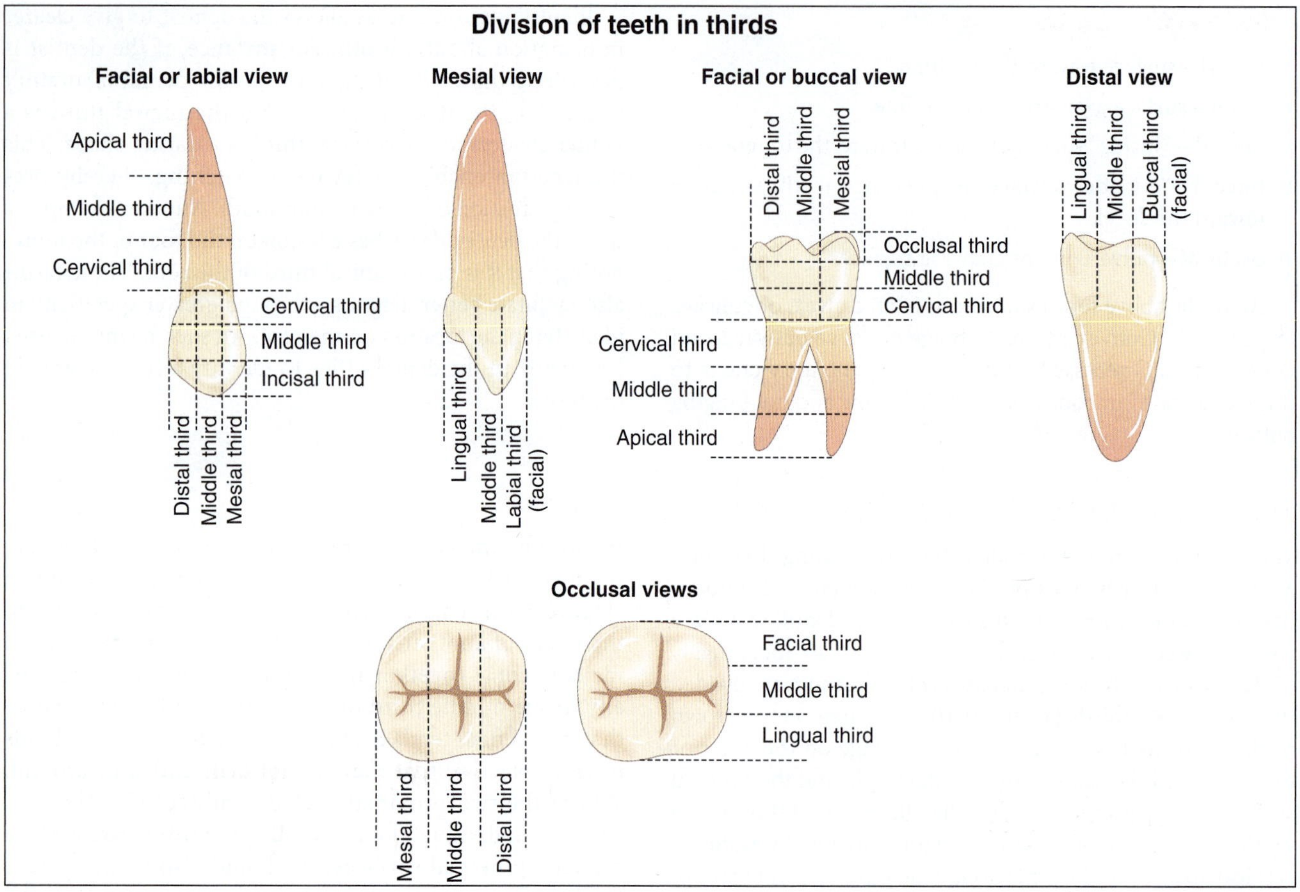

FIGURE 9-10

The crown and the root is divided into proximal thirds from all surfaces.

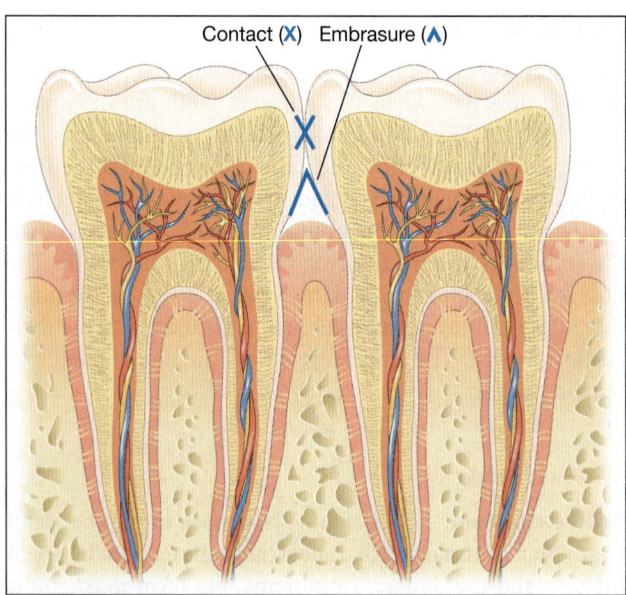

FIGURE 9-11

Contact area and embrasure shown on two adjacent teeth.

such as: Condoleezza Rice (former U.S. secretary of state), Jorja Fox (CSI star), David Letterman (late-night talk-show host), and singers such as Madonna and Elton John.

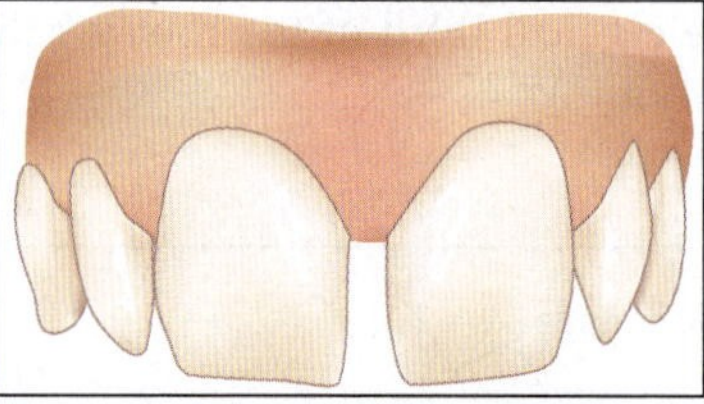

FIGURE 9-12

Diastema shown between maxillary central incisors.

Anatomical Structures

It is important to be able to identify landmarks on each individual tooth. Each area's name should be used when identifying the anatomical structures.

- **apex**—at or near the end of the root (Figure 9-13).
- **apical foramen**—opening in the end of the tooth through which nerve and blood vessels enter (Figure 9-13). There may be more than one opening at the end of the root.
- **bifurcated**—when there are two roots on one tooth, they are said to be bifurcated, or branched in two (*bi* means two and *furca* means fork) (Figure 9-14).

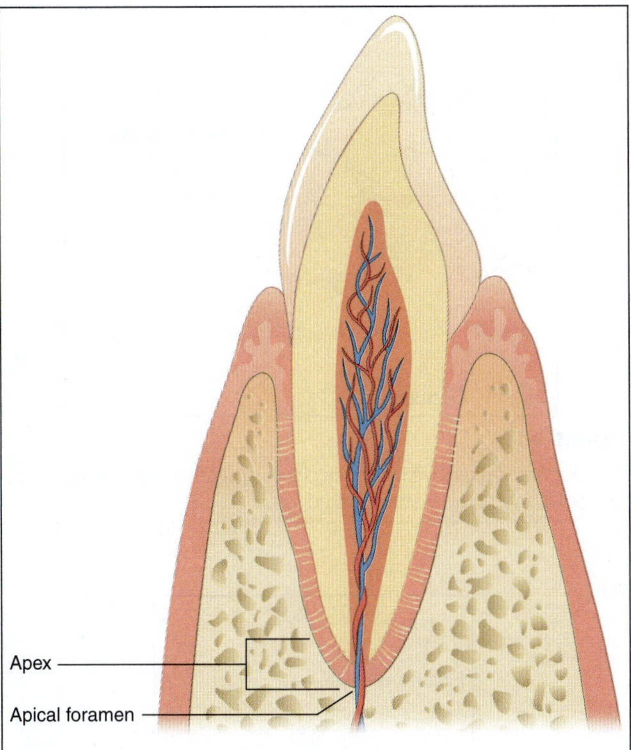

FIGURE 9-13
Apex and apical foramen of a tooth.

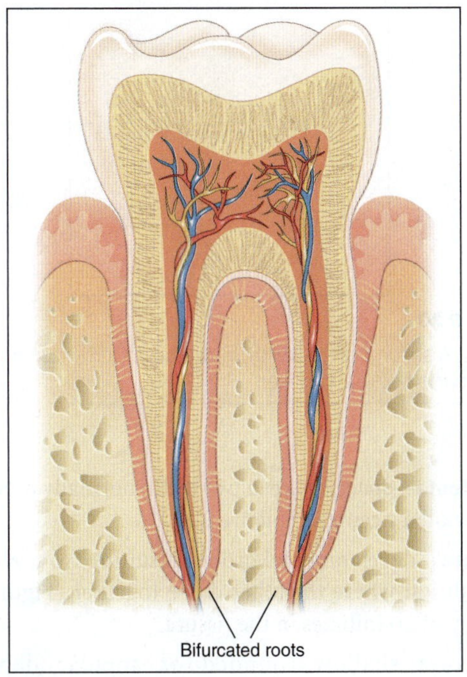

FIGURE 9-14
Mandibular molar showing bifurcated roots.

- **buccal groove**—linear depression forming a groove that extends from the middle of the buccal surface to the occlusal surface of the tooth (Figure 9-15).
- **central groove**—the most prominent developmental groove on the occlusal surface of the posterior teeth. It usually divides the occlusal surface from the medial to the distal.
- **cingulum**—convex area on the lingual surface of the anterior teeth, near the gingiva (Figure 9-16).
- **cusp**—pointed or rounded mound on the crown of the tooth (Figure 9-17).

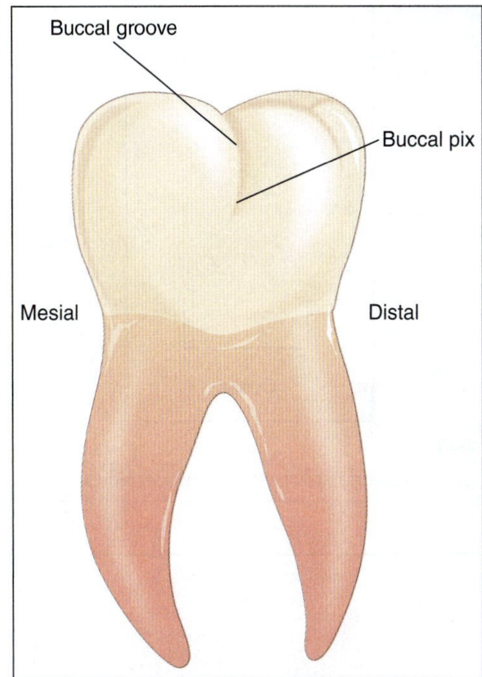

FIGURE 9-15
Mandibular molar with buccal groove identified.

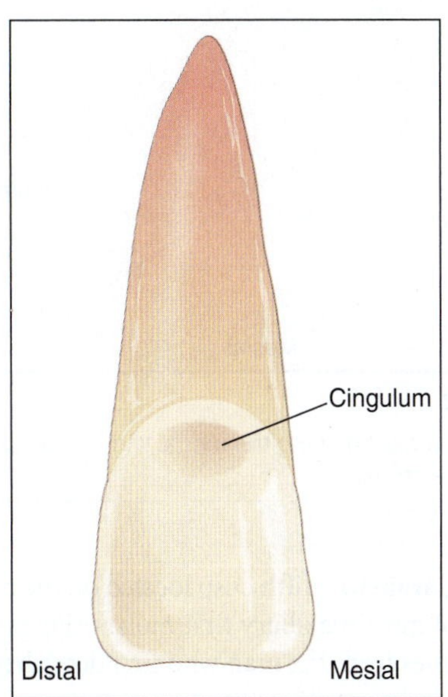

FIGURE 9-16
Lingual surface of a central incisor with the cingulum shaded.

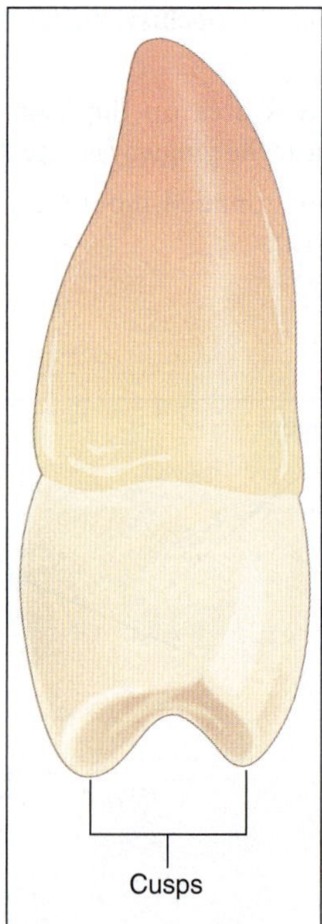

FIGURE 9-17

Maxillary second premolar with the cusps identified.

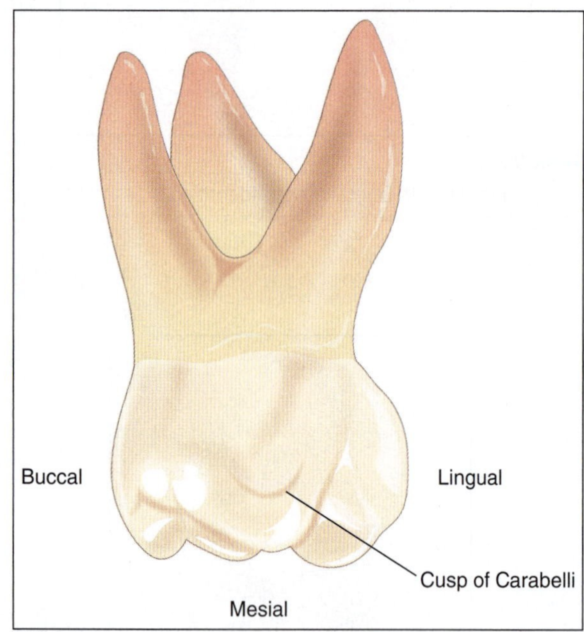

FIGURE 9-18

Maxillary first molar showing the mesial lingual side with the cusp of Carabelli identified.

- **cusp of Carabelli**—fifth cusp located on the mesial lingual surface of most maxillary first molars (Figure 9-18). (The name comes from the man who first described it.)
- **developmental groove**—groove formed by the uniting of lobes during development of the crown of the tooth (Figure 9-19).

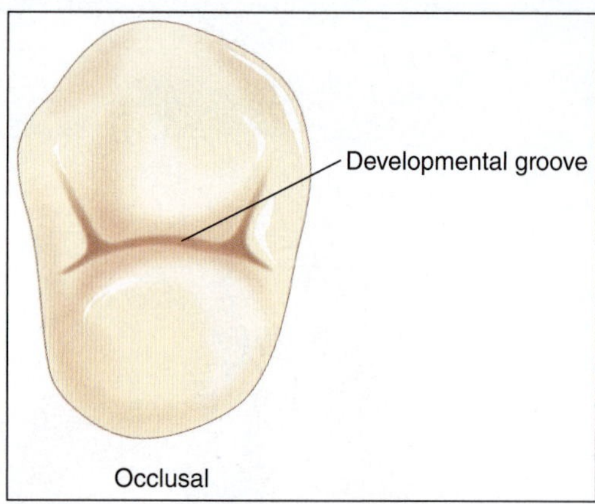

FIGURE 9-19

Developmental groove on the occlusal surface of the maxillary first premolar where lobes were united.

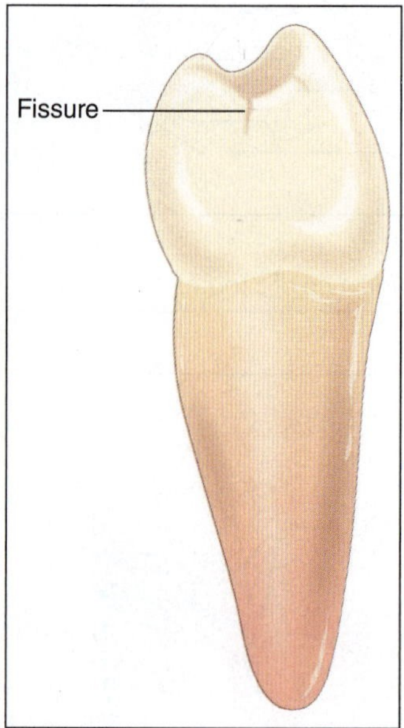

FIGURE 9-20

Mandibular second premolar showing the imperfect union or fissure on the occlusal surface.

- **diastema**—space between two teeth, normally in reference to maxillary centrals (Figure 9-12).
- **fissure**—developmental groove resulting from an imperfect union where the lobes come together (Figure 9-20). Decay often initiates in the fissure.
- **fossa**—a shallow rounded or angular depression (Figure 9-21).
- **furcation**—dividing point of a multirooted tooth (Figure 9-22).
- **lobes**—separate parts that come together to form a tooth (Figure 9-23). In the molars, the lobes often become cusps.
- **mamelons**—three bulges on the incisal edge of the newly erupted central and lateral incisor (Figure 9-24). Mamelons normally disappear due to normal wear.

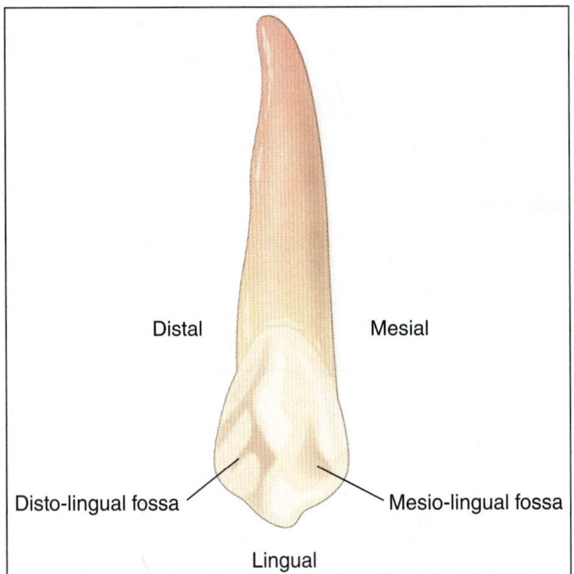

FIGURE 9-21

Lingual view of a maxillary canine with the mesio-lingual fossa and disto-lingual fossa shaded.

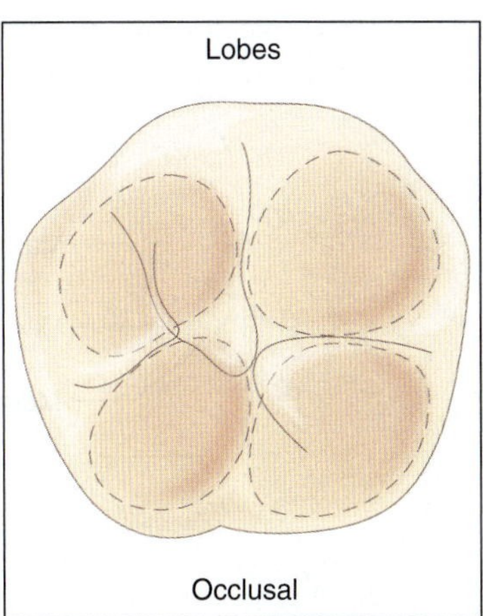

FIGURE 9-23

Occlusal view of the maxillary first molar showing the lobes and how they come together.

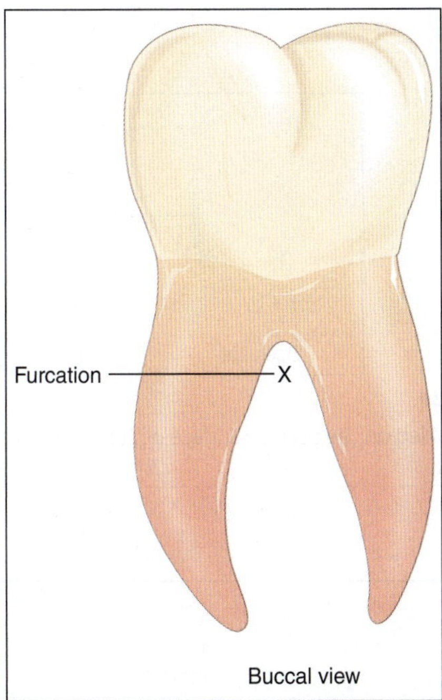

FIGURE 9-22

Mandibular first molar from the buccal side showing the furcation or dividing area where the roots fork off.

(A)

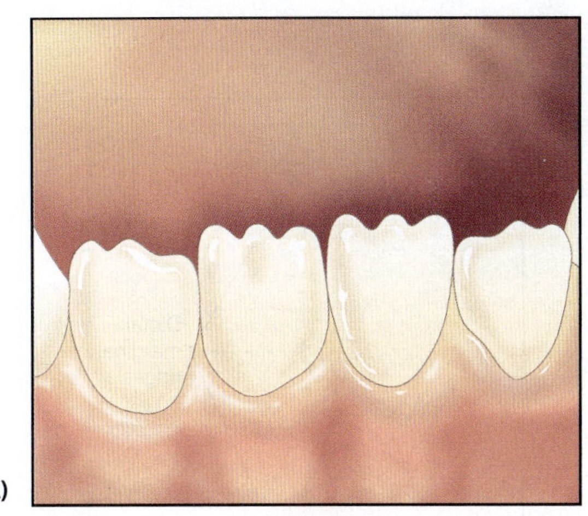

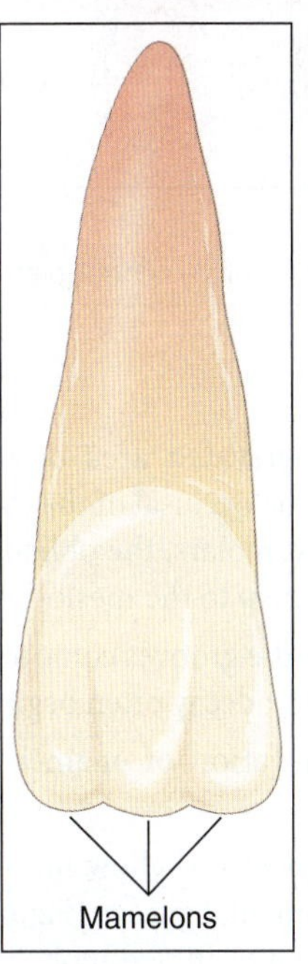

(B)

FIGURE 9-24

(A) Newly erupted maxillary incisors and laterals showing the three bulges on the incisal edge, called mamelons. (B) Mamelons shown on the anterior of the maxillary dentition.

- **marginal groove**—the developmental groove that provides a spillway for food to escape during chewing. (Figure 9-25).
- **marginal ridges**—elevated area of enamel that forms the mesial and distal borders of the lingual surface of the anterior teeth and the mesial and distal borders of the occlusal surface of the posterior teeth (Figure 9-26).

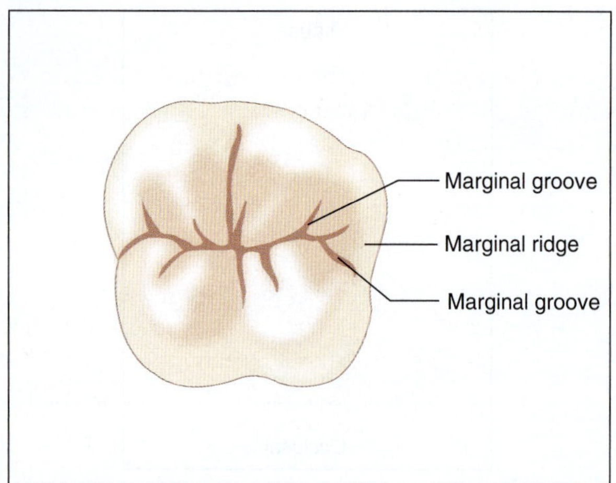

FIGURE 9-25
Mandibular first molar showing the marginal ridge and two marginal grooves.

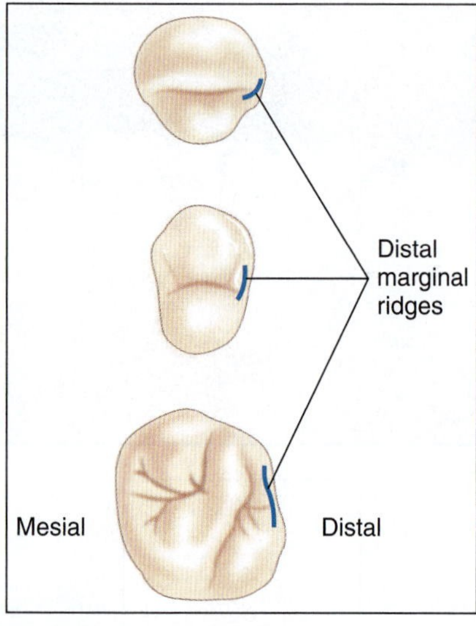

FIGURE 9-26
Marginal ridges of the maxillary central, premolar, and molar.

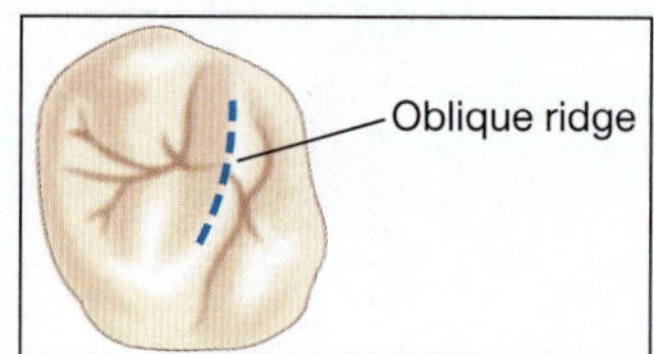

FIGURE 9-27
Maxillary first molar with the oblique ridge identified.

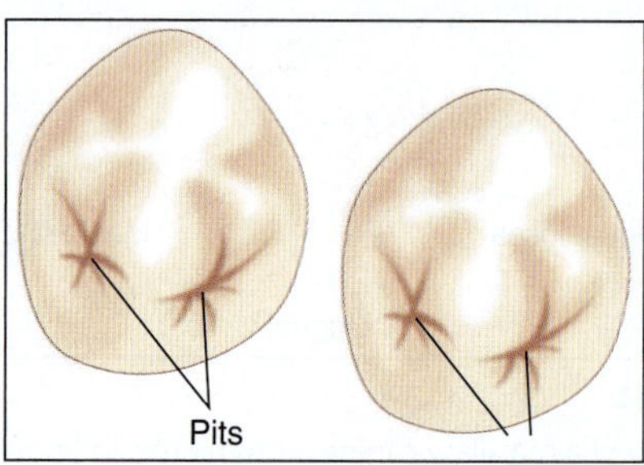

FIGURE 9-28
Permanent mandibular first premolar showing the occlusal view with pits identified.

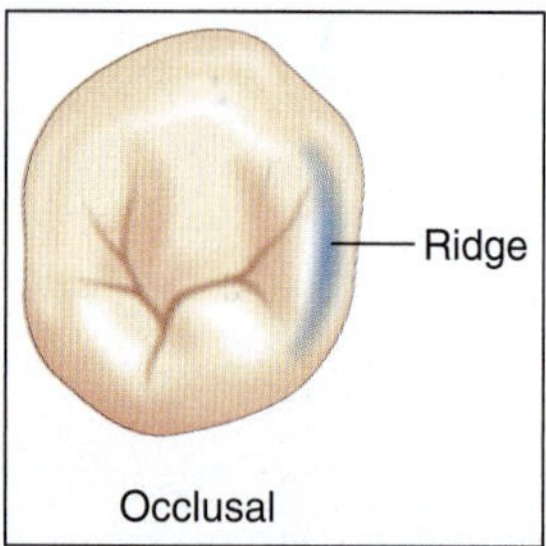

FIGURE 9-29
Ridge identified on the occlusal surface of the mandibular second premolar.

- **oblique ridge**—elevated area of enamel that extends obliquely across the occlusal of the tooth (Figure 9-27); on the maxillary first molars, the oblique ridge extends from the disto-buccal cusp to the mesio-lingual cusp.
- **pit**—place where the grooves come together or the fissures cross (Figure 9-28); decay often begins in the pit.
- **ridge**—linear elevation of enamel found on the tooth (Figure 9-29).
- **supplemental groove**—shallow, linear groove that radiates from the developmental groove (Figure 9-30); it often gives the tooth surface a wrinkled look. These grooves do not denote major divisions of the tooth.
- **transverse ridge**—union of two triangular ridges that produces a single ridge of elevation across the occlusal surface of a posterior tooth (Figure 9-31).

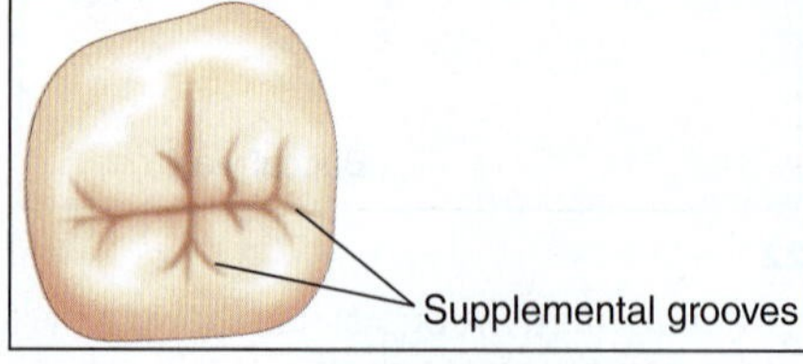

FIGURE 9-30
Occlusal surface of the mandibular second molar showing shallow linear grooves, which are called supplemental grooves.

- **triangular ridge**—ridge or an elevation that descends from the cusp and widens as it runs down to the middle area of the occlusal surface (Figure 9-32).
- **trifurcated**—three roots (*tri* means three) coming from the main trunk of the tooth (Figure 9-33).

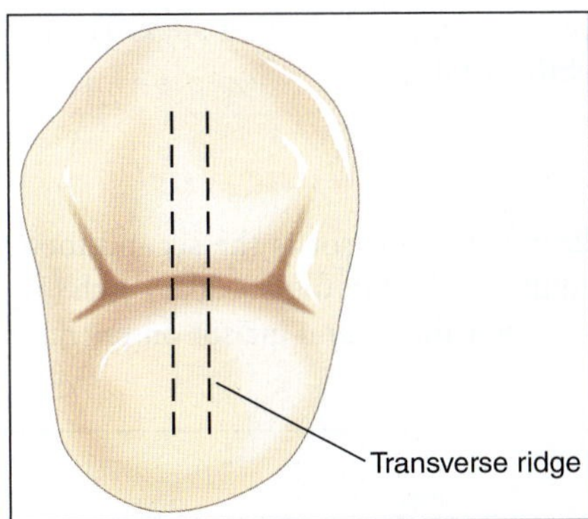

FIGURE 9-31

Maxillary right first premolar occlusal view showing transverse ridge.

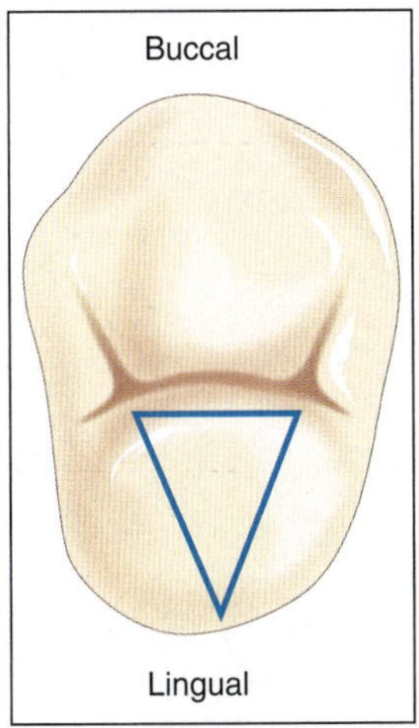

FIGURE 9-32

Triangular ridge identified on occlusal surface of a maxillary second premolar.

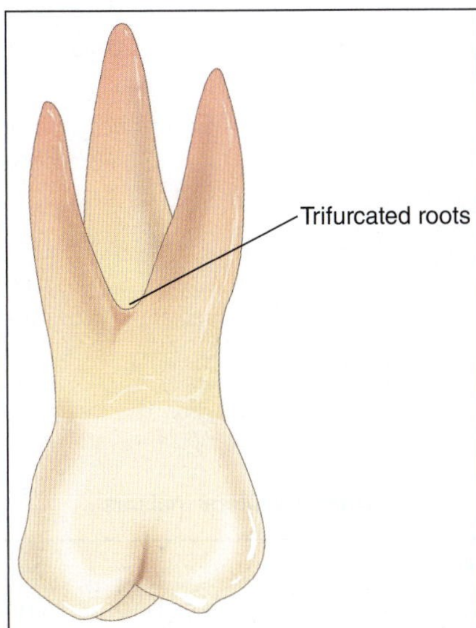

FIGURE 9-33

Maxillary first molar, buccal surface, showing the roots as trifurcated (three roots forked off from the main trunk).

Permanent Teeth

Each type of tooth in the permanent dentition serves a specific function, and the size and shape of the tooth are related to that function. A working knowledge of each type of tooth is useful for the dental assistant.

Maxillary Central Incisor

The maxillary central incisor is the first tooth closest to the midline (Figure 9-34). These teeth, along with the lateral incisors, play an important part in a person's appearance. Their

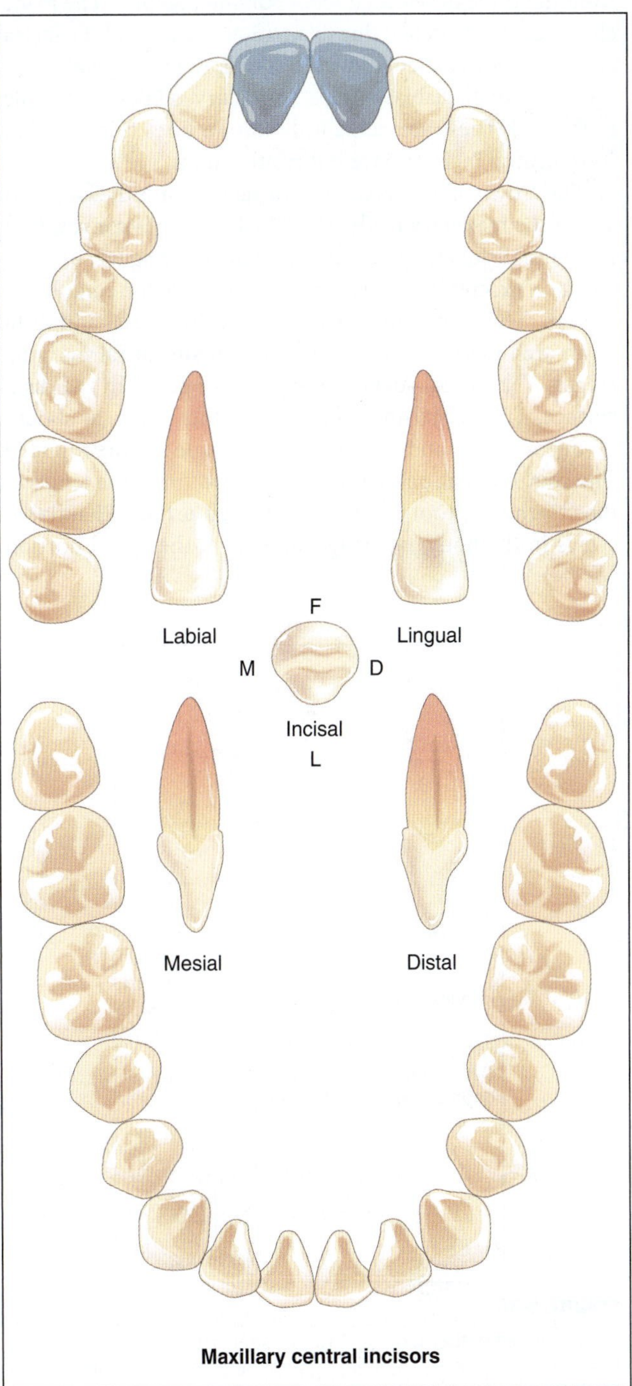

FIGURE 9-34

Permanent dentition with the maxillary central incisors identified and maxillary central incisor viewed from the five surfaces.

shape, color, size, and placement directly relate to how a person looks. The position of the teeth dictates the shape of a person's profile. Normal placement will provide for correct support of the face and lips. The incisors also play an important role in speech. To execute specific sounds, such as *Ss* and *Ts*, these teeth are necessary. Additionally, the incisors have a unique incisal edge that differs greatly from the other teeth in the mouth, which all have cusps. The ridge allows for cutting food into smaller particles.

The maxillary central incisor erupts with three bumps on the incisal edge, called mamelons (Figure 9-35). They derive from the three developing lobes coming together. The mamelons become flattened due to attrition (wear), and the incisal edge becomes a flattened surface as well. At the gingival area of the crown on the labial surface, small curved lines run parallel to the CEJ. These are called **imbrication lines** (Figure 9-35). Most central incisors have imbrication lines.

The crown of the maxillary central incisor is the longest of any of the maxillary teeth. The labial surface is convex, both mesial to distal and gingival to incisal. The lingual surface is concave, except the gingival one-third where the cingulum is present. The cingulum spreads toward the mesial and distal in an arch pattern, forming the mesial and distal marginal ridges. The mesial surface is slightly longer than the distal surface. The mesial-incisal angle is rather acute, at about a 90-degree angle, and the distal-incisal angle is more rounded. The root is about one-and-a-half to two times the length of the crown. The root appears constricted at the CEJ and then swells in the body, tapering suddenly at the apical portion. Therefore, it ends in a rather blunt apex. The root tends to incline slightly distally.

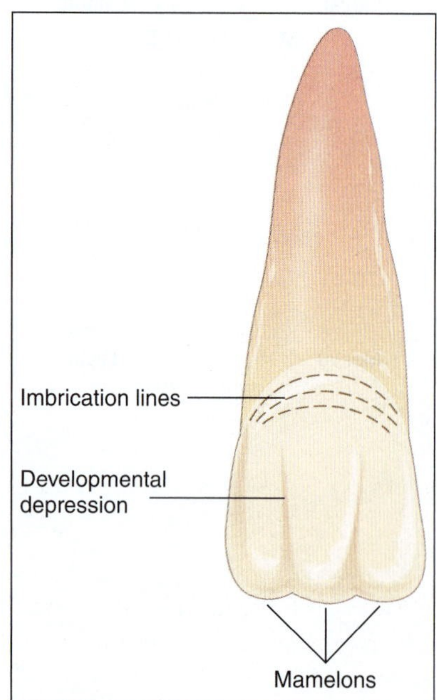

FIGURE 9-35

Labial surface of the maxillary right central incisor with the mamelons, developmental depressions, and imbrication lines identified.

Maxillary Lateral Incisor

The maxillary lateral incisor is the second tooth from the midline and the smallest in the maxillary arch (Figure 9-36). It initially contacts the central incisor on the mesial and the

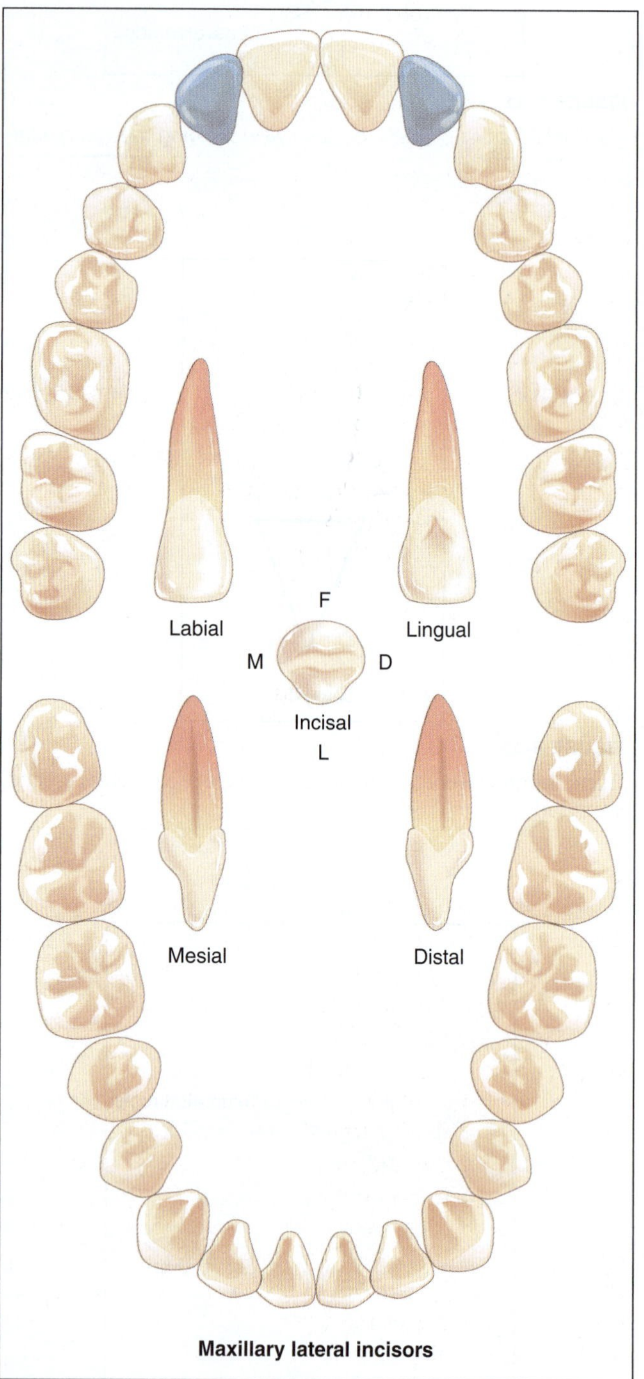

FIGURE 9-36

Permanent dentition with maxillary lateral incisors identified and maxillary lateral incisor viewed from the five surfaces.

primary canine (cuspid) on the distal. It resembles the maxillary central in most ways. The difference is primarily its size, the crown being about three-tenths smaller in all directions. The root also is smaller in all directions; however, the length has been known to be similar to that of the maxillary central. The crown of the lateral incisor appears narrower than the central, especially in females. The distal-incisal angle is more rounded than that of the central incisor, making the distal length much shorter than the mesial length.

Except for the third molars, the maxillary lateral is the tooth with the most *anomalies* (extreme variations from the norm). The most frequent is the **peg lateral**. This is a diminutive, peg-shaped crown with a smooth surface lacking contact on the mesial and distal surfaces. Maxillary laterals are sometimes congenitally missing. When the tooth buds do not form **agenesis** occurs. Roots that are curved in unusual ways and distorted crowns may appear. Many of these deviations appear generation after generation.

Maxillary Canine (Cuspid)

The canine is often called the "cornerstone of the mouth" due to its placement, which is between the incisors and the bicuspids (Figure 9-37). It is the one tooth that turns the corner for the arch. The canine's purpose is to tear the food, which is much different from the incisors, which bite or cut the food, and the premolars and molars, which chew or grind it.

The canine (cuspid) is one of the most important teeth for animals, because it tears the food. The term *canine* is derived from the Latin term for dog *(canus)*. The canines (cuspids) look much like dog's teeth and therefore are named as canines.

The canine (cuspid) is the third tooth from the midline. Because of its placement and size, it is extremely important in supporting the muscles of the face. This is due to a bony ridge covering the labial portion of the roots called a **canine eminence**, which gives the face a cosmetic manifestation and contributes to a person's appearance.

The root is the longest in the maxillary arch and therefore the most stable. The crown of the canine is convex on the facial surface, with a ridge running vertically. The incisal edge is fairly pointed and is off center, slightly toward the mesial (the name *cuspid* is derived from the long cusp that ends in a point on the incisal edge). The mesial surface of the canine (cuspid) is longer than the distal surface, and as they both turn toward the incisal edge, the angle is more rounded than that of the incisors. The lingual surface has two concave fossas, one toward the mesial and the other toward the distal, with a lingual ridge dividing them in the middle. On the outer sides of the fossa is a distal marginal ridge and a mesial marginal ridge (Figure 9-38A). On the lingual side of the tooth, toward the gingiva, is a cingulum (Figure 9-38B). The canine appears darker than the incisors because of the bulk of dentin.

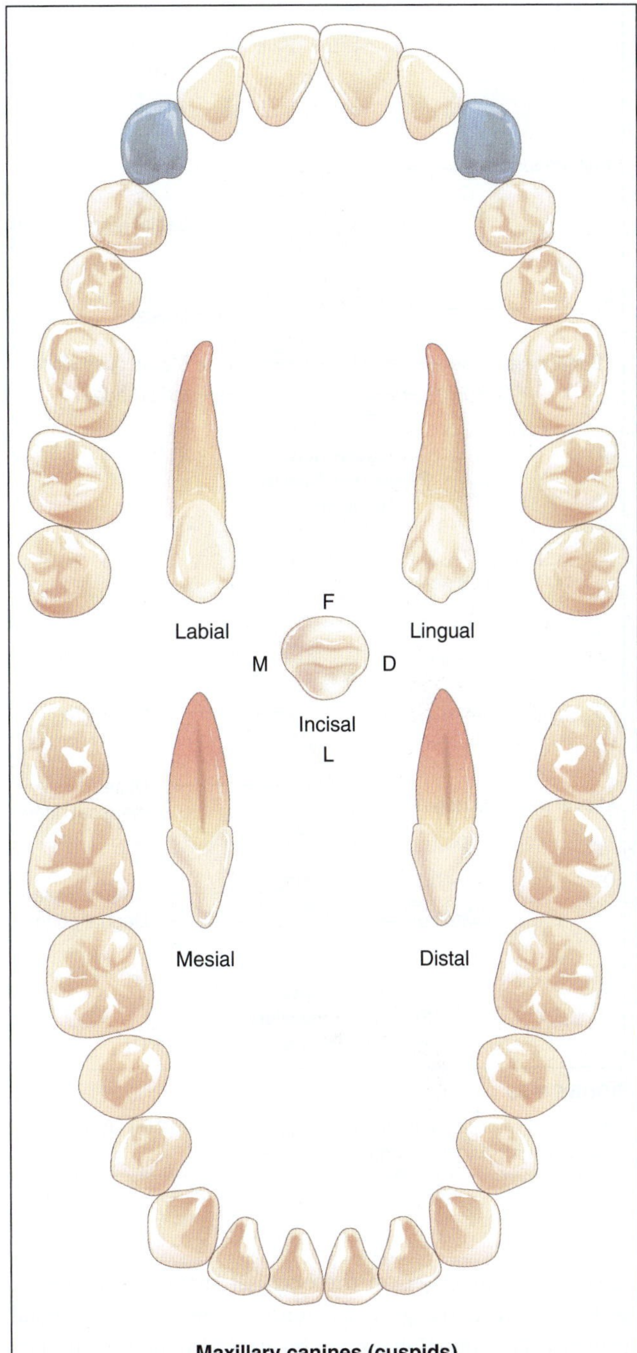

FIGURE 9-37
Permanent dentition with maxillary canines (cuspids) identified and maxillary canine viewed from the five surfaces.

Maxillary First Premolar (Bicuspid)

The facial cusp of the maxillary first premolar is much larger than the lingual cusp (Figure 9-39). It is longer and wider and appears from the facial side much like the cuspid. The

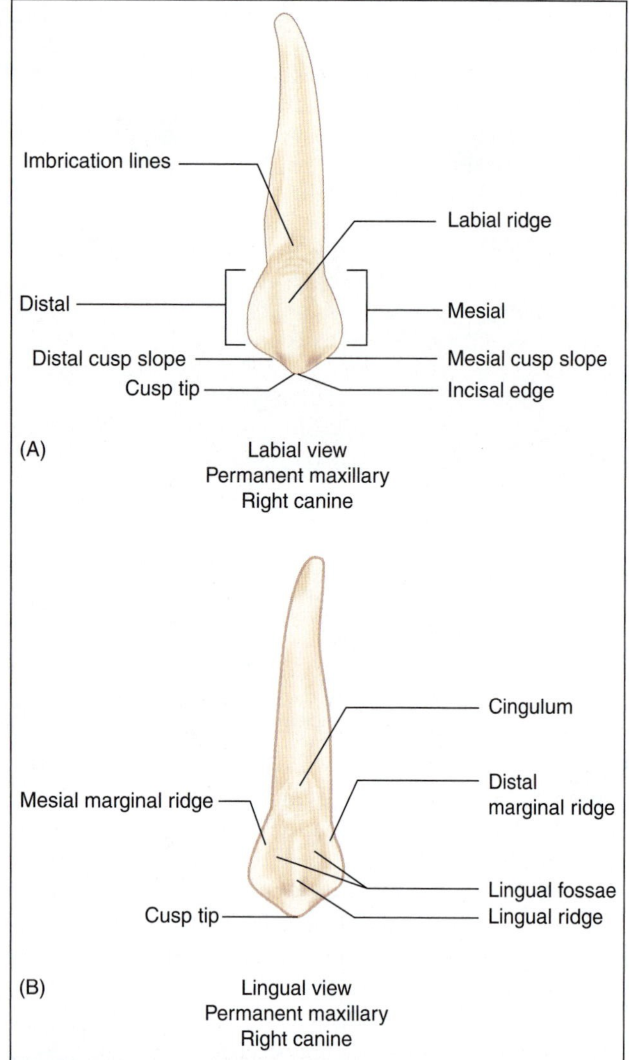

FIGURE 9-38

Permanent maxillary canine with (A) labial view and (B) lingual view, showing anatomical landmarks.

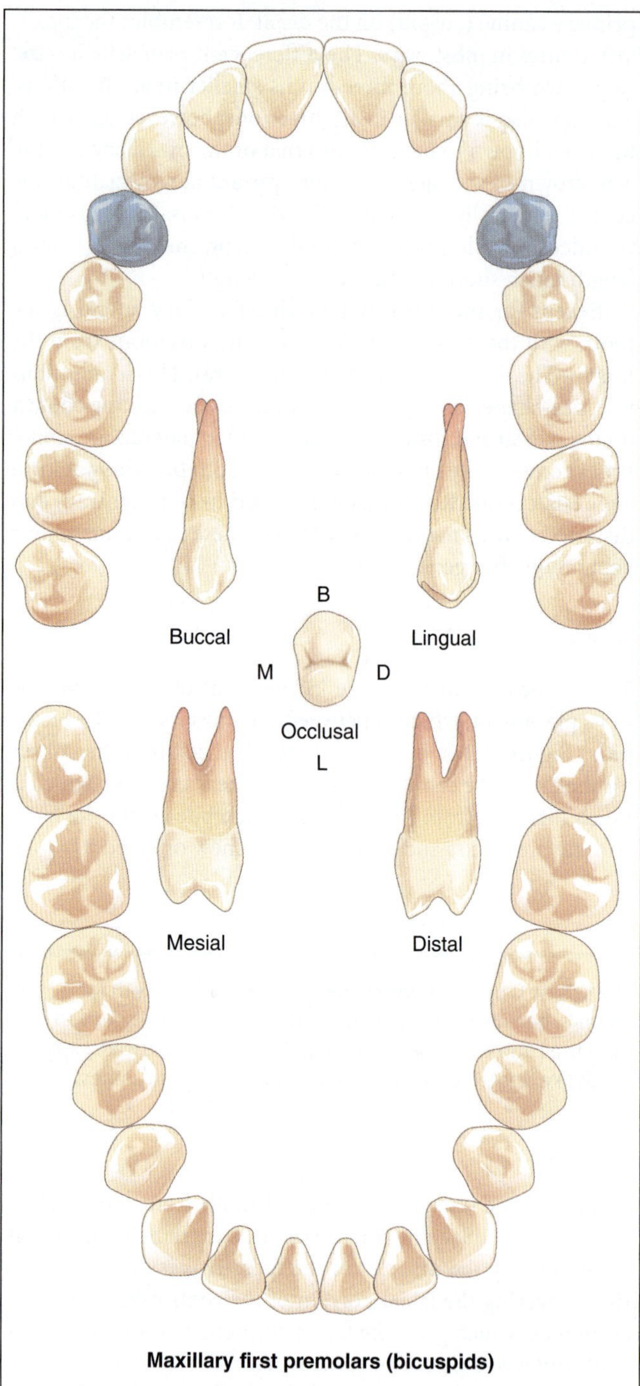

FIGURE 9-39

Permanent dentition with maxillary first premolars (bicuspids) identified and maxillary first premolar viewed from the five surfaces.

cusps come together on the occlusal surface in a central groove. This central groove extends to the mesial and distal grooves. The mesial groove is bordered by the mesial marginal ridges, and the distal groove is bordered by the distal marginal ridge. The maxillary first premolar has a bifurcated root (two roots, one buccal and one lingual) that is slightly separated. Some first premolars have roots that are fused together; thus, one root has two canals. The roots have a depression on the mesial and distal sides running from the CEJ to the root bifurcation. The roots are shorter and in this aspect resemble the roots of the molars more than they do the roots of the cuspid.

This premolar is often considered for removal if the patient's teeth are overcrowded and orthodontic treatment is needed. The position allows for movement from both anterior and posterior teeth. The orthodontist closes the space and the patient's facial appearance is not changed by the removal of this tooth. Also, the depression in the root structure makes it more susceptible to periodontal disease; therefore, it is a better choice for removal than the second premolar.

Maxillary Second Premolar (Bicuspid)

The maxillary second premolar (Figure 9-40) resembles the first in all but the following variations: The cusps, one on the buccal and one on the lingual, are more equal in length.

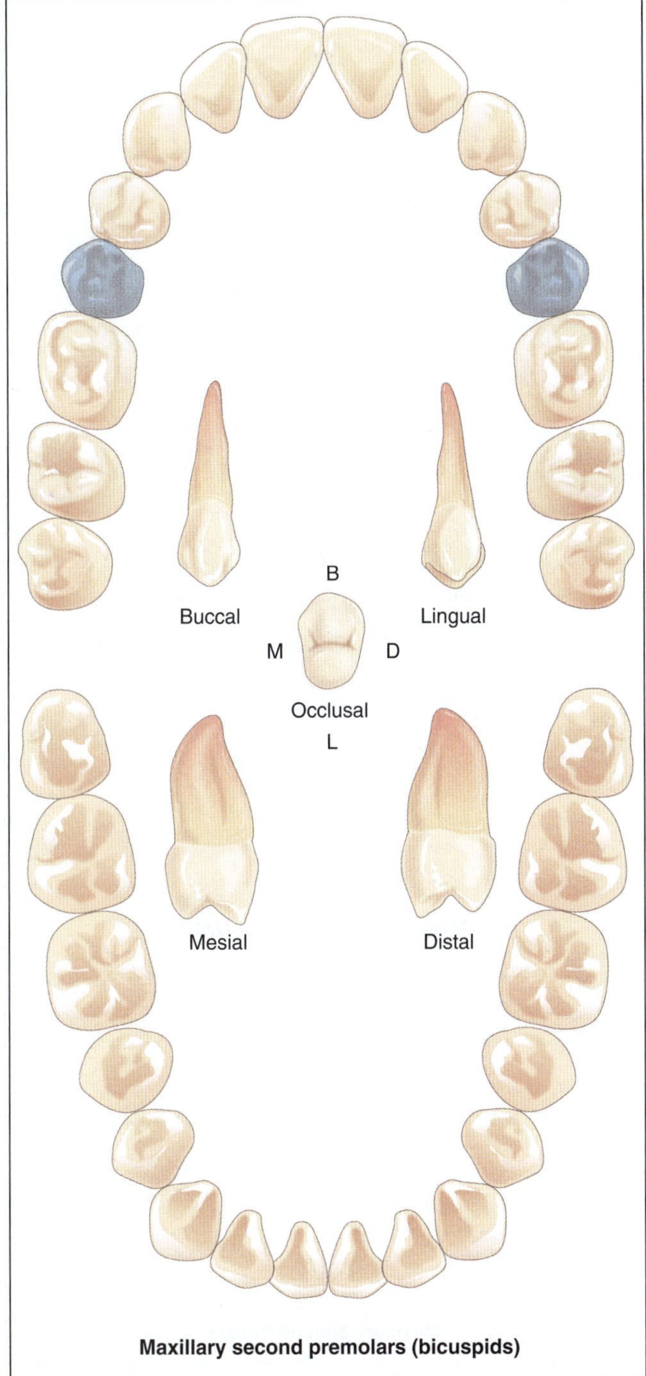

FIGURE 9-40

Permanent dentition with maxillary second premolars (bicuspids) identified and maxillary second premolar viewed from the five surfaces.

The lingual cusp is slightly shorter, but not as short as the cusp on the maxillary first bicuspid. The mesial buccal cusp slope is shorter than the distal buccal cusp slope. There is only one root and therefore only one root canal. There is a slight depression on the mesial root, but it is very shallow. The crowns of both the first and second bicuspids are wider bucco-lingually than mesio-distally. The second bicuspid is slightly more narrow mesial-distally than the first premolar.

Premolar (Bicuspid)

There are eight premolars: four in each arch, two in each quadrant. They are named the first and second premolars because of their positions from the midline. The first premolars, closest to the midline, line up in the fourth position. The second premolars line up in the fifth position from the midline. They are transitional teeth, placed between the cuspids and the molars. They look like the canines (cuspids) from the facial side; in fact, the buccal cusp functions much like a cuspid in tearing food, but the transitional teeth have an additional cusp on the lingual side (hence "bicuspids," meaning two). The additional cusp aids in further breaking down the food or pulverizing it for the molars to chew. These posterior teeth are not as critical in personal appearance because of their placement. They do not always show when smiling or talking.

Maxillary First Molar

The maxillary first molar is often referred to as the "6-year molar" because of its eruption time (Figure 9-41). Often, parents do not realize that this is a permanent tooth because of its early eruption. The crown of the maxillary first molar appears square in shape with four primary cusps present: mesio-buccal, disto-buccal, mesio-lingual, and disto-lingual. There is a fifth cusp, the cusp of Carabelli, located on the largest cusp, the meso-lingual. This cusp is located about one-third the way down from the occlusal surface and appears as a "mini" cusp. The prominence of this cusp varies from tooth to tooth.

The mesio-buccal and the disto-buccal cusps are divided by a buccal groove that extends about half the length of the crown and ends in a depression often called the buccal pit. The lingual cusps are slightly longer than the buccal cusps. The mesio-lingual cusp and the disto-lingual cusp are also divided by a lingual groove that travels about halfway down the crown on the lingual side, ending in a shallow depression called the lingual pit.

The root of the maxillary first molar is trifurcated. The first two roots, a meso-buccal root and a distal-buccal root, are placed on the buccal side. These buccal roots curve slightly toward each other. The third root is the largest and longest and is located on the lingual side. These three roots are spread out from each other and normally have one canal each.

On the occlusal surface of the maxillary first molars, the four primary cusps come together in a central fossa. There is an oblique (diagonal) ridge running across the occlusal surface that unites the distal cusp ridge of the mesio-lingual cusp and the lingual cusp ridge of the disto-buccal cusp. Another ridge, a transverse ridge, runs from the buccal cusp of the mesio-lingual cusp to the lingual cusp ridge of the mesio-buccal cusp. The occlusal surface also has a mesial ridge on the mesial of the occlusal surface and a distal ridge on the distal occlusal surface. This creates a surface with additional grooves and ridges to properly grind food.

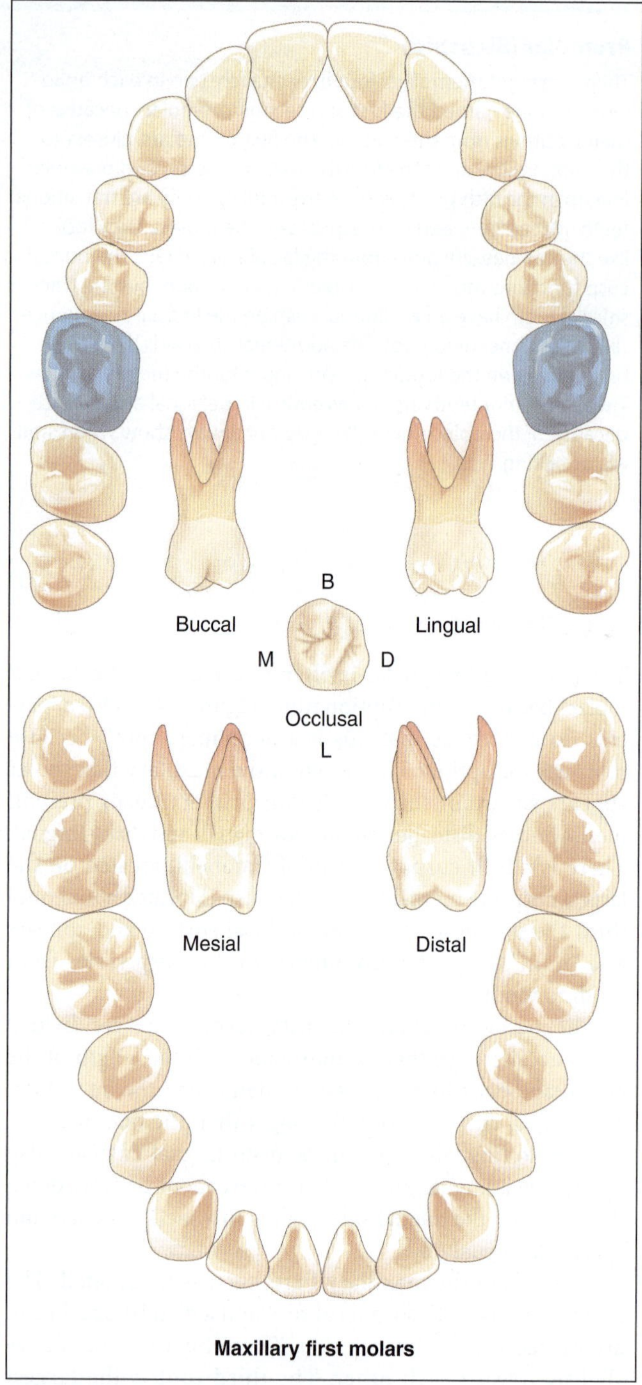

FIGURE 9-41

Permanent dentition with maxillary first molars identified and maxillary first molars viewed from the five surfaces.

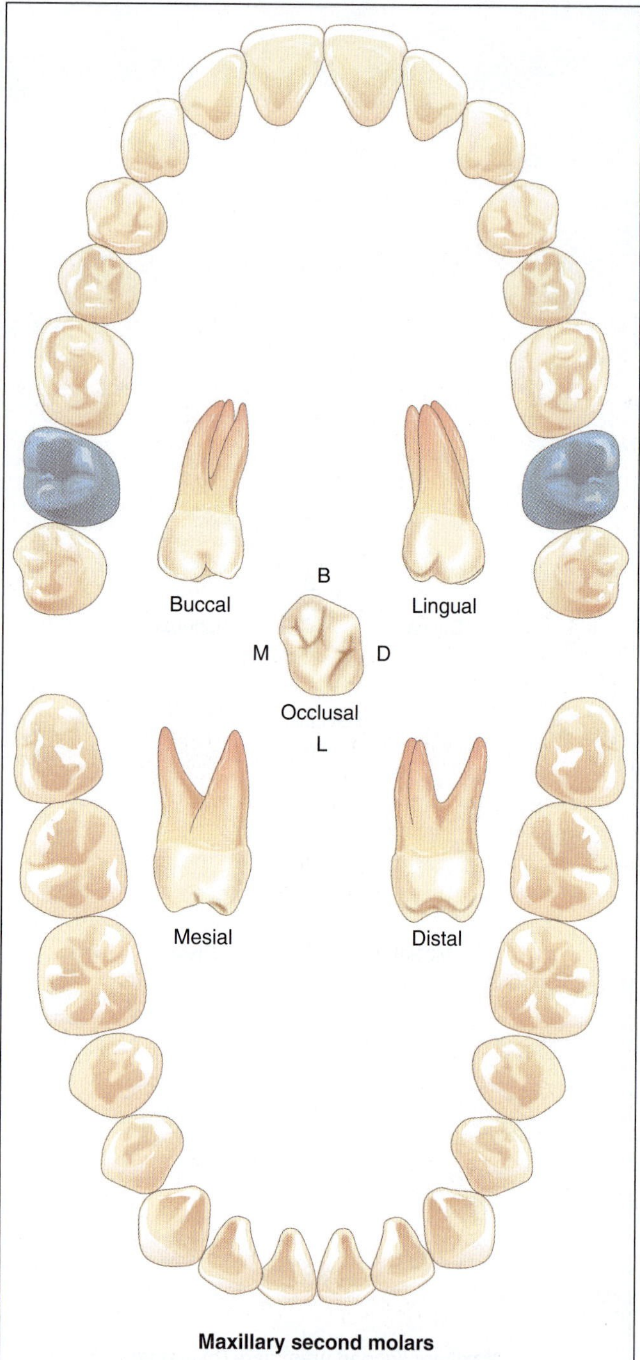

FIGURE 9-42

Permanent dentition with maxillary second molars identified and maxillary second molar viewed from the five surfaces.

Maxillary Second Molar

The second molar is called the "12-year molar" because of the time of eruption (Figure 9-42). It is similar to the first molar in many ways; however, it is smaller both in size of the crown and size of the root. The crown of the maxillary second molar has four cusps (no cusp of Carabelli). The cusps are located mesio-buccal, disto-buccal, mesio-lingual, and disto-lingual. The surface of the mesial of the tooth is greater across than the distal surface. The occlusal surface of the molars tapers down in size from the first molar toward the third molar.

The occlusal surface, although smaller, is much like that of the first molar. It has more supplementary grooves than the first molar, making it more wrinkled in appearance. The roots are the same in number but smaller in size and not as spread apart as the roots of the first molar. Each root has one canal, as in the maxillary first molar.

Maxillary Third Molar

Developmental variations make it impossible to describe exactly what the third molar looks like. The maxillary third molar is called the "wisdom tooth" because it was thought that by the time these teeth erupted into the oral cavity a person would have obtained maturity or wisdom (Figure 9-43). Many people do not develop third molars. If third molars do develop, they may not erupt into the oral cavity because of lack of space in the posterior of the arches. This is the one tooth that, after careful diagnosis, the dentist may recommend be removed.

When the tooth erupts normally, it resembles the second molar, only slightly smaller. It exhibits a more wrinkled appearance on the occlusal surface because many more supplemental grooves are usually present. The roots are normally fused together and vary in number.

Maxillary Molar

The word *molar* is derived from the Latin word *molaris*, referring to a millstone. This seems like an appropriate term for the teeth that chew, grind, or break down the food into tiny particles for swallowing. When normal eruption occurs, the molars are the first and last permanent teeth in the mouth. There are 12 molars in the oral cavity: 6 in each arch and 3 in each quadrant. They are called the first, second, and third molars because of their placement from the midline. The first molar is the closest to the midline. The molars are the strongest teeth in the arch due to the size of their crowns and the shape and size of their roots. The first molar is the largest and the strongest; this decreases toward the posterior, leaving the third molar the weakest and smallest of the molars. Just as the cuspids are considered the cornerstones of the anterior teeth, the first molars are considered the cornerstones of the developing occlusion in the posterior teeth. The molars do not replace any primary teeth and therefore are not succedaneous teeth. They erupt posterior to the deciduous dentition.

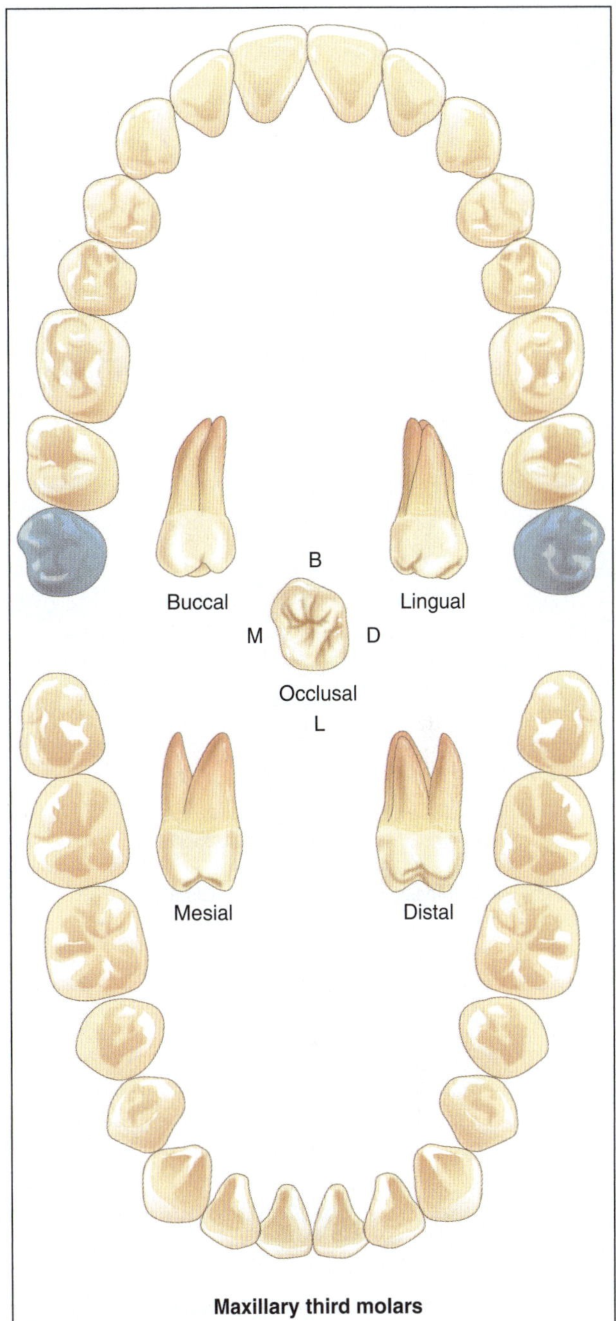

FIGURE 9-43

Permanent dentition with maxillary third molars identified and maxillary third molars viewed from the five surfaces.

Mandibular Central Incisor

The mandibular central incisor is the least variable tooth in the mouth (Figure 9-44). It is also the smallest tooth in the dentition. It is smaller than the mandibular lateral incisor, which is not the case in the maxillary arch. The maxillary central incisor is larger than the maxillary lateral incisor.

When the mandibular central incisor erupts, it has three mamelons on the incisal edge. These wear off, leaving a fairly straight incisal edge for cutting. The crown of the mandibular incisor has a labial surface that is convex but does not appear to have the developmental depressions and imbrication lines of the maxillary central. The crown is narrow and the incisal angle makes a sharp 90-degree angle as it extends down the mesial and distal surfaces. The lingual is concave and has a cingulum near the gingiva. It is relatively smooth, and the structures are not as prominent as in maxillary centrals. The root is straight and ends abruptly at the apex.

This tooth is the first from the midline; therefore, the mesial surface of each central incisor contacts its counterpart. The distal surface contacts the lateral in its prospective quadrant.

Mandibular Lateral Incisor

The anatomy of the mandibular lateral incisor so closely resembles that of the central incisor that a detailed description is unnecessary (Figure 9-45). The mandibular

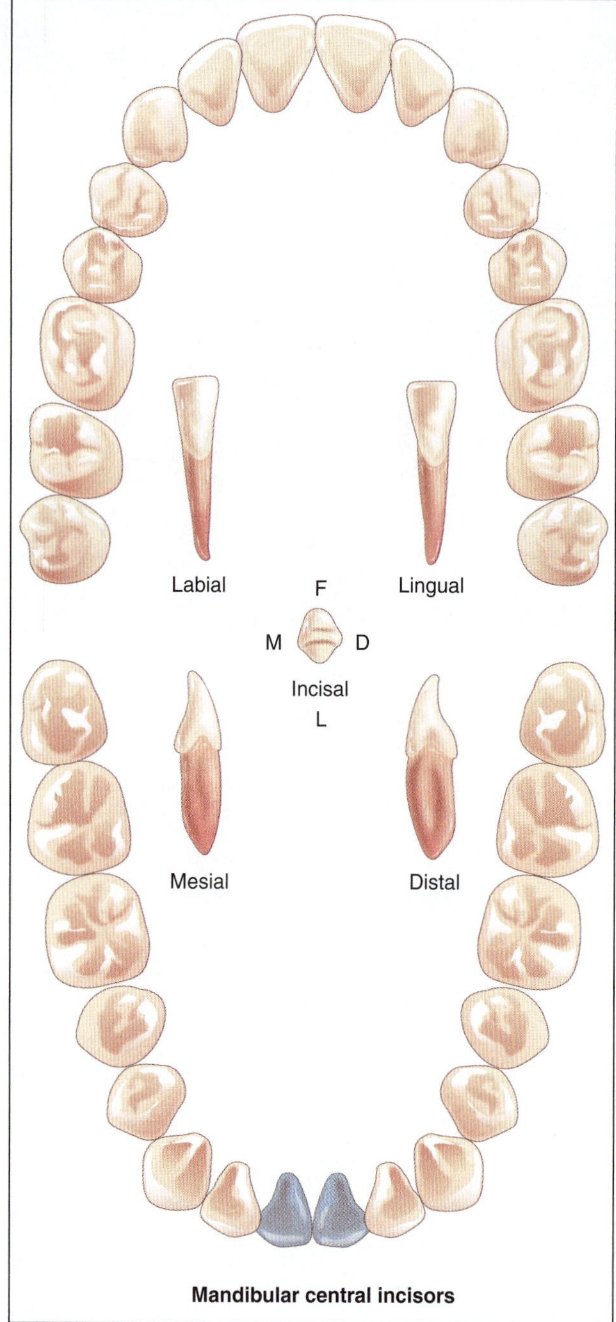

FIGURE 9-44

Permanent dentition with mandibular central incisors identified and mandibular central incisor viewed from the five surfaces.

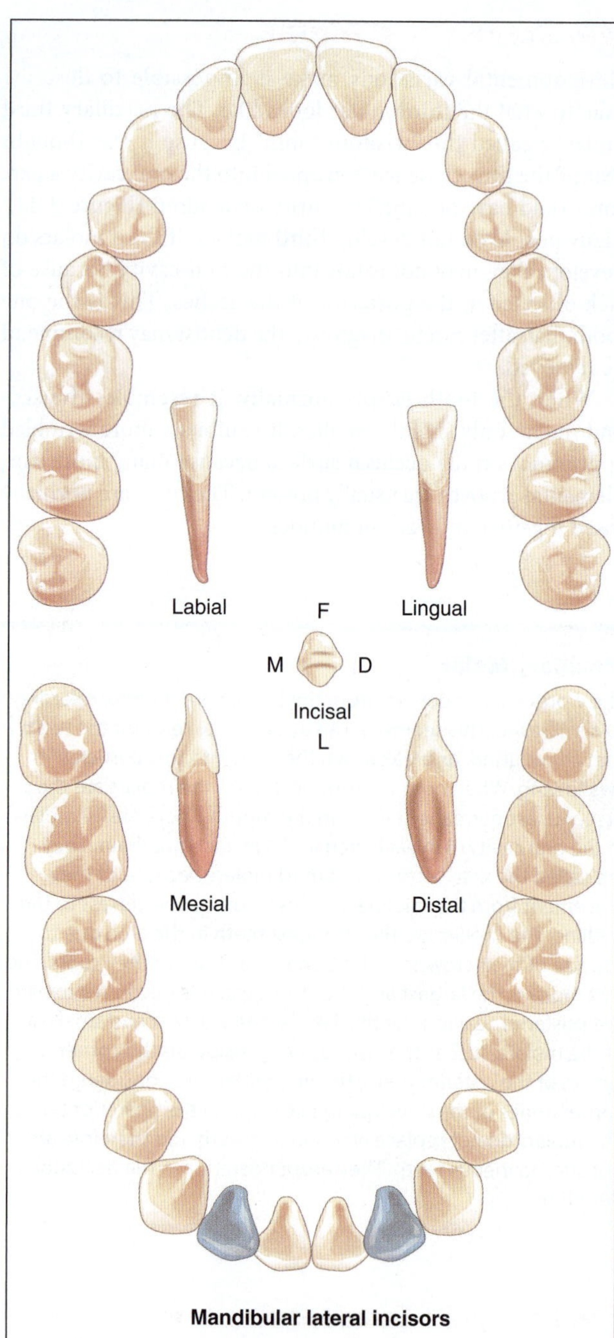

FIGURE 9-45

Permanent dentition with mandibular lateral incisors identified and mandibular lateral incisor viewed from the five surfaces.

lateral incisor is slightly larger. The root is also larger and slightly longer. Concavities may be present on the mesial and distal of the root. If these occur, the mesial concavity is shallower.

The crown of the lateral incisor is shaped the same as the central incisor except that the distal surface is not as long. The incisal distal angle is more rounded to accommodate this change in length. This tooth does not have the developmental abnormalities of the maxillary lateral.

Mandibular Canine (Cuspid)

The mandibular canine is the third tooth from the midline (Figure 9-46). It resembles the maxillary canine but is not as well developed. The crown of the tooth is approximately the same length as the maxillary canine, but the root is generally shorter (the root is still longer than the mandibular central and lateral roots). The cusp of the mandibular canine is not as well developed as the maxillary and not as sharp on the tip. The function, however, is the same: Both are designed to tear food.

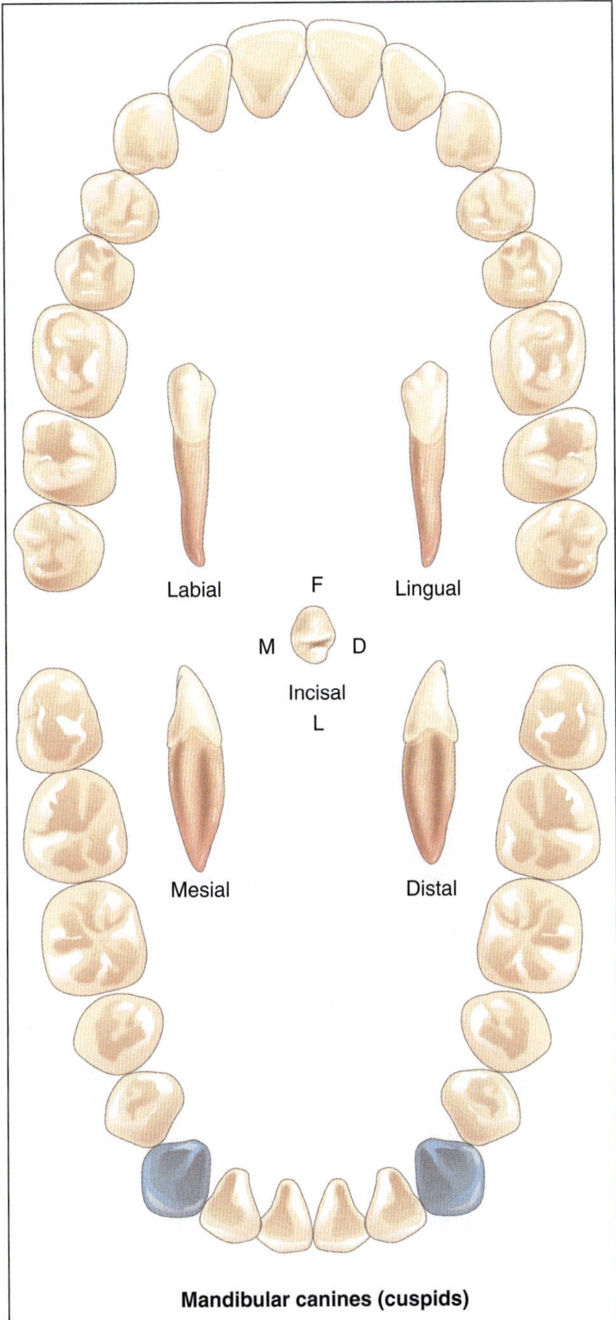

FIGURE 9-46

Permanent dentition with mandibular canines (cuspids) identified and mandibular canine viewed from the five surfaces.

The distal cusp slope is longer than the mesial cusp slope. The cingulum and marginal ridges are not as pronounced as on the maxillary canine, and the pronounced buccal ridge helps give shape to the face.

The canine is the longest tooth in the mandibular arch. The single root provides for stability; it is the cornerstone of the mandibular arch. The root, with one canal, has deep depressions on both the mesial and distal surfaces.

Mandibular First Premolar (Bicuspid)

The mandibular first premolar is much more of a transitional tooth than the maxillary first premolar (Figure 9-47). It does not resemble the mandibular second premolar as much as the maxillary first premolar resembles the maxillary second

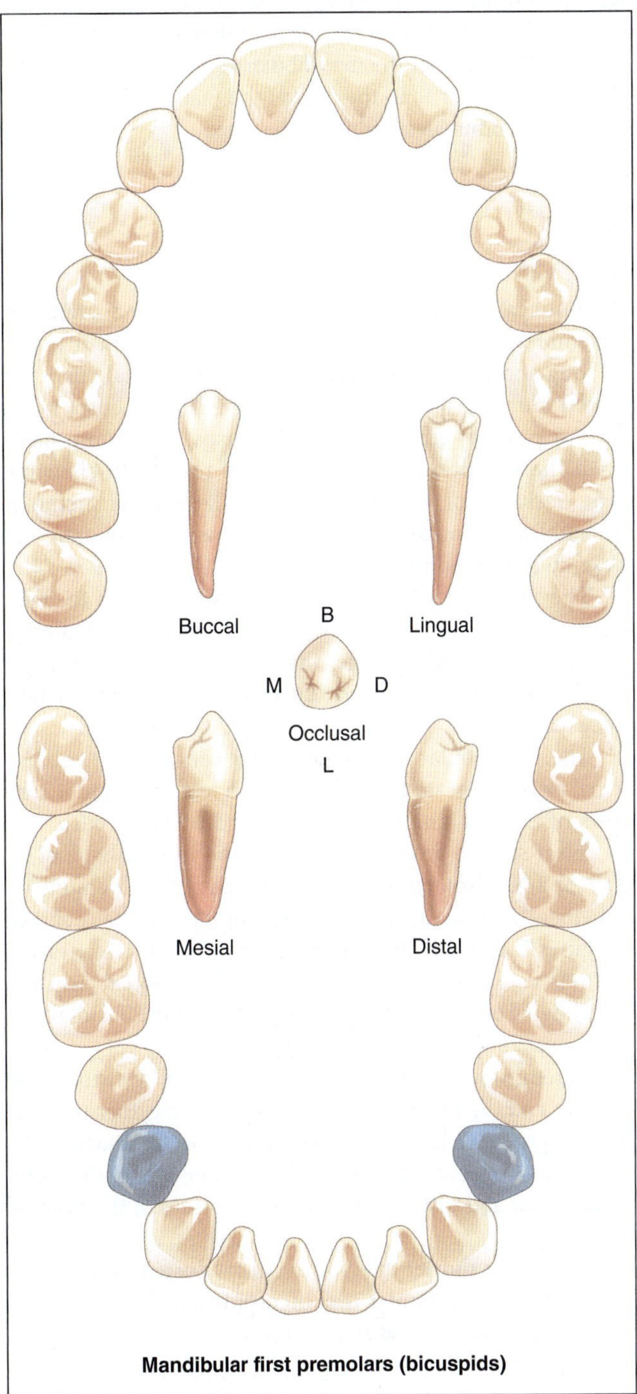

FIGURE 9-47

Permanent dentition with mandibular first premolars (bicuspids) identified and mandibular first premolar viewed from the five surfaces.

premolar. It looks much more like the mandibular canine: It has two cusps, one buccal and one lingual. The lingual cusp is often nonfunctioning; therefore, the shape is much like the canine. The buccal cusp is larger in all directions and its convex surface is more pronounced. The mesial cusp slope is shorter than the distal cusp slope.

The occlusal surface has both the mesial and distal ridges and, as the buccal and lingual cusps incline toward the occlusal groove, a transverse ridge crosses the tooth.

The single straight root of the mandibular first premolar is slightly shorter than the mandibular second premolar and a great deal shorter than the root of the mandibular canine. It sometimes bifurcates slightly at the apex.

Mandibular Second Premolar (Bicuspid)

The buccal surface of the mandibular second premolar resembles the mandibular first premolar except it is not as long and it is wider (Figure 9-48). The lingual cusps are much more developed. Instead of one lingual cusp, it has two or possibly three functioning cusps. This tooth helps with the transition from cutting and tearing to chewing. The occlusal surface of the mandibular second premolar resembles the molars, while the first mandibular premolar resembles the canine.

The cusps of the lingual surface are shorter than the buccal cusps and are divided by a lingual groove. The mesio-lingual cusp is slightly larger than the disto-lingual cusp but more equal in size than the cusps of the mandibular first bicuspid.

The mandibular second premolar can be the two-cusp type, or **bicanineate** form. This is seen less often and it consists of a larger single buccal cusp and a lingual cusp. The occulsal surface groove pattern may be in the shape of an "H" or a "U" (sometimes called a "C" pattern) depending on whether the groove pattern is straight or mesio-distally curved (Figures 9-49A and B). The three-cusp type or **tricanineate** form is seen more often and consists of one buccal cusp and two lingual cusps, and the groove pattern on the occulsal surface resembles a "Y" (Figure 9-49C).

Three grooves divide the occlusal surface. The disto-buccal groove and the mesio-buccal groove come together with the lingual groove to form a "Y" shape on the occlusal surface. All the cusps slope into these grooves in the middle of the tooth. The mesial and distal ridges outline the sides of the occlusal surface.

The root is shorter than the maxillary cuspid root but longer than the mandibular first bicuspid root. The root has a single canal and inclines slightly toward the distal.

Mandibular Molars

The mandibular molars are the largest and strongest of the mandibular teeth.

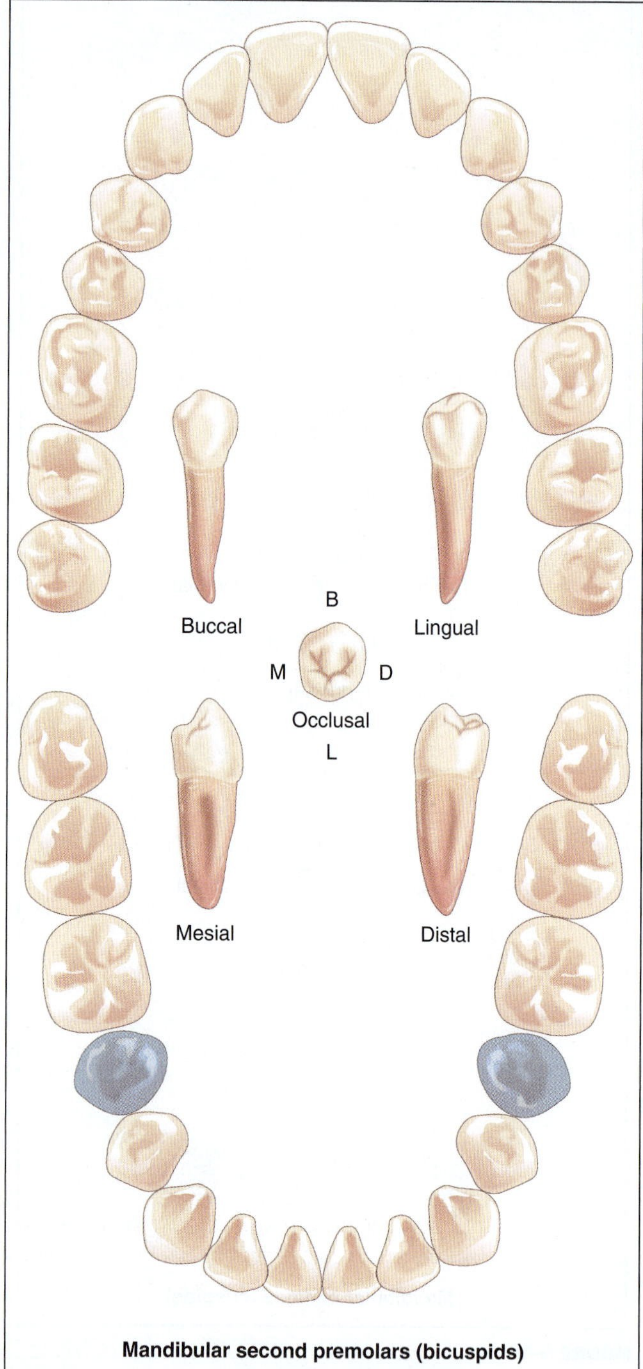

FIGURE 9-48

Permanent dentition with mandibular second premolars (bicuspids) identified and mandibular second premolar viewed from the five surfaces.

Mandibular First Molar

The mandibular first molar or "6-year-molar" (Figure 9-50) normally erupts slightly before the maxillary first molar and is thought to be the keystone of the dental arch. It has the widest crown of any tooth in the dentition and is the largest mandibular tooth.

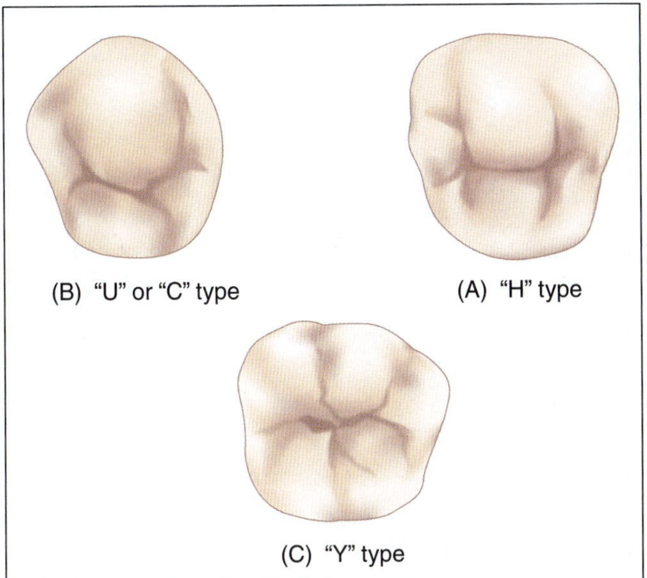

FIGURE 9-49
Different shapes of the occlusal surface of the permanent mandibular second premolar. (A) is the "H"-type shape, (B) is the "U"- or "C"-type shape, and (C) is the "Y"-type shape.

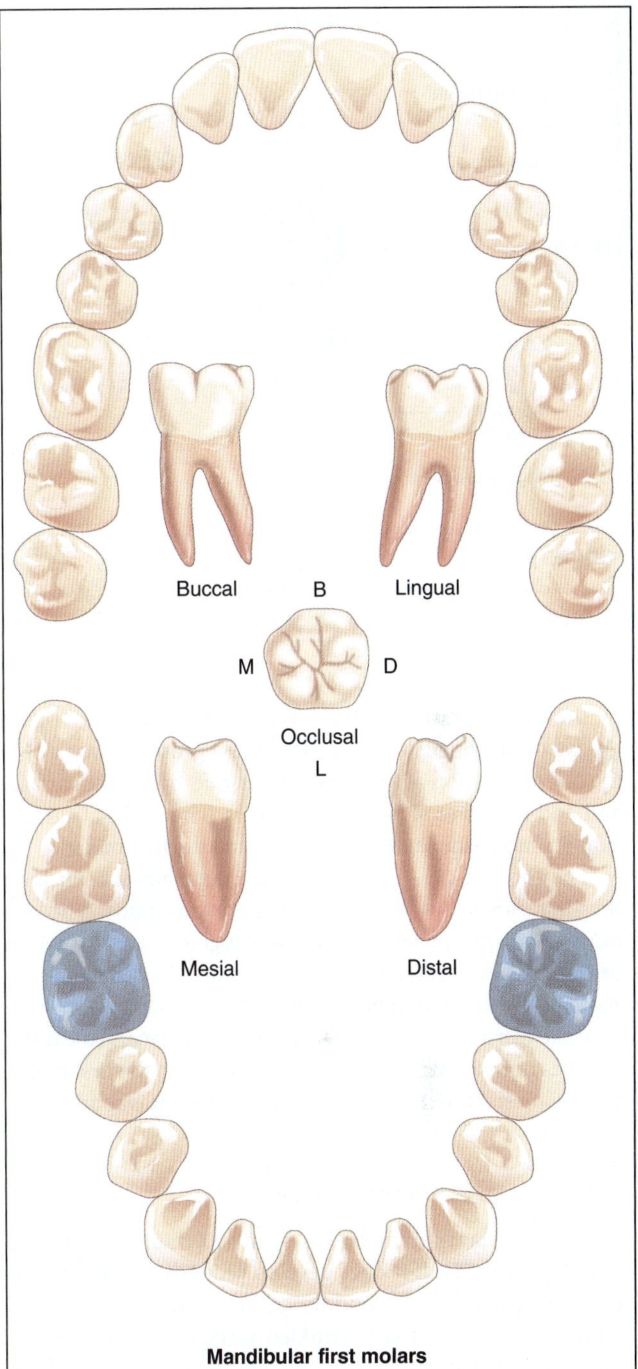

FIGURE 9-50
Permanent dentition with mandibular first molars identified and mandibular first molar viewed from the five surfaces.

There are normally five functioning cusps on the occlusal surface of this tooth (Figure 9-51). The mesio-buccal cusp is the bulkiest and the longest of the three buccal cusps; however, it is shorter than the lingual cusps. The disto-buccal cusp is a rounded cusp, found between the larger mesio-buccal cusp and the smaller distal cusp. The mesio-lingual cusp and the disto-lingual cusp are the longest and the sharpest of the five cusps. The mesio-lingual cusp may be slightly smaller than the disto-lingual cusp. All these cusps come together on the occlusal surface in the central fossa and are divided by a groove extending between one cusp and the next. For instance, the buccal groove coming from the central fossa extends between the mesio-buccal cusp and the disto-buccal cusp and ends halfway down the buccal surface of the crown of the tooth in a buccal pit (see Figure 9-15). These divisions make the occlusal surface appear as though five lobes come together. The mesial surface of the tooth is slightly concave, and the distal side is fairly straight.

The mandibular first molar has two roots: mesial and distal. The mesial root is the wider and the stronger of the two. It normally has two pulp canals, which is unusual because most of the teeth have one canal per root. The root is fairly flat in shape from the buccal to the lingual and tends to incline first toward the mesial of the tooth and then curve back toward the distal. The distal root is the smaller and weaker of the two. It is usually straight but occasionally will curve toward the mesial or the distal. It usually has a wider canal, and the outer surface of the root is more convex on the distal portion.

Mandibular Second Molar

The mandibular second molar is similar to the first molar but smaller (Figure 9-52). It has four cusps: mesio-buccal, disto-buccal, mesio-lingual, and disto-lingual. They are nearly the same size, but the mesio-buccal cusp is normally the largest and the disto-lingual cusp is normally the smallest. They are divided

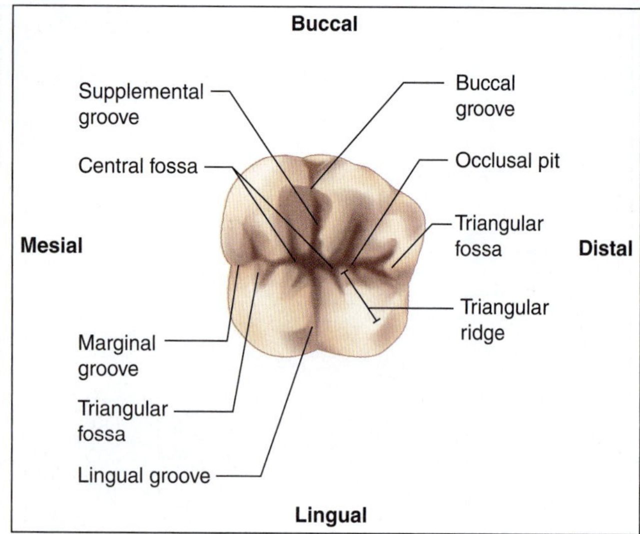

FIGURE 9-51

The permanent mandibular molar shown with the occlusal anatomy identified.

by the buccal groove on the buccal surface and the lingual groove on the lingual surface. Both these grooves travel down the outside portion of the crown, about one-half of the surface, and end in pits or shallow depressions. The occlusal surface exhibits more supplemental grooves than the first molar.

The roots of the second molar are normally shorter than the first molar, but they do have more variations. The two bifurcated roots generally are closer together and may even be fused. They normally angle more toward the distal than the roots of the first mandibular molar. The mesial root is wider than the distal root and may have one or two canals (the distal root has one canal). They are shaped similar to the first molar, but the mesial root is flatter and the distal root is rounder.

Mandibular Third Molar

The mandibular third molar has many variations in shape and size (Figure 9-53). If it does develop properly and erupt, this molar resembles the second molar but is smaller. The mandibular third molar has a wrinkled surface and the roots are often fused together. The roots tend to angle toward the distal in almost a horizontal position and may be four or more in number and fused together. These teeth, like the maxillary third molars, are referred to as "wisdom teeth" and may not develop or erupt. The dentist must determine if it is to the patient's advantage to keep these teeth. If they do erupt, they normally are difficult to keep plaque free because of their location and additional grooves.

Deciduous (Primary) Teeth

There are 20 deciduous teeth in the primary dentition: 10 in each arch, 5 in each quadrant (Figure 9-54). There is a central incisor, lateral incisor, cuspid, first molar, and second molar (there are no bicuspids in the deciduous dentition). The

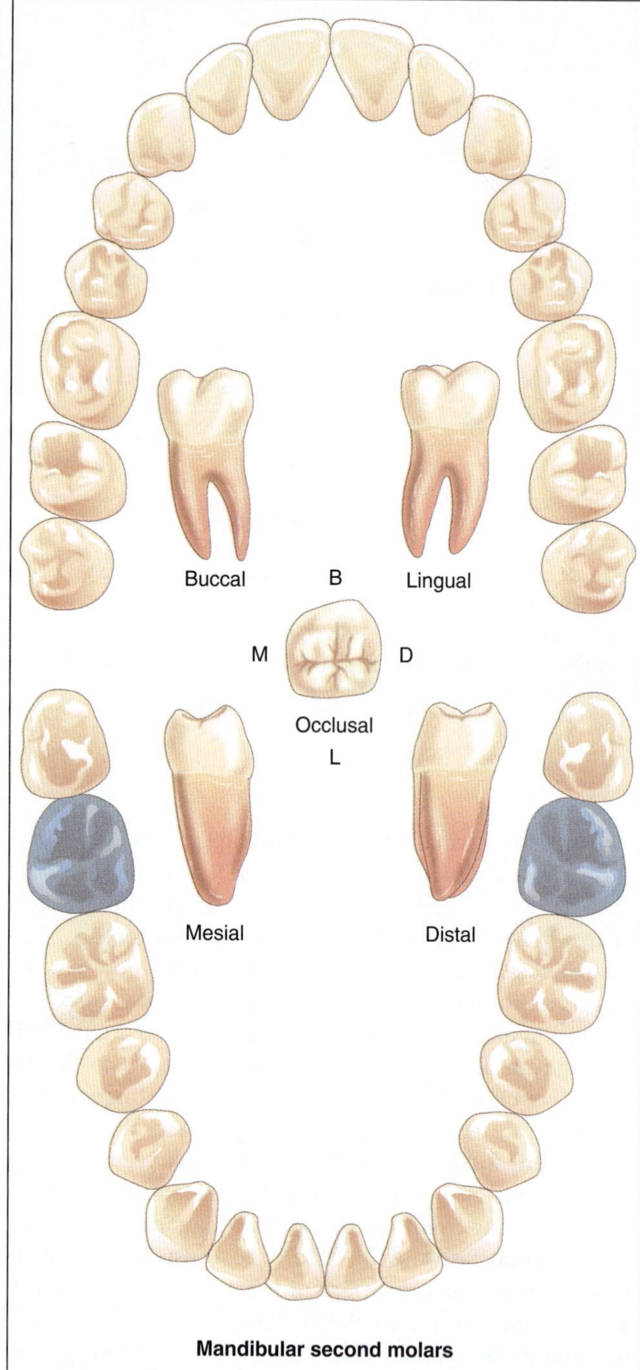

FIGURE 9-52

Permanent dentition with mandibular second molars identified and mandibular second molar viewed from the five surfaces.

primary teeth are referred to as the baby teeth, milk teeth, first teeth, or primary teeth, but the correct clinical term is deciduous teeth. They begin to erupt when the child is 6 months of age and finish erupting when the child is approximately 2 to 3 years of age.

It seems that less importance has been placed on the deciduous teeth because they are only temporary. Some patients prefer not to restore deciduous teeth and choose to have them removed, knowing they will be replaced by a permanent tooth.

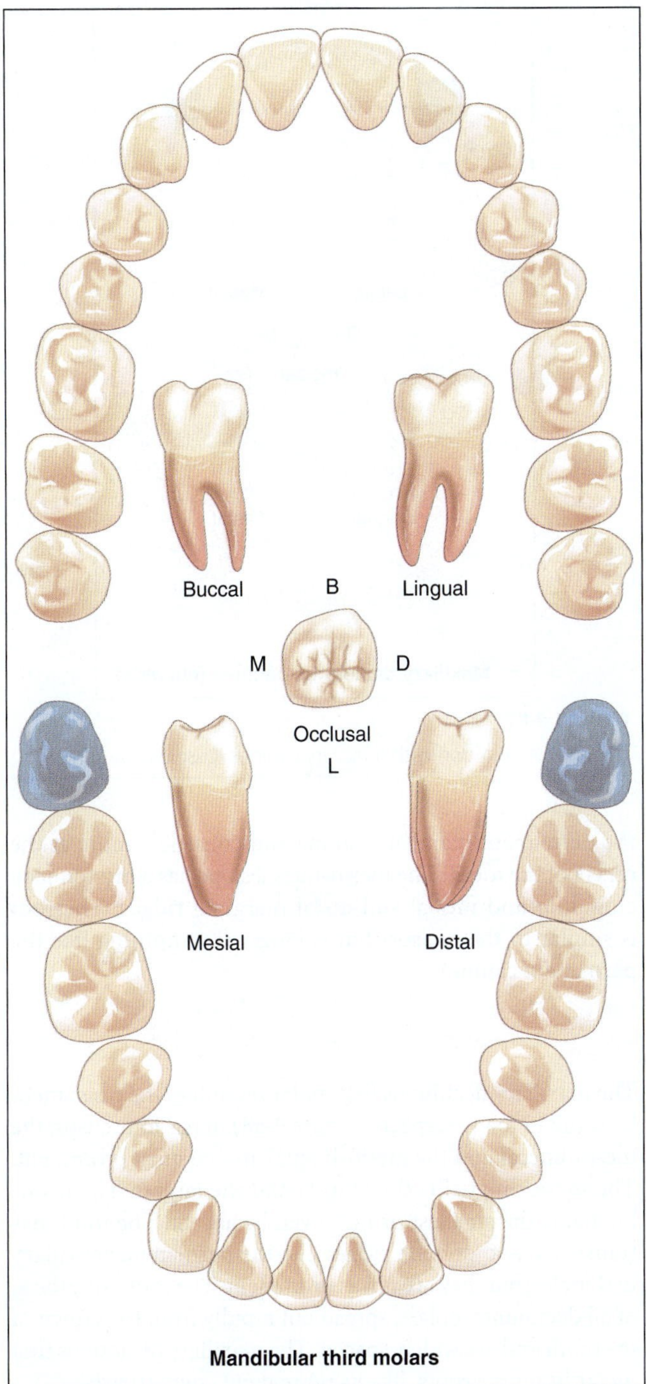

FIGURE 9-53

Permanent dentition with mandibular third molars identified and mandibular third molar viewed from the five surfaces.

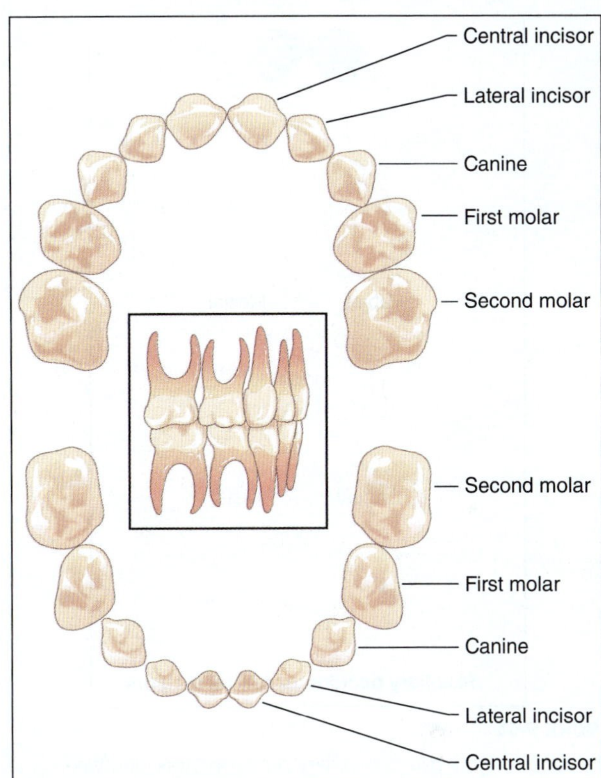

FIGURE 9-54

Deciduous dentition with tooth identification.

However, the deciduous teeth play a very important role in maintaining space for the permanent teeth, and they also aid the child in mastication and phonetics. Additionally, the appearance of the deciduous teeth plays an important role in establishing a child's positive self-image. Even though the deciduous teeth begin exfoliation by age 6, they are still an important part of facial development.

The deciduous teeth are normally smaller than the permanent teeth that replace them. The crown portion is quite short in comparison to the root, and the cervical ridge is much more pronounced. The crowns of the deciduous teeth appear more white or light bluish in color as compared to the yellow-gray color of the permanent teeth. This is because the enamel and dentin are much thinner and the pulp chamber is much larger. The deciduous molars have especially large mesial pulp horns. Knowing that the pulp is larger and closer to the surface of the deciduous tooth, a dental assistant should take great care during the coronal polish not to overheat the tooth and injure the pulp.

Maxillary Deciduous Central Incisor

The maxillary deciduous central incisor resembles the permanent maxillary central in shape (Figure 9-55). It is much smaller in size than the permanent maxillary central and has a more pronounced cervical line. The crown is the only anterior tooth in either dentition to have a shorter inciso-cervical height than the mesio-distal width. This tooth erupts with no mamelons, and the labial surface is convex and smooth.

Maxillary Deciduous Lateral Incisor

The maxillary deciduous lateral incisor is similar to the central incisor except it is smaller (Figure 9-56). Another difference is that it is longer than it is wide. The incisal edge of the deciduous maxillary lateral incisor is more rounded on the mesial and distal sides than the straight incisal edge of the central incisor.

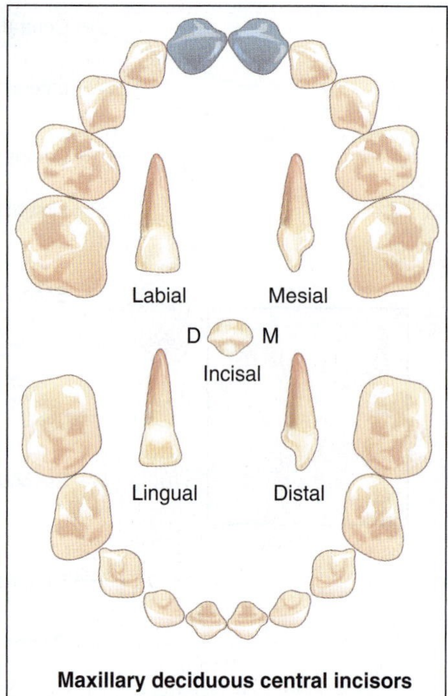

FIGURE 9-55
Deciduous dentition with maxillary central incisors identified.

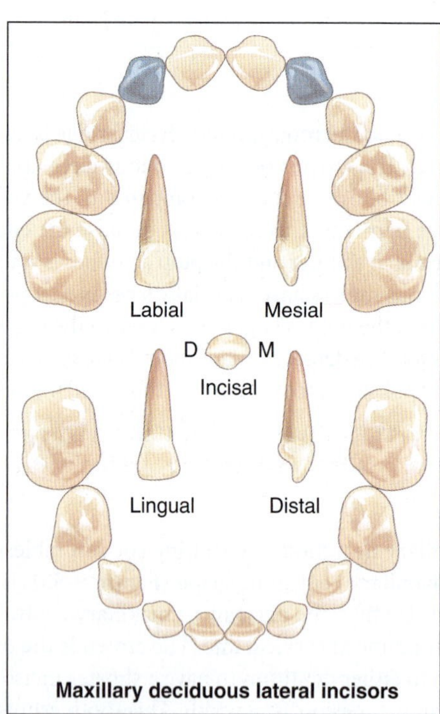

FIGURE 9-56
Deciduous dentition with maxillary lateral incisors identified.

Maxillary Deciduous Canine (Cuspid)

The maxillary deciduous canine appears to be wider than it is long; however, with the pointed incisal edge, it is slightly longer than it is wide (Figure 9-57). It is more convex than the permanent maxillary canine and constricts more at the cervix of the tooth. The mesio-incisal slope has a pronounced cingulum and mesial and distal marginal ridges. The root is similar to the incisors but is longer (but nothing like the permanent canine).

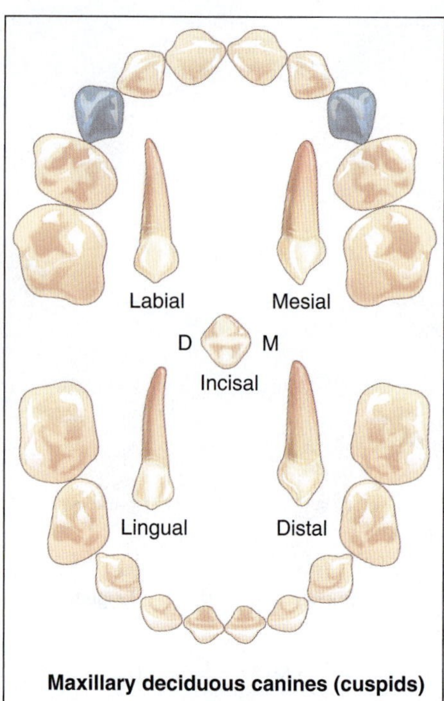

FIGURE 9-57
Deciduous dentition with maxillary canines (cuspids) identified.

Maxillary Deciduous First Molar

The maxillary deciduous first molar resembles the permanent bicuspid in many respects (Figure 9-58). It has four cusps; the mesio-buccal and the mesio-lingual are the most prominent. The mesio-lingual is the longest and the largest. The disto-lingual is the smallest or may even be absent. The tooth has transverse and oblique ridges like the permanent maxillary first molar, but they are not as prominent. The roots, like those of all deciduous molars, spread out rapidly from the crown of the tooth and are widely spaced. The maxillary deciduous first molar has three roots, like its permanent counterparts.

Maxillary Deciduous Second Molar

The maxillary deciduous second molar (Figure 9-59) resembles the maxillary first permanent molar because it has four primary cusps and may even have a cusp that resembles the cusp of Carabelli. It has three roots that are widely spaced.

Mandibular Deciduous Central Incisor

The mandibular deciduous central incisor (Figure 9-60) more closely resembles the permanent mandibular lateral incisor than its central incisor counterpart. The crown of the tooth is

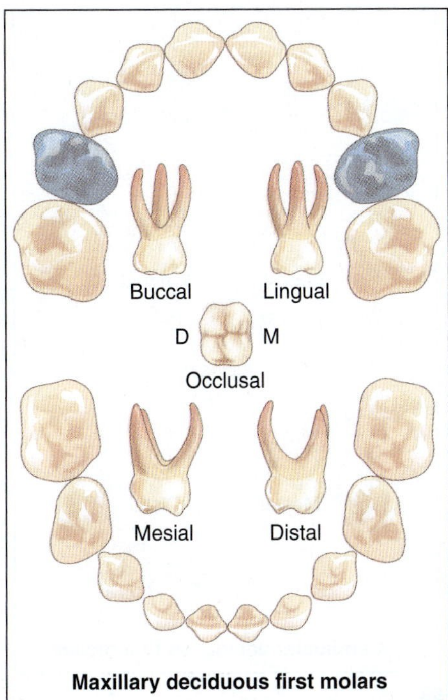

FIGURE 9-58
Deciduous dentition with maxillary first molars identified.

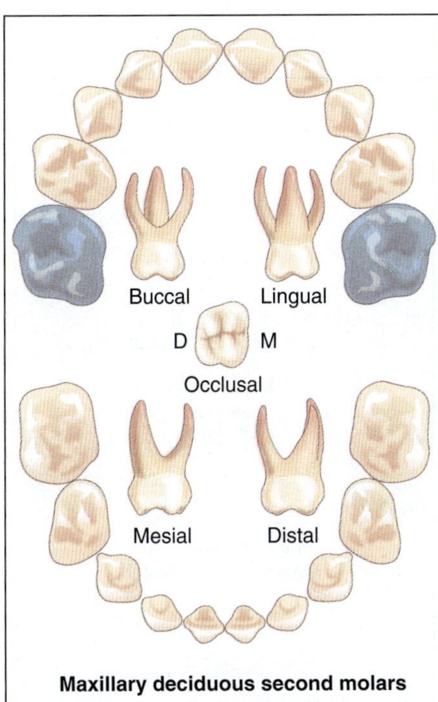

FIGURE 9-59
Deciduous dentition with maxillary second molars identified.

slightly wider than the permanent lateral incisor. The shape and form of the incisal edge is almost exactly the same as that of the permanent lateral. The root is slender and rather long. Mesial and distal surfaces of the root are flat, while lingual and labial surfaces are convex.

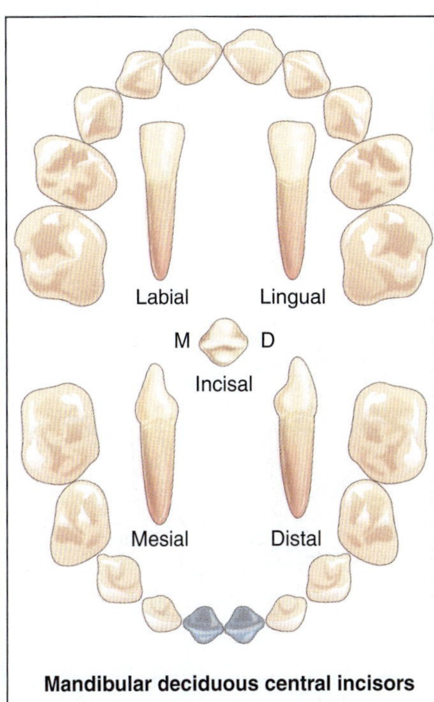

FIGURE 9-60
Deciduous dentition with mandibular deciduous central incisors identified.

Mandibular Deciduous Lateral Incisor

The mandibular deciduous lateral incisor resembles the mandibular deciduous central incisor except that it is slightly longer and wider (Figure 9-61). The cingulum and the mesial and distal marginal ridges are more pronounced and the fossa is not as shallow. The root curves toward the distal at the apex.

Mandibular Deciduous Canine (Cuspid)

The mandibular deciduous canine is much more delicate in form than that of the maxillary deciduous cuspid—even the root is not as large or long (Figure 9-62). The cingulum and the mesial and distal marginal ridges are less pronounced than those of the maxillary counterpart. The mesio-incisal slope is not as long as the disto-incisal slope; the maxillary incisal slopes are more nearly equal in length.

Mandibular Deciduous First Molar

The mandibular deciduous first molar (Figure 9-63) resembles no other permanent or deciduous tooth. It has four cusps, with the mesio-buccal the largest and the mesio-lingual next in size. The disto-buccal and the disto-lingual are much smaller. The buccal surface is longer than that of the lingual and has a very prominent cervical ridge across the gingival area, directly above where the tooth constricts at the cervix. The tooth has two roots, including a mesial root, which is much longer and wider, and a distal root. The apex of the mesial root is flattened or squared off.

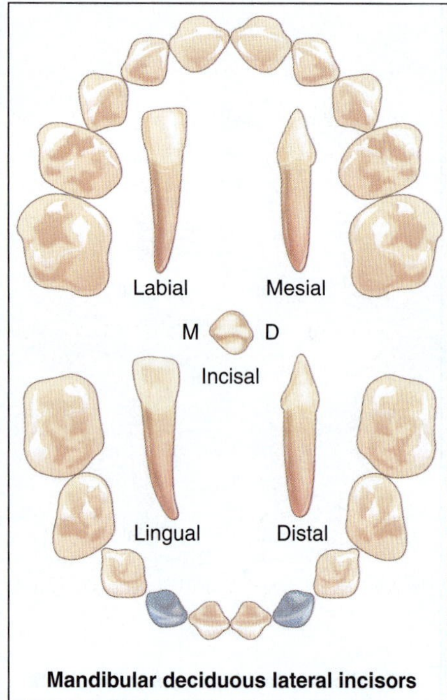

Mandibular deciduous lateral incisors

FIGURE 9-61

Deciduous dentition with mandibular deciduous lateral incisors identified.

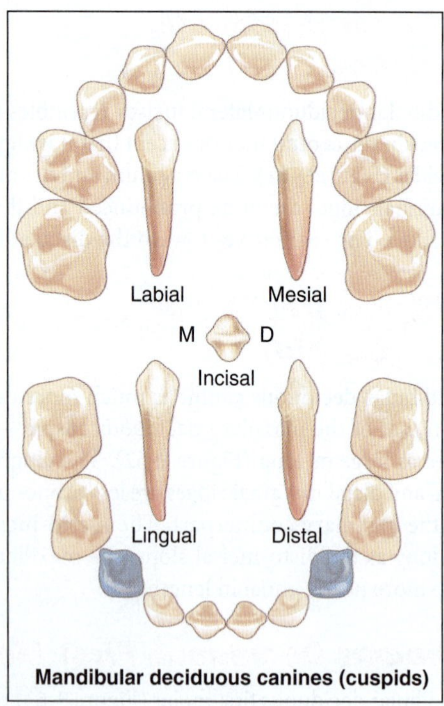

Mandibular deciduous canines (cuspids)

FIGURE 9-62

Deciduous dentition with mandibular deciduous canines (cuspids) identified.

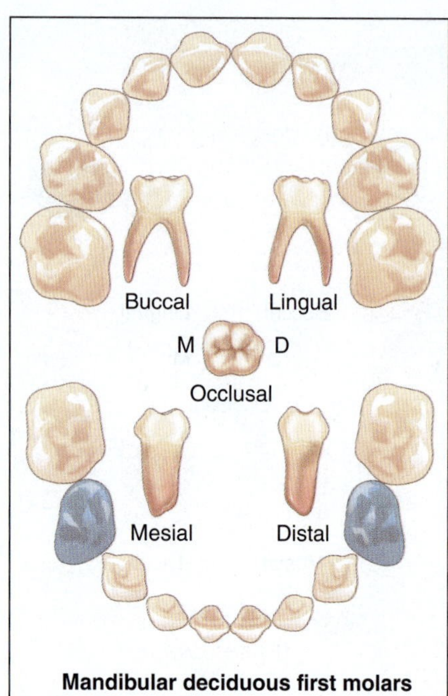

Mandibular deciduous first molars

FIGURE 9-63

Deciduous dentition with mandibular first molars identified.

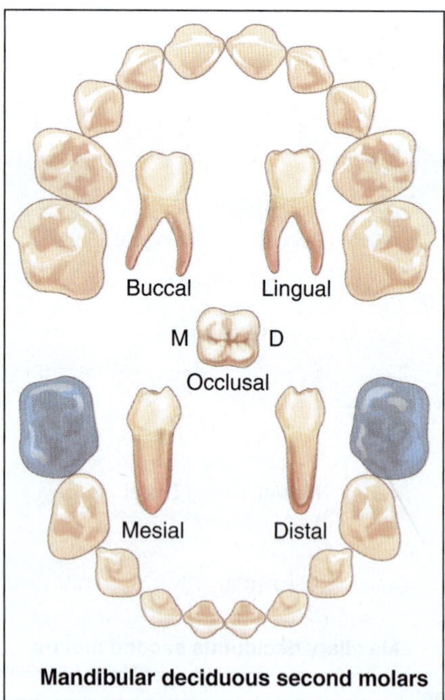

Mandibular deciduous second molars

FIGURE 9-64

Deciduous dentition with mandibular second molars identified.

Mandibular Deciduous Second Molar

The mandibular deciduous second molar closely resembles the permanent mandibular first molar (Figure 9-64). It is smaller in all dimensions, and the mesio-buccal and the disto-buccal cusps are nearly equal in size, unlike the permanent mandibular first molar. The distal root is smaller, while the mesial root is longer and wider. The permanent mandibular first molar has roots approximately the same length as this tooth.

Chapter Summary

Understanding tooth morphology will prepare the assistant to record accurately for the dentist or hygienist, contributing in a vital way to help those team members make a more accurate diagnosis. Therefore, the dental assistant will need to be able to identify each tooth from its anatomical form.

CASE STUDY

Travis Charles, age 12, complains of discomfort in the back of the mouth on both sides. The patient says it feels like the skin has broken open behind his teeth. Upon dental examination, it was noted that there was redness and edema.

Case Study Review

1. What probable condition is present?
2. Is the discomfort constant? Should Travis be concerned?
3. Does any one thing bring on the discomfort? Should Travis expect primary tooth loss in these areas?

Review Questions

Multiple Choice

1. How many teeth are in the deciduous dentition?
   a. 32
   b. 16
   c. 20
   d. 24
2. The surface of the tooth that is away from the midline is the
   a. mesial surface.
   b. distal surface.
   c. labial surface.
   d. lingual surface.
3. Three bulges on the incisal edge of the newly erupted central incisor are
   a. marginal ridges.
   b. cingulums.
   c. mamelons.
   d. fissures.
4. Except for the third molar, the maxillary tooth that has the most anomalies is the
   a. central incisor.
   b. lateral incisor.
   c. first premolar (bicuspid).
   d. second molar.
5. The cusp on the mandibular second molar that is normally the smallest is the
   a. mesio-buccal.
   b. disto-buccal.
   c. mesio-lingual.
   d. disto-lingual.
6. The cusp on the mesial lingual surface of the permanent maxillary first molar is the
   a. oblique cusp.
   b. cusp of Carabelli.
   c. cusp of succedaneous.
   d. transverse cusp.
7. The permanent teeth that replace the primary teeth are called ________ teeth.
   a. deciduous
   b. milk teeth
   c. succedaneous
   d. mamelon
8. The number of molars in a permanent dentition is
   a. 12.
   b. 8.
   c. 16.
   d. 4.
9. When there are two roots on a single tooth, they are said to be
   a. divided.
   b. trifurcated.
   c. fused.
   d. bifurcated.
10. A convex area on the lingual surface of the anterior teeth near the gingiva is called the
    a. cusp.
    b. fossa.
    c. cingulum.
    d. lobe.

Critical Thinking

1. If a patient has not formed a permanent mandibular first bicuspid on the left side, which deciduous tooth is retained in its place?
2. Which teeth in the maxillary arch are bifurcated?
3. Which surface of the anterior teeth is convex?

Web Activities

1. Go to http://www.animated-teeth.com and take the dental anatomy quiz.
2. Go to http://www.slideshare.net and find tooth morphology and review slide show and identify terms discussed in this chapter.

Section IV

Preclinical Dental Skills

CHAPTER

10

Microbiology

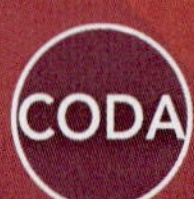

Specific Instructional Objectives

The student should strive to meet the following objectives and demonstrate an understanding of the facts and principles presented in this chapter:

1. Identify Anton Van Leeuwenhoek, Ferdinand Cohn, Louis Pasteur, Robert Koch, and Richard Petri according to their contributions to microbiology.
2. Explain the groups of microorganisms and staining procedures used to identify them.
3. Identify the characteristics pertaining to bacteria.
4. Identify the characteristics pertaining to protozoa.
5. Identify the characteristics pertaining to *Rickettsia*.
6. Identify the characteristics pertaining to yeasts and molds.
7. Identify the characteristics pertaining to viruses.
8. Describe the diseases of major concern to the dental assistant and explain why they cause concern.
9. Identify how the body fights disease.
10. Explain the types of immunity and routes of microorganism infection.

Key Terms

acquired immunity (200)
active acquired immunity (200)
aerobic bacteria (189)
allergen (200)
anaerobic bacteria (189)
anaphylactic shock (200)
antibody (200)
antigen (200)
antitoxin (200)
aphthous ulcer (197)
artificial acquired immunity (200)
bacilli (189)
bacteria (189)
bloodborne pathogens (197)
cocci (189)
cold sore (197)
conjunctivitis (197)
corneal ulcer (197)
diplococci (189)
disease outbreak (200)
endospores (189)
epidemic (200)
etiologic agent (188)
facultative anaerobic bacteria (189)
flagella (192)
fungi (193)
gram negative (188)
gram positive (188)
Gram stain (188)
gram variable (188)
herpetic whitlow (197)
hypersensitive (200)
immunization (200)
latent (194)
microbiology (187)
natural acquired immunity (200)
natural immunity (200)
normal flora (193)
pandemic (199)
passive acquired immunity (200)
pathogens (187)
Petri dish (188)
Protozoa (192)
purulence (200)
pyogenic membrane (200)
rickettsiae (192)
seroconversion (197)
spirilla/spirochetes (189)
spores (189)
sporulating (189)
staphylococci (189)
streptococci (189)
vibrios (189)
viruses (194)

Introduction

The study of microorganisms is called **microbiology**. Most microorganisms benefit humans and are often used in making vitamins, antibiotics, and food products. However, some microorganisms are harmful to humans, and these are called **pathogens** (PATH-oh-jens) (disease-producing microorganisms). In this chapter, five groups of pathogenic microorganisms are covered (bacteria, protozoa, rickettsiae, yeasts and molds, and viruses), along with the diseases they cause and the ways in which the body defends against them. Methods and instruments used to study microorganisms include the microscope, growing colonies in a culture medium, color or staining, and injection into an animal to observe the outcome.

As a dental assistant you should be able to identify common pathogenic diseases, particularly those that put the dental assistant at an increased risk through exposure. The key terms highlighted in the chapter focus on the foundations of microbiology. The terms identifying disease processes are placed in italic and should be learned as well.

Important People in Microbiology

There are several key individuals who made significant early discoveries in the field of microbiology. It is helpful to know and understand the contributions of these individuals and the impact of these discoveries on approaches to the identification and treatment of diseases.

Anton Van Leeuwenhoek

Born in Holland, Anton Van Leeuwenhoek (laye-vuhn-hook) (1632–1723) ground lenses to magnify and view things more closely. He looked at a raindrop through these lenses and found small things that moved; thus he saw microorganisms for the first time. Later, he scraped his teeth and viewed the scrapings through the ground lenses, finding a great number of moving microorganisms and referring to these single-celled organisms as "animalcules." He created over 400 different types of microscopes, several of which are still used today. They were made of hand-ground lenses in metal frames made from silver or copper.

Ferdinand Julius Cohn

Ferdinand Julius Cohn (1828–1898) was a biologist from Germany who was the first person to classify bacteria as plants. He later divided bacteria into four groups: desmobacteria, microbacteria, sphaerobacteria, and spirobacteria. His studies of the life cycle of *Bacillus* showed that it will change into an endospore from its vegetative state when it is exposed to high heat or some adverse or unfavorable environment. He understood that bacteria could go into this endospore state when being boiled and therefore the bacteria would not be killed. This has become very critical information in today's sterilization procedure. In the dental office, tests must be done to ensure that the endospores have been killed during the sterilization process.

Louis Pasteur

French microbiologist and chemist Louis Pasteur (1822–1895) (Figure 10-1) experimented with fermentation. By isolating the causative bacteria in various diseases, some affecting humans, he proved that bacteria caused disease. Pasteur found that bacteria, along with resistant spores, could be destroyed by heat. He showed that broth, when heated and kept in an airtight container, did not spoil. Pasteur suggested that food be processed by steam under pressure in an airtight container. His work led to the food-canning process used today. The sterilizers used in dental offices are based on his original premise that heat kills pathogens. Pasteur's name is noted in the pasteurization of milk, whereby the pathogens in milk are destroyed by heat. Pasteur's later work was in the area of creating vaccines. He discovered a method of using an artificially generated weak form of the disease to fight the disease or prevent its occurrence. His work has been the foundation for many of the vaccines now produced and has helped lead to

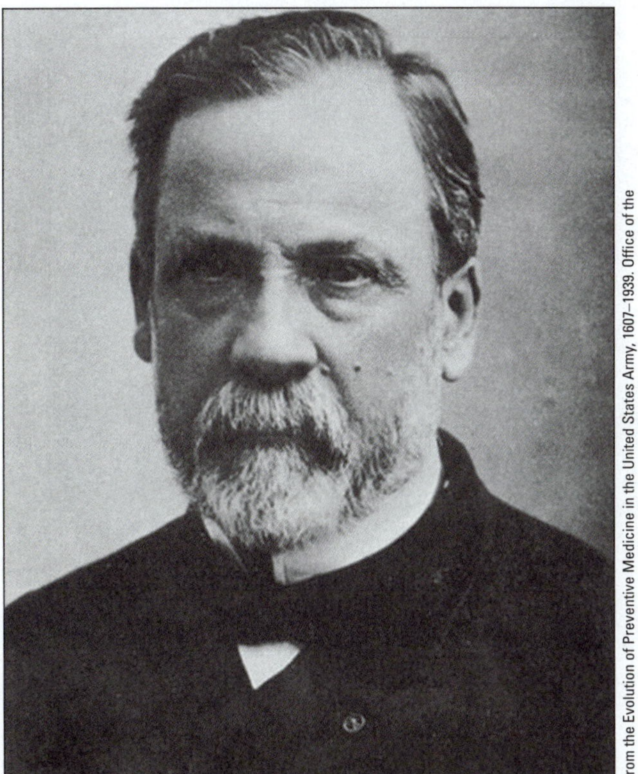

From the Evolution of Preventive Medicine in the United States Army, 1607–1939. Office of the Surgeon General Department of the Army: Washington, DC, 1968

FIGURE 10-1
Louis Pasteur.

the eradication of polio and typhus as health threats. He was noted as the "Father of Microbiology." It should be noted that Anton Van Leeuwenhoek was given this title earlier as well. Pasteur was awarded the Leeuwenhoek Medal, microbiology's highest honor, in 1895.

Robert Koch

Robert Koch (1843–1910), a German biologist (Figure 10-2), proved that a specific type of bacteria causes a specific disease; therefore, the specific bacteria is termed the **etiologic** (EE-tee-ol-OH-gic) **agent** (causative agent) of the disease. Koch was able to determine the etiologic agent for tuberculosis. He is also remembered for the "Koch Postulates," a procedure he developed to prove that a particular bacterium was the cause of a disease.

Koch's Postulates

1. The organism must be present in all cases of the disease.
2. The organism must be isolated in pure culture.
3. The organism must be able to produce the disease in another person or animal.
4. The organism must be recovered again in pure culture.

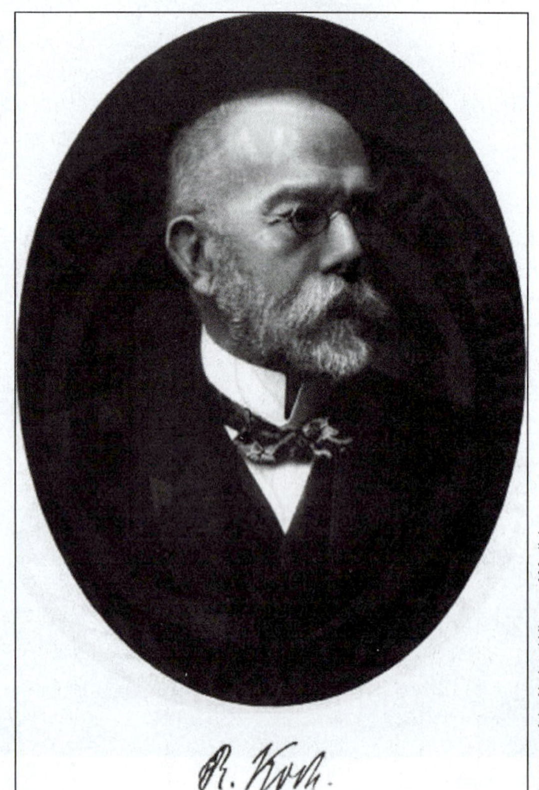

FIGURE 10-2

Robert Koch.

Richard Julius Petri

Richard Julius Petri (1852–1921) was born in Germany, and as a young adult he enrolled in training as a military physician and then received a doctorate in medicine. He worked in a research facility and was the laboratory assistant to Robert Koch. As an assistant, he realized the need for a method to easily culture bacteria for research. He devised a cylindrical, shallow dish with a clear, easily removed cover that is called the **Petri dish** or the Petri plate and is still being used in microbiology laboratories today. This dish is used with a medium of molten agar to grow or culture bacteria. Petri further developed the technique that is used today for dispensing the bacteria onto the medium (Figure 10-3). The dish bears his name and continues to enable the growth of bacteria under sterile conditions for the purpose of study and research.

Groups of Microorganisms

The two principal groups of microorganisms important to dentistry are bacteria and viruses. When looked at through a microscope, different types of bacteria are identified based on their characteristics, shapes, and sizes.

Often, bacteria cells are stained to further identify the groups. Dr. Christian Gram developed a staining procedure called the **Gram stain** to differentiate cells into two specific groups. To aid in viewing the cells, special dyes are used. The cells are placed on a slide, dried, and then stained with an alkaline solution of violet dye. The slide is rinsed with iodine and left untouched for 2 minutes. Then, the slide is gently rinsed with water and next rinsed with acetone alcohol. If the cell wall keeps the color, the cells are classified as **gram positive** and appear dark purple under the microscope. If they lose the color during the procedure, they are classified as **gram negative** and appear colorless under the microscope. The classification of bacteria that are not consistently stained are **gram variable**.

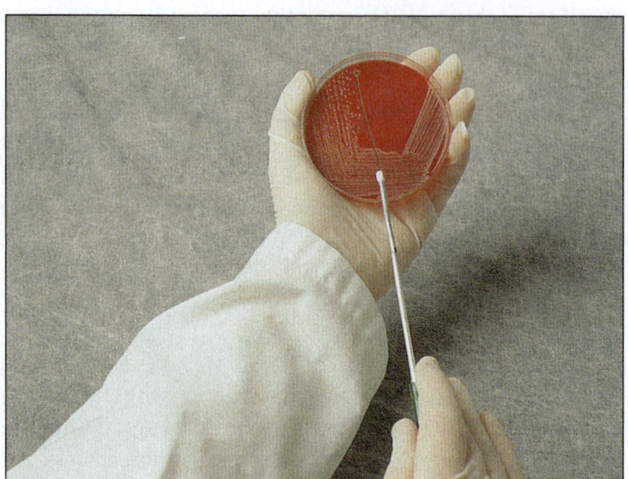

FIGURE 10-3

Microorganism being grown in a medium in a Petri dish.

Bacteria

Tiny, simple, single-celled plants that contain no chlorophyll are classified as **bacteria** (back-**TEER**-ee-uh). If an individual has 2000 bacteria lying side by side in a line, they are about the width of the period at the end of this sentence. Bacteria divide by simple fission: they elongate and divide into two separate cells, then continuously repeat this cycle. In ideal conditions (warm, dark, nutrient-rich, and moist), they divide about every 20 minutes. Bacteria are often incorrectly called "germs." Some bacteria are **sporulating**. One example is bacilli. These **spores** become enclosed in several protein coats that resist drying, heat, and most chemicals (**endospores**). They also withstand boiling. Sporulating is a means of survival for bacteria, and bacteria have been known to survive for years in this state. Later, they may land on a surface that is moist and nutrient rich, and reactivate. The process is much like a seed that floats and then lands on rich soil and begins growing.

Bacteria's Need for Oxygen

Some bacteria need oxygen to grow and live, this type of bacteria is termed **aerobic bacteria**. Most bacteria are aerobic. Other bacteria are destroyed in the presence of oxygen and live only without oxygen, this type of bacteria is termed **anaerobic bacteria**. Yet other bacteria will grow with or without oxygen, this is termed **facultative anaerobic bacteria**.

Bacteria Morphology

The shape of bacteria (morphology) is unique to this group of microorganisms (Figure 10-4). Under a microscope, the types of microorganisms are **bacilli** (rod shaped), **cocci** (round or bead shaped), **spirilla/spirochetes** (S-shaped), and **vibrios** (curved like a comma).

When the bacteria are grown in colonies, or masses, they appear differently (Figure 10-5). The prefix *diplo*, as in **diplococci**, identifies pairs of bacteria; **staphylococci** grow in clusters, much like grapes; and **streptococci** identifies chains of bacteria.

Disease Examples Caused by Bacteria

Tuberculosis. *Tuberculosis* (to-bur-kol-**O**-sis) is caused by *Mycobacterium tuberculosis* and is most often found in the lungs. Several months may pass before signs of the disease appear. Symptoms include fatigue, low-grade fever, night sweats, loss of weight, and, finally, a persistent cough. This disease is spread to others by airborne particles released through coughing, saliva contact, and, if cross-contamination occurs, dental treatment. Dental personnel must wear masks during dental procedures to protect from the handpiece spray that may contain infectious particles if the patient has tuberculosis. The disease can be detected by a skin test and/or chest x-ray. Treatment for this disease includes antibiotics and other drugs.

Legionellosis. *Legionellosis*, or *Legionnaires' disease*, obtained its name in 1976 when a large outbreak took place at an American Legion convention in the Bellevue-Stratford Hotel in Philadelphia. It received a great deal of attention in the media. This disease is caused by Gram negative, aerobic bacteria belonging to the genus Legionella. The majority of the cases are caused by *Legionella pneumophila*, which is an aquatic organism that thrives in temperatures between 55°C and 75°C. During a large outbreak, people get pneumonia that is fatal in 5 to 25 percent of the cases. It is transmitted through droplets that contain the bacteria. It may spread through central air conditioning systems, hot water systems, showers, windshield washers, spas, fountains, ice-making machines, and so on. It is often associated with hotels, hospitals, and cruise ships that may have old cooling systems. Weekly testing of water and/or cooling systems will aid in prevention. A UV light will also cause the bacteria to be inactivated. Treatment is accomplished through quick identification and prescriptions of respiratory tract antibiotics.

Diphtheria, Pertussis, and Tetanus. *Diphtheria*, *pertussis*, and *tetanus* are diseases caused by bacteria. Diphtheria, caused by the bacillus *Corynebacterium diphtheriae*, appears as a severe throat infection and fever. At one time, diphtheria took the lives of thousands. Pertussis (whooping cough) is caused by *Bordetella pertussis*. Pertussis is a disease of the respiratory system, and it mainly affects infants and young children. Tetanus is caused by spores of *Clostridium tetani*. The most common sign of tetanus is a stiffness of the jaw, commonly called lockjaw. All three of these diseases are prevented with a combined vaccination. The DPT immunization is given to children at 2, 4, and 6 months of age, and then a booster is given at 5 years of age. After age 5, tetanus boosters are given every 10 years.

Strep Throat. *Strep throat*, one of the most common bacterial diseases in humans, is a streptococcal infection. Symptoms are sore throat, fever, and general malaise. In some cases, toxins released by the bacterium can cause a rash to develop and become a condition known as scarlet fever. *Streptococcus mutans*, a species of streptococcus, has been implicated in dental caries and endocarditis. This same group of bacteria can give rise to pneumonia or rheumatic fever. Historically the ADA followed the recommendations of the American Heart Association (AHA) and had patients with certain heart diseases take antibiotics prior to dental treatment. The latest guidelines of the AHA indicate that most of these patients do not need antibiotics prior to their dental appointments and that only patients with artificial heart valves, certain specific congenital heart conditions, and those with a history of infective endocarditis should take antibiotics prior to dental appoints.

Staphylococcal Infections. *Staphylococcal infections* derive from bacteria that grow in clusters. Some diseases caused by these pathogens include the staph infection, gangrene, toxic shock syndrome, venereal diseases, and some forms of pneumonia. Antibiotics are the first line of treatment.

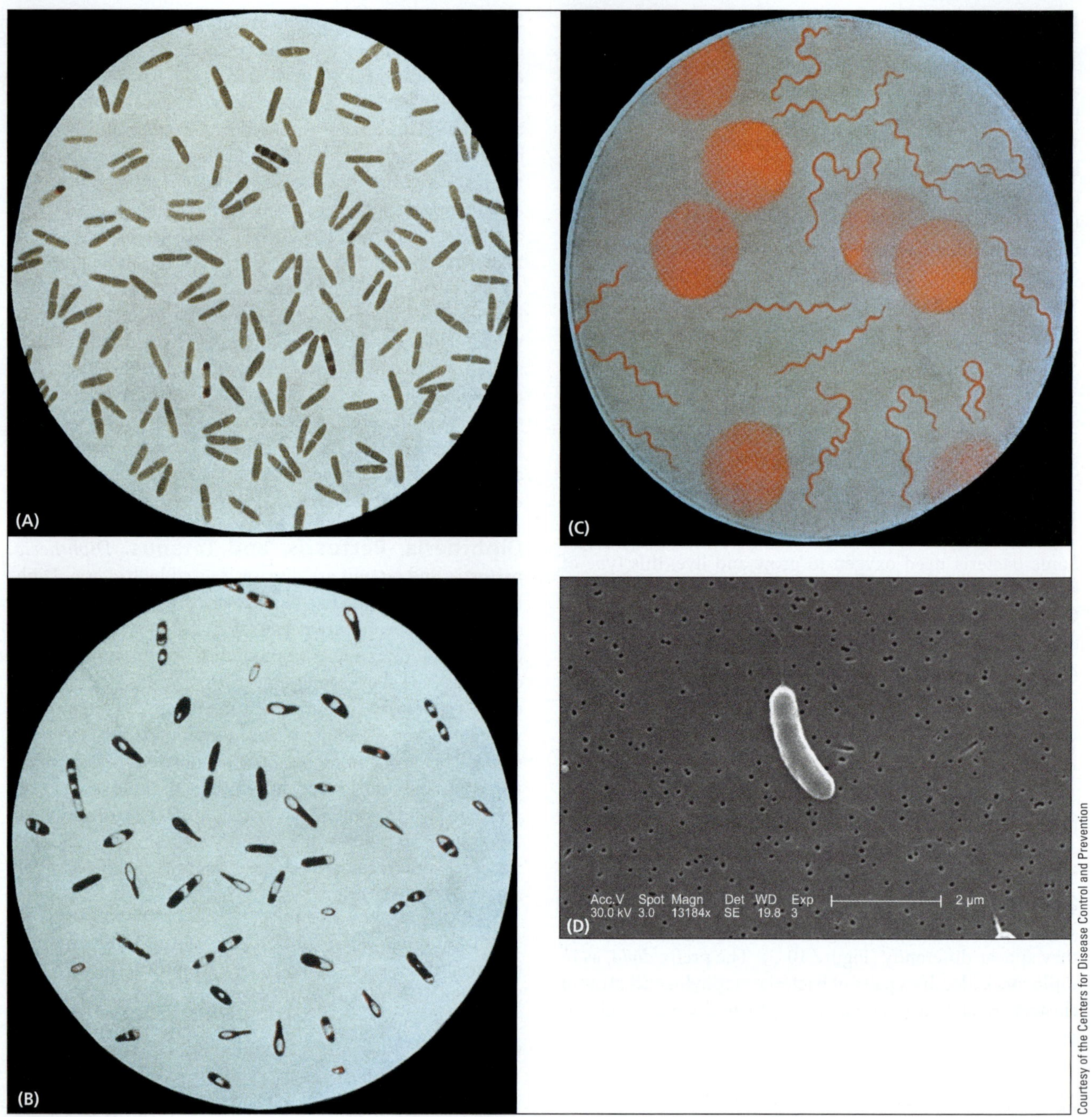

FIGURE 10-4
The unique shapes of bacteria. (A) Bacilli: rod shaped. (B) Cocci: round. (C) Spirilla: S-shaped. (D) Vibrios: curved.

Bacillus anthracis. *Bacillus anthracis*, which causes anthrax in grazing animals, including goats, sheep, and cattle, is a gram-positive bacillus that causes a lethal disease. Humans can get the disease through cuts in the skin (cutaneous anthrax) or by eating infected meat. If treatment is not administered before symptoms manifest, the disease is normally fatal. There are 100 million lethal doses in each gram of anthrax, making it 100,000 times more deadly than any other bacillus. In powder form, this bacillus can be made and disseminated easily at low cost, making it a very deadly biological weapon. Infected individuals experience symptoms within 1 to 6 days, which will start as a low-grade fever, weakness, and a dry, hacking cough. The symptoms will improve slightly before severe respiratory distress, shock, and normally death. The disease can be prevented by a vaccination or an antibiotic treatment before symptoms manifest.

Chlamydiae. Different strains of *Chlamydia trachomatis* are responsible for various genital, eye, and lymph node infections. This microorganism is the most common sexually

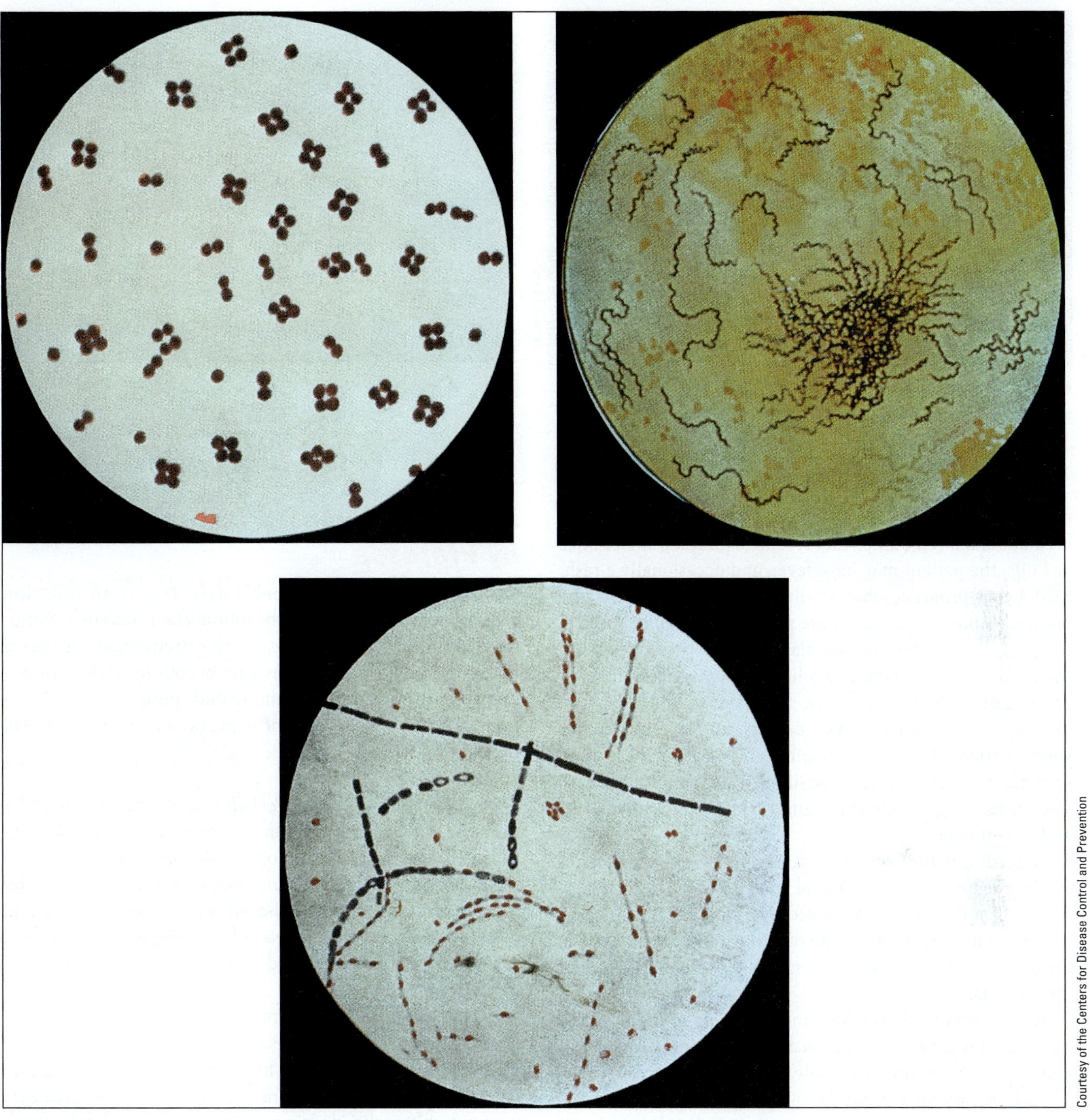

FIGURE 10-5
The pair, cluster, and chain bacterial colonies.

transmitted disease (STD) in the United States. Treatment is with antibiotics, such as tetracycline and erythromycin, and it usually succeeds quickly.

Methicillin-resistant *Staphylococcus aureus.*

Methicillin-resistant Staphylococcus aureus (MRSA) is bacteria that is resistant to commonly used antibiotics (Figure 10-6). For many years antibiotics have been used to treat colds, flu, and other viral infections. Often these viral infections don't react to these antibiotic drugs and thus have contributed to the rise of drug-resistant bacteria. Bacteria exist on an evolutionary track, so germs that survive treatment with antibiotic soon learn to resist others.

MRSA is passed from one person to another by direct contact with the infected wound or by contact with contaminated hands. Also people who carry MRSA but do not have any signs or symptoms can spread the bacteria to others. MRSA is contacted in community settings (Community Associated-CA-MRSA) and medical facilities (Health Care Associated-HA-MRSA). In community settings it causes infections

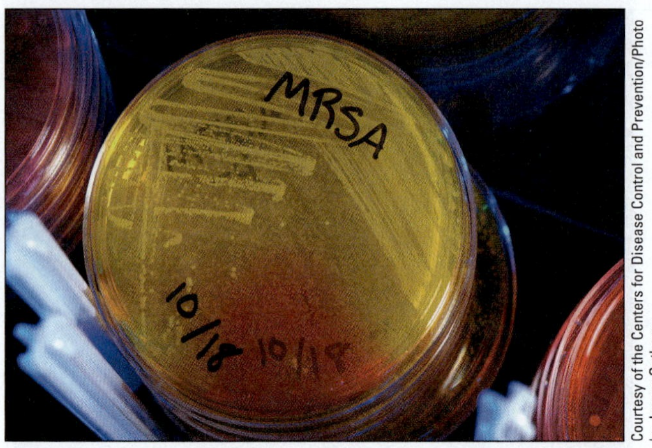

Courtesy of the Centers for Disease Control and Prevention/Photo by James Gathany

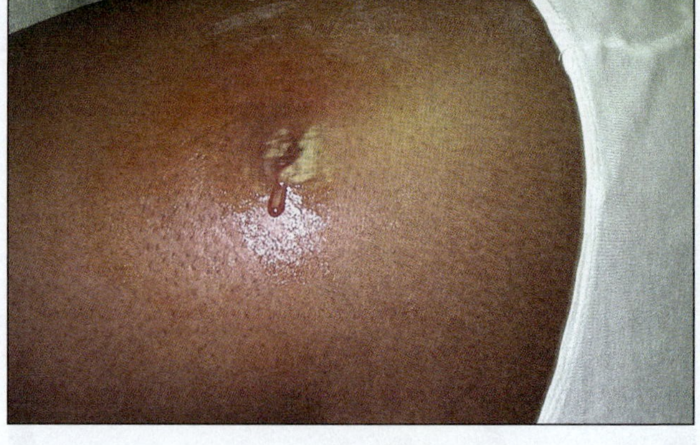

Courtesy of the Centers for Disease Control and Prevention/Bruno Coignard, M.D; Jeff Hageman, M.H.S.

FIGURE 10-6
MRSA bacterium and an example of MRSA skin lesion.

mainly in the skin. CA-MRSA symptoms on the skin may look like small red bumps that resemble pimples, spider bites or boils; the patient may have fever, and occasionally a rash. MRSA may progress substantially and within a few days, the bumps become larger and more painful and require surgical draining. Sometimes the bacteria can also progress deep into the body and cause potentially life-threatening infections in bones, joints, the blood stream, heart valves, and the lungs. In hospitals, prisons, dialysis centers, and nursing homes where patients have open wounds and weakened immune systems, HA-MRSA can cause life-threatening bloodstream infections, surgical site infections, urinary tract infections, and pneumonia.

According to the CDC, less than 2 percent of the population carries the type of staph bacteria known as MRSA. Although MRSA is still a major concern the numbers are decreasing according to CDC studies. The only way to know if MRSA is the cause of an infection is to perform a laboratory culture of the bacteria.

Risk factors for HA-MRSA include being in the hospital, having an invasive medical device (such as urinary catheters), and/or residing in nursing facility or long-term care.

Risk factors for CA-MRSA include participation in contact sports, living in crowded or unsanitary conditions (such as military training camps, child care centers, and jails), and being a homosexual male.

Protozoa

Organisms just below visibility of the naked eye (about 100 microns in size) are classified as **protozoa** (proh-tah-**ZOH**-ah) (Figure 10-7). Often called amoeba, they live in fluids in the bloodstream, mouth, and intestinal tract and survive in polluted water in pools and ponds. Protozoa are single-celled animal life, and some are sporulating. They engulf their food as they change in shape to achieve mobility. Many have a long, threadlike appendage called **flagella**. Flagella whip around and cause additional movement for the protozoa. Some protozoa contain chlorophyll, and most are aerobic.

Disease Examples Caused by Protozoa

Amebic Dysentery. *Amebic dysentery* is an infection caused by the microorganism *Entamoeba histolytica*. Symptoms include severe diarrhea and, in extreme cases, abscesses in the liver. This disease is prevalent in countries where drinking water is contaminated and overall poor hygiene conditions prevail. Drug treatment is necessary to effectively kill the parasite.

Periodontal Disease. *Periodontal disease* is caused by protozoa and bacteria. Both microorganisms are found in the inflamed tissue around the tooth. Protozoa are in the plaque in the periodontal pockets around the tooth. Treatment includes a thorough cleaning around the area to remove any plaque and diseased tissue and then impeccable oral hygiene maintenance. Periodontal disease is covered in more detail in Chapter 31.

Malaria. *Malaria* and sleeping sickness are two other diseases caused by protozoa. Both are prevalent throughout the tropics and have symptoms during the first 2 weeks, such as fever and soreness at the point of entry. Malaria is spread via mosquito bites, and sleeping sickness is spread by the tsetse fly. Both require drug therapy to kill the parasites in the bites.

Rickettsiae

A parasitic form of bacteria is classified as **rickettsiae**. Lice, fleas, ticks, and mites are often hosts to rickettsiae. They multiply only by invading the cells of another life form. The hosts then transmit the disease to humans.

Disease Examples Caused by Rickettsiae

Rocky Mountain Spotted Fever. Symptoms of *Rocky Mountain spotted fever* occur about a week to 10 days after transmission from the host and are much like those of the

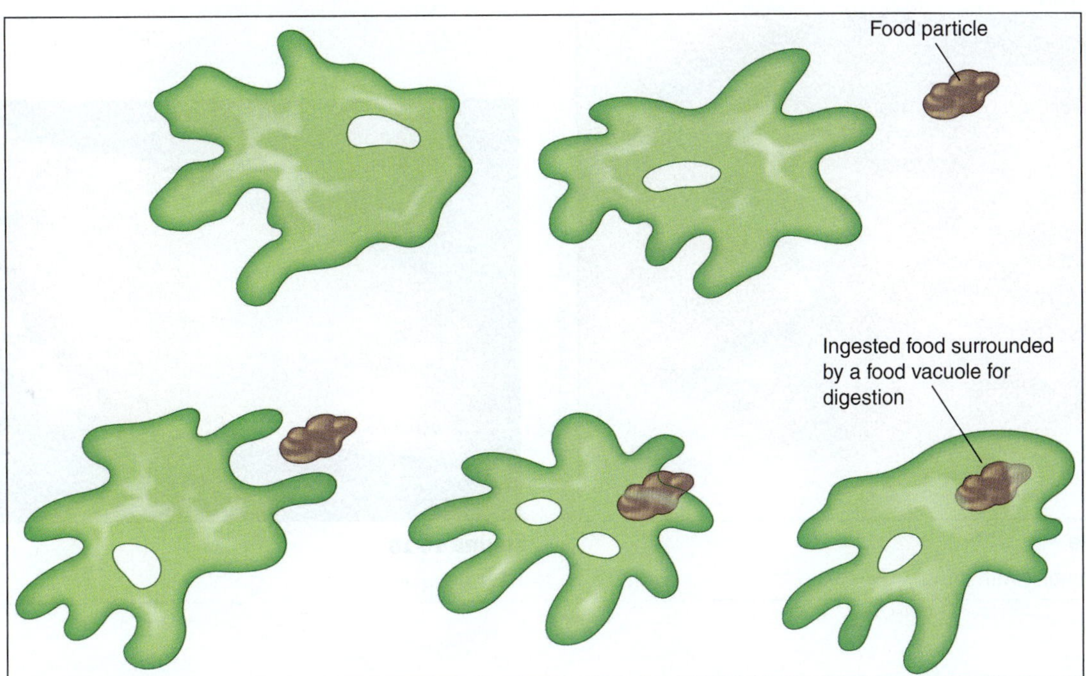

FIGURE 10-7
The protozoan changing shape as it travels to and engulfs its food.

flu. Two to 6 days after the symptoms have occurred, small pink spots appear on the ankles and wrists. The body is soon covered with these spots. Treatment with antibiotics normally cures the disease, which is rare.

Typhus. *Typhus* is another fairly rare disease, similar to Rocky Mountain spotted fever. The microorganism is spread by a host, and symptoms appear rapidly. A severe headache, back and limb pain, constipation, and high fever develop suddenly. A rash similar to measles appears, the heart beats weakly, and confusion is common. Typhus fever is treated with antibiotic drug therapy.

Head Lice. *Pediculosis* is the state of being infected with head lice. Head lice (Figure 10-8) are a common occurrence for children in schools. If one child is identified as having head lice, others should be checked carefully to stop recurrence. Lice are tiny, bloodsucking, wingless parasites that are transmitted through direct contact. Mature lice produce about six eggs every day. These eggs (nits), attached to hair shafts, are visible. Treatment consists of applying medicinal shampoo and combing to loosen the nits. Bedding, towels, brushes, combs, and clothes must also be washed with very hot water and soap. Multiple shampoo treatments may be required.

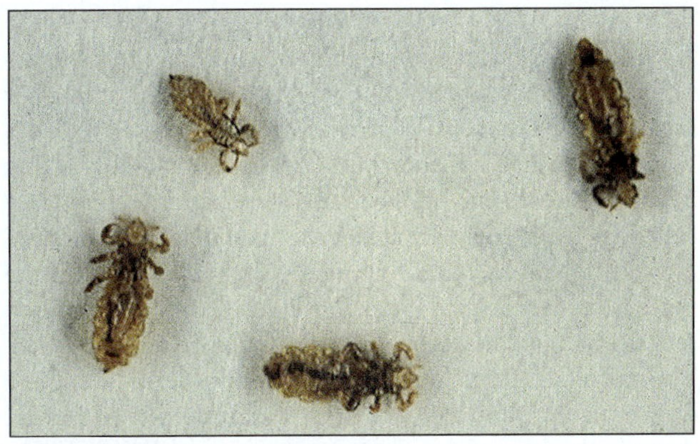

FIGURE 10-8
Greatly magnified head lice.

Yeasts and Molds

Yeasts and molds (**fungi**) are smaller than protozoa and larger than bacteria. This group of microorganisms includes bread yeast, mushrooms, and bread molds. Some are sporulating, and they reproduce by budding. They cannot be killed by the antibiotics that kill bacteria (i.e., penicillin is made from mold but does not act upon the fungi from which it is made).

Disease Examples Caused by Yeasts and Molds

Candidiasis. *Candidiasis* (kan-dih-DYE-ah-sis) is an infection by the fungus *Candida albicans*, often on areas covered with mucous membrane, such as inside of the mouth or the vaginal area. It is commonly called thrush, or moniliasis (Figure 10-9). It is kept at bay with **normal flora** (i.e., normal bacteria, in these areas). If antibiotics destroy too many of the "normal" bacteria, or if the body's immune

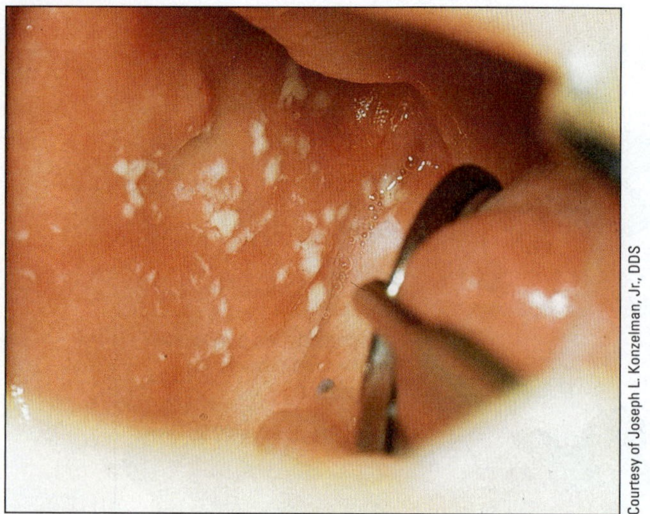

FIGURE 10-9
Patient presenting with thrush.

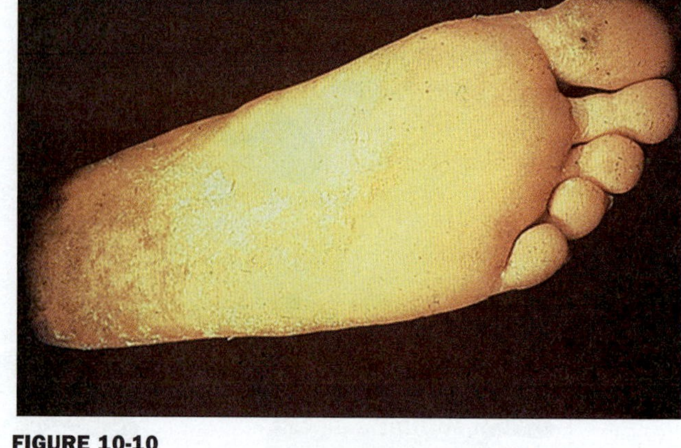

FIGURE 10-10
Tinea unguium.

system is impaired, such as is the case with acquired immunodeficiency syndrome (AIDS), then the fungi multiply and overgrow. The disease causes thick white or creamy yellow ("cottage cheese") raised patches. These patches may become irritated and cause discomfort. Treatment for candidiasis is antifungal drug therapy.

Tinea. *Tinea* includes any group of common fungal infections. They are acquired from an infected person, animal, or inanimate object such as a shower stall. Tinea pedis, which is commonly called athlete's foot, causes itching and cracking between the toes and on the foot. Tinea corporis, commonly called ringworm, usually appears as red circles with a raised edge on the body. Tinea unguium is characterized as white patches on the toe or fingernail (Figure 10-10). The location makes it difficult to treat because the fungus is under the nail. The nail may thicken, overgrow, become brittle, or be entirely destroyed. For most types of tinea, a treatment of antifungal drugs in the form of skin creams, ointments, or lotions is prescribed. Oral antifungal drugs may be necessary in persistent strains of the fungus.

Prions

Proteinaceous infectious particles called **prions** (pree-ons) are a microorganism that is an infectious agent made only of protein. All mammals have prions in the nerve cells that are normal. Prions are actually the host protein that converts normal protein molecules into abnormal structures that are responsible for a group of diseases classified as transmissible spongiform encephalopathies (TSEs). The TSEs are rare, untreatable, and deadly due to the fact that they affect the brain tissue. There is some research that identifies the prions in some fungi, but much is yet to be known about prions. Prions are associated with animal diseases such as the mad cow disease (bovine spongiform encephalopathy), and in human diseases such as Creutzfeldt-Jakob disease as well as others.

Disease Examples Caused by Prions

Mad Cow Disease. The *mad cow disease* or bovine spongiform encephalopathy (BSE) is a progressive disorder of the brain seen in cattle. The first time that cows were noted to have this disease was in the early 1970s. In the United States only one or two cases have been identified and they have been immediately contained. The fear is that a human will ingest the meat from an animal infected with BSE and that this will cause the diseased prions to react on the human's protein molecules, affecting the nerve cells that may lead to loss of brain function. Great precautions are being taken by the Centers for Disease Control and Prevention and the United States Department of Agriculture to monitor the beef industry.

Creutzfeldt-Jakob Disease. Two German neurologists, Hans Gerhard Creutzfeldt and Alfons Maria Jakob, were the first to describe *Creutzfeldt-Jakob disease.* The disease is rare, with only one case per million people in the world and only about 200 cases in the United States each year. It belongs to the TSE group of diseases. Individuals who are affected typically are around the age of 60 years of age. They present with rapidly progressing dementia, memory loss, speech impairment, involuntary jerky movements, weakness, blindness, and then coma. The disease progresses rapidly and is fatal due to the neurological deterioration. The cause of the disease is currently unknown. It is believed that this disease is related to the prion proteins, but some think that it is a slowly growing virus that is **latent**, suppressed, or dormant for a period of time. There are several variants of this disease that affect individuals earlier in life.

Viruses

The smallest microorganisms known to date are classified as **viruses.** They are tiny particles, which are one-hundredth the size of bacteria. An electron microscope must be used to observe viruses (Figure 10-11). Like rickettsiae, they are able to reproduce only inside host cells. Viruses are difficult to grow in a culture and, like bacteria, their morphology is varied. Most are easy to kill by disinfecting or exposure to air, but the hepatitis B virus is very resistant. It can live on a dry surface for up to 2 weeks. Antibiotics will not kill any true virus. Outbreaks of viruses, such as herpes simplex, can last from 10 days to 2 weeks, whether treated or not. Treatment is primarily aimed at the symptoms in order to make the patient more comfortable.

Disease Examples Caused by Viruses

Measles, Mumps, and Rubella. *Measles*, *mumps*, and *rubella* are childhood illnesses caused by viruses. Measles cause a rash and a fever, and is spread by airborne droplets of nasal secretions. An incubation period of 9 to 11 days takes place before symptoms appear. The main symptom of mumps is the swelling of the parotid (salivary) glands on one side or both sides. Mumps is spread by airborne droplets. Rubella, also known as German measles, appears as a rash on the face and may spread to the trunk and limbs. This disease is serious only if it affects women in the early stages of pregnancy, because of possible birth defects. The incubation period for both mumps and measles is 2 to 3 weeks. The MMR (measles, mumps, and rubella) vaccine is highly effective in providing long-lasting immunity and is given to all children at about 15 months of age. Treatment aims at reducing discomfort only. An analgesic such as aspirin is given for fevers, and lotion is applied to relieve itching.

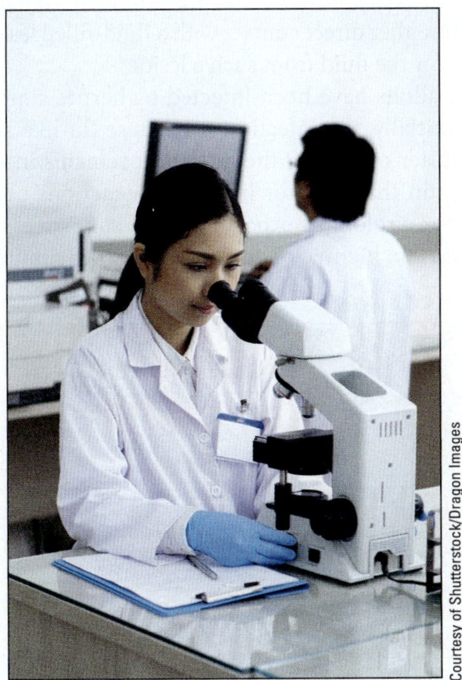

Courtesy of Shutterstock/Dragon Images

FIGURE 10-11

Viewing organism through a microscope.

Epstein-Barr Virus and Infectious Mononucleosis. *Epstein-Barr Virus (EBV)* is one of the most common viruses in humans. The Centers for Disease Control (CDC) report that close to 95 percent of adults between the ages of 35 and 40 have been infected with EBV. When infants, children, or young adults are infected, about 35 to 50 percent (according to the CDC) develop infectious *mononucleosis*. Symptoms of EBV are not much different than any other childhood illness; mononucleosis symptoms are fever, sore throat, and swollen lymph glands. Other symptoms such as liver concerns, a swollen spleen, and heart or nervous system involvement rarely occur, and this disease is almost never fatal. Laboratory tests along with the reporting of the symptoms help determine if the individual is indeed infected with the disease. The patient may need rest and the symptoms leave in about 1 to 2 months. EBV transmission occurs with intimate contact with saliva, which is why this disease is referred to as the "kissing disease." The newly infected individual will experience symptoms within 4 to 6 weeks after contact.

West Nile Virus. *West Nile Virus (WNV)* can be very serious. It is often thought of as a seasonal virus that arrives in the spring and continues until the fall. It is transmitted by means of mosquito bites and, according to the CDC, can develop into a severe illness in about one in 150 infected people. The symptoms of severe illness can include extreme high fever, neck stiffness, disorientation, headache, convulsions, tremors, muscle weakness, vision loss, coma, numbness, and paralysis lasting several weeks; however, some symptoms can become permanent. Mild symptoms occur in about 20 percent of the people infected and include fever, head and body aches, nausea, vomiting, and lymph glands that are swollen, along with a skin rash on the back, chest, and stomach. The symptoms can last from a few days to several weeks. The majority of people who were infected with West Nile Virus will not have symptoms. The CDC states that "about 4 out of 5 who are infected with WNV will not show any symptoms at all." If symptoms occur, they will develop between 3 to 14 days after the infected mosquitoes bite. No identified treatment is used to treat WNV, but symptoms are treated to make the patient comfortable.

Poliomyelitis. *Poliomyelitis* (poh-lee-oh-my-eh-**LYE**-tis), commonly called polio, attacks the central nervous system and may lead to extensive paralysis. Since the development of vaccines in the late 1950s, very few cases have been identified in the United States. The IPV (inactivated, or dead, polio virus vaccine) is given by injection; however, the IPV is not used as much as OPV (oral poliovirus vaccine), which contains live but harmless virus and is given orally at the ages of 2, 4, and 18 months. A booster dose at 5 years of age is also given.

Chickenpox. *Chickenpox* is a childhood disease caused by the varicella-zoster virus. It is characterized by a rash and slight fever. The virus remains dormant in the nerve tissue after the attack and may cause herpes zoster (shingles) later in life. Patients are contagious from about 2 days before the fever to 5 days after. The disease is spread through airborne droplets. The patient is treated for the fever but will heal within 10 days. A varicella virus vaccine is recommended for this disease, but the period of immunity is unknown. Adult symptoms are quite severe, and include pneumonia.

Common Cold and Influenza. The *common cold* and *influenza* are caused by viruses. Treatment is focused on relieving fever, upset stomach, headache, and body ache. Anti-influenza vaccines are available and are highly recommended for the elderly and medically compromised. The vaccines are successful in about 60 percent of cases. Patients are contagious from 12 to 72 hours after the symptoms appear. Colds are spread through airborne droplets, contact with contaminated objects, or hand-to-hand contact. Flu is spread through airborne droplets.

Swine Influenza. *Swine influenza* or swine-origin influenza is an infection caused by various types of swine viruses that have evolved over time. The virus originally was found in pig populations around the world. The transmission of the virus from pigs to people who have direct contact with pigs, is not common and does not always lead to human flu. However, people who are around pigs have an increased risk of contacting the swine flu. The virus evolved and is a mix of genes from swine, bird, and human flu viruses.

The Swine influenza we are most concerned with is known as H1N1 Type A swine influenza and people contact this flu from other people, not from pigs. The H1N1 virus that has been circulating for many years, the CDC calls it the "2009 H1N1 swine flu virus," is not the usual seasonal virus and most people have no natural immunity to it. The normal seasonal flu shot does not protect against this swine flu. Other strains have developed from the H1N1 strain including the H1N2 and the H2N2.

Symptoms are similar to other flu viruses, such as fever, sore throat, cough, watery eyes, body aches, headache, chills, runny nose, and in some cases diarrhea and vomiting. As with seasonal flu, H1N1 may make chronic conditions such as lung disease, diabetes, and heart disease more severe. If symptoms do not improve a health care provider should be contacted. Because these symptoms are common and hard to differentiate, the person's recent and past medical history must be evaluated for connection to swine influenza infection in people they have been in contact with. The CDC recommends an oral and nasal fluid collection in the diagnosing of H1N1 swine flu as compared to seasonal influenza.

While there is no vaccine available right now to protect against H1N1, the usual actions can help, such as avoid touching your eyes, nose, or mouth, cough or sneeze into your sleeve, or cover your nose and mouth with a tissue when you cough or sneeze, then throw the tissue in the trash, washing your hands often with soap and water or with alcohol-based hand sanitizers, and disinfect household surfaces. Avoid contact with sick people. If you become ill, stay home and limit contact with others. There are prescription antiviral drugs the health care provider can prescribe once the flu has been diagnosed as H1N1 swine flu.

Ebola. *Ebola* is a virus where the symptoms appear anywhere from 2 to 21 days after exposure. The transmission is spread through bodily fluids of a person who is sick or has died from Ebola. The symptoms include fever greater than 101 degrees, diarrhea, sore throat, severe head ache, vomiting, joint/muscle ache, abdominal pain, rash, and internal bleeding. Some individuals with the disease bleed from the eyes, nose, ears, and rectum. In 2014 Ebola affected multiple countries in West Africa and was the largest in history. There were two additional imported cases, and two locally acquired cases in health care. The highest risk is to friends and family of the infected individual and the health care workers taking care of the patient. Many new guidelines for caring for Ebola infected individuals have been put in place. The Center for Disease Control CDC is a good source for updated information.

Viral Diseases of Major Concern to the Dental Assistant

The dental assistant is at risk of exposure to a variety of infectious diseases and disorders. Some diseases pose mild risks and recovery from exposure is quick, while others may have a great risk for causing chronic illness or may even threaten the dental assistant's life. The most critical conditions to be alert to are herpes simplex, viral hepatitis, HIV, and AIDS.

Herpes Simplex

Herpes (**HER**-peez) *simplex* is a common and troublesome viral disease (Figure 10-12). *Herpes simplex virus type 1 (HSV1)* is usually associated with infections of the lips, mouth, and face; and *herpes simplex virus type II (HSV2)* is normally associated with the genital area. Type II, however, can appear in the oral cavity. Both viruses are extremely contagious and spread by either direct contact with a fluid-filled lesion, called a vesicle, or the fluid from such a lesion.

Most adults have been infected by herpes simplex virus type I. Initially, the infection may cause flu-like symptoms and a blister or sore in the mouth. It remains in the nerve cells within that area for life. HSV1 reactions often result from fever, prolonged exposure to the sun, stress, or ingestion of certain high-acid foods. These herpes simplex viruses

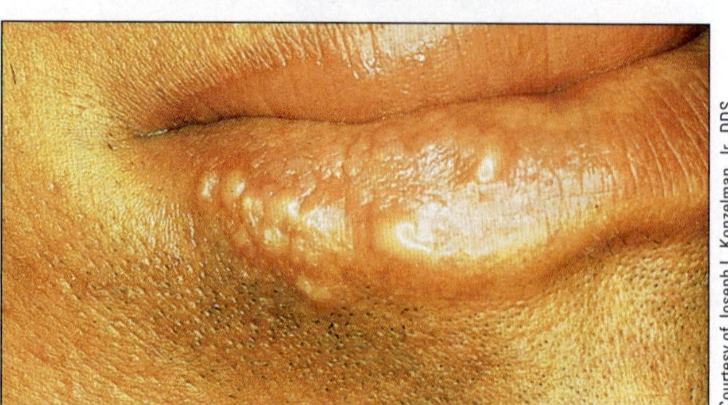

Courtesy of Joseph L. Konzelman, Jr., DDS

FIGURE 10-12
Herpetic labialis lesion.

(**cold sores** or **aphthous ulcers**) can reactivate and appear in the same general areas. The virus may infect the fingers if open sores are present; but this virus on the finger (**herpetic whitlow**) is rare, and was a greater concern to dental personnel prior to the usage of treatment gloves. The virus can be transferred to the eye and cause **conjunctivitis** or a **corneal ulcer**, which could result in blindness.

Treatment of HSV1 depends on type, site, and severity. Dental teams may suggest rescheduling the patient if the sores are apparent. This is primarily for the comfort of the patient, but it also may be office policy not to provide treatment when vesicles are present in the oral cavity. A number of topical treatments are available for patient comfort. Some people take L-Lysen, an amino acid, when they feel the symptoms coming on. Antiviral drugs such as acyclovir, the generic for Zovirax, are sometimes helpful.

HSV2 is sexually transmitted genital herpes. It displays the same vesicles, erupting on the sex organs, and may erupt orally as well. As with type 1, type 2 can recur.

Bloodborne Diseases

Bloodborne diseases, or **bloodborne pathogens** (disease-producing microorganisms), are of great concern. The Occupational Safety and Health Administration (OSHA) addresses this problem in the Bloodborne Pathogen Standard (see Chapter 11). Bloodborne diseases of concern to the dental assistant are viral hepatitis (HBV) and human immunodeficiency virus (HIV), which later develops into acquired immunodeficiency syndrome (AIDS). These diseases are transmitted directly through contaminated blood and other body fluids.

High-Risk Behavior for Acquiring Hepatitis B, HIV, and AIDS

- Injuries or sticks with sharp objects contaminated with blood or body fluid
- Multiple sexual partners, unprotected sex (homosexual, bisexual, or heterosexual)
- Sharing contaminated needles
- Exposure to non-intact skin or open wound with contaminated blood or body fluid

Viral Hepatitis

"*Hepatitis*" means inflammation of the liver and *viral hepatitis* means that it is transferred by means of a virus. Other things can cause hepatitis such as heavy alcohol use, some drugs, toxins, and bacteria. There are five primary types of hepatitis (Table 10-1). Hepatitis A and E are transmitted by person-to-person contact or by ingestion of contaminated water or food. The symptoms, which appear from 15 to 40 days after contact, range from flu-like symptoms to acute liver damage.

Hepatitis A. *Hepatitis A* (often called infectious hepatitis) is in the news when a food provider has a number of customers who become ill and the virus is identified. No long-term immunization has been available until recently. People who have possible contact with contaminated food or water are given an injection of gamma globulin within 14 days of exposure, which provides short-term immunization. In 1995, a vaccine called Havrix was licensed by the U.S. Food and Drug Administration (FDA). A paper by the Centers for Disease Control and Prevention (CDC) stated the benefits of Havrix and, in 1997, Havrix was awarded the pediatric vaccine contract. Children in areas with a high rate of hepatitis A will be given the initial and booster dose of Havrix between the ages of 2 and 18 years.

Hepatitis B. *Hepatitis B* is of major concern to dental personnel. This disease (commonly called serum hepatitis) has been recognized only since the early 1950s. Primarily transmitted through contaminated needles and syringes, the incubation period is from 50 to 180 days. Only one-third of infected people have symptoms that can be easily identified, one-third have only slight symptoms, and one-third have no symptoms at all. The symptoms include loss of appetite, digestive upset, upper abdominal pain and tenderness, fever, weakness, muscle pain, and jaundice (yellowing of the skin). According to the CDC, about 300,000 people are infected each year; of that number, 300 will die from the disease, 10,000 will be hospitalized, and 20,000 will become chronic carriers. The CDC estimates that there are over a million carriers in the United States today. The FDA approved Hepsera (adefovir dipivoxil) tablets in 2002 for treatment of chronic hepatitis B in adults. Hepsera slows the progression of chronic hepatitis B.

In 1982, a plasma-derived Heptavax-B vaccine was introduced in the United States. Since that time, Recombivax HB and Engerix-B have been licensed for use in the United States and are shown to be effective against the hepatitis B virus. Both these vaccines are administered in a series of three injections. The schedule is initially, then a month later, and then 3 months from the first vaccine administration. The vaccine is administered in the form of an injection to the deltoid muscle in the arm. It has been found that administration in the buttocks did not yield the same **seroconversion** rate (i.e., vaccine causing the development of immunity).

It should be noted that, according to OSHA standards, the employer is responsible for offering the HBV 3 series vaccination to new employees in Categories I and II within 10 days of employment at no cost to the employee. The employee can refuse the vaccine by signing an informed refusal form that is to be kept in the employee file (see Chapter 12).

After completing the three series of HBV vaccines, a blood test is performed to ensure that immunity has developed. The employer is not responsible for the blood test, because it is not noted in the OSHA standard, but it is an important step for the dental assistant to take to ensure prevention of hepatitis B. If the dental assistant tests negative for seroconversion, the physician must make a determination about additional dosages of the HBV vaccine.

TABLE 10-1 Types of Viral Hepatitis

Disease & Cause	Transmission	Symptoms	Prevention	Long-Term Effects
Viral Hepatitis A (HAV)	Human feces of persons with HAV being transmitted to oral cavity of other person. Example: not washing hands after using bathroom and then preparing food.	Fatigue, loss of appetite, fever, nausea, diarrhea, and jaundice.	• Hepatitis A vaccine recommended for people 12 months and older. • Wash hands. • Immune globulin can be taken within 2 weeks of contact.	• No chronic infection. • Have it only once.
Viral Hepatitis B (HBV)	• Blood from Infected person enters a person who is not infected. • Spread through contaminated needles, or other sharps. • Sex. • Infected mother to baby during birth.	Fatigue, loss of appetite, fever, nausea, vomiting, joint and abdominal pain, and jaundice. Approximately 1/3 of infected persons have no symptoms.	• Hepatitis B vaccine. • Use of latex condom during sexual activity. • Don't shoot drugs and share needles. • Don't share items that may have blood on them.	• 15–25% will die from chronic liver disease. • High rate of chronic liver disease in infants born to infected mothers.
Viral Hepatitis C (HCB)	• Blood from Infected person enters a person who is not infected. • Spread through contaminated needles, or other sharps. • From Infected mother to baby during birth. • It can be spread through sexual activity but that is rare.	Fatigue, loss of appetite, nausea, abdominal pain, dark urine, and jaundice.	• No vaccine. • Don't shoot drugs and share needles. • Don't share items that may have blood on them. • Wash hands.	• Chronic infection in 55–85% of infected individuals. • 1–5% may die. • Leading indication for liver transplant. • Leading indication for liver transplant. • Uncommon in the United States.
Viral Hepatitis D (HDV)	Same as viral hepatitis B: • Blood from Infected person enters a person who is not infected. • Spread through contaminated needles, or other sharps. • Sex. • Infected mother to baby during birth.	Fatigue, loss of appetite, nausea, vomiting, joint and abdominal pain, jaundice, and dark urine.	• Hepatitis B vaccine. • Education to reduce risk behaviors.	If co-infection with HBV, the individual may have more severe symptoms and is more likely to have chronic liver disease.
Viral Hepatitis E (HEV)	Same as HAV: Human feces of persons with HAV being transmitted to oral cavity of other person. Example: not washing hands after bathroom and then preparing food.	Fatigue, loss of appetite, nausea, vomiting, dark urine, and jaundice.	• No vaccine. • Wash hands.	• No long-term infection. • More severe in pregnant women in their third trimester.

This information was taken from the Centers for Disease Control Web site fact sheets for Viral Hepatitis A–E.

A booster dosage is not recommended by the CDC unless an exposure incident has occurred or a physician recommends it after testing negative for seroconversion.

Hepatitis C. *Hepatitis C*, often called non-A and non-B, reacts somewhat like hepatitis B, but there is no vaccine available currently. About 50 percent of the people infected become chronic carriers.

Hepatitis D. *Hepatitis D*, also known as the delta agent, cannot replicate on its own and requires the presence of hepatitis B. The vaccination for hepatitis B should also prevent hepatitis D.

Hepatitis E. *Hepatitis E* is found in the feces of people and animals and is therefore spread through contaminated water and food. The symptoms are loss of appetite, dark urine, fatigue, and nausea. To prevent this disease an individual should wash hands carefully when preparing food and when traveling take special care in avoiding contaminated water.

Human Immunodeficiency Virus

Human immunodeficiency virus (HIV) belongs to the class of retroviruses and is the cause of acquired immunodeficiency syndrome AIDS. It gains access to the bloodstream via sexual intercourse, transfusions, and sticks with infected needles that break the skin. Also, a fetus can be infected by its mother. HIV attacks T-lymphocytes, part of the immune system, and then multiplies. People in this stage pose no threat to the health care worker if standard precautions are followed. People who have HIV but are unaware that they carry it are called asymptomatic carriers. Some have vague complaints, such as fever, weight loss, or unexplained diarrhea. These individuals are referred to as having AIDS-related complex (ARC).

In most cases, the disease progresses and the infected individual develops some brain damage in the form of dementia. If the individual is in this state for a long period of time, more severe brain damage may occur; normally, the infected individual most likely succumbs to AIDS before this happens.

Current treatment focuses on symptoms and not the disease itself. A great deal of research is being done currently to develop a vaccine to fight this retrovirus.

Acquired Immunodeficiency Syndrome. *Acquired immunodeficiency syndrome (AIDS)* results from infection with HIV, but not all individuals infected with HIV develop AIDS. A syndrome is a group of symptoms that characterize a disease. In the United States, 100,000 cases of HIV were diagnosed in the 1980s. The first few cases were reported in 1981. The CDC was notified of a rare and unusual lung infection in young homosexual men. Also, a slow-growing skin tumor usually found in aging men, called Kaposi's sarcoma, was found to be growing aggressively in this same group of young men (Figure 10-13). Individuals with these two symptoms reported with a number of opportunistic infections, such as pneumonia.

After much research, the virus was found to be transmitted via the semen and blood of infected individuals. "Casual" spreading of the disease does not seem to happen. For example, kissing does not spread the disease. A person with full-blown AIDS exhibits cancers, infections, diarrhea, or a number of other viral diseases. The prognosis is often fatal, but life may be sustained for a number of years with appropriate diet and health measures. Through December 2009, the cumulative number of AIDS cases reported to the CDC was 1,108,611. As of 2008, the total deaths of this same group were 617,025. The majority of these diagnosed cases are in the 30- to 40-year-old age group.

There is no cure for AIDS. The complications are treated accordingly. Several antiviral drugs are used, such as zidovudine (AZT) and acyclovir. AZT has a number of side effects but has been shown to slow progression of the disease. Research continues in an effort to find a vaccine for HIV, with several drugs showing promise.

Pandemic

A **pandemic** is a wide spread epidemic of infectious disease. It may be spread worldwide or just across a large region. The disease cancer is responsible for many deaths over a large area but it is not considered to be a pandemic because it is not infectious. The flu is also not normally classified as a pandemic

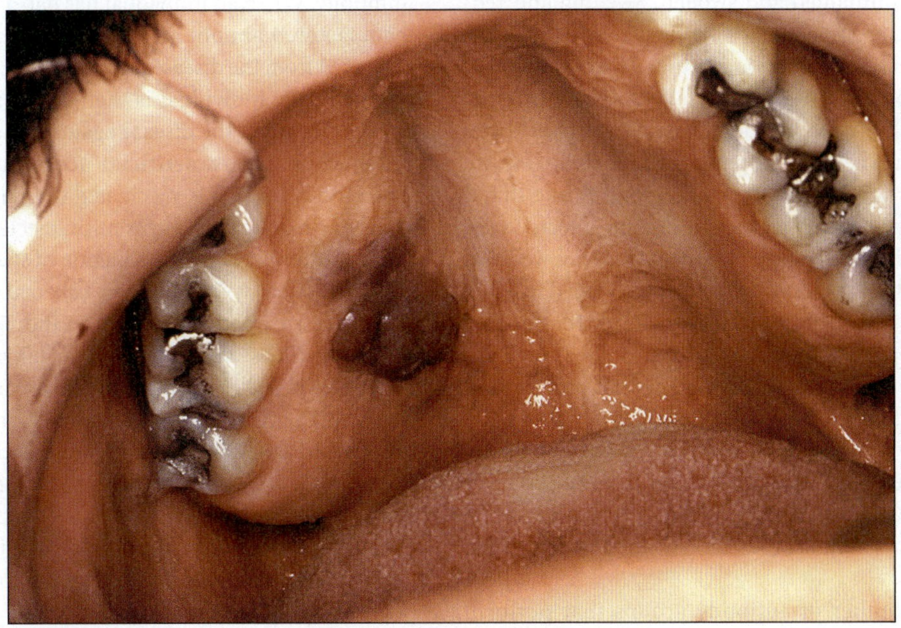

Courtesy of the Centers for Disease Control and Prevention/Sol Silverman, Jr., D.D.S., University of California, San Francisco

FIGURE 10-13

A Kaposi's sarcoma lesion on the palate.

disease because it is generally seasonal. Over the years many pandemics have occurred from diseases such as smallpox, tuberculosis, HIV, and Aids. Even a flu such as the Spanish flu of 1918–1919 was considered a pandemic because it resulted in worldwide dramatic mortality and varied from the seasonal flu. If the disease happens and it infects a greater number of individuals than expected, it is known to be a **disease outbreak**. A disease outbreak can also be a single case of a contagious disease if it is an unknown disease or a new disease to the area. An **epidemic** is when an infectious disease spreads quickly to a large number of individuals. An example is when the severe acute respiratory syndrome (SARS) epidemic took the lives of over 800 people in the world in 2003. One of the most destructive global pandemics in history was the global disease outbreak of HIV/AIDS throughout 1980–1990. There is concern about possible future pandemics occurring or reoccurring from SARS, Ebola virus, antibiotic resistance, viral hemorrhagic fevers, biological warfare, and diseases we are not currently aware of.

How the Body Resists Diseases

The body fights disease in a number of ways, such as fever or chills or localized inflammation. Before these symptoms occur, however, the pathogens must pass through other lines of defense.

Our bodies repel thousands of infections that come our way every day. Intact skin makes it impossible for a number of bacteria to enter body cells. If dust or some pathogen-laden particles get into the nose, a person sneezes. If something enters the throat, a person coughs. If spoiled food is swallowed, a person normally vomits or expels it through diarrhea.

If the pathogen gains access to the body, the second line of defense, the circulatory system, begins fighting the pathogen. The area becomes inflamed and swollen. Swelling and redness are due to the engorgement of the capillaries with blood. White cells in great numbers migrate to the area and engulf large numbers of bacteria. Many of these cells die and produce enzymes that digest the dead tissues. These mobile phagocytes or leukocytes engulf the invading pathogens and destroy them. The result of this process is **purulence** (pus). While this is going on, the body is building a dam around the infected area, called the **pyogenic membrane**. This membrane is a wall that contains the infection and does not allow it to spread to other parts of the body. If the infection can be controlled, this area fills in with connective tissue and is healed.

If the pathogens overcome the body's first and second lines of defense, the infection spreads to adjoining tissues and finally to the entire body. When this happens, the body utilizes its final defenses: antibodies. An **antibody** produces immunity against any foreign substance or pathogen. A pathogen that stimulates the production of antibodies is called an **antigen**.

There are a number of antibody groups that perform different functions in response to antigens. For instance, an **antitoxin** neutralizes the toxins given off by certain bacteria.

Infection

Another way the body fights off infection or pathogens is with fever and inflammation. Few bacteria can survive a fever of 69°C to 70°C for long. Inflammation, which is an increase in blood flow in the injured area, is characterized by four signs: erythema (redness), heat, edema (swelling), and pain. An increase in blood supply in the area causes the redness and heat and causes the walls to enlarge, allowing antibodies into the area. The swelling causes pain and pressure on nerve endings.

Immunity. The ability to resist pathogens is called immunity. People differ in their abilities to resist disease, and this resistance is stronger at various times in a person's life than at others. The two general types of immunity are natural and acquired. Humans are born with **natural immunity**. Local inflammation and blood phagocytes are part of the natural immune system.

If immunity is developed as a result of exposure to a pathogen, it is called **acquired immunity**. This also can be a borrowed immunity, called **passive acquired immunity**. This occurs when antibodies from another animal or person are injected into an individual, giving protection to the individual from a specific disease. Normally this immediate immunity only lasts up to 6 weeks. A fetus obtains temporary passive immunity from the mother through the placenta. The mother's milk also provides some passive immunity while the baby is breastfeeding.

Lasting longer and preferred over passive acquired immunity is **active acquired immunity**. The two types of active acquired immunity are natural acquired immunity and artificial acquired immunity. When an individual has had a disease, the body has manufactured antibodies to the disease, and the person has recovered from the disease **natural acquired immunity** occurs. Normally, the individual is then immune to the disease and does not contract the disease again. The second type of active acquired immunity, **artificial acquired immunity**, occurs when the individual is vaccinated (inoculated) with a specific antigen. An antigen is a substance injected into the individual in order to stimulate the production of specific antibodies. This antigen is often an expired or a weakened state of the pathogen. The process is used to increase an individual's resistance to a particular disease or to provide **immunization**.

The body itself may overreact to an antigen. If the antigen causes an allergic response, it is called an **allergen**. Individuals who are generally more sensitive to certain allergens than most people are called **hypersensitive**. In severe cases, a person's antigen-antibody response stimulates a massive secretion of histamine. This severe reaction, called **anaphylactic shock** (anaphylaxis), is sometimes fatal. It is important to take a thorough health history in order to identify individuals who are hypersensitive to one or more substances.

Chapter Summary

To safeguard against microorganism exposure in a dental office, one must understand how these pathogens pass from an infected person to a susceptible person. Therefore, within this chapter you have been given information about pathogenic microorganisms along with the diseases they cause and how the body can defend against them.

CASE STUDY

Darin Scott came down with a low-grade fever, night sweats, and weight loss. He exhibited fatigue and finally a persistent cough.

Case Study Review

1. What is one disease you would consider?
2. Is this disease common?
3. What treatment will most likely be prescribed?
4. What microorganism caused this disease?

Review Questions

Multiple Choice

1. Who developed the theory of the etiologic agent?
   a. Anton Van Leeuwenhoek
   b. Louis Pasteur
   c. Robert Koch
   d. Joseph Lister
2. Most bacteria are said to require air and is therefore called
   a. aerobic.
   b. anaerobic.
   c. facultative bacteria.
   d. gram positive.
3. Which bacteria has been implicated in dental caries?
   a. Staphylococcal
   b. *Mycobacterium tuberculosis*
   c. Bacillus *Corynebacterium diphtheria*
   d. *Streptococcus mutans*
4. The herpes simplex virus that infects the finger and was a concern before the usage of treatment gloves is called
   a. corneal ulcer
   b. herpetic whitlow
   c. tinea
   d. candidiasis
5. The name of the slow-growing skin tumor that develops from HIV is called
   a. Kaposi's sarcoma.
   b. pyogenic membrane.
   c. allergen.
   d. herpes zoster.
6. The individual credited with the creation of vaccines and the eradication of polio is
   a. Anton Van Leeuwenhoek.
   b. Louis Pasteur.
   c. Robert Koch.
   d. Joseph Lister.
7. The type of bacteria that are rod shaped is
   a. cocci.
   b. bacilli.
   c. spirilla.
   d. vibrios.
8. The bacteria that can grow with or without oxygen are termed ________
   a. aerobic bacteria
   b. anaerobic bacteria
   c. facultative anaerobic bacteria
   d. all of the above
9. The individual who was instrumental in using heat to destroy bacteria and resistant spores is
   a. Anton Van Leeuwenhoek.
   b. Louis Pasteur.
   c. Robert Koch.
   d. Joseph Lister.
10. The childhood disease that is caused by the varicella-zoster virus is ________
    a. measles
    b. mumps
    c. chickenpox
    d. poliomyelitis

Critical Thinking

1. If two individuals kiss on the lips and neither has open sores around the mouth but one of the two has AIDS, is the probability high for the other individual to acquire AIDS because of this kiss?
2. Which two of the five microorganisms are present during periodontal disease?
3. Which of the hepatitis viruses is of greatest concern to the dental assistant and why?

Web Activities

1. Go to http://www.cdc.gov and find the current statistics for HIV/AIDS mortality.
2. Go to http://www.cdc.gov and find current statistics for tuberculosis. Has the number of reported cases increased or decreased in the past 2 years? In which year was the incidence of tuberculosis the highest?
3. Go to http://www.cdc.gov and research the most recent information on Ebola and guidelines to prevent MRSA. Be prepared to discuss it in class.

CHAPTER

11

Infection Control

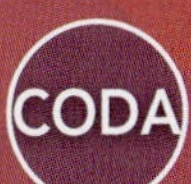

Specific Instructional Objectives

The student should strive to meet the following objectives and demonstrate an understanding of the facts and principles presented in this chapter:

1. Identify the rationale, regulations, recommendations, and training that govern infection control in the dental office.
2. Describe how pathogens travel from person to person in the dental office.
3. List the three primary routes of microbial transmission, and the associated dental procedures that affect the dental assistant.
4. Demonstrate the principles of infection control, including medical history, handwashing, personal protective equipment, barriers, chemical disinfectants, ultrasonic cleaners, sterilizers, and instrument storage.
5. List various disinfectants and their applications as used in dentistry.
6. Identify and demonstrate the usage of different types of sterilizers.
7. Demonstrate the usage of several types of sterilization monitors, such as biological and process indicators.
8. Identify and show the proper usage of preprocedure mouth rinses, high-volume evacuation, dental dams, and disposable items.
9. Demonstrate correct procedures for dental unit water line maintenance.
10. Identify and demonstrate the correct protocol for disinfecting, cleaning, and sterilizing prior to seating the patient, at the end of a dental treatment, in the dental radiography area, and in the dental laboratory.

Key Terms

aerosol (211)
agent (208)
airborne transmission (209)
alcohol-based hand antiseptic (212)
antimicrobial (211)
antisepsis (211)
asepsis (204)
aseptic technique (204)
asymptomatic (211)
barriers (223)
bioburden (227)
biofilms (240)
biological monitor (234)
bloodborne pathogens standard (205)
body substance isolation (BSI) (204)
broad spectrum activity (225)
cavitation (227)
chain of asepsis (204)
chain of infection (208)
chemical vapor sterilizer (230)
clinical contact surface (223)
compromised host (210)
contact dermatitis (216)
contact transmission (209)
cross-contamination pathways (207)
direct contact (211)
disinfection (224)
dosage indicator (234)
dry heat sterilizer (230)
emollient (212)
ethylene oxide sterilization (229)
fomite (208)
fungicidal (224)
housekeeping surfaces (223)
host (210)
indirect contact (211)
infection control (204)
inhalation (211)
integrating indicators (234)
latex allergy (216)
mechanical monitoring (233)

(continues)

Key Terms (continued)

mode of transmission (209)
multi-parameter indicators (234)
occupational exposure (206)
other potentially infectious materials (OPIM) (205)
overgloves (217)
parenteral (206)
pathogen (204)
personal protective equipment (PPE) (205)
portal of entry (209)
portal of exit (209)
process indicators (234)
reservoir (208)
residual activity (225)
reuse life (233)
sanitization (224)
shelf life (233)
single-parameter indicator (234)
splash, splatter, and droplet surfaces (223)
sporicidal (224)
spray-wipe-spray-technique (227)
standard precautions (204)
steam under pressure sterilization (231)
sterilization (224)
sterilization indicator (233)
susceptible host (210)
thermal disinfector (229)
touch surface (223)
transfer surface (223)
tuberculocidal (224)
type I allergic reaction (217)
type IV allergic reaction (216)
ultrasonic cleaner (227)
universal precautions (204)
utility gloves (217)
vector-borne transmission (209)
vehicle transmission (209)
virucidal (224)
waterline shock treatment (241)

Introduction

CDA The process of **infection control** includes methods used to reduce the transmission of infectious microorganisms. The dentist is responsible for ensuring this process is adequate. Compliance with all regulations must be accomplished on a continuing basis. Staff must be trained at the time of initial employment, when job tasks change (before the employee is placed in a position where occupational exposure may occur), and annually, thereafter. Records must be maintained for the duration of employment, plus 30 years, in accordance with regulations. Even though the dentist is ultimately responsible, often an employee (full time) is designated as the infection control and hazardous waste coordinator. This person ensures that the office is in compliance with all regulations, reads updated information on infection control and hazardous waste, and presents the information to the dental team for review. The infection control and hazardous waste coordinator schedules staff training, oversees the entire process of infection control, and makes sure that procedures ensure complete asepsis. The creation of a pathogen-free environment is termed **asepsis**. A **pathogen** is a disease-causing microorganism. In order to provide a pathogen-free environment, **aseptic technique** is required. This technique is needed for all procedures in which there is a danger of introducing infection or disease into a human's body.

Rationales and Regulations of Infection Control

All efforts are made to stop infectious diseases from spreading; adhering to routine practices eliminates mistakes. All patients are treated as if they are infectious, and, as such, **universal precautions** are implemented. Universal precautions, in addition to body substance isolation techniques termed **standard precautions**, are practiced prior to, during, and after each procedure in the dental office. Therefore, every precaution is taken to ensure that the **chain of asepsis** (aseptic procedures ensuring that no cross-contamination occurs) is not broken and that contamination does not occur.

Regulations and Recommendations for Infection Control in the Dental Office

A number of agencies have established guidelines for infection control in the dental office. These minimal standards change from time to time as the knowledge base on prevention expands. *Regulations* are made by government agencies (see following discussion) and licensing boards that have the authority to enforce compliance. If compliance is not met, dentists may be fined, lose their licenses to practice dentistry, or face imprisonment. *Recommendations* can be made by anyone, and no authority for enforcement is mandated. When regulations are introduced, the profession has a specific timeframe in which to comply. During this time, consultants, the dental association, and other groups make recommendations on the best means for compliance. See Appendix A for the addresses and phone numbers of the regulating and recommending agencies.

American Dental Association. The American Dental Association (ADA), the parent organization for dentistry in the United States, makes recommendations through its councils (see Chapter 1 Introduction to the Dental Profession) in the form of literature, videotapes, news broadcasts, manuals, brochures, the *Journal of the American Dental Association (JADA), ADA News*, and their Internet site (http://www.ada.org). The American Dental Assistants Association (ADAA), the American Dental Hygienists' Association (ADHA), and the American Dental Laboratory Association (ADLA) also provide information to their members through support services and journals.

Centers for Disease Control and Prevention. The Centers for Disease Control and Prevention (CDC) provides the basis for many of the regulations. This agency, part of the U.S. Public Health Service, a division of the U.S. Department of Health and Human Services, has developed a number of recommendations that have since been made by federal, state, and local agencies into regulations.

In 1996, the CDC issued standard precautions that augmented and synthesized the universal precautions and **body substance isolation (BSI)** techniques. BSI is a system requiring **personal protective equipment (PPE)** to be worn for protection against contact with all body fluids, whether or not blood is visible. Standard precautions, adopted by numerous health care industries, protect providers, patients, and others from infectious diseases.

National Institute of Health. The National Institute of Health (NIH) is a government agency that provides research for the expansion and implementation of knowledge for the enhancement of health, prevention of disease, the lengthening of life, and the maintenance of high professional standards. The NIH provides programs on leadership and direction in order to improve health in the United States by conducting and supporting research in the

- causes, diagnosis, prevention, and cure of human disease;
- processes of human growth and development;
- biological effects of environmental contaminants;
- understanding of mental, addictive, and physical disorders;
- direction of programs for the collection, dissemination, and exchange of information in medicine and health, including the development and support of medical libraries, and the training of medical librarians and other health information specialists.

National Institute of Occupational Safety and Health. The National Institute of Occupational Safety and Health (NIOSH) provides research and prevention programs to assist in the elimination of occupational diseases, injuries, and fatalities. NIOSH seeks to complete these tasks with high-quality research, practical solutions, partnerships, and implementing research into practice. They have worked together with the CDC to prevent occupational hazards in the healthcare environment. If a problem in healthcare arises, such as HIV/AIDS protection or latex allergies, this organization seeks answers and solutions. Some of their achievements include: means to prevent needle stick injuries, which prevents the transmission of bloodborne pathogens; development of guidelines to prevent airborne transmission of diseases, such as tuberculosis (TB); techniques and equipment to prevent back and other musculoskeletal injuries; techniques to reduce stress and fatigue; reducing hazardous chemical exposures; and reduction in the incidence of latex allergies.

Occupational Safety and Health Administration. The Occupational Safety and Health Administration (OSHA) is a regulating body that enforces requirements that state that employers must protect their employees from exposure to blood and **other potentially infectious materials (OPIM)** while employees are at work. This agency is part of the U.S. Department of Labor. Its overall mission is to protect workers in the United States from physical, chemical, or infectious hazards while in the workplace. The OSHA **bloodborne pathogens standard** became effective in 1992. This standard applies to any facility where employees are, or have the potential to be, exposed to body fluids, such as in hospitals, funeral homes, emergency medical services, medical and dental offices, and research laboratories. In 2001, the Needlestick Safety and Prevention Act was passed. This resulted in the revision of the bloodborne pathogens standard related to the use of newer, safer medical devices, and the tracking of incidents related to "sharps" injuries.

Other Potentially Infectious Materials

OSHA and the CDC define the following human fluids as blood or OPIM according to their standards:

- Blood and anything that is visually contaminated with blood
- Saliva in dental procedures
- Cerebrospinal fluid (brain and spinal fluid)
- Amniotic fluid (fluid around the fetus)
- Synovial fluid (joint and tendon fluid)
- Pleural (lung fluid), peritoneal fluid (abdominal fluid), pericardial fluid (heart fluid)
- Semen and vaginal secretions
- Unfixed tissue or organ (other than intact skin) from a human (living or dead)
- HIV-containing cell or tissue cultures, organ cultures, and HIV- or HBV-containing cultures, mediums, or other solutions
- Blood, organs, or other tissues from experimental animals infected with HIV or HBV

Compliance with OSHA standards is monitored through investigations of facilities by OSHA inspectors. If the facility fails to come into compliance, a citation resulting in a possible fine is given. If the facility continues to refuse to comply, the fine increases and additional steps are taken to ensure that noncompliant conditions are corrected. It is important for the dental office to stay up to date on changes in the recommendations and regulations related to infection control. One method to stay current on these changes is to frequently visit http://www.oshasolutions.com/osha-information/helpful-links.php.

Here you will find OSHA information for dentists and numerous other helpful links. One of the links that should be reviewed often to ensure compliance is the CDC's *Morbidity and Mortality Weekly Report* (MMWR) at http://www.cdc.gov/mmwr. These reports cover the protocols to be followed until further guidelines are released. One such report is the *Guidelines for Infection Control in Dental Health-Care settings—2003* (http://www.cdc.gov/mmwr/pdf/rr/rr5217.pdf). This report was completed by the Department of Health and Human Services' Centers for Disease Control and Prevention (CDC). The 2003 guidelines expanded on the 1993 guidelines, and gave additional information on content previously covered along with new guidelines. The CDC had experts in infection control, as well as professional organizations, public agencies, and private agencies develop the *CDC Guidelines for Infection Control in Dental Health-Care Settings*. The CDC continues to update the guidelines; for example, they have provided recent updates on infection control and isolation procedures for Ebola, due to the outbreak, which took place in 2014–2015. This content, although it is not law, represents the current standard of care.

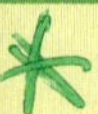

When Dental Offices Are Investigated for Compliance

- After an employee or a patient complaint is made
- In any office having 11 or more employees, randomly
- By invitation of the office requesting an inspection

All states are regulated by the OSHA standard. Twenty-four states are regulated through state agency standards that run parallel to, or are more demanding than, the federal standard; the other states are administered through regional branches of the federal OSHA.

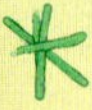

Overview of the OSHA Bloodborne Pathogens Standard

Every facility must:

- Review the Bloodborne Pathogens Standard
- Prepare a written exposure control plan outlining the means to protect and train employees
- Update the exposure control plan when changes in technology provide safer medical devices, and document the consideration and implementation of the use of these devices
- Solicit non-managerial employees to identify, evaluate, and select safer products and devices for use in the workplace
- Train all employees in a timely manner (initially, after a job task change, when new devices are implemented, and annually)
- Provide employees with everything needed in order to meet standard regulations
- Provide personal protective equipment (PPE)
- Maintain and dispose of necessary PPE
- Establish standard operating procedures (SOPs) in infection control
- Maintain a sharps injury log
- Offer the hepatitis B vaccination series to all employees
- Establish a postexposure plan, including medical evaluation and follow-up procedures (for example, occupational exposure to needlesticks)
- Provide communication on biohazards
- Establish standards for handling and disposing of hazardous waste
- Maintain records of training, hepatitis B vaccinations, and exposure incidents

Exposure Determination. In order to evaluate an employee's chances of occupational exposure to bloodborne pathogens, an exposure determination is made. An **occupational exposure** is any reasonably anticipated eye, mucosa, skin, or **parenteral** (cut, needlestick, puncture, abrasions, etc.) exposure, or any contact with blood or saliva, that may be a result of employment tasks. The determination is made based on the following three categories:

- **Category 1** includes all tasks that involve exposure to blood, body fluids such as saliva, and body tissues. (This group includes dentist, dental assistant, dental hygienist, and dental laboratory technician.)
- **Category 2** includes all tasks that involve no exposure to blood, body fluids such as saliva, or body tissues, but occasionally may involve unplanned tasks from Category 1. (This group includes the receptionist, coordinating assistant, and so on.)
- **Category 3** includes all tasks that involve no exposure to blood, body fluids such as saliva, or body tissues. (This group includes the accountant, insurance assistant, and so on.)

Written Exposure Plan. This plan documents the specific exposure determination for each employee, and identifies a schedule of implementation (how and when provisions of the standard will be implemented). This document must list how situations surrounding an exposure will be evaluated, and what measures will be taken to correct the situation (if necessary).

Step 1 All employees list tasks they perform in each job classification, and then identify which category they fall under. Any employee who may have any occupational exposure at any time is covered under the OSHA Bloodborne Pathogen standard.

Step 2 The office must have a schedule for implementation. This schedule must designate how and when each provision of the standard will be implemented.

- How and when are the hepatitis B vaccinations being offered to employees?
- How and when is communication of hazards to employees covered?
- How and when are the postexposure evaluation and office follow-up procedures accomplished?
- How and when are new devices identified and implemented?
- How and when is the recordkeeping accomplished and updated?

Step 3 A manual and procedure plan must be written to cover methods of compliance for office PPE and safety issues. For instance, the office must have written information covering all aspects of the following:

- Personal protective equipment
- Engineering controls
- Housekeeping controls
- Work practice controls

Step 4 A written policy on how exposure incidents are evaluated is required. Included in each evaluation are the circumstances that surrounded the incident and how they can be corrected. A sharps injury log must be maintained. What type of evaluation will be done by the office if an exposure incident occurs?

The Food and Drug Administration. The Food and Drug Administration (FDA), which is a division of the U.S. Department of Health and Human Services, regulates the manufacturing and labeling of medical devices and solutions. The FDA requires that certain performance standards be met prior to their use by the public. It requires that general controls be used with devices and solutions, and that labeling gives the appropriate information to the consumer. It holds manufacturers responsible for problems that develop, unless the consumer misuses the medical device or solution. In this instance, the liability lies with the user.

Items in the dental office regulated by the FDA are sterilizers; chemical and biologic indicators; cleaning solutions, such as an ultrasonic solution or cold chemicals; PPE, such as gloves, masks, glasses, and disposable clothing; sterilizing solutions; and disinfectants.

Environmental Protection Agency. The Environmental Protection Agency (EPA) is a federal regulatory agency involved in the safety and effectiveness of disinfecting and sterilizing solutions. It also regulates the disposal of hazardous waste after it leaves the dental office. All disinfecting and sterilizing solutions must be submitted by the manufacturer to the EPA for registration. After undertaking and passing specific testing requirements, and if a solution meets all the claims listed, the EPA assigns an EPA number, which must appear on its label with safety concerns noted on the container.

Organization for Safety and Asepsis Procedures. The Organization for Safety and Asepsis Procedures (OSAP), a national organization, encompasses dental health care workers, distributors of dental equipment and materials, health care instructors, dentists, and others in the field of dentistry. OSAP has regional and annual meetings that cover topics on infection control and hazard communication for dental team members. Written documentation is available from OSAP to help maintain infection control in the dental office.

OSHA-Mandated Training for Dental Office Employees

All employers must ensure that employees (full time, part time, and temporary) who fall into Category 1 or 2, whose tasks involve exposure to blood and body fluids, such as saliva or body tissues, have training. This training must be provided at no cost to the employee. The training must be given before placement in a position where bloodborne pathogens are a factor, both for all new employees and for all employees reclassifying into new positions.

The training cannot be accomplished by videos or interactive computer training programs alone. The training must be accomplished by an individual who has the background necessary to answer questions, and to supplement the training with in-office (on-site) specific information. The information must be given in a manner so that all can understand. If an employee cannot understand the content due to a language barrier or a disability, the employer must provide an interpreter, or convey this information in such a manner that the employee understands completely.

A record of the date of the training session, employees present, and qualifications of the trainer must be maintained.

OSHA-Mandated Training for Dental Employees

The following must be available to all dental employees:

- A copy of the Bloodborne Pathogens Standard and specific information regarding the meaning of the standard
- Information about bloodborne pathogens, both the epidemiology and symptoms of the diseases
- Information about the cross-contamination pathways of bloodborne pathogens
- A written copy or a means for employees to obtain the employer's/office's written exposure control plan
- Information on the tasks, category placement of employee classifications, and how each is identified in relation to bloodborne pathogens and other potentially infectious materials (OPIM)
- Information regarding the hepatitis B vaccine
- Information about exposure reduction, including PPE; work practices; standard precautions, including universal precautions; and engineering practices
- Information about the selection, placement, use, removal, disinfection, sterilization, and disposal of PPE
- Information about what to do, and whom to contact, if an emergency involving blood or OPIM arises
- Information about the procedure to follow if an incident of blood exposure occurs, how to report the incident, and what type of medical follow-up is available at no cost to the employee
- Information about the postexposure evaluation and follow-up that the employer provides
- A copy of the OSHA Hazard Communication Standard
- Safety Data Sheets (SDS) (formerly known as material safety data sheets, MSDS) as part of the Globally Harmonized System of Classification and Labeling of Chemicals (GHS)
- The opportunity for employees to ask questions of the individual giving the information

Cross-Contamination Pathways

Cross-contamination pathways are formed when pathogens travel from patients to dentists, dental assistants, dental hygienists, dental laboratory technicians, and other patients. Pathogens can also travel from dental personnel to patients. The transfer can then go to the families and friends of the dental personnel or patients.

Chain of Infection

The **chain of infection** describes the elements of an infectious process. It is an interactive process that involves the agent, host, and environment. This process must include several essential elements or "links in the chain" for the transmission of microorganisms to occur. Figure 11-1 identifies the six essential links. Without the transmission of microorganisms, the infectious process cannot occur. Knowledge about the chain of infection facilitates control or prevention of disease by breaking the links in the chain. This is achieved by altering one or more of the interactive processes of agent, host, or environment.

Agent

An **agent** is an entity that is capable of causing disease. Agents that may cause disease include:

- *Biological agents* are living organisms that invade the host, such as bacteria, virus, fungi, protozoa, and rickettsiae
- *Chemical agents* are substances that can interact with the body, such as pesticides, food additives, medications, and industrial chemicals
- *Physical agents* are factors in the environment, such as heat, light, noise, and radiation

In the chain of infection, the main concern is biological (infectious) agents and their effect on the host.

Reservoir

The **reservoir** is a place where the agent can survive. Colonization and reproduction take place while the agent is in the reservoir. A reservoir that promotes the growth of pathogens must contain the proper nutrients (such as oxygen and organic matter), maintain proper temperature, contain moisture, maintain a compatible pH level, and maintain the proper amount of light exposure. The most common reservoirs are humans, animals, environment, and fomites. A **fomite** is an object, such as instruments or dressings, that is contaminated with an infectious agent.

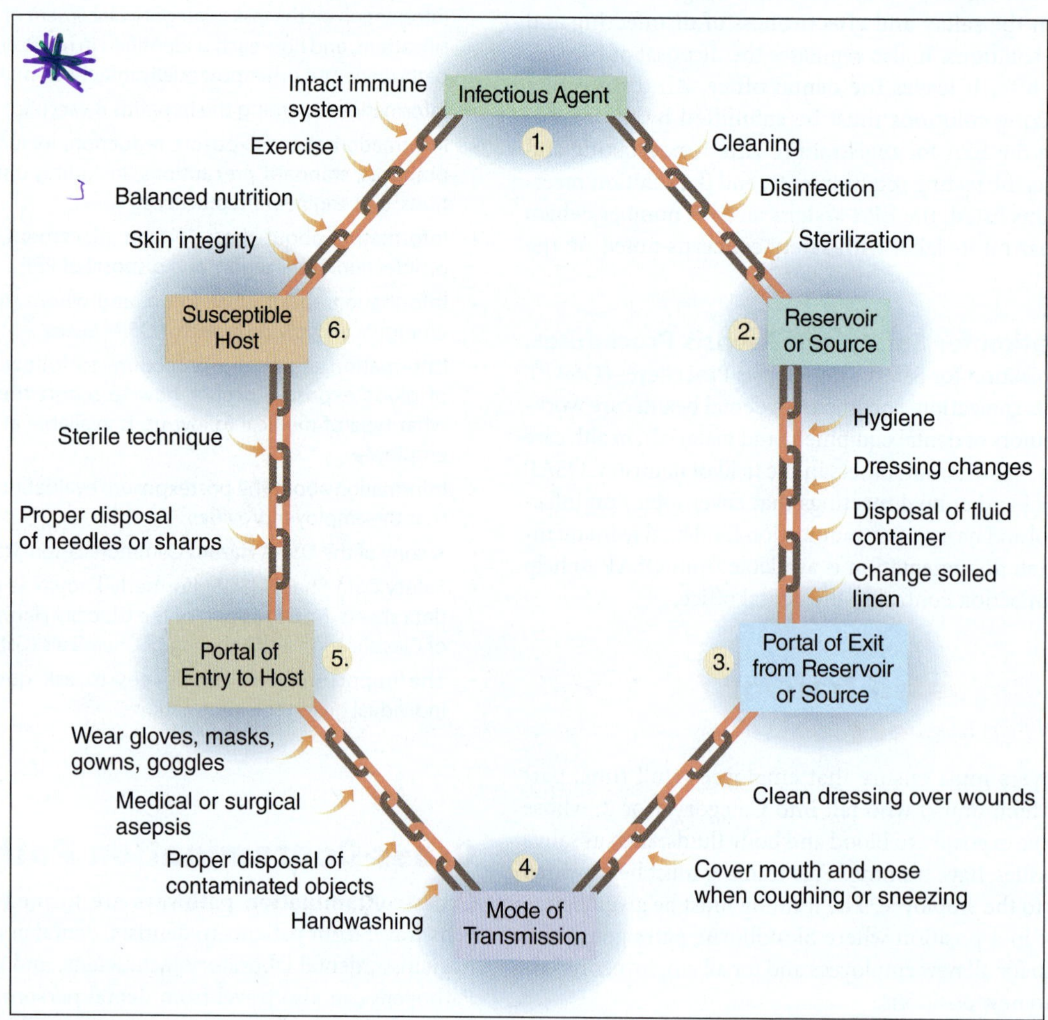

FIGURE 11-1
Chain of infection: Preventive measures follow each link.

ppe: protection equipment

Humans and animals can have symptoms of infectious agents or can strictly be carriers of the agent. Carriers have the infectious agent, but are symptom free. The agent can be spread to others in both instances.

Portal of Exit. The **portal of exit** is the route by which an infectious agent leaves the reservoir to be transferred to a susceptible host. The agent leaves the reservoir through body secretions, such as sputum, semen, vaginal secretions, urine, saliva, feces, blood, and draining wounds.

Mode of Transmission

The **mode of transmission** is the process that bridges the gap between the portal of exit of the infectious agent from the reservoir and the portal of entry of the susceptible "new" host. Most infectious agents have a usual mode of transmission; however, some microorganisms may be transmitted by more than one mode. The modes of transmission include **contact transmission**, **airborne transmission**, **vehicle transmission**, and **vector-borne transmission** and are summarized in Table 11-1.

Portal of Entry

A **portal of entry** is the route by which an infectious agent enters the host. Portals of entry include the following:

- *Integumentary system:* a break in the skin or mucous membrane
- *Respiratory tract:* inhaling contaminated droplets
- *Genitourinary tract:* contamination with infected vaginal secretions or semen
- *Gastrointestinal tract:* ingesting contaminated food or water

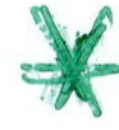

TABLE 11-1 Modes of Transmission

Mode	Definition	Examples
Contact transmission	Involves the physical transfer of an agent from an infected person to an uninfected person through direct or indirect contact with the infected person. Contact with the infected person is called direct contact. Direct contact can occur through unprotected contact with infected fluids, such as blood or salvia. Indirect contact takes place when microorganisms are transmitted to an object or surface first and then transferred to another person when the person touches the object or surface.	Examples of direct contact are sexually transmitted diseases, colds, and flu. Direct contact of health care provider with patient: • Touching • Secretions from client such as blood and saliva Indirect contact with fomites: • Clothing • Health-care equipment • Instruments used in treatments • Personal belongings • Personal care equipment • Diagnostic equipment
Airborne transmission	Occurs when a susceptible person is exposed to contaminated droplets or dust particles that are suspended in the air. The longer the particle is suspended, the greater the chance it will find an available port of entry in the human host.	Inhaling microorganisms carried by moisture or dust particles in the air: • Coughing • Talking • Sneezing • An organism that relies on airborne transmission is measles. • Spores of anthrax are also transmitted in an airborne powder form. • The dental handpiece, while in use, creates airborne droplets that can be transmitted (Figure 11-2).
Vehicle transmission	Occurs when the agent is transferred to a susceptible host by contaminated inanimate objects, such as dental instruments, water, food, meat, drugs, and blood.	Contact with contaminated inanimate objects: • Water • Blood • Drugs • Food • Urine • Salmonellosis transmitted through contaminated food
Vector-borne transmission	Occurs when an agent is transferred to a susceptible host by animate means, such as mosquitoes, fleas, ticks, lice, and other animals.	Contact with contaminated animate hosts: • Animals • Insects • Lyme disease

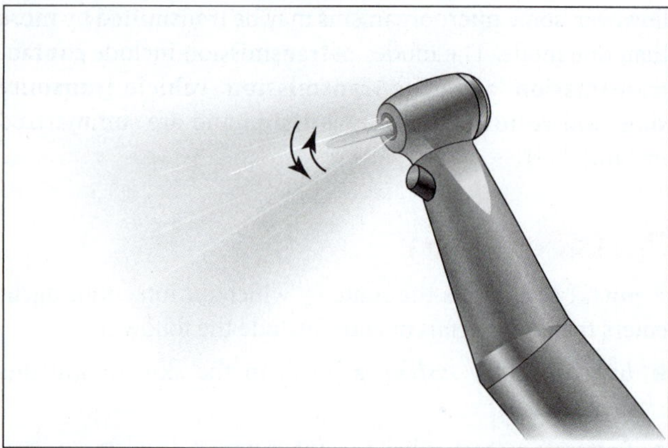

FIGURE 11-2
Airborne droplets from a dental handpiece.

- *Circulatory system:* a bite from insects or rodents
- *Transplacental:* a transfer of a microorganism from the mother to the fetus via the placenta and umbilical cord

Host

A **host** is a simple or complex organism that can be affected by an agent. As the term is used here, a host is an individual who is at risk of contracting an infectious disease. A **susceptible host** is a person who lacks resistance to an agent and is vulnerable to a disease. A **compromised host** is a person whose normal defense mechanisms are impaired and is, therefore, more susceptible to infection.

The following characteristics of the host influence the susceptibility to and severity of infections:

- *Age:* As a person ages, immunity declines.
- *Concurrent disease:* The existence of other diseases indicates susceptibility.
- *Stress:* A person experiencing a compromised emotional state has lower defense mechanisms.
- *Immunization/vaccination status:* Certain people are not fully immunized.
- *Lifestyle:* Practices, such as having multiple sex partners, sharing needles, or tobacco and drug use, can alter defenses.
- *Occupation:* Forms of employment that involve increased exposure to pathogenic sources, such as needles or chemical agents.
- *Nutritional status:* People who maintain targeted weight for height and body frame are less prone to illness.
- *Heredity:* Some people are naturally more susceptible to infections than others.

Breaking the Chain of Infection

Dental assistants focus on breaking the chain of infection by applying proper infection control practices that interfere with the spread of microorganisms. Specific strategies can be directed at breaking or blocking the transmission of infection from one link in the chain to the next. A discussion regarding each of the six links follows.

Between Agent and Reservoir

The keys to eliminating infection between an agent and a reservoir in the chain are cleansing, disinfection, and sterilization. These tactics serve to prevent the formation of a reservoir, and an environment within which infectious agents can live and multiply.

If the reservoir is an already infected individual, that individual may need to be isolated. The individual's infectious condition needs to be vigorously treated to reduce the reservoir of infectious material or eliminate the agent.

Between Reservoir and Portal of Exit

Promoting proper hygiene, maintaining clean dental operatories, and ensuring the use of clean equipment in patient care can break the chain between the reservoir and the portal of exit. The aim is to eliminate the reservoir for the microorganism before the pathogen can escape to a susceptible host.

Between Portal of Exit and Mode of Transmission

The goal in breaking the chain here is to block the exit of the infectious agent. The dental assistant must maintain clean dressings on all injuries or wounds. People should be encouraged to cover their mouths and noses when sneezing or coughing, and the dental assistant must do so as well. Gloves must be worn when caring for a person who may have infectious secretions, and care must be taken to properly dispose of contaminated articles.

Between Mode of Transmission and Portal of Entry

The goal is to break the chain of infection between the mode of transmission and the portal of entry. Dental assistants must always wash their hands between cases that may involve contact with contaminated items. Barrier protection must be worn when care involves contact with body secretions. Gloves, masks, gowns, and goggles are all forms of barrier protection.

Between Portal of Entry and Host

Maintaining skin integrity and using sterile techniques for patient contact are methods of breaking the chain between the portal of entry and the host. The goal is to prevent the transmission of infection to uninfected persons, including the dental assistant.

Between Host and Agent

To break the chain between the host and the agent, eliminate the infection before it begins. Proper nutrition, exercise, and immunization allow an individual to maintain an intact immune system, thus, preventing infection.

Routes of Microbial Transmission in the Dental Office

In dentistry, three primary routes transmit most microorganisms: direct contact, indirect contact, and inhalation or aerosol. Microorganisms may be missed because they appear as a mist, as dry, or clear on exposed surfaces. They are overlooked if careful, consistent aseptic procedures are not followed. The dental assistant is the primary caretaker of infection control practices. By using the correct barriers and PPE, as well as treating all patients as if they were infectious, and using proper disinfection and sterilization, you will break the chain of infection and eliminate cross-contamination (see also Chapter 10 Microbiology).

Routes of microbial transmission are as follows:

1. With **direct contact**, an individual has direct contact with a lesion or microorganism while performing intraoral dental procedures.
2. With **indirect contact**, an individual has contact with the microorganism through other means, such as contaminated instruments, supplies, or equipment.
3. With **inhalation** or **aerosol**, an individual contacts the microorganism through inhalation. This normally happens when the high-speed handpiece, or the ultrasonic cavitron, is used in the dental office.

Infection Control in the Dental Office

A number of steps must be followed to accomplish the goal of infection control, or asepsis. The first step is for the dental assistant to maintain good health standards. Eating and sleeping properly aid in staying healthy. Proper exercise, along with maintaining a positive mental attitude, provides the energy to attain individual goals for good overall health.

Immunizations

The dental assistant should have the immunizations necessary to fight off pathogens that are encountered because of his or her close proximity to patients during dental treatment. If the dental assistant has not had the hepatitis B series, the employer must provide information about immunizations and the available vaccine during initial training, and is also required to pay for the series. Review the employee training information regarding the hepatitis B vaccine earlier in this chapter (see also Chapter 10, Microbiology, for additional information regarding immunizations).

Medical History

Taking the patient's medical history and updating it at each appointment is a good way to gather information, but may not identify the infectious diseases that patients have. It is important to update this information, both verbally and in writing. Patients are sometimes more willing to disclose information during conversation. Most individuals infected with HBV and HIV are **asymptomatic**, meaning they have no symptoms. Therefore, a medical history may give information to the health care workers, but it cannot be used alone to identify patients who place dental personnel at high risk. Implementing standard precautions, incorporating universal precautions, and practicing infection control standards with each and every patient are essential in infection control.

Handwashing

One of the most important ways to prevent the transfer of microorganisms from one person or object to another person is handwashing. Handwashing is the vigorous rubbing together of well-lathered soapy hands (ensuring friction on all surfaces), concluding with a thorough rinsing under a stream of water and proper drying. Handwashing is both a mechanical cleaning and chemical **antisepsis** (inhibiting the growth of causative microorganisms).

Hands contain resident and transient microflora (visible by use of a microscope). The mechanical process of scrubbing removes transient microorganisms and some resident microorganisms. Transient microorganisms are fresh contaminants of brief duration. Transient microorganisms are of primary concern to the dental profession because they constitute the pathogen group that includes hepatitis. Resident microorganisms survive and multiply for a longer period, primarily in the top layers of the skin, but can also be in deeper layers of the skin. Chemical antisepsis is accomplished through the use of an antimicrobial soap. Applying the proper technique and using **antimicrobial** (microorganism growth inhibitor) handwashing products can add additional protection to ensure that microorganisms are removed each time the hands are washed.

Currently, the most beneficial antimicrobial handwashing agents include chlorhexidine digluconate, triclosan, and parachlorometaxylenol. These handwashing agents exhibit prolonged antimicrobial effects.

At the beginning of each day, every member of the dental team should complete *two consecutive 15-second handwashes*. It is important to use plenty of antimicrobial soap and water while rubbing all areas of the hands (Figure 11-3). Getting between the fingers, rubbing each finger and thumb, and cleaning beneath the fingernails is essential. Some offices provide tools that aid in scrubbing the fingernails. These tools (often made of a foam rubber pad and plastic bristles) must not be so hard that they abrade the tissue, allowing microorganisms access to the body. The tools must be disposable or autoclavable. Handbrushes are not recommended for washing the skin of the hands and arms because they may lacerate tissue, causing portals of entry. Remember, the skin is a barrier to microorganisms, and care should be taken to prevent cuts and lesions. A final rinse with cool water is used to close the pores in the skin. Dry the hands completely with paper towels, and use the paper towels to turn off the hand-controlled sink faucets and wipe the area clean. The brushes are sterilized or disposed of after each use.

A minimal 15-second handwashing should be completed before and after patient care, donning and removing gloves, breaks, ending each day, and at any other time the hands

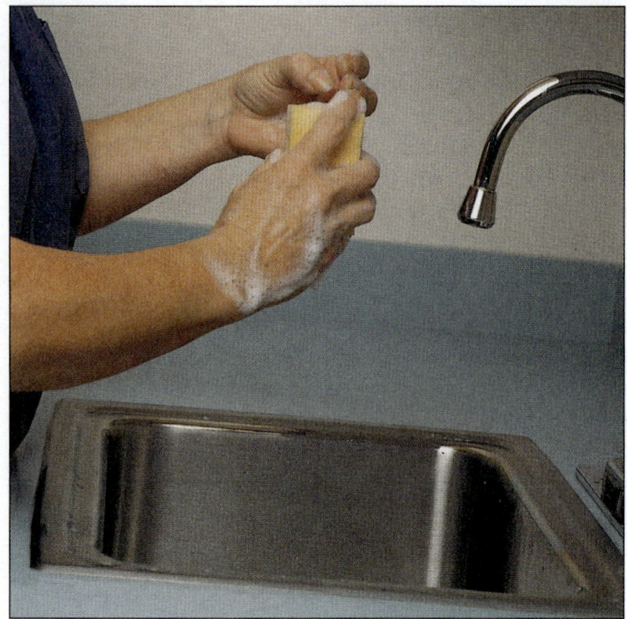

FIGURE 11-3
Dental assistant handwashing with antimicrobial soap and scrub sponge.

become contaminated. Due to constant handwashing, the hands may show effects of skin irritation. Hand lotions help to prevent hands from chapping. Procedure 11-1 presents an overview of proper handwashing technique.

Fingernail Care

- Artificial fingernails are not recommended for health professionals. Artificial fingernails have been found to exhibit high microbe counts under the nail, even after thorough handwashing.
- Wearing fingernail polish can harbor microorganisms. Wearing red fingernail polish, or other colors within that color range, can also alarm the patient if the nails pass within his or her sight. Seeing the red from the patient's point of view may appear as blood and cause the patient undue stress during treatment. It is advisable not to wear fingernail polish.
- Fingernails should be kept short enough so that they prevent glove tears and can be thoroughly cleaned. If fingernails have sharp edges or are broken, too long, and so on, they can break through the gloves. If the nail extends beyond the pad of the finger, it can tear the gloves.

The soap containers and the sink area become contaminated and should be disinfected routinely. Foot-operated soap dispensers prevent unnecessary hand contamination. The water controls should be foot or light sensor operated to cut down on contamination. Do not use reusable towels to dry hands; instead, use air or disposable towels.

Dental teams involved in oral surgery should perform a *surgical scrub* (see Chapter 25, Oral and Maxillofacial Surgery, for directions in performing a surgical scrub).

Alcohol-Based Hand Rubs

Antiseptic hand rubs are waterless agents with disinfectant properties that decrease the number of microorganisms present. They are not to be used if the hands are visibly soiled, because they do not remove organic material. To use this type of product, apply a small amount to the hands and then rub the hands together until the agent has dried (Figure 11-8). No water is needed.

Most **alcohol-based hand antiseptics** contain isopropanol, ethanol, n-propanol, or a combination of two of these products. They are available in varying concentrations, or in combination with other antiseptics. A concentration level of 60 to 95 percent is most effective. The antimicrobial activity is caused by their ability to denature proteins. Most have **emollients** (soothing to the skin) that help reduce drying of the skin. They come in gels, foams, and sanitation wipes that can be used in the dental office. Many schools and public buildings have wall-mounted dispensers. It is noted in the CDC guidelines of 2003 that alcohol-based hand rubs are the best method of reducing bacteria on hands. The benefits are rapid with effective antimicrobial action, improved skin condition (many contain aloe), and greater accessibility than sinks. The limitations to alcohol-based hand rubs are that they cannot be used if the hands are visibly soiled; the containers must be stored away from heat; and, according to the CDC, the hand softeners and glove powders may build up.

Lotions

Dental health care personnel may have difficulty with dermatitis due to the constant handwashing and wearing of gloves. Unbroken skin is a primary defense against the transmission of pathogens and infection. Using a lotion is recommended to aid with dryness and fissuring. Lotions that contain petroleum-based formulas should not be used because they weaken latex gloves and may allow permeability to occur. Use these lotions only at the end of the working day. Many lotions are on the market for dental team members to use.

Personal Protective Equipment

The dental assistant is constantly exposed to saliva and blood during intraoral/invasive dental procedures. Even with the maintenance of good health and immunizations, it is essential for dental team members to ensure better protection from microorganisms through constant use of PPE. Employers must provide this equipment according to OSHA regulations. Barriers are used to prevent potential pathogens encountered during patient care from gaining access to dental personnel. Barriers such as protective eyewear, face masks, disposable gloves, and appropriate uniforms should be used routinely to minimize exposure.

Protective Eyewear. Dental team members must wear protective eyewear during specific phases of dental treatment. The splatter of blood and saliva can transfer infectious

Procedure 11-1
Handwashing

This procedure is to be performed by all dental team members for 15 seconds before and after treating each patient (e.g., before glove placement and after glove removal); after barehanded touching of inanimate objects likely to be contaminated by blood or saliva; before leaving the dental operatory or the dental laboratory; when hands are visibly soiled; before regloving; and after removing gloves that are torn, cut, or punctured.

Source: http://www.cdc.gov/OralHealth/infectioncontrol/faq/hand.htm

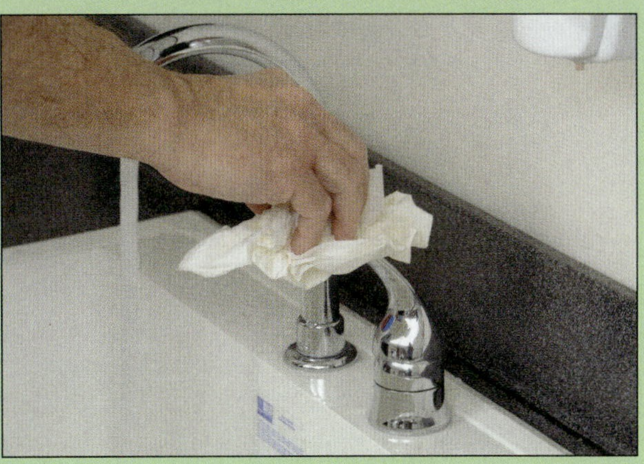

FIGURE 11-4
Turning on a faucet with a paper towel to regulate temperature and water flow.

Equipment and Supplies:

- Liquid antimicrobial handwashing agent, preferably with automatic dispensing
- Soft, sterile brush, sponge, or orange stick (optional)
- Sinks with hot and cold running water with foot control or light sensors are preferable
- Paper towels in a dispenser or a hand dryer

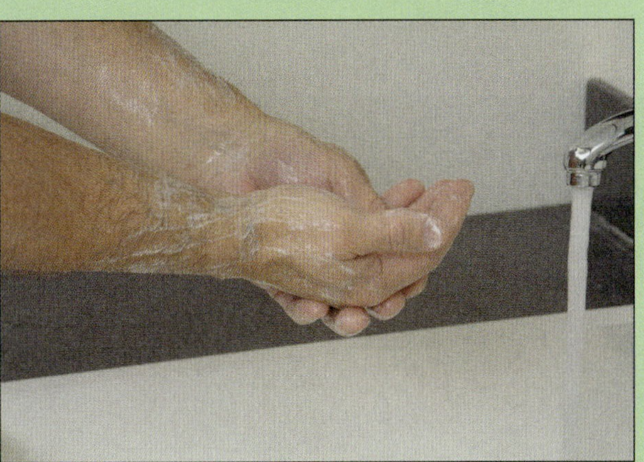

FIGURE 11-5
Scrubbing hands using the friction method.

Procedure Steps:

At the beginning of each day conduct two consecutive 15-second handwashes, and, thereafter, as required, one 15-second handwash:

1. Remove jewelry (rings and watch).
2. Adjust water flow and wet hands thoroughly. Use the foot control, light sensored control, or electronic control to regulate water flow. If these methods are not available, use a paper towel to turn on faucets and regulate temperature and water flow (Figure 11-4). Wet hands thoroughly.
3. Apply about one teaspoon of antimicrobial handwashing agent with water and bring to a lather. Hold fingertips downward and lather all parts of the hand in a circular motion. Scrub hands together and ensure that special attention is given to the area between the fingers and the thumbs, because this is the area most often missed. Scrub the backs of the hands and wrists by using the friction method, which allows contaminates to be removed from your hands and wrists (Figure 11-5). If this is the first handwashing of the day, use an orange stick under the fingernails, or a soft-bristled brush and inspect each nail to ensure that it appears clean.
4. Rinse by rubbing hands vigorously together under a stream of water until all soap has been removed, keeping the hands and fingers pointed downward (Figure 11-6).
5. Repeat steps 3 and 4.
6. The final rinse is completed, and then cool water is applied for a minimum of 10 seconds to close the pores.
7. Use paper towels to dry the hands, or allow them to air dry. When using paper towels, dry the hands thoroughly and then dry the forearms (Figure 11-7). Never use a reusable cloth towel because they contribute to the spread of

(continues)

Procedure 11-1 (continued)

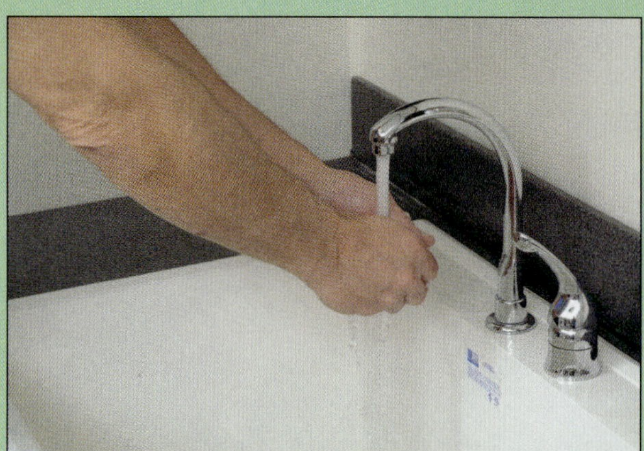

FIGURE 11-6
Rinsing hands under water flow.

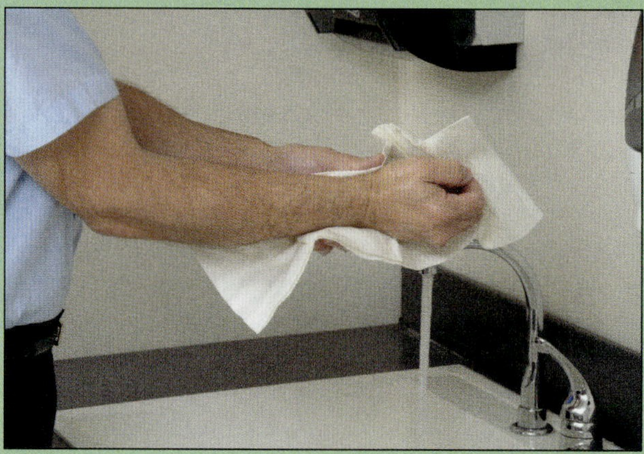

FIGURE 11-7
Using paper towels to dry hands.

microorganisms by remaining moist and being used by many people. Use a paper towel to turn off the faucets if they are not automatic. If air drying, ensure that the hands are completely dry before placing the gloves on.

Routine Handwashing: Fifteen-second handwash before and after seeing patients, donning gloves, or taking breaks. Routine handwashing must be completed at the end of each day, and any other time the hands become contaminated.

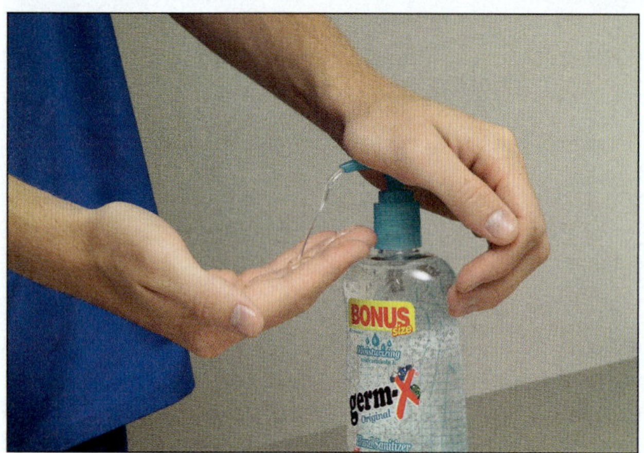

FIGURE 11-8
Placing alcohol hand cleaner in hands.

diseases, such as hepatitis and herpes simplex viruses to the mucous membranes of the eye. Aerosol droplets that contain microorganisms can cause an eye infection known as pink eye (conjunctivitis). Also, during some dental procedures, particles of gold, amalgam, and tooth fragments can be hurled into the eye, causing damage. Dental offices provide protective eyewear for patients to wear during dental treatment. These glasses, like the ones worn by the dental personnel, should be disposable, or disinfected and sterilized after use.

Protective eyewear should provide front, top, and side protection; several choices are available. The American National Standards Institute developed a standard for the design and characteristics of occupational glasses. Dental team members who wear corrective lenses may choose to wear goggles that fit over their glasses, or side shields that fit on their own eyewear (Figures 11-9A and B). Others wear glasses designed for dental personnel that incorporate top and side shields (Figure 11-9C). In addition, a face shield can be worn that covers the entire face (Figure 11-9D). A mask must still be worn with a face shield.

Eyewear is also used to protect the eyes from high-intensity lights used for curing dental materials. These glasses, or shields, are normally colored orange for protection.

At times, the eyewear becomes fogged due to warm breath coming from under the dental mask. Several antifog products are available to minimize fogging. Fog spray can be used, or the eyewear can be placed under warm water to reduce the fog problem.

Gloves. Gloves are used as a barrier to microorganisms. Any time a dental team member anticipates contact with saliva or blood, gloves should be worn. This includes saliva- or blood-contaminated surfaces, instruments, or mucous membranes. There are numerous gloves on the market that meet FDA regulations. The FDA regulates the gloves that are specific to the health care industry. The primary types of gloves that are used in the dental office are:

1. Latex gloves (nonsterile and sterile)
2. Vinyl/synthetic gloves (nonsterile and sterile)
3. Synthetic polymer gloves (nonsterile and sterile)
4. Overgloves (nonsterile)
5. Utility gloves (nonsterile)
6. Polynitrile gloves (nonsterile and sterile)*
7. Nitrile (nonsterile and sterile)*

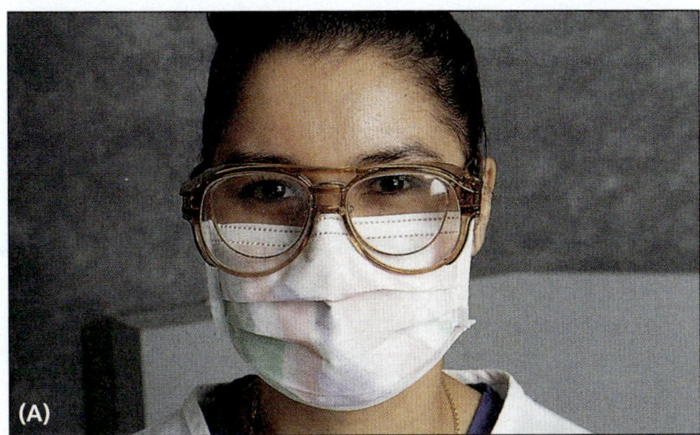

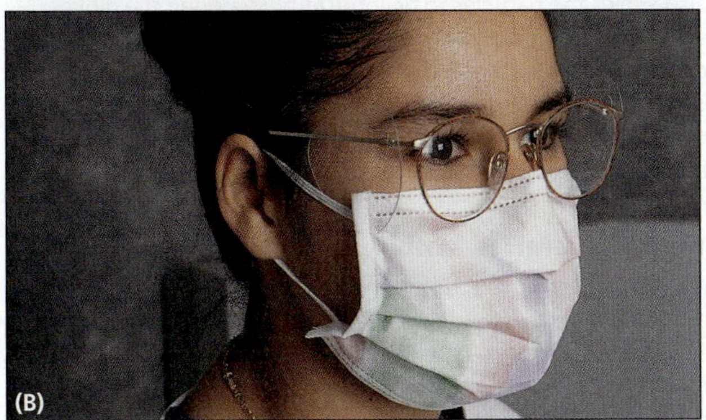

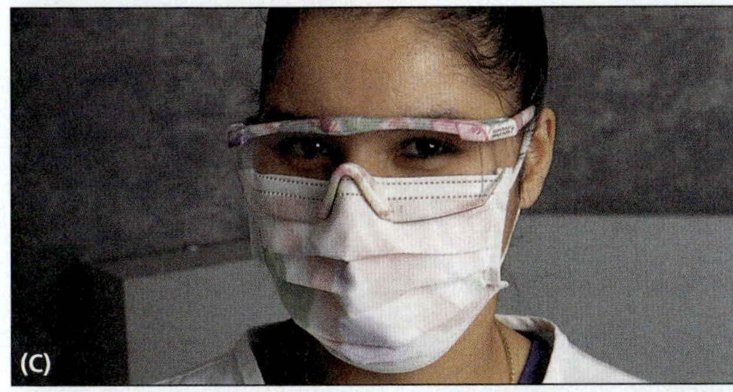

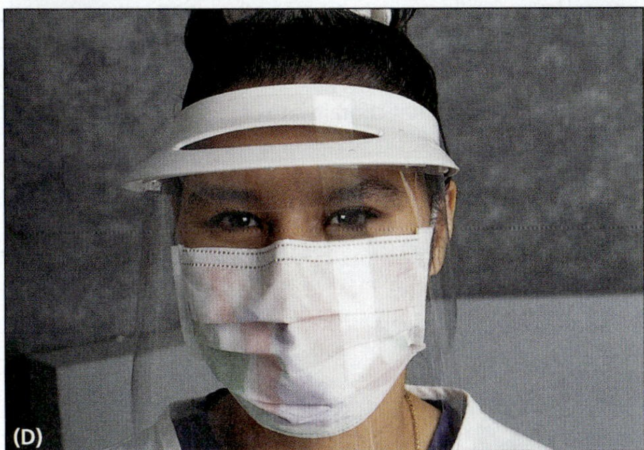

FIGURE 11-9A–D

(A) Goggles. (B) Eyewear with protective side shields. (C) Dental protective eyewear with side shields. (D) Dental face shield.

Choose gloves according to comfort, the tactile sensitivity required, and the procedure being completed. Obtaining the best quality for the greatest value is another factor in choosing gloves.

Latex, nitrile, vinyl, and synthetic polymer gloves are ambidextrous, that is, they are used interchangeably for the right or left hand (Figures 11-10A–C). To provide the proper fit and comfort for most individuals, they are supplied in a variety of sizes and flavors, they can also be chlorinated or non-chlorinated with some available with aloe and/or vitamin E. Many individuals feel that latex gloves provide a better fit. Latex-sensitive individuals use vinyl or synthetic polymer gloves as an alternative to latex or nitrile. The vinyl and synthetic polymer gloves, however, are more rigid, tear more easily, and lack tactile sensitivity. Due to increased use, however, vinyl gloves are being improved. The treatment gloves can be ordered powder free, powdered, or lightly powdered to aid in donning (placing the gloves on). Gloves are supplied as nonsterile (referred to as examination gloves) and sterile (referred to as sterile surgical gloves). Most procedures in the dental office only require the use of

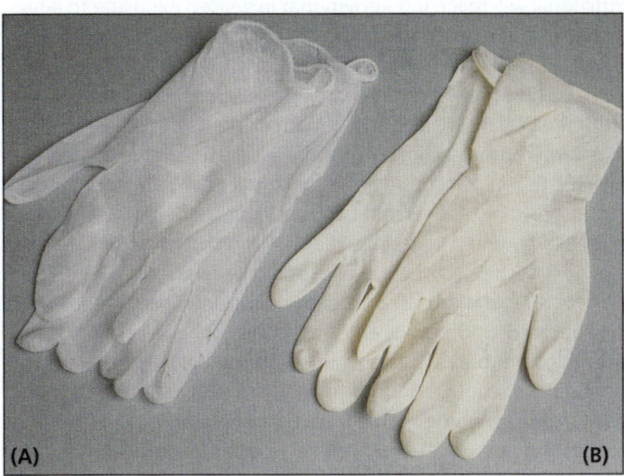

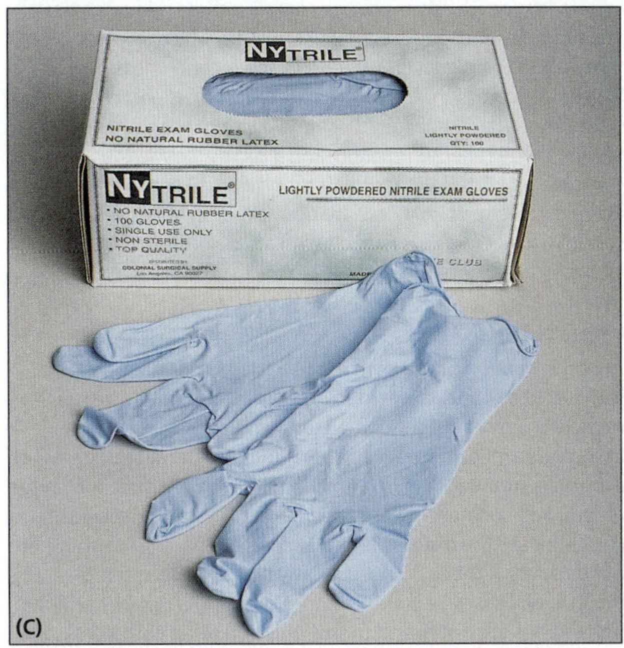

FIGURE 11-10 A–C

(a) Vinyl and (B) latex examination gloves. (C) Lightly powdered, colored nitrile examination gloves.

nonsterile gloves. They provide the minimal barrier protection needed for the dental personnel. Sterile surgical gloves are only used in specific surgical procedures requiring a sterile environment, such as oral, periodontal, and implant surgery.

Both the latex and the vinyl gloves need to be changed with each new patient. If, during the procedure, they become torn or punctured, they should be removed; the hands should be washed, and the gloves replaced with new gloves to complete the procedure. *Gloves should never be washed and reused.*

Latex Allergies

Latex is used in many of the products that are available today. In the dental office and other medical clinics, latex gloves are used routinely for patient care. This increase in latex usage has increased the number of individuals who present with latex hypersensitivity. Latex is a natural rubber that comes from a rubber tree, *Hevea brasiliensis*. It is a milky fluid that is taken from the tree, much like maple is collected for syrup, and is then manufactured. If not treated properly, the product from this tree releases proteins that can cause allergic reactions. An allergic reaction may develop after a person has had a large amount of exposure, or even a slight exposure, to latex. It is unknown how an individual will react. It is known that increased exposure to latex increases the risk of developing the symptoms of a **latex allergy**. Initially, the person normally has mild symptoms, and does not develop life-threatening responses. However, the dental assistant should be ready to aid in treating the patient who presents with allergic symptoms. The Centers for Disease Control and Prevention (CDC) sets forth guidelines for contact dermatitis and latex hypersensitivity. It says that each patient should be screened for a latex allergy when taking the medical and dental history. If a latex allergy is suspected, the patient should be referred to the physician for further medical consultation. All dental personnel should be educated on the signs and symptoms of the latex allergy, and how constant handwashing and use of latex gloves increases the possibility of contact dermatitis and latex hypersensitivity. The dental office should provide a latex-safe environment for patients and dental personnel, and provide an emergency kit containing a latex allergy reaction treatment.

Latex allergies are commonly presented in three primary types of reactions. The first one is contact dermatitis, which involves irritation only to the top layers of the skin; the second one is type IV and is the most common. A type IV allergic reaction is primarily limited to the areas that contacted the latex. The third allergic reaction to latex is a type I allergic reaction, and it can be very serious. Anyone can develop a latex allergy, but it is only a small group of individuals who actually do so. These are normally individuals who are sensitive to allergies, individuals who are in constant contact with latex products, or people who are in the rubber industry.

Contact Dermatitis

An inflammation of the skin due to a chemical irritation is referred to as **contact dermatitis**. Contact dermatitis occurs immediately, or very soon after contact. Hands that become itchy and sometimes cracked characterize it. Dental assistants are especially prone to having contact dermatitis, because they wear gloves, and constantly wash their hands. Things that increase this condition are the usage of antimicrobial agents, and washing the hands often. If the assistant uses any type of rough sponge or brush, it will increase the abrasion, and exaggerate the condition. If the hands are not rinsed thoroughly and dried completely, the chance for contact dermatitis will increase; and, if the condition is already present, it will intensify the symptoms. When wearing treatment gloves, the hands will often perspire, and this will lead to the condition, as will contact with cornstarch or powder in the gloves. The cornstarch in the powder does not have allergenic chemicals in it, but can aid in transferring the proteins and allergenic chemicals from the latex glove to the dental assistant. It also allows the particles to become airborne when the gloves are changed. These airborne particles can be inhaled, and then contact body membranes. The dental assistant should use special care to wash, rinse, and dry the hands; and then choose gloves that decrease sensitivity, change them often, and apply lotion to hands as necessary to inhibit this condition.

Type IV Allergic Reaction

A **type IV allergic reaction** to latex is also referred to as allergic contact dermatitis, delayed hypersensitivity, and chemical sensitivity dermatitis. Type IV allergic reaction is a great deal more common than a type I allergic reaction. It is the result of exposure to the chemicals added to latex during harvesting, processing, or manufacturing. A type IV allergic reaction to latex is much like an allergic reaction to poison ivy. The skin rash usually begins 24 to 48 hours after contact. It may even show up 72 hours after contact. It shows up as red areas that are itchy, and may present with oozing blisters. It normally shows up at the areas of contact, but may spread away from the initial site. It is an immune system response and is, therefore, very different from contact dermatitis. If an employee exhibits the symptoms of a type IV allergic reaction, all employees should take care and not use powdered gloves and other latex equipment. The affected employee must be provided with hypoallergenic gloves (reduced protein, powder-free gloves), or non-latex gloves or glove liners. The employer should evaluate current prevention strategies, and take steps to limit the exposure in the workplace. There are a number of items that contain latex in the office and in the home.

A few of the products that contain latex are as follows:

Office

- Treatment gloves
- Blood pressure cuffs
- Stethoscopes
- Syringe carpule stoppers
- Some goggles
- Rubber bands
- Erasers
- Dental dams
- Elastic waistbands

Home

- Hot water bottles
- Balloons
- Baby bottle nipples

- Baby bottle pacifiers
- Automobile tires
- Carpeting
- Shoe soles
- Elastic waistbands
- Many rubber devices

Type I Allergic Reaction

A **type I allergic reaction** can occur minutes after exposure to latex proteins, and can result in death if the patient has an anaphylactic reaction. This severe allergic reaction is the most serious of the allergic reactions to latex. It causes the airway to close due to swelling. A type I allergic reaction to latex is not common in the dental office, but the dental assistant should always be prepared for an emergency. The patient may show signs of coughing, wheezing, respiratory distress, and runny eyes and nose, and may become unable to breathe. Emergency medical treatment should be summoned immediately.

A type I allergic reaction is not due to the chemical additives, like with type IV; instead, it occurs in response to the proteins in the latex. The proteins can be released during contact, or they can adhere to the cornstarch or powder in the gloves and become released when the gloves are donned or removed during normal treatment. These released proteins, which are attached to the powder, then become airborne and are suspended in the air. Sensitized individuals can breathe in these proteins and a reaction may occur. Individuals who have extreme sensitivity should be treated in latex-free environments. It may be that these patients will have to seek treatment in places where latex has not been used and, thus, will not be in the air system. This is a life and death situation and should be treated as such. Individuals who have latex allergies should practice prevention and not place themselves in areas of latex usage. There is no cure available. Testing can be done to confirm that an individual is sensitive or has an allergy to latex. If a patient is sensitive to latex, non-latex gloves (vinyl) can be used as well as other non-latex products, such as rubber dam material.

Gloves in the Dental Office

- Use new gloves for each patient.
- Never wash gloves.
- If gloves become penetrated during treatment, remove gloves, wash and dry hands, and place new gloves on hands.

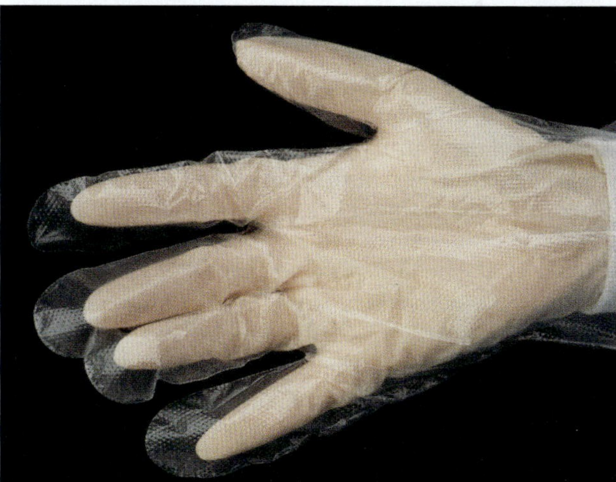

FIGURE 11-11
Overgloves used to open a drawer or write on a chart.

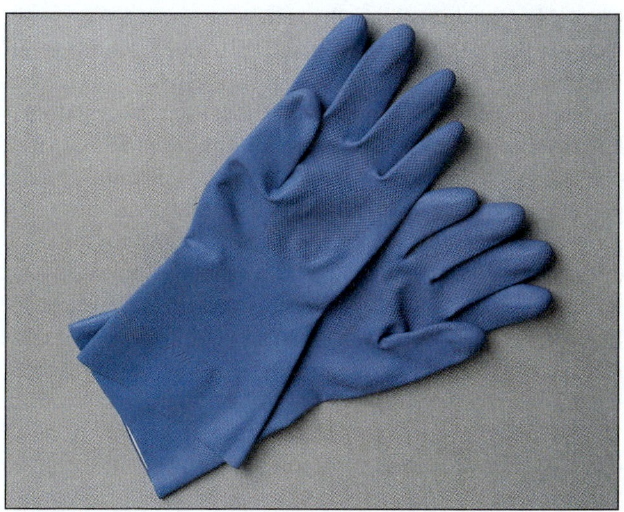

FIGURE 11-12
Utility gloves.

To prevent cross-contamination during a procedure, if the dental assistant has to reach inside a drawer, write on a chart, or touch an area that is not contaminated, **overgloves**, also known as food handlers' gloves, are placed over the latex or vinyl gloves (Figure 11-11). Overgloves are big, loose gloves that do not have the tactile touch that the latex and vinyl gloves have, however, they quickly fit over the gloves so that the user can obtain something in a sterile area. They are not to be used as examination gloves. Overgloves can be placed on rapidly to accomplish a secondary task, such as opening a container. They should be discarded after each use.

Thick **utility gloves** are used during disinfection and cleanup procedures (Figure 11-12). These gloves are used for dishwashing and, like overgloves, are not regulated by the FDA. An assistant carries the tray to the sterilization area, removes the latex or vinyl gloves, washes his or her hands, and dons the utility gloves to complete the cleanup. The utility gloves can be washed and reused. However, if they become cracked or punctured, they should be discarded and replaced.

Autoclavable utility gloves have an added benefit in that they can be sterilized in the autoclave after use. Each dental team member involved in cleanup and instrument recycling must have his or her own set of polynitrile autoclavable utility gloves.

Donning and Removal of Gloves. The donning (placement) of gloves is done after carefully washing and drying the hands. The dental assistant should not place petroleum-based hand lotion on prior to placement of gloves, because it may cause the integrity of the gloves to break down, thereby, weakening them.

When removing the gloves, tuck the fingers of one glove into the cuff of the other glove, coming from the glove side and not from the skin side. Lift it off, taking care not to touch the tissue with the gloves. It can be inverted as it is removed and remains in the palm of the gloved hand. After the first glove is removed, use the thumb of the freed hand inside the cuff (skin side) of the remaining glove and pull it down and off the hand and invert it over the first glove. Carefully dispose of the gloves into a biohazard waste receptacle (Figures 11-13A–C).

Masks. Any time that splatter or aerosol of saliva or blood can occur a mask should be worn (Figure 11-14). The dental assistant must wear a mask to protect the mucous membranes of the nose and mouth. The aerosol mist that remains suspended in the air may come from the use of the dental handpiece, the ultrasonic scaler, or the air–water syringe. At times, due to the use of the air–water syringe, splatter occurs where a concentrated amount of saliva or blood projects from the oral cavity onto the dental health worker. Proper placement of the high-volume evacuator (HVE) and the air–water syringe (see Chapter 17 Introduction to the Dental Office and Basic Chairside Assisting) aids in the reduction of splatter; however, it can still occur. Wearing a mask that covers the nose and mouth protects dental personnel in such cases.

The dental mask also protects the patient and the dental assistant from communicable diseases. The mask should be placed on, along with the eyewear, before washing hands and donning gloves (Figure 11-15). It is important that the mask be placed properly so that it fits snugly against the face, and stays in place during the procedure. Normally, the face mask has an outside and an inside (next to the face); place it according to the manufacturer's directions. Often, a color is on the outside surface for quick identification. Masks are also available in a variety of designs. For example, cartoon images are available for pediatric practices.

The mask is secured with elastic that goes around the head, over the ears, or with ties that are fastened behind the head. Some masks can be pinched above the nose to fit better and to stop the breath from fogging up the protective eyewear. Always adjust the mask to the proper position prior to the procedure. Masks should be removed after the procedure by grasping the ties or attachments. Never reuse a mask; replace it after every patient, or even during a procedure if the mask becomes moist. Never slip the mask down on the neck area, or let it dangle from the ear, after treatment is over. Remove the mask and dispose of it.

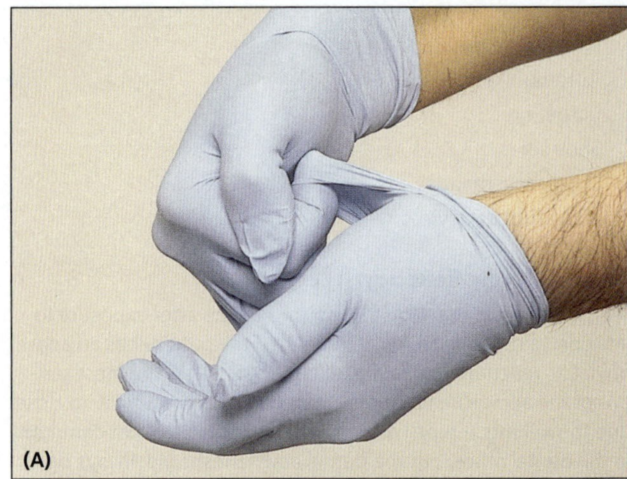
(A)

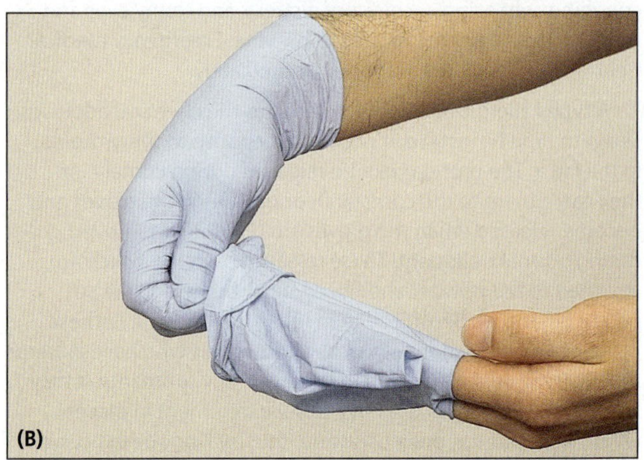
(B)

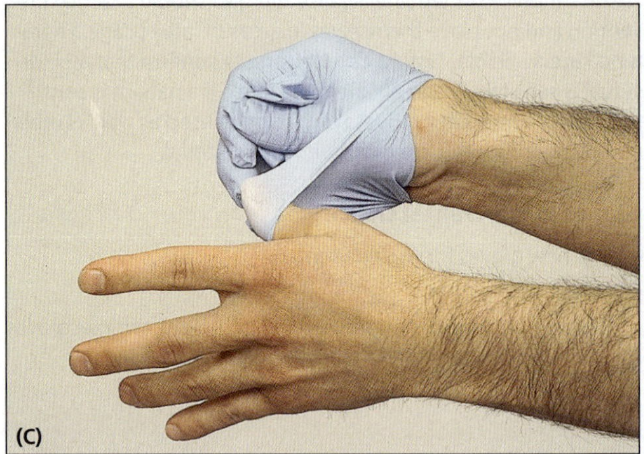
(C)

FIGURE 11-13 A–C
(A) Grasp the outside of the cuff of the first glove. (B) Invert the glove while removing, and then keep the removed glove in the palm of the gloved hand. (C) Insert the thumb of the freed hand inside the cuff of the second glove. Pull outward and over the hand while inverting the glove over the glove inside the palm, and off the second hand.

Masks During Dental Treatment

- Use a new mask for each patient.
- Replace the mask if it becomes moist or wet.
- Never let the mask dangle around the neck or from the ear; remove and discard after each use.

Protective Clothing. OSHA regulates special protective clothing worn only in the dental office. Protective clothing includes uniforms, laboratory coats, gowns, and clinic jackets. According to OSHA, the dentist must provide protective clothing that is worn in the office, and is laundered in the office or by a commercial laundering service. One uniform for each staff member each day is appropriate. Dental personnel enter the office and change into uniforms, or other PPE overgarments (Figure 11-16). The employer is required to clean, launder, and dispose of PPE at no cost to the employee. The uniforms or other PPE overgarments, such as laboratory coats, should be removed if the dental assistant is going out to lunch or going into the staff lounge for lunch.

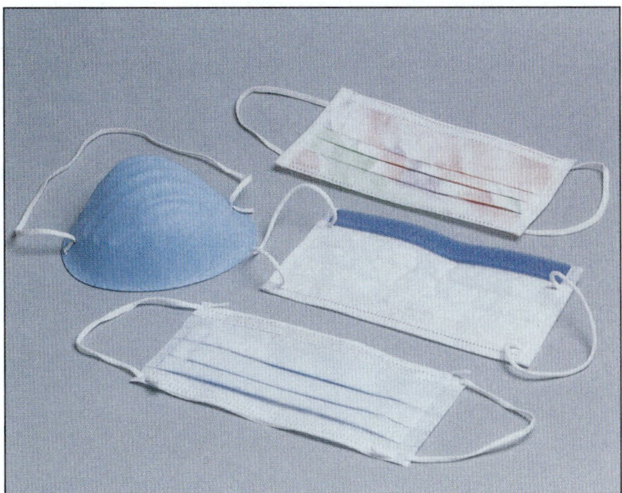

FIGURE 11-14
Face masks used in dentistry.

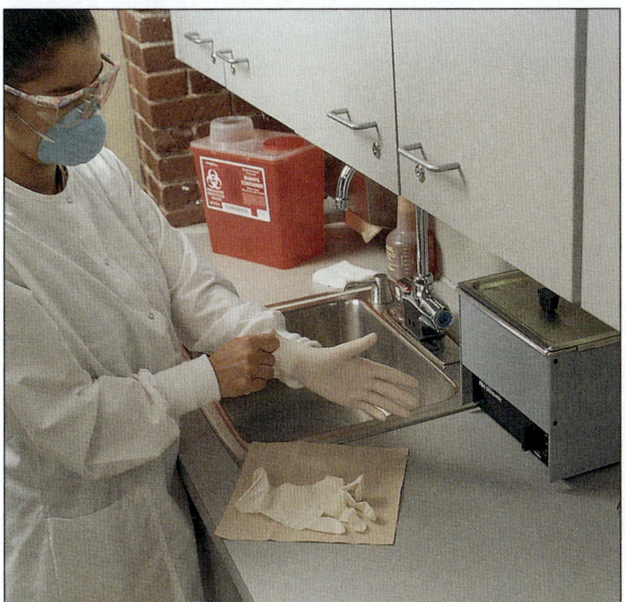

FIGURE 11-15
A dental assistant is putting on PPE before performing dental procedures.

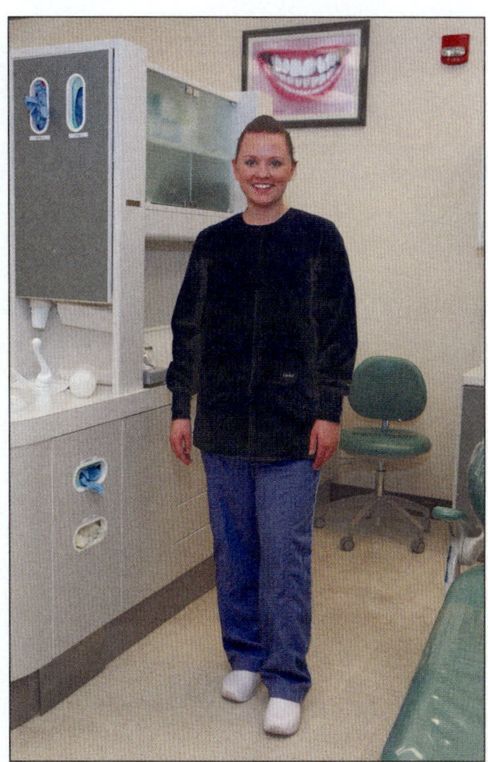

FIGURE 11-16
A dental assistant in a uniform.

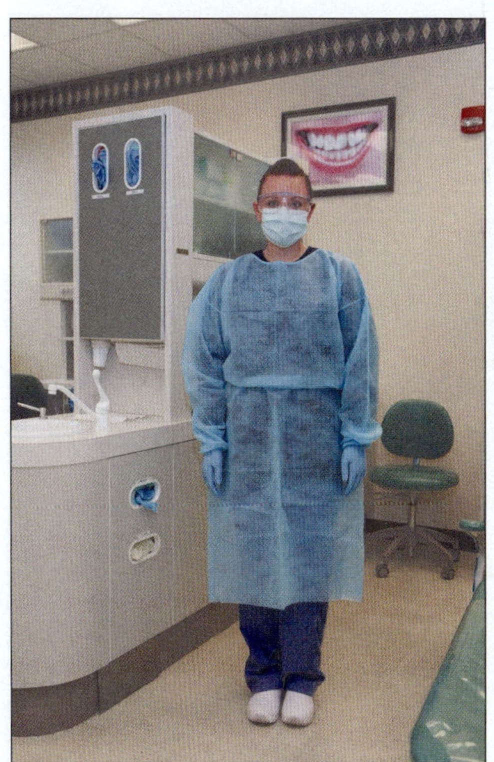

FIGURE 11-17
A dental assistant in a disposable treatment gown.

Long isolation gowns are worn by the dental team members who fall in Category 1 or 2 (Figure 11-17). Gowns and uniforms cover the arms, fit closely around the neck and wrists, and provide the greatest protection if impermeable to fluids. During the time that the gloves are on, the gloves fit over the cuffs of the uniform.

Protective clothing should be changed daily, or immediately if splattered with body fluids. Special attention to the design of the protective clothing should be taken. Any buttons, zippers, and ornamental designs should be kept to a minimum because they can harbor pathogens. Disposable outer gowns are an option for dental personnel. The specific types of uniforms or gowns worn during patient care are dictated by office policy.

When removing protective clothing, care must be taken to keep the side of the clothing that has possibly been contaminated with pathogens folded inward. The assistant should remove one arm first, then fold the clothing inward, and then slowly remove the rest of the lab coat, all the while taking special care to fold the clothing together as it is removed. OSHA notes that special care is to be taken with items that are considered potentially infectious.

Procedure 11-2
Putting on Personal Protective Equipment

This procedure is performed by the dental assistant prior to starting treatment.

Equipment and Supplies:

- Protective clothing
- Surgical mask
- Protective eyewear
- Procedure gloves

Procedure Steps:

1. Place protective clothing over your uniform, scrubs, or street cloths. It should be long sleeved, covering to the neckline, and not loose at the wrists. It can be called a lab coat, clinic gown, or clinic jacket (Figure 11-18).
2. Place surgical mask on and ensure that the nose area is tightened and adjusted so that air will not fog up the protective eyewear (Figure 11-19). Make sure that the elastic area on the ears is comfortable.
3. Place protective eyewear (Figure 11-20). Ensure that it has side shields for protection, and that it is impact resistant. Some offices use face shields or goggles, which are also acceptable.
4. After hands have been washed and dried, put on treatment gloves. Make sure that the gloves are placed on last to avoid contaminating them prior to patient contact. Hold the glove at the cuff and allow the opposite hand to enter the glove, pulling it completely into place. Moist hands will make this placement difficult. Hold the other glove at the cuff with the gloved hand and place the ungloved hand into the glove (Figure 11-21).

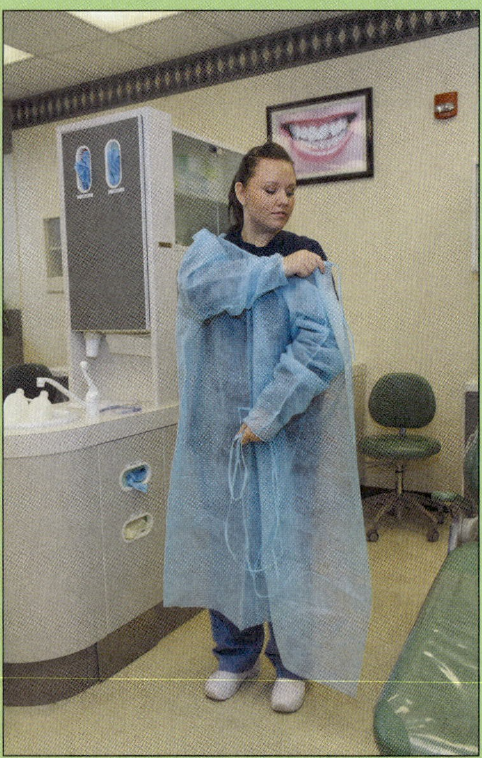

FIGURE 11-18
Placing a clinic gown on.

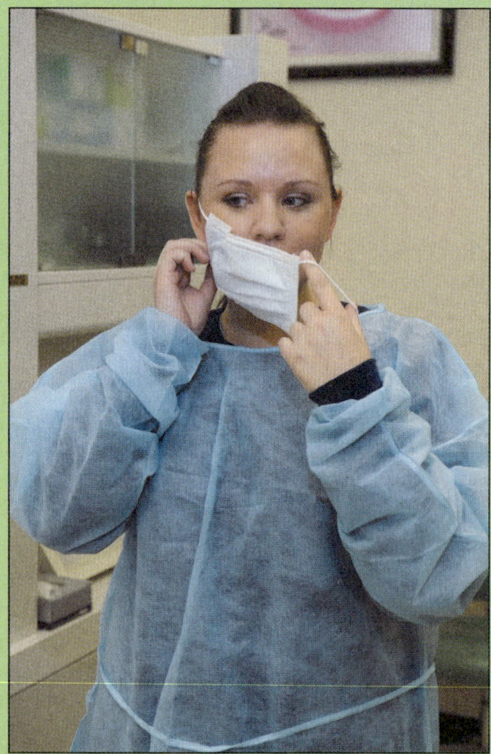

FIGURE 11-19
Placing a surgical mask on.

(continues)

Procedure 11-2 (continued)

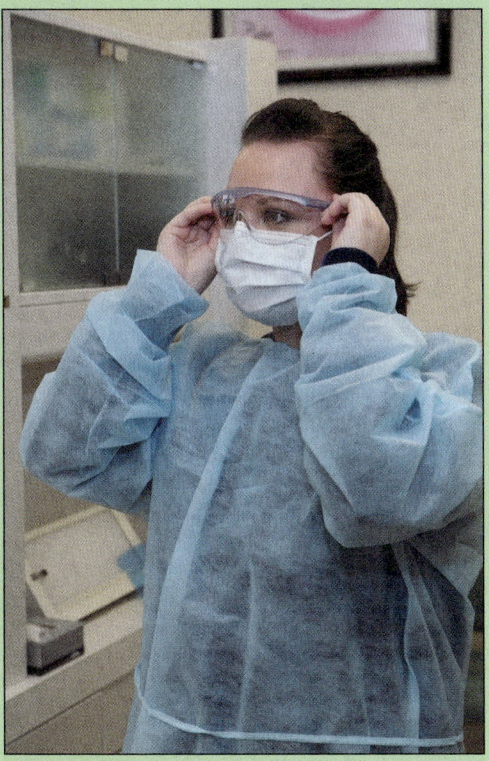

FIGURE 11-20
Placing protective eyewear on.

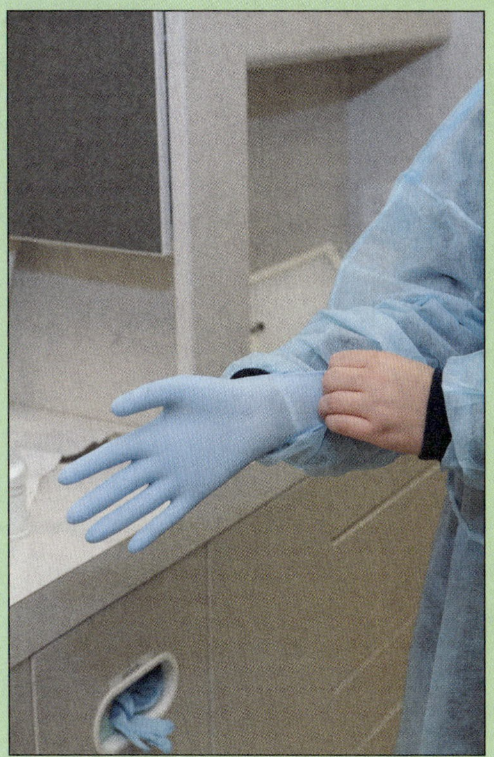

FIGURE 11-21
Placing treatment gloves on.

Procedure 11-3
Removing Personal Protective Equipment

The procedure is performed by the dental assistant after each patient treatment is completed.

Equipment and Supplies:

- Protective clothing
- Surgical mask
- Protective eyewear
- Procedure gloves

Procedure Steps:

1. Remove the treatment gloves following the steps identified in Figure 11-13 A–C.
2. Wash and dry hands completely.
3. Remove the protective eyewear by touching the sides called the ear rests. Hold the ear rests, raising them from the face (Figure 11-22). Place the eyewear on a paper towel, or on the tray until it can be disinfected.

(continues)

Procedure 11-3 (continued)

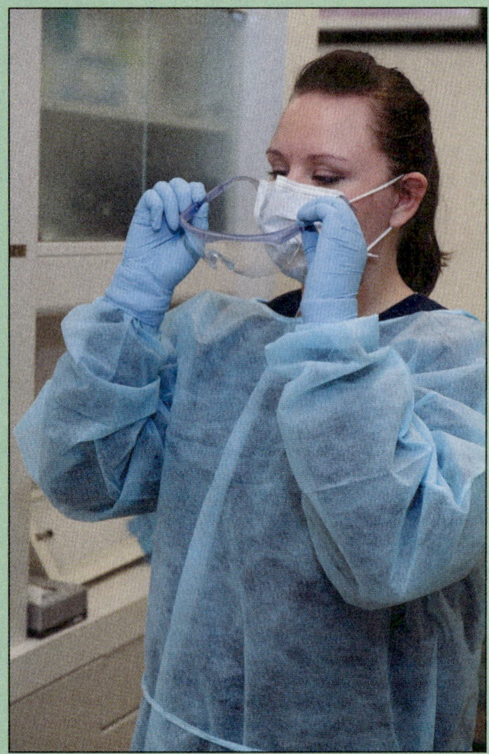

FIGURE 11-22
Removing protective eyewear.

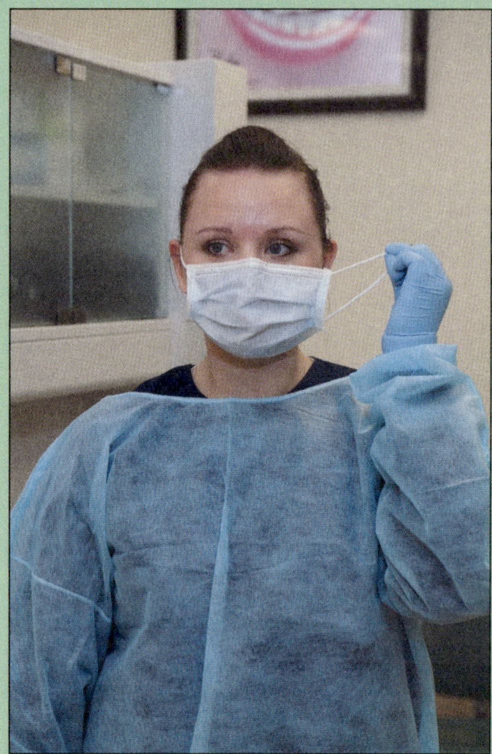

FIGURE 11-23
Removing surgical mask.

4. To remove the mask, slide the fingers of each hand under the elastic ear strap, or untie the tie straps without touching the hair or anything else, and then lift the strap from around the ear, releasing it, and removing it from the face (Figure 11-23). Dispose of the face mask in the waste receptacle.
5. Remove the gown by turning it inside out as it comes off (Figure 11-24). Do not allow the outside of the gown to touch underlying cloths or skin. Dispose of gowns in a waste receptacle daily, or more often if they become soiled.

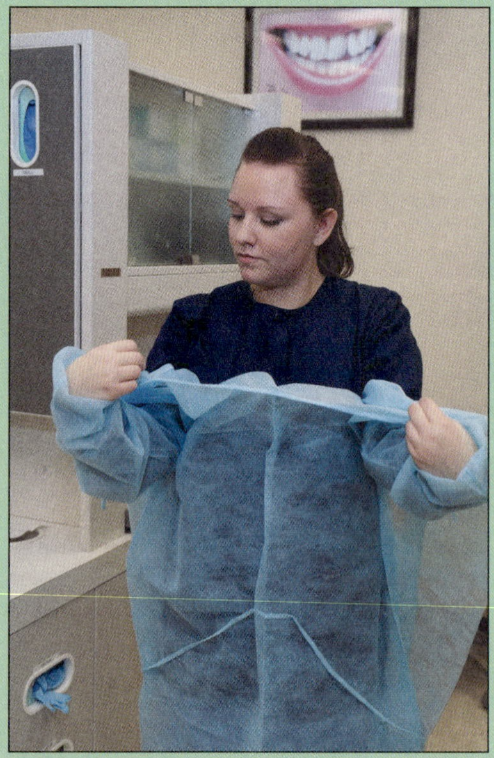

FIGURE 11-24
Removing treatment gown.

Protective Clothing in the Dental Office

- Worn only in the dental office (not in staff lounges or lunch rooms)
- Must close tightly at neck and around cuff area
- During a high-risk procedure, must be knee length when sitting
- Must be removed at the end of the day, prior to going home
- Must be laundered in the office, or sent to a laundry service

Barriers

Coverings or **barriers** are used wherever possible in all aspects of the dental office. Inside the operatory, barriers cover the patient dental chair, light (handles and operating switch), handpieces, air–water syringe, high-volume evacuator, saliva ejector, tubing, writing utensils, and surfaces (Figures 11-25 A and B). Any area where contamination is possible during dental treatment that can be covered should be covered. Barriers have been made specifically for areas that have been hard to disinfect or sterilize in the past, such as tubing and hoses for the handpieces. The patient should wear protective eyewear, and a patient napkin or bib for protection from splatter and debris (Figure 11-26).

Recommendations for Environmental Infection Control by the CDC

The CDC made recommendations for environmental infection control in dental health care settings. They identified two areas of environmental surfaces: the clinical contact surface and the housekeeping surface. The **clinical contact surface** was further identified as three areas of concern by OSAP. The **touch surface** is the area that is directly touched and contaminated during dental treatment procedures, such as light handles, unit controls, material containers, dental trays, pens, drawer handles, and so on. The **transfer surface** is not directly touched, but are areas or items that are indirectly contaminated, such as air–water syringe holders, dental trays, handpiece holders, and so on. The **splash, spatter, and droplet surfaces** are areas that dental personnel do not actually contact, but still may be contaminated. Examples of this type of surface are the counter tops or front of the dental light.

The **housekeeping surfaces** include the floors, walls, sinks, windows, and in the general overall patient care areas.

Using disposable light covers for the dental light and handles provide a barrier to the entire light. The dental chair can be covered with plastic dry cleaning bags to shield it from contaminants. Dry cleaning bags are fairly inexpensive and can be purchased on a roll. After the procedure is completed, the bag is turned inside out (contamination inside), and all disposable supplies are placed in the bag for easy cleanup. Dental chair covers are also available from dental supply companies.

Disinfection

Areas that do not lend themselves to the use of barriers in the dental office need to be disinfected if they cannot be sterilized. Some dental offices use barriers, and also disinfect. As long as all surfaces are disinfected or protected by a barrier, the requirement of asepsis is met.

Using paper mixing pads makes proper disinfection difficult. However, the plastic ends in the dental x-ray film boxes can be used to mix some cements. These ends can be cleaned and placed in a submersion sterilization solution and reused.

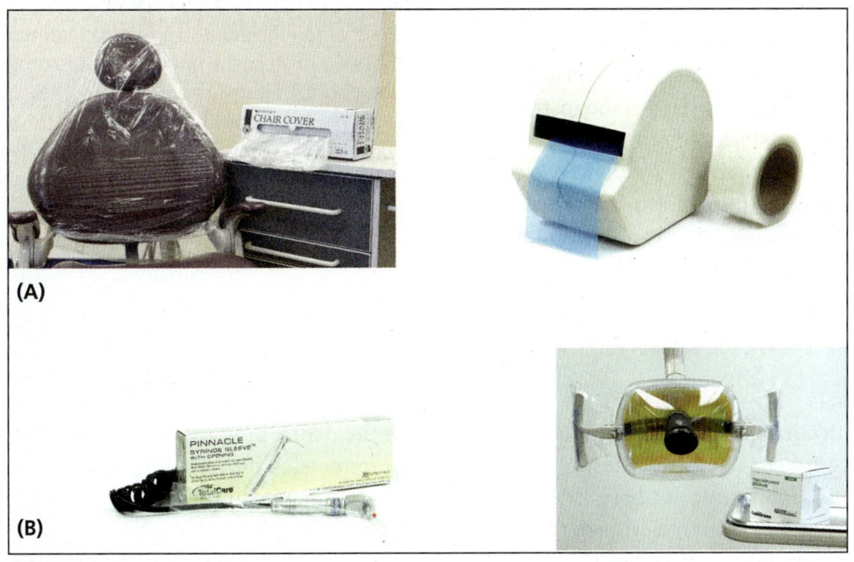

FIGURE 11-25 A & B

(A) Barriers placed on dental unit. (B) Samples of various dental barriers.

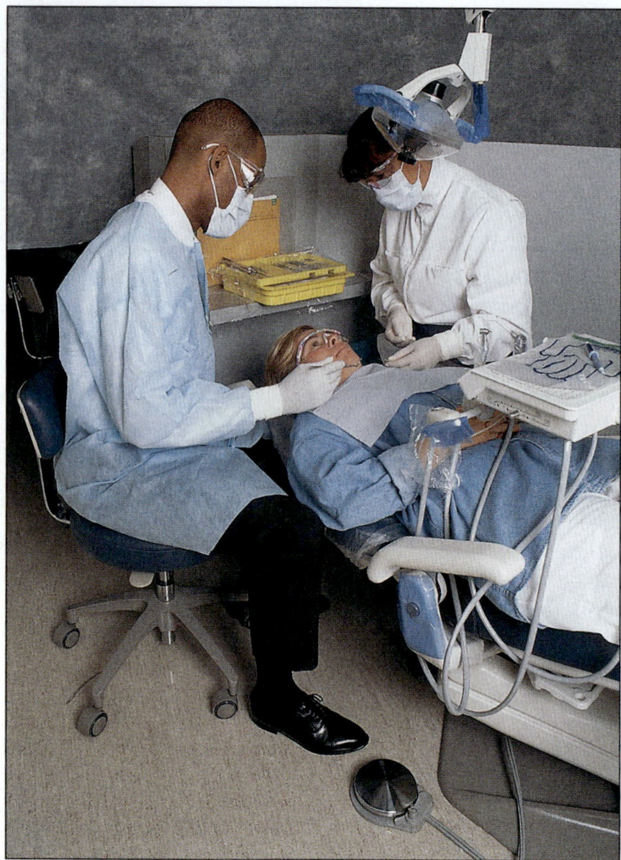

FIGURE 11-26

Barriers in place in a dental treatment room. Doctor, patient, and assistant with PPE.

Cleaning the Area

All areas where dental procedures are performed must be cleaned prior to disinfection and sterilization. *Cleaning* is the physical removal of organic matter such as blood, tissue, and debris. The process of cleaning decreases the number of microorganisms in the area and removes substances that may hinder the processes of disinfection and sterilization. This process is much like washing off dishes before placing them in the dishwasher. If the substances stay on the instruments, they cannot be disinfected or sterilized properly.

If something is sanitized, the process is much like cleaning. When an area receives **sanitization**, it means that the area has been decontaminated, but it does not mean that all microorganisms in the area have been destroyed.

Environmental Protection Agency Approval

The EPA registers disinfection and sterilization solutions only after the products have undergone careful testing. The disinfecting and sterilization solutions must have EPA approval on their labels. Each product registered with the EPA must have determination as to whether a solution sterilizes or disinfects, and what types of microorganisms it will destroy. When all forms of microorganisms are destroyed **sterilization** has been achieved. When *some* microorganisms are destroyed **disinfection** occurs. The contact time needed for each product is also defined on the label. Some products disinfect after ten minutes but need to have ten hours of submersion in order to sterilize. Disinfection levels are rated according to the EPA as high, intermediate, and low.

- *High-level disinfection* refers to a **tuberculocidal** that kills most, but not all, bacterial spores. If it is extremely strong and can kill all the bacterial spores, it is noted as a **sporicidal** on the label.
- *Intermediate-level disinfection* refers to a tuberculocidal that normally does not kill bacterial spores.
- *Low-level disinfection* (designated by the EPA as hospital disinfectants) kills some viruses and fungi, and most of the bacteria microorganisms. It does not kill tuberculosis or bacterial spores. A **fungicidal** is a biological organism or biological chemical compound used to kill or inhibit fungi or fungal spores. A **virucidal** is an agent that neutralizes or destroys viruses. This agent is different from antiviral drugs, which inhibits the development of a virus. A virucide kills MSRA and influenza.

When choosing products for disinfection and sterilization for the dental office, be aware that no one product meets all needs. Each product has advantages and disadvantages for use with specific materials. The degree of staining and corrosiveness to instruments and equipment, along with the toxicity of the material, should be considered when choosing solutions. Read labels carefully to gain the information needed about product effectiveness. Dental personnel are assisted in choosing the proper solutions for the dental office by reading the information recommended by the dental organizations, or by asking the dental supply representative for information.

Greener Infection Control

Practicing efficient and effective infection control techniques that also protect the environment is known as greener infection control. There are various programs and products available to help reduce harmful chemicals in the environment, reduce waste, and conserve water and energy. Dental office personnel can strive to be environmentally friendly, and follow greener infection control protocol.

Chemical Disinfectants

There are many solutions that can be used for disinfection. The dental assistant should be familiar with the solutions used in the dental practice. These solutions can be used as surface or immersion disinfectants, or sterilants. This includes becoming familiar with the properties of the solutions, the proper uses of the solutions, the time required for the solutions to be effective when used, and the proper storage and disposal of the solutions. The dental office should maintain SDS forms for each solution used in the practice.

Surface Disinfectants. Surface disinfectants are used on counter tops, trays, the dental unit, dental chair, x-ray equipment, and most items that cannot be disposed of, immersed, or go into the sterilizers, but are in the treatment area. The ideal surface disinfectants are odorless, cost effective, rapidly kill a broad range of microorganisms, have minimal toxicity, are easy to use, do not damage the surface being disinfected, and have **residual activity**, where the effect continues long after initial application. At this time there is not one surface disinfectant that meets all of these ideal criteria. When selecting a surface disinfectant read carefully all of the advantages and disadvantages of each product and select the one that meets the individual needs of the office. You can also refer to the manufacture's information, often they will make a suggestion as to the type of surface disinfectant that works best with the dental unit or other surfaces.

Sanitation/Disinfection Wipes. Many offices use a wipe that sanitizes and disinfects. It comes in an air-tight dispensing container with towelettes (Figure 11-27). The towelettes are presaturated with a disinfectant that is effective against tuberculosis, bacteria, fungi, and viruses. They are ideal for hard, non-porous surfaces, and equipment. The surface contact time ranges from one to ten minutes. Many of the towellettes meet the EPA, CDC, FDA, and OSHA requirements. Assistants like them because they are efficient and disposable.

Sodium Hypochlorite. Sodium hypochlorite can be obtained in a number of different concentrations. The concentration referred to here is the same as household bleach, which is 5.25 percent sodium hypochlorite. The desired concentration for use in the dental office is a 1:10 dilution. This is obtained by placing one cup of household bleach in one gallon of water. The mixed solution is ready for use. It is highly effective for intermediate-level disinfection, and is effective against a broad spectrum of microorganisms. A 1:100 dilution of ¼ cup bleach to one gallon of water is used for general-purpose disinfection. Sodium hypochlorite works rapidly (within ten minutes) on surfaces. The solution is extremely unstable and has to be mixed daily. It is also extremely corrosive to metals. Sodium hypochlorite is irritating to the eyes and skin, and can harm clothing. PPE should be worn while using all cleaning and disinfection solutions. Good ventilation is essential when using sodium hypochlorite, and caution should be used when mixing it with other cleaning agents because it can become extremely toxic.

Iodophor. Iodophor is used as an intermediate-level disinfectant. Care should be used when diluting the solution to procure the correct concentration. One of the active ingredients in iodophor is iodine. The iodine in this solution can stain white countertops and light-colored vinyl with repeated use. Iodophor works rapidly, taking 5 to 25 minutes of surface contact to be effective. It is used as a holding solution for dental impressions before they are poured or sent to the dental lab. It is corrosive to some metals and has a short life span. Solutions should be changed every three days, at a minimum, to remain active. Iodophor can be irritating to skin; thus, utility gloves should be worn while disinfecting surfaces.

Phenolics. Phenolics, or synthetic phenolics, are used for intermediate-level disinfection (Figure 11-28). They have **broad spectrum activity**, meaning that they kill a wide range of microbes.They can be irritating to the skin and eyes but often they are mixed with synthetic detergents in a non-alkaline formula to reduce the toxicity. Follow the manufacturer's directions when diluting the solution. The surface contact time is normally ten minutes. Many phenolics come in individual packets that are put in spray or pump containers to mix and dispense. They also are available as wipes dispensed in easy to use pop-up containers. Over time they can be destructive to some plastic surfaces, but overall are effective surface disinfectants.

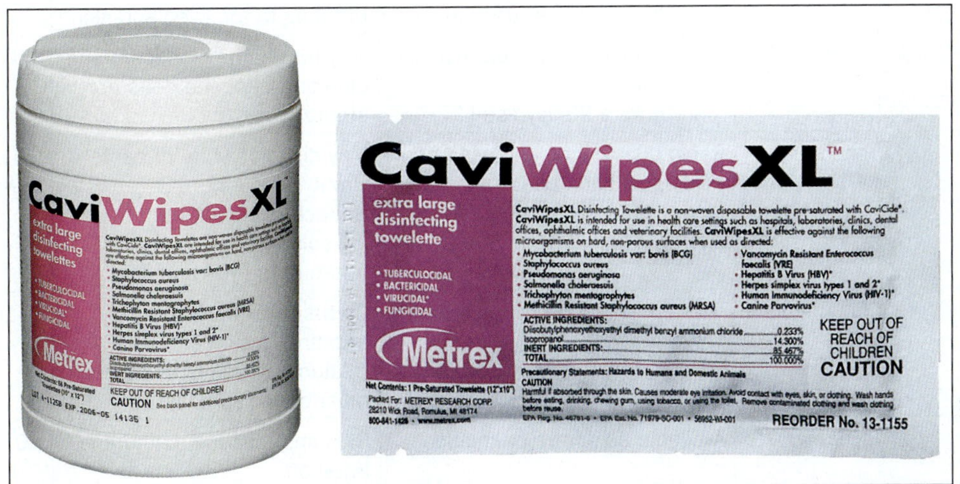

FIGURE 11-27

Disinfecting wipes for use on multiple surfaces.

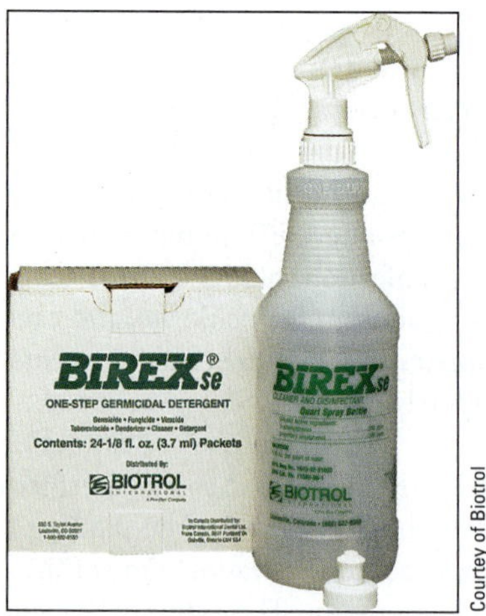

FIGURE 11-28

Synthetic phenol disinfecting solutions and wipes.

Alcohol. Isopropyl alcohol was used routinely for disinfection prior to the 1980s. Essentially, it cleaned the areas and had some disinfecting qualities, but it provides limited benefits. *Alcohol is no longer recommended for disinfection in the dental office.* Alcohol evaporates so quickly that it is difficult to have surface contact for the length of time necessary to be effective.

Table 11-2 compares commonly used disinfectants in the dental office.

Immersion Disinfectants. Immersion disinfectants, or sterilants, are used when instruments are placed into the chemical solution. Most immersion disinfectants have a time that is used for low- and high-level disinfection, as well as sterilization. The time of immersion indicates the level of either disinfection or sterilization. Review the manufacturer's directions on preparation, time, and use life. Heat sensitive instruments are used in immersion disinfectants. They are placed in a covered instrument container with an immersion tray to minimize exposure to fumes and handling (Figures 11-29A and B). After use, the instruments are rinsed with water.

Chlorine Dioxide. Chlorine dioxide (EPA registered) is a high-level disinfectant that should be used only on items not subject to corrosion. Any materials made of, or having parts made of, stainless steel, carbide steel, copper, or brass will corrode if chlorine dioxide is used. The solution should be stored only in glass or plastic containers. Follow the manufacturer's directions for dilution and contact time. Normally, disinfection is rapid, but sterilization takes 6 to 10 hours. Proper ventilation is necessary when using this product.

Glutaraldehyde. Glutaraldehyde (EPA registered) is used for high-level disinfection and sterilization. Some of the solutions are corrosive to metals. Read the manufacturer's directions regarding the dilution and contact time for disinfection and sterilization. Time for disinfection is normally 10 to 90 minutes, and for sterilization is normally 6 to 10 hours. Whenever

TABLE 11-2 Disinfectant Comparisons

Disinfectant	Level	Advantages	Disadvantages	Time Required for Effectiveness
Chlorine dioxide	High	Rapid disinfection	Corrosive to metals Requires ventilation Irritating to eyes and skin	5–10 minutes
Glutaraldehyde	High	Used for low- and high-level disinfection and sterilization Many have a 28-day use life	Some are corrosive to metal Requires ventilation Irritating to the eyes and skin	10–90 minutes
Ortho-Phthalaldehyde	High	Used to disinfect without causing sensitivity Many have a 28-day use life	May turn some plastics blue or green, and does not sterilize	10–12 minutes
Iodophor	Intermediate	Rapid disinfection and used as holding solution for impressions	May discolor white or pastel vinyls Surface disinfectant or holding solution Irritating to eyes and skin	10 minutes on surfaces
Sodium hypochlorite	Intermediate	Rapid disinfection	Corrosive to metals Irritating to skin and eyes Diluted solution is unstable, must be mixed daily	5–10 minutes
Phenolics	Intermediate	Available as sprays or liquids	Skin and mucous membrane irritation Cannot be used on plastics	10 minutes
Alcohol	Cleaner only	N/A	N/A	N/A

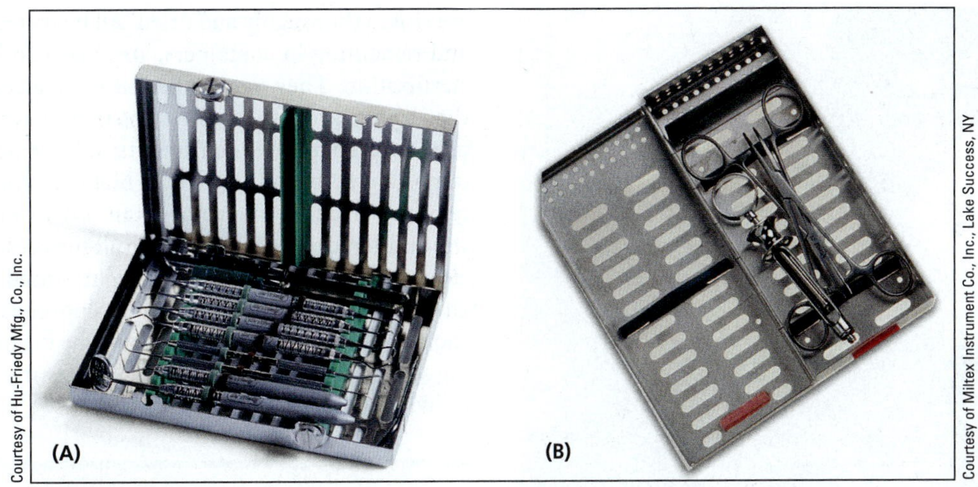

FIGURE 11-29

Disinfectant/sterilant immersion containers. (A). Larger container. (B). Smaller container.

additional instruments are added to the solution, the time countdown must be started over. Therefore, most sterilization done with glutaraldehyde must be done overnight, and is more efficiently done in a steam or autoclave sterilizer. Some glutaraldehydes, once activated, are only effective for 28 days. Fumes from glutaraldehyde are toxic and can irritate the skin and eyes, so proper ventilation is essential

Ortho-Phthalaldehyde. Ortho-Phthalaldeyde (OPA) is used as an alternative for dental assistants who have sensitivity to glutaraldehyde. This chemical is a high-level disinfectant. It comes premixed, and it disinfects in 10–12 minutes at room temperature. It is very compatible with heat sensitive instruments. It is effective against MRSA, VRE, TB, HIV, and hepatitis viruses. It reduces the risk of irritations and sensitivities of the respiratory track, eyes, and skin. Disadvantages of OPA include staining of the skin and fabrics, and a blue green coloration to some plastics.

Surface Disinfection Technique

A universally accepted technique for cleaning and disinfecting surfaces is the **spray-wipe-spray technique**. First, the surface is sprayed, then wiped to eliminate debris, accomplishing initial surface cleaning. The second spray, which must be done with a surface disinfectant, is left on the item or surfaces for the specific time indicated by the manufacturer (normally ten minutes), and then items and surfaces are wiped and items are put away. The ideal surface disinfect has residual activity, meaning that it continues to remain effective long after initial application.

Ultrasonic Cleaning

If the dental assistant is not able to recycle the instruments immediately after the procedure, the instruments may be submerged in a holding bath (*pre-cleaning*), a solution that loosens hardened debris from the instruments prior to cleaning and sterilizing. It also prevents contamination from airborne bacteria and begins the process of disinfection. The instruments remain in the holding bath until the dental assistant is ready to proceed with the processing.

The number of microorganisms, such as blood, saliva, and other body fluids contaminating an object, that has not been sterilized is referred to as a **bioburden**. The term is most often associated with bioburden testing, which is done on medical devices and pharmaceutical products for quality control. The purpose of bioburden testing is to measure the total number of microorganisms, and then use this number to determine the correct parameters for sterilization. The testing is done before sterilization to ensure the safety and effectiveness of the sterilization process.

After dental assistants have removed the treatment tray from the operatory, disinfected the area, and placed the instruments in a holding bath, they return to the sterilizing area to process the instruments. Utility gloves remain on during this procedure, as the dental assistant takes the instruments from the tray or holding bath and places them in an **ultrasonic cleaner**. Metal or plastic containers are sometimes used to hold instruments as they pass from the tray to the different solutions for processing, and then to storage (Figure 11-30). In the past, the dental assistant hand scrubbed the instruments with soap & water, rinsed them, and then placed the instruments in the sterilizer for processing. The chance of being punctured with a contaminated instrument was much greater than it is today. Instruments are now placed into a cassette and then into the ultrasonic unit for cleaning before being sterilized. The use of the utility gloves and containers along with the use of ultrasonic cleaning, instead of hand cleaning, significantly reduces the risk to the dental assistant. The ultrasonic cleaning device uses sound waves that travel through glass and metal using

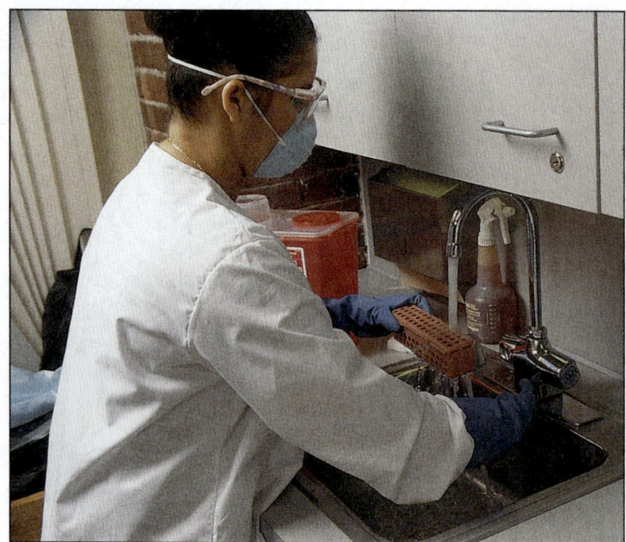

FIGURE 11-30

A dental assistant using plastic instrument cassettes for an ultrasonic cleaning procedure.

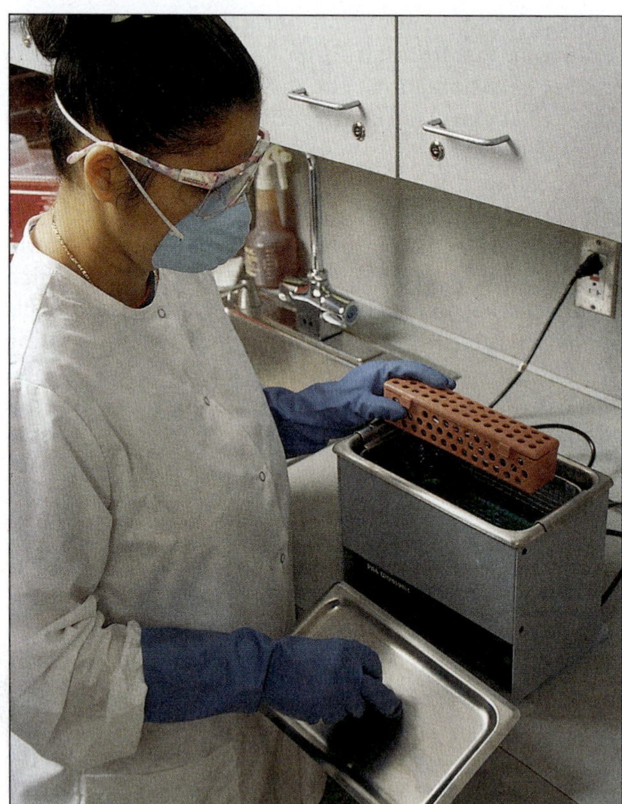

FIGURE 11-31

A dental assistant using the ultrasonic cleaning unit.

a special solution that cleans the debris from the instruments (Figure 11-31). This **cavitation** process (whereby bubbles are formed) takes three to ten minutes to complete. During that time, the bubbles implode (burst inward), and produce a cleaning effect on anything within the solution. When the ultrasonic cleaning is complete, the instruments are rinsed thoroughly and dried. All instruments, both loose and remaining in containers, are rinsed and dried prior to sterilization. They may be placed in an alcohol bath to aid the drying process. It does not matter which method is used to prepare the instruments for sterilization. What is important is that all the debris, blood, saliva, and tissue are removed from the instruments in order to ensure that the sterilization can be completed on all surfaces. The ultrasonic cleaner should be drained each night, rinsed out with water, and refilled with new ultrasonic solution each morning. It should be emptied and refilled any time the ultrasonic cleaning solution becomes exhausted, which varies depending on individual offices.

To determine whether the ultrasonic cleaner is working properly, take a small piece of aluminum foil and submerge it in the solution vertically and then run the ultrasonic for 30 seconds. Remove the foil from the ultrasonic solution, and hold it up to the light for examination. It should have no area larger than a half square inch without holes in it. This indicates whether the cleaner is operating properly. If the ultrasonic unit is not operating properly, the assistant should have it tested and repaired.

Washer-Disinfector Devices

Washer-disinfector devices have been developed for use in dental offices (Figure 11-32). These devices clean dental instruments, and some models may provide a high-level

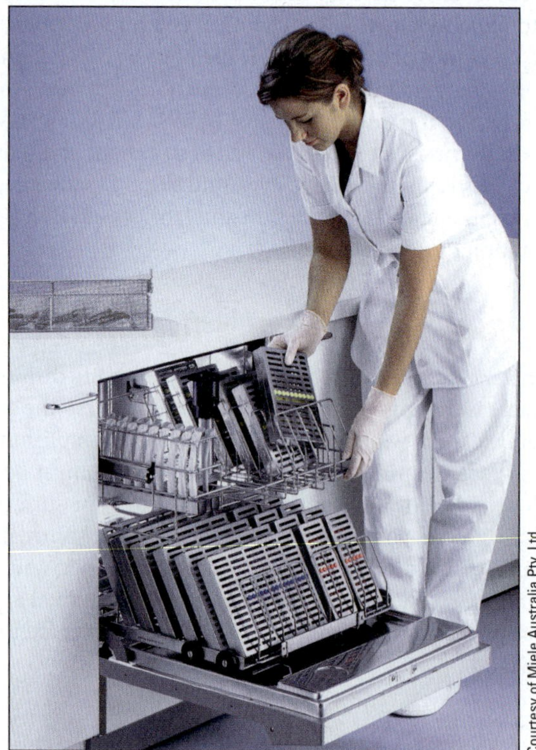

Courtesy of Miele Australia Pty. Ltd.

FIGURE 11-32

A dental washer-disinfector.

of disinfection. Those that perform high-level disinfection must be FDA 510(k) cleared in order to market. The washer-disinfector replaces the ultrasonic cleaner. Because a washer-disinfector is an automated process (i.e., the time, temperature, and chemical dispensing is all automatic) that repeats in a consistent manner, it reduces human error. It washes, disinfects, and dries (dependent upon the instrument type). The instruments come out ready to be placed into the sterilizer, or ready to be wrapped, and then sterilized. The detergents used in the units come in either liquid or powder form, and have been developed and geared toward the cleaning of blood, proteins, and tissue without damaging the instruments. An example of washer-disinfector devices is the Miele Washer-Disinfector that is available for cleaning and thermal disinfection of dental instruments, and may be seen in some dental offices. Washer-disinfectors work much like a home dishwasher; however, a home dishwasher normally heats up to 90°C/194°F, and this washer-disinfector device heats up to 93.5°C/200.3°F and keeps this temperature for over ten minutes in order to provide disinfection, in conjunction with the detergents that are used. This is called a **thermal disinfector** because the heat will kill most vegetative microorganisms. Most units come with baskets and specific racks that allow for cassettes to be cleaned, therefore, cutting down on the handling of sharps, and the chance of sharps injuries.

Sterilization

All forms of microorganisms are destroyed in the process of sterilization. The dental assistant most often is the person who ensures that all items used in intra-oral procedures are sterile. Any items that touch the skin or mucosa, or are involved in invasive procedures, must be sterilized. Several choices are available for sterilization (Table 11-3).

Liquid Chemical Disinfectant/ Sterilization

Many of the disinfecting solutions can be used for *immersion sterilization* or as an *immersion disinfectant.* The items to be sterilized are placed in the liquid for six to ten hours to ensure that all microorganisms are destroyed. The instruments are then rinsed off thoroughly, dried, and stored. Some of the items used in the dental office cannot endure heat sterilization, and must be placed in a cold sterile solution. This is the primary reason for using cold sterilizing. The disadvantages to this type of sterilant are the time involved, and the limited shelf life of the solution. Cold sterilizing is difficult to monitor for effectiveness, and the solution may be toxic to the skin and if inhaled, therefore, requiring proper ventilation. Another disadvantage is that, when the sterilizing procedure is complete, the instruments are rinsed with water that is not sterile and left unwrapped for storage; therefore, they are not maintained in a sterile state.

Ethylene Oxide Sterilization

Sterilization in the dental office can be accomplished by using an **ethylene oxide sterilization** unit (Figure 11-33). There are two different types of ethylene oxide sterilizers: the heated unit, which is fairly expensive, and a unit that can be used

TABLE 11-3 Sterilization Methods

Sterilization	Temperature/Time	Ability to Monitor	Special Considerations
Liquid chemical sterilization	Room temperature/6–10 hours	Difficult	Proper ventilation required Does not remain sterile after process
Ethylene oxide sterilization	Heated unit 120°F/48.8°C for 2–3 hours Room temperature/12 hours	Difficult	Proper ventilation Additional 24 hours to dissipate gas after sterilization
Dry heat sterilization	340°F/171°C for 1 hour	Easily monitored	Limited rust or corrosion of equipment Not for use with plastics or paper
Chemical vapor sterilization	270°F/132°C for 20 minutes	Easily monitored	Proper ventilation Special solution required
Steam under pressure sterilization	250°F/121°C for 30 minutes wrapped	Easily monitored	Requires distilled water May corrode instruments Not for use with many plastics
Steam (flash) autoclave sterilization	270°F/132°C for 3 minutes unwrapped	Easily monitored	Requires distilled water May corrode instruments Not for use with many plastics

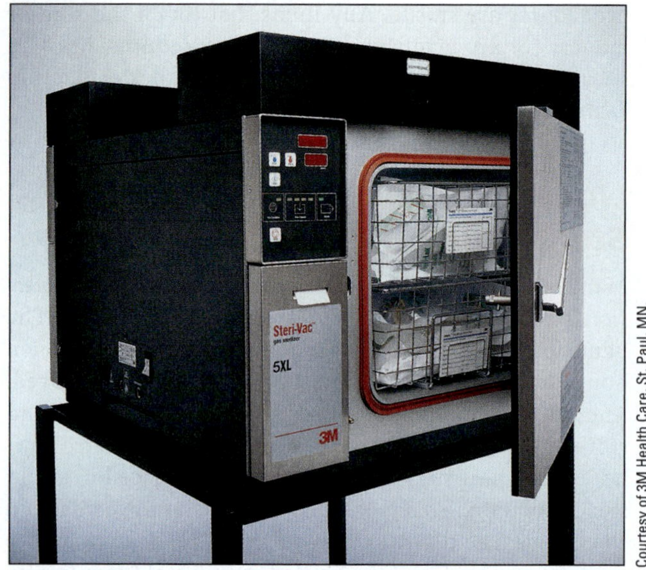

Courtesy of 3M Health Care, St. Paul, MN.

FIGURE 11-33
An ethylene oxide sterilizer.

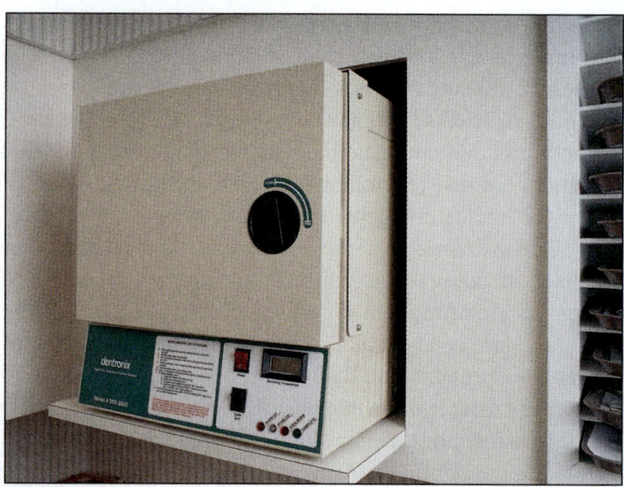

FIGURE 11-34
A dry heat sterilizer.

at room temperature. Both units are reliable for sterilization, but, as with all equipment, always follow the manufacturer's directions for use. Most heated units sterilize at 49°C (120°F) for two to three hours. Plastics and other instruments can be sterilized in this low-temperature unit. The room temperature unit takes 12 hours to complete sterilization. It is less expensive, but not as efficient as the heated unit. One disadvantage, besides the long processing time, is the toxicity of the ethylene oxide gas. Adequate ventilation is required, and any porous material requires an additional 24 hours for the gas to dissipate from it prior to use.

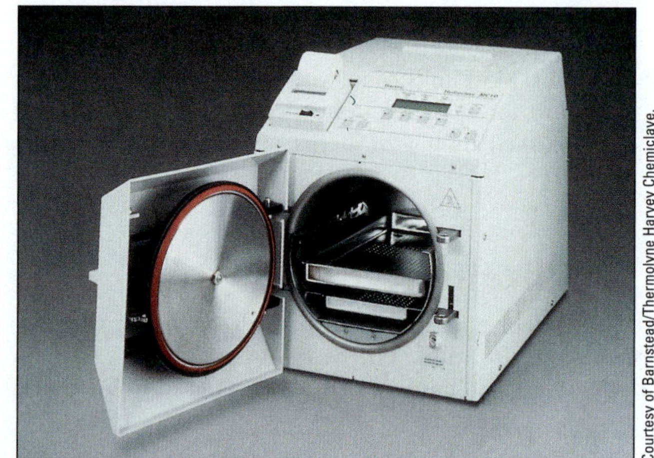

Courtesy of Barnstead/Thermolyne Harvey Chemiclave.

FIGURE 11-35
A chemical vapor sterilizer.

Dry Heat Sterilization

A **dry heat sterilizer** unit requires little maintenance, and is easy to use (Figure 11-34). Another advantage is that when dry instruments are placed into the unit, they do not experience corrosion or rust. Instruments that are very delicate, or have movable joints, will not become rusty or lose their cutting edges as rapidly. After an initial pre-heat time of 20 minutes, this unit uses heat at 171°C (340°F) for one hour to sterilize. Several units are on the market, some use the long electromagnetic waves of radiation, while others use heated moving air convection or conduction (direct contact with the source of heat). Be sure to follow the manufacturer's directions to ensure proper sterilization. This unit can be monitored for effectiveness, and is very reliable.

The high heat of the dry heat sterilizer can be a disadvantage because plastic items and some solder joints melt, and fabric chars. Loose or wrapped instruments can be placed in this unit. It requires that loads be carefully organized in the unit to allow for the circulation of air and complete sterilization.

Chemical Vapor Sterilization

The **chemical vapor sterilizer** uses a pressurized gaseous vapor of formaldehyde and alcohol for sterilization (Figure 11-35). The unit must be at 132°C (270°F) for 20 minutes in order to sterilize either loose or wrapped instruments. It is very reliable, and the effectiveness of the unit can be monitored. It is used frequently in the dental office due to its efficient sterilization time, and because it causes very little rust and corrosion on metals. A special solution must be purchased for use in this unit, and it requires good ventilation. The high temperature causes plastic and some other materials to be destroyed during the sterilization process.

Like all sterilizers, the manufacturer's directions must be followed to ensure proper technique in the sterilization process.

Badges, similar to the radiation badges, that monitor the formaldehyde levels in the area of the chemical vapor sterilization unit can be purchased. The employee would wear this badge, and it would be routinely sent to a company that measures personal exposure to formaldehyde for a specific period of time. This laboratory analysis report would be sent back to the employee with another badge for further monitoring.

Many of the new chemical vapor sterilization units are equipped with a filtration device that reduces the chemical vapor, or formaldehyde, remaining in the chamber after each cycle. This inhibits some of the odor that escapes the unit when the chamber is opened. Older units may be retrofit with a filtration device.

Steam Under Pressure Sterilization

The **steam under pressure sterilization** unit (Figure 11-36) is easy to use and easy to monitor. It uses distilled water, and in many of the units the reservoir fill port and drain tube are in the front of the sterilization unit for easy usage. The fill port notates the level of the fluid, and, if the fluid is low, the LCD display will indicate that the unit needs to be filled; and it will not begin until the fluid is filled. The display at the top front of the unit prompts the user in selecting the proper sterilization process. It can be used with wrapped or unwrapped packs, or hand-pieces. It has four preselected cycles that can be chosen. Unwrapped instruments can be sterilized at 132°C/269.6°F for 3 minutes, pouched instruments at 132°C/269.6°F for 5 minutes, packs at 121°C/249.8°F) for 30 minutes, and handpieces at 132°C/269.6°F for 6 minutes. The cycle choices are on the top or front of the unit. The LCD display will indicate the mode selected, where the unit is in the process, the remaining time, temperature and pressure of the unit, and the time for the drying cycle. When the sterilization cycle is completed, the door automatically opens and the steam begins to escape; then the drying cycle begins, which goes for 60 minutes. If the door is not closed properly, the unit will indicate the problem and will not start until the problem is corrected. Because of the steam, instruments may corrode if drying is not completed. It is not for use with many of the plastics in the dental office; therefore, always check the manufacturer's directions.

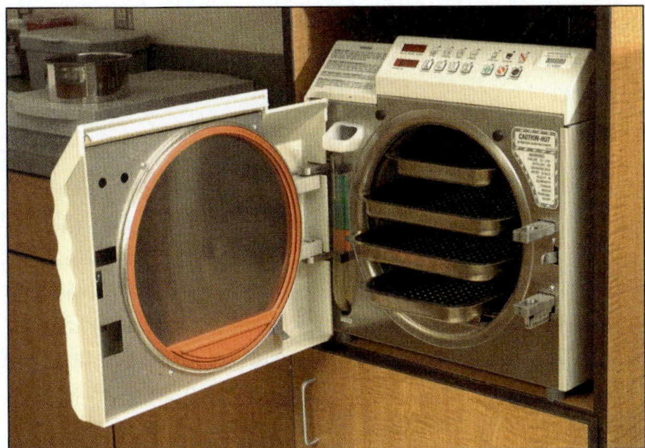

FIGURE 11-36
A steam sterilizer.

Steam Autoclave (Flash) Sterilization

Most dental offices have a steam autoclave sterilizer. These autoclave units use steam under pressure to quickly sterilize items. The effectiveness of this unit can be monitored and it is very reliable. The new steam units have a touchscreen display that displays messages and information on the current cycle. It is connected through the network portal of the dental office, where the information can be obtained on the cycle history. The office can obtain the sterilization records and verification of cycle effectiveness. If errors occur, this information can be directed to the dealer where a service technician can address the issue. All information on the sterilization process with this unit is available and stored, so that the patients and office are protected. Items can be loose or wrapped during the process. If items are loose they should be placed in pouches with forceps and sealed to remain sterile after removing them from the sterilizer. Items that are wrapped or bagged are removed from the sterilizer and place in designated storage area. The assistant should wash their hands and use forceps to handling the sterilized instruments. The unit takes 15 minutes at 121°C (250°F) at 15 pounds of steam pressure at sea level. Careful packing of the unit, so that the steam can penetrate all areas, is essential. The steam pressure, along with the temperature, allows for much more rapid sterilization to occur. When unwrapped at 132°C (270°F) at 15 pounds of steam pressure, sterilization for immediate use can be accomplished in three minutes.

After repeated use, the high temperature, along with the steam, results in melted plastics, corrosion and rust, and dull instruments. Most dental offices sterilize only dental handpieces in the steam sterilizer. The handpieces should be properly lubricated and wrapped prior to sterilization if they are going to be stored. Improper care of the dental handpiece diminishes its useful life. Because dental equipment is relatively expensive, a rapid sterilization turnaround time is beneficial so that multiple handpieces do not need to be purchased. Many of the steam sterilization units require distilled water to be used in the machine. Always read the manufacturer's directions when using any sterilization equipment.

Equipment Maintenance

Sterilization equipment, like all equipment, must be maintained in order to function properly. The chambers should be cleaned out monthly, if not more frequently. Some sterilizers have special cleaners that must be used for this process. Other sterilizers require that the used solution be drained at the end of each day. A removable tray or drainage hose facilitates this process. Some sterilizers indicate when solutions are low; others must be checked frequently to ensure that they are full. *Making sure that the right solution is used in the appropriate machine is essential.* Using the wrong solution may cause the machine to break down, resulting in costly repair charges.

Many of the machines have gaskets around the door to seal the chamber during the sterilization process. If the machine is losing pressure and/or making a hissing sound, the dental assistant should check the gasket. This is an inexpensive item, and it can be replaced quite easily.

Continued maintenance allows equipment to work at capacity longer. The dental assistant can set up a maintenance program so that each item is routinely checked.

Handpiece Sterilization

Dental handpieces are very expensive, and it is important that they are sterilized properly, and that the sterilization procedure does not extensively shorten the life of the handpieces. Always read the manufacturer's directions for sterilizing handpieces, and then form a protocol for sterilizing handpieces after each patient. After a patient has been dismissed, attach the handpiece to the unit with the bur in place, wipe all visible debris from the handpiece, and run it for 20 to 30 seconds to flush any debris, water, and air from the inside lines. Remove the bur from the handpiece, remove the handpiece from the unit, and take it to the sterilization area. The handpiece should be scrubbed with water, manufacturer-recommended soap, and a brush. For some handpieces, manufacturers recommend that parts or the entire handpiece be cleaned in an ultrasonic unit. If the manufacturer notes that an ultrasonic unit should be used, do so, but only when recommended by the manufacturer.

The next step is lubricating the handpiece. Not all manufacturers recommend this step. It is critical that the manufacturer's recommendations be followed or the warranty may be invalidated. If lubrication is recommended, use the proper lubricant for the handpiece. Never use the lubricant from another handpiece.

After lubricating, place the handpiece back on the unit with a blank bur in the chuck, and then run the handpiece to remove any excess lubrication.

Dental Fiber Optics. Clean the dental fiber optics of the handpiece with a swab moistened with isopropyl alcohol. This removes any film or debris from the optic surfaces, and helps keep the fiber optic bundle bright and clear. To complete the sterilization of the handpiece, dry the handpiece if moist, place it in a sterilization pouch, and sterilize it according to the manufacturer's directions. See Chapter 18, Basic Chairside Instrument and Tray Systems for additional information.

Packaging and Loading Sterilizers

Most of the sterilizers can be loaded with loose instruments, and obtain effective sterilization. Problems occur after the instruments come out of the sterilizer, and are stored, as they may become contaminated there. If they are sterilized in a labeled bag, then, after the sterilization cycle is completed, the instruments can stay in the labeled and sealed bag until used, thereby, maintaining their sterile condition. Labeling of the bag is normally done in pencil so that, when moisture occurs in the steam and chemical sterilizers, the information remains readable. Special preprinted indicator tape is designed for identification of instrument setups in the sterilizing bag. Tape with preprinted labels, such as exam, amalgam, and prophy, could be used (Figure 11-37 A–C).

Many dental offices use the cassette instrument sterilizing system. The instruments from a procedure are kept in a cassette during the ultrasonic cleaning, rinsing, and drying, and the cassette is then wrapped in impenetrable paper, or biofilm or paper pouches, sealed, and sterilized. The bags are heat sealed or taped because using staples or pins makes holes, thereby, allowing microorganisms to enter. This cassette, often labeled or color coded for the procedure, is removed after the sterilization cycle, and is ready to be placed on a treatment tray to be opened at the chairside for use during the next dental procedure. This keeps the instruments in a sterile state, ready for immediate use at the dental chair.

The dental assistant must ensure that the sterilization bags are not overfilled, hampering proper sterilization. It is also important that the sterilizing units are not over packed. Use a **sterilization indicator** routinely to ensure that errors in this area do not happen.

Instrument Storage

The best way to store instruments is in the packages in which they were sterilized. Limit the amount of package handling after sterilization. If packages become torn, wet, or contaminated in any manner, they need to be reprocessed. It is also important that *clean surfaces* and *contaminated surfaces* in the sterilization room be identified. To avoid contamination, nothing from the contaminated, or dirty side, should be placed on the clean side. This helps maintain sterilization integrity.

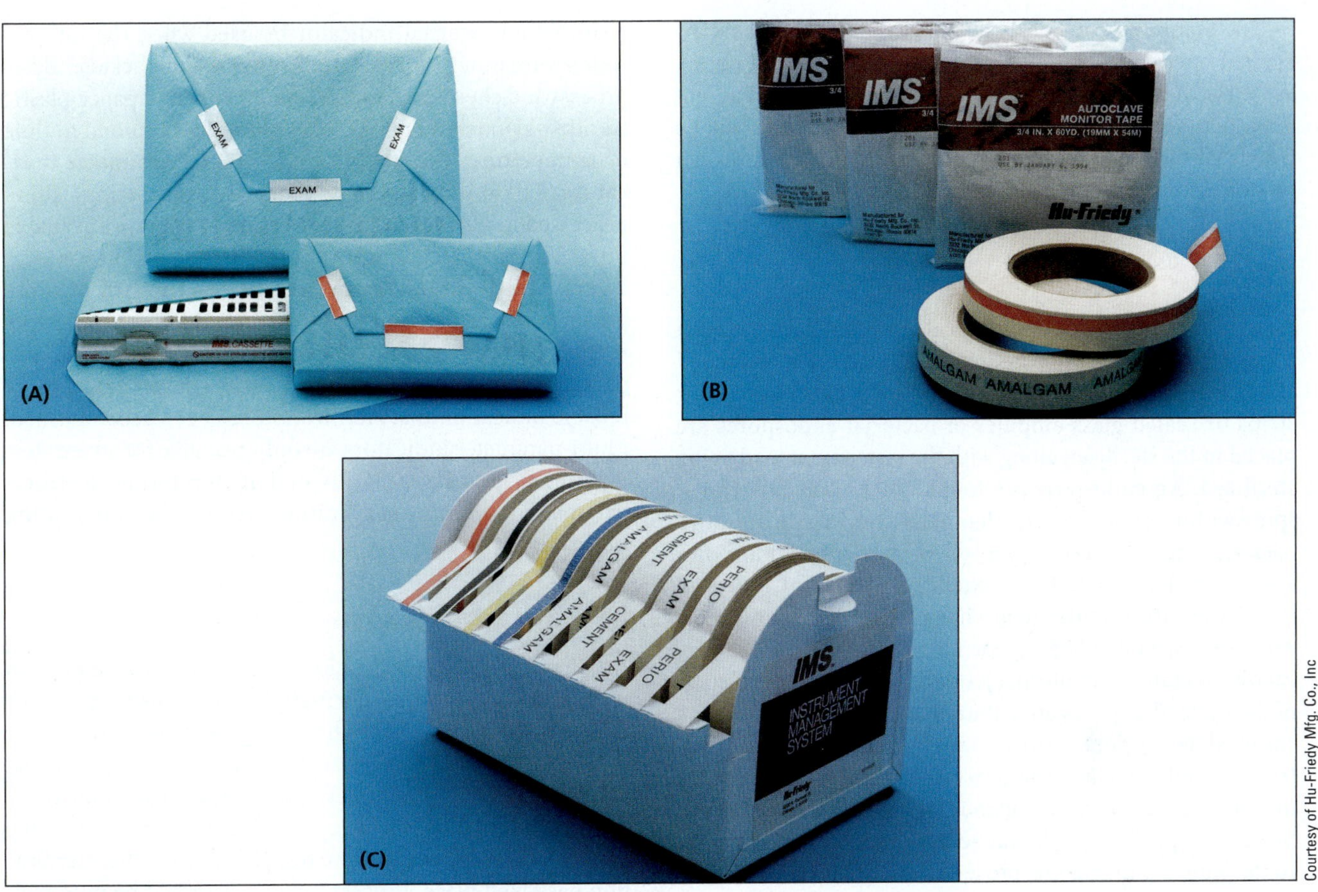

Courtesy of Hu-Friedy Mfg. Co., Inc

FIGURE 11-37 A-C

A cassette instrument sterilizing system. (A) Cassettes wrapped for sterilization. (B) Autoclave monitor tape. (C) Instrument management system tape.

Sterile packs should be stored in a dry, cool (up to room temperature) area that has protection from recontamination. Normally, instruments used in dentistry have a quick turnaround time due to high cost and limited quantities. The **shelf life** of packages is indefinite as long as the packaging material remains intact and uncontaminated. The **reuse life** is the time period that a disinfectant remains effective.

Sterilization Monitoring

Heat sterilizers are normally very reliable. It is important, however, that the sterilization process be monitored continually due to many factors that can diminish effectiveness. For example, the dental assistant could wrap instruments improperly, overload the unit, improperly set the time and temperature, or the sterilizer could malfunction.

The CDC notes in its guidelines for sterilization monitoring that mechanical, chemical, and biological monitoring should be used, and that manufacturer's instructions be followed to ensure the effectiveness of the sterilization process. Ongoing monitoring of the sterilization process is important to ensure proper technique and operation. The date that monitoring was concluded, as well as the outcome, must be documented. The records for each sterilizer should be maintained. Several types of monitors are available: mechanical monitoring, biological monitors, process indicators, and dosage indicators.

Mechanical Monitoring

Some sterilizers have gauges that monitor sterilization, and provide ongoing reports, which is called **mechanical monitoring**. The information covered is normally the temperature of the cycle, the pressure, and exposure time. The disadvantage to mechanical monitoring is that it indicates the temperature of the chamber and not the temperature in the sterilization bag of instruments. Overloading or improper placement of pouches in the chamber would not necessarily be detected.

The Statim G4, for instance, allows the operator to view current operations in real time through a networked portal, as well as the cycle history. Information can be printed or sent directly to the dealer if errors occur, and technicians will be contacted for repairs. All of the monitoring information can be stored for the lifetime of the unit.

Biological Monitors

A commercially prepared **biological monitor** offers the most accurate way to assess whether sterilization has occurred (Figure 11-38). Biological monitors in the form of paper strips or sealed glass ampules of bacterial endospores are placed in the sterilizer, along with the instrument load being sterilized. An endospore is a tough, thick walled, dormant spore within certain bacteria. It often occurs in gram-positive bacteria, and is activated by a lack of nutrients. Endospores are able to lay dormant for extended periods of time and then, when the environment changes, they become active. They are resistant to high temperatures, extreme cold, chemical disinfectants, and ultraviolet radiation. After completion of the cycle, the spores are cultured to determine if any have survived. Many dental offices have incubators for culturing. If one is not available, the processed monitors can be sent to a laboratory for culturing and the result of the data. Both incubation processes will take several days to obtain results, so this must be an ongoing procedure, normally done weekly. The CDC, ADA, and OSAP recommend biological monitoring done weekly, and some states have very specific monitoring criteria. There are many mail-in monitoring services that handle the culturing process and provide information on the results.

Chemical Monitors

The CDC recommends that the dental staff receive training to properly interpret positive and negative chemical monitoring results. They also recommend that internal process and chemical indicators are placed in every package, and also that an external indicator be used when the internal indicator cannot be seen from outside the package. Basic process and chemical monitors are on paper, or paper-plastic sterilizing pouches or bags. These monitors respond to time or temperature, and are known as **single-parameter indicators**. These indicators are very useful in distinguishing processed items from unprocessed items. They are available for steam, dry heat, and unsaturated chemical vapor sterilizers. **Multi-parameter indicators** react to two or more parameters, such as time and temperature. These indicators reference the exposure of dental instruments to the desired parameters during a sterilization cycle, and provide a more reliable indication that sterilization has been accomplished. Multi-parameter indicators are only available for steam sterilizers (i.e., autoclaves). A method of monitoring all critical parameters covering a sterilization cycle is called **integrating indicators**.

Process Indicators

Another method of sterilization monitoring is called **process indicators**. These are normally heat-sensitive tapes or inks printed either on sterilization packaging materials, or on sterilization tape that can be placed on any packaging (Figure 11-39). They contain dyes that change color upon quick exposure to sterilizing cycles. They indicate whether the packages have been exposed to heat, but not whether sterilization has taken place. Process indicators should be used with biological monitoring to ensure effectiveness of the sterilization process.

Dosage Indicators

A method of sterilization monitoring that works in much the same manner as a process indicator is a **dosage indicator**. Dyes are placed in the sterilization packing,

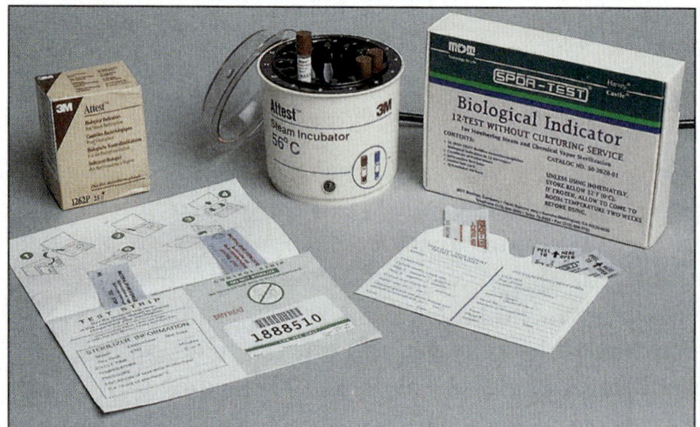

FIGURE 11-38

Biological monitors.

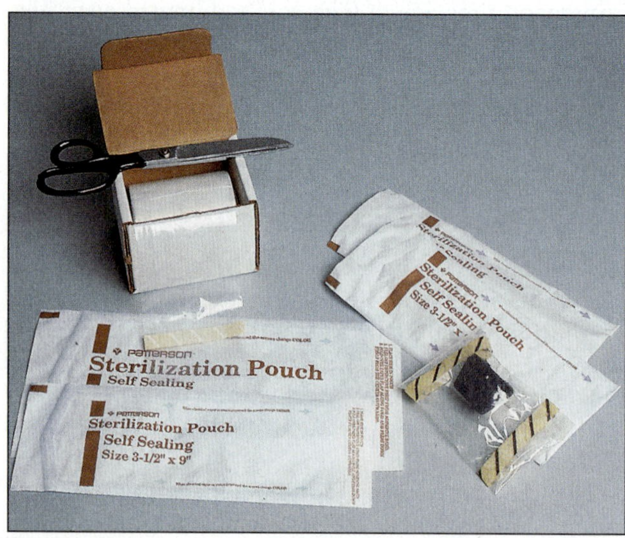

FIGURE 11-39

Process indicators used for dental sterilizers.

and they change color when exposed to dry heat, chemical vapor, or steam for a specific amount of time. They indicate whether correct conditions were present for sterilization to take place. Dosage indicators must also be used with biological monitoring.

Monitors for Liquid Disinfectants/Sterilizers
Monitors are not available to effectively determine whether proper sterilization was achieved in a liquid sterilizer. Several strips can be placed in the solution to test for the proper concentration. Using these strips, an EPA-registered solution, and closely following the manufacturer's directions, ensure that the process is effective.

Techniques and Aids for Infection Control

Several techniques and aids are effective in infection control, if practiced routinely. The dental office can continue to seek means to help reduce the exposure to microorganisms during invasive procedures. Staff training is essential to ensure that all procedure guidelines are followed.

Preprocedure Antiseptic Mouth Rinses

Using a preprocedure antiseptic mouth rinse is not a regulation, but a recommendation. A patient who rinses before treatment reduces the total number of microorganisms in his or her oral cavity. Reducing the microorganisms in the mouth leads to fewer microorganisms coming from the mouth during indirect contact through splatter and aerosols. Patient mouth rinsing helps prevent diseases from passing from the patient to dental team members.

An antimicrobial rinse often used is 0.12 percent chlorhexidine gluconate, which is effective up to five hours. Some procedures benefit from the rinse more than others. For instance, prophylaxis cleaning and ultrasonic scaling allow for the splattering of microorganisms into the air in the form of mist, unlike restorative procedures in which a dental dam (which is a barrier) can be used.

High-Volume Evacuation

The high-volume evacuator is an extremely effective way to minimize the spray coming from a high-speed rotary handpiece or an air–water syringe. (See Chapter 17, Introduction to the Dental Office and Basic Chairside Assisting, for correct placement of the HVE for maximum efficiency.) Evacuation systems use tips that are sterilizable or disposable. Most evacuation units have disposable traps that need to be cleaned routinely. Dental assistants must wear PPE while performing the cleaning procedure. Running water and specialized detergent deodorizers through the HVE at the end of each day helps reduce microorganisms in the hoses and the trap.

Dental Dam Usage

The dental dam is routinely used as a barrier from fluids and microorganisms in the oral cavity. If placed correctly, contact with saliva and oral debris is greatly reduced. However, the dental dam does not act as a perfect seal; thus, the use of gloves, glasses, and a mask is required. Using the dental dam with the HVE significantly minimizes dental splatter and aerosols during dental procedures.

Disposable Items

Many disposable, or single-use items, are available for the dental office. They are disposed of after one use to prevent microorganism transfer from one patient to another. These disposable items should not be reused under any circumstances. They are not designed to be sterilized and often do not tolerate heat or chemicals. Disposable items are usually made from plastic, paper, or low-grade metals. From the infection control standpoint, they are the most effective way to eliminate cross-contamination; however, functionally, they may not be as efficient as reusable items, and they are more expensive overall.

Clinical Asepsis Protocol

Routine steps should be followed in all treatment areas in order to maintain clinical asepsis. Shortcuts should never be an option for asepsis in dentistry. The dental assistant must ensure that infectious diseases are not spread from patient to patient, healthcare worker to patient, patient to healthcare worker, or healthcare worker to family members.

Treatment Area Protocol for Disinfecting and Cleaning

As stated earlier, surfaces in the treatment area can be protected with barriers, disinfected, or both. When a barrier is dislodged or torn, microorganisms are allowed to pass through to the surface beneath the barrier. This surface must then be disinfected. Procedures 11-4, 11-8 highlight the steps involved in preparing the treatment room, as well as disinfection and sterilization procedures to follow after treatment.

Dental Unit Waterlines

The profession of organized dentistry continues to use all means to assess and improve the quality of dental care given to patients. This includes guidelines and assessment for the

Procedure 11-4
Preparing the Dental Treatment Room

This procedure is performed by the dental assistant prior to seating the dental patient in the treatment room. By following a routine procedure that meets the regulations and protocols set forth by the dentist and regulatory agencies discussed earlier in this chapter, the dental assistant prepares the operatory and equipment.

Equipment and Supplies

- Patient's medical and dental history (including dental radiographs)
- Barriers for dental chair, hoses, counter, light switches, and controls
- PPE for dental assistant (protective eyewear, mask, gloves, and overgloves)
- Patient napkin, napkin chain, and protective eyewear
- Sterile procedure tray

Procedure Steps (*Follow aseptic procedures*)

1. Wash hands.
2. Review the patient's medical and dental history, place the radiographs on the viewbox or bring them up on a computer screen, and identify the procedure to be completed at this visit. Patient's medical and dental history can be placed in a plastic envelope barrier or under a surface barrier.
3. Place new barriers on all surfaces that can be contaminated (e.g., dental chair, hoses, counter, light switches, and controls) (Figure 11-40).
4. Bring the instrument tray with packaged sterile instruments into the operatory with patient's napkin and protective eyewear.
5. Put on PPE (protective eyewear, mask, gloves, and overgloves).
6. Ensure that handpieces and three-way syringe are working properly.

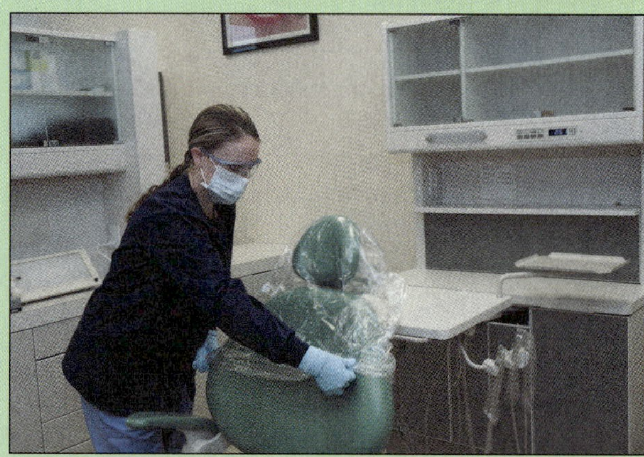

FIGURE 11-40
A dental assistant placing barriers.

Procedure 11-5
Completion of Dental Treatment

This procedure is performed by the dental assistant at the completion of the dental treatment. By following a routine procedure that meets the regulations and protocols set forth by the dentist and regulatory agencies discussed earlier in this chapter, the dental assistant completes the procedure and dismisses the patient.

Equipment and Supplies

- Patient's medical and dental history (including dental radiographs)
- Barriers for dental chair, hoses, counter, light switches, and controls
- Dental handpiece
- Air–water syringe tip (disposable)
- Patient napkin
- Contaminated instruments on tray, including HVE tip

(continues)

Procedure 11-5 (continued)

Procedure Steps (*Follow aseptic procedures*)

1. Remove handpieces, HVE tip, and air–water syringe tip and place on treatment tray.
2. Put on overgloves to document information on the chart or via computer, and assemble radiographs and chart, preventing cross-contamination (Figure 11-41).
3. Remove patient napkin and place over the treatment tray prior to dismissing patient (see Chapter 17).
4. With gloves in place, complete Steps 5 through 9.
5. Place the handpiece, HVE, and air–water syringe back on the unit and run for 20 to 30 seconds to clean the lines or flush the system. Remove handpiece and air–water syringe and return to treatment tray.
6. Place sharps in puncture-resistant sharps disposal container if disposal containers are kept in the dental treatment room (waist level). Sharps should be discarded in the treatment room or sterilization area.
7. Remove the chair cover from the patient dental chair, inverting it so that any splatter or debris remains on the inside of the bag.
8. Remove all barriers and place them in the inverted bag. All disposables can be placed in the bag as well (Figure 11-42).
9. Carry treatment tray, with all items from the treatment area, into the sterilizing area. All items to be sterilized are removed from the operatory at this time.
10. Remove treatment gloves and place them in the inverted bag. Dispose of the bag.
11. Wash hands.

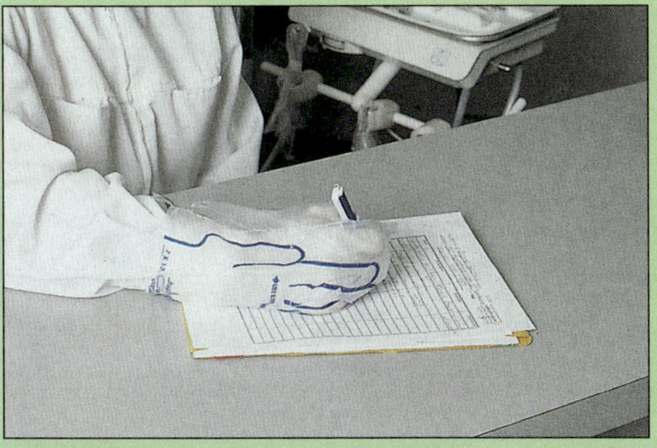

FIGURE 11-41
Dental assistant wearing overgloves while writing on a patient's chart.

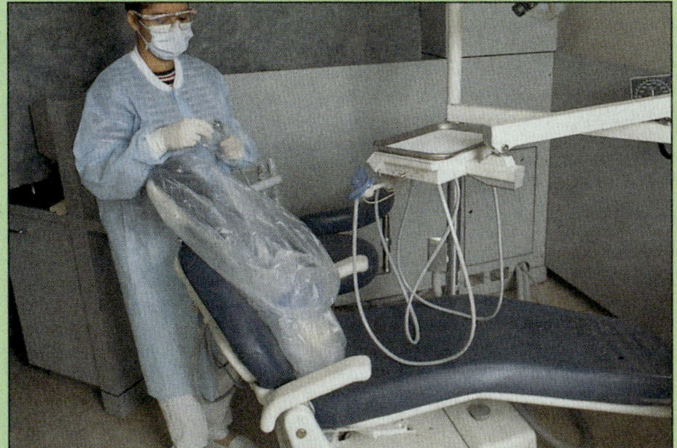

FIGURE 11-42
Post-dental treatment barriers being removed and placed in an inverted bag for disposal.

Procedure 11-6
Final Treatment Room Disinfecting and Cleaning

This procedure is performed by the dental assistant after the treatment has been completed and the patient has been dismissed. This routine procedure meets the regulations and protocols set forth by the dentist and regulatory agencies discussed earlier in this chapter.

Equipment and Supplies

- Utility gloves
- Necessary disinfecting solutions (intermediate level)
- Wiping cloths
- 4 by 4 gauze

(continues)

Procedure 11-6 (continued)

Procedure Steps (*Follow aseptic procedures*)

1. Wash hands, and pull on utility gloves.
2. Bring the necessary solutions and wiping cloths, including 4 by 4 gauze, to the operatory.

Use a small utility carry tote to hold and transport the items, such as disinfecting solutions, HVE solution, 4 by 4 gauze, towels, and chair disinfectant.

3. Have a routine procedure established for disinfection to ensure that nothing is missed. All surfaces need to be sprayed and cleaned first, then wiped to remove debris (Figures 11-43A and B). The surfaces are then sprayed a second time and the solution is left on the surfaces for a designated time, according to the manufacturer's directions (normally about ten minutes). After about ten minutes, wipe the surfaces again.
4. Another method to accomplish the initial spray and wipe is to use saturated wiping devices. Lay out several pieces of 4 by 4 gauze on the counter, spray them with disinfectant, and wipe each surface carefully.
5. Spray on the disinfectant and leave it for the correct time to accomplish disinfection (normally ten minutes).
6. Rewipe all surfaces.
7. It is critical that all surfaces that could have been contaminated are disinfected. Areas that are sometimes missed include the amalgam cradle (i.e., the holding device for the amalgam capsule in the triturator), chair adjustments, curing light, and the radiographic viewbox switch. Take care when spraying disinfectants near switches.

Disinfecting Procedure

- Spray.
- Wipe. (The spray and wipe technique can also be accomplished by wiping with a disinfectant-saturated wiping device.)
- Spray and leave (normally ten minutes).
- Rewipe.

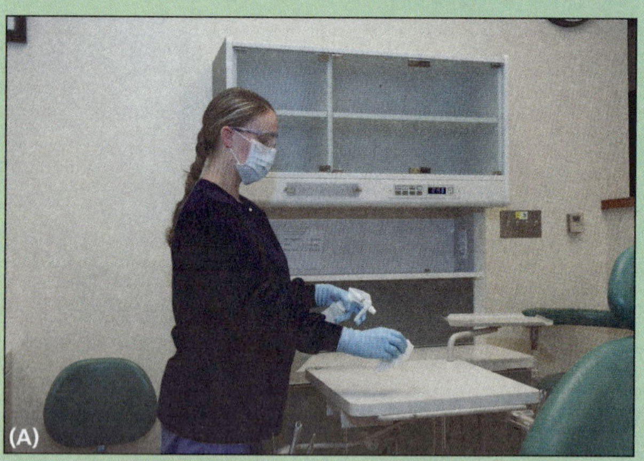
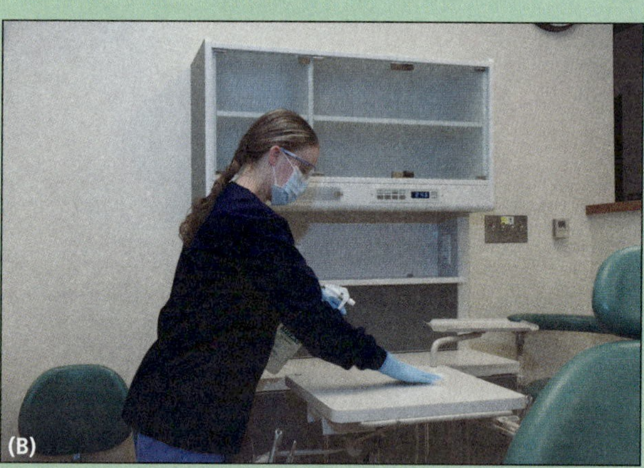

FIGURE 11-43 A & B
(A) Spraying the area. (B) Wiping and spraying the area with disinfectant again.

Procedure 11-7
Treatment of Contaminated Tray in Sterilization Center

This procedure is performed by the dental assistant in the sterilization center. By following a routine procedure that meets the regulations and protocols set forth by the dentist and the OSHA regulatory agencies discussed earlier in this chapter, the dental assistant completes the procedure.

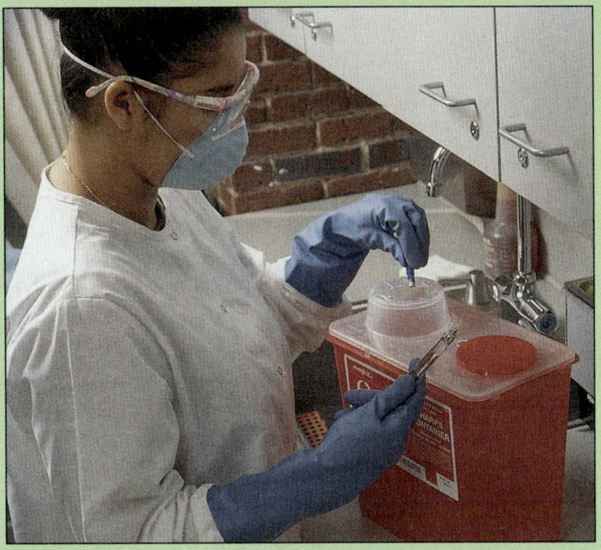

FIGURE 11-44
A dental assistant placing sharps in a sharps container.

Equipment and Supplies

- Utility gloves
- Necessary disinfecting solutions
- Wiping cloths
- 4 by 4 gauze
- Contaminated procedure tray

Procedure Steps (*Follow aseptic procedures*)

1. Place the treatment tray in the contaminated area of the sterilization center immediately following dental treatment. Sterilization can be taken care of immediately, or after the operatory is disinfected and prepared for another patient.
2. If a long time will elapse before the tray is decontaminated, immerse the instruments in a disinfecting holding solution. This prevents debris from drying, begins the process of killing the microorganisms, and prevents airborne microorganisms from being transmitted.
3. Wear utility gloves during the entire procedure.
4. Sharps are disposed of in a sharps container, if not already done while in the dental operatory (Figure 11-44).
5. All disposable items are discarded. If they are bio-hazard waste, they must be placed in an appropriately labeled waste container. (See Chapter 12, Management of Hazardous Materials, for further information.)
6. Place instruments in the ultrasonic cleaner using either the open method or a cassette. A small strainer is used for items that may become lost. Normally burs, dental dam clamps, and other such items are placed in this small container. After the timed cleaning is accomplished in the ultrasonic unit (three to ten minutes), rinse the items thoroughly.
7. After the instruments are rinsed, towel dry, separate according to the sterilizing technique, place the instruments for immersion into the cold disinfectant/sterilant solution, and note the time. Other instruments for heat sterilization are bagged and placed in the appropriate sterilizer (Figures 11-45A and B), and the door is sealed and the unit is activated. Remember that if they are in a cassette, they can be dipped in an alcohol bath and left to air dry before being placed in a sealed bag, and in the sterilizer.
8. Rinse or wipe off the dental high-speed handpiece with isopropyl alcohol. Then it must be lubricated, bagged in an instrument pouch with indicator tape, and placed in the sterilizer (follow manufacturer's directions). The steam under pressure sterilizer is normally used, due to its quick turnaround time.
9. The tray and other items on the tray need to be sprayed, wiped, sprayed again, left for ten minutes—or a time designated by the manufacturer of the disinfectant—and wiped again, before assembling them for another tray setup.
10. Clean all contaminated areas, wash and dry the utility gloves, remove them, and then wash and dry hands.

(continues)

Procedure 11-7 (continued)

11. After the sterilizer indicates that the time has lapsed, and that the instruments are sterile, they can be removed from the sterilizer with forceps. When the time has elapsed for the cold disinfectant/sterilant, the instruments are rinsed off, dried, and put away.

PPE for a Contaminated Tray

- Utility gloves are required when handling contaminated trays.
- Protective eyewear is required when handling contaminated trays.
- Masks are only required if cleaning will cause splash, aerosols, or splatter.

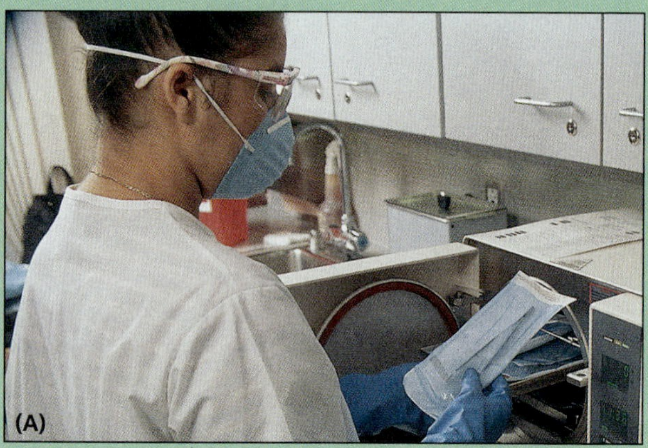
(A)

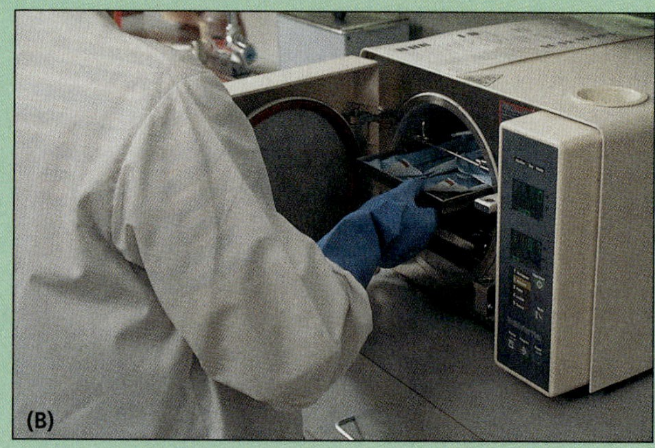
(B)

FIGURE 11-45 A & B

(A) A dental assistant placing bagged instruments in a sterilizer. (B) Sliding a tray with bagged instruments into the sterilizer.

treatment of the dental unit waterlines. Dental units are usually connected to community water lines. It is very important that uncontaminated water is used during dental procedures. Certain bacteria from the water can contaminate the dental waterlines and cause disease.

Dental unit waterlines are the small tubes that connect the water supply to the air–water syringe, high-speed dental handpieces, and ultrasonic cleaners. Water normally contains bacteria and fungi. Over time, they form thin layers on practically any surface. For instance, they can be found in showerheads, fountains, and sink faucets, as well as in dental unit waterlines. Microbes attach themselves to the sides of the tubes and grow. A buildup of these slime layers of microbes becomes an ideal environment for the growth of **biofilms**, microscopic communities that allow bacteria, fungi, and viruses to multiply. When biofilms are passed to the patient, they increase disease susceptibility.

In the United States, water quality is measured by the number of coliform bacteria. The ADA set a goal in 1995 that all dental offices, by 2000, would provide no more than 200 colony-forming units per milliliter (CFU/mL) in unfiltered water. Quality can be monitored using a water quality indicator (WQI). The ADA recommends that dental offices follow CDC, OSHA, and ADA guidelines for infection control of dental water lines. The water quality should be equivalent to the existing quality assurance standard utilized in hemodialysis units. These guidelines include flushing waterlines at the start of each day and between patients, and they recommend installing, and maintaining, anti-retraction devices.

Preventing cross-contamination, or potential aspiration of oral fluids through the high-speed handpiece or the air–water syringe (backflow), is another concern. The risk of backflow contamination is extremely low, but the ADA agrees that backflow prevention devices should be considered in the dental office.

The CDC recommends that "all dental instruments that use water should be run to discharge water for 20 to 30 seconds after each patient and for several minutes before the start of each clinic day. This practice will help to flush out any patient materials that may have entered the waterlines." Therefore, each handpiece should be flushed with air–water syringe for 20 seconds between patients to help reduce patient-borne microbes that may have been sucked back into the handpiece during use in the oral cavity. Also, waterlines should be disinfected by running them for several minutes before the start of each clinic day, and weekly, to remove biofilm.

Numerous types for water line disinfection are available. Solutions specifically developed to penetrate and remove biofilms from dental unit water lines are available. There is a shock solution or tablet that is used to clean and disinfect the lines. After the lines are purged with air and the handpieces removed, the lines can be filled with this disinfectant. Allow the solution to remain in the lines overnight, or through the weekend. These solutions are then used weekly to maintain disinfection. Some ask for a shock treatment to be done each time a new box of the product is used. When using other disinfectants, follow manufacturer's directions. For instance, there is a pink solution that is run through the system until the pink solution appears at the end of the air–water syringe and handpiece lines. This solution remains in the lines overnight. Early the next day, the solution is discarded and flushed with hot water until the pink color is gone. If not using the unit, leave after purging; if ready to use the unit, install a disinfected bottle filled with treatment water on the unit. Run the unit for 20 to 30 seconds with a steady stream of treatment water coming from the handpiece and syringe. After running the unit, it will be ready for use.

Monitoring Dental Unit Waterlines

To ensure that the waterlines meet the regulatory standards of the Environmental Protection Agency (EPA) for drinking water, it is prudent to test the waterlines routinely. This can be done by an outside agency, where water is sent to them for testing and the report is sent back, or the office can purchase waterline testing kits to evaluate the water quality. Either method that is used ensures that the collection process does not allow for further contamination. The CDC recommends that the dental office follow the recommendations of the treatment product, or the manufacturer of the dental unit, as to how often the waterlines should be monitored. Procedures 11-8, 11-9 and 11-10 outline waterline treatment and testing procedures.

Procedure 11-8
Treatment of Dental Unit Waterlines

This procedure is performed by the dental assistant at the dental unit. By following the regulations and protocols set forth by the dentist and the OSHA regulatory agencies discussed earlier in this chapter, the dental assistant completes the routine procedure.

Equipment and Supplies

- Utility gloves
- Necessary disinfecting solutions or tablets

Procedure Steps (*Follow aseptic procedures*)

1. Empty water from the bottle on the dental unit.
2. Read the manufacturer's directions.
3. Place the liquid or tablet into the bottle. Note: The initial tablet is called the **waterline shock treatment** (the initial treatment).
4. Add warm or hot (manufacturer's directions) distilled water to the bottle (Figure 11-46). If using the tablet, drop it into the water and allow 60 seconds for it to dissolve. Many offices have additional water bottles for the dental unit for this procedure.
5. Swirl the solution to clean and disinfect the inside of the bottle.
6. Connect the bottle to the dental unit and run lines until color appears (Figure 11-47). Usually the color is orange, blue, or pink according to the manufacturer.
7. Leave the treated water in the water lines overnight, or over the weekend.
8. Following the designated time, empty the solution from the bottle and replace with water. Then purge waterlines until color dissipates. Patient care can occur after the color is gone.

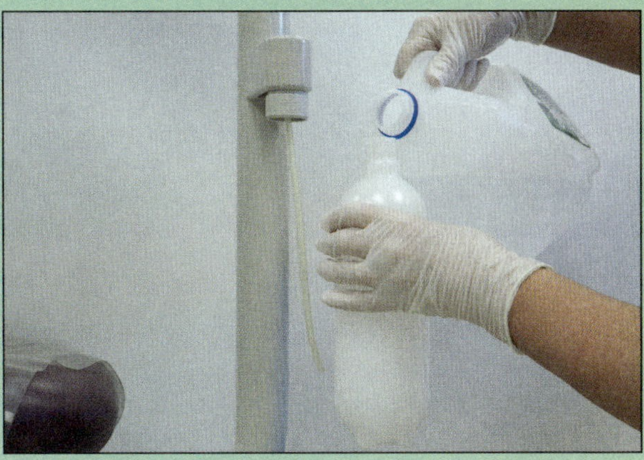

FIGURE 11-46
Pour distilled water into the water bottle.

(continues)

Procedure 11-8 (continued)

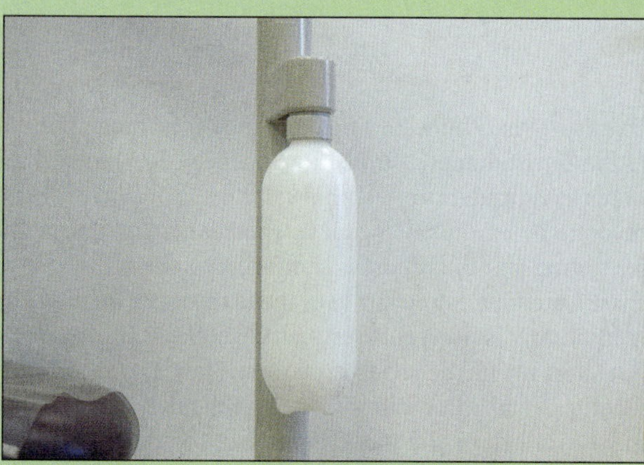

FIGURE 11-47
Attach the bottle to the waterline.

9. Some manufacturers indicate that the shock treatment be performed several additional times to ensure that odor-causing bacteria is eliminated.
10. Regular treatment of water lines occurs weekly. Follow steps one through eight using a regular tablet or solution. These tablets may be another color.
11. Test the water.

Procedure 11-9

Treatment of Dental Unit Waterlines with Microfiltration Cartridge

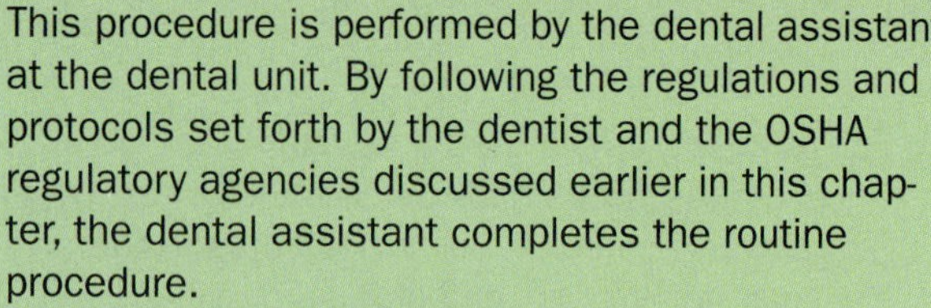

This procedure is performed by the dental assistant at the dental unit. By following the regulations and protocols set forth by the dentist and the OSHA regulatory agencies discussed earlier in this chapter, the dental assistant completes the routine procedure.

Equipment and Supplies

- Utility gloves
- Microfiltration cartridge
- Antimicrobial bottle that fits on a dental unit

Procedure Steps (*Follow aseptic procedures*)

1. Remove the water bottle from the unit.
2. Remove the existing pickup tube, and install the new pickup tube with the microfiltration cartridge.
3. Place the new tube with cartridge on the barb fitting.
4. Most microfiltration cartridges include an initial shock treatment upon use.
5. The microfiltration system should be replaced according to the manufacturer's directions. Example: every three months to once a year.
6. Microfiltration cartridges may come with a total dissolved solids (TDS) meter, or test strip, to ensure that you have installed the cartridges properly, and to test the water quality.

Procedure 11-10
Testing the Dental Waterlines

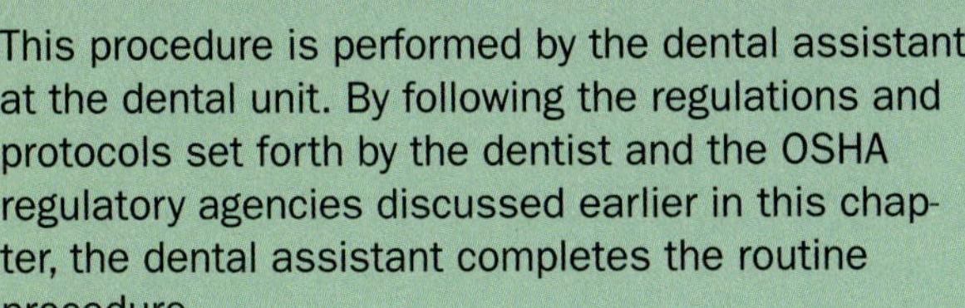

This procedure is performed by the dental assistant at the dental unit. By following the regulations and protocols set forth by the dentist and the OSHA regulatory agencies discussed earlier in this chapter, the dental assistant completes the routine procedure.

Equipment and Supplies (*Waterline Testing Service*)

- Treatment gloves
- Waterline testing kit and instructions
- Separate sterile test vial, refrigerant icepack, styrofoam mailer (if needed)

Procedure Steps (*Follow aseptic procedures*)

1. Follow the manufacturer's directions.
2. Place refrigerant pack in the styrofoam lid and freeze overnight.
3. Label each of the water sample collection vials, and identify which dental unit was sampled.
4. Complete the sample submission form to enclose with the samples.
5. Flush waterlines for a minimum of two minutes prior to taking the water samples.
6. Fill the sterile collection vial ¾ full with sample water. Ensure that contamination of the vial, or the tip of the syringe, has not occurred.
7. Place the vials into the styrofoam shipper with the submission form, and seal for shipment.
8. Samples are processed immediately, and results should be received within four days.

Dental Radiography Room and Equipment

So much attention is paid to treatment rooms that often the separate radiography rooms and radiography darkrooms, among other rooms, are missed during infection control. When dental assistants expose and process radiographs, infection control practices must be followed. The room must first be prepared, much like a treatment room, with appropriate barriers. Upon completion of the procedure, the radiography room must be disinfected in the same manner, disinfecting all surfaces that were contaminated (See Chapter 22, Production and Evaluation of Dental Radiographs). The radiographs that were placed in the mouth must be cared for properly, and all the equipment must be disinfected. Procedure 11-11 outlines infection control procedures for the radiography room.

Dental Laboratory

The dental laboratory should be disinfected in the same manner as other rooms. Use the spray-wipe-spray technique on all surfaces. If the dental assistant is polishing with pumice on the rag wheel, PPE should be worn. Extra care is necessary when wearing gloves while using the rotary equipment for polishing, because gloves can easily become caught in the wheels or motors.

After polishing, discard the pumice, and disinfect the pan. (Some dental offices mix the pumice with disinfectant.) Rinse off the rag wheel, and cycle it through the autoclave. Many disposable buffing wheels are now available, and can be discarded after use.

Thoroughly disinfect any contaminated dental laboratory cases before being handled in the office or sent to an outside laboratory. One effective way to achieve this is to place all acrylic appliances in a diluted sodium hypochlorite disinfection solution. Cases with any metal parts need to be placed in another solution, such as glutaraldehyde. Check the manufacturer's directions to identify solutions that will meet the criteria for this process.

Dental impressions must also be disinfected prior to sending them out. Check the manufacturer's directions regarding the correct procedure to accomplish this task. Alginate impressions cannot be immersed in any solution, because this can cause distortion. Alginate impressions must be sprayed, and then placed in a sealed bag.

Final impression materials, such as polysulfide and silicone, can be immersed in most disinfecting solutions according to the manufacturer's directions without distortion. Procedures for disinfecting polyether and polysiloxane impression materials vary. Some of the polyether impressions cannot go through the disinfecting procedure until a final set time of 30 minutes has elapsed. If the impression has not been disinfected prior to sending it to the dental laboratory, place it in a leak proof bag with a biohazard label for transport, and indicate that it has not been disinfected.

Procedure 11-11
Dental Radiology Infection Control Protocol

This procedure is performed by the dental assistant in the dental radiography room, if it is a separate area, or at the dental unit, if radiographs are taken in the same location as the dental treatment. By following the regulations and protocols set forth by the dentist and the regulatory agencies discussed earlier in this chapter, the dental assistant completes the routine procedure.

Equipment and Supplies

- Utility gloves
- Barriers
- Necessary disinfecting solutions
- Wiping cloths
- 4 by 4 gauze

Procedure Steps (*Follow aseptic procedures*)

1. Wash hands and place the barriers. The x-ray head fits into one of the dental chair bags. Using this type of barrier is much easier than trying to get into all of the x-ray's areas to disinfect. It will also not be as hard on the equipment (spraying the disinfecting solution can destroy electrical equipment over time).
2. The x-ray room must have a lead-lined door and walls. Both sides of the door handle need barriers. Sandwich bags work well for this type of barrier. If the switches for use of the dental radiography machine are located in another area, place a barrier over them. The chair can be covered, although no splatter or spray is anticipated (unless the patient vomits).
3. Dental x-rays can be placed in barriers at this time (see Chapter 22, Production and Evaluation of Dental Radiographs, for more information about dental x-ray barriers).
4. Put on PPE as the patient is seated. Place the lead apron on the patient.
5. After each of the x-rays is taken, place the x-ray film in a disposable cup outside the x-ray room.
6. After the procedure is completed and the patient is dismissed, remove the barriers and dispose of them, along with the treatment gloves. If the x-rays have been in a barrier, remove the barrier carefully while allowing the untouched x-rays to fall into a clean disposable cup, then remove the treatment gloves.
7. Disinfect any areas not covered by barriers.

NOTE: The lead apron is often missed during disinfection.

8. X-rays are then processed. If barriers on the dental x-ray packets have not been used, special attention should be taken not to cross-contaminate. Either new gloves must be donned as the x-rays are removed from the infected packets, or a two-cup method must be used. Careful attention to aseptic techniques will ensure that the x-rays are not re-contaminated prior to putting them through the processor.
9. One frequently contaminated area is the sleeves of the daylight processor. Place two cups inside the processor (one with contaminated x-rays in it and one with nothing in it). Don new gloves prior to placing hands through the sleeves of the processor. Open the contaminated x-rays and place them in the clean cup. Remove the gloves and place them in the contaminated cup before using clean hands to place the uncontaminated dental film through the processor. Take clean hands out of the sleeves of the daylight processor and lift the lid. Remove the two cups from the daylight loader, touching only the outside of each cup. There are a number of other ways to accomplish this task without cross-contaminating, such as using overgloves and packet barriers.

Chapter Summary

Staff must be trained for a safe workplace. Compliance with all regulations must be accomplished to ensure that the process of infection control will be adequate. Training will occur at initial employment, when job tasks change, and annually thereafter.

CASE STUDY

Victoria Scott, a dental assistant, received a personal telephone call during patient dental care. She left the dental treatment room, removed her latex gloves, and answered the telephone in the sterilization area. While in the area, she looked up another telephone number in the phone book, put instruments from the ultrasonic unit in water to rinse, and then placed them into the sterilizer, and then returned to the treatment room. Knowing that leaving the treatment area during patient care is not advocated, and focusing on asepsis, answer the following questions.

Case Study Review

1. What (if any) areas were contaminated?
2. What procedures should have been followed to prevent cross-contamination?
3. Identify the glove(s) that should have been used during each procedure.

Review Questions

Multiple Choice

1. Ultimately, the responsibility for infection control lies with the
   a. patient.
   b. dentist.
   c. dental hygienist.
   d. dental assistant.
2. A regulating body that enforces the regulation that employers protect their employees from exposure to blood and OPIM is the
   a. Centers for Disease Control.
   b. Environmental Protection Agency.
   c. Food and Drug Administration.
   d. Occupational Safety and Health Administration.
3. Dental assistants fall into which category of job classifications for exposure determination?
   a. 1
   b. 2
   c. 3
   d. 4
4. Personal protective equipment includes all the following except
   a. face masks.
   b. eyewear.
   c. ear plugs.
   d. uniforms.
5. The gloves most frequently used during dental patient care are
   a. latex gloves.
   b. overgloves.
   c. utility gloves.
   d. rubber gloves.
6. The term that refers to all patients being treated as if they were infectious is
   a. asepsis.
   b. aseptic technique.
   c. standard precautions.
   d. universal precautions.
7. The federal regulatory agency involved in the safety and effectiveness of disinfecting and sterilizing solutions is the
   a. Food and Drug Administration.
   b. Environmental Protection Agency.
   c. Organization for Safety and Asepsis Procedures.
   d. Occupational Safety and Health Administration.
8. The antimicrobial handwashing agents that are the most beneficial include
   a. chlorhexidine digluconate.
   b. triclosan.
   c. parachlorometaxylenol.
   d. all of the above.
9. The symptoms of redness, initial itching, and vesicles that appear on the areas of contact to latex within 24 to 48 hours, followed by dry skin with fissures and sores, are related to a condition known as
   a. irritant contact dermatitis.
   b. type IV hypersensitivity (delayed hypersensitivity).
   c. immediate-type hypersensitivity.
   d. type I hypersensitivity.
10. The type of gloves that are used during disinfection and clean up procedures are called
    a. overgloves.
    b. latex gloves.
    c. vinyl gloves.
    d. utility gloves.

Critical Thinking

1. If a small dental office with only four employees routinely follows infection control guidelines, would a surprise OSHA inspection be anticipated?
2. If a problem develops after a dental assistant misuses a dental solution, with whom does the liability lie?
3. During the use of a high-speed handpiece, the dental assistant should be concerned with what primary route of microbial transmission?

Web Activities

1. Go to http://www.epa.gov and find the listing of registered tuberculocide or antimicrobial products. For three of them, write down the product name, EPA registration number, manufacturer name, approval date, and active ingredients.
2. Go to http://www.osha.gov and identify the bloodborne pathogen standards. Read the section that addresses PPE, and be prepared to discuss this in class.
3. Go to http://www.ada.org and read the article under oral health topics about dental waterlines and biofilms, and be prepared to discuss this in class.

CHAPTER 12

Management of Hazardous Materials

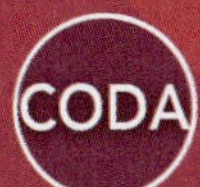

Specific Instructional Objectives

The student should strive to meet the following objectives and demonstrate an understanding of the facts and principles presented in this chapter:

1. Identify the scope of the OSHA Bloodborne Pathogens Standard and the Hazardous Communication Standard.
2. Explain the purpose of the Hazardous Communication Standard (HCS).
3. Identify the three major changes of the HCS to align with the Globally Harmonized System of Classification and Labeling of Chemicals (GHS).
4. Identify physical equipment and mechanical devices provided to safeguard employees.
5. Demonstrate safe disposal of sharps.
6. Describe the purpose of safety data sheet manuals.
7. Describe the required format of the new safety data sheets.
8. Identify the nine HCS pictograms.
9. Describe the employee training that is required to meet the OSHA standard for hazardous chemicals.

Key Terms

Globally Harmonized System of Classification and Labeling of Chemicals (GHS) (256)
National Fire Protection Association's color and number method (257)
Needlestick Safety and Prevention Act (248)
parenteral (252)
pictogram (256)

Introduction

Infection control and the standards that relate to it are discussed in Chapter 11, Infection Control. This chapter discusses the requirements of the Occupational Safety and Health Administration (OSHA) Bloodborne Pathogens Standard and Hazardous Communication Standard to manage biohazardous waste and hazardous materials, such as engineering controls, labeling, safety data sheets (SDSs), housekeeping, laundry, and the disposal of hazardous materials. Dental assistants must understand the entire standard and how compliance is accomplished (Figure 12-1). Dental assisting students do not fall under OSHA guidelines because they are not employees; however, following the same safety standards that are practiced in the workplace is preparation for employment. The scope of the standards cover:

- employee training, safety, and documentation requirements;
- exposure determination;
- infection control, universal precautions, and standard measures used to control possible exposures;
- postexposure follow-up;
- labeling/SDSs;
- housekeeping/laundry; and
- disposal of biohazardous waste.

OSHA's Bloodborne Pathogen Standard Revision

In 1991, OSHA published the Occupational Exposure to Bloodborne Pathogens Standard. However, needlesticks and other sharps injuries continued to occur frequently causing serious health effects. In 2001, according to OSHA, the CDC estimated that health care workers sustained nearly 600,000 percutaneous injuries annually, involving contaminated sharps. Due to this information, the U.S. Congress passed the **Needlestick Safety and Prevention Act**, which directed OSHA to revise the bloodborne pathogens standard. The standard was revised and became effective in April 2001.

Exposure Control Plan Additions

Two new requirements were added to the standard. First, the employer must solicit input from employees involved in direct patient care. These employees should be nonmanagerial, and the selection should be from a wide range of direct patient care interaction positions. Annually, the representative number of employees will give input after the employer has requested it.

The employer must document this input in the exposure control plan, as well as how, and from whom, they solicited said input. According to the *Revision to OSHA's Bloodborne Pathogens Standard, Technical Background and Summary*, the dentist can show that they are meeting the standard by:

- listing the employees involved and describing the process by which input was requested; or
- presenting other documentation, including references to the minutes of meetings, copies of documents used to request employee participation, or records of responses received from employees.

The employer must also:

- consider innovations in medical procedure and technological developments that reduce the risk of exposure; and
- document the use of appropriate, effective, and commercially available safer devices, and the considerations used to evaluate those devices.

The employer must select devices that are based on reasonable judgment:

- will not jeopardize patient or employee safety or be medically inadvisable; and
- will make an exposure incident involving a contaminated sharp less likely to occur.

Another addition to the standard is that, in addition to maintaining a log of occupational injuries and illnesses, the employer under the new revision must maintain a sharps injury log. As with all other employee records, this log must be kept in protection of the employee's privacy. The sharps injury log must contain the type and brand of the device involved in the incident, the location of the incident, and a description of the incident. The format of the log is set by the employer and may contain additional comments as long as the privacy of the employee is maintained.

Under engineering controls in the OSHA standard, the revision now specifies that "safer medical devices, such as sharps with engineered sharps injury protections and needleless systems" constitute an effective engineering control and must be used where feasible.

"Sharps with engineered sharps injury protections" is a new term that includes non-needle sharps or needle devices that contain built-in safety features, and are used for collecting fluids, administering medications or other fluids, or any other procedures involving the risk of sharps injury. This covers such devices as a syringe with a sliding sheath that shields the attached needle after use, and needles that retract into the syringe after use.

"Needleless systems" is a new term for devices that provide an alternative to needles for various procedures. This term is currently used more in medicine than in dentistry. It refers to such devices as a jet injection system or an IV medication system in which a port is used instead of a needle.

OSHA Compliance Directive

OSHA will continue to revise and create compliance directives to further protect employees and clarify new standards for employers. These directives are a way to clarify the intent of

Scope and Application
• The Standard applies to all occupational exposure to blood and other potentially infectious materials (OPIMs) and includes part-time employees, designated first aid providers, and mental health workers, as well as exposed medical personnel. • OPIMs include saliva in dental procedures, cerebrospinal fluid, unfixed tissue, semen, vaginal secretions, and body fluids visibly contaminated with blood.
Methods of Compliance
• General—Standard precautions. • Engineering and work practice controls. • Personal protective equipment (PPE). • Housekeeping.
Standard Precautions
• *All* human blood and OPIMs are considered infectious. • The *same* precautions must be taken with all blood and OPIMs.
Engineering Controls
• Whenever feasible, engineering controls must be the primary method for controlling exposure. • Examples include needleless IVs, disposable needle recapping devices, self-sheathing needles, sharps disposal containers, covered centrifuge buckets, aerosol-free tubes, and leak-proof containers. • Engineering controls must be evaluated and documented regularly.
Sharps Containers
• Readily accessible and as close as practical to work area. • Puncture resistant. • Properly labeled or color coded. • Leak proof. • Closeable. • *Routinely replaced* so there is no overflow.
Work Practice Controls
• Handwashing following glove removal. • No breaking or bending of needles. • When needle recapping is necessary use single-handed scoop method or use a needle guard. • No eating, drinking, or smoking in work area. • No storage of food or drink where blood or OPIMs are stored. • Minimize splashing, splattering of blood, and splashing of OPIMs. • No mouth pipetting. • Specimens must be transported in leak-proof, labeled containers. They must be placed in a secondary container if outside contamination of primary container occurs. • Equipment must be decontaminated before servicing or shipping. Areas that cannot be decontaminated must be labeled.
Personal Protective Equipment
• Includes eye protection, gloves, protective clothing, protective face masks, and resuscitation equipment. • Must be readily accessible and employers must require their use. • Must be stored at work site.
Eye Protection
• Is required whenever there is potential for splashing, spraying, or splattering to the eyes or mucous membranes. • If necessary, use eye protection with a mask, or use a chin-length face shield. • Prescription glasses may be fitted with solid side shields. • Decontamination procedures must be developed.

FIGURE 12-1

Understanding OSHA's bloodborne pathogen and hazardous materials standard.

(continues)

(continued)

Gloves
• Must be worn whenever hand contact with blood, OPIMs, mucous membranes, non-intact skin, or contaminated surfaces/ items or when performing vascular access procedures (phlebotomy). • Must be changed if punctured or torn. • Type required: — Vinyl or latex for general use. — Alternatives must be available if employee has allergic reactions (e.g., powderless, nitrile). — Puncture resistant utility gloves for surface disinfection and handling of contaminated materials and instruments. — Puncture resistant when handling sharps (e.g., Central Supply).
Protective Clothing
• Must be worn whenever splashing or splattering to skin or clothing may occur. • Must be changed when clothing becomes soiled. • Type required depends on exposure. Prevention of skin and clothes contamination is the key. • Examples: — Low-level-exposure lab coats. — Moderate-level-exposure, fluid-resistant gown. — High-level-exposure, fluid-proof apron, head and foot covering. • *Note*: If personal protective equipment (PPE) is considered protective clothing, then the *employer must launder it*.
Housekeeping
• There must be a written schedule for cleaning and disinfection. • Contaminated equipment and surfaces must be cleaned as soon as feasible for obvious contamination or at end of work shift if no contamination has occurred. • Protective coverings may be used over equipment.
Regulated Waste Containers (Non-Sharp)
• Closeable. • Leak proof. • Labeled or color coded. • Placed in secondary container if outside of container is contaminated.
Laundry
• Handled as little as possible. • Bagged at location of use. • Labeled or color coded. • Transported in bags that prevent soak-through or leakage.
Laundry Facility
• Two options: 1. Standard precautions for all laundry (alternative color coding allowed if recognized). 2. Precautions only for contaminated laundry (must be red bagged or biohazard labeled). • Laundry personnel must use PPE and have a sharps container accessible.
Hepatitis B Vaccination
• Made available within 10 days to all employees with occupational exposure. • Free to employees. • May be required for student to be admitted to a college health program, as well as to an externship. • Given according to U.S. Public Health Service guidelines. • Employee must first be evaluated by a health care professional. • Health care professional gives a written opinion. • If the vaccine is refused, the employee signs a declination form. • Vaccine must be available later if initially refused.

Courtesy of POL Consultants

FIGURE 12-1

Understanding OSHA's bloodborne pathogen and hazardous materials standard.

(continues)

(continued)

Postexposure Follow-Up
• Wash thoroughly with antimicrobial soap. • Have a blood draw as soon as possible or within 2 hours. • Document exposure incident. • Identify source individual (if possible). • Attempt to test source if consent is obtained. • Provide results to the exposed employee.
Labels
• Biohazard symbol and word *Biohazard* must be visible. • Fluorescent orange/orange-red with contrasting letters may also be used. • Red bags/containers may be substituted for labels. • Labels are required on: — Regulated waste. — Refrigerators/freezers with blood of OPIMs. — Transport/storage containers. — Contaminated equipment.
Information and Training
• Required for all employees with occupational exposure. • Training required initially, annually, and if there are new procedures. • Training material must be appropriate for the employees' literacy and education levels. • Training must be interactive and allow for questions and answers.
Training Components
• Modes of HIV/HBV transmission. • Explanation of exposure control plan. • Explanation of engineering, work practice controls. • Explanation of bloodborne standard. • Epidemiology and symptoms of bloodborne disease. • How to select the proper PPE. • How to decontaminate equipment, surfaces, and so on. • Information about hepatitis B vaccine. • Postexposure follow-up procedures. • Label/color code system.
Medical Records
Records must be kept for each employee with occupational exposure and include: • A copy of employee's vaccination status and date. • A copy of postexposure follow-up evaluation procedures. • Health care professional's written opinions. • Confidentiality must be maintained. • Records must be maintained for 30 years, plus the duration of employment.
Training Records
Records are kept for 3 years from date of training and include: • Date of training. • Summary of contents of training program. • Name and qualifications of trainer. • Names and job titles of all persons attending.
Exposure Control Plan Components
• A written plan for each workplace with occupational exposure. • Written policies/procedures for complying with the standard. • A cohesive document or a guiding document referencing existing policies/procedures.

Courtesy of POL Consultants

FIGURE 12-1

Understanding OSHA's bloodborne pathogen and hazardous materials standard.

(continues)

(continued)

Exposure Control Plan
• A list of job classifications where occupational exposure control occurs (e.g., medical assistant, clinical laboratory scientist, and dental hygienist). • A list of tasks where exposure occurs (e.g., medical assistant who performs venipuncture). • Methods/policies/procedures for compliance. • Procedures for sharps disposal. • Disinfection policies/procedures. • Procedures for selection of PPE. • Regulated waste disposal procedures. • Laundry procedures. • Hepatitis B vaccination procedures. • Postexposure follow-up procedures. • Training procedures. • Plan must be accessible to employees and be updated annually.
Employee Responsibilities
• Go through training and cooperate. • Obey policies. • Use universal precaution techniques. • Use PPE. • Use safe work practices. • Use engineering controls.
Employee Responsibilities
• Report unsafe work conditions to employer. • Maintain clean work areas. Cooperation between employer and employees regarding the Standard will facilitate understanding of the law, thereby benefiting all persons who are exposed to HIV, HBV, and OPIMs by minimizing the risk of exposure to pathogens. Meeting the OSHA standard is not optional, and failure to comply can result in a fine that may total $10,000 for each employee.

FIGURE 12-1
Understanding OSHA's bloodborne pathogen and hazardous materials standard.

the standard and the enforcement procedures for compliance. Employers and employees should continue to stay abreast of standards and requirements. The OSHA (http://www.OSHA.gov) and ADA (http://www.ADA.org) websites are good sources of information pertinent to dentistry.

Engineering/Work Practice Controls

The physical equipment and mechanical devices that employers provide to safeguard and protect employees at work are known as engineering and work practice controls. Examples of these would be splash guards on model trimmers, puncture-resistant sharps containers, and ventilation hoods for hazardous fumes. The employer must provide this equipment to meet OSHA standards, and provide a safe environment for employees. The employer must ensure that employees wash their hands immediately after gloves are removed and flush their eyes with water at an eye-wash station if contact with microorganisms or hazardous materials is suspected (Figure 12-2). The employer must ensure that employees flush any mucous membranes, immediately, if there has been possible contact with blood or other potentially infectious materials (OPIMs) in the office.

The employer sets up work practice controls to diminish harmful occupational exposure. OSHA defines occupational exposure as reasonably anticipated eye, skin, mucous membrane, or parenteral contact with blood or other OPIMs that may result from the performance of an employee's duties. It further defines **parenteral** as a means of piercing mucous membranes or the skin barrier through such events as needlesticks, cuts, and abrasions.

Sharps

The dentist may purchase needle guards for dental needles to protect employees from unnecessary sticks. Several types are available. Needles should never be recapped using the two-hand technique, because it is easy to stick the opposing hand or the other person's hand. Instead, a scoop method using one hand must be followed during the recapping procedure (see Chapter 20, Anesthesia and Sedation).

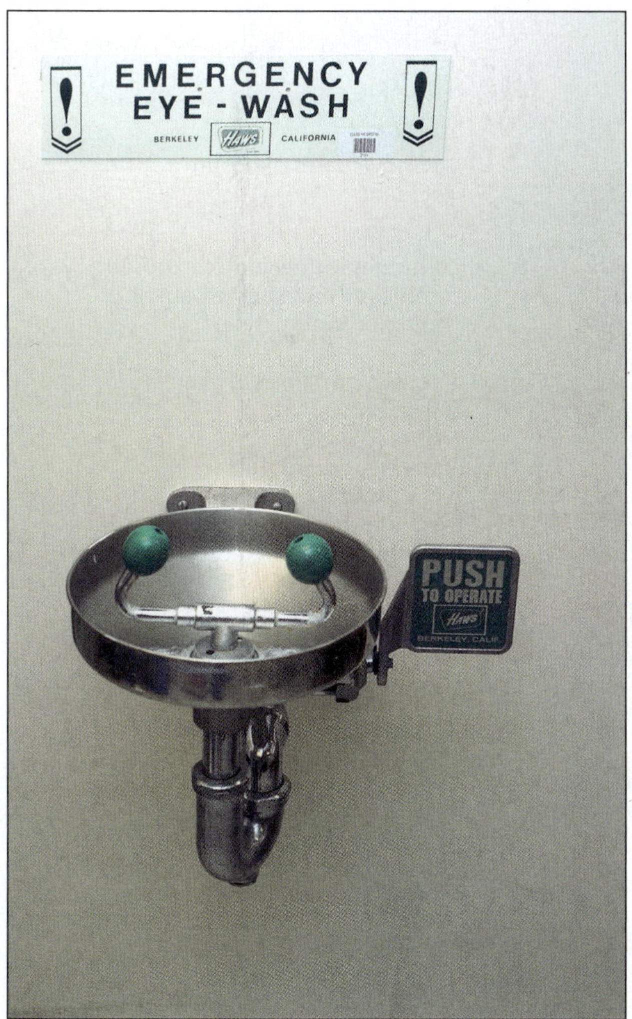

FIGURE 12-2
Eye-wash station.

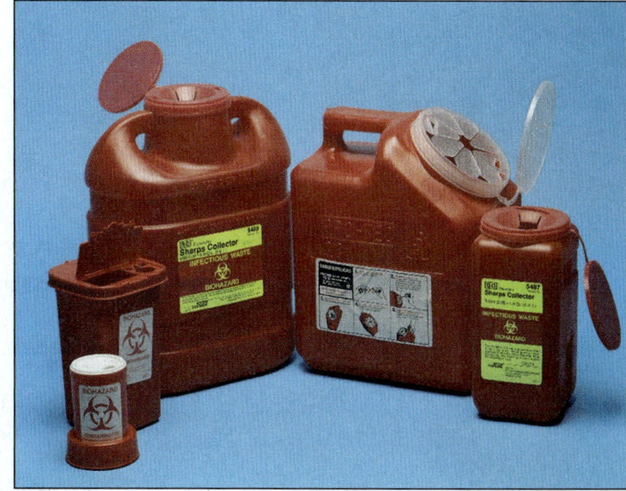

FIGURE 12-3
Puncture-resistant sharps containers.

Upon completing a procedure, contaminated sharps and needles must be placed immediately in a labeled, leak-proof, puncture-resistant container (Figure 12-3). Other sharps that are placed routinely in the sharps disposal containers are blades from knives used in surgery, broken glass, anesthetic capsules, and orthodontic wires. When the sharps disposal containers are full, they are sealed, sterilized using an autoclave if possible, and sent to an outside biohazard agency for safe disposal.

Occupational Exposure to Bloodborne Pathogens

Any employee who has an occupational exposure incident must report it immediately (Figure 12-4). The employer must immediately make available to the exposed employee a confidential medical evaluation and follow-up. The medical evaluation and follow-up are made available to the employee at no cost. The dentist refers the exposed employee to a licensed health care professional to have the most current medical evaluation and procedures performed in accordance with the U.S. Public Health Service regulations. OSHA standards do not dictate the procedures to be performed, but allow for the most current recommendations to be applied. Reporting the incident immediately allows the dentist to carefully evaluate the circumstances surrounding the incident and to find ways to prevent the situation and exposure incident from happening again.

Documentation of Exposure Incident. The dentist documents the information from the exposure incident on a report. This report includes the route(s) of exposure, the circumstances that surrounded the exposure incident, and (if known) the identity of the source patient. The exposure incident report is placed in the employee's confidential medical record and a copy of this report is provided to the health care professional who is providing the evaluation.

The employer is required to provide the licensed health care professional with a description of the employee's job duties and their relation to the incident; information about the route of the exposure; the circumstances surrounding the incident; relevant employee medical records, including vaccination status; a copy of the bloodborne pathogen standard; and the results of the source patient's blood testing (if available).

If the employer has 11 or more employees, the employer may be required to complete OSHA Form 200 (Log and Summary of Occupational Injuries and Illnesses) and Form 101 (Supplemental Record of Occupational Injuries and Illnesses) to meet the recordable occupational injury requirement.

In the case of a bloodborne pathogen exposure, the dentist must identify and document, in writing, the source patient, if known. Furthermore, the dentist must contact the source patient and request his or her consent to be tested for HBV and HIV, as well as to disclose the results of these tests to the exposed employee. If the source patient does not give consent for the testing, the dentist must document this on the report of the exposure incident. If the source patient agrees to be tested, the tests

Exposure incident occurs

⇓

Employee		Employer		HCP evaluates exposure incident
Employee reports incident to employer	⟹	Employer directs employee to health-care professional (HCP)	⟹	HCP evaluates exposure incident
		Sends to HCP: • Copy of standard job description of employee • Incident report (route, etc.) • Source patient's identity and HBV/HIV status (if known) • Employee's HBV status and other relevant medical information		Arranges for testing of exposed employee and source patient (if not known already) Notifies employee of results of all testing Provides counseling Provides postexposure prophylaxis, if medically indicated
		Document events on OSHA 200 and 101 (if applicable)		Evaluates reported illnesses (Items above are confidential) ⇓
		Receives HCP's written opinion	⟸	Sends (only) the HCP's written opinion to employer: • Documentation that employee was informed of evaluation results and the need for any further follow-up; and • Whether HBV vaccine was received.
		⇓		
Receives copy of HCP's written opinion	⟸	Provides copy of HCP's written opinion to employee (within 15 days of completed evaluation)		

Prepared by the American Dental Association in cooperation with the Occupational Safety and Health Administration (December 1997). This document is not considered a substitute for any provisions of the Occupational Safety and Health Act of 1970 or for any standards issued by OSHA.

FIGURE 12-4

Flowchart for occupational exposure to bloodborne pathogens.

should be completed as soon as feasible. When the results are disclosed to the exposed employee, information regarding the source patient's rights to disclosure must be discussed.

Exposed Employee Blood (Collection and Testing). The employee has the right to decline testing after an exposure incident or to delay the testing for up to 90 days. The employee may consent to have a baseline blood test that will determine the HBV and HIV serological status. The employee may choose to be tested only for HBV and not give consent for HIV testing at that time. The employee's blood sample must be saved for 90 days in case the employee elects to consent to the HIV testing. All tests must be performed by an accredited laboratory at no cost to the employee. The health care professional will notify the employee directly of all test results.

Postexposure Follow-Up Procedures. The employer must provide the exposed employee counseling, prophylaxis to prevent sexual transmission of any possible infection, and evaluation of reported illnesses. The provided counseling will aid the employee in interpretation of all tests, discussions about the potential risk of infection, and the need for further postexposure prophylaxis. The employee should also be counseled on the necessary use of protection during sexual contact.

Postexposure prophylaxis is provided according to the current recommendations of the U.S. Public Health Service. OSHA did not define this procedure in the bloodborne standard, due to ongoing changes that have developed in this area.

Treatment may include, but is not limited to, an HBV vaccine if the employee has not had it, or chemoprophylaxis for high-risk cases of HIV transmission.

The health care professional also evaluates any reported illnesses that the exposed employee develops. The health care professional can evaluate the symptoms in relation to HBV and HIV infections. This allows the exposed employee to have immediate medical evaluation and referral for medical treatment, so that the treatment can be started as soon as possible. This does not mean that the employer is responsible for any costs associated with the treatment of the disease.

The health care professional sends the dental employer a written opinion about the evaluation, as well as notification that the employee was informed of the test results of the evaluation and of further follow-up. The dentist provides the employee with a copy of this written opinion and evaluation of the exposed employee within 15 days of the completion of the evaluation. The original document is placed in the employee's confidential record. The employer must maintain employee records in a confidential manner for the duration of employment plus 30 years, in accordance with OSHA's standard on Access to Employee Exposure and Medical Records, 29 CFR 1910.20.

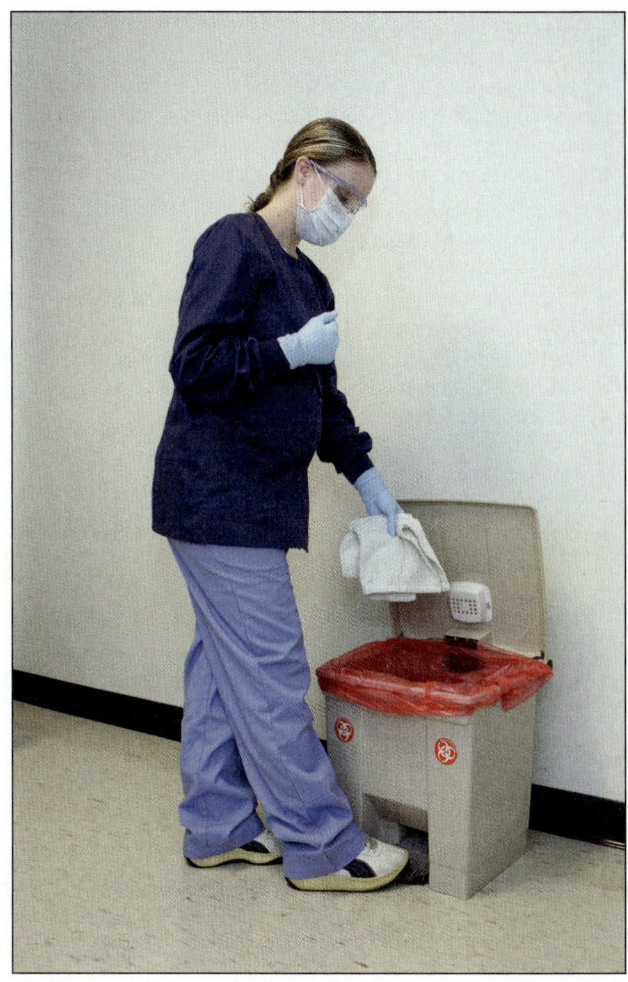

FIGURE 12-5
Proper disposal of contaminated laundry.

Employee Work Site

The employer must provide a work site that is clean and sanitary. Each office must have a written schedule for infection control and decontaminating procedures for each area. Wastepaper baskets, floors, and all other surfaces that may have been contaminated with blood or OPIM must be included. The assistant must wear utility gloves while cleaning contaminated surfaces. All disposable items that are contaminated, including gloves, must be discarded in a biohazard container.

Broken Glass. Broken glass must be cleaned up with a broom (or brush) and dust pan (or cardboard). Dental assistants must never touch broken glass with bare hands or gloved hands, due to the risk of puncture. Broken glass must be placed in a leak-proof sharps container, labeled "biohazard."

Laundry. Contaminated laundry must be handled as little as possible. Gloves must be used when placing it in a biohazard container, or a red bag that is labeled with a biohazard symbol (Figure 12-5). If the laundry is damp or wet, it must first be placed in a plastic bag to prevent blood or OPIM from seeping through it.

Laundry that is sent off site for cleaning is placed in a red biohazard bag for transportation. Dental assistants should take special care when removing protective clothing, especially items that are taken over the head. The chance for contamination of the face can take place if the outside surface of the clothing makes contact with it.

Hazardous Chemicals

The OSHA hazard communication standard is set up so that employees receive training about the risks of using hazardous chemicals, and the safety precautions required when handling them. Employees must be trained in the identification of hazardous chemicals, and the personal protective equipment to be utilized for each chemical. This training must occur within 30 days of employment or prior to the employee using any chemicals, and annually thereafter (Figure 12-6).

Employees must have a certificate available, or in their personnel files, that shows they have had the proper training. The certificate must identify that the employer has trained the employee in the proper handling of hazardous substances in the dental office (Figure 12-7).

SAFETY TRAINING FORM

All employees receive safety training before those employees assume responsibilities that involve exposure to body fluids or chemicals or within 30 days of employment. Items that must be covered in the training session are as follows:

- Overall explanation of OSHA laws
- Explanation of the epidemiology and symptoms of HBV and HIV/AIDS
- Discussion about who is at risk in the dental office
- Transmission modes of microorganisms
- Methods of infection control in the workplace
- Universal/Standard Precautions
- Personal protective equipment
- Handwashing
- How spills are to be cleaned
- Postexposure incident procedure
- Coverage of the Hazardous Communication Standard
- Chemical labels and how to read them
- How to read SDSs, how to get SDSs, where SDSs are kept in the office, and interpretation of warning signs on SDSs
- How chemicals are to be stored and inventoried
- Hazardous waste laws and how to comply
- How to use sharps containers
- How to keep and who keeps records
- Medical consent forms
- HBV forms
- Engineering control records
- Safety training certification and when training is to take place

FIGURE 12-6

Safety training form.

OSHA HAZARD COMMUNICATION AND BLOODBORNE PATHOGEN STANDARD TRAINING CERTIFICATE

This certificate indicates your successful completion of the OSHA Hazard Communication and Blood-borne Pathogen Standard Training in the office of ______________________. The program instructed you of your rights as a worker, the responsibilities of your employer, and the proper knowledge and handling of hazardous substances and bloodborne pathogens in this dental office.

Date of employment ______________________

Date of training ______________________

Instructor's signature ______________________

Employee's signature ______________________

Employer's signature ______________________

FIGURE 12-7

Sample training form.

As with the Bloodborne Pathogen Standard, a written plan identifying employee training and detailing specific control measures used in the workplace must be compiled for the management of hazardous chemicals. If the office is not in compliance, penalties may be imposed on the employer.

All hazardous chemicals must be identified on a written form, such as a chemical inventory form (Figure 12-8). Other information required about the chemicals includes the quantity stored (each month or year), the physical state of the substance (liquid, solid, or gas), the hazardous class (health problem, fire hazard, and reactive), what PPE is required, and the manufacturer's name, address, and phone number.

Hazardous Communication Standard (HCS)

The Hazardous Communication Standard, which is part of the Employee Right-to-Know Law, was revised in 2012. This revision included the adoption of the **Globally Harmonized System of Classification and Labeling of Chemicals (GHS)**. This means that chemicals and materials are classified and labeled the same way internationally, regardless of where the chemicals are manufactured, sold, or used.

Safety Data Sheets

Part of the 2012 revision to the HCS now requires manufacturers and employers to use specific criteria for classification of health and physical hazards; a label that includes a harmonized signal word, **pictogram**, and hazard statement for all categories; and a new 16-section format safety data sheet (SDS, formerly material safety data sheet).

Every office must have a safety data sheet manual that is alphabetized, indexed, and available to all employees. These manuals can be in hard copy or on a computer. The manual contains the SDSs. These sheets come from the manufacturer. If SDSs are unavailable, the employer, or a designated employee (the safety assistant), must request it from the manufacturer, or it can be easily found on the manufacturer's website. The SDS form must include the following 16 sections, of which 12 are enforced by OSHA (Figure 12-9):

1. Description
2. Hazards
3. Composition
4. First aid
5. Fire fighting
6. Accidental release measures
7. Handling and storage
8. Exposure controls
9. Physical and chemical properties
10. Stability and reactivity
11. Toxicology

Chemical Inventory Form

Date updated ______

Dental office ______

Chemical Name	Hazard Class				Physical State	Manufacturer	Comments
	(H)	(F)	(R)	(P)			

(H) Health
0—Minimal
1—Slightly
2—Moderate
3—Serious
4—Extreme

(F) Fire Hazard
0—Will not burn
1—Slight
2—Moderate
3—Serious
4—Extreme

(R) Reactivity
0—Stable
1—Slight
2—Moderate
3—Serious
4—Extreme

(P) Protection
A—Goggles
B—Goggles/gloves
C—Goggles/gloves/clothing
D—Goggles/gloves/clothing/mask
E—Goggles/gloves/mask
F—Gloves
G—Face shield/gloves

FIGURE 12-8

Sample chemical inventory form.

12. Ecology*
13. Disposal*
14. Transport*
15. Regulatory*
16. Other information

*These sections are enforced by agencies other than OSHA.

Harmonized Label

All labeling must now be done in the GHS format. The harmonized label includes a hazard statement that describes the hazard, a signal word that indicates the severity of the hazard, and an OSHA designated pictogram that indicates the type of hazard (Figure 12-10). There are nine pictograms that may be used; and OSHA enforces the use of eight of those. The pictograms communicate:

- health hazard (carcinogen and toxicity to organs or body systems);
- flame (flammable);
- exclamation mark (irritant or sensitivity);
- gas cylinder (gas under pressure);
- corrosion (skin, eye, or metal);
- exploding bomb (explosive or reactive);
- flame over circle (oxidizer);
- environment (non-mandatory); and
- skull and crossbones (acute toxicity or fatal).

The **National Fire Protection Association's color and number method** is used to easily identify information about various hazardous ingredients on the SDS and product labels. While this labeling is not required, it may still be used along with the harmonized label.

Chemical Warning Label Determination. The National Fire Protection Association's color and number method is used to signify a warning to employees using chemicals (Figure 12-11). Four colors are used:

1. Blue identifies a health hazard,
2. Red identifies a fire hazard,
3. Yellow identifies the reactivity or stability of a chemical, and
4. White indicates that PPE is needed when using the chemical.

MERCURY

Safety Data Sheet

according to the federal final rule of hazard communication revised on 2012 (HazCom 2012)

Date of issue: 11/19/2013

SECTION 1: Identification of the substance/mixture and of the company/undertaking

1.1. Product identifier

Trade name : MERCURY

CAS No : 7439-97-6

Other means of identification : Colloidal Mercury, Quick Silver, Liquid Silver, NCI-C60399, Hydrargyrum

1.2. Relevant identified uses of the substance or mixture and uses advised against

Use of the substance/mixture : Variety of industrial, analytical and research applications.

1.3. Details of the supplier of the safety data sheet

ABC Pharmaceuticals

1234 Chemcial Way
Amalgam Center, AL 31313

1.4. Emergency telephone number

Emergency number : 1-800-555-5656

SECTION 2: Hazards identification

2.1. Classification of the substance or mixture

GHS-US classification

Acute Tox. 1 (Inhalation:dust,mist)	H330
Repr. 1B	H360
STOT RE 1	H372
Aquatic Acute 1	H400
Aquatic Chronic 1	H410

2.2. Label elements

GHS-US labelling

Hazard pictograms (GHS-US) :

GHS09

Signal word (GHS-US) : Danger

Hazard statements (GHS-US) : H330 - Fatal if inhaled
H360 - May damage fertility or the unborn child
H372 - Causes damage to organs through prolonged or repeated exposure
H400 - Very toxic to aquatic life
H410 - Very toxic to aquatic life with long lasting effects

Precautionary statements (GHS-US) : P201 - Obtain special instructions before use
P202 - Do not handle until all safety precautions have been read and understood
P260 - Do not breathe vapors, gas
P264 - Wash skin, hands thoroughly after handling
P270 - Do not eat, drink or smoke when using this product
P271 - Use only outdoors or in a well-ventilated area
P273 - Avoid release to the environment
P280 - Wear eye protection, protective clothing, protective gloves, Face mask
P284 - [In case of inadequate ventilation] wear respiratory protection
P304+P340 - IF INHALED: Remove person to fresh air and keep comfortable for breathing
P308+P313 - IF exposed or concerned: Get medical advice/attention
P310 - Immediately call a POISON CENTER/doctor/...
P314 - Get medical advice and attention if you feel unwell
P320 - Specific treatment is urgent (see First aid measures on this label)
P391 - Collect spillage
P403+P233 - Store in a well-ventilated place. Keep container tightly closed
P405 - Store locked up
P501 - Dispose of contents/container to comply with applicable local, national and international regulation.

2.3. Other hazards

other hazards which do not result in classification : When inhaled, Mercury will be rapidly distributed throughout the body. During this time, Mercury will cross the blood-brain barrier, and become oxidized to the Hg (II) oxidation state. The oxidized species of Mercury cannot cross the blood-brain barrier and thus accumulates in the

FIGURE 12-9

Sample SDS.

(continues)

(continued)

MERCURY

Safety Data Sheet

according to the federal final rule of hazard communication revised on 2012 (HazCom 2012)

brain. Mercury in other organs is removed slowly from the body via the kidneys. The average half-time for clearance of Mercury for different parts of the human body is as follows: lung: 1.7 days; head: 21 days; kidney region: 64 days; chest: 43 days; whole body: 58 days. Mercury can be irritating to contaminated skin and eye. Prolonged contact may lead to ulceration of the skin. Allergic reactions (i.e. rashes, welts) may occur in sensitive individuals. Mercury can be irritating to contaminated skin and eyes. Short-term over-exposures to high concentrations of mercury vapors can lead to breathing difficulty, coughing, acute, and potentially fatal lung disorders. Depending on the concentration of inhalation over-exposure, heart problems, damage to the kidney, liver or nerves and effects on the brain may occur.

2.4. Unknown acute toxicity (GHS-US)

No data available

SECTION 3: Composition/information on ingredients

3.1. Substance

Not applicable

Full text of H-phrases: see section 16

3.2. Mixture

Name	Product identifier	%	GHS-US classification
Mercury	(CAS No) 7439-97-6	100	Acute Tox. 2 (Inhalation), H330 Repr. 1B, H360 STOT RE 1, H372 Aquatic Acute 1, H400 Aquatic Chronic 1, H410

SECTION 4: First aid measures

4.1. Description of first aid measures

First-aid measures general : Never give anything by mouth to an unconscious person. If exposed or concerned: Get medical advice/attention.

First-aid measures after inhalation : Remove to fresh air and keep at rest in a position comfortable for breathing. Assure fresh air breathing. Allow the victim to rest. Immediately call a POISON CENTER or doctor/physician. In case of irregular breathing or respiratory arrest provide artificial respiration.

First-aid measures after skin contact : Wash immediately with lots of water (15 minutes)/shower. Remove affected clothing and wash all exposed skin area with mild soap and water, followed by warm water rinse. Seek immediate medical advice.

First-aid measures after eye contact : Rinse immediately and thoroughly, pulling the eyelids well away from the eye (15 minutes minimum). Keep eye wide open while rinsing. Seek medical attention immediately.

First-aid measures after ingestion : Immediately call a POISON CENTER or doctor/physician. Rinse mouth. If conscious, give large amounts of water and induce vomiting. Give water or milk if the person is fully conscious. Obtain emergency medical attention.

4.2. Most important symptoms and effects, both acute and delayed

Symptoms/injuries after inhalation : Short-term over-exposures to high concentrations of mercury vapors can lead to breathing difficulty, coughing, acute, chemical pneumonia, and pulmonary edema (a potentially fatal accumulation of fluid in the lungs) . Depending on the concentration of over-exposure, cardiac abnormalities, damage to the kidney, liver or nerves and effects on the brain may occur. Long-term inhalation over-exposures can lead to the development of a wide variety of symptoms, including the following: excessive salivation, gingivitis, anorexia, chills, fever, cardiac abnormalities, anemia, digestive problems, abdominal pains, frequent urination, an inability to urinate, diarrhea, peripheral neuropathy (numbness, weakness, or burning sensations in the hands or feet), tremors (especially in the hands, fingers, eyelids, lips, cheeks, tongue, or legs), alteration of tendon reflexes, slurred speech, visual disturbances, and deafness. Allergic reactions (i.e. breathing difficulty) may also occur in sensitive individuals.

Symptoms/injuries after skin contact : Symptoms of skin exposure can include redness, dry skin, and pain. Prolonged contact may lead to ulceration of the skin. Allergic reactions (i.e. rashes, welts) may occur in sensitive individuals. Dermatitis (redness and inflammation of the skin) may occur after repeated skin exposures.

Symptoms/injuries after eye contact : Symptoms of eye exposure can include redness, pain, and watery eyes. A symptom of Mercury exposure is discoloration of the lens of the eyes.

Symptoms/injuries after ingestion : If Mercury is swallowed, symptoms of such over-exposure can include metallic taste in mouth, nausea, vomiting, central nervous system effects, and damage to the kidneys. Metallic mercury is not usually absorbed sufficiently from the gastrointestinal tract to induce an acute, toxic response. Damage to the tissues of the mouth, throat, esophagus, and other tissues of the digestive system may occur. Ingestion may be fatal, due to effects on gastrointestinal system and kidneys.

Chronic symptoms : Long-term over-exposure can lead to a wide range of adverse health effects. Anyone using Mercury must pay attention to personality changes, weight loss, skin or gum discolorations, stomach pains, and other signs of Mercury over-exposure. Gradually developing syndromes ("Erethism" and "Acrodynia") are indicative of potentially severe health problems. Mercury can cause the development of allergic reactions (i.e. dermatitis, rashes, breathing difficulty) upon prolonged or repeated exposures. Refer to Section 11 (Toxicology Information) for additional data.

FIGURE 12-9

Sample SDS.

(continues)

(continued)

MERCURY

Safety Data Sheet

according to the federal final rule of hazard communication revised on 2012 (HazCom 2012)

4.3. Indication of any immediate medical attention and special treatment needed

Treatment for Mercury over-exposure must be given. The following treatment protocol for ingestion of Mercury is from Clinical Toxicology of Commercial Products (5th Edition, 1984).

SECTION 5: Firefighting measures

5.1. Extinguishing media

Suitable extinguishing media	: Foam. Dry powder. Carbon dioxide. Water spray. Sand.
Unsuitable extinguishing media	: Do not use a heavy water stream.

5.2. Special hazards arising from the substance or mixture

Fire hazard	: Not flammable. Mercury vapors and oxides generated during fires involving this product are toxic.
Reactivity	: Stable. Reacts with (some) metals. Mercury can react with metals to form amalgams.

5.3. Advice for firefighters

Firefighting instructions	: Use water spray or fog for cooling exposed containers. Exercise caution when fighting any chemical fire. Prevent fire-fighting water from entering environment. Do not allow run-off from fire fighting to enter drains or water courses.
Protective equipment for firefighters	: Do not enter fire area without proper protective equipment, including respiratory protection.
Other information	: Decontaminate all equipment thoroughly after the conclusion of fire-fighting activities.

SECTION 6: Accidental release measures

6.1. Personal precautions, protective equipment and emergency procedures

General measures	: Uncontrolled release should be responded to by trained personnel using pre-planned procedures. Evacuate area. Evacuate personnel to a safe area.

6.1.1. For non-emergency personnel

Emergency procedures	: Evacuate unnecessary personnel.

6.1.2. For emergency responders

Protective equipment	: Equip cleanup crew with proper protection. In the event of a release under 1 pound: the minimum level "C" Personal Protective Equipment is needed. Triple-gloves (rubber gloves and nitril gloves over latex gloves), chemical resistant suit and boots, hard-hat, and Air-Purifying Respirator with Cartridge appropriate for Mercury. In the event of a release over 1 pound or when concentration of oxygen in atmosphere is less than 19.5% or unknown, the level "B" Personal Protective Equipments which includes Self-Contained Breathing Apparatus must be worn.
Emergency procedures	: Ventilate area.

6.2. Environmental precautions

Prevent entry to sewers and public waters. Notify authorities if liquid enters sewers or public waters. Avoid release to the environment.

6.3. Methods and material for containment and cleaning up

For containment	: For larger spills, dike area and pump into waste containers. Put into a labelled container and provide safe disposal.
Methods for cleaning up	: There are a variety of methods which can be used to clean-up Mercury spills. Use a commercially available Mercury Spill Kit for small spills. A suction pump with aspirator can also be used during clean-up operations. For larger release, a Mercury vacuum can be used. Calcium polysulfide or excess sulfur can be also used for clean-up. Mercury can migrate into cracks and other difficult-to-clean areas; calcium polysulfide and sulfur can be sprinkled effectively into these areas. Decontaminate the area thoroughly. The area should be inspected visually and with colorimetric tubes for Mercury to ensure all traces have been removed prior to re-occupation by non-emergency personnel. Decontaminate all equipment used in response thoroughly. If such equipments cannot de adequately decontaminated, it must be discarded with other spill residue. Place all spill residues in an appropriate container, seal immediately, and label appropriately. Dispose of in accordance with federal, state, and local hazardous waste disposal requirements. (Refer to Section 13 of this SDS).

6.4. Reference to other sections

See Heading 8. Exposure controls and personal protection.

SECTION 7: Handling and storage

7.1. Precautions for safe handling

Additional hazards when processed	: Supervisors and responsible personnel must be aware of personality changes, weight loss, or other sign of Mercury over-exposure in employees using this product; These symptoms can develop gradually and are indicative of potentially severe health effects related to Mercury contamination.

FIGURE 12-9

Sample SDS.

(continues)

(continued)

MERCURY

Safety Data Sheet

according to the federal final rule of hazard communication revised on 2012 (HazCom 2012)

Precautions for safe handling : As with all chemicals, avoid getting Mercury ON YOU or IN YOU. Do not handle until all safety precautions have been read and understood. Obtain special instructions before use. Wash hands and other exposed areas with mild soap and water before eating, drinking or smoking and when leaving work. Provide good ventilation in process area to prevent formation of vapor. Report all Mercury releases promptly. Open container slowly on a stable surface. Drums, flasks and bottles of this product must be properly labeled. Empty containers may contain residual amounts of Mercury and should be handled with care.

Hygiene measures : Do not eat, drink or smoke when using this product. Always wash hands and face immediately after handling this product, and once again before leaving the workplace. Remove contaminated clothing immediately.

7.2. Conditions for safe storage, including any incompatibilities

Technical measures : Follow practice indicated in Section 6. Make certain that application equipment is locked and tagged-out safely. Always use this product in areas where adequate ventilation is provided. Decontaminate equipment thoroughly before maintenance begins.

Storage conditions : Keep container tightly closed. Store drums, flasks and bottles in a cool, dry location, away from direct sunlight, source of intense heat, or where freezing is possible. Store away from incompatible materials. Material should be stored in secondary container or in a diked area, as appropriate.

Incompatible materials : Acetylene and acetylene derivatives, amines, ammonia, 3-bromopropyne, boron diiodophosphide, methyl azide, sodium carbide, heated sulfuric acid, methylsilane/oxygen mixtures, nitric acid/alcohol mixtures, tetracarbonylnickel/oxygen mixtures, alkyne/silver perchlorate mixtures, halogens and strong oxidizers. Mercury can attack copper alloys. Mercury can react with many metals (i.e. calcium, lithium, potassium, sodium, rubidium, aluminum) to form amalgams.

Prohibitions on mixed storage : Mercury can attack copper alloys. Mercury can react with many metals (i.e. calcium, lithium, potassium, sodium, rubidium, aluminum) to form amalgams.

Storage area : Storage area should be made of fire-resistant materials.

Special rules on packaging : Inspect all incoming containers before storage to ensure containers are properly labeled and not damaged.

7.3. Specific end use(s)

No additional information available

SECTION 8: Exposure controls/personal protection

8.1. Control parameters

Mercury (7439-97-6)		
USA ACGIH	ACGIH TWA (mg/m³)	0,025 mg/m³
USA OSHA	OSHA PEL (Ceiling) (mg/m³)	0,1 mg/m³

8.2. Exposure controls

Appropriate engineering controls : Ensure adequate ventilation. Ensure exposure is below occupational exposure limits (where available). Emergency eye wash fountains and safety showers should be available in the immediate vicinity of any potential exposure.

Personal protective equipment : Avoid all unnecessary exposure. Gloves. Protective clothing. Safety glasses. Mist formation: aerosol mask.

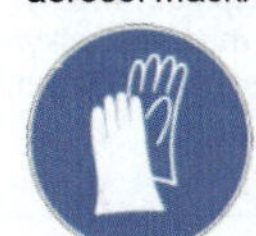

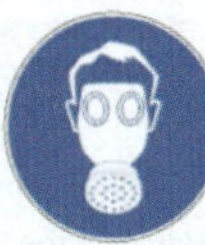

Hand protection : Wear neoprene gloves for routine industrial use. Use triple gloves for spill response, as stated in Section 6 of this SDS.

Eye protection : Splash goggles or safety glasses. For operation involving the use of more than 1 pound of Mercury, or if the operation may generate a spray of Mercury, the use of a faceshield is recommended.

Skin and body protection : Wear suitable protective clothing.

Respiratory protection : Maintain airborne contaminants concentration below provided exposure limits. If respiratory protection is needed, use only protection authorized in 29 CFR 1910.134 or applicable state regulations. Use supplied air respiration protection if oxygen levels are below 19.5% or are unknown.

Other information : Do not eat, drink or smoke during use.

SECTION 9: Physical and chemical properties

9.1. Information on basic physical and chemical properties

Physical state : Liquid

Colour : Silver white.

FIGURE 12-9

Sample SDS.

(continues)

(continued)

MERCURY

Safety Data Sheet

according to the federal final rule of hazard communication revised on 2012 (HazCom 2012)

Odor	: Odorless.
Odor threshold	: Not applicable
pH	: Not applicable
Relative evaporation rate (butylacetate=1)	: No data available
Melting point	: No data available
Freezing point	: -38,87 °C (-37.97 F)
Boiling point	: No data available
Flash point	: Not applicable
Self ignition temperature	: Not applicable
Decomposition temperature	: No data available
Flammability (solid, gas)	: No data available
Vapour pressure	: 0,002 mm Hg at 25°C
Relative vapor density at 20 °C	: 6,9 (Air = 1)
Relative density	: No data available
Relative density of saturated gas/air mixture	: 13,6
Solubility	: No data available
Log Pow	: No data available
Log Kow	: No data available
Viscosity, kinematic	: No data available
Viscosity, dynamic	: No data available
Explosive properties	: No data available
Oxidizing properties	: No data available
Explosive limits	: Not applicable

9.2. Other information

No additional information available

SECTION 10: Stability and reactivity

10.1. Reactivity

Stable. Reacts with (some) metals. Mercury can react with metals to form amalgams.

10.2. Chemical stability

Not established.

10.3. Possibility of hazardous reactions

Not established. Hazardous polymerization will not occur.

10.4. Conditions to avoid

Direct sunlight. Extremely high or low temperatures.

10.5. Incompatible materials

Acetylene and acetylene derivatives, amines, ammonia, 3-bromopropyne, boron diiodophosphide, methyl azide, sodium carbide, heated sulfuric acid, methylsilane/oxygen mixtures, nitric acid/alcohol mixtures, tetracarbonylnickel/oxygen mixtures, alkyne/silver perchlorate mixtures, halogens and strong oxidizers. Mercury can attack copper alloys. Mercury can react with many metals (i.e. calcium, lithium, potassium, sodium, rubidium, aluminum) to form amalgams.

10.6. Hazardous decomposition products

If this product is exposed to extremely high temperature in the presence of oxygen or air, toxic vapor of mercury and mercury oxides will be generated.

SECTION 11: Toxicological information

11.1. Information on toxicological effects

Acute toxicity	: Fatal if inhaled.
Skin corrosion/irritation	: Not classified pH: Not applicable
Serious eye damage/irritation	: Not classified pH: Not applicable
Respiratory or skin sensitisation	: Not classified
Germ cell mutagenicity	: Not classified Based on available data, the classification criteria are not met
Carcinogenicity	: Not classified

FIGURE 12-9

Sample SDS.

(continues)

(continued)

MERCURY

Safety Data Sheet

according to the federal final rule of hazard communication revised on 2012 (HazCom 2012)

Mercury (7439-97-6)	
IARC group	3

Reproductive toxicity : May damage fertility or the unborn child.
Based on available data, the classification criteria are not met

Specific target organ toxicity (single exposure) : Not classified

Specific target organ toxicity (repeated exposure) : Causes damage to organs through prolonged or repeated exposure.
Based on available data, the classification criteria are not met
Causes damage to organs through prolonged or repeated exposure

Aspiration hazard : Not classified
Based on available data, the classification criteria are not met

Potential adverse human health effects and symptoms : Based on available data, the classification criteria are not met. Fatal if inhaled.

Symptoms/injuries after inhalation : Short-term over-exposures to high concentrations of mercury vapors can lead to breathing difficulty, coughing, acute,chemical pneumonia, and pulmonary edema (a potentially fatal accumulation of fluid in the lungs) . Depending on the concentration of over-exposure, cardiac abnormalities, damage to the kidney, liver or nerves and effects on the brain may occur. Long-term inhalation over-exposures can lead to the development of a wide variety of symptoms, including the following: excessive salivation, gingivitis, anorexia, chills, fever, cardiac abnormalities, anemia, digestive problems, abdominal pains, frequent urination, an inability to urinate, diarrhea, peripheral neuropathy (numbness, weakness, or burning sensations in the hands or feet), tremors (especially in the hands, fingers, eyelids, lips, cheeks, tongue, or legs), alteration of tendon reflexes, slurred speech, visual disturbances, and deafness. Allergic reactions (i.e. breathing difficulty) may also occur in sensitive individuals.

Symptoms/injuries after skin contact : Symptoms of skin exposure can include redness, dry skin, and pain. Prolonged contact may lead to ulceration of the skin. Allergic reactions (i.e. rashes, welts) may occur in sensitive individuals. Dermatitis (redness and inflammation of the skin) may occur after repeated skin exposures.

Symptoms/injuries after eye contact : Symptoms of eye exposure can include redness, pain, and watery eyes. A symptom of Mercury exposure is discoloration of the lens of the eyes.

Symptoms/injuries after ingestion : If Mercury is swallowed, symptoms of such over-exposure can include metallic taste in mouth, nausea, vomiting, central nervous system effects, and damage to the kidneys. Metallic mercury is not usually absorbed sufficiently from the gastrointestinal tract to induce an acute, toxic response. Damage to the tissues of the mouth, throat, esophagus, and other tissues of the digestive system may occur. Ingestion may be fatal, due to effects on gastrointestinal system and kidneys.

Chronic symptoms : Long-term over-exposure can lead to a wide range of adverse health effects. Anyone using Mercury must pay attention to personality changes, weight loss, skin or gum discolorations, stomach pains, and other signs of Mercury over-exposure. Gradually developing syndromes ("Erethism" and "Acrodynia") are indicative of potentially severe health problems. Mercury can cause the development of allergic reactions (i.e. dermatitis, rashes, breathing difficulty) upon prolonged or repeated exposures. Refer to Section 11 (Toxicology Information) for additional data.

SECTION 12: Ecological information

12.1. Toxicity

Ecology - water : Very toxic to aquatic life. Toxic to aquatic life with long lasting effects.

Mercury (7439-97-6)	
LC50 fishes 1	0,5 mg/l (Exposure time: 96 h - Species: Cyprinus carpio)
EC50 Daphnia 1	5,0 µg/l (Exposure time: 96 h - Species: water flea)
LC50 fish 2	0,16 mg/l (Exposure time: 96 h - Species: Cyprinus carpio [semi-static])

12.2. Persistence and degradability

MERCURY (7439-97-6)	
Persistence and degradability	May cause long-term adverse effects in the environment.

12.3. Bioaccumulative potential

MERCURY (7439-97-6)	
Bioaccumulative potential	Not established.

12.4. Mobility in soil

No additional information available

12.5. Other adverse effects

Other information : Avoid release to the environment.

FIGURE 12-9

Sample SDS.

(continues)

(continued)

MERCURY

Safety Data Sheet

according to the federal final rule of hazard communication revised on 2012 (HazCom 2012)

SECTION 13: Disposal considerations

13.1. Waste treatment methods

Waste disposal recommendations	: Dispose in a safe manner in accordance with local/national regulations. Waste disposal must be in accordance with appropriate federal, state, and local regulations. This product, if unaltered by use, should be recycled. If altered by use, recycling may be possible. Consult Bethlehem Apparatus Company for information. If Mercury must be disposed of as hazardous waste, it must be handled at a permitted facility or as advised by your local hazardous waste regulatory authority.
Ecology - waste materials	: Hazardous waste due to toxicity. Avoid release to the environment.

SECTION 14: Transport information

In accordance with DOT

14.1. UN number

UN-No.(DOT)	: 2809
DOT NA no.	UN2809

14.2. UN proper shipping name

DOT Proper Shipping Name	: Mercury
Department of Transportation (DOT) Hazard Classes	: 8 - Class 8 - Corrosive material 49 CFR 173.136
Hazard labels (DOT)	: 8 - Corrosive substances 6.1 - Toxic substances

DOT Symbols	: A - Material is regulated as a hazardous material only when be transported by air, W - Material is regulated as a hazardous material only when be transported by water
Packing group (DOT)	: III - Minor Danger
DOT Packaging Exceptions (49 CFR 173.xxx)	: 164
DOT Packaging Non Bulk (49 CFR 173.xxx)	: 164
DOT Packaging Bulk (49 CFR 173.xxx)	: 240

14.3. Additional information

Other information	: No supplementary information available.

Overland transport

No additional information available

Transport by sea

DOT Vessel Stowage Location	: B - (i) The material may be stowed "on deck" or "under deck" on a cargo vessel and on a passenger vessel carrying a number of passengers limited to not more than the larger of 25 passengers, or one passenger per each 3 m of overall vessel length; and (ii) "On deck only" on passenger vessels in which the number of passengers specified in paragraph (k)(2)(i) of this section is exceeded.
DOT Vessel Stowage Other	: 40 - Stow "clear of living quarters",97 - Stow "away from" azides

Air transport

DOT Quantity Limitations Passenger aircraft/rail (49 CFR 173.27)	: 35 kg
DOT Quantity Limitations Cargo aircraft only (49 CFR 175.75)	: 35 kg

SECTION 15: Regulatory information

15.1. US Federal regulations

Mercury (7439-97-6)	
Listed on the United States TSCA (Toxic Substances Control Act) inventory Listed on SARA Section 313 (Specific toxic chemical listings)	
EPA TSCA Regulatory Flag	S - S - indicates a substance that is identified in a proposed or final Significant New Uses Rule.
SARA Section 313 - Emission Reporting	1,0 %

15.2. International regulations

CANADA

FIGURE 12-9

Sample SDS.

(continues)

(continued)

MERCURY

Safety Data Sheet

according to the federal final rule of hazard communication revised on 2012 (HazCom 2012)

Mercury (7439-97-6)	
Listed on the Canadian DSL (Domestic Sustances List) inventory.	
WHMIS Classification	Class D Division 1 Subdivision A - Very toxic material causing immediate and serious toxic effects Class D Division 2 Subdivision A - Very toxic material causing other toxic effects Class E - Corrosive Material

EU-Regulations

Mercury (7439-97-6)
Listed on the EEC inventory EINECS (European Inventory of Existing Commercial Chemical Substances) substances.

Classification according to Regulation (EC) No. 1272/2008 [CLP]

Classification according to Directive 67/548/EEC or 1999/45/EC

Not classified

15.2.2. National regulations

Mercury (7439-97-6)
Listed on the AICS (the Australian Inventory of Chemical Substances) Listed on Inventory of Existing Chemical Substances (IECSC) Listed on the Korean ECL (Existing Chemical List) inventory. Listed on New Zealand - Inventory of Chemicals (NZIoC) Listed on Inventory of Chemicals and Chemical Substances (PICCS) Poisonous and Deleterious Substances Control Law Pollutant Release and Transfer Register Law (PRTR Law) Listed on the Canadian Ingredient Disclosure List

15.3. US State regulations

Mercury (7439-97-6)				
U.S. - California - Proposition 65 - Carcinogens List	U.S. - California - Proposition 65 - Developmental Toxicity	U.S. - California - Proposition 65 - Reproductive Toxicity - Female	U.S. - California - Proposition 65 - Reproductive Toxicity - Male	No significance risk level (NSRL)
	Yes			

SECTION 16: Other information

Other information : None.

Full text of H-phrases: see section 16:

Acute Tox. 1 (Inhalation:dust,mist)	Acute toxicity (inhalation:dust,mist) Category 1
Acute Tox. 2 (Inhalation)	Acute toxicity (inhalation) Category 2
Aquatic Acute 1	Hazardous to the aquatic environment — AcuteHazard, Category 1
Aquatic Chronic 1	Hazardous to the aquatic environment — Chronic Hazard, Category 1
Repr. 1B	Reproductive toxicity Category 1B
STOT RE 1	Specific target organ toxicity (repeated exposure) Category 1
H330	Fatal if inhaled
H360	May damage fertility or the unborn child
H372	Causes damage to organs through prolonged or repeated exposure
H400	Very toxic to aquatic life
H410	Very toxic to aquatic life with long lasting effects

NFPA health hazard : 3 - Short exposure could cause serious temporary or residual injury even though prompt medical attention was given.

NFPA fire hazard : 0 - Materials that will not burn.

NFPA reactivity : 0 - Normally stable, even under fire exposure conditions, and are not reactive with water.

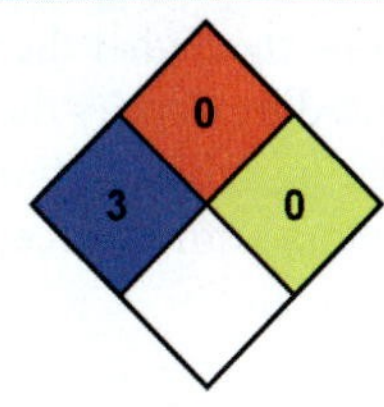

SDS US (GHS HazCom 2012)

This information is based on our current knowledge and is intended to describe the product for the purposes of health, safety and environmental requirements only. It should not therefore be construed as guaranteeing any specific property of the product

FIGURE 12-9

Sample SDS.

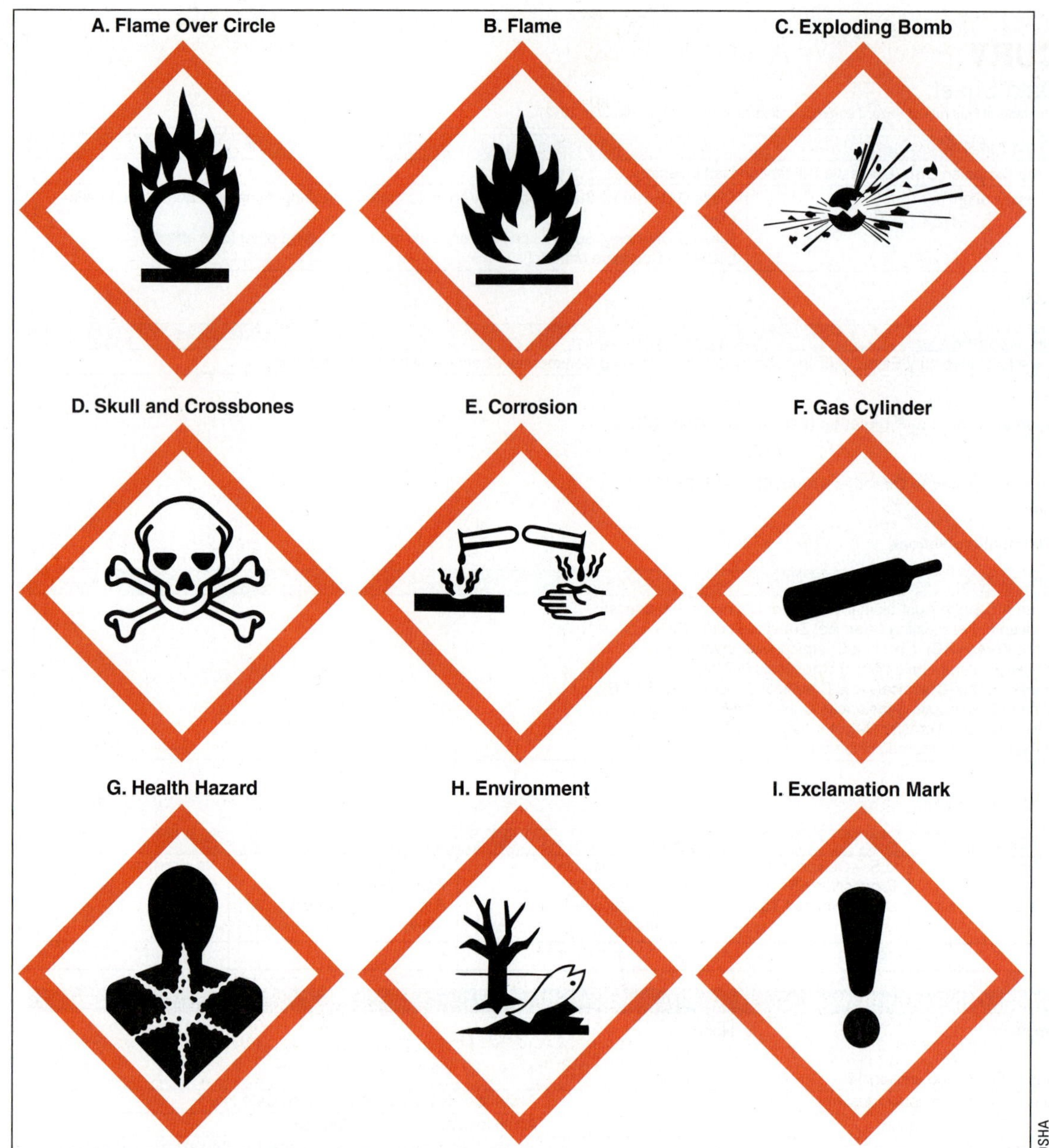

FIGURE 12-10

Hazard communication pictogram.

The level of risk for each category is indicated by the use of numbers, zero to four—the higher the number, the greater the danger. Letters are used to identify the PPE needed.

A chemical warning label, a diamond-shaped symbol, displays the four colors with a place for the numbers to be written on each (Figure 12-12). The employee can quickly identify the hazard category, the risk for each, and the PPE equipment required. All hazardous chemicals must be labeled unless they are poured into separate containers for immediate use (Figure 12-13).

RED: FIRE HAZARD	YELLOW: REACTIVITY
4 = Danger: Flammable gas or extremely flammable liquids	4 = Danger: Explosive at room temperature
3 = Warning: Flammable liquid	3 = Danger: May be explosive if spark occurs or if heated under confinement
2 = Caution: Combustible liquid	2 = Warning: Unstable or may react if mixed with water
1 = Caution: Combustible if heated	1 = Caution: May react if heated or mixed with water
0 = Noncombustible	0 = Stable: Nonreactive when mixed with water
BLUE: HEALTH HAZARD	**WHITE: PPE**
4 = Danger: May be fatal	A Goggles
3 = Warning: Corrosive or toxic	B Goggles, gloves
2 = Warning: Harmful if inhaled	C Goggles, gloves, apron
1 = Caution: May cause irritation	D Face shields, gloves, apron
0 = No unusual hazard	E Goggles, gloves, mask
	F Goggles, gloves, apron, mask
	X Gloves

Courtesy of POL Consultants

FIGURE 12-11

National Fire Protection Association's color and number method.

Chemical Warning Label Determination

The Hazard Communication Act contains specific labeling requirements. Labels must be on all hazardous chemicals that are shipped to and used in the workplace. Labels must not be removed. Material safety data sheets for all chemicals will be available to employees.

Manufacturer Requirements: Chemical manufacturers are required to evaluate chemicals, determine status as hazards, provide material safety data sheets (MSDSs), and label all shipped chemicals properly. Manufacturer labels must never be removed. The best way to determine the hazards of the chemical is to read the MSDS, obtain an OSHA designated list or State Hazardous Substance list. For most mixed chemicals, it is necessary to contact the manufacturer for MSDS.

Office Chemicals: Search through your office and write down all chemicals you have in the office. Most pharmaceuticals and common household products do not come under this standard. Ingredients can then be compared to a list of regulated substances or MSDSs will provide necessary information.

Employer's Responsibility: Any hazardous chemical used in the workplace that is not in its original container **must** be labeled with the identity of the chemical and hazards. "Target Organ" chemical labels may be used. The label must include the chemical and common name, warnings about physical and health hazards, and the name and address of the manufacturer. The employer is to compile a chemical inventory list that is to be updated as needed. MSDS information should be located in a place where it is accessible to all employees. Label and MSDS information should be provided during the safety training program.

Identity: The term *identity* can refer to any chemical or common name designation for the individual chemical or mixture, as long as the term used is also used on the list of hazardous chemicals and the MSDS.

Note: If a chemical is poured into another container for immediate use, it does not need to be labeled.

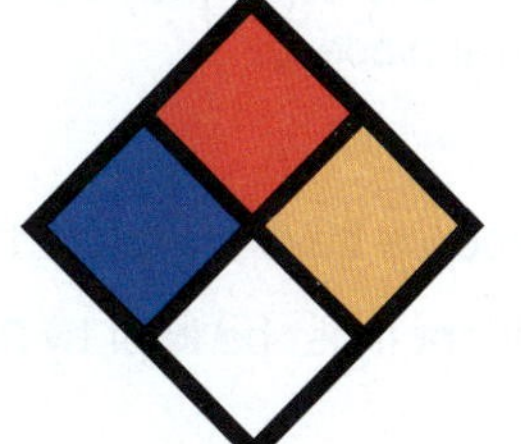

Chemical name ____________

Common name ____________

Manufacturer ____________

Courtesy of POL Consultants

FIGURE 12-12

A chemical warning label.

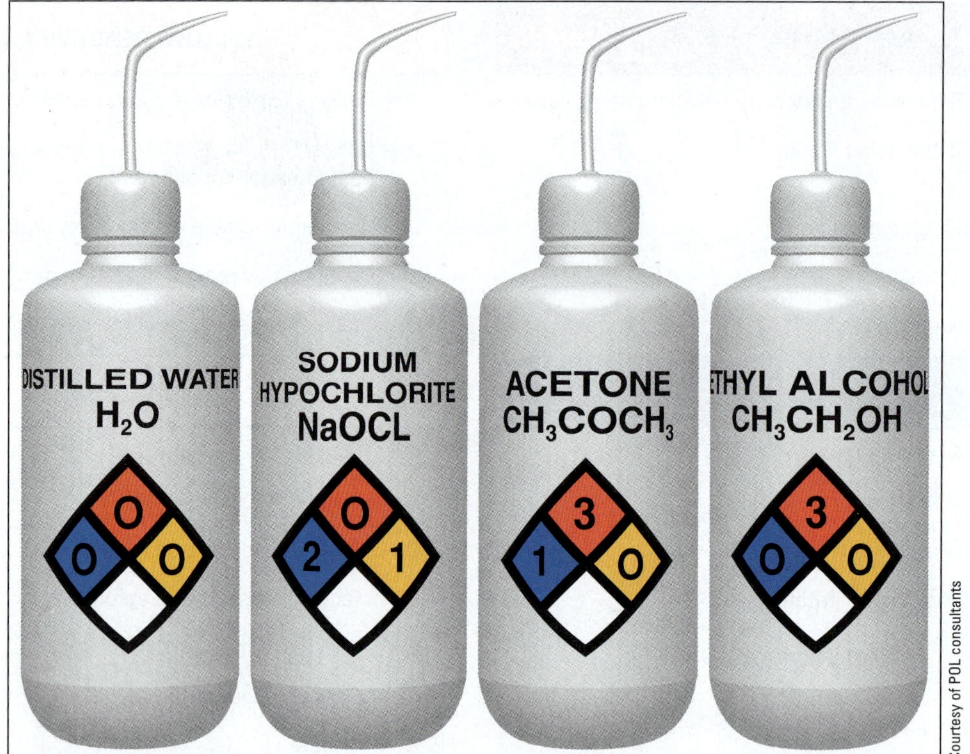

FIGURE 12-13

Containers with chemical warning labels.

Chapter Summary

OSHA regulations, including the hazard communication standard, are intended to require the employer to provide a safe work environment for all employees. The dental assistant must completely understand the entirety of the standard, and how compliance is accomplished. Staff must be trained for a safe workplace. Compliance with all standards must be accomplished to ensure a safe workplace.

CASE STUDY

Rebecca Thomas, a 25-year-old, is a newly hired employee in the office of Dr. Charles. She is working as a chairside dental assistant. She will be completing her first month of employment. A fellow employee is discussing a case with Rebecca and accidentally knocks over a glass container. It breaks into several pieces.

Case Study Review

1. What training should Rebecca have completed?
2. What records of the incident must be kept by Rebecca's employer? For how long must they be kept?
3. What must be used to clean up the broken glass?
4. Where should the pieces of broken glass be disposed?

Review Questions

Multiple Choice

1. The Bloodborne and Hazardous Materials Standard covers all the following *except*
   a. housekeeping.
   b. laundry.
   c. hours of employment.
   d. safety data sheets.
2. An example(s) of engineering or work practice controls is (are)
   a. personal protective equipment.
   b. splash guards on model trimmers.
   c. gloves, masks, and glasses.
   d. dental uniform.
3. After an exposure incident, the employer provides a copy of the health care professional's written opinion within ________days of a completed evaluation.
   a. 5
   b. 10
   c. 15
   d. 30
4. The color and number method often used to label various chemicals was developed by the
   a. Occupational Safety and Health Administration.
   b. American Dental Association.
   c. Environmental Protection Agency.
   d. National Fire Protection Association.
5. A skull and crossbone pictogram indicates
   a. a health hazard.
   b. acute toxicity or fatal.
   c. corrosion.
   d. PPE is needed.
6. Broken glass must be cleaned up and placed in ________.
   a. a plastic bag
   b. a leak-proof sharps container
   c. a cardboard container
   d. a garbage container
7. Yellow on the chemical warning label determination identifies a
   a. fire hazard.
   b. health hazard.
   c. PPE is needed.
   d. reactivity or stability of a chemical.
8. The OSHA hazard communication standard is set up so that the________ receives training about the risks of using hazardous chemicals and the safety precautions.
   a. employee
   b. employer
   c. patient
   d. both a and b
9. The following are accepted work practice controls *except*
   a. no two-handed recapping.
   b. no bending of needles.
   c. mouth pipetting.
   d. handwashing following glove removal.
10. The housekeeping area of the OSHA Bloodborne and Hazardous Materials Standard shows that all of the following must be done *except*
   a. following a written schedule for cleaning and disinfection.
   b. protective covering may be used over equipment.
   c. carpets in all operatories.
   d. If no contamination has occurred, the equipment and surfaces must be cleaned at the end of the work shift.

Critical Thinking

1. Would the scope of the OSHA Bloodborne and Hazardous Materials Standard cover the employee while traveling to the place of employment?
2. Employees have a lunchroom that becomes untidy and disorderly. The dentist never uses the lunchroom. If one of the employees has an accident in the room, who is responsible?
3. Standard precautions are issued by whom? To protect whom?

Web Activities

1. Go to http://www.osha.gov and find information on SDSs and print the two pages of requirements for the OSHA 174 document.
2. Go to http://www.osha.gov and find information about biohazardous waste. Have there been any changes in this area since the publication of this textbook? If so, note these changes and bring information to class for discussion.
3. Go to the Web and identify a source with a list of SDSs. Find two chemicals that are used in the school clinic. Were they on the list you found? What information did you find on the SDSs for the two identified chemicals?

CHAPTER 13

Preparation for Patient Care

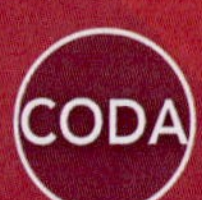

Specific Instructional Objectives

The student should strive to meet the following objectives and demonstrate an understanding of the facts and principles presented in this chapter:

1. Explain how the patient record is developed and the importance of the personal registration form, medical and dental information, clinical evaluation, and the extraoral and intraoral examinations.
2. Describe how the patient record may be called into litigation or used in a forensic case.
3. Perform or assist the dentist in an extraoral and an intraoral evaluation including lips, tongue, glands, and oral cavity.
4. Explain how a diagnosis and treatment plan is developed.
5. Perform vital signs on the patient, including both oral and tympanic temperature, pulse, respiration, and blood pressure.
6. Document the vital signs and be alert to any signs that are abnormal.
7. Identify the five Korotkoff sounds, the two that are used in recording blood pressure, and the man who described them in 1905.

Key Terms

antecubital space (284)
antipyretic (278)
arrhythmia (283)
assessment (275)
asymmetric (275)
baseline vital signs (278)
blood pressure (284)
brachial artery (284)
bradycardia (283)
bradypnea (284)
carotid pulse (281)
Celsius (278)
chronic (271)
chronological order (271)
commissures (276)
consent form (275)
dental history (274)
demographic (271)
diagnosis (278)
diastolic blood pressure (286)
exhalation (284)
Fahrenheit (278)
fever (278)
forensics (271)
hypertension (286)
hypotension (286)
hypothermic (280)
inhalation (284)
Korotkoff sounds (286)
litigation (271)
medical history (271)
palpate (276)
pulse rate (283)
pulse rhythm (283)
pulse volume (283)
radial pulse (281)
referral (275)
registration form (271)
respiration depth (284)
respiration rate (284)
respiration rhythm (284)
smile line (276)
sphygmomanometer (284)
stethoscope (284)
symmetric (275)
systolic blood pressure (286)
tachycardia (283)
tachypnea (284)
temperature (278)
temporal pulse (281)
thermometer (278)
treatment plan (278)
tympanic membrane (280)
tympanic thermometer (280)
vermilion border (276)
vital signs (278)

Introduction

Preparing for patient care is an important part of providing quality dental service to each patient. The dental assistant can begin the process of patient preparation by obtaining personal, medical, and dental history from each patient. After history forms are completed, the dental assistant reviews the information and alerts the dentist to any areas of concern.

Once the patient is in the treatment room, the dental assistant performs or assists the dentist in an evaluation of the patient. This clinical evaluation includes obtaining vital signs and performing both an internal and an external oral evaluation.

Patient Record

Dental team members must thoroughly review a patient's medical history in order to treat the patient effectively. The information must be reviewed and updated at each visit. Most dental offices have a questionnaire for patients to complete. The information is confidential and should be as thorough as possible so that the best possible care is rendered. Sensitive topics may be discussed, such as medications being taken, medical treatment, and other factors contributing to the patient's health. Certain patients may be identified for "premedication" status before dental treatment.

Every dental employee should remember that this record is the primary source of information about this patient and the dentist will use it for developing the diagnosis to provide the patient with the highest standard of dental care. It should be kept extremely accurate and up to date. It could be used in **litigation**, the act or process of seeking or contesting a lawsuit. This patient record could be brought forth in a lawsuit and will reflect on the dental office and employees as well as the patient care that was provided. It could also be used in **forensics**, where the identity of the patient is established though scientific methods by using the charting and radiographs. The record can be either in paper copy or on the computer (Figures 13-1 A & B).

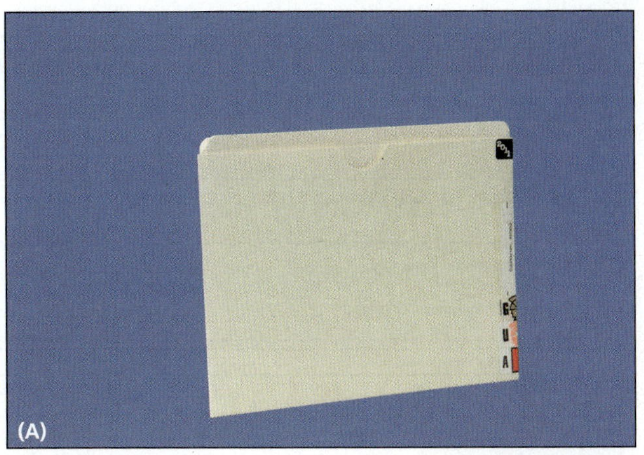

(A)

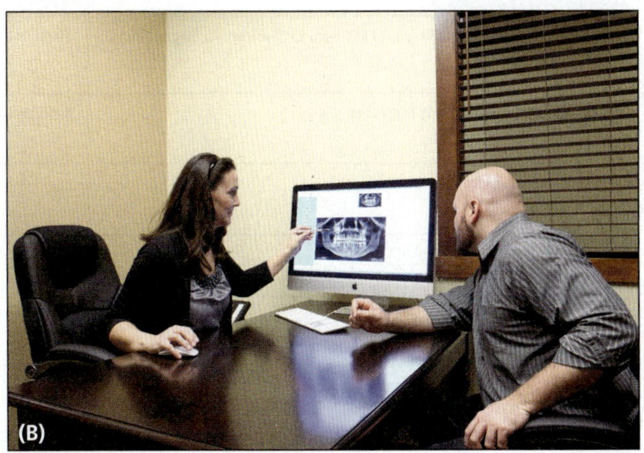

(B)

FIGURE 13-1

(A) File folder of a patient's record and (B) electronic copy of a patient's record.

Patient Registration Form

One of the first steps in caring for patients is to have them complete a patient registration form. It can be either electronic or paper. The paper form consists of a file folder which is identified with the patient's first and last name. The standard folder is 8 1/2 × 11 with a system that fastens the patient forms in place within the folder. Many come with pockets or areas to hold the radiographs. The American Dental Association (ADA) has a form that can be purchased for use in the dental office which covers the medical and dental health history information thoroughly (Figure 13-2). The electronic file mirrors the paper folder in content. However, accessing the information is achieved through a computer search using the patient's name.

Using either the paper or electronic form, the patient is requested to fill out a **registration form**. This includes information on **demographics**, which is a personal history including the following: full name, address, phone number, work number, Social Security number, insurance, emergency contacts, and physician's name and his or her phone number. The registration form also provides financial information about the patient and identifies the individual responsible for payment of the dental services. The dental auxiliary is responsible for ensuring that all information is completed by the patient before any treatment occurs. Some patients may present with a **chronic** condition, which is a medical or dental condition that has lasted a long period of time and may cause long-term changes in the body. Noting this on the chart in a **chronological order** (dates in order of occurrence) and noting the specific details will aid in future research and diagnosis. Also the HIPAA consent forms should be signed at this time (see Chapter 3, Ethics, Jurisprudence, and the Health Information Portability and Accountability Act [HIPAA]).

Medical Information

The patient is also requested to fill out a medical history. The **medical history** contains questions about past surgeries, systemic diseases, injuries, and allergies (Figure 13-2). It is critical for the dental team to know about any allergies that may affect treatment. Normally, the allergies of concern are related to anesthetics, latex, and antibiotics. The patient also should disclose any medical concerns such

Date ____________________

PATIENT NAME	SOCIAL SECURITY NUMBER	HOME PHONE ( )
Home Address	City, State, Zip	Birthdate / /
Marital Status ❑ Single ❑ Married ❑ Divorced ❑ Separated	❑ M ❑ F	Drivers License and State

Primary Insurance Company ____________ Group ____________ Subscriber ____________

Secondary Insurance Company ____________ Group ____________ Subscriber ____________

Responsible Party

NAME	SOCIAL SECURITY NUMBER	HOME PHONE ( )
Home Address	City, State, Zip	Birthdate / /
Marital Status ❑ Single ❑ Married ❑ Divorced ❑ Separated	Relationship to Patient	Drivers License and State
Responsible Person's Employer	Occupation	Work Phone ( )
Business Address	City	State Zip
Spouse's Name	Social Security Number	Birthdate / /
Spouse's Employer	Spouse's Occupation	Spouse's Work Phone ( )
Spouse's Business Address	City	State Zip

How did you hear about our Office?
(check only one)

Who selected this Office? ❑ Self ❑ Spouse ❑ Parent ❑ Employer

Where did you find the Phone Number to this Office?____________

❑ Referred by a friend	❑ Yellow Pages	❑ Relative	❑ Insurance Plan	❑ Welcome Wagon
❑ Other ________	❑ TV/Radio Ad	❑ Newspaper Ad	❑ Direct Mailing	❑ Sign by Building

If you were referred, whom may we thank for referring you?____________

CONSENT

- I will answer all health questions to the best of my knowledge ________
Initial

After explanation by the doctor, I hereby authorize the performance of dental services upon the above named patients and whatever procedures that the judgements of the doctor may decide in order to carry out these procedures. I also authorize and request the administration of any anesthetics and x-rays as may be deemed necessary and advisable by the doctor.

Signature Date Relationship to Patient

TERMS AND CONDITIONS

This office depends upon reimbursement from the patient for the costs incurred in their case. The financial responsibility of each patient must be determined before treatment.
As a condition of treatment by this office. I understand financial arrangements must be made in advance. All emergency dental services, or any dental service performed without prior financial arrangements, must be paid for at the time the services are performed.
I understand that dental services furnished to me are charged directly to me and that I am personally responsible for payment. If I carry insurance, I understand that this office will help prepare my insurance forms to assist in making collections from insurance companies and will credit such collections to my account. However, this dental office cannot render services on the assumption that charges will be paid by a insurance company.

Assignment of Insurance: I hereby authorize releases of any information needed and also authorize my insurance company to pay directly to this Office benefits accruing to me under my policy. I understand that the fee estimate listed for this dental care can only be extended for a period of 90 days form the date of the patient's examination. I also understand that in order to collect my debt, my credit history may be checked through the use of my Social Security Number or any other information I have given you. I agree that in the event that either this office or I institute any legal proceedings with respect to amount owed by me for services rendered, the prevailing party in such proceedings shall be entitled to recover all costs incurred including reasonable attorney's fees.
I grant my permission to you, or your assignee, to telephone me at home or at my work to discuss matters related to this form. I have read the above conditions and agree to their content.

Signed ____________________ **Date** ____________

There may be a charge for any missed appointments or appointments not cancelled 48 hours before the appointment time.

FIGURE 13-2

Dental and medical history.

(continues)

(continued)

PATIENTS DENTAL HEALTH

Why have you come in to see us today? (e.g.: pain, checkup, etc.) ____________

Previous Dentist ____________ Last Visit ____________ Date of last cleaning ____________

Reasons for changing dentists: ____________

What problems have you had with past dental treatment? ____________

Are you nervous about seeing a dentist? ❑ Yes! ❑ No If yes, please tell us why: ____________

How often do you brush? ____________ Do you floss? ❑ Yes ❑ No How often? ____________

(please circle each)

Y N I clench or grind my teeth during the day or while sleeping.
Y N My gums bleed while brushing or flossing.
Y N I like my smile.
Y N I prefer tooth-colored fillings.
Y N I avoid brushing part of my mouth due to pain.
Y N My gums feel tender or swollen
Y N I have problems eating.
Y N I have had orthodontics.
Y N I have had a facial or jaw injury.
Y N I want my teeth straight.
Y N I want my teeth whiter.

What are your dental priorities? ____________
(e.g.: apprentice, dental health, financial considerations, etc.)

PATIENTS MEDICAL HISTORY

I consider my health to be *(please check one)* ❑ Excellent ❑ Good ❑ Fair ❑ Poor

Do you or have you had any of the following? *please circle Y for yes or N for no.*

Doctor Notes Only:

1. Y N Heart Disease
2. Y N Heart Murmur/Mitral Valve Prolapse
3. Y N Stroke
4. Y N Congenital Heart Lesions
5. Y N Rheumatic Fever
6. Y N Abnormal Blood Pressure
7. Y N Anemia
8. Y N Prolonged Bleeding Disorder
9. Y N Tuberculosis or Lung Disease
10. Y N Asthma
11. Y N Hay Fever
12. Y N Sinus Trouble
13. Y N Epilepsy/Seizures
14. Y N Ulcers
15. Y N Implants/Artificial Joints: ❑ Hip ❑ Knee ❑ Other
16. Y N I smoke or use tobacco. If yes, how much per day? _______ How many years?______
17. Y N I have consumed alcohol within the last 24 hours.
18. Y N I usually take an antibiotic prior to dental treatment.
19. Y N Have you ever taken Fen-Phen or Redux?
20. Y N I have had major surgery: Year ________ Type of operation: ____________ Year ______ Type of opeartion: ____________
21. Y N Do you have any other medical problem or medical history NOT listed on this form? ____________
22. Y N Liver Disease
23. Y N Jaundice
24. Y N Hepatitis Type ______
25. Y N Diabetes
26. Y N Excessive Urination and/or Thirst
27. Y N Infectious Mononucleosis (Mono)
28. Y N Herpes
29. Y N Arthritis
30. Y N Sexually Transmitted/Venereal Disease
31. Y N Kidney Disease
32. Y N Tumor or Malignancy
33. Y N Cancer/Chemotherapy
34. Y N Radiation Treatment
35. Y N History of Drug Addiction
36. Y N AIDS
37. Y N Immune Suppressed Disorder
38. Y N Hearing Loss
39. Y N Fainting Spells
40. Y N Glaucoma
41. Y N History of Emotional or Nervous Disorders

WOMEN

42. Y N Are you taking birth control medication?
43. Y N Are you or could you be pregnant or nursing?

Are you allergic to any of the following?
Please circle Y for yes or N for no

44. Y N Aspirin
45. Y N Ibuprofen
46. Y N Sulfa Drugs/Sulfites/Sulfides
47. Y N Penicillin
48. Y N Codeine
49. Y N Latex, Metals, Plastics
50. Y N Local Anesthetics (Novocaine)
51. Y N Other Medications - Which ones? ____________

Please list all medications you are currently taking:

Medicine ____________ Condition ____________
Medicine ____________ Condition ____________
Medicine ____________ Condition ____________
Medicine ____________ Condition ____________
Physician's Name____________ Phone ____________
Address ____________ Fax ____________

In the event of an emergency please contact:

Name ____________ Relationship ____________ Phone ____________
Name ____________ Relationship ____________ Phone ____________

Initial medical/dental health reviewed by:

X ____________ / ____ / ____ X ____________ / ____ / ____
Doctor's Signature — Date — Patient's Signature — Date

Periodic medical/dental health reviewed by:

X ____________ / ____ / ____ X ____________ / ____ / ____
Doctor's Signature — Date — If patient is a minor: Parent/Guardian's Signature — Date

FIGURE 13-2

Dental and medical history.

as epilepsy, diabetes, or a heart condition. Allergies and medical alerts are to be noted on the inside of the patient record to bring them to the attention of dental team members (Figure 13-3). Any drugs the patient has taken recently or is currently taking should be recorded on the medical history. Often, a variety of questions are asked to gain the information needed. The assistant should tactfully question any abnormalities. Usually, any "yes" answers on a questionnaire require further inquiry. Computerized software programs automatically print copies of the medical alert when the daily schedule prints. Numerous icons and colors are used on the medical history to identify concerns. This provides added notification of patients who may require special accommodations.

Dental Information

Questions regarding the patient's **dental history** (Figure 13-2) are included in the patient's record. This information alerts the dental assistant to any concerns the patient has regarding his or her current dental health. It also gives insight into any concerns the patient may have had regarding previous dental care.

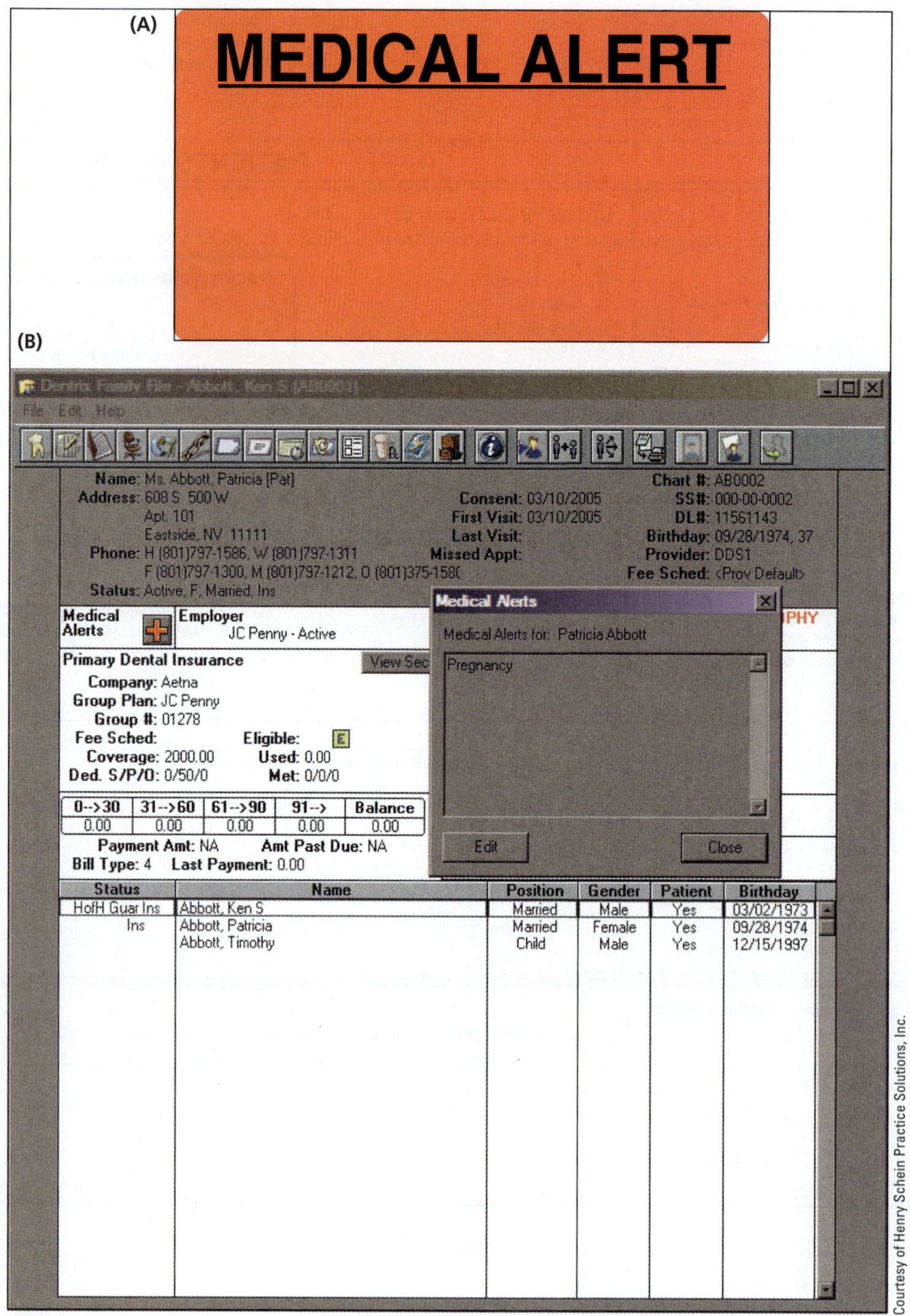

Courtesy of Henry Schein Practice Solutions, Inc.

FIGURE 13-3

(A) Allergy and medical alert sticker. (B) Electronic medical alert.

The last dental examination is noted, as well as the patient's last dental appointment and how often the patient seeks dental treatment. Some questions are asked regarding the patient's attitude toward dentistry and how he or she maintains his or her own personal oral health care.

Upon completion of the patient history, the patient signs and dates the form. This record provides the dentist and staff with useful information so that they may provide better care for the patient. The dentist and/or dental assistant will review the answers prior to initiation of treatment. The personal and medical history should be reviewed prior to each treatment series. It is the dentist's ethical and legal responsibility to gain information about the patient's medical history prior to dental treatment. The highest degree of confidentiality must be maintained by the dental team regarding the patient's history.

After thoroughly reviewing the patient's personal and medical/dental history and collecting the appropriate data, the patient is seated.

Clinical Observation and Physical Assessment

The dental assistant observes patients as they are escorted into the treatment room. If the patient displays any deviation from normal, such as walking with an abnormal gait, further probing into the health history may be required. The assistant may notice speech or behavior problems that should be brought to the dentist's attention. Looking at the patient's face for symmetry is the first step in the oral inspection. Although most individuals do not have faces that are totally **symmetric** (meaning that if the face was divided in half, the other half would be a mirror image), each side of the face should look fairly similar. If one eyelid droops, for example, or if the face is **asymmetric**, this should be noted on the patient's chart. The dental assistant also evaluates the patient's eyes and facial skin for any scars or abnormalities in color or texture. An overall **assessment**, a judgment about the patient's health based on an understanding of the situation and the upcoming treatment, is completed by the auxiliary and the findings are reported to the dentist. In most states the dental assistant is allowed to perform the initial intraoral and extraoral dental examination; however, most often the dentist performs this with the auxiliary's assistance during the initial comprehensive examination.

Clinical Setting

When the patient is brought into the dental operatory in the clinical setting, he or she is made comfortable. If the patient is going to have a general anesthetic or an invasive procedure performed, it is necessary for the patient to sign a **consent form**. By signing a consent form the patient gives formal permission for treatment. Implied consent is given if the patient is coming in for an initial examination. If the patient has been referred from another dentist for treatment, the dental team needs to have the **referral** (Figure 13-4). A referral occurs when a patient is sent to another dentist, usually a dental specialist, for a consult or treatment. The referral should be reviewed carefully to ensure that the recommended treatment is followed. The dentist may have the auxiliary proceed with dental radiographs, which can be taken with either standard radiography or digital radiography.

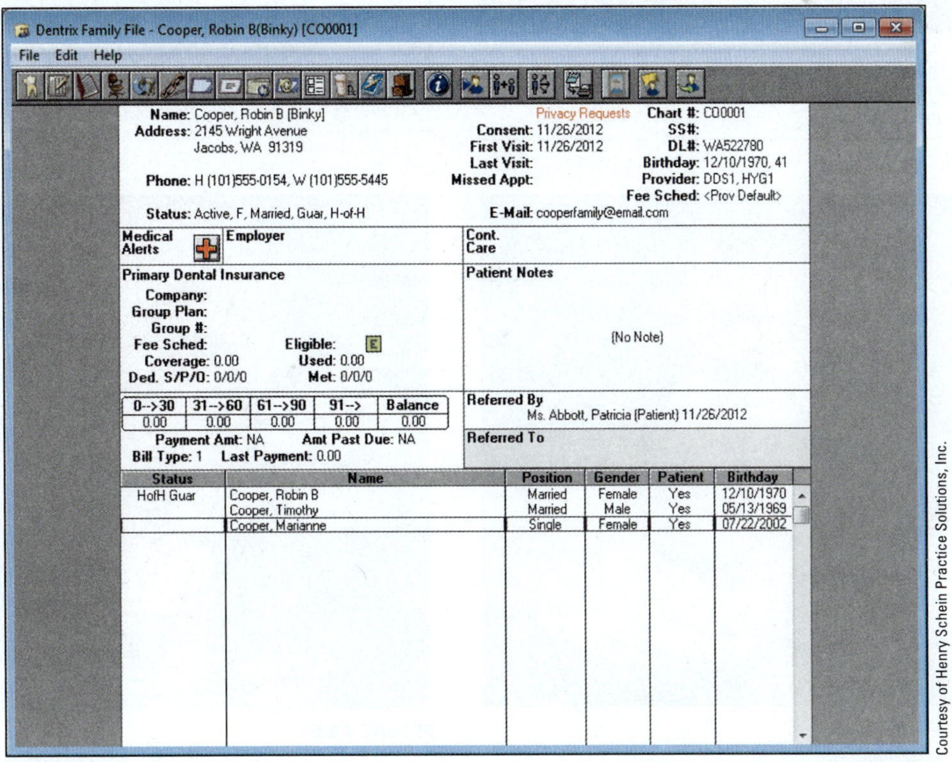

Dentrix Family File - Cooper, Robin B(Binky) [CO0001]

File Edit Help

Name: Cooper, Robin B [Binky]
Address: 2145 Wright Avenue
Jacobs, WA 91319
Phone: H (101)555-0154, W (101)555-5445
Status: Active, F, Married, Guar, H-of-H

Privacy Requests
Consent: 11/26/2012
First Visit: 11/26/2012
Last Visit:
Missed Appt:
E-Mail: cooperfamily@email.com

Chart #: CO0001
SS#:
DL#: WA522780
Birthday: 12/10/1970, 41
Provider: DDS1, HYG1
Fee Sched: <Prov Default>

Medical Alerts | Employer | Cont. Care

Primary Dental Insurance
Company:
Group Plan:
Group #:
Fee Sched: Eligible: E
Coverage: 0.00 Used: 0.00
Ded. S/P/O: 0/0/0 Met: 0/0/0

Patient Notes
(No Note)

0-->30	31-->60	61-->90	91-->	Balance
0.00	0.00	0.00	0.00	0.00

Payment Amt: NA Amt Past Due: NA
Bill Type: 1 Last Payment: 0.00

Referred By
Ms. Abbott, Patricia (Patient) 11/26/2012

Referred To

Status	Name	Position	Gender	Patient	Birthday
HofH Guar	Cooper, Robin B	Married	Female	Yes	12/10/1970
	Cooper, Timothy	Married	Male	Yes	05/13/1969
	Cooper, Marianne	Single	Female	Yes	07/22/2002

FIGURE 13-4

Electronic referral form.

Courtesy of Henry Schein Practice Solutions, Inc.

Clinical Examination

Examine the lips for cracking and dryness. The dental assistant also observes the **smile line** (where the lips are when the patient smiles), the **vermilion border** (the line around the lip), and the **commissures** (the corners of the lips) (Figure 13-5). Any deviations from normal are noted on the patient's chart. The assistant may place an accepted lip lubricant on the patient's lips prior to the examination to ensure the patient's comfort.

The next area to be examined is the external floor of the mouth and the cervical lymph nodes. The floor of the mouth is examined with the patient's mouth closed. The dental assistant palpates the soft tissues in the area with the fingers, checking for any abnormalities (Figure 13-6).

The cervical lymph nodes are examined by having the patient turn his or her head to the side. The dental assistant gently feels the chain of lymph nodes from the ear to the collar bone. This is done on the opposite side of the neck as well (Figure 13-7).

The last external area to be examined is the temporomandibular joint (TMJ). The dental assistant sits behind the patient's head to **palpate** (feeling with the fingers or hand) the joint as the patient opens and closes his or her mouth. Also, the dental assistant places a finger from each hand just anterior to the tragus of each ear and has the patient open and close his or her mouth (Figure 13-8). The operator listens for any noise in the TMJ, such as clicking, and feels for any catching as the patient's mouth opens. Any symptoms, pain, or tenderness is noted on the patient's chart.

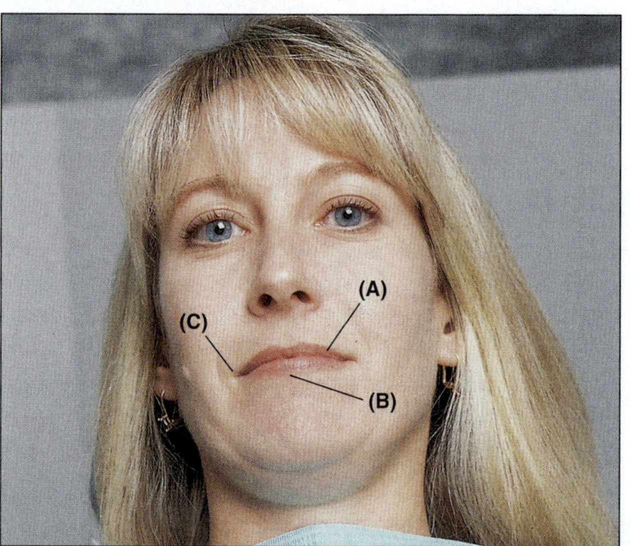

FIGURE 13-5
Visually examining (A) the smile line, (B) the vermilion border, and (C) the commissures of the lip.

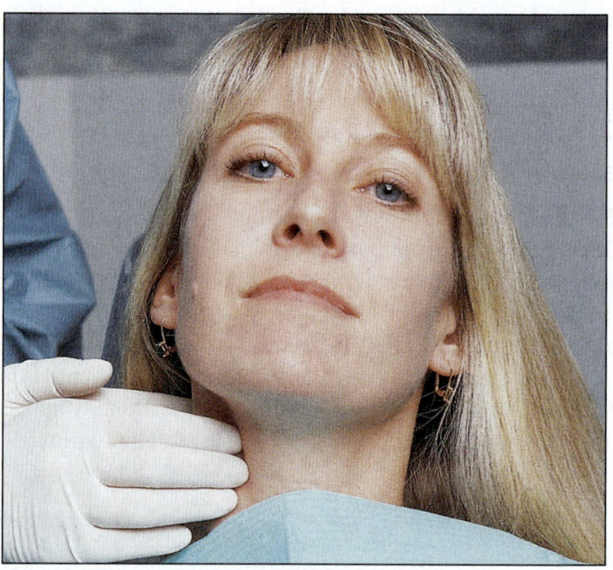

FIGURE 13-7
Examining the cervical lymph nodes.

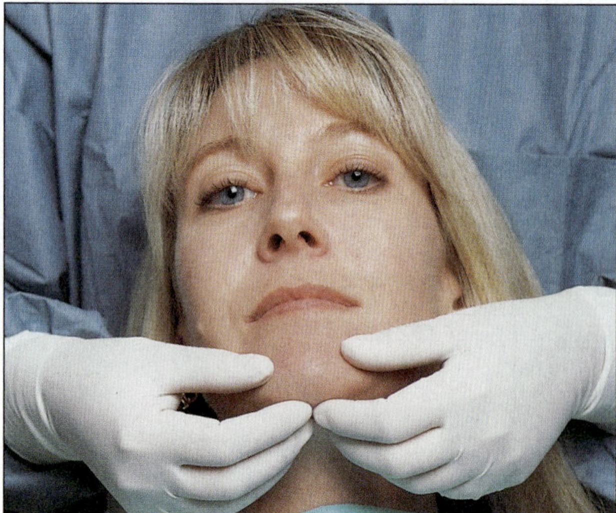

FIGURE 13-6
Examining the external tissues of the mandible and the floor of the mouth.

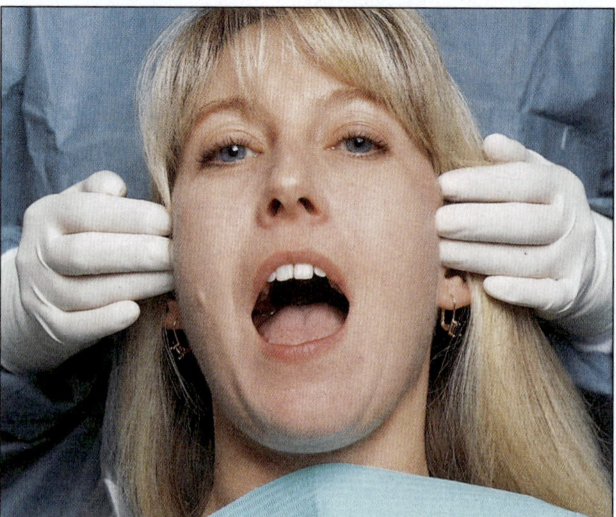

FIGURE 13-8
Examining the temporal mandibular joint as the patient opens and closes her mouth.

At the beginning of the internal oral examination, the operator first does a quick visual assessment, looking for any obvious problems. Problems could include lesions in the mouth, abscessed teeth, or color changes in the oral mucosa. The operator examines the tissues of the floor of the mouth. This is accomplished by supporting the mandible with one hand while gently palpating with the fingers of the other hand on the ventral sides of the tongue and the floor of the mouth (Figure 13-9). The mucosa and the frena of the upper and lower lips are examined by gently pulling the lips out and inspecting the area (Figure 13-10). The mouth mirror is used in the maxillary and mandibular buccal area. Using the mirror, the palate and the posterior of the tongue are examined visually (Figure 13-11).

The last area in the oral cavity to be examined is the tongue. A gauze sponge is needed to grasp the tongue. Placing the gauze around the tip of the tongue, the operator pulls to the side to visually inspect the posterior area on each side and then lifts to examine the under portion of the tongue (Figure 13-12). During this time, the patient is asked to say "ah-ah," therefore allowing the operator to examine the uvula and the tissues of the oropharynx.

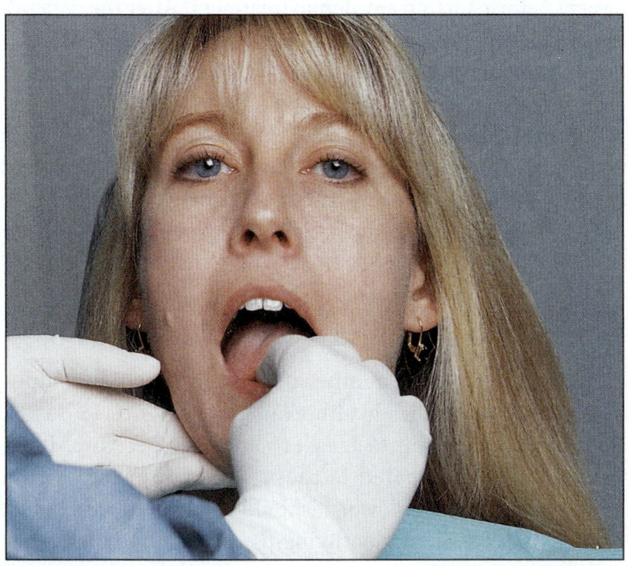

FIGURE 13-9

Operator (dentist or dental assistant) performing an intraoral examination of the floor of the mouth.

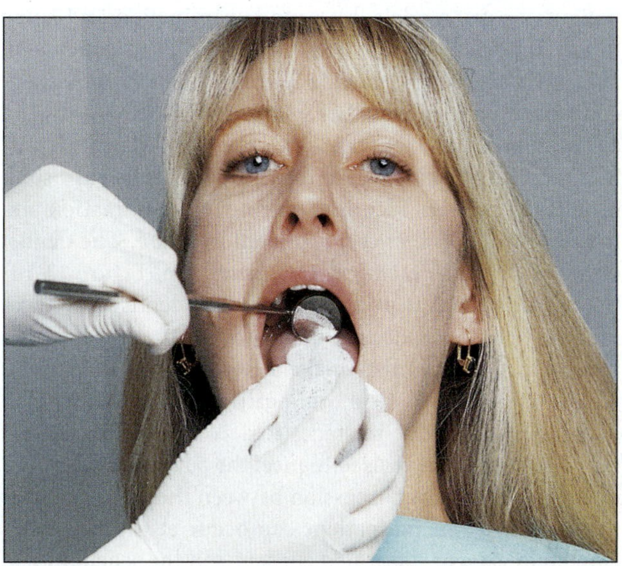

FIGURE 13-11

Examining the palate and the posterior of the tongue using a mouth mirror.

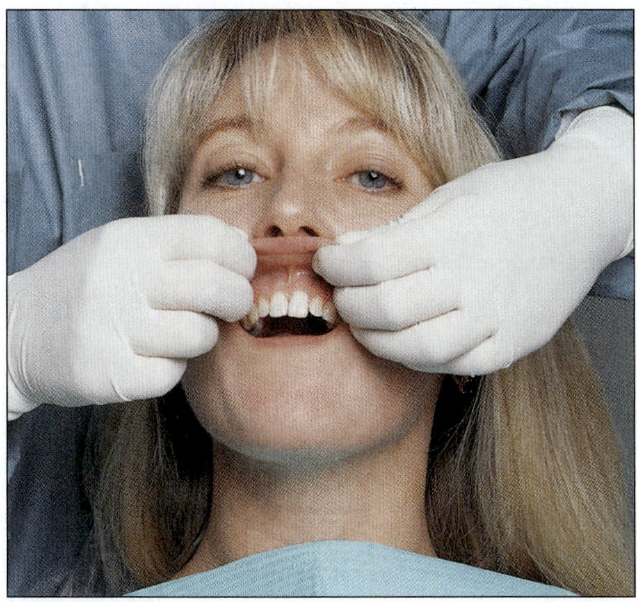

FIGURE 13-10

Examining the oral mucosa and the frenum.

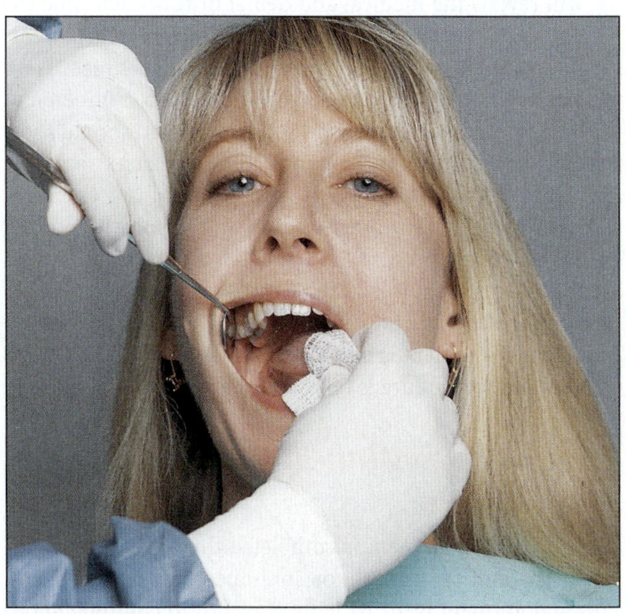

FIGURE 13-12

Examining the tongue using a gauze sponge on the tip of the tongue.

After completion of the extraoral examination, the intraoral examination begins along with dental charting (see Chapter 14, Dental Charting). Each tooth is evaluated by the dentist and the findings are noted on the dental chart portion of the dental record. In addition, periodontal charting is completed to establish the health of the gum and bone tissue (see Chapter 31, Periodontics). The dentist may order additional diagnostic items such as study models or bites that will aid in giving the patient a complete diagnosis.

Diagnosis and Treatment Plan

The dentist will evaluate the information obtained from the patient, x-rays, models, bites, and examination and come to a **diagnosis**. The diagnosis is a decision or conclusion reached by the dentist that identifies any dental problems or concerns for the patient. The treatment will be identified in a **treatment plan** (Figures 13-13A and B), where the dentist will record the plan of care for this patient. It will list all problems that were identified during the examination and the review of all other diagnostic information. The dentist or auxiliary will present the treatment plan (Figure 13-14) to the patient and answer questions. The dentist may show models, books, or videos to the patient indicating expected outcomes. Most dentists make a treatment plan that will restore the patient's ideal oral health. The treatment plan may have to be done in stages to accomplish this task. It may also have to be revised to meet the patient's budget and insurance concerns. Discussion between the dentist and/or the auxiliary and the patient can occur at the treatment plan appointment. Informed consent and the scheduling of appointments usually occur at this time.

Treatment Notes

As the treatment takes place, the dental assistant and dentist will review the medical and dental history each time the patient visits, update the information, and proceed with treatment. Treatment notes are entered on the patient's record and usually begin with the current date, the tooth number, and the specific treatment that occurred. This record should show the anesthetic given, any reactions, and the dental treatment (i.e., what was done during this appointment). Any entries in this area must be very precise, clear, and legible. If entering on the computer, be sure to include all aspects of the treatment that was completed. The dentist and auxiliary should sign the treatment notes in ink and date the information. Each time the patient is in for dental treatment, the record is updated and procedure is followed.

Recall or Continued Care Appointment

After the final treatment is completed the office will schedule the patient for a recall, or continued care appointment. This appointment is for patients of record to continue under the care of the dentist. Most offices schedule patients in 3 to 12 months for their next appointment to make sure that this follow-up will help the patient maintain his or her oral health (see Chapter 40, Dental Office Management).

Vital Signs

The **vital signs** are the basic signs of life. They include body temperature, pulse, blood pressure, and respiration rate. The initial measurements of vital signs are **baseline vital signs**. Baseline vital signs help the dentist compare subsequent measurements with the initial measurements.

The measuring and recording of vital signs is an important part of the health evaluation, and should be done with every patient before starting any dental treatment. After the patient's history is completed and the patient is seated, the dental assistant can obtain vital signs. Vital signs give the dental operator specific information about the physical and emotional condition of the patient. They may point out previously undetected abnormalities. Vital signs, along with the overall patient health information and any pain that the patient reports to the dentist, aid in planning the patient's dental treatment and are essential during emergency treatment.

Body Temperature

Measurement of body **temperature** is an essential component of every patient's health evaluation (Figure 13-15). A **thermometer** is used to measure body temperature. Body temperature is compared to the normal body temperature range and, if higher or lower, it should be further investigated. A range is used when identifying the normal body temperature, because temperature varies from person to person and throughout the day. It is well known that after exercise, emotional excitement, and even eating, temperature rises. A person's face may turn red and blush due to excitement, increasing body temperature. Temperature in young children and young infants will vary more than in adults.

Normal Temperature Ranges

Normal range in Fahrenheit	99.5°
	98.6° (average)
	96.0°
Normal range in Celsius	37.5°
	37.0° (average)
	35.5°

On the **Fahrenheit** scale, the freezing point of water is 32°F and the boiling point of water is 212°F. On the **Celsius** scale, the freezing point of water is 0°C and the boiling point of water is 100°C.

The patient has a **fever** if he or she is above the normal range. An **antipyretic**, often used to reduce fever, could include cold packs, alcohol rubs, acetaminophen, nonsteroidal

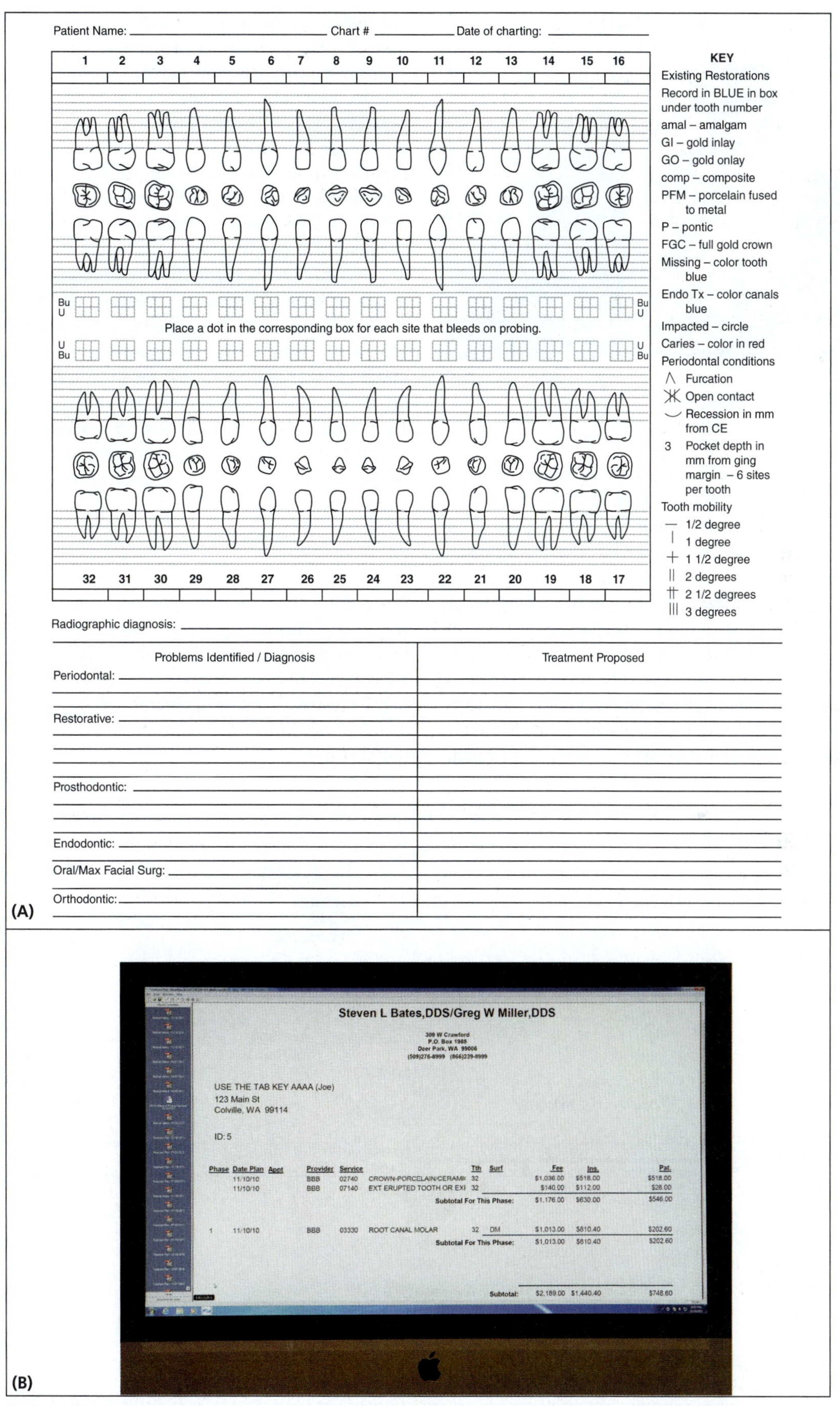

(A)

Patient Name: ______________ Chart # __________ Date of charting: __________

1 2 3 4 5 6 7 8 9 10 11 12 13 14 15 16

Bu U

Place a dot in the corresponding box for each site that bleeds on probing.

U Bu

32 31 30 29 28 27 26 25 24 23 22 21 20 19 18 17

KEY

Existing Restorations
Record in BLUE in box under tooth number
amal – amalgam
GI – gold inlay
GO – gold onlay
comp – composite
PFM – porcelain fused to metal
P – pontic
FGC – full gold crown
Missing – color tooth blue
Endo Tx – color canals blue
Impacted – circle
Caries – color in red
Periodontal conditions
Λ Furcation
Open contact
Recession in mm from CE
3 Pocket depth in mm from ging margin – 6 sites per tooth
Tooth mobility
— 1/2 degree
| 1 degree
+ 1 1/2 degree
|| 2 degrees
╫ 2 1/2 degrees
||| 3 degrees

Radiographic diagnosis: ______________

Problems Identified / Diagnosis	Treatment Proposed
Periodontal:	
Restorative:	
Prosthodontic:	
Endodontic:	
Oral/Max Facial Surg:	
Orthodontic:	

(B)

Steven L Bates,DDS/Greg W Miller,DDS

309 W Crawford
P.O. Box 1988
Deer Park, WA 99006
(509)276-8999 (866)239-8999

USE THE TAB KEY AAAA (Joe)
123 Main St
Colville, WA 99114

ID: 5

Phase	Date Plan	Appt	Provider	Service		Tth	Surf	Fee	Ins.	Pat.
	11/10/10		BBB	02740	CROWN-PORCELAIN/CERAMI	32		$1,036.00	$518.00	$518.00
	11/10/10		BBB	07140	EXT ERUPTED TOOTH OR EXI	32		$140.00	$112.00	$28.00
					Subtotal For This Phase:			$1,176.00	$630.00	$546.00
1	11/10/10		BBB	03330	ROOT CANAL MOLAR	32	DM	$1,013.00	$810.40	$202.60
					Subtotal For This Phase:			$1,013.00	$810.40	$202.60
					Subtotal:			$2,189.00	$1,440.40	$748.60

FIGURE 13-13

(A) paper treatment plan for the patient record and (B) electronic treatment plan as part of the patient record.

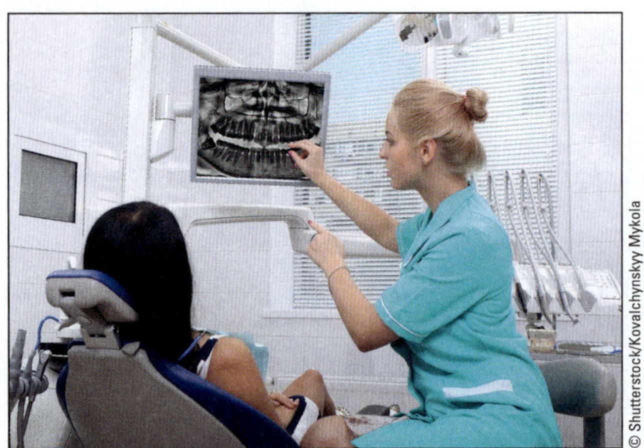

FIGURE 13-14
Dentist or auxiliary reviewing treatment plan with patient.

anti-inflammatory over the counter (OTC) drugs, or an aspirin. A patient is said to be **hypothermic** if the body temperature is below normal. Hypothermia could be caused from prolonged exposure to cold and/or an overdose of antipyretic drugs, such as aspirin.

Temperature can be measured using either a manual or digital thermometer. Procedure 13-1 presents an overview of how to measure temperature using a digital thermometer. If the manual thermometer is used, place it under the tongue to remain in place with the lips closed for 5 minutes. The manual thermometer is filled with mercury, which is a hazardous chemical; if breakage occurs, it must be disposed of properly.

If a digital thermometer is used to obtain the temperature, dispose of the probe cover in a biohazard waste container.

A **tympanic thermometer** (an ear thermometer) (Figure 13-16) has become very popular for taking a temperature, especially on young children. It is placed gently in the ear canal, an infrared signal is bounced off the **tympanic membrane** or the ear drum, and the reading appears within a few seconds. This procedure (Procedure 13-2, Taking a Tympanic Temperature) is easily performed because it does not involve an open mouth, congestion in the nasal cavity, difficulty breathing through the nose, length of time to obtain the reading, and the many other contraindications for taking an oral temperature. The only contraindication for the tympanic thermometer is that too much ear wax will not allow for a correct reading. Dental offices do not routinely take a temperature unless the situation arises where the information is needed; however, it is always beneficial to have knowledge and an understanding of temperature, the role it plays in health, and the normal temperature ranges.

Pulse

The pulse is the intermittent beating sensation felt when the fingers are pressed against an artery. A pulse rate is determined by palpation. Do not use the thumb to palpate, because it has a pulse of its own and could throw off the readings. Pulse may be palpated on one of several arteries: the radial, carotid, or temporal. The dental assistant most commonly uses the radial artery.

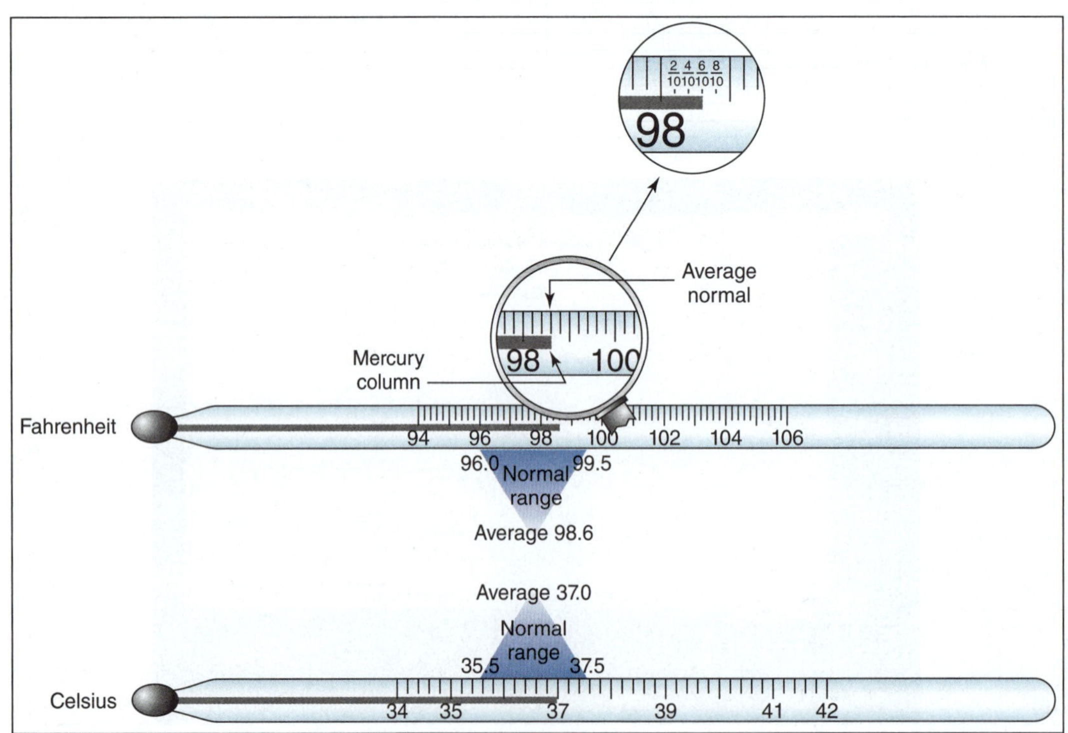

FIGURE 13-15
Fahrenheit and Celsius thermometers with the normal ranges indicated.

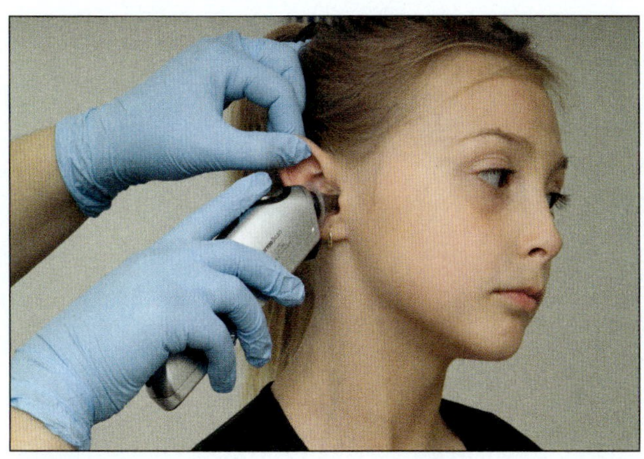

FIGURE 13-16
Tympanic thermometer.

Radial Pulse Site. The **radial pulse** site is located on the radial artery, on the thumb side of the wrist (Figure 13-20). It can be found approximately one inch above the base of the thumb. This is the most common site used for obtaining pulses in the dental office.

Carotid Pulse Site. The **carotid pulse** site is located on the carotid artery in the neck just below the angle of the mandible (Figure 13-21). It is normally large and therefore easy to locate.

Temporal Pulse Site. The **temporal pulse** site is over the smaller temporal artery located in the temporal fossa, which is a slight depression just in front of the ear at about the level of the eyebrow (Figure 13-22). The temporal pulse is more difficult to locate than the radial or carotid.

Procedure 13-1
Taking an Oral Temperature Using a Digital Thermometer

This procedure is performed by the dental assistant in order to obtain the patient's body temperature.

Equipment and Supplies

- Digital thermometer
- Probe covers
- Biohazard waste container

Procedure Steps (*Follow standard precautions*)

1. Wash hands.
2. Assemble the thermometer and probe cover.
3. Seat the patient in the dental treatment room and position him or her comfortably in an upright position.
4. Verify that the patient has not had a hot or cold drink or smoked within the last half hour. (This may give a false temperature reading.)
5. Explain the procedure to the patient.
6. Verify that the thermometer is at 0. Position the new probe cover on the digital thermometer (Figure 13-17).
7. Insert the probe under the tongue to either side of the patient's mouth.

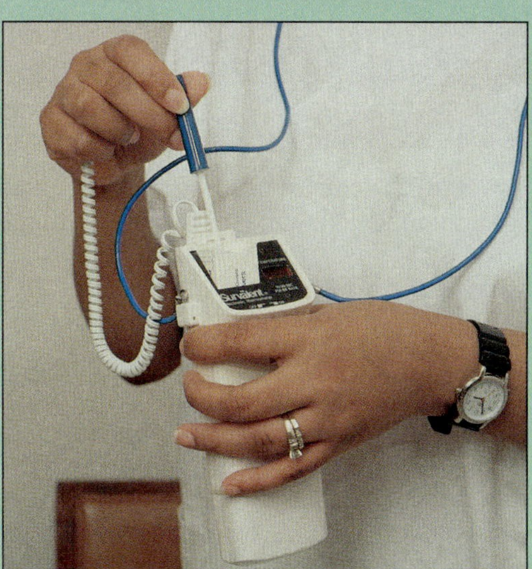

FIGURE 13-17
Slide the probe into the disposable cover, adjusting if necessary.

8. Instruct the patient to carefully close his or her lips around the probe without biting down on it (Figure 13-18).
9. Leave the probe in position until the digital thermometer beeps.
10. Remove the probe from the patient's mouth.

(continues)

Procedure 13-1 (continued)

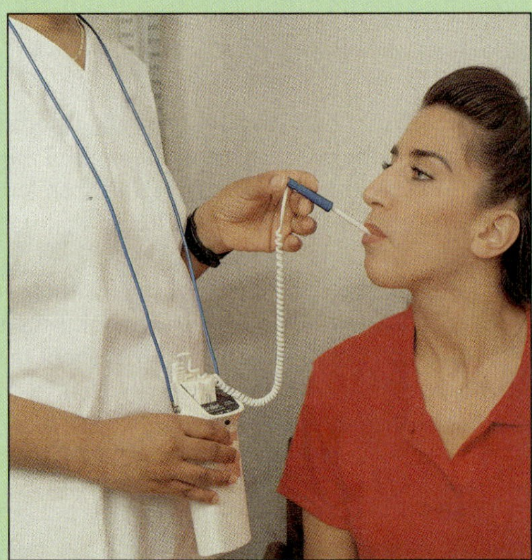

FIGURE 13-18
Insert the thermometer under the tongue and instruct the patient to close the lips around it.

11. Read the results from the digital thermometer display window.
12. Dispose of the probe cover in a hazardous waste container.
13. Wash hands.
14. Document the procedure and record the results on the patient's chart.

Procedure 13-2
Taking a Tympanic Temperature

This procedure is performed by the dental assistant in order to obtain the patient's body temperature.

Equipment and Supplies

- Tympanic thermometer
- Probe covers
- Instructions for thermometer. There are so many on the market that it is important to read the instructions before using the thermometer that was purchased. Normally the following steps are used.

Procedure Steps (*Follow standard precautions*)

1. Take the thermometer out of its holder.
2. Place a new, disposable probe cover on the tip of the thermometer.
3. If taking a child's temperature, hold the head so it does not move; adults should hold their head stable.
4. For children, gently pull the ear straight back and for an adult, gently pull the ear up and then back and gently place the probe of the thermometer in the canal of the ear (Figure 13-19). Do not force the probe, because it is not to touch the ear drum.

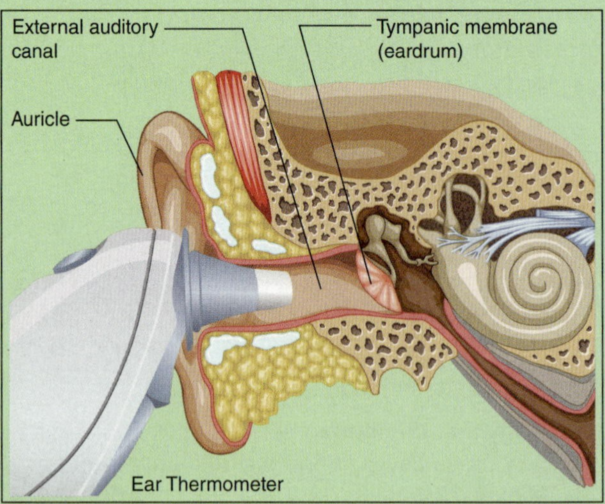

FIGURE 13-19
Gently enter the ear canal with a tympanic thermometer.

(continues)

Procedure 13-2 (continued)

5. Press the button to turn on the thermometer. Most thermometers have the button held until it beeps. If this is not the directions on the thermometer that is being used, follow the manufacturer's directions.
6. After the beep, remove the thermometer from the ear opening. The temperature should be displayed in the window on the device.
7. The temperature can be written down and the time noted and dated.
8. Dispose of the probe cover, and place the thermometer back into its holder.

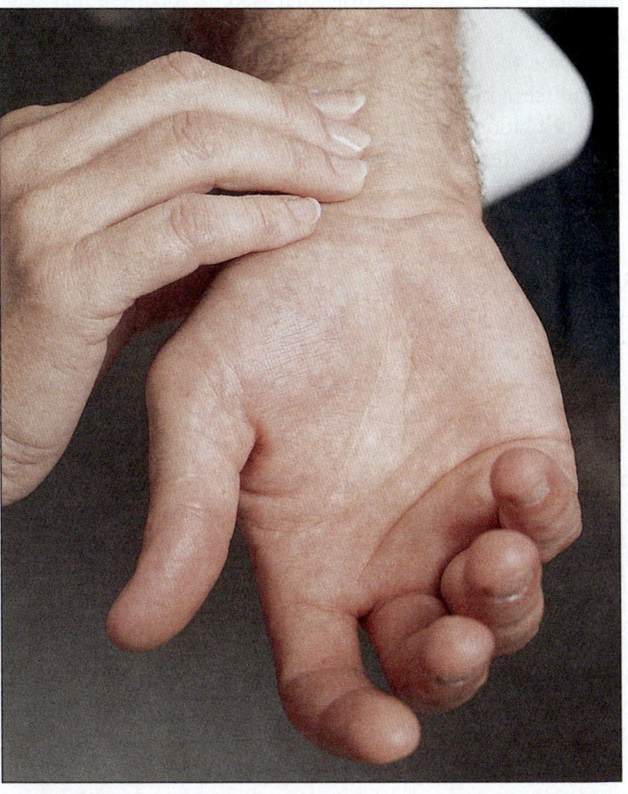

FIGURE 13-20
Radial pulse site.

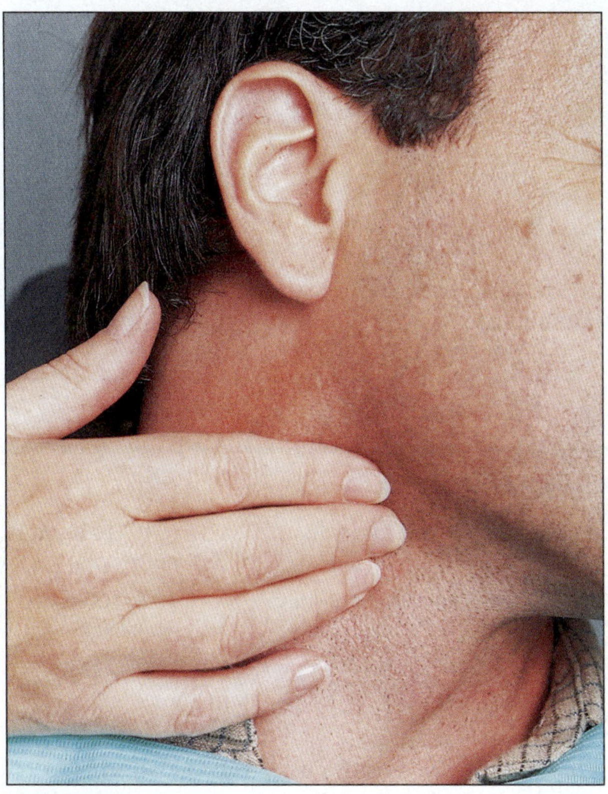

FIGURE 13-21
Carotid pulse site.

Pulse Characteristics. When a pulse is taken and documented there are several characteristics that can be noted. The **pulse rate**, or beats per minute, is always noted on the chart. The **pulse rhythm**, which notes the regular expansion and contraction of an artery caused by the heart pumping blood through the body, may also be described. It is often described as irregular, slow, or rapid. The term used when describing the strength of the pulse is the **pulse volume**. The dental assistant would say that the pulse has either a strong or a weak beat.

Taking a Pulse. After locating the pulse site, the dental assistant determines the number of beats per minute. This varies depending on the patient's age, sex, and physical and mental conditions. It is expressed in a range without an absolute number. An abnormally rapid resting pulse rate is called **tachycardia** and **bradycardia** is an abnormally slow resting heart rate.

The dental assistant must ensure that the patient is positioned with his or her arm level or lower than the level of the heart to get an accurate reading. Ensure that the arm is supported and extended. Most operators take the pulse for at least 30 seconds and then double that noted rate. Anything less than 30 seconds will not allow the operator to determine any **arrhythmia** (irregular) heartbeat patterns.

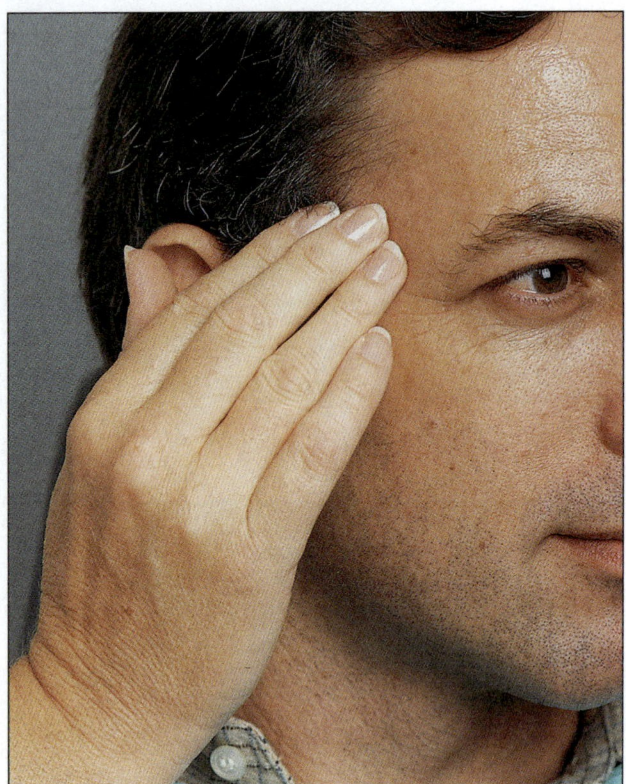

FIGURE 13-22
Temporal pulse site.

Normal Pulse Rates

- Normal pulse rate for adults 60 to 100 beats per minute
- Normal pulse rate for children 70 to 100 beats per minute

Respiration

Respiration is one breath taken in (**inhalation**) and one breath let out (**exhalation**). To ensure an accurate reading—during which the patient is unaware that respiration is being measured—take it after obtaining the pulse rate. Leave the fingers over the pulse site and count the breaths in and out for one minute; this provides the patient's **respiration rate**. The patient will assume that the pulse is still being taken. An abnormally rapid resting respiratory rate is called **tachypnea** and **bradypnea** is an abnormally slow resting respiratory rate. There are similarities in respiration and pulse rates. Children have a more rapid respiration rate; generally—as with the pulse rate—the younger the child, the faster the rate.

Along with the rate of respirations, the dental assistant should record the **respiratory rhythm**, or the breathing pattern, and the **respiration depth**, the amount of air that is inhaled and exhaled, which is recorded as shallow, deep, and so on. Other notations about the breath sounds that are heard, such as raspy, wheezy, and so on, should be documented on the chart.

Normal Respiration Rates

- Normal respiration rate in adults 12 to 18 respirations per minute
- Normal respiration rate in children 20 to 40 respirations per minute

Procedure 13-3 overviews the steps used in obtaining a pulse and a respiration rate.

Blood Pressure

A patient's **blood pressure** is an important indicator of the health of a patient's cardiovascular system. A patient may have heart disease and still feel good and look outwardly healthy. However, the fear of dental treatment may be stressful enough to induce a heart attack. Therefore, taking and recording a patient's blood pressure are very important. It is not done in all offices today, often because the dental assistants have not been trained to perform this skill. Take time to learn this skill!

Some dental offices have purchased automatic blood pressure machines that record blood pressure digitally. A number of models on the market today require very little training. One that works well is placed on the wrist and inflates and records readings readily.

Blood pressure is measured by placing a **sphygmomanometer**, a "blood pressure apparatus," (Figure 13-24) around the **brachial artery**. This apparatus is a cloth-covered inflatable rubber bladder used to control the flow of blood in the artery. There is a rubber hand bulb and pressure control valve attached to one tube and a pressure gauge attached to a second tube. The brachial artery is palpated. It is located at the inside of the elbow in the **antecubital space**, the indented area, as the arm is stretched straight.

Position the arm at the patient's heart height. After the brachial artery is located, the cuff of the sphygmomanometer can be placed one inch above the bend in the elbow and secured. The dental assistant then uses the **stethoscope**, an instrument used to hear and amplify the sounds produced by the heart (Figure 13-25). The stethoscope has two earpieces that must be placed in the ears in a forward position. At the end piece of the stethoscope is a diaphragm, which does the amplification and sends the sounds up the tubing to the ears. The dental assistant pumps up the cuff, which closes off the blood in the artery, and then slowly lets the air escape.

Before taking the patient's blood pressure, the assistant should estimate the systolic pressure using the "palpate, inflate, obliterate, deflate" method. While listening with the stethoscope, the assistant places the cuff on the patient's arm above the antecubital space and palpates the radial pulse. Then the assistant slowly inflates the cuff just until the pulse is obliterated, memorizes the number (mm Hg), and releases the pressure in the bulb. Next the assistant adds 30 mm Hg to the number representing the pulse obliteration point. This number is an estimate of the systolic pressure and gives a target point to inflate the cuff. It is best not to overinflate the cuff

Procedure 13-3
Taking a Radial Pulse and measuring the Respiration Rate

This procedure is performed by the dental assistant in order to obtain the patient's pulse and respiration rate.

Equipment and Supplies

- Watch with a second hand

Procedure Steps (*Follow standard precautions*)

1. Wash hands.
2. Position the patient in a comfortable position, upright in the dental chair (same position used for taking the temperature).
3. Explain the procedure.
4. Have the patient position the wrist resting on the arm of the dental chair or counter.
5. Locate the radial pulse by placing the pads of the first three fingers over the patient's wrist.
6. Gently compress the radial artery so that the pulse can be felt.
7. Using the watch with the second hand, count the number of pulsations for one full minute (Figure 13-23).
8. Note any irregular rhythm patterns.

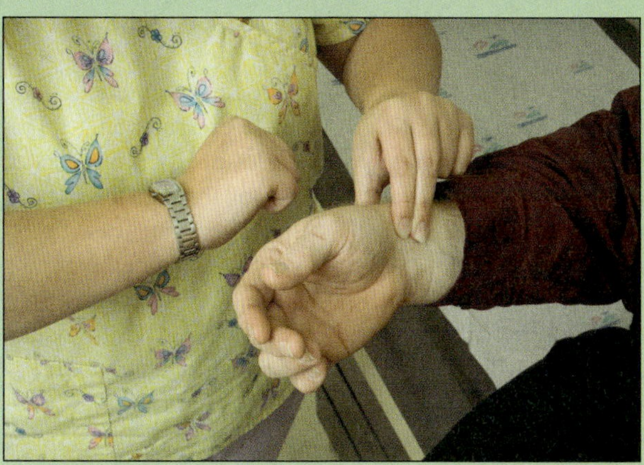

FIGURE 13-23
Taking patient's radial pulse and respiration.

9. While still keeping the finger pads placed on the radial pulse, count the rise and fall of the chest wall for one minute. This allows the patient to breathe normally due to the fact that he or she believes the pulse is still being recorded.
10. Record the number of respirations per minute. Note any irregularities in the breathing.
11. Wash hands.
12. Document the procedure and the pulse and respiration rates on the patient's chart.

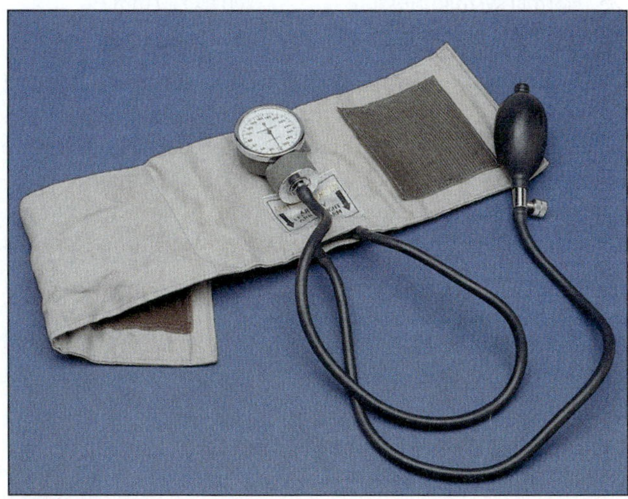

FIGURE 13-24
Aneroid sphygmomanometer.

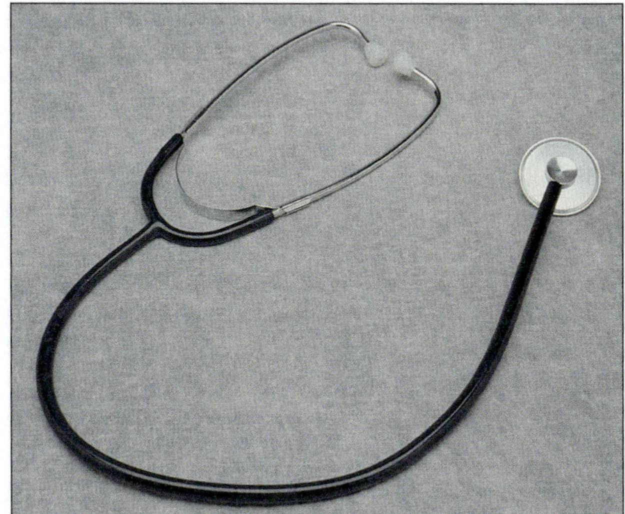

FIGURE 13-25
A single-head stethoscope, which is used with a sphygmomanometer to measure blood pressure.

and cause any additional discomfort to the patient's arm. The dental assistant should then wait one minute before reinflating. (For example, if the pulse obliterates at 120 mm Hg, add 30 for an estimated inflation of 150 mm Hg. This technique is accurate about 95 percent of the time.)

The dental assistant is now ready to begin taking the blood pressure and inflates the cuff to the estimated pressure. While listening carefully to the sounds, the assistant slowly deflates the cuff.

The assistant listens to the first pulsation sound and notes where the needle is indicating on the pressure gauge. This first sound indicates **systolic blood pressure**, which is created when the heart contracts and forces blood through the arteries. Listening carefully, the dental assistant then watches the pressure gauge until the pulsation sound disappears. This reading is noted on the gauge as the **diastolic blood pressure**. The diastolic blood pressure is created as the arteries return to their original state when the heart relaxes between contractions.

Many fully automatic, one-button operation units are available for easy use. They can come with the arm cuff or the wrist cuff. Most units have automatic inflation and deflation control. The display shows the systolic, diastolic, and pulse reading simultaneously with date and time stamp. They require batteries and, depending on the unit, store from 10 to a 100 readings for later review. The wrist units (Figure 13-26) are often used in dental offices because of convenience and time savings.

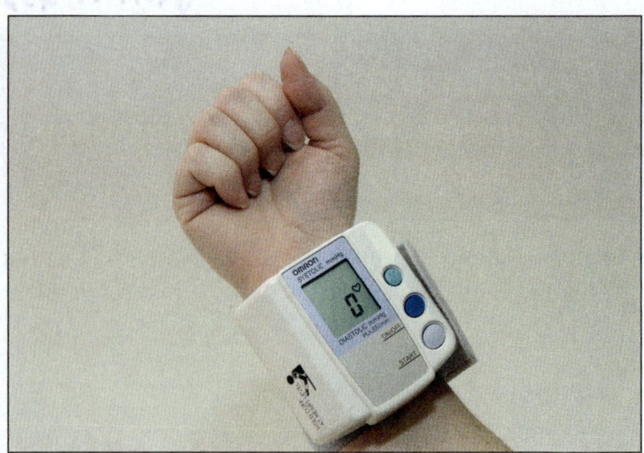

FIGURE 13-26
Wrist unit for measuring blood pressure and obtaining a pulse.

The Five Korotkoff Sounds. In 1905, a Russian physician, Dr. Nikolai Korotkoff, described the sounds that are heard when medical personnel listen through a stethoscope while they are taking blood pressure, using a non-invasive procedure. These sounds (called **Korotkoff sounds**) are not audible if the patient is without arterial disease; nor are they audible if the cuff is inflated above the systolic blood pressure, because that would mean that the blood flow is occluded, much like when pinching a rubber hose closed so that water is not allowed to flow through it. As the blood begins to flow in spurts it results in a turbulence that produces an audible sound. As the pressure in the cuff becomes less, thumping sounds continue to be heard, and then as the cuff pressure continues to go down the sounds change, become muted, and then disappear altogether when the diastolic blood pressure is noted. This is where the cuff is no longer restricting the flow of blood.

Korotkoff described the five types of sounds he heard between the systolic blood pressure and the diastolic blood pressure:

1. The first Korotkoff sound is the snapping sound first heard at the systolic pressure. Clear, repetitive, tapping sounds for at least two consecutive beats are considered the systolic pressure.
2. The second sounds are the murmurs heard for most of the area between the systolic and diastolic pressures.
3. The third sound was described as a loud, crisp, tapping sound.
4. The fourth sound, at pressures within 10 mm Hg above the diastolic blood pressure, was described as "thumping" and "muting."
5. The fifth Korotkoff sound is silence as the cuff pressure drops below the diastolic blood pressure. The disappearance of sound is considered the diastolic blood pressure—2 mm Hg above the last sound heard.

The second and third Korotkoff sounds have no known clinical significance.

Recording Blood Pressure

Two measurements are always recorded when taking blood pressure. They are recorded as a fraction—the systolic pressure is the upper figure and the diastolic pressure is the lower figure. They are always recorded in even numbers (the gauge has indications for even numbers only). There is no absolute number for normal blood pressure; it is recorded in ranges, much like other vital signs. Children normally have lower pressure and, as adults age, the blood pressure goes up. Some, however, use 120 over 80 as an average for an adult. This means 120 systolic over 80 diastolic pressure, recorded as 120/80. Normal blood pressure range is as follows:

- Normal systolic pressure 100 to 140 mm Hg
- Normal diastolic pressure 60 to 90 mm Hg

A higher-than-normal blood pressure is called **hypertension**, and a lower-than-normal blood pressure is called **hypotension**. An increase in the diastolic pressure is more significant than an increase in the systolic pressure, because it indicates that the heart is working harder. Procedure 13-4 presents the steps involved in measuring a blood pressure.

Normal Blood Pressure Readings

Child 10 years of age	100/66
Adolescent 16 years of age	118/76
Adult	Systolic below 140
	Diastolic below 90

Procedure 13-4
Obtaining Blood Pressure from a Patient

This procedure is performed by the dental assistant in order to obtain the patient's blood pressure.

Equipment and Supplies

- Stethoscope
- Sphygmomanometer
- Disinfectant and gauze

Procedure Steps (*Follow standard precautions*)

One of the best resources to review for updates on procedures on measuring blood pressure is the American Heart Association (AHA). See http://www.heart.org.

1. Wash hands.
2. Assemble the stethoscope and sphygmomanometer and disinfect the earpieces of the stethoscope.
3. Position the patient in a comfortable position, upright in the dental chair (same position used for taking the temperature).
4. Explain the procedure.
5. Have the patient position the arm resting at heart level either on the counter or on the arm of the dental chair.
6. Have the patient remove any outer clothing that is restrictive to the upper arm. Bare the upper arm and palpate the brachial artery (Figure 13-27).
7. Center the bladder of the cuff securely, about one inch above the bend of the elbow. Inflate the cuff slowly and palpate the radial pulse until the pulse is obliterated. Release the pressure. Add 30 mm Hg to the number representing the pulse obliteration point. Wait one minute before reinflating the cuff.
8. Position the earpieces of the stethoscope in a forward manner into the ears.
9. Place the diaphragm of the stethoscope over the brachial artery and hold it in place with a thumb. Place other fingers under the elbow to hyperextend the artery. (By extending the elbow, the artery can be accessed more easily and enable better reading of the blood pressure.)
10. Inflate the cuff using the bulb and the control valve on the sphygmomanometer. If the cuff is not inflating, recheck the control valve on the sphygmomanometer to ensure that it is closed. Air should not be escaping. The inflation should be to a level identified in Step 7 during the "palpate, inflate, obliterate, and deflate" technique.
11. Deflate the cuff at a rate of 2 to 4 millimeters of mercury per second by rotating the control valve just slightly (Figure 13-28).
12. Listen for the first sound and note its measurement on the scale.

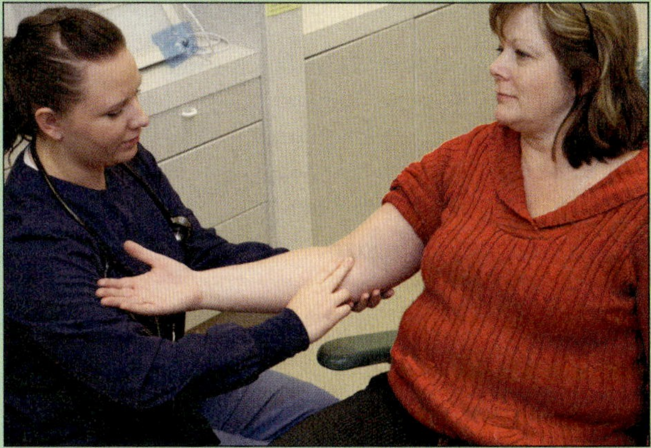

FIGURE 13-27
Palpating patient's brachial artery.

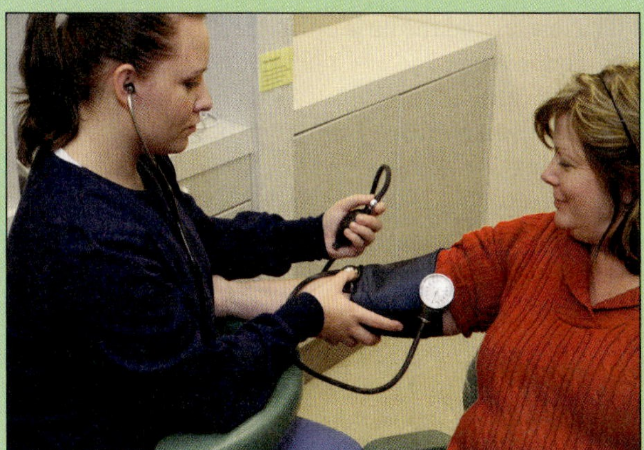

FIGURE 13-28
Taking a patient's blood pressure.

(continues)

Procedure 13-4 (continued)

13. Continue to deflate the cuff and listen to the pulsing sounds. Note when all sounds disappear. Continue deflating for another 10 millimeters to ensure that the last sound has been heard.
14. The cuff can then be deflated rapidly and removed from the patient's arm.
15. Disinfect the earpieces of the stethoscope.
16. Wash hands and record the procedure and the measurement on the patient's chart. (Remember that blood pressure is recorded in even numbers in a fraction format with the systolic measurement on top.)

Chapter Summary

The health condition of a dental patient must be kept private and confidential and updated at each visit. To treat a patient effectively, the patient's chart should include personal history, medical information, dental history, clinical observation, clinical evaluation, and vital signs.

CASE STUDY

Dwayne Allen, a 50-year-old male, was in the dental office for a dental examination. Upon taking his blood pressure, the dental assistant documented that Dwayne had a systolic pressure of 150 and a diastolic pressure of 90.

Case Study Review

1. Is Dwayne's blood pressure within the normal range?
2. Should the blood pressure be retaken to ensure that it was completed accurately?
3. Should this reading be brought to the attention of the dentist?

Review Questions

Multiple Choice

1. The line around the lip is called the
   a. commissure.
   b. smile line.
   c. vermilion border.
   d. frenum.
2. The corners of the lips are called the
   a. commissures.
   b. smile lines.
   c. vermilion borders.
   d. frena.
3. The initial measurement of vital signs are the
   a. pulse.
   b. respiration.
   c. fever.
   d. baseline.
4. The normal range in body temperature, in Fahrenheit, is
   a. 95°–100°.
   b. 96°–99.5°.
   c. 97°–99°.
   d. 96.5°–98.5°.
5. An average range for a child's pulse rate is
   a. 60 to 90 beats per minute.
   b. 70 to 100 beats per minute.
   c. 80 to 110 beats per minute.
   d. 90 to 120 beats per minute.
6. An antipyretic is used to
   a. evaluate pulse rate.
   b. evaluate blood pressure.
   c. locate the temporal pulse site.
   d. reduce fever.
7. If a patient is said to be hypothermic, the body temperature is
   a. above normal.
   b. below normal.
   c. not affected.
   d. none of the above.

8. Bradypnea is an abnormally
   a. rapid resting respiratory rate.
   b. slow resting respiratory rate.
   c. higher than normal blood pressure.
   d. lower than normal blood pressure.
9. The normal range for systolic blood pressure is
   a. 100 to 140 mm Hg.
   b. 100 to 120 mm Hg.
   c. 60 to 90 mm Hg.
   d. 80 to 100 mm Hg.
10. The normal range for diastolic blood pressure is
   a. 120 to 140 mm Hg.
   b. 100 to 120 mm Hg.
   c. 60 to 90 mm Hg.
   d. 80 to 100 mm Hg.

Critical Thinking

1. What temperature would constitute a fever for a child? What effects on dental treatment would a fever pose?
2. A patient has had a negative experience with his or her teeth in the past. What impact could this have on the current treatment? What role can the dental assistant play in making this a positive experience for the patient?
3. If a dental assistant observes a patient walking with an unsteady gait to the dental treatment room but finds no indication of this symptom in the patient's medical and dental history, what should the assistant do?

Web Activities

1. Go to http://www.ada.org, click on *Oral Health Topics*, and locate "Canker Sores, Cold Sores & Common Mouth Sores." Be prepared to come to class and discuss the differences between the canker sores and the cold sores.
2. Go to the Web and complete a search for medical thermometers. Identify several new models on the market and bring this information back to class for a discussion on which one would be best utilized in the dental office.
3. Go to http://www.ada.org, click on *Oral Health Topics*, and locate the topic of "TMJ" (Temporal Mandibular Joint) and identify what percent of American adults suffer from chronic facial pain.

CHAPTER

14

Dental Charting

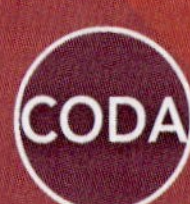

Specific Instructional Objectives

The student should strive to meet the following objectives and demonstrate an understanding of the facts and principles presented in this chapter:

1. Explain why charting is used in dental practices.
2. Identify charts that use symbols to represent conditions in the oral cavity.
3. List and explain the systems used for charting the permanent and deciduous dentitions.
4. Define G. V. Black's six classifications of cavity preparations.
5. List common abbreviations used to identify simple, compound, and complex cavities.
6. Describe basic dental charting terminology.
7. Explain color indicators and identify charting symbols.

Key Terms

abscess (297)
abutment (298)
bridge (297)
cantilever bridge (298)
caries (296)
crown (298)
denture (298)
diastema (298)
drifting (298)
Fédération Dentaire Internationale (FDI) system for numbering (291)
furcation (298)
gingival recession (298)
gold foil (298)
incipient (298)
Maryland bridge (298)
mobility (298)
occlude (291)
overhang (298)
Palmer System for numbering (291)
partial dentures (298)
periodontal pocket (298)
pontic (298)
restoration (298)
root canal (298)
sealant (298)
Universal/National System for numbering (291)

Introduction

CDA Recording the conditions in the patient's oral cavity on a document using symbols, numbers, and colors is a shorthand technique called charting. Charting, either manual or computer, is used in all dental offices. Numerous symbols and various types of charts are used; therefore, the dental assistant must identify the doctor's preferred system to ensure accurate charting. Charting is part of the patient's legal record maintained in the office. As with all legal and medical records, each patient's chart should be complete and correct. The initial charting is normally accomplished during the patient's first examination. Dentists dictate their findings to dental assistants, who chart them on a tooth diagram or by computerized charting. The doctor indicates existing conditions, dental services that have been completed, and dental services that have not been completed. The patient's dental record (chart) is used for billing purposes, diagnosis, and consultation. Forensic dentistry also uses the patient's dental record to provide information and to identify individuals involved in homicides, abuse, or other tragedies.

Dental Charts

There are several types of dental charts. Each chart has an area designed for dental charting and an area in which to record treatment. The most commonly used chart is one with diagrams of the teeth that may show an anatomic or a geometric representation of the teeth. Most charts show both the permanent and the primary dentition. The anatomical charts show either the crown of the tooth, the crown and a small portion of the root, or the crown and the complete root (Figure 14-1A). The geometric charts show the teeth as circles. Each circle represents one tooth and is sectioned into five areas indicating the corresponding surfaces of the tooth (Figure 14-1B). Each dental office chooses the chart deemed best for its current needs.

Numbering Systems

Dental offices have several numbering systems available for their use, and dentists indicate the preferred systems to be used in their offices. All patient records in a given office are documented according to a single numbering system to prevent confusion.

Universal/National System for Numbering

In 1968, the American Dental Association (ADA) adopted the **Universal/National System for numbering**. This numbering system is currently the most commonly used in the United States (Figure 14-2). Each permanent tooth has its own number, starting from the maxillary right third molar as #1 and moving clockwise to the maxillary left third molar as #16. The mandibular left third molar is #17, and the mandibular right third molar is #32. Therefore, #1 and #32 **occlude** together (normal contact with another tooth on the opposite arch when the mouth is closed) and #16 and #17 occlude together. Always remember that teeth #1 and #32 are located on the patient's right side, so that they are not reversed during charting. The primary teeth are each given either a letter or a "d" preceded by a number. The maxillary right deciduous second molar is lettered "A" or "1d," and this continues across the maxillary arch, with the maxillary left second deciduous molar identified as "J" or "10d." The mandibular left second deciduous molar is "K" or "11d," and this continues across the mandibular arch, with the mandibular right second deciduous molar lettered as "T" or "20d." Most standardized charts in the United States come with diagrams of the primary and permanent teeth using the Universal System for numbering (Figure 14-3).

Fédération Dentaire Internationale (FDI) System for Numbering

The International Standards Organization (ISO) Technical Committee (TC) 106 designated a system for identifying teeth and areas of the oral cavity. TC 106 is the technical committee of the ISO that deals with dentistry. It is widely used in Canada and European countries. This system is designed to provide an international system for coding teeth and the oral cavity. In 1996, the ADA adopted this system and the Universal System for tooth numbering. The **Fédération Dentaire Internationale (FDI) system for numbering** can be adapted easily to the computer and is widely used in most other countries (Figure 14-4). With this system, each quadrant is assigned a number. The oral cavity is given two digits. If 00s are noted, the whole oral cavity is designated. If 01 is used, it designates the entire maxillary arch; 02 designates the entire mandibular arch. For example, a full denture on the upper (maxillary) arch is noted as "denture 01."

The permanent dentition is identified by a 1 for the upper right quadrant, 2 for the upper left quadrant, 3 for the lower left quadrant, and 4 for the lower right quadrant. The deciduous dentition is assigned 5 through 8 for the corresponding quadrants. Each quadrant is numbered from 1 to 8, starting with the centrals and ending with the molars. The primary teeth are numbered from 1 to 5 in the same manner (Figure 14-5). When the FDI system is used, the quadrant number is recorded first. For example, the maxillary right lateral incisor is numbered 12 in the permanent dentition, and the maxillary right lateral incisor in the deciduous dentition is 52.

Palmer System for Numbering

The **Palmer System for numbering** and lettering the teeth is used in some dental offices (Figure 14-6). With this system, the permanent teeth are numbered 1 through 8 in each quadrant. The centrals are 1 and the third molars are 8. With each number, a quadrant bracket is used to denote which quadrant it is referring to. For example, the maxillary right first bicuspid is charted as 4. The deciduous teeth are identified in a similar manner except that the teeth are lettered "A" through "E" for each quadrant. "A" represents the central incisors and "E" represents the primary second molars. Again, the quadrant bracket is used to denote which quadrant it is referring

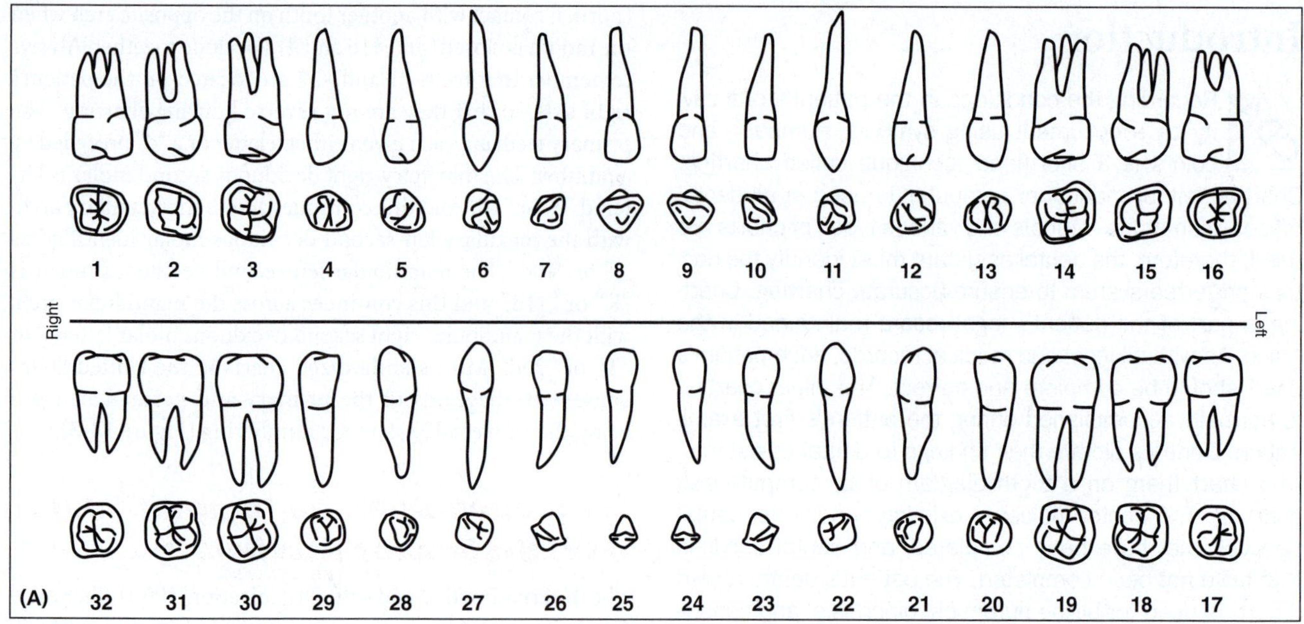

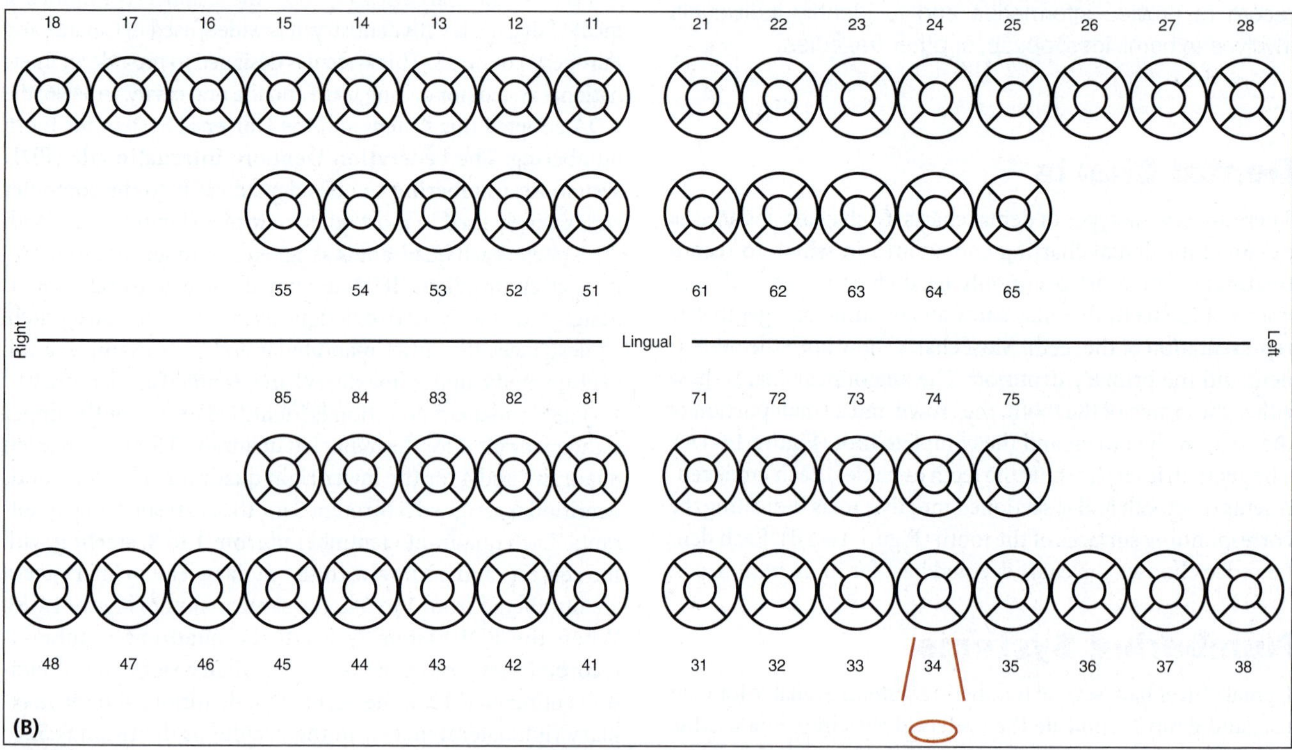

FIGURE 14-1

(A) Example of an anatomical dental chart and (B) Example of a geometric dental chart.

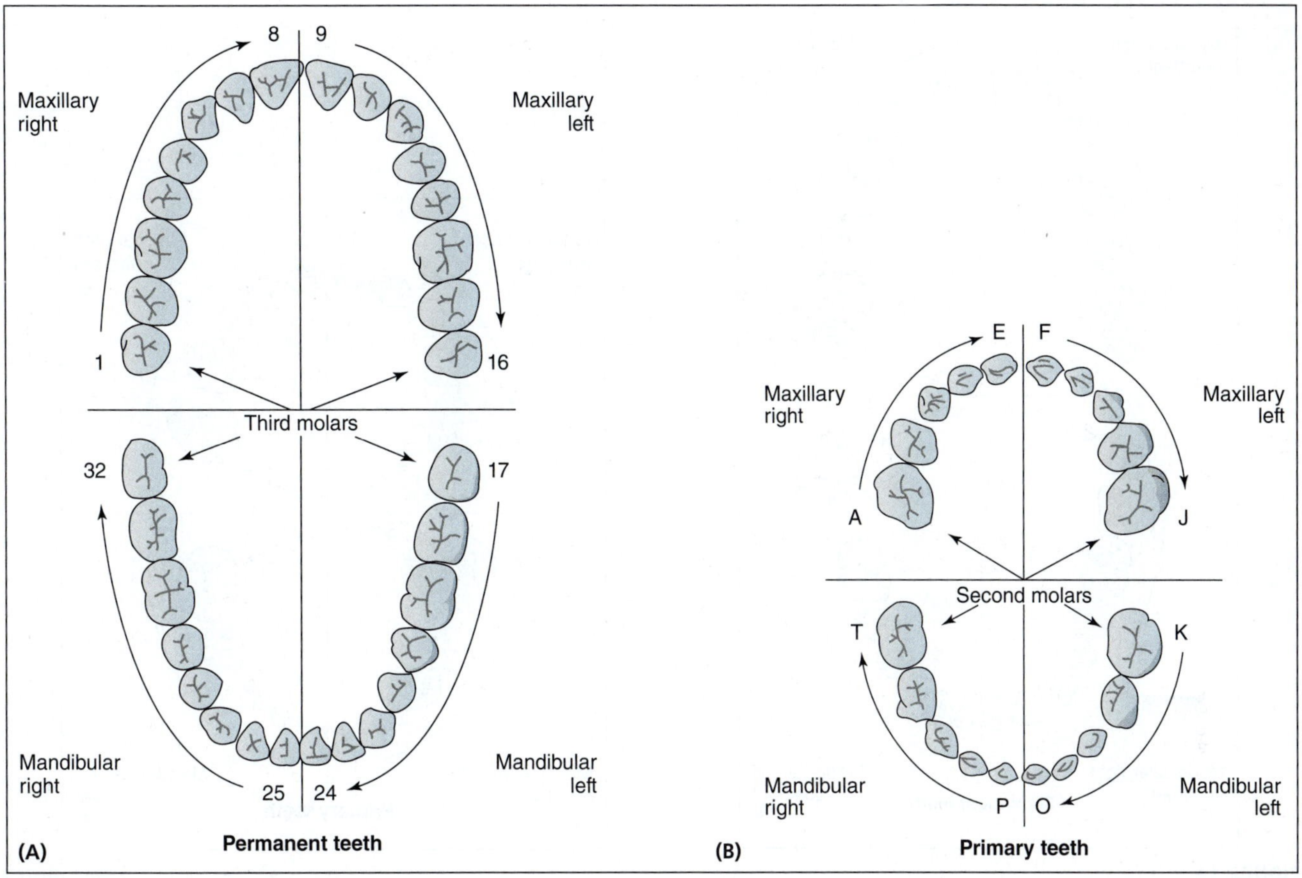

FIGURE 14-2

(A) Permanent and (B) primary dentition showing the Universal/National numbering and lettering system.

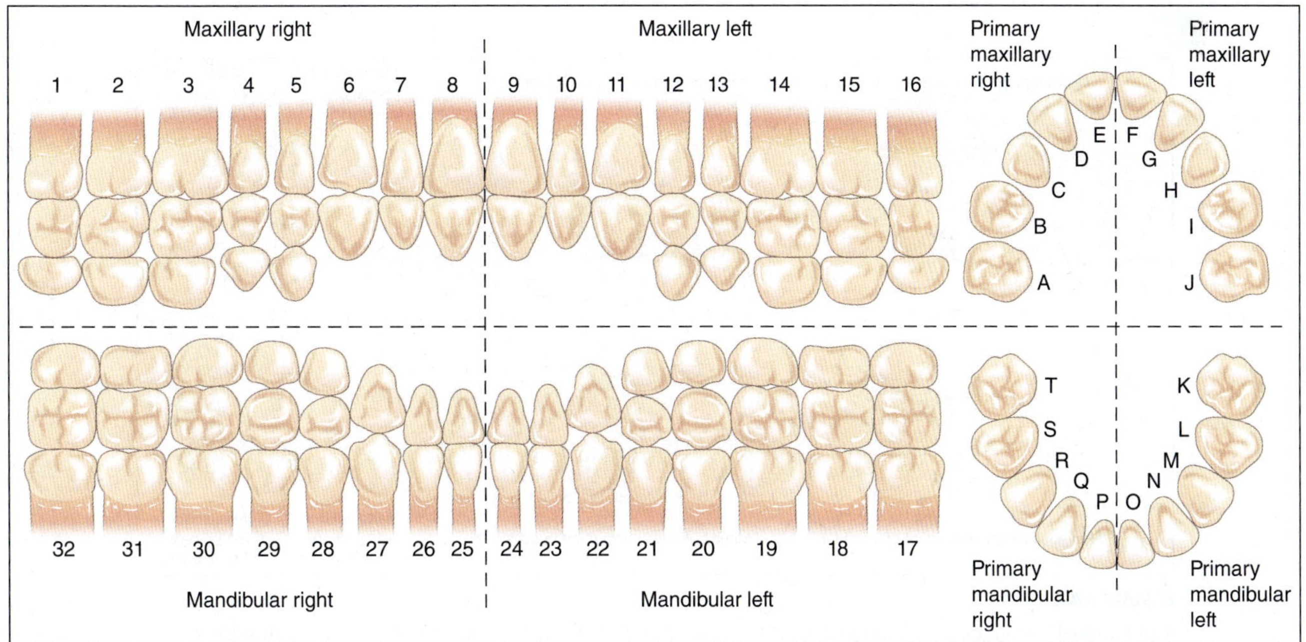

FIGURE 14-3

Universal numbering system for both permanent and deciduous teeth with identifying numbers and letters.

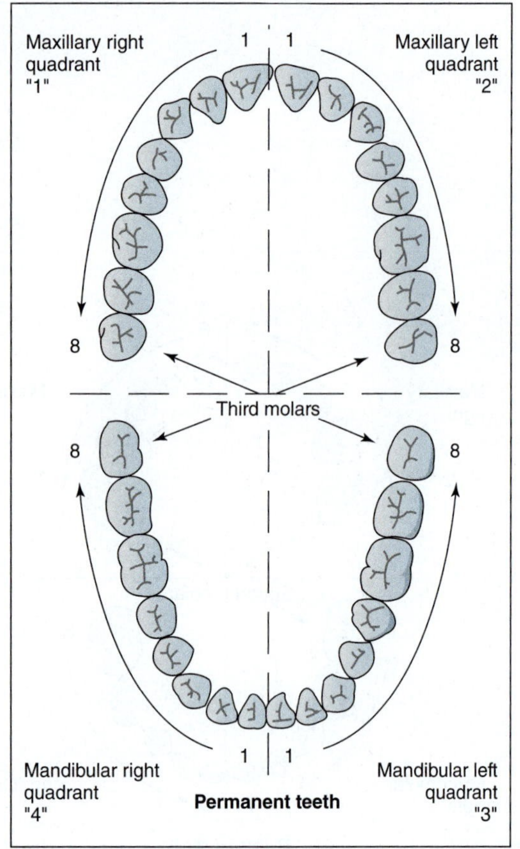

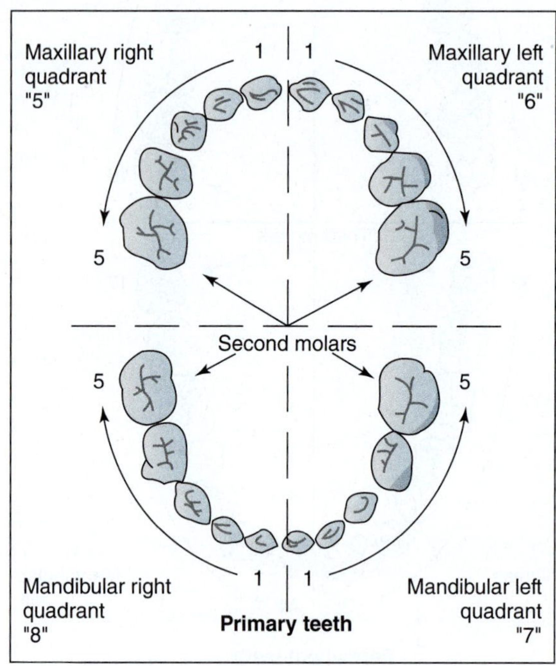

FIGURE 14-4

Permanent and primary dentition showing the International Standards Organization (ISO) TC 106 Designation System/Fédération Dentaire Internationale system.

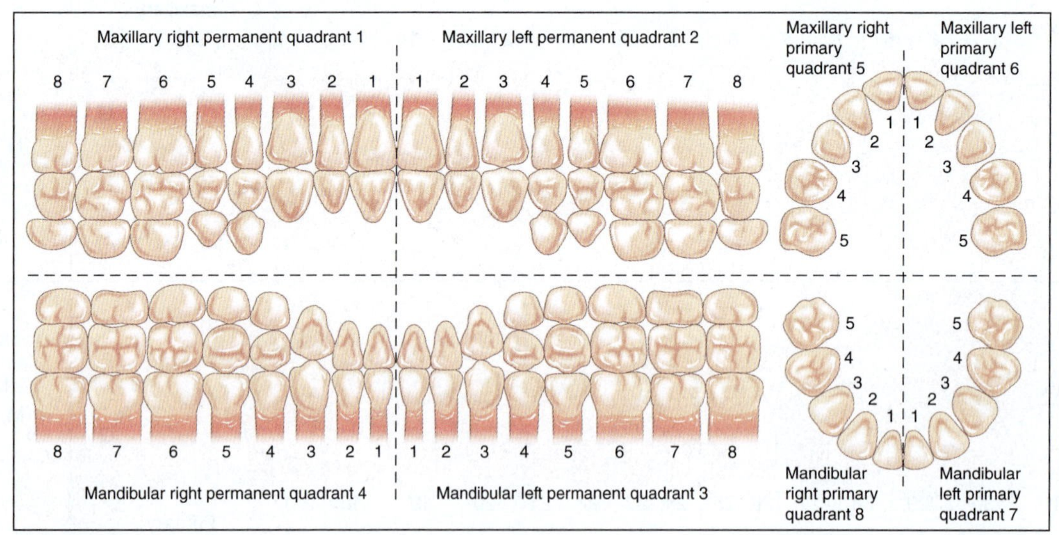

FIGURE 14-5

International Standards Organization (ISO) TC 106 Designation System/Fédération Dentaire Internationale numbering system for both permanent and deciduous teeth with identifying numbers.

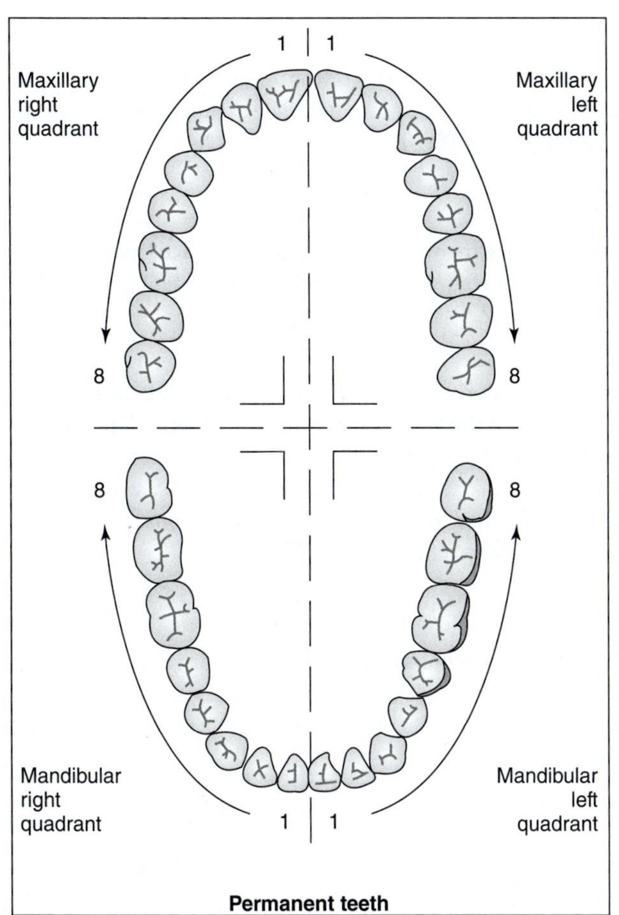

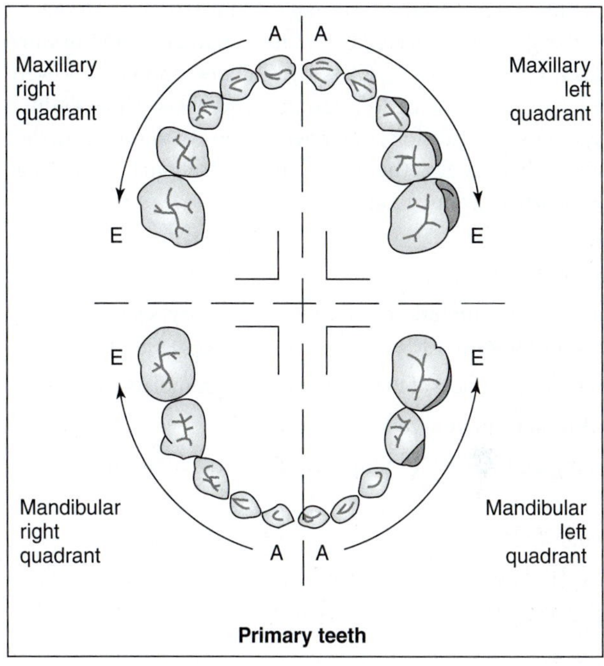

FIGURE 14-6

Permanent and primary dentition with the Palmer numbering and lettering system.

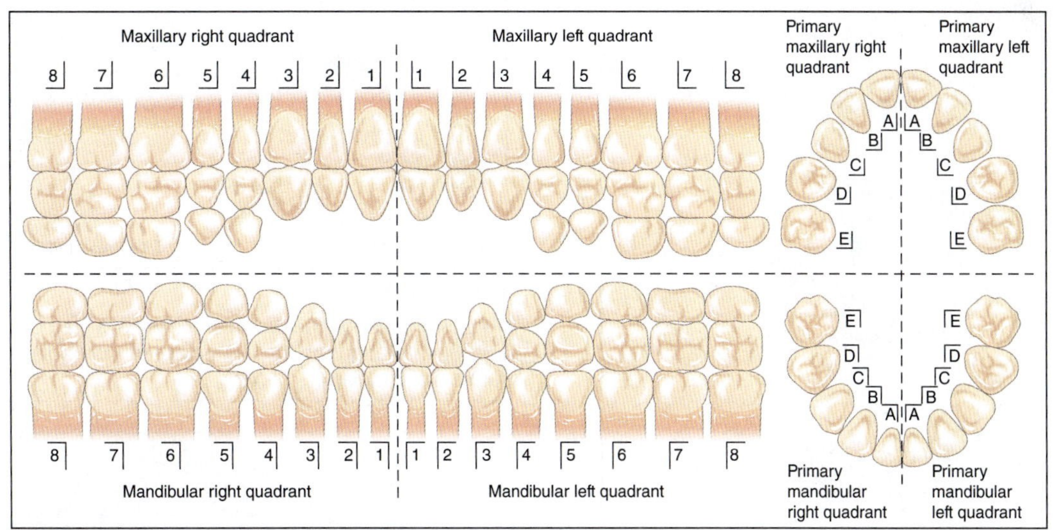

FIGURE 14-7

Palmer numbering system for both permanent and deciduous teeth with identifying numbers and letters and brackets shown.

to (Figure 14-7). For example, the deciduous mandibular right central incisor is charted as A.

Cavity Classifications

The original classification system, which is still used widely today, is based on the location of the **caries** (cavities) on the tooth. Initially the classifications, which were developed by G. V. Black (the "grand old man of dentistry"), were placed into five groups, indicated by a Roman numeral and the word "Class." Class I, Class II, Class III, Class IV, and Class V were used to describe the carious lesions. Later Class VI was added to Black's Classifications of Caries Lesions to describe further cavities that involve the incisal or occlusal surface that has been worn away due to attrition.

Class I

Class I caries include the following three types of developmental cavities in the pit and fissures of teeth (Figure 14-8):

- Occlusal surfaces of the posterior teeth (premolars and molars)
- Buccal or lingual pits on the molars
- Lingual pit near the cingulum of the maxillary incisors

Class II

Class II caries are on the proximal (mesial or distal) surfaces on the posterior teeth (premolars and molars) (Figure 14-9).

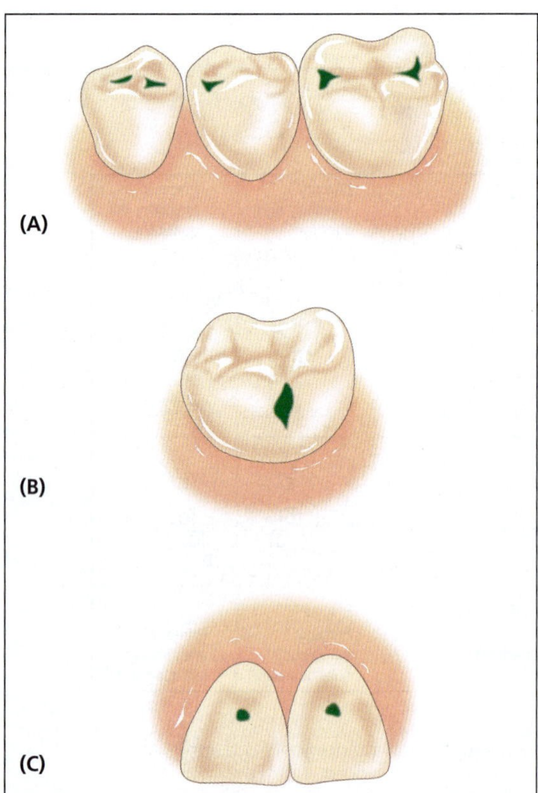

FIGURE 14-8
Class I caries on the (A) occlusal surfaces of the premolars and molars, (B) buccal surface on the molar, and (C) lingual surface on the maxillary incisors.

Class III

Class III caries are on the interproximal surface (mesial or distal) of anterior teeth (canines, lateral incisors, and central incisors) (Figure 14-10).

Class IV

Class IV caries are on the interproximal surface (mesial or distal) of anterior teeth and include the incisal edge (Figure 14-11).

Class V

Class V caries occur on the cervical third of the facial or lingual surface of the tooth (Figure 14-12). Often, Class V caries occur because the patient regularly sucks on sweets. Additionally, the dental assistant may see several Class V caries in one quadrant because the patient takes medications, chews gum, or drinks sodas over long periods of time.

Class VI

Class VI caries were not part of the original standard classification of cavities developed by G. V. Black (Figure 14-13). They were later identified to more clearly label cavities that

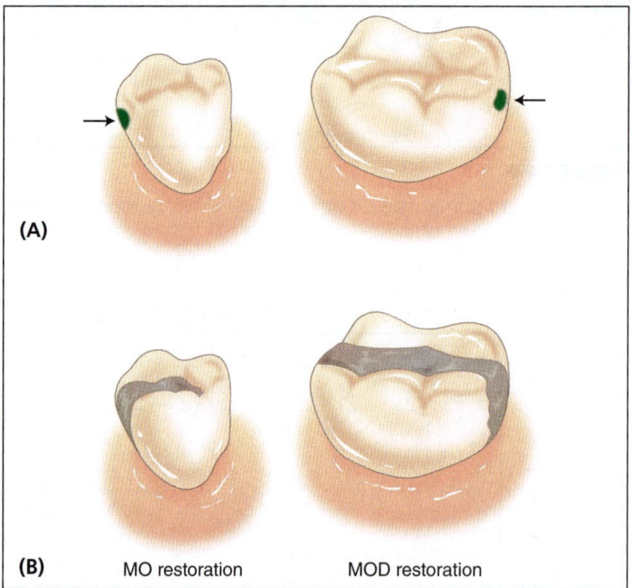

FIGURE 14-9
(A) Class II caries on the proximal surface of a premolar and a molar and (B) restorations on the MO surface of a premolar and the MOD surfaces of a molar.

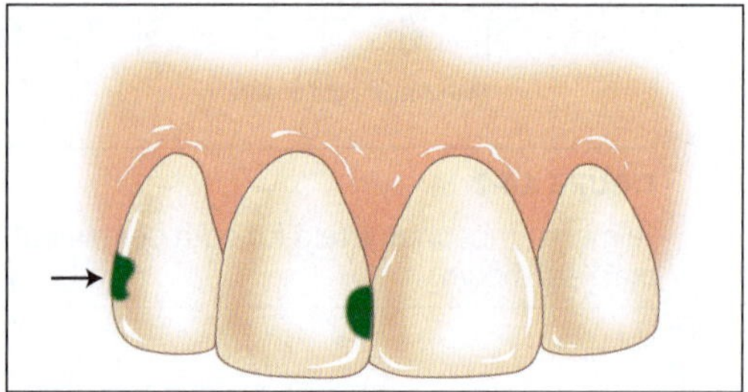

FIGURE 14-10
Class III caries on the proximal surfaces of an incisor and a cuspid.

involve the incisal or occlusal surface that has been worn away due to abrasion.

Abbreviations of Tooth Surfaces

Terms such as simple, compound, and complex are used in cavity classification. A simple cavity involves only one tooth surface, a compound cavity involves two surfaces, and a complex cavity involves more than two surfaces (Table 14-1).

When documenting the chart to record the surfaces of the teeth that need to be restored or that have been restored, the dental assistant abbreviates the notations. Each surface is abbreviated using the first letter of the surface, capitalized. For instance, an abbreviated form of a mesial restoration on tooth #8 is "#8 M." If two or more surfaces are restored, then a combined word is used. The "al" is normally dropped and "o" is substituted on the first word. For example, to identify the restoration on the distal and occlusal surfaces, the term used is disto-occlusal restoration or DO restoration. If three surfaces are combined, the same principle is applied to the second word as well. If the tooth has a mesial-occlusal-distal restoration, the correct term is mesio-occluso-distal or MOD restoration. If a mesial surface of the tooth is restored with another surface, it is always used first. Occlusal and lingual normally fall in the last position.

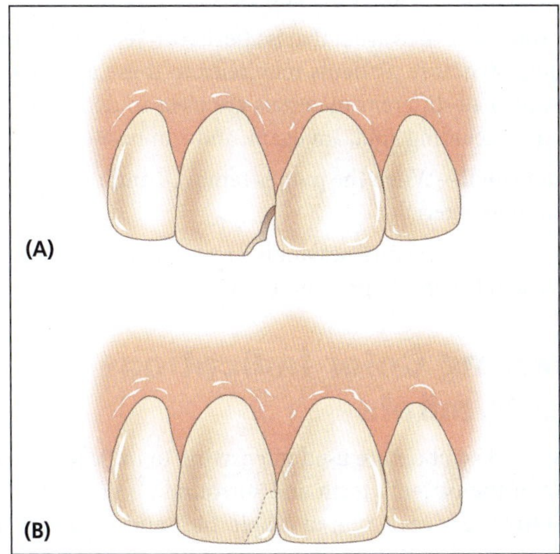

FIGURE 14-11
Class IV (A) fractured area on the proximal incisal surface of the incisor and (B) a completed restoration on the central incisor.

Basic Charting Terms

- **abscess**—Localized area of infection.
- **bridge**—Prosthetic device placed in the mouth where a tooth is missing, normally attached on each side and

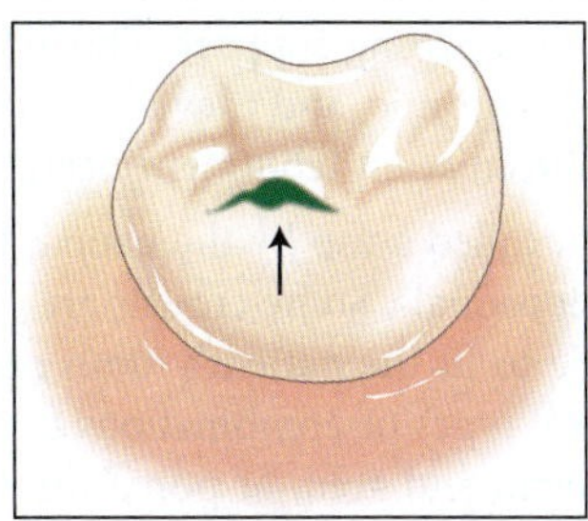

FIGURE 14-13
Class VI caries on the occlusal surface of a mandibular incisor due to abrasion.

TABLE 14-1 Abbreviations for Cavity Restorations

Abbreviations for Single-Surface Restorations (Simple Cavity Restorations)	
I	Incisal
M	Mesial
D	Distal
B	Buccal
O	Occlusal
F	Facial
Abbreviations for Two-Surface Restorations (Compound Cavity Restorations)	
OB	Occluso-buccal
MO	Mesio-occlusal
DO	Disto-occlusal
DI	Disto-incisal
DL	Disto-lingual
MI	Mesio-incisal
LI	Linguo-incisal
Abbreviations for Three or More Surface Restorations (Complex Cavity Restorations)	
MOD	Mesio-occluso-distal
MODBL	Mesio-occluso-disto-bucco-lingual

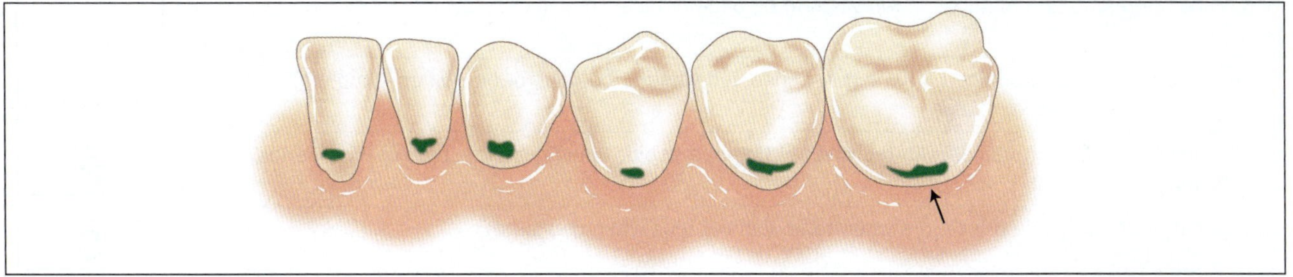

FIGURE 14-12
Class V caries on the gingival buccal areas of the teeth.

covering the space created by the missing tooth. The attaching sides are called **abutments** and the middle area, or the area where the tooth is missing, is called the **pontic**. A **cantilever bridge** is attached on only one side. This type of bridge is useful in an area that has little stress, such as a missing lateral. The abutment side could then be on the canine, which is a strong support. The **Maryland bridge** has wings on the pontic, and they are attached to the lingual sides of the adjacent (abutment) teeth.

- **crown**—Often called a cap by the patient but not usually by dental professionals. Some crowns are cast in a laboratory and made to fit the patient's tooth exactly. They are made of several types or combinations of materials, such as gold, porcelain and gold, or porcelain. Crowns can be permanent or temporary or made for the anterior or posterior. Preformed (temporary) crowns are manufactured in quantities. The dentist sizes and forms the crown to fit the tooth. These crowns are usually made from stainless steel or plastic. All crowns are "fixed" or cemented into place in the patient's mouth and are not removable like partial and full dentures. Crowns cover the complete tooth, as in a full crown, or three-quarters of the tooth, as in a three-fourths crown.
- **denture** (complete and partial)—A full denture replaces the complete arch of a patient's dentition. Patients sometimes refer to full dentures as their upper or lower plates. If all the natural teeth in one arch are missing, a full denture is needed. If some of the natural teeth are missing, a partial denture (artificial teeth mounted on a metal framework) can be used.
- **diastema** (di-a-STE-ma)—The space between the maxillary central incisors in humans. The word *diastema* could also be used to denote a space between two adjacent teeth in the same dental arch.
- **drifting**—All teeth are supported by each other in the dentition. If a maxillary tooth is removed, then the opposing mandibular tooth may drift, or overerupt, into the space. Also, the teeth adjacent to the space created by the removed tooth can drift into the space.
- **furcation**—Dividing point of a multi-rooted tooth.
- **gingival recession**—loss of gingival tissue, exposing the underlying cementum/dentin, usually seen on the facial surface.
- **gold foil**—A restoration created when several layers of pure gold are placed in the preparation. This restoration is not commonly used today.
- **incipient**—Beginning decay that has not broken through the enamel. Incipient appears as a chalky area on the tooth. It is not yet decay, but the surface has begun to decalcify. Some doctors note this on the chart by placing the word "watch" on that area. Other doctors use a series of red dots, a symbol that represents an incipient area.
- **mobility**—When the tooth moves in the socket, normally due to periodontal disease or trauma, a numbering system is used to indicate how many millimeters the tooth moves, which is recorded in Roman numerals, or I to IV.
- **overhang**—Excessive restorative material normally found interproximally near the gingiva.
- **partial dentures**—Prosthetic devices that replace missing teeth. They have a metal framework and artificial teeth.
- **periodontal pocket**—The space in the gingival sulcus created by periodontal disease. It is measured by a periodontal probe in millimeters. A healthy sulcus depth is 1 to 3 millimeters; beyond this depth it is a periodontal pocket. See Chapter 29, Periodontics and Coronal Polish.
- **restoration**—An agent that is effective in replacing missing tooth structure. Patients may refer to these as fillings. A number of different materials are used in dental restorations, including gold, amalgam, and composite.
- **root canal**—When the pulp is removed and replaced with a filling material.
- **sealant**—An enamel sealant is a resin material used to seal pits and fissures to prevent decay.

Charting Color Indications and Symbols

Colors and symbols are used in charting to indicate the condition of the patient's teeth and surrounding tissues and the restorative services required (Table 14-2 and Figure 14-14).

TABLE 14-2 Color Indications and Charting Symbols of Completed Work

• Amalgam restoration (outlined and filled solid blue when complete or red when to be done)	
• Composite restoration (outlined in red when to be done or blue when complete)	
• Gold restoration (area outlined with diagonal lines, red when to be done or blue when complete)	
• Porcelain restoration (outlined with red when to be done or blue when complete and/or *P* inside the outline)	P
• Sealant (S on occlusal surface, red when to be done or blue when complete)	S
• Stainless steel (outlined with swervy lines through it or two Ss inside it, red when to be done or blue when complete)	

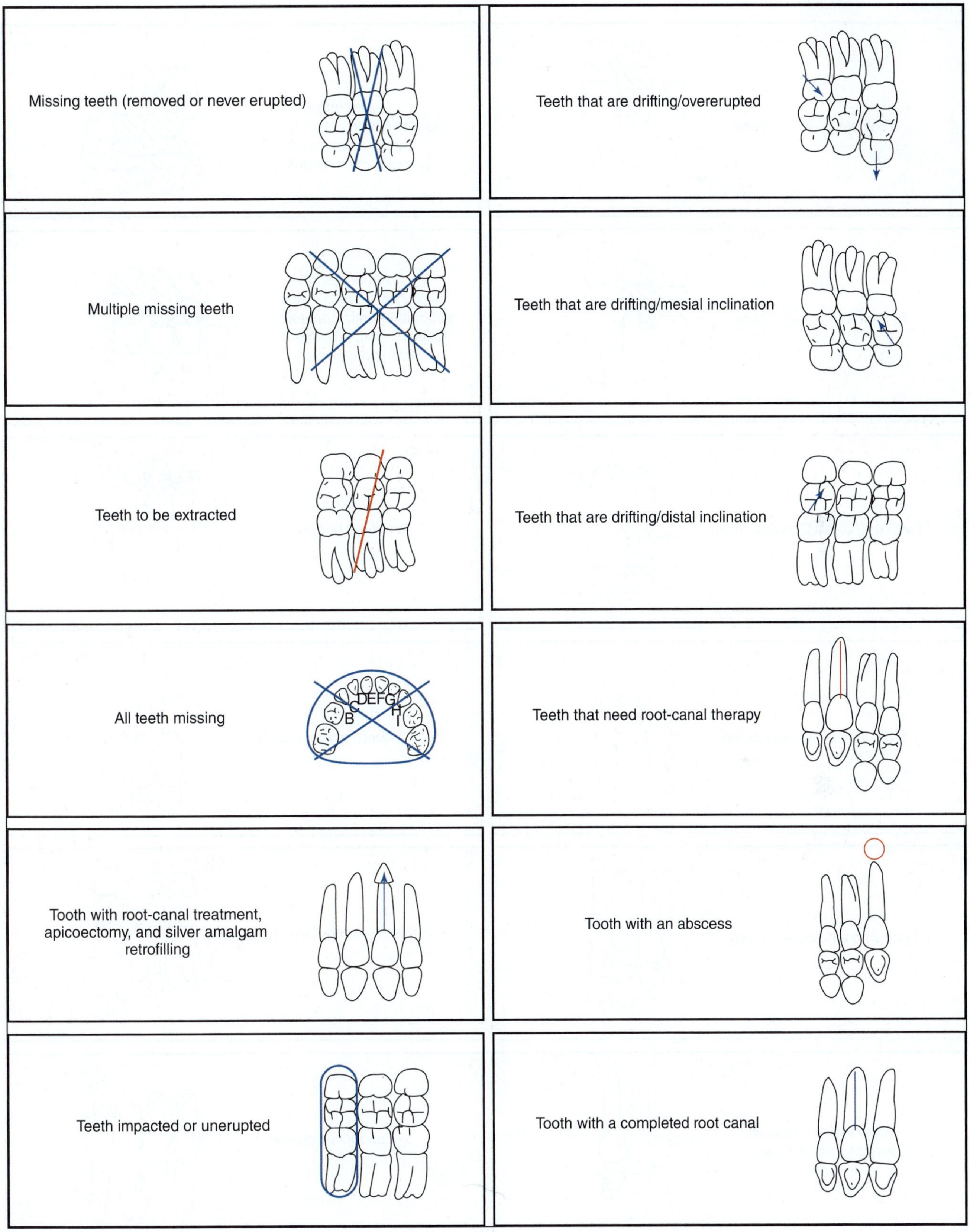

Missing teeth (removed or never erupted)

Teeth that are drifting/overerupted

Multiple missing teeth

Teeth that are drifting/mesial inclination

Teeth to be extracted

Teeth that are drifting/distal inclination

All teeth missing

Teeth that need root-canal therapy

Tooth with root-canal treatment, apicoectomy, and silver amalgam retrofilling

Tooth with an abscess

Teeth impacted or unerupted

Tooth with a completed root canal

FIGURE 14-14

Charting symbols.

(continues)

(continued)

Tooth with full gold crown 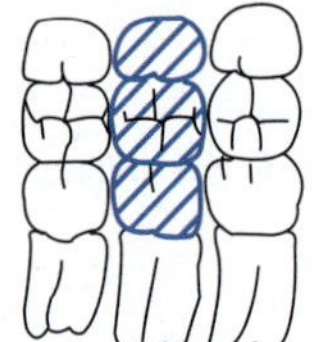	Fixed bridge (abutment porcelain fused to gold crown-pontic-full gold-abutment full gold) 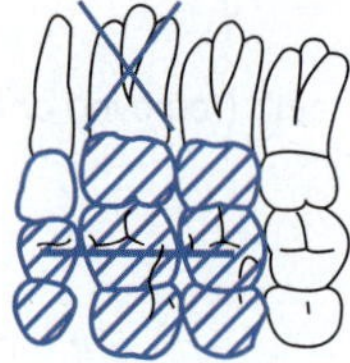
Tooth with a 3/4 gold crown 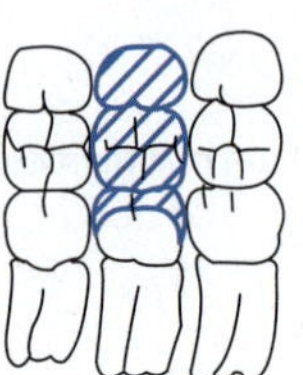	Fixed bridge (porcelain fused to metal abutment-pontic-porcelain fused to metal-abutment full gold crown) 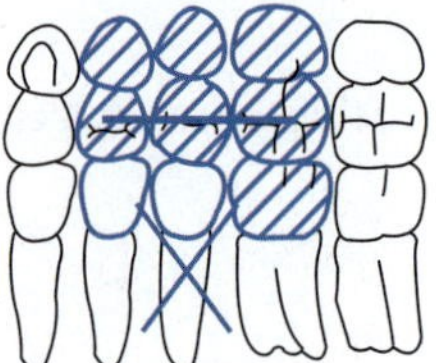
Tooth with an MOD onlay crown 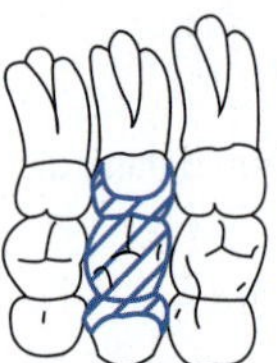	Maryland bridge 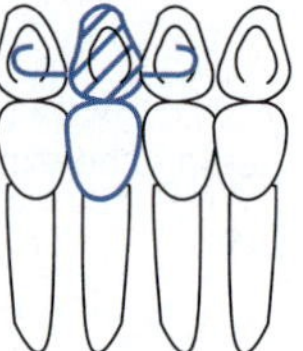
Tooth with a DO inlay crown 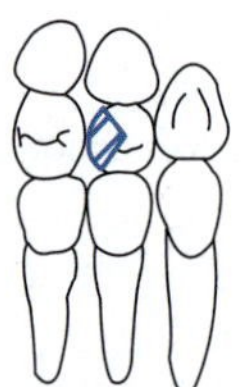	Supernumerary tooth 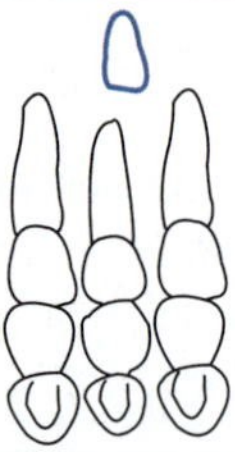
Tooth with a porcelain crown 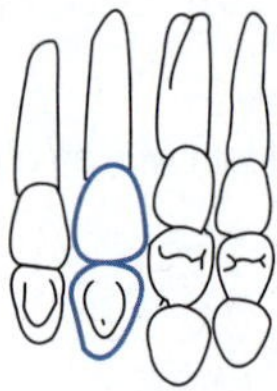	Tooth with a temporary restoration 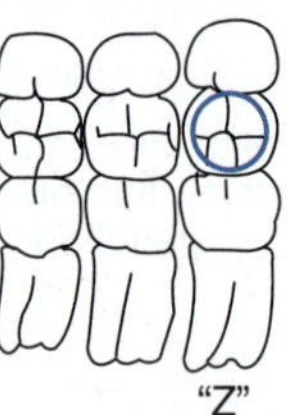
Tooth with a porcelain fused to metal crown 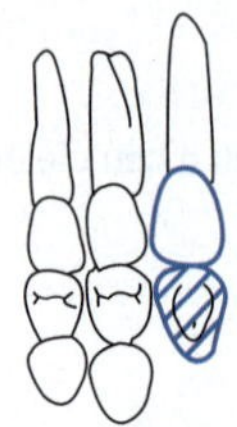	Periodontal pocket 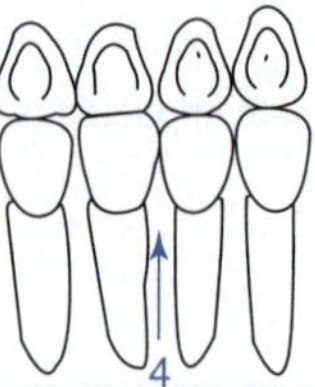

FIGURE 14-14

Charting symbols.

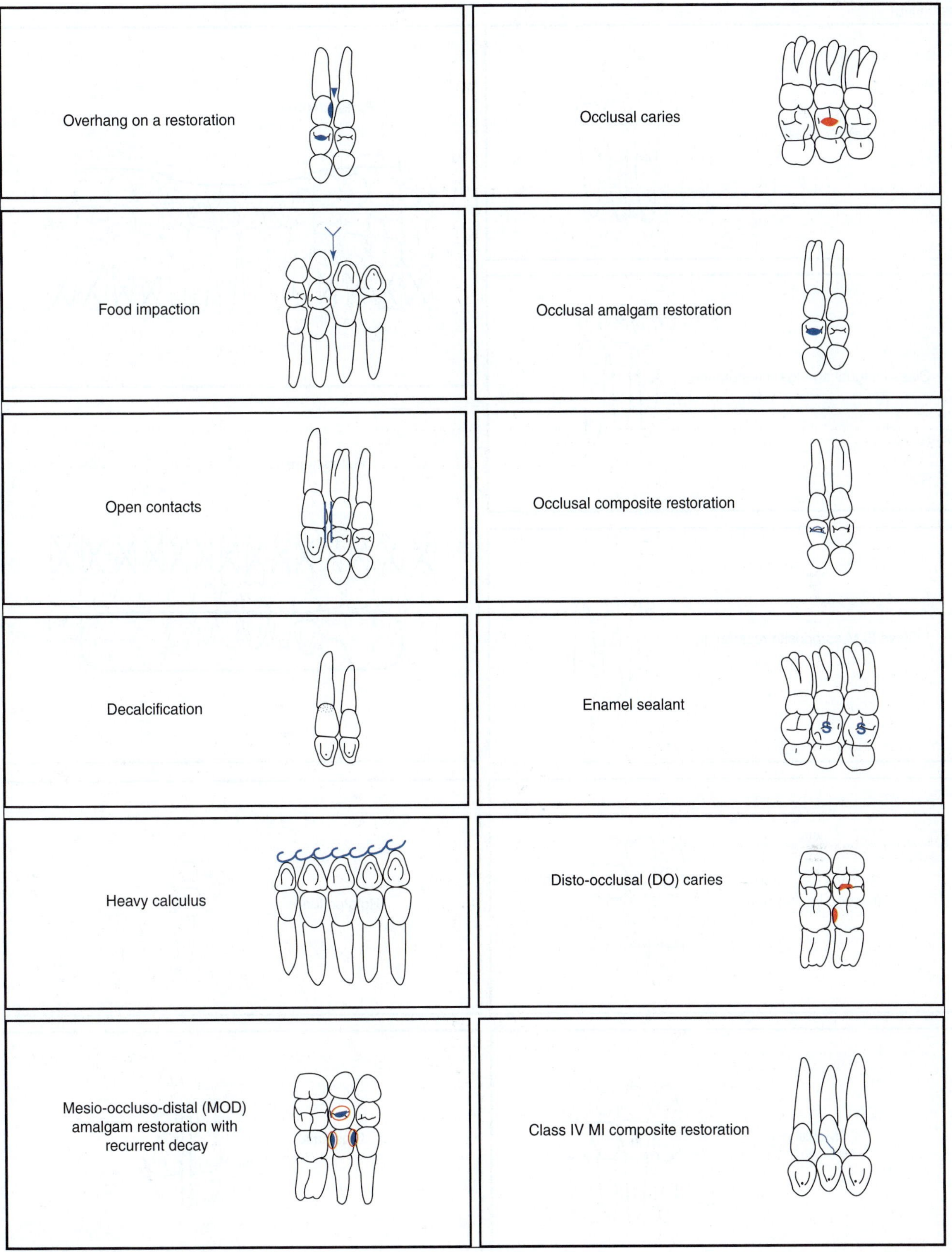

FIGURE 14-14
Charting symbols.

(continues)

(continued)

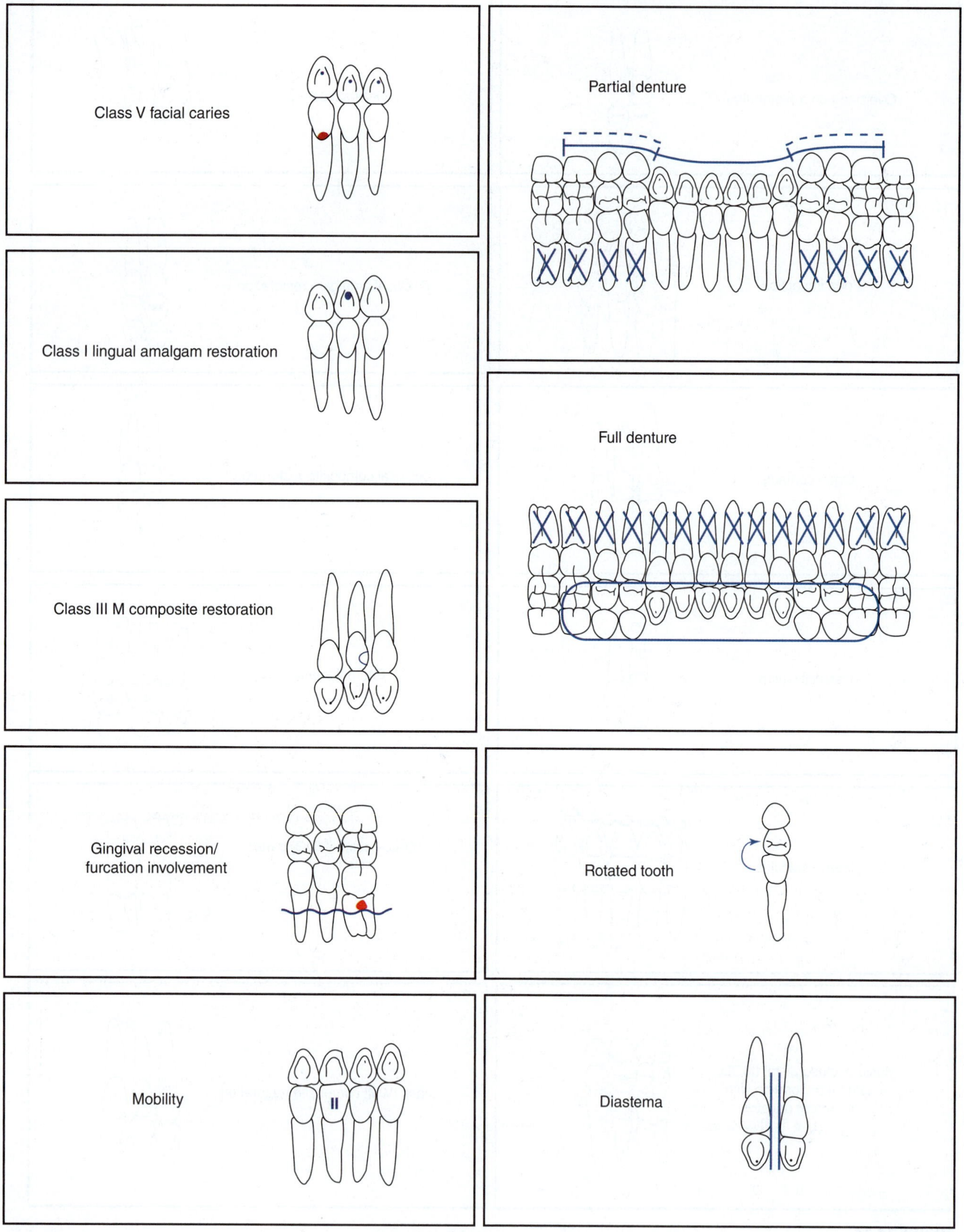

Class V facial caries

Partial denture

Class I lingual amalgam restoration

Full denture

Class III M composite restoration

Gingival recession/
furcation involvement

Rotated tooth

Mobility

II

Diastema

FIGURE 14-14

Charting symbols.

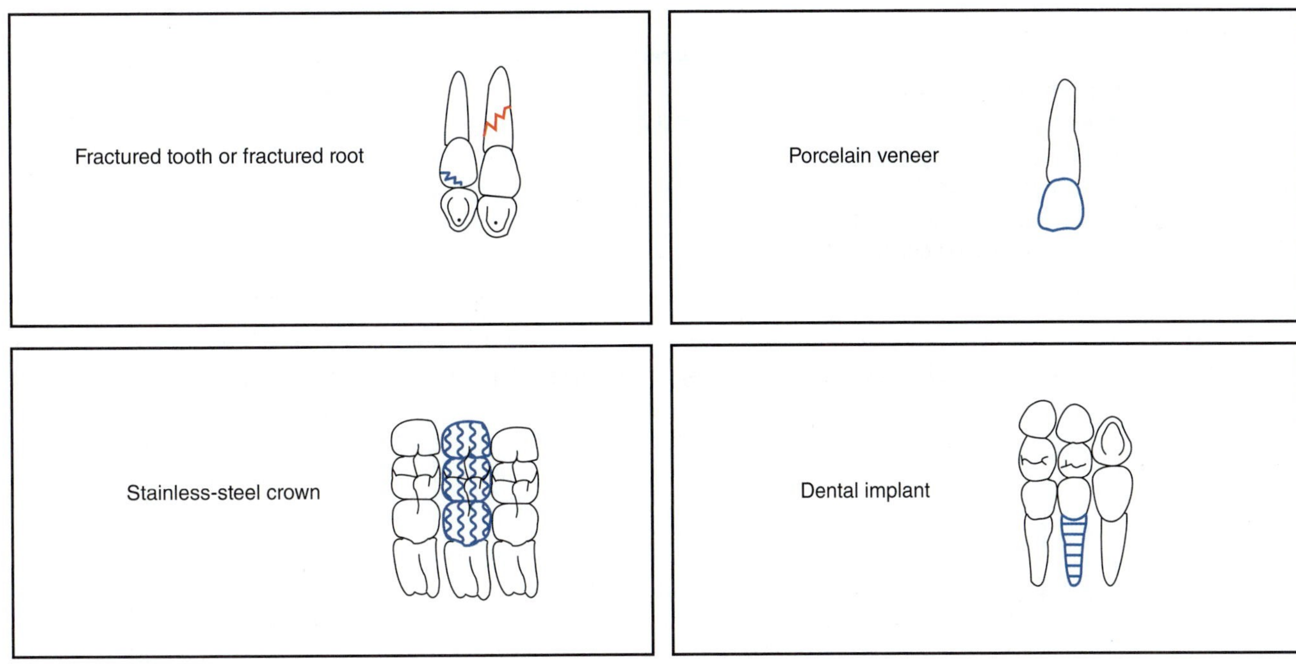

FIGURE 14-14
Charting symbols.

Some symbols allow for common references when interaction takes place between dental professionals.

Red represents the dentistry that needs to be done, and blue indicates the work that has been completed. Some symbols can be charted in either color. For instance, if a tooth is fractured but causing no discomfort to the patient or not affecting the patient's appearance, the dentist may decide not to restore it. A notation is made on the chart that nothing is to be done at this time and it is charted in either color.

Many offices are now using computerized or automated dental charting instead of, or in addition to, manual charting. Computerized dental charting increases efficiency and fosters standardization. Some offices will use voice-activated systems with their software. These systems are designed to recognize a voice and record the information. Often, voice systems confirm findings before charting them. This helps prevent mistakes. When not using a voice-activated system, the dental assistant can enter the information into the computer by keyboard or light pen. When keyboarding, the keyboard must be covered so that cross-contamination does not occur. The light pen can also be covered with a barrier for use. The light pen looks like a writing pen and is sometimes attached by a cord to the monitor. It is touched to the screen to activate a command. If, for example, the dental assistant wanted to note a composite restoration that was placed in the mouth, the assistant would touch the light pen to the screen over the tooth, highlighting the tooth. After highlighting the tooth, the assistant would move the light pen to the side of the screen and select composite restoration and the surfaces to be included. Finally, the dental assistant would touch the light pen to "existing" or "needs to be completed." The computer program would then put the color coding and/or symbol on the dental chart on the correct tooth and make a notation on the patient's chart under findings or treatment plan (Figure 14-15).

Dental software programs work differently but are learned easily. Offices evaluate which systems meet their needs before purchase. Many offices have computers or computer monitors in each operatory for the auxiliary to chart findings and complete the notations and services rendered. (For more information about computer use in the dental office, see Chapter 40, Dental Office Management.)

Dental assistants can become very proficient at computer charting (Figure 14-16). The software programs for computer charting can record "Periodontal" charting (see Chapter 31, Periodontics, for periodontal charting), conditions of the dentition, tissue, occlusion, or any notations the dentist or auxiliary would like to make.

Chart

Patient: Patricia Abbott
Birthdate: 09/30/1963
Chart #: ABB102
Date: 01/22/2003
SS#:

Provider: Dennis D. Smith D.D.S.
Phone: (801)763-9300
Office: 732 E. Utah Valley Drive # 500
American Fork, UT 84003

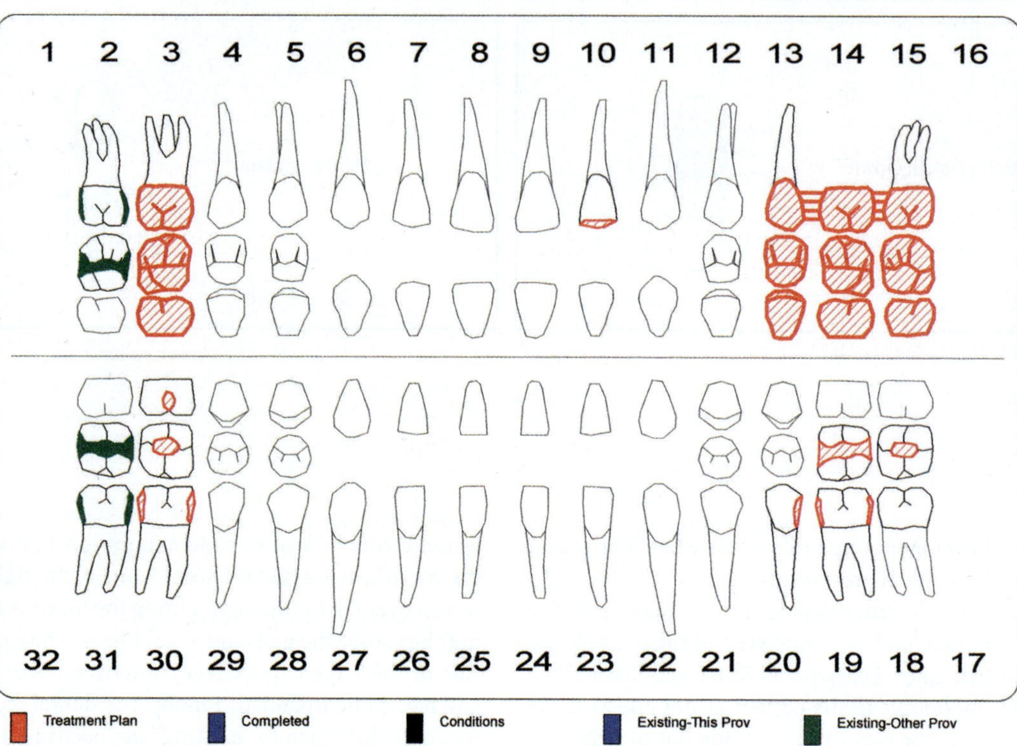

Treatment Plan Estimate

Tooth	**Description**	**Amount**	**Pat.**	**Dental Ins.**
3	Crown-porc fuse high noble mtl	613.00	306.50	306.50
3	Crown buildup, includ any pins	149.00	29.80	119.20
3	Permanent Insert	0.00	0.00	0.00
10	Resin-one surface, anterior	71.00	14.20	56.80
13	Retainer crn-porc fused-hi nob	613.00	306.50	306.50
14	Pontic-porcelain fused to hnob	613.00	306.50	306.50
15	Retainer crn-porc fused-hi nob	613.00	306.50	306.50
18	Resin-1 surface, post-permanent	80.00	16.00	64.00
19	Resin-3 surface +, post-perm	146.00	29.20	116.80
20	Resin-1 surface, post-permanent	80.00	16.00	64.00
30	Resin-3 surface +, post-perm	146.00	29.20	116.80
	Treatment Plan Totals	3124.00	1360.40	1763.60

* Treatment Plans Are Estimates Only

FIGURE 14-15
Sample computer chart.

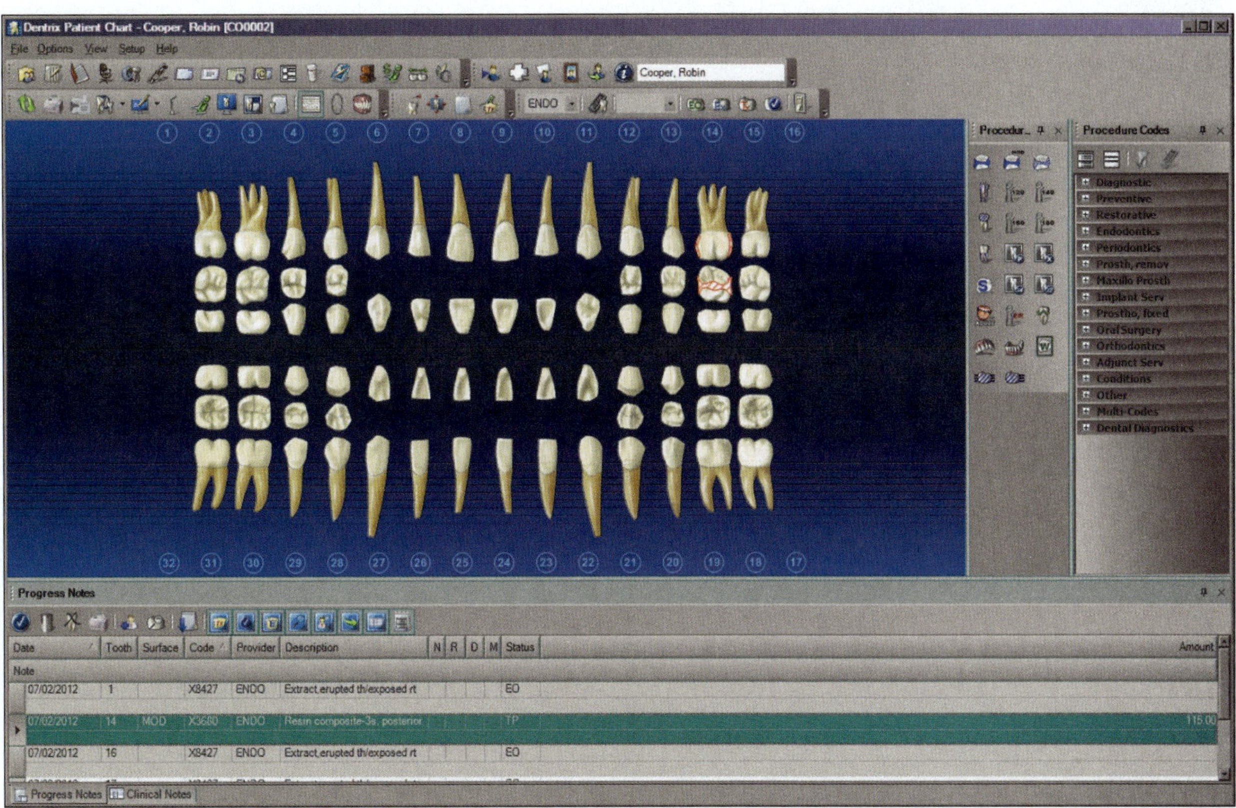

FIGURE 14-16

Sample computer chart.

Chapter Summary

Dental charting provides legal documentation of the patient's oral cavity. The correct numbering system and charting symbols ensure proper documentation. Therefore, accuracy in charting is critical.

CASE STUDY

Charting Using the Anatomical Representation of the Teeth and the Universal System for Numbering (Figure 14-17).

Tooth		
	#1	Impacted
	#2	Class II DO amalgam restoration present
	#4	Class II MOD amalgam restoration present
	#6	Class III M composite restoration present
	#8	Class IV MIFL composite restoration present
	#8 #9	Diastema present
	#9	Class III M decay
	#13	Class II MOD amalgam restoration with recurrent decay
	#14	Class II MO amalgam restoration present; food impaction between 13 and 14
	#16	Has been removed
	#17	Partially impacted and must be removed
	#19	Bridge present, abutment full gold crown
	#20	Bridge present, pontic porcelain with gold
	#21	Bridge present, abutment porcelain with gold
	#24	Mobility of III, periodontal pocket on M and D of 4 mm each, heavy calculus from mandibular left cuspid to mandibular right cuspid

(continues)

CASE STUDY

#25	Periodontal pocket on M and D of 3 mm each
#28	Needs a full gold crown with a porcelain facing
#28	Has a completed root canal
#30	Class I O decay
#31	Class II MO amalgam restoration present
#32	Has been removed

Case Study Review

1. Which tooth has a class III M caries?
2. How many teeth are restored?
3. Which tooth is a pontic?

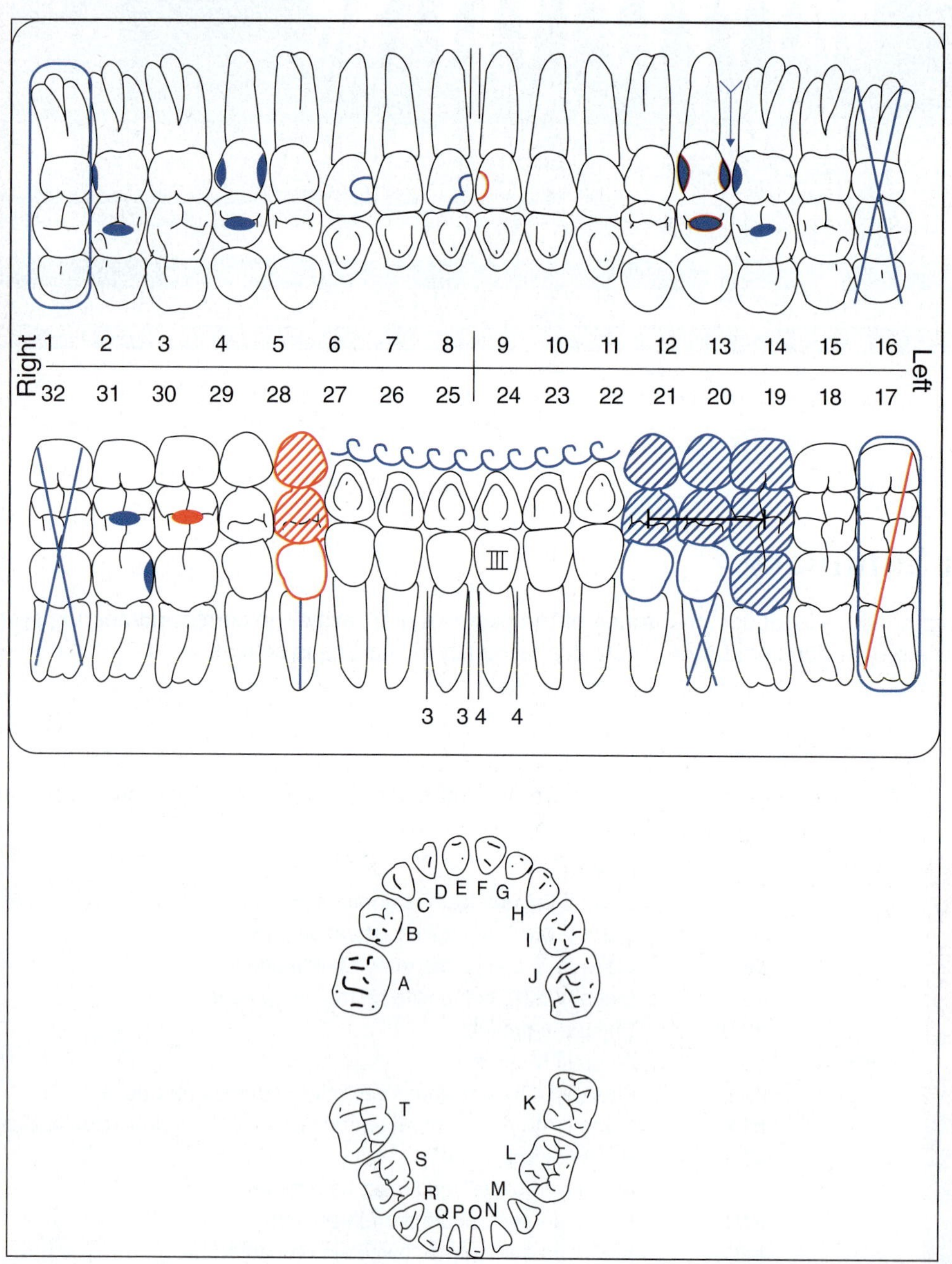

FIGURE 14-17

Charting using the anatomical teeth and the Universal/National System for numbering.

(continues)

CASE STUDY

Charting Using the Geometric Representation of the Teeth and the ISO System for Tooth Identification (Figure 14-18).

Tooth		
	#18	Impacted
	#16	Full porcelain with gold crown present
	#15	Class II MO amalgam restoration present
	#14	Class I O sealant present
	#12	Class III M composite present with recurrent decay
	#11	Class I L composite present
	#24	Bridge present, abutment full porcelain with gold
	#25	Bridge present, pontic full porcelain with gold
	#26	Bridge present, abutment full porcelain with gold
	#28	Has been removed
	#38	Has been removed
	#36	Has a full gold crown
	#34	Has an abscess and needs a root canal
	#33	Is missing and the deciduous tooth is retained
	#31	Class IV MI composite restoration present
	#42	Has a fracture on the MI edge
	#45	Class II DO amalgam restoration with an overhang
	#47	Has been removed
	#48	Mesial inclination

Case Study Review

1. Which tooth has an enamel sealant?
2. Which primary tooth is in the patient's mouth?
3. Which tooth needs endodontic therapy?

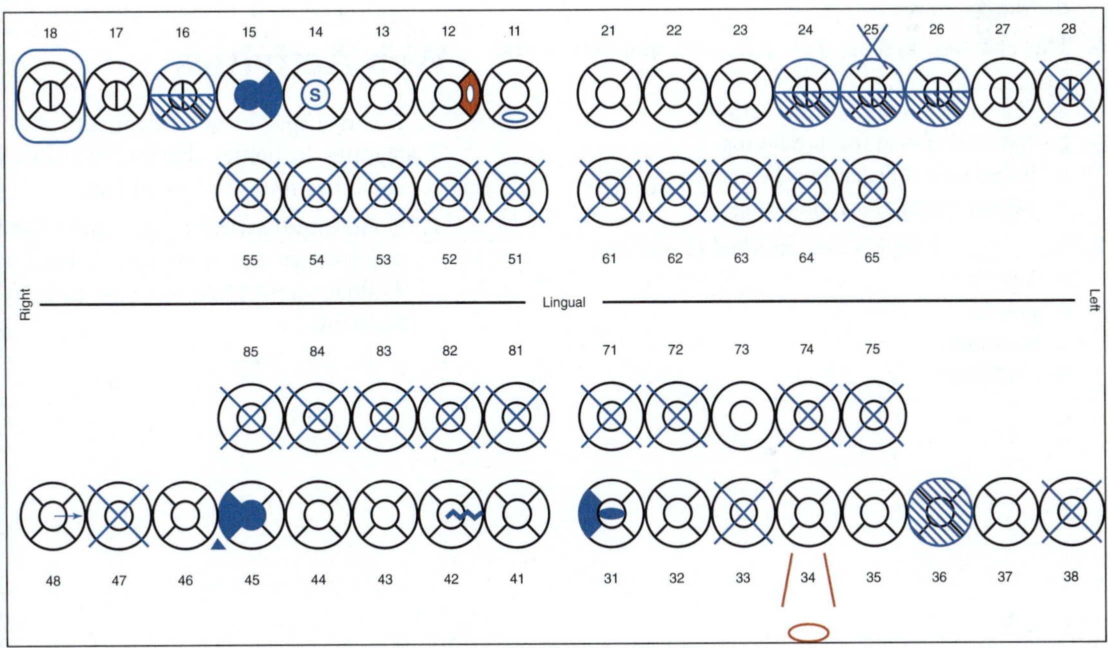

FIGURE 14-18
Charting using the geometric representation of the teeth and the ISO TC 106 designation system for the teeth.

Review Questions

Multiple Choice

1. Which of the following charting systems uses brackets?
   a. Universal System for numbering
   b. National System for numbering
   c. International Fédération Dentaire
   d. Palmer System for numbering
2. Cavities on the interproximal surface of the anterior teeth that do not include the incisal edge are
   a. Class I.
   b. Class II.
   c. Class III.
   d. Class IV.
3. Excess restorative material found near the gingival tissue is
   a. sealant.
   b. overhang.
   c. drifting.
   d. gold foil.
4. Restorations that need to be completed are charted in which color?
   a. Yellow
   b. Black
   c. Red
   d. Blue
5. Gold crowns are charted with which symbol?
   a. Diagonal lines
   b. Crosshatch lines
   c. Multiple dots
   d. Swervy lines
6. The charting system that uses only numbers is the ________
   a. Universal System for numbering.
   b. National system for numbering.
   c. International Fédération Dentaire.
   d. Palmer System for numbering.
7. A ________ bridge is only attached to one side.
   a. Maryland
   b. pontic
   c. abutment
   d. cantilever
8. The space between the maxillary central incisors in humans is the ________
   a. sealant.
   b. diastema.
   c. bridge.
   d. overhang.
9. Teeth that are impacted or unerupted have the symbol of ________
   a. circle around the tooth.
   b. "X" over the tooth.
   c. arrow pointing in the apical direction.
   d. a small circle at the apex of the tooth.
10. The dental implant is noted on charting by ________
    a. swervey lines on the crown of the tooth.
    b. root area completely filled in.
    c. parallel lines across the crown of the tooth.
    d. parallel lines across the root of the tooth.

Critical Thinking

1. The five surfaces on a posterior tooth are mesial, distal, occlusal, lingual, and buccal. What are the five surfaces on an anterior tooth? Which of these surfaces is the same for both anterior and posterior?
2. A young adult broke his upper teeth at a drinking fountain, from the middle of the biting edge to the middle of each front tooth in an upside-down V pattern. Which surfaces, classifications, and teeth numbers would be involved if using the Universal System for numbering? The ISO or FDI system? The Palmer System?
3. If an anterior tooth is fractured and does not need to be restored, which color would it be charted in and why?

Web Activities

1. Go to http://www.softdent.com and look at the new features in dental charting available on the Soft-dent computer software for dentistry.
2. Go to http://www.cengage.com/us/ and locate MindTap and identify any study cards related to dental charting. Evaluate how MindTap would help you as a dental assistant.

CHAPTER

15

Pharmacology

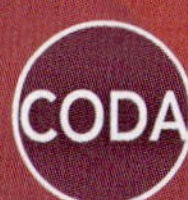

Specific Instructional Objectives

The student should strive to meet the following objectives and demonstrate an understanding of the facts and principles presented in this chapter:

1. Identify terms related to drugs, pharmacology, and medicines.
2. Identify the difference between drug brand names and generic names.
3. Identify the parts of a written prescription.
4. Identify the texts pertinent to pharmacology.
5. Give the English meanings of the Latin abbreviations used for prescriptions.
6. Specify the drug laws and who enforces them.
7. Identify the schedules for the Comprehensive Drug Abuse Prevention and Control Act of 1970.
8. Identify the routes through which drugs can be administered.
9. Demonstrate an understanding of the drugs used in dentistry, and the ways in which they are used.
10. Summarize the uses and effects of nicotine, caffeine, alcohol, marijuana, and cocaine.
11. Summarize information about heroin, morphine, and codeine.
12. Supply information about amphetamines.
13. Demonstrate an understanding of hallucinogenic drugs such as LSD, PCP, and mescaline.
14. Demonstrate an understanding of barbiturates.

Key Terms

(continues)

Key Terms (continued)

oral (316)
over-the-counter (OTC) drug (310)
patent medicine (310)
pharmacology (310)
pharmacokinetics (315)
Physician's Desk Reference (PDR) (311)
prescription (310)
prophylactic (318)
psychologically dependent (310)
the Pure Food and Drug Act (313)
rectal (316)
scored (311)
side effect (310)
signature (313)
stimulant (323)
subcutaneous (316)
sublingual (316)
subscription (312)
substance abuse (317)
superscription (312)
systemic drugs (316)
tolerance (325)
topical (316)
transdermal (317)
ulcer (323)
withdrawal (310)

Introduction

The terms *pharmacology* and *drugs* are normally associated with treating a disease, but in reality they cover a much broader aspect of chemically induced changes in the body. The study of all drugs, their properties, how they react with each other, and the actions of the drugs within the body is referred to as **pharmacology**. Pharmacology is constantly changing due to the constant new information and knowledge gained about drugs, new drugs being created, and drugs being altered. A **drug** is a substance that can change life processes within the body. Any drug that is used to treat a disease is referred to as a **medicine**.

Drugs have never been as widely used and misused as they are today. The dental assistant needs to pay attention to patients' medical and dental histories, and must carefully document the drugs used by each patient. The dental assistant must have knowledge about pharmacology, the side effects of drugs, and the interactions that take place when more than one drug is used. When a drug causes an unintended result, this result is called a **side effect**. For example, if a patient is taking antihistamines and decongestants to clear up the symptoms of a cold and the patient becomes tired, fatigue is a side effect.

At times it is necessary to take more than one drug at a time. This can be dangerous and should be avoided if the patient taking the drugs is not knowledgeable about their interactions. When one drug changes the effect of another drug by increasing or decreasing the intended result a **drug interaction** occurs. The risk of combining the drugs (the synergistic effect) is much greater to the person than the risk of taking either one of the drugs alone.

Some drugs are addictive. When a person has an **addiction**, he or she is physically dependent on a drug. Being physically dependent means that the addict must continue to take the drug in order to avoid withdrawal symptoms. The symptoms that occur when a drug addicted person stops taking a drug are called **withdrawal**. Nervousness, stomach cramps, diarrhea, shaking, and depression are symptoms of withdrawal.

Some people become **psychologically dependent** on a drug. This means that the person taking the drug has developed a strong emotional need to take that drug. It is similar to a craving. This person may not have any physical need for the drug but becomes psychologically dependent on it. The drugs that cause psychological dependence are referred to as **habit forming**.

Legal drugs are classified according to their availability to the public and their potential for abuse. Drugs with the inscription, "Federal law prohibits dispensing without prescription," must be prescribed by a licensed medical professional and dispensed by a pharmacist. Drugs without the inscription are referred to as an **over-the-counter (OTC) drug** or **patent medicine**.

Drug Names

When filling a **prescription** (a written order for a specific drug) for a dentist, the pharmacy identifies whether the drug is to be filled with a drug brand or with a generic substance. The generic substance has a similar composition to the drug brand and often does not affect the outcome for the patient. A prescription (also called an ethical drug) can only be signed by a professional who is legally authorized to prescribe medications. These professionals have been issued a Federal Drug Enforcement Agency (DEA) identification number. Dental assistants are not permitted to prescribe medications, only the dentist. Dental assistants can dispense the medications according to the precise instructions of the dentist and under their direct supervision.

Brand Names

The manufacturer of a drug assigns a **brand name** to the drug they created. These brand names, often referred to as trade names, are always capitalized and have registered trademarks. These names are controlled by the manufacturer. For example, Bayer™ is a brand name for aspirin.

Generic Names

A **generic name** of a drug is not capitalized and is not patent protected. Generic names refer to the chemical composition of the drug, and are less expensive than brand-name drugs. For example, acetylsalicylic acid (aspirin) is a generic name.

Prescriptions

Only physicians, dentists, and physician assistants are legally allowed to write prescriptions. This limits the dispensing of controlled substances to those trained and licensed to provide patients with drugs. *Ethical drugs* are dispensed only when a customer gives the pharmacist a correctly written prescription signed by a doctor with his or her **Drug Enforcement Agency (DEA) number** on it. In the past, a prescription had a form with the recipe for the needed drug on it. Today's medicines are packaged in correct **dosage** amounts preformulated for dispensing. Oral drugs come in numerous forms. They can be scored or unscored, **enteric-coated** (coating that resists breaking down by the gastric juices and dissolves in the intestines) or not, or in gelatin or in time-released capsules (Figure 15-1). When a capsule is **scored** (cut superficially to allow it to separate or break apart more easily) the patient can divide the dosage if directed to do so by the provider. Therefore, the doctor can simplify the prescription, asking for the number of tablets, pills, capsules, or liquid amount, and not indicating dosage amounts. This ensures that the patient receives the proper dosage each time the drug is taken, and the correct packaging saves time for the doctor and the patient.

All dentists have the legal obligation to use due care while treating their patients. They must have a complete health history on the patient and must be knowledgeable about the drugs they prescribe to the patient. The American Dental Association's **Council on Dental Therapeutics** gathers information about the drugs used in dentistry, and this information is given to the dentist to assist him or her in gaining necessary information about the use of new therapeutic agents. A recent publication of accepted dental therapeutics can be obtained from the ADA. The dentists can call the ADA with questions concerning accepted dental therapeutics, or if questions arise regarding any drug or chemical used in the office. Dentists can also obtain information about drugs from several texts. The most commonly used text in the dental office is the ***Physician's Desk Reference (PDR)***. The *PDR* is printed annually and has the drugs listed by trade or product name, generic and chemical names, and by category. The *PDR* is available both in book form and as a CD-ROM. Information about the drug includes the chemical description, indications and use of the drug, contraindications of using the drug, warnings and precautions related to use of the drug, and adverse drug reactions. Information about the recommended drug dosages and how the drug is supplied is also listed in the *PDR* (Figure 15-2). Many of the drugs are packaged with inserts that list the same information contained in the *PDR* about the drug. These inserts usually are not given to the patient but are retained by the pharmacist. Many drugs now have inserts that give clear instructions to the patient as well as warnings. These are given to the patient with the prescription unless the physician or dentist specifies on the written prescription not to do so. Pharmacists use two main references that have detailed information about each drug. These are the *United States Pharmacopoeia (USP)* and the *National Formulary (NF)*.

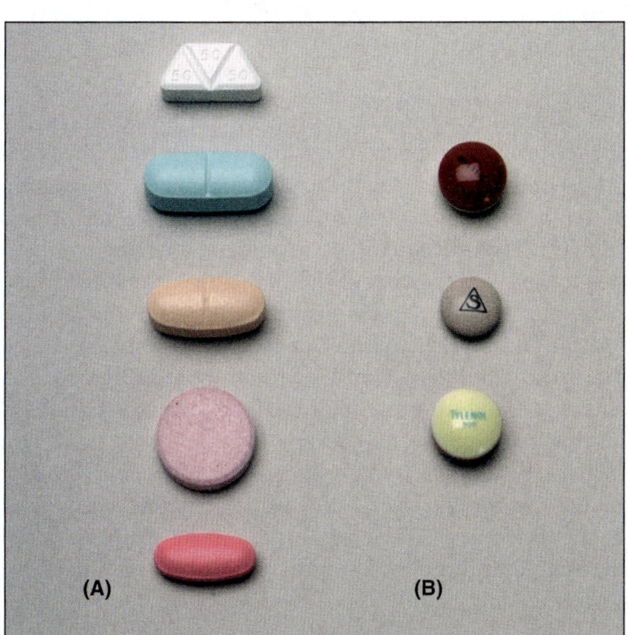

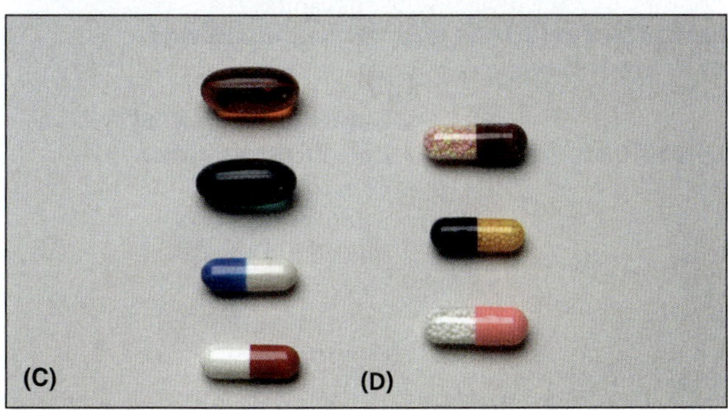

FIGURE 15-1

Tablets and capsules come in different colors, sizes, shapes, and forms. (A) Scored and unscored tablets; (B) enteric-coated tablets; (C) gelatin capsules; and (D) time-release capsules.

Parts of a Prescription

A prescription is written in several parts (Figure 15-3). All information must be completed to ensure that the correct drug is being dispensed in the correct manner, according to the directions of the dentist. Being thorough and writing clearly

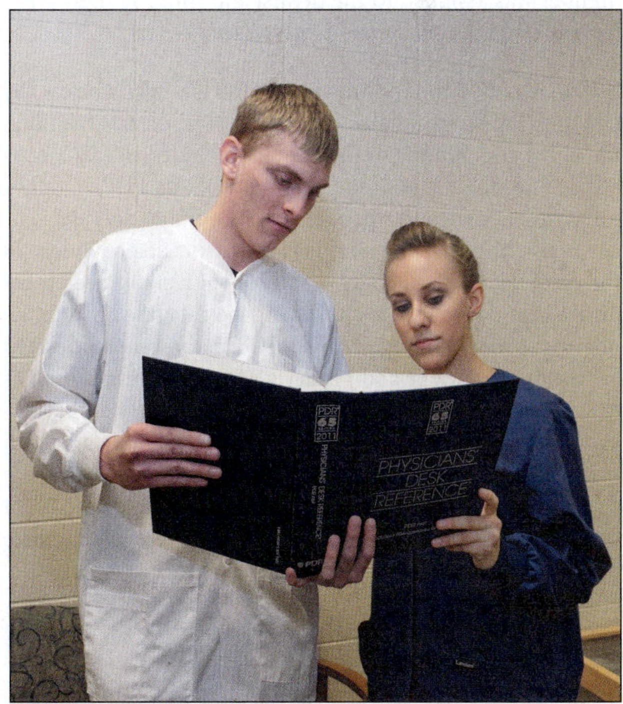

FIGURE 15-2

Dentist and dental assistant using the *Physician's Desk Reference (PDR)* to obtain information about a medication.

Parts of a Prescription

1. The heading includes the dentist's name, address, telephone number, and registration number.
2. The superscription includes the patient's name, address, and the date on which the prescription is written.
3. The *subscription* that includes the symbol Rx ("take thou").
4. The *inscription* that states the names and quantities of ingredients to be included in the medication.
5. The *subscription* that gives directions to the pharmacist for filling the prescription.
6. The *signature* (Sig) that gives the directions for the patient.
7. The dentist's signature blanks. Where signed, indicates if a generic substitute is allowed or if the medication is to be dispensed as written.
8. REPETATUR 0 1 2 3 p.r.n. This is where the dentist indicates whether or not the prescription can be refilled.
9. ☐ LABEL Direction to the pharmacist to label the medication appropriately.

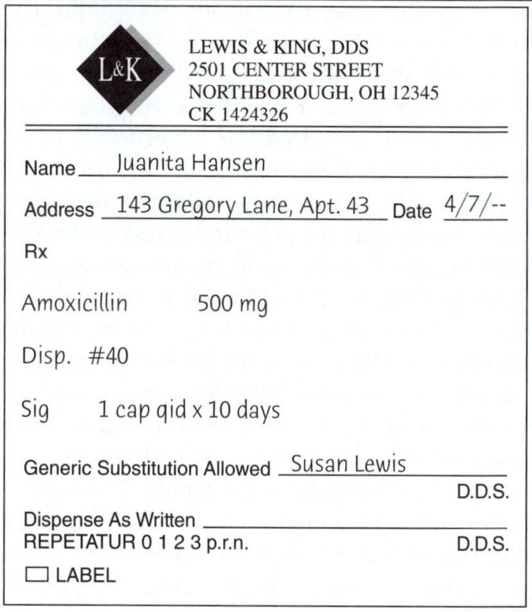

[1] L&K LEWIS & KING, DDS
2501 CENTER STREET
NORTHBOROUGH, OH 12345
CK 1424326

[2] Name Juanita Hansen
Address 143 Gregory Lane, Apt. 43 Date 4/7/--

[3] Rx

[4] Amoxicillin 500 mg

[5] Disp. #40

[6] Sig 1 cap qid x 10 days

[7] Generic Substitution Allowed Susan Lewis D.D.S.
Dispense As Written ______ D.D.S.

[8] REPETATUR 0 1 2 3 p.r.n.

[9] ☐ LABEL

FIGURE 15-3

Prescription with parts identified. (1) heading, (2) superscription, (3) Rx symbol, (4) inscription, (5) subscription, (6) signature, (7) signature for generic, (8) refills, and (9) labeling.

will assist in accuracy and quality control. It is recommended that a copy of the prescription be placed in the patient's chart for future reference.

Heading. The **heading** includes the dentist's name and degrees, office address, and phone number. The dentist's DEA number must be printed in this area or near the signature. This number was assigned to the dentist and must be used every time a controlled substance is prescribed.

Superscription. The **superscription** is directly below the heading. This area has blank lines where the dentist can fill in the name and address of the patient. Included in this area is a space for the date that the prescription was written. Other information, such as the patient's phone number, age, and gender, is also helpful to the pharmacist. Patients do not always fill the prescriptions immediately and may in fact not need them until a later date or not at all. Having the date filled in aids the pharmacist in obtaining pertinent information about the need for the drug. The age and gender give further information as to the dosage amount needed by the patient. The pharmacist has extensive training about each drug and is a helpful member of the health care team. The pharmacist may call the dentist and consult about a prescription, or about a patient obtaining prescriptions from numerous offices. Health care providers must work together in discouraging drug abuse.

Body of the Prescription. The body of the prescription is labeled with the Rx symbol and has both the inscription area and the **subscription** area. In the **inscription** area, the doctor inscribes or writes the name and strength of the drug being prescribed, the dose, and in what form the drug is to be dispensed. He or she specifies the number of doses and directions on how the drug should be taken. In the **subscription** area special directions are written to the pharmacist on how to prepare the medication and the designation of the form (pill, powder, and solution) in which the drug is be made. The office may have several pre-stamped prescription tablets with the drug of choice that the dentist can use to save time in writing, and to ensure that it can be easily read. If not, the prescription is written or completed on the computer. The writing of the body of the prescription is often done in an abbreviated format. Many Latin abbreviations are used for this. For example, the prescription might read as follows: "Sig: 1 tab q.i.d. for 2 wks." This means take one tablet four times a day for two weeks. When a prescription is dispensed by the pharmacist, it is a law that the name of the drug and the directions be put on the label of the drug container.

Latin Abbreviations and English Meanings of Prescriptions

Latin Abbreviation	English Meaning of Latin Abbreviation
a.a.	Of each
a.c.	Before meals
b.i.d.	Twice a day
t.i.d.	Three times a day
q.i.d.	Four times a day
q.h.	Every hour
q.4.h.	Every four hours
q.8.h.	Every eight hours
Sig	Take
p.c.	After meals
p.r.n	When necessary or as needed

Closing of the Prescription. The **closing** of the prescription is where the dentist signs his or her name, noting their **signature**, authorizes whether the prescription can be refilled and how many times, and checks whether a generic brand of this medication can be dispensed in place of the one written.

Many offices have prescription pads that are numbered sequentially, and the information regarding the office and doctor's name and address is preprinted on them. They may have them printed in triplicate so that a copy of each written prescription can be kept in the corresponding patient's chart, or on the pad according to the number. Routinely, prescriptions are now done on the computer, and a printed copy will be given to the patient and the electronic copy will be entered into the patient's computerized file. Either way, a notation should be written on the patient's chart about the prescription and the instructions given. The prescription pads must be kept in a secure place to prevent theft.

Drug Laws

In 1906, the U.S. government passed **the Pure Food and Drug Act.** This law was enacted to control and regulate the composition, sale, and distribution of drugs. Prior to 1906, drugs were not regulated, and drugs of varying compositions and purity were sold. Many of these drugs were harmful for human consumption.

Other laws were passed to control the sale of narcotic drugs in the early twentieth century. **The Federal Food, Drug, and Cosmetic Act** was passed in 1938. This allowed only the United States' **Food and Drug Administration (FDA)** to have control of all food, cosmetics, and drugs sold. The drugs and cosmetics must pass standards set by the FDA and obtain approval prior to sale. The FDA also controls the advertising for all food, drugs, and cosmetics. This act was amended in 1951 and 1965 to establish additional regulations to prevent tampering with foods, drugs, and cosmetics. It also required that certain preparations have warning labels such as: "This product may cause drowsiness," or "Do not drive while taking this product." This act also includes a clause that states that any nonprescription or prescription drug must be shown to be effective as well as safe. Products may note on their packaging that they have met the rigid standards set by the FDA.

The Comprehensive Drug Abuse Prevention and Control Act of 1970

The **Comprehensive Drug Abuse Prevention and Control Act of 1970** was established to identify drugs according to five schedules of abuse potential. Title II of this act deals with the control of drugs and enforcement of drug laws. The **Controlled Substances Act** gives the power of enforcement of this act to the DEA, which is part of the U.S. Department of Justice. Individuals who dispense drugs must have DEA-issued numbers to prescribe drugs. Dentists who dispense controlled substances improperly can have their offices closed and their licenses revoked. The dental assistants and the dentist must carefully check patients' medical and dental histories prior to writing any prescription.

Schedule number "I" has a higher abuse potential and is more dangerous than schedule number "V." Drugs are added and subtracted to this schedule (Table 15-1) as well as moved from one schedule number to another. This is dependent upon

TABLE 15-1 Five Schedules of Controlled Substances

Schedule Number	Abuse Potential and Legal Limitations	Examples of Substances
1. C	High abuse potential Not approved for medical use in the United States	Heroin, LSD, and mescaline
2. CII	High abuse potential May lead to severe dependence Written prescription only No phoning in of prescription by office health care worker No refills May be faxed, but original prescription must be turned in to pick up prescription In emergency, physician may phone in, but handwritten prescription must go to pharmacy within 72 hours	Morphine, codeine, methadone, Percocet, Tylox, Dilaudid, Ritalin, Oxycontin, and meperidine (Demerol)
3. CIII	May lead to limited dependence Written, faxed, or verbal (phoned-in) prescription, by physician only May be refilled up to five times in 6 months	Marinol, Tussionex, and Tylenol with codeine
4. CIV	Lower abuse potential than above schedules Prescription may be written out by health care worker, but must be signed by the physician Prescription may be phoned in by health care worker or faxed May be refilled up to five times in 6 months	Valium, Ativan, Xanax, phenobarbital, Librium, Darvocet, Restoril, and Ambien
5. CV	Low abuse potential compared to above schedules Consists primarily of preparations for cough suppressants containing codeine and preparations for diarrhea (e.g., paregoric and opium tincture)	Phenergan with codeine, Robitussin-A-C, Tussi-Organidin, N.R., Donnagel-PG, and Lomotil

Note: Some states may have stricter schedules than the federal regulations. You must be aware of the regulations in your state.

incidences of overdose, or if a drug becomes more of a societal problem. The schedule numbers are referenced with Roman numerals; and, often, these Roman numerals are inside the capital C on drug packages and inserts, as well as other drug information resources (Figure 15-4).

- Schedule I drugs have a high potential for abuse, and no accepted medical use. Drugs in this schedule include mescaline, heroin, and hallucinogens such as LSD.
- Schedule II drugs have a high potential for abuse but also have accepted medical uses. These drugs lead to physical and psychological dependence. Drugs in this schedule include narcotics such as morphine, codeine, barbiturates such as tranquilizers, and amphetamines. Prescriptions in this schedule cannot be refilled.
- Schedule III drugs have a lower potential for abuse than those in Schedule II and have accepted medical uses. Compounds from this category are used in several drugs routinely prescribed in the dental office. The drugs in this category may lead to chemical dependence and include barbiturates, stimulants, and depressants not in Schedule II, and a number of compounds such as Tylenol III.
- Schedule IV drugs have less potential for abuse than those in Schedule III and also have acceptable medical uses. Schedule IV drugs have limited dependence risk. Drugs in this schedule include antidepressants, antianxiety drugs, and sedative drugs not included in the first three schedules.
- Schedule V drugs have the least potential for abuse and may consist of a compound from other schedules in small amounts. The drugs in this schedule may be antidiarrheal medicines or cough medicines. The drugs in this group are also called OTC drugs.

Dental Assistants and the Law

It is often the responsibility of the dental assistant to keep accurate records of the drugs dispensed; and the information that was given to the patient should be recorded as well.

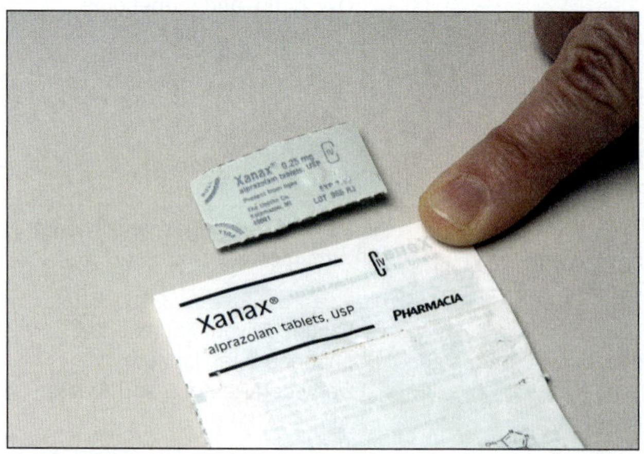

FIGURE 15-4

(A) Drug packages and (B) drug inserts showing the controlled substance schedule numbers. They are also found in numerous drug reference books.

They may write many of the prescriptions manually, or on a computer, which the doctor reviews and signs, obtaining the forms that the prescriptions were written on and insuring that the prescription pads were not left out in the open. They may also be involved in placing controlled substances in locked cupboards and insuring that certain medications are kept in stock. Dental assistants play a large role in making sure that drug samples are left in a designated area when pharmaceutical representatives leave them for the dentist to try. The dental assistant may also be the representative of the office whom the pharmacist communicates concerning patient prescriptions and questions. It is important that the following guidelines are followed in the dental office:

1. Controlled substances, if used in the office, must be locked and kept secure at all times. Records of these substances must be maintained. These records should show what was received by the office, when this occurred, and what and to whom this substance was dispensed. There must be notation of any substance that was destroyed by the office. These records, and the records of the past two years, have to be available to the DEA at any time when requested.
2. A current drug reference should be available at all times. There are a number of books available that pertain primarily to dentistry, as well as a DVD and online service that is updated regularly.
3. Update knowledge on any changes in the scheduled drugs. Check with the DEA, FDA, and the ADA for updates on drug usage and routes of administration.
4. Get to know the pharmacist who is recommended by the office, as well as other pharmacists in the area. Establish a working rapport with them and utilize their knowledge to aid the dentist in dispensing prescriptions. The pharmaceutical sales representative is also a tremendous resource for information about drugs and their usage in patient care.
5. Place prescription pads, computer-generated prescription applications, and the dentist's DEA registration number out of public areas. Keep this information concealed and safe to ensure that fraud and drug tampering do not occur.
6. Most states have an updated drug labeling law. It covers how drugs should be labeled if given out to patients. Dental assistants may be directed to give the patients medication or a few tablets to take home. They need to know what information and labeling should occur on the bottle or packet containing the medication to meet the state guidelines. Go to the state (where the office is located) department of health to find this information.
7. Keep accurate records! In most cases it is advisable to make a copy of the prescription for the patient's records. It must also be noted, along with the date, after the record of the treatment that the patient received. Many of the computer software programs allow for this information to be attached to the patient's computer record.

Pharmacokinetics

The study of the stages of drug action in the body is called **pharmacokinetics**. It refers to the ability of the body to intake a drug, and the action of the drug until it exits the body. It goes through four stages: absorption, distribution, metabolism, and excretion (Figure 15-5).

The ability of the body to take in the drug from the site of administration is **absorption**. The route impacts the speed of the absorption. Rapid absorption would occur through intravenous administration and slow absorption occurs during oral administration. After the drug has entered the body, the chemical compound of the

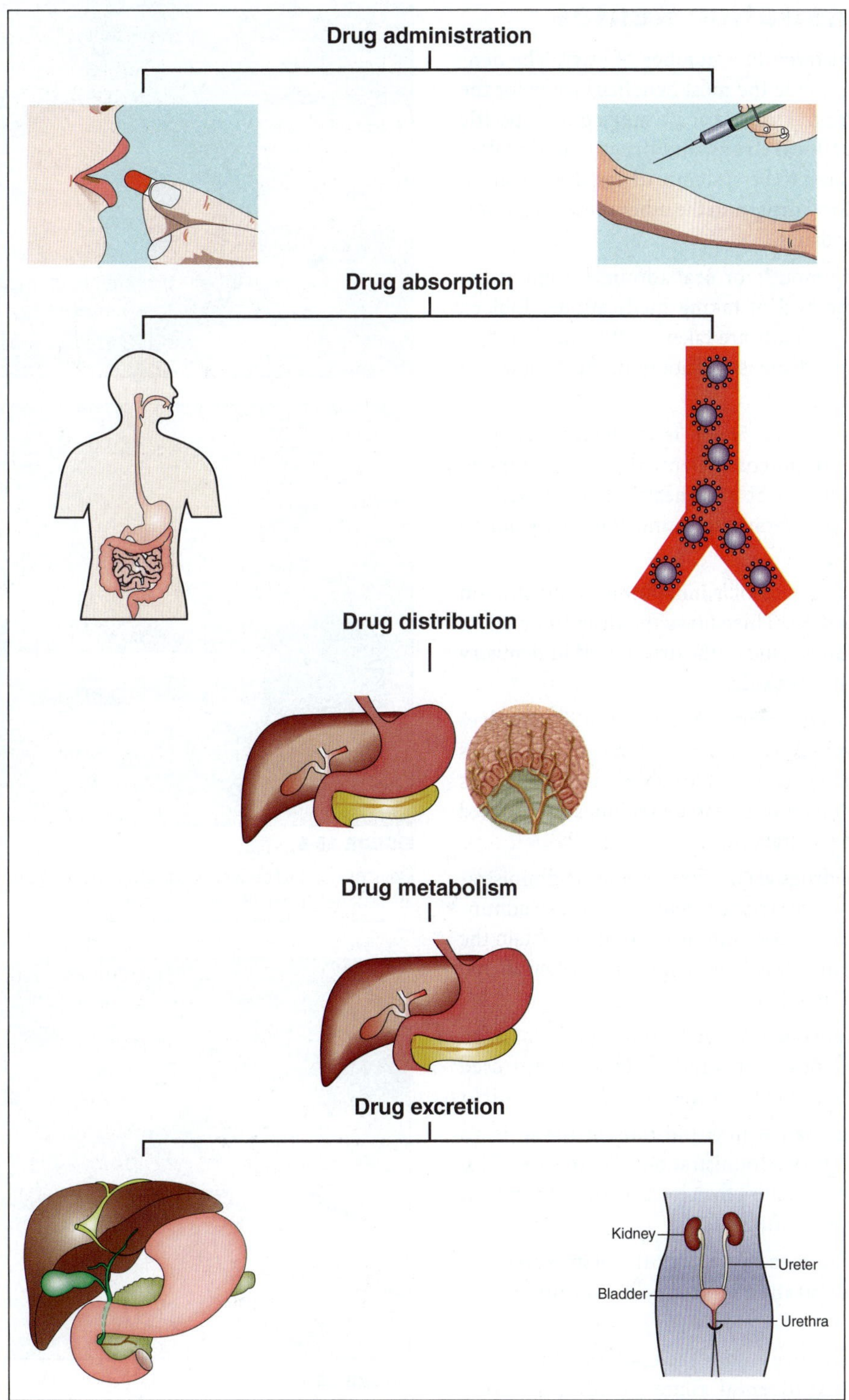

FIGURE 15-5

Pharmacokinetics: the stages of drug action in the body.

drug attaches to the protein in the blood and circulates throughout the body, affecting the destination area, this is called **distribution**. When the chemical transforms and acts on the cells of a living organism this is called **metabolism**. Excess drug is excreted through the liver or kidneys through **excretion**.

Drug Administration Routes

Drugs can be administered in a number of ways. The dentist will evaluate and decide the most beneficial route for the patient to take the drug. Drugs that are applied in a specific area are termed to be **local drugs**; and drugs that are taken internally are considered to be **systemic drugs**. Topical anesthetic is termed as a local drug, and the other routes of administration are systemic drugs.

- Administration by mouth, or **oral** administration, is the most common method of taking medications. Tablets, capsules, pills, and liquids are taken in this manner. The patient swallows the dispensed amount of the drug with a glass of water.
- Ointment, lotion, gel, or cream is applied topically to the skin surface or mucosa. Dentistry uses a **topical** drug to prepare for local anesthesia. It is applied on the oral mucous membrane to numb the area prior to injection.
- To breathe in a gas or aerosol is **inhalation** administration (Figures 15-6A and B). This allows the drug to be taken quickly into the lungs. One of the drugs used in dentistry by inhalation is nitrous oxide.
- Placement of medication under the tongue until it dissolves is **sublingual** administration. For example, if a patient is experiencing angina pectoris, a nitroglycerin pill or spray is administered sublingually. Drugs are seldom administered by this route in the dental office.
- Administration of drugs via the **rectal** route of administration in the dental office is nonexistent. Patients can administer enemas or suppositories in this manner to obtain the effects of drugs in this class. This route is used when an oral route is not recommended.
- Injection of a substance directly into the vein is an **intravenous** route of administration. This route is used for immediate drug response (Figure 15-7).
- Injection of a substance into the muscle tissue is an **intramuscular** route of administration (Figure 15-8). This route gives a slower response than intravenous administration but has a longer-lasting effect.
- Injection of a substance just under the skin, above the muscle, is a **subcutaneous** route of administration (Figure 15-9).
- Injection of a substance under the epidermis (top layer of skin) is an **intradermal** route of administration (Figures 15-10A and B).

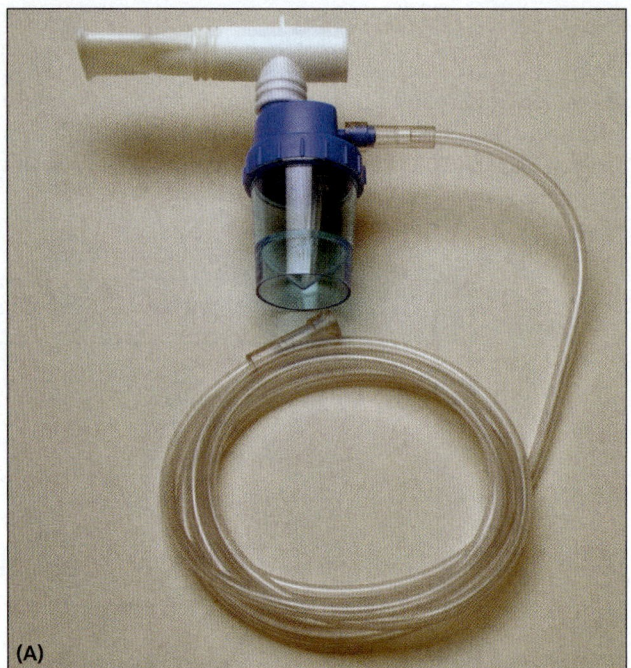

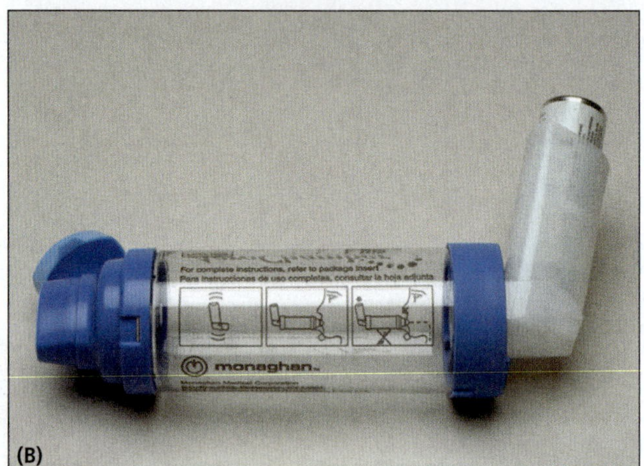

FIGURE 15-6
Devices used to deliver medication via inhalation. (A) Small volume aerosol nebulizer. (B) Metered dose inhaler.

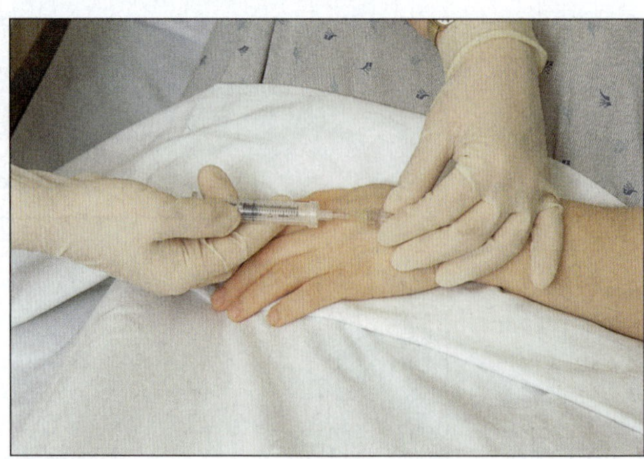

FIGURE 15-7
Administering a drug through an intravenous route.

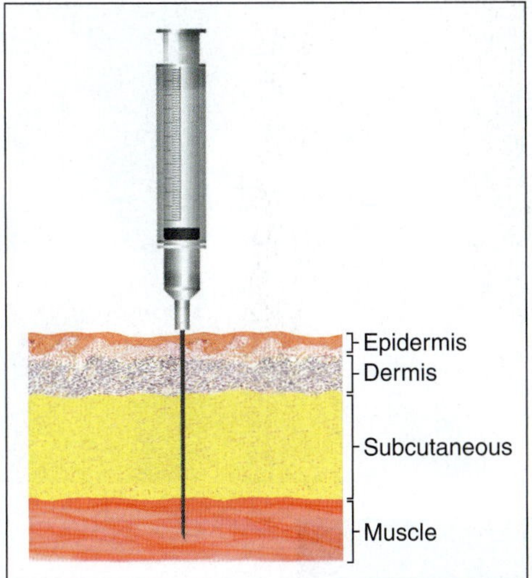

FIGURE 15-8
Administering an intramuscular injection.

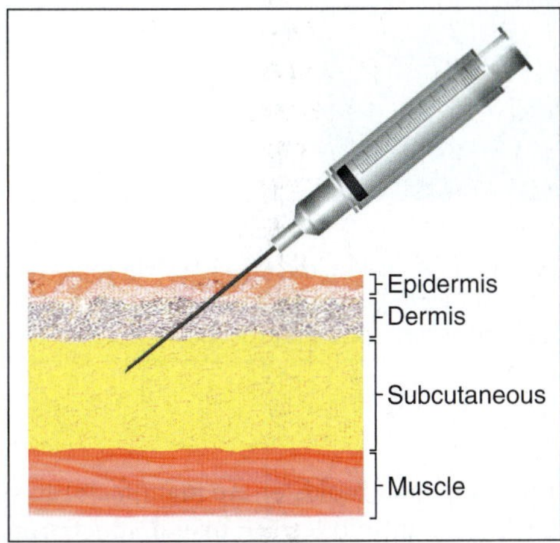

FIGURE 15-9
Administering a subcutaneous injection.

- Administration of a drug through a drug reservoir in a patch applied to the skin in a consistent, controlled manner is a **transdermal** route of administration (Figures 15-11A to C).

Drugs

The following section covers both illegal and prescription drugs. Dental assistants are concerned with prescribed drugs, but must also have knowledge about illegal drugs that patients may be using, and must understand what can happen if the drugs interact. There is an increasing rise in **substance abuse** and **drug abuse** (using drugs for other than medicinal purposes) in today's society. More and more individuals are seeking drugs for thrills or for coping with daily life. It is important that the caregiver pays special attention to the patient and listens to the information that the patient provides. It is also important to know the signs and symptoms that individuals may present if they are under the influence of drugs. Having background knowledge about drugs and their effects helps the dental assistant provide better patient care.

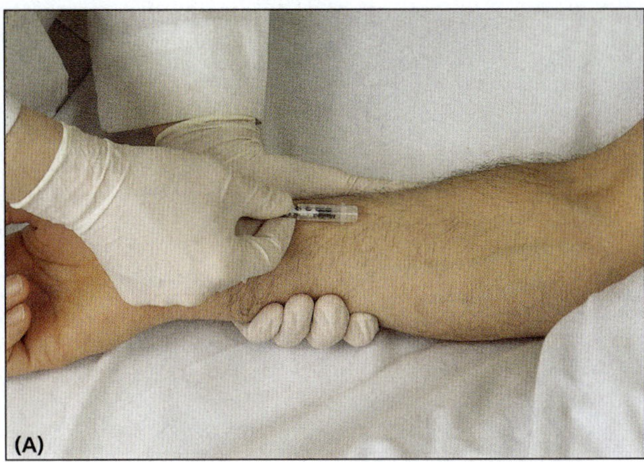

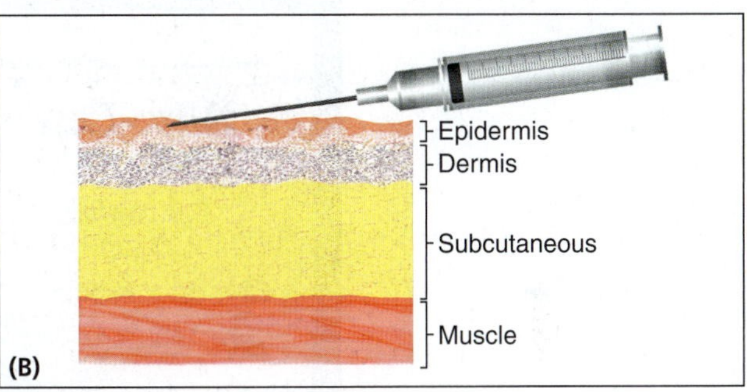

FIGURE 15-10
Administering an intradermal injection. (A) The needle is held almost flat against the skin with the bevel up, during an intradermal injection. (B) The injection must be done slowly so that the skin does not bubble up. It is just slightly under the epidermis of the skin.

Prescribed Drugs by Drug Classification

Dentists take great care in administering drugs. After discussing the condition with the patient, the dentist may prescribe or administer certain medications to alleviate treatment anxiety and discomfort. The patient's dental record must show all prescriptions given to the patient, the route administered, and the information the doctor and assistant gave orally to the patient at the time of dispensing. A copy of the prescription should be placed in the patient's record indicating the dosage amount. Any OTC drugs the dentist recommended to the patient should be noted on the patient's record as well. In addition to the drugs that the dentist prescribes, the patient may have other drugs that he or she is taking that may cause interactions or complications during dental treatment. The dentist must understand all of the drugs, their classifications, their uses, and the side effects

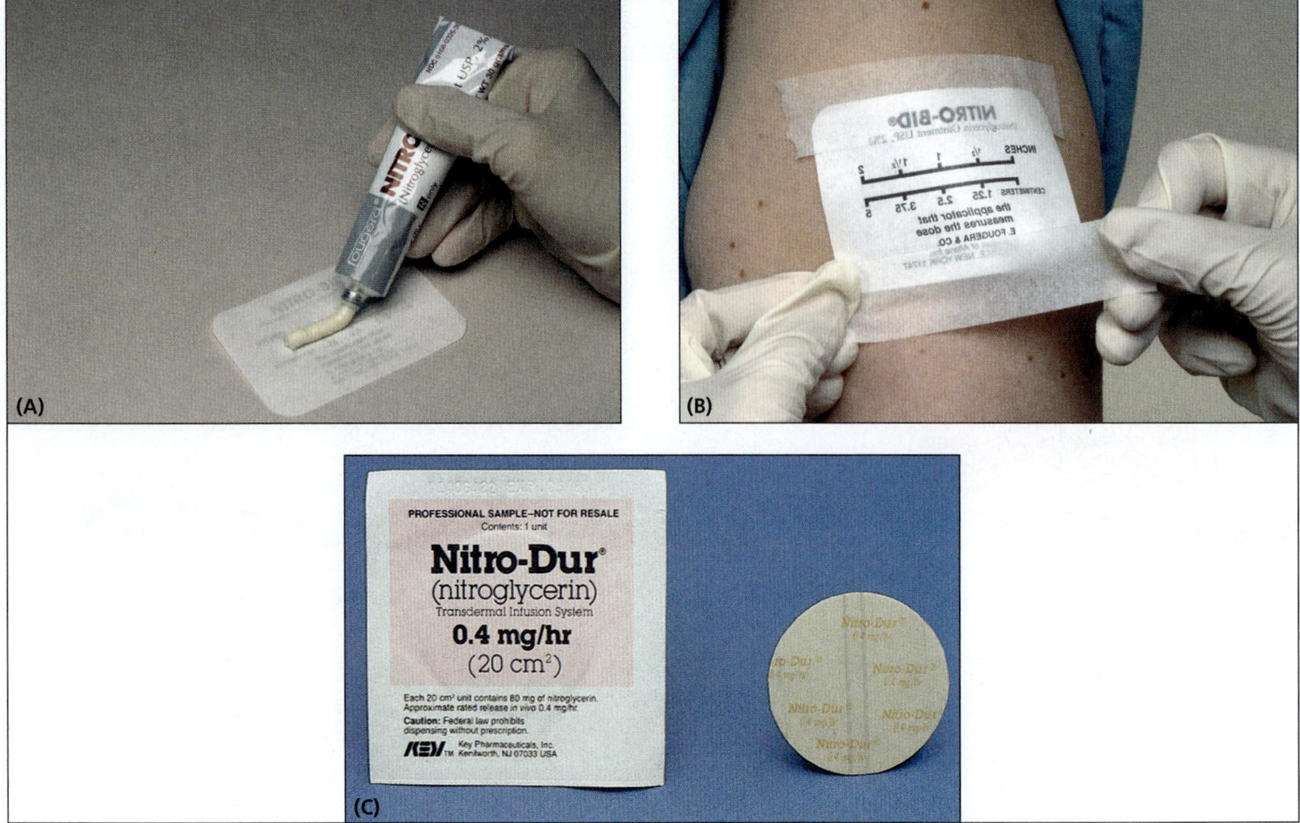

FIGURE 15-11

Transdermal administration of nitroglycerin ointment. (A) Ointment is applied on an application ruler on the paper. (B) The application paper is then inverted and the ointment contacts the skin; it is attached with paper tape. (C) Nitro-Dur® is a transdermal system of delivering medication (nitroglycerin) to manage angina pectoris. It is also available in a pre-dispensed sealed application as shown.

of each. Table 15-2 contains certain drugs, their uses, and some possible side effects.

Analgesics. An **analgesic** drug (anesthesia) causes loss of pain but not a loss of all sensation. Drugs that relieve pain can be non-narcotic, such as aspirin, ibuprofen, and acetaminophen, or narcotic, such as codeine and morphine. The non-narcotic analgesics are useful in the treatment of mild or moderate pain. If severe pain persists, a stronger narcotic analgesic is prescribed. Aspirin normally is not prescribed after a dental extraction because of its ability to thin blood and inhibit clotting. This effect is contraindicated for healing the socket area following an extraction. Other side effects of aspirin are stomach irritation and nausea. Patients must be instructed to take aspirin with a large glass of water to ensure that the pill dissolves and does not irritate the stomach lining in a concentrated form.

Side effects of narcotic analgesics, such as nausea, vomiting, constipation, and breathing difficulties, are minimal but may still occur.

Antibiotics. An **antibiotic**, such as aminoglycosides, cephalosporins, penicillins, tetracyclines, and others, is given to patients to treat infection (Figure 15-12). These drugs are derived from fungi and molds or are manufactured synthetically. Some of the antibiotics are **broad spectrum**, meaning they are effective against a wide range of bacteria, while some treat only one type of bacteria. More than one type of antibiotic may be prescribed to increase the probability of success in disease treatment. A culture can be taken to further identify the specific type of bacteria to be treated. Antibiotics are ineffective against viruses.

Normally, antibiotics are taken to treat infections, but they are often prescribed as a **prophylactic** measure to prevent infection. Any patient who has had rheumatic fever, joint replacement, heart valve replacement, or a heart murmur should take a dose of antibiotics prior to dental treatment to reduce the risk of endocarditis (inflammation of the lining of the heart).

Resistance to antibiotics can develop. This often occurs when the user fails to take the antibiotic drug as directed. The patient begins to feel better and stops taking the antibiotic before all the disease-causing bacteria have been killed. The bacteria then return stronger and more resistant to the antibiotic.

Adverse side effects of antibiotics include nausea, diarrhea, and an allergic rash. They can also kill normal body flora, causing oral, intestinal, or vaginal candidiasis (thrush). Some people also have severe allergic reactions with a rash, itching,

TABLE 15-2 Drug Classifications

Drug Type	Examples	Some Uses of the Drug	Action of the Drug	Some Possible Side Effects
Analgesic	Acetaminophen, aspirin, Dilaudid, Percodan, Tylenol, Bufferin, Panadol	Control pain	Pain therapy	GI distress, bleeding, and bruising
Antibiotic	Keflex, amoxicillin, tetracycline, penicillin G	Treatment of infection	Treats streptococcal, some staphylococcal, and meningococcal infections	Electrolyte imbalance, hypersensitivity reaction
Anticholinergic	Atropine, propantheline bromide	Treatment to reduce secretions	Treats bradycardia, dilates the pupil for ophthalmic examination, inhibits the flow of saliva	Mouth dryness, blurred vision
Anticoagulant	Coumadin, aspirin, heparin	Prevents the formation of blood clots	Embolism control	Hemorrhage, blood in urine, minor bleeding
Anticonvulsant	Zarontin, Klonopin, Depakene, Dilantin	Reduces the number and severity of seizures	Epileptic seizure control	Irritability, GI distress, sedation
Antidiabetic	Glucophage, Avandamet Dymelor, Glucotrol	Regulates blood sugar	Diabetes control	GI distress, dermatological effects
Antidepressant	Prozac, Tofranil, Elavil	Treats depression, stabilizes moods	Elevates mood	Mouth dryness, increased appetite, drowsiness, constipation, confusion
Antifungal	Mycostatin, nystatin	Used as a fungicide	Treats candidiasis (thrush)	Nausea (rare)
Antihistamine	Benadryl, Tavist Allergy, Phenergan	Provides relief of allergic symptoms caused by histamine release	Treats allergies, conjunctivitis, and rash	Drying of secretions, sedation
Antihypertensive	Tenormin, methyldopa hydralazine	Slows heart rate, inhibits arteries from closing	Treats hypertension and elevated blood pressure	Hypotension, GI symptoms
Anti-inflammatory	Motrin, Advil, prednisone, cortisone, ibuprofen	Treats inflammation	Reduces the inflammation process	GI ulceration or bleeding, heartburn, headache
Antilipemic/statins	Lipitor, Zocor, Advicor, Niaspan	Transports cholesterol and other fats through the bloodstream	Treatment of high cholesterol levels	Muscle weakness, mild GI distress, headache, elevated liver enzymes
Antithyroid	Synthroid, Levoxyl, Levothroid	Used to relieve symptoms of hyperthyroidism	Treats symptoms of hyperthyroidism	rash, fever (rare)
Bronchodilator	Albuterol sulfate, Primatene Volmax	Relaxes the smooth muscles of the bronchial tree	Relieves bronchospasm, treats asthma	Hypoventilation, GI distress, hypertension
Contraceptive	Provera, Ovrette, progestin	Prevents ovulation	Birth control	Fluid retention, weight gain or loss, migraine headaches
Decongestant	Afrin, Allerest, Sudafed	Constricts blood vessels in respiratory tract	Treats congestion and opens airways	Anxiety, hypertension
Diuretic	Lasix, Aldactone, Dyrenium	Increases the excretion of water, sodium chloride, and potassium	Treats edema and electrolyte imbalance	Fluid and electrolyte imbalance, dehydration, hypotension
Hemostatic	Gelfoam	Induces clotting	Used for dry socket	Rare

(continues)

TABLE 15-2 Drug Classifications (continued)

Drug Type	Examples	Some Uses of the Drug	Action of the Drug	Some Possible Side Effects
Hormone replacement	Estrogen, Estratest, Humulin	Hormone regulator	Maintains hormone levels and treats menopause symptoms	Hypertension, GI effects, skin disorders
MAOIs	Marplan, Nardil, Parnate	Anticonvulsants and antiparkinsonian drugs	Controls convulsing behavior	Interacts with many foods and other drugs, nervousness, headache, hypertension, tachycardia
Nitrates	Nitrostat, nitroglycerin, Nitrolingual spray	Used to dilate blood vessels	Treats angina pectoris and chest pain	Headache, hypotension, dry mouth
Tranquilizer/ antianxiety	Xanax, Librium, Valium (diazepam), Serax	Promotes relaxation	has a calming effect, minor tranquilizer	Drowsiness, dizziness

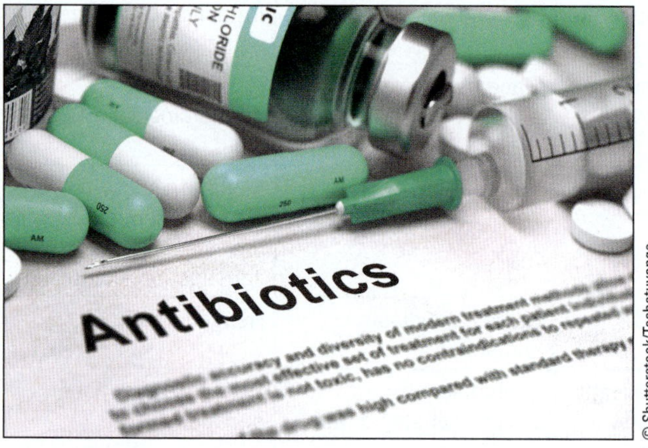

© Shutterstock/Tashatuvango

FIGURE 15-12

Various forms and types of antibiotic medications.

swelling, and difficulty breathing. If this happens, an antihistamine is used to counteract the reaction of the allergen.

- *Penicillin* was the first group of antibiotic drugs to be discovered. It is still used in the treatment of many diseases, including tonsillitis, bronchitis, and pneumonia. Side effects of the drugs in this category are allergic reactions. If an individual becomes allergic to one type of penicillin, others in this group, or any derivatives, must be administered with great caution.
- *Penicillin V*, or phenoxymethyl-penicillin, is limited to gram-positive bacteria, such as ulcerative gingi-vostomatitis and streptococcal infections.
- *Penicillin G benzathine* is often the drug chosen for a variety of infections, including pneumococci, gonorrhea, syphilis, streptococci, and meningococcal meningitis.
- *Amoxicillin* is another broad-spectrum antibiotic. Like most antibiotics, it is important to take the entire prescription to avoid antibiotic resistance. Watch for any allergic reaction as with penicillin.
- *Ampicillin*, also a broad-spectrum antibiotic, is often used for dental patients at risk for bacterial endocarditis, and is given prior, during, and after an invasive dental procedure.
- *Cloxacillin*, *nafcillin*, and *oxacillin* are primarily used to treat *Staphylococcus aureus* infections.
- *Erythromycin* is an antibiotic much like penicillin that can be used by individuals who are allergic to penicillin and by children as a substitute for tetracycline. It is a coated tablet, therefore, it is not destroyed by the acid in the stomach when taken orally. It can be given in capsule or liquid form, injected, or by ointment. Side effects include stomach pain, nausea, vomiting, and diarrhea. It can produce a rash if the individual becomes hypersensitive to the substance.
- *Tetracycline* is a broad-spectrum drug that kills a wide range of bacterial microorganisms. It must be taken with care, taking one tablet 1 hour before meals or 2 hours after a meal. The drug becomes useless if taken with some foods or dairy products. Tetracycline must not be given to children under 12 or to pregnant women because it discolors developing teeth. People with poor kidney function should not take tetracycline antibiotics, because they may cause kidney failure. Side effects of tetracycline are much like those of other antibiotics: nausea, vomiting, diarrhea, and possible rash if allergic.

Anticholinergics. Anticholinergic drugs are used as premedications before general **anesthesia** to reduce secretion from the lungs, and as emergency drugs to treat people with abnormally slow heart rates (bradycardia). They are also used to dilate the eyes during an ophthalmology examination.

- *Atropine Sulfate* and *propantheline bromide* are anticholinergic drugs used in dentistry to inhibit the flow of saliva. A patient who produces excessive saliva may make it difficult for the dental team to obtain a good impression for crown or bridge treatment. If atropine is taken a couple of hours prior to treatment, the patient will have a dry mouth, which allows for a clearly defined impression to be obtained. This effect will disappear in four to six hours after the drug has been administered.

Anticoagulants. Anticoagulant medication prevents **coagulation** (i.e., it prevents the blood from clotting). Normally it takes over 48 hours for the effect of an anticoagulant to develop, except when using heparin, and then it occurs quickly. Heparin is used around medical devices to prevent blood or plasma from clotting in or on the medical device. Anticoagulants are taken to reduce blood clotting and, thereby, prevent pulmonary embolism, strokes, and myocardial infarctions (heart attacks) from occurring. The disadvantage of these drugs is that the patient taking them may be especially susceptible to bleeding complications. The dental assistant should ensure that the dentist is made aware that a patient is taking these drugs, if he or she updates the patient's health or medical history. If surgery is the treatment that the patient is having, the dentist may make adjustments.

Anticonvulsants. An anticonvulsant is used to suppress the rapid and excessive firing of neurons that initiate a patient having a seizure. Patients with epileptic seizures take anticonvulsants. One of the effects of anticonvulsant drugs, such as Dilantin, is that they cause gingival hyperplasia, or the overgrowth of gingival tissue. (See Chapter 26, Oral Pathology, for a discussion of Dilantin hyperplasia.) Anticonvulsants are used for bipolar disorder to stabilize moodiness.

Antidiabetic Medication. Antidiabetic medications lower the glucose levels in the blood and aid in the treatment of diabetes mellitus. Many different types of antidiabetic drugs are on the market; and the physician will select the appropriate one dependent upon the type of diabetes, and the age and weight of the patient along with other factors. Diabetes mellitus type 1 and 2 are discussed in Chapter 16, Emergency Management.

Antidepressant Medication. Individuals with major depression, anxiety disorders, social anxiety disorders, and mood swing disorders may be taking an antidepressant medication. Some of the most frequently televised antidepressant medications include: Prozac, Lexapro, Cymbalta, and Zoloft. These psychiatric medications stabilize moods but may cause confusion and dry mouth, to name a couple of the side effects that affect dentistry. Make sure the pre- and post-operative instructions are clear. During the treatment the patient may want to have their mouth rinsed occasionally. The patient may share other things that may help lower the anxiety in regards to their care. For example, it may be beneficial to schedule the patient immediately after lunch, or as the first appointment in the morning, so that they can come back for treatment without causing undue stress due to having to wait.

Antifungal Agents. Drugs prescribed to treat infections caused by fungi are antifungal agents (Figure 15-13). They are available in a number of forms, such as tablets, suspensions, creams, injections, and vaginal suppositories. Preparations applied to the skin may show adverse reactions by increasing irritation. Preparations taken orally may, in rare cases, show serious side effects such as liver or kidney damage.

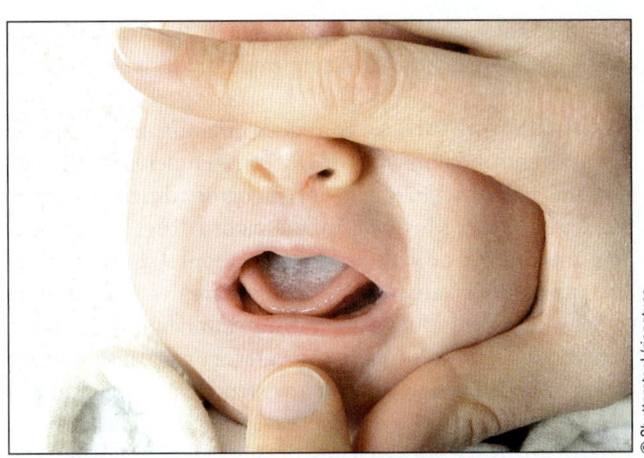

FIGURE 15-13
Oral thrush found in an infant is treated with antifungal agent.

- *Nystatin* is an antifungal drug used in dentistry to treat candidiasis (oral thrush). The suspension, administered orally, is held in the mouth prior to swallowing. It is safely taken during pregnancy. Patients should continue to take it 48 hours after the last sign of infection is apparent. Extremely high doses taken orally may cause nausea, vomiting, and diarrhea. Nystatin ointment can be used for angular cheilitis (see Chapter 27, Oral Pathology). The ointment is applied to the lesion four times a day until healed.
- *Flucinonide gel* is applied by a cotton swab to affected areas twice daily to treat mild to moderate lichen planus, a condition in the oral cavity that often presents as a lacy network of white spots covering the lining of the cheeks (see Chapter 27, Oral Pathology). Mild allergic reactions may be treated with diphenhydramine HCl, 50 mg, which is dispensed every four hours as needed. Herpetic infections are often treated with a drug called penciclovir one percent cream, which is applied to affected areas every two hours while awake.

Antihistamines. Antihistamines are taken to provide relief of allergic symptoms, conjunctivitis, and rash. They contend for the histamine receptor sites, and prevent the histamine from causing allergic symptoms such as a runny nose, sneezing, and runny eyes. Most individuals take them continuously throughout the allergy season if they have allergies. Most antihistamine drugs are available over the counter or without a prescription. A couple of the side effects are drowsiness and dry mouth.

Antihypertensives. Antihypertensive drugs are used to treat hypertension, or high blood pressure. They help slow down the heart rate and inhibit the arteries from closing. They reduce the occurrence of dementia and heart disease. Antihypertensives are often called beta blockers; examples include

Toprol, Levatol, and Zebeta. To stimulate the heart, digitalis medications are given. An example of digitalis is Digoxin.

Anti-inflammatories. To reduce inflammation, a patient may take anti-inflammatory drugs. The commercials on television show many types of anti-inflammatory drugs that are on the market today. Most anti-inflammatory drugs are available over the counter or without a prescription. Aspirin, ibuprofen, and naproxen are some common examples. Brand names such as Advil and Motrin are anti-inflammatory drugs taken to reduce pain. Most drugs in this category can cause stomach ulcers or bleeding if taken over an extended period of time.

Antilipemic Drugs. Drugs in this category are used to lower abnormally high blood levels of lipids or, to use the term heard more often, to treat high cholesterol. Lifestyle changes, such as weight loss, proper diet, and exercise, along with antilipemic medications, also called statins, can lower cholesterol scores and decrease lipid levels. Lipitor and similar drugs are included in this medication group.

Antithyroid Agents. Antithyroid drugs are taken to act upon thyroid hormones and treat hyperthyroidism. It is also used in the treatment of Grave's disease. Grave's disease is diagnosed by several methods to rule out other disorders. The functioning of the thyroid is one of the areas to check for Grave's disease. Some individuals have a bulging of the eyeballs (called **exophthalmos**). The doctor will check for hyperthyroidism and, if indicated, will conduct additional tests. The most common side effect of taking antithyroid medication is having a rash.

Bronchodilators. Bronchodilators are commonly used for asthma and similar respiratory problems (Figure 15-14). Children who have wheezing problems often carry with them a bronchodilator to improve breathing. When discussing this in the office with the patient, they may indicate that they need to use the bronchodilator prior to treatment to ensure that they won't have to stop treatment. Most individuals using a bronchodilator know when they need to use it and how it is to be used. See the discussion of asthma in Chapter 16, Emergency Management, for further information.

Contraceptives. When taking a medical history, female patients often do not put down the contraceptive drugs they are taking. They do not think of it as a medication. The birth control pill, often simply called "the pill," has been used for many years to prevent ovulation and, thereby, prevent pregnancy. It is advantageous to have all medications noted on the medical history to allow for the best possible treatment and care possible for all patients. One of the side effects of contraceptive drugs is fluid retention.

Decongestants. Decongestants are taken to reduce inflammation and mucus formation along with treating congestion by opening the airways. Side effects may include anxiety, nervousness, and dizziness. The patient may come across as agitated. Most drugs from this classification are over-the-counter drugs, or are purchased without a prescription.

Diuretics. There are a number of diuretics on the market. They all increase the excretion of water from the body and are used to treat edema (swelling) (Figure 15-15). Physicians prescribe diuretics for congestive heart failure, high blood pressure, glaucoma, edema, and so on. If a patient is taking a diuretic, the assistant should remember that the patient is going to need to go to the restroom often. They may also see swollen ankles on the patient if they have been standing or sitting up for some period of time. When the patient is laid back in the chair the fluid from the ankles may decrease. This patient may want their head elevated during their treatment.

Hemostatics. Hemostatics are used to stop the bleeding process and initiate blood clotting. In dentistry, these drugs can be used in surgery for numerous procedures,

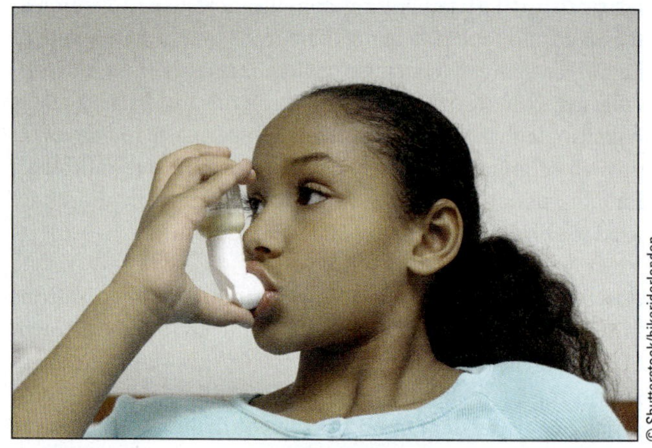

FIGURE 15-14
A bronchodilator is used to treat bronchial restriction in asthma.

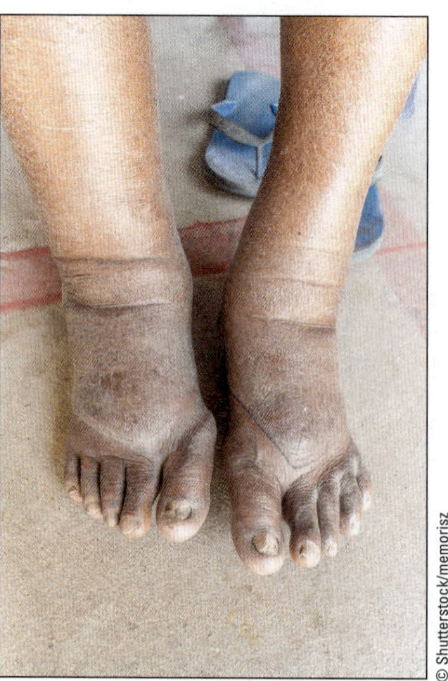

FIGURE 15-15
A swollen ankle on a patient needing a diuretic.

such as in a dry socket (where the socket does not heal after a tooth has been removed), to inhibit bleeding and form a clot; or in the retraction cord (a chemical treated cord that is used between the tooth and tissue during a crown procedure) around a newly prepared tooth to stop any bleeding, in order to make certain that a clear, accurate impression can be obtained. Hemostatic agents can form a clot that seals the hole until tissues are repaired, causing temporary blockage of a break by a platelet plug or through vasoconstriction.

Hormone Replacement Drugs. Drugs taken for hormone replacement therapy are recommended for the treatment of menopause and menopausal symptoms. They are also taken for the treatment of osteoporosis and heart disease. During and after menopause, hormone replacement therapy supplements the body with estrogen alone, or estrogen and progesterone in combination, because the ovaries are no longer producing adequate amounts of these hormones. Estrogen helps the body use calcium, which is an important mineral in bones and teeth. It also helps maintain healthy levels of cholesterol in the blood. Hormone replacement therapy also helps treat hot flashes, which women may encounter during menopause.

Monoamine Oxidase Inhibitors (MAOIs). MAOIs are drugs taken for the treatment of depression. They are also often used as anticonvulsants and antiparkinsonian drugs. Some of the side effects are nervousness, headaches, hypertension, and tachycardia.

Nitrates. Nitrates are prescribed to prevent angina attacks or relieve the symptoms of chest pain when an attack occurs. They cause the blood vessels to dilate (widen), which make it easier for the heart muscle to work. Side effects are headache, hypotension, and a dry mouth. Patients with heart disease may carry nitroglycerin pills with them, which will need to be placed under the tongue if angina occurs. They may tell you where they are located so the dental team members can help them obtain a pill or tablet if an attack takes place. They can also be prescribed as an ointment with skin patches.

Tranquilizer/Antianxiety Drugs. Drugs that provide a sedative effect are called tranquilizers. Tranquilizers relieve anxiety and allow the patient to undergo a procedure with reduced tension. Valium (diazepam) is often given orally a half-hour before a procedure to calm and relax the patient.

Drugs Not Prescribed by the Dentist

Many people think that nicotine and alcohol are not drugs, but they do change life processes within the body, and they are not usually taken to reduce diseases. Patients may be nervous about their treatment and drink alcohol or take some other drugs unknown to the dentist and staff. This may affect how well the patient does during treatment, especially if other drugs are given to the patient during the treatment. The dental team must watch the patient for any complications that can occur during the treatment. Being alert and ready for any emergency during any patient treatment is a good idea. Listen to what the patient says and document everything on the chart that pertains to the patient's health and treatment.

Nicotine. People often do not associate tobacco with drugs, but tobacco contains nicotine. Nicotine is a **stimulant**; it speeds up metabolic activities. The drug nicotine is not used for any purpose to treat disease and, therefore, is not a medicine. It has been shown that tobacco is harmful to the health of smokers as well as to others who may breathe in the secondary smoke. Cancer, lung, and heart disease are much more prevalent in smokers than non-smokers. A smoker has 10 times the risk of developing lung cancer than non-smokers. Tobacco smoke contains carbon monoxide (the same gas found in car exhaust). This gas does not allow the blood to obtain the correct amount of oxygen in the cells and, therefore, the heart and circulatory system have to work harder. This leads to heart disease, the number one cause of death in the United States today. Federal law requires that every package of cigarettes carry a warning indicating the health hazards of smoking.

Smokeless tobacco (chewing tobacco) causes some of the same problems that smoking does. Chewing tobacco adds a high risk factor for oral cancer. Both smoking and chewing tobacco are causative factors in tooth staining, periodontal disease, and halitosis.

Many dental offices are reluctant to hire a dental assistant who smokes. The dental office is a health facility where the promotion of good health habits is essential. Dental assistants should seriously consider smoking cessation. A number of measures are currently available as aids toward smoking cessation.

Caffeine. Caffeine is a habit-forming stimulant. It can be found in a number of sources, including coffee, espresso, tea, soft drinks, chocolate, and cocoa (Figure 15-16). This habit-forming drug also has side effects that may be harmful. Because it is a stimulant, caffeine causes the heart to work harder and may affect the nervous system. It may cause or irritate open sores (an **ulcer**) in the wall of the stomach. Teeth are often stained by caffeine use. Too much caffeine can be toxic. If an individual were to drink 30 double shots of espresso, or 70 to 100 cups of coffee, the result could be fatal. However, under normal use, coffee and espresso are safe to drink.

Caffeine Count

Source	Mg of Caffeine
Cocoa (1 cup)	13
Tea (1 cup)	30–45
Coffee (1 cup)	40–150
Espresso (1 shot)	60–175
Carbonated diet soft drink (one 8-oz glass)	30–50
Carbonated regular soft drink (one 8-oz glass)	35–65

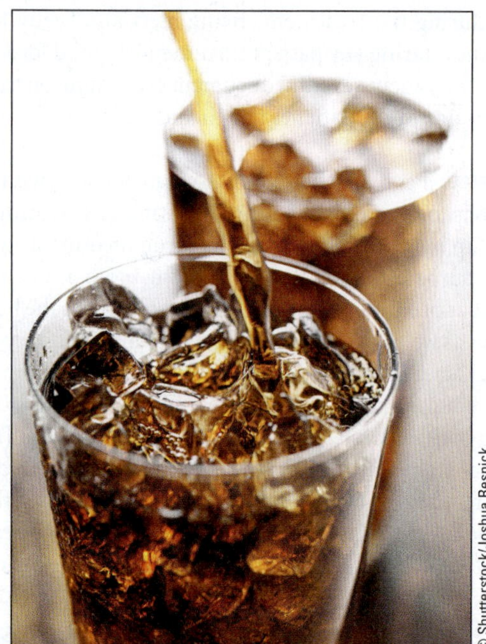
© Shutterstock/Joshua Resnick

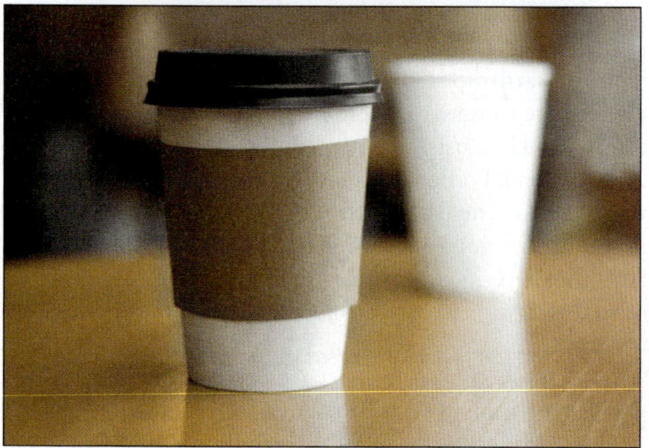
© Shutterstock/vit-plus

FIGURE 15-16

A variety of caffeinated drinks.

Alcohol. One of the oldest known drugs is ethyl alcohol, which is found in alcoholic beverages, such as wine, beer, and whiskey. Alcohol is a **depressant**, a drug that slows down body processes. This habit-forming drug has the opposite effect of stimulants. It affects the body functions rapidly because it is absorbed directly into the blood, and is then carried throughout the body. A 0.08–0.10 percent alcohol level is considered legal intoxication in most states. At 0.05 percent, an individual experiences loss in judgment and coordination, and exhibits slowed reactions and slurred speech. **According to the "National Highway Traffic Safety Administration (NHTSA) every day 28** people are killed by **an alcohol-impaired driver** unable to respond to situations while behind the wheel of their car. This statistic represents about half of all automobile accident fatalities. A person can become both physically and psychologically dependent on alcohol. Some people cannot stop at one drink and become alcoholics, unable to control their drinking. Some people are more likely to experience this disorder than others. Genetics and body weight play a role in the likelihood of alcoholism. One side effect of this drug is liver deterioration, called **cirrhosis**. The liver eventually stops working and death results. A pregnant woman who drinks large amounts of alcohol may cause birth defects in the fetus. Patients may take alcohol to overcome the fear of dentistry. Dental assistants must be alert to this because of possible harmful interaction between alcohol and other drugs used in dentistry. Alcoholics feel full and satisfied and do not seek a well-balanced diet, often resulting in malnutrition.

Marijuana. Assistants should watch for signs of drug abuse, and must have a basic knowledge of drugs and how they affect body functions in order to help if an emergency should arise. One drug that acts as both a stimulant and a depressant is marijuana. Marijuana is considered a legal drug in a few states, and should be noted on the patient's chart for patient care. Marijuana contains a number of drugs, one of the most active being tetrahydrocannabinol (THC). Some side effects of marijuana use include increased heart rate (as much as 50 percent), lung tissue damage due to smoking, and reproductive system disorders (abnormal hormonal levels, abnormal sperm production, and, in some cases, defects in the developing fetus).

The nervous system of regular marijuana users is affected. They are not able to speak and think as clearly, coordination deteriorates, and they seem to lose the motivation to be productive without marijuana use. Individuals who use the drug daily have 10 percent more THC in their body tissues than monthly users. A person is unlikely to become physically dependent on marijuana, but often becomes psychologically dependent.

A marijuana derivative is used as a medicine to treat patients taking other drugs in cancer therapy. It seems to decrease nausea and regurgitation.

Cocaine. Cocaine, a very habit-forming drug, makes the user feel in control, as if he or she has tremendous power. This drug is often referred to as the "rich man's drug" because a day's dosage can cost hundreds or thousands of dollars. Side effects of this stimulant are heart problems, mental disorders, violent behavior, and death. Long-term users suffer from great anxiety and are restless and irritable.

Cocaine is often mixed with other drugs to boost the high. Sometimes, a mixture of heroin and cocaine (called a *speedball*) is injected intravenously. The result can be fatal. Purified cocaine that resembles a crystalline rock is called *crack*. This substance is smoked in a pipe or sprinkled on tobacco and smoked. The powder form of cocaine is inhaled into the nose or rubbed into the mucosa. Intraorally, this may appear much like toothbrush abrasion but over a wider area; this is because the substance is abrasive and wears on the tooth structure as it is rubbed back and forth into the tissue. If the person inhales cocaine, permanent damage occurs to the nasal mucosa over time.

Due to the abuse of this drug, its use as a medical treatment has been reduced. Cocaine causes both a physical and a psychological dependency. Physical dependency may occur after only one or a few uses. This dependency varies with each individual according to the quantity used, frequency, and sensitivity of the person to the drug. If the person tries to stop usage, withdrawal symptoms such as craving the drug, intense anxiety, and mental illness, such as depression, are common.

Narcotics. Narcotics are addictive depressants used to relieve pain. They have been in use for about 7,000 years. For centuries, they were the most useful painkillers available to physicians. Morphine and codeine are made from the opium poppy plant. Heroin is made from morphine. All drugs in this classification cause strong psychological and physical dependency and have been replaced for medical use by less addictive drugs.

Heroin. An individual who uses heroin regularly and tries to stop will become sick within 12 hours. Symptoms include hot and cold flashes with goose bumps, stomach cramps, vomiting, diarrhea, nervousness, shaking, muscle and bone pain, and an intense craving for the drug. The intensity of the withdrawal is dependent on how much the individual has been using. It does not take long for a person who uses heroin to develop a **tolerance** to the drug. This tolerance causes the person to need larger amounts of the drug in order to produce the same effect. The desired effect is loss of pain, a high, or a feeling of euphoria and drowsiness.

Side effects include addiction, loss of appetite, constipation, and decreased respiratory and heart rates. The drug can be taken intravenously, injected subcutaneously, or inhaled. Drug users who share needles run the risk of contracting contagious diseases such as hepatitis B and HIV (human immunodeficiency virus).

Heroin is the most addictive of the narcotic drugs. A person may become addicted the first time he or she uses the drug. Overdoses cause the user to vomit, experience diarrhea and decreased respiratory and heart rates, followed by symptoms of shock and possible coma. The patient should be taken immediately to a hospital for treatment. If heroin overdose is diagnosed, a narcotic antagonist will be given to reverse the effects of the heroin. An untreated overdose can be fatal. Newborns of addicted mothers show symptoms of addiction and will die if not treated properly.

Morphine. Morphine is one of the best-known narcotic analgesic (pain killer) drugs. Medically, it is given intravenously to relieve severe pain caused by myocardial infarction (heart attack). It is administered intramuscularly to control postoperative pain. It can also be given orally to patients who are terminally ill. Possible side effects include constipation, nausea, vomiting, and confusion. Long-term use leads to addiction and an increased level of tolerance. Due to physical dependence, if the drug is stopped suddenly, the person experiences symptoms of withdrawal, such as sweating, stomach and body cramping, and flu-like manifestations.

Codeine. Used since the early 1900s, codeine has been an effective analgesic drug (painkiller). Dentistry uses it in combination with other drugs to relieve mild to moderate pain. Other medical uses for codeine are as a cough suppressant (because it suppresses the part of the brain that triggers coughing) and as an antidiarrheal drug (it acts in the intestinal wall to slow down muscle contractions).

Codeine induces drowsiness, especially if taken with alcohol. Other side effects are constipation, if taken over a long period of time, and physical and psychological dependence.

Amphetamines. Amphetamines are stimulants that increase the heart and respiratory rates and blood pressure. They were used in the past to treat obesity because they caused a loss of appetite along with side effects of nervousness and restlessness. The street name for these drugs is uppers. Taking amphetamines leads to poor judgment and violent behavior. Prolonged use causes physical dependence and tolerance to the drug.

Medically, amphetamines are used to treat narcolepsy (abnormal daytime sleeping) and children with attention deficit hyperactivity disorder (ADHD). Amphetamines have an opposite effect on hyperactive children. Rather than causing restlessness, the drug has a calming effect. There are few other medical uses for amphetamines.

Methamphetamines. Methamphetamines are commonly called the street names of *ice*, *meth*, *crystal meth*, *crank*, *quartz*, *crystal*, *speed*, or the *poor man's cocaine*. The use and production of methamphetamine, a strong stimulant drug, is becoming a serious problem in America. Use of this drug is becoming widespread as more and more people are becoming addicted. This is a very strong stimulant drug that may have the temporary effect of euphoria, high self-esteem, increased libido, and heightened alertness. The use of methamphetamines can cause serious health problems, as well as serious problems to the mouth and teeth. Research shows that about 20 percent of methamphetamine addicts develop a psychosis resembling schizophrenia that can last six months or more after methamphetamine use has been discontinued. Methamphetamine causes many oral problems for the users. When high, the user craves sugar and carbonated beverages, and flossing and brushing often does not occur. Methamphetamine also has high acid content because it is made from antifreeze, over-the-counter cold medications with ephedrine, drain cleaner, lye, iodine, lantern fuel, battery acid, and numerous other acidic products that are terrible for teeth. This drug also decreases the saliva that helps protect the teeth from this acid; in addition, users often clench their teeth, causing additional harm. The patient presents with "Meth Mouth," which is a term used to describe the mouth of a methamphetamine user because of the rampant tooth decay that often occurs with the use of this dangerous drug. These patients must overcome the desire to use this drug, or any corrective dentistry will be destroyed again with continued usage. See Chapter 27, Oral Pathology, for more information.

Hallucinogens. Hallucinogens are drugs that cause people to see and hear images and sounds that do not exist (**hallucinate**). An individual using a hallucinogen may experience a mild effect where colors simply change, or more severe effects causing emotional extremes such as terror. Sometimes, a person under the influence of a hallucinogen becomes so frightened that he or she reacts in an extreme manner—doing anything to escape the hallucination. This loss of control over one's emotions or actions is due to a change in brain activity.

Hallucinogenic recreational drugs, also called psychedelic drugs, include LSD, PCP, mescaline, and psilocybin. Marijuana and alcohol, when taken in large amounts, have also been reported to cause hallucinogenic symptoms.

Lysergic Acid Diethylamide (LSD). LSD is a synthetic drug made from ergot, a fungus that grows on rye and wheat. LSD has a high potential for abuse and no medical uses. Minute amounts of LSD can produce a "bad trip," where the user has a serious personality breakdown (including violence), which may last up to 12 hours. Flashbacks from these bad trips may occur up to several years after the user has taken LSD. There is no scientific evidence proving that LSD causes mental illness, but it is thought that it may induce psychosis, and, thus, predispose the user to mental illness. A habitual user may become both physically and psychologically addicted to the drug. Psilocybin is a hallucinogenic drug similar to LSD that originates from mushrooms.

Phencyclidine (PCP). One of the most dangerous hallucinogenic drugs is phencyclidine, called PCP. This drug is often given the name of angel dust because users often think they can fly when under its influence. It is ingested by eating, smoking, or sniffing, and is either a stimulant or a depressant. As it scrambles the brain's messages, it causes the user to become violent. Adverse side effects include violent behavior, respiratory depression, agitation, nausea, vomiting, and convulsions. Memory loss that can last for weeks often results from PCP drug use.

Mescaline. The hallucinogenic drug mescaline is obtained from the peyote cactus. It produces psychosis and effects similar to LSD that last for four to eight hours. The likelihood of bad trips is not as prevalent with mescaline. However, this addictive drug may leave the user with permanent psychosis and a constant craving for the drug.

Barbiturates. Barbiturates are sedative drugs that depress brain activity. If used over a long period of time, physiological and physical dependency develops, along with tolerance for the drug. If withdrawal occurs, after four weeks of use the user experiences stomach cramps, nausea, vomiting, twitching, convulsions, weakness, and insomnia. An overdose of the drug can result in delirium and a comatose state; it can also be fatal. If barbiturates are used with alcohol, the outcome is particularly harsh.

Barbiturates, such as amobarbital, pentobarbital, and secobarbital, are used today to treat sleeplessness and anxiety. Phenobarbital sometimes is given to dental patients who exhibit severe anxiety during dental treatment. This is especially true when treating children. It is dispensed in a liquid and taken orally. Pentobarbital is also used in the treatment of epilepsy because it reduces the sensitivity of the brain to the abnormal electrical activity that brings on seizures.

Herbal and Other Alternative Medications

Dental assistants may be asked about herbal or other alternative medications. If this occurs, it is advisable to consult the dentist and it may be prudent to refer the patient to some reliable sources for further information. There are herbal and alternative medications that can be helpful for patient care, but much of the information is not based on facts (Figure 15-17). Patients should be cautioned when taking medications that are not approved by the FDA and the ADA.

The FDA has published a report titled *An FDA Guide to Dietary Supplements*. This guide helps answer many of the questions that patients may have. Dietary supplements, such as herbal and other alternative medications, do not have to follow the same regulations as other medications; therefore, the labeling may mislead the individual consumer. For instance, if a label says "natural" it does not guarantee that the product is safe. Consumers have to seek out factual information, and then evaluate if it meets their needs. There are several online sources that provide scientific data for consumers to review. The FDA Consumer (a magazine) is available at: http://magazine-directory.com/FDA-Consumer.htm. A free, online database of herbs, providing scientific data behind the use of herbs for health, is available from HerbMed® at http://www.herbmed.org. Patients can be given these sites for their review and evaluation.

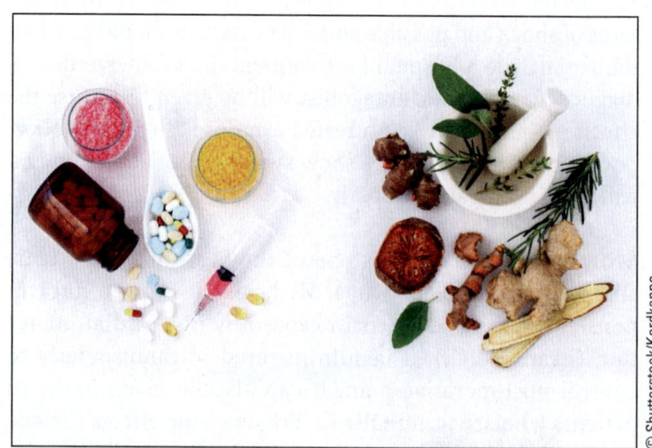

FIGURE 15-17
Sources of herbal medications.

Chapter Summary

At no other time have drugs been as widely used and misused as they are today. The dental assistant will need to pay attention to the patient's medical and dental history and carefully document the drugs used by the patient. The dental assistant will have to become knowledgeable about pharmacology, the side effects of drugs, and drug interactions. Dental assistants are concerned with prescribed drugs, but they must also have knowledge about the illegal drugs that patients may be using, and what will happen if the two types of drugs interact. It is also important to know the signs and symptoms that individuals may experience if under the influence of drugs. Background knowledge about drugs and their effects aids the dental assistant in providing better patient care.

CASE STUDY

Jordan Taylor, a 20-year-old male, comes in because an upper anterior tooth is abscessed. He is a smoker and has just had four shots of espresso (coffee) in a drink. He seems nervous about the upcoming treatment. Further information obtained from Jordan is that he has also had two regular soft drinks and a candy bar in the past two hours.

Case Study Review

1. What reaction should the dental team expect from Jordan due to the drugs he has ingested recently?
2. Are these drugs stimulants or depressants?
3. Would giving other drugs to Jordan be a problem?

Review Questions

Multiple Choice

1. The most commonly used resource to obtain information about drugs in the dental office is [the]
   a. *United States Pharmacopoeia.*
   b. *National Formulary.*
   c. *Dental Therapeutics.*
   d. *Physician's Desk Reference.*
2. Dental ointment that is placed on the mucosal surface is administered by which route?
   a. Sublingual
   b. Oral
   c. Topical
   d. Intravenous
3. Addictive depressants used to relieve pain are
   a. narcotics.
   b. amphetamines.
   c. hallucinogens.
   d. barbiturates.
4. The legislation that was established to identify drugs according to five schedules of abuse potential is the
   a. Pure Food, Drug, and Cosmetic Act.
   b. Comprehensive Drug Abuse Prevention and Control Act of 1970.
   c. Occupational Safety and Health Act.
   d. Controlled Substances Act.
5. If an antibiotic is said to be broad spectrum, it means that
   a. a culture can be taken to identify the type of microorganism.
   b. many microorganisms resist it.
   c. it causes side effects, such as nausea or an allergic rash.
   d. it is effective against a wide range of bacteria.
6. The drug schedule number that has the highest abuse potential, and is more dangerous is
   a. Schedule I.
   b. Schedule II.
   c. Schedule III.
   d. Schedule IV.
7. The route of administration of a drug that is delivered right under the skin level is
   a. intravenous.
   b. intramuscular.
   c. subcutaneous.
   d. intradermal.
8. Tylenol with codeine is under which schedule number of controlled substances?
   a. Schedule I
   b. Schedule II
   c. Schedule III
   d. Schedule IV

9. Percodan is an ________ drug type.
   a. antibody
   b. analgesic
   c. anticholinergic
   d. anticoagulant
10. A drug used to treat thrush or candidiasis could be_______.
   a. Prozac
   b. Benadryl
   c. glucophage
   d. nystatin

Critical Thinking

1. How does knowledge of illegal drugs help the dental assistant's career?
2. What are some of the side effects of tetracycline, and when is it contraindicated?
3. If a patient has a heavy flow of saliva, what drug classification, and which specific drug, may be used during the impression phase of a crown preparation procedure?

Web Activities

1. Go to http://www.ada.org and then find "Dental Therapeutics." Read the prescription tips and be prepared to discuss them in class.
2. Go to http://www.rxlist.com and look up tetracycline. Write down the drug's indications, dosage, side effects, drug interactions, warnings, and precautions.
3. Go to http://www.fda.gov and read the "Hot Topics." Report on one hot topic of interest to you.

CHAPTER

16

Emergency Management 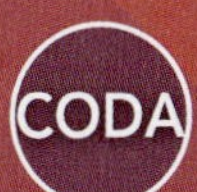

CODA

Specific Instructional Objectives

The student should strive to meet the following objectives and demonstrate an understanding of the facts and principles presented in this chapter:

1. Describe several emergency situations that may take place in the dental office. Explain how dental assistants can be prepared for these possibilities.
2. Describe the CAB approach to CPR and demonstrate the associated skills.
3. Define the terms and anatomy used in CPR delivery. Determine if the patient is unconscious and demonstrate knowledge of how to open the airway, as well as when and how to deliver chest compressions.
4. List and describe several causes of airway obstructions in the dental office. Demonstrate the ability to open the airway and to perform the Heimlich maneuver.
5. List and describe the signs and treatments for syncope, asthma, allergic reactions, anaphylactic reaction, hyperventilation, epilepsy, diabetes mellitus, hypoglycemia, angina pectoris, myocardial infarction, congestive heart failure, and stroke/cerebrovascular accident.
6. List and describe several dental emergencies that a patient may have, such as an abscessed tooth, alveolitis, avulsed tooth, broken prosthesis, soft tissue injury, broken tooth, and loose crown.
7. Explain how a pulse oximeter, capnography, and electrocardiography work, and how they can be used in the dental office.

Key Terms

abscessed tooth (347)
alkalosis (342)
allergic reactions (342)
alveolitis (347)
angina pectoris (345)
angioedema (342)
antihistamine (341)
avulsed tooth (347)
capnograph (349)
capnometry (349)
cardiopulmonary resuscitation (CPR) (332)
cerebral embolism (347)
cerebral hemorrhage (347)
cerebral infarction (347)
congestive heart failure (346)
convulsion (343)
defibrillation (334)
diabetic acidosis (344)
edema (342)
electrocardiography (349)
epilepsy (342)
erythema (342)
fistula (347)
foreign body airway obstruction (FBAO) (336)
galvanometer (349)
generalized hypoxia (349)
gingival hyperplasia (344)
grand mal seizure (343)
Heimlich maneuver (337)
hemiplegia (347)
hyperglycemia (344)
hypersensitive (341)
hyperventilation (342)

Key Terms (continued)

hypoglycemia (345)
hypoxia (349)
immunotherapy (341)
inhaler (341)
insulin (344)
insulin shock (345)
isosbestic (349)
Jacksonian epilepsy (344)
myocardial infarction (345)
orthostatic hypotension (340)
partial seizure (344)
petit mal seizure (343)
pulse oximeter (348)
status epilepticus (343)
stroke (347)
syncope (338)
tissue hypoxia (349)
transient ischemic attack (347)
traumatic intrusion (348)
Trendelenburg position (339)
universal distress signal (337)
urticaria (342)

Introduction

Emergencies can happen at any place and any time. Even though members of the dental profession try to make dentistry as comfortable as possible, patients feel stress about dental care, which can increase the possibility of an emergency occurring in the dental office. Other factors that did not exist to the same degree in the past that may increase the incidence of emergencies include: advancements in medical care, an increase in drug therapy, the increase in street drugs and opioid abuse, elderly patients seeking dental treatment, and longer dental appointments.

Advances in medical care have allowed treatments that were not available in the past. A patient seeking dental treatment may have a heart or liver transplant, a pacemaker, or be taking any number of drug therapies. Many patients, especially older patients, take more than one drug. Other patients take one or more street drugs prior to dental treatment. Any drugs given in the dental office for treatment may interact with the drug therapy or street drugs taken by the patient, thereby causing an emergency situation. Another contributing factor to the increased likelihood of emergencies is the length of appointments. Most patients would rather sit for longer appointments and have more complex dentistry completed at one time to accommodate their busy schedules. Dental offices are also more productive when longer appointments are scheduled, because less time is wasted removing barriers and practicing aseptic techniques before and after several shorter appointments. These lengthy appointments may overtax the patient's ability to remain comfortable, therefore, causing more anxiety and stress, and possibly leading to an emergency situation.

Even though the number of emergencies in a dental office is not high, the dental assistant must always be observant of the patient and be prepared to deal with an emergency. Additionally, emergencies may happen to the dentist and to other dental assistants and staff.

Prevention of Emergencies

The dental assistant and dental team should take proactive steps to decrease the chances of a medical emergency occurring in the dental office. One of the most important steps to take is to thoroughly review each patient's chart and health history prior to his or her dental appointment. The assistant should identify all noted health conditions, plan preventive measures into the appointment, and then share this information with the dentist. This may include a blood pressure check, modifications in the materials or anesthesia used during a procedure, or a consultation with the patient's physician.

Routine Preparedness for Dental Team Members

When an emergency arises, the dental team must react with an automatic response. Any hesitation at such a time could cost a life. A routine response should be established. Details, such as who should call for emergency help and written directions on how to locate the office, should be predetermined and posted close to the phone. Providing medical response teams with specific directions regarding the office location, including which door to enter, will save valuable time during the emergency response.

The Dental Assistant's Role in Emergency Care

The dental assistant has a vital role in the prevention of emergencies and in emergency care. First, the assistant closely observes the patient while escorting him or her from the waiting room to the dental treatment room. Does the patient have difficulty moving? Do the patient's eyes respond to light? Is the patient's speech slurred? Does the patient indicate anxiety about the dental treatment? Look for signs of concern that the patient has or seems to have. Many of these signs will be covered up after the patient is seated with the anesthetic given and the dental dam in place. Any areas of concern should be reported to the dentist prior to starting dental care. The patient's medical history should be reviewed as a matter of routine procedure. It is crucial that the dental team have knowledge of any changes in the patient's health. The dental assistant must be alert to any area of concern, because he or she will more than likely be the first one to suspect a possible emergency.

Another role of the dental assistant is to stay well trained for an emergency. Ideally, the dentist and dental assistants will establish a definitive plan to render treatment in an emergency situation. Often, this training takes place in a staff meeting or at a seminar. All members of the dental team should have current cardiopulmonary resuscitation (CPR) cards, and have continued training and updated knowledge of emergency situations. The dental assistant should know the answers to the following questions in order to ensure competency in dealing with emergencies:

- Where is the emergency kit and who will retrieve it?
- Who will take and monitor vital signs?
- Who will retrieve and administer oxygen?
- When will the call for help be placed and by whom?
- Who will perform basic life support, if needed?
- Who will review the medical history of the individual?

If any of these questions cannot be answered quickly by the dental team, training is needed. Once the emergency takes place, attention to the patient's condition will take precedence. All personnel must perform their tasks in a timely manner to ensure that the best treatment is administered.

Dental Office Emergency Kit

Every dental office should have an up-to-date emergency kit (Figure 16-1). A dentist may choose to design his or her own. This kit must be arranged for the specific needs of the practice. Other kits are manufactured for use in dental offices and can be obtained from a dental supply company. These are normally color coded for easy equipment and drug access. All dental emergency kits should include the following:

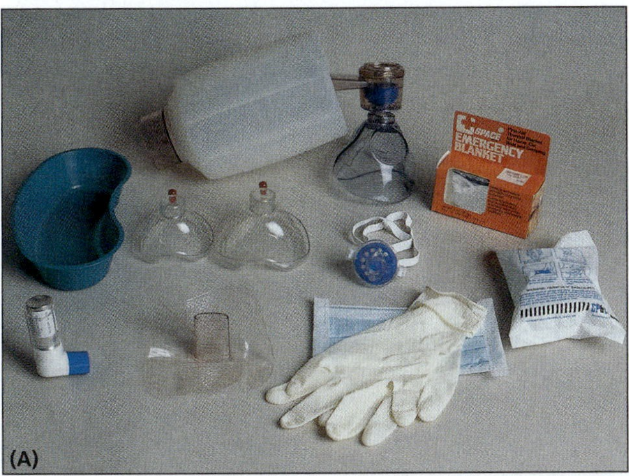

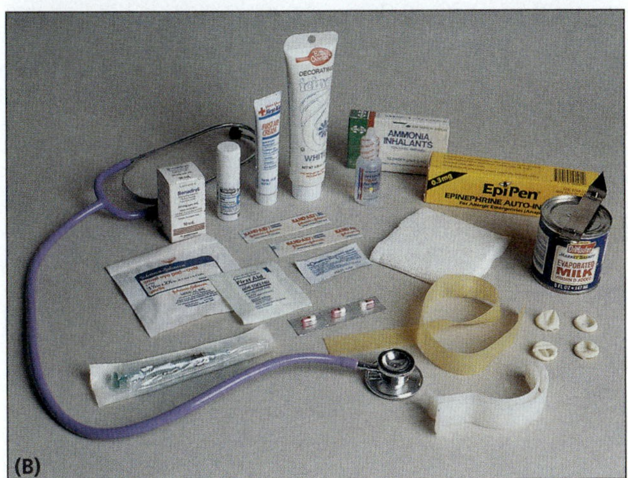

FIGURE 16-1
Sample dental office emergency kit.

- Sterile syringes, tourniquets, tracheotomy needle, barrier devices for delivery of CPR, and several oral airway devices
- Oxygen inhalation equipment, if the office does not have nitrous/oxygen equipment in each treatment room (Figure 16-2)
- Stimulants (ammonia inhalants, i.e., thin glass vials of ammonia covered with a strong gauze fabric that can be broken easily)
- Vasodilators that will increase oxygenated blood supply to the heart, such as nitroglycerin, translingual nitroglycerin, or amyl-nitrite inhalants)
- Antihistamine drugs, such as adrenaline-epinephrine, Benadryl-antihistamine™, solu-corticosteroid, or aminophylline-bronchodilator; and an epipen (a two-dose syringe of epinephrine) is recommended for quick and easy delivery
- Vasopressor to increase blood pressure (such as Wyamine™)
- Analgesics for pain (such as Talwin™)
- Depressants for convulsions (such as diazepam)
- Vagal blockers to increase pulse rate (such as atropine)

This kit should be labeled and located in an easily accessible place so that it can be quickly obtained. A crash cart with oxygen and emergency equipment can be utilized for quick access. If the emergency kit contains controlled substances, it must be kept locked up and have a log that indicates when the substances were delivered and used. This log should also note if any substances were lost or stolen. Time is an extremely important factor in treating emergencies. The kit should be

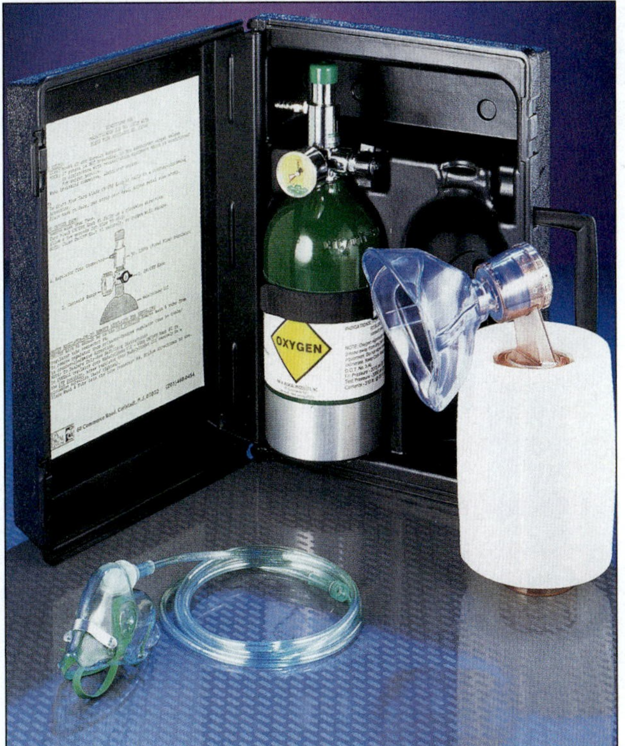

FIGURE 16-2
Oxygen inhalation equipment for use in dental emergencies.

well organized so that the assistant or dentist can find the necessary items at a glance. All items should be labeled with information pertinent to their uses and dosages. A periodic inspection of the emergency items is essential. Many of the drugs have limited shelf lives and need to be replaced as medications reach their expiration date. A sphygmomanometer and stethoscope, or digital blood pressure monitor, are essential parts of the emergency kit for monitoring vital signs.

Oxygen inhalation equipment must be readily available as well. The oxygen cylinders are green and must be stored upright and secure. Administration of oxygen may be the most important factor in caring for the patient until medical help arrives. The steps for administering oxygen are presented in Procedure 16-1. Even though the dental team is well trained to act in emergencies, a medical response team should be contacted immediately if the patient becomes unconscious.

Cardiopulmonary Resuscitation

If the patient has a sudden cardiac arrest or progresses to this condition, **cardiopulmonary resuscitation (CPR)** is necessary to help the person survive. If the adult patient becomes unconscious, the first step is to immediately call for emergency medical care. *Phone first and phone fast!* Rescuers will often be able to activate an emergency response without leaving the victims side by using a mobile phone. After calling for help, start CPR. The technique of CPR is easy to remember if you follow CAB method (see next section). Regardless of the victim's age, begin CPR with 30 chest compressions followed by 2 breaths. The likelihood of infants responding within the first 2 minutes is greater than adults.

Note: Dental assistants must take a formal CPR training program every 2 years from the American Red Cross or the American Heart Association (AHA) at the health care provider level to be proficient in emergency management.

AHA Guidelines for CPR

In 2015, the American Heart Association (AHA) revised the guidelines for cardiopulmonary resuscitation (CPR) and emergency cardiovascular care (ECC). These updates are mainly focused on chest compressions and still follow the CAB (chest compressions, airway, and breathing) approach. Recent research indicates compression depths greater than 2.4 inches may produce adverse outcomes from the procedure, and, therefore, are not recommended. Any patient experiencing a cardiovascular incident will need high-quality CPR provided by trained individuals.

Procedure 16-1
Administration of Oxygen

Many dental assistants may routinely administer oxygen in conjunction with nitrous oxide gas under the supervision of the dentist. This system is most often brought into the dental treatment room through a wall-piped system. In some instances, the tanks may be on a mobile unit that is brought into the treatment area. The dental assistant should know where the system is located and how to administer oxygen during an emergency. Oxygen should be administered to any patient in respiratory distress with the exception of hyperventilation.

Equipment and Supplies

- Oxygen cylinder with gauge regulator at the top, or gauge in the dental treatment area
- Oxygen mask and tubing

Procedure Steps *(Follow aseptic procedures)*

1. Position the patient comfortably in a supine or Trendelenburg position (see Figure 16-10).

NOTE: The Trendelenburg position is a supine position with the feet elevated above chest level.

2. Explain the procedure to the patient and reassure the patient that everything is being taken care of (if an emergency should occur).
3. Place the oxygen mask over the patient's nose and drape the tubing on either side of the face. The mask may need to be adjusted so that it is secure over the nose.
4. Start the flow of oxygen immediately. It should flow at 6 liters per minute and 2,000 pounds per square inch, per the pressure gauge.
5. Instruct the patient to breathe through his or her nose and have the mouth remain closed.
6. Continue to calm the patient by talking softly in reassuring tones.
7. Document the emergency information and procedure on the patient's chart.

A manual defibrillator, or an Automated External Defibrillation (AED) Unit equipped with a pediatric dose attenuator, is preferred; however, if neither is available, an AED without a pediatric dose attenuator can be used to save a life.

The 2010 guidelines have also done away with the "look, listen, and feel" step. It is thought that this takes up valuable time. When a victim is found to be in distress, a quick assessment is performed and if the patient is not responsive and not breathing, or is not breathing normally and has no pulse, chest compressions should begin and the emergency response system activated.

Adult CPR

It is critical to make sure the scene is safe for both the patient and rescuer before beginning CPR. Proceed to tap the patient's shoulder while asking, "Are you alright?" and at the same time looking for breathing. If there is no response and the patient is not breathing, or is not breathing normally, activate the emergency response system and get an AED if available and return quickly to the patient. It is recommended that lone health care providers tailor the sequence of actions for the most likely cause of arrest in the patient's age group. The rescuer should follow the CAB method of CPR.

Locate the trachea, using two or three fingers into the groove between the trachea and the muscles at the side of the neck, to feel for a carotid pulse. Do not use the thumb because it has a pulse of its own. Check the pulse for at least 5 seconds, but not more than 10 seconds, and if there is no pulse, begin CPR.

Compressions. Compressions (C) are first. The rescuer should position him- or herself at the patient's side. The patient should be placed face up on a firm, flat surface. If the patient is not face up, secure the head, neck, and torso and carefully roll the patient to a face up position. If the patient is in the dental chair, adjust the chair to a correct height for providing CPR and to clear access to the patient.

Place the heel of one hand on the center of the patient's chest on the lower half of the sternum (breastbone). Place the heel of the other hand directly on top of the first hand and straighten the arms while positioning the shoulders directly over the hands. Begin cycles of 30 chest compressions and 2 breaths, if alone. The compressions should be at a rate of 100, minimum, per minute. Press straight down, no more than 2.4 inches in compression depth, on the chest bone. It is important to allow the chest to recoil after each of the compressions. Counting "one and two and three" and so on, helps establish a rhythm and a total count. After every set of 30 compressions, deliver 2 slow breaths. Repeat this cycle four times and then check for a pulse. This process continues until additional help arrives. Procedure 16-2 presents an overview of the proper method to deliver CPR to an adult patient by a lone health care provider.

Airway. *Check the airway (A).* The rescuer needs to ensure that air exchange can occur. If the patient is not breathing, hold the patient's airway open using the "head tilt, chin lift" technique. Pinch the nose closed with the thumb and index finger placing the hand on the forehead (Figure 16-3).

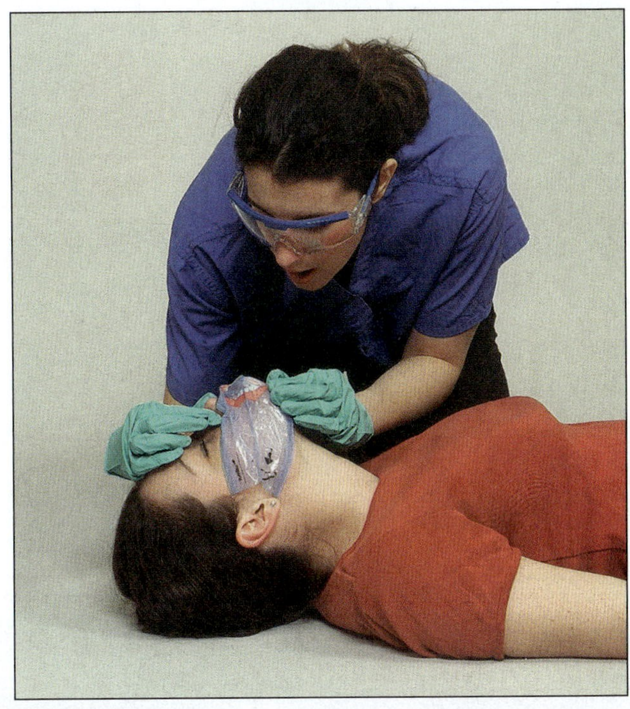

FIGURE 16-3
Tilt the patient's head back, lift the chin, and pinch the nose closed.

Breathing. *Provide rescue breathing (B).* It is advisable to use a barrier device, if one is available, when administering rescue breathing. There are a variety of barrier devices on the market (Figure 16-4). The American Dental Association has small barriers in key chains that are ready and available when the rescuer needs one. The American Heart Association and the American Red Cross have devices that are available for purchase. It is important when providing rescue breathing to create a good seal around the mouth. It is common for the patient to vomit; the rescuer will need to wipe the mouth clean and clear of secretions and then return to providing compressions and breaths.

The patient may begin breathing, but, if not, the rescuer administers 2 slow breaths (2 seconds per breath for an adult, and 1 to 1½ seconds per breath for a child). The rescuer watches for the chest to rise and waits for the exhalation

One Rescuer

- Use a 30:2 compression-to-ventilation rate for patients of all ages.

Two Rescuers

- Use a 30:2 compression-to-ventilation rate for adult patients.
- Use a 15:2 compression-to-ventilation rate for infants and children.

If more than one rescuer is available, the second person should activate the emergency response system and get the AED while the first person begins CPR.

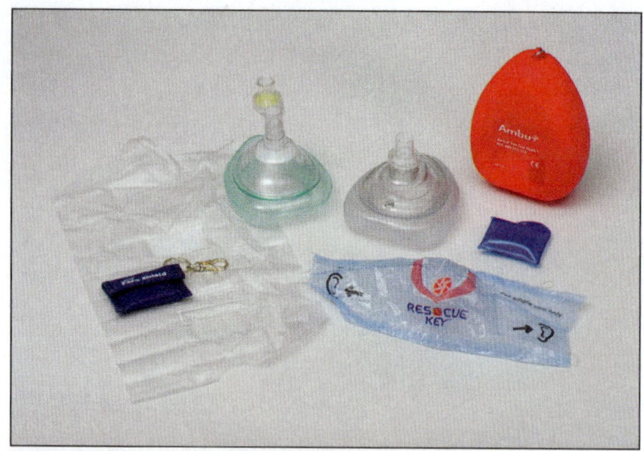

FIGURE 16-4

Examples of barrier devices used during CPR.

between breaths. The proper steps for administering rescue breaths are outlined in Procedure 16-3.

With recent advances in technology, automated **defibrillation** is used and requires additional equipment (Figure 16-6). If the site has an automated defibrillator, it increases the chances of survival for patients who have cardiac arrest. AEDs are available at many sites. Airlines, shopping centers, schools, and other sites have AEDs available. It is advisable to check the sources close to the dental office or purchase one to have it available when needed. It has been found to be extremely helpful for successful, basic life support. The equipment guides the user. The equipment's voice system indicates when and where the electrodes are to be placed. The electrodes are placed only if the patient is unconscious, not breathing, and has no pulse. The steps required for AED use are outlined in Procedure 16-4.

Procedure 16-2
CPR for an Adult, One Rescuer

If an emergency occurs, the dental assistant must be prepared to respond to breathing and/or cardiac arrest, and perform CPR or to assist the dentist in performing CPR.

Equipment and Supplies

- Resuscitation mouthpiece or other oral barrier
- Gloves (latex or vinyl)

Procedure Steps (*Follow aseptic procedures*)

1. Assess the patient's condition. Ask the patient, "Are you okay?" while at the same time looking for breathing.
2. If he or she gives no response, have someone call emergency services. (If no one is available, call for emergency services immediately; stay with patient if using a mobile phone and obtain the AED, then return to the patient.)
3. Wash hands (if possible). Put on gloves (if possible).
4. Check the pulse (for 5 to 10 seconds) at the carotid artery.
5. If the patient does not have a pulse, start chest compressions.
6. Position hands on top of each other and position your shoulders over your hands. Compress the chest 30 times at a rate of 100 per minute (minimum) (Figure 16-5).

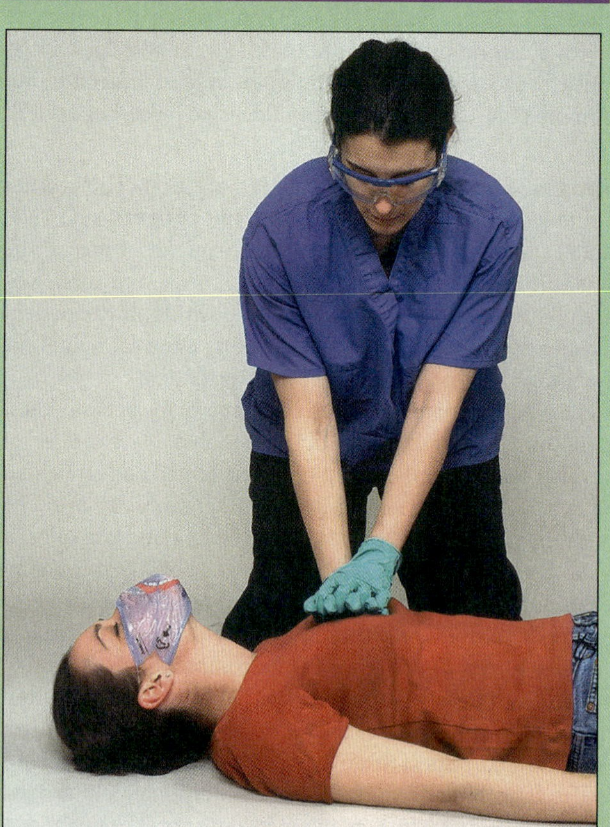

FIGURE 16-5

Position the hands on top of each other and position your shoulders over your hands, compress the chest 15 times, and follow with 2 slow breaths.

(continues)

Procedure 16-2 (continued)

7. If the patient is not breathing, tilt the head back and lift the chin. Insert the mouthpiece or barrier and pinch the nose closed (see Figure 16-4).
8. Make sure the mouthpiece or your mouth seals the oral cavity. Give two breaths and watch the chest rise.
9. Continue for four cycles of breaths and compressions.
10. Check the pulse at the carotid artery. If no pulse is apparent, continue for four cycles and then repeat checking for a pulse and four cycles of breaths and compressions.
11. Continue until the patient is revived or another person takes over.
12. Dispose of the resuscitation mouthpiece in a biohazard container.
13. Document the emergency information and procedure on the patient's chart.

Procedure 16-3
Rescue Breathing for Adults

If an emergency occurs, the dental assistant must be prepared to respond to a patient who ceases breathing and/or to assist the dentist in rescue breathing for a patient.

Equipment and Supplies

- Resuscitation mouthpiece or other oral barrier
- Gloves (latex or vinyl—optional)

Procedure Steps (*Follow aseptic procedures*)

1. Determine if the patient is responding. Ask, "Are you okay?" while looking for breathing.
2. If the patient gives no response, have someone call emergency services. (If alone, call quickly and return to the patient.)
3. Wash hands and don gloves (if possible).
4. If the patient is not breathing, hold the patient's airway open with a head tilt and chin lift. Pinch the nose closed with the thumb and index finger (placing the hand on the forehead) (Figure 16-3).
5. Position the resuscitation mouthpiece or barrier on the patient, take a regular breath, and seal your lips around the patient's mouth or barrier, creating an airtight seal. Give one breath for about 1 second and watch for the patient's chest to rise as the breath is given.
6. If the chest does not rise, reposition the patient's airway by attempting to reopen it by readjusting the head tilt and chin lift.
7. Give another breath, not deep, just a regular breath, for 1 second and watch for the patient's chest to rise.
8. Check the pulse on the carotid artery on the side closest to you. Use the forefinger and middle finger to palpate a pulse.
9. If the pulse is present but the patient is not breathing, give one breath every 5 to 6 seconds (about 10 to 12 breaths per minute). Each breath should result in a visible chest rise and last 1 second. Check the pulse every 2 minutes.
10. Continue rescue breathing for as long as the pulse remains. If the pulse ceases, begin CPR. If the pulse remains, continue rescue breathing until breathing is restored, or until someone else arrives and takes over.
11. Dispose of the resuscitation mouthpiece or barrier in a biohazard container. Remove gloves and wash hands.
12. Document what was done on the patient's chart.

Procedure 16-4

Operating an Automated External Defibrillation (AED) Unit

Health professionals may have a defibrillator available within the facility for emergencies.

Equipment and Supplies

- Gloves (latex or vinyl—optional)
- Automated external defibrillation (AED) unit (Figure 16-6)

Procedure Steps (*Follow aseptic procedures*)

- If there is no pulse, follow CAB method for CPR.
- Perform CPR until the defibrillator is attached.

1. Press "analyze" on the defibrillation unit.
2. Follow each step as the unit instructs.
3. Attach the AED to the patient as indicated by the instructions on the lid of the unit.
4. State loudly, "Everybody clear of the patient!" Verify that everyone is clear of the patient and press the analysis control switch on the AED. The assessment takes 10 to 20 seconds depending on the brand of AED. Everyone should remain clear during this time.
5. If the device indicates that a shock is not advised, resume CPR.
6. Once the unit begins charging, a synthesized voice message or light indicator indicates that it is charging. Assume that ventricular fibrillation is present, and that the AED will indicate the need to deliver a shock.
7. Verify that everyone is clear of the unit. The AED delivers shocks without additional actions from the operator. It may indicate, "shock now."
8. "Give three consecutive shocks."
9. Check the pulse.
10. If a pulse is present, assess the vital signs, support airway, and check breathing.
11. If no pulse is present, give CPR for 1 minute.
12. Check the pulse. If it is not present, press "analyze" on the AED.
13. Defibrillate up to three times.
14. If ventricular fibrillation persists after nine shocks, repeat sets of three shocks with 1 minute of CPR between each set until the "no shock indicated" message is received on the AED, or until the patient is revived.

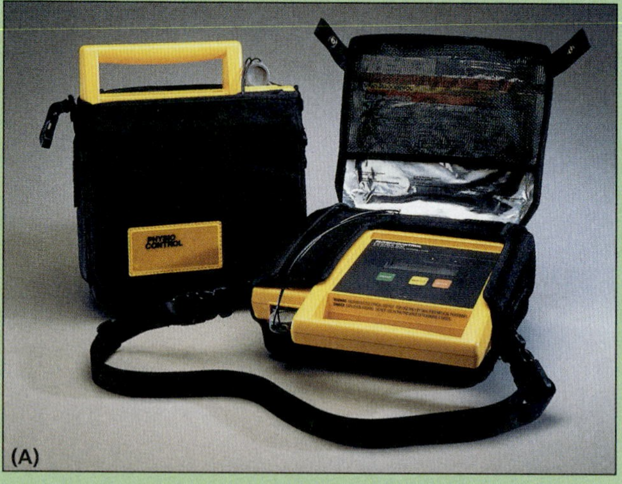

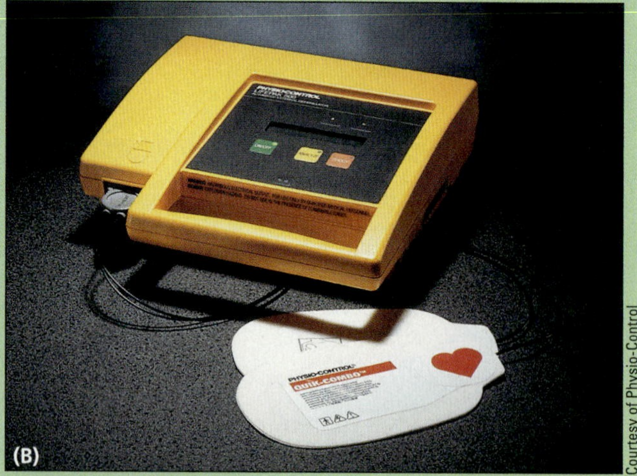

Courtesy of Physio-Control

FIGURE 16-6
An automated defibrillator increases the chances of survival for patients who experience cardiac arrest.

Foreign Body Airway Obstruction

The body depends on oxygen availability to function. Oxygen is an odorless, tasteless, and colorless gas that is essential for life. In the dental office, incidents of airway obstruction are more likely than other possible emergencies. The patient is lying in a supine position, therefore allowing objects to be propelled naturally down the throat. The moisture from saliva and blood makes objects more slippery and harder to hold. Also, the use of a number of items and materials in the mouth allows for a greater possibility of **foreign body airway obstruction (FBAO)**. A patient may take a breath at a time when a tooth is being removed, thereby dislodging it from the forceps and allowing it to fall directly into the airway. Other items causing FBAO are crowns, amalgam, composite, cotton rolls, gauze, endodontic instruments, and impression material. The person may begin choking and clutch the throat with the hands, which is the **universal distress signal** (Figure 16-7). Ask, "Are you choking?" The first action is to stop treatment, sit the patient upright, and encourage him or her to cough. Quickly evaluate the patient for a non-productive cough and listen for a high-pitched breathing sound or any other signs of respiratory distress. If the patient cannot speak, cough, or breathe and cannot expel the foreign body, the rescuer goes behind the patient and wraps his or her arms around the patient's waist. Tightly wrap one hand over the other fisted hand and, with a quick movement, give upward thrusts into the patient's abdomen. This procedure was formerly referred to as the **Heimlich maneuver** but is now known as subdiaphragmatic thrusts. The proper steps for performing this maneuver are outlined in Procedure 16-5. If the patient is in the final stages of pregnancy or obese, the rescuer stands behind, wraps his or her arms under the patient's armpits, and gives quick, inward chest thrusts. If the rescuer is unable to do this technique and the patient is still conscious, have the patient lie over a chair back to force air from the abdomen and help him or her expel the foreign body.

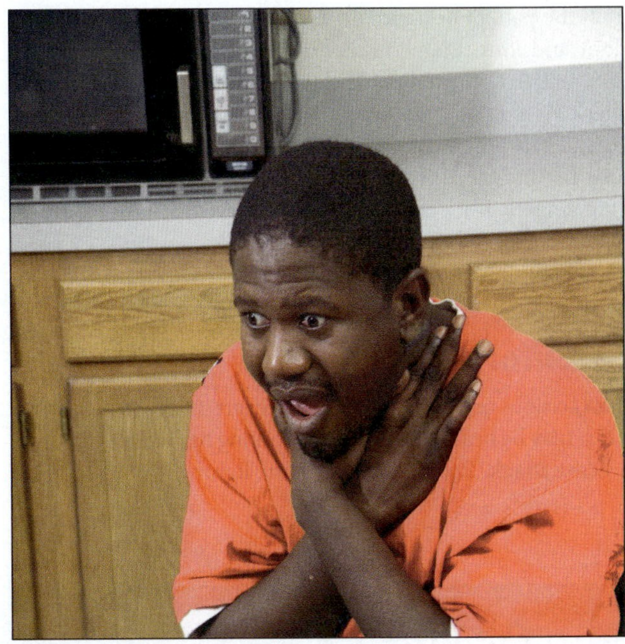

FIGURE 16-7
Holding the hands to the throat is the universal distress signal for choking.

Procedure 16-5
Subdiaphragmatic Thrusts for a Conscious Adult

If an adult is still conscious and has a blocked airway, the rescuer can talk to him or her and perform subdiaphragmatic thrusts to open up the blocked airway.

Equipment and Supplies

- No equipment required

Procedure Steps (*Follow aseptic procedures*)

1. Verify that the patient is choking. Ask, "Are you choking?"
2. If the patient is standing, tell him or her what the procedure is going to involve, position yourself behind the patient, and proceed to wrap arms around the patient's abdomen.
3. Place the thumb side of a fisted hand against the middle of the abdomen, just above the umbilicus and below the sternum.
4. Grasp hands together, keeping one hand fisted and the other wrapped on top of it.
5. Give quick, upward thrusts with hands against the abdomen (Figure 16-8).

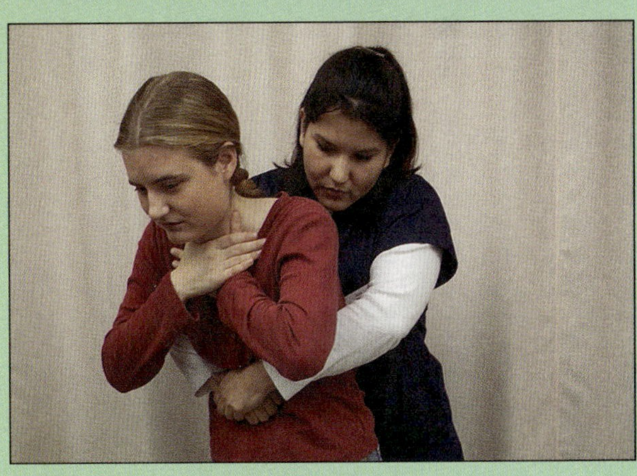

FIGURE 16-8
Place the thumb side of your fist against the middle of the person's abdomen, just above the umbilicus. Give quick, upward thrusts against the person's abdomen.

6. Repeat the procedure until the patient expels the object or the patient becomes unconscious.
7. Wash hands.
8. Document the procedure.

If the patient becomes unconscious, lay the patient on the floor and immediately activate emergency medical services (EMS). Lower the patient to the floor and begin CPR. Do not check for a pulse, start compressions immediately. Remember CAB. Each time breaths are given open the mouth wide and look for an object. If it can be easily removed, remove it with your fingers. If it cannot be easily removed continue on with CPR. See Procedure 16-6.

Causes, Signs, and Treatment of Emergencies

If an anxious or a fearful patient has heart problems, his or her heart may be beating rapidly and working harder, precipitating a heart attack. Patients may become lightheaded as they see instruments in the dental treatment room and anticipate the procedures. These patients may react by **syncope** (fainting).

Dental assistants may use preventive measures to render patients less likely to exhibit syncope. It is important that assistants are aware of anxiety-provoking events and ensure that patients do not encounter them. Talk to patients, and assure them that everything is all right. Help them overcome the apprehension and fear of treatment. In addition, keep instruments, needles, and blood out of the patient's sight. If patients are undergoing long treatments, make sure they have eaten and allow them to get up occasionally. Patients may complain of feeling flushed, having upset stomachs, and having racing heart rates; and they may appear to have pale skin. Blood pressure may also decrease. Be aware of the signs and symptoms and try to prevent syncope through close observation of the

Procedure 16-6
Adult with Airway Obstruction

If an adult is unconscious and has a blocked airway, the rescuer performs CPR.

Equipment and Supplies

- Gloves
- Resuscitation device

Procedure Steps (*Follow aseptic procedures*)

1. If the patient is unresponsive, activate EMS immediately.
2. Lower the patient to the ground and begin CPR. Do not check for a pulse, start compressions. Remember CAB.
3. Each time breaths are given, open the mouth wide and look for an object (Figure 16-9). If it can be easily removed, remove it with the fingers. If it cannot be easily removed, continue on with CPR.

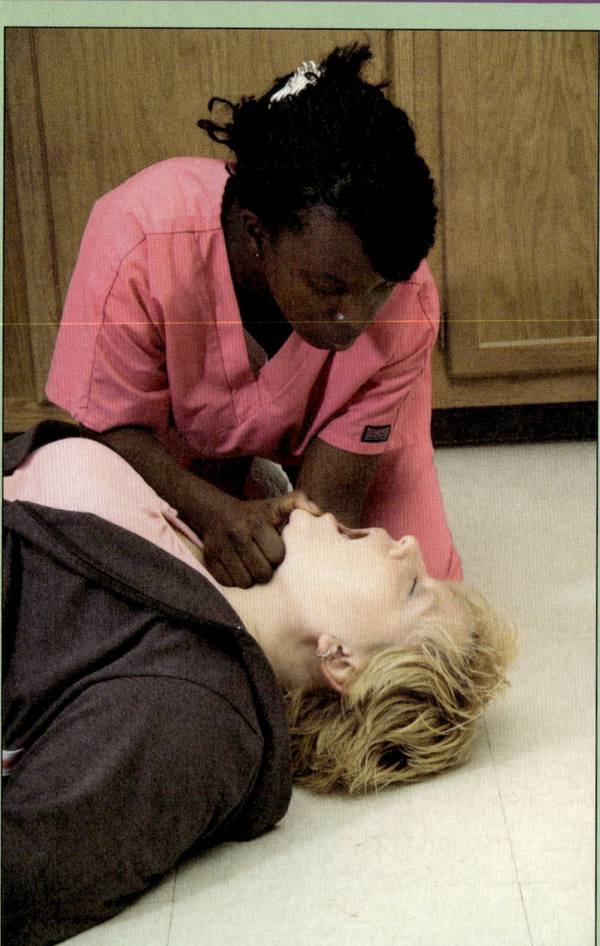

FIGURE 16-9
Open the mouth wide and look for any objects; if unable to retrieve them, begin compressions again.

patient and preventive techniques. Syncope and other common emergencies that may present in the dental office are outlined in Table 16-1.

Syncope

The most common and least life-threatening emergency that may occur in the dental office is vasodepressor syncope, commonly known as fainting. This loss of consciousness is caused by a decrease in blood flow to the brain. Syncope is normally caused by some form of stress—emotional, physical, or both. When a patient experiences stress, the body reacts by pumping large amounts of blood into the arms and legs. This response (often referred to as the "fight or flight syndrome") occurs so that the patients can quickly respond by moving their bodies. Dental patients often remain motionless, so their blood pools in the arms and legs, and the cerebral blood flow is diminished. As a result, the brain is deprived of oxygenated blood and the patient becomes unconscious—unable to respond to any sensory stimulation.

The patient may feel dizzy, nauseated, or extremely weak prior to syncope. The patient appears pale and clammy and breathes in shallow gasps. If the patient indicates that he or she is feeling faint, remain calm, quickly sit the patient down, and lean his or her head forward and place it between the knees. If a fainting person is unconscious and breathing normally, lay him or her down in the **Trendelenburg position** (Figure 16-10). This position allows the blood to flow back to the head. If the patient is not breathing normally, establish an airway by tipping the head back and performing a chin lift. At this time, any tight, constricting clothing or jewelry can be loosened or removed around the neck area.

Administer oxygen and monitor vital signs. The patient will generally resume breathing normally in less than 10 seconds. If the patient exhibits signs or symptoms of syncope, break a vial of spirits of ammonia and pass it under the patient's nose. The strong odor of the ammonia causes the patient to quickly inhale, which stimulates breathing. This gauze-covered ammonia vial is very strong, so only pass it under the patient's nostrils a couple of times, and *do not* leave it in a place where

TABLE 16-1 Emergency Conditions, Symptoms, and Treatments

Condition	Symptom(s)	Treatment
Syncope	Loss of consciousness	Lower the head to increase blood flow to the brain
Orthostatic hypotension	Loss of consciousness when standing upright, light-headed	In the dental office, have the patient sit upright before standing*
Asthma	Breathlessness	Administer patient's bronchodilator (inhaler)
Allergic reaction	Edema, erythema, urticaria	Remove irritant, administer an antihistamine if needed
Anaphylactic reaction	Blood pressure drops, airways constricted	Injection of epinephrine
Hyperventilation	Quick breathing, nervousness, faintness	Calm patient, have patient breathe in paper bag or cupped hands
Epilepsy Grand mal Status epilepticus Petit mal seizure Partial seizures	Seizure lasting 2 to 5 minutes, body jerking, twitching Continuous seizures Blank stare Simple/patient conscious, complex/patient unconscious, involuntary twitching	Remove items that may harm patient, make patient comfortable after seizure Summon emergency services No treatment necessary No treatment necessary
Hyperglycemia—Diabetic coma	Thirst, frequent urination, disorientation, nausea/vomiting, fruity or acetone breath, abdominal pain, fatigue, rapid heartbeat	Administer patient's insulin
Hypoglycemia	Nervousness, trembling, weakness, cold sweats	Administer orange juice or other source of sugar, such as cake icing gel, in buccal mucosa, or administer injection of glucagon
Angina pectoris	Pain in chest/base of neck	Administer nitroglycerin pills or spray
Myocardial infarction	Possible pain in chest, ashen color, diaphoresis (sweating profusely)	Position patient with head slightly elevated, administer oxygen and nitroglycerin pills, summon medical services
Congestive heart failure	Difficulty breathing, swollen ankles and legs	Elevate the head and heart, allow frequent restroom breaks
Stroke	Loss of speech, dizziness, weakness on one side of body	Administer oxygen, take vital signs, summon medical services

* If it is a fall in blood pressure due to other underlying issues, the patient needs to consult a physician.

it can cause irritation to the membranes in the nasal passage. The patient will normally revive totally within a couple of minutes but may remain weak. It is best to reschedule dental treatment and contact someone to drive the patient home. If the patient does not revive from the unconscious state, call for emergency help, closely monitor breathing, and begin CPR, if necessary, until help arrives. Procedure 16-7 presents the steps to follow in the event that a patient has a syncopal event in the dental office.

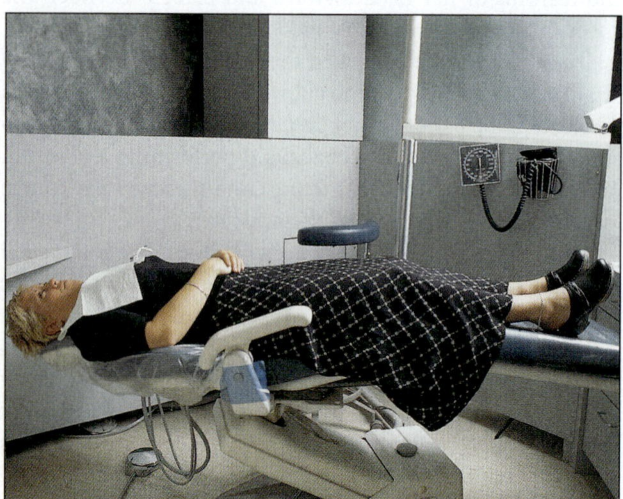

FIGURE 16-10
The Trendelenberg position (supine position with the feet elevated slightly).

Orthostatic Hypotension

A condition referred to as **orthostatic hypotension**, also known as postural hypotension, occurs when an individual loses consciousness or a level of consciousness when he or she sits in an upright position rapidly. It happens often in the dental office if the patient has been lying in a prone position for a long period of time during dental treatment, and then tries to sit up rapidly or rises to the feet immediately. It occurs from a lack of blood flow to the brain. Patients may say that they feel "light-headed." This feeling lasts only a few seconds and then the patient feels better.

It is advisable to have the patients rise up with the chair and sit in that position for a few minutes before standing. It is also best to ask the patient how he or she feels before attempting to get up out of the chair. Often, the dental assistant can write on the chart and then dismiss the patient. During this time, the patient's blood flow to the brain will return to normal. Patients

Procedure 16-7
Treatment of a Patient with Syncope

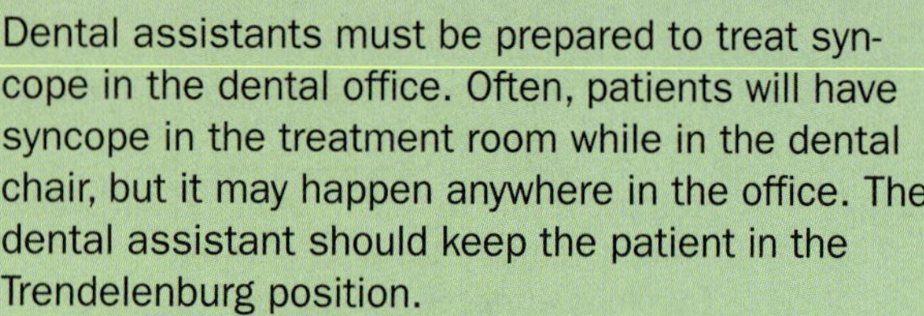

Dental assistants must be prepared to treat syncope in the dental office. Often, patients will have syncope in the treatment room while in the dental chair, but it may happen anywhere in the office. The dental assistant should keep the patient in the Trendelenburg position.

Equipment and Supplies

- Oxygen tank with gauge at top or gauge in the dental treatment area
- Oxygen mask and tubing
- Spirits of ammonia

Procedure Steps (*Follow aseptic procedures*)

1. Position the patient in a supine or Trendelenburg position (supine with feet elevated to increase blood flow to the brain). If the patient is wearing a dress or other garments that are misplaced during the syncope, attend to modesty issues as soon as possible.
2. Establish that the airway is open. If it is not, perform the head-tilt and chin-lift to open the airway.
3. Breathing normally begins spontaneously within the first 10 to 15 seconds.
4. Administer oxygen as a precautionary treatment only.
5. If the patient has not revived within the first 15 seconds, remove the oxygen mask (if one has been placed) and pass a broken ammonia gauze sponge under the patient's nose for 1 or 2 seconds only. Holding the ammonia for a long period of time under the patient's nose may cause undue irritation.
6. The patient will normally respond rapidly to the pungent odor of the ammonia, and take in a breath of air, thereby, receiving oxygen.
7. Full revival of the patient should occur within a minute or two.
8. If revival of the patient does not occur, follow the guidelines for CPR.
9. Postpone dental treatment and call for patient transportation.

who are given nitrous oxide or oxygen, patients who have been in the dental chair for long periods in a prone position, women who are pregnant, and patients who have had intravenous sedation are more prone to having orthostatic hypotension.

Asthma

Recurrent attacks of breathlessness accompanied by wheezing while breathing out and, often, by a dry cough are symptoms of asthma. The wheezing and breathlessness are due to the narrowing of the small airways in the lungs (bronchioles). When a patient with asthma exhales, the lungs collapse to expel the air, thereby causing the bronchioles to further narrow, making it even more difficult to breathe. If the lining of the bronchioles is inflamed, sputum (phlegm) is produced, which further obstructs the bronchioles and increases breathing difficulty. Refer to Procedure 16-8 for the steps for treating a patient with asthma.

Asthma is becoming more prevalent. Normally, the disease occurs during childhood, but the symptoms improve in adulthood. Approximately one in ten children in the United States have asthma. Heredity is a major factor in the development of the disease. Asthma may be caused by an allergy to a substance. An allergy is an exaggerated reaction of the immune system to an offending agent. Upon the first contact with the agent, the body becomes sensitized to it and develops antibodies (also called immunoglobulins) to fight these antigens (foreign bodies). The second or subsequent time that the body has contact with these offending agents, it overreacts in a **hypersensitive** manner. The most common allergens (the antigens that trigger the allergic reaction) responsible for asthma are animal fur, house dust, pollens, tobacco smoke, feathers, food, and drugs.

Asthma attacks are more frequent in the morning and vary from slight breathlessness to respiratory failure. There is no cure for asthma, but tests are available to identify what causes the most severe reactions in an individual so that the individual can avoid it. A treatment called **immunotherapy** (injection of the allergen) is an option, and corticosteroid drugs also provide successful therapy.

An **antihistamine** is often used to treat the physical symptoms produced by the antigen. These drugs counteract the body's production of histamine. They are administered with a rescue **inhaler**, a pressurized canister with a mouthpiece (Figures 16-11A and B). The patient carries an inhaler and, when an asthma attack is anticipated, the drug can be dispensed. The patient who suffers from asthma should be advised to bring an inhaler to any dental treatment appointment. If the patient has an attack and an inhaler is unavailable, the dentist may use the bronchodilator from the emergency kit. The drug of choice in this bronchodilator (inhaler) is albuterol, because it widens the bronchioles and improves airflow, but does not stimulate the cardiovascular system like the drug epinephrine would. To use the bronchodilator, the patient exhales first, and then takes a slow, deep breath while releasing the drug as the canister is depressed. After two dispensed amounts are taken, breathing should improve within 15 minutes. If the patient does not improve, the inhaler is used again. If this does not alleviate the condition, emergency services should be deployed to take the

Procedure 16-8
Procedure to Treat a Patient with Asthma

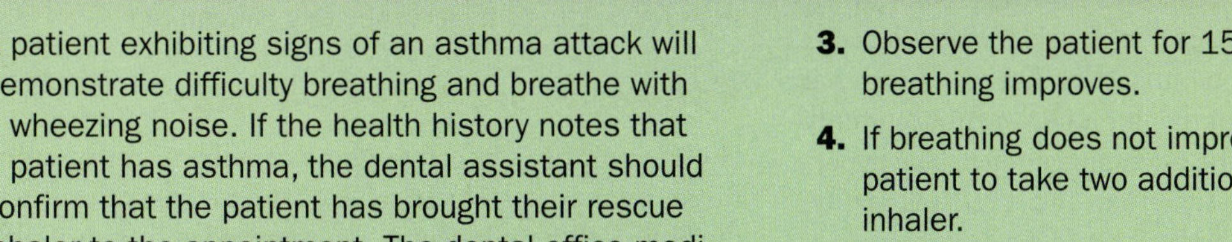

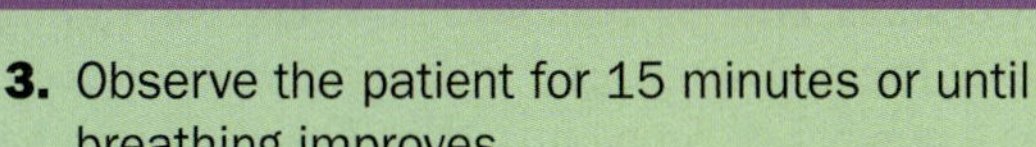

A patient exhibiting signs of an asthma attack will demonstrate difficulty breathing and breathe with a wheezing noise. If the health history notes that a patient has asthma, the dental assistant should confirm that the patient has brought their rescue inhaler to the appointment. The dental office medical emergency kit will also contain an inhaler.

Equipment and Supplies

- Bronchodilator inhaler

Procedure Steps

1. Position the patient upright in the dental chair.
2. Instruct the patient to exhale, and then instruct the patient to inhale slowly while depressing the canister. Repeat this process for a total of two breaths.
3. Observe the patient for 15 minutes or until breathing improves.
4. If breathing does not improve, instruct the patient to take two additional breaths of the inhaler.
5. The patient should be observed for an additional 15 minutes.
6. If breathing does not return to normal, emergency services should be deployed.
7. Begin administering oxygen to the patient while reassuring and keeping the patient calm.
8. Dental treatment should be postponed until the patient is evaluated by his or her physician.
9. Document emergency information and procedure on the patient's chart.

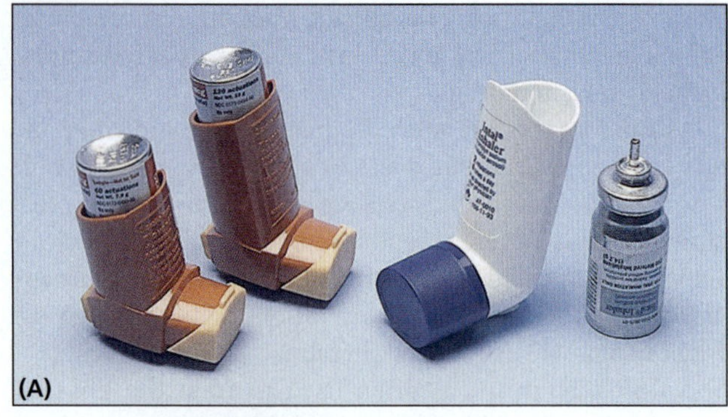

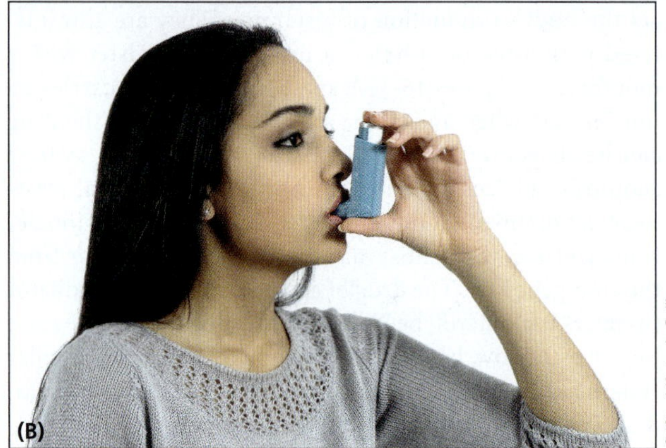

© iStock/Antonio Guillem

FIGURE 16-11

(A) Inhalers or nebulizers, and (B) inhalation of bronchodilator drug from an inhaler.

patient to the hospital. While waiting for the emergency services, the dental-office team should administer oxygen and reassure and calm the patient. The patient should also be instructed to see his or her general physician.

Allergic Reactions

A number of other **allergic reactions** may take place in the dental office. The body may react to drugs, toothpaste, latex protein, or a number of dental materials. Keep in mind that these exaggerated reactions of the immune system occur only subsequent to exposures to the offending antigen. The hypersensitive reaction may vary in symptoms and severity. It may be localized or cover the entire body. It could occur immediately or several hours after exposure to the antigen. Dermatitis, or skin reaction, may occur. If a skin reaction is apparent, dental treatment ceases until the irritant is removed.

Examples of skin reactions include the following:

- **edema** (eh-**DEE**-mah), or swelling
- **erythema** (er-ih-**THEE**-mah), or redness vesicle formation
- **urticaria** (ur-tih-**KAY**-ree-ah), or hives
- Giant urticaria, or **angioedema** (an-jee-oh-eh-**DEE**-muh), poorly defined, single, swollen areas

Treatment for both urticaria and angioedema is to remove the irritant. In some cases, the dentist will administer an antihistamine to reduce the edema.

Anaphylactic Reaction

An anaphylactic shock is a severe allergic reaction that is life threatening. It occurs in people who are extremely sensitive to a particular allergen. This may happen, for example, to a patient who is allergic to latex or has taken penicillin. Once the allergen is in the bloodstream, the body produces large amounts of histamine and other chemicals. The blood pressure drops, bronchospasm (constriction of the airways in the lungs) occurs, the tongue and throat swell, and the person experiences stomach pain. All of these symptoms come on rapidly, and an injection of epinephrine must be administered immediately to save the patient's life. Patients who know they are extremely sensitive to some allergens (e.g., bee sting venom) may carry antihistamine drugs and take immunotherapy treatment to desensitize for the allergen.

Hyperventilation

Dealing with the patient's anxiety prior to treatment alleviates fear and distress and hopefully reduces the chance of **hyperventilation**. Patients may try to hide their fears about dental treatment, and their anxiety can result in hyperventilation. They start to breathe deeply and rapidly, not realizing that they are breathing differently. As they continue breathing in this manner, they experience numbness in the extremities, faintness, and a sense that they are unable to take in a full breath. A loss of carbon dioxide from the blood occurs, causing **alkalosis** (an increase in blood alkalinity). The patient panics and breathing speeds up.

To treat the patient, first stop all dental treatment. Sit the patient upright to allow for easier breathing, and then calm him or her. Tell the patient what is happening and encourage him or her to breathe in and hold it several seconds before exhaling. This process allows more carbon dioxide to enter the bloodstream. If the patient is too agitated to follow instructions, instruct the patient to breathe into cupped hands or a paper sack (Figure 16-12). This allows the levels of carbon dioxide and oxygen to return to normal. Procedure 16-9 presents the steps for treating a hyperventilating patient.

Epilepsy/Seizure Disorder

Human emotions and thoughts normally occur in an organized, methodical, electrical excitation of nerve cells within the brain. With **epilepsy**, an unorganized and chaotic electrical discharge occurs. Seizures may appear spontaneously or as a result of a stimulus, such as a flashing light. Symptoms of the seizures may range from insignificant to severe. It is estimated that 1 person in every 200 suffers from epilepsy. Many wear bracelets or carry identification cards. Epileptics should advise colleagues about what to do in the case of a seizure.

The dentist will utilize fixed appliances (e.g., crowns or bridges, see Chapter 33; Fixed Prosthodontics and Gingival Retraction), if feasible, when treating patients who experience seizures due to epilepsy. During an epileptic seizure, the muscles tighten and the person has no control over movements. A loose dental appliance may become dislodged or broken, obstructing the airway during a seizure.

Procedure 16-9
Procedure to Treat the Hyperventilating Patient

The fearful patient may experience extreme anxiety during a dental procedure. This can lead to hyperventilation and alkalosis. The dental assistant should calm and reassure the patient prior to the procedure, reducing the chances of hyperventilation.

Equipment and Supplies

- Paper bag

Procedure Steps

1. Speak to the patient in a low calm voice.
2. Stop the dental procedure and sit the patient upright in the dental chair.
3. Explain to the patient what is happening and ask the patient to breathe in deeply and slowly and hold breaths in for a few seconds before exhaling.
4. If the patient continues to hyperventilate, instruct him or her to breathe into a small paper bag or cupped hands until the carbon dioxide level returns to normal (Figure 16-12).
5. It may be necessary to reschedule the patient if the hyperventilation cannot be controlled.
6. Document emergency information and procedure on patient's chart.

Some identified causes of epilepsy are head injury, infections, fever, brain tumor, strokes, metabolic imbalance, and drug and alcohol withdrawal states; it may also be triggered by stress. However, the causes of the majority of cases are unknown. Heredity is known to play a role. Types of seizures are classified in three general categories: grand mal, petit mal, and partial seizures.

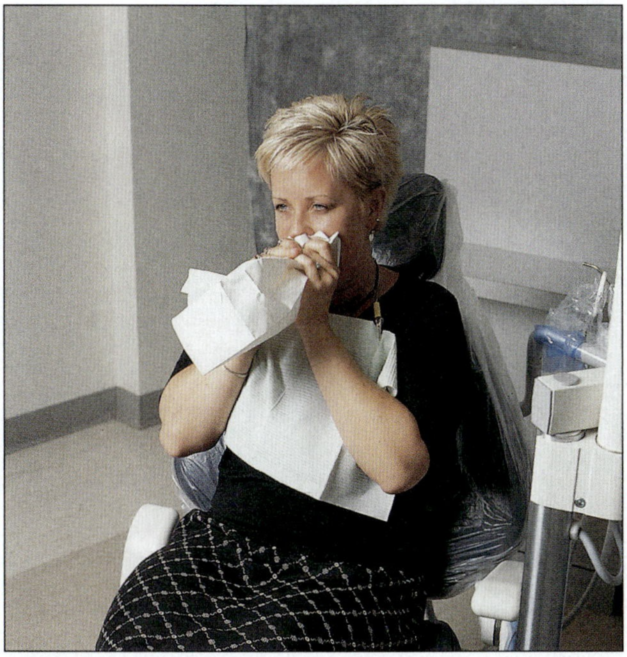

FIGURE 16.12
Patient breathing into a paper bag to increase carbon dioxide in the body.

Grand Mal Seizure. The **grand mal seizure** (tonic clonic seizure) is the most common. During this 2 to 5 minute seizure or **convulsion**, the person becomes unconscious and the body jerks, twitches, and stiffens. Breathing is often irregular. Once the seizure subsides, bladder and bowel control may be lost as the muscles relax. The person may be disoriented and exhausted, normally with no memory of the seizure. He or she may want to sleep. After the seizure, reassure the patient. If the patient experiences one seizure after another, which is called **status epilepticus** (continuous seizures), emergency services should be summoned.

Note: About 10 percent of patients experiencing status epilepticus will die due to the body's inability to deal with this overexertion.

Petit Mal Seizure. The **petit mal seizure** (absence seizure) occurs when a person experiences a momentary loss of consciousness. The patient may exhibit a blank stare or blinking of the eyes that lasts 5 to 10 seconds. Others around the person may not be aware of the seizure because of the lack of abnormal movements. The person may appear inattentive or seem to be daydreaming. Absence seizures occur in children and normally decrease in frequency with age. The absence seizure may occur several times a day and with other forms of seizures. Often, before a grand mal seizure, a petit mal seizure may be experienced first, as a warning. A person can then alert someone prior to the loss of consciousness.

Partial Seizure. A **partial seizure** can be classified into two categories: simple (person remains conscious) and complex (person becomes unconscious). A simple, partial seizure is referred to as **Jacksonian epilepsy**. As twitching occurs and spreads slowly from one part of the body to another on one side, the person remains conscious and is able to recall details of the event. During a complex seizure, the person remembers very little and exhibits involuntary actions, such as lip smacking, as the twitching spreads from one part of the body to another on the same side. If the seizure develops into a total body seizure, it is then referred to as a grand mal seizure.

To prevent seizures, a person should try to eliminate extreme stress and fatigue. Anticonvulsant drugs are the first line of treatment for epilepsy and may minimize seizures. Side effects of the drugs are fatigue and loss of concentration. Some of the drugs (such as Dilantin) cause **gingival hyperplasia**, or overgrowth of gingival tissue. This thick, granular tissue may cover the teeth and have to be surgically removed.

Treatment for Patients Who Experience Seizures. When patients experience seizures, stop dental treatment and remove everything from the oral cavity. Also, remove items from the area that could harm the person. Normally, no further action is necessary. The seizure runs its course. Do not restrain the person or place anything in the patient's mouth. Once the seizures have ceased, place the patient in the recovery position: on the right side with the airway open. Always be cognizant of the person's dignity and treat him or her in a considerate manner. The patient may feel embarrassed and reassurance is important. If the seizures continue for more than 5 minutes, or continue one after another, summon emergency help and reassure the patient.

Diabetes Mellitus

The cause of diabetes mellitus was discovered in the 1920s: the pancreas either does not produce or produces an insufficient amount of **insulin**: the hormone responsible for absorbing glucose into the cells for energy, and into the liver and fat cells for storage. Therefore, the level of glucose in the blood becomes too high, which causes thirst and excessive urination. In addition, the body cannot store glucose for the vast number of cells in the body that need glucose to survive. The body normally experiences weight loss and fatigue. Diabetes mellitus is classified into two categories: Type I and Type II.

Disturbances in the balance of glucose intake and insulin can result in **hyperglycemia** (too much glucose in the blood). The onset is slow and the person experiences early symptoms days prior to the onset, such as increased thirst, increased urination, nausea/vomiting with abdominal pain, loss of appetite, fatigue, and pain. If these patients (possibly undiagnosed diabetics) are having dental treatment, they could go into diabetic comas. If a patient reacts in this manner, stop dental treatment; if the patient is conscious, have him or her administer an insulin shot. If the patient becomes unconscious, call for emergency help and transfer him or her to a medical facility as soon as possible. One of the most serious consequences of hyperglycemia, a condition in which the patient goes into a coma and dies if not treated, is **diabetic acidosis**. This condition occurs when the patient has too much sugar (glucose) and not enough insulin. The body in this condition produces acids, and the body's pH is lowered. The body's pH range is 7.35 to 7.45. If the body's pH drops below 7.0, diabetic acidosis may occur.

Procedure 16-10
Procedure for Treatment of a Patient Experiencing Seizures

Episodes of epilepsy and seizures vary in strength and duration. Patients with epilepsy may experience a slight warning just before their seizures occur but will rarely have time to warn anyone. It is important to recognize the signs and symptoms of a seizure.

Equipment and Supplies

- There is no specific equipment necessary for this.

Procedure Steps

1. Stop all dental procedures as soon as a seizure is recognized.
2. Remove any dental items from the oral cavity.
3. Remove any items from the immediate area that could injure the patient.
4. Stay with the patient and allow the seizure to run its course.
5. Once the seizure has stopped, place the patient on their side with the airway open.
6. Allow the patient some space and reassure them that everything is okay. Be sensitive to the fact that they will feel embarrassed about the seizure.
7. If the seizure continues for more than 5 minutes, activate emergency medical services.
8. Document emergency information and procedure on patient's chart.

Hypoglycemia

Too little glucose or sugar causes a person to experience **hypoglycemia**. This condition comes on rapidly and the patient becomes nervous, shows signs of trembling and weakness, and has cold sweats. The patient becomes hungry and shows signs of a personality change. If the patient remains conscious, stop dental treatment and give him or her a sugar source, such as orange juice. If the patient becomes unconscious, terminate dental treatment, summon medical assistance, perform basic life support, and, if necessary, give the patient an injection of glucagon or a sugar source, such as cake icing gel placed in the buccal mucosa. If this condition happens frequently, the individual's physician may prescribe antidiabetic drugs to stimulate the pancreas to produce more insulin. Normally, however, the condition arises only when the person misses a meal, is overexerted, or is in a situation that causes emotional stress. Due to the stress patients experience during dental treatment and long appointment times, most dental offices have orange juice or other sources of sugar available for patients feeling changes in their blood sugar levels. Severe hypoglycemia causes **insulin shock**, manifested by tremors, sweating, and nervousness, and is soon followed by delirium, seizure-like jerkings, and collapse. Treatment requires administration of glucose intravenously. Procedure 16-11 walks through the steps to take in the event that a patient experiences hypoglycemia.

Cardiovascular Emergencies

A patient may experience angina pectoris and, if the vessel is totally occluded, the patient may experience a myocardial infarction.

Angina Pectoris. A Latin phrase meaning "strangling the chest," **angina pectoris** causes pain in the chest area. Pain may radiate into the jaw area from the base of the neck; this continuous jaw pain may be the first indication of heart disease. The chest pain normally lasts for 5 minutes. During that time, the person wants to remain motionless and stop all activity. The person may experience an increase in blood pressure and pulse rate, have a feeling of impending doom, and become pale and clammy. If this is not the first indication of the disease, the patient may be under the care of a physician. If the patient is under the care of a physician, he or she has nitroglycerin pills or spray. The small nitroglycerin pills are placed sublingually (under the tongue) to allow them to dissolve and be absorbed rapidly. Nitroglycerin spray (sprayed translingually into the oral cavity) can also be used. Nitroglycerin helps dilate the coronary arteries, allowing the heart to receive more oxygenated blood. This rapid-action drug is the accepted remedy for angina pectoris. Each patient is given a very specific dosage, because some individuals are more susceptible to the drug. If the condition arises in a dental office, all dental treatment stops. The dental team remains calm and reassures the patient. Any items that may increase stress for the patient are removed from sight. Oxygen can be administered while the patient takes the first dosage of nitroglycerin. A second dose can be administered within 3 to 5 minutes if the patient is feeling no relief while at rest. A final, third dose can be administered 3 to 5 minutes following the second dose. If the pain is not alleviated, the dental team can assume that the patient is experiencing myocardial infarction and emergency help should be summoned to transport the patient to a medical facility. Procedure 16-12 outlines the steps for treating a patient with angina.

Myocardial Infarction. A condition known as **myocardial infarction**, commonly known as a heart attack, occurs when the coronary arteries are blocked or severely narrowed (Figure 16-13). It causes sudden death of part of the heart tissue and may be precipitated by angina pectoris, or may occur

Procedure 16-11

Procedure for Hypoglycemic Patient

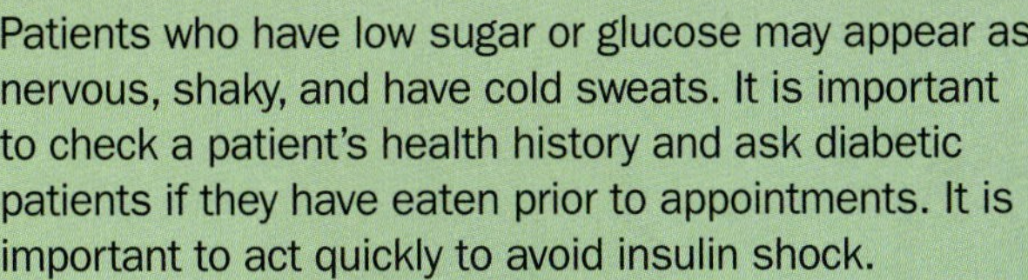

Patients who have low sugar or glucose may appear as nervous, shaky, and have cold sweats. It is important to check a patient's health history and ask diabetic patients if they have eaten prior to appointments. It is important to act quickly to avoid insulin shock.

Equipment and Supplies

- Sugar source such as juice, cake frosting, glucose gel tube, sugar packet, or sugar cube

Procedure Steps

1. Stop dental procedure immediately and position the patient comfortably in the chair.
2. Ask patient when they had their last meal.
3. Administer sugar source inside patient's mouth on their buccal mucosa.
4. Make a new appointment with the patient to complete the dental procedure.
5. If patient does not respond or symptoms worsen, activate emergency medical services.
6. Document emergency information and procedure on patient's chart.

Procedure 16-12
Procedure to Treat Angina Pectoris

Angina pectoris causes pain in the chest and is an early warning of heart disease. Patients who suffer from angina will carry a bottle of small pills, called nitroglycerine, that are taken under the tongue. Nitroglycerine is also available in spray form.

Equipment and Supplies

- Nitroglycerine
- Oxygen

Procedure Steps

1. Keep the patient in a supine position in the chair.
2. Administer specified dose of nitroglycerine.
3. The dental team should remain calm, reassuring the patient. Begin monitoring vital signs.
4. A second dose of nitroglycerine may be administered 3–5 minutes after the initial dose.
5. Begin administering oxygen.
6. A third dose can be given if symptoms persist.
7. If the pain is not alleviated, activate the emergency medical system and continue to monitor vital signs.
8. Document emergency information and procedure on patient's chart.

in a person who never had any prior symptoms. In about one-third of the cases, the person will die from myocardial infarction. The signs of a heart attack are similar to those of angina pectoris, but the pain may be increased and is not alleviated by nitroglycerin pills. A number of risk factors for the disease can be identified:

- Males are more likely to exhibit heart attacks than females.
- Smokers have a higher incidence of heart attacks than nonsmokers.
- Increased age; specific diseases, such as diabetes mellitus; and heredity are uncontrollable factors.
- Diet, stress level, high blood pressure, and exercise levels are controllable factors.

The dental team should remain calm, stop all dental treatment, reassure and reposition the patient in a comfortable position (normally the head is elevated slightly), and remove any items that may increase stress. Administer oxygen and nitroglycerin pills or spray, and summon medical emergency help immediately.

Congestive Heart Failure. As the heart weakens, a person may experience **congestive heart failure**. The weakened heart is not able to pump the fluids around the body as it should. When the person stands or sits for long periods, this fluid collects around the ankles and legs. The person may appear with swollen ankles and legs, and report indigestion and difficulty breathing. Many older patients show signs of heart weakening. When they lie in bed, these patients report difficulty breathing

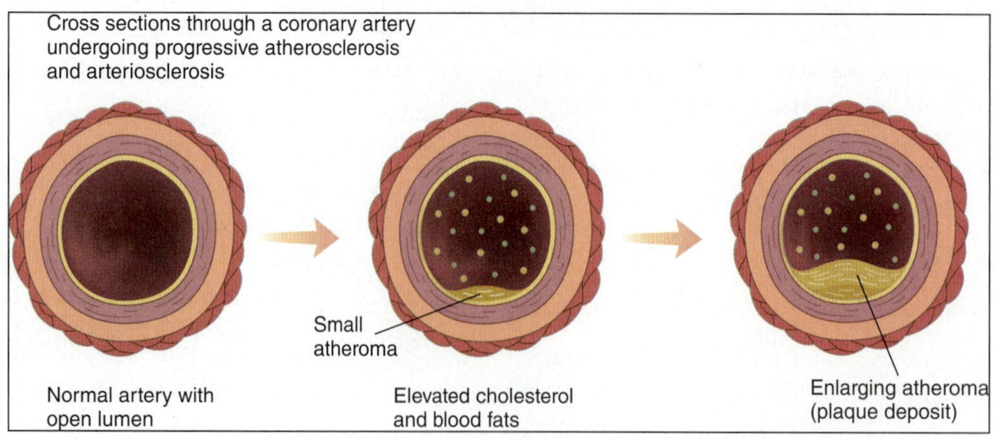

FIGURE 16-13
The progression of coronary heart disease.

and need to have large pillows to keep the head and heart elevated. This occurs because the fluids from the feet, legs, and other parts of the body gravitate toward the heart and lungs. The medical treatment for this patient is diuretic drugs that rid the body of excess fluid by increasing the output of urine. In some cases, these patients take other drugs to strengthen the contractions of the heart. While congestive heart failure may not result in a medical emergency, the dental assistant should be alert to how to make this patient more comfortable when receiving dental treatment. Be sure that these patients are seated with their heads elevated to eliminate discomfort, and reduce undue stress. Allow them to visit the restroom as needed.

Stroke/Cerebrovascular Accident. **Stroke** is a leading cause of disability and death for Americans. This condition has a sudden onset and is caused by a **cerebral infarction**, or the blood supply to the brain being interrupted by a blockage, such as a **cerebral embolism** (blood clot), or a **cerebral hemorrhage** (rupture of a blood vessel). Strokes happen to people of all ages, but occur primarily in older people. The person may have an intense headache, loss of speech, unexplained dizziness, **hemiplegia** (weakness, numbness, or paralysis on one side of the body), and loss of consciousness. An average of 200 people per 100,000 suffer strokes annually in the United States and Canada, according to the Centers for Disease Control (CDC). This figure rises with age; men have more strokes than women, and African Americans suffer more strokes than Caucasian Americans. If the person has diabetes mellitus or if the person has had a prior stroke, the risk is greater. Heredity is also a risk factor. Controllable risk factors are cigarette smoking, high blood pressure, and heart disease. Some people experience **transient ischemic attacks** (stroke-like symptoms that disappear within 24 hours). They should seek medical attention, because these are strong predictors of an impending stroke. A person may be given a blood thinner to prevent blood clots from forming and, thus, prevent the onset of a stroke.

Damage to an area of the brain may impair body sensation, function, or movement. The cerebral hemisphere in the brain on the left side controls the functions on the body's right side and vice versa. This one-sided weakness or paralysis is known as hemiplegia and it is one of the most common effects of a stroke. If a patient has had a stroke the dental assistant may observe the patient walking with an abnormal gait. If the patient has not indicated anything on the medical history about this, the dental assistant can request information from the patient. The patient may not understand that this information is important to his or her dental treatment and may feel that he or she is making a strong recovery, thus thinking that it is insignificant to his or her dental medical history. It is not only important that the dental assistant obtain the information from the patient, but that he or she is also observant when seating the patient. The doctor does not have this opportunity to view the patient as he or she is coming in for treatment.

If a patient has a stroke in the dental office, stop all dental treatment and remove any items from the patient's mouth. Position the patient so that his or her head is slightly elevated. Administer oxygen and monitor vital signs while emergency medical help is summoned. Calm the patient and provide CPR as needed.

Dental Emergencies

Patients may call the office about any number of dental emergencies. Most offices will reserve time in the schedule for emergencies. Some emergencies require the rescheduling of other patients and giving specific instructions for the patient seeking dental treatment. Several possible patient emergency situations are mentioned here. After the dentist sees each patient, a diagnosis is made and treatment rendered.

Abscessed Tooth

One of the most common emergencies for which patients seek dental care is an **abscessed tooth**. The patient's symptoms include pain from pressure, swelling, and severe responses to heat. The tooth has become infected, and as the abscess grows, it places a great deal of pressure in the area because the fluid has no place to escape in the bone. If the abscessed tooth goes untreated long enough in this painful state, the infection process may create a fistula in the bone and through the oral mucosa near the root end of the tooth. This **fistula**, an abnormal, tube-like passage at the end of the tooth to the outside surface in the oral cavity, allows the fluid to be discharged and the pressure to be released slightly. The fistula normally closes after the tooth is treated, after which the infection is reduced or eliminated.

Alveolitis

An **alveolitis** (al-vee-o-**LIGH**-tis; alveolar osteitis), a condition commonly known as a dry socket, happens after a tooth has been removed. This condition occurs when a blood clot does not form or is washed out of the socket, allowing the nerve endings over the bone to become exposed. This condition increases the chance of infection in the area. Alveolitis causes great discomfort. It is treated by gently rinsing the socket with saline solution to remove any debris and then packing a medicated iodoform gauze strip that is cut in a sufficient length into the socket. The medicated iodoform gauze treatment, which is only palliative, may have to be repeated every day or two until the pain diminishes. The patient may be given analgesics to relieve additional discomfort.

Avulsed Tooth

A patient may call the dental office and report that one tooth has been forcibly misplaced (avulsed). This **avulsed tooth** (also spelled *evulsed*) can be replanted into the socket and have a fairly high success rate if handled quickly. The patient should immediately wrap the tooth in clean, wet gauze, place it in the mucosa between the teeth and the lip, or place it in milk while transporting it to the office. The area where the tooth came out can be packed with gauze and pressure applied to control the bleeding. The outcome correlates greatly with the time that has elapsed. Getting the patient to the office and under the dentist's care quickly is essential. The dentist replants the tooth in the socket and secures it to the adjacent teeth. The dentist may perform immediate root canal therapy on the avulsed tooth prior to replanting it in the socket or complete the endodontic treatment 6 to 8 weeks after reimplantation.

Follow-up care is necessary until the tooth is reattached. There are individual emergency tooth avulsion kits available through dental suppliers and pharmacies.

Broken Prosthesis

A patient may call with a broken prosthesis. Normally, the patient is not in any physical pain but needs help due to appearance concerns and loss of function. The broken prosthesis can be repaired in the office by the dentist or sent to the dental laboratory. Additional treatment is scheduled at a convenient time for the patient and dental office. The length of time for prosthesis repair varies. It may be necessary to perform temporary repairs in the interim, until the permanent treatment can be completed.

Soft Tissue Injury

Patients experience a number of soft tissue injuries. Running with sharp or blunt objects or falling down with something in their mouth may cause a number of oral facial injuries. Electrical burns in the oral cavity can result from an individual biting into an electrical cord. Children can also fall and push newly erupted teeth back down/up into the sockets, which is called **traumatic intrusion**. Sports injuries result in soft tissue damage. The dental office should be contacted when such soft tissue injuries occur.

Soft tissue injury can occur in the dental office during any intraoral dental procedure. The oral cavity is moist and slippery, the patient may move suddenly, and dental instruments and equipment can easily become displaced, causing injury.

Broken Tooth

A patient may call with a broken tooth. Anterior teeth are commonly fractured at drinking faucets, on steering wheels, or on diving boards. The dental receptionist discerns whether the patient needs to be scheduled immediately by gaining information from the patient as to the level of discomfort, whether there are sharp edges, and how extensive the broken area is. In most offices, the patient is seen for an initial appointment on an emergency basis to determine the treatment needed.

Loose Permanent or Temporary Crown

A patient's crown may become loose or come off, requiring recementation. The patient may be in discomfort if the pulp is exposed or if the restoration has sharp edges. If the patient is out of town and unable to get dental care, petroleum jelly or orthodontic wax can be used to temporarily keep the crown in place. The patient will have to exercise extreme care while eating. If the patient can get to the dental office, treatment consists of recementing the crown with temporary or permanent cement, as indicated.

Monitoring the Patient's Health during Treatment

Dental procedures are becoming more complex with the new technologies utilized in dentistry. Patients are having longer procedures that are more invasive. More and more patients are having implants and surgeries to maintain their oral health as well as for cosmetic reasons. Older patients still have their teeth and many are having comprehensive dentistry. Additionally, the option of having mild or moderate sedation during procedures is becoming more popular. This leads to the necessity to ensure that these procedures can be completed in a safe manner and that the dental team is prepared for emergencies. Dental offices are now using a pulse oximeter and a capnograph to give the dentist additional information about the health of the patient during treatment. Some offices are also using an electrocardiogram (ECG) that provides additional health information for the dentist. Dental assistants will need to be knowledgeable and skilled with this equipment.

Pulse Oximeter

A **pulse oximeter** is a device used to indirectly measure the oxygen saturation of a patient's blood and changes in blood volume in the skin, and also to record the pulse (Figure 16-14). Most of these medical devices display pulse rates and blood oxygen levels, and have a pulse-strength indicator. It is often attached to a medical monitor so that the dental staff can view the patient's oxygenation at all times during the procedure. The real benefit of using this device is that it is a non-invasive procedure used instead of directly measuring through a blood sample. The typical procedure method is to place a portable saturometer on the fingertip.

Pulse oximeters come in both pediatric and adult sizes. A pediatric pulse oximeter is for children who weigh less than 100 pounds. A finger pulse oximeter is a small unit that can easily be placed in the pocket and used for spot checking the patient. The device is placed on the fingertip, and the reading

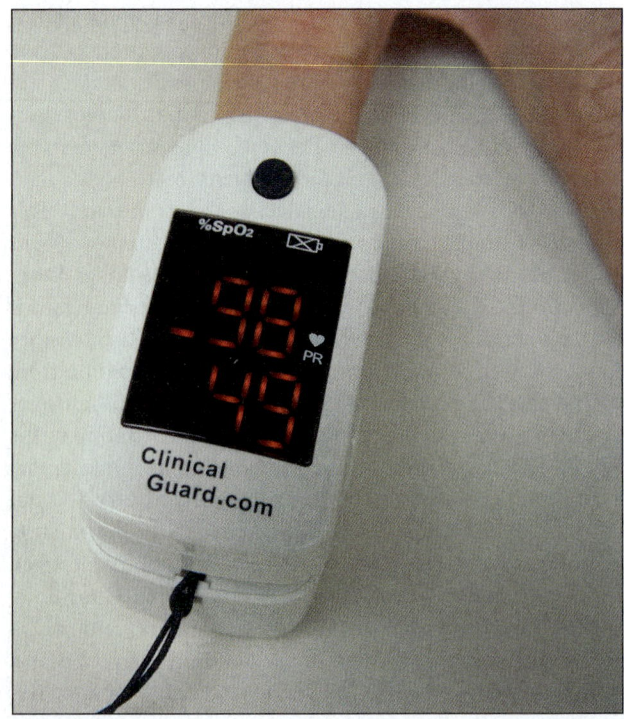

FIGURE 16-14
Example of a finger pulse oximeter.

displays on a screen on the top of the device. A handheld pulse oximeter comes with a small unit that fits over the fingertip and, normally, is attached to an easy-to-read liquid crystal display (LCD). The handheld units can be used for spot checking, or for continuous monitoring. Pulse oximeters are used almost universally in the care of critically ill patients in an intensive care unit and operating room. These units are attached to a medical monitor for the display of arterial hemoglobin in the oxyhemoglobin configuration. Normal ranges are from 95 to 100 percent; but 90 percent is common. The fundamental oximeter technology is based upon the measurement of the ratio of light absorption of red and infrared light as transmitted through the thin part of a patient's anatomy (e.g., fingertip [most common], earlobe, or the bottom of the feet on a child). Typically, the units have a pair of small, light-emitting diodes (LEDs) facing through a translucent part of the patient's body. One LED is infrared light with a wavelength of 850–1,000 nm, and the other is red light with a wavelength of 660–750 nm. The body absorbs these wavelengths differently between its deoxygenated form and its oxyhemoglobin form. Therefore, by using a ratio of the absorption of the infrared and the red light, the oxy/deoxyhemoglobin ratios can be calculated and viewed on the display. If the absorption level of the two is the same, it is at the **isosbestic** point. During the heartbeat, the arterial blood vessels expand and contract, and this signal bounces in time with each pulse rate. Oxygenated hemoglobin absorbs more infrared light and allows more red light to pass through it. The opposite is true for deoxygenated (or reduced) hemoglobin; it absorbs more red light and allows more infrared light to pass through it. The wavelength is measured in direct correlation to the pulse.

A pulse oximeter is also used in the diagnosis of sleep apnea. (Note: Once diagnosed, dental treatments that can help patients with sleep apnea include: soft-tissue palate lifts and the designing and fabrication of devices that help patients who exhibit snoring). Many of these patients have decreased intake of oxygen and report to be tired all the time. The pulse oximeter readings become the quantitative indicator of hypoxia. The condition called **hypoxia** is a pathological condition in which either the whole body (**generalized hypoxia**) or tissue limited to a region of the body (**tissue hypoxia**) is deprived of adequate oxygen supply. Pulse oximeter readings may be quantified as mild to moderate hypoxia if presented by a pulse oximeter reading of 90 to 95 percent. Moderate to severe hypoxia is represented by a pulse oximeter reading of 80 to 90 percent. Severe hypoxia is anything less than 80 percent, although the accuracy of pulse oximetry generally decreases below about 70 percent. Pulse oximetry is a relatively easy procedure to perform, but the operator must understand that the devices have limitations in their application. The dental team must be trained to do a complete patient assessment and not rely totally on one medical device. It is to be used along with other information for the doctor to make a diagnosis. The probe should be the correct size for the patient. It is intended for multiple-patient usage, but should be cleaned between patient applications according to the manufacturer's recommendations. The external monitor should also be cleaned when soiled, or a barrier can be used to protect it from any potentially transmissible organism.

Capnography

A **capnograph** is a medical device that is used to measure the carbon dioxide (CO_2) concentration in an air sample. The capnograph measures the absorption of infrared light. It is absorbed exceptionally well by carbon dioxide. A capnograph is not normally used by patients who are critically ill, but is used by patients who are hemodynamically stable. It detects changes in carbon dioxide concentrations by using an infrared beam of light on concentrations of respired gas. It is often part of the pulse oximeter device. Many of these devices can be attached to an external printer. The measurement and numerical display of maximum inhalation and expiratory CO_2 concentrations during a respiratory cycle is called **capnometry**. The normal level is around 24. The normal range in the body is 22–30 mEg/L. Both oxygen and carbon dioxide compete for a space within a cell. If the CO_2 is up, then the O_2 is down, and vice versa. If a nervous patient in the dental office is hyperventilating and, thereby, taking in oxygen too rapidly, it will show as a decrease in CO_2. Care of the capnograph is the same as for the pulse oximeter. It is intended for the use of multiple patients and must be cleaned according to the manufacturer's instructions.

Electrocardiography

The recording of the electrical activity of the heart for a period of time by way of skin electrodes is called **electrocardiography** (Figure 16-15). Using skin electrodes allows this procedure to be done in a non-invasive manner, instead of puncturing the skin and taking blood from the body and measuring the oxygen level. This procedure is painless and provides a great deal of information on how the cardiovascular system is working. The etymology of the word is derived from the Greek word for heart, *cardi*, and the Greek word meaning to write, *graph*. The outcome is a written document providing information on how the electrical activity of the heart is functioning (Figure 16-16).

The equipment needed for electrocardiography is the electrograph machine, the lead wires, sensors, and the electrocardiography paper. The machine is designed to amplify the electrical activity that comes from the body. The voltage is changed into mechanical motion by a **galvanometer**, an instrument for detecting and measuring electric current. This information is then recorded on graph paper by a heated stylus (writing utensil) in response to the electric current flowing through its coil. The sensors or electrodes are devices that measure a physical quantity and convert it into a signal that can be read by an instrument or by an operator. The sensors are made of metal or other conductive material and detect the electrical impulses on the skin. The sensors are attached to cables or lead wires, which also attach to the ECG machine. Most operators use disposable sensors that have a layer of electrolyte gel on them; they attach to the surface of the skin by means of

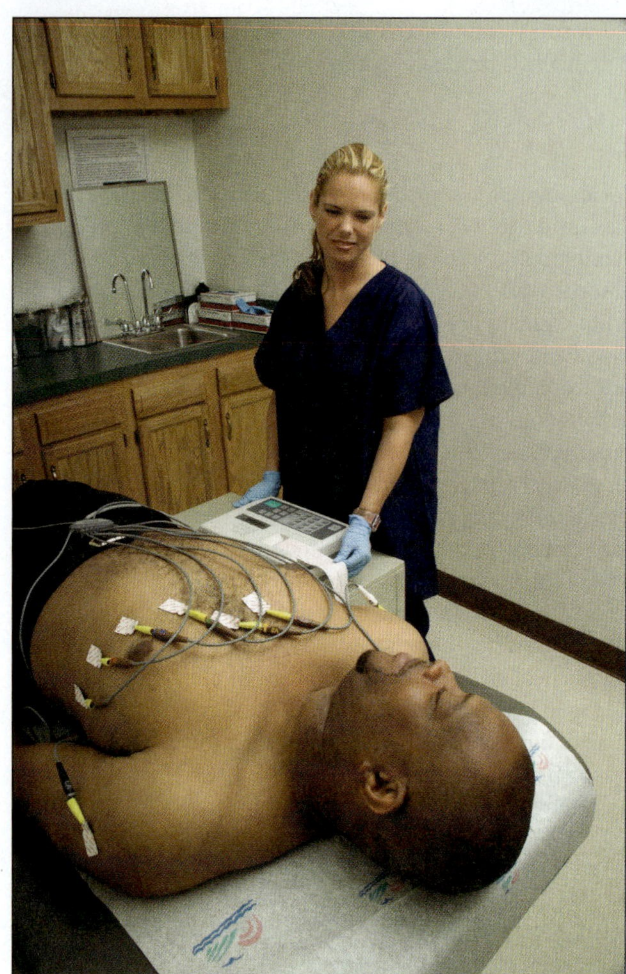

FIGURE 16-15

An electrocardiograph is useful for capturing information on the electrical activity of the heart.

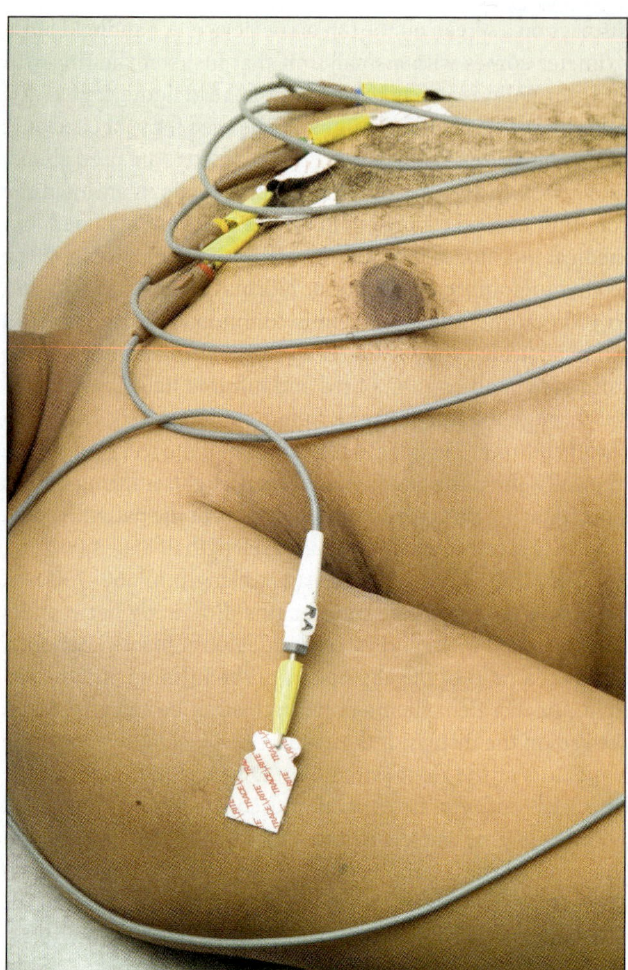

FIGURE 16-17

Lead wires attached to sensors that obtain an electrocardiograph.

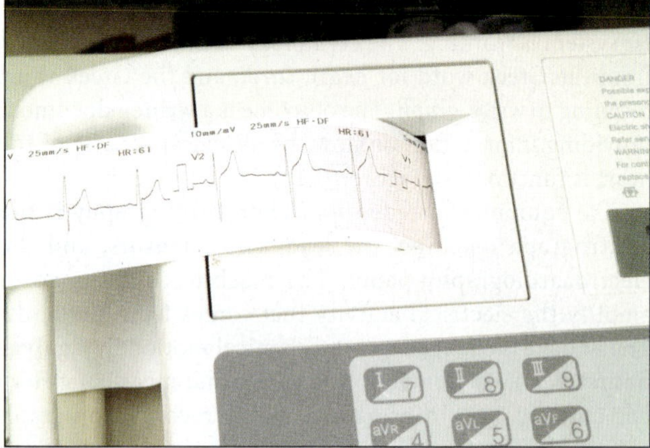

FIGURE 16-16

The reading from an electrocardiograph machine.

an adhesive. They are disposed of after each patient use. The lead wires are attached to the sensors with small clips referred to as alligator clips (Figure 16-17). They securely grasp the tabs on the sensors and ensure that a complete circuit from the patient to the machine is established. These leads are attached to the ECG machine at the other end. The lead wires are placed neatly and loosely on top of or beside the ECG machine after the disposable sensors have been removed from the patient. The paper is divided into 1 mm small squares and 5 mm larger squares (Figure 16-18). Each large square consists of 25 small squares and is 5 mm high by 5 mm wide. On the horizontal line, one small square represents 0.04 of a second. On the vertical line, one small square represents 1 mm of voltage. Therefore, each large square on the horizontal line represents 0.2 of a second (i.e., 5 × 0.04 of a second equals 0.2 of a second). It should be noted that on every fifth line, both the horizontal and vertical lines are darker to allow for easier interpretation of the information. The graph paper is available in variable colors, but it is often seen in red or black. Some are ordered in wax or with plastic coating, and more are heat and pressure sensitive. The heat of the stylus on the electrocardiograph can be adjusted to obtain a sharp tracing. Regardless of the type of electrocardiograph used, the basic components of the standard electrocardiograph procedure remain the same. Patient preparation, placement of leads, and attachment of lead wires vary little from one electrocardiograph to another. Before performing the procedure, dental assistants must be familiar with the electrocardiograph machine in

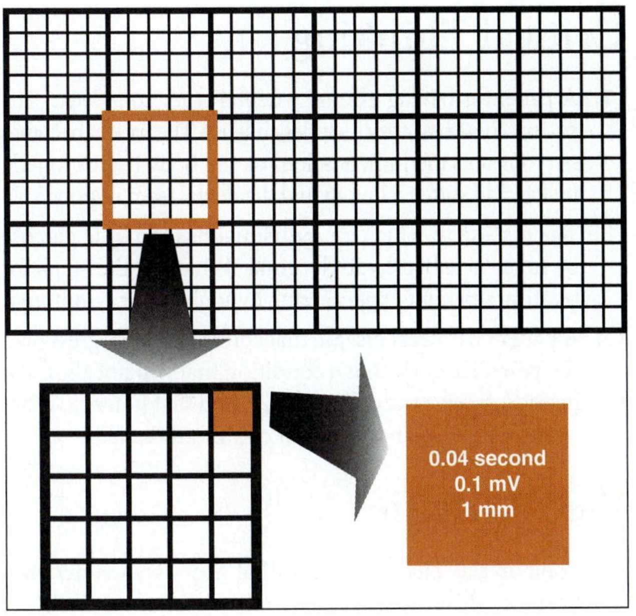

FIGURE 16-18
Example of the graph paper used for an ECG.

their facility, have further training, and should thoroughly review the manufacturer's instruction manual that accompanies the machine.

Chapter Summary

Even though the number of emergencies is not high in a dental office, the dental assistant must always observe the patient and be prepared to prevent and/or respond to emergencies. Emergencies may also happen to the dentist and to other dental auxiliaries.

When an emergency arises, the dental team must react automatically. Any hesitation at such a time may cost a life. It is best if a routine is established so that everyone can ensure that everything is addressed. The assistant has a vital role in the prevention of emergencies and in emergency care. Patient observation at all times assists in the evaluation for prevention.

CASE STUDY

Thelma Lynd, a 46-year-old woman, is seated in the dental treatment room. She indicates that she has not been feeling well recently. As she continues to talk, she experiences loss of speech, dizziness, and weakness on one side of her body. Her vital signs are elevated and she cannot respond.

Case Study Review

1. What probable condition is Thelma experiencing?
2. What should the dental assistant do in this situation?
3. Is reassurance for the patient important in this case? Why?

Review Questions

Multiple Choice

1. An exaggerated reaction by the immune system is called an
   a. allergy.
   b. antibody.
   c. antigen.
   d. allergen.
2. Asthma attacks are more frequent in the
   a. late evening.
   b. afternoon.
   c. morning.
   d. nighttime hours.
3. A medical term for giant hives is
   a. edema.
   b. erythema.
   c. urticaria.
   d. angioedema.
4. A seizure in which a person experiences a momentary loss of consciousness is called a
   a. grand mal seizure.
   b. petit mal seizure.
   c. partial seizure.
   d. status epilepticus.
5. Type ________ of diabetes mellitus is often termed juvenile diabetes due to the age at which it commonly affects people.
   a. I
   b. II
   c. III
   d. IV
6. Traumatic intrusion is the term for a newly erupted tooth being ________.
   a. removed
   b. pushed back into the socket
   c. decayed
   d. knocked out

7. Angina pectoris causes pain in the ________.
   a. legs
   b. left arm
   c. stomach
   d. chest
8. An average of ________ people per 100,000 suffer strokes annually in the United States and Canada.
   a. 100
   b. 200
   c. 300
   d. 400
9. A continuous seizure is called ________.
   a. grand mal seizure
   b. status epilepticus
   c. petit mal seizure
   d. partial seizure
10. A condition commonly known as a dry socket is called ________.
   a. alveolitis
   b. avulsed
   c. angina pectoris
   d. abscessed

Critical Thinking

1. A patient is having extensive dental work completed. The patient's health history includes epilepsy. The patient becomes nervous and then unconscious as the body begins to jerk, twitch, and stiffen. How should the dental team respond?
2. The disease in which an individual has too little glucose or sugar is called hypoglycemia. What are the steps for treating a patient experiencing hypoglycemic symptoms?
3. A patient has heart disease that continues to progress over the years. He or she has a condition that will not allow the heart to receive the oxygenated blood that it needs. What is the condition and what is it commonly called?

Web Activities

1. Look up the "chain of survival" at http://www.americanheart.org. List the four steps in the chain of survival.
2. Go to http://www.redcross.org and find the address and phone number of the Red Cross office closest to you.
3. Go to http://www.americanheart.org and look up recent discoveries supported by the AHA. Complete a one-page report on one recent discovery.

Section V

Clinical Dental Procedures

CHAPTER 17

Introduction to the Dental Office and Basic Chairside Assisting

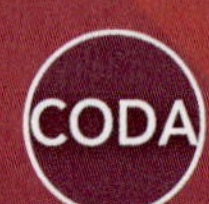

Specific Instructional Objectives

The student should strive to meet the following objectives and demonstrate an understanding of the facts and principles presented in this chapter:

1. Describe the design of a dental office, explaining the purpose of each area.
2. Describe the equipment and function of the equipment in each area.
3. Describe the daily routine to open and close the dental office.
4. Explain the basic concepts of chairside assisting.
5. Identify the activity zones and classifications of motion.
6. Describe the necessary steps to prepare the treatment room.
7. Explain the necessary steps to seat the patient for treatment.
8. Describe the ergonomics of the operator and the assistant at chairside.
9. Describe the necessary steps to dismiss the patient after treatment is finished.
10. Identify the special needs of certain patients.

Key Terms

activity zones (370)
administrative area (357)
air compressor (369)
air-water syringe (361)
amalgamator (367)
argon laser (366)
assistant's cart (360)
assisting zone (370)
central vacuum system (369)
classifications of motion (371)
condensation (369)
consultation room/area (359)
curing light (365)
darkroom (358)
dental unit (360)
ergonomics (373)
four-handed dentistry (370)
front delivery system (360)
handpieces (362)
hands-free communication system (367)
high-volume evacuator (HVE) (363)
intraoral camera (368)
laboratory (357)
light emitting diode (LED) (366)
lumbar (363)
mobile cart (360)
napkin (372)
operating light (364)
operating zone (370)
operator's cart (360)
operatory (359)
plasma arc (PAC) (366)
radiometer (light meter) (367)
rear delivery system (360)
reception room (355)
rheostat (362)
saliva ejector (363)
side delivery system (360)
six-handed dentistry (370)
static zone (370)
sterilizing area (357)
subsupine position (359)
supine position (359)
transfer zone (370)
treatment room (357)
triturates (367)
tungsten halogen (366)
ultrasonic scaler (363)
upright position (359)
water reservoir (362)

Introduction

Dental offices have numerous designs, including a single building, a medical/dental complex of individual units, a remodeled home, a suite in an office building, or space in a mall. Dental professionals go to great lengths to ensure that their offices are clean and convenient and offer pleasant settings for patients. The dentist's vision and expectations are reflected in the office design, which should always consider the patients the dentist serves. The practice may serve families, primarily children, or primarily adults and may be in a rural or an urban setting. The most successful practices encompass all facets into a welcoming atmosphere where dental treatment can be provided.

The appearance of the dental office makes a statement about the dentist, the dental staff, and the quality of the dental care. The following information describes the rooms in the dental office, the specific equipment used by dental professionals, and the concept of chairside assisting.

Dental Office Design

The dental office has several basic components designed to meet the dentist's individual preferences and needs. The office may be small with two or three treatment rooms or it may have a clinic setting with any number of treatment rooms (Figure 17-1). Most offices are designed with a reception area, a business area, treatment rooms, a sterilizing area, a laboratory, an x-ray processing room, a restroom, and the dentist's office. The sizes and numbers of these rooms vary (Figure 17-2). Dental offices may also include the following: consultation rooms/areas, a staff lounge, a patient education area, a storage area, an office for the office manager, space for a panoramic radiograph machine, a shower/change room, and a laundry room. OSHA requirements have changed the office by requiring a room for staff to change and store uniforms. Some offices have added laundry facilities. In addition, dental offices are requiring more space in the business office to accommodate high-technology equipment and to facilitate increased dental insurance processing.

Privacy for patient conversation is an aspect that is considered in the design of the dental office. There should be privacy for the patient at the front desk where they check in and fill out paper work and in the consultation and financial room/area where treatment and financial arrangements are discussed. The patient should feel comfortable when talking to the dentist and the dental auxiliary.

Innovations in dental offices include more open designs with partial walls and greater access to the treatment rooms, sterilizing area, and so on. Higher ceilings, open doorways, and more windows also create the feeling of openness for the patient and the dental team. The office should have a climate-control system that remains at a comfortable temperature throughout the year, regardless of the weather conditions. Architects and decorators often work with dental professionals to achieve the look the dentist desires.

Reception Room

The **reception room** is the area the patient initially enters and therefore gives the first impression of the office. It is important that this room be pleasing and comfortable as well as neat and clean (Figure 17-3). The dental staff should tidy this room

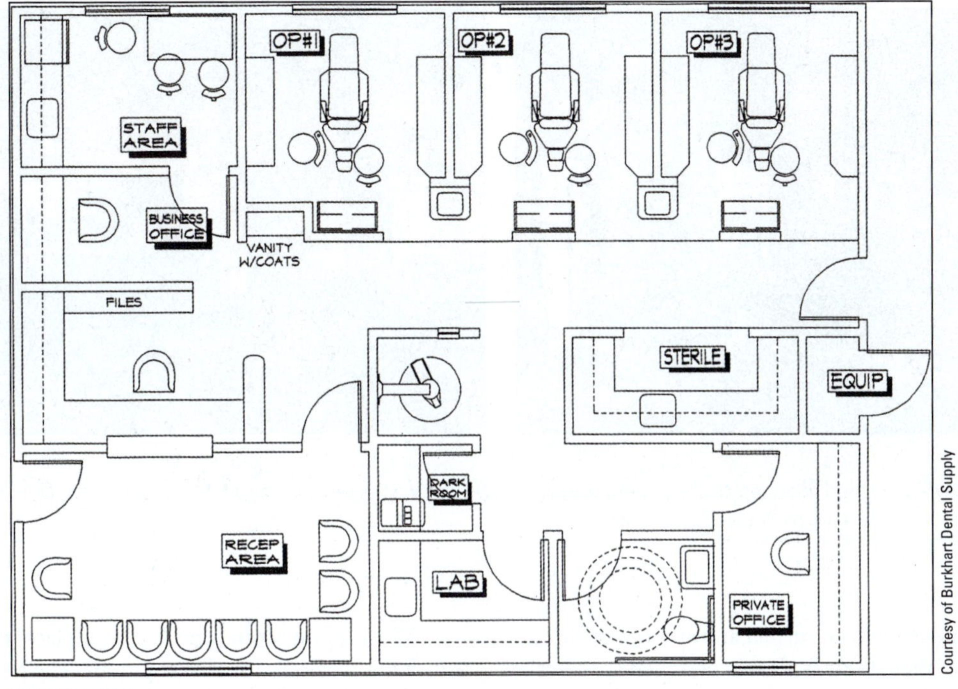

FIGURE 17-1
Small dental office blueprint.

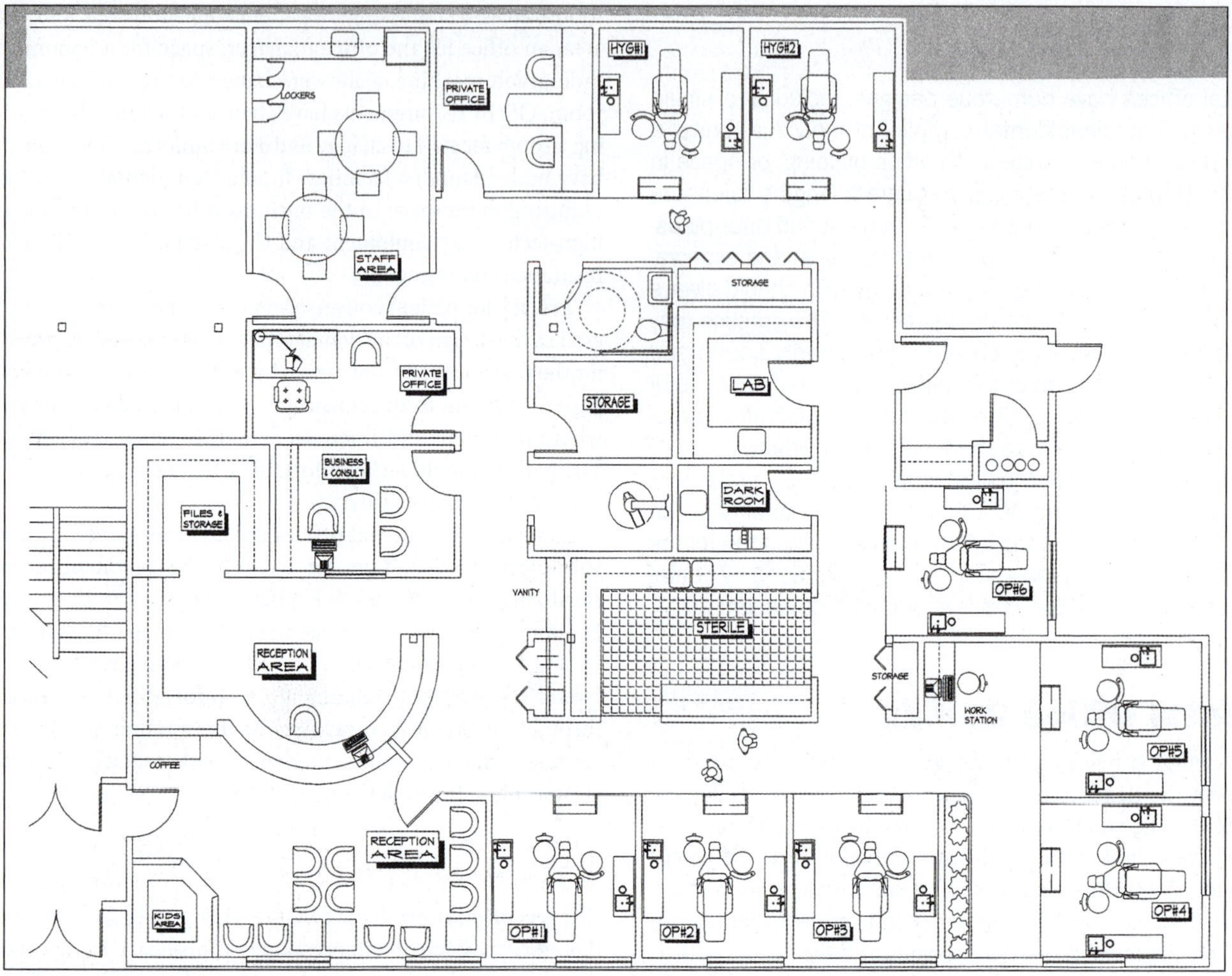

Courtesy of Burkhart Dental Supply

FIGURE 17-2

Large dental office blueprint.

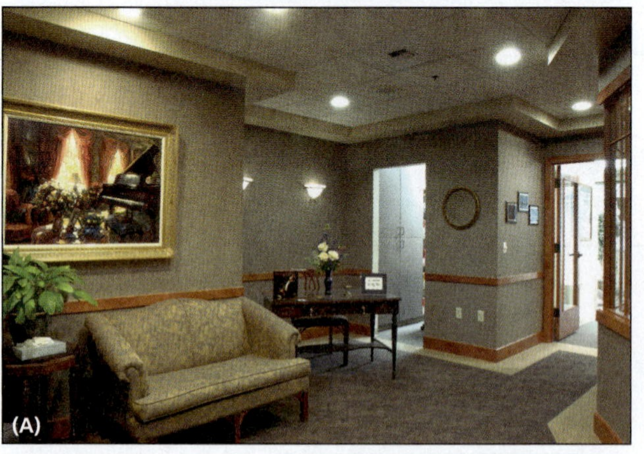

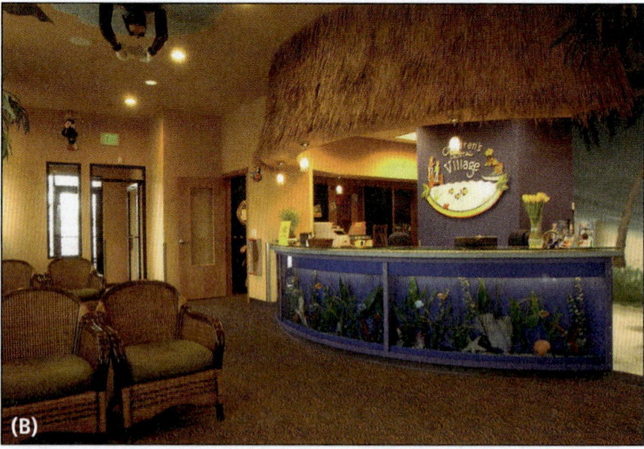

FIGURE 17-3

Reception areas can be designed to appeal to the patient population. (A) The waiting area in the cosmetic dentistry office of Dr. Charles Regalado. (B) The pediatric dental practice of Dr. Jay Enzler.

regularly. Magazines should be current and appropriate for the dentist's clientele. Often, there is an area designed specifically for children with a table, chairs, and activities to keep them occupied while they wait.

The reception room is an excellent place to provide patient education materials for all age groups. The decor of this room should be changed as often as needed to keep the atmosphere friendly and positive for the patients as they enter the dental office.

Reception Desk and Business Office

The reception desk and business office is often part of or adjacent to the reception room, so that patients can be greeted as they enter the office (Figure 17-4). This area is where patients are received when they first arrive at the office.

Appointments are made here, telephone calls are received, and patient records are updated and stored. This area includes counter space, desk space, adequate lighting, an accessible filing system, access to computer terminals, and telecommunication systems (Figure 17-5). The counter space should be designed to allow some privacy for the business office staff and provides a space for patients to schedule appointments, update information, and pay bills. Some offices have an **administrative area** where the office manager or business assistant manages the business part of the dental practice. This area is close to the front of the office and has a desk, computer system, copier, phone system, and the business files. It provides an area of privacy to conduct the financial arrangements and concerns of the practice. There is sometimes a conference room or an area somewhere close to the business office for private conversations with patients. Because the reception area is where the staff makes the first and last contacts with the patient, it should reflect a positive image of the qualities of the dental practice.

Sterilizing Area

The **sterilizing area** should be near the **treatment rooms** and should be neat and clean at all times (Figure 17-6). The sterilizing room should have good air circulation to protect everyone from the chemical fumes and exhaust from the sterilizers. In this area is a sink, counter space, a sharps container, a hazardous waste container, ultrasonic equipment, a handpiece cleaner/lubricating machine, sterilizing equipment, and storage. OSHA has specific requirements for this area so that instruments, trays, and so on flow from dirty areas to clean areas to minimize the chance of cross contamination.

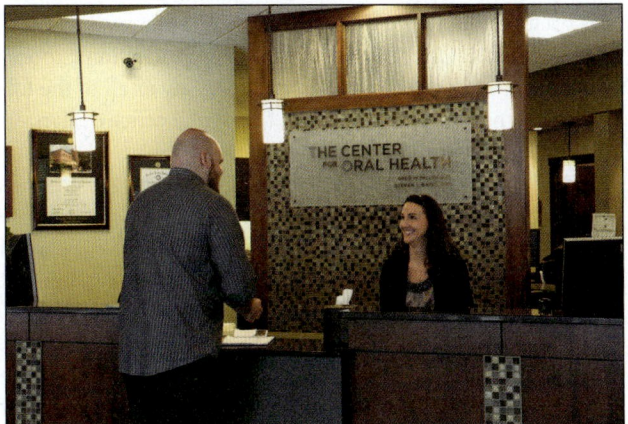

FIGURE 17-4
Reception Desk and Business Office of Dr. Charles Regalado.

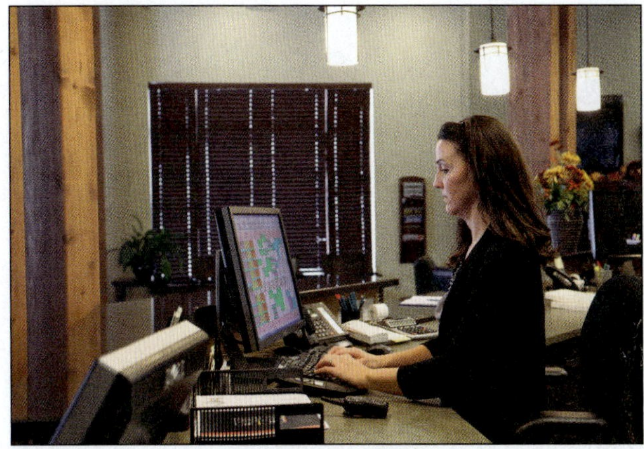

FIGURE 17-5
The reception desk should have adequate space and lighting.

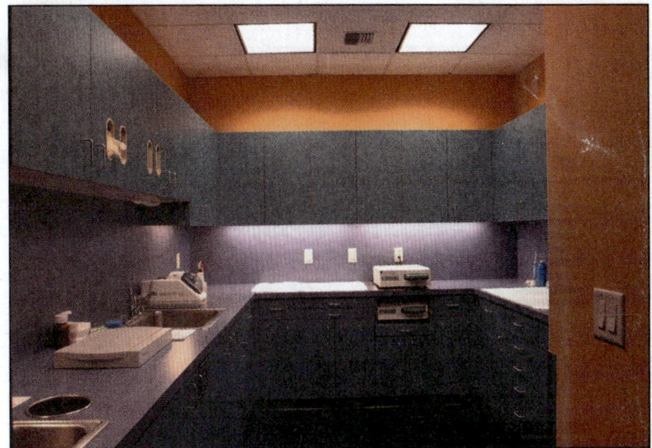

FIGURE 17-6
Sterilizing area with sink, counter space, storage, ultrasonic unit, handpiece maintenence unit, and sterilizing unit in the office of Dr. Jay Enzler.

Upon completion of sterilization, trays are set up and sometimes stored in this area. Infection control supplies, procedure supplies, and hazardous waste supplies are stored in the sterilization area. (The sterilizing equipment is discussed in Chapter 11, Infection Control.)

Dental Office Laboratory

The dental office **laboratory** is a separate area that is also well vented (Figure 17-7). The amount of lab work done in the office depends on the dentist's preference. If the dentist's practice includes a number of patients needing prosthodontic treatment, a lab technician and a lab is set up in the office. In other offices, the dental lab may be used for finishing or adjusting crowns, bridges, partials, or dentures and for pouring impressions, trimming models, polishing removable appliances, and making custom trays. (See Chapter 39 Laboratory Equipment, Materials, and Techniques.)

The dental laboratory may contain a vibrator, a model trimmer, a laboratory handpiece, a vacuum former, a sink, an exhaust fan, plaster and stone storage bins, a heat source, and a dental lathe. Cupboards provide storage for instruments such

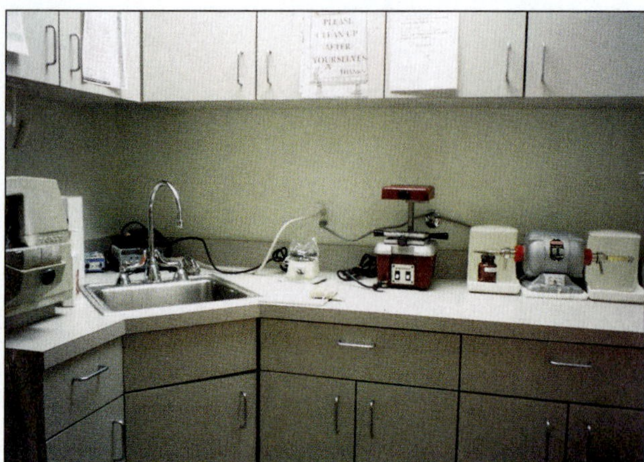

FIGURE 17-7
Laboratory area of the office of Drs. Rodney Braun and Chris Chaffin.

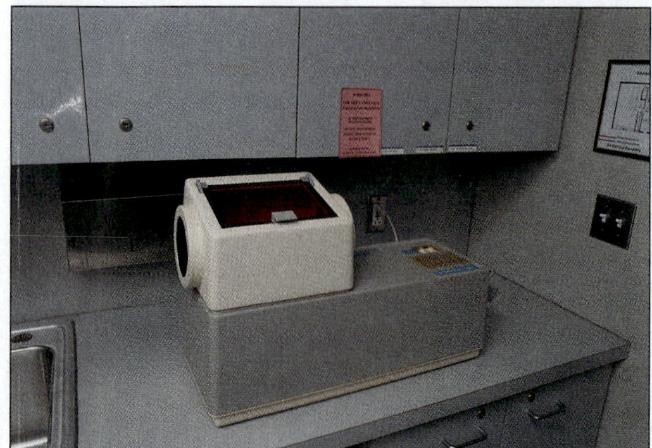

FIGURE 17-8
X-ray processing area with sink, counter space, storage, and automatic processing unit with daylight loader.

as lab knives, spatulas, and rubber bowls. All aseptic precautions must be followed when working in this setting, because often the materials have been in the patient's mouth before coming to the lab. The staff should wear protective glasses and masks to prevent dust and debris from causing injuries when working with the equipment.

X-Ray Processing Room

The x-ray processing room or **darkroom** is a small room near the treatment rooms (Figure 17-8). This room contains a sink, a manual processing tank, drying racks, space for storage, safelights, and counter space for processing and mounting radiographs. With the use of automatic processors with daylight loading, the need for this space has changed. The automatic processor may be in the processing room or in treatment rooms, the sterilizing area, or an open area in a hall space. (This room and the equipment are described in detail in Chapter 21, Introduction to Dental Radiography and Equipment.)

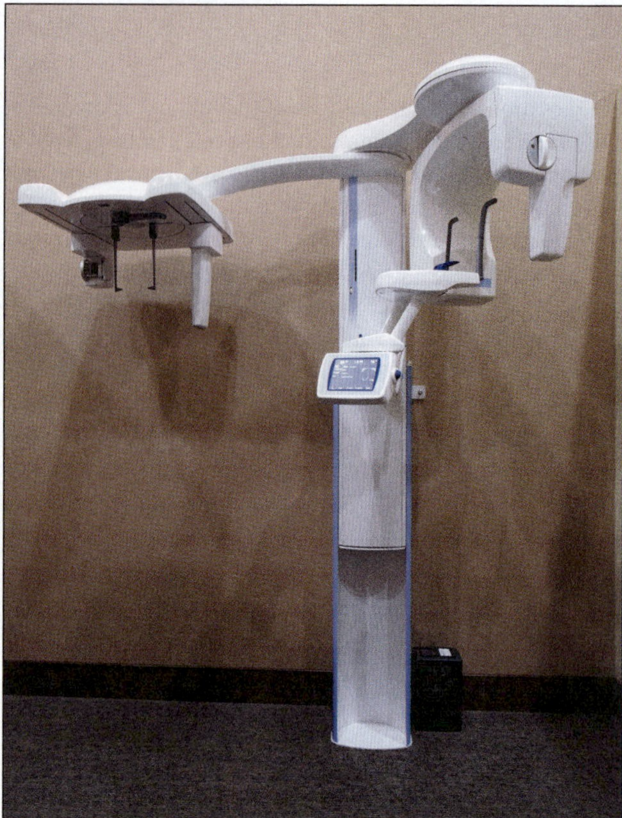

FIGURE 17-9
Panoramic x-ray machine area.

Radiography Room

In most dental offices, radiograph machines are in each treatment room for intraoral x-rays. The extraoral radiographic equipment is in a radiography room. This room must provide occupational safety from ionizing radiation and be large enough to house this equipment. Guidelines come from the state health department, and periodic inspections may be required by state agencies (Figure 17-9).

Optional Rooms in the Dental Office

Optional rooms in the dental office are dictated by the dentist's preference, patient usage, amount of space available, and practice budget. Often the office is built with additional rooms available for later growth in the practice. Any or all of the following rooms may be included in the dental office design.

Dentist's Private Office. The dentist's private office is designed according to the individual taste of the doctor. The dentist's private office is where the dentist conducts personal and professional business. This office may be used to consult with patients privately or for staff meetings.

Staff Lounge. A staff lounge is a place for staff to have lunch, and relax. This area may also be used as a room for staff meetings. In the staff lounge are a sink, refrigerator, microwave, coffee machine, table and chairs, storage cupboards, and countertop space. A washer and dryer may also be in this area.

Patient Education Area. A patient education area is a very functional and diverse area in the dental office. With each type of practice, its use may vary; for example, in the orthodontic office, the space may be furnished with mirrors and sinks where patients can practice home-care techniques. The patient education area may be an information center containing a variety of information on dental care and treatments available to patients, such as bleaching treatments or dental implants.

Often this room has a sink, a counter or table with chairs, and multimedia equipment including a television and DVD equipment. This area is also used for consultations with the patient or for the patient to wait, if necessary.

Consultation Room/Area

Some dental offices will have a **consultation room/area** where the dentist can sit down with the patient and discuss the treatment plan and financial arrangement. This room will have a table, chairs, viewbox, computer, possible models, anything to assist the dentist in explaining the treatment to the patient. This area is private and away from the main flow of the office.

The Treatment Rooms and Dental Equipment

The dental treatment room is also called an **operatory** (Figures 17-10 and 17-11). Each dentist usually has a minimum of three treatment rooms. The type and size of practice dictate the number of operatories. The treatment rooms in a general practice are usually designated for operative dentistry or hygiene and are equipped accordingly. They can be individual rooms or open spaces divided by walls and/or equipment. The rooms need to be large enough to contain the necessary equipment while still allowing for easy access to it. The treatment rooms should be designed for maximum efficiency.

A dental treatment room contains a dental chair, dental unit, operating stools, cabinets, sinks, x-ray machine, x-ray viewbox or computer screen, and mobile carts. There are many manufacturers and designs of equipment to choose from to meet office requirements. Dental equipment is expensive and, with careful maintenance, is meant to last for years. Someone in the office often is assigned to perform the routine maintenance of the equipment. A dental equipment technician is called when more substantial problems occur.

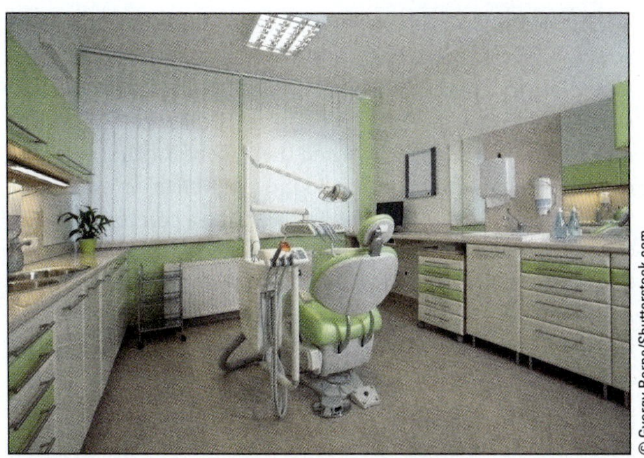

© Gyorgy Barna/Shutterstock.com

FIGURE 17-10

Dental treatment area: counter space and storage, patient chair, dental light, dental unit with handpieces, air-water syringe, high-volume evacuator (HVE), and rheostat.

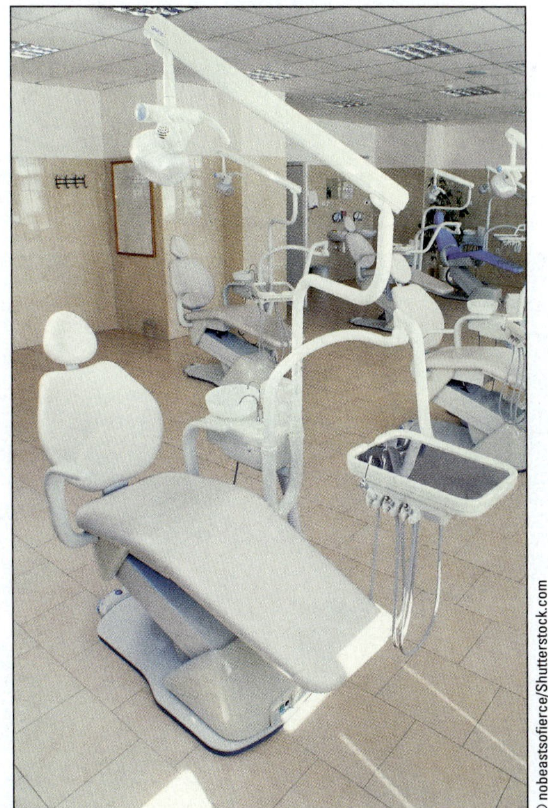

© nobeastsofierce/Shutterstock.com

FIGURE 17-11

Treatment rooms with the open concept.

The Dental Chair

The dental chair is the center of all clinical activity. The chair is designed for the operator and the assistant to provide patient treatment comfortably and efficiently. The dental chair supports the patient's entire body in either an **upright position** (back of chair is in a 90-degree angle, a **supine position** (reclined position with the nose and knees on the same plane) or a **subsupine position** (reclined position with the head lower than the feet) (refer to Figures 17-35A and B). The type of procedure, the dentist's preference, and the area of the mouth that is being treated determines the position of the chair. The upright position is used when seating and dismissing the patient, taking radiographs, and taking impressions. The supine position places the patient in a reclined position where the patient is almost laying out flat. Most dental procedures are performed with the patient in this position. It provides easy access to the different areas of the patient's mouth and the assistant can also see and have access while assisting the dentist. With the subsupine position the patient's head is lower than the feet. This position is used for emergency treatment and for the unconscious patient.

The dental chair is designed to accommodate children and adults. The head rest is narrow to allow the dentist and the assistant to be close to the patient's head and is adjustable to provide support. The dental chair has arm rests that are designed to lift or move out of the way when the patient is being seated or dismissed. It also has controls to move the chair up and down, recline the back rest, and raise the seat, and a combination button that automatically reclines or raises the patient. The controls are either on the sides of the chair back or on the floor (the floor controls are becoming more popular because they eliminate the need for infection control barriers) (Figures 17-12A and B).

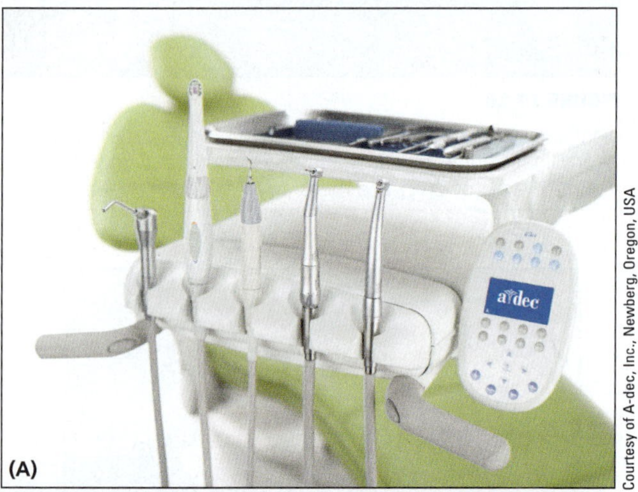

(A)

Courtesy of A-dec, Inc., Newberg, Oregon, USA

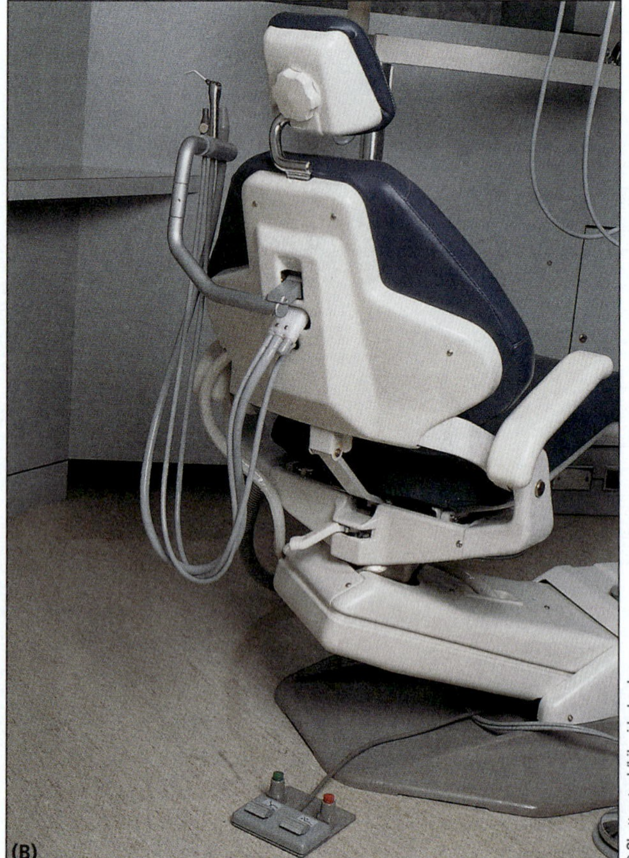
(B)

© Shutterstock/bikeriderlondon

FIGURE 17-12

(A) Digital controls for adjusting the dental chair position.
(B) Dental chair with foot controls for adjusting the chair.

The chair also has a control on the floor that allows it to be rotated left and right. To prevent cross-contamination, the head rest and controls on the chair are covered with barriers.

The dental chair is upholstered in a material that is comfortable, easy to clean, and coordinates with the office color theme. The base of the chair is sometimes secured to the floor. The chair base should be cleaned and disinfected routinely.

The Dental Unit

The **dental unit** consists of handpieces, an air-water syringe, a saliva ejector, an oral evacuator (HVE), an ultrasonic scaling unit, and numerous other options. The dental unit may be fixed to the wall, the cabinets, or on mobile carts. The unit is positioned according to the preference of the dentists, whether the dentists are left- or right-handed, whether they routinely work with assistants, and according to the design of the treatment room. The dental unit is available in three basic modes of delivery:

1. The **rear delivery system** is designed with the equipment behind the patient's head (Figure 17-13).
2. The **side delivery system** is designed with the equipment on the dentist's side. The unit is mounted to a moveable arm or mobile cart (Figure 17-14).
3. The **front delivery system** is designed so that it can be pulled over the patient's chest and is between the dentist and the assistant (Figure 17-15).

Mobile Carts. Sometimes, a **mobile cart** is used to hold delivery systems, including the air-water syringe, oral evacuator, handpieces, and saliva ejector (Figure 17-16). One cart may be used by both the operator and the dental assistant with the instrumentation on the appropriate side. Two carts, one on each side of the dental chair, may be equipped and used. The **operator's cart** is usually set up for two or three dental handpieces, rheostat, an air-water syringe, and sometimes a HVE and saliva ejector. The **assistant's cart** is usually set up with the air-water syringe, saliva ejector, and HVE. Carts are

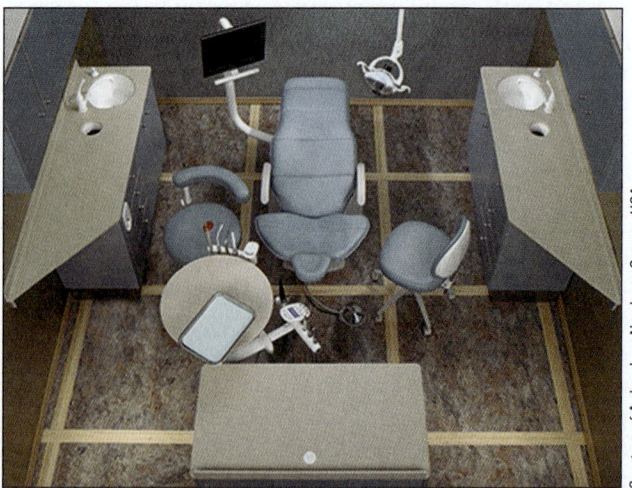

Courtesy of A-dec, Inc., Newberg, Oregon, USA

FIGURE 17-13

Rear delivery system.

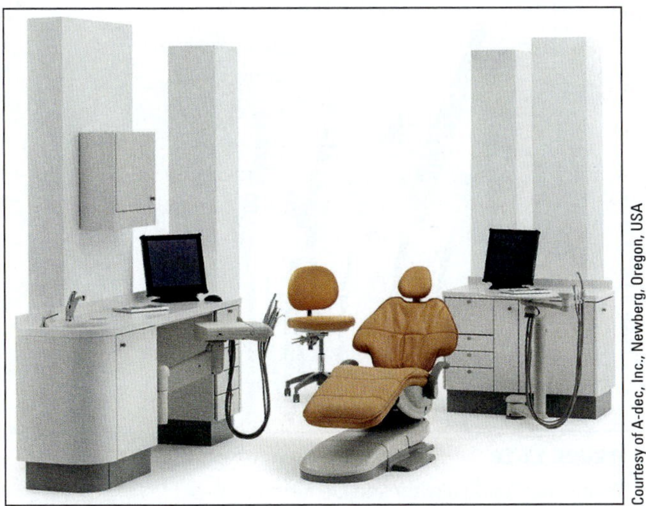
Courtesy of A-dec, Inc., Newberg, Oregon, USA

FIGURE 17-14
Side delivery system.

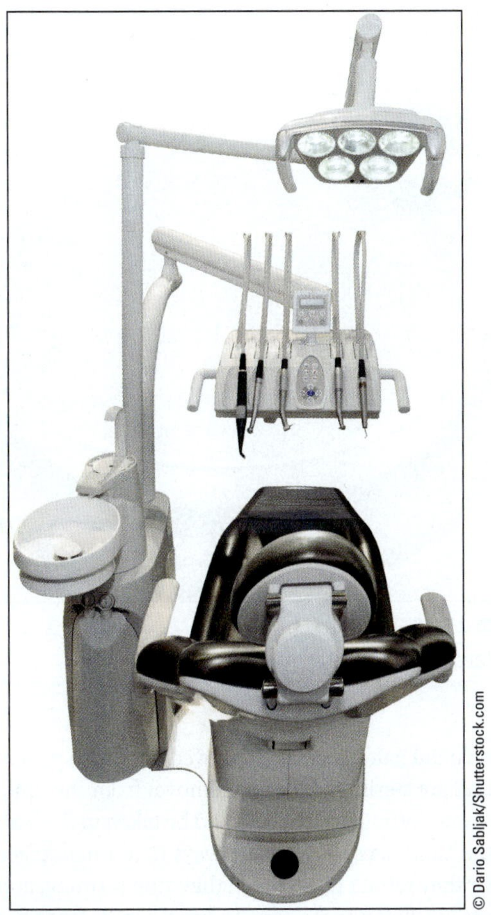
© Dario Sabljak/Shutterstock.com

FIGURE 17-15
Front delivery system.

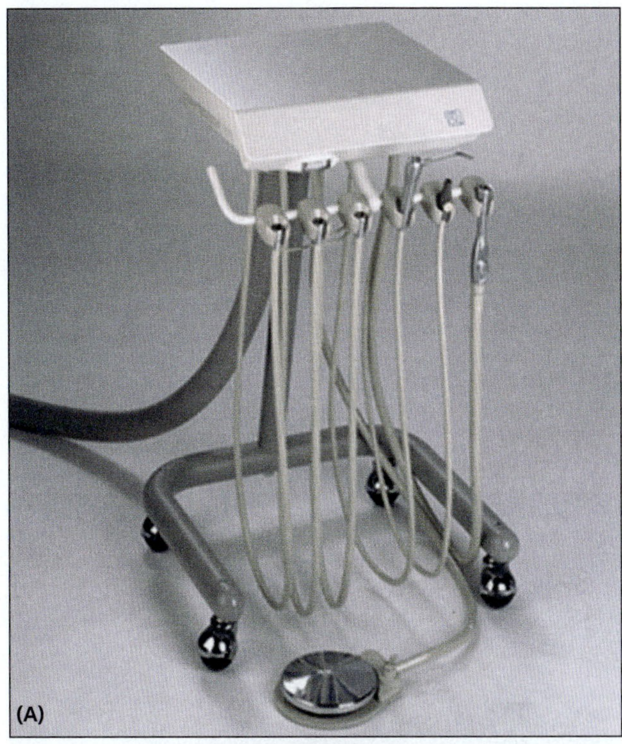
(A)

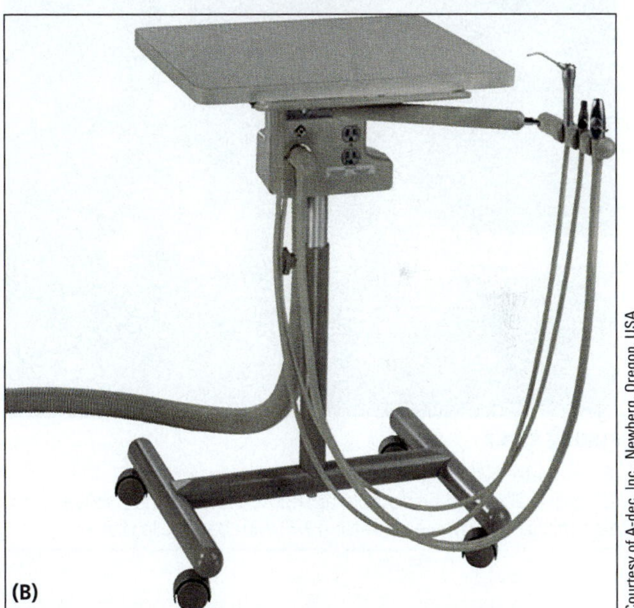
(B)
Courtesy of A-dec, Inc., Newberg, Oregon, USA

FIGURE 17-16
(A) Operator's cart with dental handpieces and air-water syringe. (B) Assistant's cart with saliva ejector, high volume evacuator (HVE), and air-water syringe.

designed to be moved easily, provide a work space and some storage, and hold basic instruments.

Air-Water Syringe. The **air-water syringe** provides air, water, or a combination spray of air and water (Figure 17-17A). The tip of the syringe is removable and made of disposable plastic or autoclavable metal. New barriers are placed on the syringe handle and the tubing for each patient (Figure 17-17B). The controls for the syringe are on the handle and should be easy to operate with the thumb of one hand. Air, water, and the combination spray help keep the oral cavity clean and dry and protect the tooth from the heat produced by the handpieces. For easier use, the syringe tips come in several lengths and are slightly angled. To reduce the risk of retaining oral fluids, flush

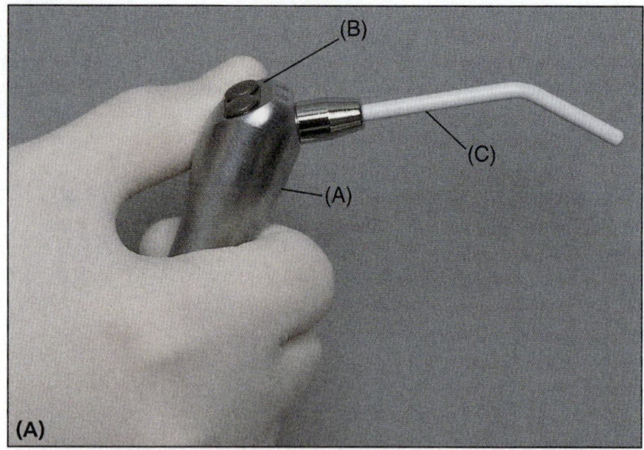

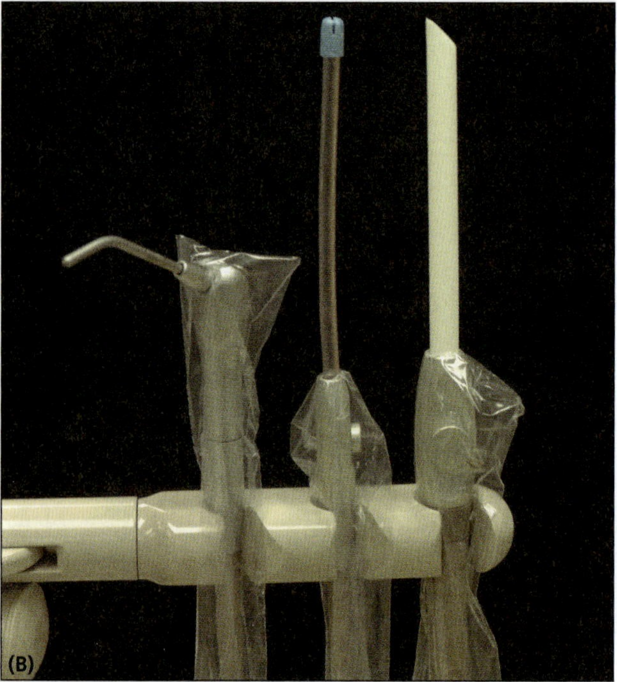

FIGURE 17-17

(A) Air-water syringe. (A) Handle. (B) Air-water controls. (C) Removable and disposable tip. (B) Air-water syringe, saliva ejector, high-volume evacuator (HVE) with barriers in place.

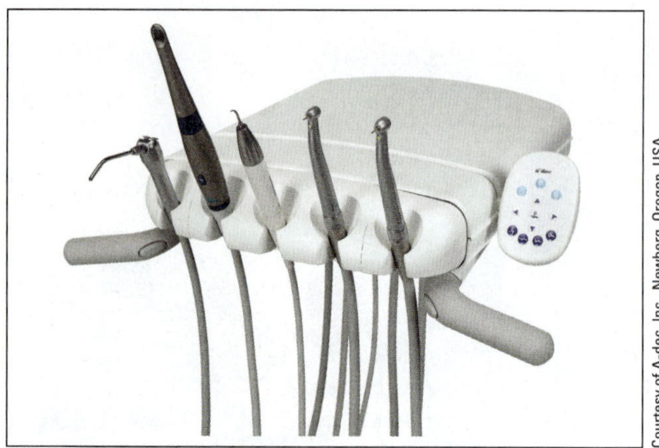

FIGURE 17-18

Dental unit: Saliva ejector and Dental handpieces.

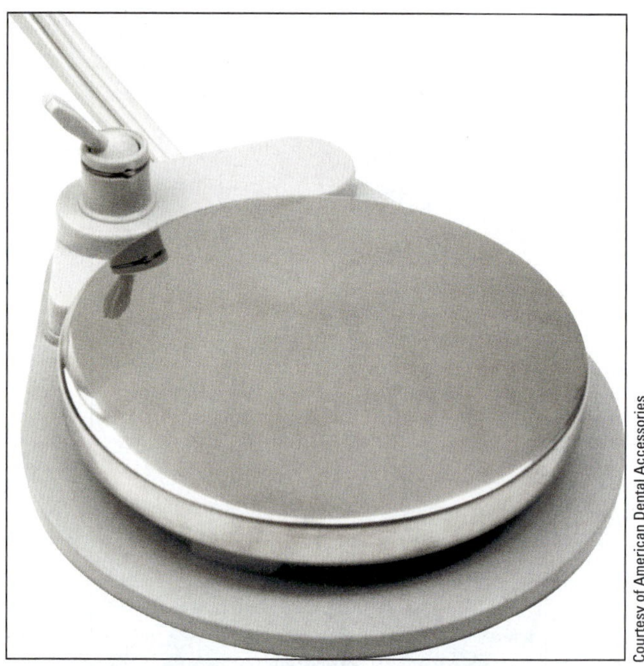

FIGURE 17-19

Rheostat showing water control switch.

the air-water syringe with water between patients and at the beginning and end of the day.

Dental Handpieces. There are usually two dental **handpieces**: low and high speed (Figure 17-18). The handpieces are attached to hoses that are part of the dental unit. It is important that these hoses are not bent or tangled. Each handpiece has two controls. First, the hose attachment on the dental unit has a control switch to prevent more than one handpiece from running at once. Second, the speed of the handpiece is controlled by a foot pedal called a **rheostat** (REE-oh-stat) (Figure 17-19). The rheostat is the round disk as seen on the floor in Figures 17-15 and 17-16A. There is also a switch on the rheostat that controls the water flow to the handpiece. The rheostat is used with both high- and low-speed handpieces.

The dental handpieces are removed after each patient's treatment and are sterilized. (Before removal from the unit, as with the air-water syringe, caution should be taken to flush oral fluids from the handpieces.) There are ways to test handpieces to see whether they retract fluids when they stop running, and manufacturers are designing means to prevent this from occurring. At the beginning and end of the day, the handpiece should be flushed for several minutes. Between patients, run the handpieces for at least one minute to flush the system. Some dental manufacturers provide a self-contained water system. Each unit has a water reservoir that supplies water for the dental handpieces and the air-water syringes. The **water reservoir** is maintained daily. Distilled water is often used to prevent tap-water deposits from building up in the water lines. (Refer to Dental Water lines discussed in Chapter 11, Infection Control.)

Ultrasonic Scaler. The **ultrasonic scaler** is attached to the dental unit. The scaler is used during prophylaxis and periodontal procedures. Small tips attach to the ultrasonic scaler. The scaler has a vibrating action that removes hard deposits, such as calculus, and other debris from the teeth. (The Ultrasonic Scaler is also discussed in Chapter 31, Periodontics).

Saliva Ejector. The **saliva ejector** is used to remove saliva and fluids from the patient's mouth slowly. It has a low-volume suction that is used during certain procedures, such as fluoride treatments and under rubber dams. The saliva ejector tip is a thin, flexible, plastic tube that is disposed of after each patient's treatment (Figure 17-20). This plastic tip slides into the opening of the saliva ejector hose that is part of the dental unit. There is a small trap in the saliva ejector that must be cleaned routinely.

High-Volume Evacuation (HVE). The **high-volume evacuator (HVE)** is also called the oral evacuator (Figure 17-21). It is used by the assistant to remove fluids from the patient's mouth. Evacuation tips are wider tubes that are often beveled at both ends. Some of the tips are metal and can be sterilized, but most offices use plastic tips that can be sterilized or disposed of. The evacuation tips fit into the handle of the hose, which is covered with a protective barrier during procedures. The on/off control for the HVE is on the handle. Each unit has a trap that collects debris from the evacuator (Figure 17-22). This trap must be changed or cleaned weekly or as needed. The HVE is flushed after each patient and there are cleaning systems available to flush and to do a thorough cleaning of the HVE at the end of the day and week.

Dental Stools

Dental stools are required by the operator and the assistant during most procedures. Ergonomic studies have resulted in the improved design of dental stools to provide comfort and

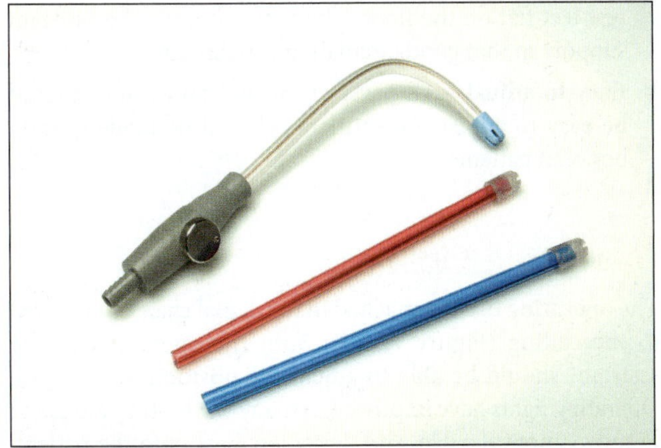

FIGURE 17-20
Saliva ejector hose with saliva ejector tips.

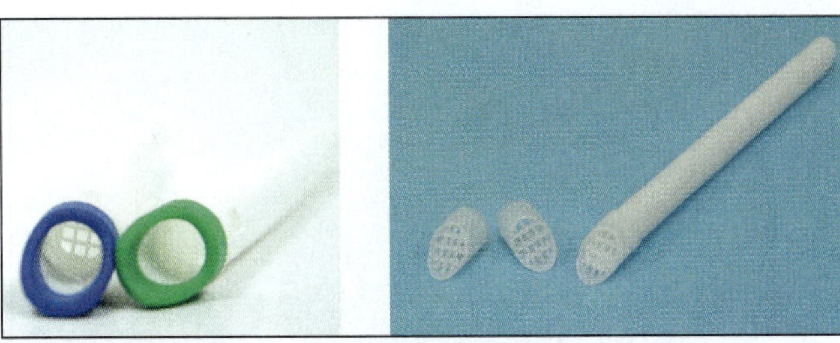

FIGURE 17-21
Evacuator (HVE) tips.

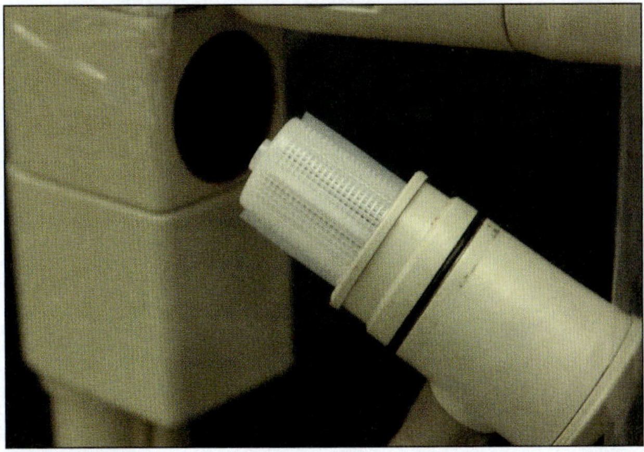

FIGURE 17-22
High-volume evacuator disposable trap.

prevent fatigue during dental procedures. When selecting stools, the dentist and staff should try a variety of stools to find the one that meets their requirements, provides good support, and is comfortable. There is more information on ergonomics and the dental team later in this chapter. The operator's and assistant's stools have some similarities but also have several differences (Figures 17-23 and 17-24).

Operator's Stool. The operator's stool has the following ergonomic characteristics:

- **Adjustable height**—The stool should have adjustment for height so that the operator's feet can be flat on the floor and the thighs can be parallel to the floor when seated.
- **Adjustable back rest**—The stool should have a back rest that is adjustable, both vertically and horizontally, to provide support and comfort. The back rest should support the **lumbar** region (lower region of the back) of the operator's back.
- **Comfortable seat**—The stool seat should be broad with firm padding and have no seams or edges to restrict circulation in the legs and feet. The seat also should be covered with a material that is easy to clean.
- **Mobility**—The stool should move easily and freely on four to five casters, even on floors with carpet.
- **Broad base**—The stool should have a broad, heavy base to prevent tipping, especially during movement. The base stabilizes the stool for the operator.

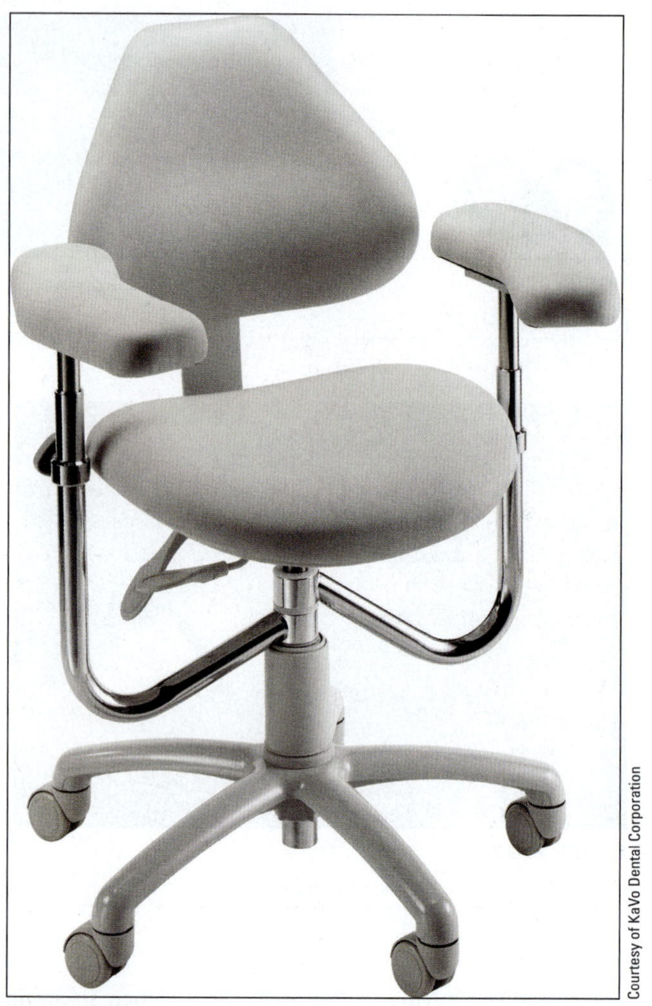

FIGURE 17-23

Operator's stool with back support, broad base, comfortable seat, and casters.

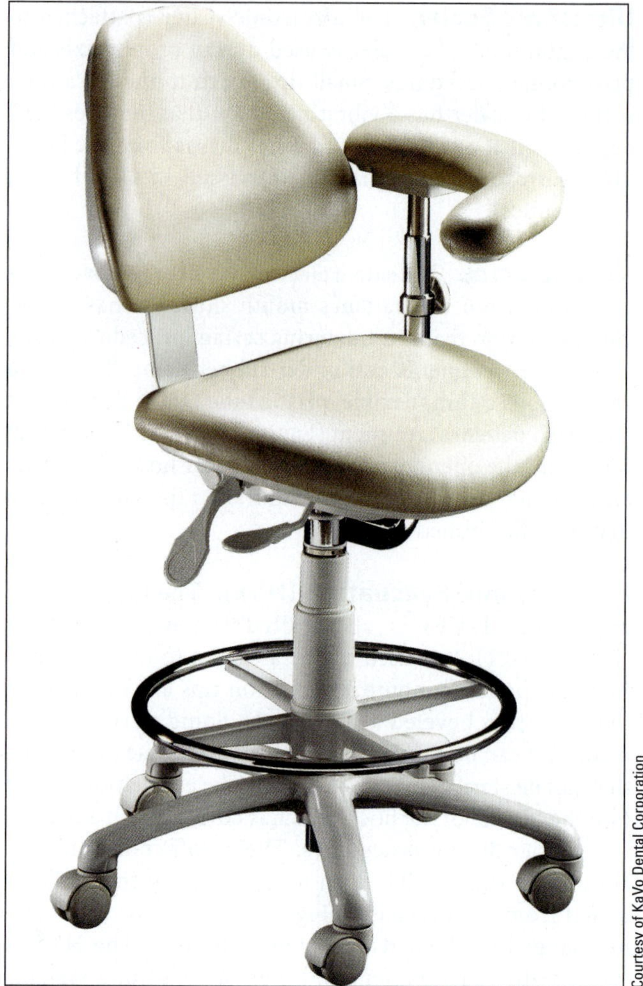

FIGURE 17-24

Assistant's stool with front arm support, comfortable seat, broad base, foot rest, and casters.

Dental Assistant's Stool. The dental assistant's stool has the following ergonomic characteristics:

- **Adjustable height**—The stool should adjust to a variety of different levels to accommodate the height of the assistant. The assistant is positioned 4 to 8 inches higher than the operator, with feet resting on the foot ring and thighs parallel to the floor.
- **Adjustable back rest/extended arm**—The stool back rest should provide support for the lumbar region and be easily adjustable. Some stools have an extended arm for support of the abdomen or side areas. The arm moves easily into place and locks to stabilize the assistant when leaning or reaching.
- **Comfortable seat**—The seat of the stool has the same criteria as the operator's stool: a broad, flat surface with no seams or hard edges.
- **Mobility**—The assistant's chair should be designed to move freely. Usually, five casters are recommended to provide stability.
- **Broad base**—The base of the stool should be broad and well balanced. It should be heavy and stable to prevent tipping.
- **Foot rest**—The assistant is usually positioned higher than the operator, so it is difficult to sit correctly on the stool and rest feet flat on the floor. The foot rest gives the assistant support so that good circulation is maintained.
- **Easy to adjust**—All parts of the assistant's stool should be easy to adjust. Adjustments should be made quickly between patients.

Operating Light

The **operating light** is attached to the dental chair or mounted to the ceiling (Figure 17-25). Both the operator and the assistant should be able to adjust the position of the light. Operating lights have improved in many ways—they are easier to move, more flexible, and direct less heat onto the patient. The light has a control switch for high and low intensities, an

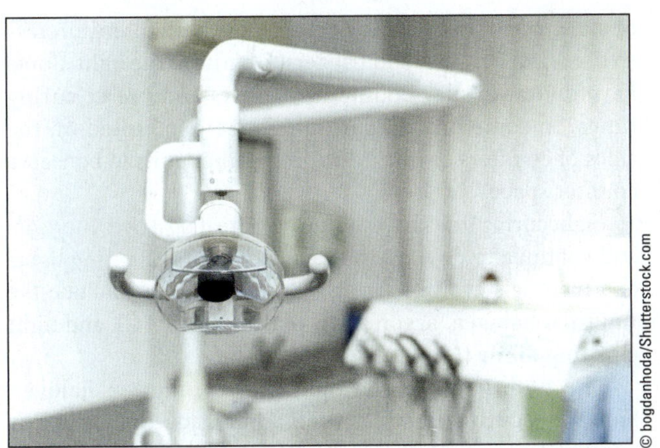

FIGURE 17-25
Dental operating light that would be attached to the dental chair.

on/off switch, and handles on both sides. The light is attached to extension arms for positioning over the patient's face to view the maxillary or mandibular arch.

The handles and on/off switch are covered with barriers during procedures. The barriers are changed between each patient. Maintenance includes changing the lightbulb occasionally and keeping the heat shield clean. It is important to follow the manufacturer's instructions for both of these procedures.

Always allow the lightbulb and the shield to cool before cleaning or changing the bulb. If a halogen bulb is used it should never be directly touched so the dental assistant should wear gloves or use a tissue when handling.

Cabinetry

Most treatment rooms have some type of cabinetry for storage of supplies and materials used during treatment. Some dental units are designed in fixed cabinets that surround the patient, operator, and assistant. These units include cupboards that open from the front and the back for treatment trays, drawers for materials frequently used, and sinks for the operator and the assistant (see Figures 17-13 and 17-14). The amount of cabinetry depends on the size of the room and the dentist's preference.

Mobile cabinets are also used in the treatment room. These cabinets come in a variety of designs and are used for storage and as work spaces. The mobile cabinet is stored against the wall and then pulled into position after the patient is seated.

Sink

The treatment room should be designed with sinks in convenient locations for the dentist and the assistants. Some treatment rooms have two sinks, one on each side of the dental chair. Other treatment rooms have one sink that is located centrally behind the dental unit for both the dentist and assistant to use.

The water controls on the sink should be operated by wrist, foot, or knee controls (this prevents the hands from becoming contaminated after hand washing by turning off the water controls). There are light and motion sensor devices that turn the water on and off automatically when standing in front of the sink.

The sinks should be easy to clean and have an area nearby for soap and towel dispensers.

Dental X-Ray Unit

A dental x-ray unit used to expose intraoral radiographs is part of most treatment rooms. Sometimes the x-ray tubehead is housed between two rooms with doors on both sides for the x-ray tubehead to slide out into either room. The controls are found outside the room so that the dental assistant is not exposed to radiation. (Further information about the x-ray unit can be found in Chapter 21, Introduction to Dental Radiography and Equipment.) The panoramic machine for exposing extraoral radiographs is usually in a separate area outside the treatment room.

Small Equipment Found in the Treatment Room

There may be a variety of small equipment in the treatment room depending on the primary use of the room. Most rooms have an x-ray viewbox, a curing light, an amalgamator, a communication system, a computerized intraoral dental camera, and (typically) a computer linked to the office local area network.

X-Ray Viewbox. The x-ray viewbox is used to read traditional radiographs (Figure 17-26). The viewbox may be placed on a counter or in a wall or cabinet. It consists of a bright light source covered with a frosted surface. X-rays are placed on the frosted surface for clear viewing.

Dental Curing Light. A dental **curing light** is used to "cure" or "set" light-cured materials (Figure 17-27A). Many

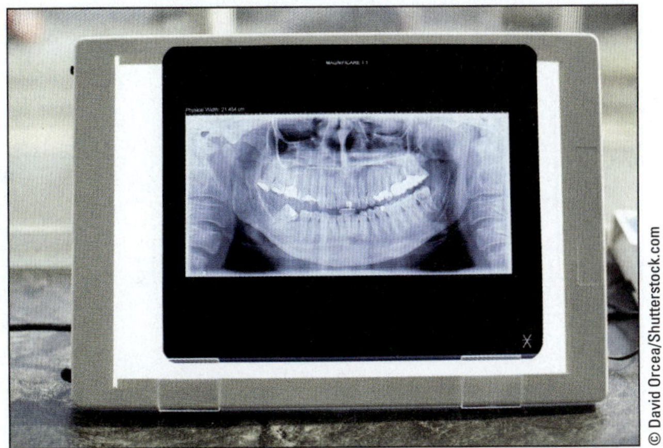

FIGURE 17-26
X-ray viewbox.

dental products are now light cured. There are various types of curing lights dentists may choose from depending on the types of materials they use and their preferences. Dentists evaluate the characteristics of curing lights needed according to the intensity and spectrum of the light, the speed of the cure, the heat that is generated, and whether they are lightweight and ergonomic in design, quiet, portable, durable, and reliable. Most curing lights have small motors or sometimes fans, wands, or tips; some have filters, protective shields, handles, and triggers to activate the light. Some have digital display countdown timers and preset curing times. In some offices, curing lights are mounted on the sides of counters or integrated into dental units to conserve counter space.

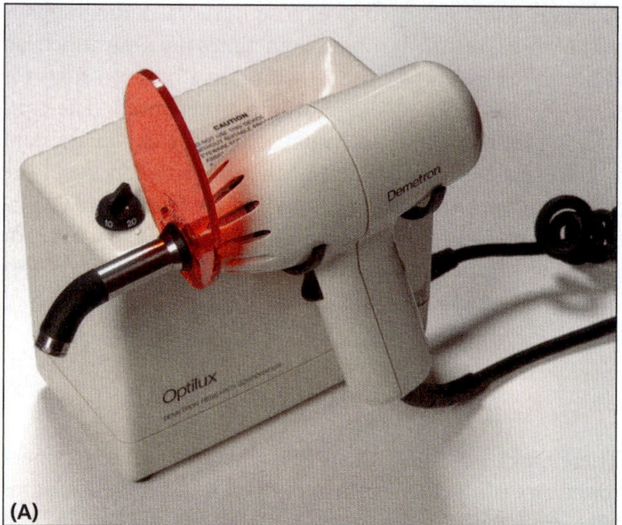

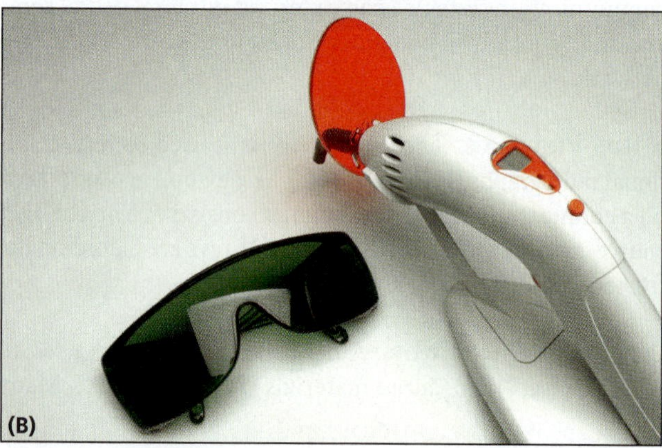

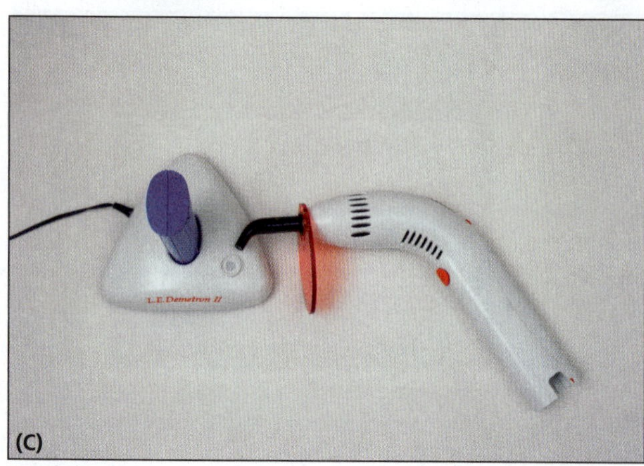

FIGURE 17-27

(A) Halogen curing light. (B) LED curing light. (C) Curing light with radiometer.

Light curing units have advanced a great deal over the years and continue to do so as the technology for the curing lights and materials evolve. Curing light technologies include the **tungsten halogen**, **argon laser**, **plasma arc (PAC)**, and **light emitting diode (LED)**.

The traditional curing light uses a tungsten halogen bulb. This curing light has been around for a while and is durable, less expensive, cures relatively quickly, and is fairly effective. It does give off some heat, uses a filter to remove useless energy emitted by the halogen bulb, and the unit is not portable.

The halogen curing lights do have a fan to cool the unit; thus it is important to remember not to turn off the unit until the fan has stopped. Light intensities can vary and change with use. To determine if the light is working at full capacity, the curing light should be tested monthly.

The argon laser (light amplification by stimulated emission of radiation) technology produces a relatively high-intensity light that does not generate noticeable heat. The speed of curing ranges from moderate to fast. The argon laser lights are not compatible with some dental materials. The laser light will not cure some materials due to the type of photo-initiator used in the materials. The argon laser curing lights are much more expensive than other types of curing lights. (*Note:* The photo-initiator is the substance added to a dental material that reacts to light and acts as a catalyst to initiate the setting [polymerization] process.)

The ultrafast and powerful PAC curing lights are more expensive. Some are large units that are not portable. Because these lights produce significant amounts of light that are not useful in the curing process, many of the PAC lights offer multiple setting tips that are filtered. The light tips filter the light to match that of the photo-initiator in the dental material. The PAC units produce a high level of heat that is a concern in some cases.

The LED curing lights are lightweight; some are ergonomically designed and have cordless portability. Some curing lights are mounted on the sides of counters or integrated into the dental unit to conserve counter space. These units are durable, produce minimal heat, have no bulbs, and are quiet because there is no need for a fan. This technology is rapidly changing to improve light performance (Figure 17-27B).

It is not as important to check the corded LED light units with a radiometer as it is with the halogen lights. But the cordless LEDs that are battery powered need to be checked according to the manufacturer's recommendations. The batteries wear down and the light output decreases. Some curing light units now have light meters built in, so the light can be tested more conveniently (Figure 17-27C).

The LED lights are still changing and improving. These lights are so convenient that more and more dental offices are purchasing them. As with all the other curing lights there are pros and cons, so before an office purchases a new light it should check the manufacturer for the procedures that the lights are most effective with.

Curing light technology is rapidly changing to improve curing intensities and speed. Materials manufacturers are evaluating their photo-initiator systems. One initiator for photo-curable dental materials being reevaluated is Camphorquinone (CPQ). This photo-initiator system works with a variety of curing lights.

If light guides come in contact with any materials during the curing process, immediately wipe them off; alternatively, the dental assistant can place a sleeve cover over the light guide to protect it or use some acetone to remove any residue that may have formed on the end of the guide.

Curing Light Radiometer. Curing lights should be tested periodically with a **radiometer (light meter)** because the light bulbs will deteriorate over time and not produce an adequate cure. Small handheld meters are available to test the halogen curing lights (Figure 17-28). The light guide is positioned over a small area on the meter and then turned on. A reading is given to determine the intensity of the light and the need to replace the bulb.

Amalgamator. The **amalgamator** is a small machine that mixes (**triturates**) dental amalgam and some dental cements. It is placed near the assistant, either on the counter or in a drawer (Figure 17-29). (The amalgamator is discussed further in Chapter 38, Restorative Materials and Matrix and Wedge.)

Communication System. The communication system is a color-coded light system or intercom system the office uses as a method for the staff and the dentist to communicate with each other. Usually, the system is found on the walls in the treatment rooms, sterilization area, laboratory, and staff lounge. It is made of a series of colored buttons that light up when pushed or an intercom/phone system. The system can designate a specific message or call a member of the dental team. For example, the hygienist lets the dentist know the patient is ready for examination or the receptionist tells everyone that the next patient has arrived. These systems can be customized for the individual needs of an office.

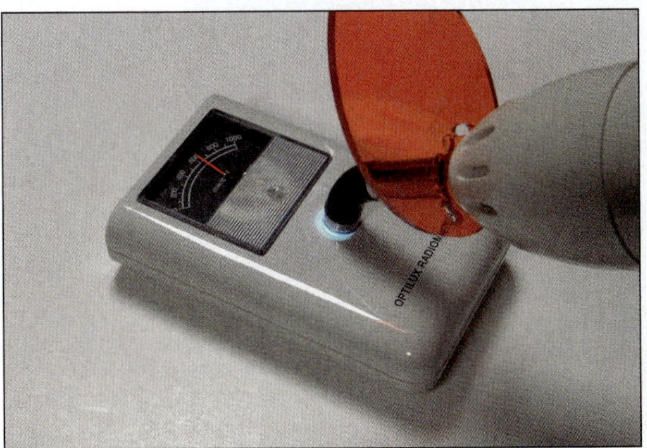

FIGURE 17-28
Halogen curing light being tested for accuracy with a radiometer.

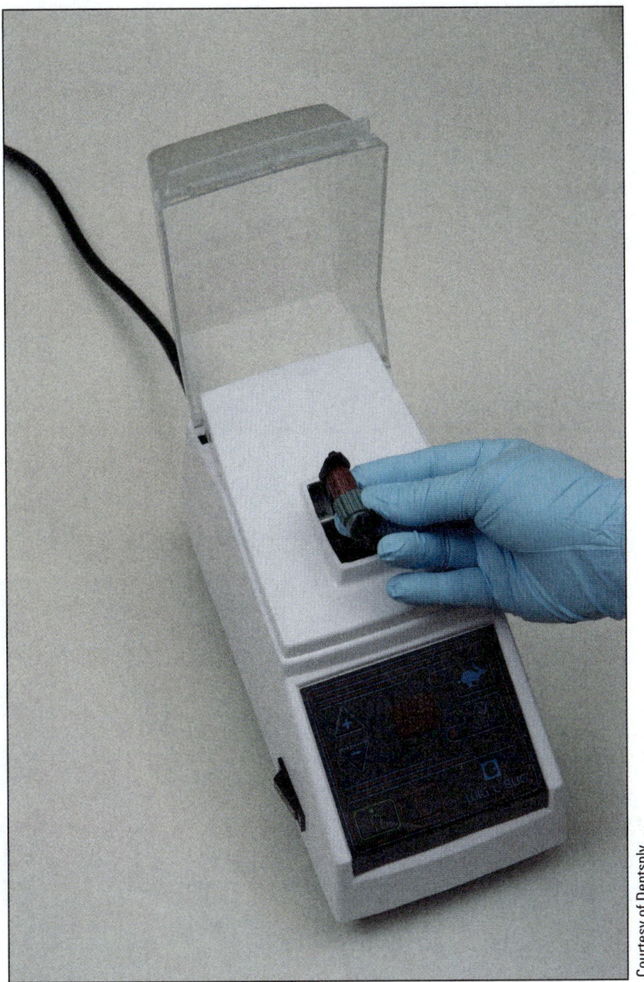

Courtesy of Dentsply

FIGURE 17-29
Dental amalgamator with digital controls.

The **hands-free communication systems** are rapidly gaining popularity. With these systems a hands-free ear piece is used by the dental team. There are many types of systems with features that work in smaller dental offices with a few staff members as well as features that work in large dental clinics. (Figure 17-30).

These systems allow the office staff to directly contact and communicate with one another using headsets that are linked over a wireless local area network. Some of the characteristics of these systems are that they are lightweight and can be easily worn by the user. Systems allow users to make outgoing calls, pick up incoming calls, and communicate with other staff members. They are also great for maintaining privacy and prevent cross-contamination since there is no need to push buttons on the colored light systems. Offices have found that with the hands-free communication system there is faster and immediate communication among the whole dental team, so they can provide superior service to the patients.

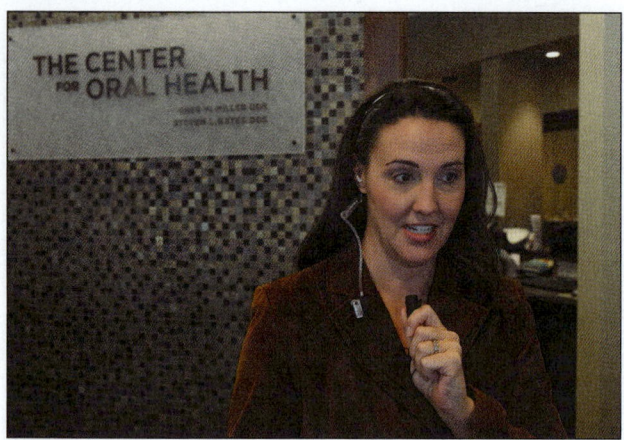

FIGURE 17-30

Business Assistant using headset for a hands free communication system.

Computerized Equipment. Computerized equipment includes an **intraoral camera** and a computer terminal. The intraoral wand contains a small camera that transmits to the computer monitor (Figure 17-31). The wand is placed in the patient's mouth, and the image is displayed on the monitor. The computer freezes a picture on the screen or prints it out. The intraoral camera allows the patient to see areas and conditions in their mouth while the dentist is discussing them.

Many offices are computerized with terminals in the treatment rooms as well as the business office. Computer systems allow the office to be "paperless" and to be more efficient at completing specific tasks, such as billing. Some systems allow the dentist and staff to enter treatment plans, chart the condition of the patient's mouth, make the patient's next appointment, bill the insurance company, and give information and instructions. The number of

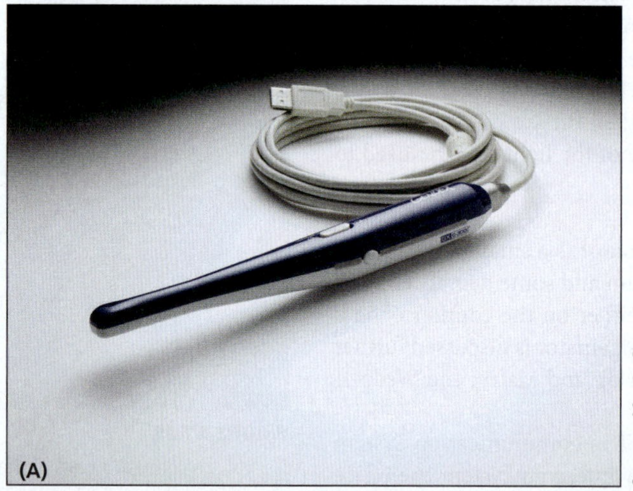

Courtesy of Gendex Dental Systems

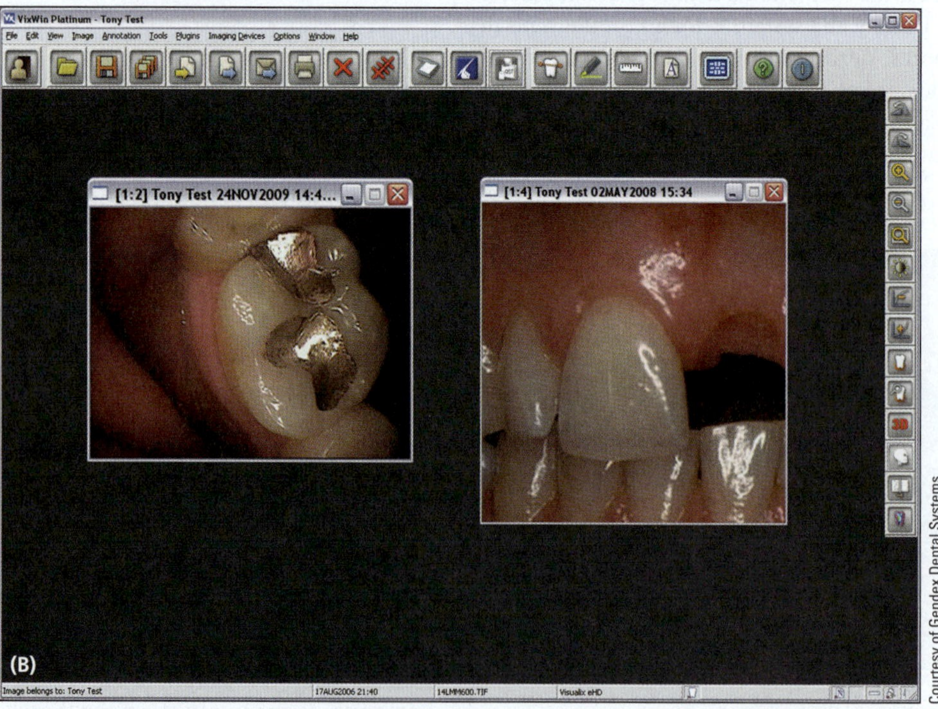

Courtesy of Gendex Dental Systems

FIGURE 17-31

(A) Intraoral camera. (B) Pictures inside the oral cavity using the intraoral camera.

computers and the programs/systems used in the office are determined by the dentist. To use the computers efficiently and effectively, additional training and cooperation of all staff members are required.

Digital radiography equipment is also part of the technology found in the dental office. (Digital radiography equipment is discussed in Chapter 23, Extraoral and Digital Radiography.)

Dental Air Compressor and Central Vacuum System

The **air compressor** provides compressed air for the handpieces and air for the air-water syringes. The size of the air compressor depends on the number of dental units used by the office. Usually, the compressor is stored away from the main office because of its size and noise level. Ongoing maintenance for the air compressor is critical. It is important that the filters be changed routinely and the compressor be checked for **condensation** in the lines. If condensation occurs, the line may have particles, moisture, and algae. These contaminants may work their way into the dental handpieces and the oral cavity. If condensation is apparent, call for dental service to correct the problem.

The **central vacuum system** provides suction for saliva ejectors and oral evacuators at each dental unit. The filters or traps must be cleaned regularly to keep this system working to capacity. This system is also stored away from the main office.

Dental office staff and dental service companies must follow manufacturer instructions for maintenance and repairs on the air compressor and the vacuum system. Both units may be set up on time clocks to run only when the office is open and operating.

Routine Office Care

With the amount of equipment being operated in the dental office, a routine schedule needs to be in place to ensure proper maintenance control. Often this responsibility is given to the dental assistants. Usually, the office is cleaned professionally, but the assistant should periodically check the overall appearance of the office.

Daily, weekly, or monthly maintenance tasks might include changing x-ray processing solutions, cleaning the inside of the sterilizers, changing ultrasonic solutions, performing monitoring activities to check the effectiveness of the sterilizers, and making miscellaneous repairs. It is necessary to keep replacement parts on hand for equipment that needs routine care (e.g., the O-rings in the air-water syringe, which must be changed when air or water leaks).

Opening and Closing the Dental Office

The daily routine of opening and closing the dental office usually falls to the dental assistants. These tasks are sometimes divided, with one assistant opening the office and the other closing the office. If there are numerous staff members these responsibilities are often divided by the week or month.

Whoever is responsible to open the office in the morning usually arrives 30 to 45 minutes early and completes the routine (Procedure 17-1) before the other staff members arrive.

To close the office, the responsible person stays after the last patient and makes sure that everything is turned off and the office is ready for patients the next day (Procedure 17-2).

Procedure 17-1
Daily Routine to Open the Office

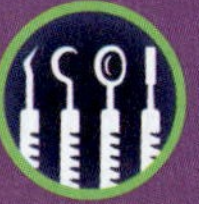

These tasks are done by the assistant each morning. The assistant arrives at the office early to open the office and prepare for the day's schedule.

Procedure Steps

1. Turn on master switches to lights, each dental unit, the vacuum system, and the air compressor.
2. Check the reception room, turn on lights, straighten the magazines and the children's area, and unlock the patients' door to the office.
3. Turn on the communication system, check the answering machine or the answering system, start the computers, unlock the files, and organize the business area.
4. Post copies of patient schedules in designated areas throughout the office according to HIPAA regulations.
5. Turn on all equipment in the x-ray processing area. Change the water in the processing tanks and replenish solutions, if necessary.
6. Change into appropriate clinical clothing, following OSHA guidelines.
7. Review the daily patient schedule.
8. Prepare treatment rooms for the first patients. Check supplies, place barriers, fill water reservoirs, and review patient records. Then, prepare the appropriate trays and lab work for the first patients.
9. Turn on any sterilizing equipment and check solution levels. Prepare new ultrasonic and disinfection solutions. Complete overnight sterilization procedures.
10. Replenish supplies needed for the day.

Procedure 17-2
Daily Routine to Close the Office

These tasks are done by the assistant at the end of the day. The office evening routine includes closing the office for the evening and preparing for the next day. As with the opening routine, the assistants usually share the responsibility of closing the office. Each office has specific details, but the following are general tasks.

Procedure Steps

1. Clean the treatment rooms. This may include an in-depth cleaning of the dental chair and dental unit. Flush the handpieces and air-water syringes, run solutions through the evacuation hoses, clean traps/filters, and maintain water reservoirs.
2. Position the dental chair for evening housekeeping.
3. Turn off all master switches.
4. Process, mount, and file x-rays. Follow the manufacturer's instructions to shut down automatic processors. Turn off water supply to manual processing tanks.
5. Wipe counters and turn off the safe light.
6. Sterilize all instruments and set up trays for the next day. Empty ultrasonic solutions and turn off all equipment. Restock supplies.
7. Make sure all laboratory cases have been sent to the lab and early-morning cases have been received from the lab.
8. Confirm and complete appointment schedule for the next day, insurance forms, and daily bookkeeping responsibilities. Pull charts for the next day or review patient information on computer.
9. Turn off business office equipment and turn on the answering machine or service. Lock patient and business office files.
10. Straighten the reception room. For the security of the office, all doors and windows should be locked.
11. Change from uniform to street clothes, following OSHA guidelines.
12. Turn off machines in the staff lounge and clean tables and counters.

Concepts of Dental Assisting

Originally, the dentist and the dental assistant worked standing on either side of the dental chair. Although some dentists still may stand occasionally, both the dentist and assistant now sit during procedures most of the time. Many studies and research in ergonomics found that sit-down dentistry was the best for both the dentist and the assistant, creating less strain and increasing efficiency. When the dentist and assistant are working at the dental chair together, it is called **four-handed dentistry**. The assistant assists the dentist throughout the entire procedure, passing instruments, mixing materials, and watching the patient. Sometimes, an additional assistant is needed to bring items to the treatment room, assist the assistant in mixing materials, or help with a patient. This is called **six-handed dentistry**. Four- and six-handed dentistry have proven to be efficient and effective in providing patients with quality care.

Activity Zones

When the dentist and the assistant are positioning themselves around the patient, the following are vital:

- Good visibility of the patient's mouth
- Easy access to all areas of the patient's mouth
- Easy access to dental equipment, instruments, and materials
- Safety and comfort for the patient, the operator, and the assistant

The area around the patient's mouth is divided into four **activity zones: operating zone, assisting zone, static zone,** and **transfer zone**. These activity zones are determined by visualizing the patient's head as the center of a clock (Figures 17-32 and 17-33).

The operating zone is the area where the operator is positioned to access the oral cavity and have the best visibility. For right-handed operators, this area extends from the 7 to 12 o'clock position. For left-handed operators, this area extends from the 12 to 5 o'clock position. The operator moves within the zone depending on which arch, quadrant, or surface of the patient's teeth the operator is working on.

The assisting zone is the area in which the assistant is positioned to easily assist the dentist and access instruments, evacuator, and dental unit or cart without interference. The assistant's zone for a right-handed operator is 2 to 4 o'clock and for a left-handed operator 8 to 10 o'clock.

The static zone extends from 12 to 2 o'clock for a right-handed operator and from 10 to 12 o'clock for a left-handed operator. Rear delivery systems are found in the static zone, along with dental instruments and equipment used at the chair.

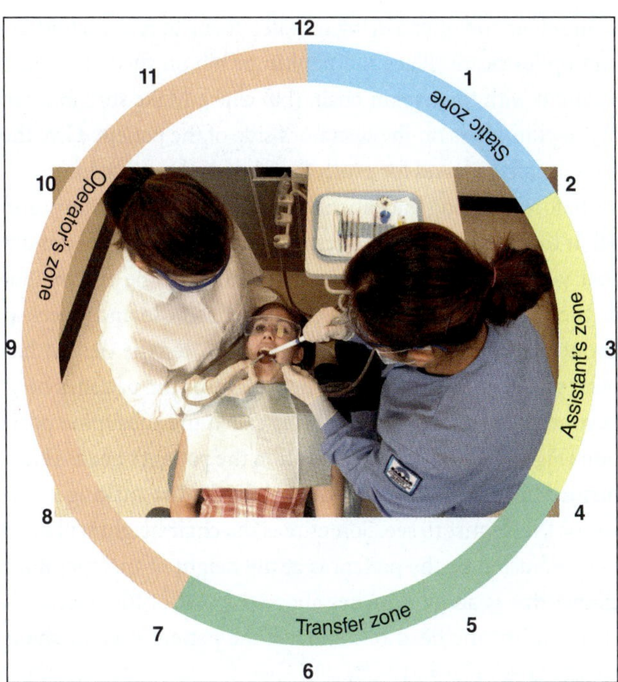

FIGURE 17-32

Activity zones for a right-handed operator, with the assistant on the left.

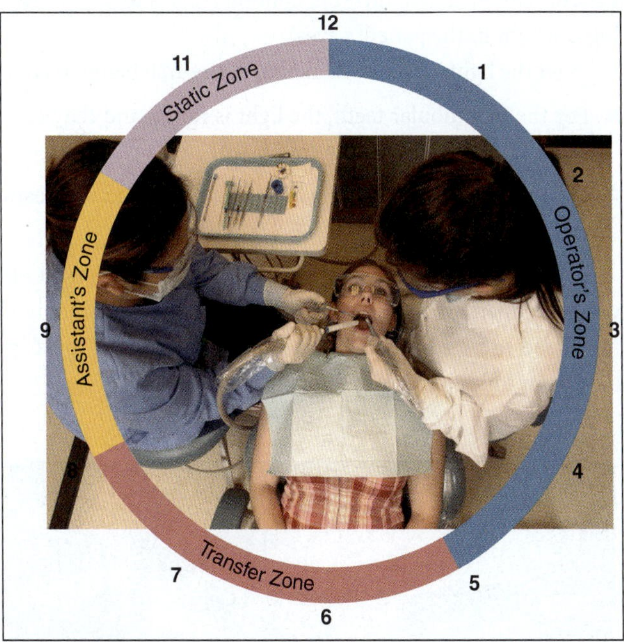

FIGURE 17-33

Activity zones for a left-handed operator, with the assistant on the right.

The transfer zone is the area below the patient's nose where instruments and materials are passed and received. Usually, the operator and the assistant transfer instruments between the area that is below the patient's nose and above the upper chest. To follow the clock concept, this would be between 4 and 7 o'clock for a right-handed operator and 5 and 8 o'clock for a left-handed operator.

Classifications of Motion

There are five **classifications of motion** to describe the dental team's range of motion:

1. **Class I motion** involves only finger movement. An example of Class I motion is picking up an instrument from the tray.
2. **Class II motion** involves movement of the fingers and wrist. An example of Class II motion is mixing dental cement on the tray.
3. **Class III motion** involves finger, wrist, and elbow movement. An example of Class III motion is transferring an instrument to an operator or removing excess cement from a crown seated in the patient's mouth.
4. **Class IV motion** involves movement of the entire arm and shoulder. An example of Class IV motion is taking dental radiographs or taking dental impressions.
5. **Class V motion** involves movement of the arm and twisting of the body. An example of Class V motion retrieving instruments and miscellaneous items from counter near the dental assistant or adjusting the dental light.

Ideally, for proper ergonomics the operator and the assistant should be positioned to stay in class I, II, and III motion ranges. The dental unit, counter space, instruments, and equipment should all be close enough to avoid class IV and V motions for the majority of dental treatment.

Preparing the Treatment Room

The dental assistant prepares the treatment room for each patient. The room is cleaned and disinfected after each patient, and new barriers are placed on the dental unit, dental chair, counters, and dental light switches (see Chapter 11, Infection Control). After all the barriers are placed, the room is tidied so that no obstacles are in the patient's path upon entering the treatment room. The rheostat is placed behind the dental chair, and the operator and dental assistant's chairs are moved out of the way. Mobile carts are pulled out of the patient's path, and the dental light is raised out of the patient's way as he or she sits in the chair. The arm of the dental chair is raised or turned for easy access for the patient. The dental chair is positioned about 15 to 18 inches from the floor, and the chair is tilted back slightly.

Patient records are reviewed to double-check the procedures to be done, and the medical/dental history for each patient is examined for any previous problems or alerts. The x-rays are placed on the viewbox, and the charts/records are located away from the treatment area or covered with a barrier. If the office is computerized, the dental assistant should open the patient's file to have the information, chart, and x-rays ready for the dentist. Any model or lab work is brought into the treatment room. The tray is set up, and accessory items for specific procedures are prepared.

Seating the Dental Patient

One of the important roles the dental assistant plays is to put the patient at ease and to begin to establish a rapport with the patient. This begins when the dental assistant seats the patient in preparation for treatment.

Greet and Escort the Patient

Greet the patient by stepping into the reception area and identifying him or her by name. Then, tell the patient that you are ready for him or her now. If you have not met the patient before, introduce yourself, and, before leaving the reception area, ask the patient if he or she wants to hang up his or her coat. Then, ask the patient to follow you into the treatment room.

When escorting the patient back to the treatment room, it is a good idea to identify the room by number, color, or location. Make sure that all obstacles are out of the way, and offer assistance if the patient appears to need it. For example, patients who have trouble getting up out of chairs or patients who walk with canes or walkers may need assistance.

Once in the treatment room, as a courtesy to the patient and for infection control, ask the patient if he or she would like to rinse his or her mouth with mouthwash before he or she sits down. Then, offer to store any personal items, such as a purse or briefcase, on a counter or shelf. These items should be placed where they are in the patient's view but not interfering with the treatment.

It is important to establish rapport with the patients and make them feel welcome and at ease. Remember to talk to the patients and show an interest in what they have to say. Ask them about subjects they are involved with and are comfortable discussing. People like to talk about themselves, their families, work, vacations, and hobbies. Note points of interest on the treatment chart so continued reference can be made. Often, patients will ask questions about dental concerns. General information can be given by the dental assistant. The dentist can answer specifically when he or she comes into the treatment room. Communication with patients begins when they walk into the office and should continue until they leave.

Seat and Prepare the Patient

Ask the patient to be seated in the dental chair. The patient's back should be against the back rest and his or her legs completely supported. Once the patient is in the chair, lower the arm of the chair and offer a drink of water, tissue to remove lipstick, and lip lubricant. Place the **napkin** or bib on the patient and secure it with the napkin chain (bib clips). Make sure more of the napkin/bib is on the operator's side of the patient. Give the patient safety glasses for protection during the procedure.

Before reclining the patient, review the medical history and ask if the patient has any questions. Then, inform the patient that you are going to recline the chair. Recline the patient to the supine position, with the patient's nose and knees at about the same level (Figure 17-34A). After the dentist has been seated sometimes he or she will lower the patient's head beyond the supine position; this is called the subsupine position (Figure 17-34B). In this position the patient's head is back further and slightly tilted up toward the dentist, making it easier for the dentist to see. Sometimes the chair height will need to be adjusted so the patient is at the height of the operator's elbow; this is about 8 inches above the seat of the operator's chair. Adjust the head rest and ask the patient if he or she is comfortable (Figure 17-35).

Position the dental light for maximum illumination of the area where the dental procedure is being performed. This is accomplished by bringing the light about 3 to 5 feet from the patient's mouth and tilting the light downward toward the patient napkin. Then, turn the light on (this is to avoid shining the light in the patient's eyes).

After the light is on, slowly raise it to the arch being treated:

- For the mandibular teeth, the light is raised and the beam is directed downward (Figure 17-36).
- For the maxillary teeth, the light is lowered and the beam is directed upward (Figure 17-37).

After the light is adjusted, the assistant turns the light off until the operator is seated. During the procedure, the light may need to be adjusted periodically. The assistant must be observant to keep the field of operation well lit.

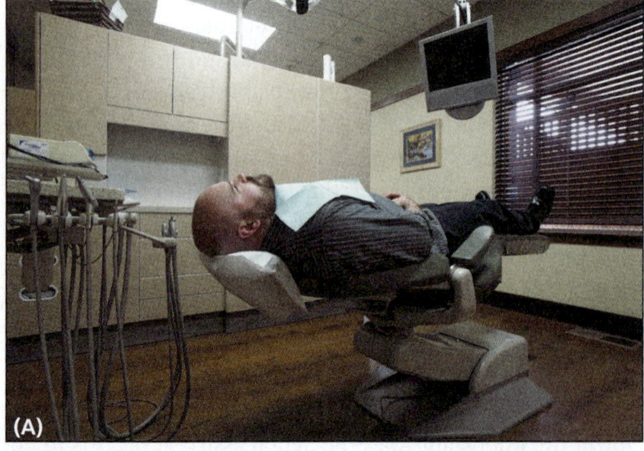

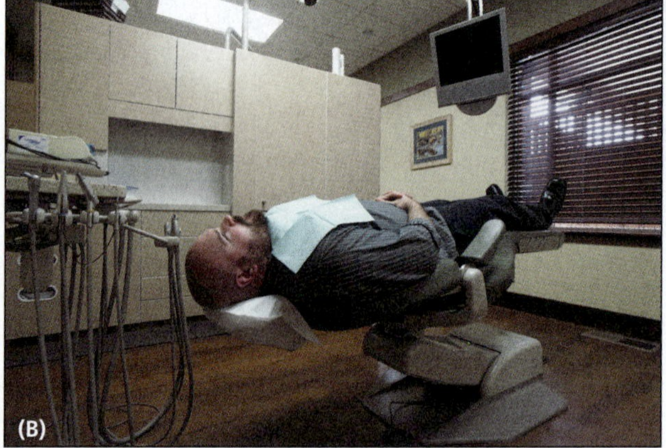

FIGURE 17-34

(A) Patient in the supine position with nose to knees level. (B) Patient in the subsupine position with the head below the plane of the nose to knees.

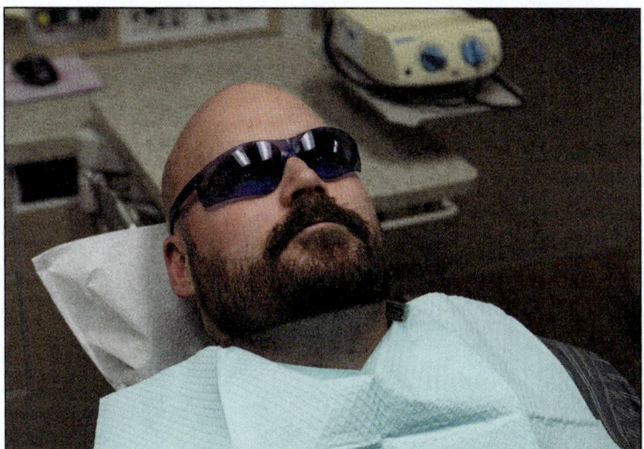

FIGURE 17-35

Patient prepared for treatment with protective glasses and napkin in place.

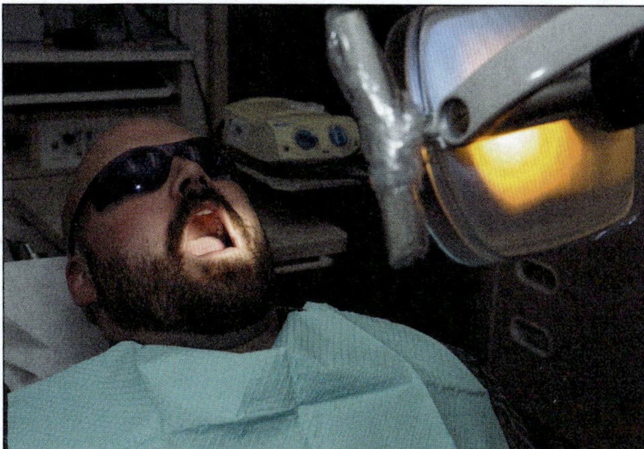

FIGURE 17-37

Patient seated and light adjusted for the maxillary arch.

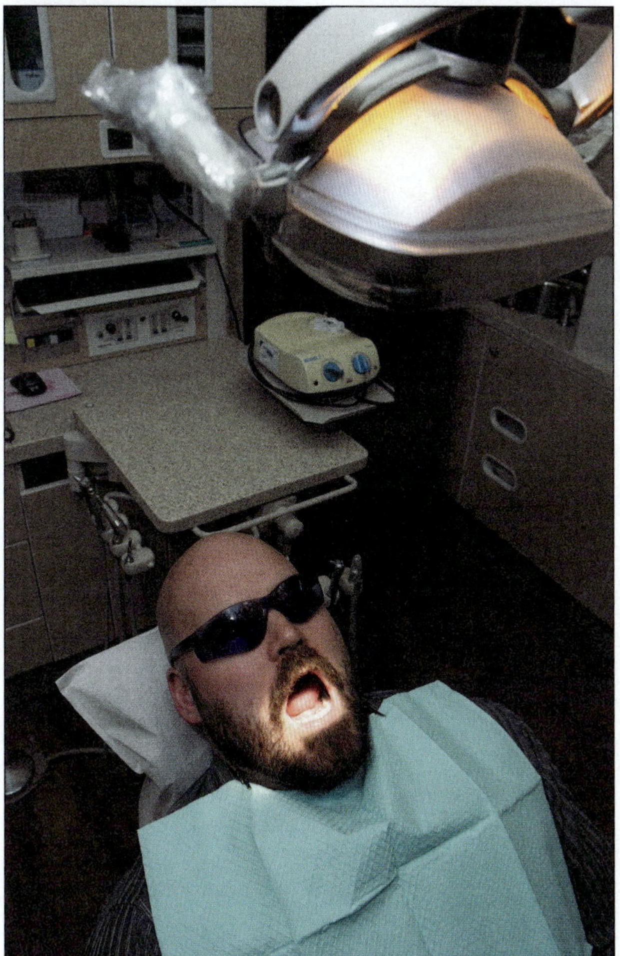

FIGURE 17-36

Patient seated and light adjusted for the mandibular arch.

Ergonomics for the Operator and the Assistant

As individuals stay in the profession of dentistry for a number of years and seek to improve the working environment and reduce stress, dental ergonomics has become an important issue. The term **ergonomics** refers to the study and analysis of human work, including the anatomic and psychological aspects of people and their work environments. Ergonomics must be learned and then applied to benefit individuals. All members of the dental team should be involved in applying ergonomic concepts in the dental office.

Correct ergonomic practices for the operator and the assistant can save time and prevent muscle strain and fatigue. In four-handed, sit-down dentistry, it is ideal when the equipment and materials are as close as possible to the operator and the assistant. This allows the dental team to function as a coordinated and organized unit. Both the operator and the assistant are seated according to the operating zones previously discussed. (For additional information see Chapter 40, Dental Office Management.)

> To prevent back strain and fatigue, evaluate the comfort and function of the operator's and dental assistant's stools. The stools should be well padded and easy to adjust to different positions. The seat upholstery material should be easy to clean and maintain.

Ergonomics for the Operator

The operator's position is key to the arrangement of the patient, assistant, and equipment. The operator must be seated in a comfortable position to perform the dental procedure efficiently, with easy access to the oral cavity and a clear view of the operating field. The following are characteristics for proper positioning for the operator:

- The operator is positioned squarely on the seat of the operator's stool, with his or her weight evenly distributed.
- The operator's thighs are parallel to the floor and the feet are flat on the floor. The stool should be adjustable to accommodate varying heights.
- The operator's back is supported in the lumbar region. The back and neck are in an upright position with the top of the shoulders parallel to the floor.

Procedure 17-3
Seating the Dental Patient

This procedure is performed by the dental assistant to prepare the patient for the dental treatment. The dental assistant has reviewed the patient's medical and dental records, cleaned and prepared the treatment room with appropriate barriers, readied the tray setup, and removed any possible obstacles from the patient's pathway. After being greeted by name in the reception area, the patient is escorted to the treatment room by the dental assistant.

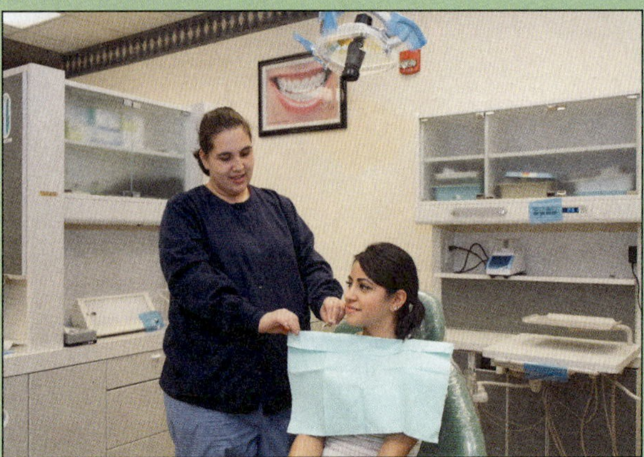

FIGURE 17-38
Dental assistant placing napkin and eyewear on the patient once he or she is seated in the dental chair.

Equipment and Supplies

- Patient's medical and dental records (updated)
- Basic setup: mouth mirror, explorer, and cotton pliers
- Saliva ejector, evacuator (HVE), and air-water syringe tip
- Cotton rolls, cotton-tip applicator, and gauze sponges
- Lip lubricant
- Patient napkin and napkin clip
- Tissue
- Safety glasses

Procedure Steps (*Follow aseptic procedures*)

1. Greet and escort the patient to the treatment room. Show the patient where to place personal items, such as a purse, backpack, or coat so it is in the patient's view. Some offices offer mouthwash to the patient at this time.
2. Seat the patient in the dental chair. Have the patient sit all the way back in the chair. (At this time, the dental assistant may offer the patient a tissue to remove lipstick and ask if he or she would like lubricant for his or her lips.)
3. Place the napkin on the patient, and give the patient safety glasses to wear during the procedure (Figure 17-38).
4. Review the patient's medical history for any changes since his or her last visit. Ask the patient if he or she has any questions, and give a brief explanation or confirmation of the dental treatment to be completed at this appointment. Place x-rays on the viewbox.
5. Position the patient for treatment, adjust the head rest until the patient's head is well supported and the patient is comfortable, and adjust the dental light for the appropriate arch.
6. Position the operator's stool and the rheostat.
7. Position the assistant's stool. Put on mask and protective eyewear, and then wash hands and place on gloves before being seated at chairside.
8. Position the tray setup. Prepare the saliva ejector, evacuator tip, air-water (three-way) syringe tip, and dental handpieces.

- The operator's elbows are close to the body.
- The patient's chair is lowered over the operator's thighs, to about the same level as the operator's elbow.
- The distance between the operator's face and the patient's oral cavity is approximately 14 to 18 inches.
- The operator moves freely in the operator's zone (Figure 17-39).

Ergonomics for the Assistant

The assistant is positioned across from the operator on the opposite side of the patient. The assistant must also have good visibility and easy access to the oral cavity. The tray setup and other necessary instruments should be close at hand. The following are characteristics of proper positioning for the dental assistant:

- The assistant's stool is positioned 4 to 6 inches above the operator's for good visibility (Figure 17-40).

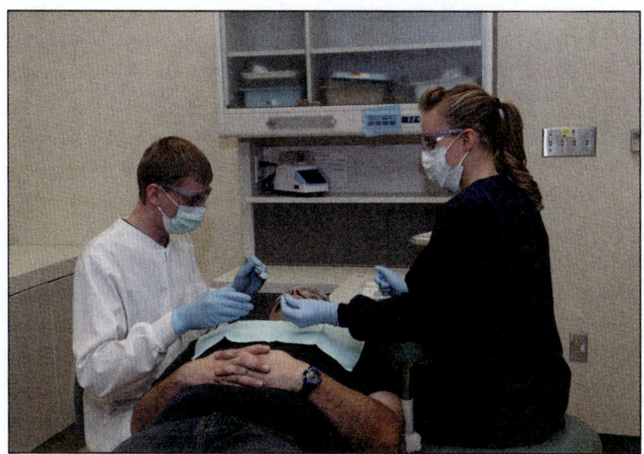

FIGURE 17-39

Operator and assistant positioned for proper ergonomics with patient reclined and ready for treatment.

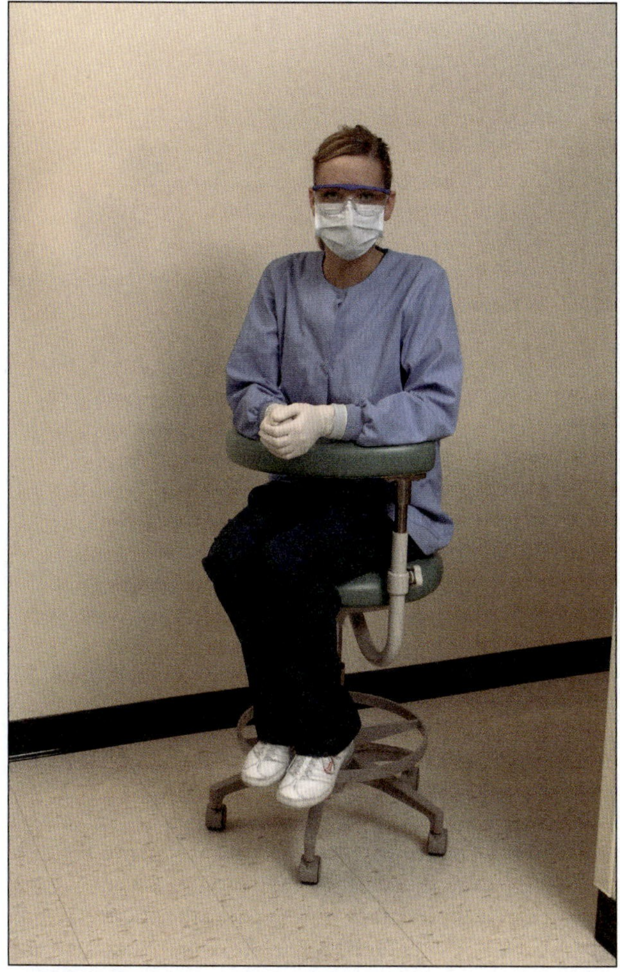

FIGURE 17-40

Dental assistant properly positioned on a stool with feet resting on foot rest, thighs parallel to the floor, and back upright.

- The assistant is positioned on the stool so that his or her weight is distributed evenly over the seat.
- The front edge of the assistant's stool is even with the patient's mouth.
- The assistant's feet are resting on a flat ring or tabular bar around the base of the stool just above the casters (wheels), and his or her thighs are parallel to the floor.
- The assistant is positioned as close as possible to the side of the patient.
- The assistant's back is straight, with support in the lumbar region; on some assistant's chairs there is a side support that extends around in front of the assistant. This extension supports the assistant when he or she leans forward slightly or when reaching. The side support is adjusted to fit the assistant at the level of the abdomen.
- After the assistant is correctly positioned on the chair, the cabinet top or mobile cart is placed over the thighs as close as possible for convenience and efficiency.

Dismissing the Patient

After the treatment is completed, the light is turned off and moved out of the way. The dentist leaves and the assistant begins the process of dismissing the patient. The assistant raises the dental chair to an upright position. The patient is asked to remain seated for a minute, in case he or she is a little light-headed from being in the supine or subsupine position during treatment.

The HVE tip, saliva ejector, and syringe tip are removed and placed on the tray. During this time, the assistant wipes any debris from the patient's face and removes the napkin. The tray can be covered with the patient's napkin.

The dental assistant should put on overgloves or remove treatment gloves and wash hands before documenting the procedure and escorting the patient to the reception area.

The rheostat and the operator's chair should be moved out of the patient's way. The right arm of the chair is raised so the patient can stand easily. Ask the patient if he or she has any questions, and give postoperative instructions at the dentist's directions. Return any personal items to the patient, and escort him or her to the reception area.

The dental assistant gathers the patient's records, including the x-rays, to give to the receptionist or enters the information in the computer. The receptionist can make future appointments and complete the financial arrangements (Figure 17-41).

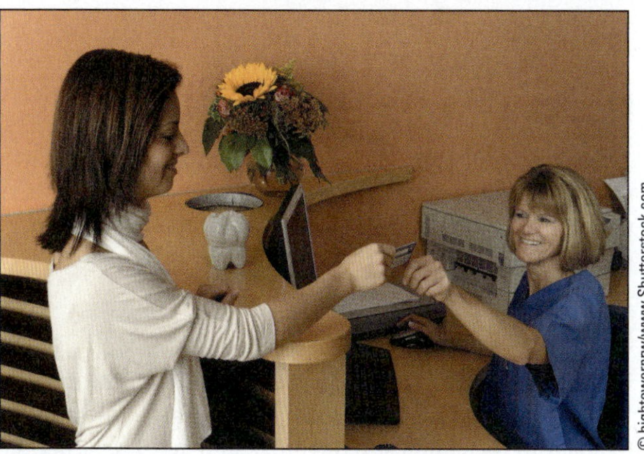

FIGURE 17-41

Patient making final arrangements at reception desk before leaving the office.

Procedure 17-4
Dismissing the Dental Patient

This procedure is performed by the dental assistant after the dental procedure has been completed.

Equipment and Supplies

The following items were set up for the procedure and now must be handled as the assistant dismisses the patient.

- Patient's medical and dental records
- Basic setup: mouth mirror, explorer, and cotton pliers
- Saliva ejector, evacuator (HVE), and air-water syringe tip
- Cotton rolls, cotton-tip applicator, and gauze sponges
- Lip lubricant
- Patient napkin and napkin clip
- Tissue
- Safety glasses

Procedure Steps (*Follow aseptic procedures*)

1. When the operator is finished with the procedure, rinse and evacuate the patient's mouth thoroughly. The dental light is positioned out of the patient's way.
2. The patient is returned to an upright position and asked to remain seated. Remove any debris from the patient's face. (The patient can double-check in a mirror before leaving the office.)
3. The napkin is removed from the patient and is placed over the tray setup. The patient's safety glasses are removed (Figure 17-42).
4. The evacuator (HVE) tip, saliva ejector, and air-water syringe tip are removed and placed on the tray.
5. The operator's stool and the rheostat are moved out of the patient's way.
6. After removing treatment gloves and washing hands or donning overgloves, the procedure is documented on the patient's chart or in the computer terminal. The patient's chart and x-rays are gathered.
7. Postoperative instructions are given to the patient.
8. The patient's personal items are returned and the patient is escorted to the reception area.

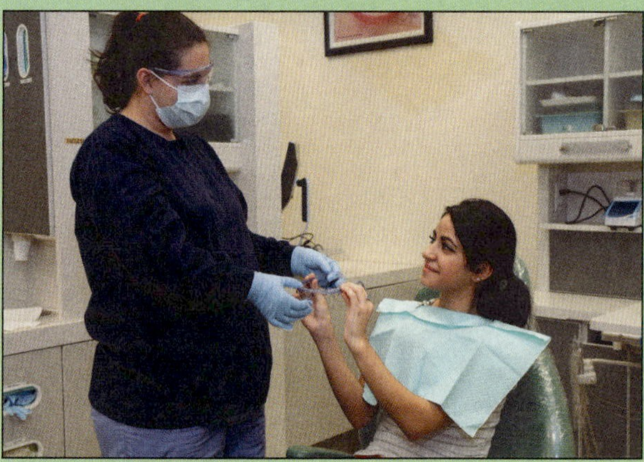

FIGURE 17-42
Dismissing the dental patient after treatment.

Patients with Special Needs

Although most patients can be seated in a routine manner, some patients need special considerations. With most of these patients, planning and preparing before their appointment eliminates problems.

Child Patients

Many of the skills in seating a child patient are the same as when seating an adult. However, some changes are needed to adapt to the child's size, maturity, and age. Preparing the patient's records is the same, except the child's parent or guardian should be consulted when reviewing the medical history. The dental chair is lowered to accommodate the child. A booster chair, pillow, or cushion may be used to elevate the child in the chair. If the child is too small to reach the head rest, some operators just remove or reposition it so that it does not interfere with treatment or the patient's comfort. To prevent the child from sliding down in the dental chair, have him or her sit with legs crossed (Figure 17-43).

When the dental assistant steps into the reception room, it is important to greet both the parent and the child, but the focus should be on the child. Kneel down to the same level as the child and greet him or her. Escort the child to the treatment room, and assist him or her into the dental chair, if necessary. Answer questions the child has, using language appropriate to his or her level of understanding. More information on dealing with the child patient appears in Chapter 29, Pediatric Dentistry. Once

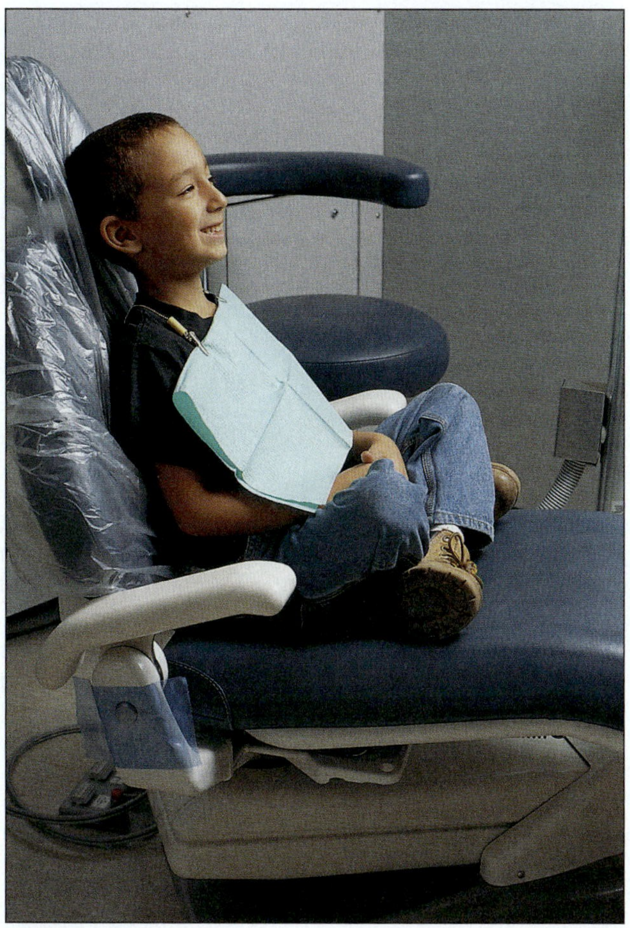

FIGURE 17-43
Child patient seated with legs crossed to prevent them from sliding down in the chair.

the procedure is completed and the child is dismissed, escort him or her to the reception area and inform the parent/guardian about the treatment performed. Postoperative instructions for the child should be repeated to the parent/guardian.

Senior Patients

With senior patients, assistance may be needed. The dental assistant should be careful not to offend these patients by challenging their ability to take care of themselves. Usually, the older patient will ask for help if it is needed. Review the medical history for any changes in health and medication. Treatment can be broken into shorter segments to accommodate restroom and stretching breaks. The senior patient may not be comfortable in the reclined position for long periods, so the dental assistant should position the patient upright whenever possible.

Pregnant Patients

When a pregnant woman is sitting in a reclined position, it may be difficult for her to breathe. The dental assistant can allow her to sit upright until the dentist is ready to begin the procedure. During the first trimester of pregnancy, women may find dental treatment uncomfortable because of nausea. The safest and most comfortable time to schedule dental appointments is during the second trimester of pregnancy. Restroom breaks may become more necessary for women in the third trimester of pregnancy.

Hearing-Impaired or Blind Patients

When a patient has hearing difficulties, the dental assistant must be in a position where the patient can observe lip movement and facial expression. Remove the mask and speak normally but slowly; make eye contact and ask questions to be sure the patient understands. To make the patient feel comfortable and show that the assistant really cares about him or her, the assistant may consider learning a few words in sign language.

The patient who is blind may be escorted by someone, but he or she is often very independent. Good communication requires information about his or her abilities and concerns. The dental assistant should talk to the blind patient throughout the procedure and explain what is happening or what is about to be done.

Patients with Wheelchairs or Walkers

If a patient comes into the office in a wheelchair or using a walker, he or she may need some assistance getting into the dental chair. The pathway to the treatment room should be cleared as much as possible. If the patient is using a walker, give assistance when needed. Usually, the patient has a routine and will tell you if help is needed. The wheelchair patient often needs someone to lift or move him or her from the wheelchair to the dental chair (Figure 17-44).

Patients with special needs know their abilities. Communicate with them to understand their needs and treat them the same as all other patients.

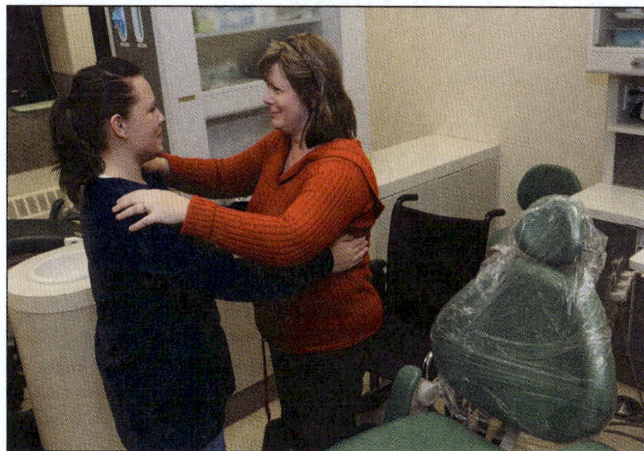

FIGURE 17-44
Patient being transferred from wheelchair to the dental chair.

Non English Speaking Patients

Some dental practices have patients who neither speak English nor do they understand the procedures. The dental staff needs to assist these patients in any way they can. Sometimes an interpreter, a relative, a friend, or someone from a church or social agency comes with the patient. This is very helpful, especially during the first several visits. The staff may try to learn key words in the patient's language to assist in communication as well as to show that the office cares and is making an effort to understand the patient. The dental staff may research and find information about the patient's country or culture to identify something in common with the patient. Pictures help when trying to make the patient understand what is involved in a procedure and what to expect.

Finding means of communicating with patients from other cultures who speak languages other than English is important. Placing yourself in that situation should help you imagine how you would feel if you have a dental problem when traveling or living abroad. Think of ways to work with these patients.

Chapter Summary

It is important for the dental assistant to understand the various dental office designs and how each area relates to patient care. Each dentist lays out his or her office to meet the needs of the practice. The assistant learns the function of each area in the dental office and the equipment that is used in this area. Responsibilities and the job description of the dental assistant are discussed in relation to preparing for the patient and seating and then dismissing the patient. Concepts of assisting are described including assisting for a left- or right-handed dentist. Dental health professionals go to great lengths to ensure patient and employee safety and an ergonomic work environment.

Examining the needs of various special needs patients gives the dental assistant the information to plan and prepare for these patients to eliminate problems and make their experience a positive one.

CASE STUDY

Mrs. Maxine Rose, age 77, had several restorations completed during her hour-long appointment. She is in good health but was in the supine position for most of her appointment.

Case Study Review

1. What can the dental assistant expect will happen once the procedure is complete and the patient is again seated upright?
2. How can the assistant aid Maxine before escorting her to the reception area?
3. Is there anything the dental assistant can do to prevent patients from experiencing discomfort resulting from positioning during treatment?

Review Questions

Multiple Choice

1. There are four activity zones. Which zone extends from 12 to 2 o'clock for a right-handed operator?
   a. Operating zone
   b. Assisting zone
   c. Static zone
   d. Transfer zone
2. After the treatment is completed and before the patient is dismissed, all of the following are removed from the unit and placed on the procedure tray *except*
   a. high-volume evacuator tip.
   b. overhead dental light.
   c. saliva ejector.
   d. air-water syringe tip.
3. In which of the following areas would a dental unit be located?
   a. Reception area
   b. Dental treatment room
   c. Sterilizing area
   d. Processing room
4. When seating a dental patient, where does the dental assistant place the patient's personal items?
   a. In the reception area
   b. In the treatment room where the patient can see them
   c. In the lounge
   d. In the dentist's office
5. The ultrasonic equipment would be located in which of the following areas?
   a. Treatment room
   b. Sterilizing area

c. Laboratory area
d. X-ray processing area

6. The patient is in the supine position when
   a. the patient is sitting upright.
   b. the patient is reclined so the head is lower than the rest of the body.
   c. the patient's nose and knees are on the same plane.
   d. the patient's nose is a foot above the feet.
7. The front delivery systems are
   a. pulled over the patient's chest and between the dentist and the assistant.
   b. located behind the patient's head.
   c. located on the dentist's side of the dental unit.
   d. located on the assistant's side of the dental unit.
8. The function of the rheostat is to
   a. control the air-water syringe.
   b. regulate the water reservoir.
   c. control the speed of the dental handpieces.
   d. control the overhead light.
9. The saliva ejector is used
   a. during fluoride treatments.
   b. under rubber dams.
   c. for low-volume suction.
   d. All of the answers are correct.
10. Tungsten halogen, argon laser, plasma arc, and light emitting diode are
   a. dental amalgamators.
   b. dental curing lights.
   c. computer communication systems.
   d. intraoral cameras.

Critical Thinking

1. List ways a dental assistant can create an atmosphere that would put patients at ease and give them the impression that this office is competent and provides quality dentistry.
2. Explain what is necessary to be effective and efficient when the dentist and the assistant are positioned around the patient.
3. Identify methods to ensure comfort for a patient having dental treatment while in the third trimester of pregnancy.

Web Activities

1. Go to http://www.ada.org and search for the ADA's stand on OSHA's ergonomics regulations.
2. Go to http://www.A-dec.com and view a line of dental chairs, units, and accessories.
3. Visit http://www.hspinc.com, and click on the link for the four-handed dentistry training manual. Review the benefits and concepts behind the technique.

CHAPTER 18

Basic Chairside Instruments and Tray Systems

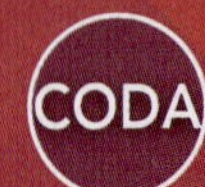

Specific Instructional Objectives

The student should strive to meet the following objectives and demonstrate an understanding of the facts and principles presented in this chapter:

1. Identify the parts of an instrument.
2. Describe how instruments are identified.
3. Identify the categories and functions of dental burs.
4. Describe the types and functions of abrasives.
5. Explain the various handpieces and attachments.
6. Describe the types of tray systems and color-coding systems.

Key Terms

Abrasive rotary instrument (401)
acrylic bur (397)
air abrasion (406)
amalgam carrier (391)
amalgam condenser (391)
amalgam gun (391)
angle former (386)
bevel (381)
bi-beveled (381)
binangle (383)
Black's formula (384)
blade (381)
bur (395)
bur block (403)
burnisher (393)
carborundum disc (401)
carver (392)
cement spatula (394)
chisel (384)
chuck (404)
composite instrument (390)
cone socket handle (382)
contra-angle (404)
cotton plier (390)
crown and collar (bridge) scissors (394)
cutting edge (381)
cutting instrument (000)
Dycal instrument/small-balled instrument (391)
electric handpiece (405)
excavator (387)
explorer (389)
fiber-optic light source (404)
file (393)
finishing knife (393)
frictional heat (402)
friction-grip shank (396)
gingival margin trimmer (GMT) (385)
hatchet (385)
high-speed handpieces (404)
hoe (385)
Jo-dandy disc (401)
laboratory spatula (394)
laser handpiece (406)
latch-type shank (396)
low-speed handpieces (404)
mandrel (399)
manufacturer's number (384)
microetcher (407)
monangle (383)
mouth mirror (387)
nib (381)
noncutting instrument (000)
periodontal probe (390)
plane (384)
plastic filling instrument (391)
plastic spatula (394)
preset tray system (408)
revolutions per minute (rpm) (404)
rheostat (404)
rotary instruments (395)
separating disc (401)
serrated (381)
shaft (382)
shank (382)
small-balled instrument/Dycal instrument (391)
straight shank (396)
ultrasonic handpiece (405)
vulcanite bur (397)
working end (381)
XTS composite instrument (390)

Introduction

Dental instruments are continually developing as technology changes and dental materials require instruments of specific designs or materials. Most instruments are made of stainless steel, and a few consist of a high-tech plastic/resin or anodized aluminum. Manufacturers of dental instruments provide many designs and sizes and make improvements as new materials become available. Dentists select the instruments that they feel the most confident and comfortable using. Each procedure requires special instruments to accomplish the task. For example, when examining the pits and grooves of the teeth, the dentist uses an explorer. The ends of all explorers are pointed and sharp but designed with different angles to reach all surfaces of the tooth.

The dental assistant is responsible for keeping the instruments sterilized and in working condition. The dental assistant orders new instruments as needed and keeps the instruments in sequence while assisting during the procedure.

Instruments are generally categorized into hand instruments and rotary instruments. Hand instruments are manually operated and are categorized by procedure. In this chapter, the basic instruments used in general dental procedures are discussed, including common cutting and noncutting instruments.

Instruments for Basic Chairside Procedures

Learning the parts of dental instruments will aid in the understanding of how and where the instrument is used. Dental instruments are also classified in several different ways including number of working ends, their function, manufacturer's number, and Black's formula. The classifications make it easier to remember each instrument's name and function.

Instruments for basic chairside procedures include the basic setup found on all trays. This basic setup includes the mouth mirror, explorer, and cotton pliers. Sometimes a periodontal probe is included in this setup. Instruments that are found on restorative tray setups such as for composite and amalgam procedures will also be discussed in this section. Instruments used for specialty procedures will be found in the specific specialty chapters; for example, the root canal instruments will be found in Chapter 24, Endodontics.

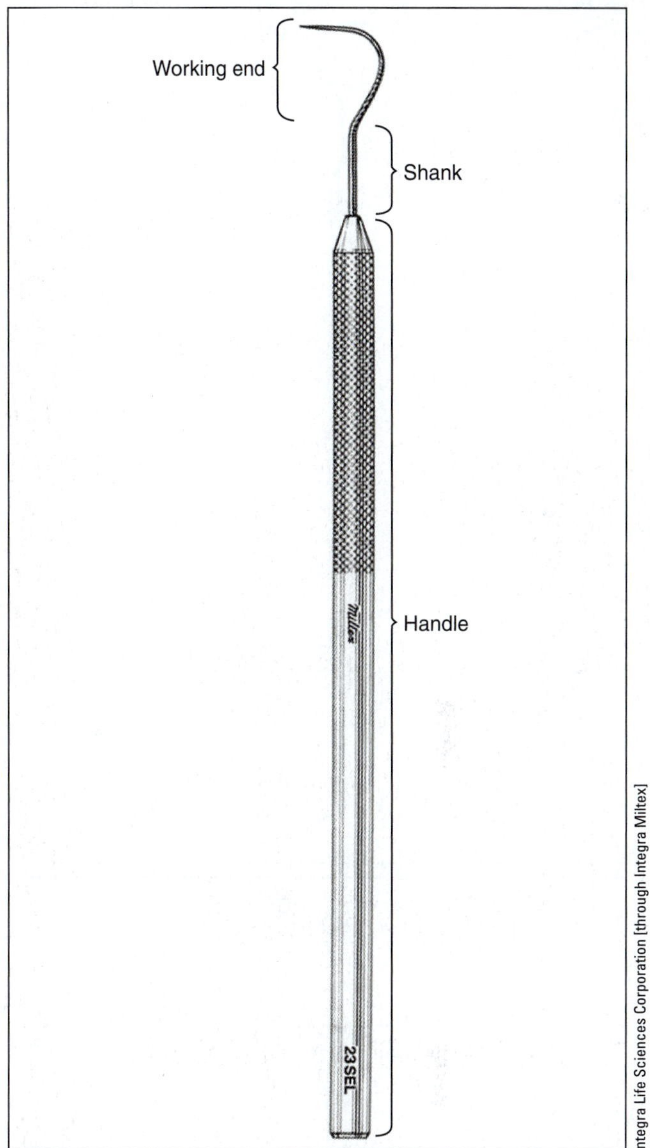

FIGURE 18-1
Parts of the single-ended dental instrument.

Basic Structural Parts of Dental Hand Instruments

The dental instrument is generally 6 inches long and is single or double ended. The parts of the dental hand instrument include the working end, shank, and handle (Figure 18-1).

The Working End of an Instrument. The **working end** performs the specific function of the instrument. The working end may be a point, blade, or nib. A point is sharp and is used to explore, detect, and reflect materials. The **blade** may be flat or curved and have a rounded or cutting edge. The **cutting edge** is formed by a **bevel** (slanted edge or side) on the working end of the instrument. The blade may also be **bi-beveled** (beveled on both sides of the blade). A **nib** is the blunt end of an instrument that is **serrated** or smooth (Figures 18-2A–C).

The working ends of instruments may also be beaks or rounded ends. The beaks may be smooth, serrated, or grooved, depending on their functions. The rounded ends come in different sizes and shapes and are used to smooth surfaces.

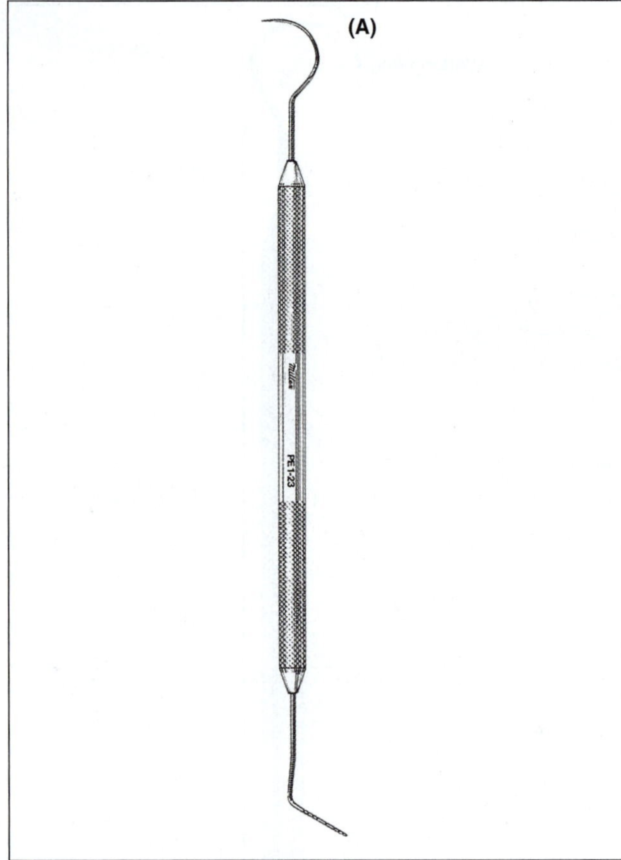

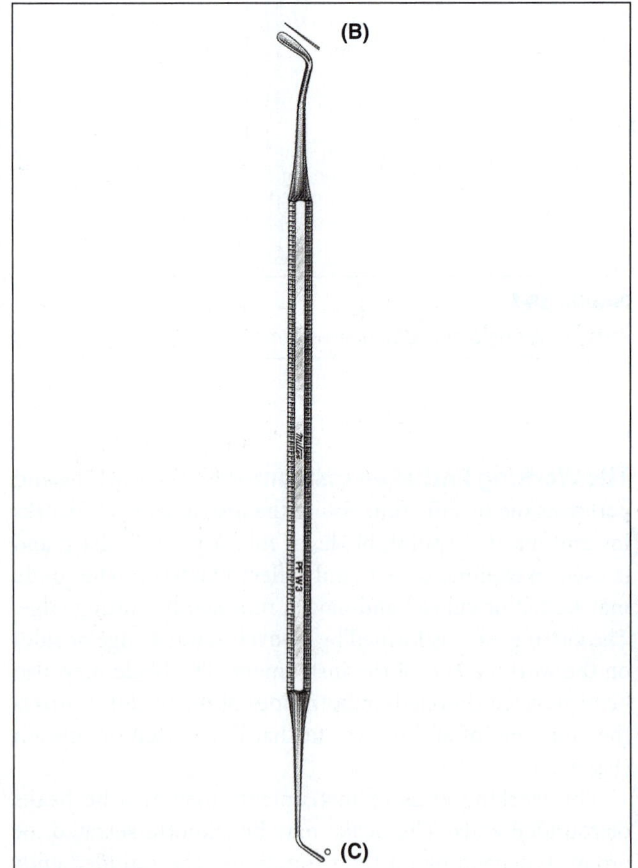

FIGURE 18-2

Various working ends. (A) Point. (B) Blade. (C) Nib.

The Handle (Shaft). The handle, or **shaft**, of an instrument is where the instrument is held by the operator. The handle may be serrated or smooth. It is usually hexagonal (six sided), which provides for a better grip. Some handles are ergonomically designed, which means they are made larger and designed with finger rests and grooves. Other handles are covered with a soft, rubber-like material that makes the instruments easier to hold and grip. These instruments are sterilizable and durable. A few instruments are designed with a **cone socket handle**, which allow the working ends to be replaced (Figures 18-3A–I).

The Shank. The **shank** connects the handle to the working end. It narrows or tapers from the handle to the working end. The shank may be angled to reach particular areas of

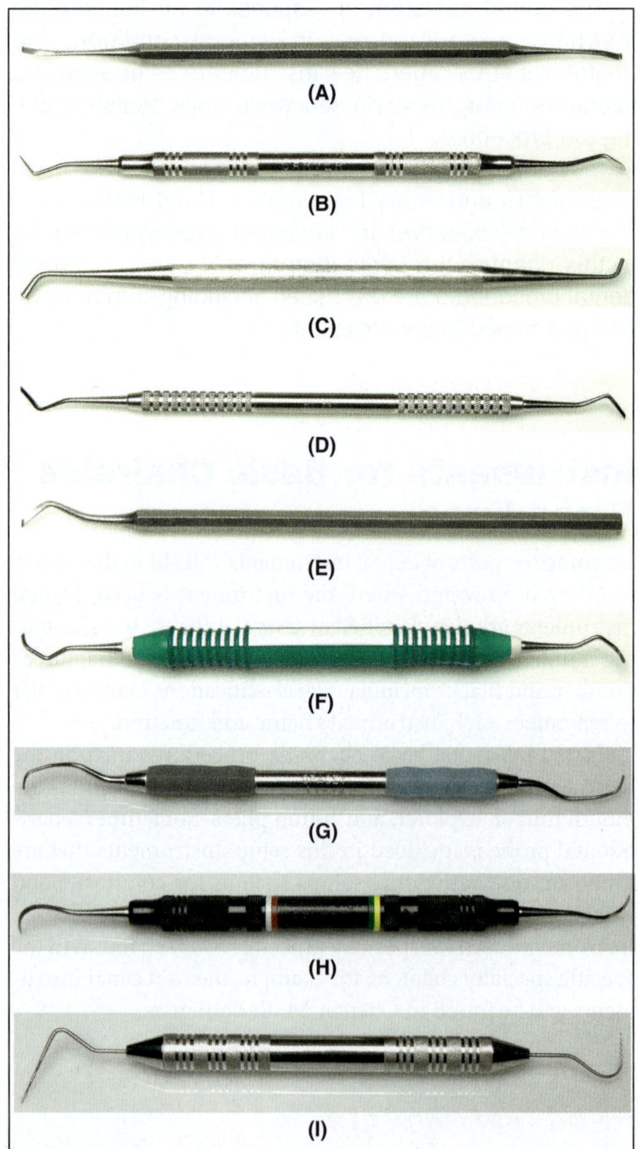

FIGURE 18-3

(A–E) Various instrument handle styles. (F–I) Ergonomically designed handles.

the mouth. Usually, instruments that are used in the posterior areas of the oral cavity have more angles, while instruments with fewer angles are used in anterior areas. Shanks of dental instruments are formed in the following ways: straight (no angles), curved (slightly bent), **monangle** (one angle), **binangle** (two angles), or triple angle (three angles) (Figures 18-4A–E).

Basic Classification of Dental Instruments

Dental instruments are classified in many ways, including by number of working ends, function, manufacturer's name and number, and Black's number formula.

Number of Working Ends. The number of working ends on an instrument falls into two categories: single-ended and double-ended instruments (Figure 18-5). Single-ended instruments have only one working end and long handles. Double-ended instruments have two working ends in the following combinations:

- The two ends have similar functions, but one end is larger than the other (e.g., an amalgam condenser).
- The two ends are paired right and left for preparing the right or the left side of a cavity preparation (e.g., a gingival margin trimmer).
- The two ends have a combined function in which the ends are used for the same procedure but each end has a different use (e.g., a plastic filling instrument).

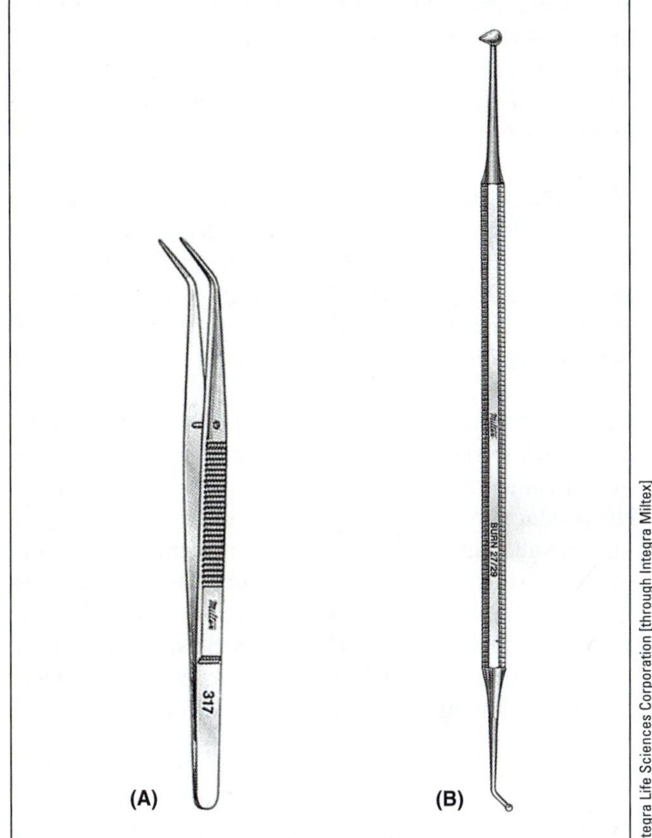

FIGURE 18-5
Working ends of (A) cotton pliers for transporting materials and (B) burnishers for smoothing materials.

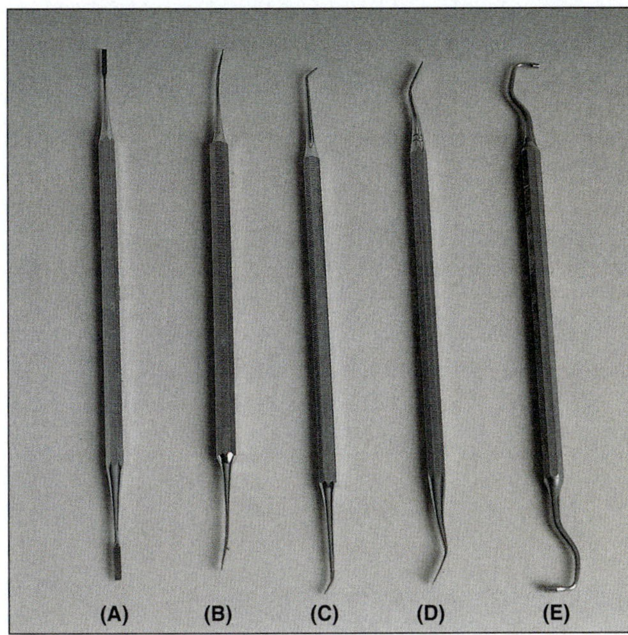

FIGURE 18-4
Instrument shanks. (A) Straight. (B) Curved. (C) Monangle. (D) Binangle. (E) Triple angle.

Cutting and Noncutting Instruments

Cutting Instruments

- Angle formers
- Chisels
- Excavators
- Gingival margin trimmers
- Hatchets
- Hoes

Noncutting Instruments

- Basic instruments (mouth mirror, explorer, and cotton pliers)
- Burnishers
- Carriers
- Carvers
- Composite instruments
- Condensers
- Files
- Finishing knives
- Plastic filling instruments

Instruments Classified by Function. Instruments are classified by function. Operative hand instruments are categorized as cutting and noncutting. Other instruments are classified according to a specialty, use with a specific material, or a procedure.

Manufacturer's Number. The **manufacturer's number** is found on the handle of the instrument. This number, used when ordering the instrument, indicates the instrument's placement in a set of instruments. Some instruments are named or classified by the name of the individual who designed the instrument.

Black's Formula. **Black's formula** was developed by G.V. Black to standardize the exact size and angulation of an instrument. This formula minimizes discrepancies in the production of instruments from one manufacturer to another and simplifies ordering instruments. Black's formula for hand cutting instruments includes the size of the blade and the angle at which it is positioned to the handle. Some instruments, such as chisels, hatchets, and hoes, have a series of three numbers and some, such as angle formers and gingival margin trimmers, have four numbers.

Black's Three-Number Formula

1. The first number (Figure 18-6) is the width of the blade in tenths of a millimeter. In the formula 20 9 14, the first number (20) indicates that the blade is 2.0 mm wide.
2. The second number is the length of the blade in millimeters. In the formula 20 9 14, the second number (9) indicates that the blade is 9 mm long.
3. The third number gives the angle of the blade to the long axis of the handle, in degrees centigrade. In the formula 20 9 14, the third number (14) indicates that the instrument has a blade at an angle of 14/100 of a circle.

Black's Four-Number Formula

1. The first number (Figure 18-7) is the same as that in the three-number formula, representing the width of the blade in tenths of a millimeter. In the formula 15 85 8 12, the first number (15) indicates that the blade is 1.5 mm long.
2. The second number, differing from that in the three-number formula, represents the degree of the angle of the cutting edge of the blade to the handle of the instrument. In the formula 15 85 8 12, the second number (85) indicates that the cutting edge forms an 85-degree C angle with the handle.
3. The third number is the same as the second number in the three-number formula. Using the formula 15 85 8 12, the third number (8) indicates that the blade is 8 mm long.
4. The fourth number is the same as the third number in the three-number formula. Using the formula 15 85 8 12, the fourth number (12) indicates that the blade forms a 12-degree C angle with the handle of the instrument.

Cutting Instruments

Hand cutting instruments are used to assist in the design of the cavity preparation. They refine and define the cavity walls and margins. There are six hand cutting instruments: chisels, hatchets, hoes, gingival margin trimmers, angle formers, and excavators. Review Procedure 18-1: Identify hand cutting instruments.

Chisels. A **chisel** is used to shape and **plane** (make surface flat or level) enamel and dentin walls of the cavity preparation. The blade of the chisel is straight and has a cutting edge with a one-sided bevel. The chisel is usually a double-ended instrument—one end with a standard bevel on the blade and one end with a reversed bevel on the end of the blade (Figures 18-8A and B). Chisels have several different shanks, which is where they get their names.

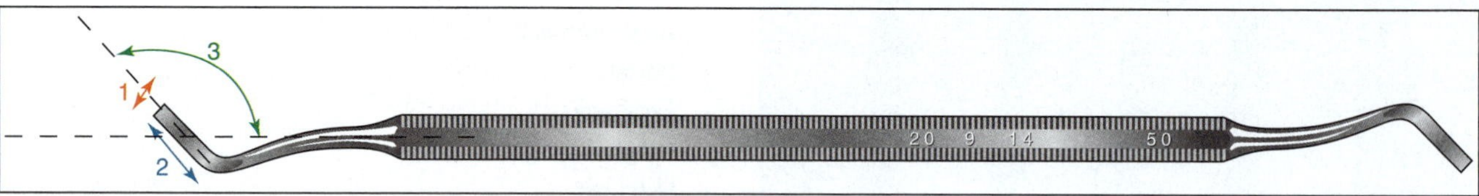

FIGURE 18-6
Instrument with Black's three-number formula.

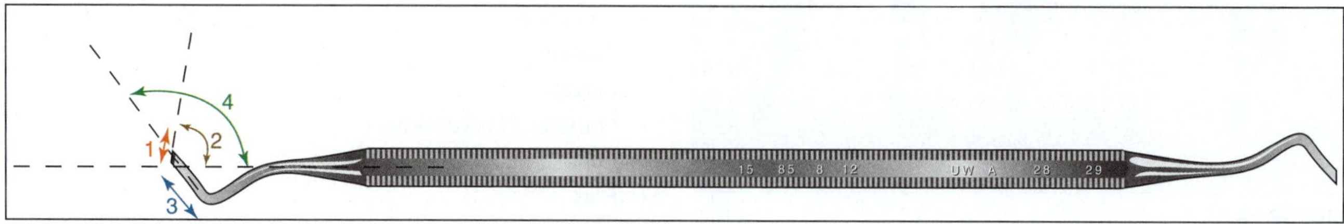

FIGURE 18-7
Instrument with Black's four-number formula.

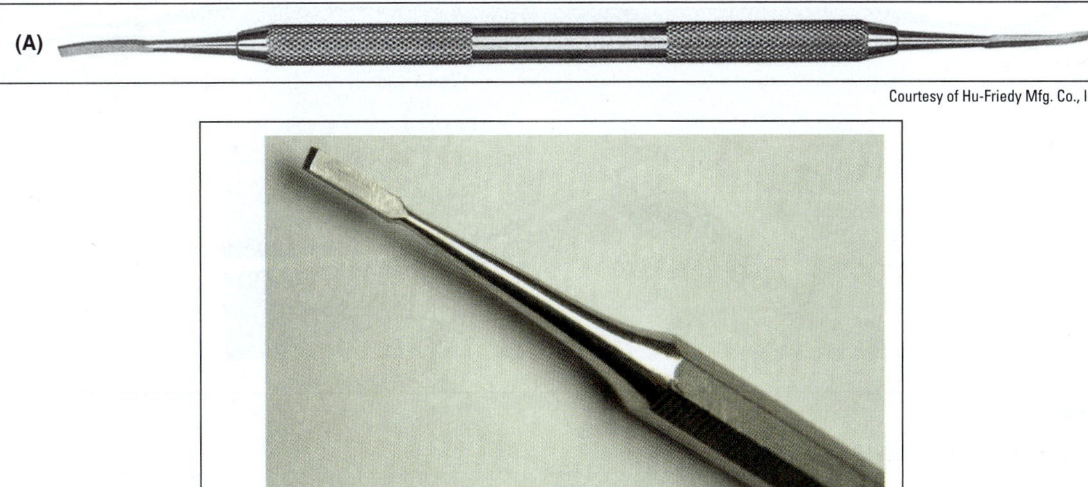

Courtesy of Hu-Friedy Mfg. Co., Inc.

FIGURE 18-8

(A) Chisel with standard and reverse bevel. (B) Close-up view of the working end of the chisel.

- *Straight chisels* have no angle in the shanks and are used on maxillary and mandibular teeth in class III or IV cavity preparations (Figure 18-9A). Straight chisels are used with a mallet to remove fixed prosthetics.
- *Wedelstaedt chisels* have slightly curved shanks and are used for class III and IV cavity preparations (Figures 18-9B and D).
- *Binangle chisels* have two angles in the shanks of the instruments and are used in Class II cavity preparations (Figure 18-9C).

Hatchets. A **hatchet**, sometimes called an enamel hatchet, is similar to the hatchet used to cut wood. There is an angle in the shank of a hatchet and the blade is flat. Hatchets are paired left and right, with a bevel on one side of the blade on one end of the instrument and on the reverse side of the blade on the other end. The hatchet is used in a downward motion to refine the cavity walls and to obtain retention in the cavity preparation (Figures 18-10A and B). Sometimes, hatchets are marked with rings on the handles to indicate left and right ends.

Hoes. A **hoe** is an instrument that is used in a pulling motion to smooth and shape the floor of the cavity preparation. A hoe is shaped like a garden hoe, with straight and angled shanks. All hoes have blades that form cutting edges (Figure 18-11).

Gingival Margin Trimmers. The **gingival margin trimmer (GMT)** is similar to the hatchet regarding the position of the blade to the handle, but there are two distinct differences. First, the blade on the GMT is curved, not flat like the hatchet. Second, the cutting edge is at an angle, not straight across like the hatchet. The GMT is a double-ended and paired instrument. With the double ends of the instrument, one end curves toward the left and the other end

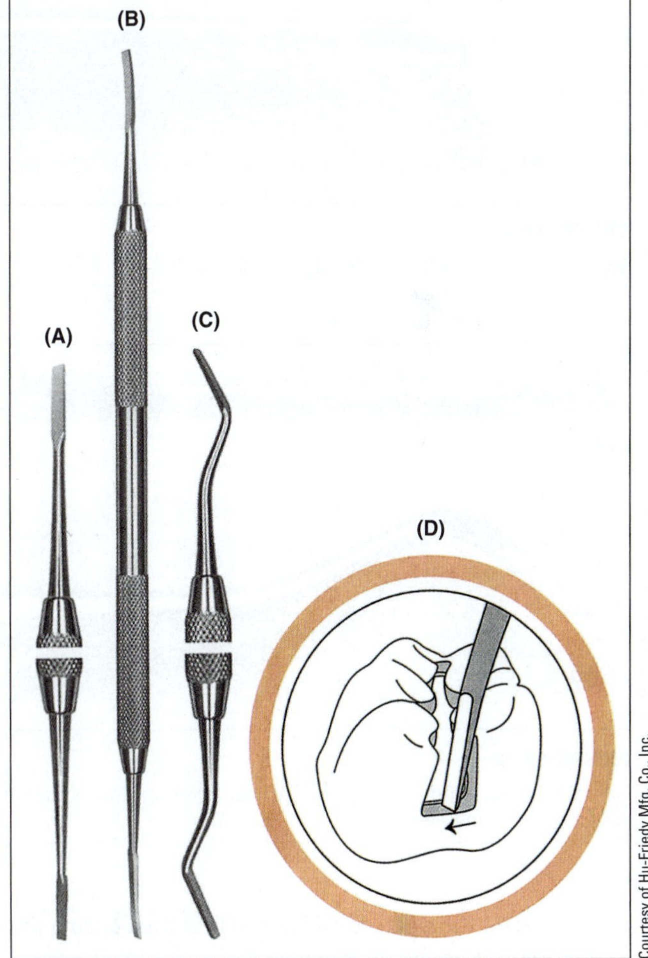

Courtesy of Hu-Friedy Mfg. Co., Inc.

FIGURE 18-9

Chisels. (A) Straight. (B) Wedelstaedt. (C) Binangle. (D) Chisel being used to prepare cavity.

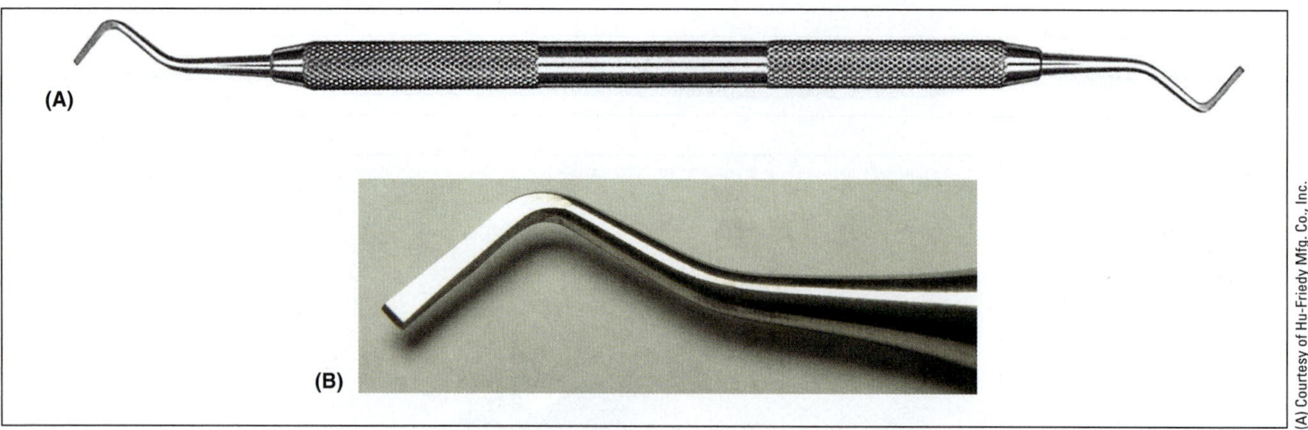

FIGURE 18-10

(A) Hatchet. (B) Close-up view of the working end of the hatchet.

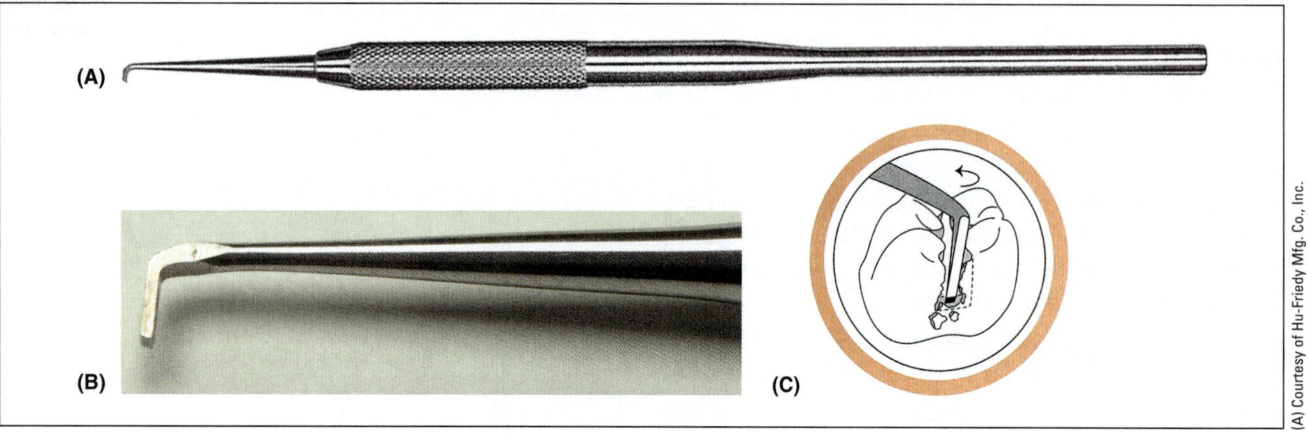

FIGURE 18-11

(A) Hoe. (B) Close-up view of the working end of the hoe. (C) Fracturing away the undermined enamel with a hoe.

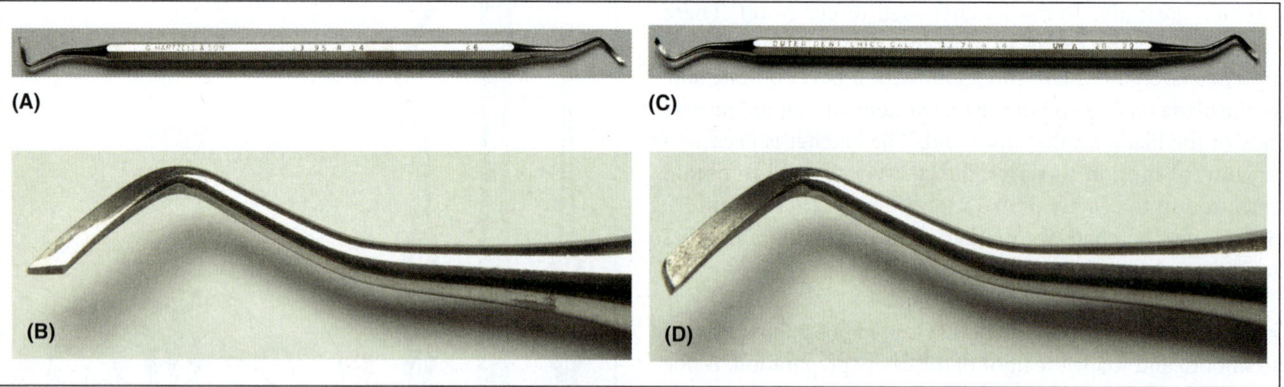

FIGURE 18-12

Gingival margin trimmers. (A) Distal GMT. (B) Close-up view of the working end of the Distal GMT. (C) Mesial GMT. (D) Close-up view of the working end of the Mesial GMT.

curves toward the right. A pair of GMTs is used during the cavity preparation, because one instrument is for the distal surfaces and another is for the mesial surface (Figure 18-12). The GMTs are used to bevel the gingival margin wall of the cavity preparation.

Angle Formers. The **angle former** is used in a downward pushing motion to form and define point angles and to sharpen line angles. The angle former is similar to the hoe, except the cutting edge is angled like the gingival margin trimmer. Therefore, this also is a four-numbered

Gingival Margin Trimmer Identification

To distinguish between the mesial and the distal GMT, consider the following:

1. *The number on the handle.* This is a Black's four-numbered instrument, so the second number in the series on the handle indicates the angle of the blade. If this number is 90 or above, it is used on the distal surface of the cavity preparation; if it is 85 or below, it is used on the mesial surface.
2. *Hold the instrument upright.* If the cutting edge forms a line that is parallel to the handle, it is used on the distal (down for distal). If the cutting edge does not form this line, it is used on the mesial.

instrument. This instrument is double-ended, so it can be used on either the left or right surfaces of a cavity preparation (Figure 18-13).

Excavators. An **excavator**, also known as a "spoon excavator," is an instrument used to remove carious material and debris from the teeth. This instrument is also used for numerous other tasks, including removing excess dental cement, tucking rubber dam material, and packing gingival retraction cord. The excavator is similar to the GMT with the curved blade, but the difference is that the cutting edge of the excavator is rounded all the way around the periphery of the blade (Figure 18-14).

Noncutting Instruments

Noncutting instruments include basic examination instruments and instruments used to insert and finish amalgam and composite restorative materials. Examples of noncutting instruments include basic examination setup instruments, plastic instruments, amalgam carriers, condensers, carvers, burnishers, files, and finishing knives. Review Procedure 18-2: Identify non-cutting dental instruments.

Basic Examination Instruments. The basic examination setup instruments are used for examining the teeth but are also common to all tray setups. All procedures begin with the operator examining the teeth, so the mouth mirror, explorer, and cotton pliers are the first three instruments on a procedure tray setup. The periodontal probe is an optional instrument in the basic examination setup.

Mouth Mirrors. The **mouth mirror** is a single-ended instrument made of metal or plastic. It may have a handle with a "cone socket" for easy replacement of the mirror head

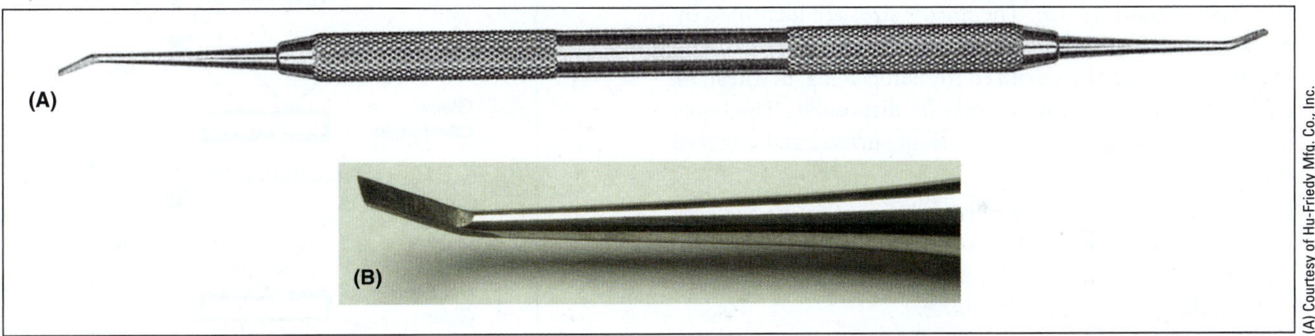

(A) Courtesy of Hu-Friedy Mfg. Co., Inc.

FIGURE 18-13

(A) Angle former. (B) Close-up view of the working end of the angle former.

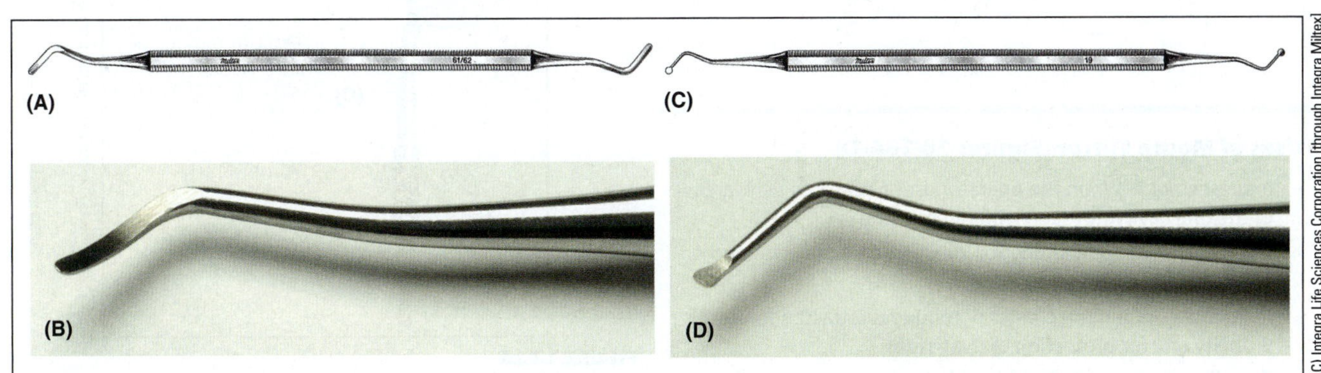

(A,C) Integra Life Sciences Corporation [through Integra Miltex]

FIGURE 18-14

Excavators. (A) Blade. (B) Close-up view of the working end of blade excavator. (C) Spoon. (D) Close-up view of the working end of the spoon excavator.

Procedure 18-1
Identify Cutting Instruments

This procedure is performed by the dental assistant to identify the hand cutting instruments, explain their function and numbering system, and list the procedure(s) where they are used.

Equipment and Supplies

- Angle formers
- Chisels
- Excavators
- Gingival margin trimmers
- Hatchets
- Hoes

Procedure Steps

1. Hold the instrument and examine the instrument closely.
2. Identify the instrument by name.
3. Explain the function of the instrument and how it is used.
4. Explain the numbering system identified on the instrument.
5. List the procedure(s) where the instrument may be used.

or come in one piece. Mirrors are available in various sizes and types (Figure 18-15). The mirror sizes are identified by number; the most commonly used are numbers 4 and 5. The mouth mirror may be sterilized (by autoclaving, dry heat, or cold chemical sterilizing) or may be disposable. The types of mirrors are the plane surface, front surface, and concave surface.

- *Plane or regular surface mirrors* have reflective surfaces (silver coatings) on the backs of the glass (Figure 18-15A). This gives the image a "ghost image" as the light reflects from the glass and the silver layer.
- *Front surface mirrors* have reflective coatings (rhodium) on top of the glass. This coating eliminates the "ghost image"; it reflects only once to give a clear view free of distortion (Figure 18-15B).
- *Concave surface mirrors* magnify the image.

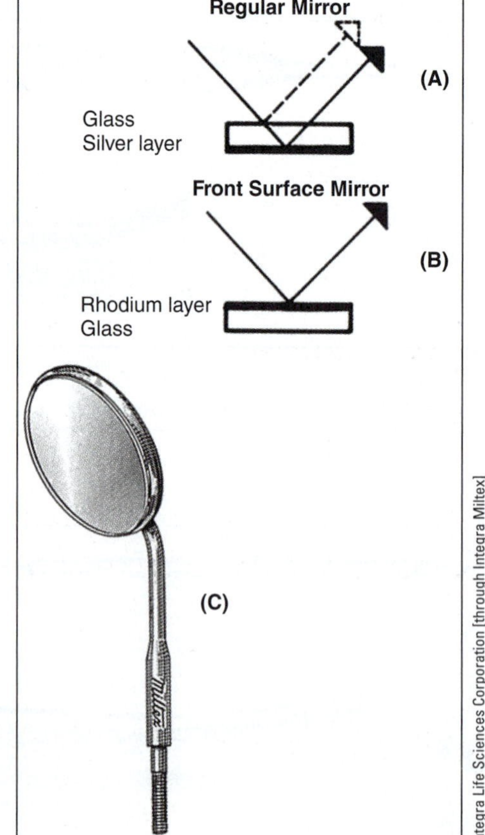

FIGURE 18-15

(A) Plane (regular) surface mirror. (B) Front surface mirror. (C) Cone socket mirror.

Uses of Mouth Mirror (Figures 18-16A-D)

- *Indirect vision*—When the operator uses a mirror to view areas of the oral cavity not seen with direct vision
- *Reflection of light*—Illumination of an area being examined or treated
- *Retraction*—When the cheeks or tongue is retracted for better visibility and for protection of the tissues
- *Transillumination*—Reflection of light through the tooth surface to detect fractures

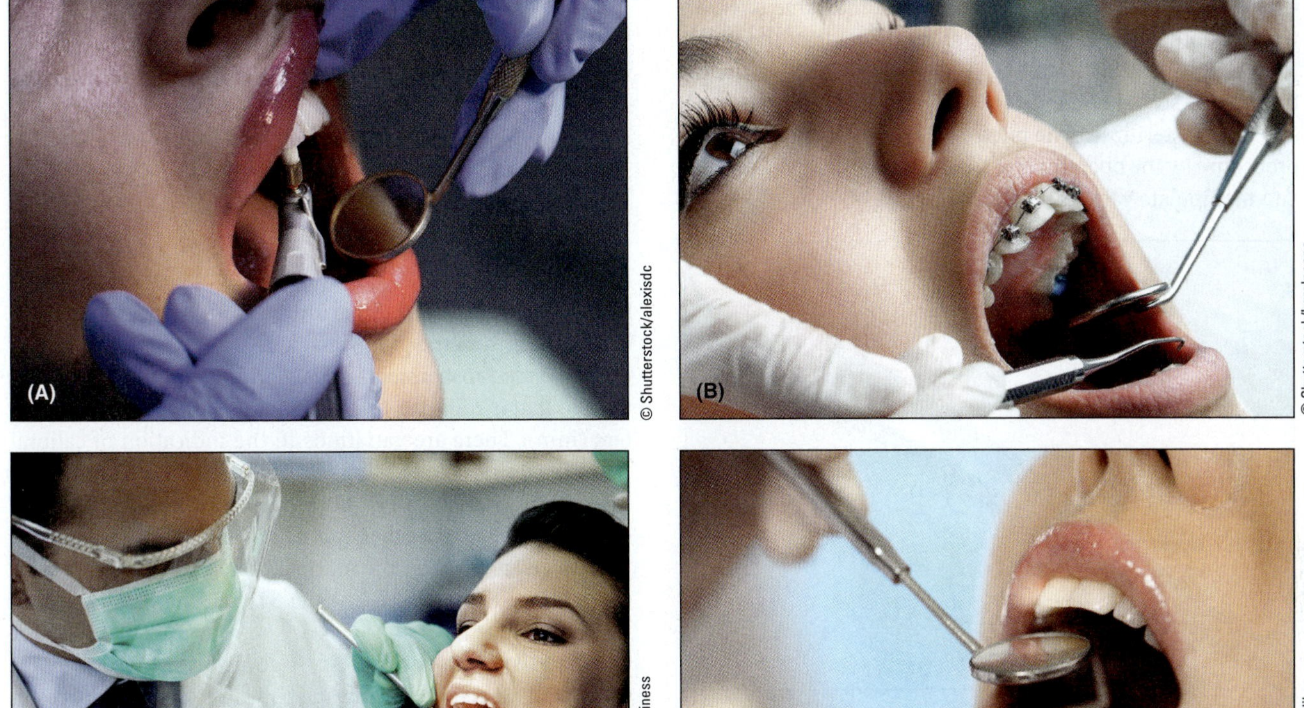

FIGURE 18-16

Uses of the mouth mirror. (A) Using the mouth mirror for indirect vision gives the operator a view of areas of the oral cavity not seen with direct vision. (B) Reflecting the light from the overhead dental light to illuminated areas in the oral cavity. (C) Retracting with the dental mirror to hold the tongue and/or cheeks away from the working area during a procedure. (D) Transillumination, is shown here with the mirror reflecting the light through a tooth surface as well as using reflection, retraction, and indirect vision.

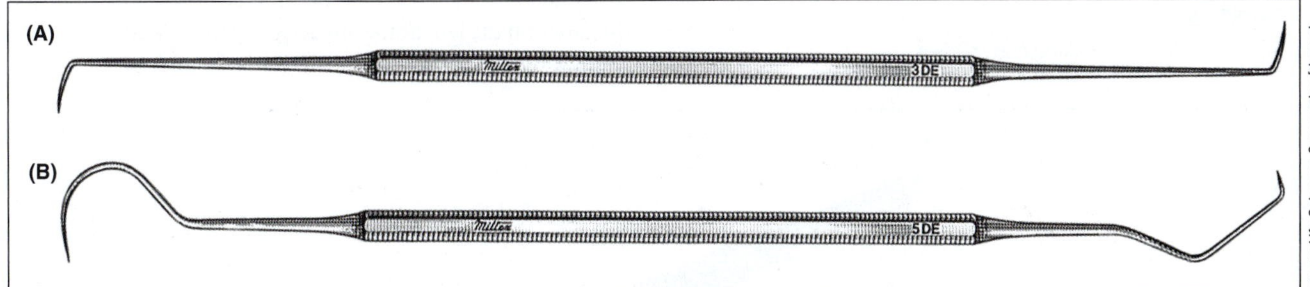

FIGURE 18-17

Types of explorers. (A) Pigtail. (B) Shepherd's hook and #17.

Explorers. An **explorer** is a single- or double-ended instrument. The working end is a thin, sharp point of flexible steel. This allows the operator to examine surfaces of the teeth to detect any irregularity. There are a variety of angles of explorers, and often the ends are different so that the operator can access various areas of the mouth. Several common shapes include the pig tail, shepherd's hook, right angle, and #17 (Figure 18-17).

Uses of Explorers

- *Examination of the tooth structure* for defects or areas of decay
- *Examination of restorations* to check for faulty margins or fractures
- *Removal of excess materials* from around the margins of restorations or from bases and liners in the cavity preparation

Cotton Pliers. A **cotton plier** is shaped like large tweezers with smooth surfaces or serrations on the ends of the beaks. They are available with locking or nonlocking handles, and the tips may be straight or angled. They are made of stainless steel and can be sterilized. The pliers are used frequently during a procedure by the operator and the dental assistant to transport and manipulate various materials (Figure 18-18).

Uses of Cotton Pliers

- *To place* and remove items from the oral cavity, such as cotton rolls, cotton pellets, wedges, and large pieces of debris
- *To grasp* and transfer materials to and from the oral cavity
- *To retrieve* materials from drawers, cupboards, and so on to avoid contamination

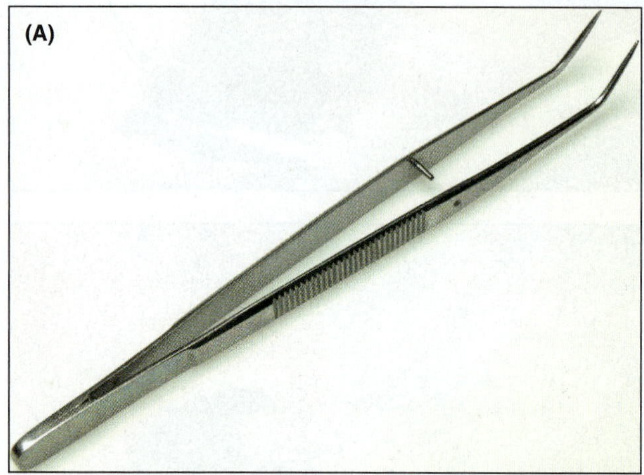

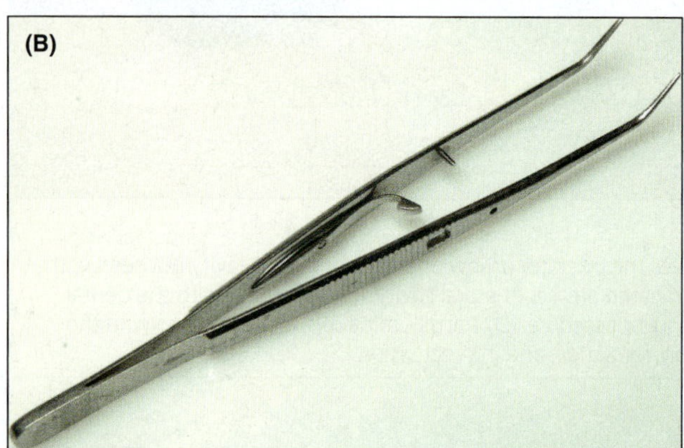

FIGURE 18-18
(A) Cotton pliers. (B) Locking cotton pliers.

Periodontal Probes. A **periodontal probe** is used to measure the depth of the gingival sulcus. They may be single- or double-ended instruments. The working end of the probe is a blade that is rounded or blunted and is marked in millimeters (mm). There are variations in the indication of calibrations, including color coding (Figure 18-19A). A combination instrument that has an explorer tip on one end and a periodontal probe on the other end is known as an *expro*. It is very functional and reduces the number of instruments on the tray (Figure 18-19B) (also see Chapter 31, Periodontics).

Composite Instruments. A **composite instrument** is used in all aspects of placing and finishing a composite restoration. They are double-ended instruments made of stainless steel or stainless steel with an anodized aluminum coating. The aluminum-titanum nitride (XTS) instruments are nonadhering, hard, and scratch resistant. An **XTS composite instrument** has ergonomically designed handles and black working ends for contrast with the tooth surface.

Composite instruments come in a wide variety of shapes that are designed for the different functions required when doing a composite filling. These include placement, condensing, carving, contouring, and burnishing the composite or other tooth-colored materials (Figure 18-20). The instruments may have the same shape on each end but different sizes or they may be designed so that one end is used on the right and the other on the left. Some are designed to be used on anterior restorations and others for posterior restorations.

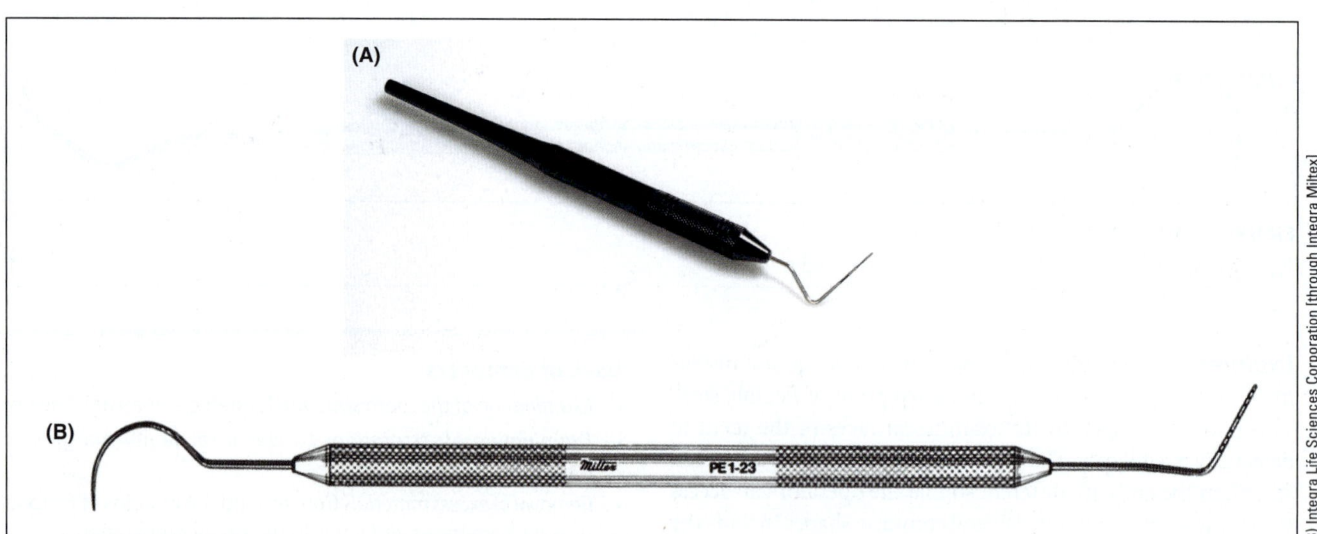

(B) Integra Life Sciences Corporation [through Integra Miltex]

FIGURE 18-19
(A) Periodontal probe. (B) Expro with explorer (1) and periodontal probe (2).

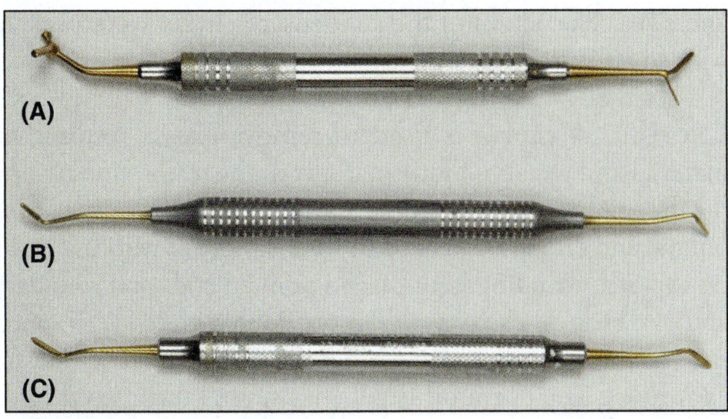

FIGURE 18-20

Composite Instruments. (A) IPC. (B) Tindilly - XTS. (C) Garrison's Universal.

The XTS composite instruments are not placed in the ultrasonic but are instead cleaned separately with mild detergent. Check the manufacturer's information.

Plastic Filling Instruments. A **plastic filling instrument** is used to place and condense pliable restorative materials and to place cement bases in the cavity preparation. These instruments are made of plastic or metal and are usually double-ended. One of the most common plastic instruments has a paddle on one end and a small condenser on the other end (Figure 18-21).

The **small-balled instrument/Dycal instrument** is usually a smaller instrument in size than the plastic filling instrument and has a small ball tip on the working end. It is used to place dental liners in the cavity preparation (Figure 18-21D).

Amalgam Carriers. An **amalgam carrier** is designed to carry and dispense amalgam or composite into the cavity preparation. The carriers may be single- or double-ended with small and large ends. Most carriers are made of stainless steel, and some have Teflon or coated barrels to prevent clogging. The dental assistant loads both ends of the carrier with the restorative material and either passes it to the operator or places the amalgam in the cavity preparation and then refills the carrier as needed (Figure 18-22A).

A spring-action **amalgam gun** is used to carry and place composites, glass ionomers, and amalgam alloys. It is single-ended and made of high-grade plastic (Figure 18-22B).

Amalgam Condensers (Pluggers). An **amalgam condenser**, or plugger, is used to pack amalgam into the cavity preparation. There are hand condensers and mechanical condensers. The hand condensers are usually double-ended and are available in a wide variety of working ends. The locations and designs of cavity preparations have required that condensers be diverse in design. The working ends may be plain (smooth) or serrated. They may be round, ovoid, rectangular, diamond, or cone shaped (Figure 18-23). The shanks of condensers may be monangled, binangled, or triple angled.

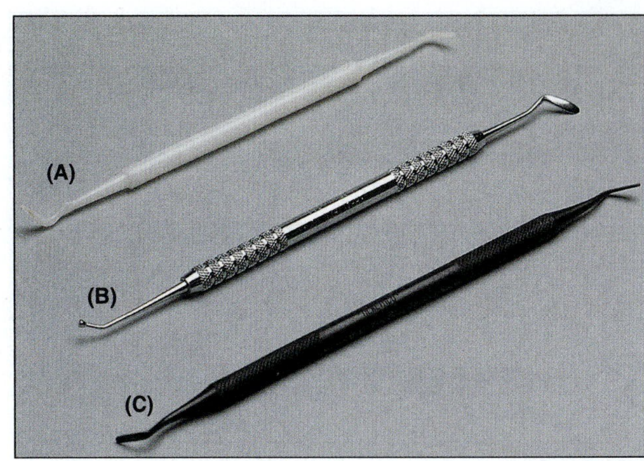

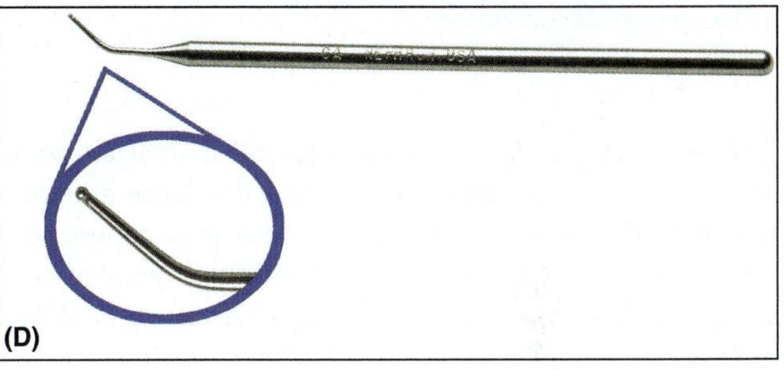

FIGURE 18-21

(A) Plastic filling instrument. (B) Woodson instrument. (C) Composite instrument. (D) Small-balled/Dycal instrument.

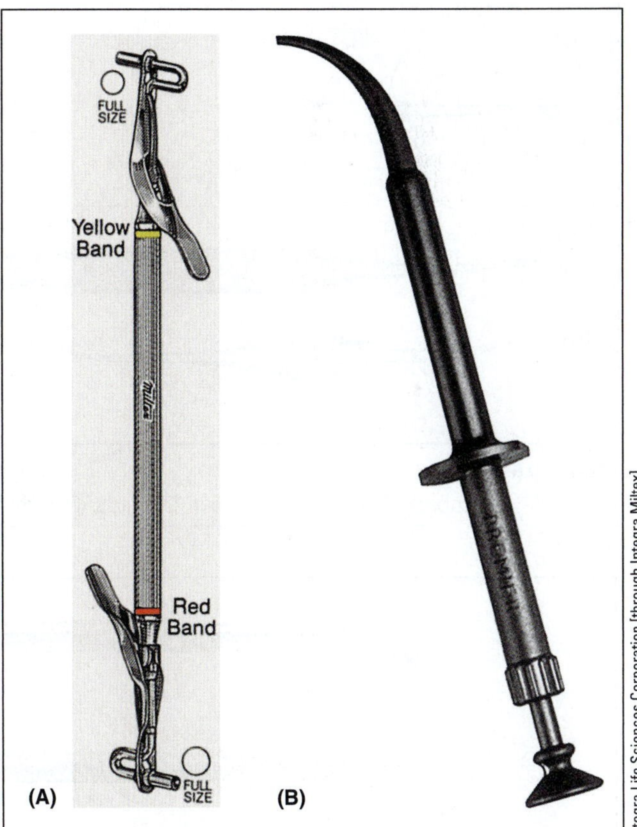

FIGURE 18-22

(A) Double-ended amalgam carrier. (B) Amalgam gun.

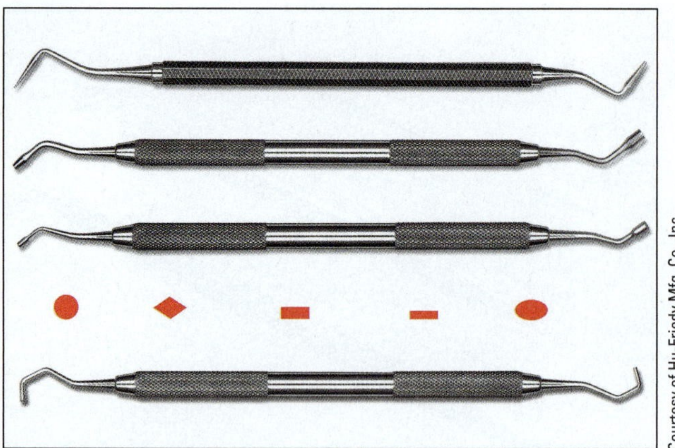

FIGURE 18-23
Various shapes of condensers.

Mechanical condensers, sometimes called amalgam packers or vibrators, are used to pack and condense amalgam through vibrations into the cavity preparation. These condensers are attached to the dental unit and operated with compressed air. Packing points come in a variety of shapes and sizes. The action of the condenser is like a woodpecker, with short, quick movements.

Carvers. A **carver** is used to remove excess restorative material and to carve tooth anatomy in the restoration before the material hardens. Carvers are also used to carve wax inlays, onlays, and crowns. There are a wide variety of working ends on carvers, including long-bladed pointed ends and rounded and oval shapes. Usually, carvers are double-ended with some ends having sharp edges and others rounded blades similar to excavators. The operator usually has several favorite carvers, which often include the Hollenback and the cleoid-discoid. The Hollenback is a long-bladed carver used to shape the restoration, and the cleoid-discoid carver is used to shape amalgam restorations. The cleoid end looks like a claw, and the discoid end is shaped like a round disc (Figure 18-24). The T-3 carver has one end shaped like a disc and the other end is a blade. It is used to remove excess restorative material and to carve and shape occlusal anatomy. Another carver is the Interproximal Carver Instrument (IPC) which has long thin blades on each end that is placed at different angles. It is used to trim excess filling material in the interproximal surface and to carve and smooth interproximal surfaces (Figures 18-25A and B).

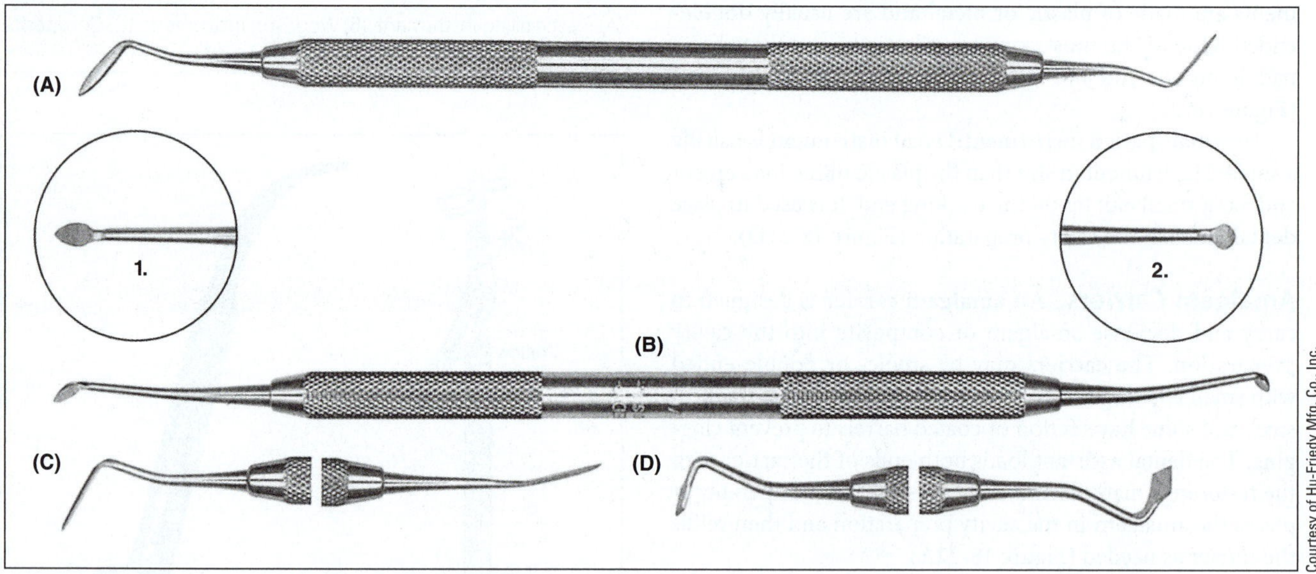

FIGURE 18-24
Carvers. (A) Hollenback. (B) 1. Cleoid; 2. Discoid. (C) Ward's. (D) Frahm.

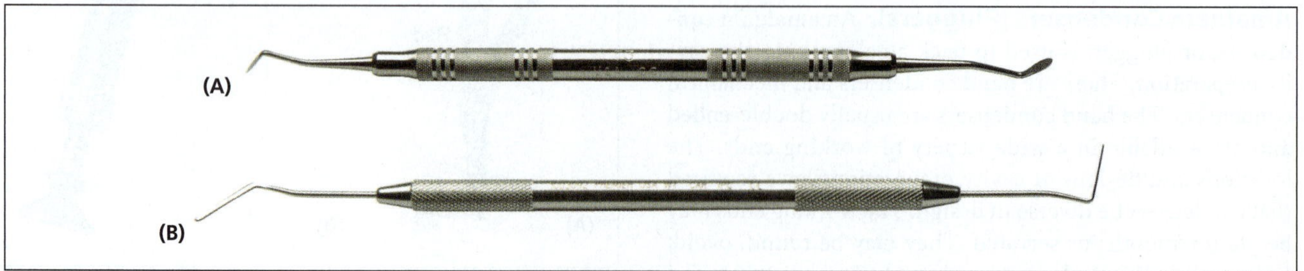

FIGURE 18-25
(A) T-3 carver. (B) IPC.

Burnishers. A **burnisher** is used to smooth rough margins of the restoration and to shape metal matrix bands. Burnishers are blunt, rounded instruments that come in a variety of shapes, including ball shaped, T-ball, and the acorn. The acorn burnishers are very popular to smooth composite and amalgam restorations. Burnishers may be single- or double-ended instruments (Figure 18-26A–F).

Files. A **file** is used to trim excess filling material and to smooth the restoration, especially the margins. They come in a variety of shapes, with a serrated surface on one side of the blade. The working end is often thin and small enough to reach interproximal spaces. Files are available as single- or double-ended instruments (Figure 18-27).

Finishing Knives. A **finishing knife** is used to trim excess filling material. The working ends of the finishing knives have sharp, knife-like blades. Finishing knives come in a variety of shapes and angles to access restoration margins (Figure 18-28).

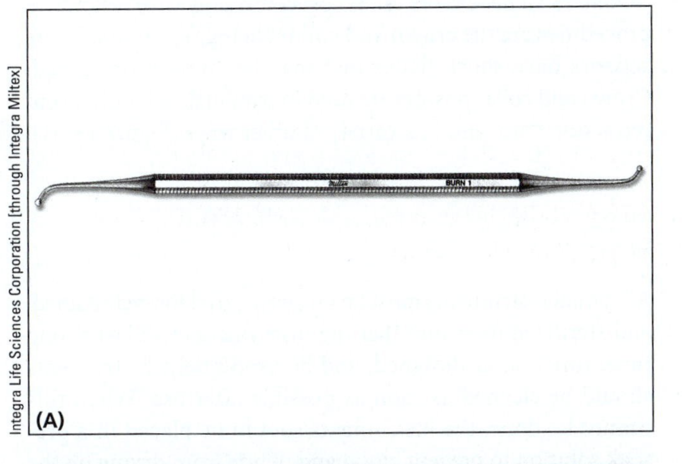

Integra Life Sciences Corporation [through Integra Miltex]

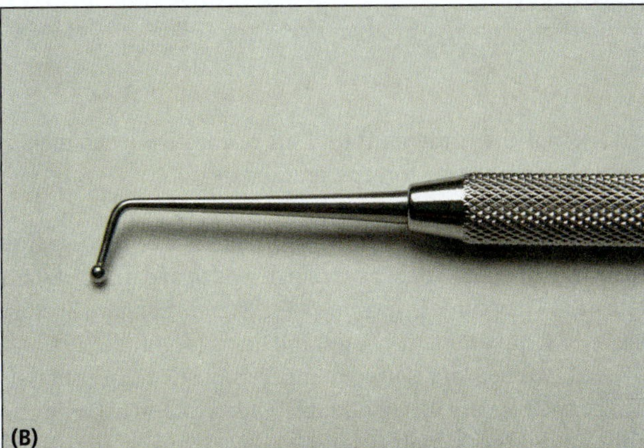

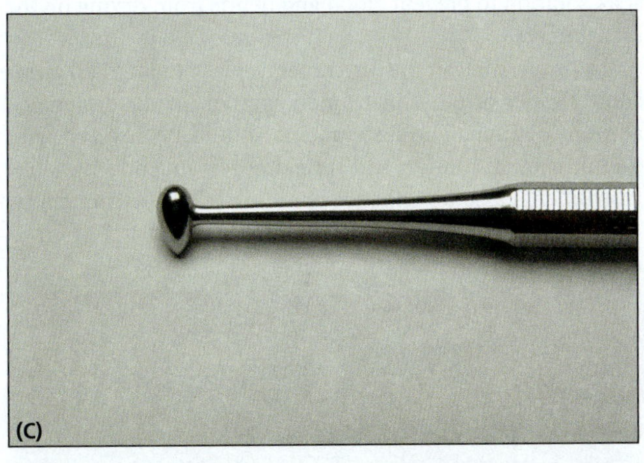

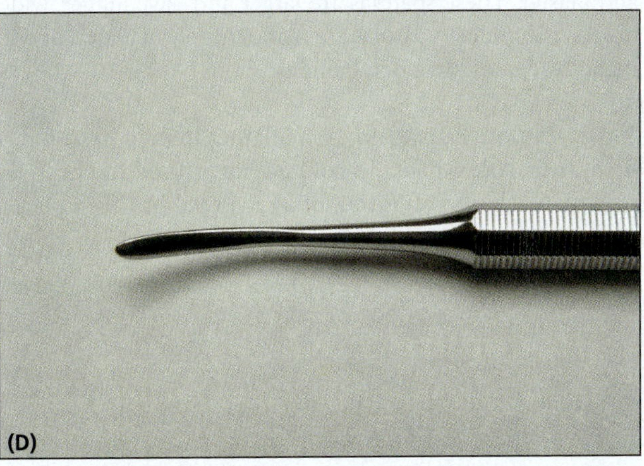

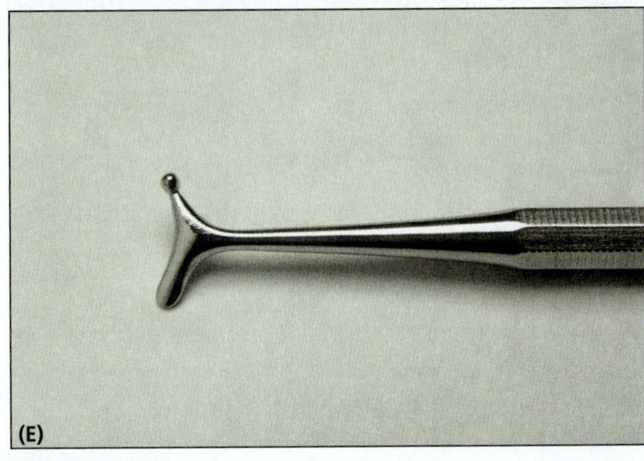

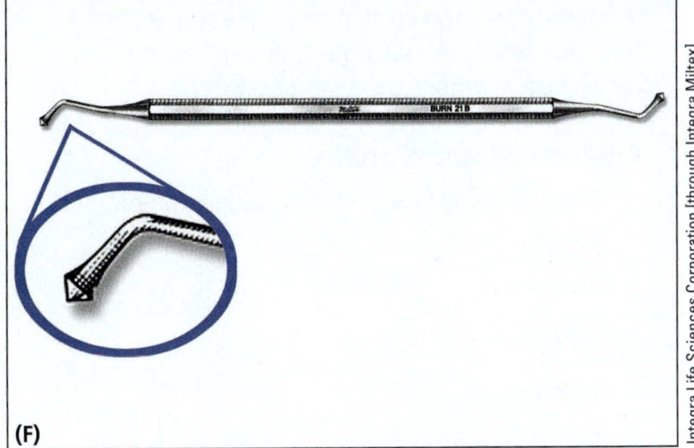

Integra Life Sciences Corporation [through Integra Miltex]

FIGURE 18-26
(A) Burnisher. (B) Ball burnisher. (C) Football burnisher. (D) Beaver tail burnisher. (E) T-Ball burnisher. (F) Acorn burnisher.

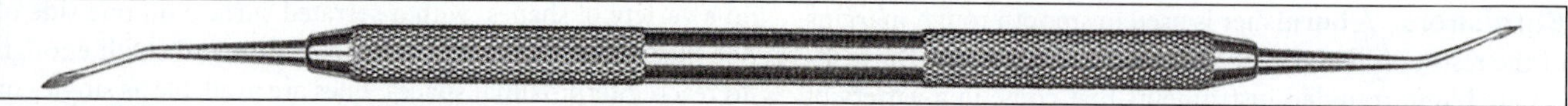

Courtesy of Hu-Friedy Mfg. Co., Inc.

FIGURE 18-27
File.

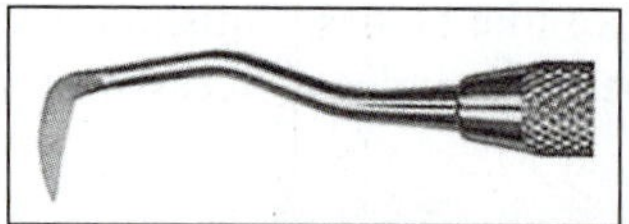

Courtesy of Hu-Friedy Mfg.Co., Inc.

FIGURE 18-28
Finishing knife.

Miscellaneous Instruments

Additional instruments found on restorative trays include spatulas, articulating forceps, and scissors.

Spatulas. During restorative procedures, a **cement spatula** may be used. These spatulas are single-ended and made of stainless steel. They come in a variety of sizes and strengths. Spatulas are used to mix cements, bases, and liners (Figure 18-29).

A **plastic spatula** is used to mix composite resin materials. These spatulas are usually double-ended and may be disposable. A **laboratory spatula** is used to mix impression materials and plaster. These spatulas are larger and have longer, wider blades. Laboratory spatulas are made entirely of plastic or with metal blades and wooden handles.

Articulating Forceps. Articulating forceps are used to hold articulation paper, a colored paper used to check the patient's occlusion after the filling material has been placed. The forceps are made of stainless steel or disposable plastic and are opened and closed by placing pressure on the handle (Figure 18-30). Sometimes cotton pliers, especially locking cotton pliers, are used in place of articulating forceps.

Scissors. The scissors used most commonly with restorative procedures are the **crown and collar (bridge) scissors.** These scissors have short blades that may be straight or curved. Crown and collar scissors are used to trim matrix bands, to cut retraction cord, and in a variety of other ways (Figure 18-31).

Instrument Care, Maintenance, and Sterilization

All dental instruments must be properly cared for, maintained, and sterilized to ensure that the instruments will last a long time, function as designed, and be used safely. Instruments should be cleaned as soon as possible after use. When this cannot be done, the instruments should be placed in a presoak solution to prevent blood and debris from drying on the instruments.

To properly clean the instruments, place them in an ultrasonic cleaner or other instrument washer for the designated amount of time. The instruments should be covered with the ultrasonic solution and spread out as much as possible. Instrument cassettes enhance handling of the instrument by

Procedure 18-2
Identify Non-Cutting Instruments

This procedure is performed by the dental assistant to identify the non-cutting instruments, explain their function, how the instrument is used, and list the procedure(s) where they are used.

Equipment and Supplies

- Basic instruments (mouth mirror, explorer, and cotton pliers)
- Burnishers
- Carriers
- Carvers
- Composite instruments
- Condensers
- Files
- Finishing knives
- Plastic filling instruments

Procedure Steps

1. Hold the instrument and examine the instrument closely.
2. Identify the instrument by name.
3. Explain the function of the instrument and how it is used.
4. List the procedure(s) the instrument may be used.

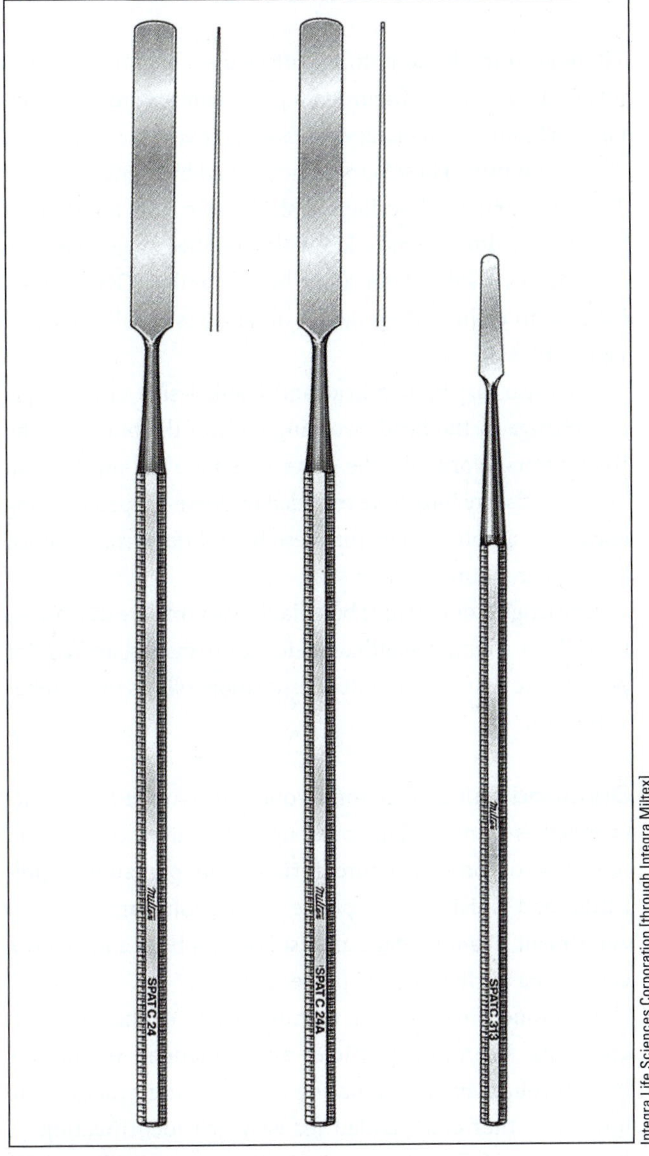

FIGURE 18-29
Cement spatulas.

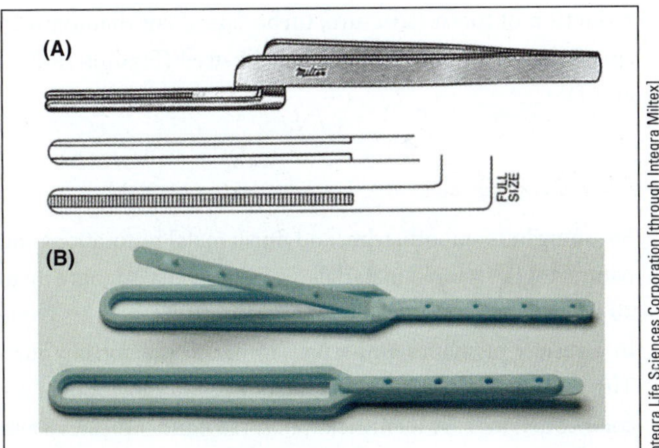

FIGURE 18-30
(A) Articulating forceps. (B) Disposable articulating forceps.

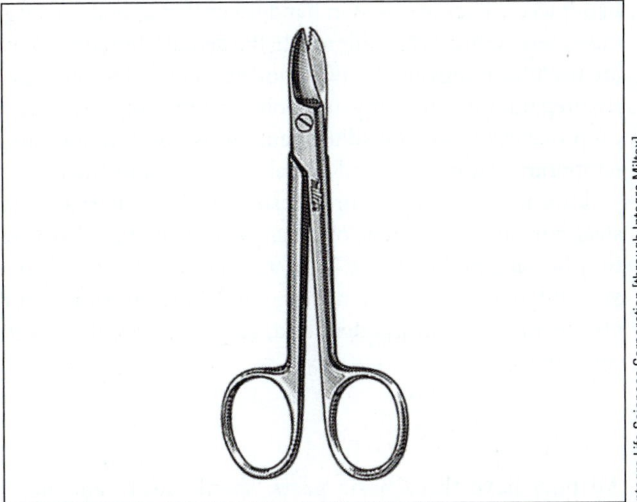

FIGURE 18-31
Straight crown and collar (bridge) scissors.

reducing the possibility of damage to the instrument and providing more organization and efficiency. The cassettes also reduce the risk of injury to the dental assistant during the cleaning and sterilization of the instruments.

Hinged instruments should always be cleaned and sterilized in the open position, because doing so prevents debris from gathering in the hinges and keeps the instruments functioning smoothly. Following the manufacturer's directions when lubricating hinged instruments after cleaning (but before sterilizing) will increase the longevity of the instruments.

When instruments are removed from the ultrasonic bath, they should be rinsed thoroughly under running water and then dried before being prepared for sterilization. After sterilization, instruments should be dried completely before being stored. When instruments are not dried before being stored, corrosion and staining could occur. When the sterilization bags in which the instruments are processed are not completely dry, they become a source of bacterial contamination and they also tear more easily. In some cases, this would mean that the instruments should be resterilized. For more information, refer to Chapter 11, Infection Control.

The dental assistant should examine all instruments carefully. Check for corrosion, stains, broken tips, and sharpness. Check that hinged instruments open and close smoothly and have no excess lubricant near the hinges. This evaluation step allows time for the manufacturer's recommended maintenance and/or for replacement instruments to be ordered.

Dental Rotary Instruments

A dental **bur** is part of a group of instruments referred to as **rotary instruments**. Rotary instruments also include discs and stones and are designed to be used with dental handpieces. They are used in handpieces that operate at various speeds, both at chairside and in the dental laboratory. Burs are used for removing decay, removing old restorations, cavity preparations, finishing and polishing restorations, surgical procedures, occlusal adjustments, finishing and polishing temporary restorations, and dental appliance adjustments.

Burs are made of steel or tungsten carbide materials. The steel burs are not used as often as the carbide burs because they become dull very fast. Tungsten carbide burs are stronger and remain sharper during cavity preparations. Bur groups include cutting, diamond, surgical, laboratory, and finishing.

Parts of the Bur

All burs have three basic parts: shank, neck, and head (Figure 18-32A).

Shank. The shank of the bur is inserted into the handpiece. To accommodate various dental handpieces, there are three styles of bur shanks (Figure 18-32B):

- The **straight shank** (designated HP when ordering), or long shank, functions with the straight, low-speed handpiece.
- The **latch-type shank** (designated RA) is shorter than the straight-shanked burs. On the latch-type shank is a notch that fits into the contra-angle/right-angle handpiece and latches securely in place.
- The **friction-grip shank** (designated FG) is short, small, and smooth. These burs are used in friction-grip, high-speed handpieces.

Neck. The neck of the bur is the tapered connection of the shank to the head.

Head. The head is the working end of the bur. There are many shapes and sizes of heads on dental burs. A variety of burs are needed to perform the multiple tasks in restoring teeth and in specialty procedures.

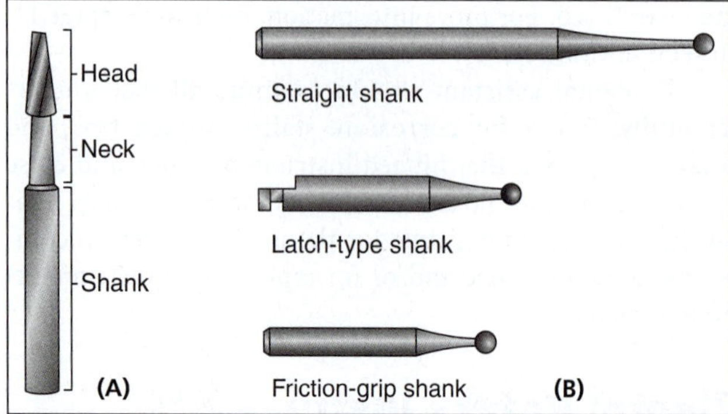

FIGURE 18-32

(A) Parts of a bur. (B) Different shanks: straight, latch type, and friction grip.

Cutting Burs

There are nine basic cutting bur shapes, including round, inverted cone, plain fissure straight, plain fissure cross-cut, tapered fissure straight, tapered fissure cross-cut, end-cutting, wheel, and pear. These burs are identified by number ranges. The bur numbers describe the shape, size, and variation of the bur. It is important to know the number ranges, because dentists often will ask for a bur by its number. Cutting burs have six to eight cutting blades or surfaces (Table 18-1 and Figure 18-33).

Burs also vary in both head and shank design. An example of a change in the head (working end) of the bur is on the fissure burs. Normally, the fissure burs are flat on the end, but some fissure burs have rounded or dome-shaped working ends. The number range for these burs differs from that for the regular fissure burs.

The lengths of the three bur shanks vary and are designated by an *L* for a longer length, an *S* for short shanks, and a *P* for pedodontic shanks. The letter designation follows the number of the bur.

Diamond Burs. Diamond rotary instruments are categorized as diamond burs or stones. They are used for rapid reduction of tooth structure during cavity preparation, polishing and finishing composite restorations, and occlusal adjustment. Diamond burs are also used for bone and gingival contouring during surgical procedures.

Diamond burs come in a wide variety of shapes, sizes, and grits. Diamond particles are embedded in the bur head through an electroplating or a bonding process. The burs are either color coded for easy grit identification or have letters following the bur numbers to indicate the grit (Figures 18-34A and B). These burs may be specifically designed for a certain procedure, such as finishing, trimming, or composite restorations. For increased cutting reduction of tooth structure, turbo/speed cut diamonds in spiral shape or dual cross cut may be used (Figures 18-34C and D).

Finishing Burs

Finishing burs smooth, trim, and finish metal restorations and natural tooth–colored materials. Finishing burs can have up to 30 blades ("flutes") for ultra-fine finishing. These burs come in a variety of shapes and sizes, similar to the cutting burs. They are identified by the manufacturer's number. Some are color coded for easy identification. A red band indicates 8 and 12 blades on the finishing bur. A yellow band indicates 16 and 20 blades, and a white band indicates a 30-blade finishing bur (Figure 18-35).

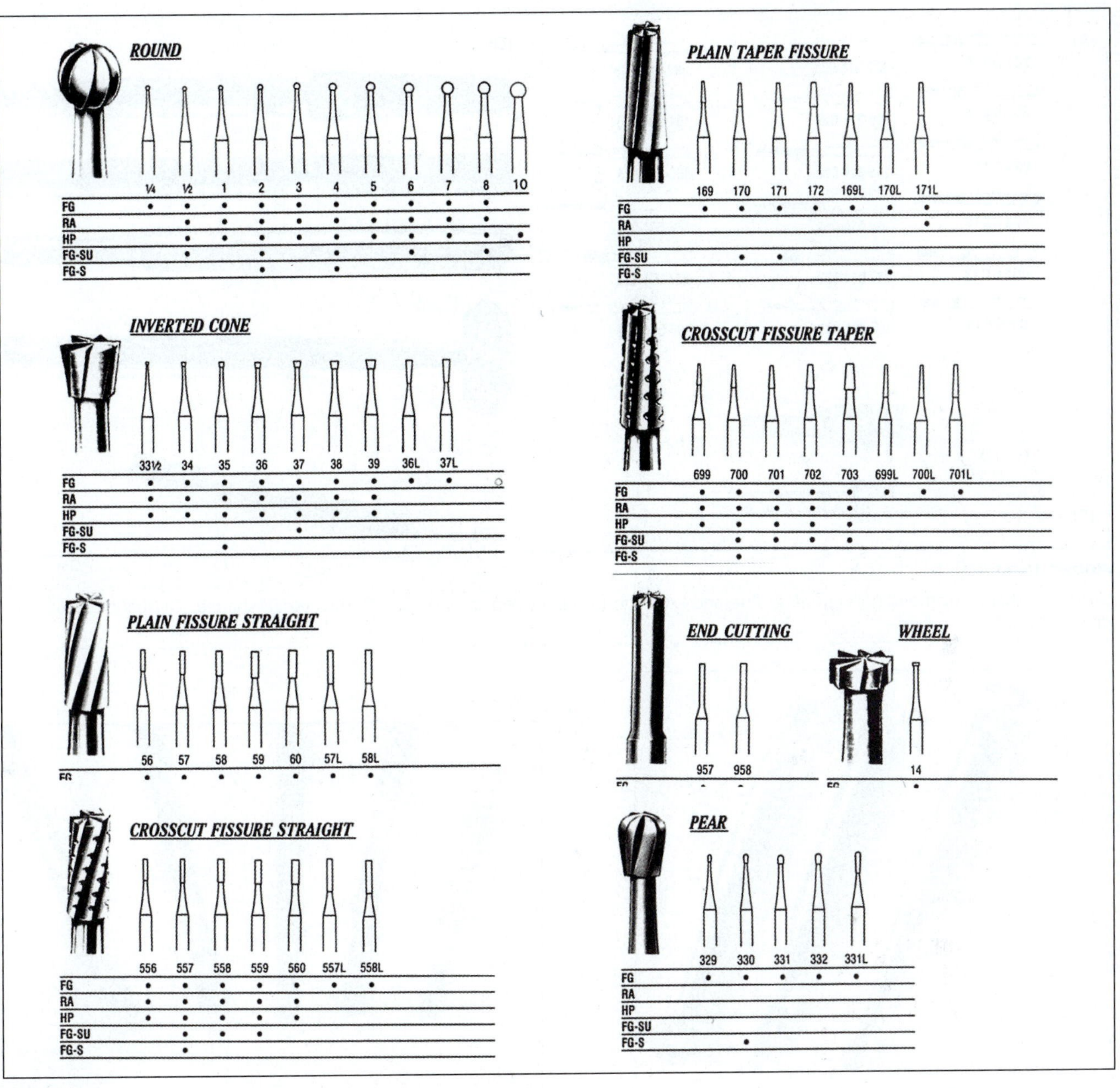

Integra Life Sciences Corporation (through Integra Miltex)

FIGURE 18-33

Bur shapes and number ranges.

Surgical Burs

Surgical burs are used in a low-speed handpiece to reduce and contour the alveolar bone and tooth structure. The heads of surgical burs come in various sizes and shapes and have long shanks (Figure 18-36).

Laboratory Burs

Laboratory burs are used to adjust acrylic materials, such as partials, dentures, and custom trays. They are also used on plaster, stone, and metal materials. Laboratory burs have long shanks and large working ends. These burs come in a variety of sizes and shapes. Sometimes they are referred to as a **vulcanite** or **acrylic bur** (Figure 18-37).

Fissurotomy Burs

Fissurotomy burs are extremely small (0.33 mm). Made of carbide, they are used to explore the occlusal surface and to allow for effective diagnoses and treatment while preserving healthy tooth structure. These burs cut quickly, leaving a smooth, minimally invasive groove in suspicious pits and fissures. Fissurotomy burs are designed as depth gauges, giving the burs minimal access to the fissures and permitting virtually pain-free fissure cavity preparation (Figure 18-38).

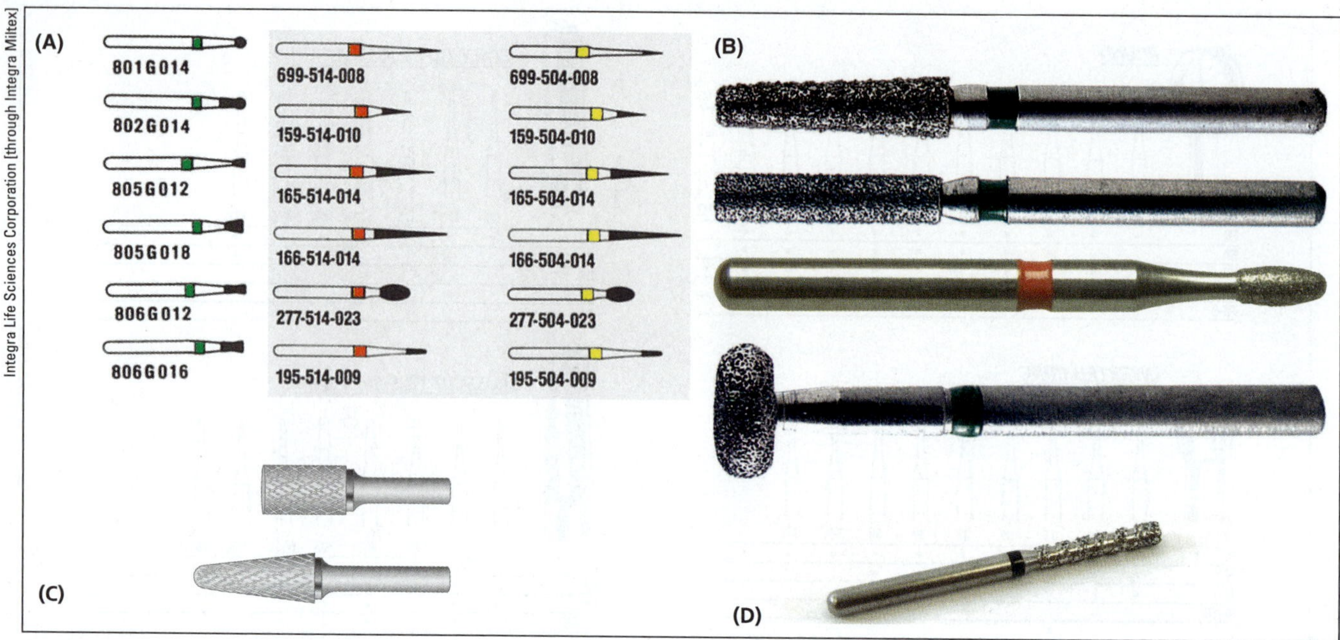

Integra Life Sciences Corporation [through Integra Miltex]

FIGURE 18-34

(A) Various shaped diamond burs in: coarse, fine, and extra fine. (B) Variety of diamond burs. (C) Turbo spiral shaped. (D) Dual-crosscut diamond burs.

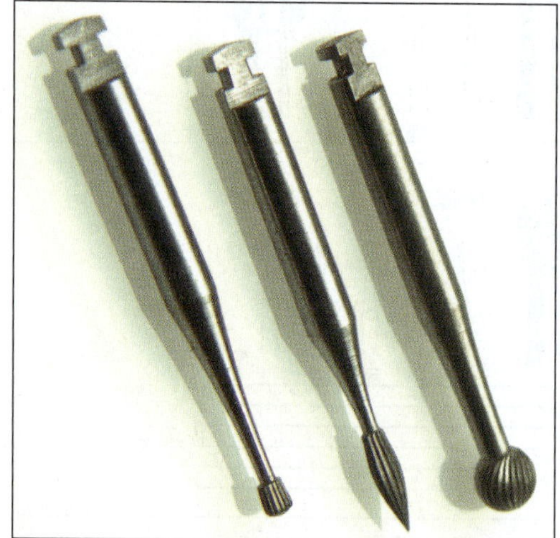

FIGURE 18-35

Finishing burs in various shapes.

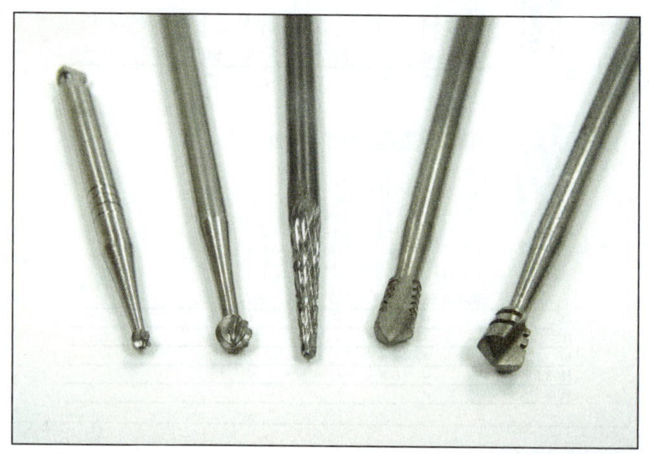

FIGURE 18-36

Surgical burs.

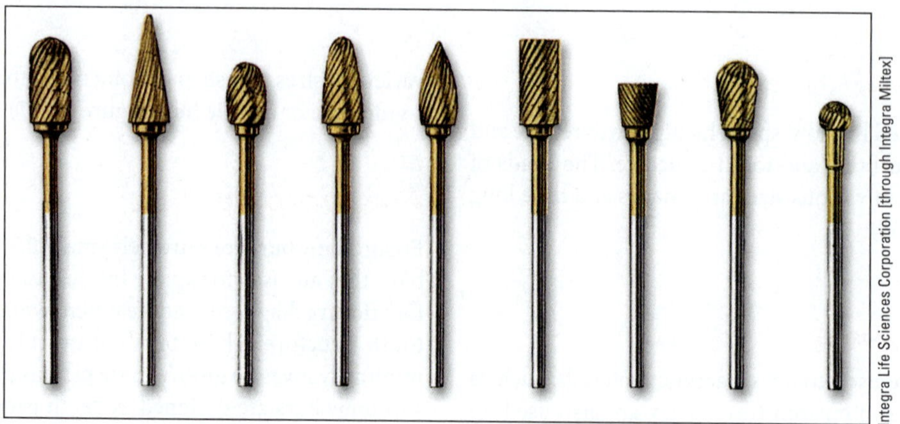

Integra Life Sciences Corporation [through Integra Miltex]

FIGURE 18-37

Laboratory burs.

TABLE 18-1 Burs and Their Functions

Name	Function	
Round bur	Used first to open the cavity and remove carious tooth structure.	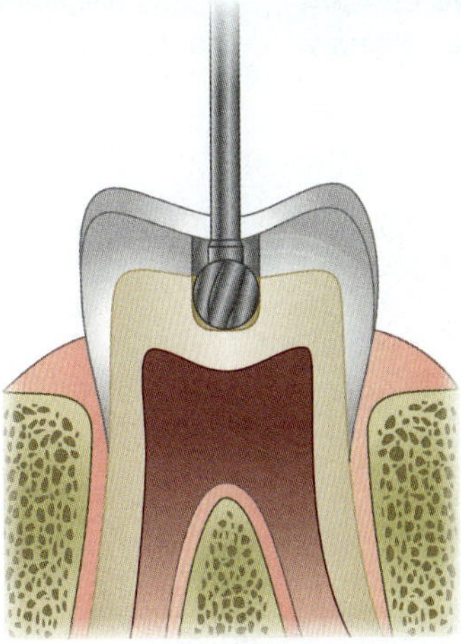
Inverted cone bur	Removes caries and makes undercuts in the preparation.	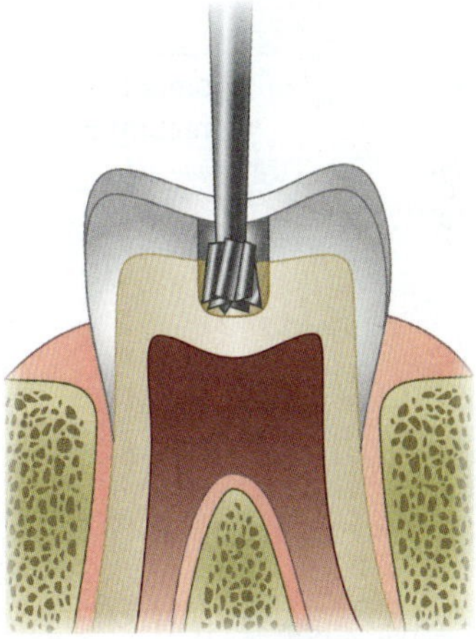
Plain fissure straight bur and plain fissure cross-cut bur	Forms the cavity walls of the preparation.	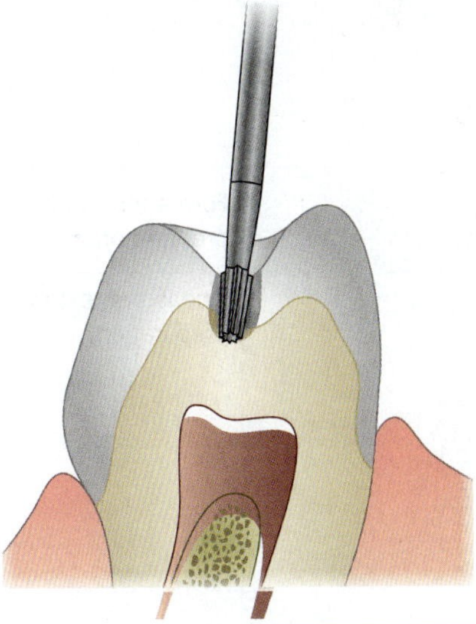

(continues)

TABLE 18-1 Burs and Their Functions (continued)

Name	Function	
Tapered fissure straight bur and tapered fissure cross-cut bur	Forms divergent walls of the cavity preparation.	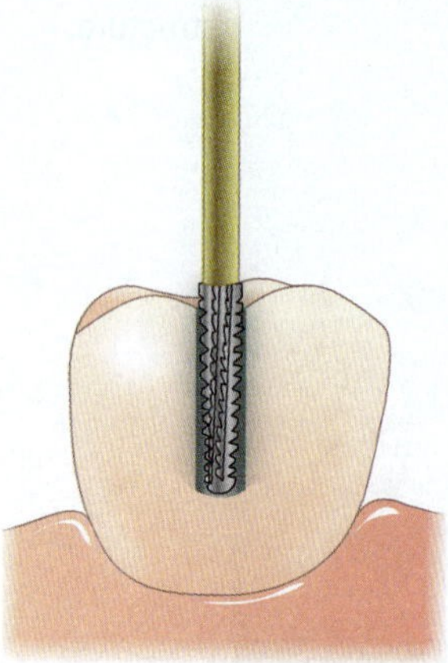
End-cutting bur	Forms the shoulder for crown preparations.	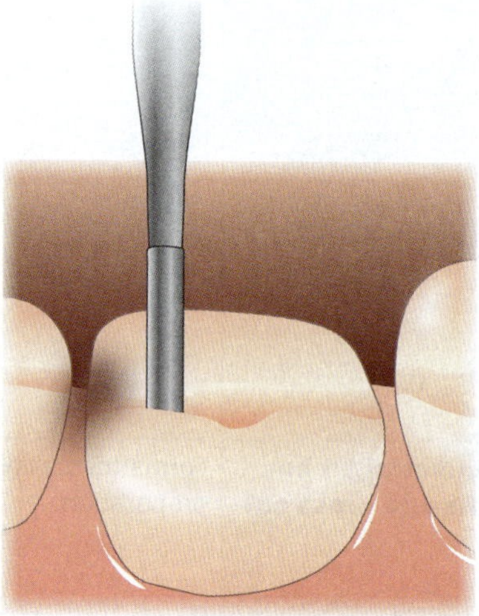
Wheel bur	Forms retention in preparations.	
Pear bur	Opens and extends the cavity preparation.	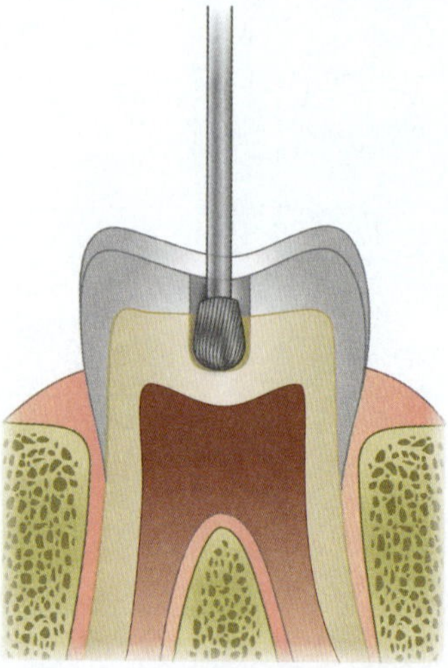

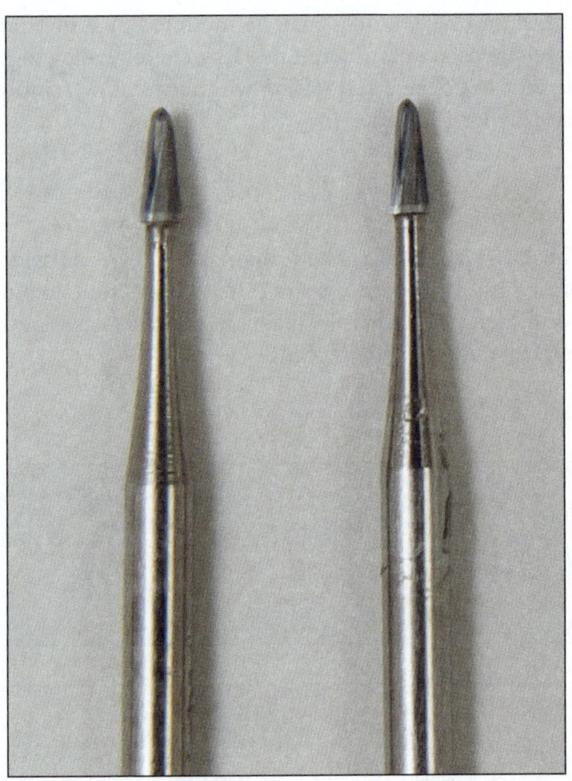

FIGURE 18-38

Fissurotomy burs.

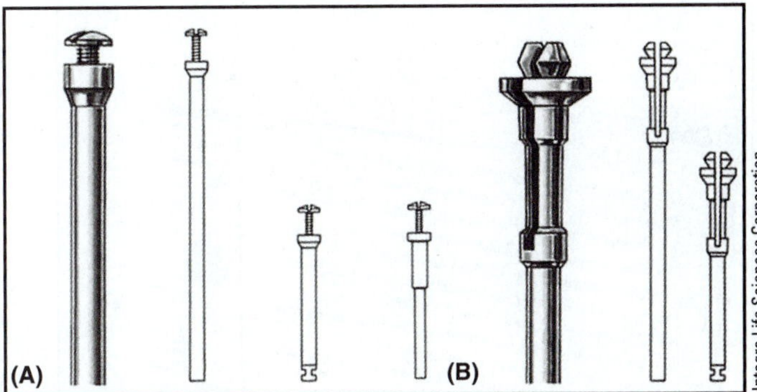

FIGURE 18-39

Mandrels with different heads and shanks. (A) Screw-type mandrels. (B) Snap-on mandrels.

Abrasive Rotary Instruments

An **abrasive rotary instrument** is a non-bladed instrument used to finish and polish restorations and appliances. Some abrasives are also used for cutting. Abrasives come in a wide variety and are categorized by their shapes, such as discs, points, and wheels. Abrasives are also categorized by the materials they are made of, such as rubber, stone, and sandpaper. Some restorative materials come with select abrasives that are designed to give the restoration a premium finish.

Mandrels

A **mandrel** is a rod (they come in various lengths) used in low-speed handpieces with various abrasives. The abrasives are either permanently attached (mounted) to a mandrel or separate and placed on a mandrel (unmounted). Mandrels are available in three shanks: latch, friction grip, or straight. The head of the mandrel, where the abrasives attach, is available in snap-on, screw-on, or pin designs (Figures 18-39A and B).

Discs

Discs are used to polish, smooth, and adjust restorative materials and dental appliances. Discs are circular, abrasive instruments that are usually designed to be mounted to mandrels. The abrasive agents are bonded on one or both sides of paper, metal, or plastic. The discs may be rigid or flexible, and are available in a variety of sizes and grits. The abrasive material may be made of several different materials, such as garnet, diamond, quartz, sand, and carborundum. When ordering abrasives, the size, grit, abrasiveness, and mandrel type must be specified.

Sandpaper Discs. Sandpaper discs are used to finish and polish all types of restorations and appliances. They are available in a wide variety of sizes, grits, and abrasive materials, including garnet, sand, emery, and cuttlefish. These materials are mounted on one side of the paper disc. Sandpaper discs are flexible and are applied to surfaces on one side only. They come with metal or pin-hole centers (Figure 18-40).

Diamond Discs. Diamond discs have diamond particles or chips bonded to both sides of steel discs. They are used for rapid cutting.

Carborundum Discs. A **carborundum disc**, also known as a **Jo-dandy disc** and **separating disc**, is a thin, brittle disc that breaks easily. They are double-sided and are used primarily in the dental laboratory to cut and finish gold restorations, but they can be used intraorally as well (Figures 18-41A and B).

Cuttlefish. Cuttlefish (cuttlebone) comes in a variety of shapes. It adheres to discs, points, and wheels and is used for finishing and polishing restorations (Figure 18-42A).

Stones

Stones are available in many sizes, shapes, and grits, similar to discs. They are used for cutting, polishing, and finishing amalgam, gold, composite, and porcelain restorations. Stones are used in the laboratory to adjust and polish appliances

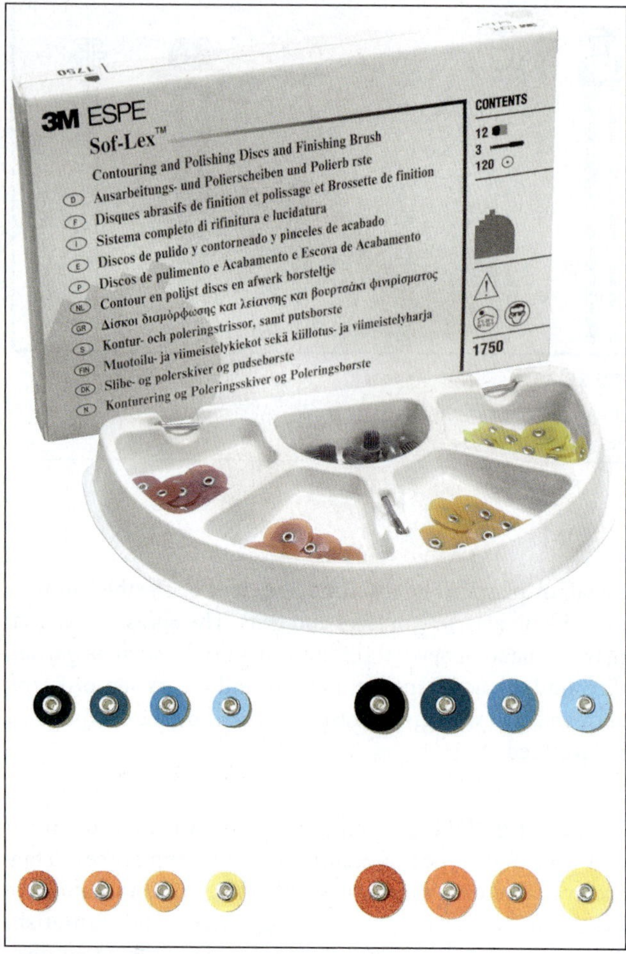

Courtesy of 3M ESPE Dental

FIGURE 18-40

Sandpaper discs in various shapes, types, and grits.

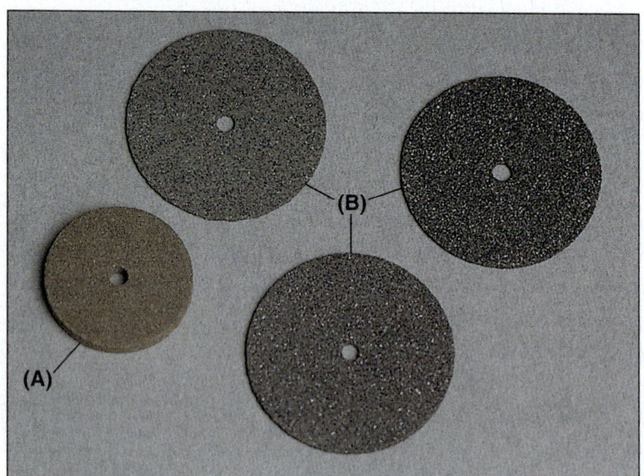

FIGURE 18-41

(A) Rubber wheel. (B) Carborundum discs.

and custom trays. The type of abrasive material and the grit control the cutting or polishing action of the stone. The abrasive materials include silicon carbide, garnet, and aluminum oxide. Stones may be mounted or unmounted. Some stones are considered heatless, thereby allowing the operator to polish a restoration without creating **frictional heat** (Figure 18-42B).

Rubber Wheels

Wheels are made of rubber material impregnated with an abrasive agent (Figures 18-41–18-43). They come mounted and unmounted and are available in various grits. They are used for finishing and polishing.

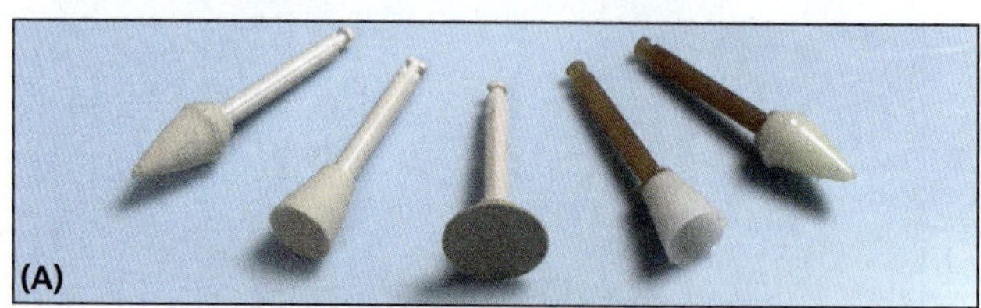

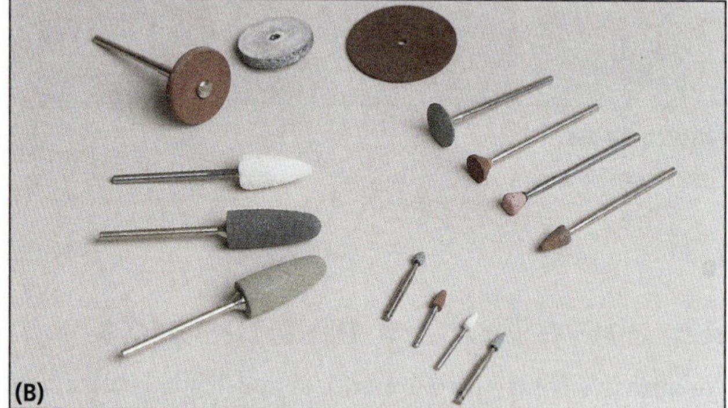

FIGURE 18-42

(A) Various points, cups, and wheels to define, polish, and finish composite restorations. (B) Various types and grits of stones, wheels, and points.

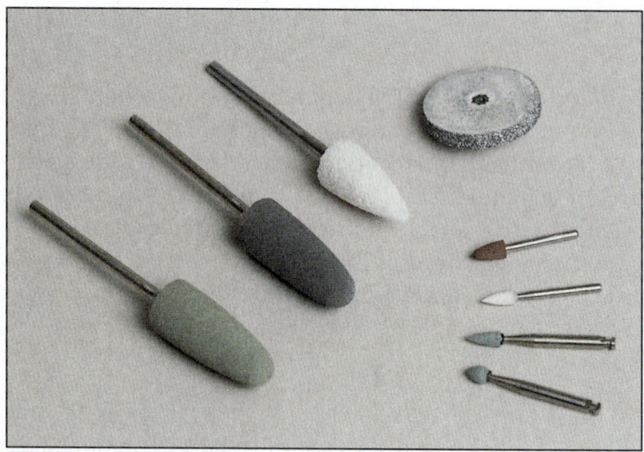

FIGURE 18-43

Wheel and points.

Rubber Points

Rubber points come in a variety of sizes and grits. They are made of rubber material impregnated with abrasive agents. Points are used to polish and are especially adaptable when defining anatomy in the restoration (Figures 18-42 and 18-43). Rotary instruments are sterilized or disposed of after each use in the oral cavity. Burs that are sterilized are first scrubbed or placed in an ultrasonic unit to remove debris from the blades; when debris remains between the blades, a wire brush is used to remove the embedded materials. The burs are then rinsed and sterilized according to the manufacturer's instructions.

Bur Blocks

Rotary instruments are stored in a **bur block**. There are many variations and designs, such as round or rectangular shapes. Bur blocks come with covers and may be magnetic. Both friction-grip and latch-type burs can be stored in bur blocks. They are made of metal or plastic (Figure 18-44).

Some bur blocks can be sterilized with the burs they hold. If the bur blocks cannot be sterilized, the burs are placed in a mesh holder that looks like a tea strainer. The burs are placed in this holder and run through the ultrasonic cleaner, and then placed in the sterilizer.

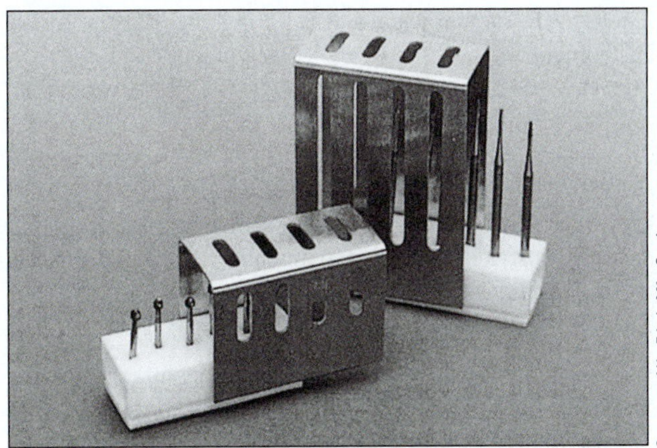

Courtesy of Hu-Friedy Mfg. Co., Inc.

FIGURE 18-44
Bur block with covers, magnetized and made of metal.

Dental Handpieces

A wide variety of dental handpieces are available to meet the needs of dental procedures, both in the oral cavity and in the laboratory. Handpieces are used to remove dental decay and to prepare the tooth for a restoration; to polish the teeth; to polish and finish dental restorations; and to cut, finish, and polish dental appliances, models, and trays. Review Procedure 18-4: Identify Dental Handpieces, Demonstrate Attaching

Procedure 18-3
Identification of dental rotary instruments and abrasives

This procedure is performed by the dental assistant to identify the rotary instruments and abrasives, identify their category, and explain their function.

Equipment and Supplies

- Cutting burs
- Diamond burs
- Finishing burs
- Surgical burs
- Laboratory burs
- Fissurotomy burs
- Abrasives
- Mandrels
- Discs
- Stones
- Rubber wheels
- Points

Procedure Steps

1. Hold the instrument and examine the instrument closely.
2. Identify the instrument by name.
3. Explain the function of the instrument and how it is used.
4. List the procedure(s) where the instrument may be used.

Them to the Dental Unit, and Selecting and Placing Rotary Instrument.

The Parts of the Dental Handpiece

All dental handpieces have the following basic parts:

- *Working end (head)*—Where burs, discs, stones, and other rotary instruments and attachments are held and the cutting and polishing are accomplished.
- *Shank*—The handle portion of the handpiece.
- *Connection end*—Where the handpiece attaches to the power source. The forward and reverse controls may be located here.

Dental handpieces are often divided into two categories: **high-speed handpieces** and **low-speed handpieces**. The high-speed handpieces operate at up to 450,000 **revolutions per minute (rpm)** and higher (Figure 18-45A). The low-speed handpieces operate up to 30,000 rpm (Figure 18-45B).

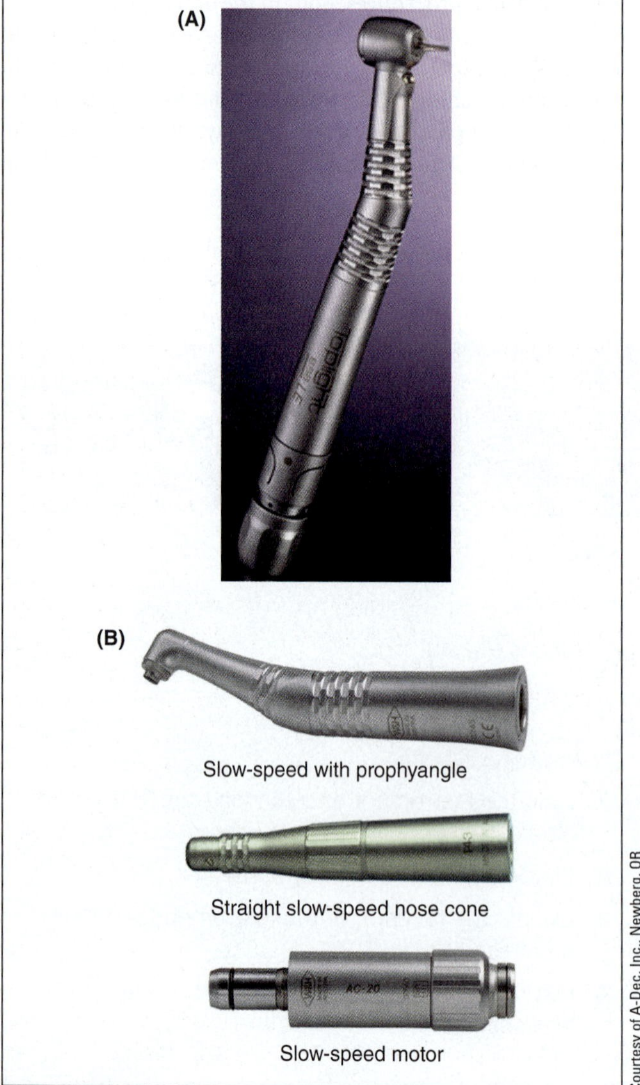

FIGURE 18-45

(A) High-speed handpiece. (B) Low-speed handpiece.

High-Speed Handpiece

The high-speed handpiece is used to rapidly cut tooth structure and finish restorations. Because of the high speed of this handpiece, frictional heat is produced. Frictional heat can cause pulpal damage to the tooth, so to reduce the frictional heat of the handpiece, a coolant such as air, water, or an air–water spray is used. These coolants also provide the operator with better vision by removing debris and tooth structure from the preparation.

The high-speed handpiece design is a smooth, one-piece design, usually a **contra-angle**, with the head slightly angled to the shank of the handpiece (Figure 18-46A). The high-speed handpiece does not hold any attachments but does hold burs and other rotary instruments. To hold these rotary instruments, the head of the handpiece has a small, metal cylinder called a **chuck**. The chuck holds the shank portion of the bur in place. To tighten or loosen the chuck, either a bur tool/wrench or a button/release lever on the back of the head of the handpiece is used (Figure 18-46B). The manufacturer provides the specific bur tool with the handpiece (Figure 18-46C). The head of the handpiece comes in standard and pediatric sizes. The pediatric handpiece is used for easier access with children and adults with small mouths.

The power source for the dental handpiece comes from the dental unit. Compressed air drives the turbines in the handpiece. To activate and control the speed of the handpiece, a **rheostat** (foot control) is operated, much like the accelerator on a car.

High-speed handpieces are available with a **fiber-optic light source**. Fiber-optic systems greatly improve visibility of the treatment area for the operator. The fiber-optic light is carried along optical bundles in the tubing of the handpiece. The light source is either a separate control box or a bulb behind the handpiece in the dental unit.

Low-Speed Handpiece

The low-speed handpiece is often referred to as the straight handpiece because the shank and head are in a straight line. These handpieces are used in both the dental operatory and the laboratory. At the dental unit, the low-speed handpiece is used to polish teeth and restorations, remove soft carious material, and define cavity margins and walls.

In the dental laboratory, this handpiece is used to adjust, finish, and polish appliances. Usually, the low-speed handpiece does not have or need a water supply, but in some procedures the dental assistant periodically applies air or water to the tooth or restoration to prevent any heating of the tooth.

The low-speed handpiece is a little bulkier than the high-speed handpiece. The straight handpiece is used with long-shank rotary instruments, such as burs, discs and stones, and with attachment heads such as the contra-angle and the right-angle (Figures 18-47A–D).

- The contra-angles are usually latch type, but they also come in friction grip. The contra-angles hold burs, discs, stones, rubber cups, and brushes for intraoral and extraoral procedures.

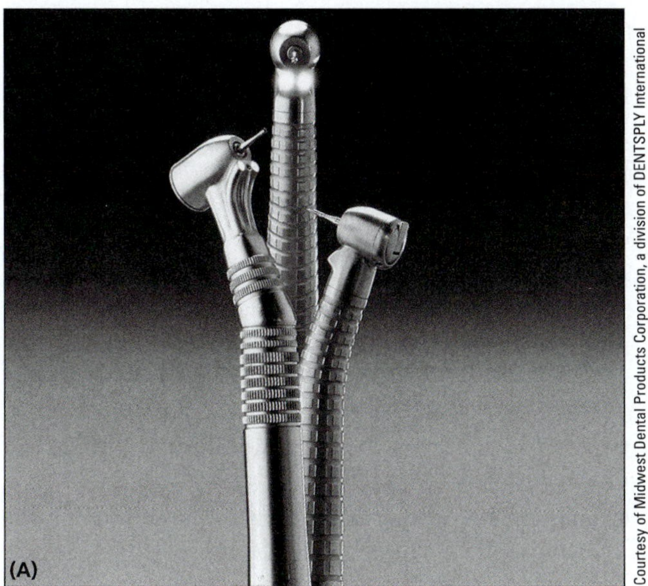

(A)
Courtesy of Midwest Dental Products Corporation, a division of DENTSPLY International

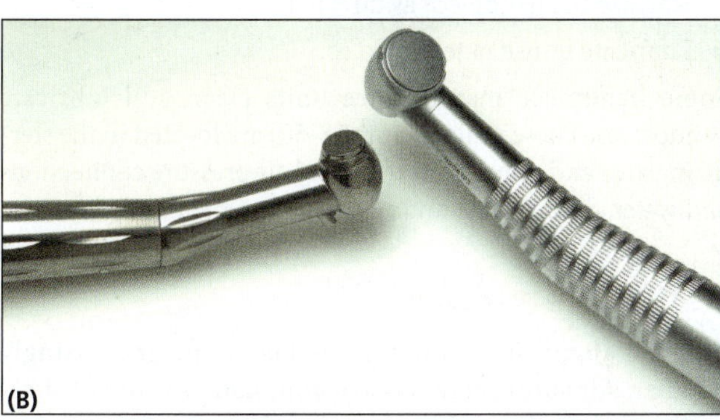

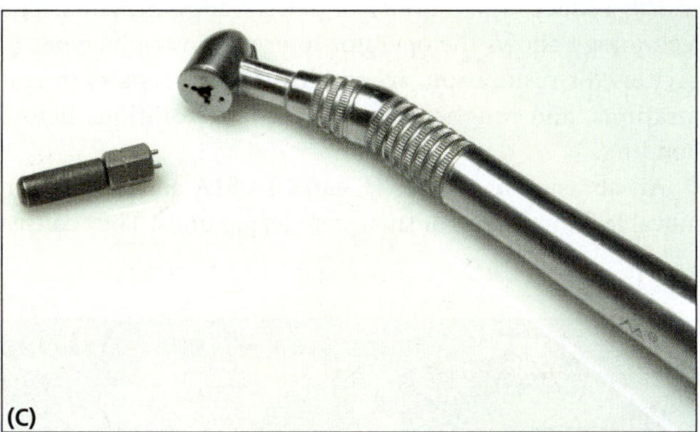

FIGURE 18-46

(A) High-speed handpieces with fiber optics. (B) High-speed handpieces with push-button back to place and remove the bur. (C) Handpiece with a bur tool to place and remove the bur.

- The right angles or prophy angles are used to polish the teeth with rubber cups or brushes.

On the shank of the low-speed handpiece is a mechanism to lock the rotary instrument or the attachment onto the handpiece. This may be a tightening knob or a snap-on apparatus. Also on the shank near the connecting end there may be a reverse and forward control. The power source for controlling the speed of the low-speed handpiece is the rheostat.

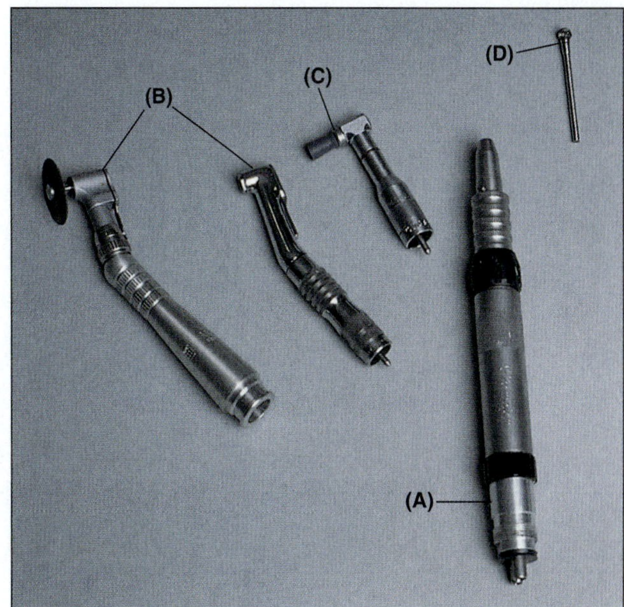

FIGURE 18-47

(A) Low-speed handpiece with nose cone and attachments for the low-speed handpiece. (B) Contra-angle with and without a disc. (C) Right angle or prophy angle, with rubber cup. (D) Round bur with long shank to be placed in nose cone of the straight low-speed handpiece.

Electric Handpiece

An **electric handpiece** is an alternative to the air-driven handpieces mainly used by dentists today. The electric handpieces have greatly improved and are becoming more popular in the dental office. The units can be calibrated to be used with existing air pressure and rheostats. They can be used for all high- and low-speed needs, operating at a speed range of 27,000–200,000 rpm with various attachments. Procedures they are used for include cavity preparation; endodontic procedures; dental implants; contouring and trimming provisional crowns and bridges; adjusting crowns, bridges, and permanent restorations; prophylaxis; and composite polishing. There is also an interproximal head for interproximal polishing, cleaning, and preparation. The electric handpieces are quiet, vibration free, efficient, and sterilizable. They allow for smoother cuts and refined margins with higher torque and precision.

The high-speed electric handpiece has a push-button auto chuck that firmly grips the bur and a lightweight cellular optic rod that delivers illumination and reduces eye fatigue. The low-speed electric handpiece has several attachments and is available in either the contra-angle or the straight handpiece style (Figure 18-48).

Ultrasonic Handpiece

The **ultrasonic handpiece** is mainly used for scaling procedures and root canal therapy but also may be used to remove bonding materials after cementing crowns and orthodontic appliances. The handpiece is attached to the ultrasonic scaler unit. The unit converts electrical energy into ultrasonic vibrations that are transmitted to the

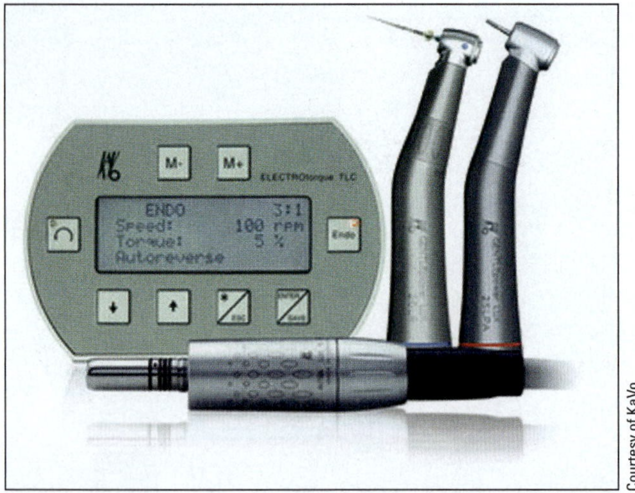

Courtesy of KaVo

FIGURE 18-48

Electric handpiece.

handpiece. There are specific connections on the dental unit for the electrical and water needed for the ultrasonic unit. Ultrasonic handpieces are controlled by a foot pedal. (Figure 18-49).

Dental Laser Handpiece

The dental **laser handpiece** is used to cut and remove both hard and soft tissue, control bleeding (cauterize), and biopsy tissue. The handpiece is similar to other dental handpieces in size and shape and comes with a variety of tips. The handpiece is attached to a unit with a fiber-optic cable and has water and air to cool the tooth and tissues. The laser unit has the controls for the handpiece. Some newer units do not require a cable and the handpiece is thinner and more flexible. It is important not to touch the exposed fiber-optic cable and to keep the cable as straight as possible to prevent damage to the fiber-optic cables. (See Chapter 31 Periodontics for more information.)

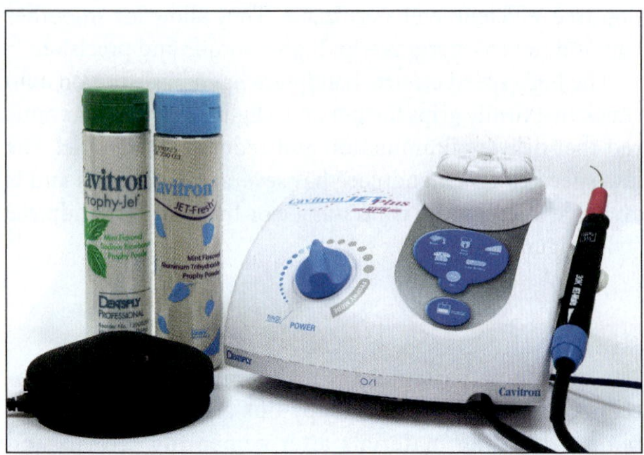

FIGURE 18-49

Ultrasonic handpiece.

Maintenance and Sterilization of Dental Handpieces

The manufacturer's directions for maintaining and sterilizing the handpiece should be followed carefully. Handpieces that are used for patient treatment must be sterilizable; disinfecting handpieces is not acceptable. General guidelines include the following:

- While the handpiece is attached to the tubing and a bur is still in the handpiece, flush the handpiece by running it for 20 to 30 seconds. Follow the manufacturer's instructions for specific flushing and for the use and maintenance of waterlines and check valves.
- Scrub the handpiece to remove debris. Rinse and dry it if manufacturer instructions include this step.
- Lubricate the handpiece if it is not lube free. Use only the manufacturers' suggested lubricants. This must be done before the handpiece is sterilized.
- Sterilize the handpiece as directed.
- Lubricate if instructed to do so.

Some handpiece maintenance units clean and lubricate handpieces. These units (Figure 18-50) are located in the sterilizing area and require electrical and air pressure connections and water. Some of the units also sterilize the handpiece.

Air Abrasion Unit

The **air abrasion** technology is becoming increasingly popular. Air abrasion reduces or eliminates the use of anesthetics and drilling with dental handpieces. This shortens and/or reduces the number of patient appointments. The technology allows the operator to prepare various types of cavities for restoration, accomplish special repairs in restorations, and roughen the insides of restorations before bonding.

Air abrasion base units (Figures 18-51A and B) come in movable floor models or small countertop units. They consist

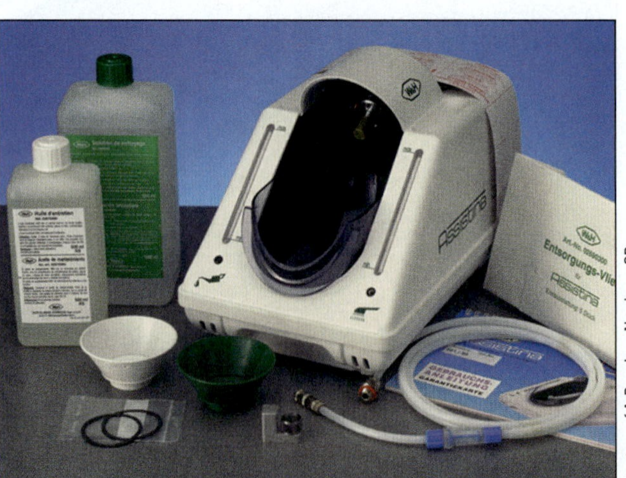

Courtesy of A-Dec, Inc., Newberg, OR

FIGURE 18-50

Handpiece cleaner and lubricant maintenance unit.

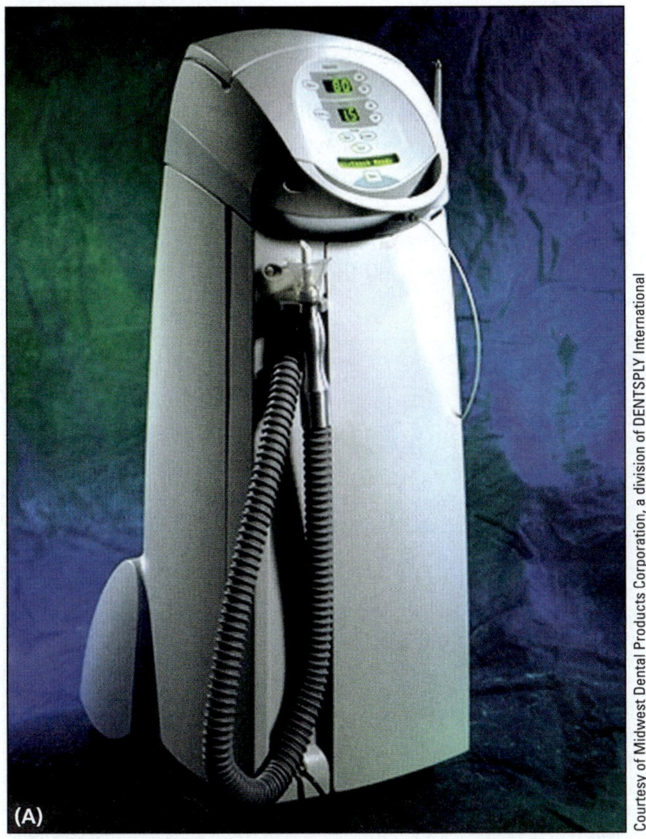
Courtesy of Midwest Dental Products Corporation, a division of DENTSPLY International

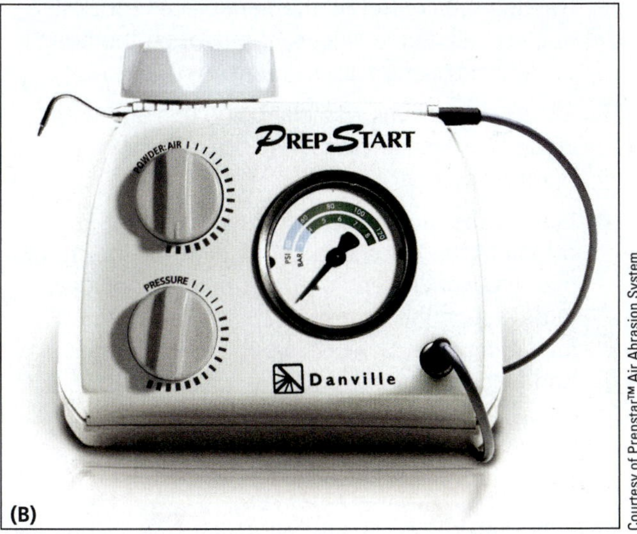

Courtesy of Prepstar™ Air Abrasion System

FIGURE 18-51
(A) Air abrasion unit. (B) Air abrasion table unit.

of the base unit, control panel, foot switch, air pressure gradient (varies the pressure in small increments), handpiece and handpiece nozzler, abrasive flow control, and external suction device. Each unit requires an air pressure source (most can use air lines to the dental unit) and the abrasive. The abrasive is aluminum oxide. The particle size varies, with 27 or 50 microns most commonly used, but more variations are being developed for specific tasks.

During use, the dental team and the patient should wear protective eyewear. The dental assistant uses the HVE in addition to external suction to remove debris.

Routine maintenance is important and the manufacturer's directions should be followed.

Microetcher

The **microetcher** is a smaller version of the air abrasion units. They are used for intraoral sandblasting and dentin bonding. Microetchers are used for many procedures, including:

- Removal of occlusal stains from deep occlusal grooves
- Pit and fissure sealant preparation
- Denture repairs
- Etching of existing amalgam, composites, and porcelain restorations
- Roughening the surface for bonding of orthodontic bands and brackets
- Roughening the surface of crowns, bridges, and posts for maximum bonding

The microetcher looks like and is about the size of a pen and it has an abrasive reservoir with an interchangeable jar. The reservoir is attached to the microetcher and holds the abrasive. The microetcher comes with several different tips called nozzles (Figure 18-52). It can be hooked up in an operatory or a lab where there is an air line for compressed air of 40 to 100 psi.

Microetcher Abrasives. The abrasives used with the microetcher should be dry and clean. Since abrasives are hygroscopic (water loving) they should be kept in a tightly sealed container to keep them dry and clean. Some of the abrasives used include:

- Aluminum oxide, 90 micron, tan, for rapid removal of cements and etching of metals to prepare for bonding
- Aluminum oxide, 50 micron, white, for preparation of amalgam, composite, and porcelain bonding

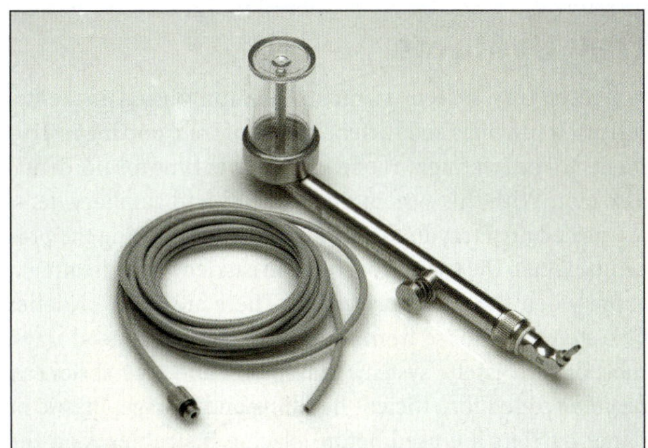

FIGURE 18-52
Microetcher with hose and abrasive reservoir.

- Microprophy B, white, for stain removal
- SA-85 to remove resin
- Glass beads, 90 micron, white, to clean dentures

The jar on the microetcher should be filled to about three-quarters full to allow the abrasive to move easily in the jar.

Operation, Safety, and Sterilization. When using the microetcher, the dentist and assistant should wear protective eyewear and a mask. The patient should have protective eyewear on and a rubber dam should be placed on the patient.

The microetcher can be sterilized if used intraorally. A plastic barrier can be placed over the microetcher with only the tip exposed to avoid contamination by the patient. To prepare for sterilization, remove the abrasive jar and then allow the compressed air to flow through the unit. Remove any debris from the microetcher and the nozzle and then sterilize.

Procedure 18-4

Identify Dental Handpieces, Demonstrate Attaching them to the Dental Unit, and Selecting and Placing Rotary Instrument

This procedure is performed by the dental assistant to identify various dental handpieces, demonstrating how to assemble and attach to the dental unit, and placing a rotary instrument.

Equipment and Supplies

- High-speed handpiece
- Low-speed handpiece
- Contra-angle/latch attachment
- Prophy/right-angle attachment
- Variety of dental rotary instruments

Procedure Steps

1. Identify the high-speed handpiece, attach to the dental unit, and be careful to align the receptors properly so the handpiece fits securely.
2. Select the correct bur and place in working end of the handpiece (This step will vary depending on the design of the handpiece). Check to be sure that the bur is secure.
3. Identify the low-speed handpiece, attach to the dental unit, and be careful to align the handpiece with the receptors so the handpiece fits securely.
4. Identify the contra-angle attachment and attach to the low-speed handpiece by slipping it over the working end of the straight handpiece and twisting the control on the handpiece to lock it in place. Slide the lever to the right on the head of the contra-angle attachment.
5. Select a latch-type bur, insert the bur, and then close the lever, and check to be sure that the bur is secure.
6. Identify the prophy/right-angle attachment and attach to the low-speed handpiece by slipping it over the working end of the straight handpiece and twisting the control on the handpiece to lock it in place. Select a prophy cup or brush and place on prophy angle.

Tray Systems

A **preset tray system** is most commonly used in dental offices. It provides an efficient means of transporting instruments to the treatment room, which saves time for the dental assistant. With this system, instruments and auxiliary items are placed on a tray in the order of their use during the procedure. Then the tray is covered and carried to the treatment room when the patient is seated. There are many varieties of systems to choose from, including plastic or metal trays, tubs, or the cassette system. Trays, tubs, and accessories can be color coded for efficient handling and storage. Plastic or paper barriers are used before placing instruments on the tray, especially for ribbed trays. These barriers help with tray disinfection.

Positioning on Trays

Every operator has preferences on the instrumentation for a procedure. However, there are some basic considerations:

- Clear plastic tray barriers may be placed.
- Instruments are placed in order of use, beginning on the left and moving to the right.
- The basic tray setup (mouth mirror, explorer, and cotton pliers) is placed first on the left side.
- Instruments should be grouped according to functions; for example, all the carvers are placed together.
- Cotton supplies are usually arranged across the top of the tray.
- Scissors, hemostats, or other hinged instruments are placed on the far right of the tray for easy access.

- Return instruments to their original positions after receiving them from the operator. This ensures that an instrument can be found easily if the operator needs to use it again.
- Keep instruments clean and free of debris before returning them to the tray. Gauze sponges on the tray aid with the immediate removal of cement, blood, or debris, which will harden on the instrument after use.

Cassette System for Instruments

Cassette systems are designed to carry instruments for use in treatment rooms, through the cleaning and sterilizing processes, and then into storage (Figure 18-53). Instruments for a certain procedure are color coded and then placed in a cassette. The cassette provides an efficient and safe means for handling instruments. Also, when the cassette is open, it provides its own tray. After being used for a procedure, the cassette is carried to the sterilization area. Here the instruments are reorganized and placed in the cassette. When the cassette is closed, the instruments remain securely in place. The cassette is then placed in the ultrasonic or instrument washer. When this process is complete, the cassette is rinsed thoroughly, and then wrapped or packaged and labeled, sterilized, and stored until needed. In the treatment room, the cassette is unwrapped on the counter top or cart, ready for use. The wrap acts as a barrier between the tray and the counter (Figure 18-53).

The cassette system efficiently keeps instruments together at all times. It increases safety by reducing the possibility of puncture injuries during cleaning and sterilizing. The cassettes come in different sizes and can be stored vertically or horizontally because the instruments are held into position. The wrapped cassettes are labeled with tape that is premarked for all procedures performed in the office. This makes it easy to identify the tray set that is needed in the treatment rooms. For more information, refer to Chapter 11, Infection Control.

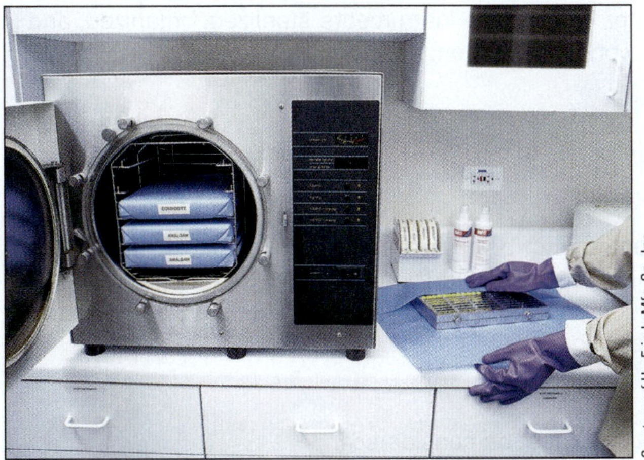

Courtesy of Hu-Friedy Mfg. Co., Inc.

FIGURE 18-53

Cassette system. Cassettes are wrapped in paper and taped with label tape and then placed in sterilizer.

Color-Coding Systems

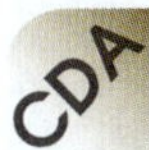

Color coding is a method for easily identifying instruments and trays (Figure 18-54).

The color coding may be set up to indicate the following:

- Procedures, such as amalgam or composite.
- Treatment rooms, where the instruments are stored or used.
- Additional sets of instruments (there may be four composite setups, each marked for the procedure and then a second color for the set).
- Individual operators. The dentist may have two tray setups for prophylaxis and the hygienist may have four additional prophylaxis tray setups. Color coding keeps the dentist and the hygienist tray setups separate.
- Sequence. Instruments can be color coded diagonally to indicate the sequence of use.
- Any combination of these.

Types of Color-Coding Materials. There are several different types of materials used to color code dental instruments, including plastic rings and colored coding tape. Color-coding tape may also be used to color code tubs and trays, bur blocks, and tray mats. Also available are color-coded systems where the tubs, trays, tray mats, bur blocks, and mouth mirrors are all one color. Color-coding materials must be autoclavable and durable (Figures 18-55A–C).

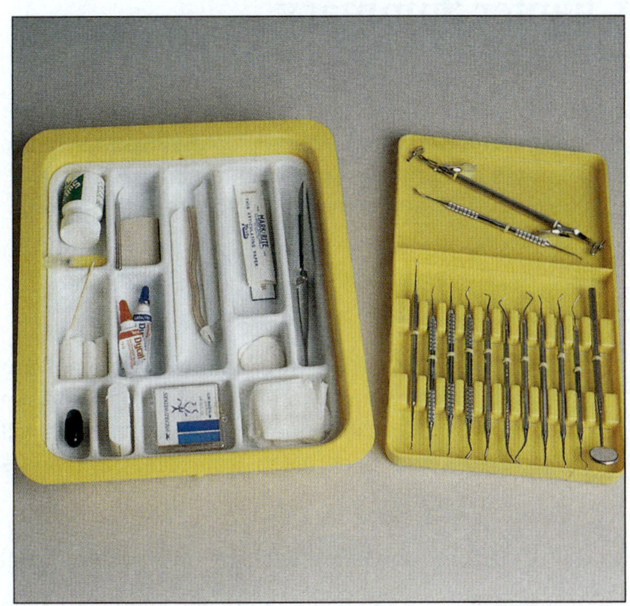

FIGURE 18-54

Tub, tray, and instruments, all color coded.

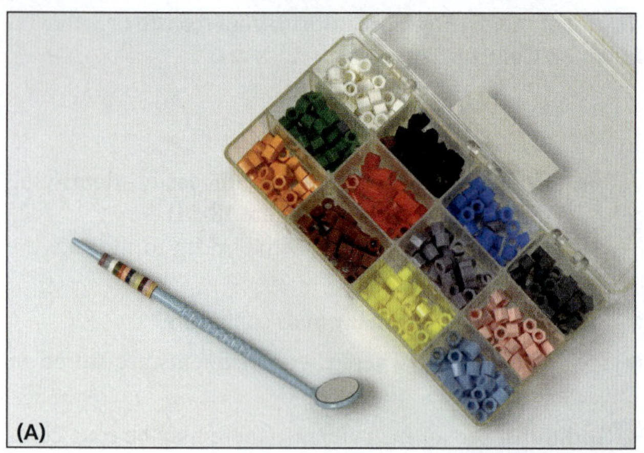
(A)

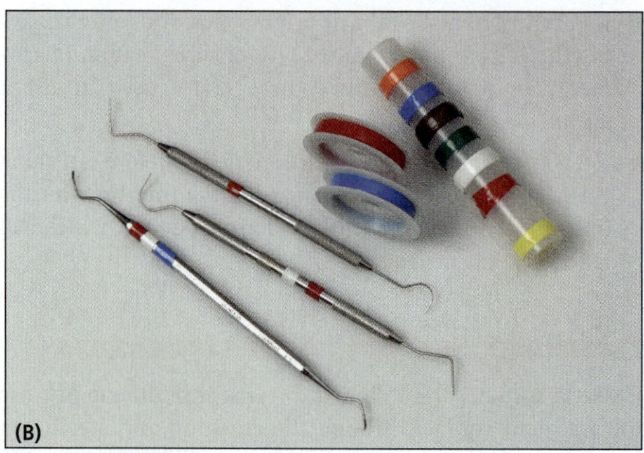
(B)

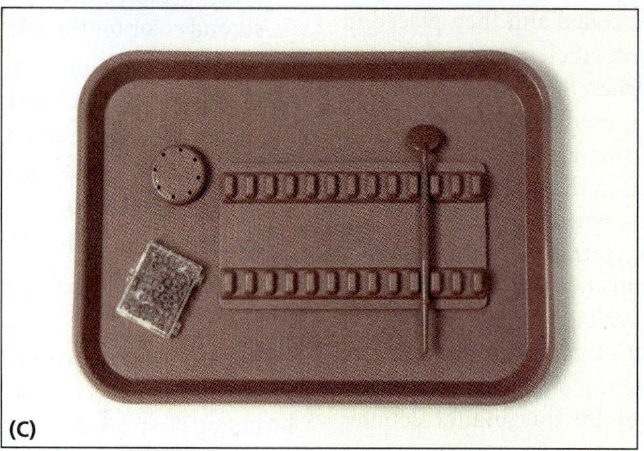
(C)

FIGURE 18-55

Color-coding materials. (A) Plastic rings. (B) Tape. (C) Tray, instrument mat, mouth mirror, bur block, and colored rings all color coordinated.

Chapter Summary

The basic instruments used in general dental procedures include common cutting and noncutting instruments. Instruments are generally categorized as hand instruments and rotary instruments. Each procedure requires special instruments to accomplish specific tasks. Various dental handpieces are identified and their functions are discussed. The assistant is responsible for keeping the instruments sterilized, organized, and in working condition.

CASE STUDY

Dr. Charles Thomas has been practicing dentistry for 5 years, and his practice has grown to the point where his tray setup system must be changed. Dr. Thomas has three treatment rooms and one hygiene room. He is willing to finance the necessary updating and would like to color code his instruments, trays, and so forth.

Case Study Review

1. Before deciding on a system, what factors must be considered?
2. Suggest some color-code combinations.
3. What are the benefits of an office in which a color-coding system is effectively used?

Review Questions

Multiple Choice

1. The part of the dental instrument that is straight, curved, monangle, binangle, or triple angle is called the
   a. handle.
   b. shank.
   c. working end.
   d. shaft.
2. Which of the following instruments has a four-number formula?
   a. Chisel
   b. Angle former
   c. Spoon excavator
   d. Hoe
3. The mouth mirror uses include all of the following except
   a. indirect vision.
   b. light reflection.
   c. retraction.
   d. direct vision.
4. The ________ bur is used for rapid reduction of tooth structure and ________ burs are used to reduce and contour the alveolar bone and tooth structure.
   a. diamond–surgical
   b. diamond–laboratory
   c. cutting–finishing
   d. fissurotomy–cutting
5. The rotary instrument also known as a "Jo-dandy" is the
   a. diamond bur.
   b. sandpaper disc.
   c. carborundum disc.
   d. rubber wheel.
6. Which of the following handpiece types would accept a notched bur?
   a. The friction grip handpiece
   b. The screw-on right angle
   c. The straight handpiece
   d. The latch contra-angle
7. The end of the handpiece where discs, burs, stones, and other rotary instruments and attachments are held is called
   a. the working end of the handpiece.
   b. the shank of the handpiece.
   c. the connecting end of the handpiece.
   d. the plunger.
8. The shank of the chisel may be ________
   a. straight only.
   b. straight or curved only.
   c. straight, curved, or binangle.
   d. binangle only.
9. Egg shaped, t-ball, football, acorn, and beavertail are all shapes of ________
   a. finishing knives.
   b. burnishers.
   c. plastic filling instruments.
   d. gingival margin trimmers.
10. Color-coding systems are set up to indicate all of the following *except*
   a. procedures.
   b. which dental arch/tooth the instrument is used on.
   c. treatment rooms.
   d. individual operators.

Critical Thinking

1. What information does a bur number provide about the bur?
2. Which handpiece would the dental assistant select if the procedure included polishing the patient's teeth? Would an attachment be required?
3. List the basic hand instruments that would be necessary for an amalgam restoration procedure.
4. Using the color-coding system, describe how to color-code restorative and hygiene instruments when there are two dentists, two hygienists, two sets of instruments for each procedure, and they need to be in order.

Web Activities

1. Go to http://www.agd.org and search for information on dental lasers used in dental procedures.
2. Dental rotary instruments can be ordered from numerous sources. Visit http://www.dental-burs.com and look up the price of diamond burs and carbide burs.
3. Go to http://www.kavousa.com and find out how to care for dental handpieces between patients as well as weekly or as needed.

CHAPTER 19

Instrument Transfer and Maintaining the Operating Field 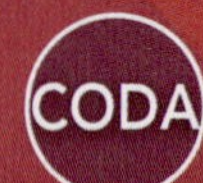

CODA

Specific Instructional Objectives

The student should strive to meet the following objectives and demonstrate an understanding of the facts and principles presented in this chapter:

1. Describe the transfer zone.
2. Define a fulcrum and tactile sensation.
3. Describe the grasps, positions, and transfer of instruments for a procedure.
4. List the eight rules for instrument transfer.
5. Understand instrument transfer modification.
6. Describe and demonstrate how to maintain the oral cavity.
7. Explain the equipment used in the treatment of the oral cavity.
8. Describe techniques for moisture control and isolation.

Expanded Functions

9. Explain the expanded functions performed by the dental assistant.
10. Explain the purpose of the dental dam and identify who places it on a patient.
11. List and explain advantages and contraindications of the dental dam.
12. Identify the armamentarium needed for the dental dam procedure and explain the function of each.
13. Explain how to prepare the patient for dental dam placement and how to determine the isolation area.
14. Describe and demonstrate how dental dam material is prepared.
15. List and demonstrate the steps for placing and removing the dental dam.
16. Explain and demonstrate the dental dam procedure for the child patient.

Key Terms

air–water syringe (425)
anchor tooth (431)
cervical clamps (433)
dental dam clamps (431)
dental dam forceps (433)
dental dam frame (431)
dental dam napkin (430)
dental dam punch (431)
dental dam scissors (434)
dry angle (428)
expanded functions (429)
fulcrum (413)
high-volume evacuator (HVE) (421)
interseptal (434)
inverting (433)
Isolite system (427)
key hole punch (435)
ligature (433)
malaligned (430)
modified pen grasp (414)
mouth prop (426)
Ostby frame (431)
palm grasp (414)
palm–thumb grasp (415)
pen grasp (414)
punch table/punch plate (431)
quickdam (444)
radiotransparent (431)
reflux (426)
reverse palm–thumb grasp (415)
saliva ejector (422)
septum (435)
stamp (431)

(continues)

Key Terms (continued)

tactile (413)
template (431)
thumb-to-nose grasp (415)
transfer zone (413)
U-frame (431)
winged clamps (433)
wingless clamps (433)
Young frame (431)

Introduction

In this chapter, the dental-assisting student will learn the critical skills needed when assisting the dentist. Maintaining the operating field and the transfer of instruments are very important aspects of four-handed, sit-down dentistry. Failure to master these basic skills may result in injury to the patient, dentist, or the assistant and/or loss of production for the office. It is the responsibility of the assistant to think ahead and have everything ready for the dentist as the procedure progresses.

The dental assistant will learn how to grasp the different instruments, and then how to transfer the instruments to the dentist. Instruments can be transferred with one or two hands. Both of these methods are discussed, as well as modifications to these methods when passing two instruments at a time, hinged instruments, dental handpieces, and the air–water syringe.

In order to maintain the operating field, the assistant must adjust the dental light; evacuate the area with the HVE and the saliva ejector; use mouth props; retract the cheeks, lips, tongue, and tissue; know how to place and remove isolation systems; and know when and where to place cotton rolls and dry angles. Placing and removing the dental dam is also used to maintain the operating field, and the dental assistant is usually responsible for this skill. This may be an expanded function in some states, be aware of your dental practice acts.

These skills take practice and knowledge about how the dentist wants things to be done. Once the assistant has mastered the basic skills, he or she can adapt to different dentists and/or hygienists fairly easily. By being organized and comfortable with maintaining the operating field and transferring instruments, the assistant can make the procedure go smoother and faster.

Instrument Transfer

Instrument transfer or exchange is one of the basic functions in four-handed, sit-down dentistry. The assistant must learn to pass and receive instruments to and from the operator with confidence and skill. Efficient instrument transfer allows the operator to keep his or her eyes focused on the oral cavity, and requires little movement of the operator's hand. A smooth transfer of instruments and materials occurs when the assistant is able to anticipate the operator's needs. This takes practice and cooperation between the operator and the assistant. Once the transfer skills are accomplished, the operator and assistant work as one. The following occurs when proper instrument transfer is accomplished:

- The operator's view remains on the oral cavity.
- Stress and fatigue for the operator and the assistant are reduced.
- Safety and comfort are maintained for the patient.
- Productivity is increased using less time and motion.

The transfer of instruments between operator and assistant takes place in the **transfer zone**, the area just below the patient's nose, near the chin. The assistant brings the instrument to the operator so that the operator will not have to move his or her hand from the established **fulcrum** to exchange the instrument. The fulcrum is a finger rest that assists in stabilizing the operator's hand. The fulcrum should be established on a firm surface, such as the teeth, and be positioned on the same arch and as close to the area you are working on as possible (Figure 19-1). See Chapter 32 Coronal Polish for examples of how a fulcrum is used. The **tactile** sensation allows the operator to know that the exchange has taken place without his or her eyes moving from the area. The assistant should pass the instrument with pressure firm enough for the operator to feel the instrument in his or her hand.

Fulcrum

A fulcrum is a point of rest on which the fingers are stabilized, and from which they can pivot. For example, when working on the mandibular first molar, the fingers rest on the occlusal surface of the mandibular bicuspids, providing the fulcrum.

Tactile Sensation

Tactile sensation is the feeling sensed by touch. For example, the pressure of the instrument exchanged during an instrument transfer is tactile sensation.

Transfer Hand

To aid the assistant in the delivery of instruments, the fingers and thumb of the hand are identified as follows: the thumb, the index finger or the first finger, the middle finger or the second finger, the ring finger or the third finger, and the little finger or the fourth finger (Figure 19-2).

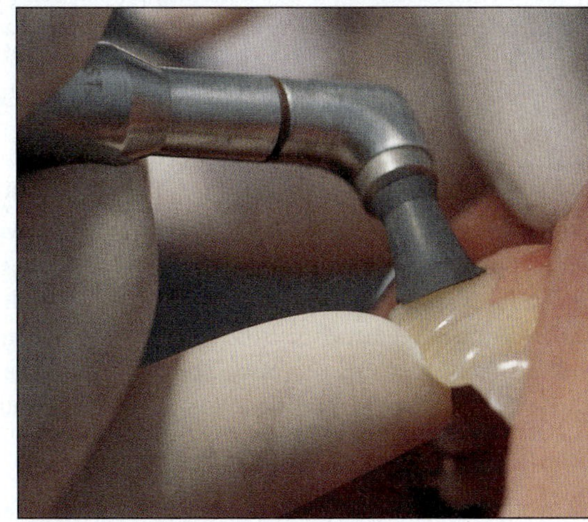

FIGURE 19-1
Note the use of the fulcrum.

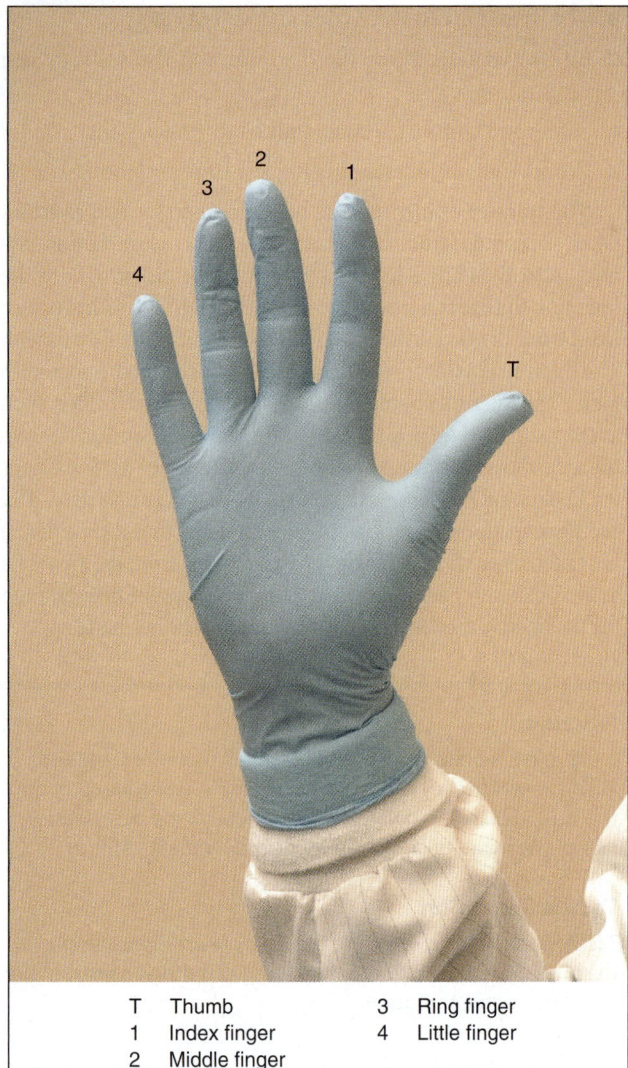

FIGURE 19-2
Fingers of the hand are labeled for instrument transfer reference.

The assistant passes and receives instruments with the left hand when working with a right-handed dentist, and with the right hand when assisting a left-handed dentist. Using one hand for instrument transfer frees the other hand for evacuation and retraction.

Instrument Grasps

The way an instrument is held influences how efficiently the instrument can be used. Selecting the correct grasp allows the operator control of the instrument and greater tactile sensitivity, and reduces fatigue to the operator's fingers and hand. The way an instrument is grasped also dictates how it is exchanged. Several different instrument grasps are commonly used in operative dentistry: pen, modified pen, palm, palm-thumb, and reverse palm-thumb.

Pen Grasp. The **pen grasp**, as the name indicates, is when an instrument is grasped in the same manner as a pen or pencil (Figure 19-3). The instrument is held between the pad of the thumb and the pad of the index finger, with the side of the middle finger on the opposite side of the thumb. With the pen grasp, the instrument is held at the junction of the shank and handle of the instrument (see Chapter 18, Basic Chairside Instruments and Tray Systems). The pen grasp is used to hold instruments that have angled shanks.

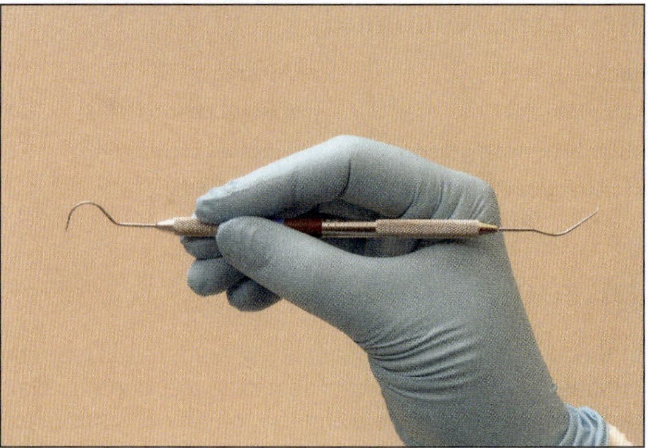

FIGURE 19-3
Pen grasp.

Modified Pen Grasp. The **modified pen grasp** is similar to the pen grasp. The instrument is held with the same fingers as the pen grasp, except that the pad of the middle finger is placed on the top of the instrument with the index finger (Figure 19-4). The modified pen grasp is preferred by some operators and provides more control and strength in some procedures. This grasp also lessens operator fatigue. The modified pen grasp is used with the same instruments as the pen grasp—those with angled shanks.

Palm Grasp. With the **palm grasp**, the operator holds the instrument in the palm of the hand and fingers grasp the handle of the instrument (Figure 19-5). The palm grasp is used with surgical pliers, rubber dam forceps, and other forceps. In some procedures, the palm is up when the operator is working on the maxillary teeth and the working end of the instrument is pointed

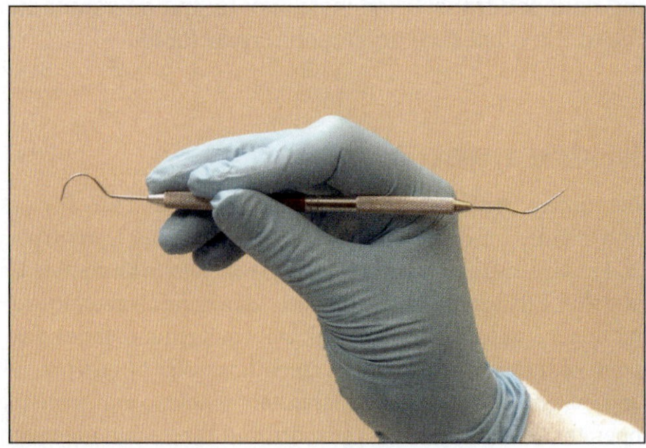

FIGURE 19-4
Modified pen grasp.

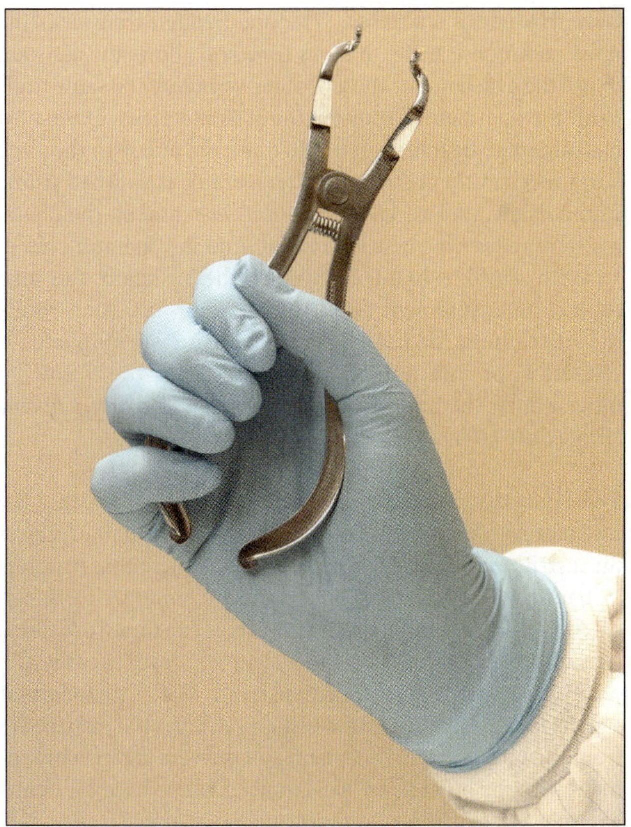

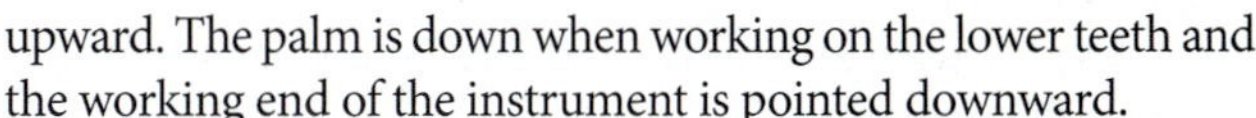

FIGURE 19-5
Palm grasp.

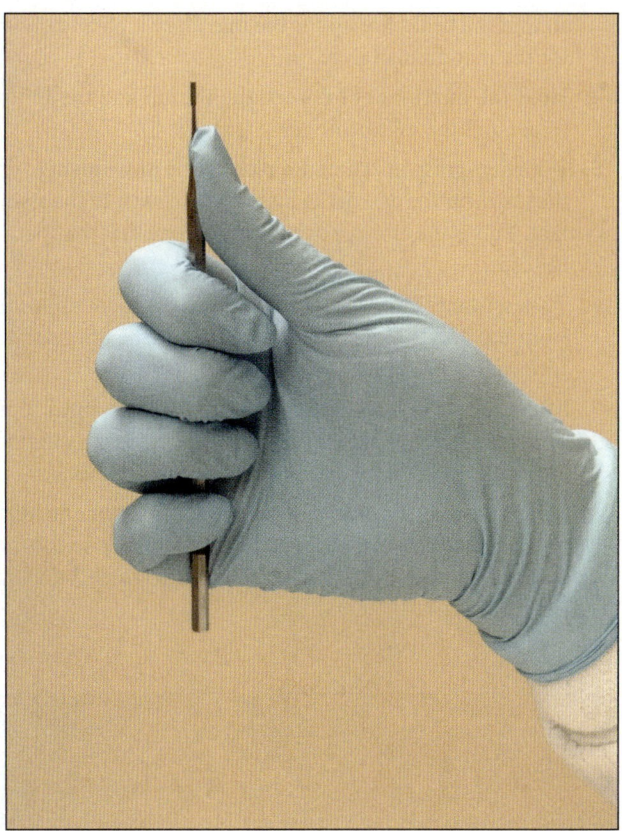

FIGURE 19-6
Palm–thumb grasp.

upward. The palm is down when working on the lower teeth and the working end of the instrument is pointed downward.

Palm–Thumb Grasp. For the **palm–thumb grasp**, the operator grasps the handle of the instrument in the palm of the hand with the four fingers wrapped around the handle while the thumb is extended upward from the palm (Figure 19-6). The palm–thumb grasp is used with instruments having straight shanks and blades, such as the straight chisel or the Wedelstaedt chisel.

Reverse Palm–Thumb Grasp. The **reverse palm–thumb grasp** is a variation of the palm-thumb grasp that is frequently used to hold the evacuator tip in the patient's mouth. The reverse palm-thumb grasp is sometimes called the **thumb-to-nose grasp**. With this grasp, the evacuator tip is held in the palm of the hand with the thumb directed toward the assistant instead of toward the patient, as with the palm-thumb grasp (Figure 19-7).

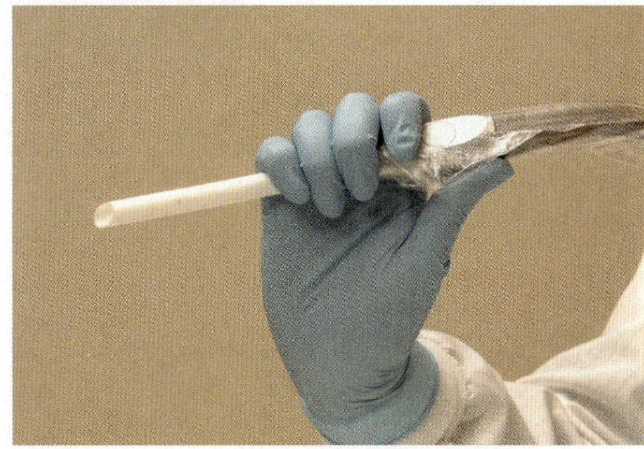

FIGURE 19-7
Reverse palm–thumb grasp.

Instrument Transfer Methods

The assistant selects the next instrument and holds it ready for transfer until the operator signals for the exchange. Usually, this signal occurs when the operator tilts the instrument back away from the patient while still maintaining the fulcrum. The assistant removes the used instrument from the operator's hand and places the new instrument in it.

Eight Basic Rules for Instrument Transfer.

1. With angled-shank instruments, the primary working end should be placed away from the assistant on the tray.
2. With straight-shank instruments, the primary working end should be placed toward the assistant on the tray.
3. With hinged instruments, the beaks are placed toward the assistant. Once the instrument is picked up, it is rotated

so that the beaks are up for the maxillary arch and down for the mandibular arch.

4. Hold the instrument between the thumb and the index finger and the middle finger (Figure 19-8).
5. With pen-grasp instruments, pick up the instrument from the tray near the end of the instrument closest to the assistant. This is the end opposite from the one that the operator uses.
6. The assistant's hand is placed on the instrument opposite from the end the operator uses to allow the operator to receive the instrument (Figure 19-9).
7. Rotate the working end of the instrument until it is directed toward the dental arch being treated, positioned upward for maxillary and downward for mandibular.
8. Hold the instrument parallel to the instrument held by the operator. Instruments are held as close to one another as possible, without becoming tangled during the transfer.

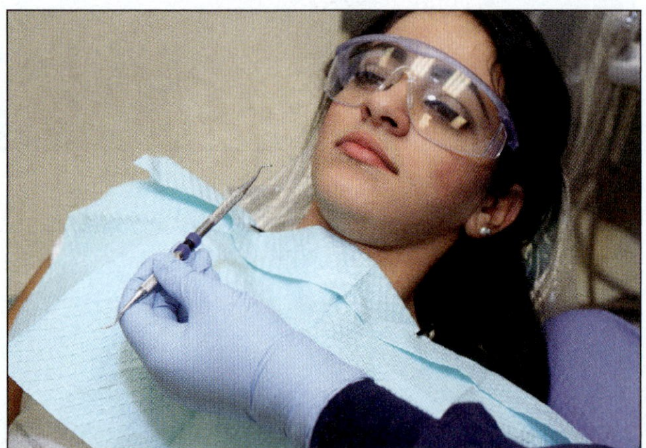

FIGURE 19-8
Instrument correctly held for transfer.

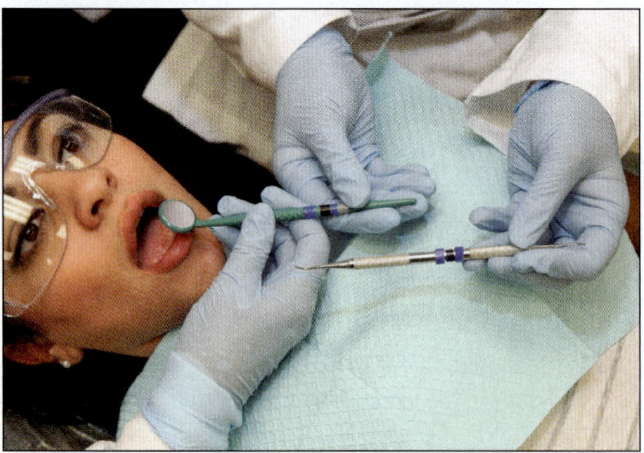

FIGURE 19-9
Two-handed transfer: The assistant uses one hand to receive an instrument from the operator and the other hand to pass a new instrument.

One-Handed Transfer. The one-handed transfer is the most common transfer. It saves time and allows the assistant to use the evacuator or the air–water syringe at the same time. With the one-handed transfer, the assistant picks up the next instrument to be transferred with one hand and with the same hand receives the instrument the operator is finished using. Immediately after receiving the used instrument, the dental assistant rotates the new instrument into the operator's hand.

With the one-handed transfer, the assistant can also receive an instrument from the operator and then rotate the instrument for use with the opposite working end. A sequence for instrument transfer includes the following movements: the approach, the retrieval, and the delivery (Procedure 19-1).

Two-Handed Transfer. With the two-handed transfer, the assistant uses both hands for the transfer. One hand receives the instrument from the operator and the other passes the next instrument. This transfer is used most commonly for surgical forceps or when both hands are free. For the two-handed pass, the assistant picks up the instrument from the tray and positions it for delivery with one hand. When the operator signals for an exchange, the assistant retrieves the instrument from the operator with one hand and delivers the new instrument with the other hand. This transfer is also used for dental handpieces and the air–water syringe.

The two-handed exchange follows the same steps as the one-handed exchange: the approach, followed by the retrieval, and then the delivery (Figure 19-9). The two-handed transfer requires the assistant to use both hands for the exchange—one to receive the used instrument and one to pass the new instrument to the operator.

Instrument Transfer Modifications

There are times when the transfer must be modified. The operator may have to move away from the mouth to receive some instruments, or the size or weight of some instruments may require the transfer to be modified.

The Mirror and Explorer Transfer. At the beginning of the procedure, the operator needs the mirror and the explorer to examine the area to be treated. The assistant picks up the mirror in the right hand and the explorer in the left hand to transfer to a right-handed operator. The operator signals readiness by putting his or her hands in position. The assistant then simultaneously places both instruments in the operator's hands (Figure 19-14).

The Cotton Pliers Transfer. When nonlocking cotton pliers are used to transfer small items, a one-handed transfer can be accomplished with slight modifications. The assistant must hold the pliers closer to the working end; this way, the item remains secure in the pliers during the transfer. When the pliers are returned to the assistant, he or she receives them at the working end to avoid dropping any materials (Figure 19-15).

Procedure 19-1
One-Handed Instrument Transfer

This procedure is performed at the dental unit by the dental assistant and the operator. In this procedure, the dental assistant uses his or her left hand to transfer instruments for a right-handed dentist. This is reversed for a left-handed operator. The dental assistant's free hand may hold the evacuator or retract oral tissues.

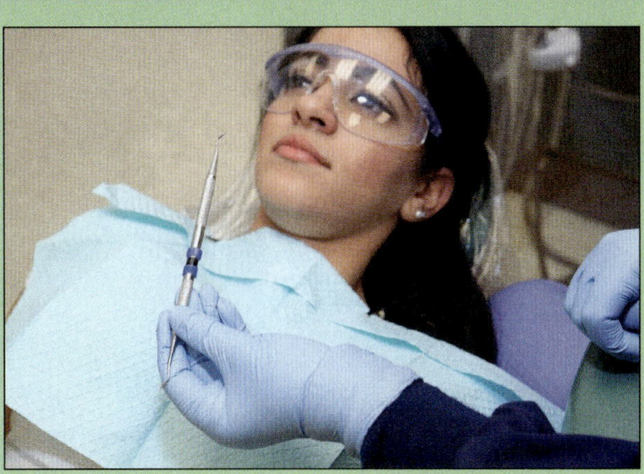

FIGURE 19-11

The assistant carries the instrument and approaches the operator for the exchange.

Equipment and Supplies

- Basic setup: mouth mirror, explorer, and cotton pliers
- Spoon excavator (for pen or modified pen grasp)*
- Straight chisel, forceps, or elevators (for palm grasp)[1]

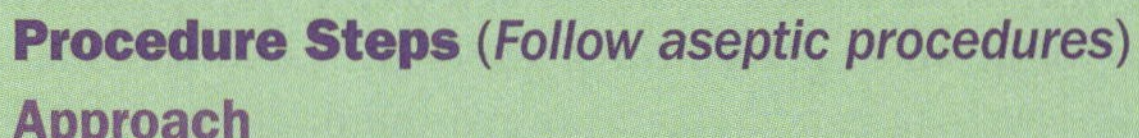

Procedure Steps (*Follow aseptic procedures*)

Approach

1. Lift the instrument from the tray using the thumb, index finger, and second finger, holding it near the nonworking end (Figure 19-10).
2. Turn the palm upward into passing position, rotating the nib toward the correct arch (Figure 19-11).
3. Move toward the operator's hand.

Retrieval

4. Extend the little finger and/or the ring finger and close around the handle of the instrument the operator is holding (Figure 19-12).
5. Lift the instrument out of the operator's hand and pull this instrument toward the assistant's palm and wrist.

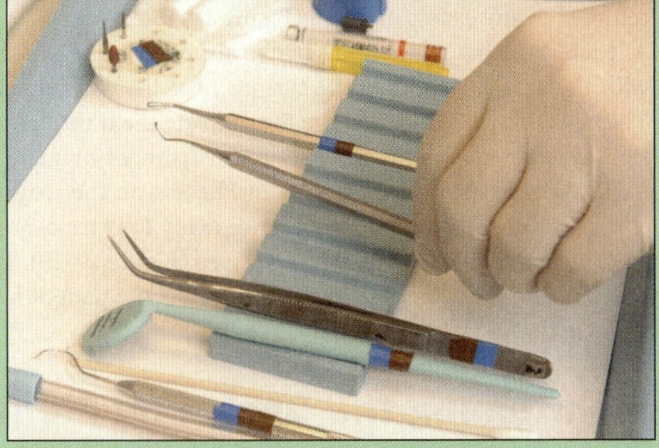

FIGURE 19-10

Instruments on tray in order of the procedure sequence. The assistant picks up the instrument at the end closest to the edge of the tray.

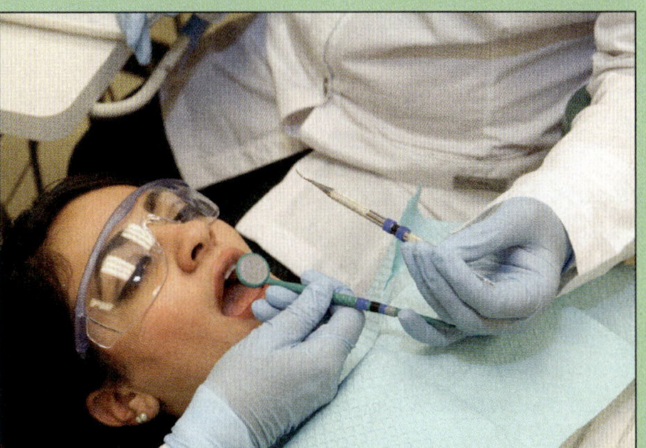

FIGURE 19-12

The operator signals when ready for an exchange. The assistant retrieves the instrument.

*Any instrument combination can be used to provide a variety of instrument grasps and transfers.

(continues)

Procedure 19-1 (continued)

Delivery

6. Rotate the hand toward the operator and place the instrument in the operator's fingers (Figure 19-13).
7. Once the operator has the new instrument, rotate it to the delivery position for use again or return it to the tray.

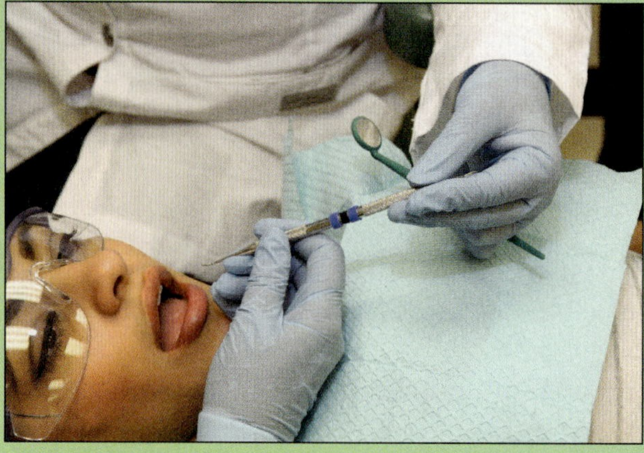

FIGURE 19-13
The assistant places the new instrument in the operator's hand.

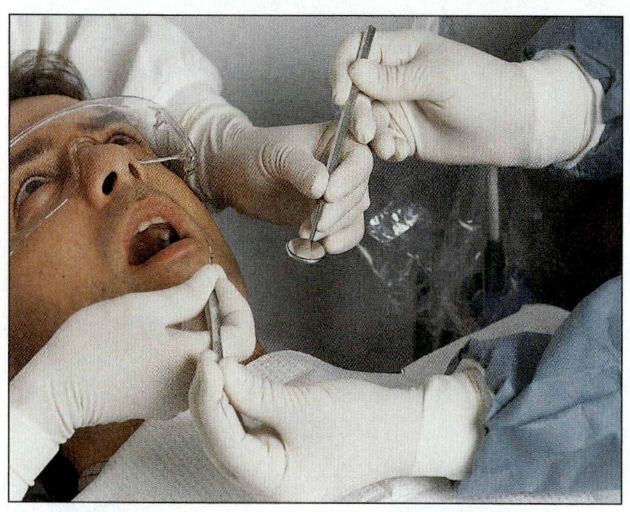

FIGURE 19-14
Mirror and explorer being transferred to the operator at the same time.

Scissors Transfer. Modifications are required for both the assistant and the operator when transferring scissors. The assistant picks up the scissors, slightly open, at the hinge near the working end. The operator's hand is moved away from the oral cavity and positioned with thumb and fingers apart to receive the scissors. When finished with the scissors, the assistant receives the scissors near the hinge and the working area (Figure 19-16).

Dental Handpieces. Dental handpieces are bulky, but they can be transferred with the one-handed transfer. The assistant picks up the handpiece near the hose attachment, away from the working end. Handpieces are heavier and, with the hose attachment, are difficult to transfer, but with time and practice the transfer will be smooth and manageable. If both hands are free, use the two-handed pass to transfer the handpieces (Figure 19-17).

Air–Water Syringe Transfer. To pass the air–water syringe, the assistant holds the end of the syringe covering the nozzle and tip with the palm of the hand. The handle of the syringe is projected toward the operator for easier grasping. The operator receives the syringe at the handle. For the return transfer, the assistant receives the syringe in the same manner it was passed, by covering the nozzle and tip with the palm of the hand. This process can be accomplished by either the one- or two-handed exchange (Figure 19-18).

Miscellaneous Items. The dental assistant transfers dental materials close to the operator's reach, usually near the patient's chin. If the material is on a paper pad, the assistant holds the pad near the patient's chin and holds gauze for the removal of any excess material (Figure 19-19).

Materials that come in a syringe are passed like scissors, with the assistant holding the syringe near the working end. The operator grasps the handle to complete the transfer.

Any time the operator passes an instrument or material back to the assistant with blood and debris on the working end, the assistant should have a gauze ready to place over the working end as the instrument is received (Figure 19-20). This contains the blood and debris, and prevents the patient from viewing them.

Maintaining the Operating Field

Maintaining the operating field is the process of keeping the area directly involved in the treatment clean, visible, as accessible as possible, and comfortable for the patient. A well-maintained field is essential for the procedure to be performed safely.

The requirements of maintaining the operating field are determined by the type of procedure, the tooth or teeth being treated, the oral anatomy of the patient, and the preferences of the operator.

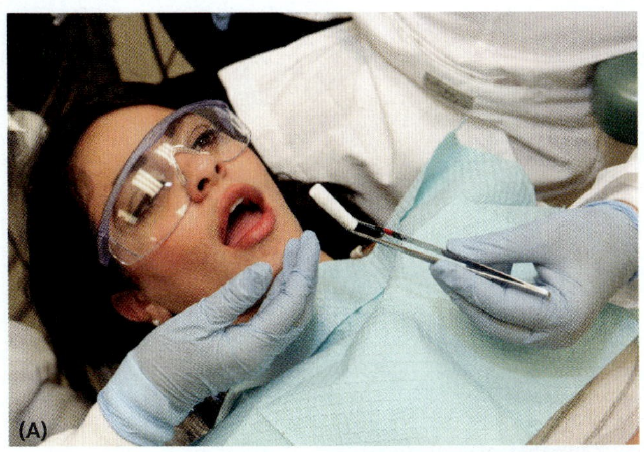

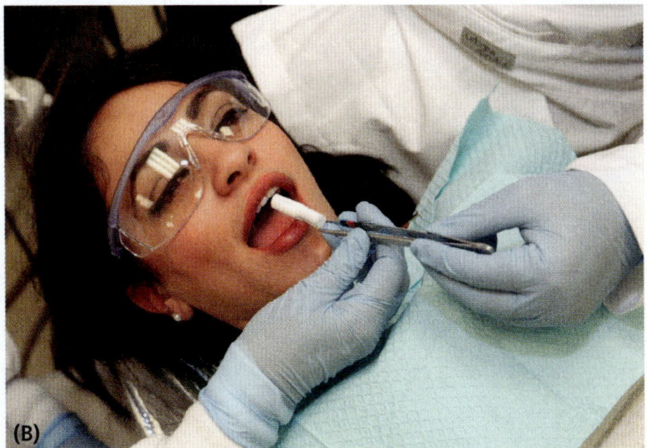

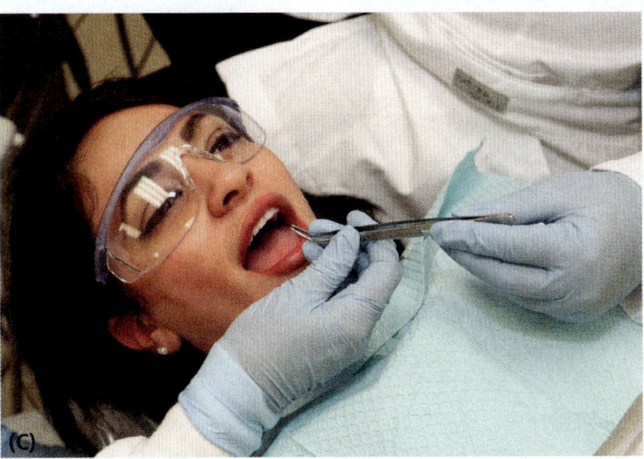

FIGURE 19-15

Cotton pliers transfer: (A) Cotton roll in nonlocking cotton pliers ready for transfer. (B) Operator receiving cotton pliers. (C) Operator returning cotton pliers to the assistant.

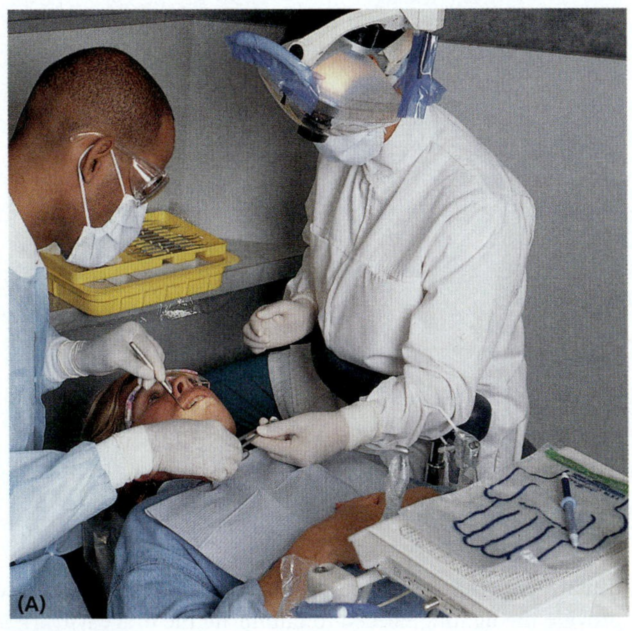

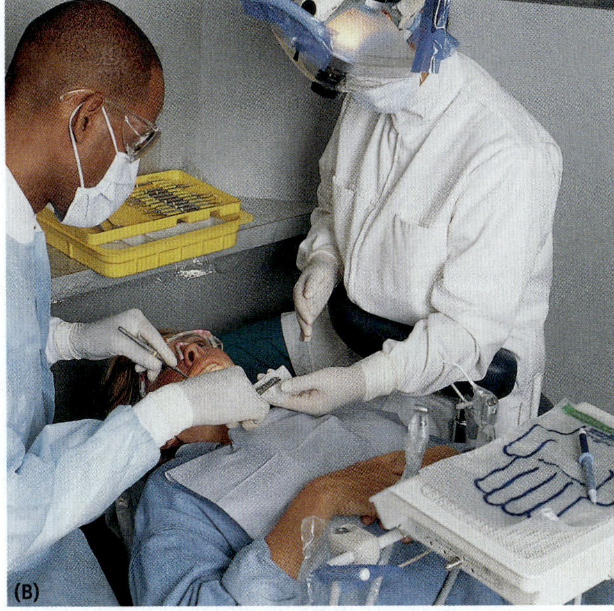

FIGURE 19-16

Scissors transfer: (A) The operator receives the scissors. (B) The operator comes away from the oral cavity to return the scissors to the assistant.

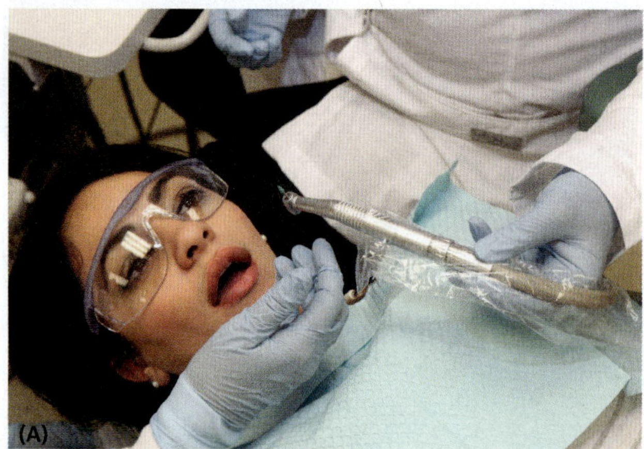

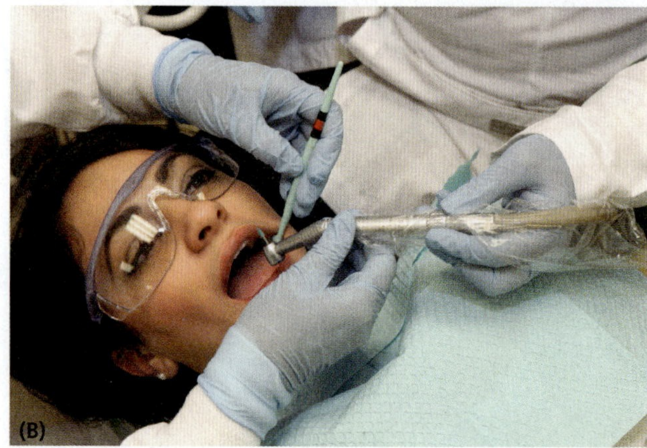

FIGURE 19-17

Dental handpiece transfer: (A) The dental handpiece is prepared for transfer. (B) The operator receives the handpiece.

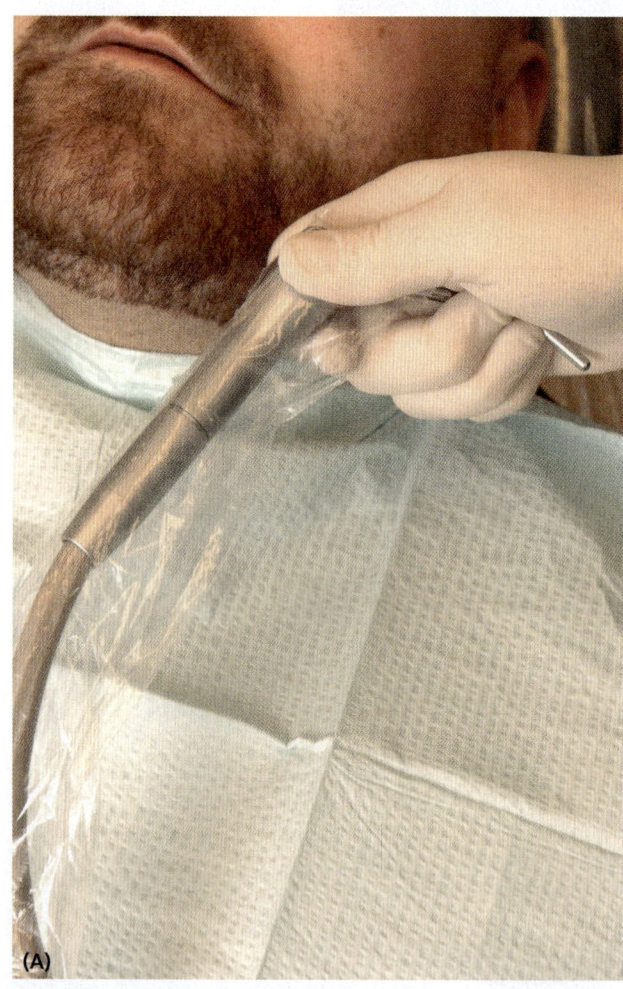

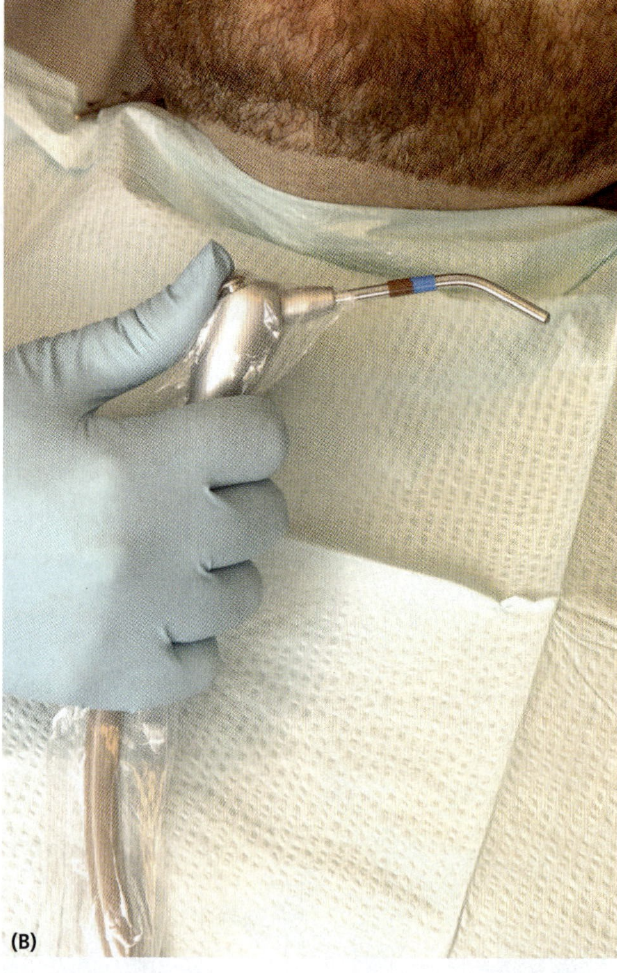

FIGURE 19-18

Air–water syringe transfer: (A) The assistant holds the air–water syringe near the handle in transfer position. (B) The operator receives the syringe handle with the tip in position for use.

Lighting

The operator must be able to see the area of the oral cavity that is receiving treatment. Part of the dental assistant's responsibility is maintaining the operating field by positioning the dental light throughout the procedure. The dental light, the illuminated dental mouth mirror, and the fiber optics on the dental handpiece provide the lighting needed to illuminate the oral cavity. (For more information, refer to the section on Seating and Preparing the Patient in Chapter 17, and the fiber-optic handpiece discussed in Chapter 18, Basic Chairside Instruments and Tray Systems.)

Maintenance of the Operating Field

The dental assistant is primarily responsible for ensuring that:

- the operator's vision and access are not obscured by oral tissues, moisture, or debris;
- fluids do not interfere with the application of dental materials;
- there are no fluids or materials for the patient to swallow or aspirate;
- there is no interference with the manipulation of the handpiece and the instruments being used by the operator.

Maintaining the Operating Field is Accomplished by a Combination of the Following Techniques:

- Use of the dental dam or cotton rolls to isolate the field
- Use of an isolation system
- Use of high-volume evacuator and the air–water syringe to rinse and clean the oral cavity
- Retraction of oral tissues for clear vision

The Following Items are used by the Dental Team for Maintaining the Operating Field:

- Dental lighting
- High-volume evacuator
- Low-volume saliva ejector
- Air–water syringe
- Retractors and mouth props

The Evacuation System

The evacuation system is designed to remove fluids and debris from the oral cavity. Dental handpieces require the use of a water coolant to reduce the frictional heat that is produced while cutting tooth structures. Because there is a considerable amount of water released from the handpiece during this phase of the procedure, a **high-volume evacuator (HVE)** is used to remove the water, saliva, blood, and debris. This system eliminates the need for the patient to sit up and empty his or her mouth.

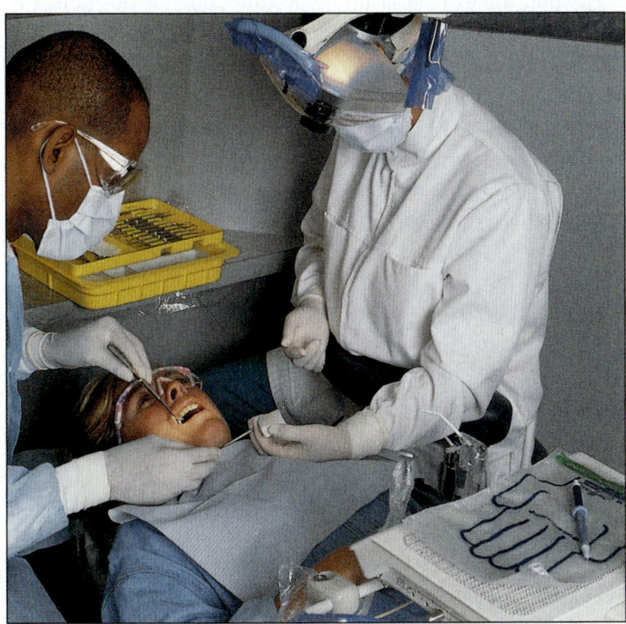

FIGURE 19-19

The dental assistant holds a paper pad with mixed cement close to the patient's chin, ready for the operator's use.

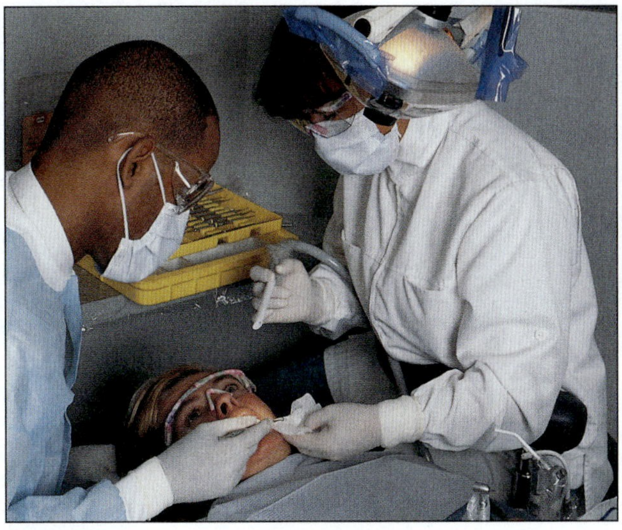

FIGURE 19-20

The assistant holds 2 × 2 gauze open to receive the instrument with debris on the working end.

Parts of High-Volume Evacuation System.

- **Hose**—The hose is flexible tubing that connects to the unit at one end and to the handle at the other end. The hose must be long enough for the assistant to reach the patient's oral cavity without restrictions.
- **Evacuation tip**—The evacuation tip is a plastic or metal tip that fits into the handle/hose of the evacuation system. These tips come in a variety of lengths and shapes and can have beveled ends. They may be straight or slightly bent, and they are either disposable or can be sterilized. Some tips may have the working end of the evacuator rubber coated for patient comfort. Some evacuator tips come with screens incorporated within them, or they can be added to the working end of most evacuators. (Figures 19-21 A through D). Some procedures require a tip that is very narrow on one end. These are used during surgical procedures to allow evacuation in a restricted area.
- **Handle**—The handle is where the evacuation tip is inserted and the on/off controls are located. The control switch may be a dial, switch, or button—there are many variations. The assistant should be able to operate the control switch with the hand that holds the evacuator (Figure 19-21B).

In Which Hand Is the Evacuator Positioned?

The evacuator is held in the assistant's right hand when assisting a right-handed operator and in the left hand when assisting a left-handed operator.

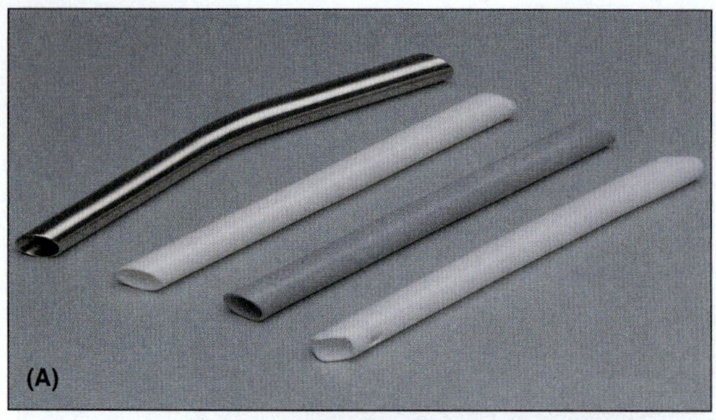

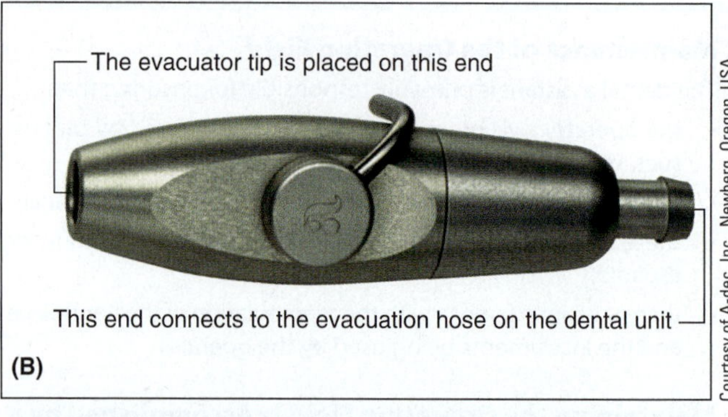
The evacuator tip is placed on this end
This end connects to the evacuation hose on the dental unit
Courtesy of A-dec, Inc., Newberg, Oregon, USA

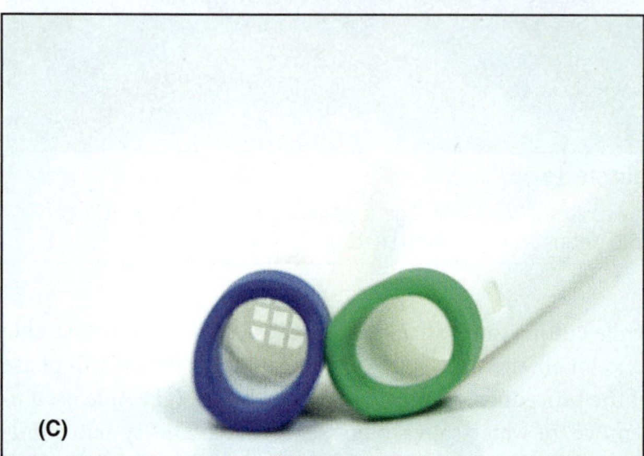

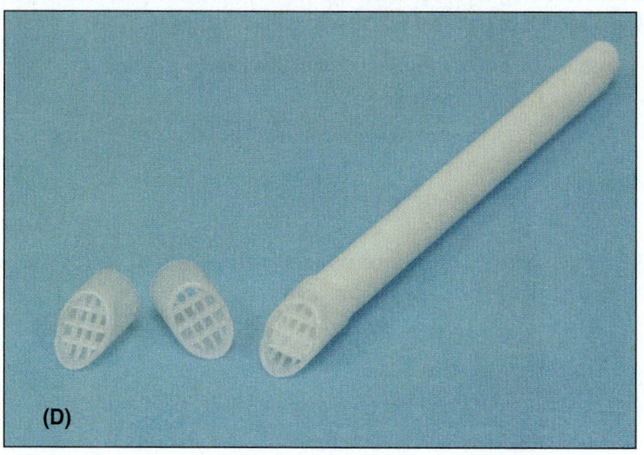

FIGURE 19-21

(A) Several types of evacuator tips (curved metal tip and a variety of plastic tips). (B) Evacuator (HVE) handle. (C) Rubber coated tips. (D) Tip covered with screen.

Grasps for Oral Evacuation. There are several ways to grasp an evacuator tip. Which grasp to use is determined by where the tip is placed; whether it is used to evacuate fluids, retract tissue, or both; and how comfortable the assistant feels with the grasp. The grasps most commonly used are the pen, modified pen, thumb-to-nose, and the reverse palm–thumb. The pen grasp or the modified pen grasp are used when working on the anterior maxillary and mandibular teeth, or when using the narrow surgical tip. The thumb-to-nose grasp is used for maxillary and mandibular posterior teeth. When using the thumb-to-nose grasp, the assistant has greater control, and better retraction of the cheeks and tongue, which causes less strain on the assistant's hand.

Tip Placement for Evacuation of the Oral Cavity. Knowledge and skill regarding the placement of the evacuator tip is essential for the dental assistant. Each area of the mouth requires a different tip placement. Procedure 19-2 illustrates the proper positioning of the evacuator in each mouth quadrant.

Saliva Ejector

The **saliva ejector** is the low-volume evacuation system. It is a flexible, plastic tube about one-third the size of the high-volume evacuation tube. The saliva ejector is bent and then positioned between the tongue and the mandibular teeth or between the cheek and the mandibular teeth.

General Guidelines for Oral Evacuation Tip Placement

- Carefully place the evacuator tip in the patient's mouth. Avoid bumping the teeth, lips, or gingiva.
- Position the evacuator tip before the operator positions the handpiece or an instrument.
- Place the evacuator tip approximately one tooth distal to the tooth being worked on.
- Hold the bevel of the evacuator tip parallel to the buccal or lingual surface of the teeth.
- The middle of the evacuator tip opening should be even with the occlusal surface. Position the tip far enough away from the handpiece so that it does not draw the water coolant away from the bur.
- Hold the evacuator tip still while the handpiece or instrument is being used. Any movement may startle the operator or the patient, and may cause the handpiece or instrument to be bumped.
- Rest the tip on cotton rolls, not the gingival tissue. Cotton rolls are placed in the vestibular area near the tooth being worked on before the evacuator tip is placed.
- Avoid placing the evacuator tip on the soft palate, the back of the tongue, or the anterior pillar/tonsilar area. Allowing the tip to contact any of these areas could cause the patient to gag.
- Keep the evacuator tip far enough away from the mucosal tissue to prevent it from being sucked into the tip and making a noise. If this does occur, either turn it off or rotate the tip to break the seal, and avoid saying "Oops" or "I'm sorry." Just go on with the procedure.

Procedure 19-2
Specific Tip Placements for Evacuation of the Oral Cavity

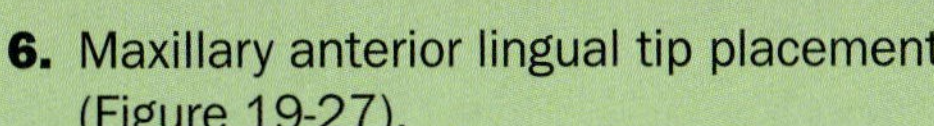

This procedure is performed by the dental assistant during dental treatment. The oral cavity is maintained to keep the area clear and clean for the operator and for the comfort of the patient. Each area of the mouth requires different evacuator tip positioning. The following illustrates how to position the tip for each quadrant when assisting a right-handed operator.

Equipment and Supplies

- Basic setup: mouth mirror, cotton pliers, and explorer
- HVE tip and air–water syringe tip
- Cotton rolls
- Dental handpiece

Procedure Steps (*Follow aseptic procedures*)

1. Maxillary right posterior tip placement (Figure 19-22).
2. Maxillary left posterior tip placement (Figure 19-23).
3. Mandibular right posterior tip placement (Figure 19-24).
4. Mandibular left posterior tip placement (Figure 19-25).
5. Maxillary anterior facial tip placement (Figure 19-26).
6. Maxillary anterior lingual tip placement (Figure 19-27).
7. Mandibular anterior facial tip placement (Figure 19-28).
8. Mandibular anterior lingual tip placement (Figure 19-29).

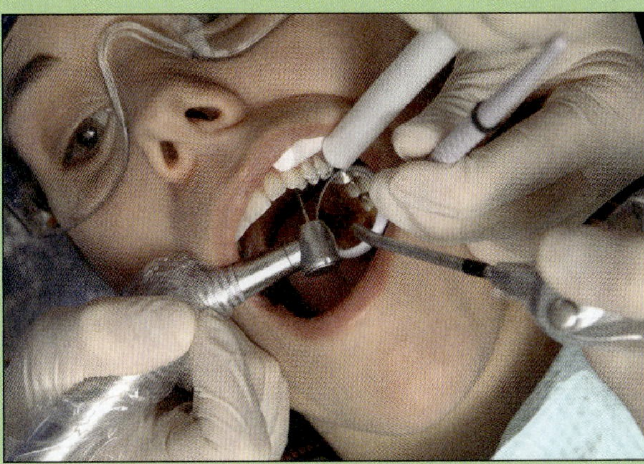

FIGURE 19-23
Evacuator tip in position with cotton rolls. Also, the handpiece and mouth mirror are in position with the air–water syringe tip. The evacuator tip is positioned parallel to the buccal surface of the teeth and is resting on a cotton roll.

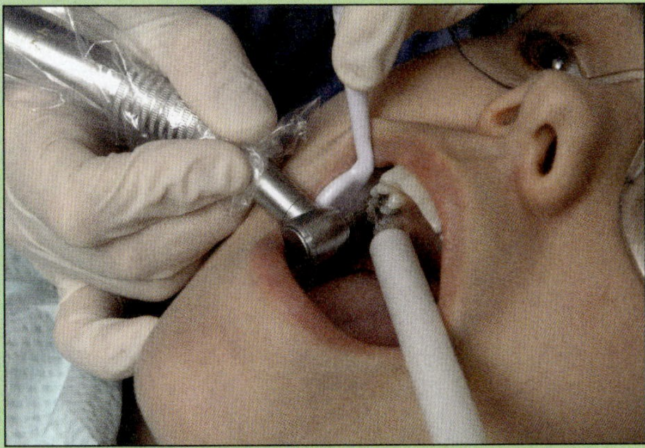

FIGURE 19-22
The tip is placed near the lingual surface, just distal to the tooth being worked on. The bevel of the tip is parallel to the lingual surface of the teeth. Notice that the tip is resting on the teeth in the maxillary left quadrant.

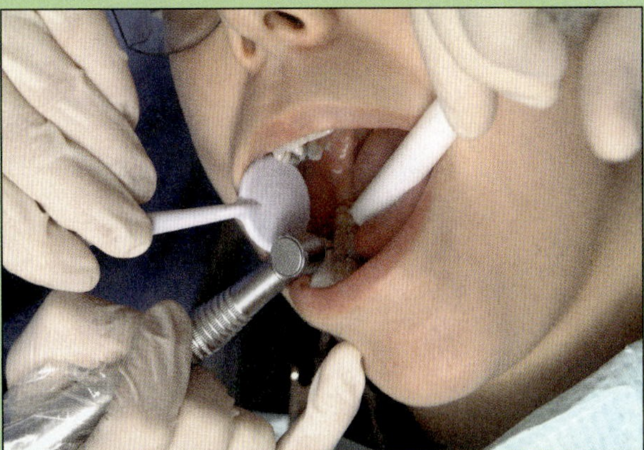

FIGURE 19-24
Evacuator tip in position with handpiece and mouth mirror. The tip comes across the mandibular left teeth and is positioned between the lingual surface of the teeth and the tongue. The tip is parallel to the lingual surface of the teeth. A cotton roll can be used to retract the tongue.

(continues)

Procedure 19-2 (continued)

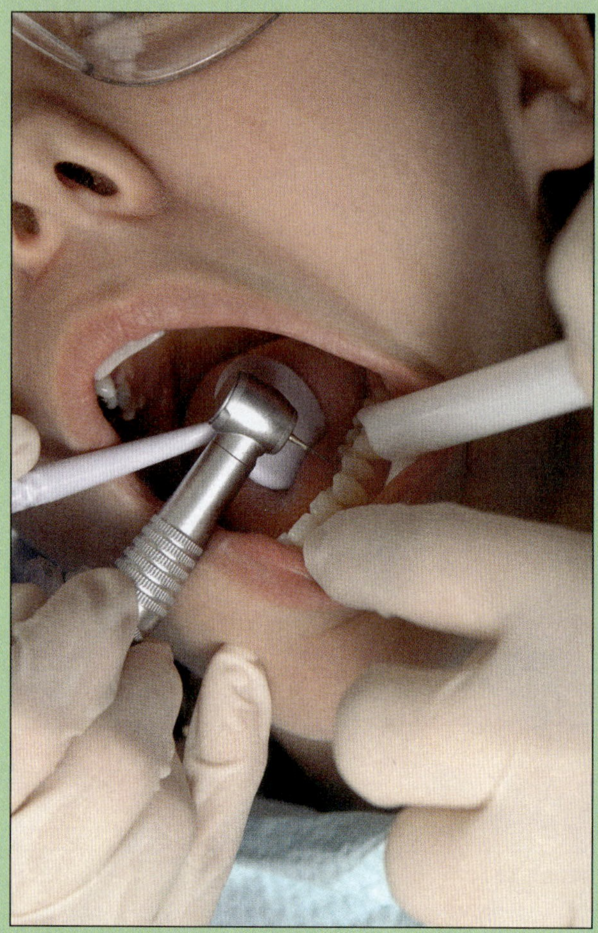

FIGURE 19-25

The evacuator tip is placed and the handpiece is positioned. The tip of the bevel of the evacuator tip is positioned parallel to the buccal surface of the teeth. A cotton roll can be placed to assist in the retraction of the cheek.

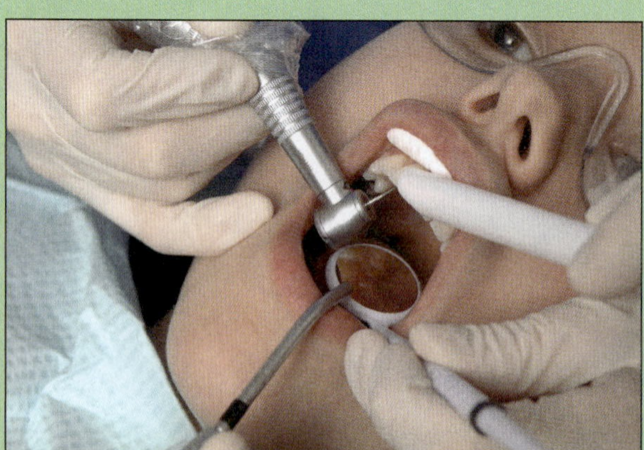

FIGURE 19-26

The evacuator tip is placed with the handpiece positioned. For the anterior facial tip placement, the operator positions the handpiece toward the facial surface. The evacuator tip is placed near the lingual surface of the maxillary anterior teeth with the beveled tip rotated to catch the water near the facial surface with the bevel of the tip rotated toward the incisal edge of the maxillary teeth.

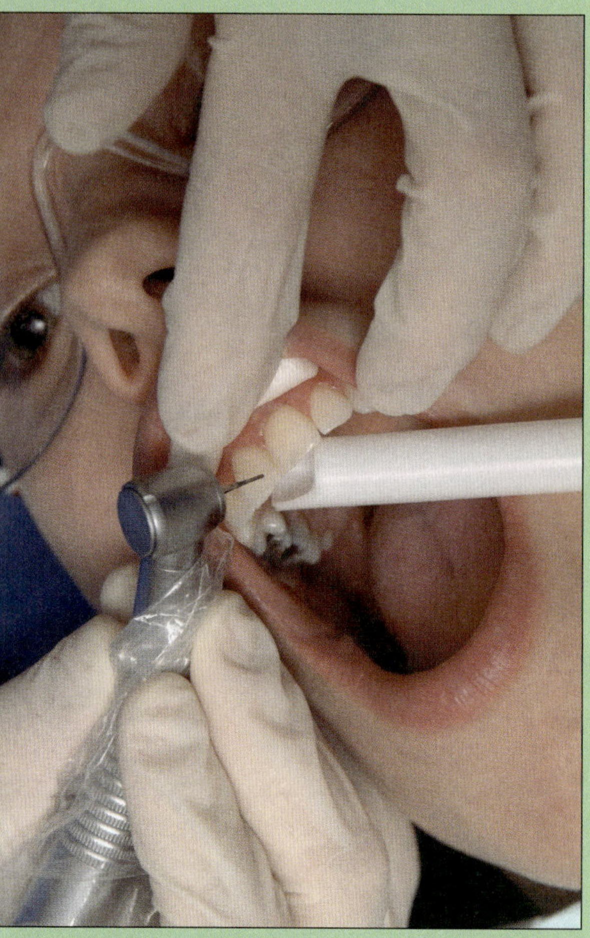

FIGURE 19-27

The evacuator tip is placed with the handpiece, mouth mirror, and air–water syringe tip. The tip is placed on the lingual surface, out of the operator's way. Optional tip placement would be from the facial surface.

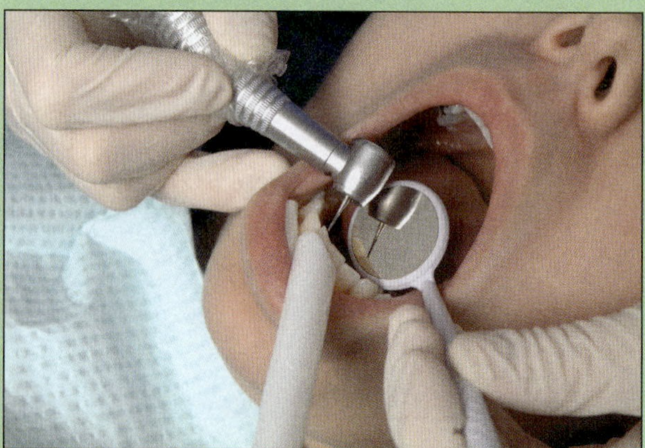

FIGURE 19-28

The tip is placed and the handpiece and mouth mirror are in position. The evacuator tip is positioned on the cotton roll near the facial surface of the teeth. The lip is retracted with a cotton roll and the bevel surface of the evacuator tip is parallel to the facial surface.

(continues)

Procedure 19-2 (continued)

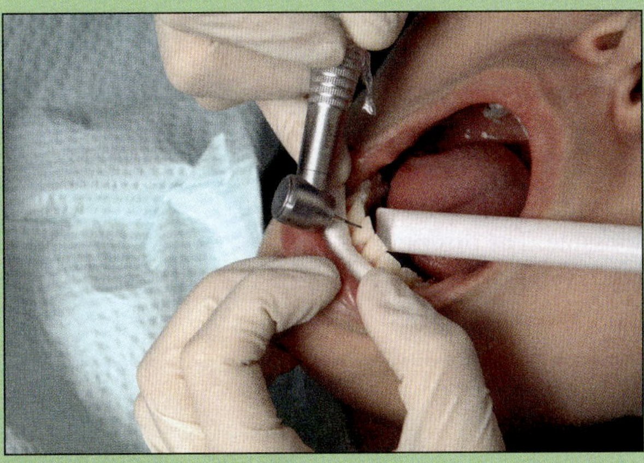

FIGURE 19-29

The tip is placed and the handpiece is positioned. The evacuator tip is positioned parallel to the lingual surface of the teeth.

Parts of the Saliva Ejector.

- **Plastic tube** or a metal "shepherd's hook" tube—The plastic tube is the most common, although stainless-steel tubes are available. The plastic saliva ejectors are less expensive and are disposable. The end placed in the patient's mouth has a guard cover to prevent large particles of debris from becoming lodged in the tube.
- **Handle**—The plastic tube is inserted in the handle, which is connected to the hose. The handle has an on/off control and also a small screen that acts as a filter, located near the tube end of the handle.
- **Hose**—The hose end attaches to a low-volume vacuum source in the unit. The saliva ejector is used during procedures that do not require removal of large amounts of fluids, such as during fluoride treatments, under the rubber dam, or during a coronal polish (Figure 19-30).

For a review on how to maintain the high-volume evacuator (HVE) and saliva ejector, refer to Chapter 11, Infection Control. It is important for the dental assistant to establish a routine for maintaining these systems.

The Air–Water Syringe

The **air–water syringe**, also referred to as the three-way syringe, emits water, air, or a combination of both in a spray. The patient's mouth is rinsed with the air–water syringe and simultaneously evacuated. The assistant can dry an area or keep the mirror clean with air for the operator to have clear vision. The air–water syringe is held in the assistant's left hand for a right-handed operator and in the right hand for a left-handed operator.

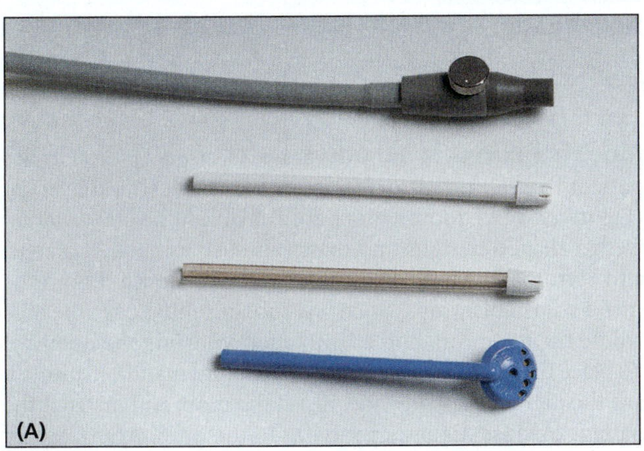

(A)

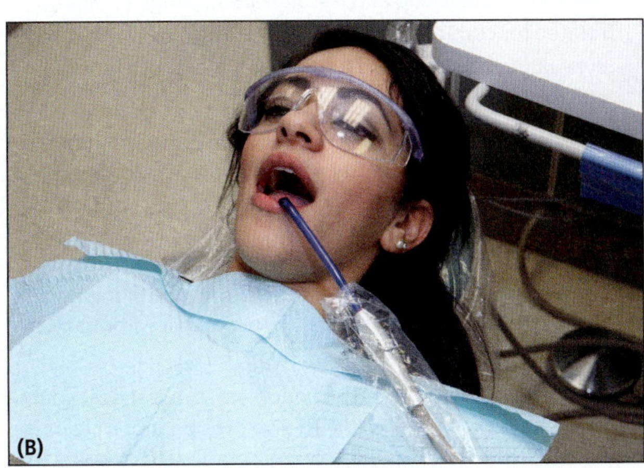

(B)

FIGURE 19-30

(A) Saliva ejector hose with controls and attachment with several different types of saliva ejectors. (B) Saliva ejector in the patient's mouth. Notice the handle control on the hose and the flexibility of the saliva ejector, which is bent to stay in the patient's mouth.

Parts of the Air–Water Syringe.

- **Handle**—The handle is connected to a hose, which in turn is connected to the unit. The top of the handle is called the nozzle area and has buttons for the water and the air. If the buttons are pressed simultaneously, a spray of water and air is released (Figure 19-31A). In the handle, there are O-rings that may have to be changed if the syringe begins to leak.
- **Syringe tip**—The syringe tip directs the air, water, or spray. The tips are either metal and can be removed and sterilized, or plastic and disposable. The tips can be rotated for positioning toward the maxillary or mandibular teeth (Figure 19-31B).

Courtesy of A-dec, Inc., Newberg, Oregon, USA

FIGURE 19-31

Parts of the air–water syringe: (A) Handle. (B) Syringe tip. (C) Air control. (D) Water control. Both controls are pressed simultaneously for air–water spray.

Reflux with the Three-Way Syringe Tip

When the water button is released, the normal action on the three-way syringe tip causes "suck back" or **reflux** to occur. This action allows contaminated fluids to retract back into the tip due to negative water pressure. By using disposable tips, possible cross-contamination is eliminated.

Retraction of Tissues

Retraction of the tongue, cheeks, lips, and tissue is used to increase the field of vision in the oral cavity. There are several types of retractors used, including the mouth mirror, the rubber dam, the evacuator tip, cotton rolls, cotton gauze, and specially designed tissue retractors. Retractors are used during any procedure to allow for better access and lighting, and to prevent injury to the tissues (Figures 19-32A and B).

Guidelines for Use of the Air–Water Syringe

1. The most effective way to use the air–water syringe is with the air–water spray. A spray is effective and easier to control (Figure 19-33A). However, the spray creates aerosol, and so some dentists prefer water followed by air.
2. When rinsing a patient's mouth, use the evacuator tip to follow the spray. The patient's mouth is rinsed in quadrants, and the evacuator tip and the air–water syringe tip are rotated for correct placement (Figure 19-33B). Rinsing and evacuating the patient's mouth requires practice to achieve efficiency and control.
3. When the operator is using the handpiece and a mirror for indirect vision, water from the handpiece falls onto the mirror and distorts the operator's view. The assistant will be expected to keep the mirror's surface dry and free from debris. To accomplish this, the assistant places the tip of the air–water syringe close to the edge of the mouth mirror, and directs the air across the surface of the mirror without interfering with the operator's view.
4. When the operator stops the handpiece, the assistant completes a quick "rinse and dry" to give the operator a clean, dry mirror for good vision. This is accomplished by using the spray, followed by air.

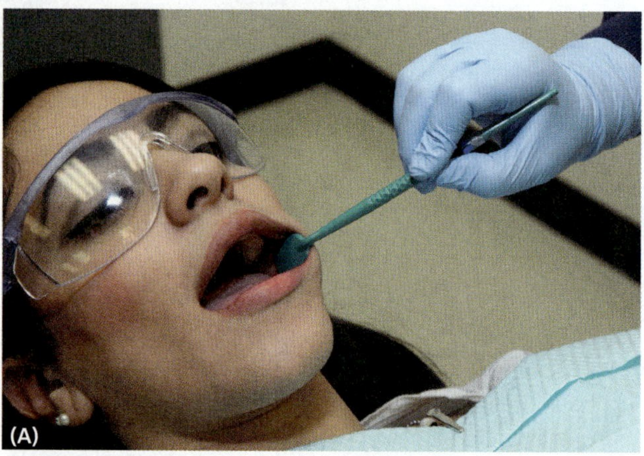

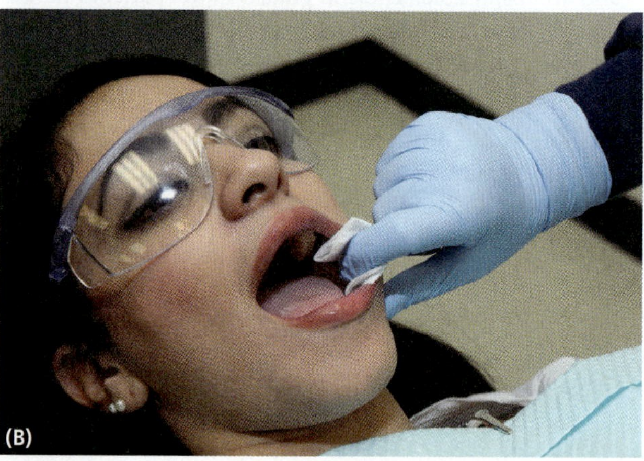

FIGURE 19-32

(A) Retraction using a mouth mirror. (B) Retraction using cotton gauze.

Mouth Props. A **mouth prop** is used to assist the patient in keeping his or her mouth open during treatment (Figure 19-34A). Mouth props are available in several different wedge-shaped designs and materials such as rubber, plastic, and Styrofoam. Another distinctive type of mouth prop is the metal adjustable prop, which has rubber tubing over the area where the teeth rest, and a handle for adjusting the opening. To place the prop between the maxillary and mandibular teeth, ask the patient to open wide, insert the prop, and instruct the patient to close his or her mouth on the prop. After placing the prop, ask if the patient is comfortable and adjust the prop, if necessary (Figure 19-34B).

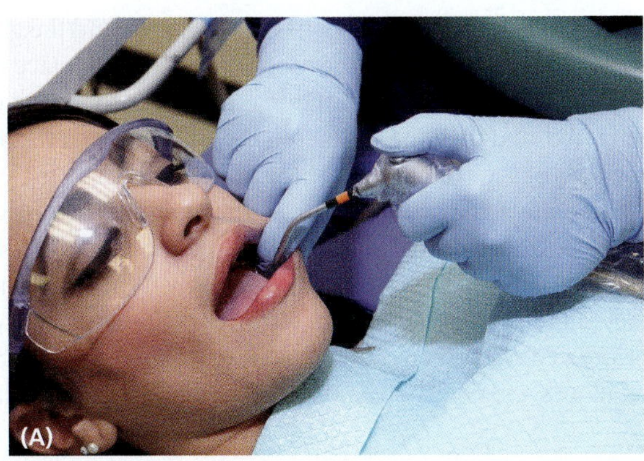

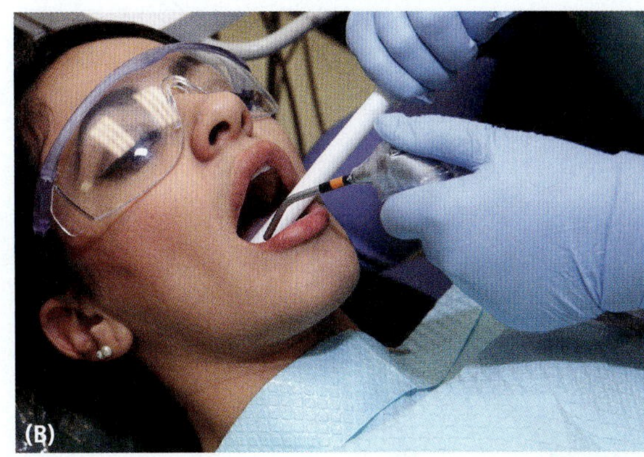

FIGURE 19-33

(A) Assistant using the air–water syringe. (B) Assistant using the HVE and the air–water syringe.

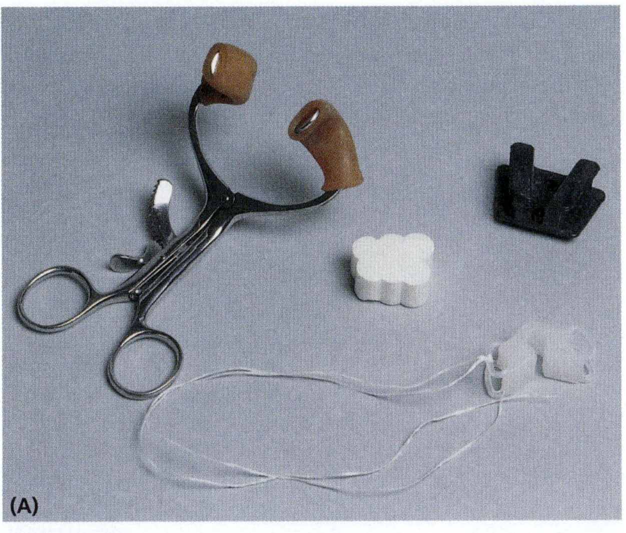

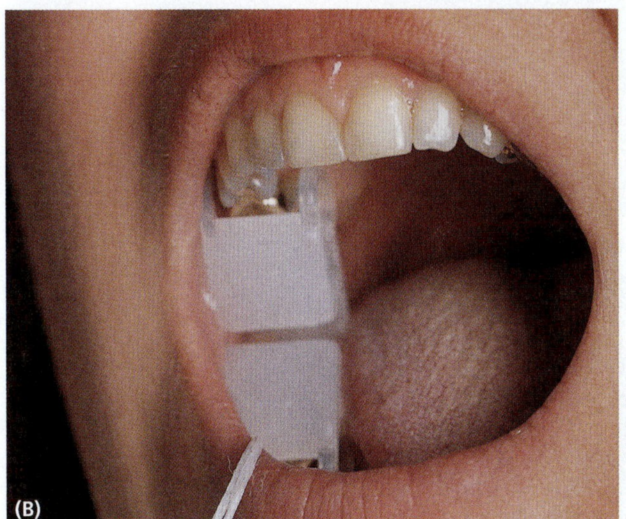

Courtesy of Isolite Systems

FIGURE 19-34

(A) Examples of mouth props. (B) A mouth prop in a patient's mouth.

Isolite System

There is another system used to maintain a clear, dry field for the operator. The **Isolite system** provides isolation, retraction, evacuation, and a light source in one piece of equipment. The system includes a titanium control head, power/vacuum hose, and a one-time-use mouthpiece. The control head contains a light emitter, a dual-channel vacuum, and controls for both. This system is connected to the dental unit's vacuum system and an electrical source. The mouthpieces are attached to the control head before each procedure, and then placed in the patient's mouth.

The mouthpiece is made of a soft flexible material and comes in a variety of sizes. The mouthpiece includes a tongue and cheek protector, throat barrier, vacuum channels, and an integrated bite block (Figures 19-35A and B). Once the mouthpiece is placed, the operator can work on either the upper or lower quadrants. The patient is comfortable with the bite block in place; and the tongue, cheeks, and throat are protected. The dental assistant is free to perform other functions during the procedure. The mouthpiece is disposed of after each use to prevent cross-contamination.

The Isolite system is used with many different procedures including: crowns and bridges, fillings, implants, sealants, veneers, CERAC dentistry, and laser dentistry, as well as some oral surgery and orthodontic and periodontic procedures. Procedure times have been reduced by over 20 percent with use of this system. It is becoming increasingly popular with dentists, dental assistants, and dental hygienists. The main disadvantage is the cost of the mouthpieces, and a learning curve.

Techniques for Moisture Control and Isolation

We have discussed the use of the saliva ejector and the HVE to control the moisture in the oral cavity, and the importance of removing fluids and keeping the area dry and free of debris. Several other techniques can assist in keeping the field dry during a procedure. These techniques include the use of cotton rolls, dry angles (absorbent wafers), and the placement of the dental dam.

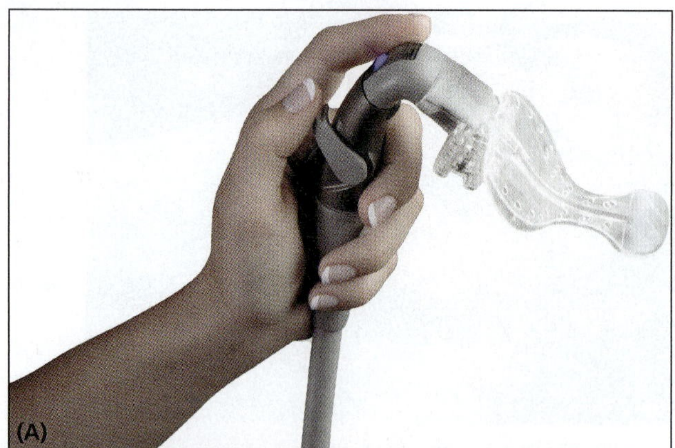

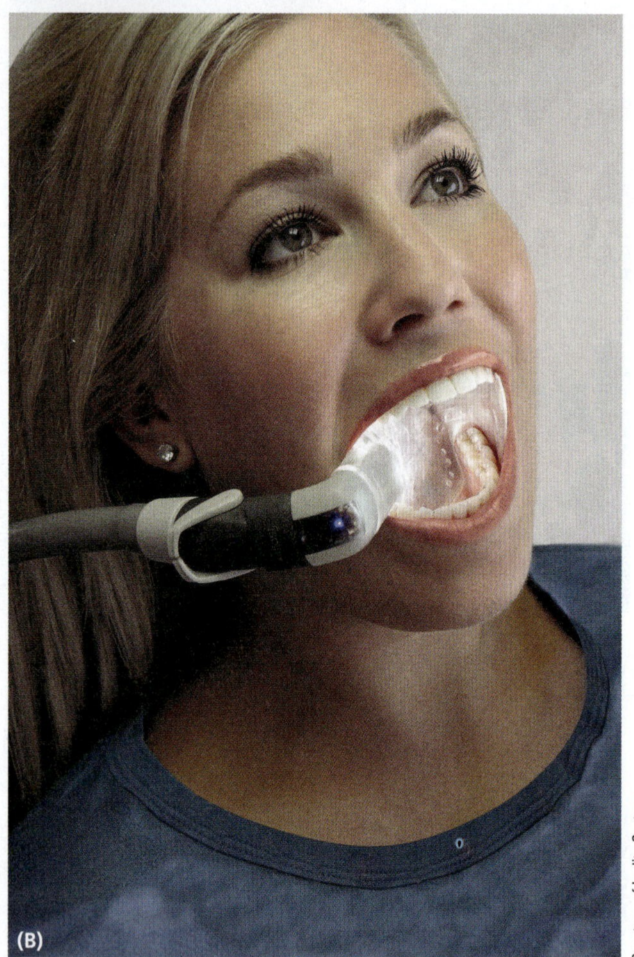

Courtesy of Isolite Systems

FIGURE 19-35

Isolite system: (A) Handle and mouthpiece. (B) Isolite placed in patient's mouth.

Cotton Rolls

Cotton rolls come in a variety of sizes and designs. They are used to isolate an area, rest the evacuator (HVE) on, place materials with, or serve as something for the patient to bite on. Cotton rolls are flexible for easy placement. They can be placed using cotton pliers or directly placed in the mouth by the dentist or the dental assistant. To place the cotton rolls on the buccal side (cheek side) of the teeth, for both the maxillary and mandibular arches, the cheek is gently pulled away from the teeth. The cotton roll is then placed in the vestibule area—the pocket formed by the soft tissues of the cheeks and the gingiva, sometimes referred to as the mucobuccal fold. To place cotton rolls on the lingual side of the mandible, the tongue is gently retracted, and then the cotton roll is placed between the lingual surfaces of the teeth and the base of the tongue.

To remove the cotton rolls from the mouth, either use cotton pliers or directly remove them from the mouth. When cotton rolls are moist, they can be removed easily. When they are dry, they should be *moistened with water* from the air–water syringe before removal. When cotton rolls are dry, they stick to the mucosal tissues and need to be moistened to prevent tissue irritation.

Dry Angles

Saliva from the parotid gland enters the mouth through the Stenson's duct. As discussed in Chapter 7, Head and Neck Anatomy, the Stenson's duct is on the buccal mucosa around the maxillary second bicuspid area. To help control the moisture from this area, **dry angles** are used. Dry angles are triangular, absorbent pads that absorb the flow of saliva and protect the cheek (Figure 19-36A). Dry angles are placed directly on

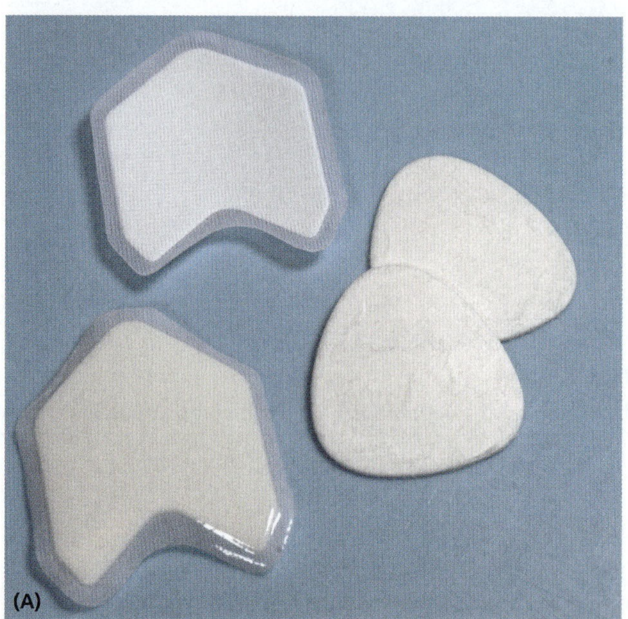

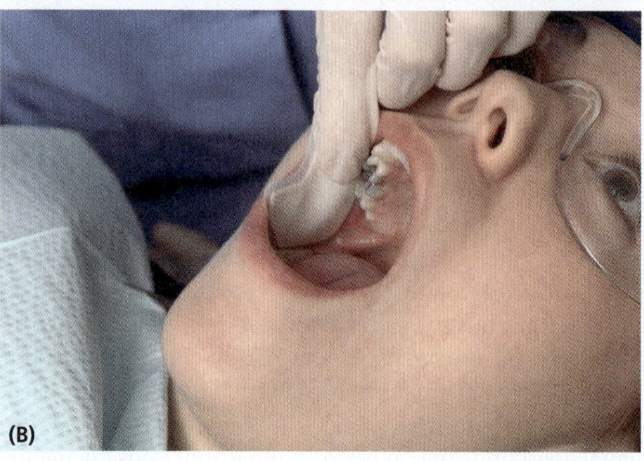

FIGURE 19-36

(A) Dry angles. (B) Dry angles placed in a patient's mouth against the cheek.

the buccal mucosa and absorb moisture as well as provide a surface for cheek retraction (Figure 19-36B). Like cotton rolls, they need to be moist before removal. Use the air–water syringe to wet the dry angle, and then remove with cotton pliers. Dry angles may need to be changed during the procedure if they become too saturated with moisture.

Advanced Chairside Functions

Dental Assistants Performing Expanded Functions

In many states dental assistants can perform **expanded functions** with additional course work, skill competency, and registration/licensure. The expanded functions are skills above and beyond the normal scope of dental assisting. When performing these skills, the assistant works alone, not under the direct supervision of the dentist. The dentist delegates the expanded functions allowed in their state to fit the needs of their office. This advanced-skilled dental assistant can increase productivity in the office by freeing up the dentist to see more patients. These expanded functions skills include: taking x-rays, placing and removing a rubber dam, coronal polish, taking study model impressions, placing sealants, making provisionals, placing bases and liners, taking photographs, many orthodontic procedures, removing sutures, and placing periodontal dressings. In some states, dental assistants can place restorations and take final impressions. Each state is different and unique with regard to the skills a dental assistant is permitted to perform, as they are regulated by each state's dental practice act.

The assistant needs to be prepared and efficient when performing chairside functions alone (Figure 19-37). When working solo, the assistant:

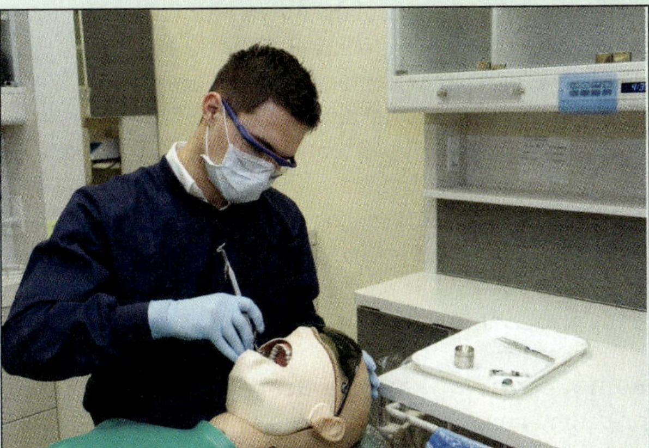

FIGURE 19-37
Expanded function dental assistant working as a solo operator.

1. sits on the operator's side of the chair depending upon whether the assistant is right or left handed;
2. uses the operator's stool rather than the assistant's stool;
3. sets up the tray and the unit to accommodate working alone;
4. places items on the tray within easy reach;
5. brings the handpieces, HVE, and air–water syringe near the patient's head, where it is convenient to use them together or alone;
6. uses the saliva ejector, and then rinses and evacuates with the HVE as needed;
7. brings the dental light within reach.

Dental Dam

Dental dam (also referred to as a rubber dam) placement is one method of isolating teeth for restoration. It can be used on almost any patient. The dental dam is a barrier that is applied by the dentist and, in some states, by the dental assistant and the dental hygienist. After the patient has received the anesthetic, the dental dam is prepared and placed. The dental assistant assists the dentist with its placement, or places the dental dam before the dentist begins to prepare the tooth. The dam can be placed to isolate one tooth, or one or more quadrants.

Advantages of Dental Dam Use

The advantages of using the dental dam are as follows:

- Greater visibility because of the contrast between the tooth and the dental dam material
- Greater accessibility to the operating field by retracting gingiva, tongue, cheeks, and lips
- Control of moisture, keeping the area dry for better vision and ensuring a dry tooth when bonding agents, etchants, and restorative materials are used
- Protection of the patient from swallowing or aspirating debris during the procedure
- Protection of the gingiva during acid-etching procedures

Advanced Chairside Functions (Continued)

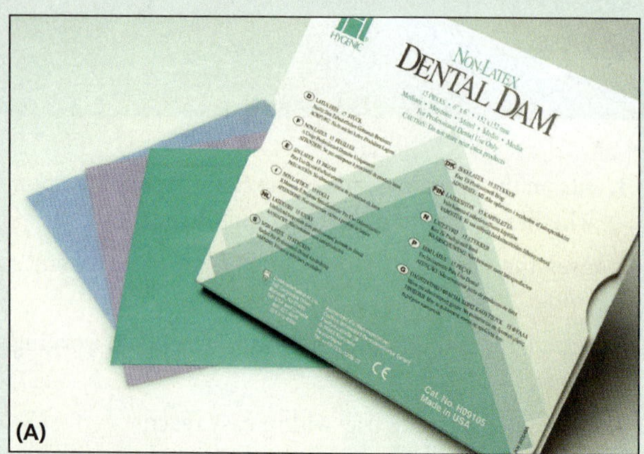

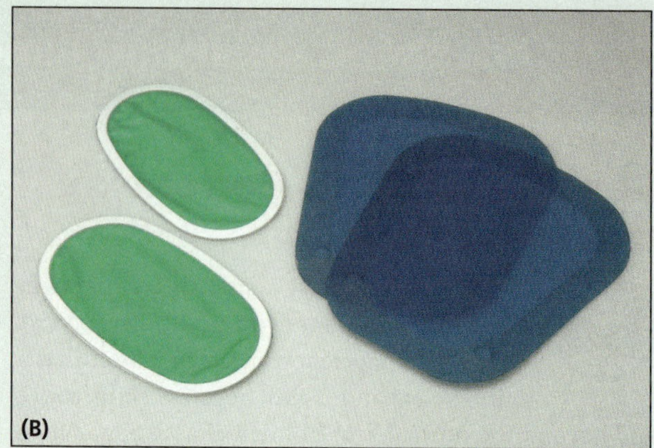

FIGURE 19-38
(A) Various colors and sizes of dental dam material. (B) Dental dam with frames.

- Improved patient management and decreased operating time due to limited patient conversation, and the maintenance of a clear, dry field
- Decreased amount of contaminated aerosol exposure

Contraindications to Dental Dam Isolation

Conditions that contraindicate dental dam use include the following:

- Physical conditions of the patient, such as asthma, respiratory congestion, allergies to latex, herpetic lesions, or lesions of the commissures (corners of the mouth)
- Concerns that the patient may have, such as if the patient is claustrophobic (cannot tolerate the dental dam), or the patient has had, or has heard of, a bad experience with the dental dam (hesitant to have the dam used for the dental procedure)
- Conditions in the oral cavity, such as partially erupted teeth or **malaligned** teeth

Materials and Equipment

The dental dam procedure requires a variety of instruments and materials. The materials and equipment may be on a separate tray stored at the dental unit, or in a tub for easy use. Materials include the dental dam material, dental dam napkin, dental floss, and tape. Specific equipment needed include dental dam clamps, forceps, frame, punching guides, and a punch.

Dental Dam Material. The dental dam is a latex or latex-free material that comes in various sizes, weights, and colors, which is selected according to an office's preference. The most common sizes of the dental dam are the 5 × 5 inch or the 6 × 6 inch precut squares. The 5 × 5 inch dental dam is used for endodontic procedures, anterior applications on adults, and for children. The 6 × 6 inch dental dam is used for adult procedures. These squares usually come in a box of 50 or more, and are lightly powdered on one side to prevent sticking. The dental dam is also available in a continuous roll of 5 inch and 6 inch widths. This material is cut to the desired length by the operator.

The dental dam is available in different weights (thicknesses), including thin, medium, heavy, extra heavy, and special heavy. The thin or light dental dam materials are passed easily through contacts, but tear easily and do not retract the tissues effectively. The medium and the heavy materials are often used because they do not tear as easily and provide greater tissue retraction. The heavier the material, the more difficult it is to place interproximal, but the retraction of the tissues is excellent (Figure 19-38).

The dental dam is available in various colors (shades), from dark gray or green to pastels. The darker shades provide more contrast with the teeth and are easier for the operator. A scented dental dam is also available and is very pleasing to the patient (in comparison to the latex smell). It may be scented with mint or fruit.

The dental dam material has no definite shelf life but is sensitive to temperature changes and, like other latex rubber, to age. For a longer shelf life, store dental dam material in the refrigerator.

Dental Dam Napkin. The **dental dam napkin** is used for patient comfort and to absorb saliva, water, and perspiration. Disposable napkins are made of a soft, absorbent fabric and are precut. They are designed to prevent the dam material from touching the face by covering the area around the mouth and the cheeks (Figure 19-39).

Advanced Chairside Functions

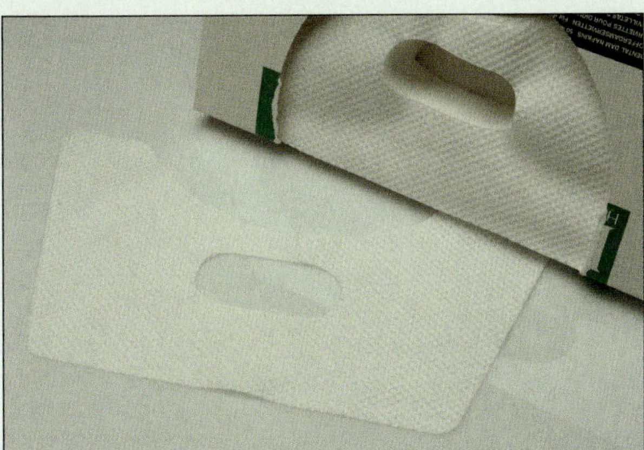

FIGURE 19-39
Dental dam napkins.

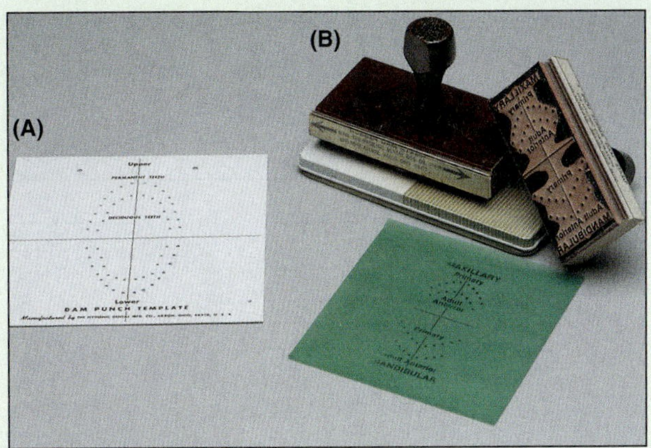

FIGURE 19-41
Dental dam punch guides: (A) Template. (B) Stamp with inkpad.

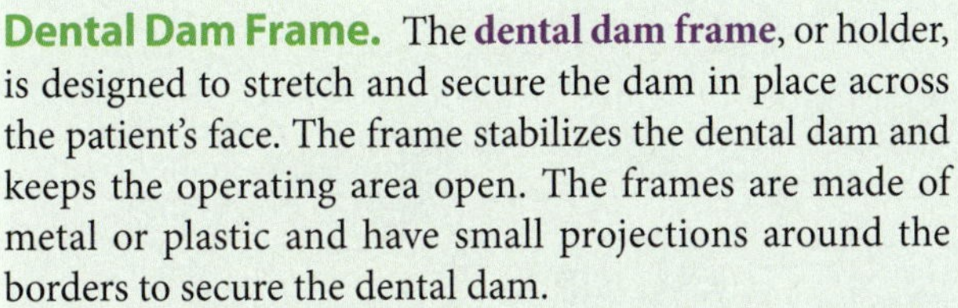

Dental Dam Frame. The **dental dam frame**, or holder, is designed to stretch and secure the dam in place across the patient's face. The frame stabilizes the dental dam and keeps the operating area open. The frames are made of metal or plastic and have small projections around the borders to secure the dental dam.

Several styles of frames are available (Figure 19-40). The metal U-shaped frame is very common and is known as the **Young frame**. It is easy to apply and comfortable for the patient. The Young frame is made of stainless steel and can be autoclaved. The plastic U-shaped frame is also common and is known as the **U-frame**. It is also easy to apply and comfortable for the patient. This plastic frame is radiolucent and autoclavable. The **Ostby frame** is an oval-shaped plastic frame that was designed to follow the shape of the lower face. Projections on the outer borders secure the dental dam. This frame is **radiotransparent**—allows radiation to pass through it so that it does not interfere with images on an x-ray—and can be autoclaved.

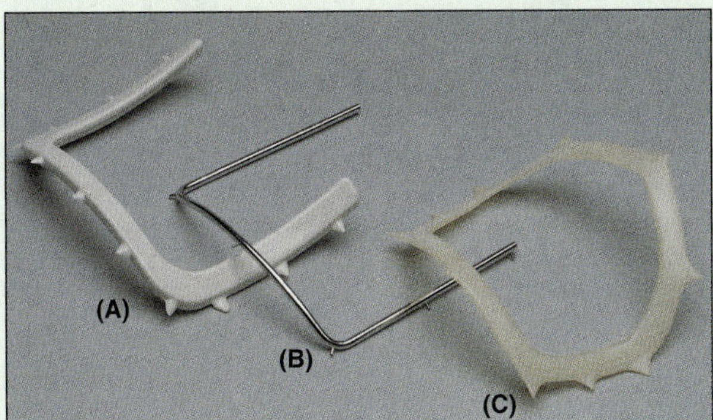

FIGURE 19-40
Dental dam frames: (A) U-frame. (B) Metal Young frame. (C) Ostby frame.

Dental Dam Punching Guides. The dental dam may be marked by using a **template** or a **stamp** of the adult and pediatric arches. Both the template and stamp are marked to indicate where the holes for the teeth should be punched. The stamp is used with an inkpad, and the dam may be stamped ahead of time. The template comes in both 5 × 5 inch and 6 × 6 inch sizes and can also be used to mark the dam ahead of time (Figure 19-41).

The dental dam guides are perfect dental arches, so they will not fit every patient. Instead, the markings act as guides. They are especially helpful when learning to punch the dental dam, but, eventually, they become unnecessary and the operator uses the patient's teeth as the guide.

Dental Dam Punch. The action of the **dental dam punch** is similar to that of the paper punch, although the design is much different. The punch has a handle and a working end (Figure 19-42A). The working end of the punch has a stylus, which is a sharp projection that punches through the dental dam, and a **punch table** or **punch plate**. The table has four or five differently sized holes, and rotates to facilitate the punching of holes for the various teeth (Figure 19-42B). The punch table should be adjusted so that the hole is centered under the stylus before the punch is made. This prevents damage to the holes of the punch table. When the punch table is rotated, it makes a clicking sound as it adjusts.

Dental Dam Clamps. The **dental dam clamps** come in numerous designs and sizes to fit around the teeth (Figure 19-43). Their purpose is to stabilize and secure the dental dam material in place. The tooth that the clamp is placed on is often called the **anchor tooth**. The anchor tooth is one, or two, teeth distal to the tooth or teeth being restored.

Advanced Chairside Functions (Continued)

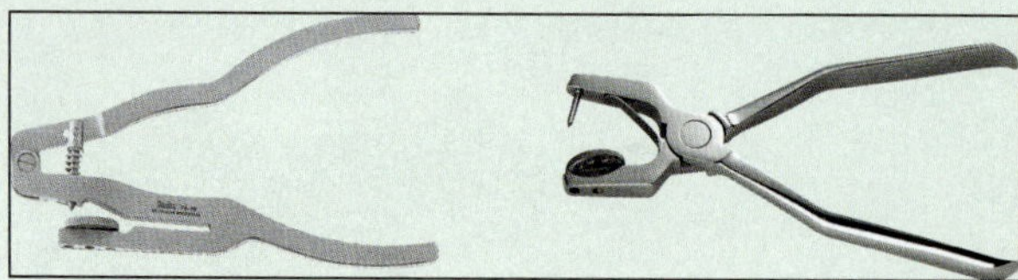

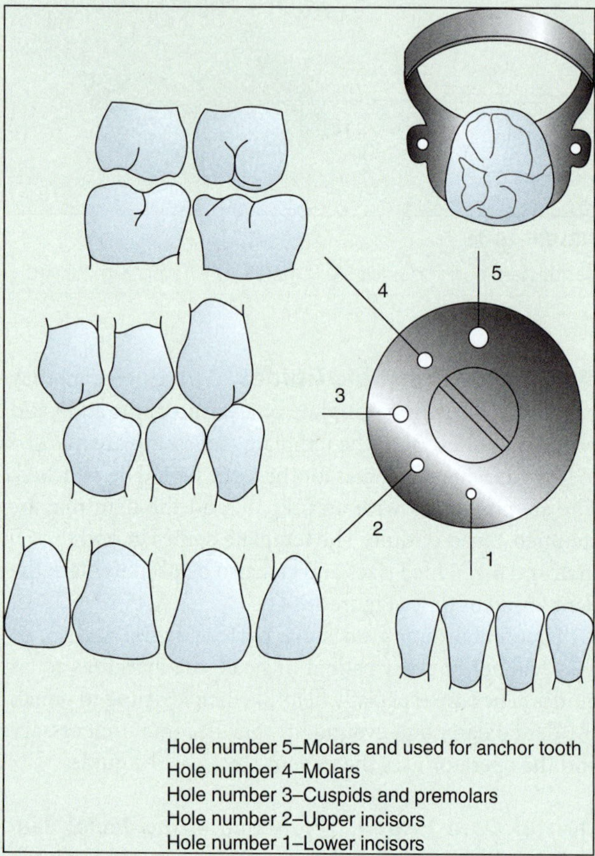

FIGURE 19-42

(A) Dental dam punches. (B) Punch table with corresponding teeth.

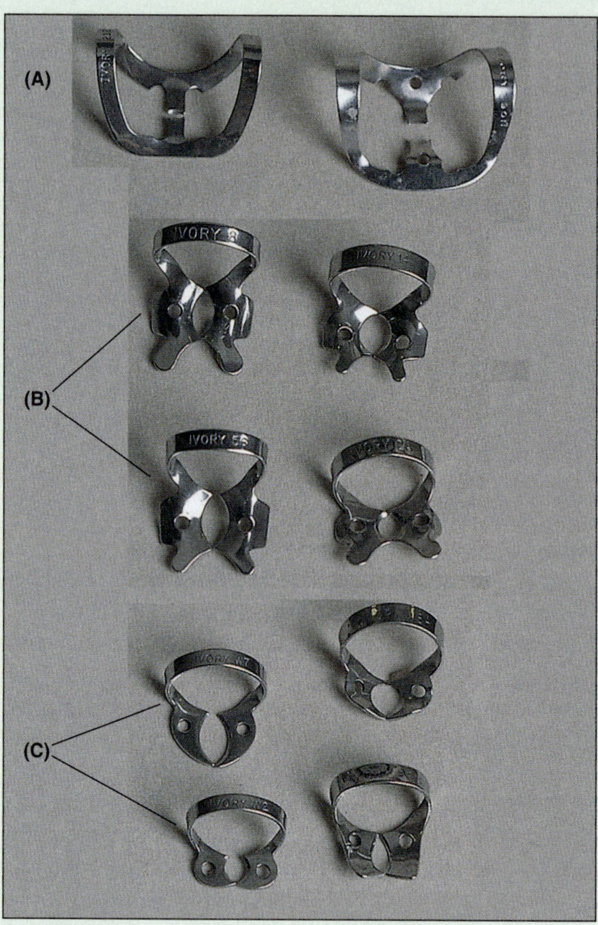

FIGURE 19-43

Assorted clamps: (A) Cervical. (B) Winged. (C) Wingless.

Dental dam clamps are made of high-quality stainless steel, and are designed to be used on specific teeth. They are identified by numbers and letters, not by the teeth they are used on. The basic parts to a dental dam clamp include the following (Figure 19-44):

- **Bow**—Arched metal joining the two jaws of the clamp.
- **Jaws**—The part of the clamp that expands to fix over the tooth, and then releases to fit on the gingival one-third of the tooth. The jaws secure the clamp to the tooth. The jaws have different sizes for different teeth in the arch. In order to improve retention, there are clamps available with serrated jaws.
- **Forceps holes**—Located on the jaws of the clamp, the dental dam forceps attach to the clamp to place and remove the clamp from the tooth at these holes.

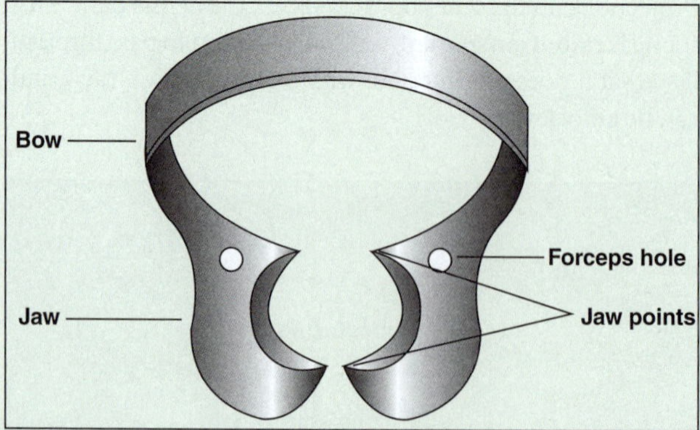

FIGURE 19-44

Parts of the dental dam clamp.

- **Points**—These are the parts of the jaws that actually contact the tooth. The points are located at different widths and angles to fit and secure the clamp on the tooth.

Advanced Chairside Functions

- The jaws of the clamp are designed to be winged or wingless. The **winged clamps** have extra projections for better retraction, and they hold the dental dam in place because the wings are angled toward the gingiva. The **wingless clamps** have the letter *W* in front of the number on the clamp and have no projections.
- Some clamps are double bowed, and they are called **cervical clamps**. These clamps are used for Class V restorations on anterior teeth. These clamps assist in gingival retraction and often must be stabilized with stick impression compound after the teeth have been exposed. Examples are the SSW 212 or the Hygienic B6 and B5.
- Dental dam clamps that have the letter "A" following the number have jaws that bend sharply downward, toward the gingiva. Clamps without the letter "A" have jaws on a flat plane.

Selecting Clamps. The tooth to be clamped must be evaluated before the clamp selection is made. The mesiodistal width at the cementoenamel junction (CEJ) of the tooth must be evaluated in order to select a clamp. The width on the tooth must be about the same as the width between the points of the jaws on the clamp. The faciolingual width at the CEJ of the tooth must also be estimated to ensure that the clamp fits tightly. Once the tooth has been evaluated, a clamp can be selected. To place the clamp, the jaws are opened wide enough to clear the height of contour, which is the widest part of the tooth. Then, the jaws are closed slowly on the tooth to fit tightly at the CEJ. The points should rest securely all around the tooth.

Dental Dam Forceps. The **dental dam forceps** are used to place and remove the dental dam clamp (Figure 19-45). The forceps have two beaks that fit into the holes of the jaws of the clamp. Once the beaks are securely in the holes, pressure is applied to the handle of the forceps and the clamp jaws are opened slightly. There is a lock (sliding bar) on the handle that keeps the clamp in this position until it is placed on the anchor tooth. When the handle is squeezed again and the lock is released, the operator has control over the clamp and can make adjustments to the clamp position. As the clamp is placed properly, the tension that expands the clamp is eased, and the clamp is secured on the tooth. Once the clamp is stable, the beaks of the forceps are removed from the clamp and the forceps are removed from the mouth.

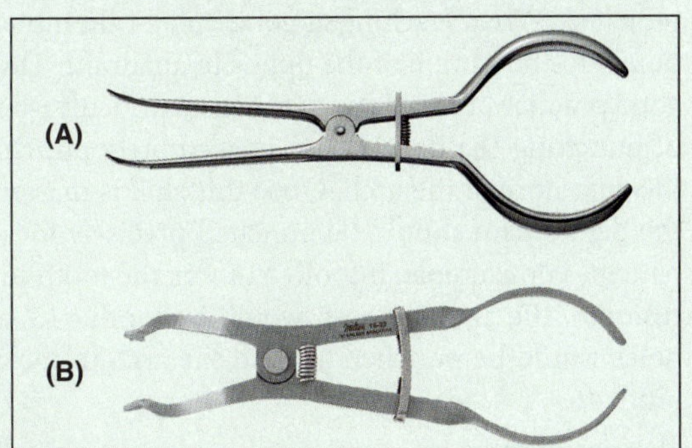

FIGURE 19-45
Dental dam forceps.

Dental Floss. Dental floss is used for a variety of reasons with dental dam isolation:

1. A piece of dental floss, about 18 inches long, is tied to the bow of the dental dam clamp before the clamp is placed. If the clamp slips off the anchor tooth, the floss makes it easy to retrieve. The floss ends are always on the outside of the mouth for quick access. Sometimes the floss is called a *ligature* or safety line.
2. The floss is used to ease the dental dam material through tight contacts.
3. The dental floss assists in **inverting**, or tucking, the dental dam material around the teeth to prevent moisture leakage.
4. The clamp stabilizes the dental dam on one end of the arch, and dental floss is sometimes used to secure the opposite end. On the distal end of the last tooth on the opposite side from the clamped tooth, a piece of floss is placed interproximally, and then looped over with a second piece of floss to secure the end of the punched dental dam (see Figure 19-50A).

Ligatures. A **ligature** is a piece of floss or a cord that stabilizes the dental dam in different applications. Ligatures are used in fixed bridge isolation, bleaching procedures, and individual tooth isolation. Sometimes, the floss is tied into a slip knot and placed over the tooth, such as for isolation when bleaching a tooth. With some patients, the floss or cord is threaded between the teeth or under the pontics for placement, and then tied into place to retain the dental dam material.

Stabilizing Cord. Stabilizing cord is an elastic cord that comes in different sizes and colors (Figure 19-46). It is stretched and then placed interproximally to secure the dental dam material. The cord is used to stabilize the dental dam placement at the opposite end of the clamp or for individual teeth. For example, instead of using a dental dam clamp, use the stabilizing cord for an anterior dental dam placement (see Figure 19-50B).

Lubricant. A small amount of lubricant is placed on the back or underside of the dental dam. This facilitates slipping the dam material over the teeth. A water-based dental

Advanced Chairside Functions (Continued)

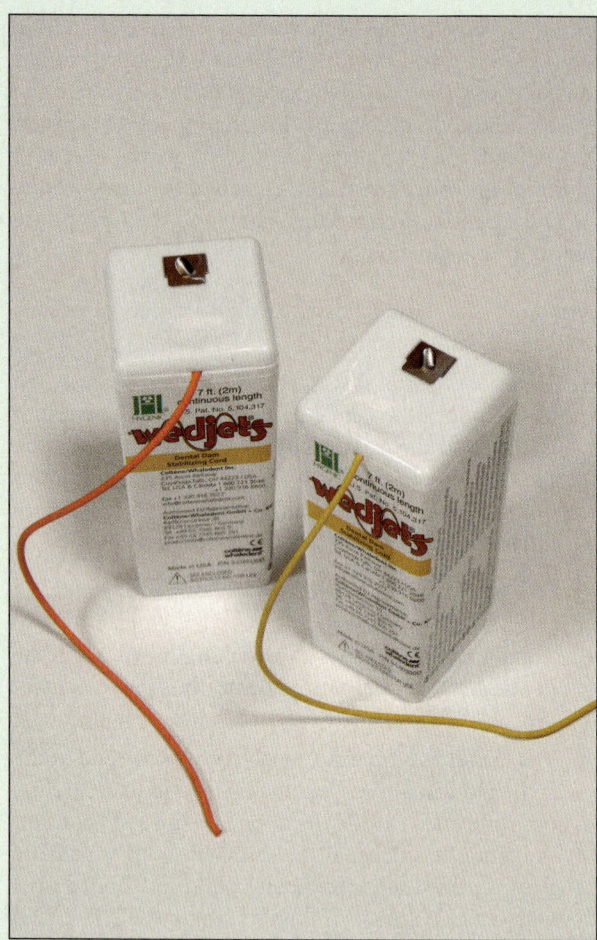

FIGURE 19-46
Stabilizing cord of various sizes.

dam lubricant works better than a petroleum base (such as Vaseline), because it does not leave a film on the teeth that makes the teeth slippery, making it difficult to hold the dental dam material in place. For the patient's comfort, a light amount of petroleum jelly, or another type of lip lubricant, can be applied to the lips prior to the placement of the dental dam.

Scissors. Scissors are used to cut the **interseptal** (between the teeth) dental dam during removal of the dam from the patient's mouth. The **dental dam scissors**, or any small pair of scissors the operator feels comfortable with, can be used. When cutting the interseptal dam material, direct the scissors away from the tissues to prevent tearing of the dam material, and to completely cut the interseptal dam.

Inverting or Tucking Instrument. The dental floss can be used to invert or tuck the dental dam, but sometimes an instrument is needed to accomplish this step. Some options include a periodontal probe, spoon excavator, or the flat side of the T-ball burnisher. These instruments are used to turn under the edge of the dental dam that is around the tooth. The instrument is started on one side of the tooth and is run at an angle to the other side. The edge of the dam is tucked under to assist in keeping the area dry.

Preparation Before Dental Dam Placement

Before the dental dam is placed, the procedure should be explained to the patient, and the operator should examine the oral cavity to determine the area of isolation.

Educating the Patient. Patients like to know what is going to happen during their appointments. The dental assistant should explain the purpose of the dental dam, and then have the patient acknowledge acceptance of this part of the restorative procedure. If the patient has had the dental dam placed before, ask whether the patient has any questions before beginning the placement. If the patient has not had a dental dam application before, explain how the dam is placed, and what to expect before beginning the placement. Some points that might be included are the pressure of the clamp on the tooth, to breathe through the nose, and that the patient can still swallow.

Determining the Area to Isolate. Before the dental dam is punched, the area to be isolated needs to be determined and then examined. Follow these steps:

1. Determine the tooth to be restored, and then determine the anchor tooth, which is usually one or two teeth distal to the tooth being restored. The number of teeth to be included in the punch is a personal preference. Some operators like only one or two teeth exposed, while others like eight or more teeth to be punched. When learning, a good rule of thumb is to punch to the canine of the opposite quadrant. This is good practice because one of the most difficult aspects of punching the dental dam is accurately punching the curvature of the arch. Once this skill is mastered, the dental dam should be punched precisely for any patient. For example, if tooth #14 was the tooth to be restored, the anchor tooth would be tooth #15, and holes would be punched around the arch to include tooth #6.
2. The size and the shape of the arch are examined so that they can be duplicated on the dental dam as closely as possible to the patient's arch.

Advanced Chairside Functions

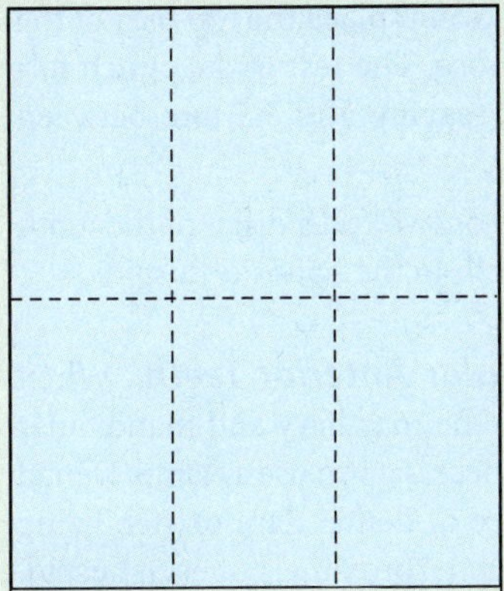

FIGURE 19-47
Dental dam divided into sixths.

3. The area is examined for missing teeth, teeth that are out of alignment, or fixed prosthetics. The dental dam can be punched and placed to accommodate most conditions in a patient's mouth.
4. The area is flossed to identify tight contacts and open spacing.

Dividing the Dental Dam. Select the dental dam with proper size and weight that best suits the patient and the procedure. (Refer to the Materials and Equipment section of this chapter to review the information on the dental dam material.) When preparing the dental dam material for punching, it is first divided into sixths (Figure 19-47). One way to mark the divisions is to fold, and then crease the dental dam. This leaves a faint mark on the dam for the operator to use when punching the dam.

To begin, fold the dam in half and then crease the fold. This horizontal line is the division between the maxillary and mandibular arches. With the dam folded in half, fold the dam vertically into equal thirds and crease along each fold. The center third is where the dam will be punched. This represents the width of the arches of most patients. Some operators prefer to divide the dam into thirds only, and some divide the dam into quarters and mark the center point as a reference point before punching.

Punching the Dental Dam. After the dental dam is divided, it is ready to be punched for placement. There are many places to begin actually punching the dental dam, so it is important for the operator to visualize the patient's arch on the dental dam. Often, the **key hole punch** is punched first. The key hole punch is the largest hole punched in the dental dam. It is the hole that slides over the clamp and onto the anchor tooth. The next holes are punched, moving forward about 3 to 3.5 mm apart. This is the amount of dental dam that slides between the teeth. It is called the **septum**. The punch table is adjusted for the size of the teeth (see Figure 19-42B).

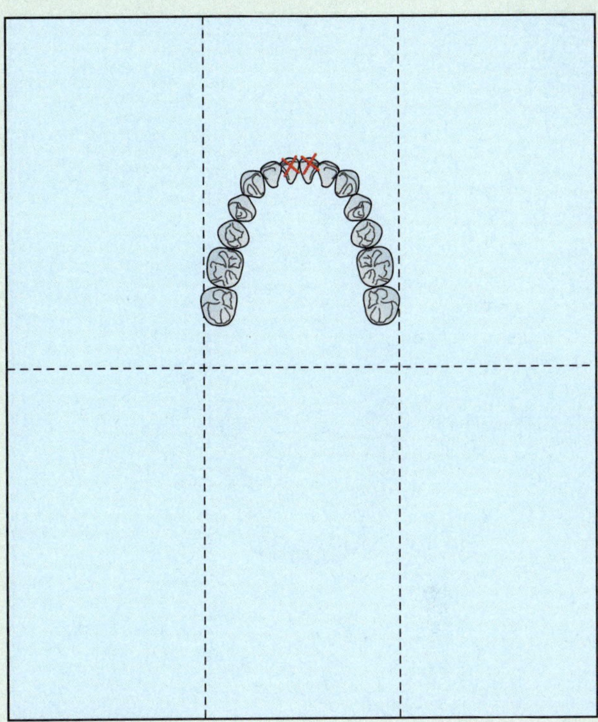

FIGURE 19-48
A maxillary arch punched for work on the maxillary central incisors.

Maxillary Arch. The maxillary arch is punched in the upper middle sixth portion of the dental dam (Figure 19-48).

- Holes punched for the anterior teeth should be 1 inch from the top edge of the dam. This assists in positioning the arch.
- Variations in this 1-inch guide are used for patients with full upper lips or mustaches, or patients with thin upper lips. The distance is increased or decreased accordingly.
- Punch the pattern to follow the patient's arch, leaving 3 to 3.5 mm between each tooth.
- The punch includes from one to two teeth distal of the tooth to be restored and then all teeth to the opposite cuspid.
- Punch the two centrals first. Then, continue to punch the remaining teeth. This centers the punch pattern on the dam.

Mandibular Arch. The mandibular arch is punched in the lower sixth portion of the dental dam (Figure 19-49).

- The first punch is the key hole punch. Teeth #17 and #32 are punched at the junction of the horizontal half and the vertical third. The more mesial the key hole punch is in the arch, the closer the punch is to the middle and bottom of the dam.

Advanced Chairside Functions (Continued)

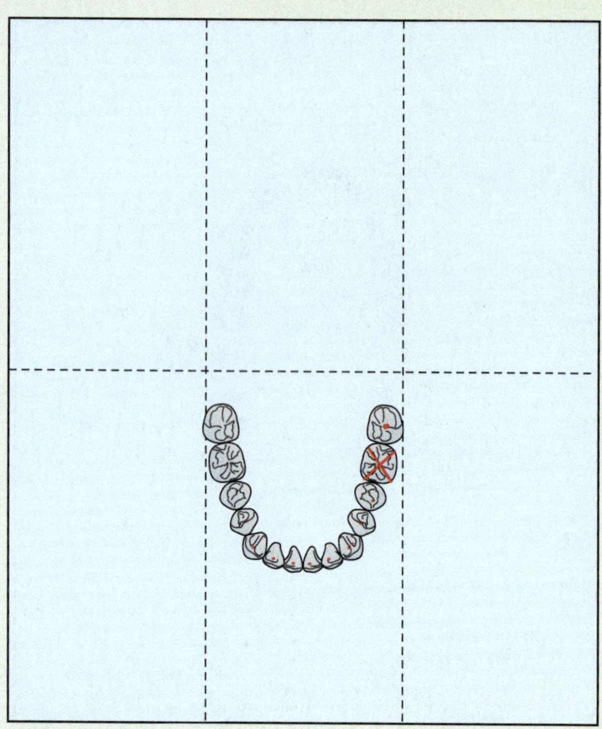

FIGURE 19-49

A mandibular arch punched for work on the mandibular left, first molar.

- Beginning with the central incisors, punch 2 inches up from the lower edge of the dental dam. Punching the holes for the central incisors 1 inch from the lower edge of the dental dam would place the top part of the dam over the patient's nose. The rest of the punch follows the patient's arch, leaving 3 to 3.5 mm between each tooth.
- The punch includes one or two teeth distal of the tooth to be restored and all teeth to the opposite cuspid.

Maxillary and Mandibular Anterior Teeth. When placing the dental dam for the maxillary and mandibular anterior teeth, it is often unnecessary to use a clamp. Dental floss is doubled and a piece of dental dam or stabilizing cord is placed in the distal interproximals of each cuspid. This is usually enough to hold the dam in place without the placement of a clamp (Figure 19-50).

- There is no key hole punch.
- The punches for the two centrals are in the middle third of the dam, 1 inch from the top edge for the maxillary and 2 inches from the bottom edge for the mandibular.

Missing or Malpositioned Teeth. Punching for patients who have missing or malpositioned teeth is accomplished by the operator following the patterns of the teeth in the patients' mouths as the dental dams are punched.

- When teeth are malpositioned (out of normal alignment or position), they often are positioned either buccal or lingual of the normal curve of the arch, so the corresponding holes must be positioned either toward the buccal or the lingual to match the arch.

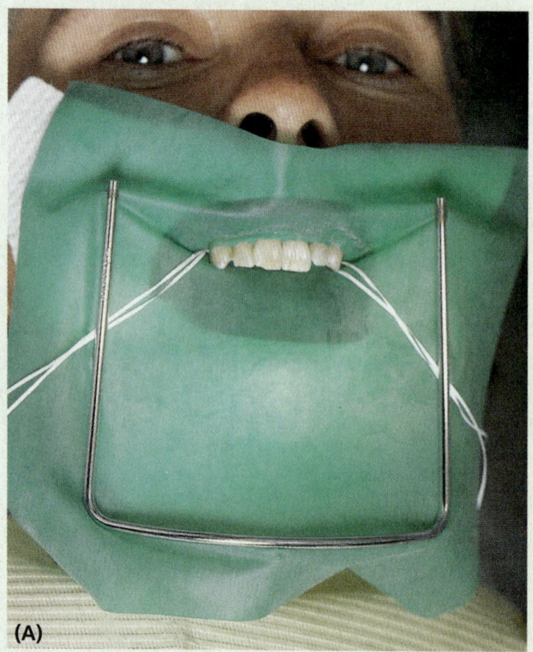

(A)

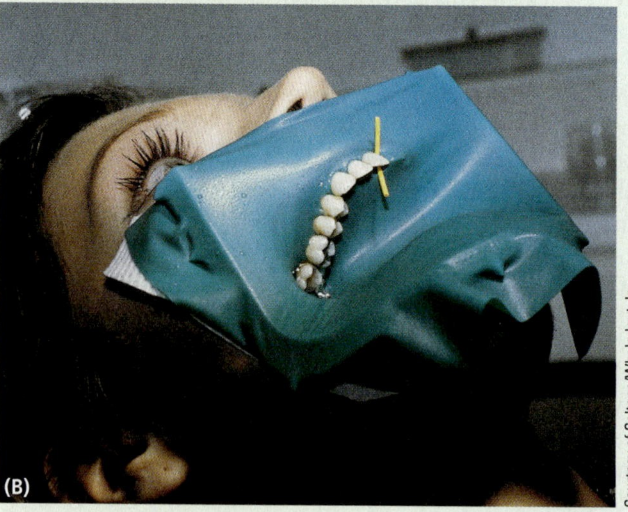

(B)

Courtesy of Coltene/Whaledent, Inc

FIGURE 19-50

(A) Maxillary anterior placement with floss used as ligatures. (B) Patient with Wedjets stabilizing cord securing dental dam in place.

Advanced Chairside Functions

- Missing teeth or edentulous areas are accommodated by leaving a space on the dam between holes punched for teeth present in the mouth. So, if tooth #5 is missing, then tooth #4 would be punched, a space would be left, and then teeth #6, #7, and so on would be punched.

Bridgework Placement. Patterns for patients with bridgework require punches similar to the punches with missing teeth. It is impossible to punch holes for the pontics (portion of a bridge that replaces the missing tooth), so the punches are made for the abutment teeth, and spaces are left for the number of pontics. Slits are cut between the holes with scissors to allow the bridges to be exposed.

Class V Restoration Placement. For a Class V restoration, the hole is punched facially to its normal position in the arch. A cervical clamp is often used with the Class V restorations because they retract the gingiva and the dam beyond the borders of the cavity. The lower the cavity is on the facial surface of the tooth, the more the punch hole is moved toward the facial. The largest hole on the punch is used for this clamp, because the double wings allow an additional 1 to 3 mm between adjacent teeth.

Common Errors When Punching a Dental Dam. The curve of the arch should match the arch curve of the patient. Punching the arch too flat or wide results in folds or bunching and stretching on the lingual; and punching the arch too curved or narrow results in folds and stretching on the facial. These errors make tucking the dental dam into the gingival sulcus difficult.

The punch table should be clean and free of previously punched dam material. Also, check for nicks in the holes of the punch table. If there are marks on the punch table, or if the stylus does not line up directly, the punched holes may leave a tag of dam material or have a tear around the hole. The dam material will tear more easily when being stretched for placement with either of these errors, and the dam may leak once in place.

The hole spacing should match the space between the patient's teeth. If the holes are too close together, there will not be enough material to seal around each tooth, but the dam will be stretched and gingival tissue will be exposed. If the holes are too far apart, there will be excess material between the teeth. It may be difficult to get all the dam material interproximal when placing the dental dam, and the bunched dental dam material may get in the operator's way during the procedure.

Placement and Removal Procedures for the Dental Dam

There are many techniques for placement of the dental dam, and the operator will find, through practice, which ones work best. Dental assistants help the dentist with the dental dam in states where it is not legal for them to place the dental dam, but in states where dental assistants can place the dental dam, the assistants punch the dam, select the clamp, and place and remove the dental dam without the chairside presence of the dentist (Procedure 19-3).

Procedure 19-3
Placing and Removing the Dental Dam

This procedure is performed by the dentist or dental assistant. The patient has been anesthetized before placement of the dental dam and before cavity preparation begins. The dental assistant has prepared all equipment and supplies needed for the entire procedure. Only the items needed for the dental dam are listed for this procedure.

Equipment and Supplies *(Figure 19-51)*

- Dental dam material (6 × 6 inch sheets)
- Dental dam napkin
- Dental dam punch
- Assortment of clamps
- Dental dam forceps
- Dental dam frame
- Dental floss
- Lubricant
- Cotton-tip applicator
- Tucking instrument (plastic instrument, T-ball burnisher, or spoon excavator)
- Scissors

(continues)

Advanced Chairside Functions (Continued)

Procedure 19-3 (continued)

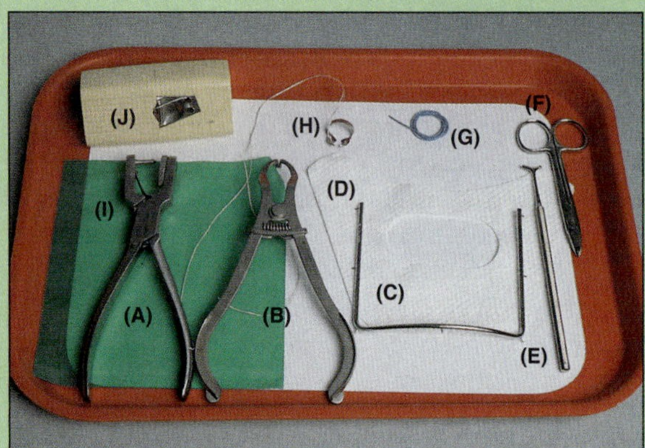

FIGURE 19-51

Dental dam tray setup (labeled): (A) Dental dam punch. (B) Forceps. (C) Frame. (D) Dental dam napkin. (E) Tucking instrument. (F) Scissors. (G) Wedjets ligature. (H) Clamp. (I) Dental dam material. (J) Floss.

Procedure Steps (*Follow aseptic procedures*)

Placement of Dental Dam

1. Inform the patient about the dental dam procedure.
2. Examine the patient's oral cavity to determine the anchor tooth, shape of the arch, tooth alignment, missing teeth, and the presence of crowns and bridges. Also, examine the gingival tissues and check for tight contacts (Figure 19-52).

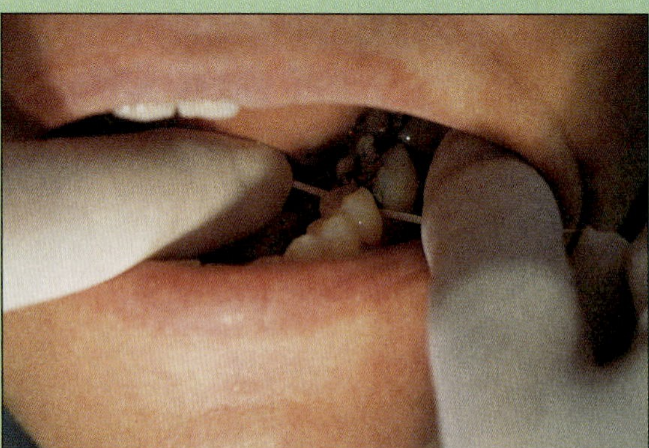

FIGURE 19-52

Dental assistant checking patient's contacts with floss.

3. Prepare the dam material by dividing it into sixths and then punch the dam, aligning the stylus and the holes carefully.
4. Center the punch in the upper or lower middle third of the dental dam. Holes are punched according to the size of the tooth, with the key hole punch being the largest to accommodate the anchor tooth and the clamp.
5. Holes are punched following the pattern of the patient's arch (Figure 19-53). Lubricate the dental dam on the tissue side of the dam with a water-soluble lubricant.

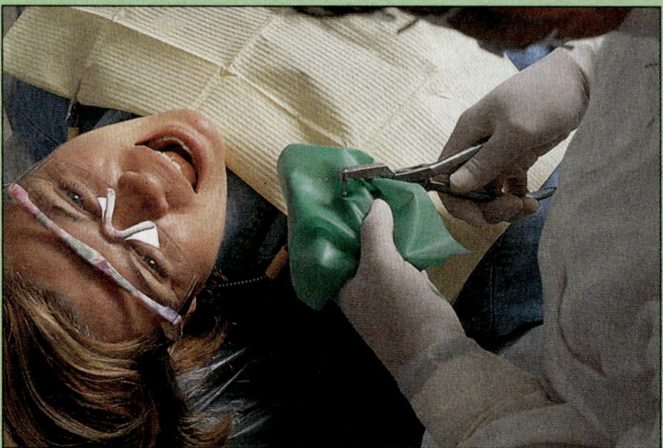

FIGURE 19-53

Dental assistant punching dental dam material.

6. Select the clamp, or several clamps, to try on the tooth. Things to consider when selecting the clamp are as follows:
   - Clamp design (if it is a winged or wingless clamp)
   - Mesiodistal width at the CEJ of the anchor tooth
   - Faciolingual width at the CEJ of the anchor tooth
   - Height of the occlusal plane of the anchor tooth
7. Attach a safety line on all clamps that are to be tried on. When trying on the clamps, keep the end of the safety line in hand (Figure 19-54).
8. Secure the clamp on the clamp forceps and spread the jaws slightly to lock the forceps.
9. Place the clamp over the anchor tooth. To widen the jaws of the clamp, squeeze the forceps handle slightly to release the locking bar (Figure 19-55).

(continues)

Advanced Chairside Functions

Procedure 19-3 (continued)

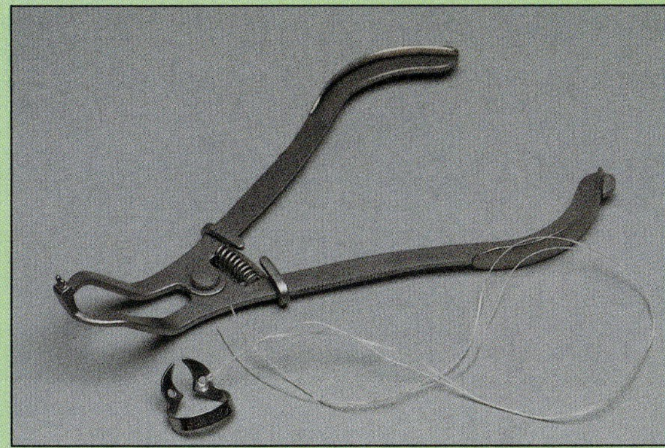

FIGURE 19-54
Clamp with floss safety ligature and dental dam clamp forceps.

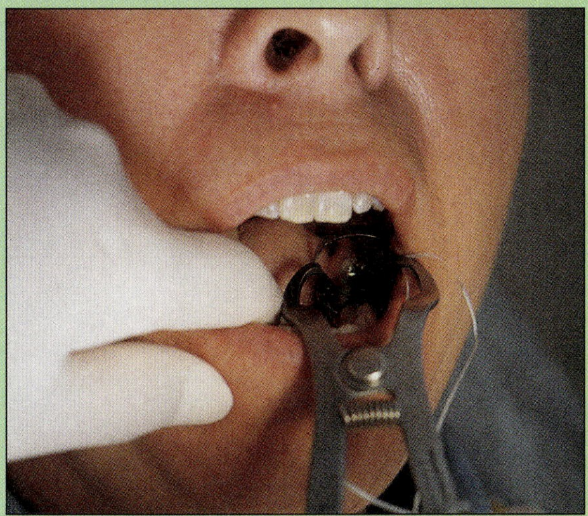

FIGURE 19-55
Dental dam clamp placed on anchor tooth.

10. Fit the lingual jaws of the clamp on the lingual side of the tooth first. Next, spread the clamp and slide the buccal jaws of the clamp over the height of contour of the buccal surface of the tooth. Release the pressure on the clamp forceps slightly against the tooth to evaluate the clamp, but do not release the clamp from the forceps.

11. The jaw points of the clamp should be at the CEJ, adapting to the gingival embrasures on the buccal and lingual. The clamp should be secure on the tooth, and not pinching any gingival tissue. The clamp may be adjusted to the tooth by moving the wrist to the left and right, and by putting more pressure on the distal or mesial side of the clamp.

12. When the clamp is in place, confirm with the patient that the clamp position is comfortable (Figure 19-56).

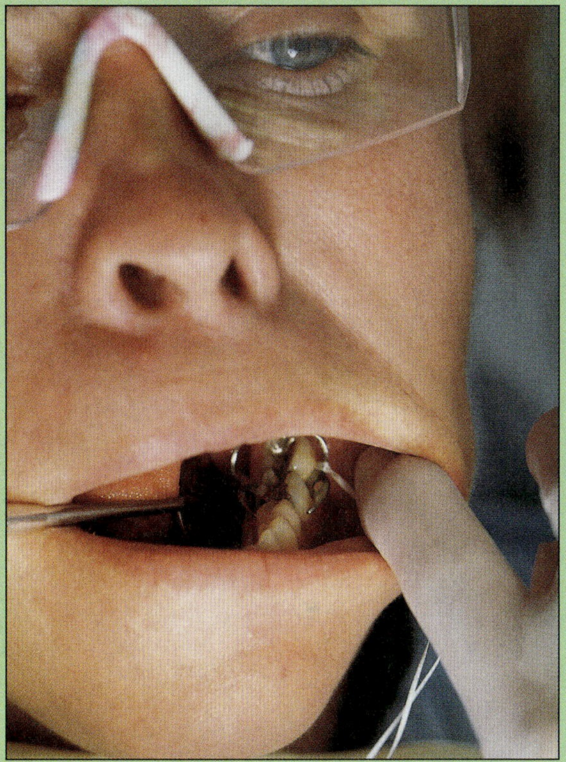

FIGURE 19-56
Evaluate clamp placement and patient comfort.

13. Place the dental dam over the clamp bow by grasping the dam material and placing the index fingers on each side of the key hole punch. Spread the hole wide enough to slip over the clamp. Stretch the hole over the anchor tooth and one side of the clamp, then expose the other clamp jaw so that the entire clamp and anchor tooth are exposed. Pull the safety line through the dam and drape to the side of the patient's mouth.

14. Isolate the most forward tooth, usually the opposite canine. The dam material is secured on the distal of this tooth with a double loop of floss, a corner cut of the dental dam material, or a stabilizing cord (Figure 19-57).

(continues)

Advanced Chairside Functions (Continued)

Procedure 19-3 (continued)

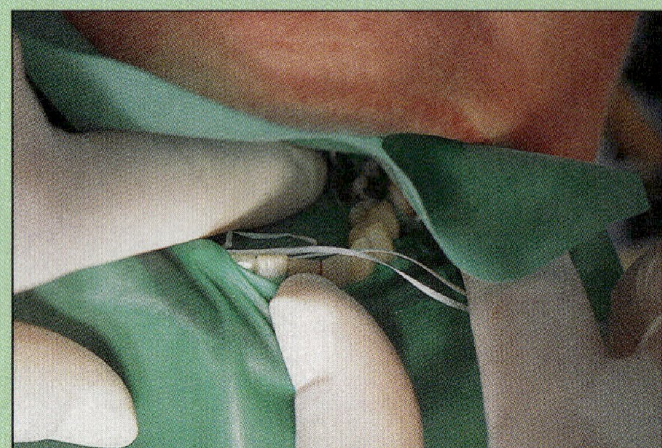

FIGURE 19-57
Clamp with dental dam material on tooth and secure to the opposite cuspid.

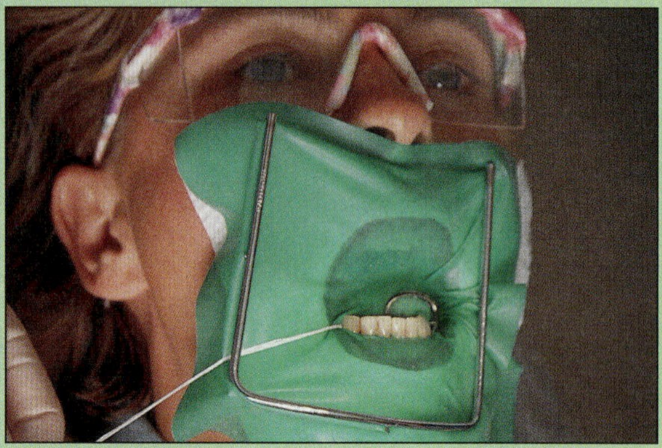

FIGURE 19-59
Frame stretching dental dam material.

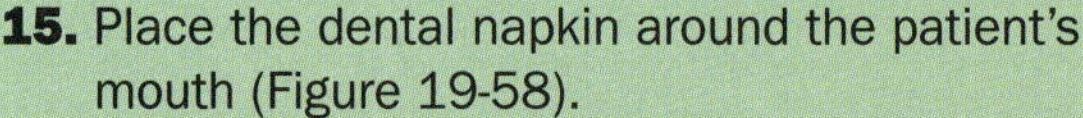

15. Place the dental napkin around the patient's mouth (Figure 19-58).

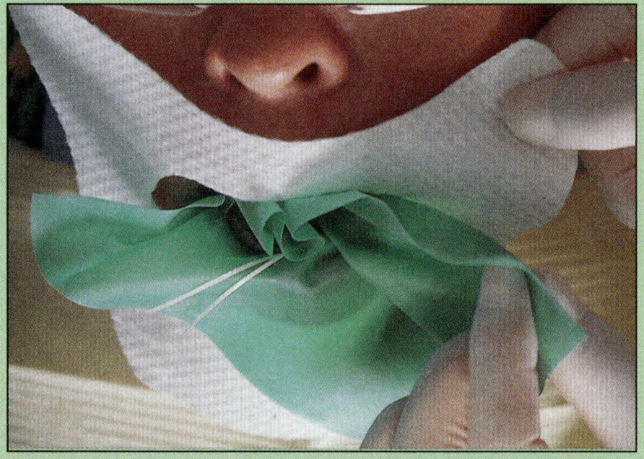

FIGURE 19-58
Dental napkin being placed around patient's mouth.

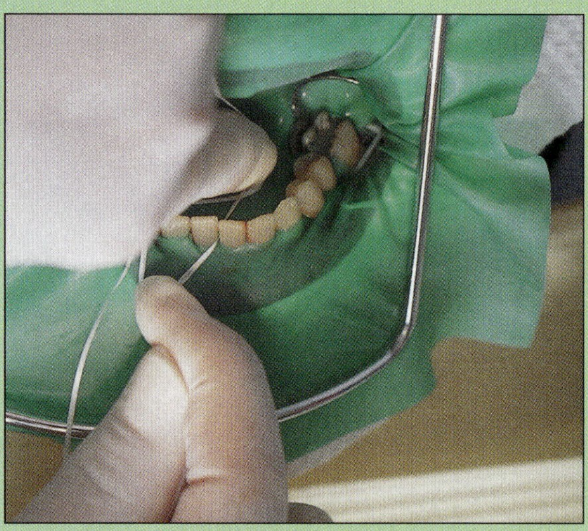

FIGURE 19-60
Dental assistant placing dam between contacts with floss.

16. Place the frame or holder to stretch the dam to cover the oral cavity. The frame can be placed either under or over the dental dam material, depending on the type of frame and the preference of the operator (Figure 19-59).

17. Isolate the remaining teeth. The dental dam is worked gently between the contacts. Dental floss is used to assist in placing the dental dam and exposing the teeth. When using the floss, catch the edge of the hole with the floss and pull it over the tooth, into and through the contact (Figure 19-60). Using the air syringe to dry the teeth at this time facilitates the placement of the dam material.

18. Invert or tuck the dam material. The edge of the dam that surrounds the tooth must be inverted or tucked into the sulcus of the gingiva to seal the tooth and prevent leakage. There are several ways this is accomplished. Carefully pull the dental dam material slightly apically; and the dam will often invert when the dam is released. When using the floss to place the dam interproximally, the dam may be inverted. Or, use a T-ball burnisher, a plastic instrument, or a spoon excavator

(continues)

Advanced Chairside Functions

Procedure 19-3 (continued)

to tuck the buccal and lingual surfaces (Figure 19-61). Use the air from the air–water syringe to dry the surface, and then invert the edge of the dam. Continue until all edges of the dam are sealed.

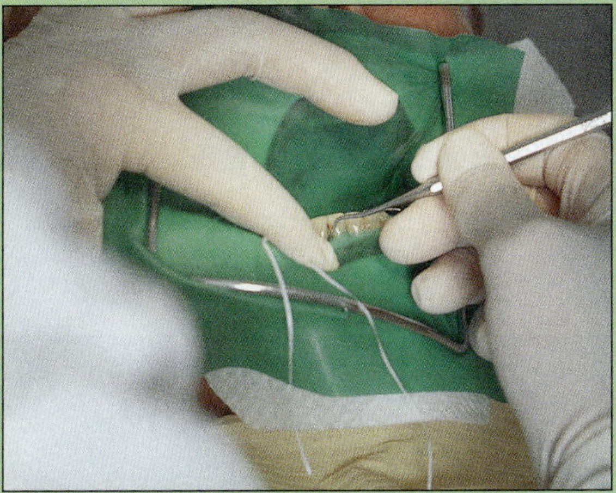

FIGURE 19-61
Dental dam is in place, and the dental assistant is tucking the dam material with a tucking instrument.

19. Coat all tooth-colored restorations with lubricant.

20. Place and position a saliva ejector and/or bite-block under the dam for patient comfort, if needed.

21. Double-check dam placement and patient comfort (Figure 19-62).

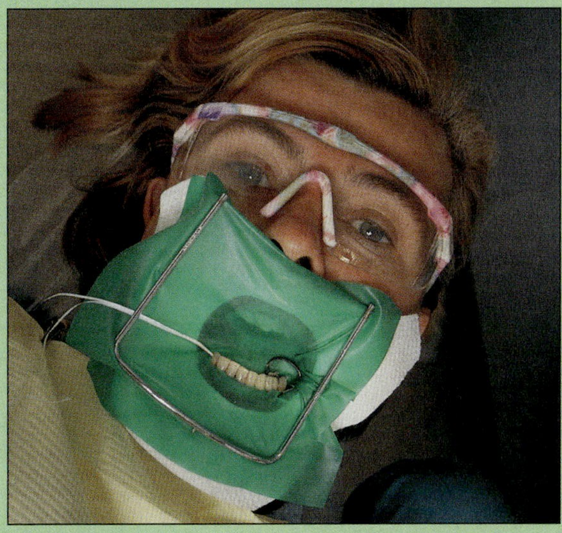

FIGURE 19-62
Patient with dental dam on and ready for dentist.

Alternate Technique for Placing Dental Dam

Some operators prefer to carry the clamp, dental dam material, and, in some placements, even the frame to the tooth when applying the clamp. This technique requires practice and confidence when placing the clamp but takes less time (Figure 19-63). The clamp is selected (usually a winged clamp) and the ligature is secured on the bow of the clamp. The bow of the clamp and the forceps holes on the jaws are exposed through the dental dam material. The clamp forceps are placed in the forceps holes and secured. The operator holds the rest of the dam material up and out of the way while placing the clamp and dam on the anchor tooth. After the clamp is secured on the tooth, the wings of the clamp are exposed and placement is completed following the procedure steps.

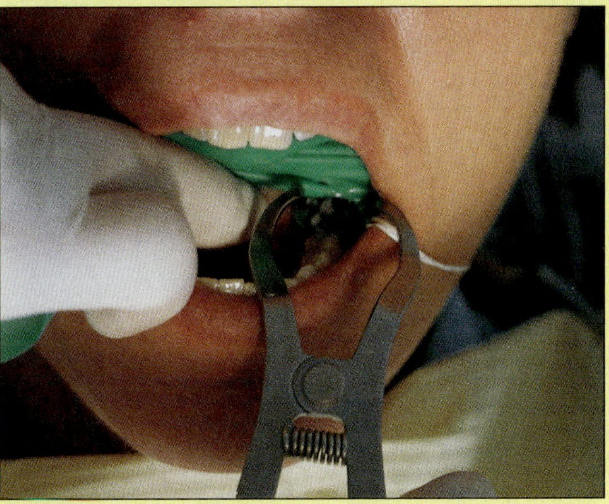

FIGURE 19-63
The dental dam clamp secured in forceps, with dental dam material in position over the bow of the clamp for placement.

Advanced Chairside Functions (Continued)

Removing the Dental Dam

When the operator is ready to remove the dental dam, the area is rinsed and dried using the evacuator and three-way syringe.

1. Explain to the patient the procedure to remove the dental dam and caution him or her not to bite down when the dam is removed.
2. Free the interseptal dam with scissors. To protect the patient, slip the index or middle finger underneath the dam material and stretch it facially, away from the tooth. Slant the scissors toward the occlusal surface, and clip each septum with the scissors (Figure 19-64). Pulling the dam material toward the facial, the operator cuts the interseptal dam.
3. Remove the dental dam clamp. Place the forceps in the clamp holes and squeeze the handles to open the clamp jaws. Usually, the clamp can be lifted straight off the tooth, but if this is not possible, rotate the clamp facially so that the jaws clear the lingual and then rotate the clamp lingually to clear the buccal (Figure 19-65).
4. Remove the frame or holder and the dam material.
5. Remove the napkin, wiping the area around the mouth.
6. Examine the dam material by spreading the dental dam material out flat and examining to make certain that all the interseptal material is present (Figure 19-66). If there are any pieces missing, floss between the teeth. This should dislodge any small segment of remaining dam.
7. Massage the gingiva around the anchor tooth to increase circulation of the area.
8. Rinse and evacuate the patient's mouth thoroughly.

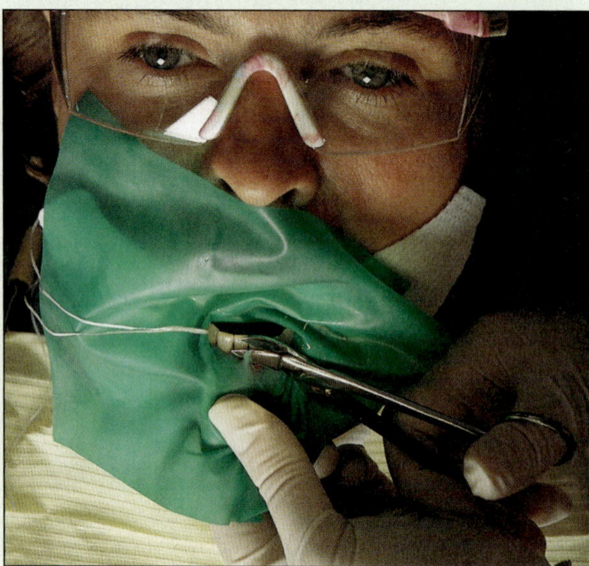

FIGURE 19-64
Pulling dental dam material toward facial, the operator cuts the interseptal dam.

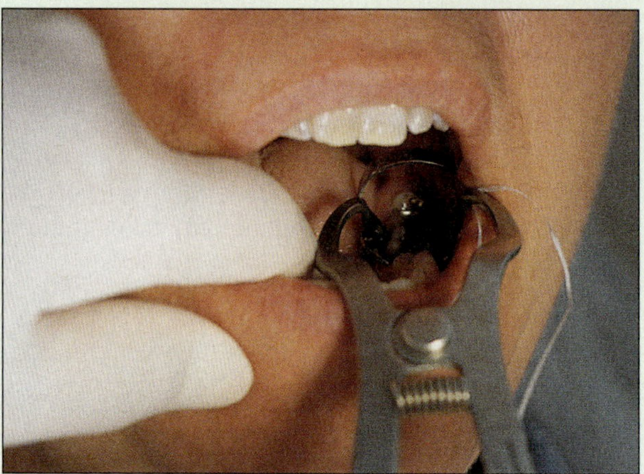

FIGURE 19-65
Clamp forceps remove the clamp from the anchor tooth.

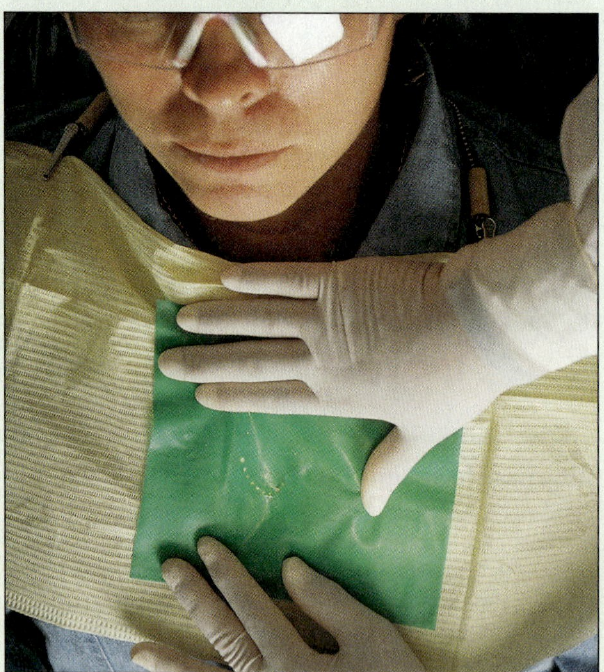

FIGURE 19-66
The dental dam material is placed on the patient's bib or tray for the operator to examine.

The Dental Dam for Pediatric Patients

Dental dams are used on children as routinely as they are on adults. The key advantages become even more important when trying to control the busy tongue and lips of a child. The basic technique is the same for both adults and children. There are, however, several modifications.

Advanced Chairside Functions

It is important to explain to the child the parts of the dental dam and the procedure. Use terminology and explanations that are appropriate for the maturity of the child. Words that are commonly used to describe the dental dam include "raincoat" or "umbrella," the clamp might be the "button" or the "tooth raincoat holder," and the frame is the "coat hanger." Explain to the children how to swallow and breathe with the dental dam in place. Let them help by holding the saliva ejector during the procedure and establish a way for them to communicate—for example, by raising a finger on the dental assistant's side. When people try to talk with the dental dam in place, it is amazing how well the dentist and the dental assistant can understand "dental dam talk."

Look at the patient's dentition and determine whether all primary teeth are present, or whether there are missing teeth, partially erupted teeth, and/or if the patient is in mixed dentition. The holes are punched according to these conditions. Generally, the holes are punched closer together and no holes are punched where teeth are missing or just barely erupted.

Placing the Dental Dam for Pediatric Patients

When placing the dental dam for the pediatric patient (Figure 19-67), punch the holes in a 5 × 5 inch dental dam in the same manner as for adult patients, with the anchor hole the same, but with smaller holes for the individual teeth (see Procedure 19-4). The arch is still punched following the pattern of the child's arch, going to the opposite cuspid. In some cases, the holes are punched only for the teeth that are directly involved. Dental dam clamps with projections are used on "short teeth" or teeth that are partially erupted. Bicuspid clamps are often used. Ligatures, on the primary first molars or cuspids, aid in retaining the dam on the tooth. Wooden wedges are also used interproximally to depress the gingiva and the dental dam.

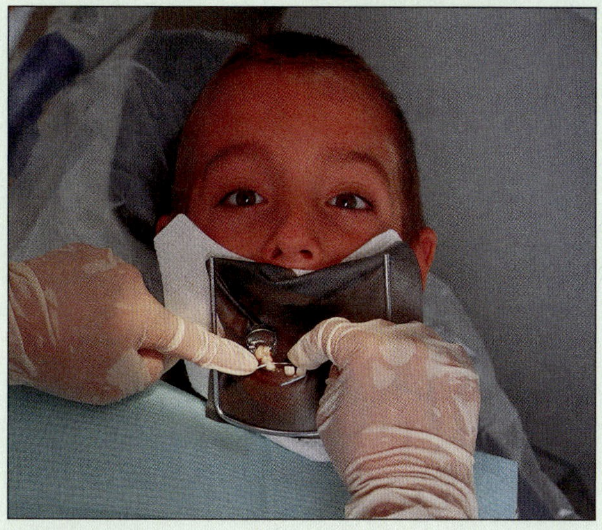

FIGURE 19-67
The dental dam is placed on a child patient.

Procedure 19-4
Rubber Dam Application for a Child Patient

The procedure is performed by the dentist or the dental assistant. The dental dam is quickly placed on the teeth. The patient's dentition must be evaluated to determine which teeth can be included in the isolation. Look for partially erupted teeth and teeth that are loose.

Equipment and Supplies

- Basic setup: mouth mirror, explorer, and cotton pliers
- Dental dam material (5 × 5 inch)
- Dental dam napkin
- Dental dam punch
- Assortment of pedodontic clamps (bicuspid clamps)
- Dental dam clamp forceps
- Dental dam frame
- Dental floss
- Lubricant
- Cotton-tip applicator
- Tucking instrument (plastic instrument, T-ball burnisher, or spoon excavator)
- Scissors

(continues)

Advanced Chairside Functions (Continued)

Procedure 19-4 (continued)

Procedure Steps (*Follow aseptic procedures*)

1. Prepare the child for the dental dam placement by explaining the materials and the procedure at a level that the child can understand.
2. Determine the number of teeth to be isolated, and the size and shape of the arch.
3. Using the 5-inch, square, heavyweight dental dam, punch the predetermined pattern. The holes are punched closer together than they would be for adults.
4. Select the clamp. Winged clamps are often selected because they retract the heavyweight rubber dam for better vision. The wings are also used to position the clamp below the height of contour of teeth that are partially erupted. Tie a piece of floss to the bow of the clamp for security.
5. The clamp is positioned on the tooth using the clamp forceps. Often, the clamp, dental dam, and frame are carried all in one for application to the tooth.
6. Check to see whether the clamp is securely positioned. Slide the dam over the wings of the clamp to expose the wings.
7. Place the dental dam over the remaining teeth.
8. A ligature of stabilizing cord or floss is placed to secure the dental dam.

Alternatives to the Full Dental Dam Placement

An alternative to the full dental dam placement is an oval piece of dental dam that has a border of flexible plastic. This dental dam comes with its own template to mark each tooth. The **quickdam** is punched using a regular punch and the same size holes (see Procedure 19-5). After the holes have been punched, the dam frame is folded and inserted into the patient's mouth, lying in the vestibular area. The dam must be fitted around the teeth to be isolated; sometimes, a ligature or dental dam clamp is used to secure the dam (Figure 19-68).

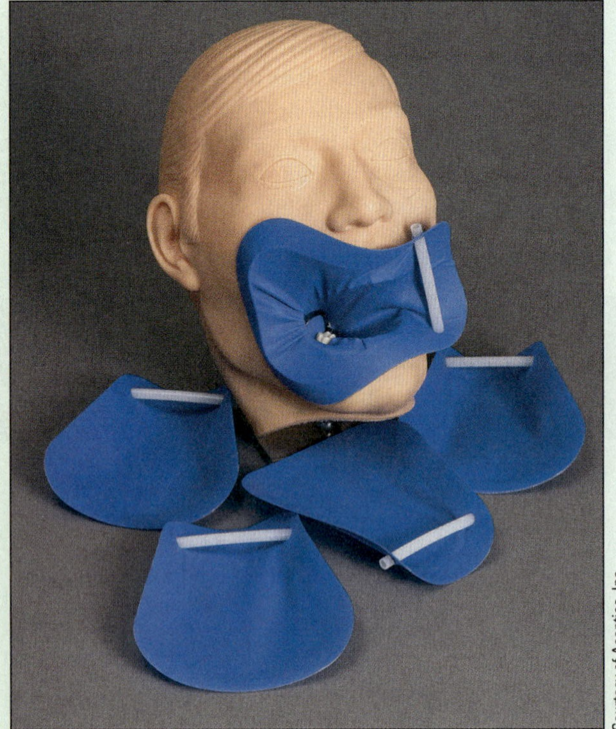

FIGURE 19-68

An alternative to a full dental dam placement.

Advanced Chairside Functions

Procedure 19-5
Quickdam Placement

This procedure is performed by the dentist or dental assistant. The patient is anesthetized, and the quickdam is placed.

Equipment and Supplies

- Quickdam
- Quickdam template
- Dental dam punch
- Dental dam clamps
- Dental dam clamp forceps
- Dental floss
- Tucking instrument

Procedure Steps (*Follow aseptic procedures*)

1. Examine the patient's dentition to determine the punch pattern. Note any malpositioned teeth and the curve of the arch.
2. Use the quickdam template to mark each tooth to be punched and allow for any deviations. Mark with a felt-tip pen.
3. Punch the marked teeth according to the corresponding hole size for each tooth.
4. The quickdam can be used with or without a dental dam clamp. Without a clamp, fold the ends of the quickdam toward each other and press the sides together. Insert the quickdam into the patient's mouth and release the sides. The quickdam fits into the patient's vestibule. Slide the dam over the teeth to be isolated. Use dental floss to tuck the dental dam, and secure the dam with floss ligatures on the distal of the last isolated teeth.
5. Select a clamp and attach a ligature to the bow of the clamp. To place the clamp and dam in one step, secure the clamp in the hole punched for the tooth to be clamped. Apply the clamp forceps, and place the clamp over the tooth. Once the clamp is securely on the tooth, remove the clamp forceps. Place the dam over the teeth to be isolated and tuck the dam.

Chapter Summary

Four handed, sit-down dentistry has changed the role of the dental assistant. Working right at the chair with the dentist or dental hygienist, the assistant has become an important aspect of performing dental procedures on patients. Transferring instruments and evacuation are skills the dental assistant will use every day with every patient. Learning how to correctly perform these tasks and understanding what needs to be done during a procedure will enable the dental assistant to be a great asset to the operator and a comfort to the patient.

Expanded Functions for dental assistants are introduced in this chapter, including what they can do, and the advantages of expanding their skills. The dental dam is an expanded function included in this chapter. The dental dam has many advantages, such as greater visibility, control of moisture, and protection for the patient. This chapter includes information on the materials and equipment needed, as well as the steps involved in the placement and removal of the dental dam.

CASE STUDY

Dr. Danton and his assistant, Kaitlin, are placing a composite filling on Chance Garrett. Kaitlin wants to prove her skills and efficiency during the procedure by having instruments ready and keeping the operating field clean and dry.

Case Study Review

1. What can Kaitlin do to prepare for the procedure so that everything will keep moving smoothly during the procedure?
2. Describe how Kaitlin should transfer instruments.
3. What is involved in maintaining the operating field?

Review Questions

Multiple Choice

1. A fulcrum is a point of rest on which the fingers are stabilized and can pivot/move.
   a. This is a true statement.
   b. This is a false statement.
2. All of the following are instrument grasps *except*
   a. the palm–index finger grasp.
   b. the modified pen grasp.
   c. the palm grasp.
   d. the pen grasp.
3. Which grasp is generally used with instruments that have plier-like (hinged) handles?
   a. Pen grasp
   b. Modified pen grasp
   c. Palm–thumb grasp
   d. Palm grasp
4. The three procedure steps in instrument transfer are
   a. approach, delivery, and return.
   b. pick-up, retrieval, and return.
   c. approach, pick-up, and retrieval.
   d. approach, retrieval, and delivery.
5. Which of the following instruments require the transfer to be modified?
   a. Cotton pliers
   b. Scissors
   c. Air–water syringe
   d. All of the above
6. To work on tooth #29 for an MO restoration, the evacuator tip (HVE) placement on the mandibular right quadrant is
   a. the bevel on the lingual surface of tooth #30.
   b. the bevel on the buccal surface of tooth #31.
   c. the bevel on the lingual surface of tooth #19.
   d. the bevel on the buccal surface of tooth #18.
7. Which of the following is used to assist the patient in holding his/her mouth open during treatment?
   a. The evacuator tip
   b. A bite block
   c. A saliva ejector
   d. An air–water syringe
8. Which of the following may be considered an expanded function of the dental assistant?
   a. Maintaining the operating field with the HVE
   b. Placing and removal of the dental dam
   c. Instrument transfer during a procedure
   d. Tray setup for a procedure
9. Which of the following is used to place and remove the dental dam clamp?
   a. Dental dam frame
   b. Dental dam punch
   c. Dental dam clamp forceps
   d. Stabilizing cord
10. All of the following are true statements about the dental dam material *except*
    a. dental dam materials are available in several sizes.
    b. dental dam material comes in various thicknesses.
    c. dental dam material is a grey color only.
    d. holes are punched in the dental dam material prior to placement.

Critical Thinking

1. How can contamination buildup in the evacuator and air–water syringe be prevented?
2. Identify ways to control moisture as well as isolation methods in the oral cavity. List the location of the salivary glands and ducts to locate areas that need moisture control.
3. How does the dentist steady his or her hand when working with a dental instrument to ensure control? In what specific areas would a dentist place his/her fulcrum and why they would choose that area?
4. List the advantages for the dental assistant when the dental dam is placed.

Web Activities

1. Go to http://www.osap.org and find the dental waterline fact sheet. Look under "How" for what you can do to prevent contamination of dental unit waterlines.
2. Go to http://www.isolitesystems.com and take the video tour to learn more about the Isolite system.
3. Look into your state's Dental Practice Act under Expanded Functions for Dental Assistants and see if placing and removing the dental dam is allowed.
4. Go to http://www.Coltene/Whaledent.com and look up the variety of dental dam clamps available.

CHAPTER 20

Anesthesia and Sedation

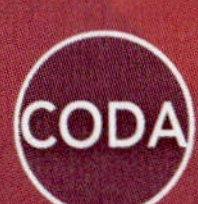

Specific Instructional Objectives

The student should strive to meet the following objectives and demonstrate an understanding of the facts and principles presented in this chapter:

1. Describe the methods used to manage the pain and anxiety associated with dental procedures.
2. Explain various topical anesthetics and their placements.
3. Describe types of local anesthetics.
4. Identify the injection sites for the maxillary and mandibular arches.
5. Describe the equipment and materials needed to administer local anesthetic.
6. List the steps for preparing for the administration of local anesthetic.
7. Identify supplemental techniques to administer anesthetics.
8. Discuss the role of nitrous oxide in the care of the dental patient.
9. Demonstrate the ability to assist in the administration of nitrous oxide.

Key Terms

analgesia (449)
analgesic (449)
anesthesia (448)
aspirates (453)
aspirating syringe (452)
carpules (450)
cartridges (450)
computer-controlled local anesthesia (462)
conscious sedation (448)
diffuses (449)
duration (450)
electronic dental anesthesia (462)
epinephrine (450)
field block anesthesia (451)
gauge (454)
general anesthesia (448)
hematoma (451)
inhalation sedation (448)
intramuscular sedation (448)
intraosseous anesthesia (461)
intrapulpal injection (461)
intravenous conscious sedation (448)
local anesthesia (449)
local infiltration anesthesia (451)
lumen (454)
National Institute of Occupational Safety and Health (NIOSH) (462)
nerve block anesthesia (451)
nitrous oxide (462)
oral sedation (448)
paresthesia (451)
periodontal ligament injection (461)
permeates (449)
sedation (449)
systemic toxicity (451)
tidal volume (465)
topical anesthetic (449)
toxic reaction (450)
vasoconstrictor (450)
Wells, Horace (462)

Introduction

One of the biggest fears for patients visiting the dentist is the injection. People have shared their "experiences with the needle" for generations. Over the years, though, many advances have been made to control patients' pain and anxiety. Improved administration techniques and equipment for managing patients' pain and anxiety continue to be focuses of research.

Because most procedures require some form of **anesthesia** (temporary loss of feeling or sensation), the dentist may select one method or a combination of methods to control pain, depending on the patient and the procedure to be completed.

Anesthetics and Sedation

The formal education a dentist has received determines the type of anesthesia and sedation he or she can administer. Guidelines are set by the American Dental Association for various levels of training and clinical experience required. Some specialties include the necessary training to administer conscious sedation, deep sedation, and general anesthesia (e.g., oral and maxillofacial surgery and periodontics). If a general dentist wishes to use conscious sedation, deep sedation, or general anesthesia, he or she must complete specific courses and programs to achieve this credential. Some dentists hire a nurse anesthetist or anesthesiologist to administer general anesthetic to their patients.

Sedation and anesthesia in dentistry include the following: conscious sedation, IV sedation, oral sedation, inhalation anesthesia, intramuscular sedation, general anesthesia, topical anesthesia, local anesthesia, and nitrous oxide.

Conscious Sedation

With **conscious sedation** the patient is placed in an altered state of consciousness. Pain relievers and sedatives are used to lower pain and discomfort for the patient. Trained professionals administer and closely control the patient who is under conscious sedation. The patient can communicate any discomfort and respond to questions or comments. This is a very safe means for patients to be free of any pain and discomfort during dental procedures. However, the patient may experience a headache, nausea, and brief periods of amnesia after conscious sedation.

Intravenous Conscious Sedation (IV Sedation)

An **intravenous conscious sedation** occurs when sedative drugs are administered directly into the patient's blood system. An IV is set up in the vein and remains throughout the procedure. A specially trained person monitors the patient's pulse and oxygen levels. IV sedation allows the patient to be conscious but in a deep relaxed state. Often the patient does not remember what took place from the time the IV drug was started until the drug starts to wear off.

This is a very common means to keep patients relaxed, comfortable, and pain free during dental procedures. More about IV sedation will be discussed in Chapter 25, Oral and Maxillofacial Surgery.

Oral Sedation

Medication for **oral sedation** is taken before the dental appointment to relieve anxiety about the dental procedure the patient is going to have done. The dentist prescribes the oral sedation drug to be taken the night before the appointment. This relieves stress for the patient and helps the patient get a good night's rest.

Benzodiazepine is a commonly prescribed drug that can be used in two ways: as a sedative hypnotic or as an anti-anxiety drug. If benzodiazepine is used as a sedative hypnotic drug the patient is calm and drowsy. If benzodiazepine is used as an anti-anxiety drug the patient will be very calm and relaxed.

Inhalation Sedation

The dentist may use **inhalation sedation** when IV sedation is difficult to administer. These potent inhalation agents are odorless and colorless gases that provide general anesthesia.

Inhalation sedation is easy to administer through a facemask, a laryngeal mask airway, or an endotracheal tube. Inhalation anesthetics relieve pain and cause sleepiness, and the patient doesn't remember much of the procedure. Patients are closely monitored, and because the agent is not long-lasting, a local anesthetic may also be administered to relieve pain after the general anesthetic wears off.

Intramuscular Sedation

With **intramuscular sedation** a needle is used to inject the sedative drug into the muscle of the upper arm or thigh. This is not a very common form of sedation, and it may be used more in the pediatric dental office with children than in the general dental practice that treats mainly adults. The effect of intramuscular sedation is to ease a fearful or anxious patient's concerns or apprehension when visiting the dentist. The patient will be totally relaxed and will remember little of the appointment. They lapse into a dreamy state and have an attitude of indifference toward their dental treatment. The injection is given at the office into the muscle of either the upper arm or the thigh.

Intramuscular drugs take longer to take effect, usually about 20 to 30 minutes before the procedure can begin.

General Anesthesia

When **general anesthesia** is administered, the patient goes into an unconscious state that is carefully controlled by an anesthetist. The anesthetic temporarily alters the central nervous system so that sensation or feeling is lost. General anesthetic is ideal for some patients for various dental surgeries and treatments.

General anesthesia is accomplished with a mixture of very potent drugs to ensure major surgeries are accomplished without pain to the patient. During general anesthesia, the patient's vital signs and fluids are closely monitored and a ventilator breathes for the patient while the patient is unconscious. The ventilator remains on until after the surgery and the patient recovers enough to breathe on his or her own.

Usually general anesthesia is given in a hospital setting but some oral and maxillofacial surgeons have "mini" operating rooms that are fully equipped to administer general anesthesia. Some dentists have received the necessary training to administer general anesthesia but often an anesthesiologist or nurse anesthetist performs this task so the dentist can concentrate on the surgery.

The dental assistant is not involved with the administration of the general anesthetic but does assist during the surgery and is responsible for dismissing and monitoring the patient during recovery. Refer to Chapter 25, Oral and Maxillofacial Surgery, for more information.

Definitions

A state of **analgesia** is defined as the absence of pain.

An **analgesic** is a drug that relieves pain.

A state of **anesthesia** is defined as partial or complete loss of sensation with or without the loss of consciousness caused by disease, injury, or injection or inhalation of an anesthetic agent. (A drug that produces loss of feeling or sensation locally or generally.)

A state of **sedation** is defined as a state of calmness or process of reducing nervous excitement.

Topical Anesthesia

Before the local anesthesia is injected, the area is numbed with **topical anesthetic**. This material desensitizes the oral mucosa for a brief period so that the patient will not feel the pinch of the needle. Topical anesthetics affect the small nerve endings in the surface of the skin and mucosa. Dental assistants must be aware of the various topical anesthetic solutions and possible patient reactions. They must know application sites and how to apply the anesthetic. In some states, the dental assistant can apply the topical anesthetic for the dentist before an injection.

Local Anesthesia

A **local anesthesia** produces a deadened or pain-free area while the dentist performs a procedure that may cause the patient uncomfortable sensations if no anesthetic were used. Sensory impulses, such as pain, touch, and thermal change, are temporarily blocked. Local anesthesia only works when it contacts the nerve fibers carrying impulses to the brain or the small nerve endings picking up sensations in the tissue. After the local anesthetic is injected into the tissue it **diffuses** (spreads) into the nerve fibers and **permeates** (spreads or covers throughout) the nerve fibers to then block the normal action of the nerves until the bloodstream carries the anesthetic away and the sensations return.

The dental assistant must be aware of the various anesthetic solutions and techniques used when administering local anesthetic. The dental assistant is responsible for preparing, safely transferring, and caring for the anesthetic syringe and accessories.

Topical Anesthetics

Topical anesthetics are placed on the surface of the oral mucosa to eliminate sensation, but they have several other uses in dental procedures, such as decreasing pain sensation for subgingival scaling, root planing, seating crowns, placing matrix bands, and performing periodontal probing. Sometimes topical anesthetic is used to depress the gag reflex that occurs when taking intraoral x-rays or impressions.

Topical anesthetics are available in gels, ointments, liquids, or metered sprays (Figure 20-1). The gels, ointments, and liquids are applied in small amounts to specific areas. The sprays are metered to control the amount of solution sprayed and to confine it to the desired area. Topical anesthetic gels are also available in single-dose packaging, where there is a swab and topical gel in a single package. There is also a gel patch for specific placement. The patch can be trimmed and shaped.

The composition of topical anesthetics is classified as the ester or amide local anesthetics. Benzocaine is an example of an ester topical anesthetic, and lidocaine is an example of an amide topical anesthetic. These classifications are according to chemical linkages, which define several properties of the anesthetics, including how the materials are absorbed into the system. The concentration of solution for topical anesthetics is greater than the concentration of solution used for local anesthetics. For example, lidocaine topical anesthetic is a 5 or 10 percent concentration, while the lidocaine used as a local anesthetic is a 2 percent concentration. Due to the higher

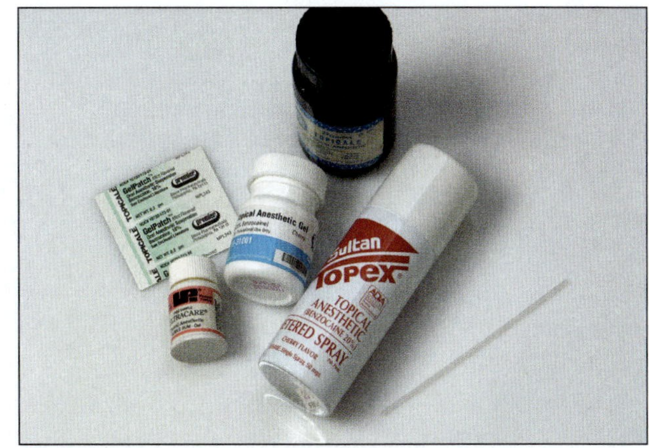

FIGURE 20-1

Examples of topical anesthetic, metered spray, gel, gel patch, and single dose.

concentrations of the topical anesthetics, there is a greater risk for allergic and/or toxic reactions to occur than there is with local or general anesthetics.

An allergic reaction is a hypersensitive reaction to the anesthetic solution. The reaction can range from mild to severe and can occur up to 24 hours or more after the application. Clinical manifestations include swelling, redness, ulcerations, and difficulty swallowing and breathing. Topical anesthetics may also contain flavorings that patients may be allergic to, such as banana, mint, or cherry.

A **toxic reaction** occurs as symptoms that appear to result from overdose or excessive administration of the anesthetic solution. The first symptom is the stimulation of the central nervous system (CNS). The patient becomes more talkative, apprehensive, and excited, with an increased pulse rate and blood pressure. This is followed by depression of the CNS as the drug dissipates.

To avoid either of these reactions, review and revise the patient's medical history at each visit, taking special care to note any allergies or allergic reactions.

The ADA recommends that topical anesthetics be left on the mucosa for 1 minute for the solution to be most effective. The dentist considers the type, concentration of the anesthetic solution, treatment location, and manufacturer's directions when applying topical anesthetic. The procedure for typical placement is described later in this chapter.

Local Anesthetics

Local anesthetics are used to manage pain for most dental procedures. The solution is injected into the soft tissues. To be effective, it must contact the sensory nerve fibers. Once the anesthetic solution anesthetizes the nerve, sensations cannot pass through to register the feeling of pain in the brain. The tissues and teeth in the affected area can be operated on without the patient experiencing pain.

The local anesthetics used for injection are available in liquid form and supplied in premeasured **carpules** or **cartridges** (Figure 20-2). They come in cans or blister packs.

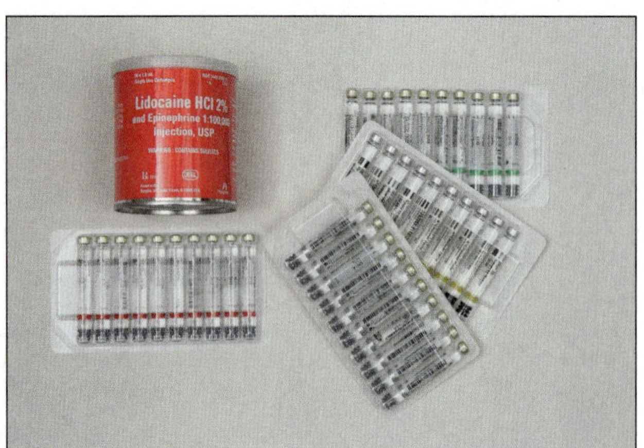

FIGURE 20-2

Various anesthetic cartridges (they come in a can or sealed package).

Local Anesthetic Agents

There are two local anesthetic solutions used for injections in dental procedures. They are amide or ester chemical compounds. Some of the available agents are as follows:

- *Amides*: lidocaine, mepivacaine, prilocaine, articaine, bupivacaine, and etidocaine
- *Esters*: propoxycaine and procaine

Patients may react to one type of local anesthetic but not to another. Specific notations should be made on the patient's chart regarding the type of anesthetic, type of injection, percent of solution, number of cartridges administered, and any reaction the patient experienced.

The **duration** is the time during which something continues or exists. Most patients want as much dental treatment completed at one time as possible. This requires an anesthetic that lasts for a long period of time. The duration of the local anesthetics, which can be divided into the three following sections, depends on the presence or absence of a vasoconstrictor.

1. *Short-duration* solutions last about 30 minutes and contain no vasoconstrictor.
2. *Intermediate-duration* solutions last about 60 minutes and usually contain a vasoconstrictor. Most anesthetics fall into this category.
3. *Long-duration* solutions last longer than 90 minutes and contain a vasoconstrictor.

Vasoconstrictors

A **vasoconstrictor** is a drug that is added to anesthetic solutions to constrict the blood vessels around the injection site and reduce blood flow in this area. Vasoconstrictors slow the absorption of the anesthetic into the bloodstream, thereby affecting the intensity and duration of the solution in the area. Adding vasoconstrictors to the anesthetic lowers the level of local anesthetic solutions in the bloodstream, which decreases the risk of a toxic reaction. Vasoconstrictors also decrease bleeding at the operating site.

The most common vasoconstrictor used in dentistry is **epinephrine**. Epinephrine is added to local anesthetics in very small amounts. The dilution of vasoconstrictors is commonly referred to as a ratio. The most common ratios are 1:20,000, 1:50,000, 1:100,000, and 1:200,000. These ratios, listed on cartridges, indicate one part vasoconstrictor to 20,000 or 100,000 parts anesthetic solution.

Sometimes other drugs that patients are taking interact with the vasoconstrictor and cause reactions. Again, this information should be highlighted on the patient's medical/dental history.

Possible Complications of Local Anesthetics

A toxic reaction is a complication that also occurs with local anesthetics. Anesthetics used for dental procedures are very safe, but the possibility exists for a toxic reaction. Reactions to the anesthetic depend on the following:

- Type of anesthetic solution
- Amount of anesthetic injected

- Rate at which the solution was injected and absorbed
- Patient's characteristics
- **Hematoma** (bruised area caused by a ruptured blood vessel)

Another complication of local anesthetic is **paresthesia**, the sensation of feeling numb. Paresthesia can last for hours or days beyond the temporary numbness experienced after an injection. Most patients who experience paresthesia regain sensation within 8 weeks without treatment. Paresthesia may be caused by:

- Trauma to the nerve sheath (covering) during the injection
- Hemorrhage into or around the nerve sheath, causing pressure on the nerve
- Injection of local anesthetic contaminated by alcohol or disinfecting solution near a nerve

Paresthesia can be permanent if the damage to the nerve is severe enough, but this rarely occurs. If the patient calls the office following a dental procedure and complains of extended numbness, the patient should speak to the dentist and be scheduled for an examination as soon as possible. In most cases, paresthesia is limited. The major concern of short-term numbness is that patients may injure themselves by biting the tongue, cheeks, or lips.

A condition of **systemic toxicity** relates to the anesthetic affecting a particular body system or the entire body. Anesthetics used in dentistry are considered extremely safe but their overall effect is always reviewed. The following are considered when any anesthetic solution is injected into the tissues: type of solution, amount of solution, rate of injection, patient's mental attitude, and other drugs that maybe in the patient's system.

Types of Injections

Three types of injections are given for dental procedures: (1) local infiltration, (2) field block, and (3) nerve block. The type of injection is determined by the injection site and the innervation of the area or specific tooth.

Local Infiltration Anesthesia. A **local infiltration anesthesia** is an injection method that places anesthetic solution into the tissues near the small terminal nerve branches for absorption (Figure 20-3). The local infiltration injections are used for various dental treatments, including root planing, soft tissue incision for a biopsy, gingivectomy, or frenectomy.

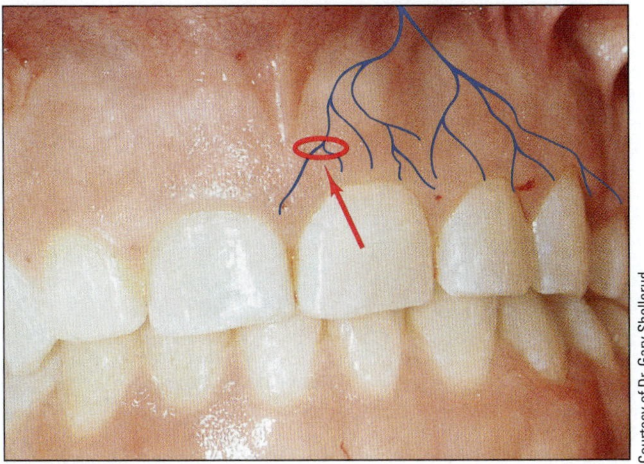

Courtesy of Dr. Gary Shellerud.

FIGURE 20-3

Local infiltration. Anesthetic is placed in the area of treatment.

Field Block Anesthesia. A **field block anesthesia** is commonly referred to as local infiltration anesthesia; however, with the field block anesthesia, the anesthetic is deposited near larger terminal nerve branches (Figure 20-4). This prevents impulses from passing from the tooth to the CNS. This anesthesia is used most often for dental procedures involving the teeth or bone on the maxillary and mandibular anterior regions. Field block anesthetic injections are given near the apex of the tooth and involve one or two teeth. Usually, the patient feels numb within 2 to 3 minutes.

Nerve Block Anesthesia. A **nerve block anesthesia** is injected near a main nerve trunk (Figure 20-5). The anesthetic prevents any pain sensation from passing from the site to the brain, including any branches of the nerve trunk.

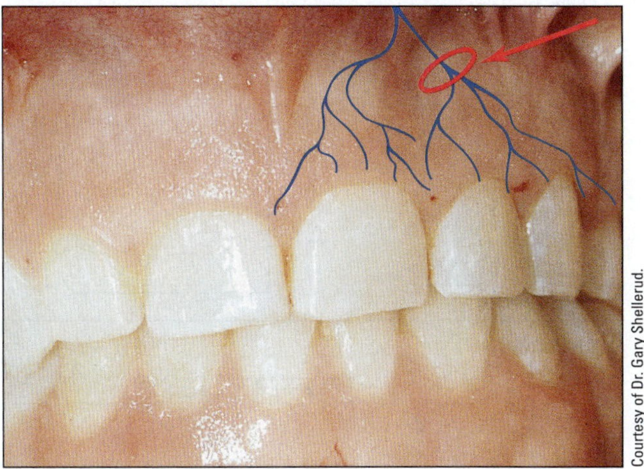

Courtesy of Dr. Gary Shellerud.

FIGURE 20-4

Field block anesthesia. Anesthetic is injected near the larger terminal nerve ending at the apex.

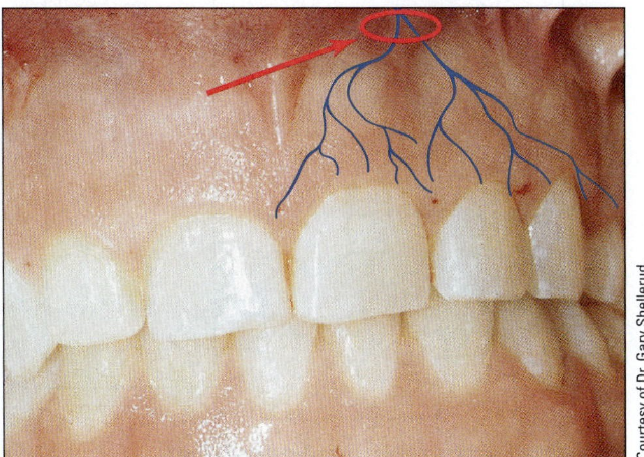

Courtesy of Dr. Gary Shellerud.

FIGURE 20-5

Nerve block anesthesia. Anesthetic is injected close to the main nerve trunk.

These injections eliminate sensations over a larger area than infiltration or field block anesthesia. Some nerve block injections numb from the posterior region of a quadrant to the midline. The nerve block injection usually takes effect within 4 to 5 minutes.

Injection Sites

To assist effectively or place the topical anesthetic correctly, the dental assistant must know the injection sites. The sites are divided between the maxillary and mandibular arches (Figures 20-6 and 20-7 and Tables 20-1 and 20-2). (Refer to Chapter 7 for divisions of the trigeminal nerve.)

Anesthetics, Syringes, and Needles

The equipment needed to administer local anesthetic includes a syringe, a needle, and an anesthetic carpule

The Anesthetic Syringe

Various types of syringes are used for dental procedures, but the most common is the **aspirating syringe**. The aspirating syringe, recommended by the ADA, is designed to allow the operator to check the position of the needle before depositing the anesthetic solution. The aspiratory syringe has a harpoon on the end of the piston. The harpoon penetrates the rubber

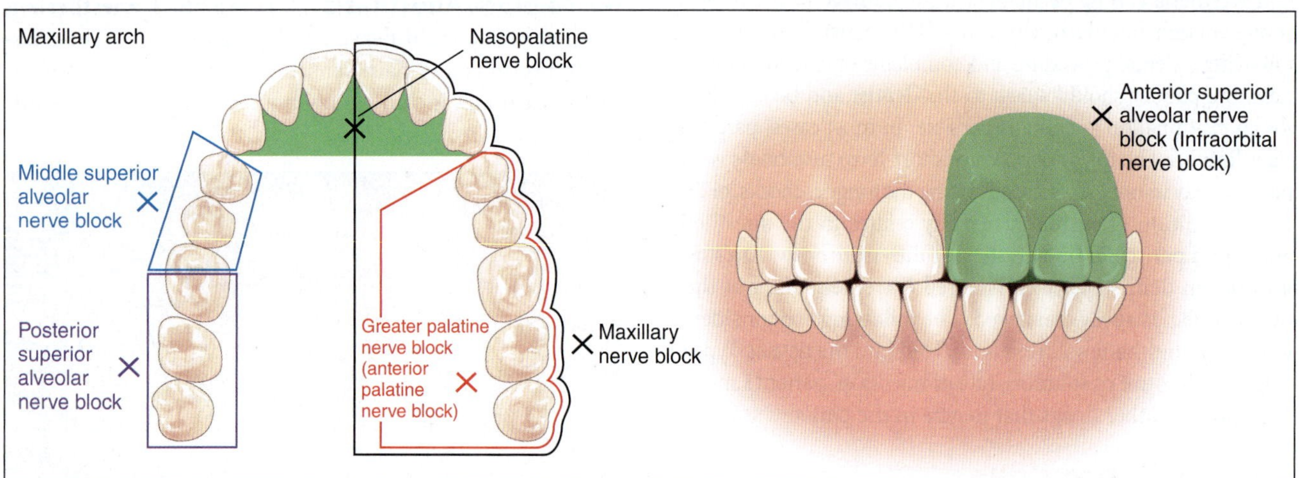

FIGURE 20-6

Maxillary arch injections and site locations.

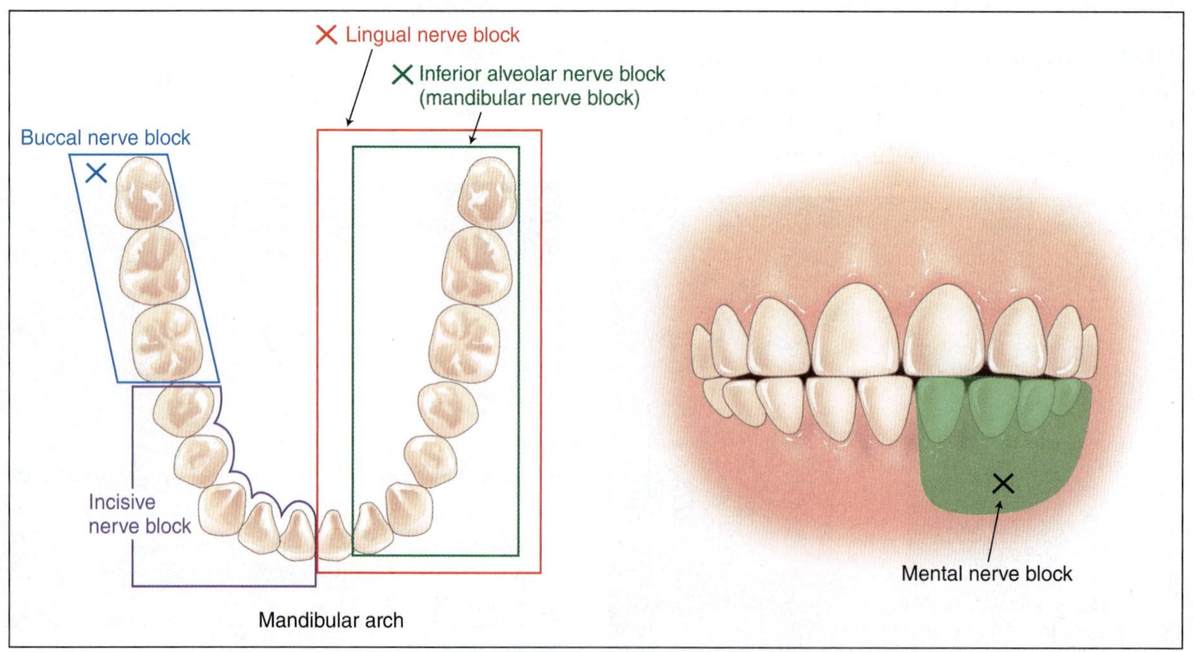

FIGURE 20-7

Mandibular arch injections and site locations.

TABLE 20-1 Maxillary Local Anesthesia Injection Sites

Name of Injection	Affected Teeth/Tissues	Location of Injection
Infiltration (field block)	Individual teeth.	Near the apex of the tooth; most commonly used on the maxillary anteriors.
Anterior superior alveolar nerve block (also referred to as the infraorbital nerve block)	Maxillary central and lateral incisors and cuspid in a single quadrant.	Height of the mucobuccal fold at the maxillary first premolar.
Middle superior alveolar nerve block	Maxillary premolars in one quadrant and mesial of maxillary first molar.	Height of mucobuccal fold at the maxillary second premolar.
Posterior superior alveolar nerve block	The maxillary second and third molars, the distobuccal and palatal roots of the first molar. The buccal tissues adjacent to these teeth.	Apex of the second molar toward the distobuccal root.
Greater palatine nerve block	The hard palate and soft tissues covering the hard palate from the distal of the canine posteriorly.	Anterior to the greater palatine foramen, middle of the maxillary second molar on the palate.
Nasopalatine nerve block	The anterior one-third of the hard palate from canine to canine.	The lingual tissue adjacent to the incisive papilla.
Maxillary nerve block	The buccal, palatal, and pulpal tissues in one quadrant. Skin of the lower eyelid, side of nose, cheek, and upper lip.	Height of the mucobuccal fold above the distal of the maxillary second molar.

TABLE 20-2 Mandibular Local Anesthesia Injection Sites

Name of Injection	Affected Teeth/Tissues	Location of Injection
Infiltration (field block)	Individual teeth.	Near the apex of the individual tooth.
Inferior alveolar nerve block (commonly referred to as the mandibular block)	A mandibular quadrant including the teeth, mucous membrane, anterior two-thirds of the tongue and floor of the mouth, lingual soft tissues, and periosteum.	Inside of the mandibular ramus, posterior to the retromolar pad, below and anterior to the mandibular foramen.
Buccal nerve block	Buccal tissue adjacent to the mandibular molars only.	Mucous membrane to the distal and toward the buccal of the last mandibular molar tooth in the arch.
Lingual nerve block	The lingual tissues and side of the tongue. Mandibular teeth to the midline.	Lingual to mandibular ramus and adjacent to maxillary tuberosity.
Mental nerve block	The mandibular premolars, canines, and facial tissues adjacent to these teeth.	Anterior to the mental foramen, between the apices of the roots of the mandibular premolars.
Incisive nerve block	Premolars, canine, lateral, and central incisors. Buccal mucous membrane from the mandibular second premolar, the lips, and chin.	At the height of the mucobuccal fold in front of the mental foramen.

end of the anesthetic cartridge. Once the needle is placed in the tissues, the operator **aspirates** (draws back) by retracting the thumb ring creating negative pressure (Figure 20-8). If the needle has penetrated a blood vessel, a thin line of blood is drawn into the cartridge. The operator then repositions the needle to avoid injecting the anesthetic into the blood vessel and retests until there is evidence that the needle is not placed in a blood vessel. The aspirating syringe allows the operator to place the anesthetic for maximum benefit.

Syringes may be metal (stainless steel) or non-metal (plastic). Metal syringes are autoclavable, while nonmetal syringes may be either disposable or autoclavable.

Parts of the Aspirating Syringe.

- *Thumb ring*—Located at one end of the syringe. A ring for the operator's thumb allows the operator to aspirate and apply force during the injection. The thumb ring loosens and should be checked and tightened as needed before every use.
- *Finger grip/bar*—Supports the index and middle fingers of the operator as the anesthetic solution is administered into the oral tissues.
- *Syringe barrel*—Holds the cartridge. One side of the barrel is open so that the cartridge/carpule can be loaded, known as a breech-loading syringe. Opposite the open side is a "window" for the operator to view the solution left in the cartridge.

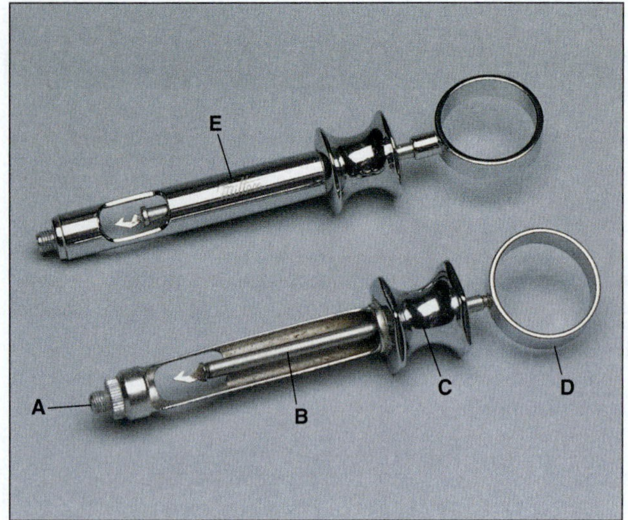

FIGURE 20-8
Aspirating syringe with parts labeled. (A) Needle adapter. (B) Piston with harpoon. (c) Finger grip. (D) Thumb ring. (E) Syringe barrel.

- *Plunger* or *piston rod*—Located inside the syringe barrel. It is a rod with the harpoon on the end. The rod is used to apply force to the rubber stopper in the anesthetic cartridge to expel the solution.
- *Harpoon*—A barbed tip at the end of the piston rod that engages the rubber end in the cartridge. The harpoon allows the operator to aspirate with the syringe. When the operator pulls the thumb ring back, the engaged harpoon pulls the rubber end of the cartridge.
- *Threaded end of the syringe*—Where the needle attaches to the syringe. This end must be checked to be sure it is secure on the syringe. Also, sometimes the needle attaches so tightly to the threaded end that this end loosens with the needle and can be discarded mistakenly.

Care and Handling of the Anesthetic Syringe. Follow the manufacturer's recommendations for the care and handling of autoclavable syringes. After each use, the harpoon is cleaned with a brush and the syringe is prepared for sterilization like other autoclavable instruments. Some syringes need periodic lubrication in the threaded joints and where the thumb ring meets the finger bar. The harpoon may need to be replaced if it becomes bent or dull and does not remain embedded in the rubber stopper.

The Needle

The needle is used to penetrate the tissues and to direct the local anesthetic solution from the carpule into the surrounding tissues. Most needles are made of stainless steel and are disposable.

One factor to consider when selecting a needle for a dental procedure is needle length. Dental needles are available in two lengths: short (1 inch) and long (1 5/8 inch) (Figure 20-9). The selection usually depends on the operator's preference, the approximate depth of the soft tissues to be penetrated, and

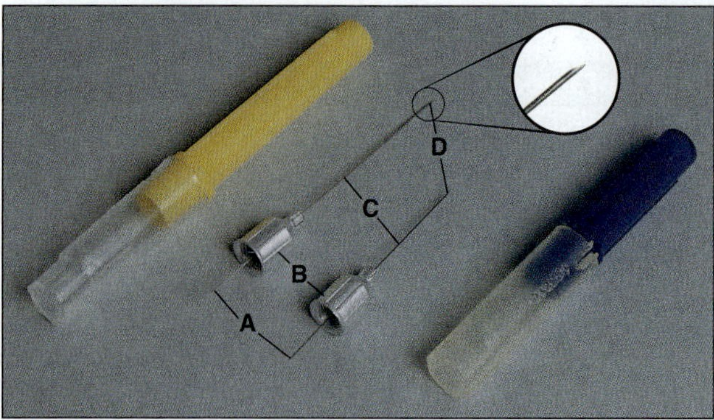

FIGURE 20-9
Needle parts labeled; short and long needles. (A) Syringe end. (B) Hub. (C) Shank. (D) Bevel.

the aspiration potential. The short needle is used for injections that require little penetration of the soft tissues, such as infiltration and field block injections and the following nerve block injections: posterior superior alveolar nerve block, incisive nerve block, and mental nerve block. Periodontal ligament injections are also often administered with a short needle.

The long needle is used for injections that require the penetration of several layers of soft tissue. The long needle is used for nerve block injections such as the infraorbital, buccal, and maxillary and mandibular nerve blocks.

Another consideration when selecting a needle is the needle **gauge** or diameter. The needles used in dentistry are 25, 27, and 30 gauge. The *smaller* the gauge, the *larger* the diameter of the needle. Both long and short needles come in all sizes. The 25-gauge needle is used when there is a high risk of positive aspiration (drawing blood into the cartridge). The internal opening of the needle, where the anesthetic solution flows through, is called the **lumen**.

Parts of the Dental Needle.

- *Bevel*—The slanted tip of the needle that penetrates the soft tissues.
- *Shank*—The length of the needle from the hub to the tip of the bevel. It is sometimes referred to as the shaft. Along the inside of the shank runs the lumen.
- *Hub*—The part of the needle that attaches to the threaded end of the syringe. The hub may be a plastic or metal piece. The hub is normally prethreaded.
- *Syringe end*—The end of the needle that punctures the diaphragm end of the anesthetic cartridge.

Care and Handling of the Dental Needle. The needle is used on a patient and then disposed of in a sharps container. If the operator penetrates the tissue with the needle more than four times during a procedure, the needle should be changed, because disposable needles become dull. When opening the needle package, a seal must be broken; if the seal is already broken, do not use the needle and dispose of the needle as if it had been used. Always be aware of the location and position of the uncovered needle tip to minimize the risk of a needlestick.

Recap the needle using the one handed scoop technique or a recapping device to place the protective covers on needles when they are not being used. Dispose of needles following OSHA guidelines placing them into a sharps container.

Needlestick Protection. There are many types of guards to protect the operator and the assistant from a needlestick. Needlesticks can occur during the transferring of the syringe or during the recapping procedure. Most devices are easy to use with one hand and involve the needle cap being securely held in position for the needle to be placed back in the cap (Figures 20-10A and B). The devices are plastic or metal and not large in size. They are located near the operator and assistant for easy placement. A stick shield may also be used for protection against a needlestick. The shield is a rectangular piece of cardboard that slips onto the needle cap. With the shield in place the assistant is protected when handling the syringe with a contaminated needle (Figure 20-10B). (In the case of a needlestick, begin treatment and report the incident immediately to the dentist. Follow guidelines discussed in Chapter 11, Infection Control.)

Procedure If Needlestick Occurs:

1. Go to a sink and wash the wound area thoroughly with soap and water.
2. Notify the dentist and find out which patient the instrument was used on.
3. Review the patient's chart and medical history.
4. Follow CDC and OSHA protocol for occupational exposure to bloodborne pathogens. (Refer to Chapter 12, Management of Hazardous Materials.)

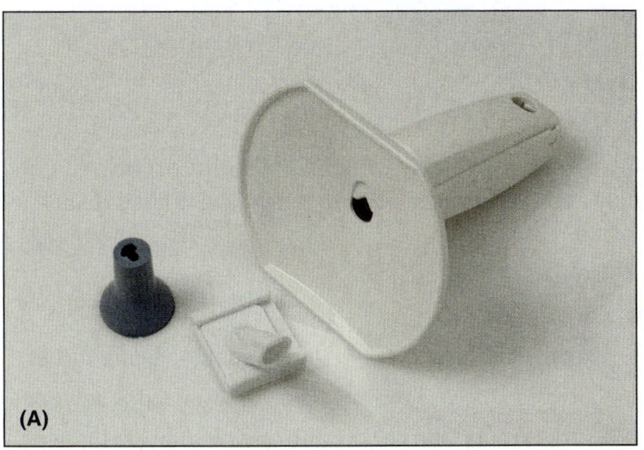

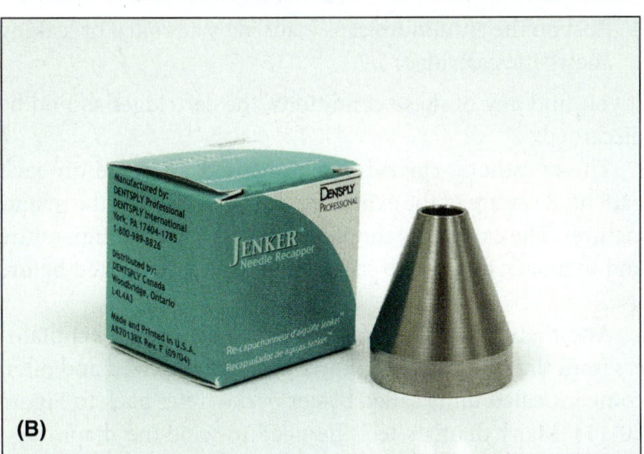

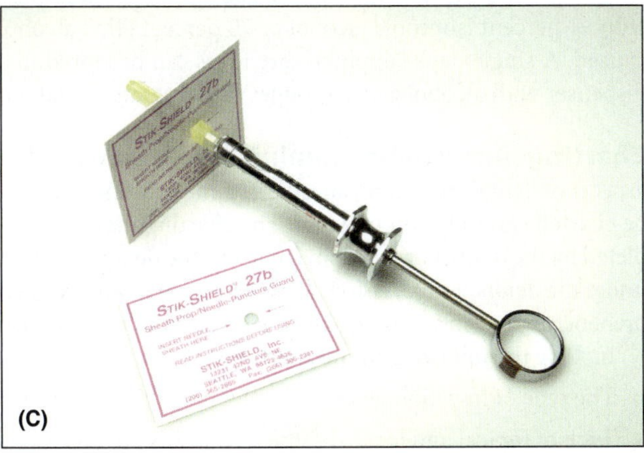

FIGURE 20-10
Needlestick protective covers.

The Anesthetic Cartridge

The anesthetic cartridge, also called the carpule, is a glass cylinder that contains the anesthetic solution (Figure 20-11).

Parts of Anesthetic Cartridge.

- *Glass cartridge*—Contains the anesthetic solution. A thin plastic label covers all glass cartridges. This provides protection to the patient, the dentist, and the assistant should the glass break. In addition, manufacturers place pertinent information on the label. This information includes the following: volume of anesthetic, brand name, solution concentration, vasoconstrictor ratio (if the anesthetic has vasoconstrictor added), lot number, and expiration date. Each anesthetic cartridge contains 1.8 mL of solution. In a 2 percent solution the volume or amount of anesthetic is 36 mg and in a 3 percent solution the volume or amount of anesthetic is 54 mg.
- *Rubber stopper or plunger*—Located in the harpoon end of the cartridge. Most stoppers are treated with silicone so that they can move along the inside of the glass more smoothly. The stopper should be slightly indented from the edge of the glass cartridge.
- *Aluminum cap*—Located at the opposite end of the cartridge from the rubber plunger. It is a silver-colored aluminum cover that fits tightly around the neck of the glass cartridge. In the center of the end is a thin diaphragm.
- *Diaphragm*—Where the syringe end of the needle penetrates the anesthetic solution. The diaphragm is made of a latex rubber.

Color Coding of Local Anesthetic Cartridges. Manufacturers of local anesthetics that want to carry the ADA Seal of Acceptance use a uniform cartridge color-coding

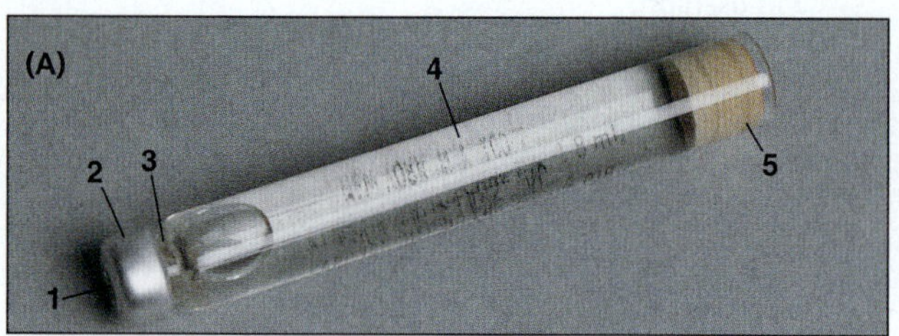

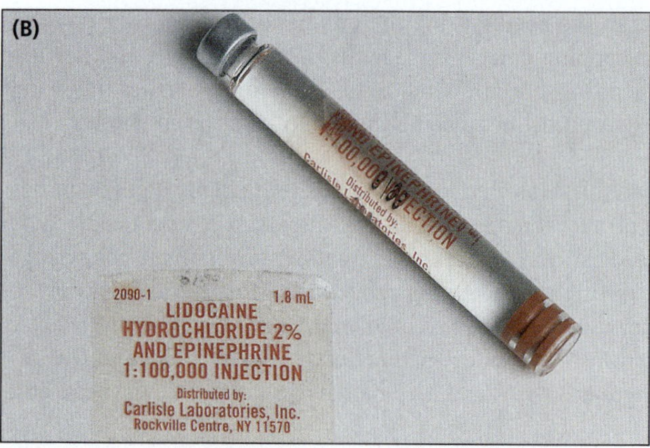

FIGURE 20-11

(A) Anesthetic cartridge with parts labeled. (1) Rubber diaphragm. (2) Aluminum cap. (3) Neck. (4) Glass cylinder. (5) Rubber stopper. (B) Anesthetic cartridge and Mylar plastic label with information identified.

system (Figure 20-12) for identifying local anesthetics and local anesthetic/vasoconstrictor combinations. This color-coding, which standardizes local anesthetics and local anesthetic/vasoconstrictor combinations from manufacturer to manufacturer, includes a band near the stopper end of the cartridge. The cap may match the ADA color-coding system or be silver. Stoppers will not be color coded and will not indicate the drug or the color code. The lettering on the cartridge is black and is durable print that is not removed with normal handling.

Anesthesia Color Coding

Anesthetic	Color
2% Lidocaine with epinephrine 1:100,000	
2% Lidocaine with epinephrine 1:50,000	
Lidocaine plain	
Mepivacaine 2% with levonordefrin 1:20,000	
Mepivacaine 3%	
Prilocaine 4% with epinephrine 1:200,000	
Prilocaine 4%	
Bupivacaine 4% with epinephrine	
Articaine 4% with epinephrine	

Preparation for Injection

- Review medical history.
- Wipe injection site with 2 x 2 gauze to remove excess saliva.
- Apply topical anesthetic and let it remain for 2 to 3 minutes.
- Assemble and hand anesthetic syringe to doctor for injection
- Most commonly used needles:
  - 30-gauge short (blue cap) for infiltrations and maxillary blocks
  - 27-gauge long (yellow cap) for mandibular blocks

FIGURE 20-12

Local anesthetic solution color codes.

Care and Handling of the Anesthetic Cartridge. Carefully examine cartridges before using them. Things to look for include:

- Expired shelf-life dates
- Large bubbles
- Extruded plungers (caused by the solution being frozen)
- Corrosion (caused by immersion in disinfecting solutions)
- Cracks around the neck region and the rubber stopper
- Rust on the aluminum caps (caused by a broken or leaking anesthetic cartridge)

If you find any of these conditions, the cartridges should be discarded.

The anesthetic cartridge is discarded after use on each patient. Be aware of the expiration date indicated by the manufacturer. The cartridges should be stored at room temperature and in a dark place. The cartridge need not be heated before use.

Anesthetic cartridges are stored in their original containers until they are used. The cartridges are sterilized and often come in sealed units called blister packs (refer back to Figure 20-11). Many dentists feel the need to wipe the diaphragm with a solution before use. A 2 × 2 gauze sponge moistened with 91 percent isopropyl alcohol or 70 percent ethyl alcohol is used. A single day's supply of cartridges can be stored in a dispenser with alcohol gauze sponges in a separate container.

Charting Anesthetic Administration. Like other aspects of dental treatment, anesthetic administration should be charted carefully and in detail. The charting may be completed by the dentist or by the hygienist or the dental assistant under the dentist's supervision. Most dentists will want a comprehensive description of the anesthetic given to the patient.

Include the following in the charting:

- The type of injection given
- Type of topical and local anesthetic administered
- If the anesthetic contains vasoconstrictor
- Percentage of solution

- Number of carpules used
- Any reactions by the patient

Some dentists also want to record the needle(s) used and the volume (in milligrams) of the solutions used.

Example of a chart notation: *R-PSANB, 2% lidocaine with 1:150,000 epi, 25-short, 1 carpule (36 mg). No complications.*

Preparing the Anesthetic Syringe and Assisting with the Administration of Topical and Local Anesthetic. Procedure 20-1 outlines the proper steps for preparation of an anesthetic syringe. Procedure 20-2 provides the steps required for assisting with the administration of local or topical anesthesia.

Procedure 20-1
Preparing the Anesthetic Syringe

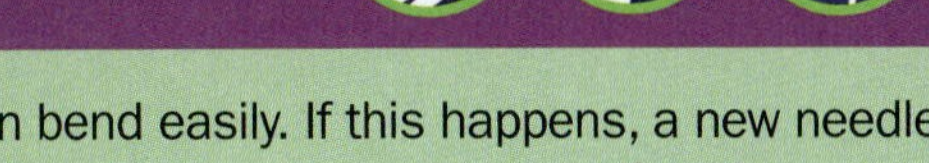

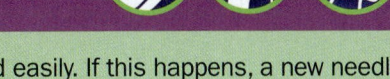

The dental assistant prepares the syringe out of the patient's view. A topical anesthetic is applied by the dentist or the dental assistant. The equipment and materials are on the procedure tray or stored at the dental unit.

Equipment and Supplies (*Figure 20-13*)

- Sterile syringe
- Selected disposable needle
- Selected anesthetic cartridge
- Needlestick protectors
- 2 × 2 gauze sponge moistened with 91 percent isopropyl alcohol or 70 percent ethyl alcohol

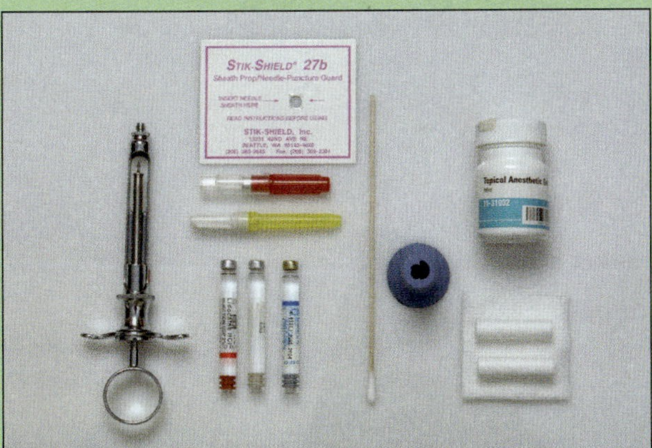

FIGURE 20-13
Equipment and supplies needed to prepare an anesthetic syringe.

Procedure Steps (*Follow aseptic procedures*)

NOTE: It is common in dentistry to first attach the needle to the syringe before placing the cartridge. Precautions should be followed with this technique, because pressure is required on the thumb ring to engage the harpoon into the rubber plunger, which can break the cartridge. Also, if the plunger is not retracted fully while placing the cartridge into the syringe, the needle can bend easily. If this happens, a new needle must be placed before the syringe can function.

This procedure is described for a right-handed person.

1. Following aseptic procedures, select the disposable needle and the anesthetic the dentist has specified for this procedure.
2. Remove the sterilized syringe from its autoclave bag or pouch. Inspect the syringe to be sure it is ready for use. Tighten the thumb bar or ring, as this sometimes is loose.
3. Hold the syringe in the left hand and use the thumb ring to fully retract the piston rod (Figure 20-14).
4. With the piston rod retracted, place the cartridge in the barrel of the syringe. The plunger end (rubber stopper end) goes in first (Figure 20-15). To prevent contamination, do not place a finger over the diaphragm while placing the cartridge in the syringe. Once the cartridge is in place, release the piston rod.
5. With moderate pressure, push the piston rod into the rubber stopper until it is engaged fully (Figure 20-16). Do not hit the piston rod to engage the harpoon, and do not hold your hand over the cartridge while engaging the harpoon.

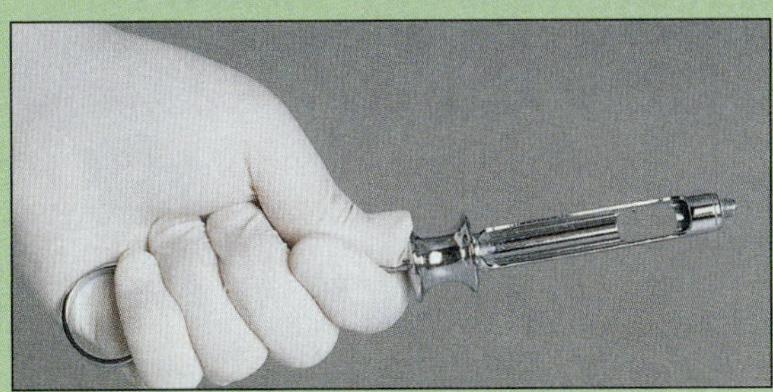

FIGURE 20-14
Left-hand retraction of the piston rod of an aspirating anesthetic syringe.

(continues)

Procedure 20-1 (continued)

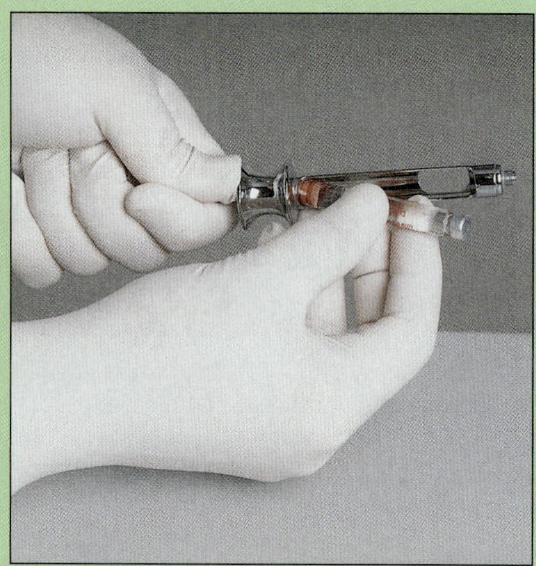

FIGURE 20-15
Technique for placing a cartridge in an aspirating syringe.

6. Remove the protective plastic cap from the syringe end of the needle, and then screw or press the needle onto the syringe depending on the type of needle hub. Make sure that the needle is secure but not too tight (Figure 20-17). A disposable needle guard is often placed on the protective cap covering the needle.
7. Carefully remove the protective cover from the needle. Holding the syringe upright, expel a few drops to ensure that the syringe is working properly. Replace the cap and place on the tray, ready for use.

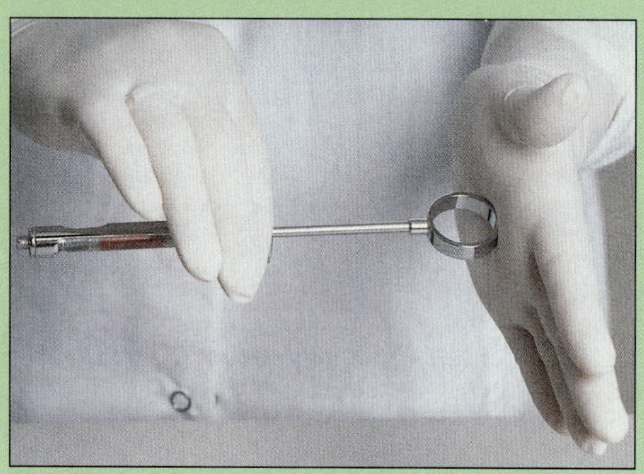

FIGURE 20-16
Engage the harpoon with pressure on the finger ring (bar).

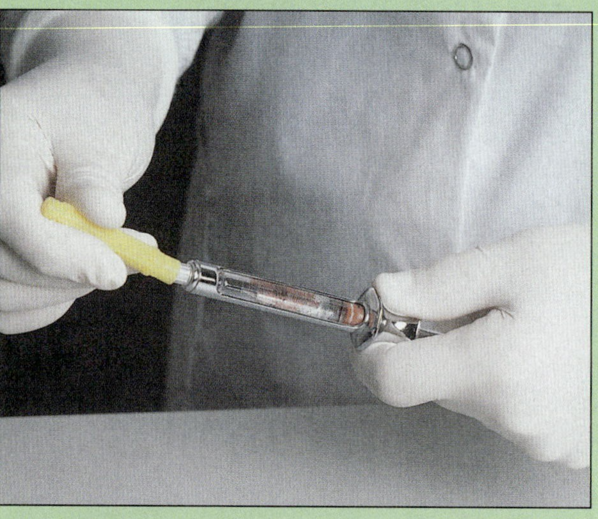

FIGURE 20-17
Open the cap on the needle.

Procedure 20-2
Assisting with the Administration of Topical and Local Anesthetics

The dental assistant checks with the dentist for instructions on the type of anesthetic and needle for the procedure. The equipment and materials are on the procedure tray or stored at the dental unit.

Equipment and Supplies *(Figure 20-18)*

- Patient's medical/dental history and chart
- Basic setup: mouth mirror, explorer, and cotton pliers
- Air–water syringe tip and evacuator tip (HVE)
- Cotton rolls, cotton-tip applicator, and 2 × 2 gauze sponges
- Topical anesthetic
- Aspirating syringe
- Anesthetic cartridge
- Selection of needles

(continues)

Procedure 20-2 (continued)

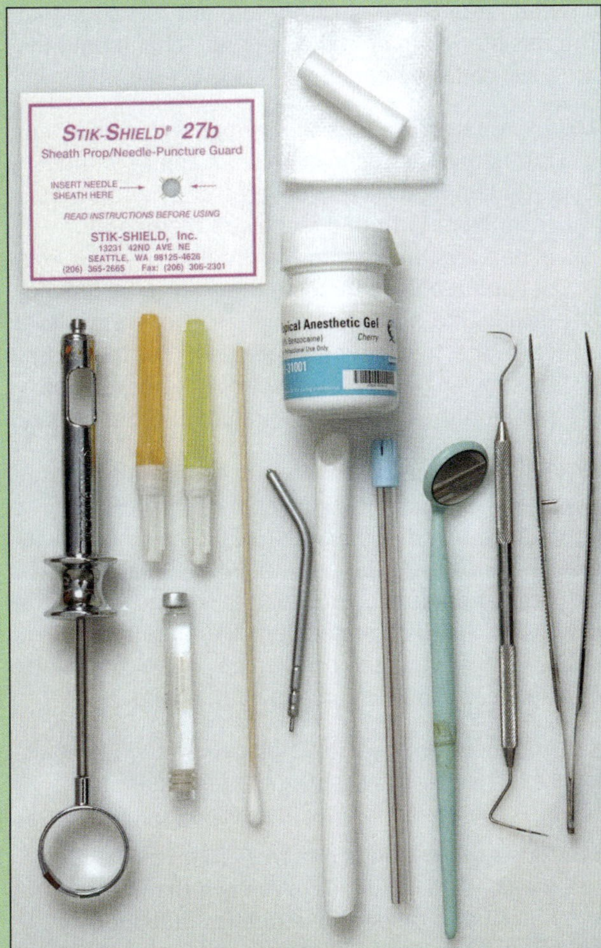

FIGURE 20-18

Equipment and supplies needed to place the topical anesthetic and pass the prepared syringe for local anesthetic administration.

Procedure Steps (*Follow aseptic procedures*)

Placing Topical Anesthetic (by the dentist or the assistant)

1. After seating the patient, review and update the medical/dental history.
2. Prepare the patient for the procedure and explain what you are doing and the tastes and sensations the patient may experience. (Explain briefly and avoid such words as "pain," "shot," and "injection.") Explain that the topical anesthetic is being applied to make the patient more comfortable during the procedure.
3. Place a small amount of topical anesthetic on a cotton-tip applicator.
4. Prepare the oral mucosa by drying with a sterile 2 × 2 gauze sponge. Keep the tissue retracted.
5. Place the topical anesthetic on the site of the injection and leave in place for the specific time allotted according to manufacturer's directions (Figure 20-19).

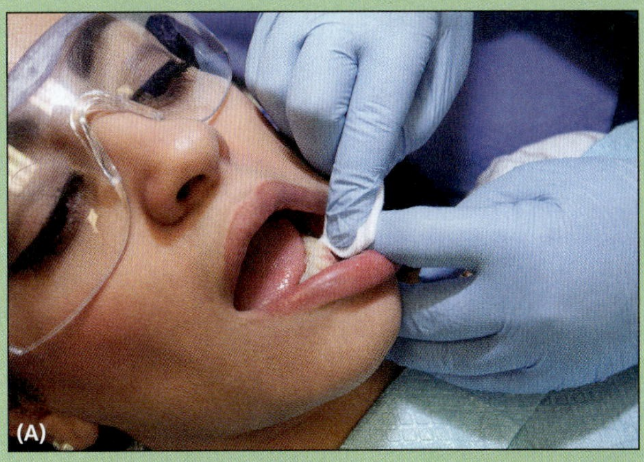

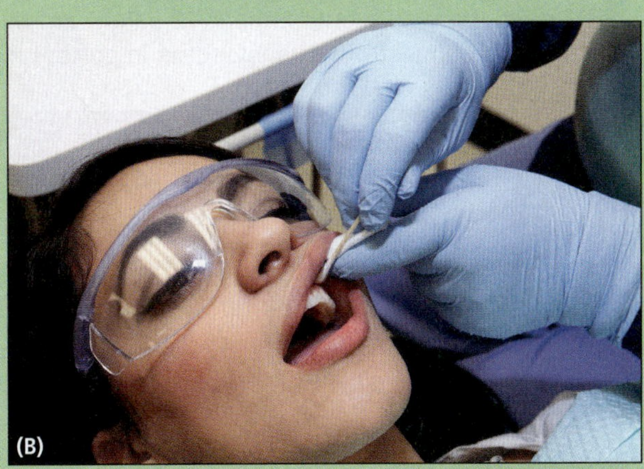

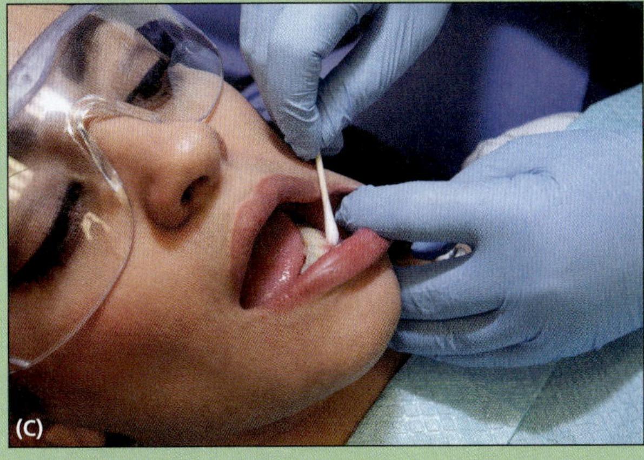

FIGURE 20-19

(A) Dry the tissue with a gauze. (B) Place the topical anesthetic on the maxillary injection site. (C) Place the topical anesthetic on the mandibular injection site.

(continues)

Procedure 20-2 (continued)

Administering the Local Anesthetic

6. While waiting for the topical anesthetic to take effect, prepare the syringe if this has not already been completed. Assemble the syringe, cartridge, and needle as described previously.
7. When the operator indicates, take the cotton-tip applicator and prepare to pass the syringe.
8. Check the needle bevel so that it is directed toward the alveolar bone, and then loosely replace the cap on the needle. The protective cap is placed on the hub of the needle so that it is secure but can be removed easily.
9. Pass the syringe below the patient's chin (or behind the patient's head), placing the thumb ring over the dentist's thumb (the dentist grasps the syringe at the finger rest and takes the syringe) (Figure 20-20). As the dentist takes the syringe, remove the protective guard. During the injection, watch the patient for any adverse signs or reactions.

NOTE: There are different methods to safely remove the cap and complete the transfer. It is important for the dentist and the assistant to establish a routine. The assistant can hold the operator's hand until they have cleared the needle.

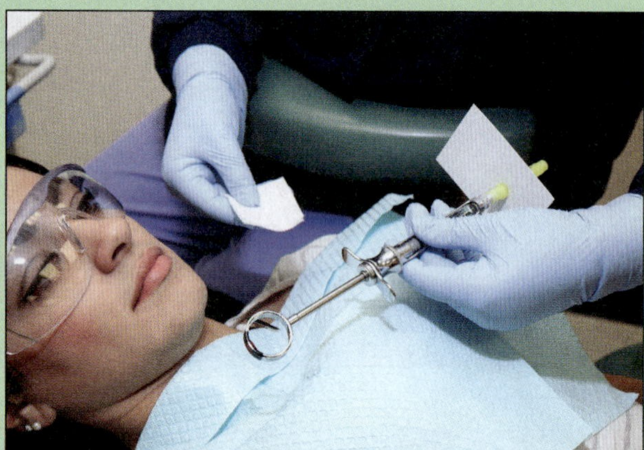

FIGURE 20-20
Pass the prepared anesthetic syringe.

10. The operator recaps the syringe with one of two methods. The technique for recapping without a recapping device is called a one-hand scoop technique. With this technique the operator slides the needle into the protective guard. The second technique uses a mechanical recapping device. If a second injection is given, remove the cartridge, insert a new cartridge, test the syringe by expelling a few drops, check the bevel, and position the needle for the dentist to retrieve.

NOTE: At this time, the syringe is contaminated. Most needlesticks occur during recapping. To prevent this from happening, the dentist should recap the needle and retrieve it after the assistant has replaced the cartridge and has repositioned the syringe on the tray or counter. A variety of needle holders are available. These devices hold the needle cap so that the needle can be recapped while protecting the hand.

11. The recapped syringe is placed on the tray, out of the way for the rest of the procedure but close in case more anesthetic is needed.
12. Rinse the patient's mouth with the air–water syringe and evacuate to remove the water, saliva, and taste of anesthetic solution.

Unloading the Anesthetic Syringe

1. After the procedure is completed and the patient is dismissed, don utility gloves, take the syringe apart, and prepare it for sterilization.
2. Retract the piston to release the harpoon from the cartridge (Figure 20-21A).
3. Remove the cartridge from the syringe by retracting the thumb ring enough to release the

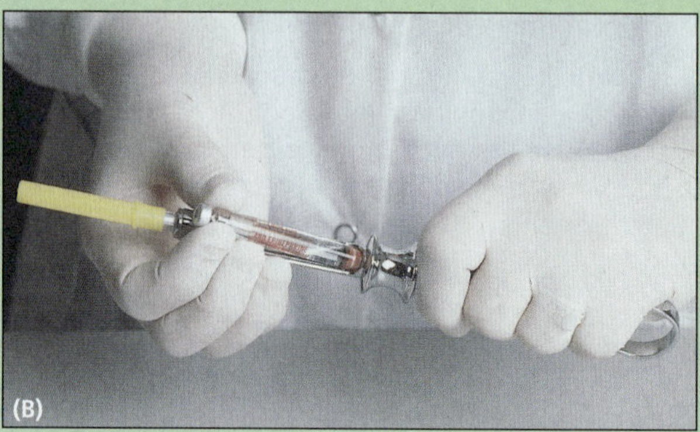

FIGURE 20-21
(A) Retract the piston to release the harpoon from the cartridge and (B) remove the cartridge from the syringe.

(continues)

Procedure 20-2 (continued)

cartridge. Turn the syringe until the cartridge is free (Figure 20-21B).

4. Carefully remove the needle with the protective cap in place. Carefully unscrew the needle. A hemostat can be used to hold the needle while it is being removed from the syringe. Also, there are mechanical devices that cut the needle from the hub; after being cut, the needle falls into a closed container. The needle is discarded in the sharps container.

NOTE: The needle can also be removed before the cartridge.

5. Prepare the syringe for sterilization.

Supplemental Anesthetic Techniques

Various techniques for administering anesthetics supplement the infiltration and block injection techniques or can be used as the only anesthetic injection technique.

Intraosseous Anesthesia

An **intraosseous anesthesia** places local anesthetic directly into the cancellous bone (spongy bone). This injection is used for anesthesia in a single tooth or multiple teeth in a quadrant. The bone, soft tissue, and root of a tooth/teeth are anesthetized by the intraosseous injection. This type of anesthetic injection is useful for patients who do not like the feeling of a numb lip and tongue. It is immediate in action and is atraumatic for patients.

The intraosseous injection requires a special system for administration. This technology has been modified with two parts:

1. A perforator, which is a solid needle that attaches to a slow-speed handpiece. The needle perforates the cortical plate of bone and leaves a very small hole for the anesthetic needle to be placed.
2. An 8-mm, 27-gauge needle that is inserted into the hole for administration of the anesthetic (Figure 20-22).

To ensure that this is a "painless" injection, a topical anesthetic is first placed on the tissues. Once the perforator (solid needle) is injected into the tissues, a small amount of anesthetic is administered to numb the nerve endings in this area.

Periodontal Ligament Injection

The **periodontal ligament injection**, or intraligamentary injection, is used for pulpal anesthesia of one or two teeth in a quadrant and sometimes as an adjunct to another injection where the patient is only partially anesthetized. It also is used as an aid for diagnosing abscessed teeth and when a patient does not want the lip and tongue to be numb.

This technique involves inserting the needle into the gingival sulcus along the long axis of the tooth to be treated on the mesial or distal or the root. The original pressure syringe used for the periodontal ligament injection was developed in 1905. This technique has become popular again, mainly because manufacturers have designed pressure syringes for easier administration (Figure 20-23).

Intrapulpal Injection

The **intrapulpal injection** technique deposits the anesthetic directly into the pulp chamber or root canal of the involved tooth. This injection may be used when there is difficulty in securing pain control. A 25- or 27-gauge short or long needle is used; sometimes, the needle is bent to access the pulp canal.

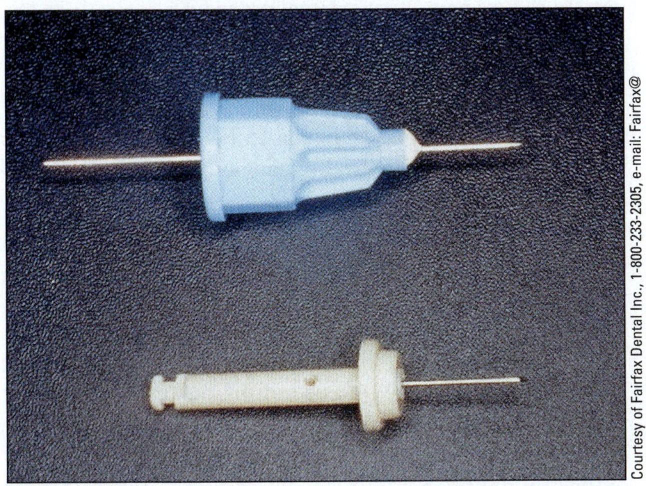

Courtesy of Fairfax Dental Inc., 1-800-233-2305, e-mail: Fairfax@stabident.com

FIGURE 20-22
Stabident system (Lasystem).

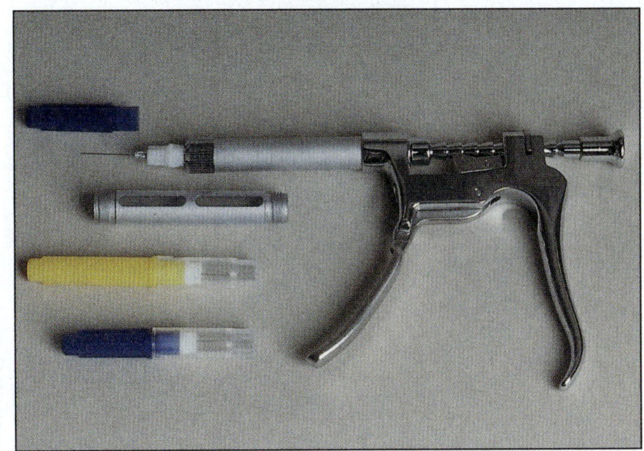

FIGURE 20-23
Periodontal ligament injection syringe and selection of needles.

Electronic Anesthesia

An **electronic dental anesthesia** has been used for a long time with low-to-moderate levels of success. When used with nitrous oxide inhalation sedation, the effectiveness is improved. It has been used in many dental procedures, such as placing restorations, muscle relaxation, and determining the patient's centric occlusion. Electronic dental anesthesia may be used when local anesthetics are contraindicated, such as with patients who are allergic to local anesthetics or who are extremely fearful of the injection.

Computer-Controlled Local Anesthesia Delivery System

A **computer-controlled local anesthesia** delivery systems promise pain-free injections. These systems can be used to administer all traditional infiltration and block injections. The computer-controlled system is a microprocessor that delivers a controlled pressure and volume of anesthetic solution at a rate that is commonly below the pain threshold. The microprocessor adjusts the pressure for low-resistant tissues to high-resistant tissues and can be used for injections on the palate and periodontal ligament.

Standard anesthetic cartridges and any size or gauge Luer Lock needle can be used with the system. On the microprocessing unit, the cartridge is twisted into place with the diaphragm end of the cartridge down and the rubber plunger up; plastic microtubing is linked from the plunger to the "handpiece" where the needle is attached. A foot control is used to activate the delivery of the anesthetic (Figure 20-24).

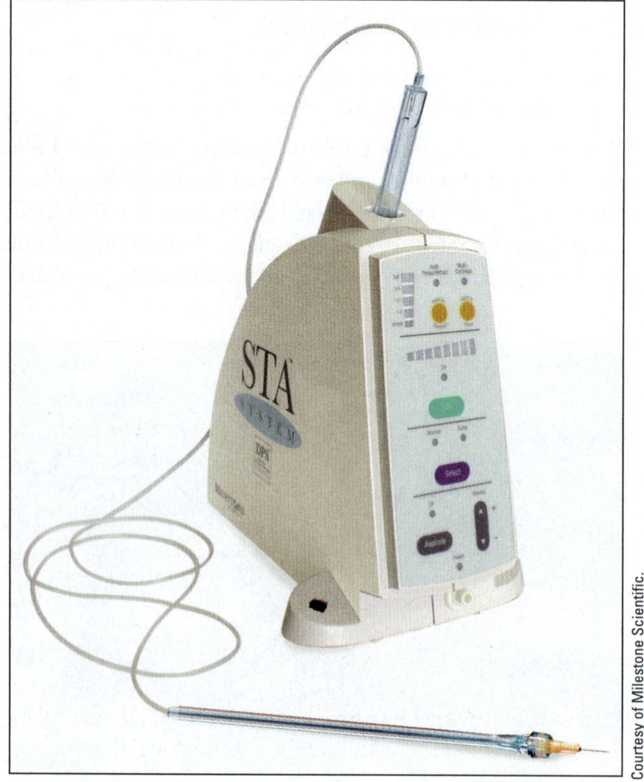

Courtesy of Milestone Scientific.

FIGURE 20-24

Computer-controlled local anesthetic delivery system (The Wand).

Nitrous Oxide Sedation

The use of **nitrous oxide** and oxygen gases are combined to provide relaxation and to relieve apprehension for patients during dental treatment. These two gases used together allow a safe method of sedation for patients who experience great fear during dental care. This gas allows patients to maintain consciousness while taking the "edge" off the pain so that relaxation can occur. Patients report a floating sensation, tingling fingers, and the feeling that time is passing quickly. Used safely, nitrous oxide can be a wonderful aid to allow patients to be comfortable and relaxed while receiving dental treatment.

Nitrous oxide is a stable, nonflammable gas. When used with oxygen, nitrous oxide is one of the safest anesthetic agents available. It is administered through a small nosepiece to the patient and has very little offensive odor. As the patient breathes in the gas, it travels through the nasopharynx and oropharynx, then down the larynx to the trachea. From the trachea, it continues into the right and left bronchi. The gas then travels through the smaller tubes, called the bronchioles, to the alveolar sacs, which consist of alveoli (see Chapter 6, General Anatomy and Physiology). The gases are then transferred across the alveoli in the lungs and blood plasma and red cells of the circulatory system. The blood carries the gas in the blood plasma and red cells to the brain, where the nitrous oxide analgesic agent takes effect. This process is much the same as breathing atmospheric air in which the body takes oxygen through the lungs and into the blood, and the blood carries the oxygen to the brain and throughout the body. The pharmacologic actions of nitrous oxide and oxygen are mild and mainly affect the central nervous system. Nitrous oxide raises the pain threshold without the loss of consciousness so that the patient can talk and follow directions.

Nitrous oxide gas was first discovered by Joseph Priestly in the early 1770s. It was thought the gas would cure diseases. **Horace Wells** (1815–48) (Figure 20-25), a Connecticut dentist, was the first to use nitrous oxide as an anesthetic during dental surgery. He immediately recognized that it could be used to reduce pain during dental procedures.

Safety and Precautions

The use of nitrous oxide needs to be monitored for the safety of both the dental health team and the patient. Excessive occupational exposure to nitrous oxide or exposure for specific populations of patients may result in adverse health effects.

Dental Office Personnel Safety. The American Dental Association (ADA) has been monitoring and pursuing information about the safe use of nitrous oxide for many years. They convened an expert panel and made a number of recommendations to ensure safe usage of nitrous oxide for dental personnel. In addition, the **National Institute of Occupational Safety and Health (NIOSH)**, which has continued activities relating to safe nitrous oxide

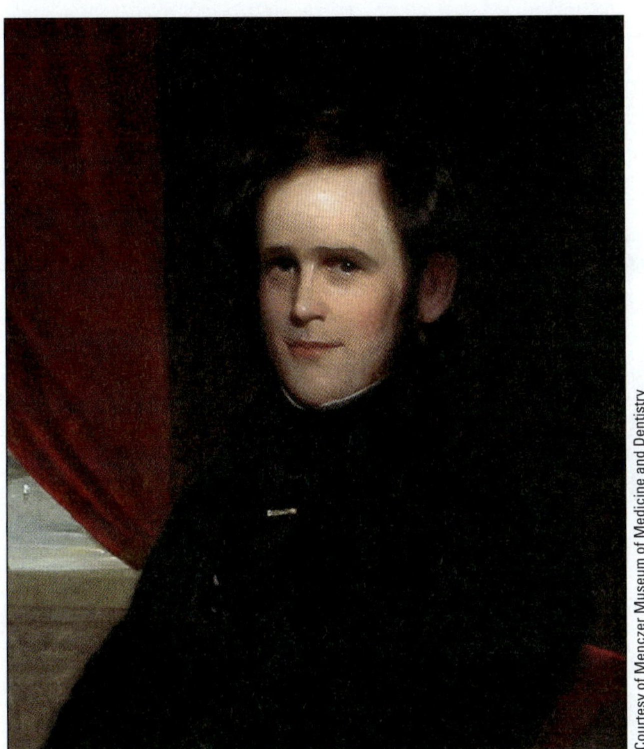

FIGURE 20-25
Horace Wells (1815–48), artist unknown, c. 1838, oil.

concentrations in the dental office, reported that the recommended exposure limit of 25 ppm can be controlled with leak-free delivery units, better-fitting masks, proper exhaust rates, and additional exhaust ventilation. OSHA protocol for personal exposure monitoring is to complete two tests more than one week apart. If both test results are low, then periodic testing should be completed at least once a year. The ADA suggested that twice a year, chairside personnel exposed to nitrous oxide be checked with diffusive samplers (dosimeters) or with infrared spectrophotometers. There are many types of badges that can be purchased that are worn by the dental auxiliary for a specific amount of time and then returned to the manufacture for evaluation and monitoring.

Patient Safety. To ensure patient safety, the patient's health history should be kept current and all known allergies and reactions should be noted. During administration of nitrous oxide sedation, the dental assistant should monitor the heart rate, blood pressure, respiratory rate, and responsiveness of the patient. Safety and precautions must be practiced with patients because of problems associated with nitrous oxide. Women in the first trimester of pregnancy, infertile people using in vitro fertilization procedures, immunocompromised people at risk of bone marrow suppression, and people with neurological complaints need special consideration. Nitrous oxide may cause fertility problems for those who work with and around nitrous oxide sedation long term.

Indications for Use of Nitrous Oxide Sedation

Patients who would benefit from nitrous oxide analgesia are as follows:

- Fear dental treatment
- Have a very sensitive gag reflex
- Can breathe through their nose
- Have a heart condition (they benefit because of stress reduction and the oxygen)
- Have a long appointment

Contraindications for Use of Nitrous Oxide Sedation

- Patients unable to breathe through their nose
- Patients involved in drugs or psychiatric treatment
- Women in the first trimester of pregnancy
- Immunocompromised people at risk of bone marrow suppression
- Infertile people using in vitro fertilization procedures
- People with neurological complaints

Equipment

Nitrous oxide is delivered to the patient through tubing connected to a nosepiece and tanks of nitrous oxide and oxygen. The gases flow through a unit with a flow meter and adjustment controls. After the adjustments are made, the gas flows through the breathing tubes to the mask. The excess gas and air exhaled from the patient flows through the scavenging nasal hood, which is a mask inside another mask. Each mask has two tubes connected to it. The inside mask receives the nitrous oxide that flows directly to the patient and from the patient to the outside mask. The outside mask is connected to the reservoir bag and the vacuum system, which carries away exhaled and additional gases from the treatment area, the patient, and dental team members (Figure 20-26).

Nitrous oxide units can be portable or wall mounted and distributed throughout the office (Figures 20-27 and 20-28). Cylinders of nitrous oxide gas are blue, and those of oxygen are green. When a wall-mounted nitrous oxide unit is used, the gas is sent from the cylinders through pressure lines to outlets in the treatment rooms.

Every day the nitrous oxide equipment should be monitored for safe operation. The control panels for the nitrous oxide and the oxygen tanks should be examined as well as the tubing and nosepieces. It is important to make certain that there are no tears or kinks and that the tubes and nosepiece are free of blockage. The nitrous oxide and oxygen equipment should be calibrated weekly and the manufacturer's directions should be followed.

Procedure 20-3 outlines the steps for administration of nitrous oxide.

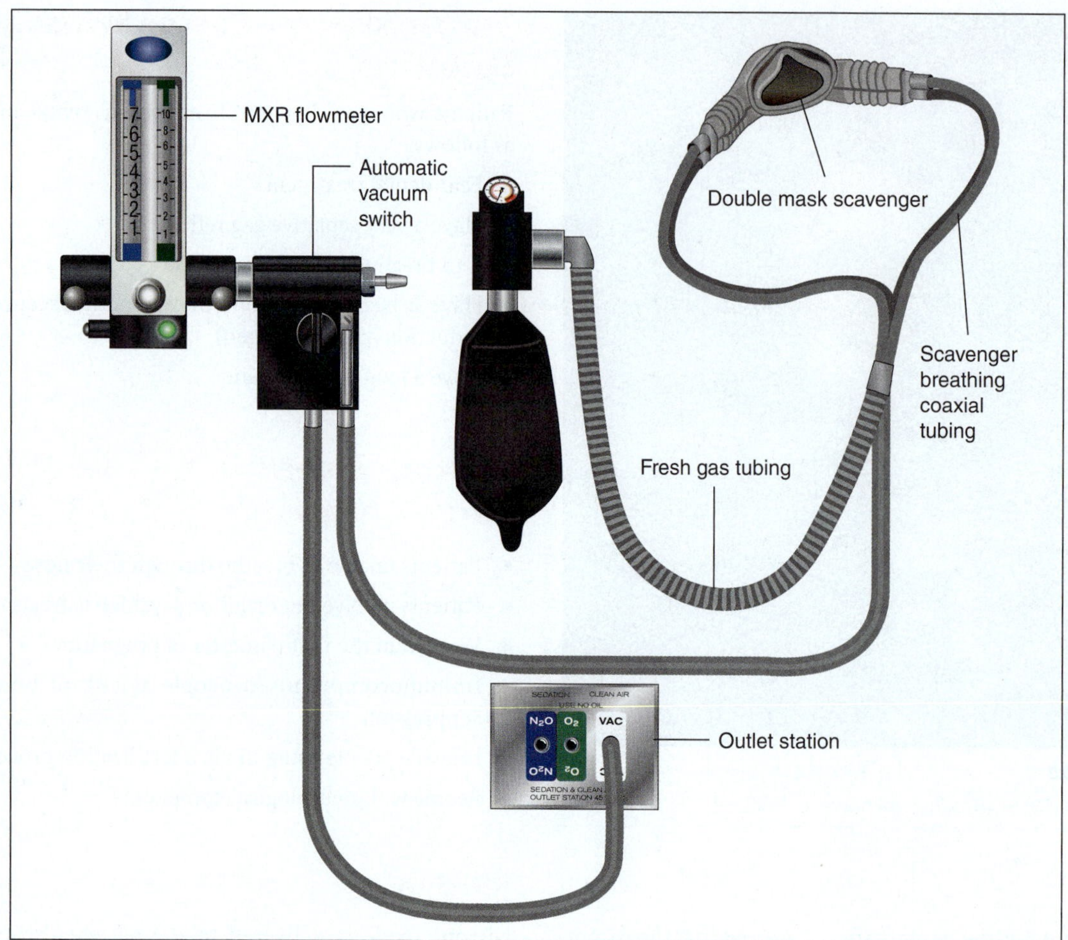

FIGURE 20-26

Parts of a nitrous oxide system.

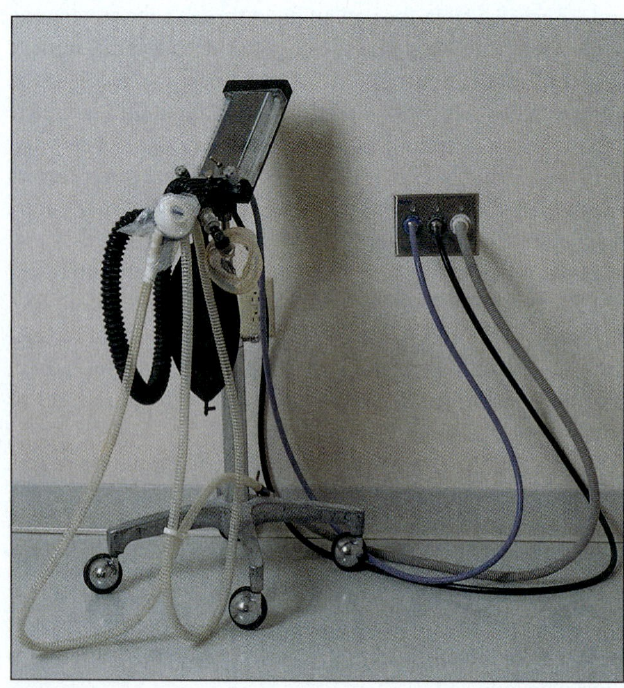

FIGURE 20-27

Portable nitrous oxide-oxygen unit.

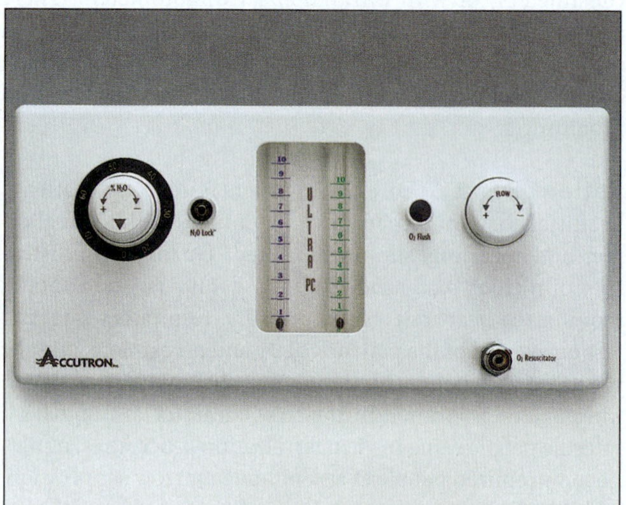

Courtesy of Accutron, Inc., Phoenix, AZ.

FIGURE 20-28

Example of a wall-mounted nitrous oxide-oxygen unit with gas cylinders in remote storage area.

Procedure 20-3
Administration and Monitoring of Nitrous Oxide Sedation

Some states allow dental assistants to perform this task under the supervision of the dentist; in other states, assistants assist dentists in administering nitrous oxide and/or monitoring nitrous oxide.

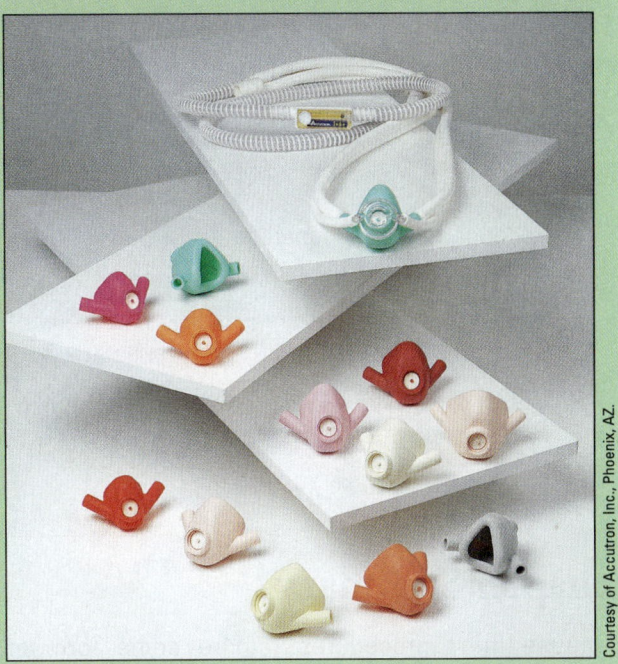

FIGURE 20-29
Nitrous oxide nasal hoods with scavenging circuit.

Courtesy of Accutron, Inc., Phoenix, AZ.

Equipment and Supplies
- Nitrous oxide unit with controls and gauges
- Tanks of nitrous oxide and oxygen
- Patient nitrous nosepieces (sterile)

Procedure Steps (*Follow aseptic procedures*)
Preparation
1. Check all equipment to verify that it is working properly.
2. Check the levels of gases to determine that the tanks are full.

Administration
1. Seat the patient and place him or her in a supine position.
2. Explain the effects, sensation, and potential hazards of nitrous oxide to the patient.
3. Have the patient give informed consent, allowing administration to continue.
4. Attach a sterile nitrous scavenger mask to the tubing (Figure 20-29).
5. Place the nosepiece mask over the nose of the patient, ensuring a proper fit, with the tubing draped to each side (Figure 20-30).
6. Instruct the patient to breathe through the nose slowly.
7. Begin the flow of oxygen (5 plus liters per minute) and nitrous oxide. (Many offices begin with the flow of oxygen for a minute before the nitrous oxide to determine the patient's **tidal volume** (normal volume of air inhaled and exhaled with each breath). This allows the patient to become accustomed to the mask and the situation before adding the effects of the nitrous oxide.)
8. Sit with the patient and monitor for any effects as the nitrous oxide is administered. Watch for Guedel's signs, stage I (Guedel's classification is a means of assessing the depth of anesthesia. Stage I is the assessment from the beginning of the administration). Talk with the patient and ask how he or she is feeling. (This allows the baseline nitrous oxide to be identified for the patient. Adjustments are made until a comfortable level of sedation is achieved. The patient does not lose consciousness and dialogue is ongoing.)
9. Watch the patient's chest and the reservoir bag rise and fall during the breathing.

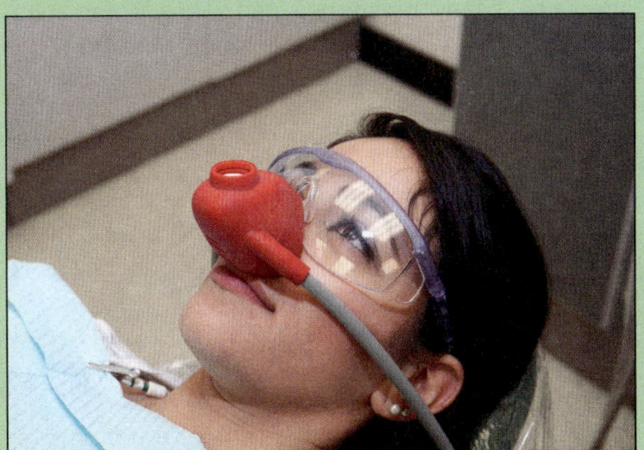

FIGURE 20-30
Nitrous oxide unit assembled and in place on patient.

(continues)

Procedure 20-3 (continued)

10. The local anesthetic solution is administered within a few minutes of nitrous oxide application. The patient is comfortable and the procedure can continue.

Recovery

1. When the dental procedure is nearing completion, turn off the nitrous oxide.
2. The patient will breathe oxygen for a minimum of 5 minutes or until all signs of the nitrous oxide sedation have disappeared.
3. Remove the nosepiece from the patient's nose.
4. Turn off the oxygen at the unit. The flow meters for the nitrous oxide and oxygen will be at zero.
5. Seat the patient upright and ask how he or she feels.
6. Ask the patient to stay seated for a minute or two until his or her head clears. (Even without nitrous oxide, rising from the supine position may make the patient feel lightheaded.)
7. Dismiss the patient when he or she feels normal.
8. Complete all documentation on the patient's chart, including notation about the administration of nitrous oxide.
9. The patient nosepiece is given to the patient for later use or disposed of. Some offices provide plastic bags for patients to save their nitrous oxide masks for repeated use to reduce disposables. Patients then bring their masks back for future appointments.
10. Disinfect the tubing.

Chapter Summary

Because most procedures require some form of anesthesia, the dentist may select one or a combination of methods to control pain, depending on the patient and the procedure. The dental assistant is responsible for preparing, safely transferring, and caring for the anesthetic syringe and accessories. During this time, the assistant must be aware of the various topical solutions, the application sites, how to apply the topical anesthetic, and possible patient reactions. In addition, the assistant follows the dentist's directions for the administration of sedation and monitoring requirements.

CASE STUDY

Chuck Thompson, 45 years old, was scheduled for a crown preparation. Topical anesthetic was placed, and Chuck became very talkative and excited. His pulse rate increased.

Case Study Review

1. Which items in the patient's medical history could be related to or cause this reaction?
2. What kind of reaction is Chuck experiencing?
3. Are there any other symptoms to watch for?

Review Questions

1. Anesthetic that produces a deadened or pain-free area is called ________ anesthetic.
   a. general
   b. local
   c. topical
   d. sedation
2. Topical anesthetics are available in all of the following forms *except*
   a. powders.
   b. gels.
   c. ointments.
   d. metered sprays.
3. An injection that deposits anesthetic near a large terminal nerve branch, and is mainly used for treatment on the maxillary or mandibular anterior regions is a(n) ________ injection.
   a. infiltration
   b. field block
   c. block
   d. periodontal ligament

4. A drug that is added to anesthetic solutions to reduce blood flow around the injection site is called
   a. paresthesia.
   b. vasoconstrictor.
   c. infiltration.
   d. nitrous oxide.
5. Which of the following best describes the injection site for the mental nerve block?
   a. The lingual tissue adjacent to the incisive papilla
   b. Halfway between the apices of the roots of the mandibular premolars
   c. The mucofacial fold adjacent to the root apex of the maxillary second molar
   d. Distal to the maxillary second molar
6. All of the following are parts of the dental needle except the
   a. bevel.
   b. syringe.
   c. plunger.
   d. hub
7. When preparing the anesthetic syringe the dental assistant should
   a. ensure the piston rod is engaged in the rubber stopper of the anesthetic carpule.
   b. ensure the syringe is working properly by expelling a few drops of solution.
   c. adjust the needle so the bevel is directed toward the alveolar bone.
   d. all of the above.
8. ________ places local anesthetic directly into the cancellous bone (spongy bone).
   a. Periodontal ligament injection
   b. Intrapulpal injection
   c. Electronic dental anesthesia
   d. Intraosseous anesthesia
9. Patients report a floating sensation, tingling fingers, and the feeling that time is passing quickly when ________ is administered to them before a dental procedure.
   a. topical anesthetic
   b. local anesthetic
   c. nitrous oxide sedation
   d. general anesthetic
10. The first dentist to use nitrous oxide as an anesthetic during dental surgery was
    a. Joseph Priestly.
    b. Pierre Fuchard.
    c. Wilhelm Roentgen.
    d. Horace Wells.

Critical Thinking

1. Which anesthetic solution provides a longer lasting pain control and promotes less bleeding for the patient?
2. What should be noted on the patient's chart regarding the local anesthetic?
3. Which types of patients benefit most from nitrous oxide analgesia?
4. If a patient becomes more talkative, apprehensive, and excited after the anesthetic solution has been administered, what would the dental assistant think is happening and what would they do in this situation?

Web Activities

1. Go to http://milesci.com and look up clinical studies on the benefits of computerized anesthetic.
2. Go to http://aamgpaloalto.com and research the role of an anesthesiologist in the dental office.
3. Go to http://www.cdc.gov and research the control of nitrous oxide in dental operatories.
4. Go to http://www.sedationcare.com and research sedation dentistry.

Section VI

Dental Radiography

CHAPTER

21

Introduction to Dental Radiography, Radiographic Equipment, and Safety Protection CDA

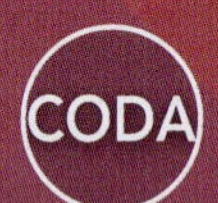

Specific Instructional Objectives

The student should strive to meet the following objectives and demonstrate an understanding of the facts and principles presented in this chapter:

1. Identify uses of dental radiography.
2. Explain the history of radiation and the use of the Hittorf-Crookes and Coolidge tubes.
3. Describe the history of dental x-ray film.
4. List the properties of radiation.
5. Describe the radiation types.
6. Identify the radiation units of measurements.
7. Explain the biological effects of radiation exposure.
8. Identify the components of a dental x-ray unit and explain the function of each component.
9. Describe safety precautions when using radiation.
10. Explain how an x-ray is produced.
11. Describe the composition, sizes, types, and storage of dental x-ray film.

Key Terms

aluminum filter (479)
American National Standards Institute (ANSI) (483)
anode (471)
as low as reasonably achievable (ALARA) (477)
atom (473)
basal cells (476)
Bremsstrahlung radiation (479)
cathode (471)
central beam (479)
collimator (479)
contrast (478)
control panel (477)
density (478)
digital imaging (473)
dosimeter (481)
electromagnetic energy (473)
electrons (473)
emulsion (483)
fluorescence (471)
focal spot (479)
focusing cup (479)
genetic effects (476)
gray (GY) (474)
halide crystals (483)
hard radiation (474)
inherent filter (479)
intensity (478)
intraoral (472)
ionization (473)
kilovoltage (kV) (478)
kinetic energy (479)

latent image (483)
latent period (477)
lead apron (476)
leakage radiation (474)
long wavelengths (474)
maximum permissible dose (MPD) (477)
milliamperage (mA) (478)
milliamperage seconds (mAs) (478)
milliroentgen (mr) (474)
mitosis (476)
neutrons (473)
position indicator device (PID) (473)
primary radiation (474)
protons (473)
radiation absorbed dose (rad) (474)
radiation monitoring device (481)
radiographs (471)
radiology (471)
radiolucent (483)
radiosensitive (476)
relative biological effectiveness (rbe) (476)
roentgen (R) (474)
roentgen equivalent man (rem) (474)
scatter radiation (474)
secondary radiation (474)
sensor (473)
short wavelengths (474)
sievert (Sv) (474)
soft radiation (474)
somatic effects (476)
thermionic emission (482)
transformers (479)
tubehead (479)
tungsten target (482)
x-rays (471)
x-ray tube (479)

Introduction

The science or study of radiation as it is used in medicine is called **radiology**. It provides the foundation for obtaining images that allow the dentist to view conditions of the oral cavity that would not otherwise be seen. The images referred to as **x-rays** or **radiographs** can be captured on film or digital sensors. Dental radiographs are an important element of patient treatment and diagnosis. Dental radiographs are used to:

- Identify dental decay and diseases in the oral cavity
- View the health of the teeth and surrounding areas
- Identify and diagnose suspicious areas of concern
- Locate abnormalities in the hard and soft tissue
- Identify foreign objects and lesions
- Record changes in trauma or periodontal health
- Obtain further information from trauma incidents
- Provide continued information during and after treatment for implants, root canals, orthodontic treatment, oral surgery, and so on
- Examine growth and development patterns
- Provide information for the preparation of treatment planning
- Provide a baseline record of the condition of the patient's oral cavity and dentition
- Used for patient identification, such as in the case of forensics, abductions, and so on

The History of Radiology

Wilhelm Conrad Roentgen (rent'-gun) discovered x-rays in 1895 (Figure 21-1). Roentgen was a professor of physics at the University of Wurzburg in Germany. During this time, he was performing experiments with a cathode ray tube called the Hittorf-Crookes tube. This glass vacuum tube had an electrical circuit connected to each end. Roentgen, as well as a number of other physicists at this time, was interested in the stream of bluish-colored light that passed from one end of the tube to the other when the electrical circuit was connected. The colored light was later discovered to be a stream of electrons that traveled from the **cathode** end to the **anode** end of the tube.

Roentgen placed an aluminum sheet with a window opening on the side of the tube to study the properties of the cathode ray. The room was darkened and a number of fluorescent screens were placed around the laboratory. While conducting his experiments, Roentgen noticed that a **fluorescence** (a glow that results when a fluorescent substance is struck by cathode rays, light, or x-rays) was occurring on the other side of the room. Because Roentgen knew that the cathode rays (negatively charged particles) could travel only a short distance outside the cathode tube in the air, he knew he was observing a new phenomenon, an unknown ray that he identified as an "x" ray, using the notation for the unknown variable in mathematics.

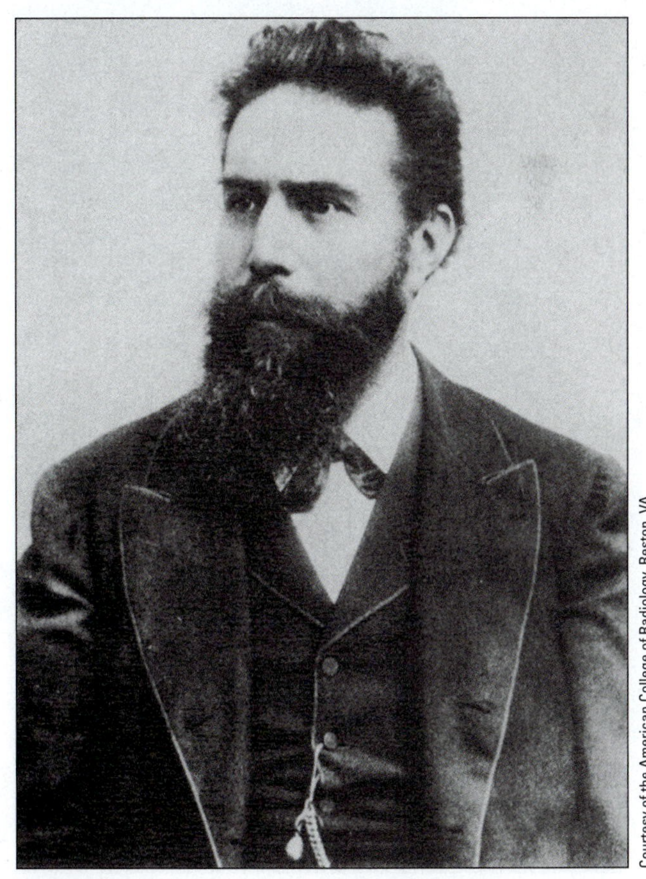

Courtesy of the American College of Radiology, Reston, VA

FIGURE 21-1
Wilhelm Conrad Roentgen (1845–1923) discovered x-rays in 1895.

Roentgen continued his experiments with the x-ray. He placed various objects in front of the beam and observed the images that were made on the fluorescent screen. For instance, when he placed metal in front of the beam, there was no visible image on the fluorescent screen. The metal blocked the beam. However, paper and wood allowed the x-ray to pass through, and the glow on the fluorescent screen changed according to the density of the object. It was while placing the objects in front of the screen that Roentgen noticed that he could see a shadow of the bones in his hand. The soft tissues of the hand allowed the x-rays to pass through, but the harder tissue of the bones stopped the x-rays.

Roentgen furthered his experiments with the x-ray and produced images on photographic plates. A couple of the first radiographs made were those of Roentgen's shotgun barrel and his wife Bertha's hand (Figure 21-2).

News of the discovery of the x-ray was soon heard around the world. Roentgen was awarded the first Nobel Prize in physics in 1901 for his work. Today, units of x-ray exposure are still expressed in roentgens in his honor.

In Germany in 1895, Dr. Otto Walkoff was the first to take a dental radiograph, just two weeks after the discovery of the x-ray. He used a small glass plate coated with photographic emulsion with an exposure time of about 25 minutes to obtain his desired result.

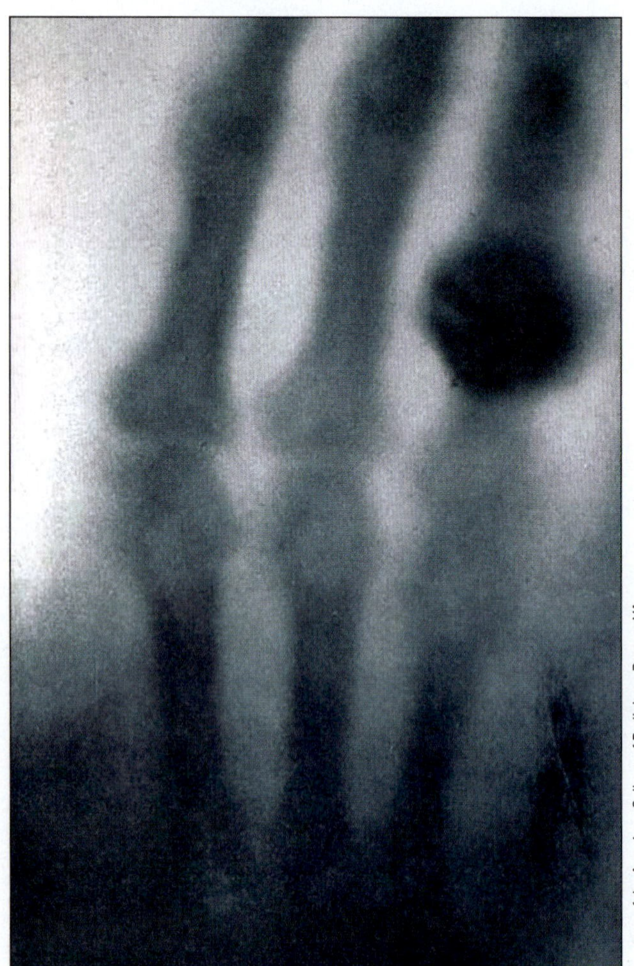

Courtesy of the American College of Radiology, Reston, VA

FIGURE 21-2
Early radiograph; thought to be of Mrs. Bertha Roentgen's hand.

In 1896, Dr. C. Edmond Kells, a New Orleans dentist, took the first **intraoral** radiograph using his own equipment and techniques. Later, he presented a clinical demonstration of dental x-rays at a dental association meeting in North Carolina. Dr. Kells used a method for adjusting the x-ray beam he called "setting the tube." In this technique, he placed his hand between the tube and the screen and adjusted the beam until he could see the bones of his hand clearly. He was unaware of the dangerous effects of radiation. Kells experienced pain and erythema (redness of the skin) on his hands from continued radiation exposure. Ongoing exposure resulted in the subsequent loss of three fingers, Kells's hand, his arm, and eventually his life at the age seventy-two.

The inventor of the first dental x-ray unit was Dr. William Rollins of Boston, Massachusetts, in 1896. He reported effects of radiation exposure, noting burning of the skin on his hands. He was an early advocate of the cautious use of "x" radiation.

Dr. William D. Coolidge, a physicist, invented the hot cathode x-ray tube in 1913. This hot filament replaced the need for the residual gas of the older model and established a standard for producing x-rays that were more uniform and, therefore, more predictable. The first American-made x-ray machine was manufactured around this time as well.

Prior to 1913, dental x-ray photographic plates were made from glass. Film was cut into the sizes needed, then wrapped with black paper and rubber. In 1913, a company named Eastman Kodak produced the first prewrapped dental intraoral films that were used in dentistry. These films replaced the hand wrapping technique used prior. In 1920, this process became further automated with the manufacturing of the first machine-made film packets.

In 1923, the Victor X-Ray Corporation, which later became known as the General Electric Corporation, developed a dental x-ray machine using the Coolidge tube in the machine head, which was cooled by oil immersion. Although the x-ray machine has been enhanced with numerous modifications to meet current application and safety requirements, this basic prototype is still used today.

Around 1905, Dr. Howard Rober and A. Cieszyski, an engineer, developed the bisecting technique. This technique applies a geometric principle, which is known as the rule of isometry (discussed later in this book).

In 1920, Frank McCormack developed an additional technique for exposing dental x-rays called the paralleling technique. This technique is often called the right-angle technique. To further improve the paralleling technique, Gordon M. Fitzgerald and William J. Updegrave developed the long cone technique and devices for positioning the x-rays, and also refined information on how to expose the x-ray properly. Over the years, the long cone technique has become simpler due to the change in the shape of the cone. Open-ended cylinders or rectangular tubes have replaced the pointed cone, allowing the operator to direct the x-rays more accurately. The open-ended tube, called the **position indicator device (PID)**, is still commonly called "the cone."

Several doctors researched the concept of rotational panoramic machines. The desired outcome was an x-ray of the entire dental arch on one film. To accomplish this, some machines rotated the film, others rotated the patient, and some rotated the x-ray beam. In 1959, the panoramic technique was developed. Dr. Y. V. Paatero was credited with developing the first orthopantomograph unit that would take acceptable panoramic radiographs. Over the next 10 years, a number of advances were made, and in 1980 the Panorex II was developed by Dr. Charles Morris. This machine allowed the operator to make a split or continuous image of the oral cavity.

Current radiographic technology uses the principles of tomography, whereby mouth structures can be visualized in a chosen layer or plane while intentionally blurring structures in other planes. This technique is not routinely used in dental offices.

X-ray film also has changed throughout history. At first, glass photographic plates were used. Later, film was cut to size in the darkroom and wrapped in paper and a rubber coating; however, this process was very time consuming. In 1913, Kodak developed the first prewrapped film packets. Today's x-ray films come in easy-to-use sizes and are of the quality we have come to expect. They also require minimal patient exposure to achieve results.

Introduced in dentistry in 1987, **digital imaging**, is currently used in many offices. Images are computer generated and, thus, are not film processed. The term "digital" comes from the use of "digits" (binary numbers), which are sent to the computer to produce an image. The information is obtained through a digital **sensor** used in place of the dental film. This technology permits numerous image adjustments and the rapid transfer of images during consultations without additional film processing or the retaking of images. Because the images are computerized, they can be integrated into paperless charts, easily stored, and require much less storage space. Digital imaging is also used at chairside to help patients understand diagnoses. (See Chapter 23, Extraoral and Digital Radiography, for additional information on digital imaging.)

Radiation Physics and Biology

Radiation is a type of **electromagnetic energy**. The most familiar forms of electromagnetic energy are radio and television waves, and visible light. All electromagnetic energy has some similar properties. First, energy travels in waves, which move in straight lines at the speed of light (186,000 miles per second). Second, the waves only consist of energy. Therefore, energy can be sent through lines to a receiver, such as a television. No mass is involved, only energy. Third, electromagnetic energy travels through space in the form of transverse waves. The wavelength, the distance between the peaks of adjacent waves, is called a cycle (Figure 21-3).

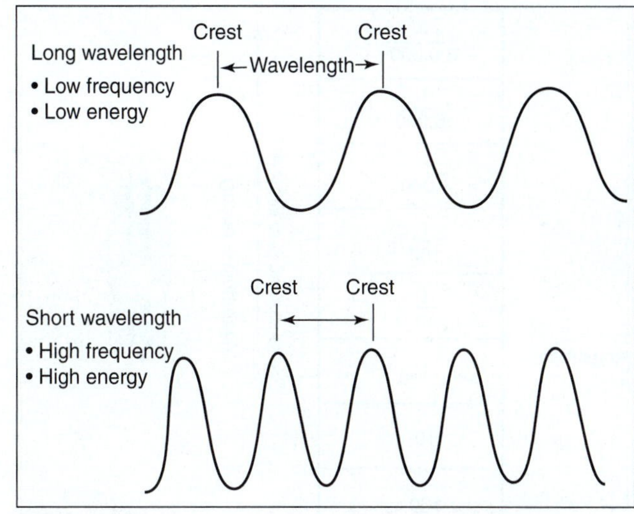

FIGURE 21-3

Wavelengths as they relate to energy, frequency, and x-rays. In dentistry, the shortest wavelength, with high frequency and energy, is used to expose dental film.

Electromagnetic energy is characterized by the length of the wavelength. Examples of electromagnetic radiation with longer wavelengths are visible light, television, and radio waves. Forms of electromagnetic radiation with shorter wavelengths are x-rays and gamma rays. The electromagnetic scale identifies the relationship between the type of energy and length of its wave (Figure 21-4). The more cycles that pass a point in a given time, the higher the frequency. Therefore,

- short wavelengths with high frequency equals more energy and
- long wavelengths with low frequency equals less energy.

It is important that individuals working with radiation understand the behavior and nature of x-rays. Visible light is the only wavelength that is detectable with human senses. Invisible x-rays, used for diagnosis in dentistry, carry 10,000 times more energy than visible light. X-rays travel in a straight line and can be deflected off an object and scatter. They can penetrate matter, whereas visible light is absorbed or reflected.

The Structure of an Atom and Ionization

Understanding the composition of an atom helps the dental assistant understand the process of **ionization**, in which atoms change into negatively or positively charged ions during radiation. Atoms make up all matter. An **atom** is composed of a nucleus, the inner core that is positively charged; and **electrons**, negatively charged particles that orbit the nucleus. The nucleus is composed of **protons** (positively charged), **neutrons** (not charged), and subatomic particles that are divided into hadrons, leptons, and quarks.

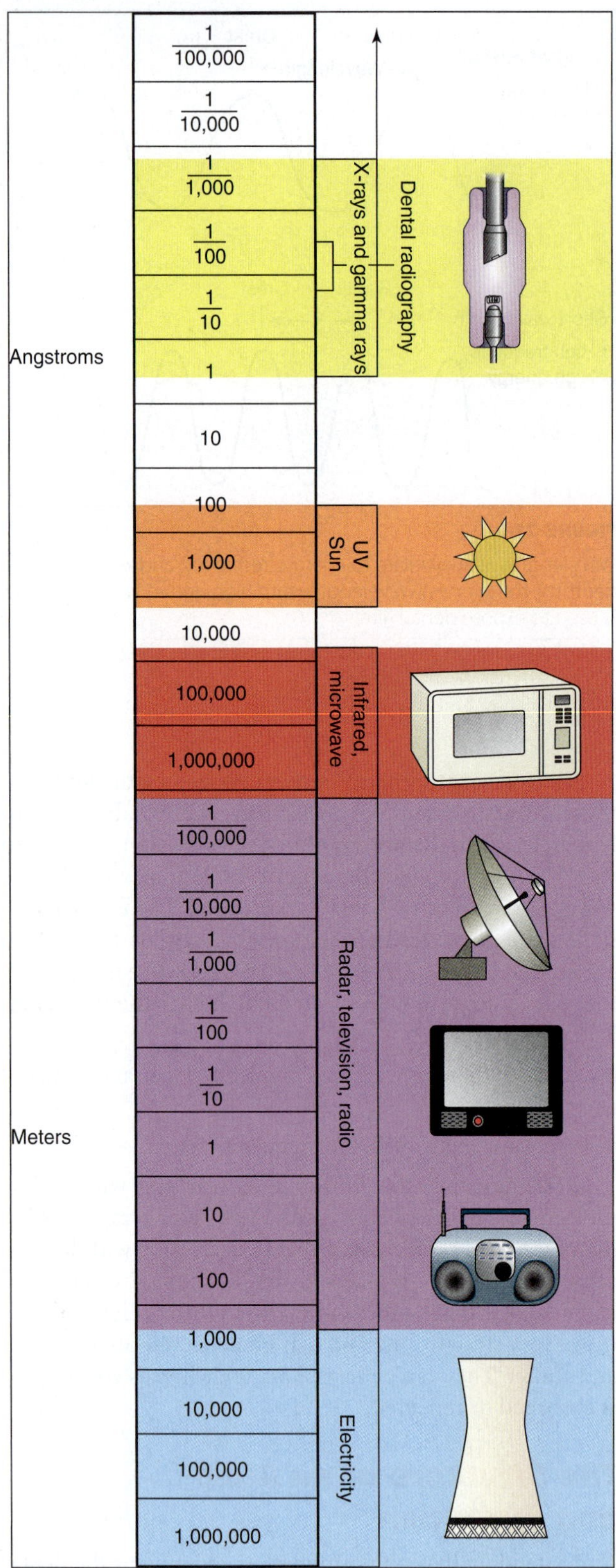

FIGURE 21-4
Electromagnetic energy spectrum and its applications.

Unless disturbed, electrons remain stable as they orbit the nucleus. If they are disturbed—for example, when x-ray photons collide with the atoms—electrons are lost and the atoms that have lost their electrons become positive ions (Figure 21-5). These positively charged ions are now able to react with atoms in tissues and other matter. This process can alter living cells and tissues and even cause permanent damage.

The patient and the operator must always be protected during exposure to ionizing radiation. Following safety guidelines, monitoring radiation, and using lead-lined protection protects individuals from the harmful effects of radiation.

Radiation Types

The wavelengths desired in dental radiographs are **short wavelengths**, or **hard radiation**. These have high frequency, high energy, and high penetrating power. On the other hand, **soft radiation**, or **long wavelengths**, have low energy, low frequency, and low penetrating power. They are unsuitable for exposing dental radiographs. These soft radiation rays are often called Grenz rays.

The four types of radiation (Figure 21-6) are the following:

1. **Primary radiation** is the central beam that comes from the x-ray tubehead. It consists of high energy, short wavelength x-rays that travel in a straight line. Primary radiation, often called the primary beam, is the useful x-ray that produces the diagnostic image on the x-ray film.
2. **Secondary radiation** forms when primary x-rays strike the patient, or contact matter (any substance). The waves are often transformed into longer wavelengths that lose their energy.
3. **Scatter radiation** is deflected from its path as it strikes matter. Often, secondary and scatter radiation are used interchangeably. This radiation scatters in all directions and, therefore, presents the most serious danger to the operator. Due to scatter radiation, the operator must stand at least 6 feet from the patient while exposing x-ray film, or stand behind structural shielding and out of the path of the primary beam.
4. **Leakage radiation** escapes in all directions from the tube or tubehead. The x-ray machine must be checked for leakage and should not be used until the problem is addressed. Leakage radiation is not useful for the diagnostic process; the long wavelengths only cause harm.

Radiation Units of Measurement

The terminology for the measurement of radiation has changed. Several new terms are replacing older, more familiar ones (Table 21-1).

In 1937, the International Committee for Radiological Units established the official definition of radiation quantity. A **roentgen (R)** equals the amount of radiation that ionizes one cubic centimeter of air. A **radiation absorbed dose (rad)** or **gray (GY)** is the amount of ionizing radiation absorbed in a substance. A **roentgen equivalent man (rem)** or **sievert**

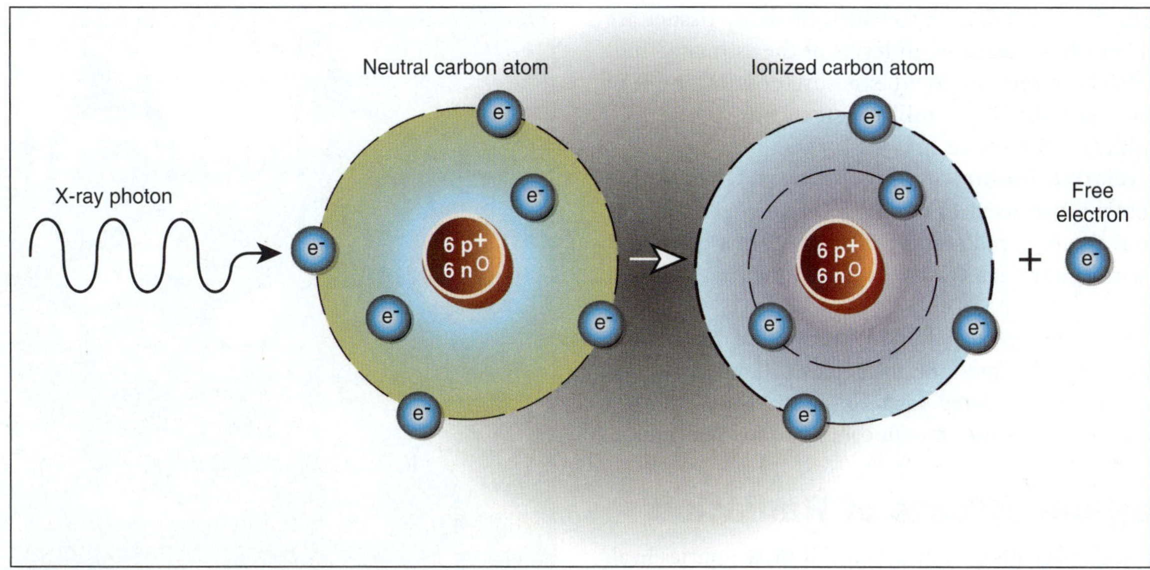

FIGURE 21-5

The process of ionization. Protons (+ charge) and neutrons (no charge) comprise the nuclei of atoms. Clouds of electrons (− charge) orbit nuclei at different energy levels (sometimes called "shells"). When an x-ray beam interacts with electron clouds, the ionization of atoms occurs.

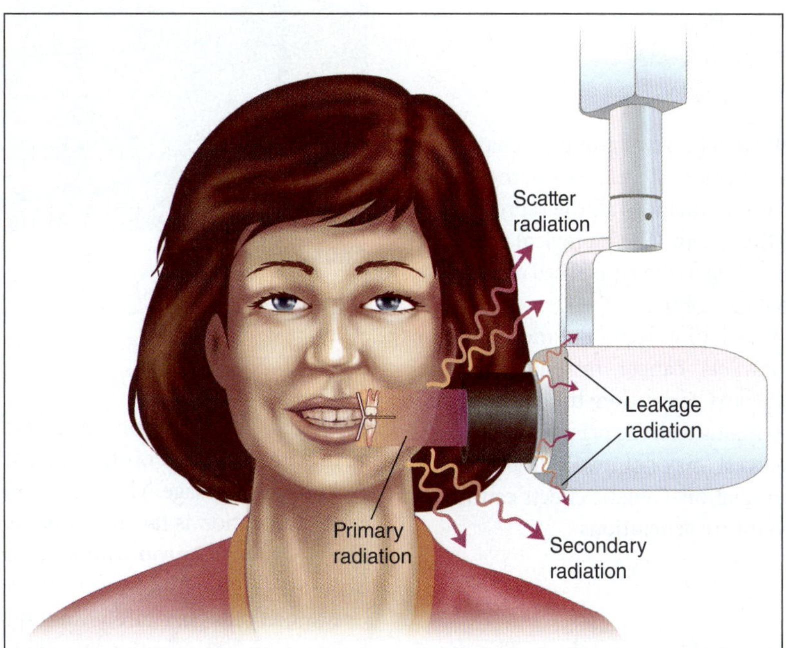

FIGURE 21-6

Primary, secondary (scattered), and leakage radiation identified on an x-ray tube and a patient's face.

TABLE 21-1 Radiation Measurement Terms

	Standard System (Traditional)	Metric Equivalent or Système Internationale (SI)
Exposure (C/kg)	Roentgen (R) 3.88 × 10 R =	Coulomb per kilogram 1 C/kg
Dose	Radiation absorbed dose (RAD) 100 rads =	Gray (GY) 1 GY
Dose equivalent	Radiation equivalent man (REM) 100 rems =	Sievert (Sv) 1 Sv

(Sv) is the dose of radiation to which the body tissues are exposed, which is measured in terms of the estimated biological effects in relation to an exposure dose of one R of "x" or gamma radiation. A **milliroentgen (mr)** is one one-thousandth (1/1,000) of an R.

The **relative biological effectiveness (rbe)** is the measurement unit used to compare the biological effects on various tissues irradiated by different forms of energy. Dental x-rays have arbitrarily been assigned an rbe unit of one.

Determine the rem by multiplying the rad by the rbe. Therefore, 100 rads times one rbe equals 100 rems. The rad and the rem are considered equal for dental x-rays; a rad is an absorbed dose, not the amount coming from the machine.

Biological Effects of Radiation

X-rays can damage body tissues. Some of these injuries heal, but some do not. If the cell is affected by direct radiation, the cell may die immediately, change immediately, change at **mitosis** (cell division in the sex cells in which the number of chromosomes in each is reduced to one-half), or remain unaffected.

Somatic and Genetic Effects of Radiation

The cells in the body are divided into two groups: somatic and genetic. The somatic group includes all cells except the reproductive cells. The genetic group includes all the reproductive cells, such as the ova and the sperm. The biological effects of radiation are classified according to the type of cell affected by the radiation, that is, somatic or genetic.

The **somatic effects** of radiation leave the individual in poor health and with cataracts, cancer, or leukemia. The effects are not passed to the next generation; the consequence of the radiation exposure remains with the primary individual. The **genetic effects**, in contrast, may not involve the primary individual exposed to the radiation. Genetic effects cannot be repaired and are passed to future generations.

Radiosensitive Cells

Some cells are more **radiosensitive** than others. The more sensitive cells are immature cells, rapidly dividing cells, and cells that do not perform specialized functions. Examples of rapidly dividing cells are the **basal cells** of the skin. They are sloughed off and continuously replaced. Therefore, a person may develop skin cancer due to prolonged exposure to sunlight, a high dosage of radiation, and/or frequent radiation exposure.

Today, people are more informed about the effects of radiation. Most patients request protection from radiation during pregnancy, because individuals understand that the embryo is very sensitive to it. Radiation of an embryo may cause death, congenital malformations, or growth retardation. The effects of radiation depend on the stage of the developing embryo and radiation dosage. Therefore, when pregnancy is suspected, every precaution is taken. All patients should receive protection with a **lead apron** with a thyroid collar during radiation exposure (Figure 21-7).

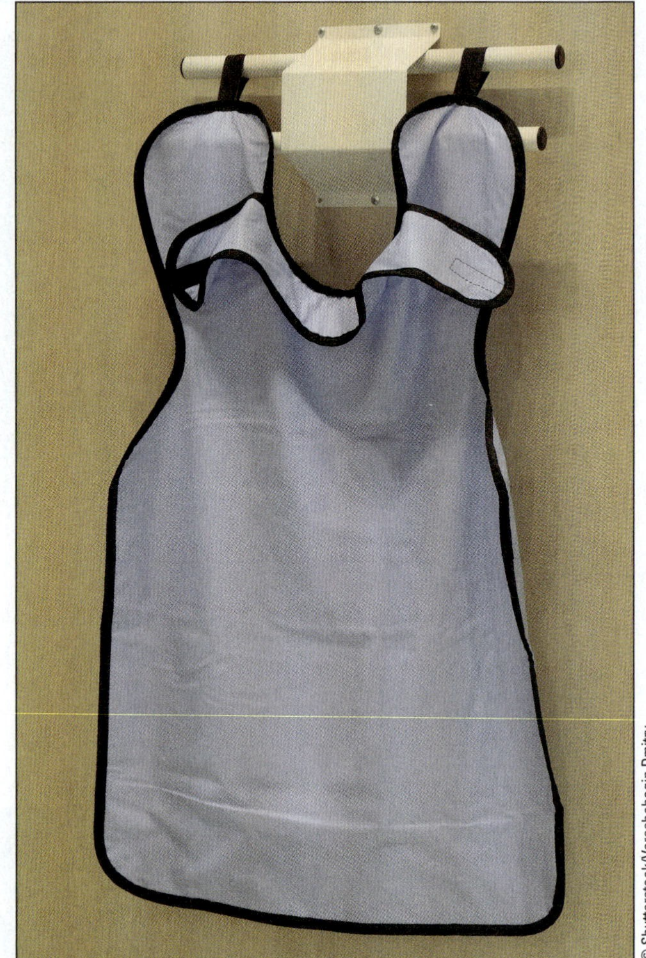

FIGURE 21-7
Lead apron with a thyroid collar.

Mature cells that rarely undergo cell divisions are *radioresistant*, or less sensitive to radiation. Examples of radioresistant cells are nerve and muscle cells. Table 21-2 shows the levels of sensitivity of different cells.

Low-level radiation normally does not cause damage that cannot be repaired within cells. Tissues that are radiosensitive in the dental region are the lens of the eye and the thyroid gland. Because of their location near the oral cavity, these tissues may be exposed to the primary beam (central beam) of the x-ray. Very high radiation dosages (not used in dentistry) have been known to cause cataracts in the eye and thyroid carcinoma. It is unlikely that dental x-rays cause one of these serious effects, but it is always

TABLE 21-2 Tissue and Organ Radiation Sensitivity

Most sensitive	Lymphoid Reproductive cells Bone marrow Intestinal epithelium Thyroid
Moderately sensitive	Skin Intestinal tract Oral mucosa
Sensitive	Connective tissue Growing bone
Less sensitive	Mature bone Salivary glands Liver
Least sensitive	Kidney Muscle Nerves

necessary to use the least amount of radiation possible. All dental personnel use the **as low as reasonably achievable (ALARA)** concept for radiation protection. Dental offices use a thyroid shield extension on the lead apron to further protect patients.

Occupational Exposure

Individuals who routinely use ionizing radiation in their occupations are regulated by dose limitations defined by the National Council on Radiation Protection and Measurements. The **maximum permissible dose (MPD)** is the maximum dose of radiation that, in light of present knowledge, would not be expected to produce any significant radiation effects in a lifetime. The MPD calls for the dose limit of occupational exposure to be at 0.05 Sv (5.0 rems) per year or 100 mrem per week for radiation workers. Nonoccupational exposure and pregnant workers are regulated at one-tenth this limit. Most resources recognize the 0.05 Sv per year maximum; however, recommendations by the International Commission on Radiological Protection call for the occupational exposure dose limits to be 20 mSv (2.0 rems).

Daily Radiation Exposure

The general population is exposed to two major categories of radiation daily: natural and artificial. Annually, a person encounters an average of 3.6 mSv (360 mrems) of radiation from all sources. Natural sources make up a large percent of radiation exposure. It comes from the earth (radon, for instance), the sun, and the atmosphere.

The rest of radiation exposure comes from artificial radiation, such as x-rays used for diagnosis, as well as from consumer products, such as television, airline travel, tobacco, and smoke alarms.

Accumulation of Radiation

The effects of radiation are cumulative, meaning that the effects of exposure increase every time the individual is exposed to radiation. This is often called the long-term effect.

The normal aging process tends to accelerate due to radiation accumulation. Most adults know that the skin of individuals who have (or had) high exposure to the sun ages at an increased rate—the higher the doses, the more rapid the effects. This period between direct exposure and the development of biological effects (or symptoms) is called the **latent period**.

Components of the Dental X-Ray Unit

The dental assistant should know and understand the components within a dental x-ray unit. The assistant may be responsible for obtaining x-rays, as well as for the care and maintenance of equipment used to obtain patient x-rays.

Control Panel

The **control panel** is where the circuit boards and controls, which allow the operator to adjust the correct setting for each patient, are located (Figure 21-8). It is where the on/off switch is located, as well as the controls for the milliamperage (mA), kilovoltage (kV), and the electronic timer.

The operator chooses settings according to the individual (e.g., children need less radiation), the area of the oral cavity needing diagnostic x-rays, exposure technique, and film speed.

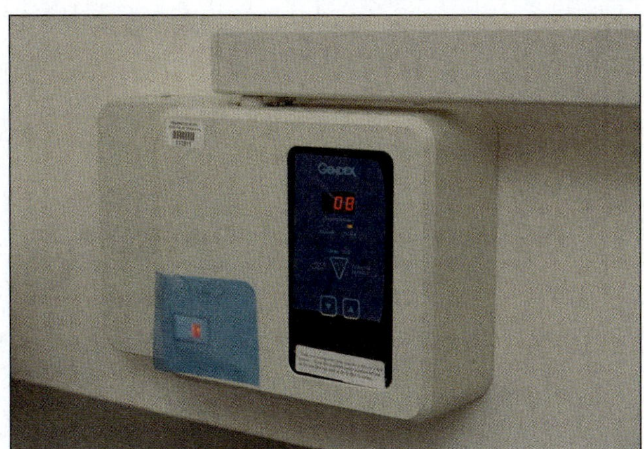

FIGURE 21-8
Control panel.

Milliamperage. The **milliamperage (mA)** determines the amount or *quantity* of electrons. Milli (1/1,000) amperage is a measurement unit for electrical current—the higher the mA, the greater the amount of radiation.

Some dental x-ray machines use 10 or 15 mA. Many machines are set up with selectors for 10 or 15 mA on the control panel. This milliamperage selector also acts as the on/off switch for the machine. Often, 10 mA is used with this type of dental x-ray machine. Radiation is not produced until the electronic timer is pushed. Some newer units are preset at 7 mA for all x-rays; they have separate on/off switches.

Milliamperage X-Ray Beam Factors

Increased milliamperage = increased density = darker images on x-ray film

Decreased milliamperage = decreased density = lighter images on x-ray film

Kilovoltage. The **kilovoltage (kV)** determines the *quality* or penetrating power of the central beam. The higher the kV, the greater the penetration power of the x-rays, and the less required exposure time. Therefore, there is less patient radiation. Higher quality of radiographs (showing a longer range of the Gray scale) are the results of higher speeds of radiation going through the tissues. A longer range of the Gray scale would show varying tissue density and provide greater diagnostic quality.

The kilovoltage meter is on the control panel. The operator adjusts the kilovoltage selector to the desired setting. The most common settings for kilovoltage are from 70 to 90 kV. On many of the digital machines, the kilovoltage is set automatically according to the area to be x-rayed.

Kilovoltage X-Ray Beam Factors

Increased kilovoltage = low contrast = increased density = dark film

Decreased kilovoltage = high contrast = decreased density = light film

Electronic Timer. The electronic timer controls the total time that rays flow from the x-ray tube. It is a rotating dial with which the dental assistant selects how many fractions of a second or impulses are needed to produce the x-ray. Thirty impulses equal one-half a second. The operator determines the number of impulses or exposure time after evaluating the technique to be used, the type of x-ray film, the target film distance, and which tissues are going to be radiographed. Again, this may be preset on the digital machines. The digital machines have touch pads and/or switches with simple drawings of adults or children on which to select patient size. By indicating patient size, the amount of kV, and the area to be radiographed, the machine sets the timer automatically.

The switch to the timer is outside the room or behind a lead barrier. The operator pushes the switch, and the timer allows the electrons to flow from the x-ray tube for the indicated time, and then it resets. The milliamperage, kilovoltage, and electronic timer components control the image quality factors of milliamperage seconds, contrast, and density.

Increased time will increase the density; and decreased time will decrease the density.

Milliamperage Seconds. The **milliamperage seconds (mAs)** determine the amount of radiation exposure the patient receives. To determine mAs, the dental assistant calculates the milliamperage times the exposure time. Once set, most offices do not change the kVp (peak kilovolts) and mAs, except for child and adult variations.

Characteristics of X-Radiation

Three primary characteristics of x-radiation are contrast, density, and intensity. These characteristics determine the sharpness and detail of the x-ray image. The detail can be determined by movement, film speeds, PID placement, and subject matter. The contrast is highly influenced by the kilovoltage settings and the density is primarily influenced by the milliamperage. The **intensity** is defined as the product of the quantity (number of photons from milliamperage) and the quality (penetration power of the photons from kilovoltage), together with the exposure time and distance.

Contrast. An x-ray is a black-and-white picture that also shows shades of gray. The **contrast** is the difference between shades of gray. The black, white, and shades of gray on an x-ray reflect the densities of the subject and the film. Contrast is controlled by the kV, the developing process (if the developing solution is old or exhausted), film fog (possibly caused by a light leak in the darkroom), and distortion (patient or cone moving).

Density. The **density** is the degree of darkness on an x-ray. Contrast is basically the difference between the densities of adjacent areas on a film. Several factors affect the density of a film, including the distance from the x-ray tube to the patient, patient tissue thickness, and the amount of radiation reaching the film. Density is controlled by mAs, developing techniques, kV, and film fog.

Intensity. Intensity is the combination of the number of photons (product of the quantity or milliamperage), and the energy of the photons (product of the quality or kilovoltage) affected by time and distance.

Arm Assembly and Tubehead

The arm assembly is attached firmly to the wall in the x-ray room (Figure 21-9A). The flexible extension of the arm allows the operator to freely position the tubehead for the various positions required for dental radiography exposures.

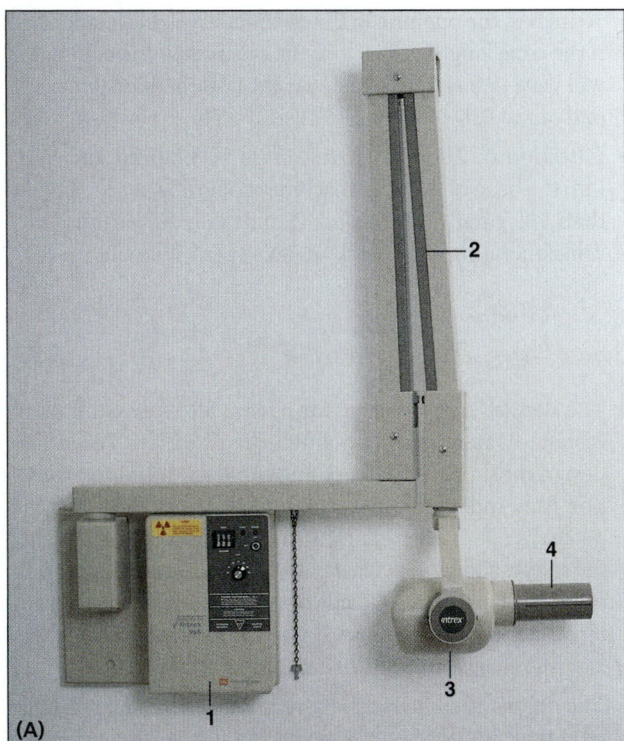

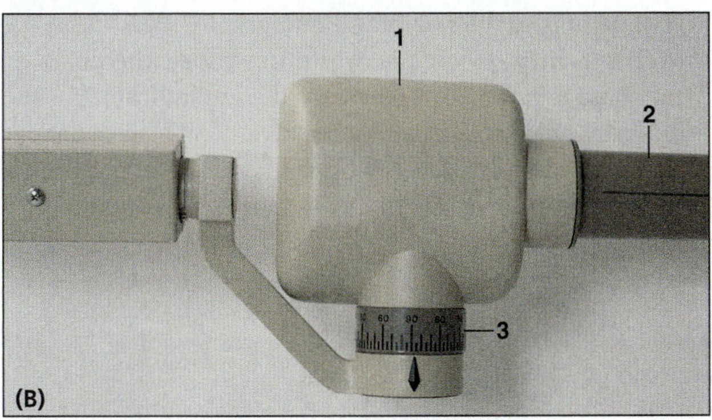

FIGURE 21-9

Parts of the dental arm assembly: (A) 1. Control panel. 2. Extension arm. 3. Tubehead. 4. Position indicator device (PID). (B) 1. Tubehead. 2. PID. 3. Vertical indicator scale.

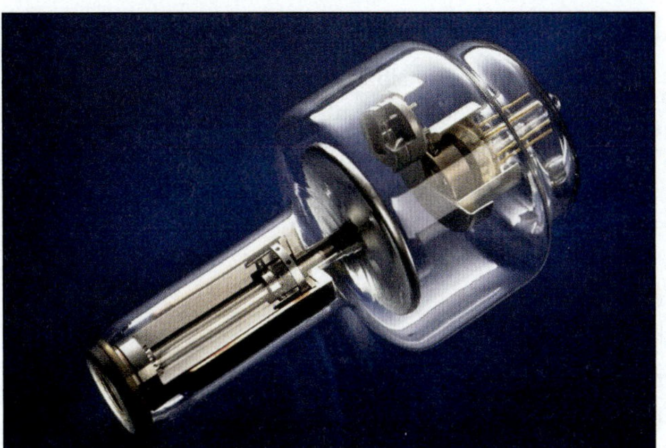

Courtesy of the Dunlee, Division of Phillips Medical Systems

FIGURE 21-10

X-ray tube.

The **tubehead** (Figure 21-9B) is where the x-ray vacuum tube and the step-up and step-down **transformers** are located. The high voltage (step-up transformer) provides the kV needed to propel the electrons, and the low voltage (step-down transformer) adjusts the voltage down to the amount of power needed to heat the filament of the cathode and produce the milliamperage. It is where x-rays are generated. The tubehead is made of a metal casing that is lead lined or made of lead to limit the amount of radiation leakage. An oil bath surrounds the components in the tubehead to provide cooling as heat is given off. The heat is derived from the production of the cloud of electrons and the manufacturing of the x-rays.

The **x-ray tube**, approximately 6 inches long and 0.5 in diameter, is often called a Coolidge tube (Figure 21-10). The tube is made from leaded glass and has a window (aperture window) of unleaded glass on the side where the x-rays exit. The tube is in vacuum (all air has been removed from the tube), so that the electrons are free to travel at the speed of light and not collide with air or gas molecules. On the cathode (−) side of the tube, a **focusing cup** made of molybdenum with a filament of tungsten is positioned. This is where the electrons originate. Tungsten is used because it has a high melting point, high ductility so it can be made into a fine wire, and a high atomic number so that a large number of electrons are ejected when it is heated. The focusing cup is designed to direct the stream of electrons to the anode. The anode (+), which is opposite the cathode, is made of a tungsten target, which is set at an angle to direct the flow of the x-rays. The small spot on the tungsten target where the electrons hit is called the **focal spot**. After the electrons hit, a great deal of heat is generated. The anode tungsten target is attached to a copper stem, which is then attached to a heat radiator that conducts the heat away from the focal spot. The heat dissipates through the copper stem, and is then cooled by the heat radiator and the surrounding oil bath.

After leaving the anode, the x-rays go through the aperture, or non-leaded window, and encounter a solid metal filter, usually made of aluminum. This **aluminum filter**, known as the **inherent filter**, is placed in the path of the x-rays to eliminate the soft x-rays (those with low penetrating power). The hard x-rays with short wavelengths, called the **central beam**, continue through the filter to the **collimator**, or lead diaphragm. The collimator is a lead disc with an opening in the middle that restructures the beam and filters out additional weak rays. The opening limits the size of the x-ray beam that is allowed to pass through the open cone and out the PID. The x-ray beam cannot exceed 2.75 inches in diameter (Figure 21-11A). Approximately 1 percent of the **kinetic energy** (energy of motion) created during the x-ray process is converted into useful x-rays. The remaining 99 percent is dissipated as heat.

Bremsstrahlung radiation is the primary type of radiation in the x-ray beam going out from the tubehead. *Bremsstrahlung* originates from a German word meaning, "braking." This braking action takes place when the electrons strike the anode target.

Safety and Precautions

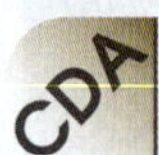

It is the responsibility of manufacturers, dental team members, and patients to follow safety and precaution measures when using radiography equipment. Steps must be taken to minimize the risk to the patient and to all dental personnel.

Manufacturer's Responsibilities

The federal government has set up safety specifications that all manufacturers of dental x-ray units must meet, they are as follows:

- The machine must have a separate control switch to cut off electricity to the machine. The exposure switch must have an electronic timer to stop the electricity automatically when the control switch is released. This "deadman" switch ensures that the exposure ends when the preset time has passed and not when the button is released.
- The PID must be lead lined, and the x-ray tube must be sealed in an oil-immersed casing.
- The control panel must have indicators that display mA, kV, and impulses per exposure time. Some models display the preset number for mA and only two choices for kV. On a digital control panel, the timer is preset, and changes on the digital panel display according to the chosen exposure area.
- The collimator, fitted directly over the opening where the x-ray beam exits the tubehead, is made of a lead plate. The opening, or hole, in the middle of the lead plate of the collimator is regulated to ensure that the useful beam does not exceed 2.75 inches in diameter. If the cone length is 16 inches, the opening in the collimator will be smaller and if the cone length is 8 inches, the opening of the collimator will have to be larger to achieve the correct diameter at the end of the PID (Figure 21-11B).
- Filtration of 2.5 mm of aluminum is required and built into the head of all x-ray machines operating at a kV higher than 70. Total filtration of 1.5 mm is required for x-ray units operating at or below 70 kVp (peak kilovolts).

Dentist's Responsibilities

- The dentist is responsible for having all x-ray equipment installed safely and to maintain it properly. The office design must provide occupants with lead filtration protection from radiation. The location of the x-ray room and the protective lead barriers must meet specific requirements for safety, allowing at least 6 feet in the opposite direction of the primary ray. X-ray machines must be inspected regularly, usually once a year, by the state regulatory agency x-ray control section to ensure proper functioning.
- The dentist must prescribe x-rays for patients responsibly, remembering that only x-rays for a proper diagnosis are necessary. The dentist is responsible for adhering to the "Guidelines for Prescribing Radiographs" (see the ADA Web site http://www.ada.org to download the chart or purchase a hard copy). These guidelines indicate that the dentist is responsible for ensuring treatment of each patient for her or his individual radiographic needs, thus, avoiding over prescription of routine x-rays for every patient.

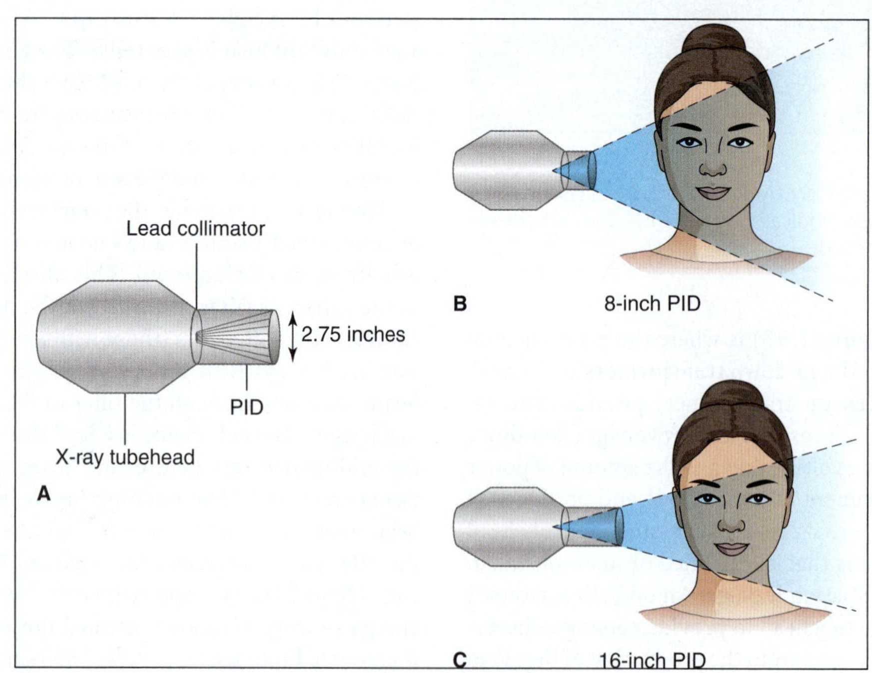

FIGURE 21-11

(A) The collimator diameter is 2.75 inches at the end of the PID. (B) An 8-inch PID versus a 16-inch PID with the correct collimation.

- Protocol for suspected x-ray machine malfunction is to stop usage immediately when a problem is apparent. It is the dentist's responsibility to repair x-ray equipment and to ensure on-going safety and compliance.
- The dentist is responsible for having dental assistants properly credentialed and trained for exposing and processing radiographs. The dentist is also responsible for supervising dental assistants in these tasks.

The Consumer Patient Radiation Health and Safety Act was enacted in 1981. This federal law requires each state to inform the Secretary of Health and Human Services how compliance with the act is accomplished.

Dental Assistant's Responsibilities

- The dental assistant must be trained in aseptic techniques, radiation hygiene, and maintenance of quality assurance and safety.
- Dental assistants must obtain proper education in exposure and processing techniques. They must understand the physics and biological effects of ionizing radiation, and use their understanding during every radiographic exposure.
- The dental assistant must understand the ALARA principle, and use a lead apron with a thyroid cervical collar for the patient's safety every time an x-ray is taken (see Figure 21-7).
- Dental assistants must properly label and store patient x-rays to prevent loss.

Patient's Responsibilities

The patient is responsible for notifying the office of any changes in health (pregnancy, for instance). Patients are also responsible for presenting, to the best of their abilities, radiation histories as part of their dental records.

Additional Notes on Reducing Radiation Exposure

- It should be noted that we currently expose patients to 2 percent of the exposure time that was used when films were first manufactured in 1920. Dental x-ray film is continually being advanced, with speed and image definition being improved. Using E-type film, which was developed in 1981, instead of D-type film, which was first developed in 1955, reduces the time of radiation exposure to the patient by up to 50 percent. There has been some resistance to changing from the standard D-type film because of quality control, but recent studies have demonstrated that E-type film is of comparable quality.
- Kodak InSight dental film is an F-speed film, developed in 2000, that reduces radiation exposure up to 20 percent compared to Kodak Ektaspeed Plus intraoral dental film, and up to 60 percent compared to D-type speed films.
- A patient having an 18-film series (full mouth) using a long, round PID without a lead apron results in a genetic exposure of 0.5 mrad; with a lead apron, the genetic exposure is approximately 0.01 mrad. If a thyroid collar is used, a 50 percent reduction is noted in the thyroid area.
- A patient having an 18-film series using a rectangular PID, instead of a round PID, reduces the radiation exposure to the patient by approximately 60 percent. (Figure 21-12).
- The National Council on Radiation Protection and Measurements (NCRP) makes recommendations on radiation protection and measurements, and disseminates information and guidance. In a report titled, "Radiation Protection in Dentistry" (Report 145), the Council stated that a lead apron is not necessary if a dental office is using F-speed film and rectangular collimation. Staying current on changes and recommendations via the ADA and NCRP is critical for a dental team using ionizing radiation. The NCRP works with the Centers for Disease Control and Prevention. To contact the NCRP, email NCRPpubs@NCRPonline.org.
- The *best* way to reduce a patient's radiation exposure is to use faster film and rectangular collimation. F-speed film is currently the fastest, and many manufacturers offer cone attachments for the dental position indicator device (PID).
- Proper filtration can reduce somatic (all tissues) exposure by 50 percent. A number of rare earth filters are being used to further reduce radiation exposure in extraoral radiography. Contact the Radiation Health and Safety Board, or the Kodak Company, for updated information on approved filters.

Any dental assistant producing radiographs should wear a **radiation monitoring device** or **dosimeter** badge (Figure 21-13) at the heart level outside of the clothing at all times while in the dental office. This badge monitors an individual's radiation exposure and accumulated dosage in the office. It is important that the badge is not be worn outside of the office, because it will produce an inaccurate reading. The badges are normally read monthly; and each employee should

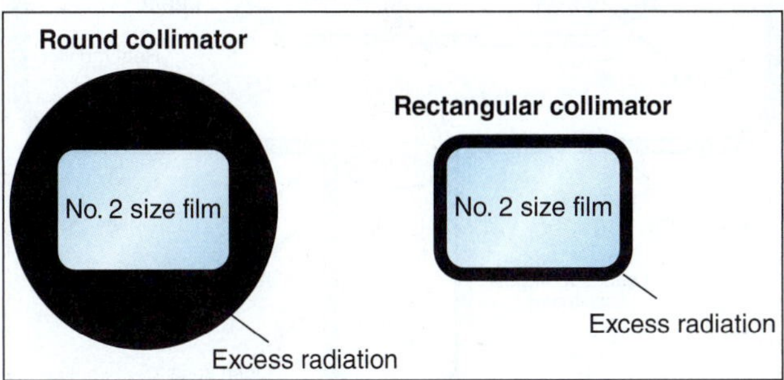

FIGURE 21-12
Compared to the rectangle collimator, the round collimator exposes the patient to greater excess radiation.

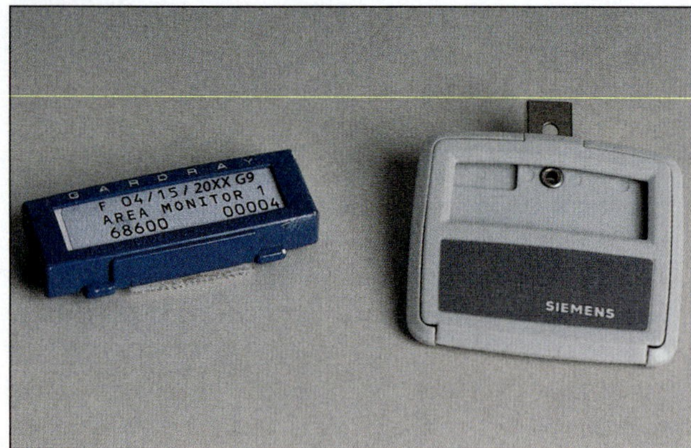

FIGURE 21-13
Operator wears a film badge to detect radiation.

be apprised of the outcome immediately, and corrective measures should be taken.

A quality assurance (QA) program should be developed for the production and processing of radiographs in the dental office.

Radiation Production

X-rays are produced when the operator depresses the exposure switch and starts generating electricity (Figure 21-14). The electricity passes to the control panel by way of the step-down and step-up transformers, where specified instructions on the quantity and the quality of x-rays have been selected. From the setting of the mA, time, and kV circuits, the electricity travels to the cathode filament. This current passes through the filament and heats it to an extremely high temperature. This process is called **thermionic emission**. When the filament reaches a certain temperature, electrons are ejected. Electrons are negatively charged, and, therefore, are attracted to the positively

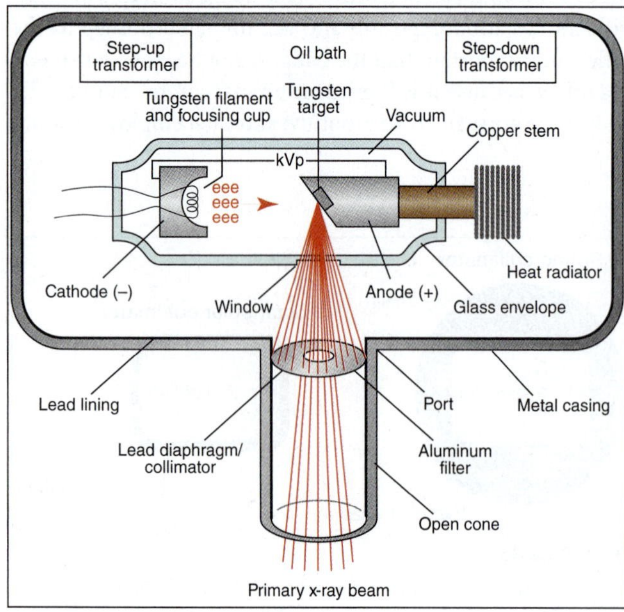

FIGURE 21-14
X-ray production in the tubehead.

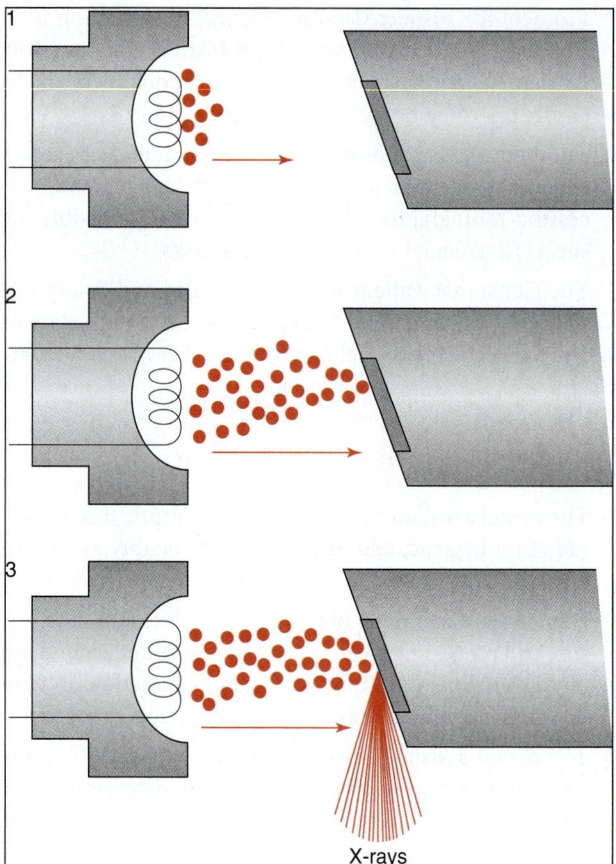

FIGURE 21-15
The production of dental images occurs in the x-ray tube. First, the filament circuit is activated, and the filament heats up causing the thermionic emission to occur. Second, when the filament reaches a certain temperature, electrons rapidly travel from the cathode to the anode. Third, the electrons contact the tungsten target, and their kinetic energy is converted into x-rays and heat.

charged anode side of the tube. The electrons rapidly travel toward the anode. The focusing cup on the cathode directs the electrons to a small area (about 1 mm^2 in size), called the focal spot, on the anode **tungsten target**. The precise moment of contact occurs when the x-rays are produced due to forceful collision of the electrons. Less than 1 percent is used for the x-ray energy or central ray. At the time of collision, the x-rays "bounce" off the tungsten target and weaker rays go in all directions, this 99 percent is lost as heat is absorbed and cooled by the copper stem, oil, and heat radiator. The useful x-rays travel through the filters and collimator, and out the PID opening (Figure 21-15).

The excess heat generated by the collision is dissipated by a heavy copper stem that takes the heat from the tungsten target and cools it in oil in the tubehead. In addition to the copper-stem cooling, a bulb also takes heat into the oil-bath chamber of the tubehead to increase cooling.

Dental Intraoral X-Ray Film

Intraoral dental x-ray film is film placed inside the oral cavity. It has emulsion on both sides of the film to reduce radiation to the patient. Intraoral films are used to diagnosis teeth and tissues. Proper care and handling of the dental x-ray film is critical to the quality of the x-rays produced. It is important to understand the qualities of the film. A sound understanding of the quality and characteristics of the film will allow the dental assistant to maintain high-quality radiographs.

Composition of Dental X-Ray Film

The film used in dental radiography is composed of a flexible, thin, polyester plastic base (about 0.2 mm thick). This semi-clear base (cellulose acetate) has a slightly bluish tint to enhance the quality of the image. The primary function of the base is to support the emulsion. It permits easy handling during the processing and makes viewing the image less difficult. The base is coated on each side by the emulsion and is attached firmly by an adhesive (Figure 21-16). The adhesive ensures that the emulsion is distributed uniformly over the base. The **emulsion** is made of a homogeneous mixture of silver **halide crystals** suspended in a gelatin. Halides are halogen compounds, such as chlorine, bromine, and iodine that combine with another element, such as silver. In dental films, silver is combined most frequently with bromine. During radiation exposure, the silver halide crystals store the energy to which they have been exposed, and react with the chemicals in the processing tank to form a black (**radiolucent**) region on the film. The silver halide crystals that have not been struck by the radiation are not energized and wash off the film when it processes.

This energy, or **latent image**, does not become visible until the film has been exposed to chemicals for a given time at a given temperature. If a film has been totally exposed to visible light, it appears black after the processing. If the film was not exposed to light or radiation, the film appears clear after processing. The emulsion washes off and appears as a semi-clear blue base. The emulsion is placed on both sides of the base to reduce the amount of radiation needed, and it means that the x-ray can be read from either side. On top of the emulsion is a protective coating that is used to protect the emulsion, especially from the rollers in an automatic processor.

It should be noted that the film base has a small raised dot on one corner of the film. This dot is used for identification and mounting of the dental radiographs after processing (see Chapter 22).

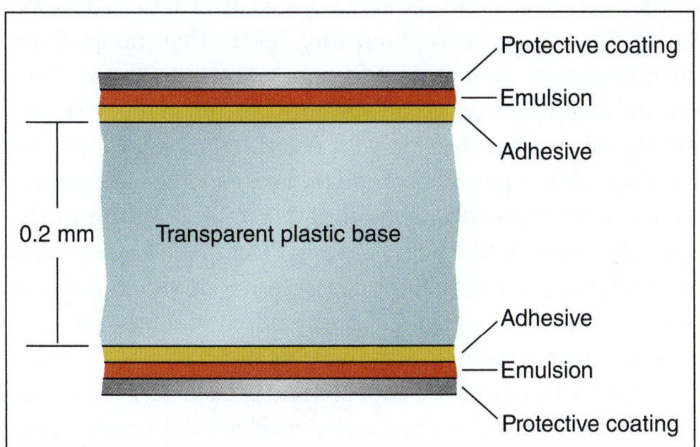

FIGURE 21-16

Composition of dental x-ray film. Transparent plastic base.

Film Speed

Crystal size in the emulsion regulates the speed of the film, normally, the larger the crystals, the faster the film. Dentists typically use one of the three dental x-ray films: D-speed film, called Ultraspeed; E-speed film, called Ektaspeed; or F-speed film, called InSight. Ektaspeed film requires approximately 40 percent less exposure time than Ultraspeed; and InSight requires 60 percent less exposure time than D-speed film and 20 percent less exposure time than E-speed film. InSight/F-speed film is the highest-speed dental film, allowing for the greatest reduction in radiation exposure for the patient. The **American National Standards Institute (ANSI)** is the organization that classifies dental x-ray film. The current classifications are the letters A–F. Currently, dental offices use the classifications D-, E-, and, primarily, F-speed.

Film Sizes

Dental intraoral film packets come in five basic sizes (Figure 21-17). Each size is used for a specific radiographic exposure, depending on the size of the patient's oral cavity and the area to be radiographed (Table 21-3 and Figure 21-18). The film is selected to produce the best radiographic results with the least radiation exposure for the patient.

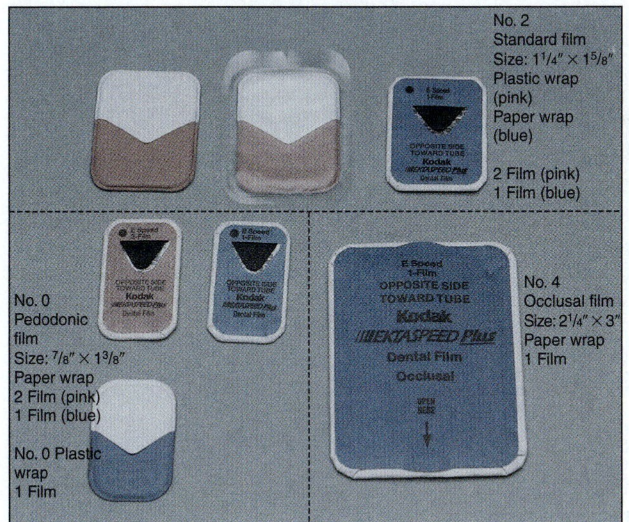

FIGURE 21-17

Sample dental x-ray films showing sizes and numbers. (Size No. 1, narrow anterior film size; and Size No. 3, long bitewing film size are not shown.)

TABLE 21-3 Intraoral Film Sizes and Uses

Film Size	Description/Use
No. 0	Child size
No. 1	Narrow anterior film size
No. 2	Adult size
No. 3	Long bitewing film size
No. 4	Occlusal film size

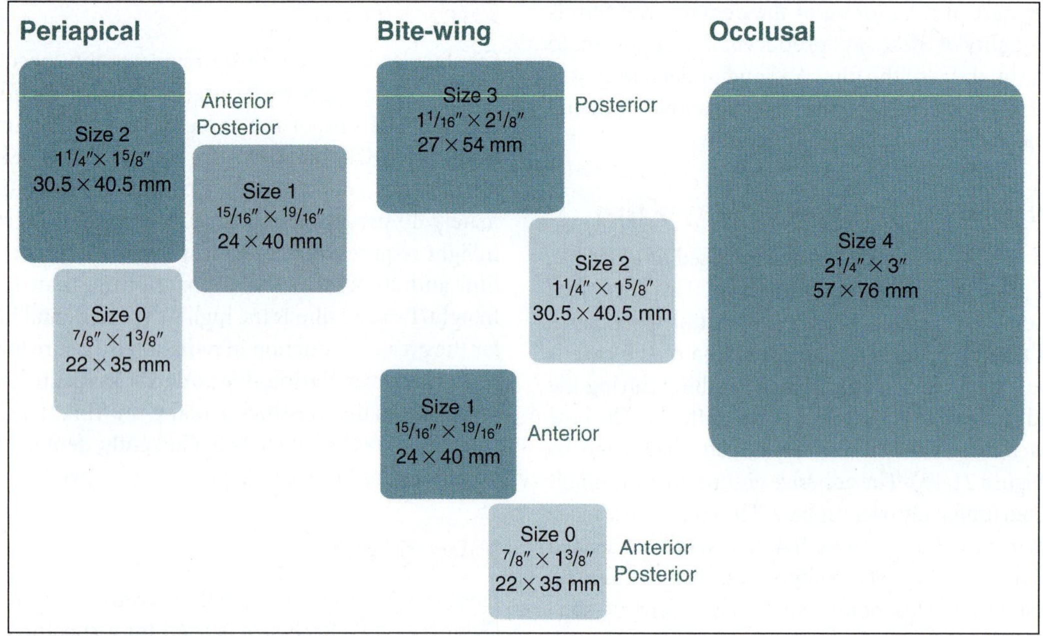

FIGURE 21-18

Dental x-ray film sizes used for periapical, bitewing, and occlusal film exposures.

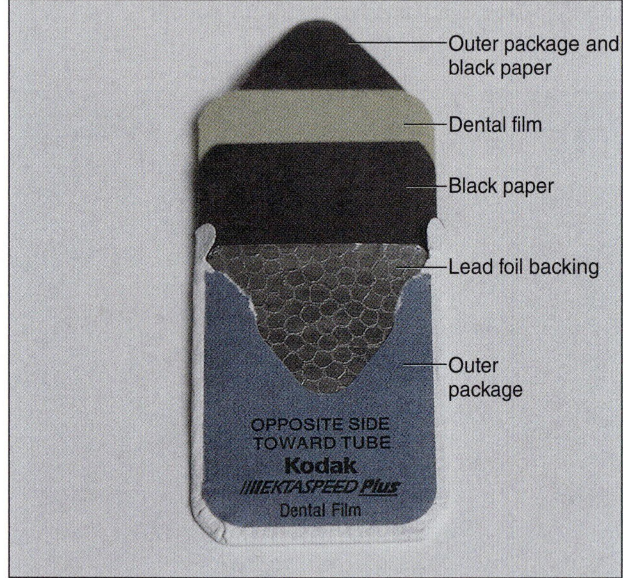

FIGURE 21-19

Parts of a dental film packet.

Dental Film Packet

Dental film is available in dental film packets that are designed to protect it from moisture and light. The intraoral film comes in boxes of 50 to 150 film packets. The boxes are labeled with the type of film, quantity of film packets, film speed, number of films in each film packet, the expiration date, and if packets have barriers.

The intraoral film packet has a sealed outer plastic wrap (Figure 21-19). Inside the wrapper, black paper is folded around the film, and a lead foil backing is placed away from the x-ray tube. The lead foil absorbs any unused radiation and the scattering of secondary radiation, and helps prevent film fogging. The outer plastic, or paper wrap, is completely sealed to prevent moisture from getting to the film. The outside film package shows where the identification dot is located. The dot is convex on the white side of the film package. The film packets also come in double packets. These film packets contain two films per packet. They take slightly more radiation for exposure, but allow both the doctor and the specialist to have an original film. Package color and numbering may differ from one manufacturer to another. Kodak numbers on the film and packet denote film speed, size, and single- or double-packet film. An example is Kodak IP-22, which indicates that the film speed is IP (F-speed or InSight Film), #2 size film, with two packets, or double-packet film. Single-packet film of the same size and speed would be labeled IP-21. Film packets may come with barriers in place. These are removed when processing.

Dental Film Storage

Before use, dental x-ray film should be stored carefully. It is sensitive to stray radiation, high temperatures, and chemicals. Ideally, unexposed film should be stored at 50°F to 70°F (10°C to 20°C) with relative humidity levels that range from 30 to 50 percent. Follow manufacturer's directions for film storage and care. Many dental offices store the film in the refrigerator. Dental assistants take only the needed films to the area, and use disposable cups to collect and transfer exposed radiographs.

The dental assistant should pay careful attention to the expiration date on the boxes of film. Placing the boxes of film in the storage area so that the oldest film is used first will prevent any film from expiring. Using expired film for a patient's radiographs may inhibit diagnostic quality.

After the film has been exposed and processed, it should be mounted and placed in a protective envelope. All x-rays should be handled with care so that the integrity of the radiograph is not compromised and they are not scratched. Radiographs are records of the patient's conditions at that time and may be used as legal documents.

Chapter Summary

This chapter examines the history of dental radiology, including the inventors and dates of their discoveries. Dental assistants must understand the physics and biological effects of ionization radiation, use their understanding during every radiographic exposure, understand the ALARA principle, and use the lead apron with cervical collar for the patient's safety every time an x-ray is taken. The assistant must label and store patient x-rays properly to prevent loss and, thereby, avoid the need for x-rays to be retaken.

CASE STUDY

In 1910, dentist Deziree Scott was very interested in radiography and had obtained a unit for her office. Every time she used it, she would test the machine by focusing it on her hand to ensure that the bones could be viewed, and to focus the x-ray tube. Her hand started turning red after a few weeks of using it this way.

Case Study Review

1. What is the damage to Dr. Scott's hand called?
2. Should Dr. Scott continue with this procedure?
3. What will occur if Dr. Scott continues to adjust the x-ray tube in this manner?
4. Would it be possible to lose her hand due to this procedure?
5. Would it be possible to lose her life from this procedure?

Review Questions

Multiple Choice

1. Physics professor ________ discovered x-rays in 1895.
   a. Dr. C. Edmond Kells
   b. Dr. Otto Walkoff
   c. Dr. William Rollins
   d. Wilhelm Conrad Roentgen
2. ________ film requires the least amount of exposure time.
   a. D-speed
   b. E-speed
   c. F-speed
   d. Ultraspeed
3. The polyester plastic base of dental x-ray film has a slightly ________ tint.
   a. green
   b. blue
   c. red
   d. orange
4. ________ invented the hot cathode x-ray tube.
   a. William Rollins
   b. Dr. Howard Rober
   c. Frank McCormack
   d. Dr. William Coolidge
5. The hot cathode x-ray tube was developed in
   a. 1895.
   b. 1896.
   c. 1913.
   d. 1920.
6. All of the following are examples of electromagnetic radiation with longer wavelengths *except*
   a. visible light.
   b. radio waves.
   c. television.
   d. x-rays.
7. ________ radiation escapes in all directions from the tube or the tubehead.
   a. Primary
   b. Secondary
   c. Scatter
   d. Leakage
8. Identify the most sensitive tissue or organ to radiation.
   a. Reproductive cells
   b. Muscle
   c. Nerves
   d. Mature bone
9. The amount of ionizing radiation absorbed by a substance is called a
   a. rem.
   b. sievert.
   c. milliroentgen.
   d. gray.

10. The quality, or penetrating power, of the central beam is determined by
    a. milliamperage.
    b. kilovoltage.
    c. the electronic timer.
    d. the collimator.

Critical Thinking

1. A patient has been exposed to a large number of radiographs due to other health issues. The dental assistant is going to take a necessary radiograph as requested by the dentist. In order to minimize radiation exposure, the dental assistant decides to reduce the kilovoltage. Is this sound thinking? Name some practices that would reduce the patient's exposure.
2. If the film badge that the dental assistant wears during radiograph exposures comes back registering a high exposure reading, what should be done initially? What questions should be directed to the dental assistant? Besides a defective x-ray machine, what could have caused the high readings?
3. A dental assistant's friend is outdoors sunbathing. After she went indoors, the sun worshipper tells the assistant that she had been in the sun for several hours and tanned very little. A few hours later the friend is in a great deal of pain and her "sun lines" are extremely red. How would you explain the minimal change in her skin tone earlier in the day, and her subsequent discomfort? Does ongoing exposure to the sun cause aging?

Web Activities

1. To find questions that patients frequently ask about dental x-rays, go to http://www.ada.org and search under x-rays.
2. Go to http://www.nrc.gov, locate the radiation protection topic, and find sources of radiation. Be prepared to share five sources of radiation with the class and instructor.
3. At the site, http://www.osha.gov, click on "Safety and Health Topics," and then, in the topics index, choose Radiation. Find the scale that shows both nonionizing radiation and ionizing radiation. Be prepared to discuss in class.

CHAPTER

22

Production and Evaluation of Dental Radiographs 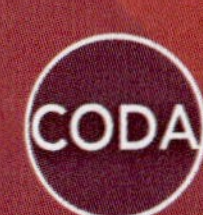

CODA

Specific Instructional Objectives

The student should strive to meet the following objectives and demonstrate an understanding of the facts and principles presented in this chapter:

1. Describe a diagnostic quality x-ray.
2. Identify the means of producing quality radiographs.
3. List and describe the types of film exposures, including periapical, bitewing, and occlusal radiographs.
4. Explain the bisecting principle and technique.
5. Explain and demonstrate the paralleling principle and techniques including a full-mouth radiographic survey and bitewing series.
6. Describe and demonstrate taking radiographs on various patients, including occlusal, pediatric, edentulous, endodontic radiographs, and special needs/compromised patients.
7. Describe manual film-processing equipment and technique. Demonstrate processing film, using the manual processing equipment.
8. List and explain the composition of processing solutions used with manual and automatic processing equipment.
9. Describe automatic processing equipment and explain the technique.
10. Explain and demonstrate how to mount dental x-rays.
11. List common radiographic errors that occur during exposure, and processing of x-ray films.
12. Explain and demonstrate how to duplicate dental radiographs.
13. Describe the storage of final radiographs.
14. Explain the legal implications, and radiology risk communication concerning dental radiographs taken in the dental office.
15. List standardized procedures, and state policies that dental offices follow to ensure quality radiographs.

Key Terms

acetic acid (521)
Angulation (492)
automatic processing (521)
bisecting technique (492)
bitewing radiograph (491)
blurred image (527)
central ray (493)
clear film (526)
cone cutting (526)
cross-section technique (507)
curve of Spee (494)
developer solution (519)
double exposure (526)
duplication technique (531)
Elon (521)
elongation (525)
film artifact (528)
fixer solution (521)
fogged film (530)
foreshortening (526)
herringbone pattern (528)
Horizontal angulation (493)
Hydroquinone (520)

(continues)

Key Terms (continued)

Introduction

Taking a quality radiograph is a skill that takes practice and patience. The dental assistant will take many different x-rays on patients of all ages; and these x-rays must be of the quality the dentist needs to provide an accurate diagnosis. The two techniques for exposing radiographs are discussed and demonstrated in this chapter. Once the radiographs are exposed the dental assistant needs to understand how they are processed and mounted. Common radiographic exposure and processing errors are identified and discussed so that the dental assistant can use the correct techniques to prevent these errors.

This chapter also discusses how and why radiographs are duplicated, and that radiographs are part of the patient's permanent record and must be properly stored and maintained.

ADA and FDA Guidelines for Dental Radiography (Adapted from the Updated Guidelines)

1. The new guidelines support the use of rectangular collimation. However, rectangular collimation is not widely used because of the view that the smaller x-ray beam area results in alignment errors, thus, requiring images to be retaken.
2. The position indicating device should be open ended and have a metallic lining that restricts the x-ray beam and reduces the area of exposure to radiation.
3. Use F-speed film to reduce exposure without compromising the diagnostic quality of the image.
4. Use film holders that align precisely with the x-ray cone.
5. Dental professionals should not hold the film holder during exposure, and only under unusual circumstances when the patient's family or caregiver must hold the film holder in place during exposure; they should wear appropriate protective shielding.
6. On the dental x-ray units, the kilovoltage should be set between 60 and 70 for optimal results.
7. Use protective aprons with a thyroid collar for protection.
8. Follow the ALARA Principle (as low as reasonably achievable) to minimize the patient's exposure.

Producing Quality Radiographs

Producing a diagnostic quality radiograph involves many steps, which are based on the dental assistant's skills in exposing the radiograph, and his or her knowledge of what the dentist needs in order to read the x-rays and make a diagnosis. The radiographs become part of the patient's records, and help the dentist to identify if there is a need for treatment. The images on the radiographs must be accurate and clear for the dentist to evaluate.

Careful attention must also be focused on preparation of the x-ray room and setting up the x-rays, film holders, and barriers for each patient: The patient is prepared in the chair, the protective apron is placed, and films are positioned for correct exposure.

What Is a Quality X-Ray?

- The desired teeth and surrounding area are on the film.
- Images are dimensionally accurate.
- The contacts between the teeth are open.
- The teeth are not elongated or foreshortened.
- The entire length of the tooth is visible, including 1 to 2 mm beyond the cusps, and 4 to 6 mm beyond the apex.
- The film has enough contrast and density to show good detail of all anatomy.
- The radiograph is free of spots, stains, handling marks, and other artifacts (black lines).

Preparing for X-Ray Exposure

The dental chair should be covered with a plastic bag, or at least have a barrier on the headrest and chair controls. The x-ray units should have barriers covering the dials, the exposure buttons, the cone, the tubehead, areas of the extension arm that could be touched, and any other areas that may be contaminated (Figures 22-1A and B). If there is a door that the dental assistant needs to open and close, a barrier should be placed on the doorknob (plastic sandwich bags work well to barrier this area). An area for clean and contaminated films should be prepared. The procedure for infection control is outlined in Procedure 22-1.

Set up the materials needed. For example, assemble the parts of the sterile Rinn XCP instruments and select the appropriate x-ray films. Also, have a tissue available for the patient, and gauze and cotton rolls for x-ray film positioning. X-ray film that is going to be used should be prepared and then kept close to the room where the x-rays will be taken, but not in the same room.

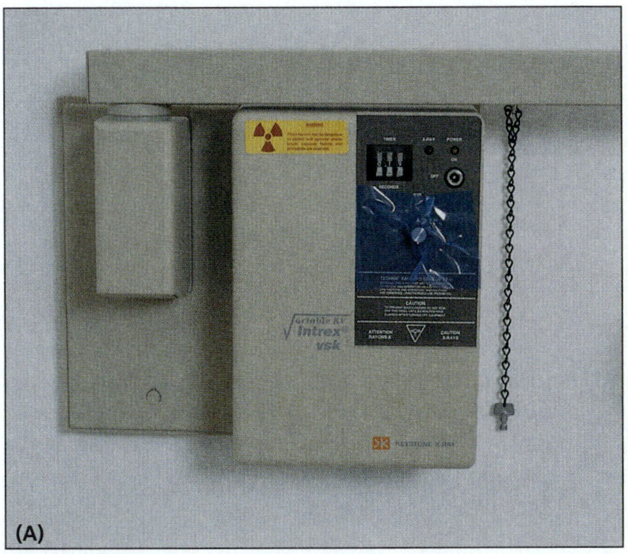

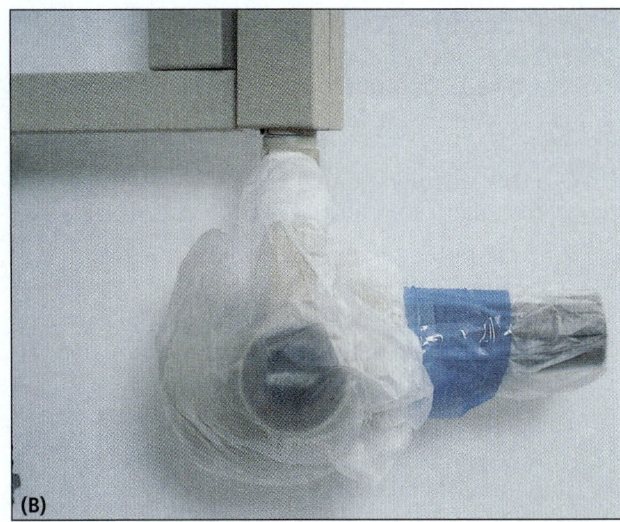

FIGURE 22-1

(A) Control panel. (B) Tubehead with barriers.

1. Wear gloves when exposing radiographs and handling contaminated film packets. Use other PPE (e.g., protective eyewear, mask, and gown) as appropriate if spattering of blood or other body fluids is likely.
2. Use heat-tolerant or disposable intraoral devices whenever possible (e.g., film-holding and positioning devices). Clean and sterilize with heat, heat-tolerant devices between patients. At a minimum, high-level disinfect semicritical, heat-sensitive devices, according to the manufacturer's instructions.
3. Transport and handle exposed radiographs in an aseptic manner to prevent contamination of developing equipment.
4. The following apply for digital radiography sensors:

   (a) Use FDA-cleared barriers.

   (b) Clean and heat sterilize or high-level disinfect between patients, barrier-protected, semicritical items. If the item cannot tolerate these procedures then, at a minimum, protect it with an FDA-cleared barrier; and then clean and disinfect it with an EPA-registered hospital disinfectant with intermediate-level (i.e., tuberculocidal claim) activity between patients. Consult with the manufacturer for methods of disinfection and sterilization of digital radiology sensors and for protection of associated computer hardware.

(Adapted from the Centers for Disease Control and Prevention: Guidelines for Infection Control in Dental Health-Care Settings—2003 Atlanta, GA, 2003, U.S, Department of Health & Human Services.)

Procedure 22-1
Radiography Infection Control

This procedure is performed by the dental assistant. The dentist designates which radiographs are needed for diagnosis. The dental assistant prepares the patient and area, takes the radiographs, and processes and mounts the films for viewing according to infection control protocol.

Equipment and Supplies

- Barriers for the x-ray room
- X-ray film (size selected accordingly)
- Rinn XCP materials (assembled for use) or other paralleling technique aids
- Film barriers (optional)
- Lead apron with thyroid collar
- Paper towel or tissue
- Container (e.g., disposable cup) for exposed film, labeled with patient's name
- Surface disinfectants
- Treatment gloves (glasses and mask are optional)

(continues)

Procedure 22-1 (continued)

Procedure Steps (*Follow aseptic procedures*)

1. Wash and dry hands.
2. Place appropriate barriers on the dental chair, film, and x-ray equipment (Figure 22-2).
3. Prepare the equipment and supplies needed for the procedure, including sterile Rinn XCP instruments, tissue or paper towel, and a cup or container with the patient's name on it.
4. After the patient is seated and positioned, wash and dry hands. Don treatment gloves. Glasses and mask may also be worn.
5. After the x-rays are exposed and removed from the patient's mouth, wipe off the x-rays and place them in a cup/container or on a covered surface.
6. When all x-ray exposures are complete, remove the lead apron from the patient. There are several ways this is done to follow aseptic protocol. The lead apron can be removed once the contaminated gloves are removed, or over-gloves can be placed over the treatment gloves before removing the lead apron. If the lead apron is removed with contaminated gloves, it must be disinfected following the procedure.
7. After the patient is dismissed, remove and dispose of all the barriers.
8. Any areas that were not covered with a barrier must be disinfected, including the x-ray film.

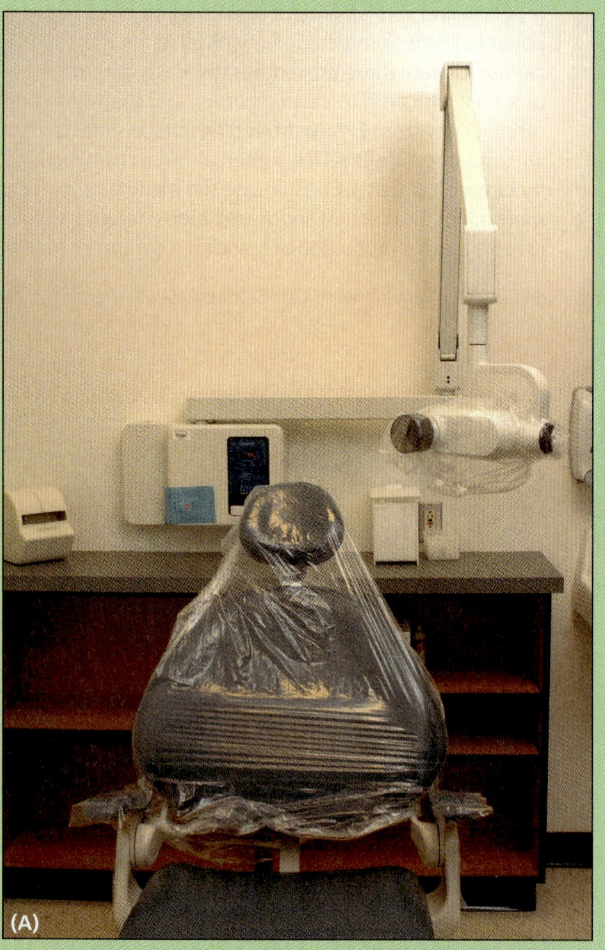

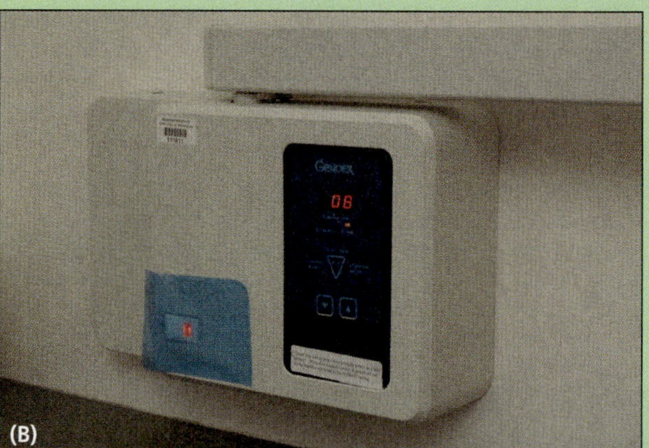

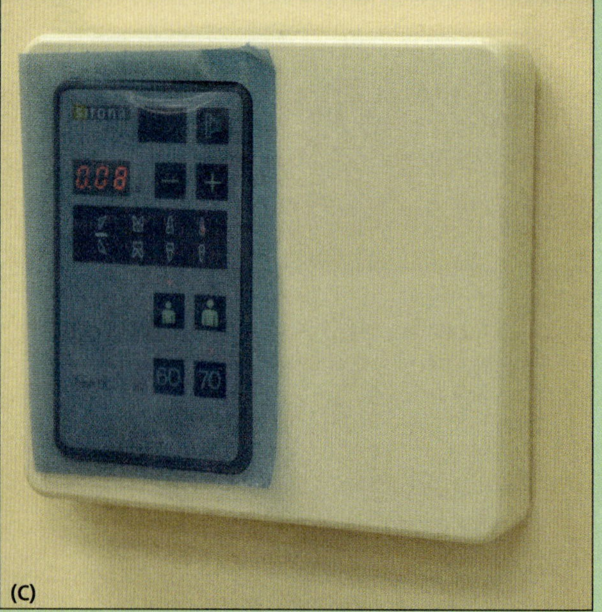

FIGURE 22-2
(A) Room prepared with barriers on the chair and tubehead. (B and C) Two control panels.

During Film Exposure

During film exposure, the dental assistant should wear gloves, protective eyewear, and a mask. After removing the exposed film from the patient's mouth, wipe the saliva from the film and place it in a paper cup or on a covered surface. Film can be purchased with a plastic barrier or separate plastic barriers can be purchased to place on the individual film packets before exposure.

Patient Exposure

Before the patient is seated, prepare the room following aseptic techniques. Review the patient's medical history and check the dental chart to confirm the number and types of x-rays the dentist has requested for diagnosis.

Establish a routine to check the x-ray machine. Check the settings for the kV, mA, and exposure time. Note that some x-ray machines are preset and require no changes. Select the x-ray unit if the control panel operates more than one tubehead.

Escort the patient into the room, seat the patient in an upright position, and position the headrest to secure the head. Ask the patient to remove eyeglasses, partials, or any metal objects that will interfere with the x-rays. Place a lead apron with a thyroid collar on the patient, making sure that it is secured and covers the patient (Figure 22-3). Explain the procedure to the patient and indicate how the patient can assist during the exposure of the x-rays. Bring the tubehead close to the working area and proceed.

After Films Are Exposed

After films are exposed, dental assistants remove their gloves or place overgloves on, remove the lead apron from the patient, and make chart notations. Films are then taken to the processing area for processing. After films are processed, they are reviewed by the dentist. The patient is dismissed. Following appropriate infection control procedures, remove the barriers from the dental chair, x-ray unit, and control buttons. Dispose of barriers after each patient and disinfect the area. When handling contaminated films without barriers, wipe or spray them with a disinfectant, and leave for 10 minutes. If film barriers are used, remove them, along with other contaminated barriers.

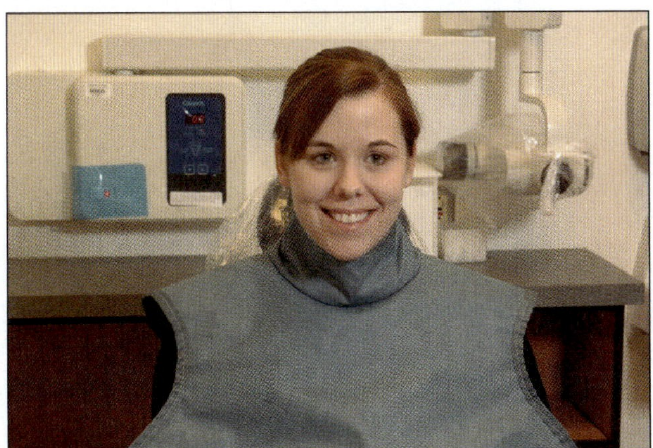

FIGURE 22-3

Barriers on a dental x-ray unit and a lead apron with thyroid collar on a patient.

Hints to Prevent Gagging

Some patients have problems with gagging. Try to get the patient to breathe through the nose and to think of something else, because psychological factors contribute to triggering the gag reflex. Talk to patients, work quickly, and have patients concentrate on breathing. If a patient still has problems, an anesthetic mouth rinse or a throat lozenge may be helpful. Position the tubehead in the approximate location for the film exposure before placing the film in the patient's mouth.

Lead Apron Suggestions

After exposing the x-ray film, remove the film, pull the x-ray tubehead out of the way, and place the film in a cup/container or on a barrier. After all films have been taken, remove the lead apron from the patient, disinfect the apron, and then place the lead apron over a bar or hang it on a hook to prevent creases or folds. If the lead apron is creased routinely, the lead may be damaged and protection from x-ray exposure would be incomplete in these areas. Protective aprons and thyroid shields should be hung or laid flat and never folded, and manufacturer's instructions should be followed. All protective shields should be evaluated monthly for damage (e.g. tears, folds, and cracks), using visual and manual inspection.

Types of Film Exposures

Three types of film exposures/radiographs are used most commonly in the dental office: the periapical, bitewing, and occlusal. The type of film used and the number of x-rays taken are determined by the dentist.

Periapical Radiographs. The **periapical radiograph** pictures the entire tooth and surrounding area (Figure 22-4A). Periapical radiographs are used to assess the health of the teeth, bone, and surrounding tissues. Tooth development and eruption stages also are seen on periapical radiographs. Abnormalities and pathological conditions are diagnosed by the dentist using these radiographs. The size of the patient's mouth usually determines the size of the x-ray film and the number of exposures.

Bitewing Radiographs. The **bitewing radiograph** pictures the crowns, the interproximal spaces, and the crest area of the alveolar bone of both the maxillary and the mandibular teeth (Figure 22-4B). Bitewing radiographs, usually taken only on the posterior teeth, are used to detect caries, faulty restorations, and calculus, as well as to examine the crestal area of the alveolar bone. The size of the patient's mouth determines the size of the film used for the bitewing x-ray.

Occlusal Radiograph. The **occlusal radiograph** pictures large areas of the mandible or maxilla (Figure 22-4C). These radiographs can be used alone or to supplement periapical or bitewing films. For adults, a No. 4 film is used, and for children, a No. 2 film may be used.

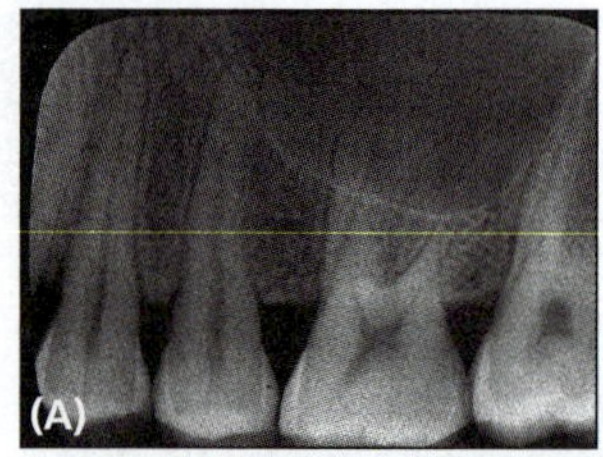

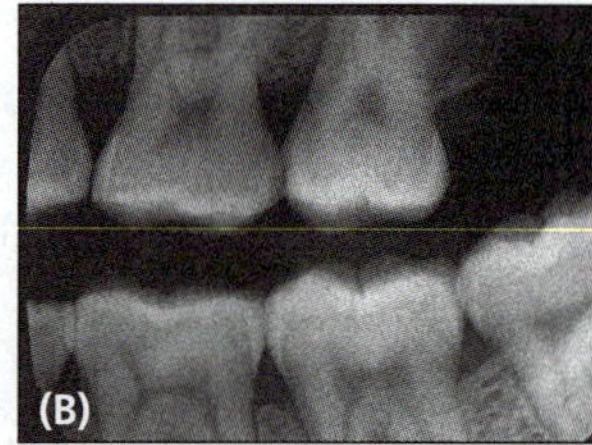

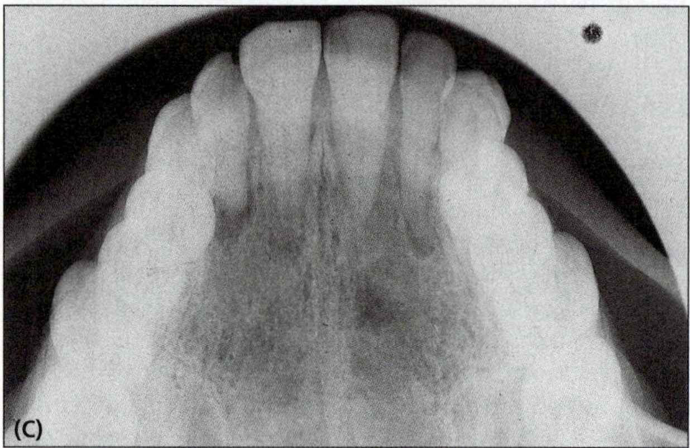

FIGURE 22-4

(A) Periapical radiography showing crowns, roots, and supporting bone. (B) Bitewing radiograph showing crowns of teeth on both arches. (C) Occlusal radiography showing entire dental arch.

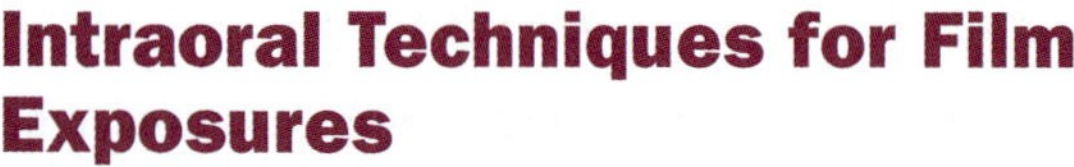

Intraoral Techniques for Film Exposures

There are two basic techniques used for film exposures in dentistry: the **bisecting technique** and the **paralleling technique**. The bisecting technique, which is used for more specific or unique radiographs rather than the routine, is the oldest technique. The paralleling technique is widely accepted because the detail of the image is more accurate. The American Association of Dental Schools, and the American Academy of Oral and Maxillofacial Radiology recommend the paralleling technique.

Terminology Used with Exposure Techniques

Angulation, in reference to dental radiology, is the alignment of the central x-ray beam in vertical and horizontal planes. Correct angulation is critical to produce quality x-rays.

Parallel lines are always the same distance apart, never intersecting (Figure 22-5 A).

Intersecting lines cross each other at some point (Figure 22-5 B).

Long axis of the tooth is a line that divides a tooth into equal halves starting from the incisal/occlusal surface and ending at the apex of the tooth (Figure 22-5 C).

Perpendicular lines form when one line is exactly vertical, and is intersected with a horizontal line to form a right angle (Figure 22-5 D).

A **right angle** is formed when two perpendicular lines form a 90 degree angle (Figure 22-5 E).

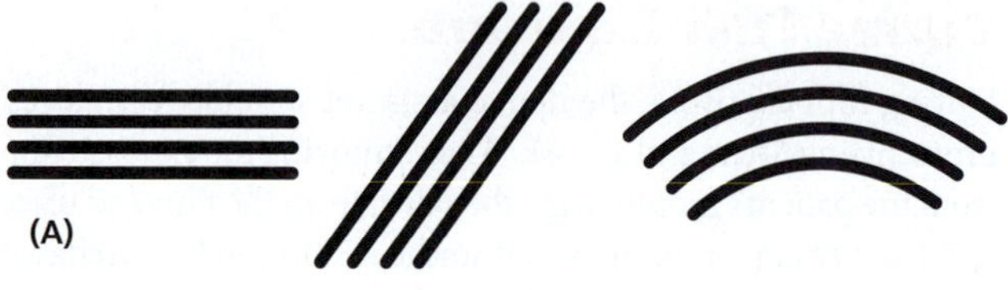

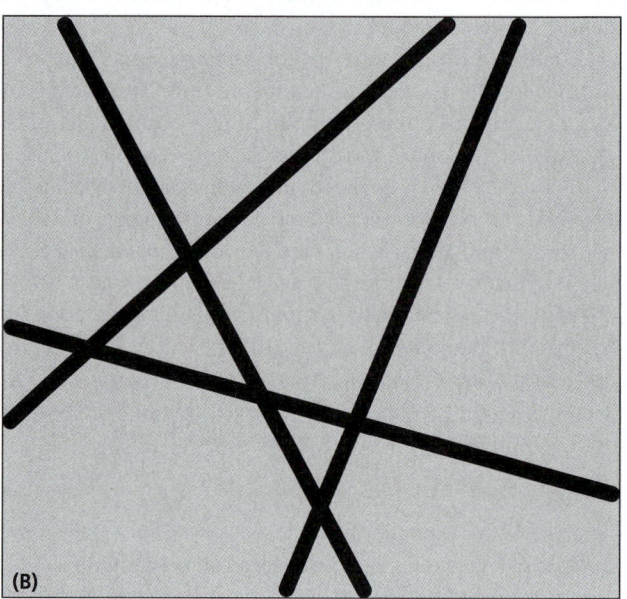

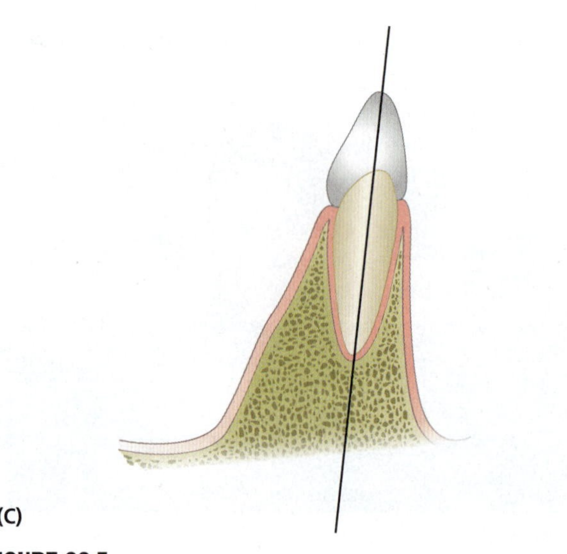

FIGURE 22-5

(A) Parallel lines. (B) Intersecting lines. (C) Long axis of tooth.

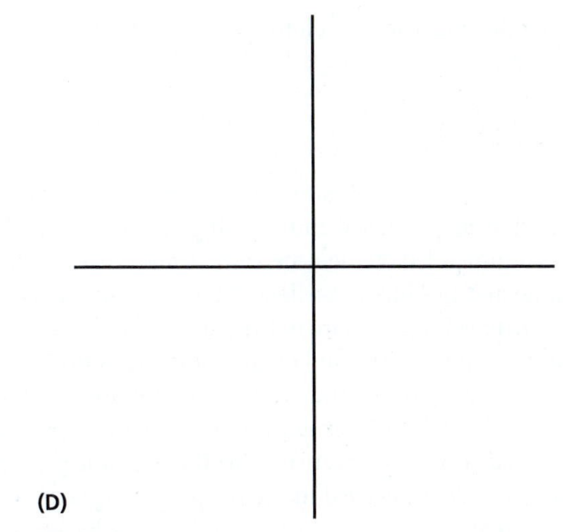

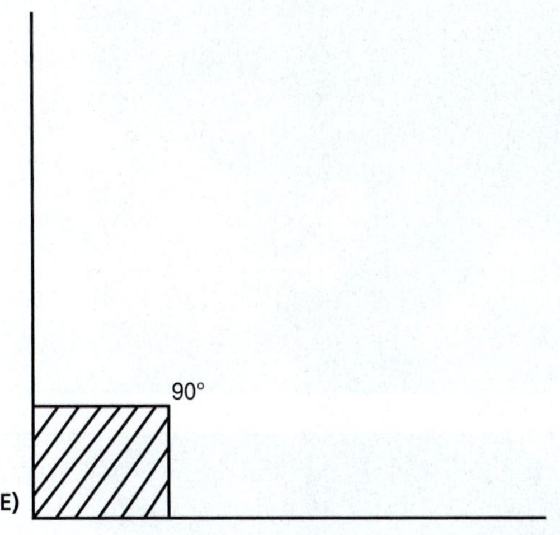

FIGURE 22-5 (continued)

(D) Perpendicular lines. (E) Right angle.

Bisecting Technique

The bisecting technique is used to expose periapical, bitewing, and occlusal radiographs (Figures 22-4A through C). In the bisecting technique, a film holder is used to secure the film close to the tissue/tooth without bending the film. In this technique, the **central ray** (x-rays at the center of the x-ray beam) is directed at an imaginary line that bisects the angle created by the length (long axis) of the tooth and the film packet. The central ray must be perpendicular to this bisecting line (the rule of isometry). The direction of the central ray creates **vertical angulation**. An average for the vertical angulation has been predetermined for this technique. The angulation works with most patients, but operators should determine the appropriate angle after the patient has been positioned and the film is in place (Figure 22-6). Table 22-1 summarizes the angulation settings.

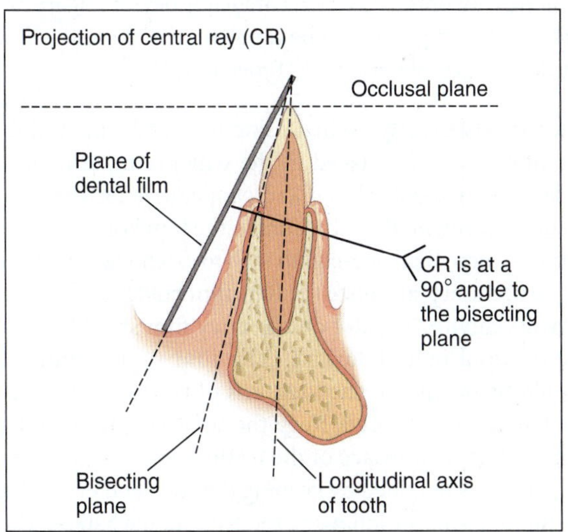

FIGURE 22-6

Principle of the bisecting technique. The central ray is directed at a right angle to the bisecting plane (imaginary bisector). The image on the film will be equal to the length of the tooth when the central ray is directed at a 90° angle to the bisecting plane.

TABLE 22-1 Vertical Angulation Table

Area	Maxillary	Mandibular
Incisors	+40°	−15°
Canines	+45°	−20°
Premolars	+30°	−10°
Molars	+20°	−25°

Principles of the Bisecting Technique. The principles of the bisecting technique include the following:

- The patient's head must be in the correct position for each arch. For the maxillary arch, seat the patient in an upright position and support the head so that the occlusal surfaces of the maxillary teeth are parallel to the floor and the patient's nose is positioned slightly downward (Figure 22-7A). For the mandibular arch, seat the patient in an upright position and support the head slightly tilted back so the occlusal surfaces of the mandibular teeth are parallel to the floor and the patient's nose is positioned slightly upward (Figure 22-7B).
- The film is placed in the patient's mouth as close to the lingual surface of the tooth as possible without bending the film.
- Various kinds of film holders can be used to hold the film. Examples include the Stabe, Snap-a-Ray, Rinn XCP, Precision, and bite blocks. As a last resort, the patient's finger can be used to hold the film in position. Be sure that the patient's finger pressure is adequate to prevent film movement during exposure, but not so firm as to cause the film to bend.
- Set the appropriate vertical angulation using the vertical angulation degree guide on the x-ray tubehead (Figure 22-8). **Horizontal angulation** is determined by directing the central ray at the teeth to be exposed, and

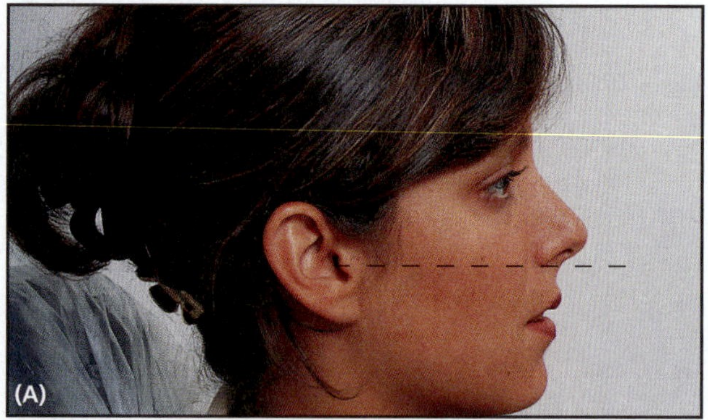

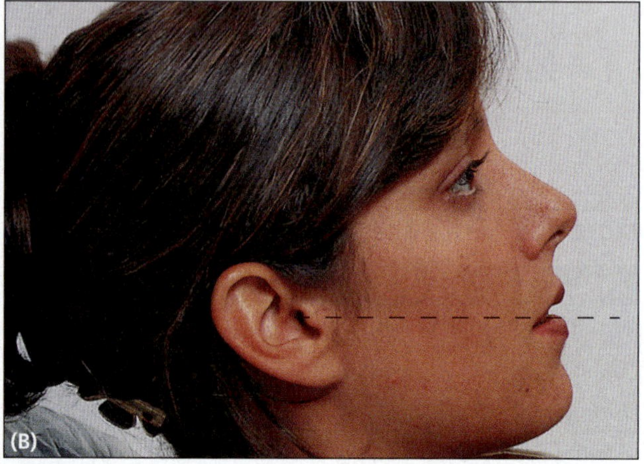

FIGURE 22-7

When exposing radiographs using the bisecting technique, the patient's head is positioned as shown for (A) the maxillary regions (tragus of the ear to the ala of the nose) and (B) the mandibular regions (tragus of the ear to the corner of the mouth).

aiming the beam directly through the interproximal spaces (contact areas) (Figure 22-9).

- The film is placed in the patient's mouth so that only an edge of the film, one-eighth of an inch, can be seen beyond the occlusal surface or the incisal edge. The cone must cover the x-ray film completely. As with other techniques, the patient and the tubehead should be still during exposure. The occlusal edge of the x-ray film should follow the "**curve of Spee**." This is a slight anatomical curve of the occlusal alignment of the teeth, beginning with the mandibular cuspids/canines and following the buccal cusps of the premolars/bicuspids and molars. Exposure time, mA, and kVp selections are determined according to the type of film, area of exposure, and dental x-ray machine being used.

Disadvantages of Bisecting Technique. Disadvantages of the bisecting technique include image distortion, guesswork with the technique, patient positioning, and increased exposure to the patient's finger and hand.

The technique is still used, however, on small children, adults with small or tender mouths, for selected endodontic exposures, and on patients who have conditions or oral anatomies that make it difficult to use the parallel positioning instruments.

Paralleling Technique

The paralleling technique is the technique most commonly used in exposing periapical and bitewing radiographs, and is highly recommended by the American Dental Association. It is accurate and produces excellent diagnostic quality radiographs. There is less exposure to the patient's head and neck, and the technique is easier and requires less guesswork. However, the paralleling technique can be uncomfortable for small children, adults with small or sensitive mouths, or for patients with low palatal vaults. Practice helps the operator gain the skills and confidence needed to use the paralleling technique with all patients.

The paralleling technique requires the film packet and the long axis of the teeth to be parallel. The x-ray beam is directed perpendicular to this parallel line formed by the teeth and the film packet (Figure 22-10). With the exception of the mandibular molars, the anatomy of the oral cavity requires the film to be placed toward the center of the mouth to keep the film packet flat and have the film parallel to the long axis of the teeth. A film holder is used for ease of technique and correct alignment.

Holders for the Paralleling Technique. Various film holders are available for use with the paralleling technique. The function of the holder is to secure the film away from the lingual surfaces of the teeth, and parallel with the long axis of the teeth. Some holders have supports to prevent the film from bending. One example is the Rinn XCP. Also, several holders have positioning rings that assist the operator in correct cone placement, and allow the patient to be in varied positions for x-ray exposure. The film holders may be simple, one-piece bite blocks (Snap-a-Rays) (Figure 22-11A); hemostats with rubber bite blocks; or they may come with several pieces, such as the Rinn XCP kit or the Precision paralleling device (Figure 22-11B and C). It is important to be familiar with these to allow for quick and accurate assembly (Procedure 22-2).

Film Positioning. When using the paralleling technique, the film should be placed in the patient's mouth with care to keep the patient relaxed and cooperative for the film and holder placement. Place the film in the film holder evenly and allow no more than one-eighth inch to extend beyond the edge of the occlusal plane once the film/film holder is placed in the patient's mouth. The dot on the x-ray film should be toward the occlusal/incisal surface. The film packet/film holder should be parallel to the long axis of the teeth, covering all the teeth to be exposed. Keep the film packet flat and away from the lingual surface of the teeth. Vertical and horizontal angulation is obtained by keeping the cone end even with the positioning ring, or following the guide of the handle with the other film holders (Figure 22-13). The positioning ring guides the cone for correct placement to ensure that the film is covered. Without the ring to act as a guide, the operator needs to visually check the film placement and direct the cone to cover the entire film.

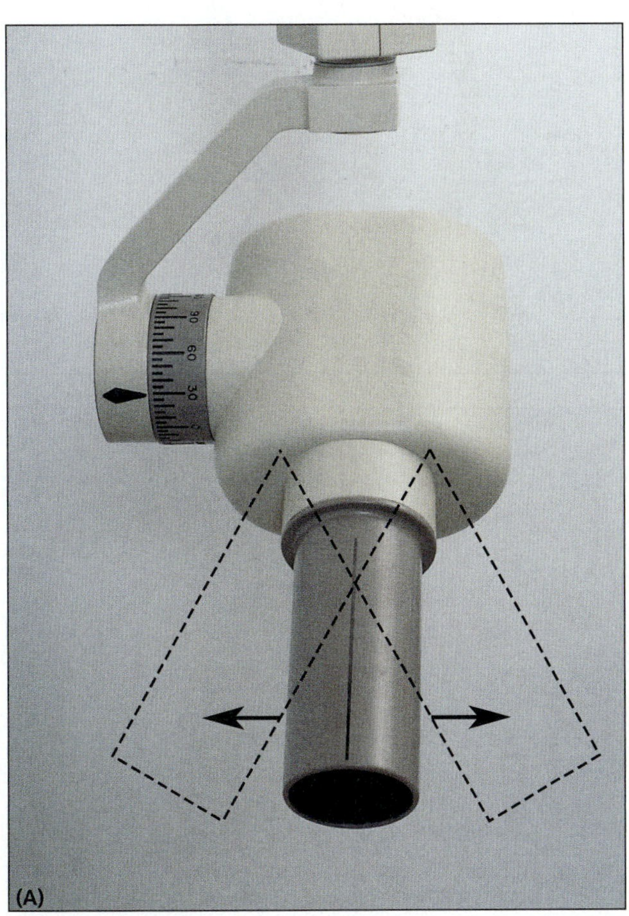

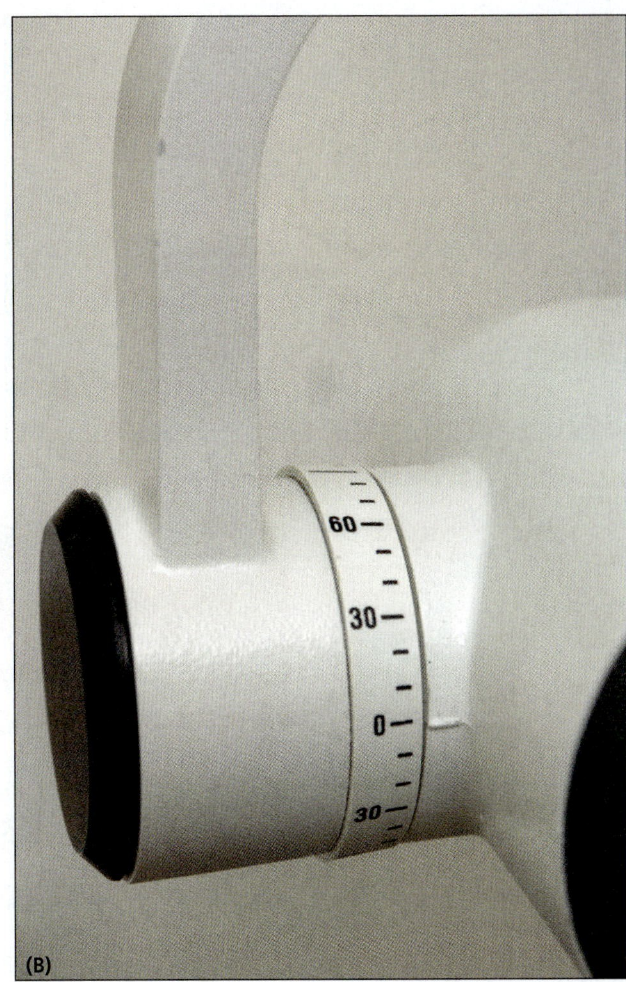

FIGURE 22-8

(A) Example of cone positioning for horizontal angulation (left and right rotation). (B) The numerical degree guide on the side of the tubehead is shown.

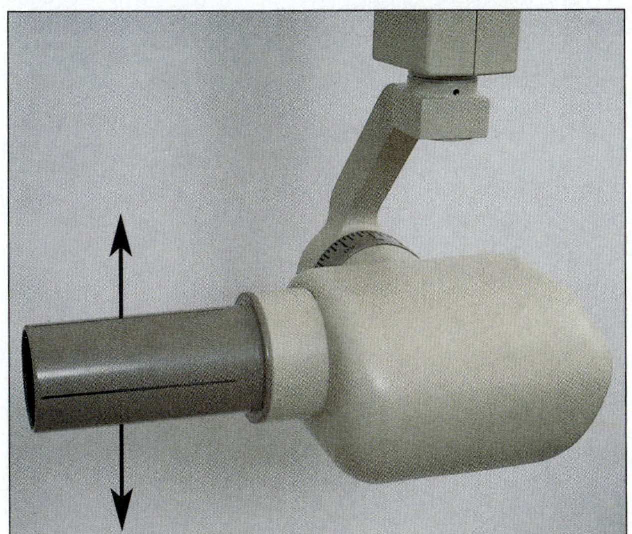

FIGURE 22-9

Example of cone positioning for vertical angulation (up and down rotation).

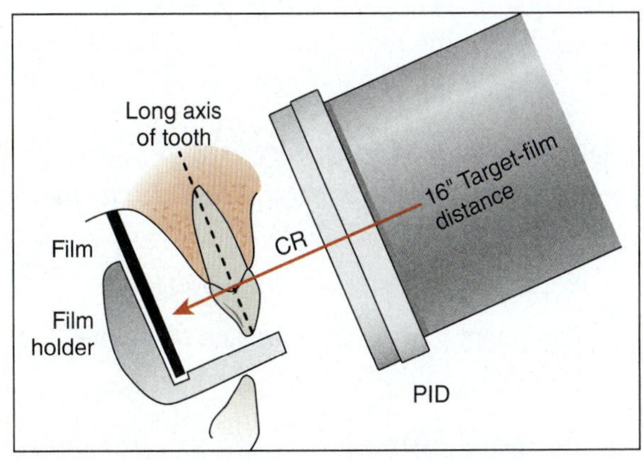

FIGURE 22-10

Position of film for the paralleling technique.

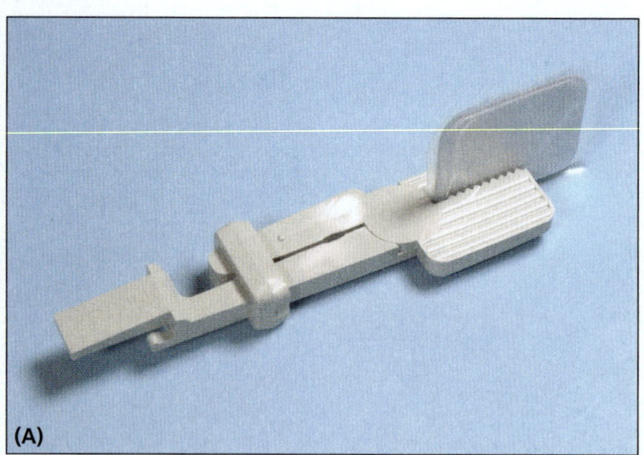

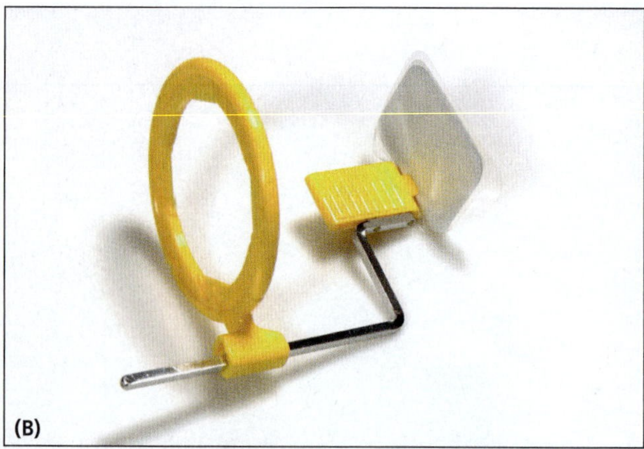

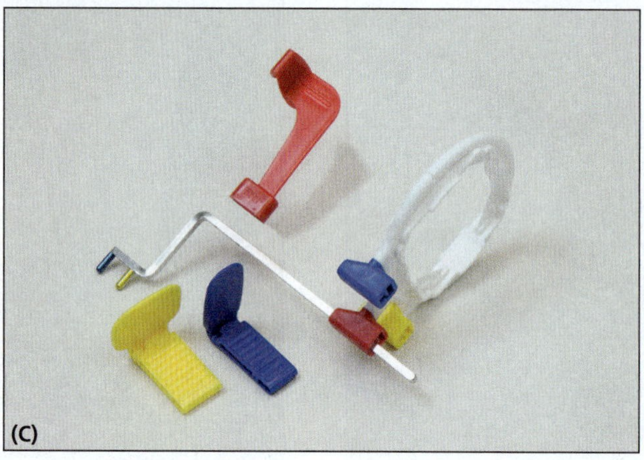

FIGURE 22-11

Film holding devices for the paralleling technique. (A) Snap-a-Ray. (B) Rinn XCP. (C) New film holding device with one aiming ring and one indicator arm for all exposures.

Procedure 22-2
Assembly of Film Positioning Devices (Extension-Cone Paralleling Instrument = XCP)

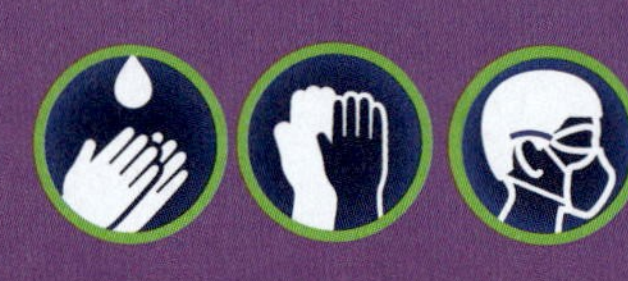

This procedure is performed by the dental assistant. The dentist designates which radiographs are needed for diagnosis. The dental assistant gathers the equipment needed and assembles the pieces according to the radiographs to be taken, following infection control protocol.

Equipment and Supplies

- Sterilized Rinn XCP materials including rings, bite blocks, and indicator arms (Figure 22-12)
- Paper towel or tray with tray cover
- Treatment gloves. Glasses and mask are optional.

Procedure Steps (*Follow aseptic procedures*)

1. Open the bag of sterilized XCP instruments and lay its contents on a paper towel.

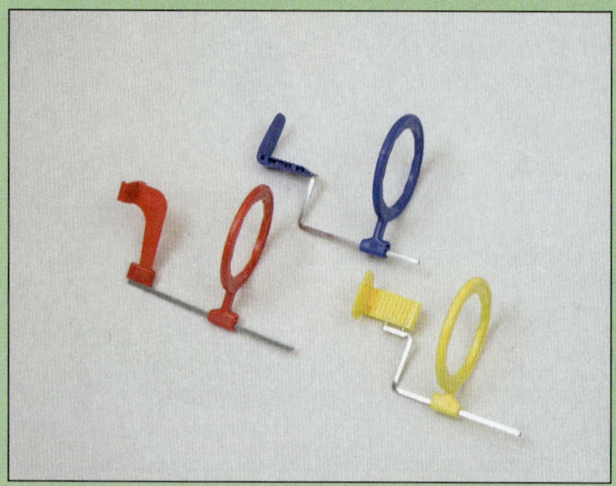

FIGURE 22-12

Rinn XCP components assembled correctly for (A) anterior exposures, (B) bite-wing exposures, and (C) posterior exposures.

(continues)

Procedure 22-2 (continued)

2. The bite blocks and aiming rings are color-coded. Gather instruments of the same color together, and select the correct aiming indicator arms for each exposure.

   Note: Blue is the universal color for the anterior XCP Instrument. Yellow is the universal color for the posterior XCP Instrument. Red is the universal color for the bitewing XCP Instrument. The indicator arms are stainless steel and come in three different angles. Lay all three indicator arms flat: the straight arm with the two prongs coming out the side is for bitewing x-rays; the indicator arm that has two angles with two prongs at the end when lying flat is for posterior x-rays; and the indicator arm with two angles and two prongs that angle upward when lying flat is for the anterior x-rays.

Anterior Assembly

1. Take the blue anterior XCP Instrument bite block and place it on the two prongs of the anterior indicator arm with the bite block aiming upward.
2. Place the blue aiming ring on the indicator arm so that it covers the bite block when you look through the ring.
3. Flex the back of the bite block for easy placement of the film.

Posterior Assembly

1. Take the yellow posterior XCP Instrument bite block and place it on the two prongs of the posterior indicator arm.
2. Place the blue aiming ring on the indicator arm so that the ring covers the bite block when you look through the ring.
3. Flex the back of the bite block for easy placement of the film.

Bitewing Assembly

1. Take the red XCP Instrument bite block and place it on the two prongs of the posterior indicator arm.
2. Place the red aiming ring on the indicator arm so that the ring covers the bite block when you look through the ring.
3. Flex the back of the bite block for easy placement of the film.

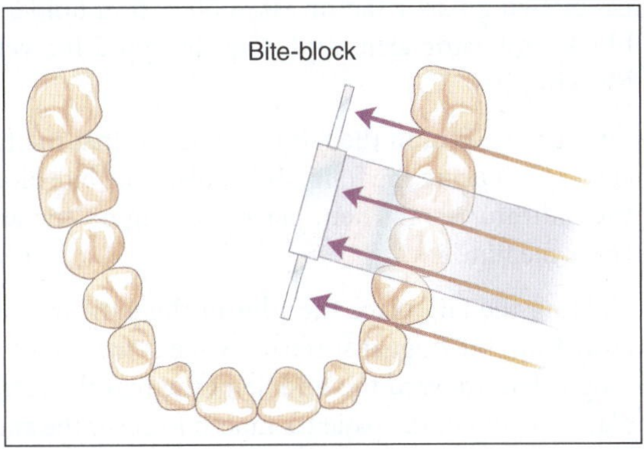

FIGURE 22-13

The correct placement of premolar bitewing film, using a film-holding device. The film is positioned such that the x-rays pass directly through the interproximal spaces to prevent the overlapping of the teeth. The curve of the patient's arch is evaluated when placing the dental film.

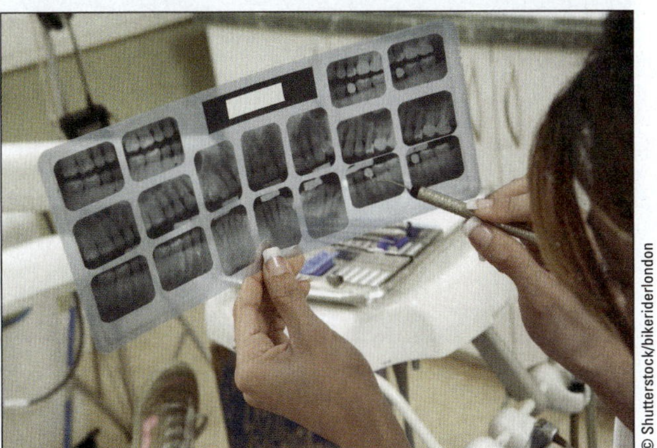

FIGURE 22-14

Full mouth set of radiographs (x-rays) includes x-rays of maxillary and mandibular teeth. This full mouth has six anterior x-rays and eight posterior x-rays with four bitewing x-rays.

Full-Mouth Radiographic Survey

A full-mouth radiographic survey (FMX) (Figure 22-14) is composed of periapical and bitewing radiographs (Procedure 22-3). This survey includes a number of radiographs that collectively display all the teeth and surrounding structures and areas. The dentist determines what is needed for diagnosis and for the patient's records.

The number and the size of radiographs taken depend on several factors, including what the dentist needs to view on the radiograph, the size of the patient's mouth, the number of teeth in the oral cavity, conditions that may interfere with film placement, and the patient's ability to cooperate. A full-mouth survey for an adult routinely includes 14 periapical and 4 bitewing films. This number may vary depending on the factors listed and the dentist's directions.

When exposing any radiographs, an order should be followed to prevent double-exposing the patient. There is no recommended sequence, so dental assistants should decide what order they are comfortable with and can follow routinely. Once films are exposed, they should be placed in a cup or on a barrier away from the unexposed film.

Bitewing Series

Bitewing radiographs are a routine part of the dental exam. They are taken as part of the full-mouth series and also at 6- to 12-month intervals. These radiographs are used specifically for caries detection but also assist in the evaluation of restorations, calculus detection, and assessment of the alveolar crestal bone, tooth eruption, occlusal relationships, and some pulpal pathology. Bitewing radiographs, also known as **interproximal** radiographs, are taken of the premolar/bicuspid area and the molar area. The film is placed most often in a horizontal position, but when the dentist wants to see more of the tooth root and alveolar bone, the film is placed vertically.

Bitewing radiographs are taken with a variety of film holders. The film holder has a wing or tab for the patient to bite on to hold the film in position. The film holder may be a loop of paper that goes around the film with a tab extending out, or a stick-on tab made of paper or Styrofoam (Figure 22-15A). The tabs that stick on the film are placed in the center of the smooth side of the film. There are also a variety of film-holding devices to use when exposing bitewing radiographs, such as the Snap-a-Ray or the Rinn XCP (Figure 22-15B).

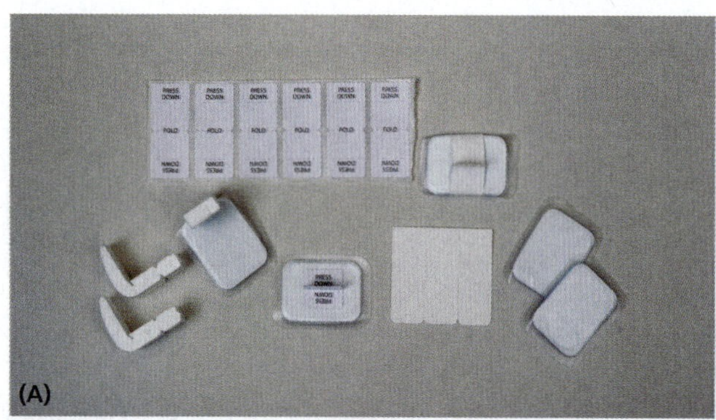

(A)

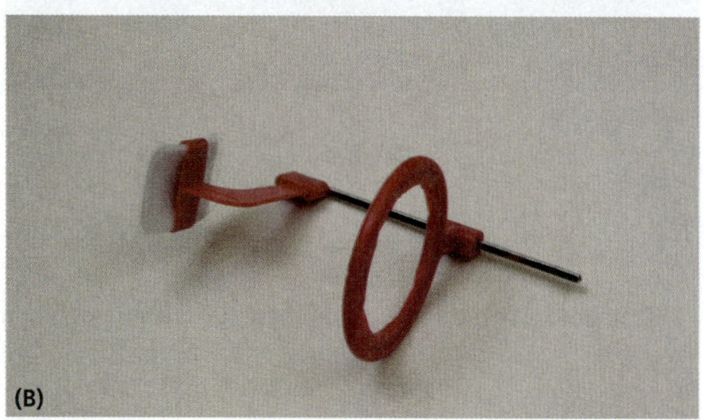

(B)

FIGURE 22-15

(A) Bitewing loops and tabs. (B) Rinn XCP holding bitewing x-rays.

- Horizontal Positioning—With adults, four No. 2 size films are taken (one premolar and one molar on each side). Some dentists choose to use the longer No. 3 size film and take one on each side, but care must be used when selecting this film size because different horizontal angulations are needed on the premolars and molars to open the contacts. With children, the size of the child's mouth determines the number and size of the film. Older children may need only one No. 2 size film on each side of the mouth, while younger children, or children with small mouths, may need two No. 0 or two No. 1 size films on each side of the mouth.
- Vertical Positioning—Vertical bitewing radiographs are requested by the periodontist as well as the general dentist. With the increase in periodontal disease, dentists are requiring bitewing radiographs that show more of the root area. Root caries, advanced periodontal pockets, and bone loss can be seen to a greater extent on bitewing radiographs if the film is placed vertically instead of horizontally. The vertical bitewing can be used in both the posterior and anterior areas. An adhesive tab or film-holding device is used to hold the film in the correct position. The film placement, and the vertical and horizontal angulation remain the same as with the horizontal bitewing radiograph (Figure 22-16).

Anterior Vertical Bitewing

1. To prepare for the anterior vertical bitewing use a vertical bitewing paper tab or assemble a film holder (bite block, indicator arm, and ring designed for vertical bitewings).
2. Position the film in the tab or holder so that the film is centered. If using the film holder, place the bite block on the indicator arm. Then, place the ring on the arm to cover the film.
3. Holding the tab, place the film in the patient's mouth, away from the lingual surfaces, while gently moving the tongue back toward the middle of the mouth. Vertically place the film in the patient's mouth to cover the anterior maxillary and mandibular teeth.
4. The vertical angulation for the anterior bitewing is set at $+10°$ so that the cone is perpendicular to the film. The maxillary anterior teeth are tilted, thus, the film is slightly bent. The horizontal angulation is directed so that the beam is between the contacts of the maxillary central incisors. Place the cone near the patient's face, covering the film and perpendicular to the film.
5. When using the positioning instrument, place it in the patient's mouth, pushing the tongue back away from the lingual surfaces; have the patient close on the bite block and slide the ring close to the patient's face, then position the tube against the ring, covering the film.

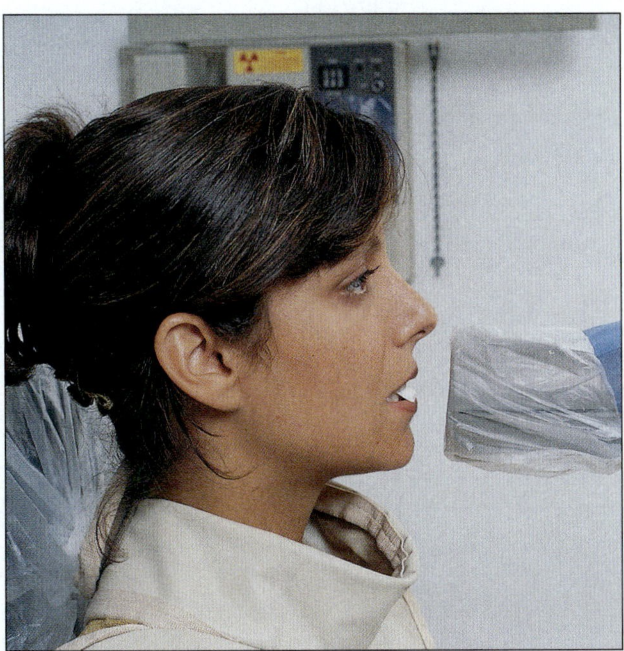

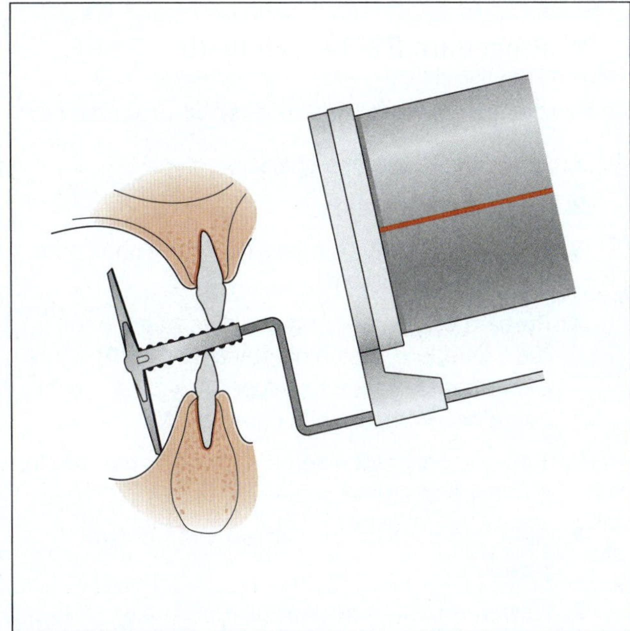

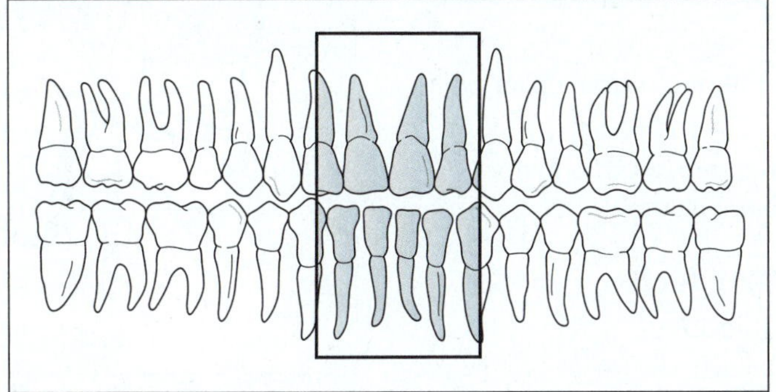

FIGURE 22-16

Anterior vertical bitewing.

Procedure 22-3

Preparation for Full-Mouth X-Ray Exposure with Paralleling Technique

This procedure is performed by the dental assistant. The dentist requests a full-mouth set of radiographs. The dental assistant prepares the equipment (Rinn XCP instruments), the area, and the patient; takes the radiographs; and processes and mounts the films for viewing according to infection control protocol.

This procedure explains film placement and exposure for the central incisors in each arch and one-half of the maxillary arch and one-half of the mandibular arch. The same technique would be used to expose the opposite arches.

Equipment and Supplies

- Patient's chart
- Barriers for the x-ray room and equipment
- X-ray film (appropriate size and number of films)
- X-ray film barriers (optional)
- Cotton rolls (optional)
- Rinn XCP materials (assembled for use) or other paralleling technique aids
- Lead apron with thyroid collar
- Container for exposed film
- Paper towel or tissue

(continues)

Procedure 22-3 (continued)

Procedure Steps (*Follow aseptic procedures*)

1. Review the patient's chart.
2. Wash and dry hands.
3. Place appropriate barriers on dental chair, film, and x-ray equipment.
4. Prepare equipment and supplies needed for the procedure, including sterile Rinn XCP instruments, tissue or paper towel, and cup or container with patient's name on it.
5. Turn the x-ray machine on and check the mA, kV, and exposure time.
6. Seat and position the patient in an upright position.
7. Have the patient remove all removable appliances, earrings, facial jewelry, or eyeglasses that may interfere with the exposing process.
8. Place the lead apron with the thyroid collar on the patient.
9. After the patient is prepared, wash and dry hands and don treatment gloves.

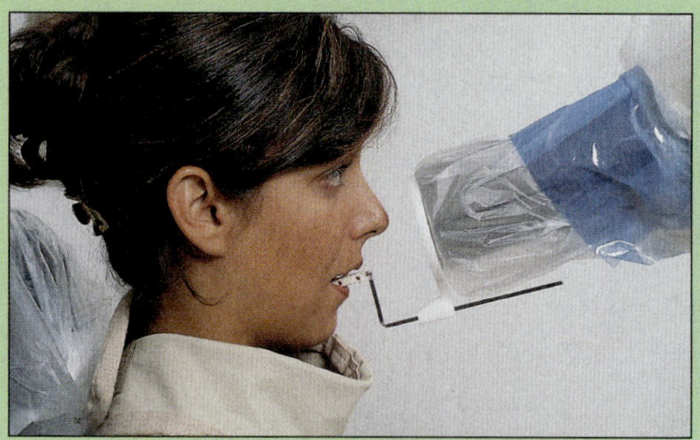

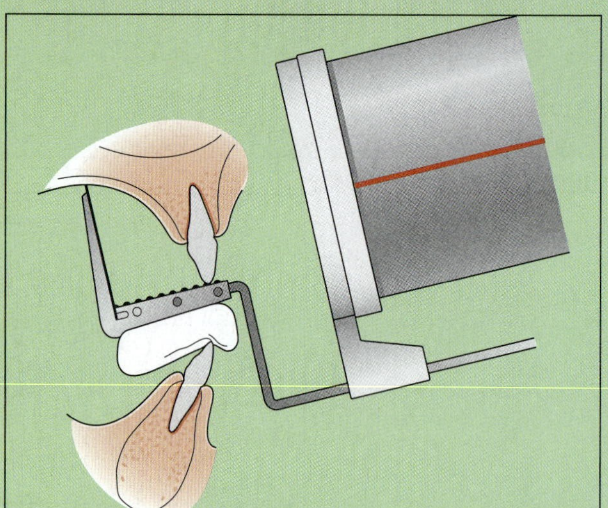

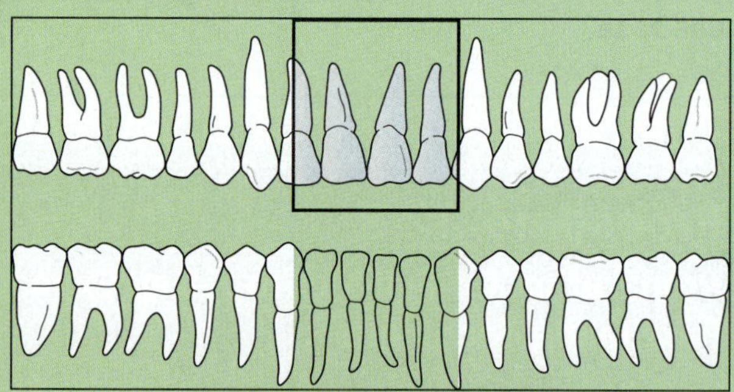

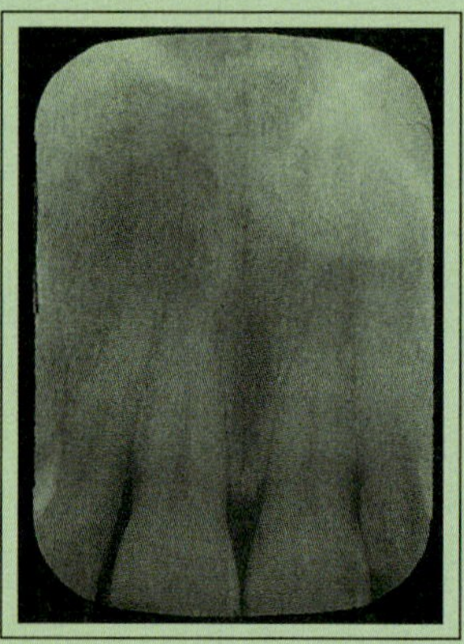

FIGURE 22-17
Maxillary incisors.

Positioning for Maxillary Arch

- Maxillary Incisors—(Figure 22-17)

1. To prepare the maxillary incisors for exposure, tilt the back of the film holder slightly and insert the film vertically into the slot on the bite block. Adjust the ring on the metal rod to cover the film. Pull the positioning ring backward on the metal rod, away from the bite block.
2. Bring the tubehead near the area of exposure.
3. Tilt the film/film holder downward to place it in the patient's mouth. Position it in the mouth away from the lingual surfaces and center it behind the incisors. Have the patient close slowly and evenly on the bite block.
4. Holding on to the metal rod, slide the positioning ring close to the patient's face. Position the cone parallel to the metal indicating rod and place it to within one-half inch of the positioning ring. The cone end should be at an equal distance from the positioning ring. This directs the central ray perpendicular to the film. The patient may help hold the metal rod to secure the film holder in position.
5. The incisal edges rest on the flat portion of the bite block.
6. The diagram shows the film, tooth, positioning ring, and open end of the cone parallel to each

(continues)

Procedure 22-3 (continued)

other. The central ray will be perpendicular to the film. No. 2 size film will show all four incisors. Teeth are centered on the radiograph, showing the apices, roots, and crowns. The bite block may be seen as a radiopaque area near the incisal edge of the film.

- Maxillary Canines—(Figure 22-18)

1. For the maxillary canines, tilt the film/film holder, place it in the patient's mouth, and position it away from the lingual surfaces. The film is placed in the mouth directly behind the center of the canine and toward the midline.
2. Have the patient close slowly and center the canine on the bite block. Holding the metal rod, slide the positioning ring toward the patient's face.
3. Bring the tubehead toward the ring, placing the cone end evenly around the positioning ring.
4. All planes are parallel so that the central ray will be directed perpendicular to the film plane. Because of the curvature of the maxillary arch, the distal sides of the canine are overlapping the first premolar on many canine radiographs. Note that the central ray is directed at the center of the canine.

- Maxillary Premolars—(Figure 22-19)

1. For the maxillary premolars, tilt the film/film holder, place it in the patient's mouth, and position it away from the lingual surfaces, toward the middle of the palate.
2. Place the anterior edge of the film behind the middle of the canine to ensure that the film will cover the area of the two premolars.
3. While holding the film in place, have the patient close slowly on the bite block. Hold the metal rod and slide the positioning ring toward the patient's face.
4. Bring the tubehead toward the ring, placing the open cone evenly around the ring. Note that the angle of the film and the film holder is positioned so that the central ray will pass through the contact point of the first and second premolars.
5. The bite block is centered on the premolars. On this radiograph, the distal side of the cuspid is visible, and the first and second premolars show that the contact between them is open.

- Maxillary Molars—(Figure 22-20)

1. For the maxillary molars, tilt the film/film holder so that it is less vertical when entering the patient's mouth. Place the film in the patient's

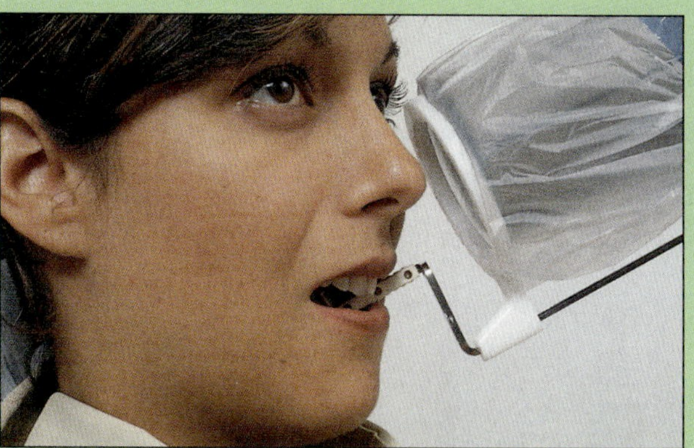

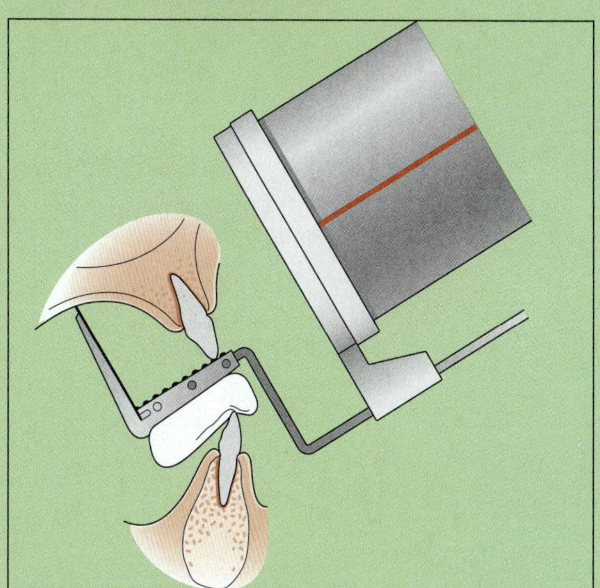

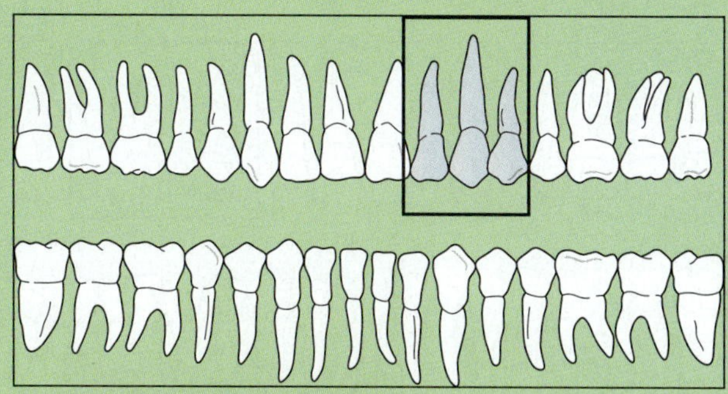

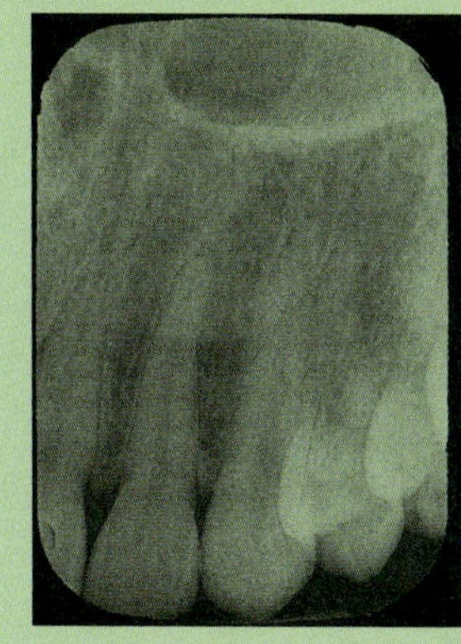

FIGURE 22-18
Maxillary canines.

(continues)

Procedure 22-3 (continued)

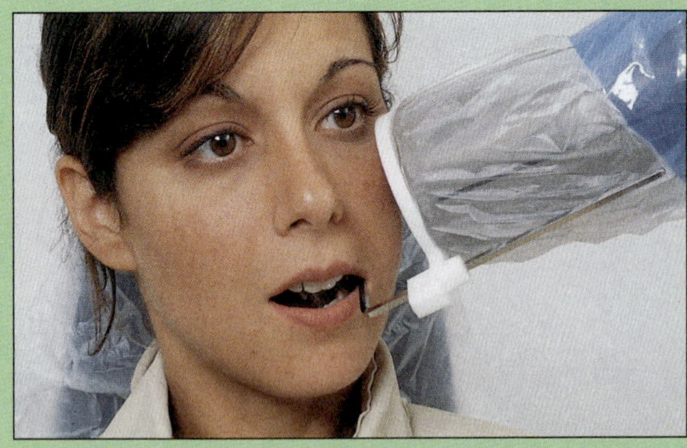

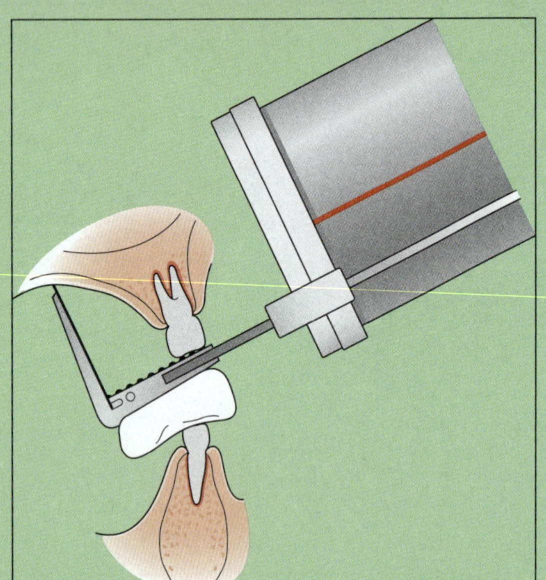

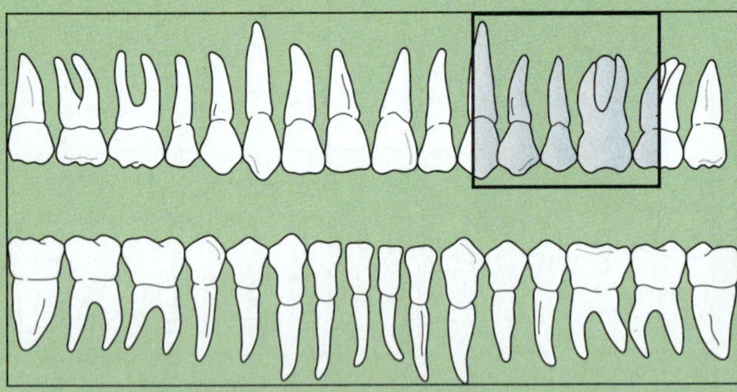

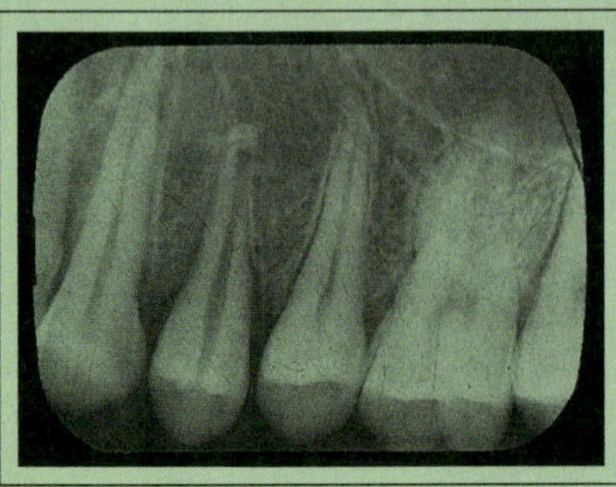

FIGURE 22-19
Maxillary premolars.

mouth and position it away from the lingual surfaces of the molars.

2. Center the bite block on the second molar. Have the patient close slowly on the bite block.
3. Bring the tubehead toward the ring, placing the open end of the cone evenly around the positioning ring.
4. The diagram in Figure 22-20 B shows the film, tooth, and cone lined up for correct direction of the central ray. This radiograph shows the open contact between the first and second molars. The distal side of the second premolar is seen. Note that the film angles are parallel to the lingual surface of the molars and placed near the middle of the palate.

Use of Cotton Rolls During X-Ray Exposure

Cotton rolls are often placed between the teeth and the bite block of the arch that is not being exposed. This technique makes it easier for the patient to close on the bite block and stabilize it to prevent movement. The cotton roll is placed over the teeth in the arch that is not going to be exposed, and then the bite block is placed on top of it. The patient is asked to close and secure the Rinn in place. This is an optional technique, and may be used for all exposures, or only for those in areas where the patient is having difficulty closing.

Positioning for Mandibular Arch

- Mandibular Incisors—(Figure 22-21)

1. The film holder is assembled in the same way for mandibular and maxillary positions. For the mandibular incisors, tilt the film/film holder and place it in the patient's mouth, gently pressing the film on the floor of the mouth behind the incisors and away from the lingual surface.
2. Have the patient close slowly on the bite block. Holding the metal rod, slide the positioning ring close to the patient's face.
3. Bring the tubehead close and place the cone parallel to the metal rod. The open end of the cone should be even with the ring.
4. The diagram in Figure 22-21 B shows how far the film needs to be placed in the mouth to see the entire length of the tooth. Sometimes the tongue is moved when the film is being placed. Being gentle with the placement will encourage patient cooperation.

(continues)

Procedure 22-3 (continued)

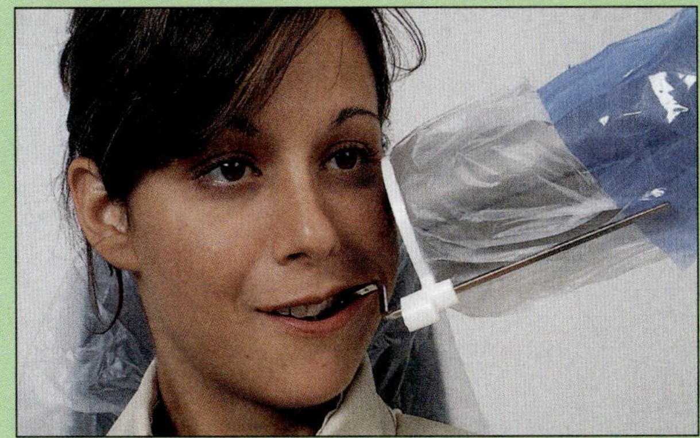

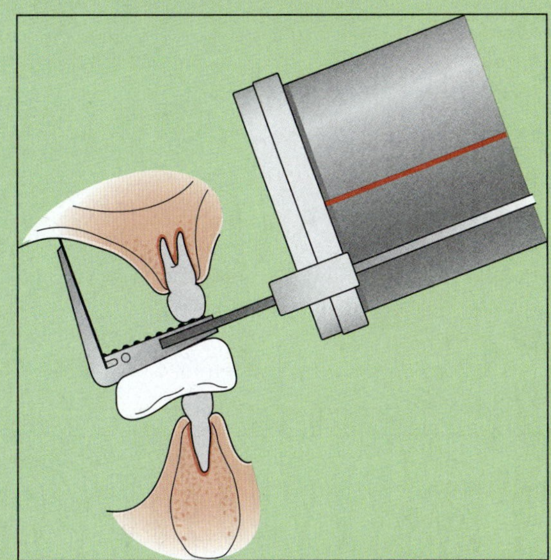

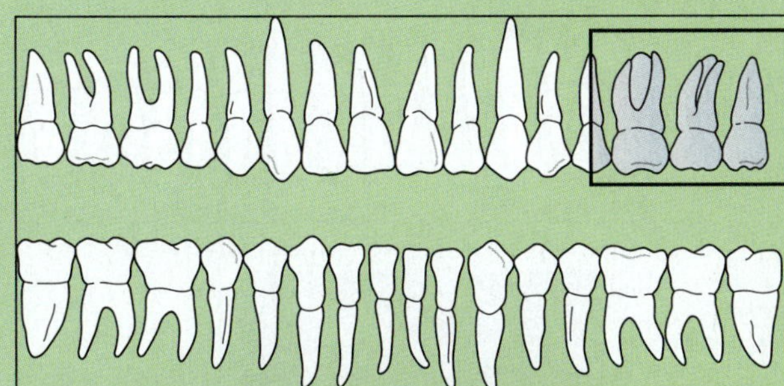

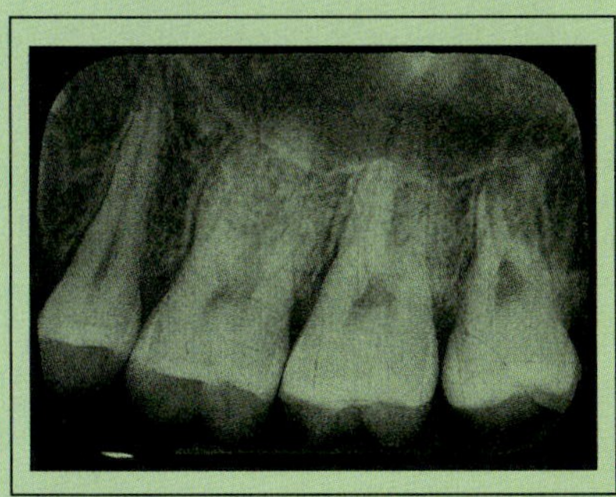

FIGURE 22-20
Maxillary molars.

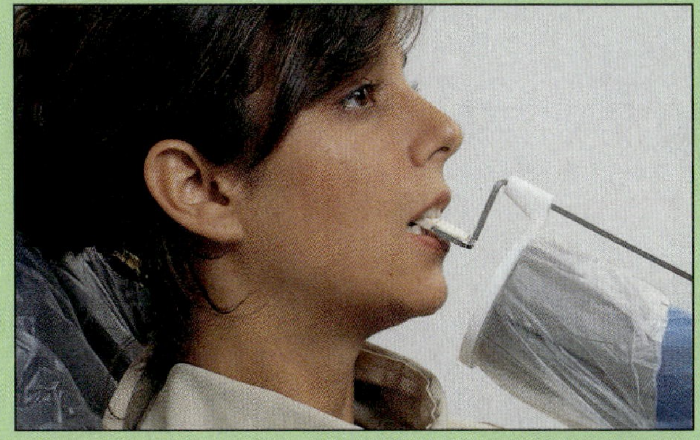

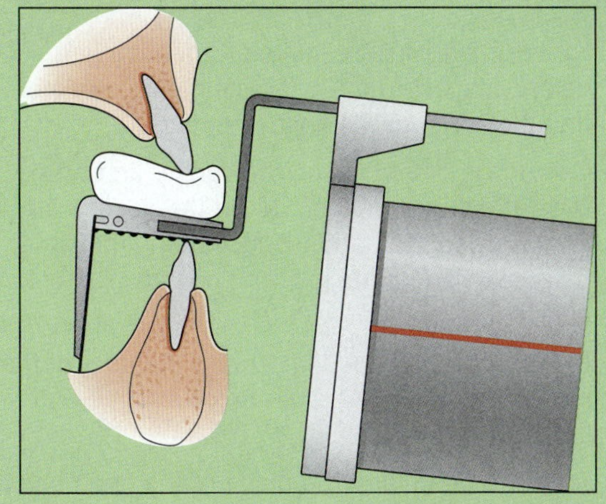

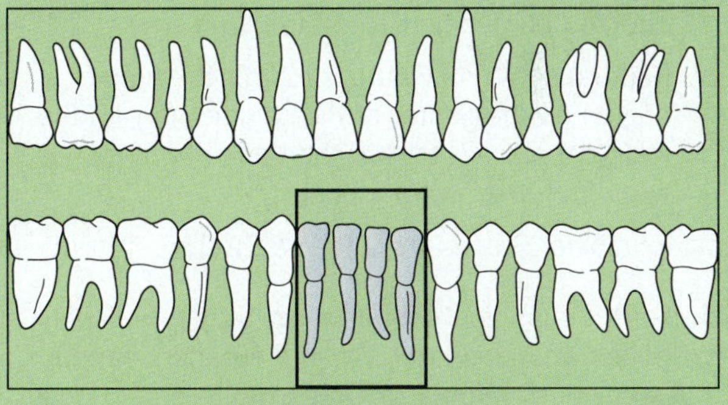

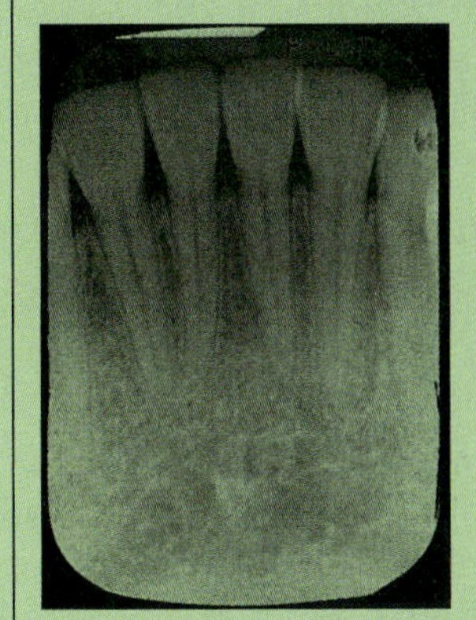

FIGURE 22-21
Mandibular incisors.

(continues)

Procedure 22-3 (continued)

5. The mandibular incisors are centered on the bite block. The incisal edges of the teeth are one-eighth inch from the top of the film.
6. The central ray is directed between the two central incisors through open contact areas. The curve of the arch will cause some overlapping on the distal sides of the lateral incisors.
7. The diagram illustrates the film placed directly behind the incisors, and as far into the mouth as the tongue attachment allows.

- Mandibular Canines—(Figure 22-22)

1. For the mandibular canine, tilt the film/film holder, place it in the patient's mouth, and position it away from the lingual surface.
2. Center the bite block on the canine and have the patient slowly close. Move the positioning ring close to the patient's face, bring the cone parallel to the metal rod, and position the open end of the cone flat with the ring.
3. Insert enough of the film toward the floor of the mouth to ensure that the film covers the entire length of the canine.
4. The film, tooth, and the plane of the open end of the cone are all parallel. The central ray will be directed perpendicular to the film plane.
5. In the diagram in Figure 22-22 B, the film is angled on the center of the canine. As with the incisors, place it toward the base of the tongue, away from the alveolar bone.

- Mandibular Premolars—(Figure 22-23)

1. For the mandibular premolars, tilt the film/film holder and place the film in the patient's mouth, gently positioning it between the lingual surface of the teeth and the tongue.
2. Place the anterior edge of the film at the middle of the canine to ensure that the film covers the area of the two premolars.
3. Have the patient close on the bite block.
4. Note the position of the film as it is placed in the space between the tongue and the mandibular arch.
5. The film, teeth, and plane of the open end of the cone are all parallel. The first and second premolars are seen on the following film with the contact points open.

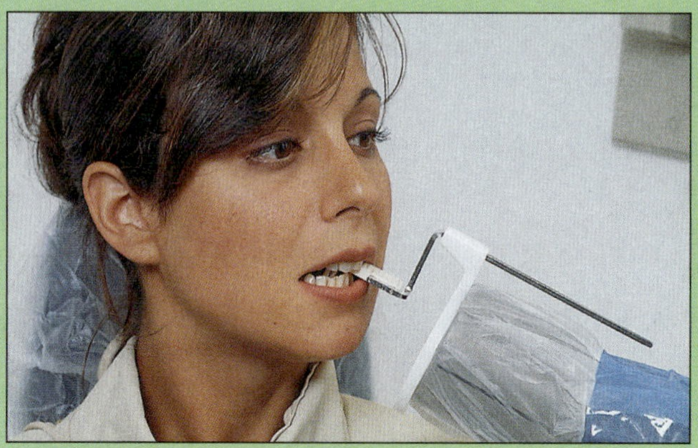

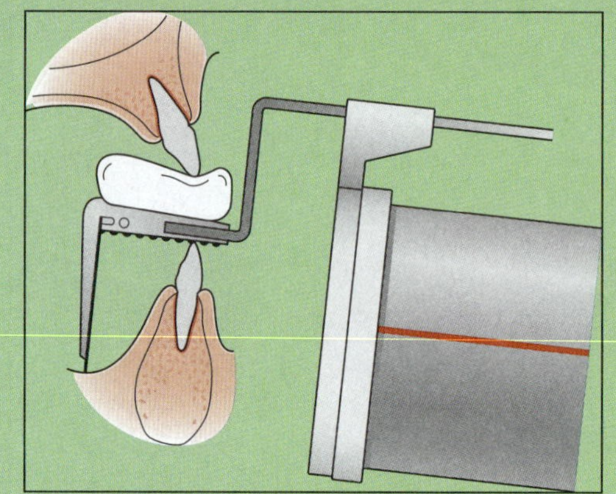

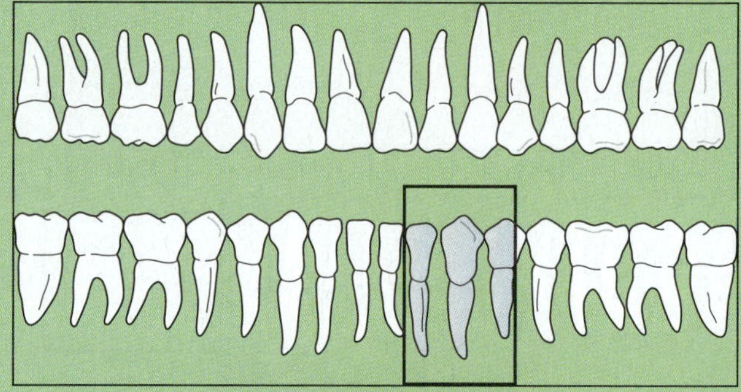

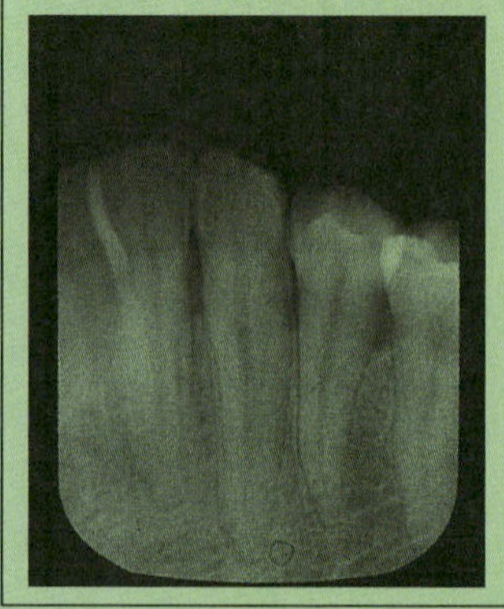

FIGURE 22-22
Mandibular canines.

(continues)

Procedure 22-3 (continued)

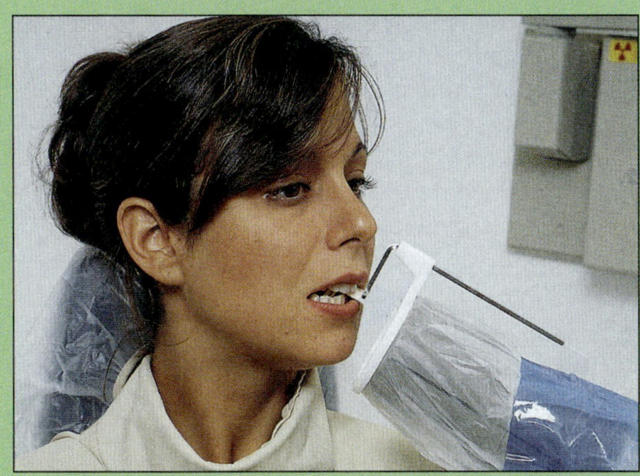

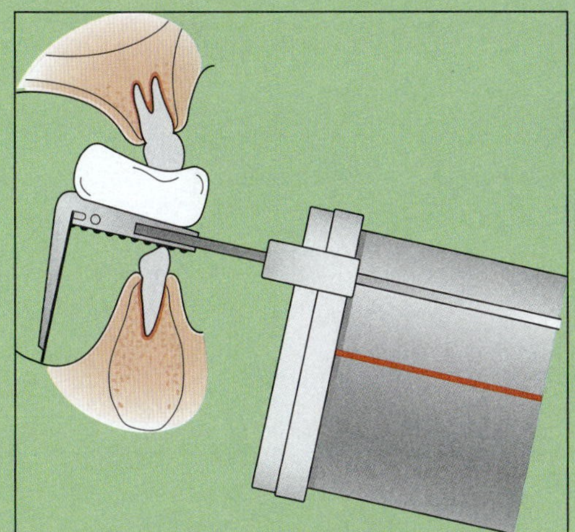

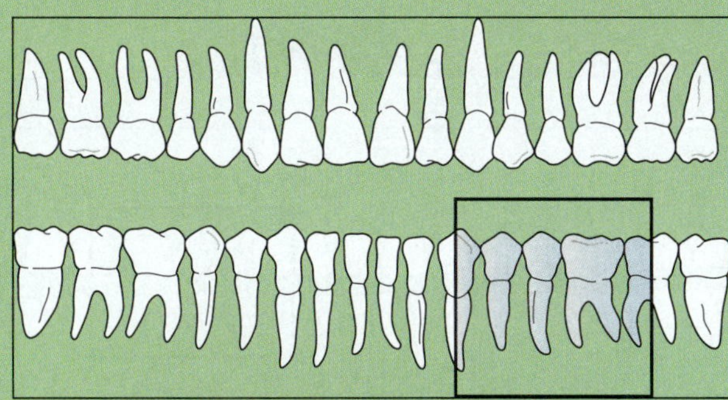

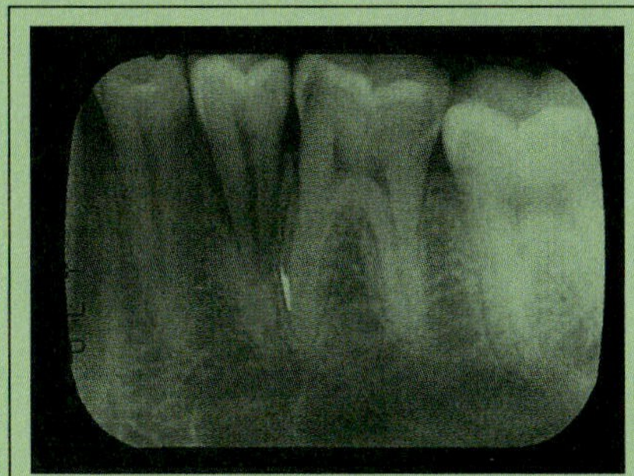

FIGURE 22-23
Mandibular premolars.

- Mandibular Molars—(Figure 22-24)

1. For the mandibular molars, tilt the film/film holder and place the film holder with the film in the patient's mouth, positioning it between the tongue and the lingual surfaces of the teeth.
2. Center the bite block over the second molar. Hold it in the desired position, and have the patient close to secure it in place.
3. Gently place the patient's cheek over the bite block, if this is more comfortable for the patient.
4. Align the positioning ring and cone.
5. Note how close the film is to the lingual surface. Move the tongue toward the center of the mouth to make this placement more comfortable for the patient.
6. The edge of the film is positioned only one-eighth inch above the occlusal edge.
7. The first, second, and third molars are seen on this film with the contacts open. The third molar may not be erupted into the oral cavity, but it will be seen on the film.
8. During placement, to prevent the film and film holder from moving forward, hold the bite block in position until the patient closes firmly on it.

- Premolar Bitewing—(Figure 22-25)

1. To position bitewing radiographs, a tab or positioning instrument is used. Tabs come with adhesive backs or with loops to surround the film. The positioning instrument comes with a bitewing holder, an indicator rod, and a positioning ring.
2. Holding the film horizontally, place the tab in the center of the film or, if using a positioning instrument, make sure the film is centered on the bitewing holder with the smooth side of the film directed toward the positioning ring.
3. The drawing and radiograph in Figure 22-25 illustrates the position of the film covering the premolars, with the front edge of the film upon the middle of the canine, while the back edge of the film may be upon the mesial side of the second molar.
4. Hold the tab and place the film near the lingual surface of the teeth in the patient's mouth, positioning the film to cover the mandibular premolars.

(continues)

Procedure 22-3 (continued)

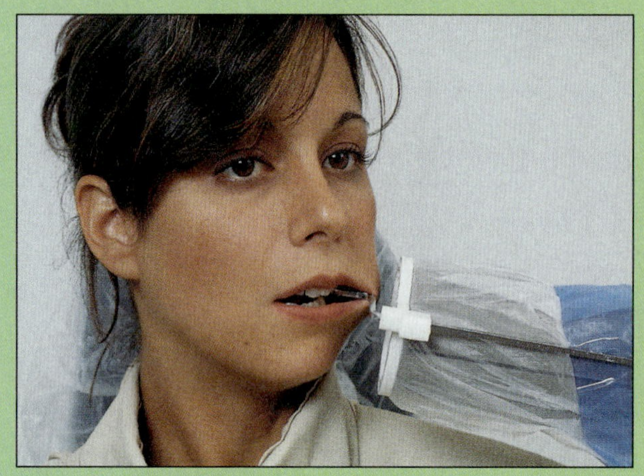

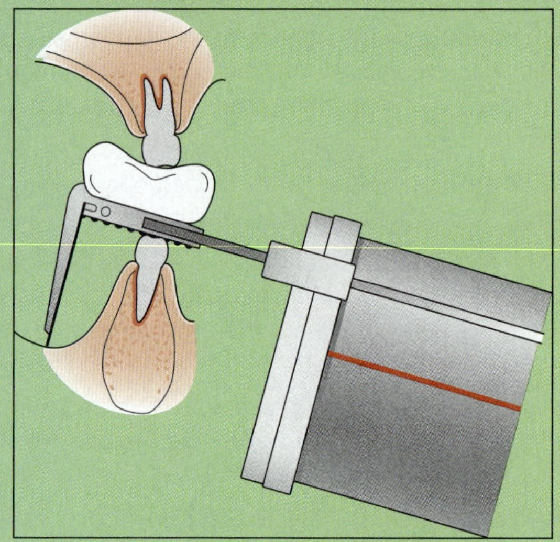

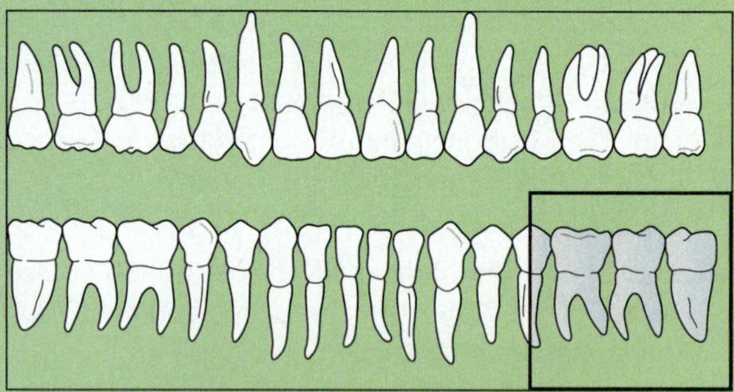

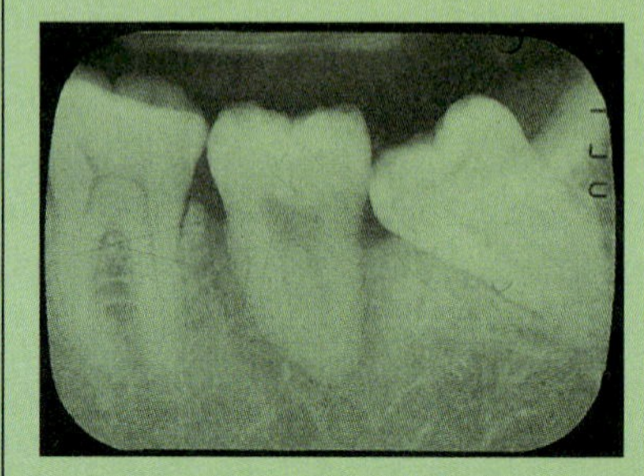

FIGURE 22-24
Mandibular molars.

5. While holding the tab in place, slowly rotate fingers out of the waym while having the patient close. When using a positioning instrument, place the bitewing holder in the patient's mouth, away from the lingual surface of the teeth. Position the film to cover the premolars and to be parallel to them. Have the patient close slowly on the bitewing holder to secure it in place.
6. The cone positioning for the premolar bitewing begins with the vertical angulation set between

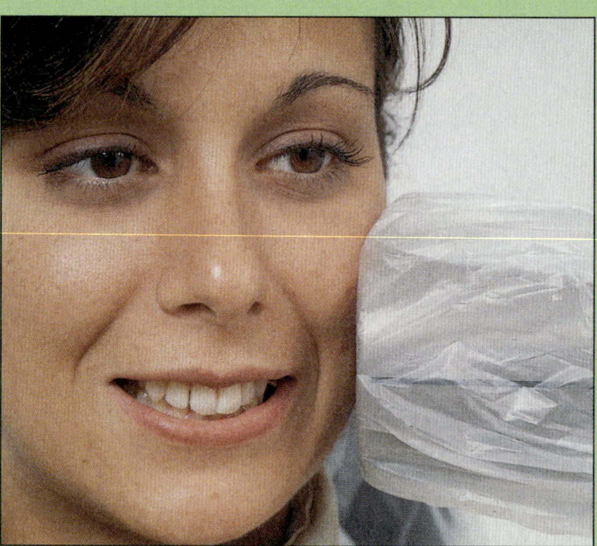

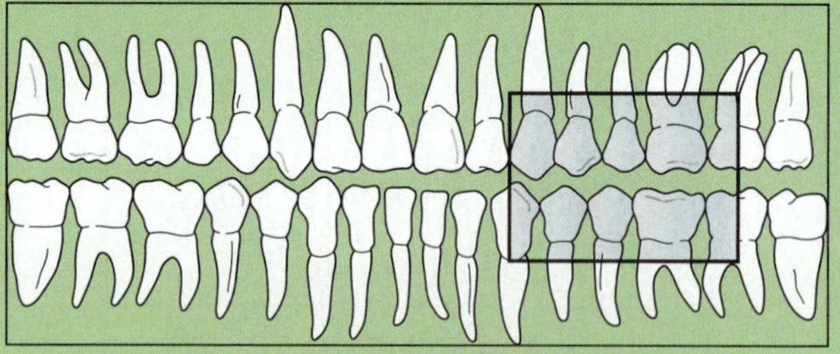

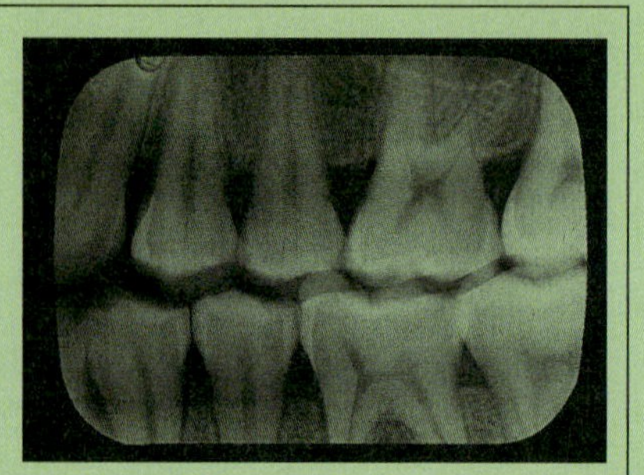

FIGURE 22-25
Premolar bitewing using a bitewing tab.

(continues)

Procedure 22-3 (continued)

+5° to +10°, depending on the slant of the film as it is positioned in the patient's mouth.

7. The horizontal angulation is positioned so that the beam is aimed directly between the contacts of the premolars, and the cone is perpendicular to the film. This film placement is sometimes uncomfortable for the patient because of the alveolar ridge curvature near the canine. Gentleness when positioning this exposure will be rewarded with patient cooperation. When using the positioning instrument, first hold the indicator rod, and then bring the positioning ring close to the patient's face.

- Molar Bitewing—(Figure 22-26)

1. Position the film to cover the molars and the distal half of the second premolar. Place the front edge of the film at the distal side of the second molar.
2. Holding the tab, place the film in the patient's mouth, away from the lingual surfaces, while gently moving the tongue toward the middle of the mouth.
3. When using the positioning instrument, place it in the patient's mouth, pushing the tongue away from the lingual surfaces.
4. The vertical angulation for the molar bitewing is set at 0° so that the cone is perpendicular to the film. The horizontal angulation is directed so that the beam is between the contacts of the first and second molars. Place the cone near the patient's face, covering the film and perpendicular to the film. Look at the curve of the patient's arch rather than the patient's face to position the cone.

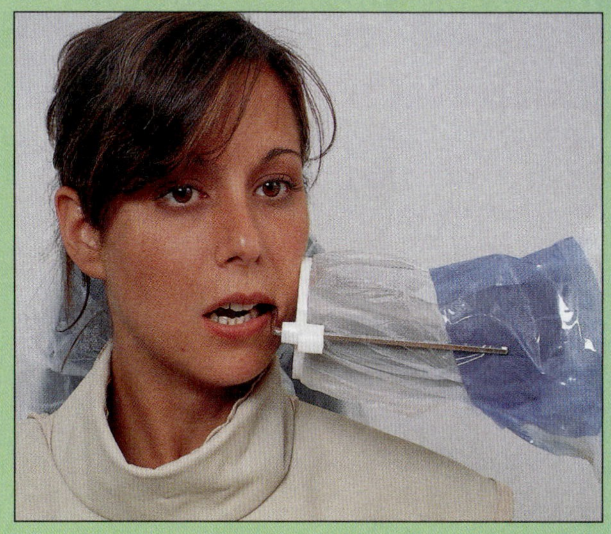

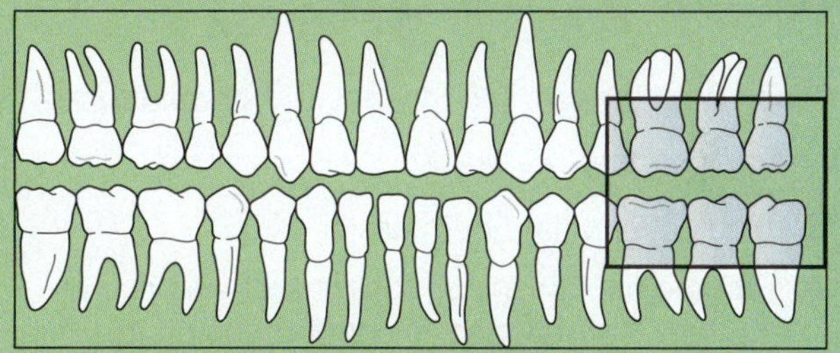

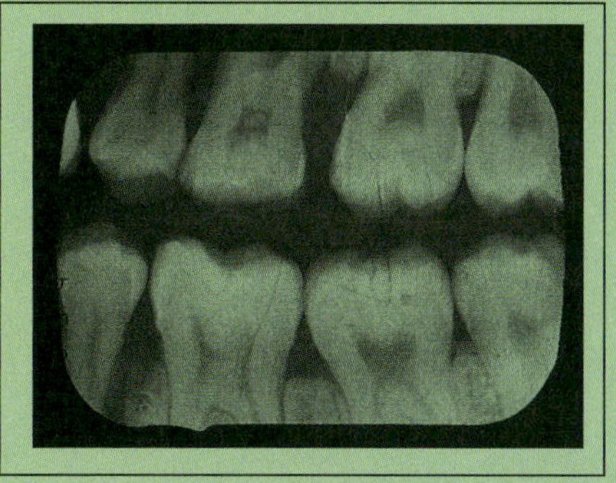

FIGURE 22-26
Molar bitewing using Rinn XCP.

Producing Special Radiographs

Special radiographs include the occlusal radiograph, radiographs on children, edentulous patients, endodontic radiographs, and radiographs on special needs patients or compromised patients. Each situation requires additional skills in working with the patient, and knowing how to correctly position the radiograph to achieve the desired results. Exposing radiographs on patients with special needs requires the dental assistant to be prepared; have a positive attitude; and be patient, understanding, and creative. It is important for the dental assistant to speak directly to the person, even if there is a caregiver present. Do not ask personal questions about the patient's condition, instead, the best method is to ask the patient what the best way is to assist them.

Occlusal Radiographs

Occlusal radiographs show a large area of the dental arch. They are used with children when periapicals are difficult to expose, and with patients who have difficulty opening the mouth or controlling muscular movement. The films are placed on the occlusal surface and then the patient closes gently on the film to hold it in place. Occlusal radiographs are used (1) to locate or define fractures, impacted teeth, foreign bodies in the bone or floor of the mouth; and (2) to identify the location of other artifacts, changes in the size and shape of the arches, supernumerary teeth, cleft palate, root fragments, cysts, malignancies, tumors (odontomas), osteomyelitis, stones in the ducts of the salivary glands, unerupted teeth, and malpositioned teeth.

Two techniques are used to expose occlusal radiographs: the **topographic technique** and the **cross-section technique**

Procedure 22-4
Exposing Occlusal Radiographs

This procedure is performed by the dental assistant at the direction of the dentist. The dental assistant prepares the equipment and supplies, the area, and the patient. The occlusal films are exposed using either the topographic or the cross-sectional technique.

Equipment and Supplies

- Barriers for the x-ray room
- Occlusal film (No. 2 size for children and No. 4 size for adults)
- Lead apron with thyroid collar
- Container or barrier for exposed film

Procedure Steps (*Follow aseptic procedures*)

1. Wash and dry hands.
2. Place appropriate barriers.
3. Prepare film, tissue or paper towel, and cup or container with patient's identification on it.
4. Seat the patient in an upright position and place the lead apron on the patient.
5. Wash and dry hands and don treatment gloves.

Topographic Technique

6. For the *maxillary view*, positioning is similar to that used for the bisecting technique. The patient is positioned so that the maxillary arch is parallel to the floor.
7. The film is placed in the mouth with the smooth/plain side toward the cone.
8. Have the patient close on the film, leaving about 2 mm of an edge beyond the incisors.
9. Move the cone to a vertical angulation of +65° to +75°.
10. Direct the cone over the bridge of the nose, with the lower edge of the cone covering the incisors (Figure 22-27).

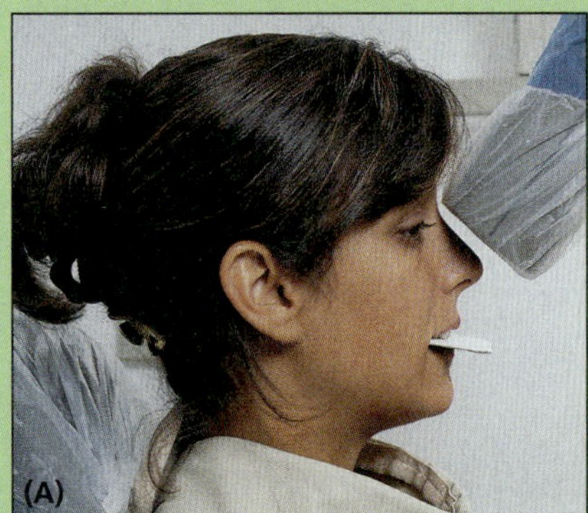

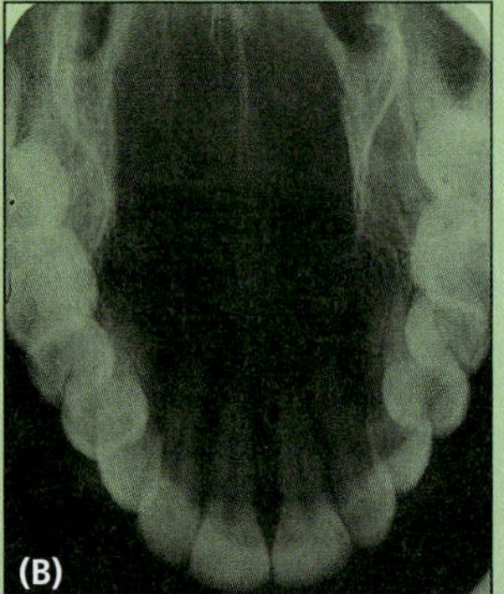

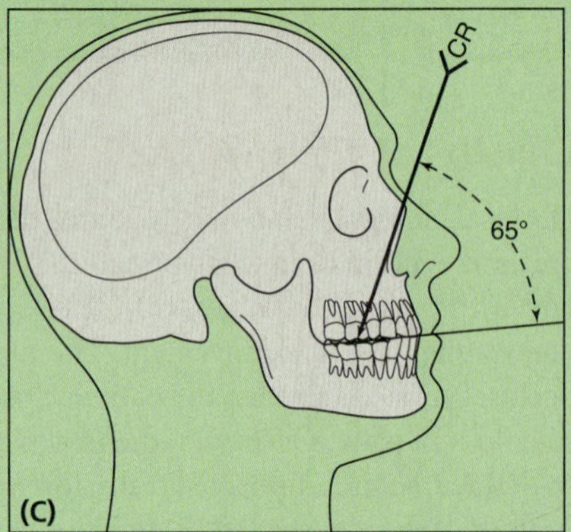

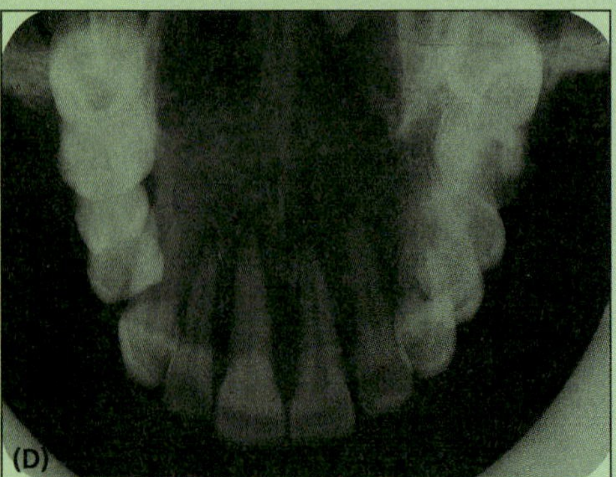

FIGURE 22-27

Topographic occlusal radiograph of the maxillary arch. (A) Vertical film placement. (B) X-ray of vertical film placement. (C) Horizontal film placement. (D) X-ray of horizontal film placement.

(continues)

Procedure 22-4 (continued)

11. For the mandibular view using the topographic technique, the patient's head is tilted back.
12. Place the smooth side of the film on the occlusal surfaces of the teeth with the central incisors at the front edge of the film.
13. Have the patient close gently on the film.
14. The vertical angulation will vary with each patient between −40° and −55°.
15. Center the cone over the film, directing the central ray at the middle and tip of the chin (Figure 22-28).

Cross-Section Technique

1. For the *maxillary view* using the cross-section technique, the patient should be in an upright position with the head tilted backward slightly.
2. The film placement is the same as with the topographic technique. The cone is positioned over the top of the patient's head with the central ray directed perpendicular to the film.
3. Be sure the cone covers the maxillary area to be exposed (Figure 22-29).

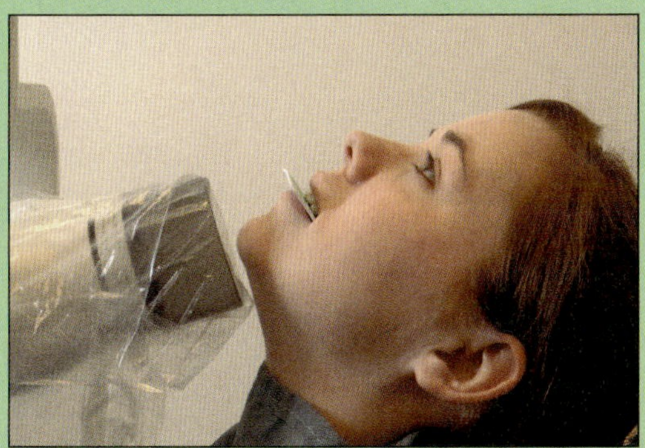

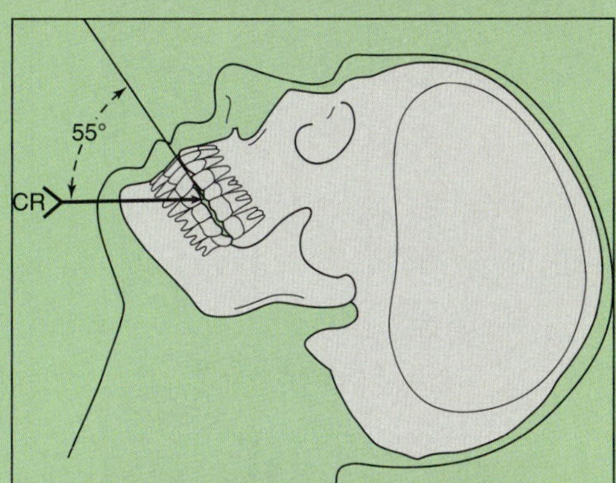

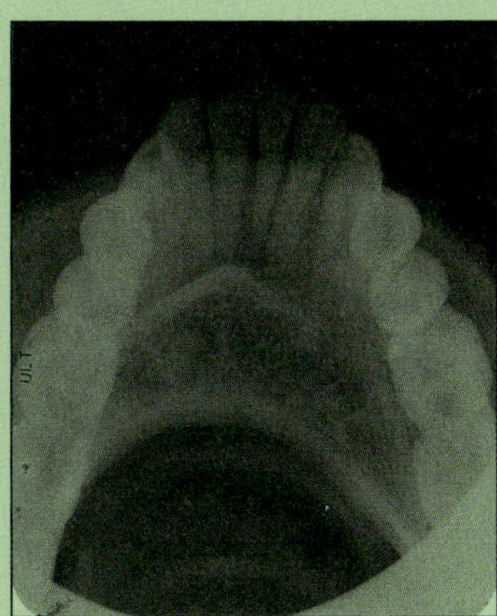

FIGURE 22-28
Topographic occlusal radiograph of the mandibular arch.

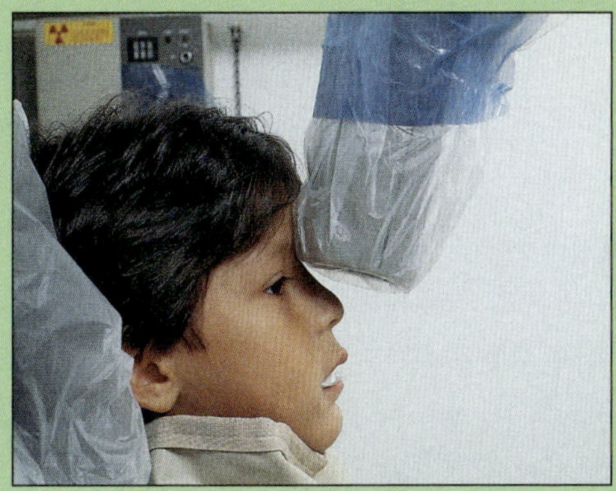

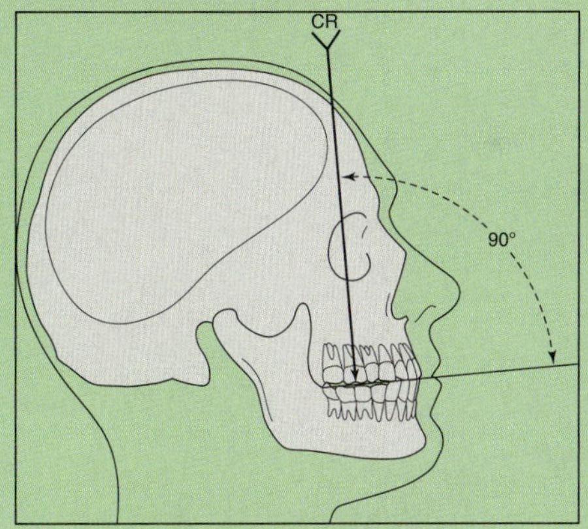

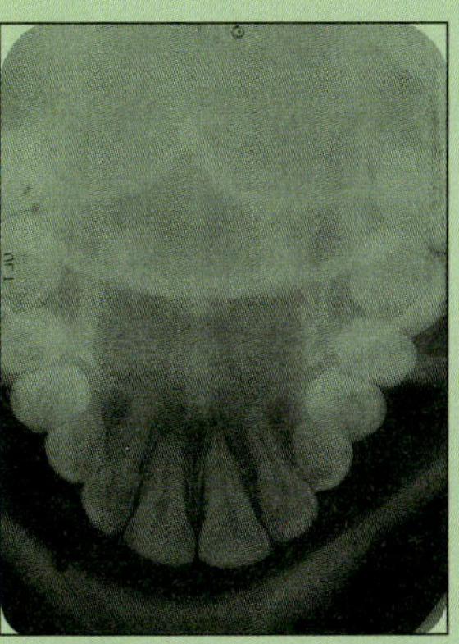

FIGURE 22-29
Cross-sectional occlusal radiograph of the maxillary arch.

(continues)

Procedure 22-4 (continued)

4. For the *mandibular view*, the patient's head should be tilted backward.
5. The film placement is the same as with the topographic technique.
6. The cone is positioned under the patient's chin with the central ray directed perpendicular to the film. The patient may have to lift the chin up in order to position the cone (Figure 22-30).

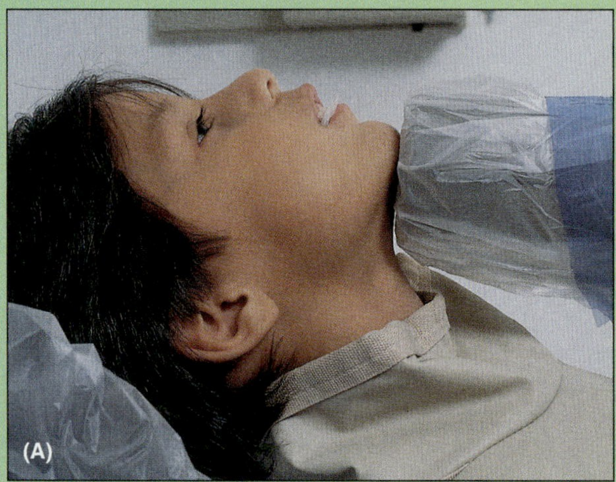

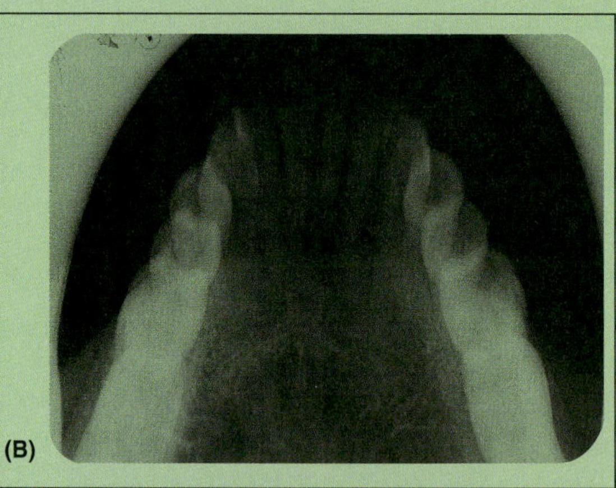

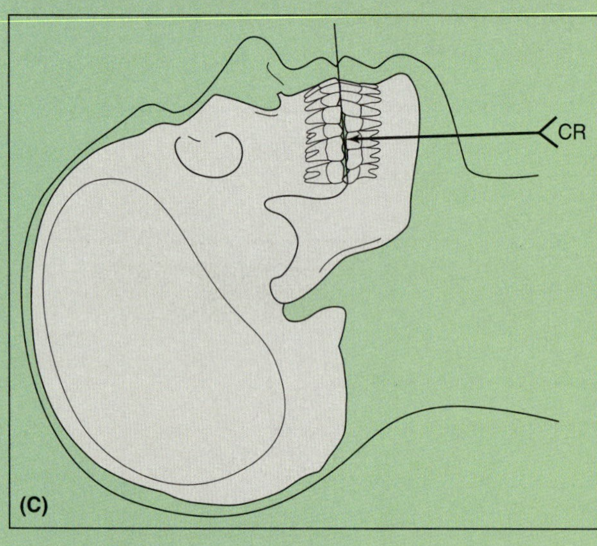

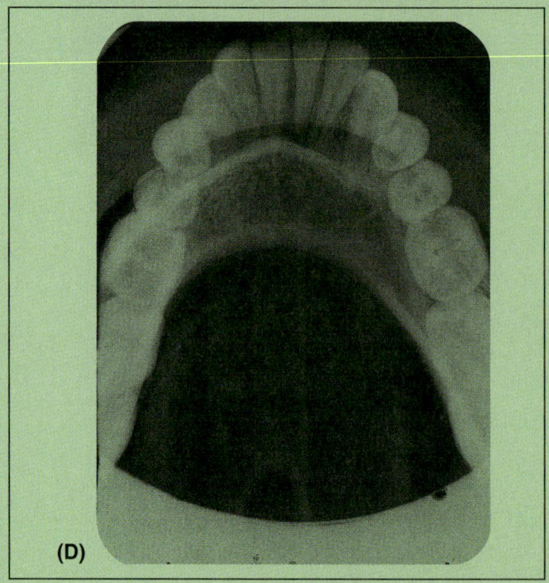

FIGURE 22-30
Cross-sectional occlusal radiograph of the mandibular arch. (A) Horizontal film placement. (B) Vertical film placement.

(Procedure 22-4). Technique selection is determined by the view the dentist needs for diagnosis. With the topographic technique, the rules of bisecting are followed: The central ray is directed perpendicular to the bisecting plane. With the cross-section technique, the central ray is perpendicular to the film.

Pediatric Radiographs

Radiographs play an important role in the dental health of children. They are used to detect caries, abscesses, cysts, anodontia, and fractures, and to evaluate eruption stages and growth patterns. Technique suggestions associated with pediatric radiographs are as follows:

- Because developing tissues are sensitive to radiation, the exposure time should be reduced and the number of radiographs should be kept to a minimum.
- The oral mucosa of young children in eruption stages is sensitive to the slightest pressure, so carefully examine the mouth for loose or erupting teeth, any parulis, pulp polyps, cold sores (herpes simplex), canker sores (aphthous ulcers), or any deviation from the normal.

- Talk to the child and demonstrate what is going to happen.
- Evaluate the child's behavior and cooperation. Having the child help often reduces apprehension.
- Work quickly and confidently, because children move constantly and become bored easily.
- Evaluate the child's mouth to determine the number and size of x-ray film to be used. Select the smallest film you can to minimize discomfort and still obtain the view needed. For preschool children, No. 0 film is most often used. Older children will vary from a No. 0 film to Nos. 1 and 2, depending on the size of the mouth, the tenderness of the tissues, and the depth of the palate and the floor of the mouth. For occlusal views, No. 2 film is used. The number of films and the size of the film used can be tailored to the child and the dentist's needs (Figures 22-31A through C).
- Take anterior films first to encourage the child's cooperation.
- The paralleling technique is most frequently used; all guidelines are the same as for adults. Procedure 22-5 outlines the steps involved in taking a pediatric full mouth exposure.

Edentulous Radiographic Survey

A series of radiographs on the edentulous (ee-**DENT**-you-lous) (toothless) or partially edentulous patient may be indicated to show cysts, impacted teeth, retained root tips or bone fragments; other pathological conditions; and normal landmarks, such as the mental foramen, mandibular canal, maxillary sinuses, and alveolar bone. As part of the routine examination, radiographs are taken before dentures and partials are made; if abnormal pathology or sensitivity is found, the patient can receive treatment before the removable prosthesis is made. Technique suggestions associated with treatment for the edentulous patient are as follows:

- A routine full-mouth survey consists of six anterior and eight posterior films, but these numbers can be reduced by taking fewer anterior films in smaller arches, thus, eliminating bitewing radiographs.
- Either the paralleling or the bisecting technique can be used, but both will need to be modified. In the paralleling technique, cotton rolls are used with the film holder to position the film parallel to the alveolar ridge. If the patient has dentures or partials, leave the appliance in the opposing arch for better support. In the bisecting technique, the film

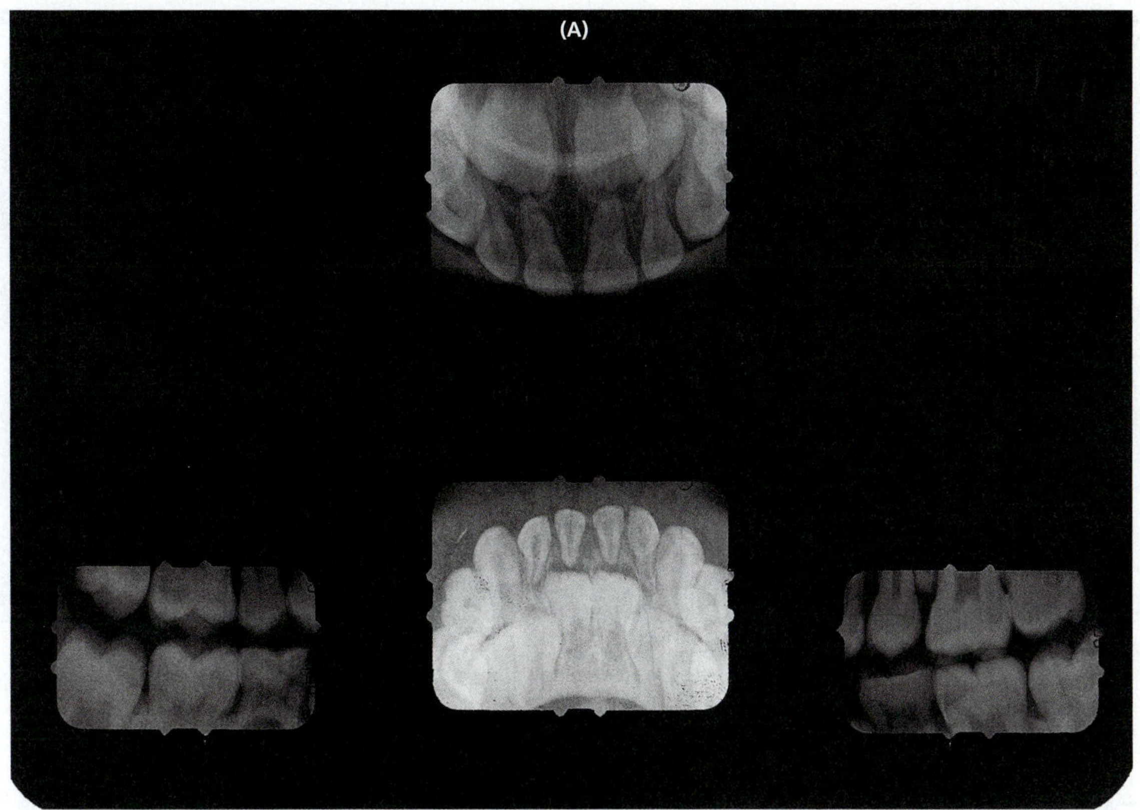

FIGURE 22-31

(A) Pedodontic full mouth survey of a 5-year-old child includes two bitewings and two occlusals.

(continues)

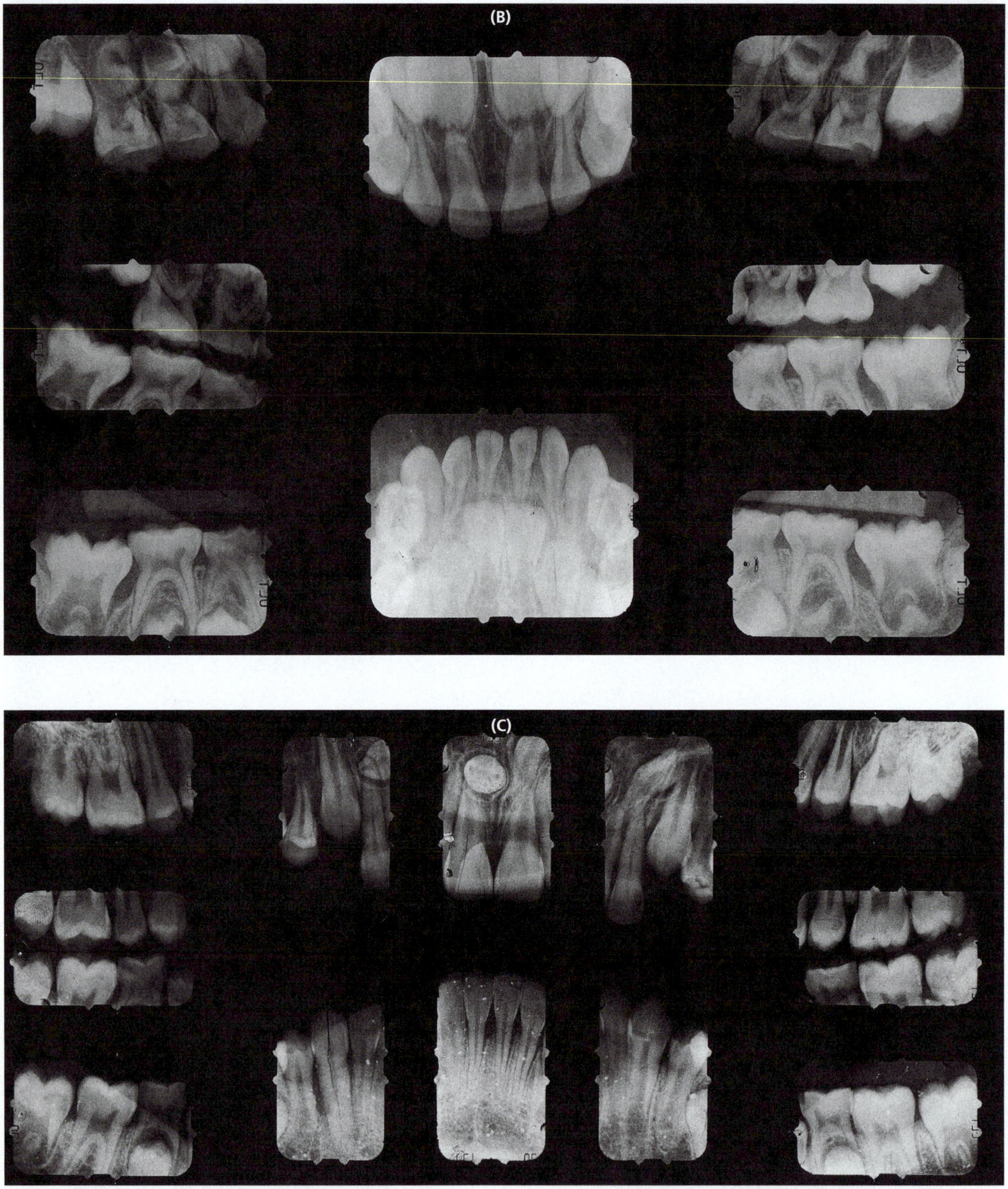

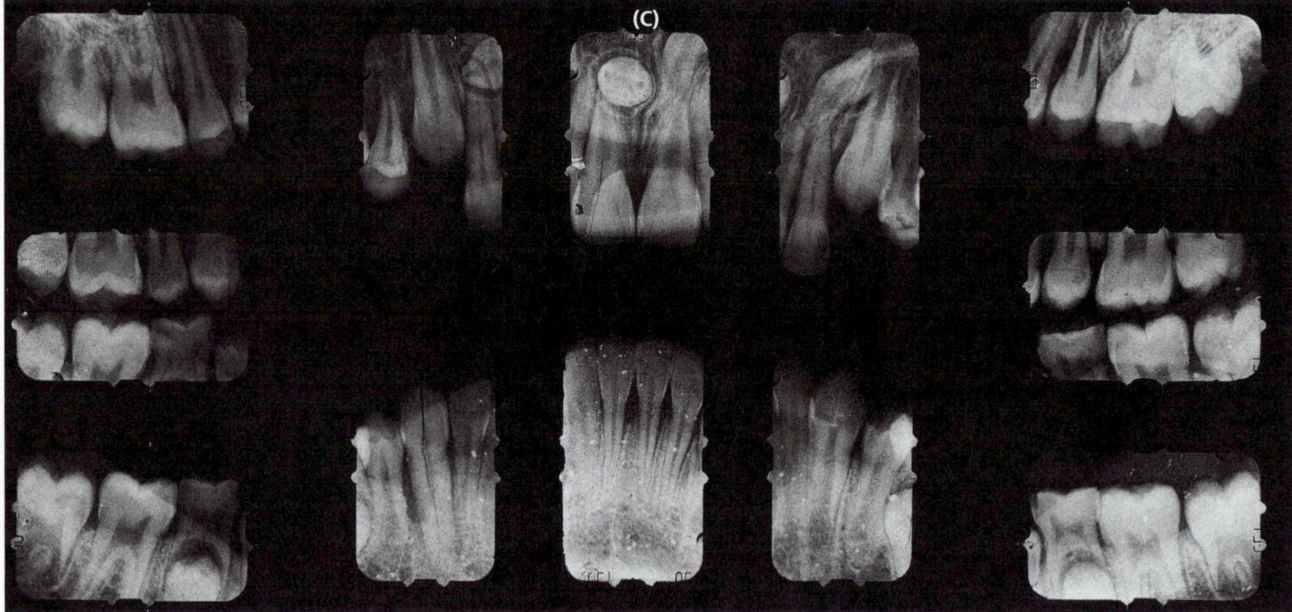

FIGURE 22-31 (continued)

(B) Pedodontic full mouth survey of a child 3 to 5 years old includes two bitewings, two occlusals, and four periapicals. (C) Pedodontic full mouth survey of a child 6 to 12 years old includes two bitewings, six anterior incisors, and four posterior periapicals.

will be almost flat. Just extend the edge of the film one-quarter inch beyond the crest of the alveolar ridge.

- The vertical angulation will be increased. Reduce exposure time by one-quarter of the normal time to prevent overexposure of an area where teeth are missing and the bone is thinner.
- Try using occlusal film and exposing individual quadrants and/or arches, take a panoramic film that includes

Procedure 22-5
Full-Mouth Pediatric X-Ray Exposure

This procedure is performed by the dental assistant. The dentist requires that a pediatric full-mouth set of radiographs be taken and identifies the eight films. The dental assistant prepares the equipment (Rinn XCP instruments), the area, and the patient; takes the radiographs; processes the films; and mounts the films for viewing according to infection control protocol.

This procedure explains film placement and exposure for the two occlusal films, maxillary and mandibular; two bitewing x-rays; and four periapical x-rays.

Equipment and Supplies

- Barriers for the x-ray room and equipment
- X-ray film, six No. 0 size films and two No. 2 size films
- X-ray film barriers (optional)
- Cotton rolls (optional)
- Rinn XCP materials (assembled for use) or other paralleling technique aids
- Lead apron with thyroid collar
- Container for exposed film
- Paper towel or tissue

Procedure Steps (*Follow aseptic procedures*)

1. Review the patient's chart.
2. Wash and dry hands.
3. Place appropriate barriers on the dental chair, film, and x-ray equipment.
4. Prepare film No. 2 for children.
5. Assemble sterile Rinn XCP instruments and prepare tissue or paper towel, and cup or container with patient's name on it.
6. Turn on the x-ray machine and check the mA, kV, and exposure time.
7. Seat the patient in an upright position.
8. Place the lead apron with the thyroid collar on the patient.
9. After the patient is prepared, wash and dry hands, and don latex treatment gloves.
10. Explain the procedure to the patient.

Maxillary Occlusal X-Ray/Topographic Technique

1. For the maxillary view, positioning is similar to that used for the bisecting technique. The patient is positioned so that the maxillary arch is parallel to the floor.
2. Place the film in the mouth with the smooth/plain side toward the cone.
3. Have the patient close on the film, leaving about 2 mm of an edge beyond the incisors.
4. Move the cone to a vertical angulation of +65° to +75°.
5. Direct the cone over the bridge of the nose with the lower edge of the cone covering the incisors.

Mandibular Occlusal X-Ray/Topographic Technique

1. For the mandibular view, the patient's head is tilted backward until the mandibular arch is parallel to the floor to allow for correct placement for the bisecting technique.
2. Place the smooth side of the film on the occlusal surfaces of the teeth with the central incisors at the front edge of the film.
3. Have the patient close gently on the film.
4. The vertical angulation will vary with each patient between −40° and −55°. Center the cone over the film, directing the central ray at the middle and tip of the chin.

Deciduous Bitewings

1. To position bitewing radiographs, a tab or positioning instrument is used. Tabs come with adhesive backs or with loops to surround the film. The positioning instrument comes with a bitewing holder, an indicator rod, and a positioning ring.
2. While holding the film horizontally, place the tab in the center of the film or, if using a positioning instrument, make sure the film is centered on the bitewing holder with the smooth side of the film directed toward the positioning ring.
3. Position the film covering the deciduous first and second molars, with the front edge of the film to the middle of the canine.

(continues)

Procedure 22-5 (continued)

4. Hold the tab and place the film near the lingual surface of the teeth in the patient's mouth, positioning the film to cover the mandibular deciduous molars.
5. While holding the tab in place, have the patient close and slowly rotate the fingers out of the way.
6. When using a positioning instrument, place the bitewing holder in the patient's mouth, away from the lingual surface of the teeth. Position the film to cover and parallel the deciduous molars. Have the patient close slowly on the bitewing holder and hold it in place.
7. The cone positioning for the premolar bitewing with vertical angulation is set to 0°.

Positioning for Maxillary Deciduous Molars

1. For the maxillary deciduous molars, tilt the film/film holder, place it in the patient's mouth, and position it away from the lingual surfaces, toward the middle of the palate.
2. Place the anterior edge of the film behind the middle of the canine to ensure that the film will cover the area of the two molars.
3. While holding the film in place, have the patient close slowly on the bite block. Hold the metal rod and slide the positioning ring toward the patient's face.
4. Bring the tubehead toward the ring, placing the open cone evenly around the ring. Note the angle of the film and the film holder, which is positioned so that the central ray passes through the contact point of the first and second deciduous molars.
5. Center the bite block on the deciduous molars. On this radiograph, the distal side of the canine is seen and the first and second deciduous molars have the contact between them open.

Positioning for Mandibular Deciduous Molars

1. For the mandibular deciduous molars, tilt the film/film holder, place the film in the patient's mouth, and gently position it between the lingual surface of the teeth and the tongue.
2. Place the anterior edge of the film at the middle of the canine to ensure that the film covers the area of the two deciduous molars.
3. Have the patient close on the bite block.
4. Note the position of the film as it is placed in the space between the tongue and the mandibular arch. The film, teeth, and plane of the open end of the cone are all parallel. The first and second deciduous molars are seen on this film with the contact points open.

both arches and the surrounding area on one film, or use periapical films if areas are of a suspicious condition (Figure 22-32).

Endodontic Radiographic Technique

Radiographs are taken periodically during the endodontic procedure (Figure 22-33A). The radiographs allow the dentist to check the progress of the procedure and take the necessary measurements. Technique suggestions associated with endodontic procedures are as follows:

- Use the paralleling technique to reduce distortion whenever possible.
- Place the film in a hemostat, Snap-a-Ray, or XCP Instrument endodontic positioning device. The endodontic film-holding device is made of plastic and aids in positioning the film while keeping the patient's mouth open. The patient needs to hold the mouth open during this time, because there is a reamer in the root canal that extends beyond the tooth. The endodontic film holder is like the Rinn film holder in that there is also a ring to line up the cone.
- Loosen the dental dam from the frame on one side and position the film on the lingual surface, parallel to the tooth. If a plastic frame is not used, the metal frame may have to be removed to prevent the frame from being exposed on the radiograph and possibly distorting the image.
- The film should cover the entire length of the tooth and the surrounding area at the apex of the root.
- Center the tooth on the film and direct the central ray perpendicular to the tooth. The patient must keep the mouth open because of protruding endodontic instruments and materials, so work quickly (Figure 22-33B).

Special Needs Patients/ Compromised Patients

Patients come to the office with a wide variety of special needs. Consideration and creativity often are required to obtain the desired radiographs. The wheelchair patient is one example where advance preparation is needed in order to have the treatment room ready (Figure 22-34). When there is a plan in place to expose the x-ray, the procedure is much easier for

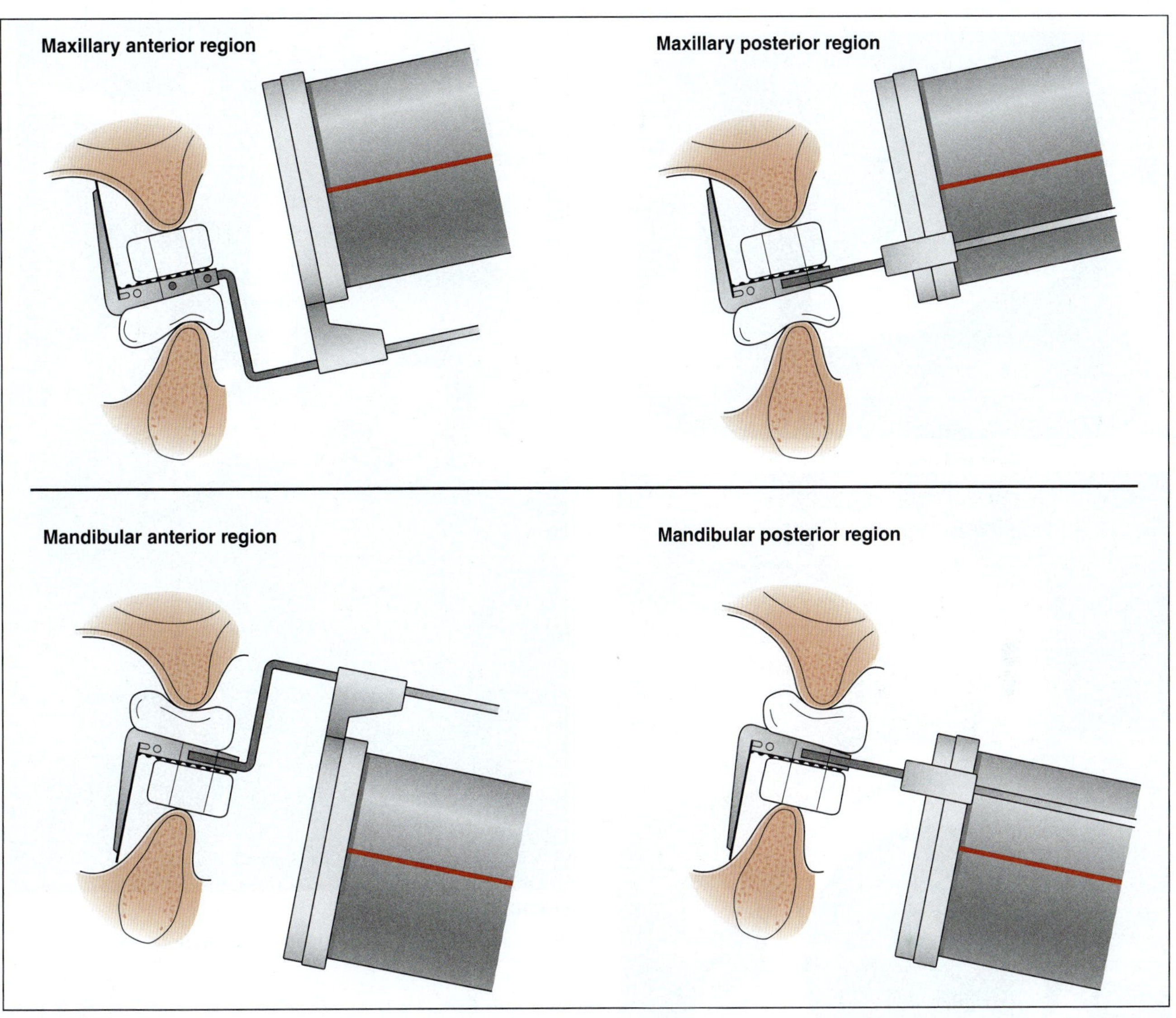

FIGURE 22-32

Radiographs of a full mouth series of an edentulous patient. Cone and film-holding device are positioned in four areas. Note: an additional bite block is secured to the Rinn bite block to provide the height that the teeth would normally provide. A cotton roll is placed on the opposite side to assist the patient in holding the bite block securely.

everyone involved. With other special needs patients, a parent or guardian may be asked to assist in holding the patient or the x-ray steady; however, every attempt should be made to expose the x-ray by another means. Work as quickly as possible. If it is impossible to expose a periapical film, an occlusal or a panoramic film may be substituted. Technique suggestions associated with treatment for special needs patients are as follows:

- Before treating special needs patients, discuss how to best handle them with the entire office. A good time to do this is during office meetings. The entire staff needs to work together to make these patients' visits as simple and comprehensive as possible.
- Prepare all areas in the office that the patient will be in before the appointment, including the reception and treatment rooms. For example, have extra radiation protection in the treatment room for the parent or guardian in case he or she has to hold the film in the patient's mouth.
- Call the patient, caregiver, or guardian in advance and ask for suggestions on how to best accommodate the patient's needs.
- Read about patients' conditions to better understand and communicate with them. For example, when working with a deaf patient, learn a few words in sign language.

Vision Impaired Patient. Patients who have vision impairment require clear verbal communications. Carefully explain exactly what is involved in the procedure, and what you are doing before you begin. Let them know anything they might feel or taste when possible. Check with them to see if they have any questions or concerns.

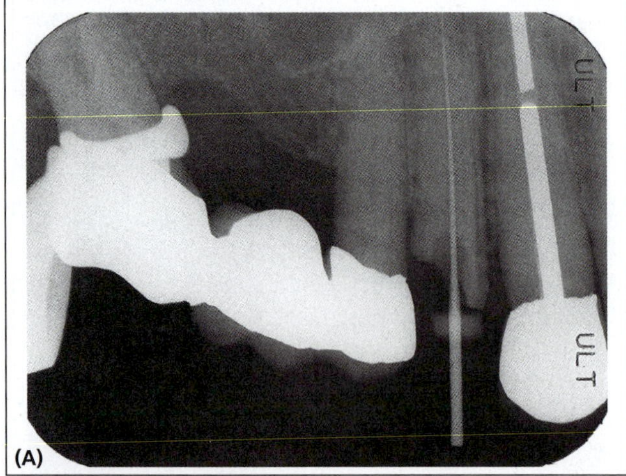

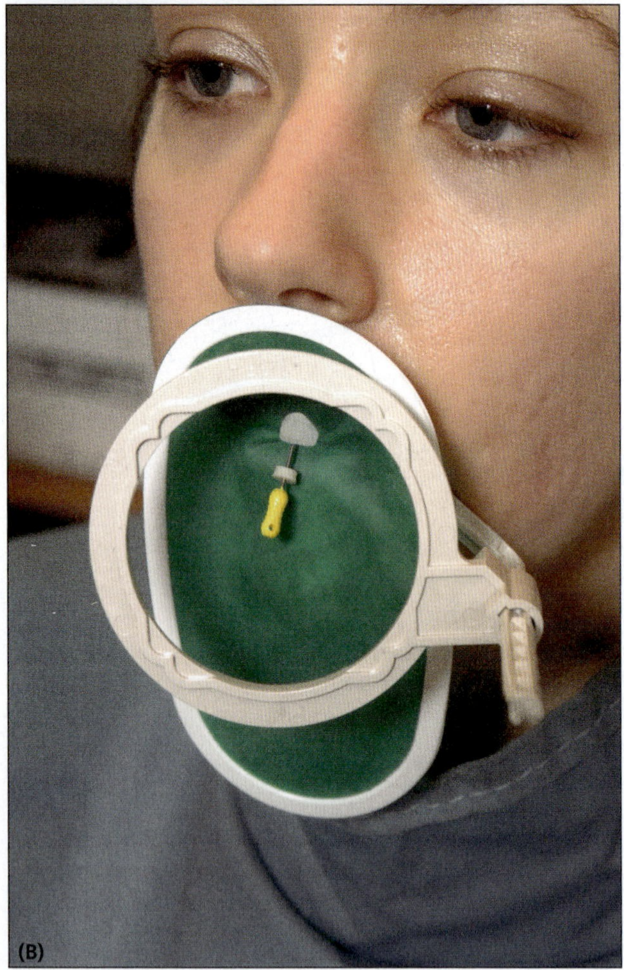

FIGURE 22-33

(A) When an x-ray is positioned for an endodontic radiograph, the patient does not close on the film holder because the reamer in the root canal is beyond the line of occlusion. The radiograph shows the reamer in place. (B) Patient with endodontic film holder positioned for exposure.

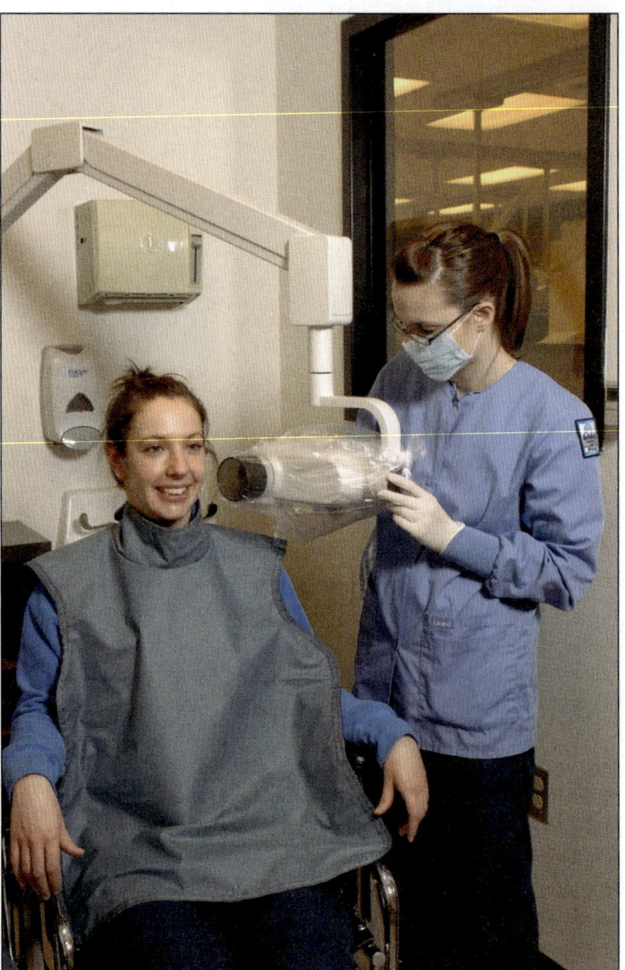

FIGURE 22-34

Wheelchair patient having intraoral radiographs taken.

Hearing Impaired Patient. Patients who have a hearing impairment may be able to lip read. If they can, remove your mask and speak slowly and clearly so that they can read your lips as you give them information. Written communication is another means for informing the patient about the procedure. Have the steps of the procedure listed for them to review, and ask if they have any questions. Learning a few terms in sign language is an excellent way to show the patient that you really care and you want to communicate something about the treatment he or she is receiving.

Processing Quality Radiographs

CDA Normally, the darkroom is in the center area of the dental office, or near the x-ray units for easy accessibility by dental assistants. It is a small room where x-ray processing (i.e., developing, fixing, and washing) can be accomplished. This room needs to be well ventilated and of an adequate size.

One of the main concerns of the darkroom is that it must exclude all white light. It is important that there is no light leaking in around doors, fans, and vents, because light harms the sensitive film emulsion during processing. Safelights must be used when the film packets are opened, when attaching the film to the racks, and during processing procedures. A safelight will not affect the film emulsion because it is in the red–orange spectrum. The film is much more sensitive to the blue–green spectrum, as the wavelengths are shorter. Safelight filters must be free of scratches and fit precisely. The safety lights should be mounted at least 4 feet from the counter surface where the films are unwrapped. A 15-watt incandescent bulb should be used. If the safelight must be mounted closer to the counter, a lower-watt bulb, such as 7.5 watts, needs to be used. When using indirect lighting, such as facing the light toward the ceiling, a 25-watt bulb may be used with the proper filters. It was once thought that the walls of the room should be painted black, but it is currently recommended that they be a light color to reflect the safelight. It is more important that the walls be washable because of the spills and splashes that take place during processing.

When processing films where an intensifying screen (a layer of fluorescent crystals found in cassettes used with extraoral films, see Chapter 23, Extraoral and Digital Radiography) has been used, a filter that eliminates more light must be used—a red filter should be used in place of the orange. Films that have been exposed with intensifying screens are more sensitive to light. Therefore, orange filters for the safelight should never be used for extraoral films. A good safelight filter to use with both intraoral films and extraoral screen films is the GBX-2 safelight filter manufactured by Kodak.

There are no recommendations for the overhead white light. It is, however, important that it provide proper illumination for the whole room, and that the switch not be placed where it could be turned on accidentally.

Many offices have viewboxes in their darkrooms so that x-rays can be read while still wet. This box should also be in an area where the switch cannot be turned on accidentally.

There may be a warning light outside the darkroom that indicates when x-ray processing is taking place. Also, it is advisable to have a lock on the door to prevent light exposure from the door being opened accidentally. A rotational darkroom door that allows access for individuals while maintaining darkness in the room can be used.

The darkroom must have a hot- and cold-water source, along with a drainage line. Thermostatic water controls are also necessary to control the intake waterline, and to enable adjustment of the water to maintain constant temperatures in the processing solutions. A large sink with a gooseneck faucet is recommended for use in replenishing and changing the processing solutions (Figure 22-35).

Manual Processing Equipment

The **manual processing** tanks should be made of stainless steel. The processing tank contains a large tank for the water bath, and two 1- or 2-gallon insert tanks (Figure 22-36). The water bath has an inlet valve where the water flows in, and an outlet valve or overflow pipe where the water escapes the tank. The tank comes with a tank cover that must be kept on

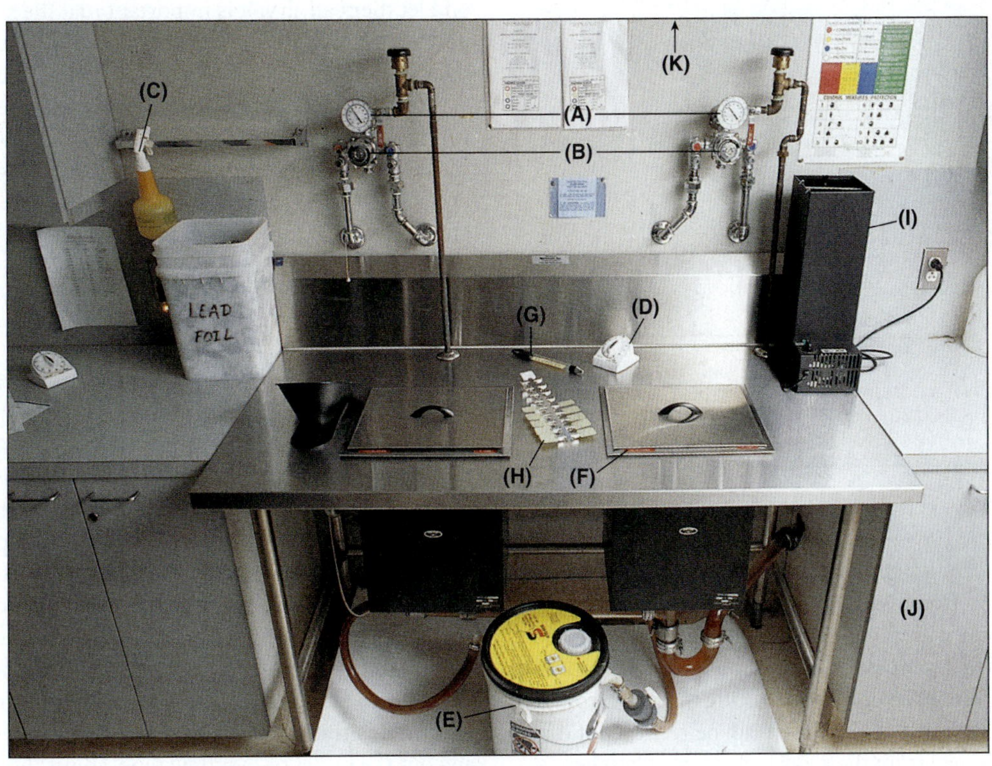

FIGURE 22-35

Manual processing room with equipment. (A) Thermostatic water gauge. (B) Thermostatic water control. (C) Disinfectant solution. (D) Timer. (E) Silver recovery unit. (F) Manual tank. (G) Floating thermometer. (H) X-rays on rack. (I) Dryer. (J) Storage for stirring rod, solutions, viewbox, and cleaning supplies. (K) The safelight is above the manual tanks.

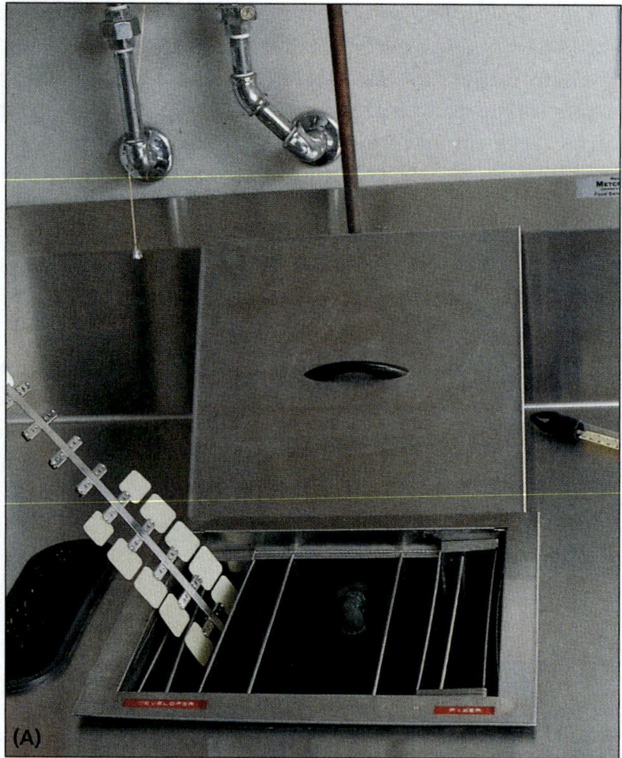

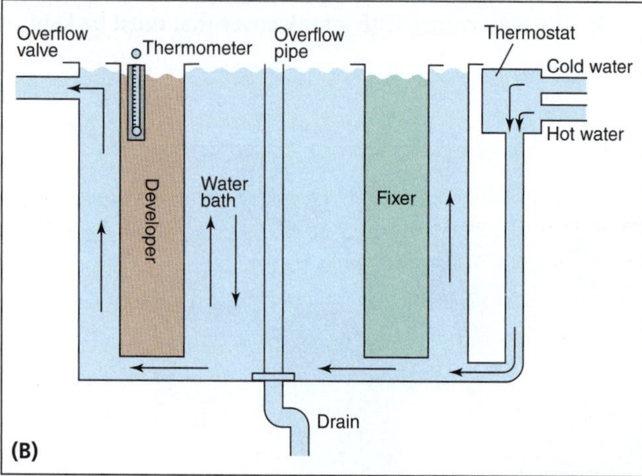

FIGURE 22-36

(A) A typical manual processing tank showing developer and fixer insert tanks in the water bath. (B) Line drawing of manual processing tank.

at all times, except when placing or removing films, to prevent the solution from oxidizing or evaporating. Many newer insert tanks come with film retrievers that slide into the insert tanks, and have bars across their tops for use in placement and removal. The film retriever is used to bring the x-ray from the bottom of the tank upward so that it can be retrieved if it has mistakenly loosened from the x-ray rack. Normally, when facing the processing tank, the developer is on the left side of the processing tank, and the fixer is on the right side. The insert tanks should never be interchanged due to the sensitivity of the processing solutions.

Other items needed in the darkroom are a thermometer, a timer, processing racks, stirring rods, a dryer, and brushes or sponges with long handles (refer back to Figure 22-35). The thermometer is designed so that it can be suspended in the developing solution. It is critical that the solution is checked before developing a set of x-rays. The dental assistant must know the precise temperature of the developer, rather than of the water surrounding the tanks or the incoming water. Because it takes time for the developer and the surrounding water temperature to equalize, it is important to check the developer solution each time.

No darkroom is complete without a timer. The correct monitoring of processing time is critical for producing quality x-rays. An accurate timer that can be set easily and has a loud alarm must be used.

Processing racks, sometimes called intraoral film hangers, come in a number of sizes, ranging from one to twenty clips. They are made of stainless steel and, except for the single film hanger, have equal numbers of clips on each side. If the film hanger has defective clips, it should be discarded, as it causes films to be lost, or it may scratch films on other racks.

Stirring rods or paddles are used first thing in the morning, and first thing in the afternoon, to stir the developer and fixer solution. They should be marked according to solution and not used interchangeably.

Dental x-ray dryers are used after the processing is complete. The x-rays are left on the racks and placed in the dryer, suspended from a rod over a fan and heat element to dry. This process takes between 15 and 20 minutes. An alternative to this procedure is to hang the x-rays from a towel rack or rod, and let them air dry. It is important that the x-rays not touch, and that the drying is out of the way in a clean area to prevent dust and other debris from collecting on the x-ray.

Long-handle brushes or sponges are used to clean the inside of the processing tanks. There should be one brush for the developing tank and one for the fixing tank. These brushes should be marked and never be interchanged. After use, they should be rinsed and stored separately.

Processing Preparation

The developing and fixing solutions are normally prepared from liquid concentrates, following the manufacturer's instructions. They come in two packs with color-coded lids and labels. Verify that the correct solution is placed in the proper tank to prevent chemical cross-contamination. After checking the date on the solution, carefully open the top and pour the developer into the developing tank. Add water, about 68°F or slightly cool to the touch, to the indicator line at the top of the tank. The fixer is prepared the same way. After the insert tanks are in the processing tank, start the water coming through the inlet valve. The water can run in fairly quickly during this time. When it is up to the point where it is flowing out the outlet or overflow pipe, adjust the water to a slow, steady flow. Then stir each insert tank with the appropriate stirring paddle to mix the chemicals completely. Check the temperature of the developing solution; if it is around 68°F, it is ready to process x-rays (Table 22-2). A time/temperature

TABLE 22-2 Processing Temperatures and Times

Time in Processing Steps Is in Minutes		
Temperature (°F)		**Developer**
Rinse	**Fixer**	**Wash**
80	5–6	2½
75	6–7	3
70	9–10	4
68	10	4½
65	10–12	6
½ for all		20 for all

chart appears on every developer/fixer solution package. Have the chart available in the darkroom for review. Charts may vary slightly from manufacturer to manufacturer.

The optimal temperature is from 68°F to 70°F. If the temperature goes 20°F up or down from the optimum, the chemicals in the solutions may be destroyed and will have to be discarded. It is necessary to change the solutions every 3 to 4 weeks to maintain optimal processing under normal use. With heavy use, change solutions more often.

Each day, a test film should be processed to compare to the film that was processed the first day the solutions were changed. If a change is seen in the processed films, then the solutions may not be effective. It is important to keep a log of the date that you last changed the solution. Also, check the solution visually to ensure that it is not cloudy or dark. This also may indicate that the solution must be changed.

Replenishing Processing Solutions. Processing solutions need to be maintained to ensure adequate strength, freshness, and solution levels. The dental assistant should **replenish** the developer and fixer solutions daily. The solution levels, especially the developing solution, are subject to reduction due to **oxidation**. Oxidation is a process where solutions combine with oxygen, which cause the solutions to lose strength and volume. Follow the manufacturer's directions to add fresh chemicals or replenishing chemistry. Replenishing the solutions will raise the solution levels and extend the life of the processing solutions. Manual processing solutions should be changed at least every 4 weeks, or as recommended by the processing chemical manufacturer.

Manual Film Processing Technique

After the solutions are stirred with the appropriate stirrers and the temperature in the developer is checked, it is ready to process x-rays (Procedure 22-6). The work area must be clean and dry. Obtain the correct processing rack, and write the patient's name, date, and number of x-rays on the identification tab at the top with a pencil. The x-rays themselves may be in a cup. If they have come directly from the patient's mouth, wear gloves while the x-rays are carefully unwrapped and placed on the racks. Do not touch any portion of the film directly. Other ways to handle the aseptic technique are to disinfect the x-rays before bringing them into the darkroom, or to use preplaced protective coverings on the films themselves, which are removed after exposure, and then to place the uncontaminated films in a cup ready for processing. It is not important which technique is used, but a standard policy must be followed so that cross-contamination does not take place.

The overhead light is turned off and the safety light is turned on. The door is locked, when possible. When the eyes are accustomed to the safety light, unwrap the film; pull back the plastic coating, the black paper, and the lead foil; and attach the film to the hanger. Hold the film by the edges to confirm that it is securely on the hanger. Place each film on the x-ray rack in the same manner. When this process is completed, lift the lid off the processor and place the rack in the developer solution. Be sure to agitate the films in the solution by quickly raising and lowering the films several times into the solution before attaching the rack to the side of the tank. This ensures that the films are bathed totally in the solution, and that no bubbles are on the surface of the film. Place the lid on the processing tank and wait for 4 minutes if the temperature is at 70°F. The timer should be set immediately after the lid is on. When the time is up, open the lid cover (safety lights only) and lift the rack from the developer. Carefully shake off excess solution, and then place the rack in the water bath solution. The x-ray films must be rinsed for at least 30 seconds in the running water (middle portion of the tank). The rinsing stops the process of the developing solution. After 30 seconds, raise the rack and let the excess water drain off. Place the film in the fixer insert tank. The tank cover is then replaced over the tank and the timer is set again. The time for processing in the fixer is twice that of the developer; therefore, process for 8 minutes at 70°F. After the fixing time is complete, the films are removed from the fixer solution and placed in the wash bath in the center of the tank for the final rinse. The films are rinsed with clear-running water for about 20 minutes. When this is complete, the films are removed and hung from a towel rack, or placed in an electric dryer for 15 to 20 minutes. The films are then ready for mounting.

Composition of Processing Solutions

Film processing involves a series of steps that convert an invisible latent image on the dental x-ray film to a visible permanent image on the dental radiograph. The diagnostic quality of the radiograph image depends on properly following the detailed steps involved in processing these films. In this section, the role of film processing solutions will be discussed, and manual and automatic processing equipment and techniques will be identified.

The Developer. The **developer solution** has a pH of above 7 and chemically reduces the exposed area of the emulsion, making it visible to the naked eye. The pH scale is from 0 to 14, with pH 7 being neutral. Anything with a pH value below 7 is considered acidic, and anything with a pH value above 7 is considered alkaline.

Procedure 22-6
Processing Radiographs Using a Manual Tank

This procedure is performed by the dental assistant. The assistant prepares the equipment, supplies, and area. The exposed radiographs are taken to the darkroom by the dental assistant to process.

Equipment and Supplies (*Figure 22-36*)

- Barriers for the darkroom counter
- Exposed radiographs
- X-ray rack
- Processing tank
- Safelight(s)
- Timer
- Thermometer
- Pencil
- Electric film dryer

Procedure Steps (*Follow aseptic procedures*)

1. Wash and dry hands (gloves must be worn if the x-rays are contaminated).
2. Make sure the area is clean and free of splashes. Place barriers on the counter in the darkroom.
3. Check the temperature of the developer with the thermometer. Also, check the processing chart for the corresponding temperature and time information.
4. Check the volumes of the processing solutions to ensure that they do not need replenishing. Replenish if necessary.
5. Stir the developer and fixer when the first processing is being completed that morning or afternoon. Stir the solutions with the corresponding stirring rods. Do not interchange.
6. Check the x-ray rack to ensure that the clips are in working order.
7. Label the x-ray rack in pencil with the patient's name, date of exposure, and the number of x-rays taken.
8. Turn on the safelights and turn off the white lights.
9. Remove the films from their wrappers and place on the x-ray racks. Use gloves if the x-rays are contaminated.
10. Check each film to make sure it is attached securely and placed in a parallel manner so that it is not touching the adjacent film.
11. Place in the developer tank and agitate the rack slightly in the developing solution to eliminate bubbles on the surface of the emulsion.
12. Place the tank cover on the processing tank. Set the timer for 4 minutes if the temperature of the developer is at 70°F. The area can be cleaned up, and the barrier and x-ray wrappers disposed of.
13. When the timer goes off, remove the x-ray rack from the developer, letting the excess solution drip into the developer prior to placing the rack in the running water (the middle area in the processing tank). Let it rinse for 30 seconds.
14. Remove the x-ray rack from the rinsing area, let the excess water drip off, and then immerse the rack in the fixing solution for 8 minutes. If the dentist must view the patient's x-rays, they can be removed after 3 minutes, and then returned to the fixer later for the remaining time.
15. Replace the processing lid and set the timer for 8 minutes.
16. After 8 minutes, remove the x-ray rack from the fixer and place it in the running water at the center of the processing tank. The final wash takes 20 minutes to complete.
17. The rack of x-rays can be removed from the water after 20 minutes and placed in an x-ray dryer for an additional 15 to 20 minutes or until drying is complete.
18. When the x-rays are dry, remove them from the rack and place them in a labeled x-ray mount.

The following components make up the developing solution: hydroquinone, elon, sodium carbonate, sodium sulfite, potassium bromide, and water.

- **Hydroquinone** is extremely sensitive to changes in temperature, and is inactive when the temperature is below 60°F. Hydroquinone is a reducing agent, or a chemical that blackens exposed silver halide crystals. Even though this chemical acts slowly, the image gains density steadily during the developing process. Hydroquinone is responsible primarily for the film contrast.

- **Elon** is a reducer that also blackens the exposed silver halide crystals. Elon is not affected greatly by temperature changes. It acts quickly, and is responsible for giving detail to the film. Reducers develop only in an alkaline medium.
- **Sodium carbonate** is often used as the alkaline medium in the developer. It softens and swells the emulsion so that the reducers can reach the silver crystals. If the solution has too much alkaline medium, over swelling of the emulsion takes place, causing blisters on the film.

The reducer and alkaline medium are affected by oxygen. The oxygen in the air and solution can spoil the developer. Therefore, a preservative is used to slow this process.

- **Sodium sulfite** prevents oxidation and increases the life span of the developing solution by 2 to 4 weeks.
- If the chemicals work too fast, a film fog appears and the x-rays are unclear. A restrainer such as **potassium bromide** is used to slow the developing process to a practical speed and prevent film fog.
- The last ingredient used to mix all these chemicals is water. Distilled water is recommended so that no additional chemicals are brought into the developing solution.

Fixer Solution. The **fixer solution** removes the unexposed and undeveloped crystals from the film emulsion, and stops the developing process. The following components make up the fixer solution: sodium thiosulfate, acetic acid, sodium sulfite, potassium alum, and water.

- **Sodium thiosulfate**, or hyposulfite, is known as the "hypo" agent. It is responsible for removing the unexposed and undeveloped crystals from the film.
- The chemical that stops the developing action, and provides the required acidity for sodium thiosulfate to work is **acetic acid**. The third chemical in the fixer is sodium sulfite, and it works much as it does in the developer, by preserving the solution and preventing oxidation.
- **Potassium alum** is the chemical that shrinks and hardens the emulsion gelatin. This hardening process protects the film from abrasion, and helps the film to dry more quickly.
- The final ingredient is water. It is used as a medium to incorporate the chemicals. It is not as critical to have distilled water in the fixer as it is in the developer.

Used fixer solution stains clothing. The silver salts accumulate in it and form spots that may not show up until after the garment is laundered. If the fixer solution has spotted the clothing before being washed, rinse it first in unused fixer solution, and then thoroughly rinse it with water before laundering. There are several products on the market for treating stains on dental uniforms.

Disposing of the Fixer and Developer (OSHA Guidelines). Disposal of the fixer and developer solution must follow OSHA hazardous waste guidelines. Silver is in the fixer solution and must be disposed of properly. It cannot be washed down the sink. Both the used developer and fixer solution should be put in a leak-proof container and disposed of by a company specializing in biohazard waste. The fixer solution can be treated in the dental office if the office has a silver recovery unit in place. The recovery units are used to remove hazardous silver ions before allowing the fixer solution to go down the drain. Used fixer solution is circulated through a cartridge within the silver recovery unit. Once the cartridge is saturated, it is removed by a commercial waste disposal company, and a new cartridge is put in place.

The lead in the film packet is also a hazardous material. The lead can be saved in a container and sold, along with the recovered silver, to a metal recycling company.

The dental office should retain receipts of developer and fixer solution disposal in order to prove proper disposal of hazardous wastes.

Automatic Processing

Automatic processors are used in most dental offices (Figure 22-37A). Automatic processors are easy to use and reduce processing time. The x-rays are consistently of a good quality. Most processors are compact and require minimal darkroom space. If space in the darkroom is a problem, some processors have daylight-loading units that can be added (Figure 22-37B). With the daylight-loading units, the processors can be placed wherever they are convenient to use. One important factor to consider when using automatic processors is that maintenance of the units and daily chemical control are essential.

Although **automatic processing** follows the same basic sequence as manual processing, the order in which the film is placed in solutions differs (Procedure 22-7). With automatic processors, a series of rollers or guides move the x-ray film through the developing compartment, the fixing compartment, the water compartment, and, last, the drying compartment before depositing it onto a tray (Figure 22-38).

The rollers/guides are moved by gears, belts, or chains that must be lubricated and maintained according to the manufacturer's instructions. The x-ray film is processed in 4 to 7 minutes, depending on the temperature of the developing solution. The temperature also determines the speed at which the rollers/guides are set. Automatic processing is done between 82°F and 95°F. This increase in temperature greatly reduces total processing time. The rollers/guides move the film through each compartment, and also squeeze off the excess solution between compartments. This prevents processing chemicals from being carried into the next stage of processing.

Automatic Processing Solutions. Automatic processing solutions are designed specifically for automatic processors and are not interchangeable with solutions used for manual processing. In automatic processing solutions, the developer has chemicals added to prevent the emulsion from becoming soft and sticking to the rollers. The solution also has an agent that reduces the swelling of the emulsion so that the films will not absorb too much developing solution. Automatic processing solutions are used to replenish the processor solutions daily. Some machines have the ability to replenish the solutions automatically each time a film is fed into the unit.

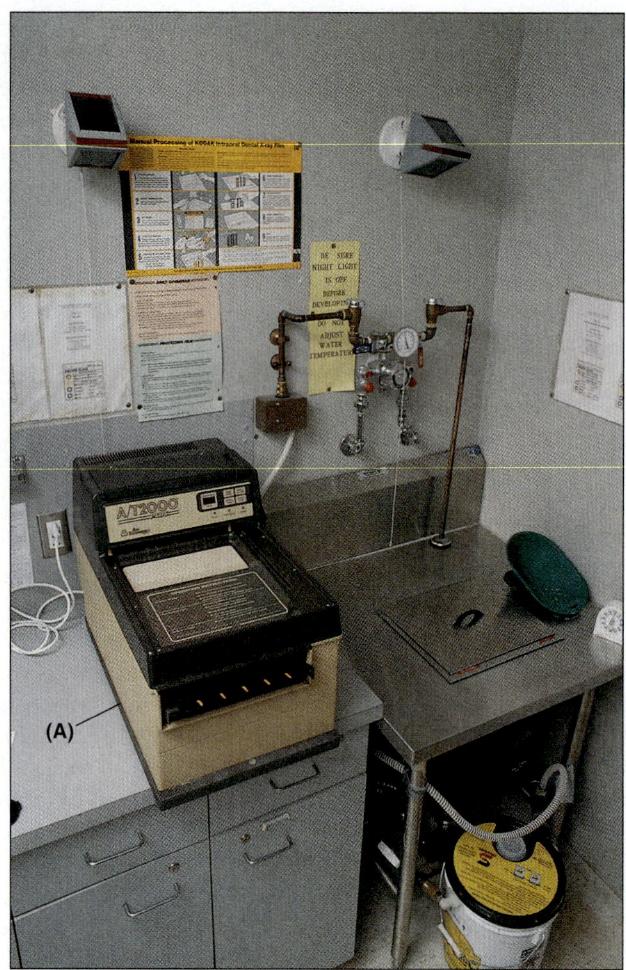

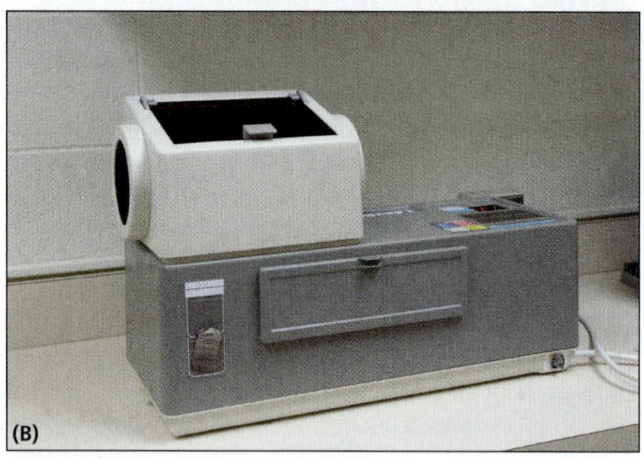

FIGURE 22-37

(A) Automatic film processor without daylight loader. (B) Automatic film processor with daylight loader.

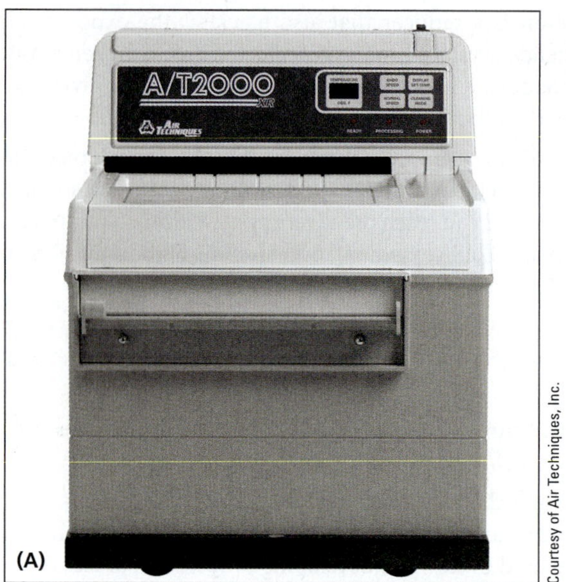

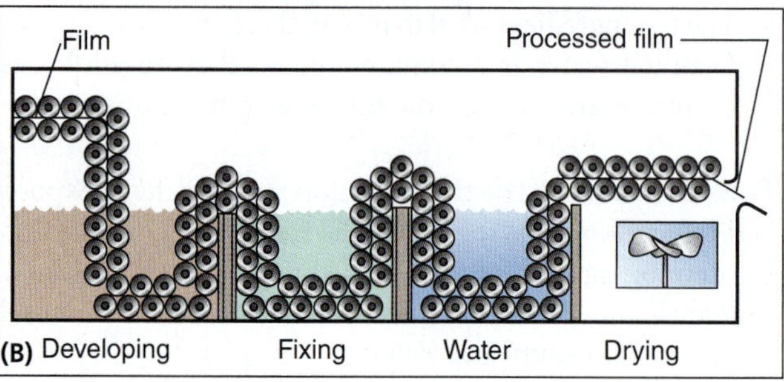

FIGURE 22-38

(A) Automatic film processor. (B) Drawing of the inside of a typical automatic film processor.

Care of Automatic Processors. Proper care of automatic processors is critical. To ensure quality x-ray film processing, daily and weekly maintenance procedures must be followed. Read the manufacturer's instructions and set a schedule for maintenance. Designate a staff member to be the "quality assurance controller" for x-ray processing. A few general guidelines are as follows:

- Every morning, check the solution levels and add solutions where needed. Turn the water on so that fresh water is running continuously, or place fresh water in those units without a water hookup. Place the lid on securely and run a panoramic film through the processor to remove any debris.
- Turn off the water every night. Lift the lid and place it slightly ajar to prevent fumes from accumulating and condensing, which can cause films to fog, and to prevent processor motor problems.
- Rinse the rollers with warm water, weekly, and then soak them as recommended by the manufacturer.
- Solutions should be changed every 2 to 6 weeks, depending on use and how often the solutions have been replenished. The cleaning solutions recommended by the manufacturer should be used routinely.
- Rinse the rollers completely before replacing them in the compartments. Each compartment has a plug that needs to be secure before the tanks are filled.

Mounting Radiographs

Each radiograph has a raised dot to facilitate the mounting process. The film pack is placed in the patient's mouth so that the raised dot, or convex side, is toward the x-ray cone. Mounting the radiographs so that the dot is toward the operator means that the operator is looking at the film as if the

Procedure 22-7

Processing Radiographs Using an Automatic Processor

This procedure is performed by the dental assistant. The dental assistant prepares the equipment, supplies, and work area. The exposed radiographs are taken to the automatic processor by the dental assistant to process.

Equipment and Supplies

- Exposed radiographs
- Automatic x-ray processor with daylight loader

Procedure Steps (*Follow aseptic procedures*)

1. Turn on the automatic x-ray processor at the beginning of each day. This ensures that it is warmed up and ready to process after the x-rays are exposed. The chemicals must be heated to the correct temperatures or the x-rays will appear light, and the diagnostic quality will be diminished.
2. Wash and dry hands.
3. Place exposed radiographs in the daylight loader with two additional containers/cups.
4. Don gloves, and position gloved hands through the sleeves of the daylight loader.
5. Remove each radiograph from its packet, and place the film in one uncontaminated container. Be careful not to touch and contaminate the film as the packet is removed.
6. Place the empty packets in the other container/cup.
7. After all x-rays are unwrapped, remove the gloves and place them in the contaminated container with the empty packets.
8. With clean hands, feed the unwrapped films into the machine slowly. Start on one side of the processor and rotate to the other side. Repeat. If using a film holder, place all films in the holder and release for processing. Continue until all films are placed in the processor. Remove your hands from the sleeves of the daylight loader.
9. Open the top of the daylight loader and carefully gather the cups with film wrappers and gloves and dispose of them.
10. Remove processed films from the outlet area, and place in a labeled x-ray mount.

operator were facing the patient. The patient's left side would be on the operator's right side facing the film mount. This type of mounting is called labial mounting (Procedure 22-8). The ADA recommends that dental offices use labial mounting. An x-ray **viewbox** may be used to mount dental radiographs. A viewbox is a lighted box that has a white, frosted surface so that x-rays can be viewed easily for diagnostic purposes (Figure 22-39).

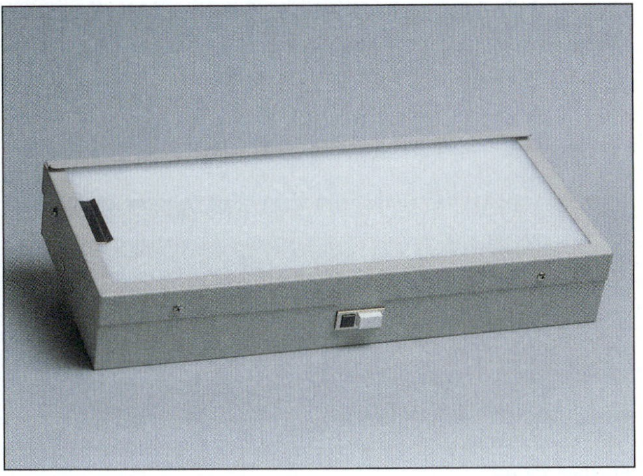

FIGURE 22-39
Dental x-ray viewbox used when mounting processed x-rays.

In the other type of mounting, called lingual mounting, the depressed dot (concave side) is toward the operator, therefore, the operator views the films from the inside out, or from a position inside the oral cavity looking outward. This type of mounting has the patient's left side on the operator's left side. Both systems of mounting are used in dental offices today; however, the labial system is more common.

A number of different mounts are available (Figure 22-40). The sizes range as follows: 1, 2, 4, 7, 14, 16, 18, 20, and 28 windows. Bitewing x-ray mounts normally come in 2 or 4 windows. The 14- or 16-window mounts are used most commonly for periapical mounts. The 18- or 20-window mounts are used most often for full-mouth (both periapical and bitewing) mounting.

Mounts can be purchased in a number of different materials. They should be stiff enough to keep the films rigid and hold them securely in place. The most commonly used mounts are made from plastic or cardboard. The plastic mounts come in clear, frosted, or dark colors. The advantage of plastic mounts is that they are water repellant and can be reused. The disadvantages are that the plastic mounts can crack or split and, if the operator uses the clear mounts, they can give off a glare around the films and inhibit diagnosis (the frosted and dark mounts cut glare).

The cardboard mount is normally less expensive than the plastic mounts and blocks out any glare around the film. It

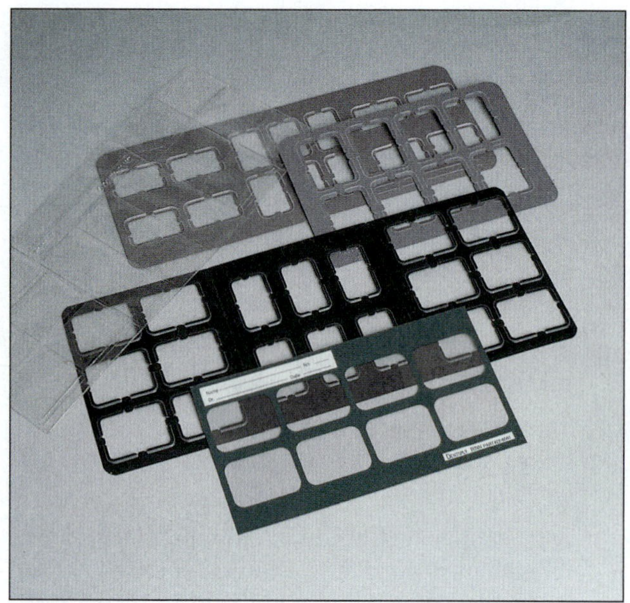

FIGURE 22-40
Various full-mouth, bitewing, and single-film mounts.

can be reused if a pencil is used to write in the patient's name. The cardboard mounts have an area for each film to slide into place. Some operators prefer one type of mount to the other. The disadvantages of a cardboard mount are that it is not water resistant, and it bends and breaks easily. The operator can determine which mount to use.

After selecting the correct mount, place the x-rays on a clean counter in front of a viewbox. If mounting a full-mouth set of x-rays, divide the x-rays into three groups: bitewings, anterior periapicals, and posterior periapicals. It is easy to identify the bitewing x-rays because they have both the crowns of the mandibular and the maxillary teeth on them. Individuals may find it easier to mount the bitewing x-rays first to reference them for the placement of the periapicals. However, there is no set pattern for which x-rays should be mounted.

The four bitewing x-rays are mounted so that the molar x-rays are on the outside and the corresponding bicuspid x-rays are on the inside, just as if looking directly at the patient (Figure 22-41). Note the curve of Spee (or formation of a smile pattern), which comes from the curvature of the mandible on correctly mounted x-rays. Check carefully that the dots are convex, the molars are on the outside, the bicuspids are on the inside, and the occlusal plane is curved in a smile pattern.

Now mount the anterior periapical x-rays. The maxillary anterior teeth are always larger and wider than the mandibular anterior teeth. The maxillary central teeth are normally the easiest to identify. Locate them and place them in the full-mouth mount in the center upper portion. They should be placed as they are positioned in the mouth, with the incisal edge in the middle of the mount and the roots toward the outside of the mount. Find the mandibular central x-rays (they will appear to have the smallest teeth on them), and place them directly below the maxillary teeth with the incisal edges toward each other. There are four canine x-rays (two maxillary and two mandibular) left to mount. Look for the maxillary canines first. They will appear larger, and may show the maxillary sinuses near the distal side of the apex of the roots. Remember that the roots always tend to curve distally. Mount both the maxillary and the mandibular canine x-rays in the correct position, with the lateral sides toward the centrals and the bicuspid sides outward. Make sure that all the incisal edges come together in the middle, just like the mouth does.

The mandibular and maxillary posterior films are differentiated from each other on the basis of root and crown shape, along with anatomic landmarks. The maxillary posterior x-rays may show the nasal cavity or sinuses. The maxillary premolars usually have two roots, and the molars have three roots. The roots of the maxillary molars may look unclear because of the lingual root showing through the mesial and distal roots. Mount the maxillary molars on the upper part of the mount toward the outside. The bicuspids will be placed between the molars and the anterior canines. The bicuspid and molar x-rays that have been placed in the mount must match each other, as should the corresponding crowns of the bitewing x-rays. Identify the same restoration in several x-rays; it may be from different angles, but it still should appear similar. The mandibular periapical x-rays should be mounted in much the same manner as the maxillary. The molars will have two roots that are more clearly defined than the maxillary; the bicuspids will have one root. After all the x-rays are in the mount, do a quick check to see whether all the x-rays are mounted similar to the position of the teeth in the mouth (Figure 22-42). Several practices may be necessary to be able to quickly identify any incorrectly mounted x-rays, and to be able to replace them correctly.

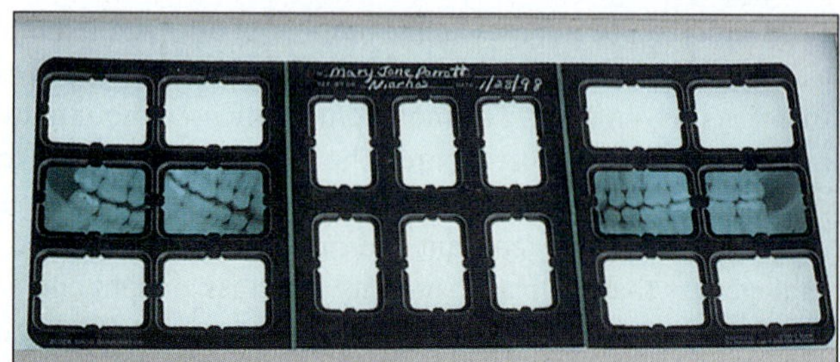

FIGURE 22-41
Full-mouth mount with bitewing x-rays in place.

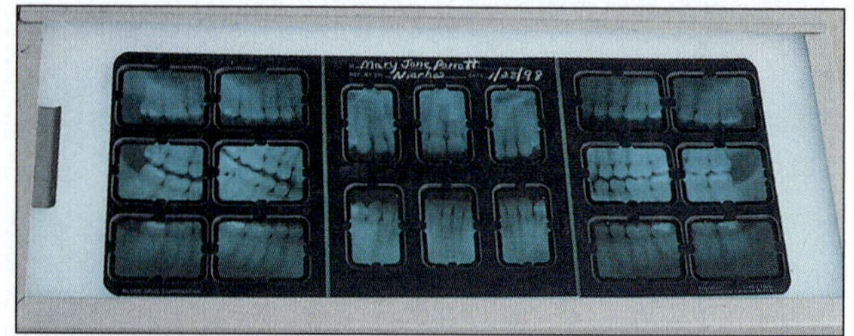

FIGURE 22-42
Full-mouth x-rays mounted with correct placement references.

Procedure 22-8
Mounting Radiographs

This procedure is performed by the dental assistant. A viewbox may be utilized when mounting the radiographs.

Equipment and Supplies

- Radiographs
- Lighted viewbox
- X-ray mount (using full-mouth, 18 x-ray mount)
- Clean, dry surface

Procedure Steps (*Follow aseptic procedures*)

1. Wash and dry hands.
2. Label the x-ray mount with the patient's name and the date of the exposure (in pencil).
3. Turn on the viewbox (optional).
4. Place the radiographs on a clean surface so that all dots are convex or outward to the viewer.
5. Using the viewbox, categorize all x-rays into three groups: bitewings (four in number), anterior (six in number), and posterior (eight in number).
6. Place the bitewing x-rays in the mount, making sure the dots remain convex, the molars are toward the outside, and the bicuspids (premolars) are toward the inside. Make sure that the x-rays are mounted according to the curve of Spee.
7. Put the anterior x-rays in place, with the maxillary above and the mandibular below. The incisal edges should be closest to each other in the mount, and the roots positioned as they grow. The centrals are placed in the middle with the canines on the outer sides. The maxillary centrals are much larger than the mandibular centrals.
8. Place the remaining posterior x-rays. The molars should be placed toward the outside, and the bicuspids (premolars) toward the inside. The maxillary molars have three roots and the mandibular molars have two roots. Both should be placed according to their position in the mouth, with the roots opposite each other and the biting surfaces more closely positioned.
9. Review the mounted x-rays to verify that they have been placed properly.

Common Radiographic Errors

Errors during exposure and processing of radiographs are inevitable, especially when learning. Understanding basic principles and practices helps to produce quality diagnostic x-rays. Practice on manikins to gain experience and prevent errors. Perfect your x-ray technique and skills in order to reduce the number of unnecessary retakes, which expose the patient to more radiation and require more time for everyone. To avoid common radiographic errors, it is necessary to understand what constitutes a quality x-ray.

Correct assembly of the film-holding device eliminates many errors. Be sure the bite block is in the correct position for the corresponding arch. Also, be sure that the film is centered in the indicating ring. Select the correct size film to cover the area that will be exposed. If the film is too small, the apex may be cut off. If the film is too large, it may be difficult for the patient to hold, and the x-ray may be distorted. When the film is placed properly in the mouth, a 1- to 3-mm edge of the film should show beyond the occlusal/incisal surface of the tooth. If a hemostat or Snap-a-Ray film holder is used, be sure to hold the film at the edge, touching it just enough to hold the film secure.

Common Exposure Errors

Common exposure errors involve positioning of the film in the patient's mouth, or the position of the cone in relationship to the teeth and the film. Other errors are nonexposure of the film or double-exposing the film. The patient needs to remain immobile during exposure to prevent a blurred image, and the x-ray machine must be set correctly to match the type of film being exposed.

Distortion. Sometimes the film will bend or curve on the palate and in the canine area on the mandible; when the film bends, the image distorts. During film placement, the film may crease. These crease marks show on the processed film as black lines (artifacts). Adjust the film position farther into the mouth, toward the midline of the palate of the maxillary, and push the tongue gently so that the film is between the tongue and the mandible (Figures 22-43 and 22-44).

Elongation. An **elongation**, a vertical angulation error, is caused by too little angulation, meaning that there is too little positive angulation on the maxillary or too little negative angulation on the mandibular. This error occurs more

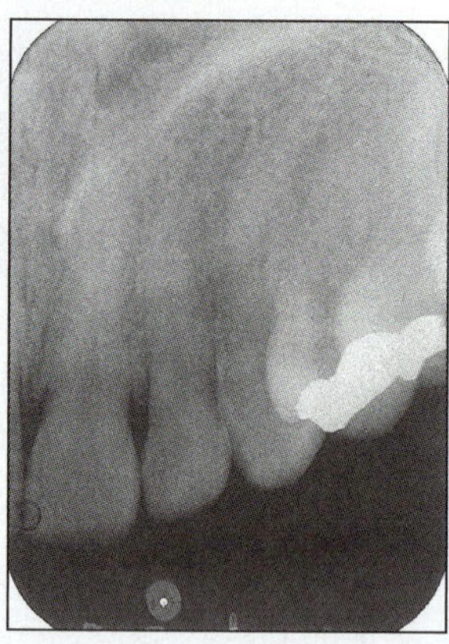

FIGURE 22-43
A curved film distorts radiograph images.

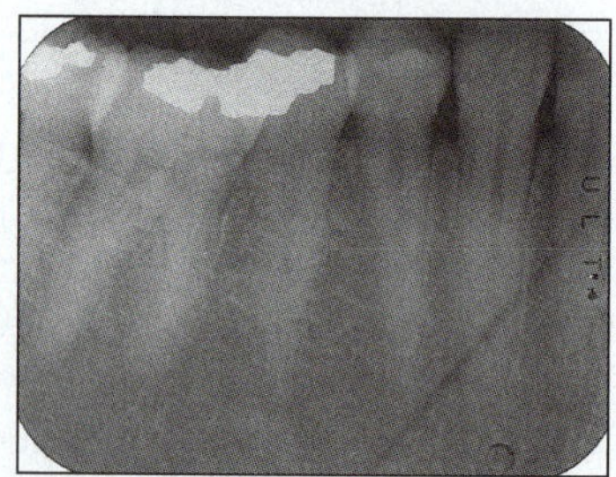

FIGURE 22-44
A bent film appears as a black crease or a thin, dark, radiolucent line.

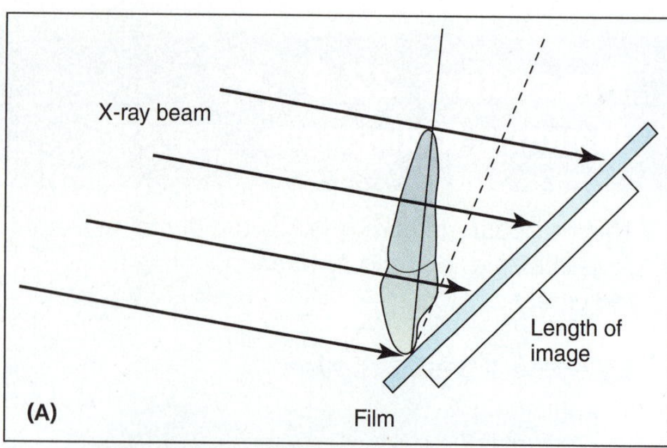

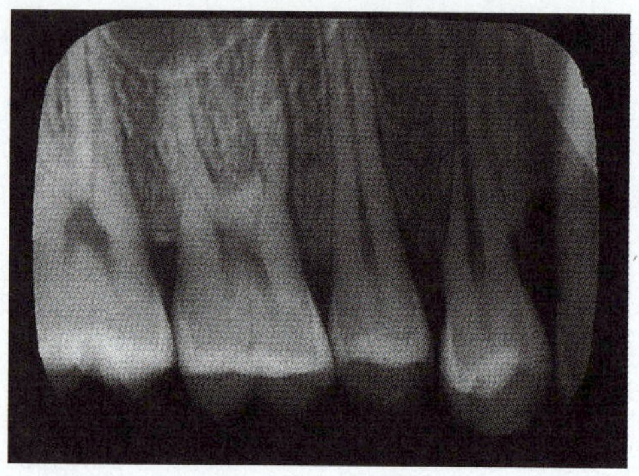

(B)

FIGURE 22-45
(A) The diagram shows how a film is elongated. (B) Elongation on a radiograph.

often when using the bisecting technique. In the paralleling technique, elongation is minimized if the cone end is positioned evenly against the indicating ring, and the film is placed correctly.

> Paralleling instruments are aids, but evaluate each cone placement. Sometimes the angulation may need to be slightly increased or decreased from the guides (Figure 22-45).

Foreshortening. A **foreshortening** is also a vertical angulation error. Foreshortening is the opposite of elongation and is caused by too much angulation. This error also occurs more often with the bisecting technique, and can be corrected by decreasing the vertical angulation. If the paralleling technique is used, align the cone with the film holder (Figure 22-46).

Overlapping. An **overlapping** is caused by incorrect horizontal angulation. When the cone is angled toward the mesial or the distal surfaces of the teeth instead of the interproximal areas, overlapping occurs. The cone/central ray should be directed straight at the teeth, and at a 90° angle to the film in order to keep the contacts open. Remember to evaluate the film placement in regard to the curve of the arch, not the contour of the patient's face (cheeks) (Figure 22-47).

Cone Cutting. A **cone cutting** error means that the x-ray beam missed part of the film, causing the film to be only partially exposed. Because the cone is lead-lined, the shape of the cone cut on the film will match the shape of the cone (either round or rectangular). Be sure that the x-ray film is placed in line with the center of the cone (Figure 22-48).

Clear Film/Absence of Image. If there is no image on the film and it is **clear film**, the film may not have been exposed (Figure 22-49). Check the x-ray machine to verify that it was turned on. If it was, then it may be malfunctioning and needs to be repaired. Another possible explanation for the clear film is that, if the exposure routine was interrupted, an unexposed film may have been placed with the exposed films. Other possible causes are that the film may have been placed in the fixer first, or, if the film had been placed in a warm water rinse, the emulsion might have dissolved. Always check to see which tank contains the developer and which one contains the fixer. Remove films from the water bath at the end of the washing period.

Double Exposure. Sometimes, inadvertently, film is exposed twice. This can be avoided by keeping exposed film separate from unexposed film. A **double exposure** results in indistinct images, or dark x-rays. When examining the film closely, two images can be seen. Establishing a routine can help avoid double-exposed films (Figure 22-50).

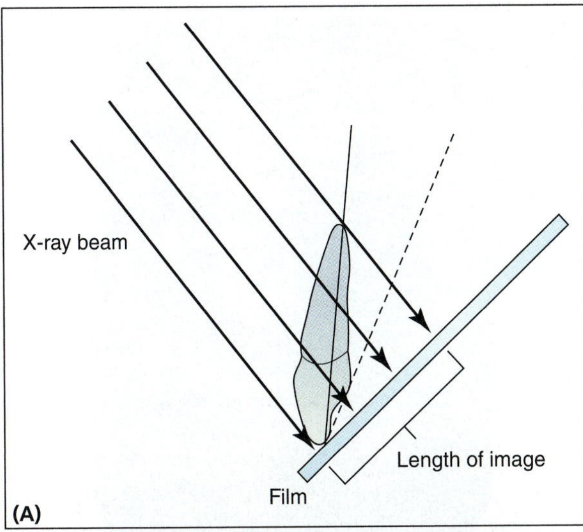

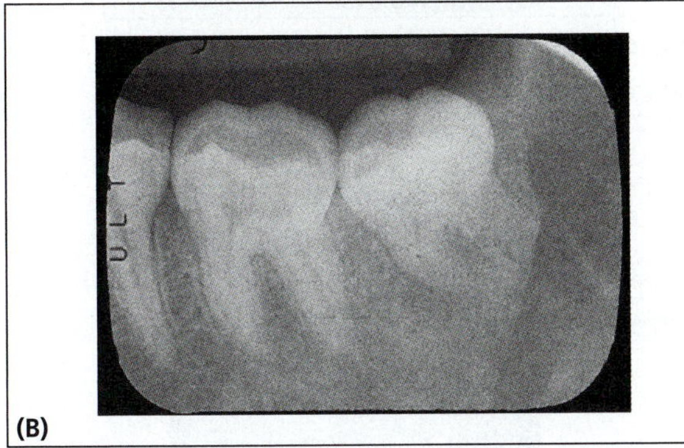

FIGURE 22-46

(A) The diagram shows how a film is foreshortened.
(B) Foreshortening on a radiograph.

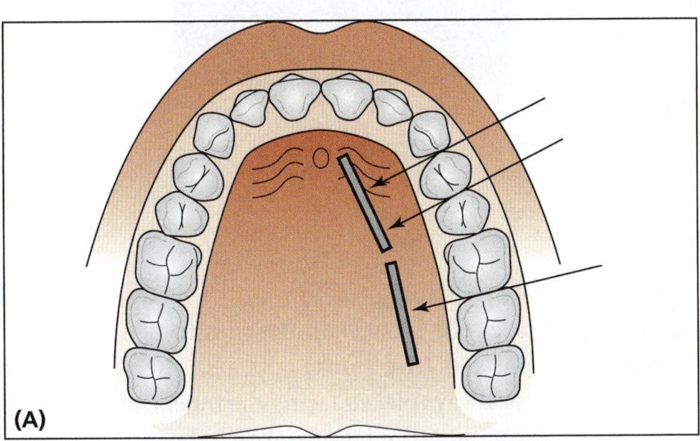

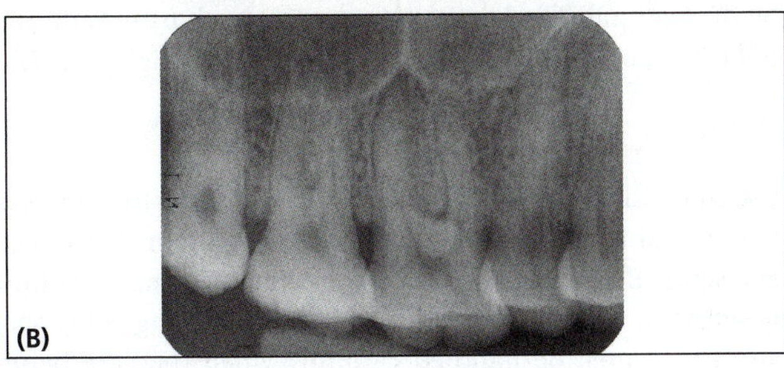

FIGURE 22-47

(A) The diagram shows the position of an x-ray beam to prevent overlapping. (B) Overlapping.

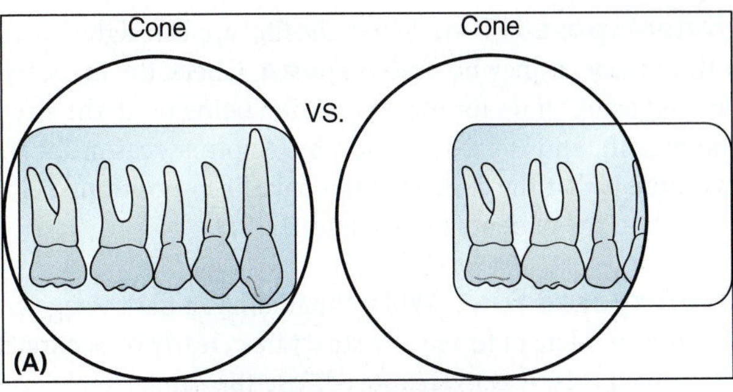

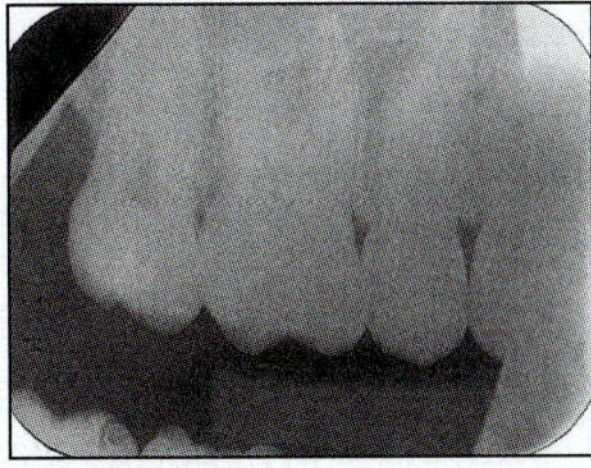

FIGURE 22-48

(A) The diagram shows correct and incorrect positions of a cone to prevent cone cutting. (B) Cone cut.

FIGURE 22-49

Clear film. This film has not been exposed to x-rays.

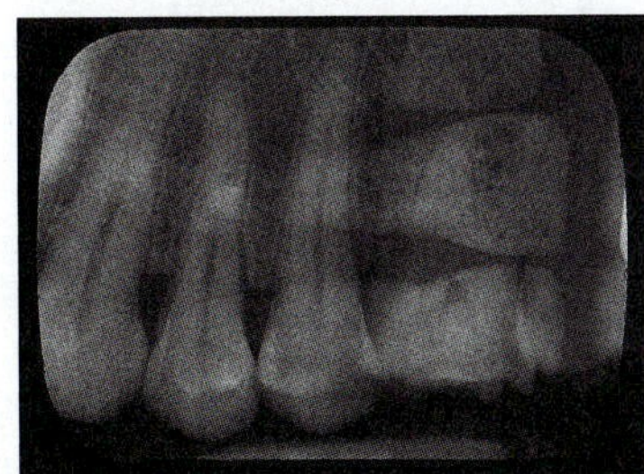

FIGURE 22-50

Double exposure. A film was exposed twice, with each exposure shown on the x-ray film.

Blurred Image. A **blurred image** results from movement of the patient's head or the tubehead, or from the x-ray film moving in the patient's mouth. The images are undefined and unclear. Be sure the patient can hold the film in place, and hold still for the exposure. Also, make sure the tubehead is still before leaving the room.

Underexposed Film. When the film appears light and has a thin image, it may be **underexposed**. Check the mAs, kVs, and exposure times for the type of film being used, the size of the patient, and the x-ray machine. Another reason for this outcome is that the cone may not have been positioned close enough to the patient's face (Figure 22-51).

Overexposed Film. When the film has a dark image and is too dark (dense) to see any structures clearly or accurately for a diagnosis, it is overexposed. Use the same checks used for light film images (Figure 22-52).

Film Artifacts. A **film artifact** is an image found on an x-ray other than normal anatomy and pathology. These images may be radiopaque or radiolucent and include the following:

- Artifacts found on x-rays include removable appliances that were not removed before exposure (e.g., partials or space maintainers). Sometimes the patient's glasses, earrings, or facial jewelry will show on the x-ray (Figure 22-53).
- Fluoride ions on gloves that are transferred to the film during handling leave dark fingerprint smudge marks (Figure 22-54).
- X-rays that overlap (touch) during processing leave an artifact on the film. The artifact will often be a straight line or in the shape of the edge or corner of the film (Figure 22-55).
- If the films are roughly handled before processing, a black crescent mark on the film may be caused by the operator's fingernail (Figure 22-56).

FIGURE 22-51
With underexposed film, the image appears light.

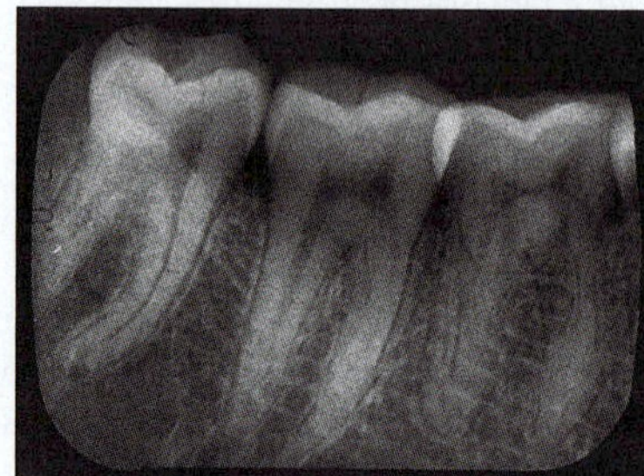

FIGURE 22-52
With overexposed film, the image appears dark.

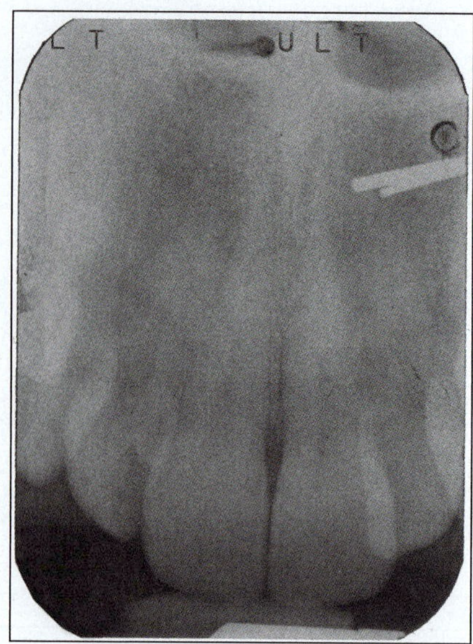

FIGURE 22-53
An x-ray with an artifact.

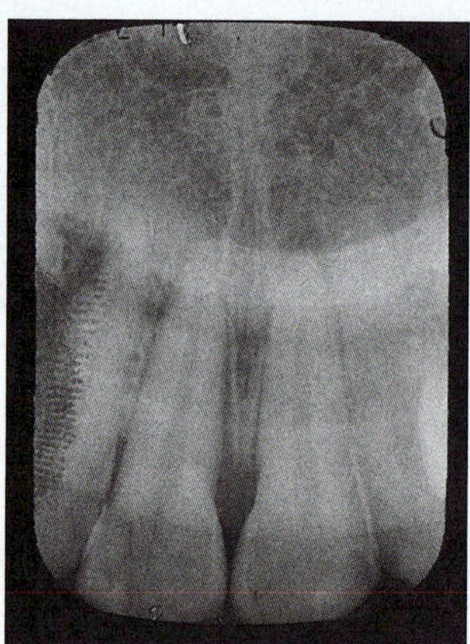

FIGURE 22-54
A fingerprint from fluoride ions on an x-ray.

Backward Film. Placing the film in the mouth backward or reversed causes the images on the film to be light, and a **herringbone pattern** (tire track) appears. The white, plain side of the film is always placed facing the tubehead. If the film is reversed, the amount of x-rays that reach the film is reduced by the lead foil. The herringbone or tire track pattern on the foil is seen on the sides of the processed x-ray (Figure 22-57).

Common Film Processing Errors

Common film processing errors result from how the film was handled during the processing stage, and the maintenance and setup of the film processing equipment. Dental x-ray film is sensitive to the temperature of the processing solutions, and films must be handled carefully when they are being unwrapped and placed in the processing machine. Maintenance of the processing machine is necessary to ensure clean films without streaks or stains.

FIGURE 22-55
X-rays that have touched or overlapped each other during processing.

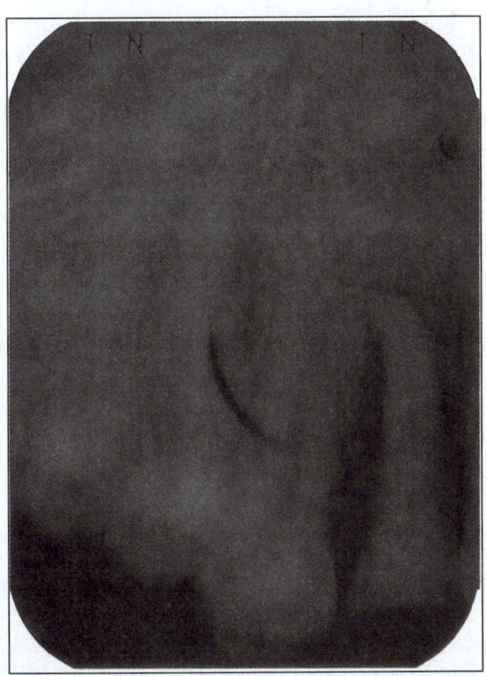

FIGURE 22-56
X-ray showing crimping, or fingernail marks.

A Light Film Image. Light and dark film images can occur not only while exposing the film, but also during processing. A light film is considered to be underprocessed. If the film is underprocessed, the developing time was too short, the developer temperature was lower than recommended, or the developing solution was "exhausted" (i.e., it is too weak from overuse and needs to be changed).

Another cause is the fixing process. If the film is not fixed completely, the emulsion will not be sufficiently hardened and will wash off in the water. With overfixation, the film is left too long in the fixer and the image bleaches out. Also, if the film

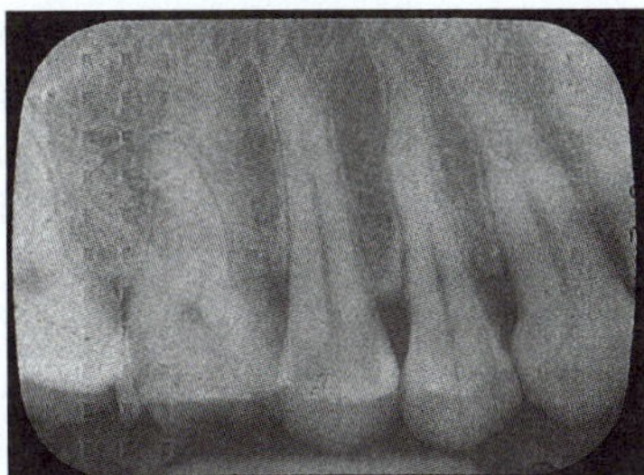

FIGURE 22-57
An x-ray where the film was placed in the patient's mouth backward. Note the herringbone pattern on the molars.

was placed in the mouth backward, the result is a lighter film (Figure 22-58).

A Dark Film Image. Dark film images can be caused by overdeveloping, the developing solution temperature being too high or the solution being too strong, or the film being left in the developer too long. Routinely check solutions and adjust processing times accordingly (Figure 22-59). Refer to the x-ray film processing section discussed earlier in this chapter for more detail on how to check the temperature of processing solutions. Several methods for monitoring film quality are discussed later in this chapter.

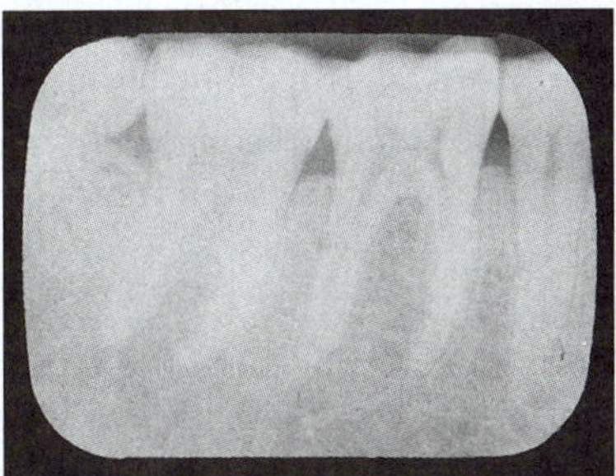

FIGURE 22-58
A light image due to a film processing error.

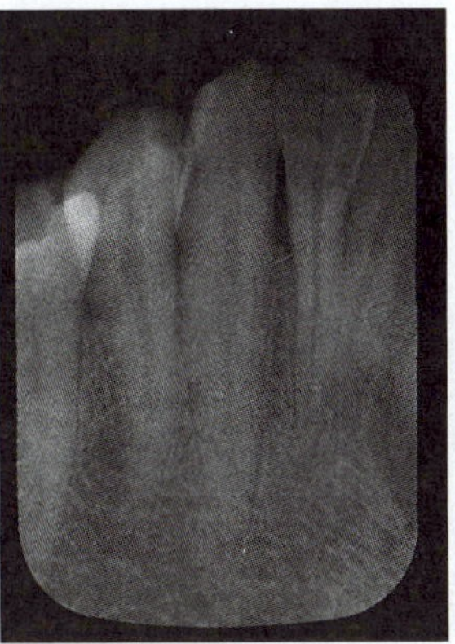

FIGURE 22-59
A dark image due to a film processing error.

Fogged Film. A **fogged film** error has a gray appearance, and there is lost image detail and contrast. It is like viewing a film image through a dense fog. Fog on films can be caused by improper storage conditions, outdated films, light leaks in the processing room, or light leaks from loose fittings on the automatic processors and daylight loaders. Also, safelights, lights with filters under which the film can be manipulated without exposing it, may need to be adjusted or changed; for example, they may be too close to the processing area, too bright, or faulty (Figure 22-60).

Partial Image. A **partial image** on the film is the result of film placement in the processing tanks when the solution levels are low. The film is not completely immersed, and a partial image results. Always check the levels of the processing solutions. Some evaporation takes place daily, and the films absorb some of the developer as well, so replenish the developer regularly (Figure 22-61). To avoid the chance of a partial image, do not use the top clips on the x-ray racks.

Spotted Films. Spots on the x-ray film result from not handling the films carefully, or not keeping the area around the processing tanks clean. As a result of these actions, the following might occur:

- Water touching unprocessed film will leave a clear area(s) on the film.
- White spots on the film may be caused by contact with the fixer. Drops of fixer may splash onto the counter around the processor, and if the unprocessed film comes in contact with the fixer, it will leave white spots on the film (Figure 22-62).
- Dark spots on the film may be caused by contact with the developer. If the unprocessed film comes in contact with the developer, it will leave dark spots on the film (Figure 22-63).
- Yellow-brownish stains on films are usually caused by improper or insufficient washing or rinsing of the film during the processing sequence. Use of exhausted developer and fixer, and insufficient fixing time may also cause a yellow-brownish stain on the x-ray films.
- Static electricity can cause black branching lines on the film. Opening a film packet too quickly can cause a small charge of electricity during times of low humidity.

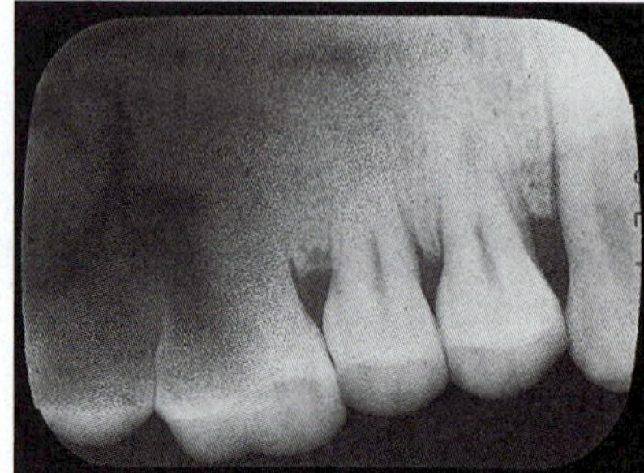

FIGURE 22-60
Fogged film.

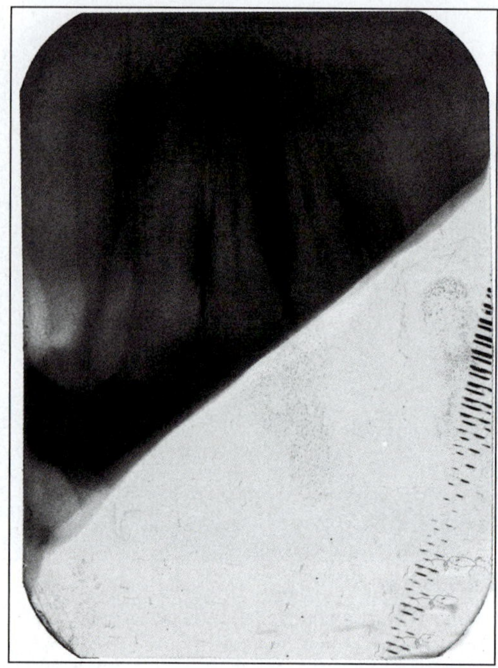

FIGURE 22-61
A partial image due to low levels of the processing solution.

Torn or Scratched Film. Rough handling of the film can lead to the emulsion on the film being torn or scratched, leaving a white area or mark on the processed film. Films can be scratched and torn if they are not handled carefully in overcrowded tanks, or during retrieval, if the film is lost off the film racks (Figure 22-64).

Air Bubbles on the Film. Air bubbles are trapped on the film if it is not agitated when placed in the processing solutions. The air bubbles leave round, white spots where they were attached to the film (Figure 22-65).

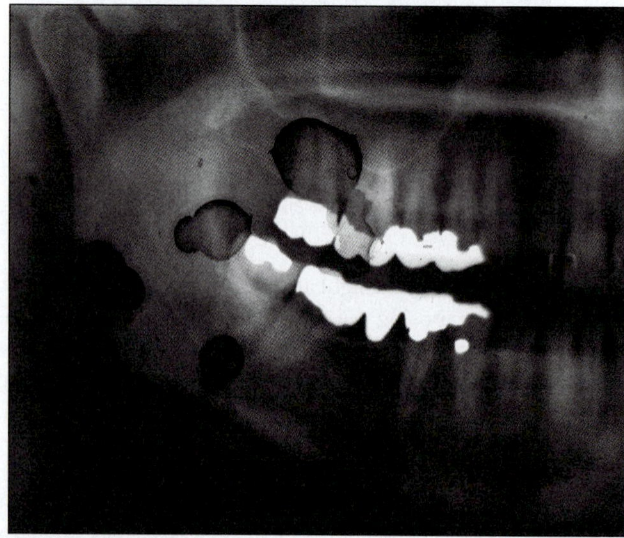

FIGURE 22-62
An x-ray with white (fixer) spots.

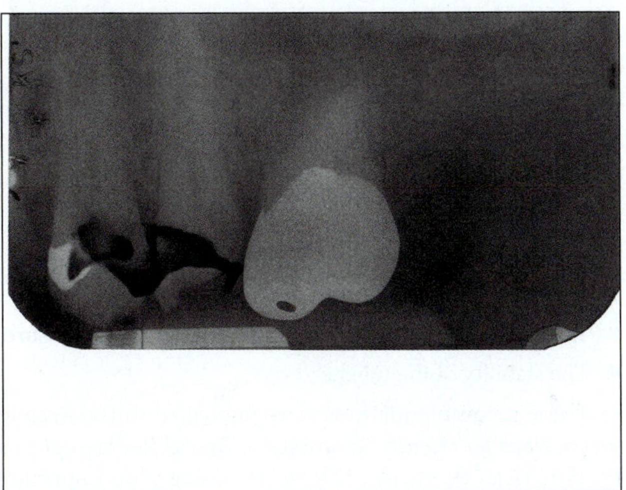

FIGURE 22-63
An x-ray with dark (developer) spots.

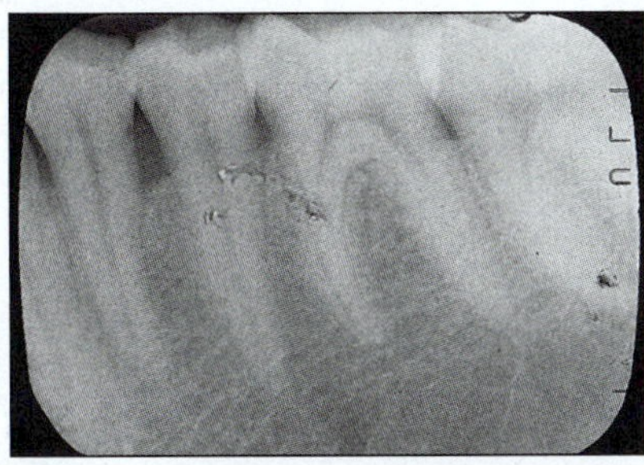

FIGURE 22-64
A radiograph with a torn or scratched emulsion.

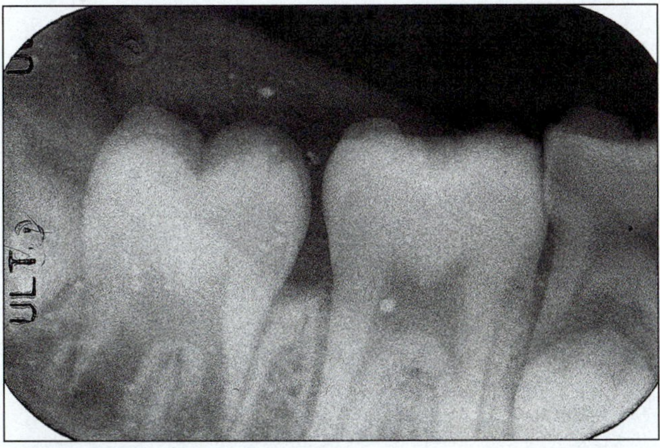

FIGURE 22-65
Films that are agitated poorly when placed in the processing solutions leave air-bubble artifacts on the processed film.

Reticulation. A **reticulation** occurs when a film has been exposed to a high temperature followed by a low temperature. The film emulsion swells and then shrinks. The film looks like it has been dried and has tiny cracks. The temperature of the solutions and the water should be monitored to ensure that they are within the recommended temperature ranges.

Streaks. Streaks on films may result from unclean rollers when using automatic processors, or from unclean x-ray racks. Debris is picked up as the films pass through the rollers, leaving a streaked appearance on the film. Streaks from unclean x-ray racks occur during the processing procedure; debris, including processing solutions, runs from the racks onto the film.

Duplicating Radiographs

Dental x-rays can be duplicated so that the originals never have to leave the office. The need for duplication is increasing; this is partly because more patients have dental insurance. Patients also request x-rays to be sent to specialists, and request them to be forwarded when patients change residence. Also, malpractice suits have increased, which require radiographs to be sent for defense support. Copies of x-rays can be made by a duplication process in the darkroom. These copies offer protection for the dentist, as well as reference sources for the patient.

The **duplication technique** requires the purchase of duplicating film and a duplication machine. The film comes in a variety of sizes and can be processed manually or with an automatic processor (Procedure 22-9). Duplicating film has emulsion on one side only and is coded with a notch in the upper right corner when the emulsion side is facing the dental assistant. Duplicating film is a direct positive film; thus, if an increase in film darkness (density) is desired, exposure time is reduced.

Duplicating machines have light sources with glass over them. The lid closes with a latch to prevent light leaks. There is a setting for viewing the x-rays and a timing selector. These machines are not large and fit conveniently on a counter top.

Storage of Patient Radiographs

Patients' radiographs are stored in the treatment record. If they are removed from the mount, they are placed in a small envelope with the patient's name, date, and number of x-rays enclosed labeled on the outside. Each state has regulations on the length of time radiographs must be saved, because they are considered legal records. Dental assistants should inquire about the pertinent statutes of limitation in their states.

The Legal Implications of Radiographs

As stated previously, x-rays are legal records and should not be destroyed. They belong to the dentist and should not be given to the patients. If a patient switches to another dentist, send a duplicate of the x-rays to the new dentist; keep the original for the office files.

Radiation Risk Communication

In radiation risk communication or management the dentist is responsible for discussing with their patients the benefits and risks of the x-ray examination. The dentist should have the policies and procedures in place to reduce the risk of a malpractice lawsuit. Patient education and accurate patient records, confidentiality, and patient informed consent are key areas to discuss in radiation risk management. There are brochures and other materials to assist the dentist with communication about this. The ADA, the Alliance for Radiation Safety, and the National Council for Radiation Protection and Measurements produce a report, "Radiation Protection in Dentistry," that outlines the risks. Individual state guidelines may also specify specific regulations in that state. Included in risk management are quality assurance procedures and policies for the assessment of radiographic equipment, film processing, image receptor devices, dark room integrity, and abdominal and thyroid shielding.

Quality Assurance

A **quality assurance (QA)** program refers to routine procedures that have been developed to ensure the highest quality x-ray with minimal risk to the patients due to radiation exposure. Under this program, equipment, solutions, and procedures are tested to ensure that consistent high quality is maintained. These **quality control tests** require several aspects of the equipment to be checked each year by state regulatory agencies:

- kV output
- mA output
- Exposure timer
- Half value layer (HVL)
- Focal spot size
- Beam alignment and beam size
- The x-ray output, and the reproducibility of the exposure
- The stability of the tubehead

These recommendations were published in the *Recommendations for Quality Assurance in Dental Radiography* by the American Academy of Dental Radiology. It is important that the date of the test, the type of the test performed, the name of the person performing the test, and the results be kept in a service log. Include documents of any service work in the log. Radiographic units are like any other equipment and must be calibrated occasionally to work optimally.

Implementation of a QA program, and assessment of the variables that affect x-ray quality, greatly benefit patients and

Procedure 22-9
Processing Duplicating Technique

This procedure is performed by the dental assistant. The dental assistant prepares the equipment, supplies, and work area. The radiographs to be duplicated are taken to the darkroom by the dental assistant to duplicate.

Equipment and Supplies

- Duplicating film and radiographs to be duplicated
- X-ray duplicating machine
- Automatic x-ray processor with daylight loader

Procedure Steps (*Follow aseptic procedures*)

1. Place the x-rays in the desired position on the duplicator (Figure 22-66). Make sure the dot on the film is upward (convex).
2. If the machine has a viewing light, turn it on to assist during placement of the x-rays.
3. Turn off the viewing light, and, under safelight conditions, place the duplicating film over the x-rays with the emulsion side facing downward so it contacts the x-rays (the notch will be in the upper left corner).
4. Cover with the lid and latch tightly. Set the timer to 4 to 5 seconds (this may vary with machines).

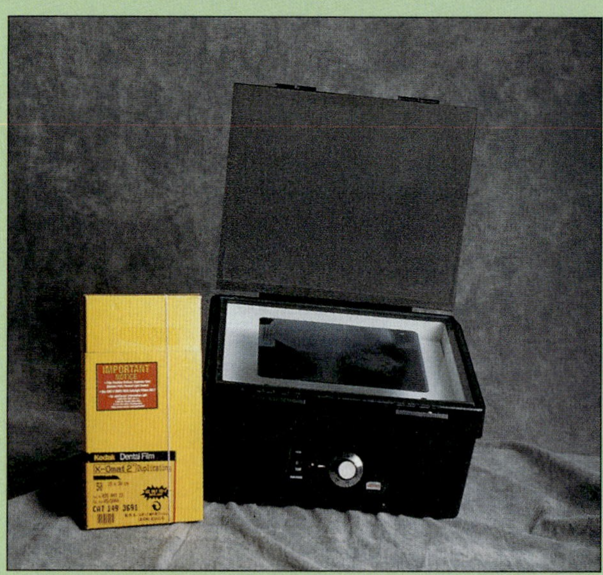

FIGURE 22-66
Duplicating machine and duplicating film used to duplicate full-mouth series and panoramic exposures.

5. Activate the machine to expose the film.
6. When completed, remove the duplicating film under safelight conditions and process the film.

operators. The tests used for routine assessment give the accuracy needed to provide good diagnostic x-rays.

- One of the most important aspects of a QA program is monitoring film processing. Make sure the lighting conditions in the darkroom are safe. Use the proper filters for the films currently in use. If faster films are used, then the red filter is correct. If in question, check with a state regulatory representative.
- White light leaks in the darkroom are another area of concern. A simple way to evaluate the darkroom for possible light leaks is to do a "coin test." On the counter in the immediate processing area, place a coin on an unwrapped, unexposed x-ray film under the safelight for 2 to 3 minutes. Then, process the film using standard procedures. If the outline of the coin is evident on the film after processing, then the safelight filtration is inadequate or a white light leak is possible (Figure 22-67). Document the results in a log and date it. Correct any problems and do the test again. This test should be performed monthly.

A technique for monitoring the quality of the processing solutions is to use a **step wedge**. Use a commercial step wedge or make a step wedge by placing several lead foil pieces from x-ray film packets together in a stair-step manner and soldering them (Figure 22-68). Expose twenty x-rays the first day the processing solution is changed. Make sure it is stirred, and check the temperature. Then, process one of the x-rays. This processed film will become a standard for evaluating the other films. Choose a density in the middle of the film to be used for comparison. Store the other nineteen exposed x-rays in a cool, dry place. Every day or two process another of the x-rays and compare it to the first one. The same middle density on these later films should be comparable to the first one. If the later film differs from the standard by two or more steps, check the processing solution.

Other areas to be checked include the last time the solution was changed or replenished, water temperature, processing time, and whether the solutions have been contaminated. After checking all possibilities and correcting the problem, process an additional test x-ray to compare to the standard film.

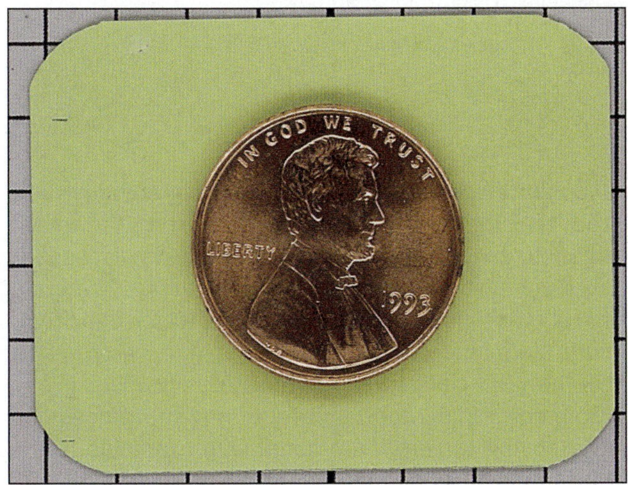

FIGURE 22-67

An unexposed film with a coin on it, demonstrating the safelight test.

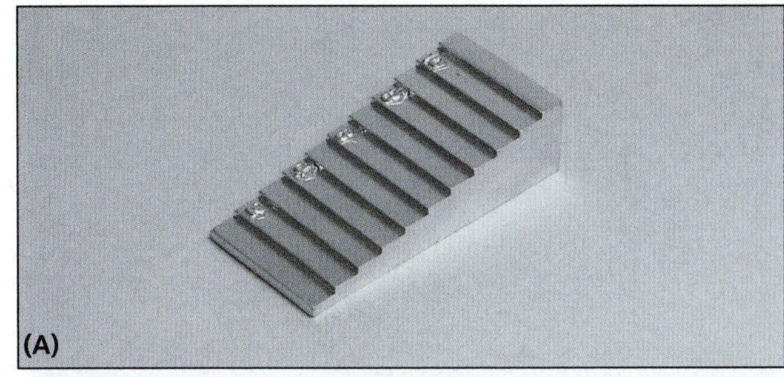

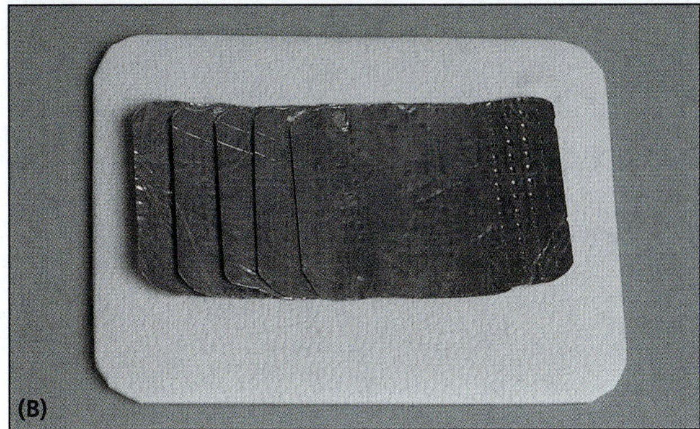

FIGURE 22-68

(A) Manufactured step wedge. (B) Step wedge made from the lead foil from x-ray film packets.

- Monthly, the x-ray machine can be checked by using several additional equipment items. To test the timer, a spin top is needed (Figure 22-69A). Place the film (normally size No. 4) on the sitting area of the x-ray chair. Select the mA and kVp values and the number of impulses to be tested. Place the spin top on the film, place the PID over the top and film, and set it to spin, make the exposure, and process the film. Count the number of dots visible on the film to interpret the results (Figure 22-69B). The number should correspond to the number of impulses selected on the machine.
- To evaluate the effectiveness of the milliamperage, use the step wedge and place it on a size No. 2 film, and position the PID so that it covers the film. Then expose the film. Do this each month; if the appearance of the corresponding shade varies more than two steps, the mA should be checked and adjusted by a qualified service person (Figure 22-70).
- To measure the kVp, a dosimeter and a charger are needed (Figure 22-71). Make sure the dosimeter is charged and at the 0 reading. Place the dosimeter on a surface, place the PID over it, and expose the dosimeter. It should show a reading of the appropriate kVp. If it does not, have it checked by a qualified service person.

If a problem is apparent, it is important that no radiographs be taken until the problem is fixed. Quality control cannot be overlooked. Each step of the procedure must be followed

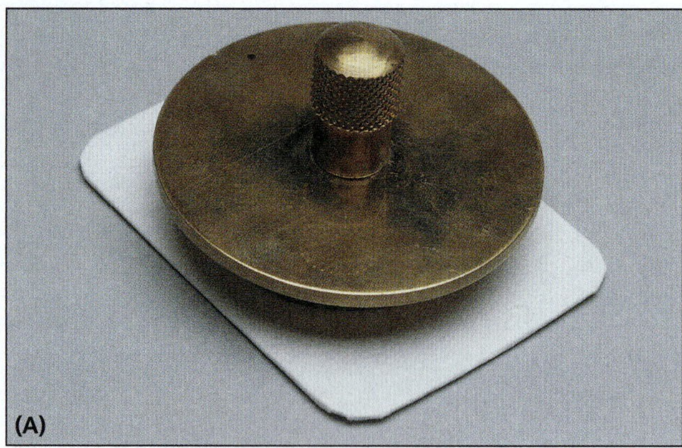

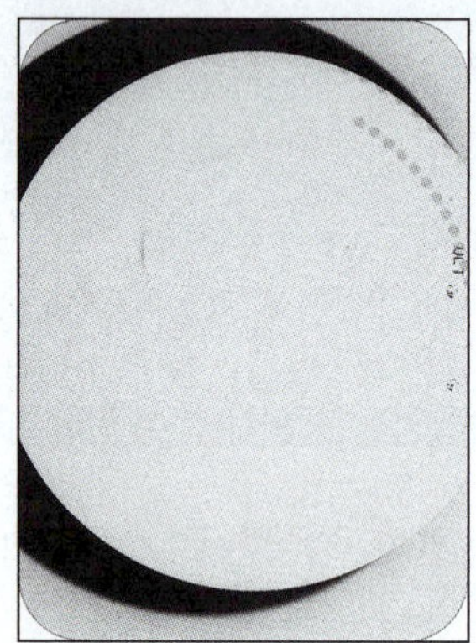

FIGURE 22-69

(A) Spin top used in checking time accuracy and an exposed x-ray showing the results of the spin top test. (B) Impulses indicated by markings on the x-ray.

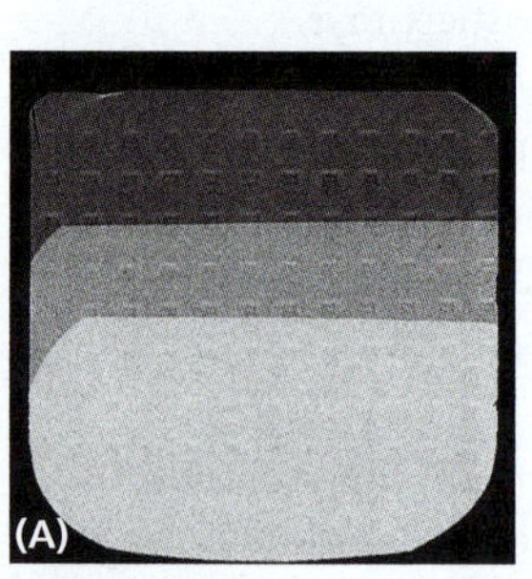

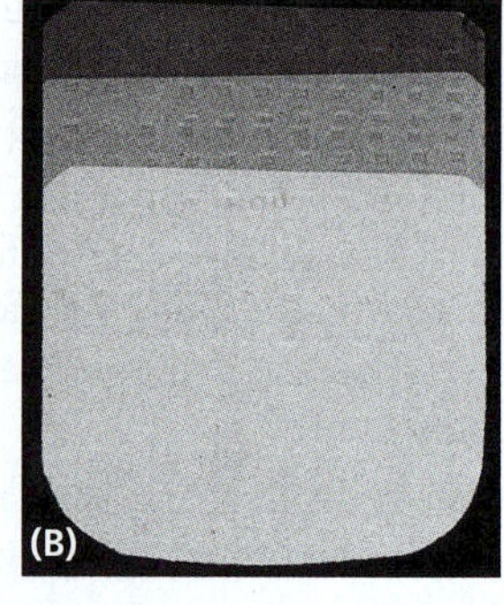

FIGURE 22-70

A comparison of two x-rays exposed using the step wedge. (A) Standard processed when the solution was first prepared. (B) Standard processed after solution replenishment.

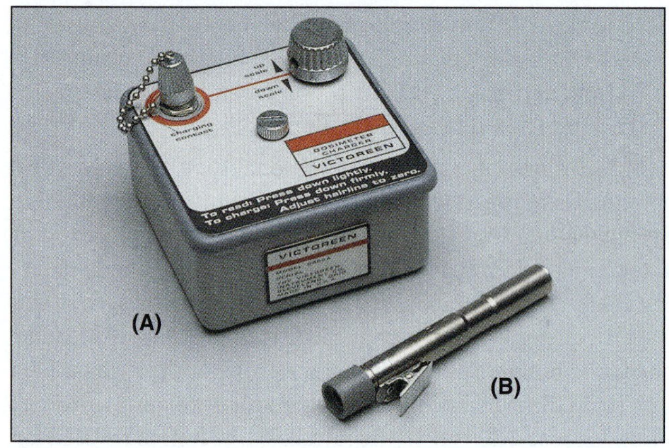

FIGURE 22-71

A dosimeter used to evaluate kilovoltage. (A) Dosimeter charger. (B) Dosimeter.

carefully, including storage of unexposed films; use of a lead apron with a thyroid collar; proper placement of the film and cone to reduce retakes; and correct, final labeling of the film mount from which the diagnosis is to be made. All of the steps in between are important for minimizing radiation exposure to the patient. It is important that each dental assistant has proper training to take x-rays. Every patient deserves competent, quality service.

1. Set high standards for quality assurance.
2. Follow a consistent procedure to maintain control.
3. Check equipment, solutions, and procedures often.
4. Keep a log of daily, monthly, and yearly procedures used to maintain quality radiographs.

Chapter Summary

The dentist uses both intraoral films, placed in the patient's mouth for exposure, and extraoral films, placed outside the patient's mouth, to produce quality radiographs used in diagnosing dental conditions. Simply, a quality radiograph facilitates accurate diagnosis.

The two techniques used to expose radiographs are bisecting and paralleling. Both techniques are described in this chapter, but the most widely used is the paralleling technique. The equipment required for the paralleling technique is demonstrated for each area of the mouth for adults and children.

Once the radiographs have been exposed, they must be processed. Manual and automatic processing equipment and techniques are described and compared. Chemical components of the developing and fixing solutions are listed, and the role they play in converting the latent image into a visible permanent radiograph is discussed.

Radiographs are then mounted for viewing. There are various types of dental x-ray mounts to choose from. Helpful hints for determining the order in which x-rays are mounted, especially when learning, are provided.

Common radiographic errors, during the processing and exposing of x-rays, are listed with examples. Careful attention to positioning during x-ray exposure, and detailed step-by-step procedures for processing can assist in the elimination of errors.

Patient radiographs are needed for many reasons. For instance, insurance companies require copies of the patient's x-rays to determine insurance coverage, and other dental offices require a copy of the patient's x-rays for their own diagnoses. Radiographs can be duplicated so that the original radiographs never have to leave the office. The special film and equipment needed for this process are discussed. Dental offices are required to properly store final radiographs to prevent losses, thereby, avoiding the need for x-rays to be retaken.

Quality assurance programs ensure that equipment, solutions, and procedures are tested to ensure high-quality radiographs and standards for the patient.

Review Questions

Multiple Choice

1. The entire tooth and surrounding area are seen on the
   a. periapical x-ray.
   b. bitewing x-ray.
   c. occlusal x-ray.
   d. none of the above.
2. Which one of the following two exposure techniques uses a vertical angulation table for proper positioning of the cone?
   a. Paralleling technique
   b. Bisecting technique
3. Occlusal radiographs are used to locate or define all of the following *except*
   a. fractures.
   b. impacted teeth.
   c. changes in size and shape of arches.
   d. a facial view of the entire mandibular arch.
4. A full-mouth survey of a child aged 3 to 5 years includes
   a. two bitewings, six anterior incisors, and four posterior periapicals.
   b. four bitewings, six anterior incisors, and two posterior periapicals.
   c. two bitewings, two anterior incisors, and four posterior periapicals.
   d. four bitewings, six anterior incisors, and eight posterior periapicals.
5. What is the optimal temperature for processing x-rays in the automatic processor?
   a. 85°F to 95°F
   b. 68°F to 70°F
   c. 100°F
   d. 75°F
6. When processing film in an automatic processor, what is the sequence of the solutions?
   a. Developer, fixer, water
   b. Developer, water, fixer
   c. Water, developer, fixer
   d. Fixer, developer, water
7. When viewing properly mounted x-rays, where or how is the dot on the film mounted?
   a. So that it is raised or convex
   b. So that it is depressed or concave
   c. In the middle of the film
   d. In any position
8. Which error results in interproximal spaces overlapping on a radiograph?
   a. Vertical angulation
   b. Horizontal angulation
   c. Improper film placement
   d. Improper film processing
9. All of the following are exposure errors *except*
   a. distortion.
   b. elongation.
   c. torn or scratched film.
   d. overlapping.
10. Duplicating film is the same type of film used to expose x-rays of the teeth.
    a. This is a true statement.
    b. This is a false statement.

Critical Thinking

1. If the radiographs were dark after processing, what areas would the dental assistant want to check to correct the problem?
2. List three primary errors that may be apparent on routine bitewing x-rays, and explain how they can be corrected.
3. Discuss how taking radiographs on children is different from exposing radiographs on adults.

Web Activities

1. To find questions that patients frequently ask about dental x-rays, go to http://www.ada.org, type in *Oral Health Topics* and look under "X-Rays."
2. Check http://www.Carestreamdental.com and learn more about Kodak *Insight* dental film and other dental radiology subjects.
3. Identify three different duplicating machines at http://www.Rinncorp.com. At this site also look at the variety of sensor holders available.

CHAPTER 23

Extraoral and Digital Radiography 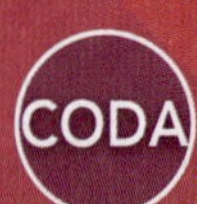

CODA

Specific Instructional Objectives

The student should strive to meet the following objectives and demonstrate an understanding of the facts and principles presented in this chapter:

1. Identify extraoral films and describe exposing techniques.
2. Identify normal and abnormal radiographic landmarks.
3. Identify imaging systems used for dental purposes.
4. Explain the fundamental concepts of digital radiography.
5. Identify and describe the types of digital imaging.
6. Identify the components of digital radiography.
7. Describe storage phosphor imaging.
8. Identify the features used to enhance a digital image with various software programs.
9. List and discuss the advantages and disadvantages of digital imaging.
10. Explain the procedure for using digital radiography.
11. Describe 3-D imaging systems.

Key Terms

3D dental imaging (558)
analog image (553)
axial plane (551)
cassette (537)
cephalometric radiograph (544)
cephalostat (544)
charge-coupled device (CCD) (553)
complementary metal oxide semiconductor (CMOS) (553)
computed tomography (CT scanning) (550)
digital image (553)
digital imaging technology (550)
digital radiology (553)
digital subtraction (554)
direct digital imaging (553)
extraoral film (539)
extraoral imaging (537)
focal trough (538)
Frankfort plane (542)
ghost image (540)
gray scale (553)
handheld intraoral radiography (560)
indirect digital imaging (555)
intensifying screen (539)
lateral jaw radiograph (545)
lead apron artifact (540)
magnetic resonance imaging (MRI) (550)
midsagittal plane (542)
panoramic radiography (537)
pixels (553)
photostimulable phosphor (PSP) (555)
radiolucency (553)
radiopacity (553)
rare earth phosphors (539)
rotational centers (538)
storage phosphor imaging (555)
tomography (538)
tragus of the ear (544)
transcranial temporomandibular joint radiograph (545)
trismus (537)

Introduction

Extraoral radiography is standard practice in the dental office and extra oral radiographs are taken routinely as part of patient records. Types of **extraoral imaging** include panoramic radiographs that are used in general and specialty dental offices, and cephalometric radiographs that are mainly taken by orthodontists. The lateral jaw radiograph and the transcranial temporomandibular joint radiograph are the other extraoral radiographs discussed in this chapter.

The dental assistant should become familiar with radiograph interpretation, because it will help them take quality radiographs and be more prepared for the selected treatment. Interpretation involves learning the terminology, and then identifying the landmark on a radiograph.

Digital radiography is becoming standard in many dental offices, and it is likely that all dental offices in the future will take and store digital radiographs. Digital equipment and techniques, and their advantages and disadvantages, will be discussed. Digital radiography equipment is changing and improving, while the technique is being made easier for the dentist and dental staff to learn and incorporate into their office routine.

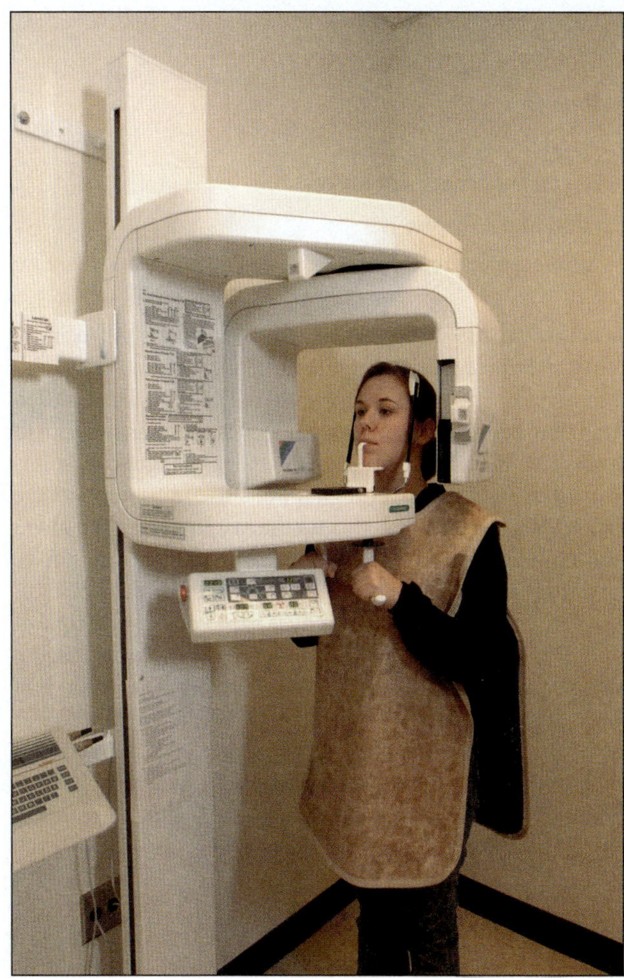

FIGURE 23-1

Patient positioned in a panoramic x-ray machine.

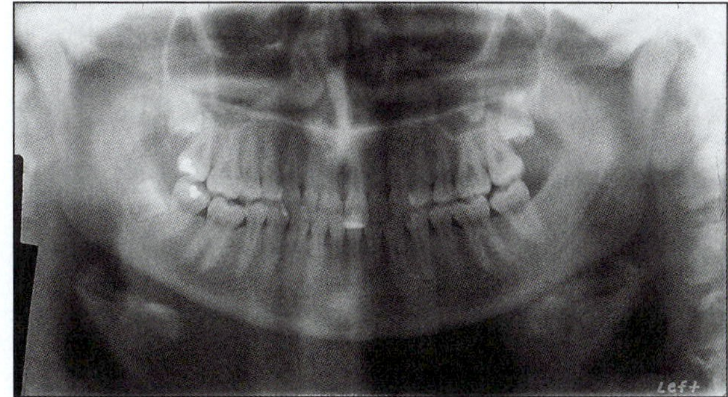

FIGURE 23-2

A panoramic radiograph.

Extraoral Radiographs

Extraoral radiographs are used by the dentist to identify large areas of the skull on one radiograph. These radiographs give the dentist an overall view of the teeth, oral cavity, and skull and are used most often in conjunction with periapical, bitewing, and occlusal radiographs. Orthodontists and oral maxillofacial surgeons routinely use extraoral radiographs, especially panoramic and cephalometric exposures.

Panoramic Radiography

Many dental offices have **panoramic radiography** machines (Figure 23-1). Panoramic machines take a radiograph that shows the entire maxilla and mandible on one film (Figure 23-2). Panoramic radiography is commonly known and named after the brand name of the panoramic x-ray machine. There are many types of panoramic machines, including film-based units and digital imaging units. With both the film-based and the digital unit, the film holder (**cassette**) and the x-ray head rotate opposite each other around the patient's head. Because they are connected by bars extending from the top of the machines, they rotate at the same speed. The result is an x-ray that extends from the condyle on one side of the patient's head to the condyle on the other side. There is some overlapping and loss of detail, but panoramic radiographs are valuable when an overall assessment of the patient is needed. Panoramic x-rays can be taken on adults, children, edentulous patients, patients who have **trismus** (lack the ability to open the mouth very wide), and patients in wheelchairs.

Panoramic x-rays give the dentist a general view of the following:

- The entire dentition
- Nasal and orbital areas
- Alveolar bone
- Carious lesions
- Fractures, cysts, and tumors

- Malocclusion
- Maxilla and mandible
- Sinuses
- Unerupted teeth
- Dental appliances and restorations
- Periodontal disease
- Temporomandibular joint

Fundamentals of Panoramic Radiography. As mentioned previously, in panoramic radiography, the x-ray tubehead and cassette film move around the patient's head. When using film-based panoramic machines it is necessary for film to be correctly placed into the cassette under safelight conditions prior to exposure. Direct digital units use phosphor storage plates (PSP) inserted directly into the cassette; therefore, there is no need for film placement. Indirect digital units must have the phosphor imaging plate placed inside the cassette prior to exposure. Panoramic radiography is based on the principle of **tomography** (meaning part). Tomography shows the imaging of one layer or section of the body while blurring images from other areas. In panoramic radiography, the image conforms to the curve of the dental arches. The patient is positioned, and when the panoramic exposure button is pushed, the tubehead rotates in one direction around the patient while the cassette rotates in the opposite direction. The patient may stand or sit in a stationary position during the exposure. The rotation is synchronized from **rotational centers**. Rotational centers vary in number and location, depending on the manufacturer of the panoramic machine. They also influence the shape and size of the focal trough. The **focal trough** (Figure 23-3), also known as the image layer or sharpness, is a three-dimensional (3-D) curved zone in which the dental arches are positioned to achieve the sharpest image. The panoramic machine will expose this selected plane of tissue, while the areas outside the selected plane will be blurred. The size and shape of the focal trough varies from one panoramic machine to another, but each machine is designed to accommodate the average person. The quality of the panoramic radiograph depends on the precise positioning of the patient's teeth within the focal trough, and the degree to which the patient resembles the average-person design of that specific machine. The manufacturer provides specific instructions for positioning the patient and for how to work with "non-average" patients.

Panoramic Unit. Panoramic units are constantly being updated and improved (Figure 23-4). They differ by the size and shape of the focal trough, the number and location of the

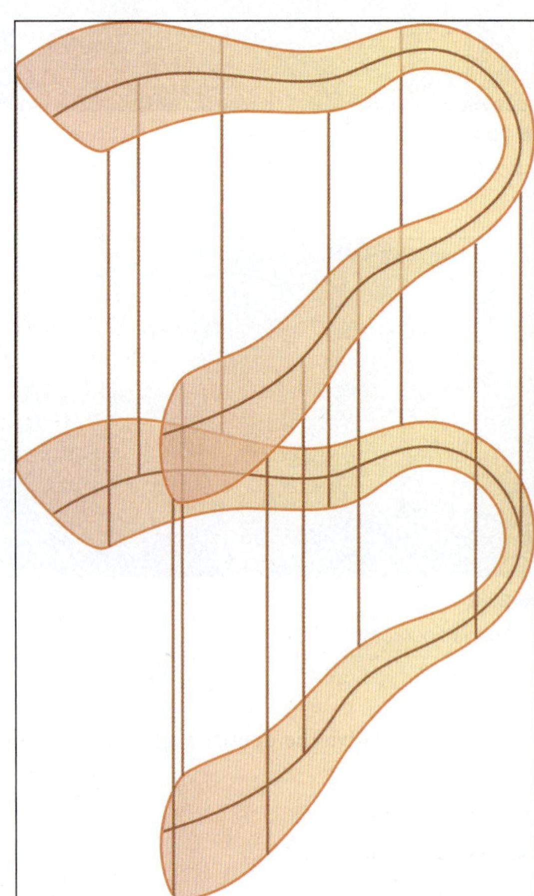

FIGURE 23-3
Focal trough or image layer.

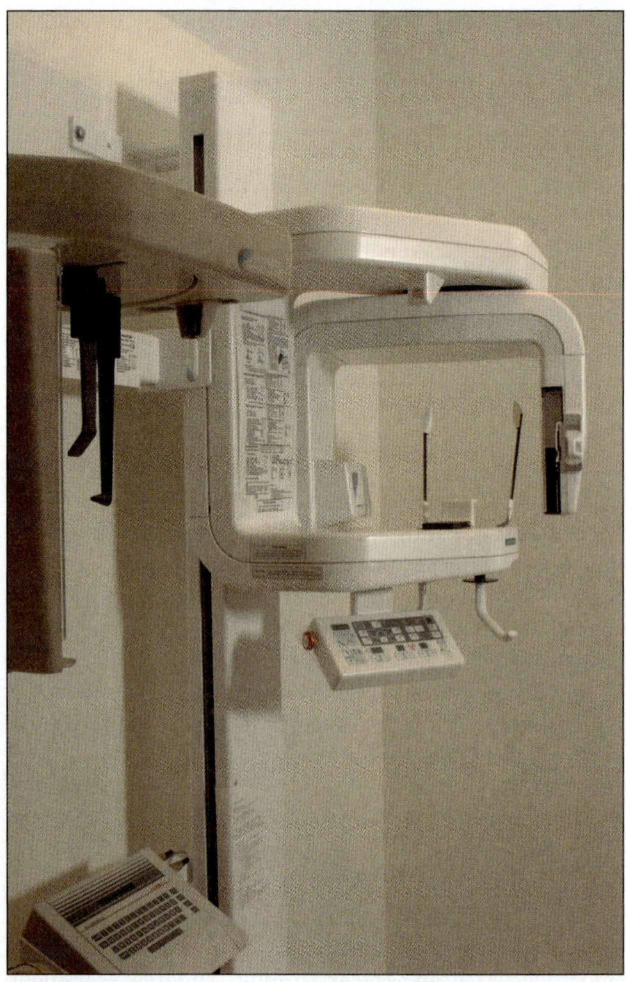

FIGURE 23-4
A panoramic unit.

rotational centers, and the type of cassette (holder) used for the x-ray film. All units, however, include the following basic components:

- Exposure controls
- Head positioner
- X-ray tubehead
- Cassette holder

Exposure Controls. The exposure controls are usually located outside the x-ray room. In cases where the controls are part of the unit, the exposure control button itself is located outside the room. The manufacturer determines many exposure factors, such as exposure time, but kilovoltage and milliamperage can be adjusted. The instruction manual provides information on variations for different exposures.

Head Positioner. The head positioner consists of lateral head supports or guides, a chin rest, a notched bite block, and a forehead rest. There are also handles for the patient to hold onto for support located near this area. Each panoramic machine is slightly different, and the operator must follow the manufacturer's instructions on how to correctly position the patient.

X-Ray Tubehead. The extraoral x-ray tubehead is similar to an intraoral x-ray tubehead; however, the collimator shape is different. The collimator used in panoramic machines has a narrow vertical slit, in contrast to the small round or rectangular shape of intraoral machines. The x-ray beam is emitted from the panoramic tubehead through the narrow slit forming a vertical band of x-rays, which pass through the patient and exposes the panoramic film through a vertical slit in the cassette holder. The patient receives minimal radiation exposure due to the collimator shape, and the amount of x-rays emitted from the x-ray tubehead.

Cassette Film Holders. Cassettes are used to hold the film or phosphor plates during exposure. Cassettes are either flat, hard containers that open on the back, or flexible, thin sleeves that open on one end (Figure 23-5). Both prevent light from entering, while allowing the x-rays to pass through. The cassettes must be marked in order to distinguish left from right because there is no raised dot on the film. With some panoramic machines, the films are labeled with the patient's name, dentist's name, date, and so on. The assistant enters the information digitally before exposure. After exposure of a film-based panoramic radiograph, and under safelight conditions, the film is run through a marking device. The film is then processed, and the information appears on the film. There is no need to load the film into the cassette when using a direct digital technique, because the imaging plate is already embedded into the cassette. If using the indirect digital technique the operator must load the phosphor plate prior to exposure. Open the patient's chart on the computer screen, select the correct radiograph to be taken, and then expose the radiograph; the image will appear on the monitor, and will need to be saved in the appropriate patient's computer chart.

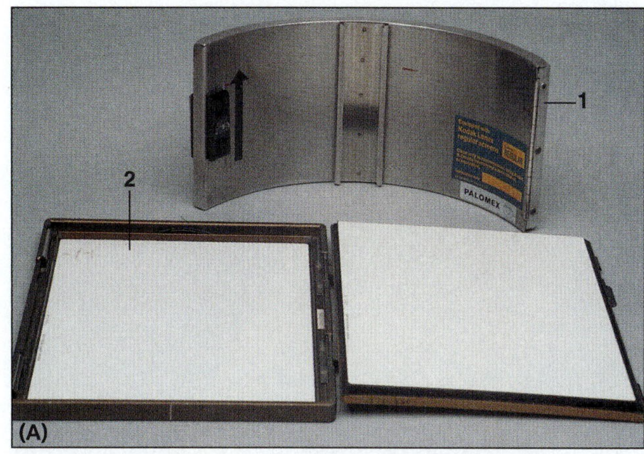

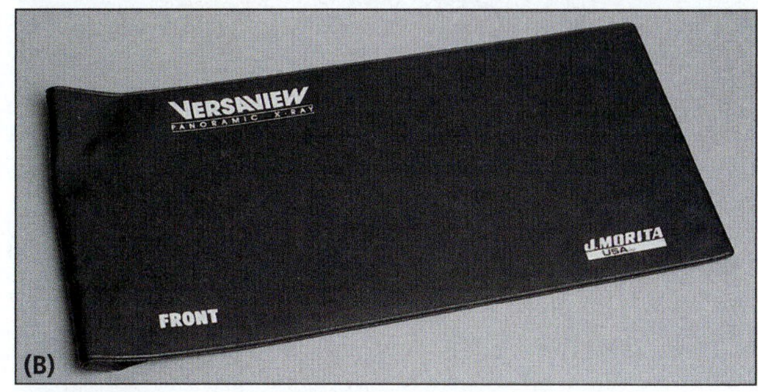

FIGURE 23-5

(A) 1. A hard cassette for a panoramic x-ray. 2. Intensifying screens on the inside of a cephalometric cassette. (B) Soft cassette.

Cassettes are usually lined with an **intensifying screen**. Care must be taken to avoid scratching the screens, and to keep them free of stains and debris. The action of the x-rays on the film is increased, or intensified, by the screens; therefore, the required exposure to the patient is decreased. A substance called phosphor is used on the screens. The phosphor emits light when struck by x-rays. Some phosphors emit blue light and others emit green light. It is important to use film that is sensitive to the kind of light the phosphor emits. The green-light phosphors are known as **rare earth phosphors** and are faster; thus, the patient receives fewer x-rays during exposure. Calcium tungstate phosphors emit blue light. These screens are not as fast, and require more x-rays to make a radiograph than the rare earth screens.

Extraoral Film. The **extraoral film** comes in a variety of large sizes, ranging from 5 × 12 inches for the panoramic to 8 × 10 inches for the cephalometric exposure. The film is not wrapped individually; it comes in a box of 50 or more sheets (Figure 23-6). Therefore, the film must be loaded into the cassettes in the darkroom under safelight conditions. The box must be closed carefully to prevent light exposure to the remaining film in the box.

Extraoral film is screen film, requiring the use of screens for exposure. The film is placed between two intensifying screens in the cassette holder. Screen film is sensitive to the light emitted from the intensifying screens rather than to radiation. The film must be sensitive to the type of light emitted by the screen

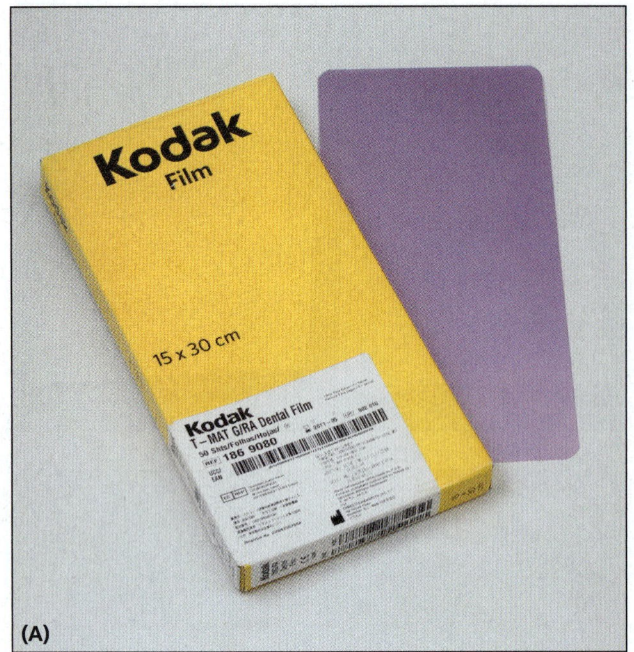

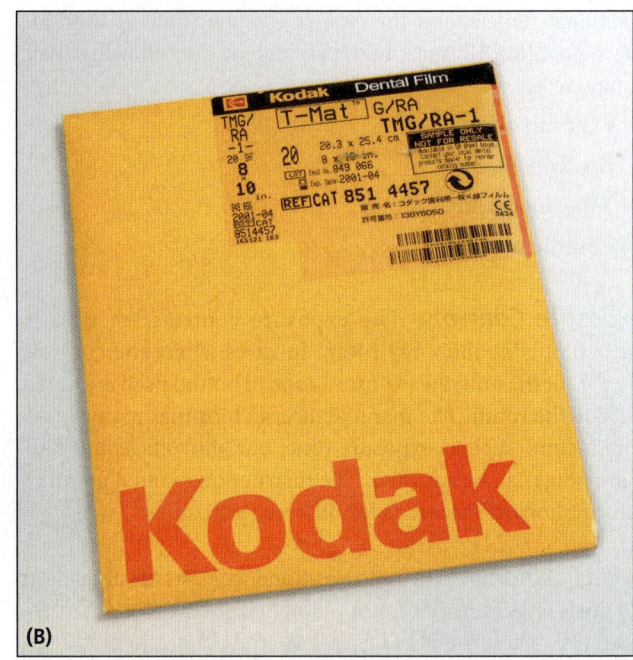

FIGURE 23-6
Extraoral film. (A) Panoramic film. (B) Cephalometric film.

particles. It is important to have extraoral film that is designed specifically for the type of intensifying screens being used.

Film-Holding Devices. Panoramic machines have cassette holders attached to them. With other extraoral exposures, the cassette holder may be attached to a wall or the patient may hold the cassette. For some extraoral exposures, the cassette is placed on a flat surface and the patient rests her or his face on it.

Panoramic Exposure Technique Suggestions. There are many types of panoramic machines and each machine has specific instructions provided by the manufacturer for successful exposures on a variety of patients. Be sure to read and follow these instructions. A few guidelines for all panoramic exposures follow:

- The patient should always wear a lead apron *without* a thyroid collar. The collar interferes with the image and, because the x-ray beam is directed upward, the x-ray exposure to the thyroid gland is minimal.
- The patient needs to be still during the entire exposure. Every machine is equipped with some type of chin rest, bite block, and head positioner to prevent movement.
- Explain the procedure to the patient, including the rotation of the machine and what to do during the exposure. Remove bulky sweaters, coats, hair clips, or anything that may interfere with the rotation of the x-ray tubehead. Remove earrings, necklaces, and dental appliances as well.
- Place the cassette in the machine, prepare the patient, carefully position the patient following the procedure steps of the panoramic unit, using the guidelines set the machine, and take the exposure. Release the patient and remove the cassette for processing and reloading (Procedure 23-1).

Common Panoramic Radiography Errors. Errors in preparation and positioning of the patient are discussed in this section.

Preparation Errors. When preparing the patient, make sure that the patient has removed all metal objects that might cast a **ghost image** on the film. A ghost image is a radiopaque artifact seen on the panoramic film that is caused by double-exposure of a dense object by the x-ray beam. A ghost image is similar to the real image but is cast on the opposite side of the x-ray and is larger, higher, and blurred. A common ghost image is produced by an earring left in one ear. All metal objects (e.g., earrings, eyeglasses, hairpins, necklaces, facial piercing, partial or removable dentures, hearing aids, and orthodontic retainers) must be removed before exposure to ensure that the radiograph is of adequate quality for diagnosis.

Adjust the lead apron correctly so that it lies flat around the patient and below the cassette and x-ray tubehead as they rotate around the patient. A **lead apron artifact** will also occur if a lead apron with a thyroid collar is used. The collar used on most people is large and closes around the chin.

Positioning Errors. The patient must be positioned correctly to expose the clearest and most accurate image possible. Panoramic radiographs show the dentist the entire dentition and related structures, from one condyle to the other condyle. The dental assistant must pay attention to every detail while positioning the patient. See Table 23-1 for common errors in positioning the patient.

Procedure 23-1
Exposing Panoramic Radiographs

This procedure is performed by the dental assistant at the direction of the dentist. The assistant prepares the cassette, panoramic machine, and patient for exposure.

Equipment and Supplies

- Mouth mirror
- Panoramic film if using a film-based machine
- Phosphor plate if using indirect digital unit
- Cassette
- Bite block
- Barrier for the bite block
- Lead apron without thyroid collar
- Panoramic machine

Preparation for Film-Based Panoramic Radiographic Exposure

1. Under safelight conditions, load the cassette in the darkroom. The cassettes are lined with two intensifying screens, and the panoramic film is placed between them. The cassette must be securely closed to prevent light leaks. With some cassettes, information can be added, such as left and right, the patient's name, the date, and the dentist's name.
2. Place the cassette into the cassette holder of the panoramic machine (Figure 23-7).
3. Prepare the bite block. A protective barrier can be placed on the bite block, such as plastic wrap. The bite blocks should be sterilized between patients.
4. Adjust the machine to the patient's approximate height, and set the kilovoltage and milliamperage according to the manufacturer's guidelines.

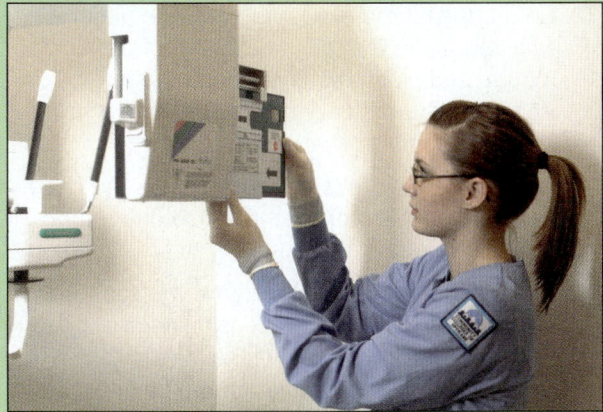

FIGURE 23-7
Placing a cassette into the panoramic machine.

Preparation for Digital Panoramic Radiographic Exposure

1. Turn on the computer and load software to enter the patient's identification information and select the type of radiograph to be exposed.

Indirect Digital Technique:

Under safelight conditions, load the cassette in the darkroom. The cassettes are lined with two intensifying screens, and the phosphor plate is placed between them. The cassette must be securely closed to prevent light leaks.

Direct Digital Technique:

There is no need to load a cassette because the phosphor plates are embedded in the cassette.

2. Place the cassette into the cassette holder of the panoramic machine (Figure 23-7).
3. Prepare the bite block. A protective barrier can be placed on the bite block, such as plastic wrap. The bite blocks should be sterilized between patients.
4. Adjust the machine to the patient's approximate height, and set the kilovoltage and milliamperage according to the manufacturer's guidelines.

Preparing the Patient for Panoramic Exposure

1. Explain the procedure to the patient, and answer any questions.
2. Ask the patient to remove eyeglasses, earrings, tongue bars, facial piercing, hairpins and clips, necklaces, hearing aids, partial and full dentures, and anything else that may interfere with the film exposure or cast a shadow on the film.
3. Place and secure the lead apron on the patient. The lead apron used for the panoramic exposures is double-sided *without* a thyroid collar (Figure 23-8). This apron is placed with one side on the front of the patient and one side on the back to protect the patient as the machine

(continues)

Procedure 23-1 (continued)

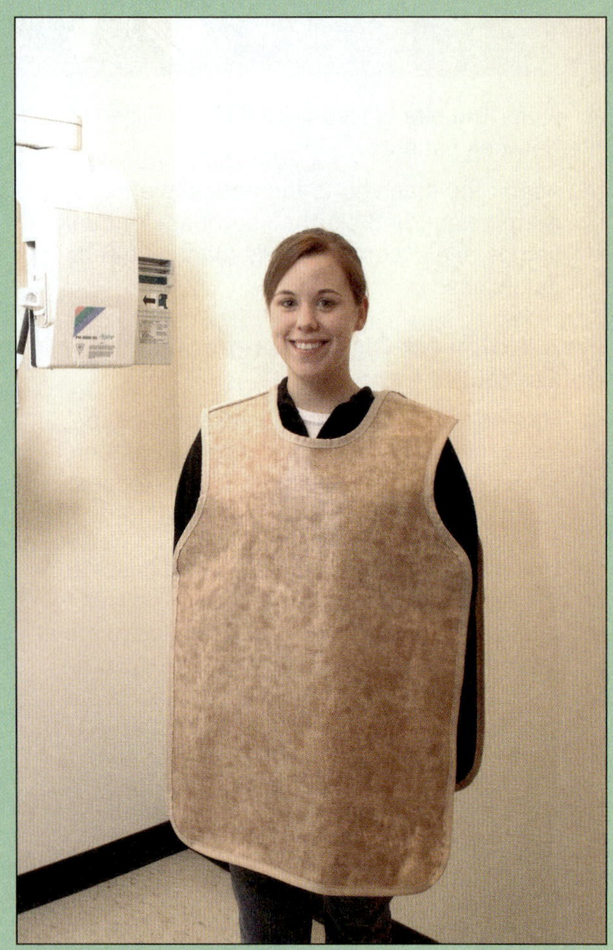

FIGURE 23-8

A patient wearing a lead apron, ready to be positioned in the panoramic machine.

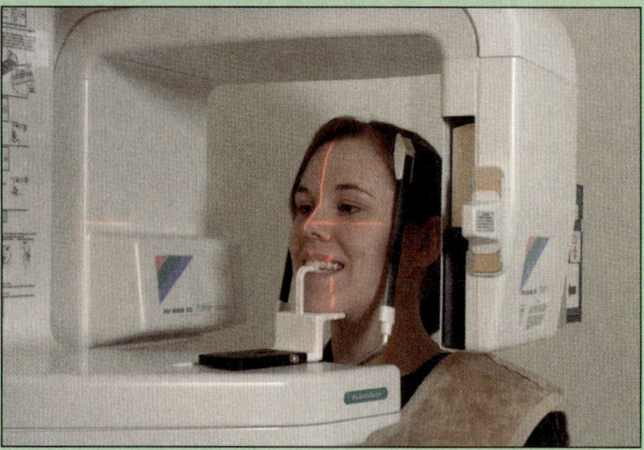

FIGURE 23-9

A patient biting on the bite block and correctly positioned for panoramic exposure. The horizontal line highlighted on the patient's face indicates the midsagittal plane and the vertical line shows the Frankfort plane.

rotates around during the exposure. The thyroid collar is not recommended for panoramic exposures because it may interfere with the exposure and block part of the x-ray beam.

4. Guide the patient into position, whether sitting or standing. Ask the patient to stand/sit up as straight as possible so that the spine is perfectly straight. If the spinal column is not straight, it will cast a white shadow in the middle of the radiograph.
5. Raise the machine to the appropriate level so that the patient can easily bite on the bite block. Have the patient move forward until the upper and lower teeth are secured in the groove on the bite block. The groove aligns the teeth in the focal trough. If the patient is edentulous, the alveolar ridges should be positioned over the grooves of the bite block. Cotton rolls can also be used to assist in positioning (Figure 23-9).
6. The **Frankfort plane** is the imaginary line drawn from the middle of the ear to just below the eye socket across the bridge of the nose. This line must be parallel with the floor, so that the occlusal plane is at the correct angle (Figure 23-10A).
7. The **midsagittal plane** is the imaginary line that evenly divides the face into right and left halves. This midsagittal plane must be perpendicular to the floor, so that the head is not tilted; otherwise, the image will be distorted (Figure 23-10B).
8. Some panoramic machines have lights to assist with the positioning of the Frankfort plane and the midsagittal plane. At this point, turn the light on and adjust the patient accordingly.
9. Before taking the exposure, have the patient swallow, place the tongue at the roof of the mouth, and close the lips around the bite block. Reassure the patient and instruct him or her to remain still during the exposure.
10. After the exposure is complete, guide the patient away from the panoramic machine and remove the lead apron.
11. For film-based machines remove the cassette and proceed with film processing as described in Chapter 22. For direct digital based techniques evaluate the image on the monitor of the patient's chart. For indirect digital techniques, remove the cassette and process it through the scanner.

(continues)

Procedure 23-1 (continued)

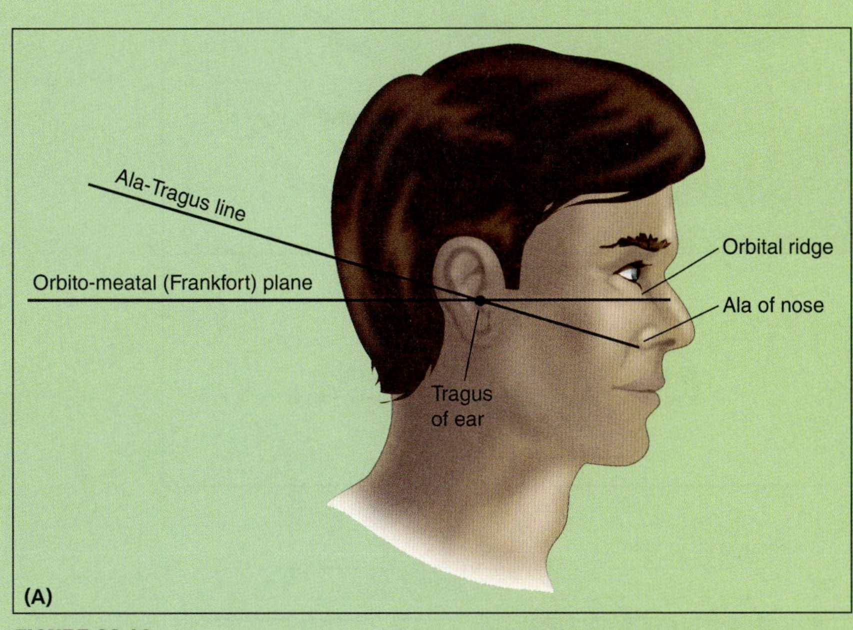

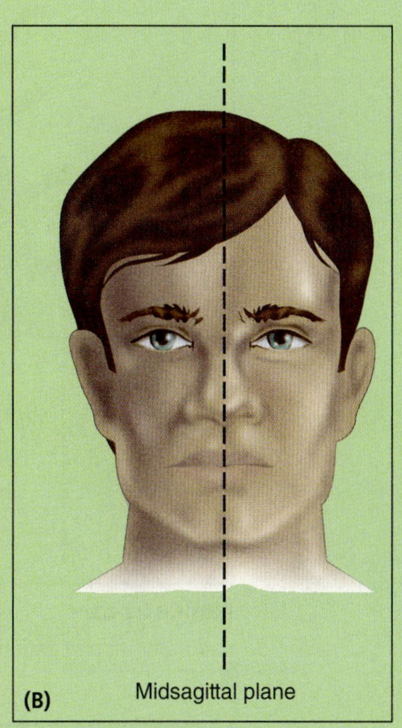

FIGURE 23-10
(A) Frankfort plane. (B) Midsagittal plane.

TABLE 23-1 Patient Positioning Errors

Problem	Correction
The patient is positioned too far forward on the bite block. The anterior teeth are not in the grooves on the bite block, but are biting in front of the grooves. The anterior teeth will be out of the focal trough, so they will be blurred. The spine is superimposed on the ramus areas of the mandible, and the bicuspids appear overlapped (Figure 23-11).	Have the patient bite in the grooves of the bite block and hold in this position. The head supports might need to be adjusted to prevent the head from moving forward.
The patient is positioned too far back. The anterior teeth are not in the grooves on the bite block but are biting too far in back of the grooves. The anterior teeth will be out of the focal trough, and, thus, will be blurred and appear wide. Ghost images of the mandible and spine will also appear (Figure 23-12).	Have the patient bite in the grooves of the bite block and hold in this position. The head supports might need to be adjusted to prevent the head from moving backward.
Frankfort plane: Patient's head is tilted downward. Apices of the lower incisors are blurred, mandibular condyles may not be seen, a shadow of the hyoid bone is superimposed over the center of the mandible, and the curve of the arch is exaggerated in an upward direction (Figure 23-13).	Carefully position the patient with the Frankfort plane parallel to the floor.
Frankfort plane: Patient's head is tilted upward. Maxillary incisors are blurred, the hard palate and floor of the nasal cavity appear superimposed over the apices of the maxillary teeth, and the curve of the arch is exaggerated in a downward direction (Figure 23-14).	Carefully position the patient with the Frankfort plane parallel to the floor.
Patient's tongue was not resting on the roof of the mouth during exposure. This will cause a dark radiolucent area above the apices of the maxillary teeth (Figure 23-15).	Instruct and watch the patient as she or he swallows, and then raises the tongue to the roof of her or his mouth and holds it there during the exposure.
Patient was not standing or sitting up straight, resulting in a ghost image of the spine superimposed on the center of the x-ray (Figure 23-16).	Position the patient so that the midsagittal plane is perpendicular to the floor and the midline is centered on the bite block.

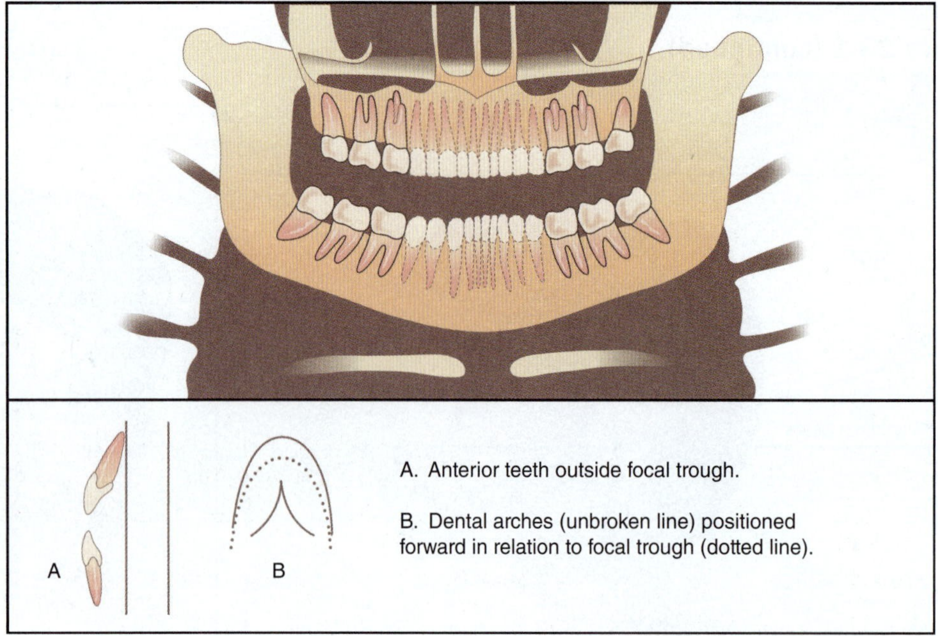

A
B
A. Anterior teeth outside focal trough.
B. Dental arches (unbroken line) positioned forward in relation to focal trough (dotted line).

FIGURE 23-11
Panoramic film of patient positioned too far forward.

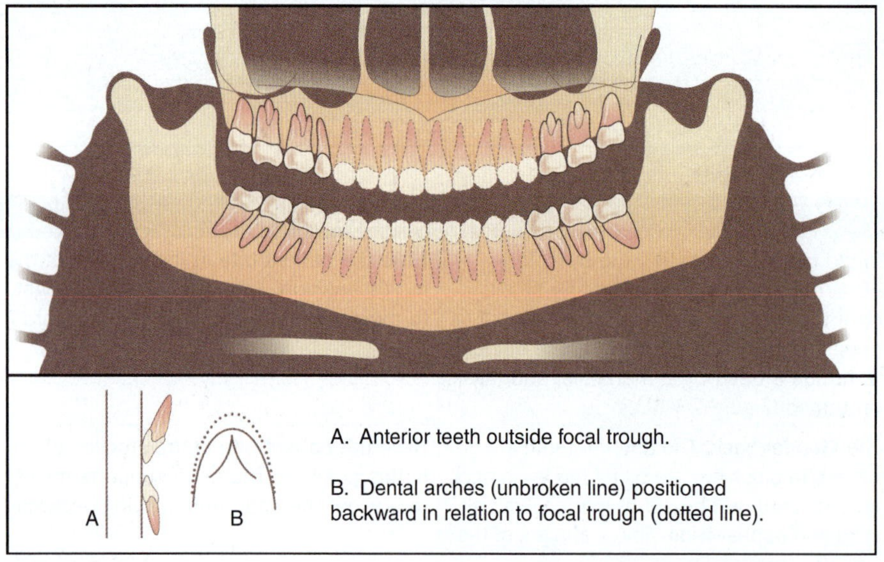

A
B
A. Anterior teeth outside focal trough.
B. Dental arches (unbroken line) positioned backward in relation to focal trough (dotted line).

FIGURE 23-12
Panoramic film of patient positioned too far back.

Cephalometric Radiographs

A **cephalometric radiograph** (*cephalo* means "head" and *metric* means "measurement") is used to assess the patient's skeletal structure and profile (Figures 23-17 and 23-18). The cephalometric radiographs are used mainly by orthodontists for treatment planning of their patients, but some oral maxillofacial surgeons and general practitioners include these radiographs for patient assessment. The patient's bony structure, as well as soft tissues, are recorded on the cephalometric radiograph. Lateral (side) or posterior anterior (back to front) views are used for orthodontic measurements, examination of the sinuses, implant evaluation, and TMJ assessment. A cephalometric unit provides a way to ensure that the patient is accurately positioned in a manner that can be duplicated as the patient grows, and as repeated radiographs are needed for comparison. The unit consists of a **cephalostat**, or head-holding device; a cassette holder for an 8 × 10 inch cassette; and an x-ray tubehead.

For lateral views, position the patient by placing the left side of his or her head against the cassette, positioned so that the midsagittal plane is parallel to the cassette. The Frankfort plane of the patient, or line from the **tragus of the ear** to the floor of the orbit, is parallel to the floor. The x-ray beam is directed perpendicular to the cassette.

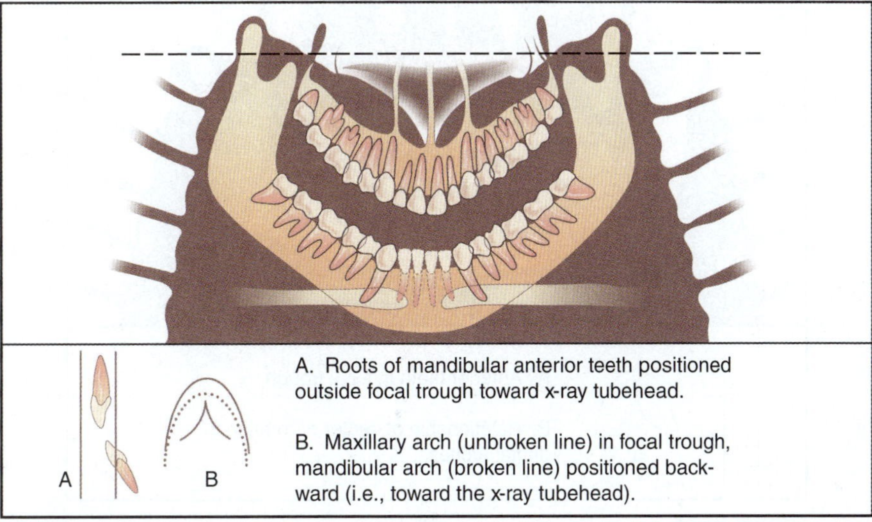

A. Roots of mandibular anterior teeth positioned outside focal trough toward x-ray tubehead.
B. Maxillary arch (unbroken line) in focal trough, mandibular arch (broken line) positioned backward (i.e., toward the x-ray tubehead).
A
B

FIGURE 23-13

Panoramic film of patient's head tilted downward. Frankfort plane adjustment needed.

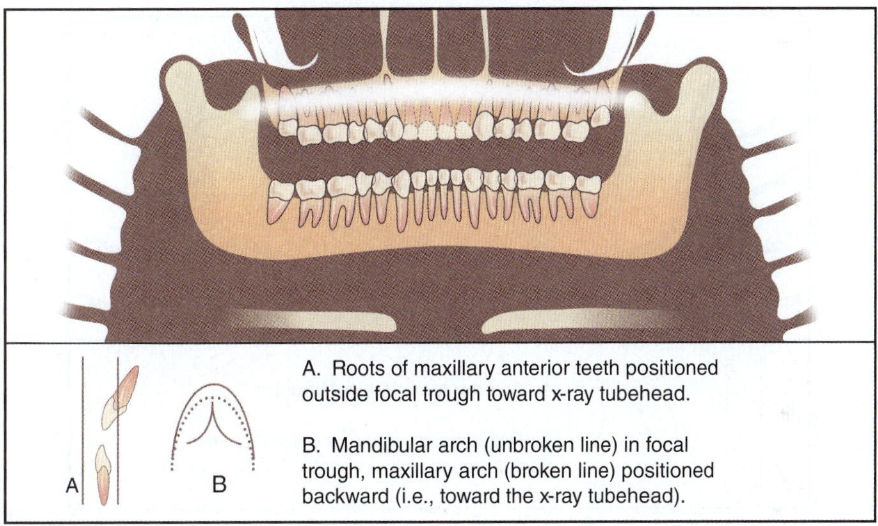

A. Roots of maxillary anterior teeth positioned outside focal trough toward x-ray tubehead.
B. Mandibular arch (unbroken line) in focal trough, maxillary arch (broken line) positioned backward (i.e., toward the x-ray tubehead).
A
B

FIGURE 23-14

Panoramic film of patient's head titled upward. Frankfort plane adjustment needed.

For posterior anterior radiograph views, the patient faces the cassette with the Frankfort plane parallel to the floor, and the x-ray beam directed at the occipital bone and perpendicular to the cassette (Figures 23-19A and B).

Lateral Jaw Radiograph. The **lateral jaw radiograph** can be used if the dental office does not have a panoramic x-ray machine. Large areas of the jaw can be radiographed by using a 5 × 7 or an 8 × 10 inch film cassette, and instructing the seated patient to hold the cassette next to his or her face and rest it on his or her shoulder. The x-ray tubehead is positioned on the opposite side, and directed so that the central ray is perpendicular to the patient's head and the cassette. The x-ray exposure time is increased because of the layers of tissue and bone. The patient's head is positioned differently depending on the area the dentist needs to view.

Transcranial Temporomandibular Joint Radiograph. The **transcranial temporomandibular joint radiograph** is taken with the patient holding a cassette against the side of the head and the cone/central x-ray positioned on the opposite side of the patient's head, slightly above and behind the external auditory meatus. Positioning devices assist in correctly aligning the head for the x-ray (Figures 23-20 and 23-21). The radiograph can be taken with the patient's mouth open or closed.

Radiographic Interpretation

Being familiar with the terminology used in radiographic interpretation will make the dental assistant better prepared to perform radiographic procedures (Table 23-2).

Learning landmarks makes radiographic interpretation much easier and more meaningful. The following structures

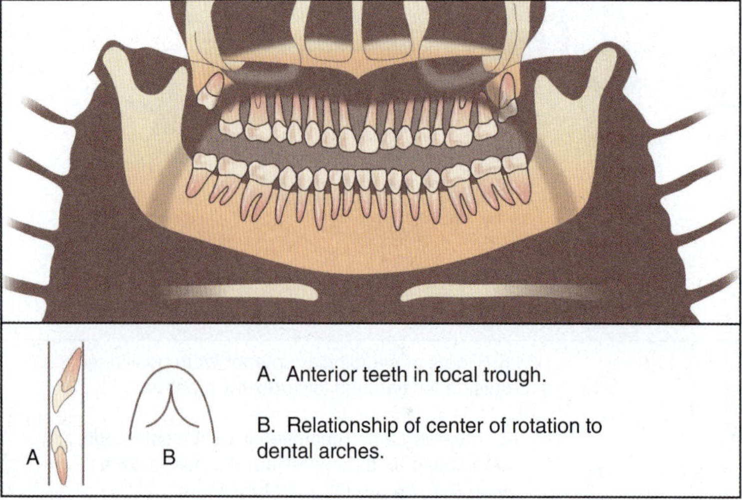

FIGURE 23-15
Panoramic film of patient's tongue not against the roof of the mouth.

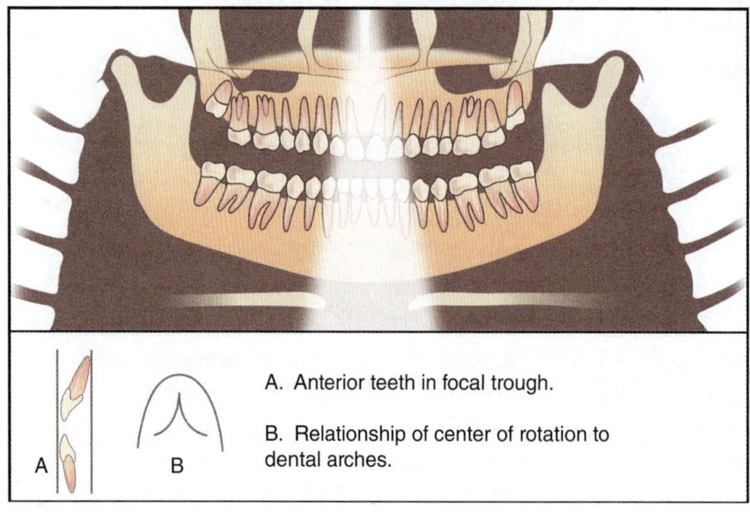

FIGURE 23-16
Panoramic film of patient not standing up straight, resulting in a midsagittal plane error.

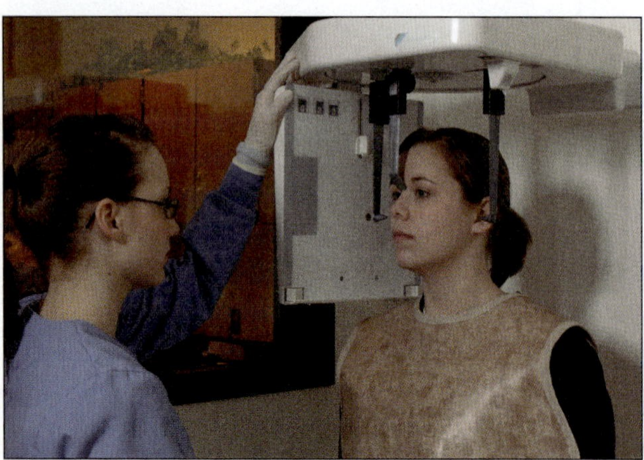

FIGURE 23-17
Patient positioned for a lateral cephalometric radiograph.

are defined and identified on radiographs and/or in diagrams, showing both normal and abnormal landmarks. The dental assistant interprets radiographs to prepare for the dentist and the procedure.

The terms begin with the tooth and the surrounding tissues, and then cover the maxilla and the mandible. Periapical, occlusal, and panoramic radiographs are used to show each term, but the landmark may be seen on more than one type of radiograph.

Tooth and Surrounding Tissues

Enamel: A radiopaque area on the crown of the teeth.

Dentin: The area just inferior to the enamel; it is less radiopaque than enamel.

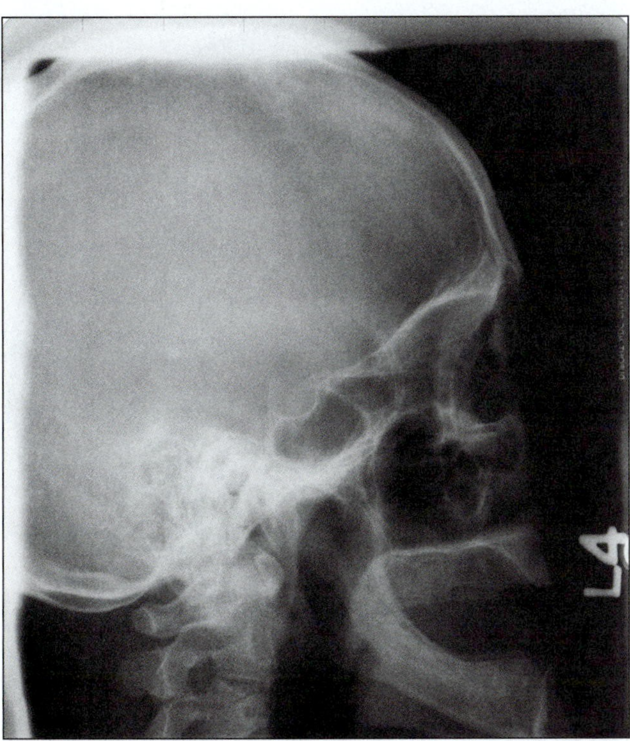

FIGURE 23-18
A lateral cephalometric radiograph.

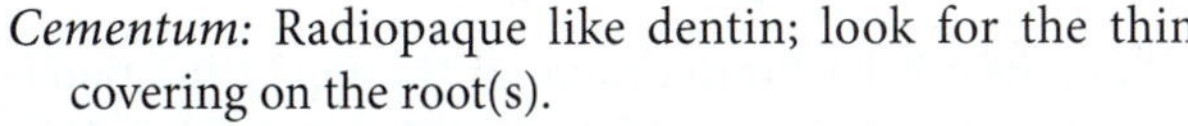

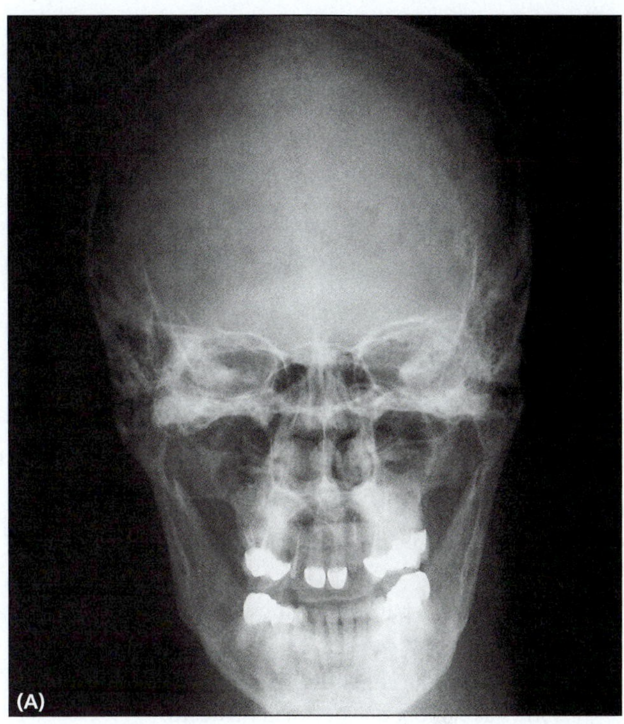

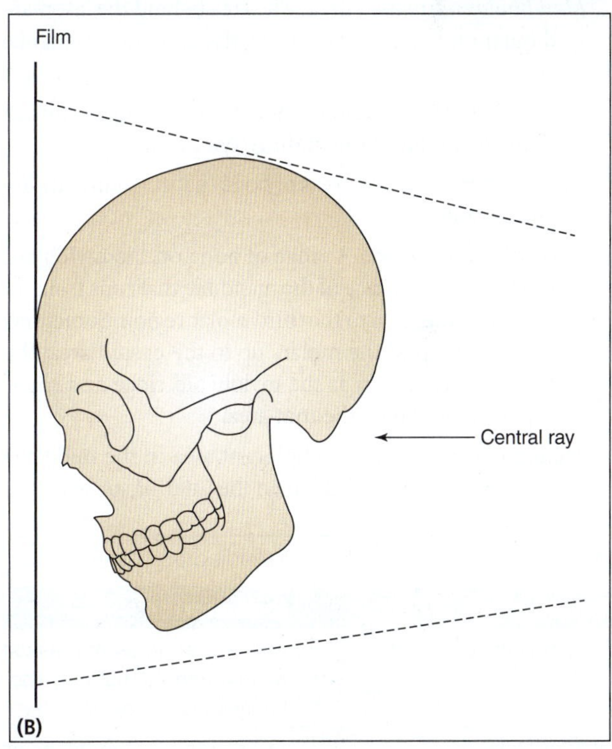

FIGURE 23-19
(A) Posterior anterior radiograph. (B) A labeled line drawing of a posterior anterior radiograph.

Cementum: Radiopaque like dentin; look for the thin covering on the root(s).

Pulp chamber: A radiolucent area surrounded by dentin; the pulp horns can be seen; these projections usually correspond with the cusps of the tooth, as seen on the x-ray.

Pulp canals or root canals: Radiolucent areas in the root, which extend from the pulp chamber to the apex of the tooth.

Periodontal ligament/space: A radiolucent area that surrounds the root(s) of the tooth.

Lamina dura: A radiopaque line of cortical bone that surrounds the root(s) of the tooth and the periodontal ligament.

Cortical plate: A dense, compact bone that forms the tooth socket.

Interradicular bone: The alveolar bone found between the roots of a tooth; it shows radiopaque on the x-ray.

Interdental bone: The alveolar bone found between two teeth; it shows radiopaque (Figure 23-22).

Mandibular Landmarks (Figure 23-23)

Mental foramen: A radiolucent area between the roots of the premolar.

Mandibular canal: The canal is radiolucent, but outlined by radiopaque lines that extend from the mandibular foramen to the mental foramen.

External oblique ridge: A ridge on the external surface of the mandible, extending from the middle of the rami to beyond the molar area. This ridge runs in an oblique line but curves more toward the middle third of the molars than the internal oblique ridge.

Trabecular patterns: Spongy or cancellous bone that surrounds the teeth and forms the mandible. The

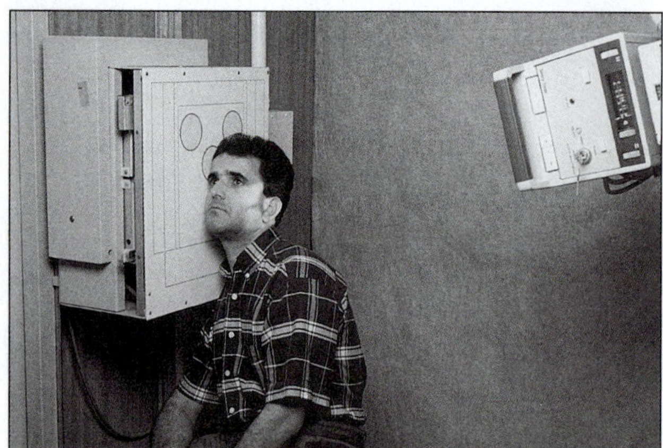

FIGURE 23-20

Patient positioned for a transcranial lateral position TMJ radiograph with the mouth closed.

spongy bone pattern is shown as radiopaque with radiolucent spaces.

Alveolar crest: The compact edge of the cortical bone that shows as radiopaque between the teeth.

Mandibular retromolar area: The area behind the last mandibular molar; it shows varying tissues in this triangular space.

Lingual foramen: A radiolucent area on the lingual surface of the mandible at the midline/symphysis.

Genial tubercle: Raised areas of bone that surround the lingual foramen.

Internal oblique ridge: A ridge of bone on the mylohyoid ridge internal surface of the mandible that runs from the middle of the rami to the third molar region. Sometimes it continues past the molars up to the cuspid area; this extension is known as the mylohyoid ridge and shows superimposed over the root area.

Mandibular foramen: A radiolucent area in the middle of the ramus of the mandible on the interior surface.

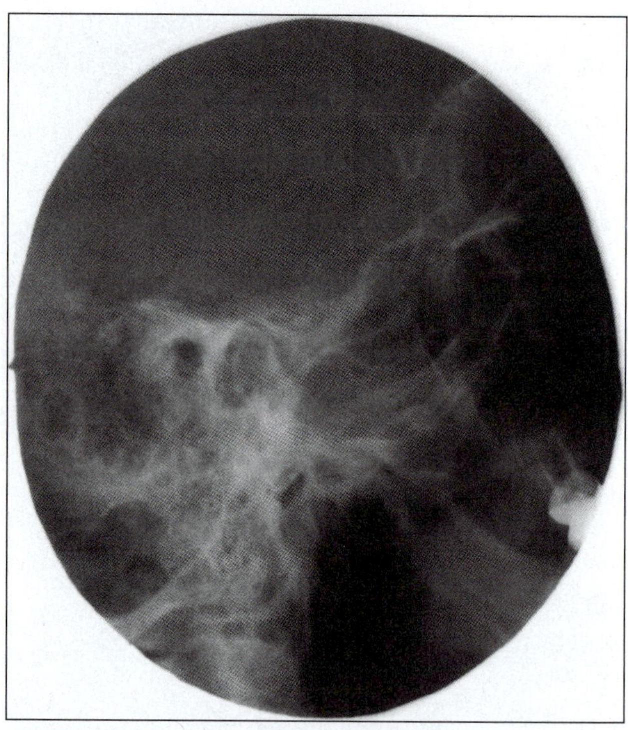

FIGURE 23-21

Transcranial TMJ radiograph with the mouth closed, showing the relationship of the condyle to the glenoid fossa.

Condyle: A back projection on the top of the ramus; it shows radiopaque and is articulated in the glenoid fossa.

Coronoid process: The front projection of the tip of the ramus; it shows radiopaque.

Medial sigmoid notch: The indented area between the condyle and coronoid processes on the ramus; also known as the coronoid notch or the mandibular notch.

Ramus: The section on each side of the mandible that runs vertically.

TABLE 23-2 Terminology Used in Radiographic Interpretation

Terminology	Explanation
Anatomical landmarks	Anatomical areas that assist in identification for mounting x-rays and communicating with the dentist and the patient. The dental assistant does not diagnose x-rays, but can interpret x-ray images and recognize what is normal and what is abnormal.
Radiopaque	Structures that are dense and do not allow rays to pass through them. The x-rays are blocked or absorbed to varying degrees depending on the density of the structure. The structures show up in light gray to white shades on the x-ray, depending on the density.
Radiolucent	Structures that show up on x-rays in shades of dark gray to black. The structure is not dense; x-rays penetrate in varying degrees.
Diagnosis	To know; the art or act of identifying disease.
Interpretation	To explain the meaning of something.
Superimposition	One structure lying over another.

Note: Radiopaque and radiolucent are comparative terms. They are used to compare one structure or substance to another.

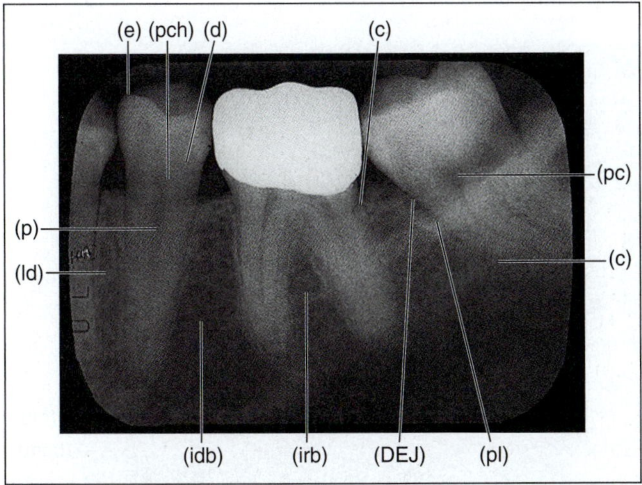

FIGURE 23-22

X-rays identifying the parts of a tooth and surrounding structures: (d) Dentin. (c) Cementum. (e) Enamel. (p) Pulp canal. (pc) Pulp chamber. (pch) Pulp chamber. (DEJ) Dentinoenamel junction. (pl) Periodontal ligament (black line). (ld) Lamina dura (white area of cortical bone). (irb) Interradicular bone. (idb) Interdental bone.

Body of mandible: The section of the mandible that runs horizontally.

Border of the mandible: The lower edge of the body of the mandible that is made of compact bone.

Symphysis: The chin area, or anterior portion of the mandible.

Hyoid bone: The U-shaped bone suspended by ligaments below the mandible, but anterior to the larynx; it is occasionally seen on dental x-rays.

Nutrient canals: The radiolucent paths that extend toward the alveolar crest.

Maxillary Landmarks (Figure 23-24)

Hard palate: A radiopaque structure that forms the roof of the mouth.

Incisive foramen: A radiolucent area at the midline of the palate posterior to the central incisors.

Maxillary suture: Also known as the median palatine suture, a radiolucent line that joins the right and left halves of the maxillary bone and palatine bones.

Zygomatic process: The process on the external surface that begins around the first molar region.

Malar: A part of the zygomatic bone that forms the cheek.

Nasal septum: A radiopaque line that divides the nasal fossae.

Nasal cavities: The two side-by-side openings of the nose.

Nasal conchae: Bony, scroll-shaped plates in the lateral walls of the nasal cavity.

Maxillary sinuses: Left and right cavities located superior to the apices of the teeth, which can extend from the canines to the molar area.

Infraorbital foramen: A radiolucent area inferior to the inferior border of the orbit (eye socket).

Orbit: The bone that circles the eyeball.

Maxillary tuberosity: A radiopaque area behind the most posterior molar on the maxilla.

Glenoid fossa: A depression on the lower border of the temporal bone where the condyloid process of the mandible articulates as the temporomandibular joint.

Mastoid process: The process of the temporal bone that lies in the lower anterior section just posterior to the ear (auditory canal).

External auditory meatus: A radiolucent area in the temporal bone for the auditory canal.

Hamular process: A slender projection of bone that lies posterior and medial to the maxillary tuberosity.

Styloid process: A projection of bone, larger than the hamular process that comes from the temporal bone and lies posterior to the glenoid fossa.

Conditions or Artifacts on X-Rays

Conditions or artifacts that may appear on x-rays (Figure 23-25):

- Dental caries
- Implants
- Impacted tooth
- Recently extracted tooth
- Root canal with reamer
- Periodontal pocket
- Orthodontic bands
- Overhang
- Calculus
- Attrition
- Abscesses
- Cysts
- Vertical bone loss
- Eyeglasses
- Amalgam shavings
- Vertebra
- Metallic restoration
- Fracture
- Mixed dentition
- Abrasion
- Drifting
- Supernumerary tooth
- Horizontal bone loss

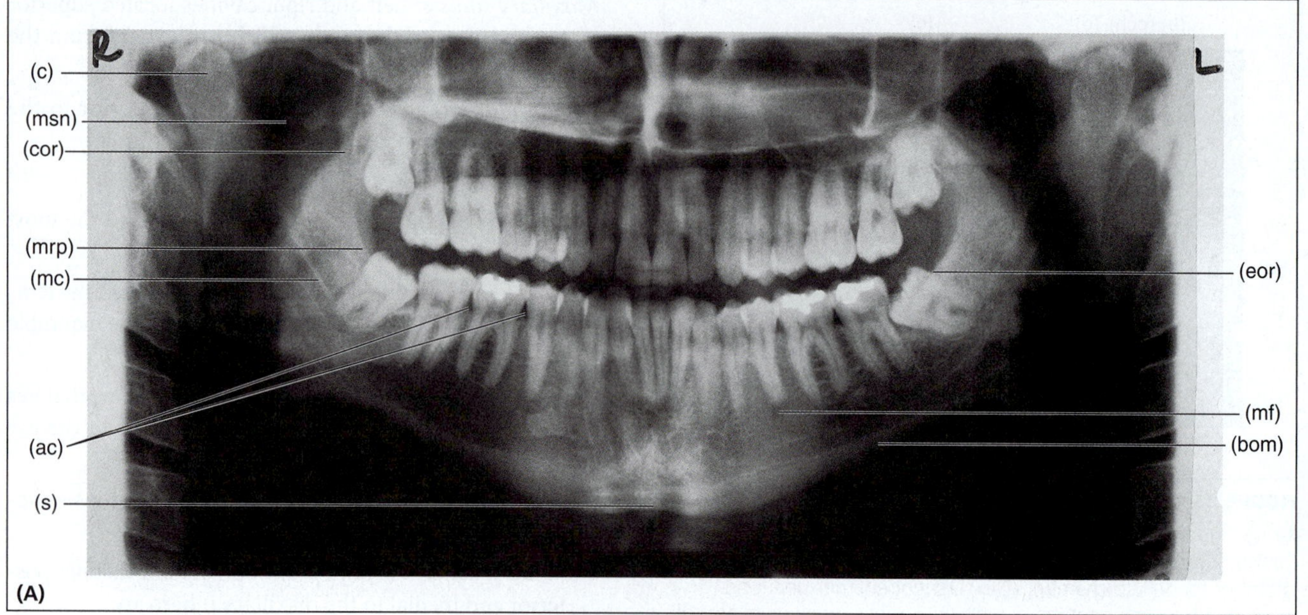

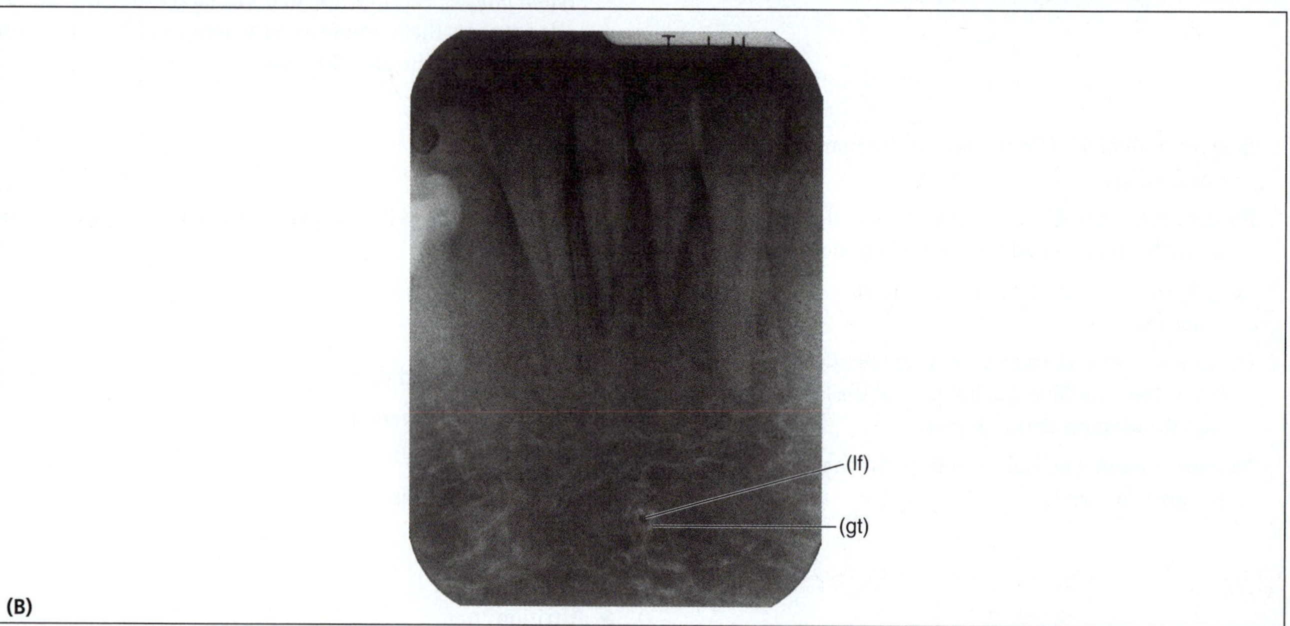

FIGURE 23-23

(A) Panoramic radiograph identifying mandibular landmarks. (s) Symphysis. (ac) Alveolar crest. (mc) Mandibular canal. (mrp) Mandibular retromandibular pad. (cor) Coronoid process. (msn) Medial sigmoid or mandibular notch. (c) Condyle. (eor) External oblique ridge. (mf) Mental foramen. (bom) Border of mandible. (B) X-ray showing lingual landmarks of the mandible. (lf) Lingual foramen. (gt) Genial tubercles.

- Bridge
- Earrings
- Edentulous patient
- Cement base/lining
- Root canal restoration
- Pins/posts
- Cervical burnout
- BBs or shrapnel
- Framework from reconstructive jaw surgery

Imaging Systems/Digital Imaging Systems

Imaging systems are used frequently by dental professionals. The systems most commonly used are **computed tomography (CT scanning)** and **magnetic resonance imaging (MRI)**. These imaging systems are found in hospitals or specialized clinics.

Advances continue to be made in **digital imaging technology**. These computerized systems are the future in dental radiology, and will be in every dental office. Dental assistants

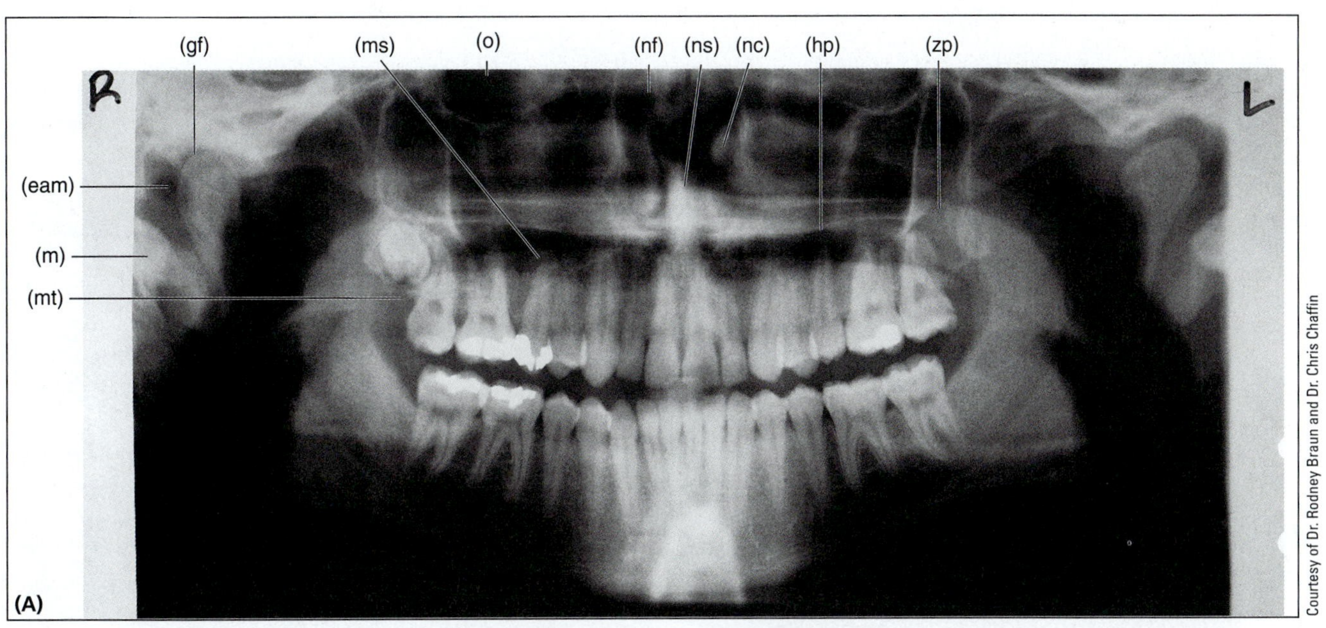

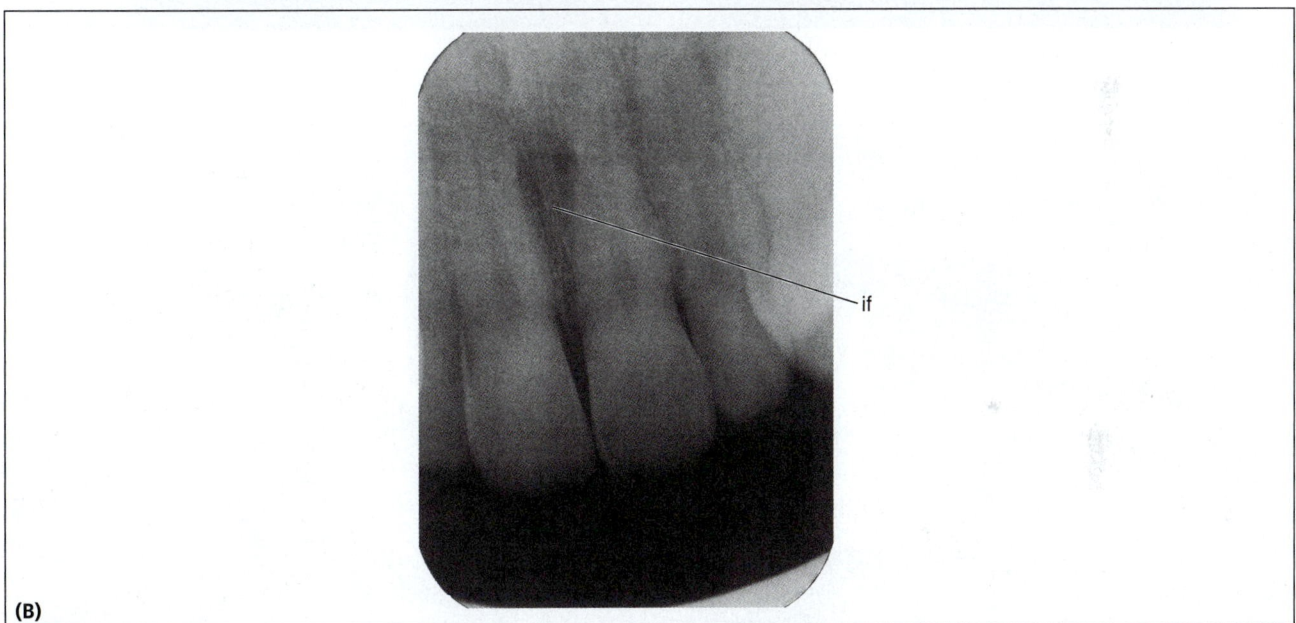

FIGURE 23-24

(A) A panoramic and periapical radiograph identifying the maxillary landmarks. (mt) Maxillary tuberosity. (m) Mastoid process. (eam) External auditory meatus. (gf) Glenoid fossa. (ms) Maxillary sinuses. (o) Orbit. (nf) Nasal fossa. (ns) Nasal septum. (nc) Nasal conchae. (hp) Hard palate. (zp) Zygomatic process. (B) (if) Incisive foramen.

continually need to be up-to-date concerning these systems as they are integrated into the dental office.

Computed Tomography (CT Scanning)

CT scanning is used to plan implant surgery, and to locate and define lesions associated with the oral cavity. Computed tomography eliminates the use of x-ray film, but still uses ionizing radiation as the source of energy. Patients are placed in a CT unit, where the radiation and image detector rotate around them. The information is transmitted to a computer, which calculates an image and displays it on a monitor. The image can be transferred to film for later study. The computer is able to produce images in all dimensions or planes, although the original image is taken in one plane: the **axial plane**. This is where the original CAT scan (computed axial tomography) came from. *CT scanning* is the accepted term for computed tomography (Figure 23-26).

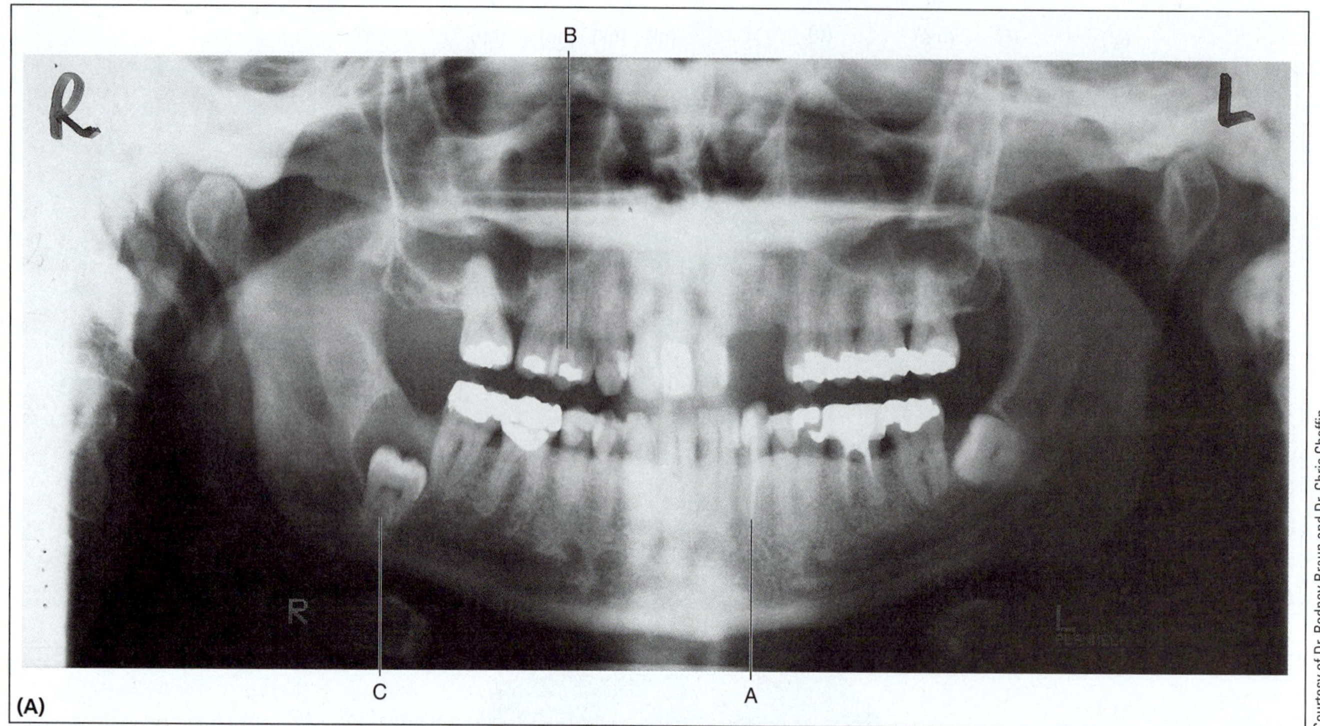

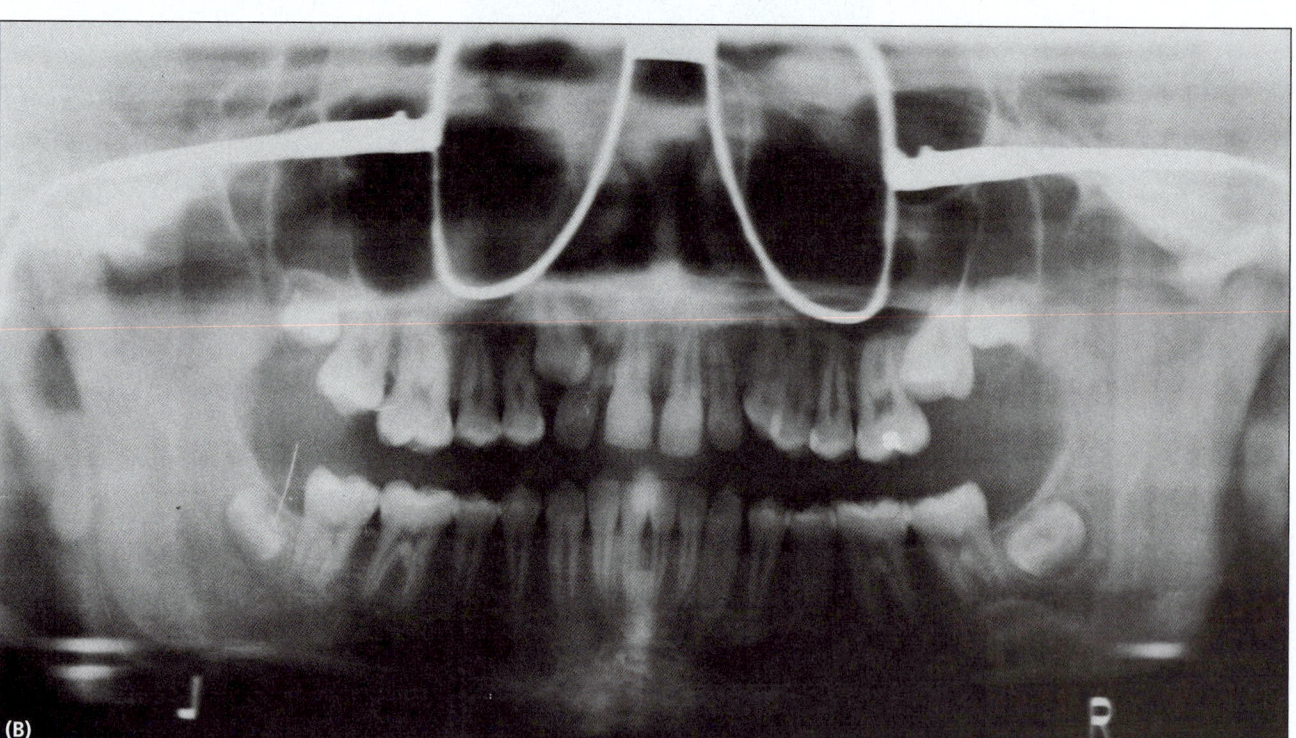

FIGURE 23-25

(A) Panoramic radiograph showing artifacts that may appear, such as (A) root canal, (B) caries, and (C) impacted tooth. (B) Panoramic radiograph showing an artifact.

Magnetic Resonance Imaging

MRI techniques are used mainly for diagnoses of temporomandibular joint (TMJ) disease. They enable the dentist and radiologist to view the soft tissues of the TMJ with very little risk to the patient. These techniques use low-energy electromagnetic radiation instead of ionizing radiation. The patient is placed in a unit that contains powerful primary and secondary coils. The primary coils produce the magnetic field, while the secondary coils maintain the magnetic field and alter the primary magnetic field to receive information from

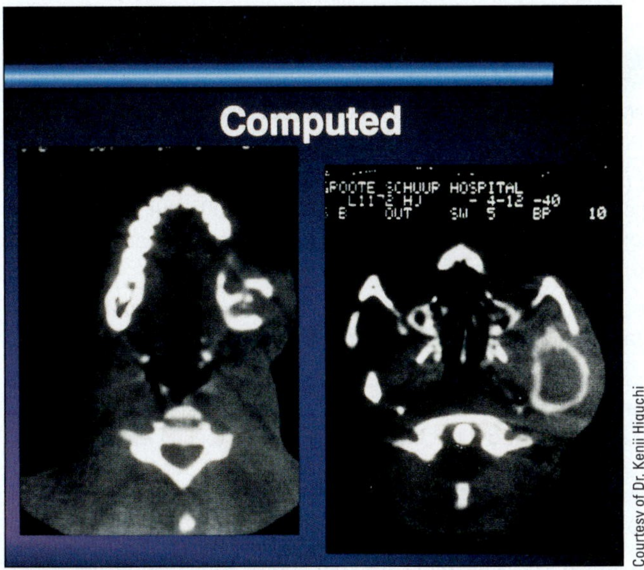

Courtesy of Dr. Kenji Higuchi

FIGURE 23-26
A CT scan of the skull on the coronal plane.

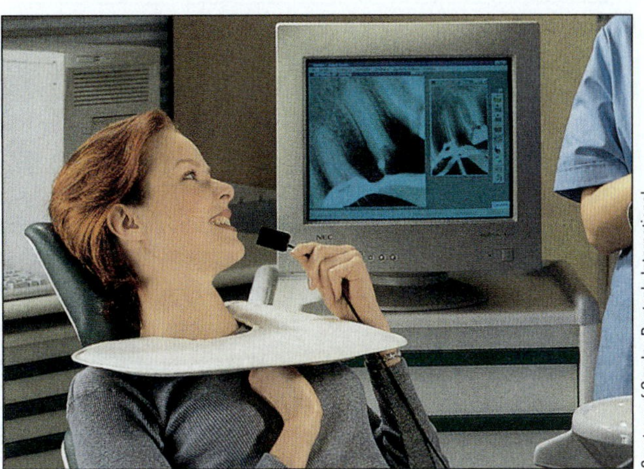

Courtesy of Gendex Dentsply International

FIGURE 23-27
An intraoral digitizing unit.

different planes of the body. The secondary coils also transmit and receive radio frequency pulses or magnetic signals.

Digital Radiography in the Dental Office

Digital intraoral imaging (**digital radiology**) is one of the many changes in dentistry that continues to develop and become the standard of practice. Digital radiography is expected to eventually replace all conventional film exposure. Digital radiology is a computerized system that allows the dentist to take an intraoral or extraoral radiograph, and then display the image on a computer screen without processing the dental film (Figure 23-27). Table 23-3 provides definitions of terminology related to digital radiography.

The Fundamental Concepts of Digital Radiography

Digital radiography breaks the radiographic image into electronic pieces and then displays them on the computer. The image can be digitized, enhanced, printed, stored, or sent to another office by email, Internet transmission modes, or portable digital storage media. In digital radiography systems, the *image* is the term used to describe the picture produced, instead of *radiograph* or *x-ray* film. Digital radiography is not limited to intraoral images; extraoral images, such as panoramic and cephalometric images, can be taken with some digital imaging systems.

In the traditional system, when the x-rays strike the film the information is recorded on the film. This is known as an **analog image**. Analog images depict a continuous spectrum of gray shades between black and white. The analog image is a smooth transition from one color/shade to another. In digital imaging, the sensor receives the analog information and converts it into a **digital image** within the computer. The digital image is like a mosaic, comprised of many small pieces known as **pixels**. Pixel is short for "picture elements". Each pixel is a small dot within a digital image—more pixels equal a higher resolution, and a sharper image. Each pixel has a distinct shade of gray, black, or white. The **gray scale** of the image is important for diagnosing the condition of the teeth, tissues, and surrounding bone. The dentist relies on the contrast—**radiolucency** and **radiopacity**—to determine the presence of disease. The computer monitor can display over 200 shades of gray, but the human eye can only detect around 32 shades of gray. Therefore, computer software is used to enhance gray shades to improve detailing and comparison.

A sensor or image detector takes the place of traditional x-ray film (Figure 23-28). This sensor is an electronic or specially coated plate that is positioned in the mouth and then exposed to x-rays. When the x-ray beam contacts the sensor, an electronic charge is produced on the surface of the sensor. This electronic form/signal is digitized, or converted into data that can be read and stored by the computer. Depending on the type of imaging system, the sensor may connect directly to the computer through a fiber optic cable or the sensor may be wireless.

Types of Digital Imaging

Currently there are both direct and indirect methods of obtaining a digital image.

Direct Digital Imaging. A **direct digital imaging** system includes the following components: x-ray machine, sensor, computer monitor, and computer software. Direct digital imaging uses a solid-state sensor that contains an x-ray sensitive silicon chip with an electronic circuit. These sensors are either a **charge-coupled device (CCD)** or **complementary metal oxide semiconductor (CMOS)** technology. Both

TABLE 23-3 Digital Radiology Terminology

Term	Definition
Analog image	An image produced by traditional film, in which there is a continuous spectrum of gray shades between black and white.
Charge-coupled device (CCD)	A solid-state detector used in many common electronic devices, such as video cameras, fax machines, and surgical microscopes. In digital radiography, the CCD is the image receptor in the intraoral sensor. This receptor converts x-rays into electrical charges, the intensity of which is related to a color (gray scale).
Digital radiography	A filmless imaging system that uses a sensor and computer to capture an image and convert it into pixels (electronic data). This image is enhanced, presented, and then stored as part of the patient's record.
Digital subtraction	This feature allows images that were taken at different times to be compared. The images are electronically merged with images that did not change, thereby, canceling each other out. The images that did change will stand out. Another feature of digital subtraction is the ability to reverse the gray scale of The image: The radiolucent images (normally black) are now white, and the *radiopaque* images (normally white) are now black.
Digitize	The conversion of an x-ray film image into a digital image that can be processed by a computer.
Direct digital imaging	A technique of exposing an intraoral sensor to radiation in order to obtain a digital radiographic image that can be viewed on a computer. This method uses an intraoral sensor, x-ray machine, computer monitor, and computer software program.
Gray scale	Shades of gray visible in an image.
Indirect digital imaging	A technique used for scanning x-ray images on pre-existing dental films into digital images before moving on to storage phosphor imaging. This method uses an intraoral sensor, x-ray machine, scanner, computer monitor, and computer software program.
Pixel	Derived from the plural of *picture* (pix) and the word *element* (el), pixels are discrete units of information that comprise an image.
Sensor	A small electronic or specially coated plate that is sensitive to x-rays. When placed intraorally and exposed to radiation, the sensor captures the radiographic image.
Storage phosphor imaging	An indirect digital imaging method of obtaining a digital image. The image is recorded on a special phosphor-coated plate, and then placed in an electron scanner. A laser scans the plate and produces an image on the computer monitor.

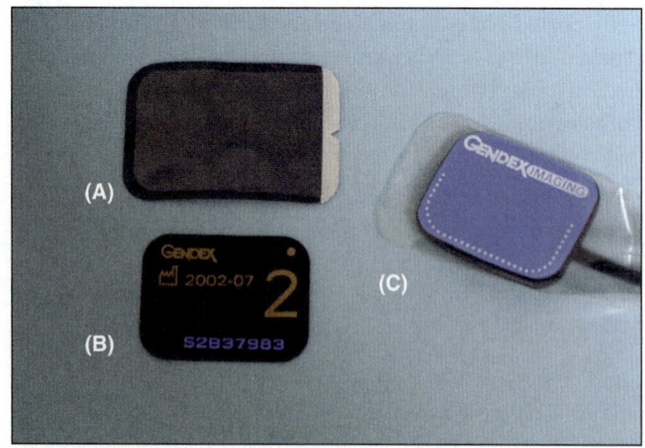

FIGURE 23-28
(A) Barrier. (B) Imaging plate. (C) Direct digital sensor.

CCD and CMOS technologies work equally well in converting x-rays into an electronic signal, which is, then, sent to the computer. The difference between the two is the design of the electronic chip. The manufacture of the sensors determines which technology to use.

The charge-coupled device (CCD) is one of the most common image receptors used in dental digital radiography. Developed in the 1960s, the CCD is used in many devices, such as fax machines, home video cameras, microscopes, and telescopes. The CCD is a solid-state detector comprised of a grid of small transistor elements that convert x-rays to electrons. The electrons produced by the x-ray are deposited in a small box or "well" known as a pixel. A pixel is the digital equivalent of a silver halide crystal used in traditional radiology. However, the arrangement of the silver halide crystals is random, unlike the pixels in digital radiography, which are structured in an ordered arrangement. The CCD is 640 × 480 individual pixels in size. Once the elements are exposed to x-rays, they are read and the electron charges are converted to form the digital image.

With the direct digital imaging the sensor is placed in the patient's mouth and exposed to x-rays. The image is produced on the surface of the sensor, digitized, and then transmitted to the computer. Almost immediately, the image appears on the monitor. Software is then used to enhance the image and store the image as part of the patient's records.

Indirect Digital Imaging. An **indirect digital imaging** system contains the following components for indirect digital imaging: image plates, dark container, a scanner with carousel computer, computer software, and a viewbox.

The **photostimulable phosphor (PSP)** plate sensor technology, also called **storage phosphor imaging,** is a wireless system that uses specially coated imaging plates instead of sensors to record the image. This system is very different than the CCD and CMOS technology. PSP sensors are similar to film in the way they look, and in the way the radiographic image is captured as an analog image and then processed. PSP technology uses plates that are coated with a phosphor layer, which, when exposed to x-rays, stores the x-ray image as a latent image, similar to the way silver halide crystals within the film emulsion stores the latent image. The image plates are covered with a barrier, and then placed in the mouth using a film-holding device. They are flexible and fit into the mouth much like intraoral film. Unlike the direct digital imaging sensors, there is no cable attached. Once the plate is exposed to x-rays, it is placed in a dark container until all films have been taken. The image plates are then placed on a high-speed laser scanner to release the energy stored on the plates, converting the information into a digital image. The computer uses the digital values to reconstruct the image on the computer. Laser scanning processing makes the PSP technology similar to film-based radiology in that both the x-ray film and the image plate must be "developed" later. Because of this extra step, which ranges from seconds to minutes, this type of digital radiography is more time consuming than direct digital imaging. After the image plates have been scanned, they must be cleared between each use by exposing them to bright light, like that on a viewbox, for several minutes. Once the image is erased from the image plates, they can be sterilized for use again.

Digital Radiography Equipment

Equipment needed for digital imaging includes a dental x-ray machine, sensor or image detector, a computer, and digital imaging software.

X-Ray Machine. A conventional x-ray machine is used with digital radiography. The x-ray machine should be capable of producing 70 kV or less, and 5 mA or less. The timer must be adapted to allow exposure in a time frame of 1/100 of a second.

Sensor (Image Detector). As previously stated, the sensor is a small detector that takes the place of traditional x-ray film. It is placed in the patient's mouth and used to capture the image. Sensors for direct digital imaging are solid-state (electronic) digital sensors and use CCD or CMOS technology. Sensors for indirect digital imaging use PSP technology with specially coated plates. Sensors for both direct and indirect digital imaging come in a variety of sizes: 0, 1, 2, and 4 x-ray films. Some of the sensors are thick, bulky, and rigid, while others are thin and flexible. The edges are sometimes too sharp to be very comfortable in the patient's mouth, but improvements are continually being made. The sensors are covered with barriers before being placed in a patient's mouth, and some can withstand cold sterilization.

The intraoral sensors used in direct digital imaging may be either *wired* or *wireless*. Wired sensors are attached to a fiber optic cable, which is connected to a computer. The sensor converts the x-rays into an electronic signal, which is then recorded by the computer. The cable varies in length from 8 to 35 ft (1.5 to 10.7 m); the shorter the cable, the more limited the range of motion. Wireless sensors are not connected directly to the computer, but transmit through radio frequency to a circuit board in the computer.

Computer and Computer Software. The computer digitizes, processes, and stores information received from the sensor or scanner. Some requirements for this computer are adequate memory for rapid conversion, and the ability to store digital radiographs while simultaneously generating high-resolution images on a monitor. The computer must be conveniently located for easy viewing by the dentist and the patient, connected to a printer for generating hard copies as needed, and linked to the Internet for electronic transferring of patients' images to insurance companies, other dentists, or dental specialists.

Software is provided by the manufacturers that offer digital imaging systems. They offer a variety of features to enhance and manipulate the images for better detection and for improved patient understanding. Some of the features offered by software systems include the following:

- Charting
- Density and contrast
- Digital subtraction
- Embossing
- Magnification
- Measuring tools
- Reversing the gray scale
- Side-by-side displays of images

Advantages and Disadvantages of Digital Radiography

Although digital radiography is continually advancing, there are advantages and disadvantages to this technology.

Advantages.

- Less exposure to radiation for the patient. Sensors are more sensitive and require less radiation, falling by 50 percent compared to using F-speed films.
- Results appear on the computer monitor almost immediately after exposure to x-rays. The dentist can then enhance, contrast, zoom, take exact measurements, make notes about the image, and alter the color and brightness/

contrast of the image, right at chairside to better evaluate the patient's condition.

- Patients can view images when the dentist is discussing areas of concern.
- Because digital images are stored on computer media, much less space is required for storage.
- The darkroom, processing equipment, and solutions are eliminated, thereby eliminating the maintenance of this equipment, and the need to deal with the storage of used chemicals.
- Digital images are quickly and easily sent via an email attachment to other dental offices, insurance companies, patients, and so on. Allowing, for example, faster processing of insurance claims.

Disadvantages.

- The main disadvantage of digital imaging is the initial expense of the equipment and software. Prices vary according to manufacturer and system quality.
- Extra time is required to become proficient in using the digital imaging hardware and software. Correctly positioning the sensor or imaging plate is still a prerequisite for a detailed, quality radiograph. Positioning technique errors are similar to traditional x-ray exposure positioning errors.
- There is a learning curve for dentists in reading and diagnosing from digital radiography, as the approach is different from that used in traditional radiography.
- Sensors are usually thicker than x-ray film packets. Placement is often uncomfortable for the patient, and sometimes causes the patient to gag. However, sensor design is improving, and these problems will sooner or later be eliminated.
- There are concerns about rapid and costly updating, computer viruses, and system failures.
- Infection control is a concern with digital radiography. The sensors are covered with barriers that can tear and are not always totally aseptic. The keyboard and mouse must also be covered, and the covers changed with each patient. Some manufacturers suggest an intermediate-level disinfectant applied with gauze pads for cleaning and disinfecting the sensor, keyboard, and mouse as needed.

Procedure 23-2
Digital Radiology Techniques

This procedure serves as a general guideline when using digital radiology. Manufacturers of digital radiography systems provide detailed instructions on preparation of the equipment and the patient, taking the exposure, and using the software.

Equipment and Supplies

- Barriers for the x-ray room and equipment
- Sensor or imaging plates
- Barriers for the sensors or imaging plates
- Cotton rolls (optional)
- Appropriate x-ray film holders (assembled for use)
- Dark container for exposed imaging plates
- Lead apron with thyroid collar

Preparation of Equipment

1. Turn on the computer and load the software to select the patient chart or identification.
2. Enter the radiology icon of the chart and enter the type of radiograph to be exposed.
3. Select a sensor that has been disinfected or sterilized, and then prepare it by placing an approved barrier over the sensor (Figure 23-29).
4. Place the sensor in an appropriate x-ray film holder (Figure 23-30).

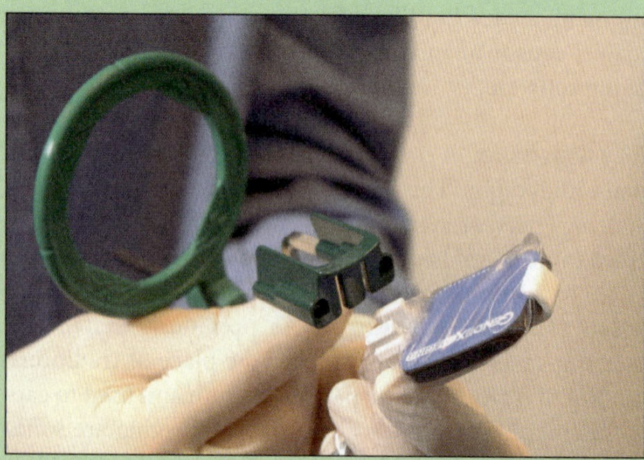

FIGURE 23-29

A sensor that has been prepared with a barrier prior to placement in the patient's mouth.

(continues)

Procedure 23-2 (continued)

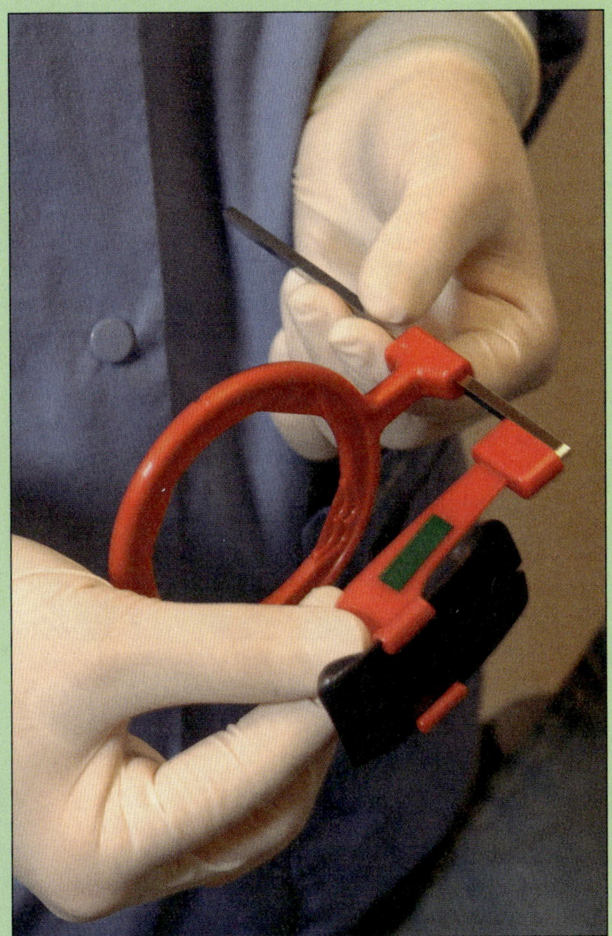

FIGURE 23-30
A sensor being placed in the Rinn x-ray film holder.

5. Prepare the x-ray machine and adjust the settings. For most digital systems, the exposure settings are half those used for F-speed x-ray film exposures. For suggestions on exposure settings, always follow the manufacturer's instructions.

Preparation of Patient

Patient preparation is virtually the same as for traditional radiograph exposure.

1. Seat the patient and have him or her sit so that the midsagittal plane is perpendicular to the floor.
2. Adjust the chair to a comfortable level.
3. Adjust the headrest to position the patient's head so that the occlusal plane is parallel to the floor.
4. Place the lead apron with thyroid collar on the patient.
5. Request the patient to remove eyeglasses, and all objects from the mouth that might interfere with the procedure.
6. Quickly inspect the oral cavity for anything that may require alteration of sensor placement, such as tori or a shallow palate.

Taking the Exposure

1. Place the sensor in the patient's mouth (Figure 23-31), and carefully move into position for exposure.
2. Align the x-ray cone and PID to direct the central rays, using the same technique for x-ray film exposure.
3. Using the keyboard or mouse, activate the sensor for exposure.
4. Press the exposure button to expose the sensor.

Direct Digital Imaging System

1. Wait until the image appears on the monitor and evaluate it (Figure 23-32). If the image is what the dentist needs for a quality diagnosis, continue on with the next image to be exposed. If a positioning error has occurred, do not remove the sensor from the patient's mouth; determine what caused the error, and correct the sensor position or realign the PID. Note: Even though the amount of radiation that the patient is exposed to is reduced, retakes should be limited, just as they are when taking traditional radiographs.
2. When the image is satisfactory, remove the sensor or reposition it for additional exposures. Repeat until all exposures are acquired.

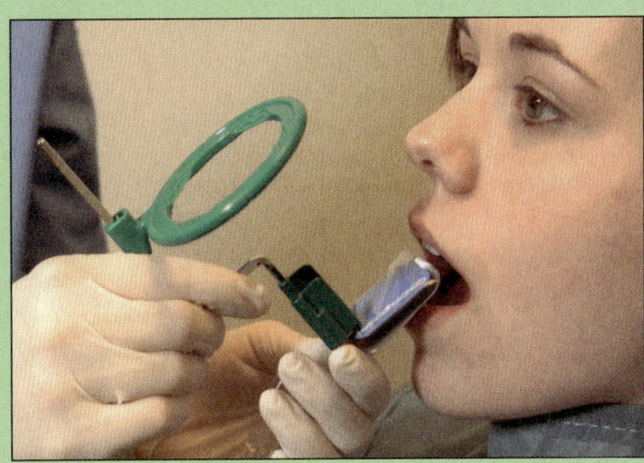

FIGURE 23-31
A sensor being placed in the patient's mouth for correct alignment.

(continues)

Procedure 23-2 (continued)

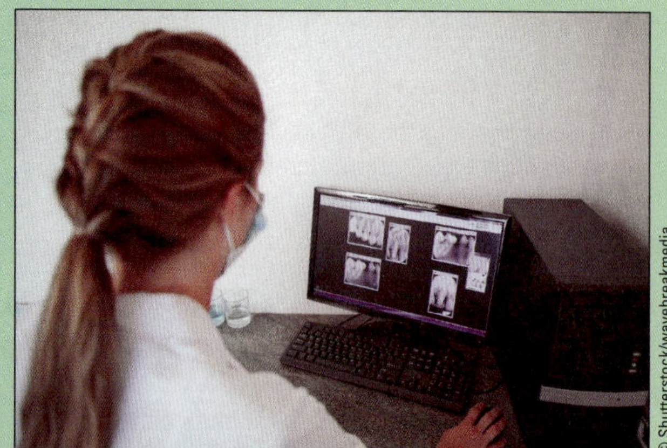
© Shutterstock/wavebreakmedia

FIGURE 23-32
A dental assistant reviewing digital radiographs on the computer.

Indirect Digital Imaging System

1. Remove the imaging plate from the patient's mouth.
2. Remove the imaging plate from the film holder and remove the plastic barrier.
3. Place the imaging plate in a dark container until all exposures have been taken.
4. After all exposures are complete, in a semi-dark room place the imaging plates on the scanner and activate.
5. The images will begin to appear on the monitor. Evaluate the images according to the requirements for quality diagnostic images. If the image does not meet diagnostic standards, erase the image from the plates and disinfect them according to the manufacturer's instructions, and then follow the same technique listed previously (Figure 23-33).

After Exposure

1. Save the patient's images and back up the file on the computer or on a supplemental storage system.

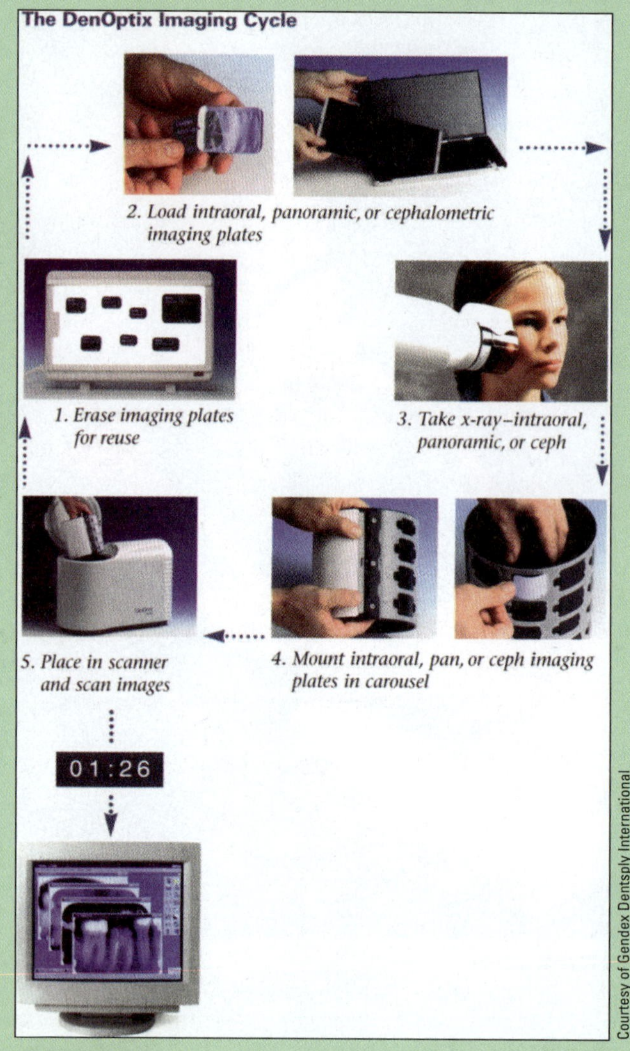

The DenOptix Imaging Cycle
2. Load intraoral, panoramic, or cephalometric imaging plates
1. Erase imaging plates for reuse
3. Take x-ray–intraoral, panoramic, or ceph
5. Place in scanner and scan images
4. Mount intraoral, pan, or ceph imaging plates in carousel
01:26

Courtesy of Gendex Dentsply International

FIGURE 23-33
An indirect digital imaging cycle.

Three-Dimensional Imaging in Dentistry

Dentistry has entered into the world of **3D dental imaging** and diagnosis. The 3-D imaging unit, which is about the size of a panoramic unit, can be placed in the dental office for dental applications. This technology offers dentists and dental specialists comprehensive diagnosis data, improves information and interpretation for multiple treatments, and enables the design of treatment plans with more predictable results. It shows more information than traditional dental x-rays or CT scans.

The 3-D dental image scan shows an immediate 3-D reconstruction of a patient's mouth, face, and jaw areas including the condyles and surrounding structures. Tooth positions are visualized to show impactions in the alveolar bone, the location of adjacent teeth, and their proximity to vital structures, such as the mandibular nerve canal and sinus walls.

This technology provides an excellent image quality with fine three-dimensional details and the lowest possible radiation dose.

What Is 3-D Imaging?

There are a number of companies that manufacture 3-D units that meet the needs of different clinic settings, and that take a variety of images, including complete or partial skull fields of view. The units are designed to produce digital panoramic and cephalometric images and 3-D photos, as well as cone beam volumetric tomography (CBVT) and cone beam volumetric imaging (CBVI). Along with the 3-D imaging units there are many advanced imaging software tools to meet the requirements of dental radiology.

With the 3-D imaging device, the x-ray beam is cone-beam shaped and aimed at a solid-state flat panel detector that covers the desired image volume (see the following Note) in a single scan. Depending on the imaging device, the image is usually captured in a single rotation around the patient's head. Traditional CT scans had a fan-shaped beam that required multiple, repeated-slice scans to accomplish a similar image volume.

The cone beam shows hundreds of isotropic images of the patient from different positions around the scan rotation. The information is transferred to the computer, which reconstructs it into the anatomical volume for the dentist to see. The measurements and information gathered are dimensionally accurate and detailed. Once the data is reconstructed, imaging software is used for the multilayer viewing of the anatomical volume. This information is then saved on a designated system in a format that specialists, dentists, and other imaging-related services can access. Wide selections of volume sizes are available to meet diagnostic needs without excess radiation outside the area of concern.

Note: What is *volume* in 3-D dental imaging? Volume equals a unit of 3-D space that a substance or shape occupies.

Which Dentists Would Use 3-D Imaging?

Three-dimensional technology is becoming more familiar with many dental professionals as it develops and more dental offices incorporate it into their diagnostic procedures. The concepts of 3-D imaging are designed to enhance dental treatment in the following areas: endodontics, periodontics, orthodontics, maxillofacial surgery, and general dentistry. Software is designed to produce the images and information each dental office needs for the treatment of their patients. Specialists and general dentists can store the scanned information for future use, and it can be sent to other dentists working with the same patient case.

Uses and Benefits

There are many applications for this technology in all aspects of dentistry. Three-dimensional dental images are recommended for the following:

- To provide data to determine bone quality and quantity
- To locate detailed anatomy
- To locate pathology, such as cysts, tumors, and bone lesions
- To evaluate deformities and pathologies
- To view critical landmarks and show minuscule detail
- The details of the scan allow for early detection and evaluation.
- Accurate planning and measuring for dental implants
- To plan virtual orthognathic surgery
- To evaluate TMD and TMJ diagnosis (analysis)
- To show the entire dentition and the whole maxillofacial and mandibular regions
- To produce complete and partial 3-D face photos
- Precise measuring tools and improved general dental imaging
- To locate and evaluate impactions and many other dental conditions
- For advance treatment planning and assisted delivery abilities, software has been designed to make custom precision surgical guides, virtual models, and laser-generated resin models
- Spinal studies
- Airway assessment

Patient Preparation. With the 3-D dental imaging machine the patient can have the scan completed right in the dental office. With the 3-D dental imaging equipment, the patient either stands or is seated comfortably in an open scanner, instead of being placed in the supine position (Figure 23-34). Once the patient is seated, images are scanned in a very short period of time that varies with each machine, usually from 8 to 20 seconds. Once the scan is complete, the

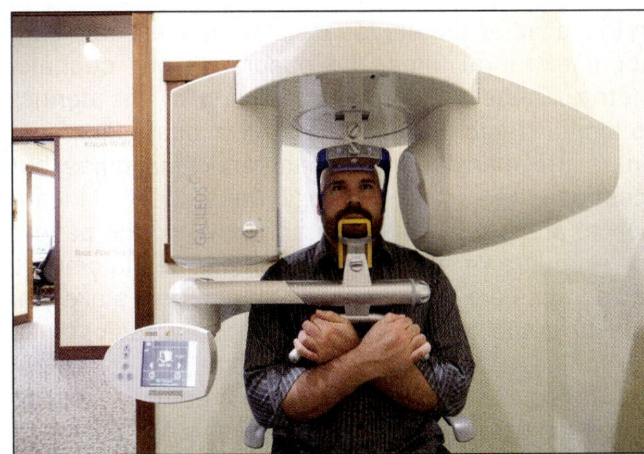

FIGURE 23-34
A patient positioned to take a 3-D image.

information is transferred to the computer through different software programs. Software is quick and effective, reconstructing critical anatomy in less than 30 seconds. The software is designed to solve dental problems through perceptive integration of diagnosis, computer-aided therapy planning, and detailed intraoperative implementation.

Once the information has been successfully scanned, the dentist can show the patient the images, and then discuss the diagnosis and give the patient an understanding of their treatment options.

Hand-held Intraoral Radiography

Another new technology is the portable hand-held dental x-ray unit. These low radiation dose, **hand-held intraoral radiography** machines are battery operated and are being purchased in increasing numbers by dental offices and clinics (Figure 23-35). They have been available in other countries for some time, and have aided in providing global access to dental care to clinics in remote areas of the world. The hand-held systems can be used in a variety of settings including the following: military bases, dental offices, clinics, teaching facilities, forensic clinics, nursing homes, and out of the office use. The units can also be used in times of power outages because they are battery operated.

The hand-held units have a digital control panel that is simple and quick to use. Selections include adult or child, anterior or posterior bitewings, and the type of exposure medium, either film, digital sensor, or phosphor plate. The panel also shows the battery status. The hand-held units are usually preset at 60 kV and 2 mA; with most x-ray units the exposures are preset, but can be adjusted and saved manually. The batteries for most units are made of lithium polymer technology and most units come with an extra battery, a battery charger, and a stand so that the unit is ready at all times. Most units take more than a 100 exposures on one battery charge.

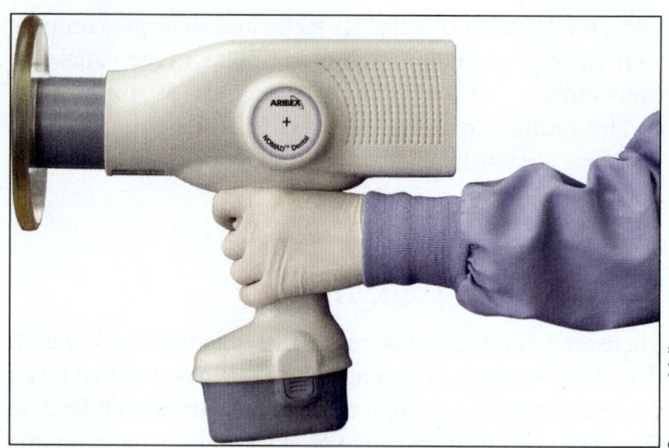

Courtesy of Aribex

FIGURE 23-35
A hand-held dental intraoral radiography machine.

Because the units are hand-held, the operator is allowed to stay with the patient, thus reducing the time necessary when exposing x-rays. The hand-held units are safe and specially designed with significantly more shielding around the x-ray tube, and a back-scattering radiation protection shield. This shield is composed of lead impregnated acrylic, which blocks scattered radiation. The position indicating device (PID) or collimator is also shielded. Its low radiation makes it safe for both the patient and user alike.

This new technology requires education, time, and a willingness to change how x-rays are routinely taken by the dental team. The hand-held x-ray unit is expensive and requires training before using. Several studies on the safety and quality of radiographs as compared to the standard x-ray machine have shown that the hand-held x-ray unit is safe and produces quality radiographs, but there is still some reservation and the need for more research.

Chapter Summary

In this chapter the dental assistant student will learn about extraoral films, the panoramic and cephalometric. These radiographs are used by the dentist to identify large areas of the skull in one radiograph. There are many types of panoramic machines but most use the same technology. The student will learn how to prepare the machine, the film, and the patient for exposure of a quality radiograph. Cephalometric radiographs are used to assess the patient's skeletal structure and profile. The cephalometric radiographs are mainly used by the orthodontists, but some oral maxillofacial surgeons and general dentists include these radiographs for patient assessment and treatment planning.

As part of the students training they will learn to examine radiographs and identify normal and abnormal landmarks. This will include the teeth, surrounding tissues, mandibular and maxillary landmarks and conditions and artifacts that are sometimes seen.

Digital radiography is identified and explained in this chapter. Digital radiography is one of the recent advancements in dentistry. Types of digital radiography are discussed as well as the equipment and techniques. The three-dimensional imaging has now entered the profession of dentistry. The 3-D dental image scan shows immediate 3-D reconstruction of a patient's mouth, face, and jaw areas. This technology shows an excellent image quality with the finest details in three dimensions and with the lowest possible radiation dose.

Another new technology introduced in this chapter is the hand-held dental x-ray unit. These machines are low radiation and are battery operated. They can be used to expose x-rays on adults and children. The hand-held units are used in various settings including military bases, dental clinics, teaching facilities, and nursing homes. This technology requires education and the willingness to change how x-rays are routinely taken.

CASE STUDY

Dr. Danton is considering changing the way his office takes radiographs. His patients have been asking about reducing radiation exposure during x-rays. Dr. Danton has been practicing for about 10 years and is comfortable with traditional x-ray film exposures for both intraoral and extraoral radiographs, but he also wants to keep up with technology and current trends in dentistry.

Case Study Review

1. Describe alternatives to traditional x-ray film exposures that Dr. Danton can explore.
2. Enumerate the advantages and disadvantages of digital technology.
3. What factors must be considered by the dental team deciding to use a digital radiography system?

Review Questions

Multiple Choice

1. Which of the following is considered extraoral film?
   a. Panoramic radiograph
   b. Occlusal radiograph
   c. Cephalometric radiograph
   d. Both A and C
2. A cassette is used to
   a. hold the film for extraoral radiographic exposures.
   b. act as a lining.
   c. intensify the x-rays.
   d. hold films during processing.
3. All of the following are true statements about panoramic exposure techniques *except*:
   a. Remove bulky sweaters, coats, and hair clips that may interfere with the rotation of the x-ray tubehead.
   b. The patient should always wear a lead apron without a thyroid collar.
   c. The film is placed in the patient's mouth, and the patient gently closes on the film.
   d. The patient is positioned in the chin rest, biting on a bite block, with the head properly positioned for the film exposure.
4. Dental assistants are allowed to diagnose dental disease by interpreting x-rays.
   a. This statement is true.
   b. This statement is false.
5. All of the following are seen as radiopaque structures on dental x-rays *except* the
   a. cementum.
   b. enamel.
   c. pulp chamber.
   d. lamina dura.
6. Which of the following radiology techniques is used mainly for diagnosis of temporomandibular joint disease?
   a. Computer tomography
   b. Magnetic resonance imaging
   c. Digital imaging
   d. None of the above
7. ________ allows the dentist and/or dental assistant to take x-rays, and then display the image on a computer monitor.
   a. Computer tomography
   b. CT scanning
   c. Digital radiography
   d. Magnetic resonance imaging
8. All of the following are part of direct digital imaging systems *except* the
   a. x-ray machine.
   b. sensor.
   c. computer software and monitor.
   d. duplicating film.
9. With which of the following systems is a scanner used after the x-rays have been exposed?
   a. Direct digital imaging system
   b. Indirect digital imaging system
10. All of the following are true statements about 3-D imaging systems *except:*
    a. can be used in maxillofacial surgery, endodontics, periodontics, orthodontics, implantology, and TMJ analysis.
    b. uses standard periapical film.
    c. permits diagnosis in detailed three dimensions.
    d. lowest possible radiation dose to the area of interest on the patient.

Critical Thinking

1. A patient appears to have a fractured mandible. The dentist requests an x-ray. What type of x-ray would be the most beneficial for diagnosing a fractured mandible? Would the dental assistant be able to obtain this x-ray clinically?
2. Name the types of radiographs in which all of the following can be seen: alveolar crest, coronoid process, maxillary retromolar pad, and the mental foramen.
3. Digital imaging is replacing conventional film exposures in dentistry. What type of exposures can be achieved using digital imaging? Discuss the advantages of digital imaging over conventional film exposures.

Web Activities

1. To study questions that patients frequently ask about dental x-rays, go to http://www.ada.org. Select "Search" and put in "digital x-rays" to learn more about the use of digital x-rays.
2. Check http://www.sirona.com to learn more about their 3-D imaging system and the latest advances in this technology. Then go to http://www.ada.org and put in "3-D imaging" to find related information from the American Dental Association.
3. To learn more on hand-held dental radiography, go to http://www.Aribex.com and the American Dental Association at http://ada.org.

Section VII

Dental Specialties

CHAPTER

24

Endodontics

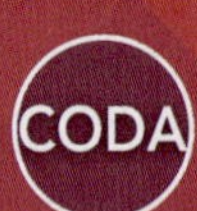

Specific Instructional Objectives

The student should strive to meet the following objectives and demonstrate an understanding of the facts and principles presented in this chapter:

1. Define endodontics and describe what an endodontist does.
2. Describe pulpal and periapical disease.
3. Identify diagnostic procedures.
4. Identify instruments used in endodontic procedures and describe their functions.
5. Identify materials used in endodontics and describe their functions.
6. Describe endodontic procedures and the responsibilities of the dental assistant.
7. Describe endodontic retreatment.
8. Explain surgical endodontic procedures and the instruments used.

Key Terms

abscess (566)
apex finder (574)
apexification (584)
apexogenesis (584)
apical curettage (581)
apical periodontitis (565)
apicoectomy (581)
barbed broach (569)
cellulitis (566)
chelating (574)
debridement (569)
electronic pulp tester (567)
endodontic bender (575)
endodontic handpiece (575)
endodontic microscope (575)
endodontic obturation system (573)
endodontics (565)
extirpate (570)
exudate (565)
files (570)
fistula (566)
flex files (570)
Glick #1 (573)
gutta percha (567)
heating unit (575)
Hedström file (570)
hemisection (584)
intracanal instruments (569)
irreversible pulpitis (565)
K-type file (570)
master cone (579)
nonvital pulp (565)
obturating (572)
osteomyelitis (566)
palpation (566)
percussion (567)
perforation (571)
periapical abscess (565)
periapical cyst (565)
periradicular (565)
periradicular abscess (565)
periradicular cyst (565)
periradicular periodontitis (565)
plugger (572)
pulpal necrosis (565)
pulpectomy (581)
pulpitis (565)
pulpotomy (581)
reamer (570)
retrograde filling (583)
retrograde restoration (581)
reversible pulpitis (565)
root amputation (584)
root canal sealer (571)
rubber stop (571)
selective anesthesia (568)
sodium hypochlorite (573)
spreader (572)
transillumination test (568)
ultrasonic unit (575)
vital pulp (565)
vitality scanner (567)

Introduction

The field of **endodontics** comprises diagnosis and treatment of diseases of the pulp and periapical (**periradicular**) tissues. Endodontic procedures include diagnosis, root canal treatment, and periapical surgery.

The endodontist has advanced education and training in the field of endodontics. General dentists, who can also treat the pulp and periapical tissues, render the same standard of care within their education and experience, but then refer the patient to an endodontist for cases requiring advanced knowledge and training.

The general dentist sends written instructions and radiographs to the endodontist to prevent miscommunication. The endodontist also often communicates with the referring dentist concerning the patient's treatment and prognosis. The patient may return to the general dentist for the final restoration after the endodontic treatment is completed by the endodontist.

Endodontic Team

The staff in the endodontist's office shares responsibilities similar to those of the general dental office staff, except that there is an increase in communication with other dental offices because most of the patients are referrals.

The endodontist is assisted by dental assistants who perform traditional assisting responsibilities in addition to expanded duties specific to endodontics as allowed by state dental practice acts.

Progress of Pulpal and Periapical Diseases

A healthy pulp is said to be a **vital pulp**. When the pulp or periapical tissues are irritated or injured, the result is inflammation and this condition is called **pulpitis**. Advanced dental decay is one of the main sources of irritation. Other irritations or injuries include heat, impact trauma, fractures, invasive restorative procedures, and adverse reactions to dental materials. The degree of pulpal inflammation depends on the severity and duration of the irritation or injury and the ability of the tissues to respond. The patient may or may not have symptoms that indicate the degree of the inflammation of the **nonvital pulp**.

Pulpitis

Pulpitis includes reversible pulpitis, irreversible pulpitis, and pulpal necrosis.

- **Reversible pulpitis**—The pulp is inflamed but able to heal when the irritant is removed. Causes include incipient caries, enamel fractures, and occlusal attrition. Symptoms include sensitivity to hot and cold. Treatment involves removing the irritant and placing sedative materials to soothe and heal the pulp.
- **Irreversible pulpitis**—The inflammation continues until the pulpal tissue cannot recover. Symptoms include pain to the patient that may be short and sharp or dull and continual. The treatment for irreversible pulpitis is root canal therapy or extraction.
- **Pulpal necrosis**—The death of the pulpal cells often results from irreversible pulpitis. Symptoms and treatment for pulpal necrosis are similar to those for irreversible pulpitis. As the pulp inflammation progresses, **exudate** (**ECKS**-you-dayt), or pus, and gas form in the pulp chamber. If the tooth is sealed and the exudate cannot escape, pulpal necrosis is rapid. If the exudate drains through caries or exposure to the oral cavity, the process is slowed. A fistula is a tubelike passage that sometimes forms to drain an abscess from the apex of a tooth to the oral cavity. The exudate in the fistula may move from an area of high concentration to an area of low concentration, forming a "gumball" on the tissue.

Periapical Diseases

When the infection in the pulp reaches the apex of the tooth, it continues into the periapical area. The intensities of the inflammation and the host response determine the extent of the infection. Periapical disease includes apical periodontitis and periapical abscess.

- **Apical periodontitis**—Also known as periapical periodontitis, AP, and **periradicular periodontitis**. Pulpal inflammation extends into the periapical tissues. This response can be either acute or chronic. The acute condition subsides if the irritation is removed. With the acute inflammation there is pain, pus formation, sensitivity to touch, and swelling. If the process continues and the irritant is not removed, the apical periodontitis becomes a chronic inflammation. This abscess is asymptomatic with little or no pain. A radiograph of the area shows an interruption of the lamina dura and destruction of the periapical tissues (Figure 24-1). The immediate area of chronic apical periodontitis is usually classified as a granuloma or a cyst. A granuloma consists of numerous cells of the inflammatory process. If a granuloma is left untreated and the irritation continues, a cyst forms. A cyst is filled with liquid and semisolid materials and is partially lined with stratified squamous epithelium (**SKWAY**-mus ep-ih-**THEE**-lee-um) and surrounded by connective tissue.
- **Periapical abscess (periradicular abscess)** (A localized destruction of tissue and accumulation of exudate in the periapical region. The patient's reaction can range from moderate to severe discomfort and/or swelling. The treatment includes releasing the pressure by creating an opening into the pulp chamber, removing the necrotic pulp, and root canal therapy.
- **Periapical cyst (periradicular cyst)**—A very common cyst of the jaw, it is the result of infection of the tooth. The infection spreads to the apex of the tooth and into the surrounding bone. The cyst is caused by pulpar necrosis that is secondary to dental caries or trauma.

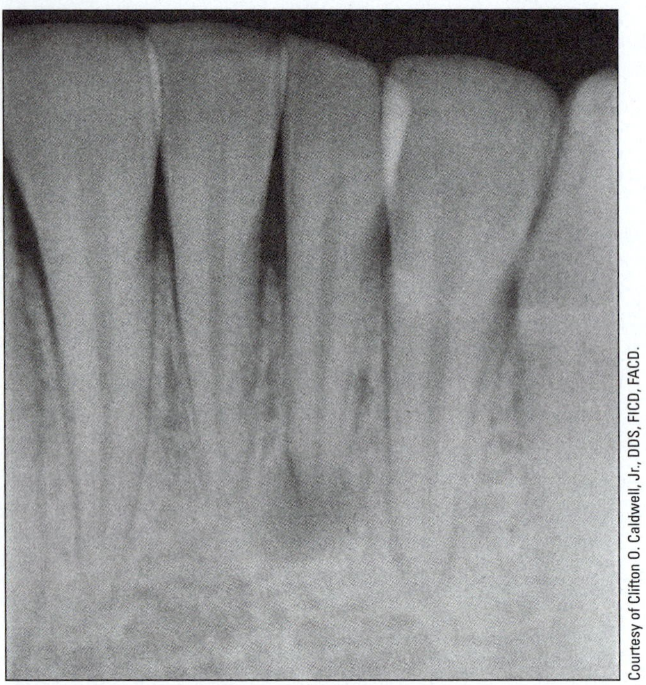

Courtesy of Clifton O. Caldwell, Jr., DDS, FICD, FACD.

FIGURE 24-1
Radiograph of tooth with apical abscess (dark shadow at the apex).

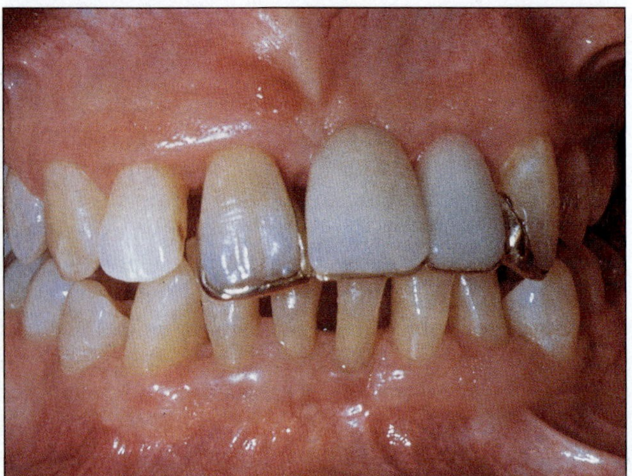

FIGURE 24-2
Patient with gingival abscess (red area above tooth #8 near frenum).

Related Terms

- **Fistula** (**FIS**-tyou-lah)—A path to the external surface, created by the body to drain the **abscess** (Figure 24-2)
- **Cellulitis** (sell-you-**LYE**-tis)—When the abscess spreads into the facial tissues, causing swelling and discomfort
- **Osteomyelitis** (oss-tee-oh-my-eh-**LYE**-tis)—An advanced stage of periapical infection that spreads into and through the bone

Endodontic Diagnosis

Endodontic diagnosis includes patient medical and dental history; clinical examination, including radiographs, pulp testing, and review of communication from the referring dentist about the case. Each office has a routine procedure that is followed carefully to ensure that all pertinent information is gathered.

Medical History

The first step is for the patient to fill out a medical history. Once completed, the history is reviewed and clarified to ensure that accurate and complete information is gathered. The medical history may reveal information that relates to previous treatment of the tooth pulp to be used in diagnosis.

Dental History

The dental history provides the endodontist dental experiences and the signs and symptoms of the current concern. The dental history opens the way for subjective examination (the problem explained in the patient's words). The patient should be allowed to describe the type of pain, sensitivity to heat and cold, duration of the condition, and any other symptoms.

Clinical Examination and Pulp Testing

The clinical examination, or the objective examination, includes evaluation of the extraoral tissues, such as facial asymmetry, swelling, redness, and external fistulas.

During the intraoral examination, the soft tissues are thoroughly evaluated and palpated, while searching for any abnormalities or signs of inflammation. Visual examination of the teeth may reveal caries, discoloration, or fractures, but clinical tests are usually performed to develop a complete diagnosis. Clinical tests are performed by the dentist to correctly diagnose the patient's situation. Selected testing procedures are described below.

Radiographs. Radiographs are often the most useful of the diagnostic tools. Radiographs are taken and processed immediately so the dentist can refer to them throughout the procedure. If the inflammation has extended beyond the apex of the tooth and has bone involvement, a radiolucent area will be apparent. Detailed periapical x-rays with accurate positioning and good contrasting qualities are necessary to view the area around the end of the tooth root. Radiographs are taken at several stages during the root canal procedure, including the initial radiograph, upon opening a canal to determine the length, upon placement of the final size files in the canals, and a final radiograph is taken once the root canal procedure is completed.

Palpation. The endodontist performs **palpation** of the soft tissues. Pressure is applied to the mucosal tissue near the apex of the root of the suspicious tooth. Normally, one or more additional teeth are palpated for comparison. Around the indicated tooth, the area may be soft and raised (pus filled).

Percussion. The endodontist will also perform **percussion** by tapping on the occlusal or incisal surface of the tooth. The handle of a mouth mirror is often used (Figure 24-3). The tapping is first done on a control tooth and then on the symptomatic tooth. The control tooth should be the same tooth in the opposite arch. The patient may experience mild to moderate pain if there is periodontal inflammation, and sharp pain if there is periapical inflammation.

Mobility. Mobility is evaluated to determine the condition and involvement of the supporting structures of the tooth. Teeth that move 2 to 3 millimeters should not have root canal therapy because they lack sufficient support. Mobility is tested by placing the handle of an instrument or a finger on the lingual surface and the handle of another instrument on the facial surface of the tooth and applying pressure (Figure 24-4).

Cold Test. Cold testing is accomplished using dry ice, ethyl chloride (Figure 24-5 A), or a piece of ice (ice is the most common and easiest to use). The tooth is isolated and dried, and then the ice (usually the water that is frozen is a sterilized, anesthetic carpule) is applied to the facial surface of the tooth (Figure 24-5 B). The ice test is more effective on the anterior teeth than the more insulated posterior teeth. A normal tooth will respond within a few seconds. If the response to the cold is intense and long lasting, irreversible pulpitis is indicated. Teeth with necrotic pulps will not respond to the cold test.

Heat Test. Heat testing uses several heat sources. Examples include a small ball of **gutta percha** heated by a flame, the heated end of a ball burnisher, or frictional heat from running a rubber cup on the tooth surface. Heat is applied to the tooth and, if the pain increases and lasts, there is a distinct chance of irreversible pulpitis (Figure 24-6).

Gutta percha is a thermoplastic material used to fill the root canal.

Electric Pulp Testing/Vitality Scanner. Electric pulp testing does not measure the degree of tooth vitality but does indicate whether the tooth is vital or nonvital. Like other pulp tests, the **electronic pulp tester** can produce a false reading (Figure 24-7 A). Therefore, other tests should be completed for comparison and thus determination of pulp vitality. Electronic pulp-testing units are usually battery operated and deliver high-frequency currents that can vary. The current creates an electrical stimulus to the tooth.

The **vitality scanner** allows the dentist to scan each tooth in minutes (Figure 24-7 B). The scanner indicates endodontic

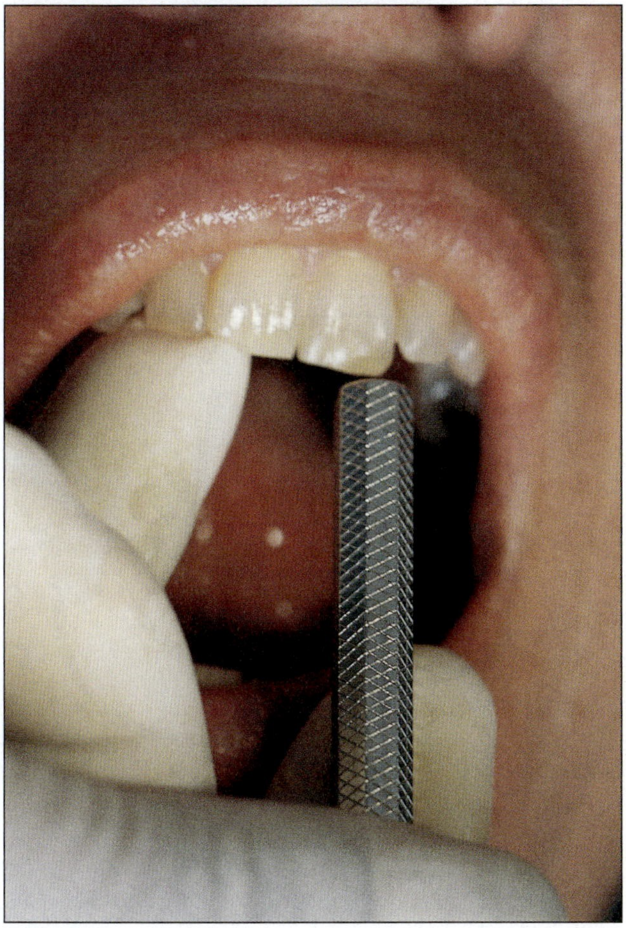

FIGURE 24-3
Percussion test with instrument handle.

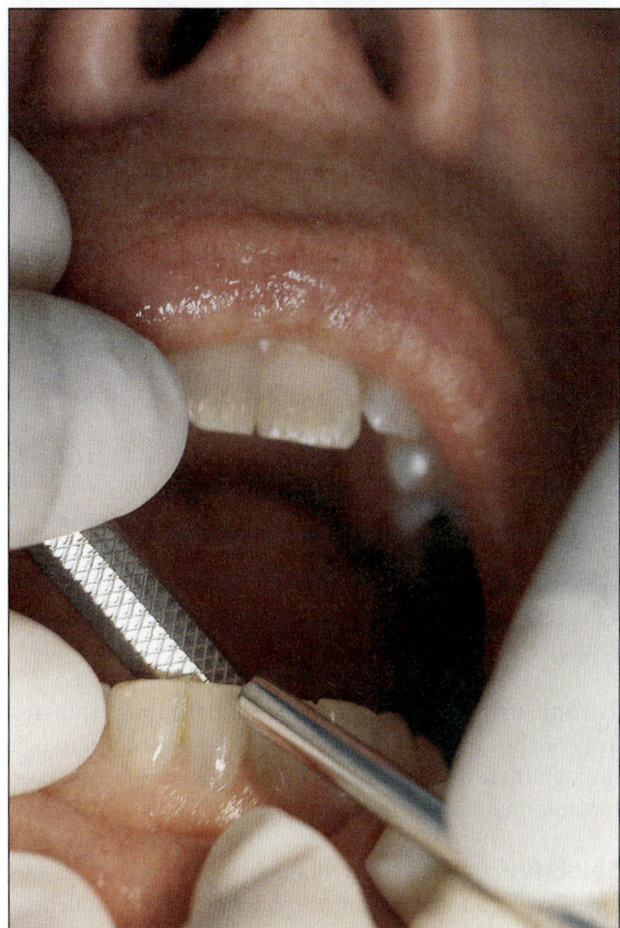

FIGURE 24-4
Mobility test using the ends of two instruments.

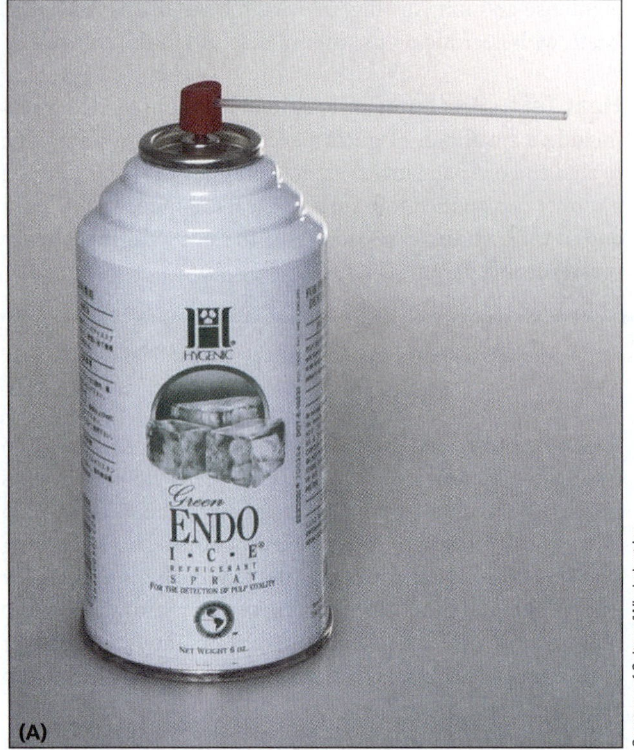

(A)

Courtesy of Coltene/Whaledent Inc.

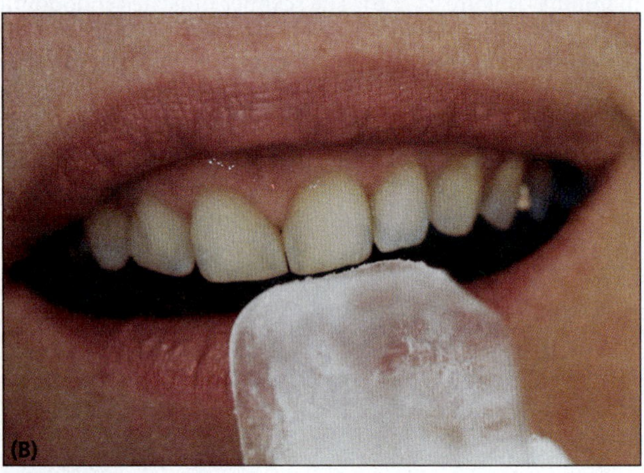

(B)

FIGURE 24-5

(A) Endo Ice used to test the vitality of a tooth. (B) Cold test on patient's tooth with an ice stick.

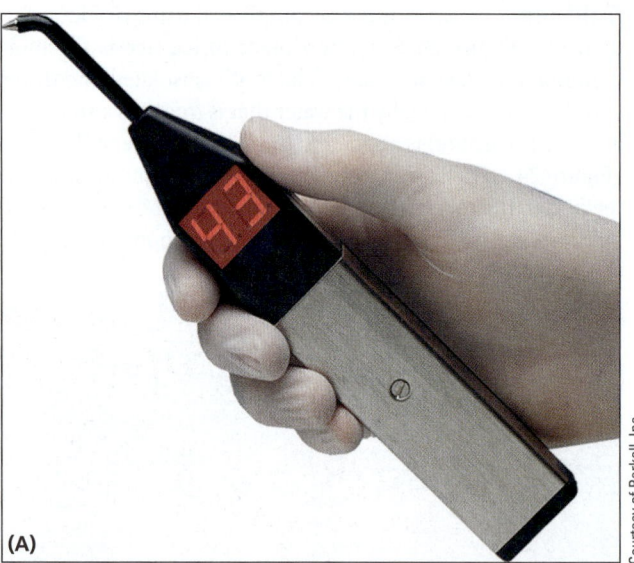

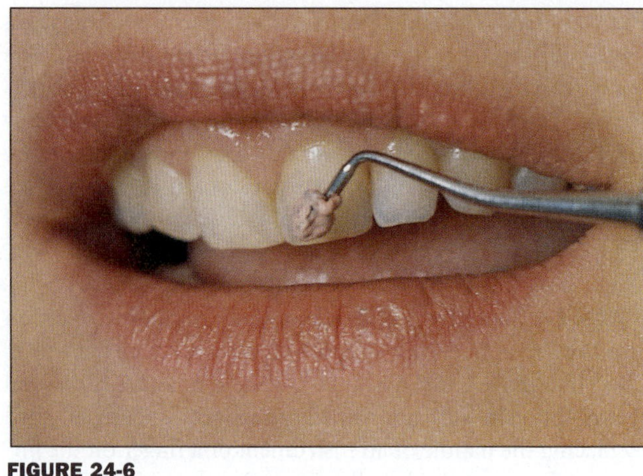

FIGURE 24-6

Heat test on patient with gutta percha ball.

(A)

Courtesy of Parkell, Inc.

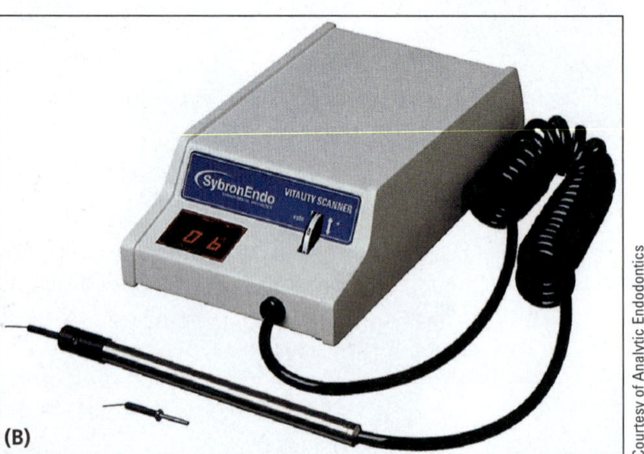

(B)

Courtesy of Analytic Endodontics

FIGURE 24-7

(A) Electronic pulp tester. (B) Vitality scanner.

problems in the early stages. The probe on the scanner records a reading and then automatically resets for the next tooth. Procedure 24-1 outlines the steps for electronic pulp testing.

Transillumination Test. The **transillumination test** involves the use of a strong fiber optic light that transmits light through the crown of the tooth. The light produces shadows that may indicate vertical fractures.

Selective Anesthesia. Sometimes the patient cannot identify which tooth or which arch is causing the problem. In these cases, after talking with the patient and completing the clinical examination, **selective anesthesia** is used. One area of the patient's mouth is selected and an injection is given. If anesthetic in this area alleviates the discomfort, the problematic quadrant has been determined. Usually, selective anesthetic is used on the maxillary teeth beginning in the most suspicious anterior area, and then progressing to the posterior area.

Procedure 24-1
Electronic Pulp Testing

Equipment and Supplies

- Basic setup: mouth mirror, explorer, and cotton pliers
- Electronic pulp tester
- Conducting medium, such as toothpaste

Procedure Steps

Follow these steps to electronically test the pulp (test control tooth first):

1. Place a small amount of toothpaste on the tip of the electrode (the toothpaste acts as a conducting medium). Dry the tooth before using the electrode.
2. Ask the patient to signal when he or she notices a sensation, which is usually a tingling or hot feeling.
3. Place the tip on the facial surface of the tooth and gradually increase the power. **Caution:** Do not place the electrode on a metal restoration, a wet surface, gingiva, or artificial crowns.
4. If the patient feels any sensation, some degree of tooth vitality is indicated. If no sensation is felt, the pulp may be necrotic.

Caries Removal. The removal of dental caries is necessary in some patients to evaluate the pulp condition. If the patient has no symptoms but the radiograph shows deep caries and the tooth responds positively to other tests, caries removal will further determine pulp status. The dentist uses the dental handpiece to remove the decay and to determine whether there is reversible or irreversible pulpitis. Depending on the prognosis for the tooth, the endodontist would place a temporary or permanent restoration.

Treatment Plan

Once all the information has been gathered and the dentist has made a diagnosis for root canal therapy, the patient is informed of the necessary treatment. The patient must sign a consent form and make appointments and financial arrangements before treatment begins. To minimize anxiety and answer questions about the upcoming procedure, endodontic pamphlets or videos may be provided.

Endodontic Instruments

Procedures performed in endodontic treatments may require the use of specialized instruments. The purpose of these instruments is for **debridement**, which is removal of diseased and necrotic tissues from the canal. The instruments then shape and smooth the canal. Once the canal is free of bacteria and debris and the walls are smooth, a filling material can be placed. The dental assistant working in an endodontic office should be familiar with the various instruments used for endodontic treatment.

Characteristics of Intracanal Instruments

Endodontic **intracanal instruments** are made of stainless steel and nickel titanium alloy wire. They are flexible, fracture resistant, smooth, able to maintain sharp cutting edges, and corrosion resistant. The wire is twisted and tapered into instruments called files and reamers. To ensure consistency in the sizes and lengths of intracanal instruments, the ADA and manufacturers have standardized a number and color-code system (Figure 24-8). Intracanal instruments have precise diameters and lengths that are consistent from manufacturer to manufacturer. Intracanal instruments range in size from 08 to 140 and in length from 21 to 25 mm.

Barbed Broaches

A **barbed broach** is made of fine metal wire with tiny, sharp projections or barbs along the instrument shaft. The barbs are angled to allow a smooth entry but to catch tissue when

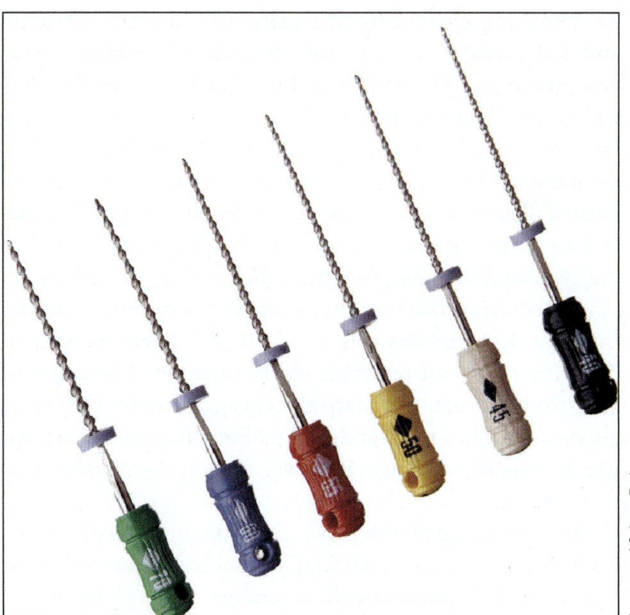

Courtesy of Sybron Endo

FIGURE 24-8
K-flex files showing standardized numbers.

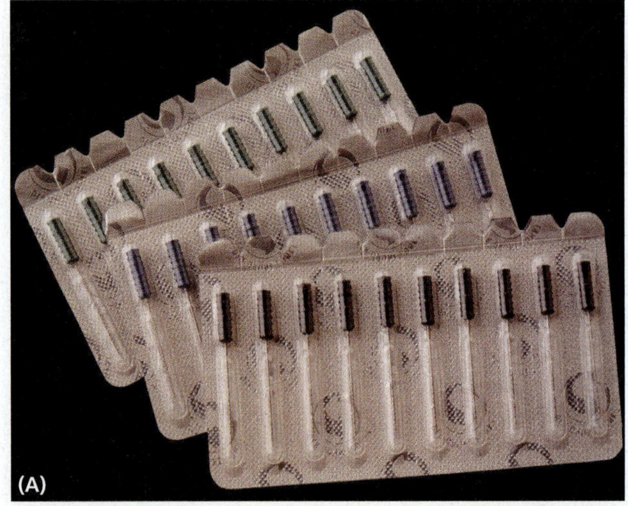

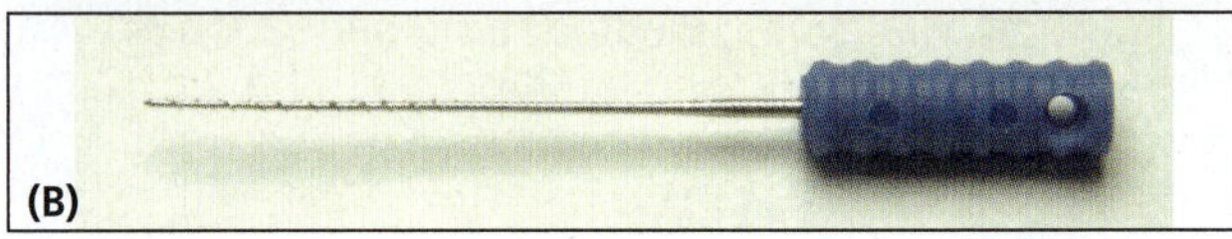

Courtesy of Sybron Endo

FIGURE 24-9

(A) Barbed broach. (B) Close-up picture of a barbed broach.

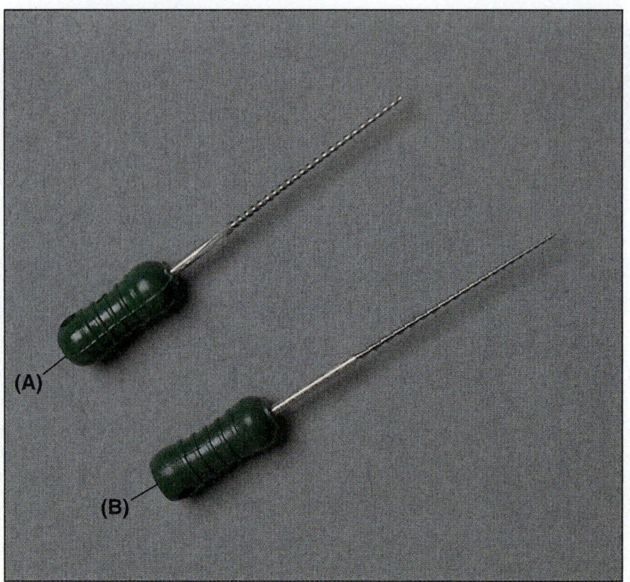

Courtesy of Sybron Endo

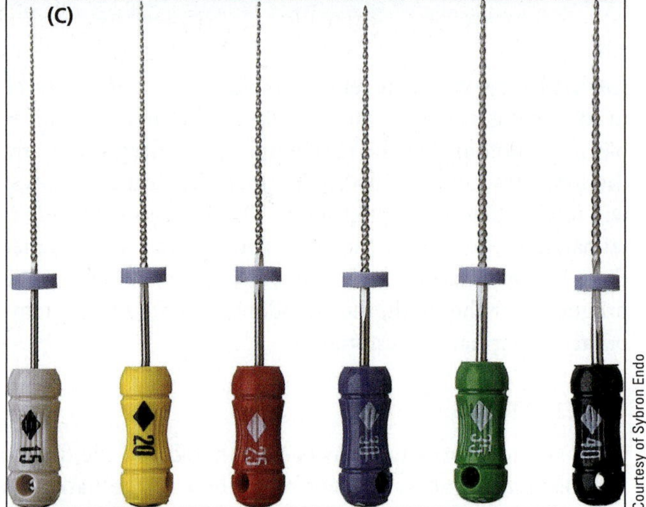

Courtesy of Sybron Endo

FIGURE 24-10

(A) K-type file. (B) Hedström file. (C) Flex files.

retracted. Broaches are used to remove soft tissue from the pulp canal (to **extirpate** the canal). The dentist selects a broach that is large enough to remove pulpal tissue but small enough so that it will not bind in the canal.

Barbed broaches are supplied in various diameters, ranging from xxx-fine to coarse. The handles are metal or plastic and are color coded (Figure 24-9).

Files

Endodontic **files** are used to enlarge and smooth the canal. They are long, tapered, twisted instruments that are moved up and down inside the canal, and are available in various diameters and types. The handles of the endodontic files are color coded according to standardized measurements. For example, a size-15 file is color coded white, and a 20 is color coded yellow.

Standard files are known as **K-type files**. These tightly twisted files are used to scrape and widen the walls of the canal and to remove necrotic tissue. The K-type file is rotated in the canal and then removed from the canal (Figure 24-10 A).

A **Hedström file** is manufactured by a different process than the K-type files (Figure 24-10 B). They are shaped like pine trees and resemble stacks of cones. The edges of Hedström files are very sharp and cut aggressively. These files are only used in a push-and-pull motion; they are not rotated like K-type files because they will bind in the canal due to their design.

Another group of files is available from many manufacturers: **flex files** (Figure 24-10 C). Flex files are made of stainless steel or nickel-titanium and are crafted for an optimal balance of flexibility, strength, and sharpness. Used for curved and narrow canals requiring flexibility to negotiate, flex files come in various sizes and in both the 21- and 25-mm lengths.

Reamers. A **reamer** is used with a "reaming" or twisting motion. Like the files, they have long, twisted shanks, but their blades are spaced much farther apart (Figure 24-11). The cutting action is completed as the reamer is revolved out of the canal. They are color coded and numbered according to size, similar to the files. Reamers are not used as frequently as files.

Rotary Intracanal Instruments

There are also broaches, files, and reamers available for use with an endodontic handpiece; these are called rotary or engine broaches, files, and reamers. These instruments have a notched end that attaches to a low-speed handpiece that is specially designed for use in endodontic procedures. The rotary intracanal instruments are numbered and color coded just like manual instruments.

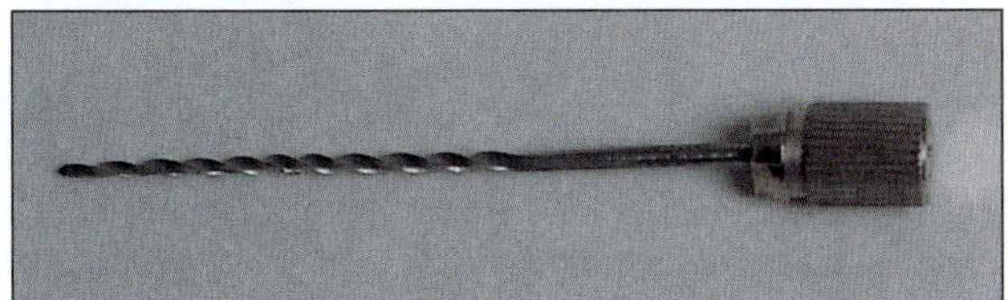

FIGURE 24-11

Close-up view of a reamer.

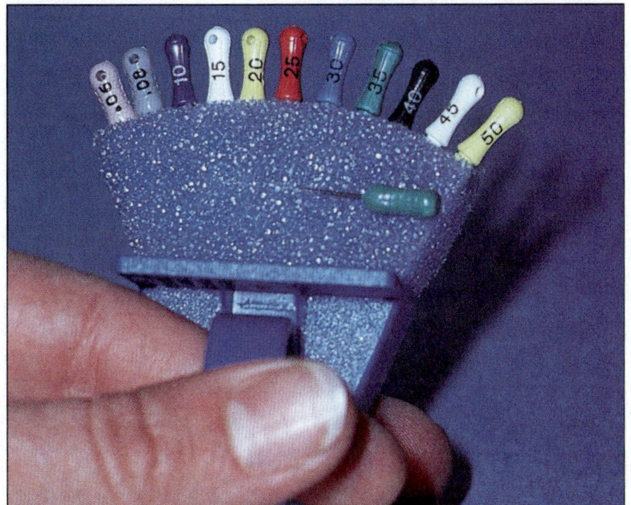

FIGURE 24-12

Various intracanal instruments in an endodontic organizer for storage and sterilization, and a sponge holder/ring for use at the chair.

Endodontic Organizers

Various methods are available to store and organize reamers and files. Some storage containers can be sterilized and are designed to hold a range of intracanal instruments. Large organizers often have built-in measuring gauges for setting stops. Finger rings are much smaller, holding only a few instruments at once (Figure 24-12). They come with disposable Styrofoam pads.

Rubber Stops

A **rubber stop** (also called a file stop, endo stop, or marker) is placed on reamers and files to mark the length of the root canal and prevent **perforation** of the apex of the tooth during treatment (Figure 24-13). These small, circular, silicone disks have prepunched holes in the center for easy application. The length is determined by holding a file with a rubber stop against a radiograph and adjusting the stop to match the incisal or cusp edge. The marked file is then measured on a small millimeter gauge. This number is recorded for reference and for marking other intracanal instruments.

Gates-Glidden Drills

Gates-Glidden drills are used with latch attachments on low-speed handpieces. These drills run in a clockwise direction; are long shanked and elliptically shaped with blunt, football-shaped ends; and they are supplied in six sizes, marked near

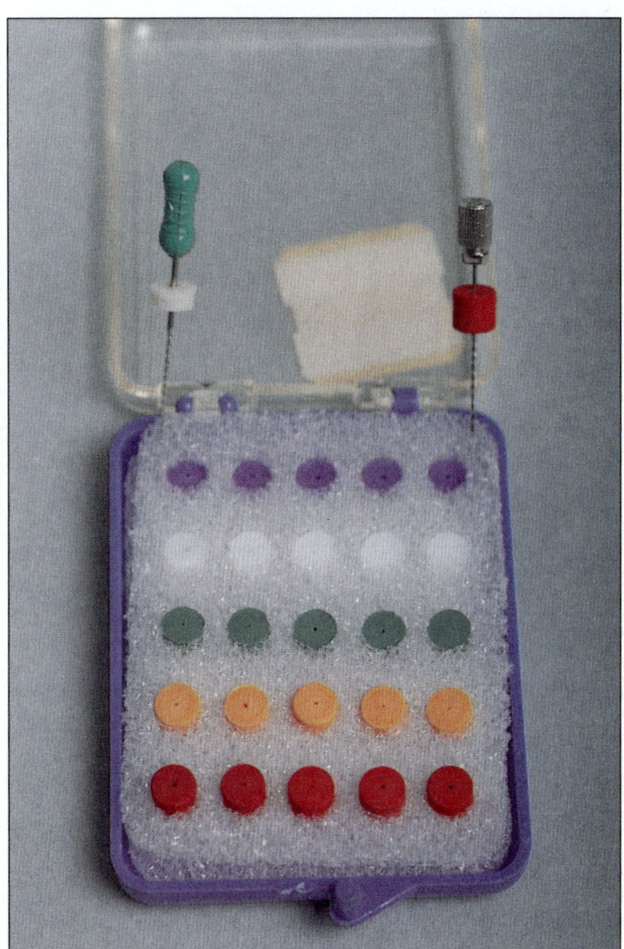

FIGURE 24-13

Examples of rubber stops and how they are positioned on files.

the notch of the shank. For example, a #1 drill has one stripe and #6 has six stripes. The #1 is equal to a size-50 K-type file, with each consecutive size increasing in diameter (Figure 24-14). Gates-Glidden drills are used in the upper portion of the canal to prepare access to the opening by removing obstructing dentin.

Peeso Reamers

Peeso reamers have parallel cutting sides rather than the elliptical shape of the Gates-Glidden drills (Figure 24-15). They are used with latch attachments on low-speed handpieces. Peeso reamers are supplied in various sizes, beginning at 0.70 mm for #1 and increasing 0.20 mm for every subsequent size, ending at #6. The handles are striped to indicate corresponding size. These instruments are supplied with or without safe tips. Peeso reamers are used to prepare the canal for a post and to reduce the curvature of the canal orifice for straight-line access.

Lentulo Spirals

The Lentulo spiral is a long, twisted, very flexible wire instrument used to spin **root canal sealer**, or cement, into the canal (Figure 24-16). The spirals are used with low-speed handpieces and latch attachments.

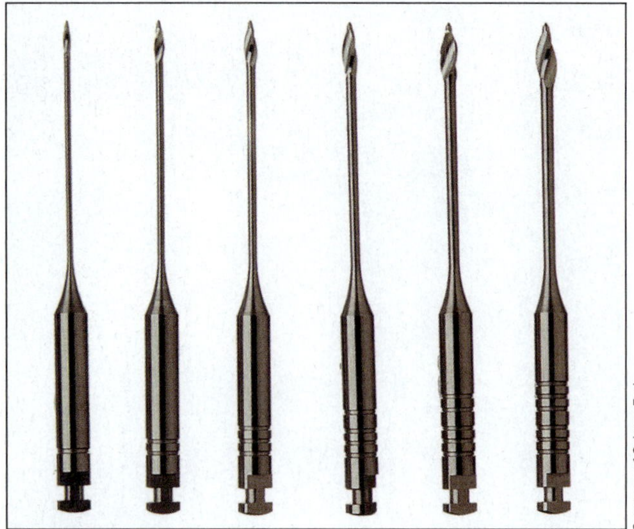

Courtesy of Sybron Endo

FIGURE 24-14

Gates-Glidden drills. The tip of the drill is elliptically shaped and has a noncutting end.

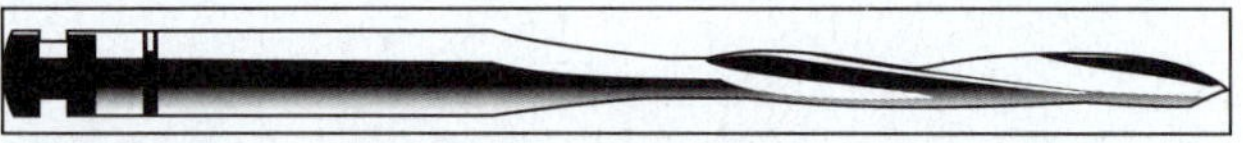

Courtesy of Premier Dental Products Company

FIGURE 24-15

Peeso reamer. The blades are long and parallel with noncutting ends.

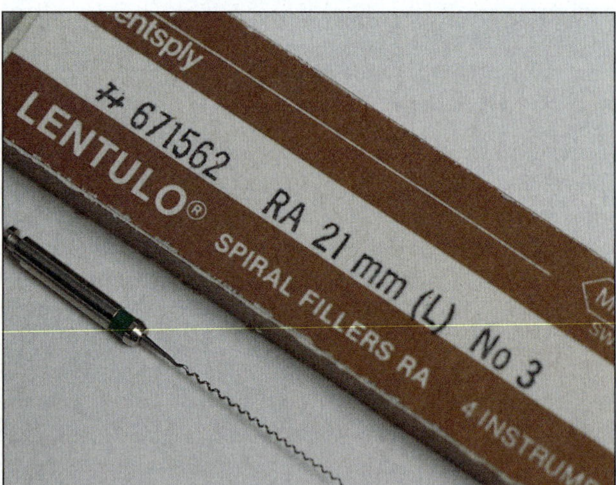

FIGURE 24-16

Lentulo spiral used to place root canal sealer in the canal.

Endodontic Spoon Excavator

The spoon excavator has a very long shank that allows the instrument to reach into the coronal portion of the tooth. The spoon-ended excavator removes deep caries, pulp tissue, and temporary cement. The double-ended instrument has right and left ends (Figure 24-17 A).

Endodontic Explorer

The endodontic explorer is designed to help locate canal orifices (openings). It is a double-ended instrument with long, tapered ends that have sharp points. This stiff-ended explorer is designed specifically for endodontic procedures (Figure 24-17 B).

Endodontic Spreaders, Pluggers, and the Glick #1

A **spreader** and **plugger** (condenser) is an instrument used to laterally condense materials when **obturating** (sealing/filling) the canal. Both these instruments have long, tapered working ends. The spreaders are pointed on the ends, while the pluggers are flat. Both these instruments have instrument metal handles or "finger-type" plastic handles (Figures 24-18 A and B). Spreaders are used to adapt the gutta percha into the canal (lateral condensation); pluggers are used to condense the filling material to provide space for additional gutta percha cones (Figure 24-18 C).

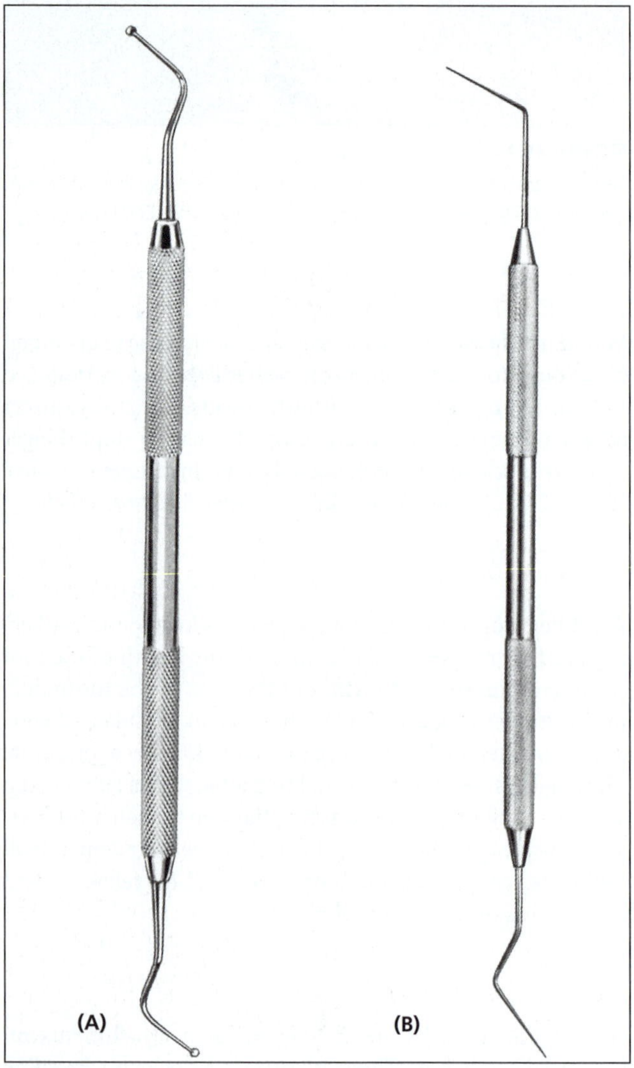

(A) (B)

Courtesy of Hu-Friedy Mfg., Co., Inc.

FIGURE 24-17

(A) An endodontic spoon excavator. (B) An endodontic explorer.

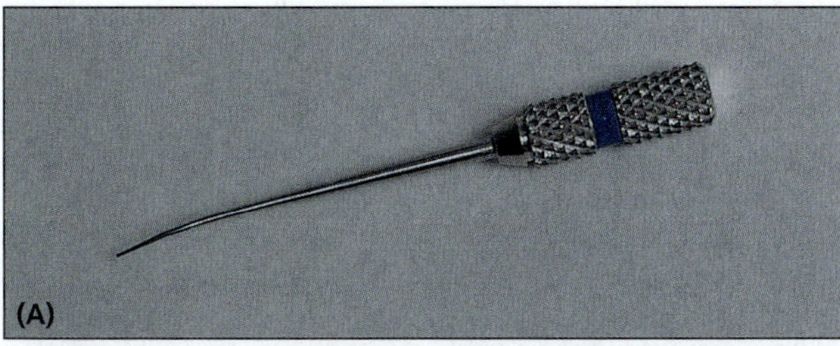

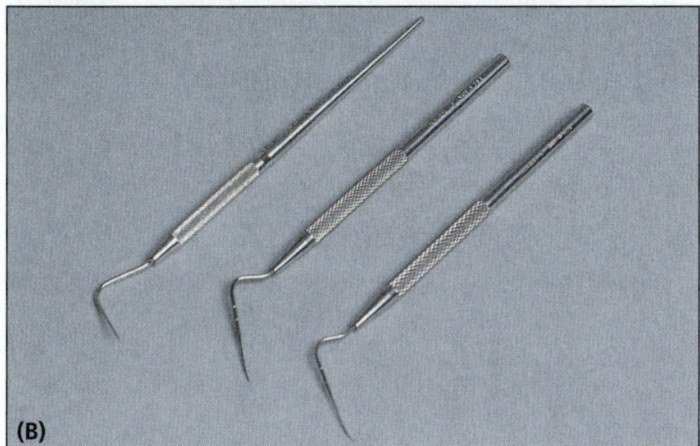

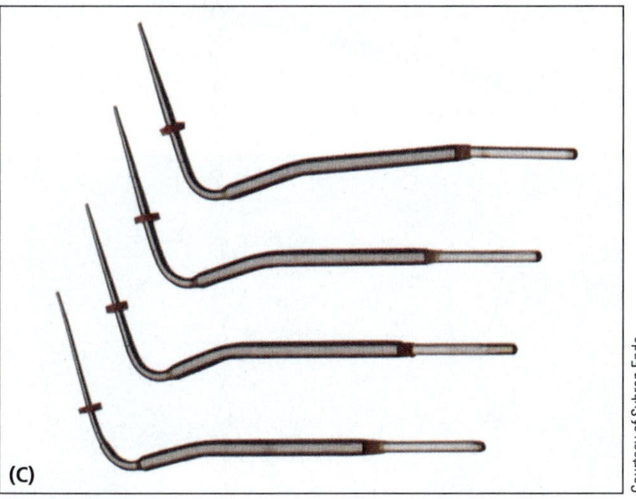

Courtesy of Sybron Endo

FIGURE 24-18

Endodontic spreaders. (A) Finger spreader. (B) Handled spreader. (C) Endodontic pluggers.

The **Glick #1** instrument is used to remove excess gutta percha from the coronal portion of the canal and to condense the remaining gutta percha in the canal opening.

Endodontic Materials

Endodontic materials are substances used in endodontic procedures to dry, fill, or treat the root canal. The dental assistant should be aware of characteristics of the various types of materials used.

Absorbent Paper Points

Paper points are used to dry canals, place medications, and take cultures of the canal (Figure 24-19). Paper points are absorbent and are supplied in various sizes, from x-fine to coarse. Also available are color-coded paper points to match the color coding of reamers and files. The colors change when they absorb moisture. They come conveniently packaged and are supplied sterile or nonsterile. Locking cotton pliers are used to transport paper points to and from the tooth being treated endodontically.

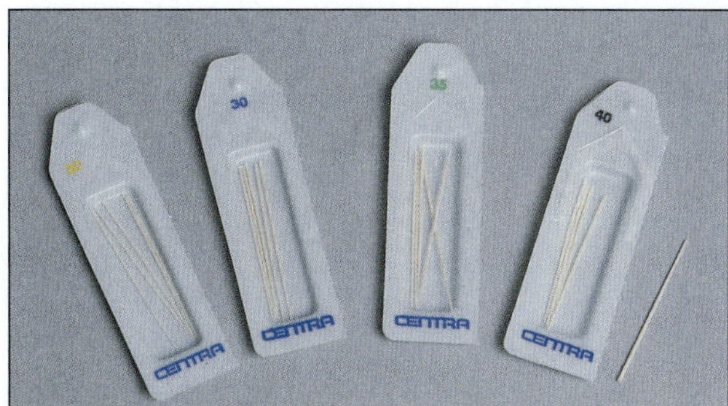

FIGURE 24-19

Examples of various sizes of paper points.

Gutta Percha

Gutta percha is used to obturate (sealing/filling) the canal. It is a thermoplastic material that is flexible at room temperature yet stiff enough to be placed in the root canal. Gutta percha cones are supplied in graduated sizes, from x-fine to large (Figure 24-20). Color-coded gutta percha is also available to match color-coded reamers and files.

Thermal gutta percha **endodontic obturation systems** (e.g., thermafil endodontic obturators) are also available. These systems include metal cores coated with gutta percha. The gutta percha and cores are heated with units specific to the system or with an open flame and then inserted by hand or with low-speed handpieces into the root canal (Figure 24-20).

Silver points are rarely used anymore to obturate the canal. They are used much like the gutta percha but are not as flexible. However, the silver points may be removed and replaced with gutta percha.

Irrigation Solutions

During root canal treatment, the root canal is irrigated frequently to remove debris. There are several solutions used to rinse and remove materials from the canal including: the biomechanical cleaner **sodium hypochlorite**, which is household bleach. This antimicrobial solution is mixed with water (50/50) and loaded into a Luer-Lock syringe. The canal is irrigated with the sodium hypochlorite/water solution, which disinfects and dissolves necrotic tissue. Care must be used not to get any of this solution on the skin as it may cause irritation or on the patient's clothing. Parachlorophenol (PCP) is a combination of 35 percent paracholorphenol and 65 percent camphor. It is used as an antimicrobial agent in the irrigating of the pulp canal. It is also administered in an irrigating syringe.

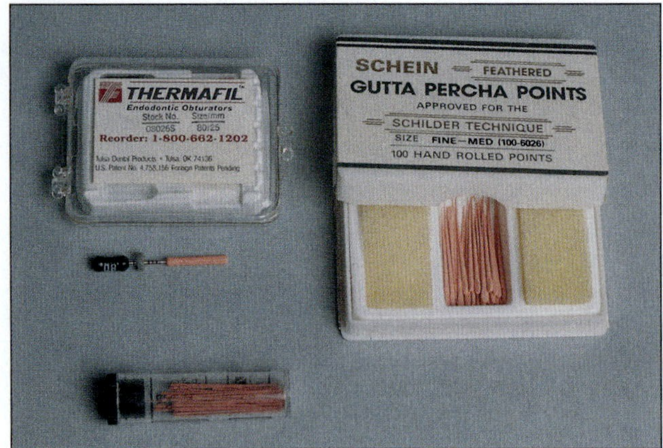

FIGURE 24-20

Thermafil obturators and gutta percha points.

With these irrigating solutions the dental assistant places the evacuator close to the tooth to remove the debris and solution.

Besides sodium hypochlorite and Parachlorophenol, other solutions used to irrigate the root canal include hydrogen peroxide, saline solutions, alcohol, anesthetic solution, and chlorinated soda.

Root Canal Disinfecting, Cleaning, and Lubricating

Dentists may sometimes want to disinfect the root canal. A small amount of disinfectant is applied to the inside of the root canal walls with an applicator tip and is left in between appointments.

Materials for cleaning the root canal come in paste or gel form. These specially formulated materials, a variety of which are available on the market, allow for a chemomechanical action that softens calcified deposits. Some materials also produce a bubbling action that flushes debris from the root canals.

A gel is sometimes used during the root canal treatment as a lubrication and **chelating** agent. Chelation is the process by which an agent encloses or grasps a toxic substance and makes it nontoxic. The lubricant acts as a conditioner to make the cleaning and shaping of the canals easier. Lubricating agents are typically available in a syringe and gel for easy application.

Root Canal Sealers/Cements

Root canal sealers used with obturating materials prevent microleakage in the canal. Various materials are used as sealers/cements, including zinc oxide-eugenol, calcium hydroxide, and glass ionomer. They are supplied in powder/liquid, paste, syringe, and capsule forms (Figures 24-21 A–C). Sealers are mixed to a thick consistency and then inserted into the canal using paper points, the Lentulo spiral, or files, or by placing the sealer directly on the gutta percha.

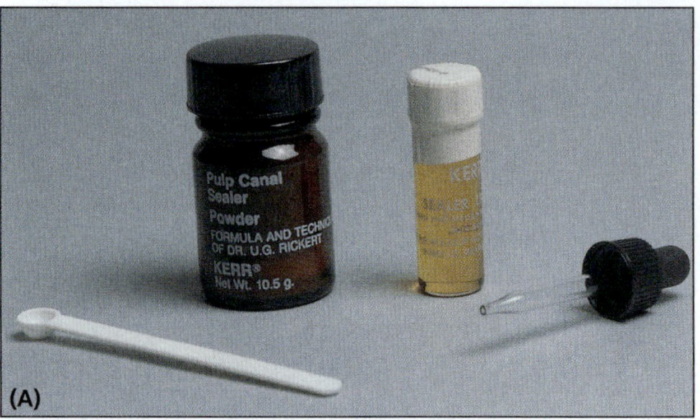

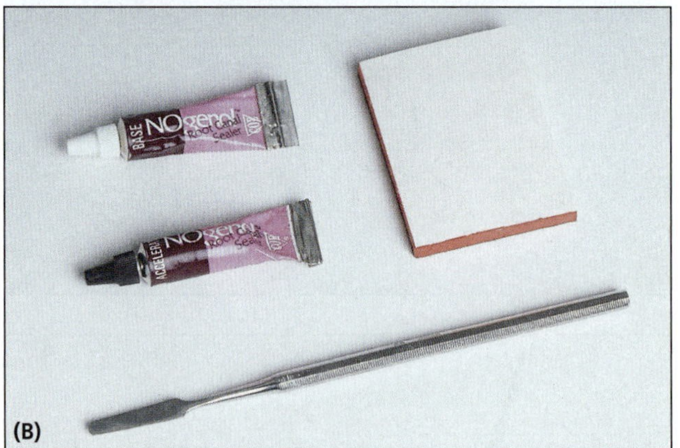

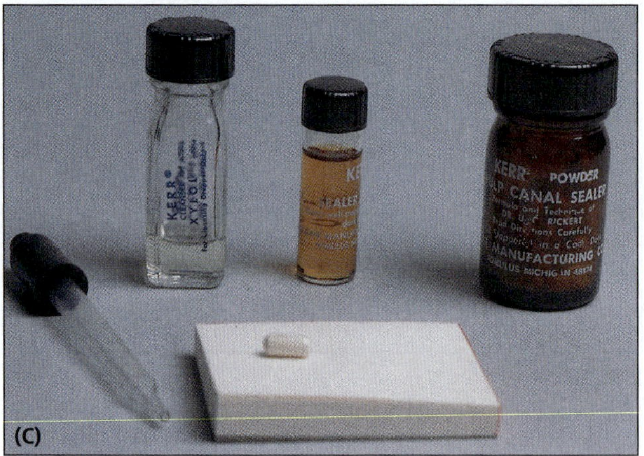

FIGURE 24-21

Root canal sealers. (A) Powder/liquid sealer. (B) Two-paste system. (C) Capsules of powder and liquid sealer.

Equipment Used in Endodontic Procedures

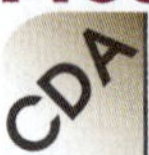

As technology advances, new equipment is being developed to assist in endodontic procedures.

- The **apex finder** measures the distance to the apex of the tooth and displays the information on a digital readout (Figure 24-22 A). Some apex finders/locators also display a graphic design of the endodontic file positioned in the root canal during treatment. The position of the file changes as the treatment progresses. As the file nears the apex, some units enlarge the image. The apex finders may have audio feedback—the unit produces a sound as it nears the apex of the root canal. The volume can be set and, on some units, the distance from the apex can be programmed.

- The **heating unit** can be controlled or continuous. It has many applications, including providing heat for vitality testing, warming the gutta percha for obturation, and providing heat for bleaching procedures (Figure 24-22 B).
- The **endodontic handpiece** is designed to provide quarter-turn motion that is consistent and even. It duplicates the manual motion needed during the cleaning and enlarging of the root canal. There are a variety of options the dentist can choose from, including a specifically designed endodontic handpiece with a torque-controlled motor or other handpiece, low-speed handpieces. A low-speed handpiece with a reduction contra angle can also be used. All of these handpieces are used with the endodontic rotary instruments that are required to prepare the root canal (Figures 24-22 C).
- The **ultrasonic unit** is designed specifically for endodontic procedures. Microprocessors operate and control the unit to deliver the right amount of power and amplitude at the tip to complete a variety of endodontic procedures. Various tips are used to perform specific tasks. This unit is used for troughing (making a groove or channel) around a post and for opening calcified canals, breaking away cement or calculus, and vibrating a post out of a canal or vibrating a crown or bridge off. Other uses include seating a crown, acting as a spreader in the root canal procedure, assisting in the retrieval of separated files that are lodged in the apical third of the canal, and preparation of root canals (Figure 24-23 A and B).
- The **endodontic bender** is designed to carefully bend endodontic reamers, files, posts, pluggers, and spreaders to conform to the shape of the root canal. They are made of stainless steel and are used instead of hemostats, cotton pliers, and fingers. The endodontic bender is autoclavable (Figure's 24-24).
- The number of endodontists using an advanced **endodontic microscope** is increasing and they are becoming an integral part of endodontic treatment (Figure 24-25). With these microscopes there is a variety of high levels of magnification, with levels ranging from 2× to 20×. There is also high-intensity illumination that adds brightness in a concentrated area and is designed to be shadow free. The microscopes come in many designs to meet the needs of different offices. They can be mounted on the wall or ceiling or can be on a base or stand.

The benefits for the dentist include the increased capability to find canals in teeth with difficult anatomies; the ability to see problems at an earlier stage; easier identification of tooth fractures; greater precision in techniques and thus fewer failures and need for retreatment; and greater success in completing more complex treatments, thus avoiding the need for surgery. The microscopes are ergonomically designed to allow the dentist to sit more upright and thus reduce neck and back strain. They are flexible and easy for the dentist to adjust.

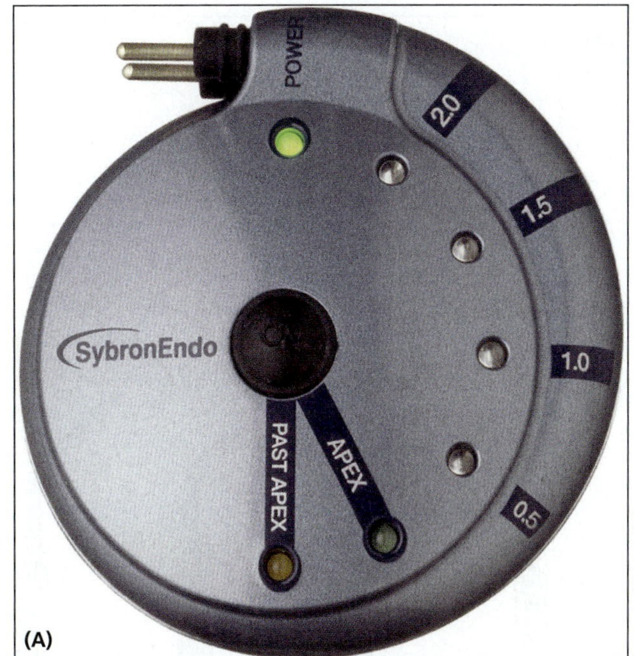

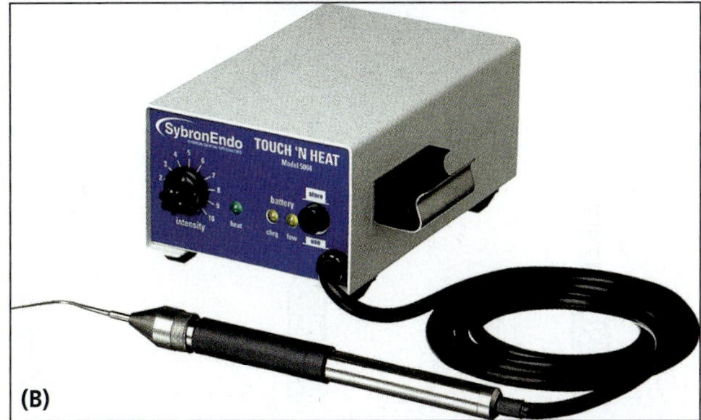

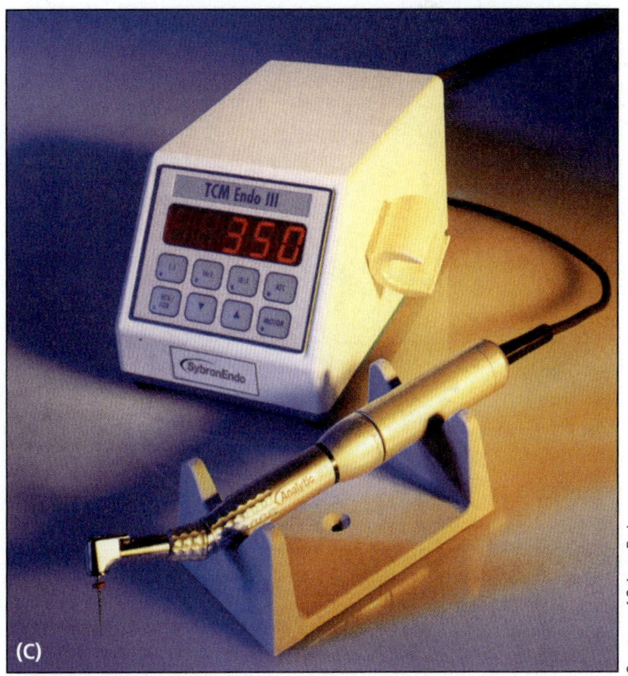

FIGURE 24-22

(A) Apex finder. (B) Touch'n Heat heating unit. (C) Endodontic handpiece.

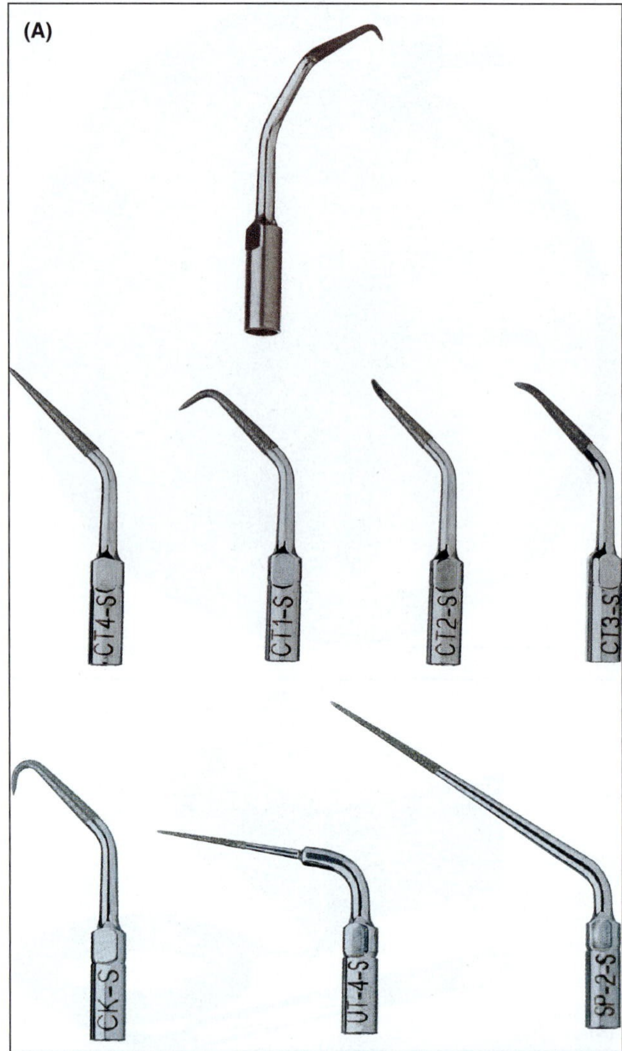

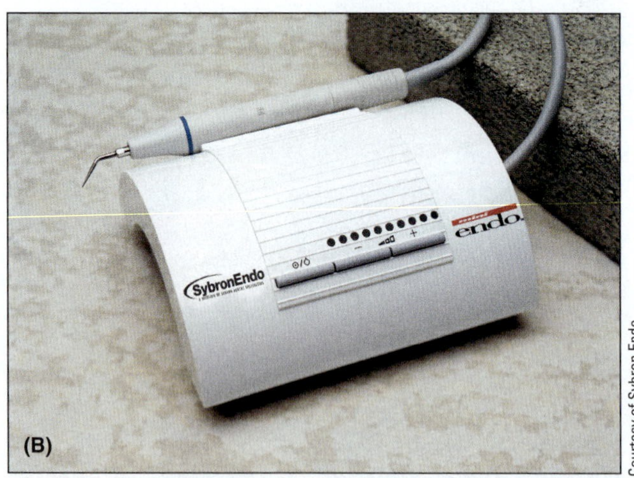

Courtesy of Sybron Endo

FIGURE 24-23

(A) Various tips to be used with the ultrasonic unit. (B) Ultrasonic unit.

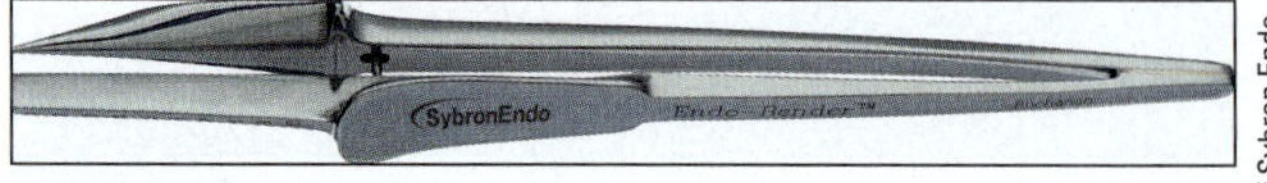

Courtesy of Sybron Endo

FIGURE 24-24

Endodontic bender.

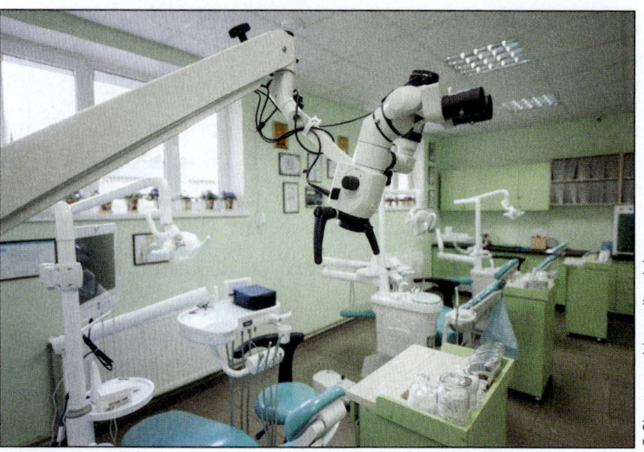

© Shutterstock/anatoliy_gleb

FIGURE 24-25

Endodontic microscope mounted in dental operatory.

Some microscopes are designed so an assistant/observer can also see what the main operator is seeing. These microscopes have a beam-splitting device; this splits the light between the dentist and an assistant/observer and can also be integrated with various types of digital recording devices. With the digital documentation capabilities, the dentist can keep working and have the assistant capture images as they proceed through the treatment. These images can be shared during examination, during the treatment, and postoperatively. The microscope with the beam-splitting device allows the assistant to see right where the dentist is at in the treatment so he or she can be prepared for the next step of the procedure. Overall improved vision with these microscopes advances patient care and aids in the education of the patient, staff, and referring dentists.

- The endodontic obturation system is a new system designed to obturate (fill) the canal once the dentist has completed the preparation. This system is powered by a cordless unit that warms the filling material (either brand name materials or traditional gutta percha) and then allows the dentist to place the material into the canal for vertical and backfill obturation.

Sterilization Procedures

Endodontic instruments must be sterilized before they are used and during the cleaning and shaping of the canal. Sometimes instruments are sterilized at chairside using a small glass bead sterilizing unit (refer to Chapter 11, Infection Control). A flame may also be used at chairside to resterilize endodontic instruments and burs.

Reamers and files are fragile and should be examined closely before use. If there is any concern about the ability of the instrument to function properly, it should be discarded. Some manufacturers recommend one-procedure use for reamers and files.

Endodontic Procedures

Common endodontic procedures that the dental assistant should be familiar with are root canal treatment, endodontic retreatment, pulpectomy, and pulpotomy.

Root Canal Treatment

Root canal treatment is usually completed in two appointments, but this varies depending on the degree of infection and the dentist's judgment. The dentist may decide to postpone filling the canal to allow more time to treat the infection. When this occurs, the canal is irrigated, sometimes medicated, and a temporary filling is placed in the coronal portion of the tooth. The patient is rescheduled for a continuation of the procedure.

The procedure begins with the dentist opening the coronal portion of the tooth with a dental high-speed handpiece and burs. This is followed by cleaning and enlarging the canal. Restoration of the canal is also known as obturation. During this phase of treatment, the pulp canal is permanently filled and sealed. The steps involved in a root canal treatment are outlined in Procedure 24-2.

General Steps in Root Canal Therapy

The following general steps in root canal therapy can be divided into two or more appointments depending on dentist preference and the extent of the infection. Steps 1 through 8 would take place on the first appointment. Steps 6, 7, and 9 would be done at the second appointment. Once completed, the patient would follow Step 10.

1. Administer the anesthetic.
2. Isolate the area.
3. Gain access to the pulp.
4. Locate the canals.
5. Remove the pulpal tissues.
6. Enlarge and smooth the root canal.
7. Irrigate the root canal.
8. Place temporary filling.
9. Obturate (seal) the root canal.
10. Refer the patient to a general dentist for final restoration.

Procedure 24-2
Root Canal Treatment

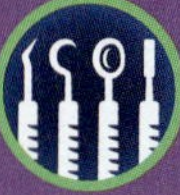

This procedure is performed by the dentist, who is assisted by the dental assistant. The following sequence will indicate steps involved in a root canal treatment that requires two appointments.

Equipment and Supplies (*Figure 24-26*)

- Basic setup: mouth mirror, explorer, and cotton pliers
- Endodontic explorer and spoon excavator
- Locking cotton pliers
- Saliva ejector, evacuator tip (HVE), air–water syringe tip
- Cotton rolls, cotton pellets, and gauze sponges
- Anesthetic setup
- Dental dam setup
- High-speed handpiece and assortment of burs
- Low-speed handpiece
- Irrigating syringe and solution (sodium hypochlorite or hydrogen peroxide)
- Barbed broach, assorted reamers and files, and rubber stops
- Paper points (assortment)
- Temporization materials
- Permanent obturating materials (gutta percha or silver points and root canal sealer)
- Heat source
- Endodontic spreaders, pluggers, and the Glick #1
- Articulating forceps and paper

Procedure Steps (*Follow aseptic procedures*)

Administer Anesthetic

1. Administer topical and local anesthetic for endodontic treatment in the same way as for restorative procedures in general dentistry.
2. Usually the dentist will anesthetize the patient at every appointment, but it is at the dentist's discretion. After the first appointment, when the pulp chamber has been opened and the canals have been cleaned, the dentist may determine that anesthetic is unnecessary.
3. Prepare the syringe and assist during the administration of the anesthetic.

(continues)

Procedure 24-2 (continued)

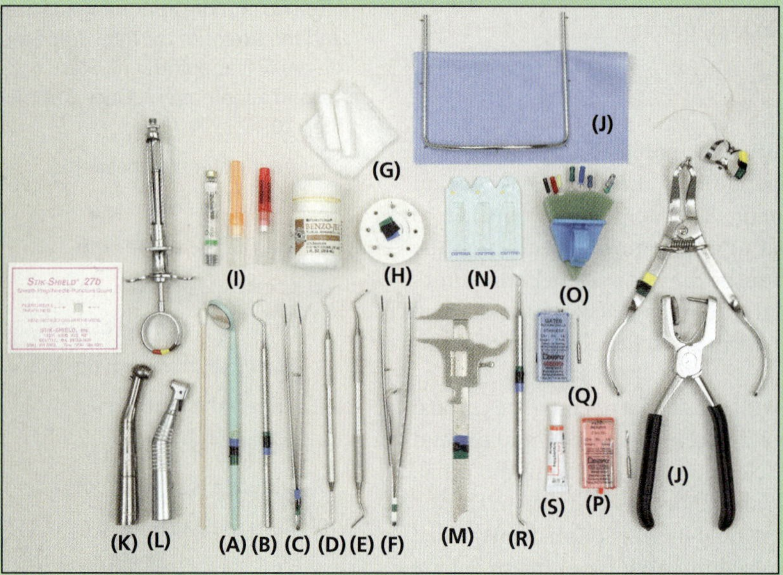

FIGURE 24-26

Root canal treatment tray setup, opening appointment. (A) Mouth mirror. (B) Explorer. (C) Cotton pliers. (D) Endodontic explorer. (E) Endodontic spoon excavator. (F) Locking cotton pliers. (G) Cotton rolls/gauze sponge. (H) Bur block. (I) Anesthetic setup. (J) Dental dam set up. (K) High-speed handpiece. (L) Low-speed handpiece. (M) Millimeter ruler. (N) Paper points. (O) Barbed broach, assorted reamers and files, with stops in endodontic organizer. (P) Peeso reamers. (Q) Gates-Glidden drills. (R) Glick endodontic instrument. (S) Temporary filling material.

Isolate Area

1. Place the dental dam, isolating the tooth being endodontically treated. Besides isolating the tooth, the dam improves visibility and protects the tooth from saliva and solutions used in endodontic treatment. The dental dam also maintains an aseptic field and protects the patient's mouth and throat.
2. Once the dental dam is placed, wipe the area with a disinfectant to remove bacterial contaminants.

Gain Access to Pulp

1. The dentist uses the high-speed handpiece and a round or fissure bur to access the pulp. The opening is made through the crown of the tooth and should be sufficient to expose the pulp chamber and permit access for intracanal instruments.
2. Evacuate and maintain good visibility for the dentist.
3. Once access to the pulp has been gained, the endodontic explorer is used to locate the main and accessory canals.

Remove Pulpal Tissues

1. The dentist inserts a barbed broach into the canal and withdraws it to remove pulpal tissues.
2. Receive the barbed broach in a gauze sponge.

Enlarge and Smooth the Root Canal

1. Using the periapical radiograph, the dentist estimates the length of the tooth root (Figure 24-27). The assistant should record the root length on the patient's chart for reference. An apex finder may also be used. Rubber stops are used to mark the tooth length on files and reamers. A series of small files are used to remove debris and enlarge the canals. Canals must be at least a #25 file before Gates-Glidden burs can be used. As the files enlarge the diameter of the canal, the size of the files and/or Gates-Glidden burs increase, respectively.
2. Prepare the stops on the files and reamers according to the dentist's instructions. This measurement must be precise for each hand instrument. (The duties of the assistant may vary greatly depending on the preferences of the

(continues)

Procedure 24-2 (continued)

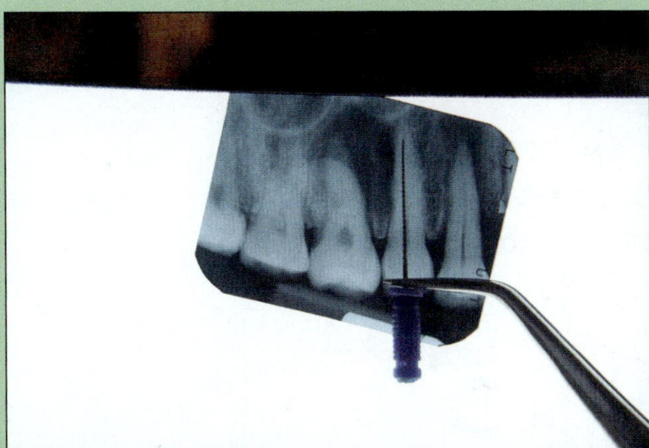

FIGURE 24-27
Measuring length of the root using a radiograph and reamer.

dentist. For example, some dentists may want the assistant to sterilize the reamers and files at chairside, or they may want radiographs taken periodically.)

3. Keep the files and reamers in order and free of debris.

Irrigate Root Canal

1. Periodically, the canal is irrigated to remove debris (Figure 24-28). After the canal is flushed, it is dried with paper points.
2. Prepare the solution in the disposable syringe and transfer it to the operator. As the operator flushes the solution into the canal, evacuate the area. Then, transfer paper points in locking pliers to the operator and receive the used saturated points in a gauze sponge. To dry the canal, measure the paper points 1 mm short of the apex.

NOTE: At this time, the dentist may decide to place a temporary restoration and reappoint the patient in several days to 2 weeks.

3. Prepare the temporary restorative materials and place the temporary or assist the dentist in placement.
4. Remove the dental dam and dismiss the patient.

Obturate Root Canal (*Figure 24-29*)

1. Obturation of the root canal is routinely performed at the second appointment. After the patient is seated, the temporary is removed and the canal is flushed to remove debris.

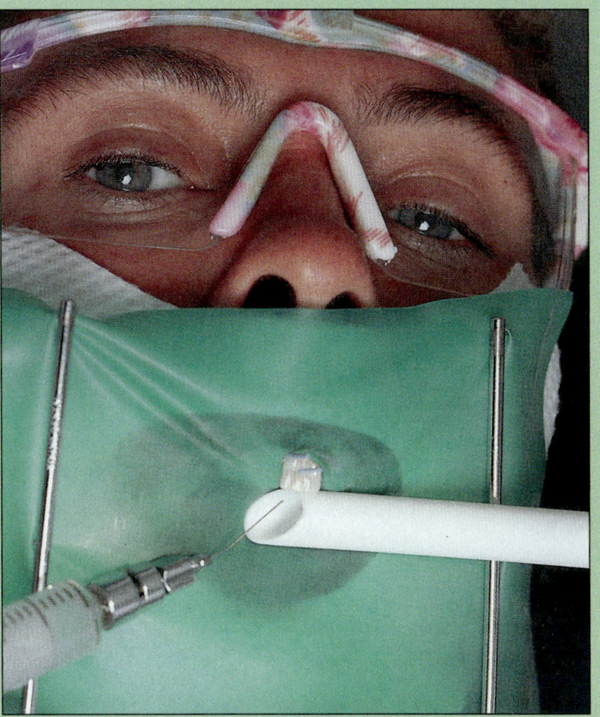

FIGURE 24-28
Irrigating the root canal.

2. Radiographs are taken periodically throughout the procedure for the dentist to evaluate the progress. Once the canal is adequately enlarged and free of disease, it is permanently filled to prevent debris, fluids, and bacteria from entering the canal. There are many materials and techniques available to fill the canal, but gutta percha materials are most common.
3. The dentist selects a gutta percha point as the **master cone**. The cone should be no more than 1 mm short of the prepared length. The dentist inserts the cone into the canal to check the fit. If the master cone is the correct length and fits snugly near the apex, the cone is removed and the root canal sealer is prepared.
4. The root canal sealer is mixed and then placed in the canal with a Lentulo spiral and/or a master cone dipped in the sealer and placed in the canal.
5. A spreader is used to create space for additional accessory gutta percha cones. Dip each accessory gutta percha cone into the root canal sealer and transfer it to the dentist for placement. Transfer the spreader to create space for the subsequent cones. Repeat this procedure until the canal is filled (Figure 24-30).

(continues)

Procedure 24-2 (continued)

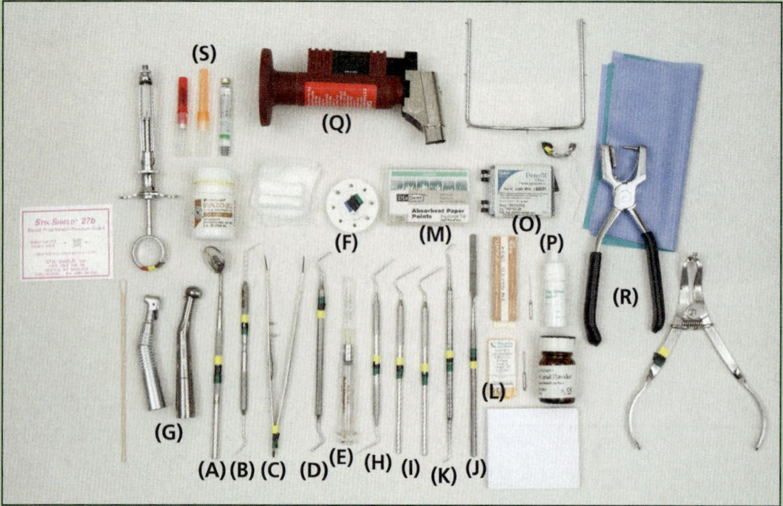

FIGURE 24-29

Root canal completion appointment tray setup. (A) Mouth mirror. (B) Endodontic explorer. (C) Locking cotton pliers. (D) Endodontic spoon excavator. (E) Irrigating syringe. (F) Burs. (G) High- and low-speed handpieces. (H) Spreaders. (I) Pluggers. (J) Spatula. (K) Glick instrument. (L) Gates-Glidden drills. (M) Absorbent sterile paper points. (N) Lentulo spiral. (O) Gutta percha. (P) Root canal sealer. (Q) Heat source. (R) Rubber dam setup. (S) Anesthetic setup.

6. Once the canal is filled, the excess gutta percha in the crown of the tooth is removed with a hot Glick #1 or a heated plugger. The warm gutta percha is condensed vertically into the cervical portion.
7. Hold a 2 × 2 inch gauze to remove any excess gutta percha from the instruments.
8. A final radiograph is taken.
9. The coronal portion of the tooth is sealed with a permanent restoration or a temporary restoration if a fixed prosthesis is the treatment choice.
10. The dental dam is removed and the patient's mouth is rinsed.
11. The patient's occlusion is checked with articulating paper.
12. Give the patient postoperative instructions and dismiss him or her.

NOTE: The patient returns to the general dentist for the final restoration of the tooth. Follow-up radiographs may be taken at 6-month and 1-year intervals.

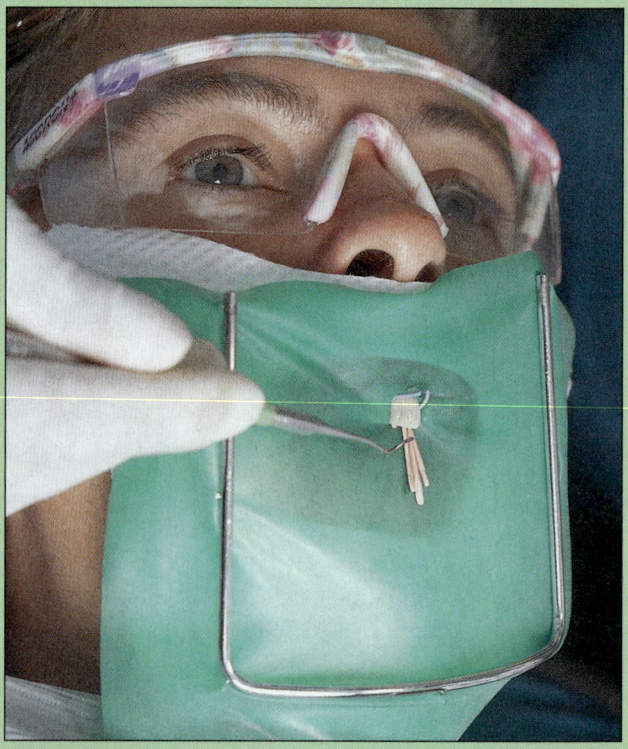

FIGURE 24-30

Root canal being filled with gutta percha cones and sealer.

Endodontic Retreatment

In most cases, teeth that have been treated endodontically will last as long as natural teeth. However, patients continue to experience sensitivity to heat and pain in some teeth. This can happen immediately after treatment or years later. If the tooth fails to heal and the disease process continues or starts again, it can be retreated and have a second chance to heal.

Root canal treatment may fail for a variety of reasons:

- Abscess did not heal.
- Narrow or curved canals were not treated during first treatment.
- New decay forms along the filling material.
- Complicated canal anatomy, such as supplemental canals, went undetected.
- Restoration was not placed soon enough after treatment.
- Restoration became loose, cracked, or broken, and exposed the tooth to new infection.

If the patient feels pain and discomfort with a tooth that has had root canal treatment, she or he should return to the endodontist and discuss treatment options. The endodontist will reopen the tooth to gain access to the root canal. This can be difficult to accomplish because the tooth may have a crown, post, and core material, and all of these have to be removed to permit access.

After removing the restorative materials, the endodontist can clean the canal and carefully examine the inside of the canal. The problem could be supplemental canals and/or unusual anatomy. After cleaning, the canal will be filled and sealed, and a temporary filling will be placed. The patient will then return to her or his general dentist for the final restoration, which may include a new post, core build-up, and crown.

Sometimes the endodontist may believe that the problem is at the apex of the tooth, and will recommend an apicoectomy (discussed later in this chapter).

Pulpectomy

A **pulpectomy** is the removal of all pulpal tissues beginning in the coronal portion of the tooth and terminating 1 to 3 mm short of the apex in the root canal of a tooth. This procedure is used in the treatment of deep caries in permanent teeth. Pulpectomy is the first stage of root canal treatment; cleaning and enlarging the canal usually follow.

Pulpotomy

A **pulpotomy** involves removing the pulp in the coronal portion of the tooth, leaving the pulp in the root canal intact and vital.

A pulpotomy is indicated for the following:

- Primary teeth with pulp exposures
- Treatment in emergency situations where there is pulpal exposure
- Teeth with deep carious lesions

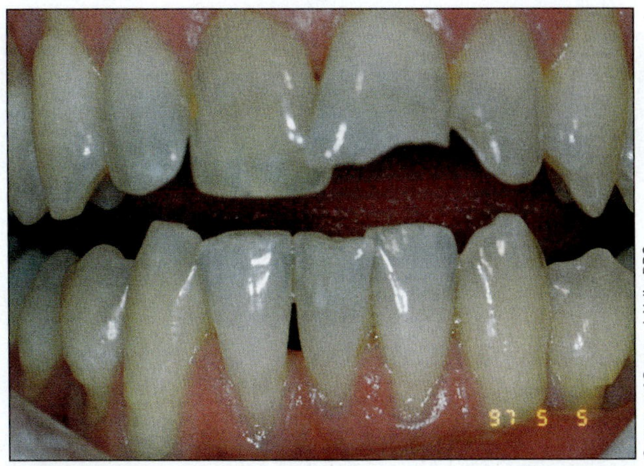

Courtesy of George J. Velis, DDS

FIGURE 24-31

Fractured central incisor with pulp exposure indicates the need for a pulpotomy.

- Apexogenesis (ay-**PECKS**-oh-jen-ah-sis) (treatment of vital tooth where the root is incompletely developed)
- Fractured anterior teeth (Figure 24-31)

Surgical Endodontics

Endodontic treatment has a high rate of success, but situations arise in which surgical endodontic treatment is necessary to prevent extraction of the involved tooth. Surgery is performed in the area surrounding the roots of the teeth. These surgeries involve a facial surface incision through the tissue to expose the underlying bone. An opening through the alveolar bone is made to expose the root area where surgical endodontic treatment is performed.

Surgical techniques include apicoectomy, root amputation, and hemisection.

Apicoectomy and Apical Curettage

One of the most common endodontic surgical procedures is the **apicoectomy**/(a-pee-koh-**ECK**-toh-me) (see Procedure 24-3). In this procedure, the apex of the root is surgically removed. Once the apex of the root has been removed an **apical curettage** may be performed. This is where the diseased tissues are removed from the area by scraping with a curette. Indications for this treatment include the following:

- Extreme curvature of the root, preventing root canal instruments from reaching the apex
- Root canal is hypercalcified, obstructing root canal therapy
- Previous endodontic treatment did not adequately seal the canal due to additional canals, fractures, or other causes of endodontic failure
- Gaining access to the apex of the root canal for examination and treatment

After the apicoectomy and apical curettage have been completed the apex of the root may be prepared to be sealed. With the **retrograde restoration** the root canal is filled with a filling material such as amalgam, composite, or gutta percha.

Procedure 24-3
Apicoectomy

This procedure is performed by the dentist, who is assisted by the dental assistant.

Equipment and Supplies (*Figure 24-32*)

- Basic setup: mouth mirror, explorer, and cotton pliers
- Endodontic explorer and spoon excavator
- Locking cotton pliers
- Saliva ejector, surgical evacuator tip, and air–water syringe tip
- Cotton rolls and gauze sponges
- Anesthetic setup
- Scalpel and blades
- Periosteal elevator and tissue retractors
- High-speed handpiece and assortment of burs (handpiece is specifically designed with a very small head)
- Surgical curettes
- Irrigating syringe and sterile saline solution
- Hemostat and surgical scissors
- Amalgam setup
- Suture setup

Procedure Steps (*Follow aseptic procedures*)

1. Anesthetic is administered to the patient.
2. The dentist makes a flap incision with the scalpel and lifts the tissue away from the bone with a periosteal elevator (Figure 24-33). Retract the tissue for the dentist throughout the procedure.
3. Transfer instruments and keep the site clear and clean using the surgical evacuator and tissue retractors.

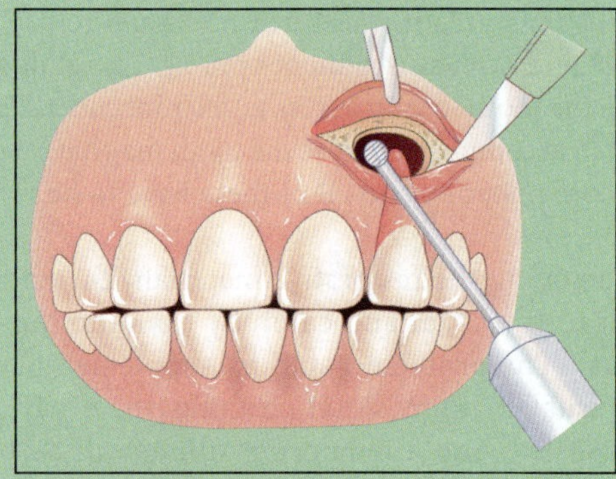

FIGURE 24-33

Apicoectomy procedure begins with a flap incision.

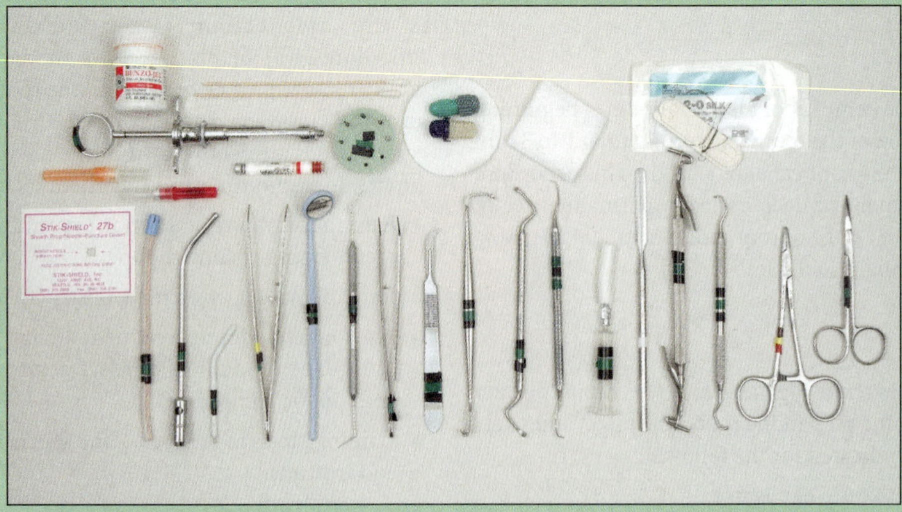

FIGURE 24-32

Apicoectomy tray setup.

(continues)

Procedure 24-3 (continued)

4. The high-speed handpiece is used by the dentist to gain access to the root apex through the bone (Figure 24-34).
5. The dentist removes debris and infection around the apex of the root with a surgical curette (apical curettage) (Figure 24-35).

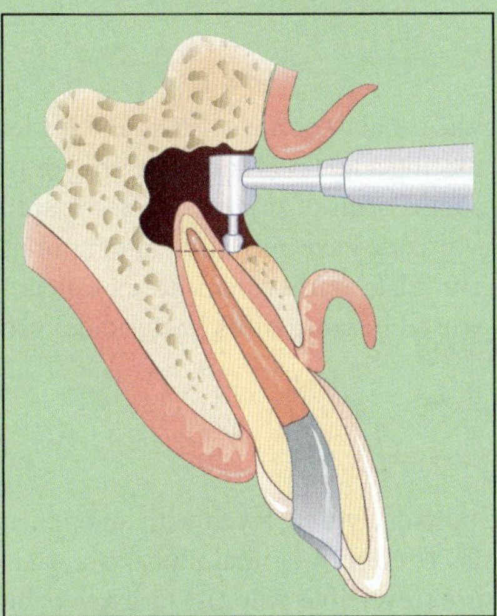

FIGURE 24-34

Dental handpiece is used to remove the bone and expose the root tip.

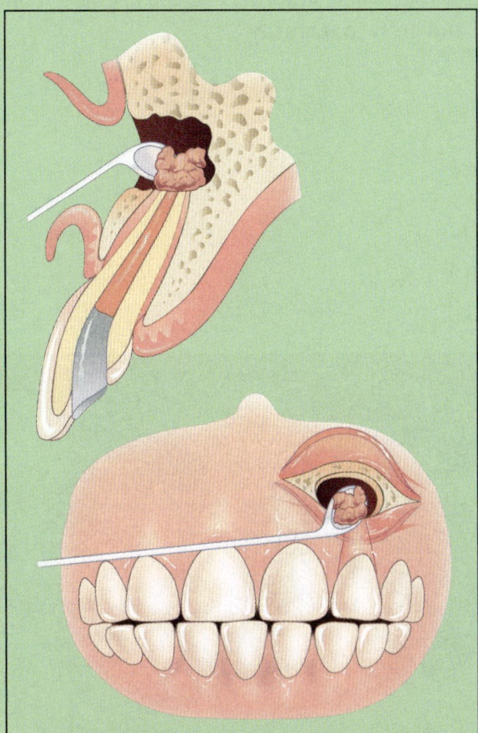

FIGURE 24-35

Apical curettage. Removing infection and debris with a surgical curette.

6. Evacuate and remove debris from instruments with a gauze sponge.
7. Prepare handpiece and sterile saline irrigation syringe.
8. The high-speed handpiece and burs are used to remove a section of the exposed root tip (Figure 24-36). The root tip is beveled to enhance access. The area is rinsed with the sterile saline to prepare the root to receive the **retrograde filling** material.
9. Retrograde filling material is placed in the prepared cavity (Figure 24-37). Amalgam is

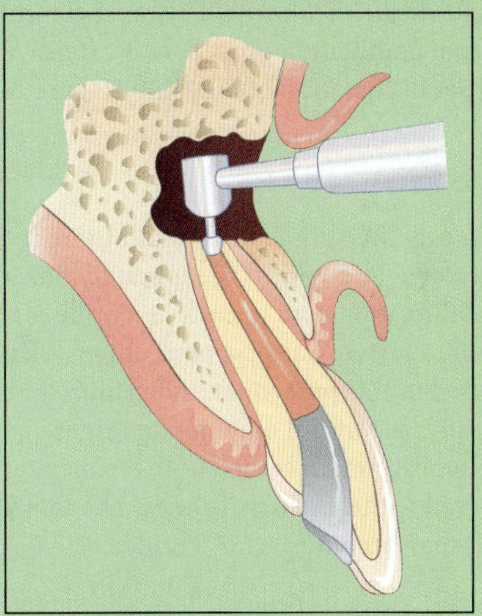

FIGURE 24-36

Opening the root apex in preparation for retrofill.

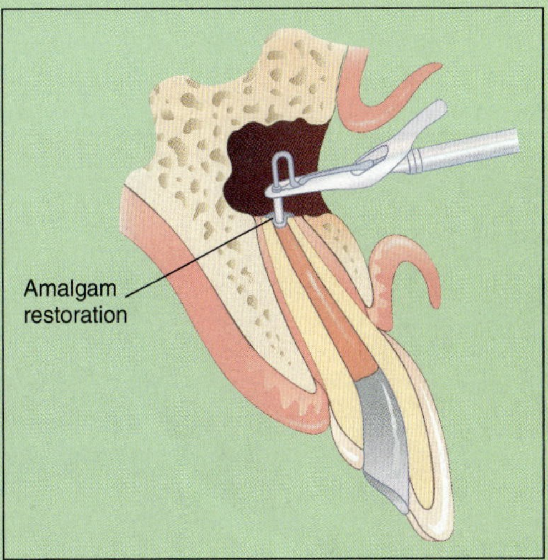

FIGURE 24-37

Retrofill being placed in the root canal at apex of the tooth.

(continues)

Procedure 24-3 (continued)

commonly used, but gutta percha, zinc oxide-eugenol, and composites are also used.

10. Flap replacement and suturing are the final steps of this procedure. The flap is returned to position and held in place for a few minutes. The dentist then sutures the flap into place.

11. Prepare sutures and assist during placement. Once suturing is complete, give the patient post-operative instructions, a prescription for pain medication, and dismiss him or her.

Root Amputation

A **root amputation** is a surgical procedure to remove one or more roots of a multirooted tooth. The root is amputated where the root meets the crown. The most common indication for the root amputation procedure is extensive bone loss around the root or furcation of the tooth (Figure 24-38).

Hemisection

A **hemisection** is the surgical removal of one root and the overlying crown. The tooth is separated buccolingually through the bifurcation, and the affected or diseased portion of the tooth is removed. Surgical burs, chisels, elevators, and forceps are used in this procedure. Indications for a hemisection are the same as for root amputation (Figure 24-39).

Once the hemisection is complete, the remaining tooth and root are restored with a fixed prosthesis. The tooth may need a crown, or it may become part of a bridge.

Apexification

An **apexification** is treatment of the root canal apex in a tooth that is necrotic. Apexification creates a calcified barrier across the open apex of the tooth. The treatment involves cleaning and shaping the canal to remove debris and bacteria, which is followed by placing a material such as a drug or paste into the canal to the apex. Forms of zinc oxide, cresol, antibiotic paste, or calcium hydroxide have been used to temporarily obdurate the canal to stimulate apical calcification. Calcium hydroxide is commonly used because of its bactericidal properties and alkaline pH.

Apexogenesis

Treating the pulp of a young tooth with an open apex is called **apexogenesis**. The tooth is vital, but has a carious or traumatic exposure (reversible pulpitis) or irreversible pulpitis. It is treated with a pulp capping or pulpotomy to permit continued closure of the open apex and growth of the root. Calcium hydroxide preparation is again indicated in this treatment. In most patients, a calcified bridge will form across the exposure; the pulp will heal and stay vital and the apex will continue to develop and grow to maturity.

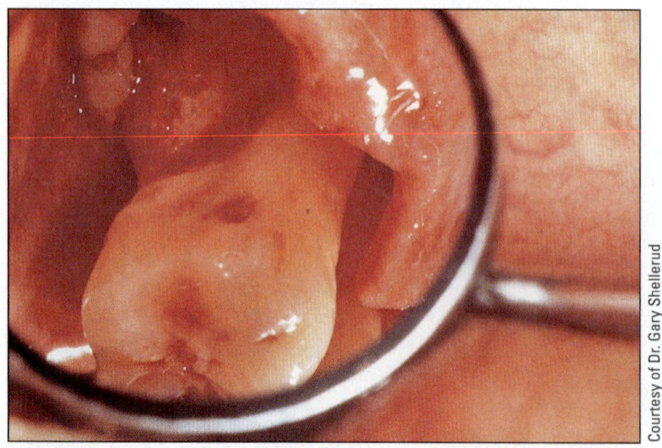

Courtesy of Dr. Gary Shellerud

FIGURE 24-38

Root amputation on a mandibular first molar. The crown is saved, but the diseased root is surgically removed.

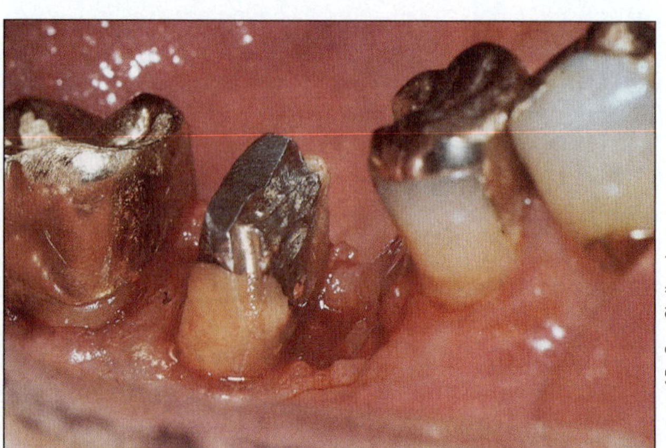

Courtesy of Dr. Gary Shellerud

FIGURE 24-39

Hemisection on a mandibular first molar. One root and half the crown over the root are removed.

Chapter Summary

Endodontics comprises the diagnosis and treatment of pulp and periapical tissue diseases. Procedures include diagnosis, root canal treatment, and periapical surgery.

The endodontist is assisted by dental assistants who perform traditional assisting responsibilities in addition to expanded duties specific to endodontics as allowed by state dental practice acts.

Endodontic diagnosis includes patient medical and dental history; clinical examination, including pulp testing; and review of communication if the patient is sent from a referring dentist.

CASE STUDY

Gerald Frank, aged 67, had an appointment with Dr. Lamb for examination of his mandibular right side. He has been experiencing pain and inflammation in this area. Upon examination, Dr. Lamb suspects that the mandibular first molar is causing Mr. Frank's problem.

Case Study Review

1. What are the key indications for treatment?
2. What clinical tests should be prepared?
3. Identify a possible treatment.
4. What information should be given to Mr. Frank concerning his treatment?

Review Questions

Multiple Choice

1. An endodontist
   a. diagnoses and treats diseases of the pulp and periapical tissues.
   b. provides treatments including root canal treatment and periapical surgery.
   c. has advanced knowledge and training in endodontic procedures compared to the general dentist.
   d. All of the above are true statements.
2. Which one of the following diseases is a localized destruction of tissue and accumulation of exudates in the periapical region?
   a. Periodontitis
   b. Apical periodontitis
   c. Osteomyelitis
   d. Periapical abscess
3. The clinical examination for endodontic diagnosis includes all of the following *except*
   a. radiographs.
   b. sweet test.
   c. mobility test.
   d. cold test.
4. Which instrument is used to enlarge and smooth the root canals?
   a. Barbed broach
   b. Endodontic reamer
   c. Endodontic file
   d. Peeso reamer
5. Peeso reamers are used during the root canal procedure to
   a. prepare the opening access by removing the obstructing dentin in the upper portion of the canal.
   b. prepare the canal for a post and to reduce the curvature of the canal orifice for straight-line access.
   c. mark the reamers and files to the length of the root canal.
   d. spin root canal sealer or cement into the canal.
6. Sodium hypochlorite is used to
   a. open the root canal at the beginning of the procedure.
   b. irrigate the canal to remove debris.
   c. fill the canal after it has been cleaned and enlarged.
   d. enlarge the canal.
7. Root canal treatment is most often completed in ________ appointments.
   a. two
   b. three
   c. four
   d. five
8. All of the following statements are true about endodontic retreatment *except:*
   a. The patient does not feel pain and discomfort.
   b. The need for retreatment can occur immediately or years later.
   c. The endodontist will reopen the tooth to gain access to the root canal.
   d. The problem could be supplemental canals and/or unusual anatomy of the canal.

9. In which of the following procedures are one root and the overlying crown surgically removed?
   a. Hemisection
   b. Root amputation
   c. Pulpotomy
   d. Apicoectomy
10. Which procedure is performed to gain access to the apex of the root canal?
   a. Pulpotomy
   b. Root canal treatment
   c. Apicoectomy
   d. Root amputation

Critical Thinking

1. Differentiate among a pulpectomy, pulpotomy, and root canal treatment.
2. Is anesthetic always administered for root canal treatment? Explain.
3. What is the difference between K-type files and Hedström files?

Web Activities

1. To see more endodontic equipment and supplies, visit http://Dentsply.com.
2. For a Web site dedicated to patients with questions about endodontic treatment, go to the American Association of Endodontists website at http://www.aae.org, then go to "Patients".
3. To learn more about the newest endodontic instruments and apex finders, vitality testers, and endodontic handpieces, go to http://www.sybronendo.com.

CHAPTER

25

Oral and Maxillofacial Surgery

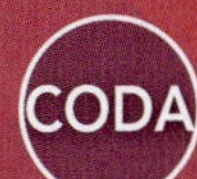

Specific Instructional Objectives

The student should strive to meet the following objectives and demonstrate an understanding of the facts and principles presented in this chapter:

1. Describe the scope of oral and maxillofacial surgery.
2. Identify the surgical instruments used in various types of surgery and describe their functions.
3. Explain the aseptic procedures followed in the oral surgeon's office.
4. Describe evaluation procedures for new patients.
5. Describe how to prepare the patient for surgical treatment.
6. Explain surgical procedures, including tray setups and assisting responsibilities.
7. List and describe cancer and oral abnormalities detection.
8. List and describe biopsy techniques.
9. List the postoperative instructions given to patients.
10. Explain postsurgical complications.
11. Describe temporomandibular joint (TMJ) disease.
12. Explain the oral surgeon's relationship with the hospital.

Advanced Chairside Functions

13. Explain the function of sutures and when they are placed.
14. List the equipment and supplies needed for suture removal.
15. Determine and identify the location and number of sutures and how to evaluate the healing process.
16. Identify the following suture patterns: simple, continuous simple, sling, continuous sling, horizontal, and vertical mattress.
17. List the basic criteria for suture removal.
18. Explain the steps of removal for identified suture patterns.

Key Terms

alveolitis (607)
alveoplasty (599)
apical elevator (593)
armamentarium (618)
articular eminence recontouring (610)
arthrocentesis (609)
arthroplasty (610)
arthroscopy (609)
biopsy (605)
cheek retractor (590)
continuous simple suture (616)
continuous sling suture (616)
crepitus (609)
debride (615)
discectomy (610)
disc repositioning (610)
dry socket (607)
elevator (593)
excisional biopsy (606)
exfoliative cytology (606)
extraction forceps (593)
hard tissue impaction (600)

(continues)

Key Terms (continued)

hemostat (590)
horizontal mattress suture (617)
incisional biopsy (605)
lip retractor (590)
luxates (600)
mouth prop (590)
mucoperiosteum (593)
needle holder (591)
oral and maxillofacial surgery (588)
oral brush biopsy (606)
orthognathic surgery (611)
paresthesia (607)
periosteal elevator (593)
plastic stint (601)
retractor (590)
rongeurs (592)
root tip pick (593)
simple suture (616)
sling suture (616)
soft tissue impaction (600)
stylet (592)
surgical aspirating tips (591)
surgical bone file (593)
surgical chisel (592)
surgical curette (592)
surgical mallet (592)
surgical rotary instruments (596)
surgical scalpel (589)
surgical scissors (591)
tinnitus (609)
tissue forceps (590)
tissue retractor (590)
TMJ replacement (610)
tongue retractor (590)
trismus (609)
universal forceps (594)
VELscope (604)
vertical mattress suture (617)
ViziLite (604)

Introduction

The branch of dentistry that focuses on the diagnosis and treatment of diseases, injuries, and malformations is **oral and maxillofacial surgery**. It involves surgery for both functional and esthetic aspects of the face, jaws, mouth, neck, and head. This specialty is sometimes called oral surgery.

General dentists refer surgical cases that go beyond their scope of training to oral surgeons. Although the general dentist studies surgical procedures, the number of surgical procedures performed in the general dentist's office depends on preference and training. Upon graduating from dental school, an oral surgeon receives a minimum of 4 more years of advanced training in anatomy, anesthesia, pain control, and surgical procedures in and out of the hospital setting before receiving a degree in oral and maxillofacial surgery.

The Oral and Maxillofacial Surgeon's Office

There are various settings for oral surgeons' offices with some offices being located close to a hospital for convenience and the doctor's preference. The oral surgeon's office includes much the same as a general dental office, with the addition of the recovery area and, in many offices, a room(s) that is/are equipped comparable to hospital operating rooms. The recovery area is usually a separate area with large reclining chairs or beds for the patient to recover from the general anesthetic. Postoperative instructions, prescriptions, and home care supplies are given to the patient or the patient's support person in this area, once the patient has recovered.

It is the trend to save the patient money and time by having some medical procedures done in "outpatient" facilities. This is also being done with oral surgery by completing some surgeries in the office operating rooms.

The Oral and Maxillofacial Surgery Team

The oral surgery office team varies according to the surgeon's goals for the practice. In addition to the oral and maxillofacial surgeon, the team usually consists of the receptionist, the business office staff, the dental assistants, and, in some offices, a nurse anesthetist or an anesthesiologist.

Oral and Maxillofacial Surgeon

The oral and maxillofacial surgeon performs the following: patient examination; diagnosis; teeth extraction; cyst and tumor removal; temporomandibular joint treatment; biopsies; and emergency, reconstructive, and implant surgeries. The oral surgeon works mainly in the office setting but also goes into the hospital to perform complicated surgeries and to treat emergencies. Like all professionals, the oral surgeon continually attends seminars and courses to advance knowledge and skills.

Receptionist and Business Staff

The receptionist and the business staff perform many of the same duties in the oral surgery office as they would in the general dental office. Because most of the oral surgeon's patients are referred by other dental and medical offices, communication and recordkeeping responsibilities increase. The patient's x-rays and written information must be received in the surgeon's office before the patient's appointment. When patients first arrive at the office, they are given forms to fill out. Appointments for treatment are scheduled and insurance claims and financial arrangements are completed before the day of the surgery.

Surgical Dental Assistant

The surgical dental assistant's responsibilities often vary depending on the size of the practice. For example, a dental assistant may be responsible for sterilization and room preparation, the seating and dismissing of patients, pre- and postoperative care, and assisting the oral surgeon during all procedures.

Typical responsibilities of a surgical dental assistant are as follows:

- Perform traditional duties, such as instrument transfer and maintaining the operating field during the procedure
- Assist with the administration of intravenous sedation and analgesics

- Take and record vital signs
- Prepare the treatment rooms
- Sterilize instruments
- Ensure that all presurgery steps are completed and that any required materials or prosthetics are ready
- Prepare the patient for treatment
- Maintain asepsis throughout the procedure
- Stabilize the patient's head and mandible during surgery, if necessary
- Provide postoperative care of the patient
- Clean the treatment room
- Remove sutures (if this is a legal expanded function)

During surgical procedures, six-handed dentistry is often practiced. The second assistant provides support in maintaining the patient's position and acts as a rover for off-tray items. The main assistant is then free to focus on assisting the dentist.

Nurse Anesthetist or Anesthesiologist

The oral surgeon makes the decision to have a nurse anesthetist or anesthesiologist as part of the surgical team. The nurse anesthetist may be a full- or part-time member of the surgical team, while an anesthesiologist is generally only part-time in the office and works with the oral surgeon with every patient in the hospital setting.

The responsibility of the nurse anesthetist varies but may include administering the anesthesia and maintaining the patient during the procedure; continuously monitoring the patient's vital signs; managing fluid therapy; providing or supervising postoperative recovery, postoperative follow-up, and patient evaluation and maintaining records.

The anesthesiologist is hired to perform preoperative evaluations and preparations, administer anesthetics, monitor patient reactions to the anesthetic and surgery, and advise the oral surgeon of adverse reactions. The oral surgeon communicates very closely with the anesthesiologist to make certain that both have all the information they need to ensure the safety of the patient and to enable the oral surgeon to successfully accomplish the procedure. The anesthesiologist relieves the oral surgeon of anesthetizing the patient so that the surgeon can concentrate on the procedure to be performed.

Oral Surgery Instruments

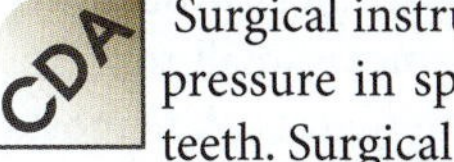

Surgical instruments are designed to apply adequate pressure in specific areas to remove bone tissue or teeth. Surgical instruments are made of stainless steel (so they can be sterilized after each use) or disposable plastics.

Scalpel

A **surgical scalpel** is a surgical knife used to incise or excise soft tissue precisely with the least amount of trauma.

Scalpels are designed in two sections: the handle and the blade (Figure 25-1). The metal handle is slim and straight and is designed to accommodate detachable, disposable blades. A common handle is the Bard Parker style. This handle is flat and has a metric ruler. The blades are very sharp and are supplied in various lengths and designs. The blades are used once and then disposed of in the sharps container. Blades are made of surgical carbon steel and are numbered according to shape. Common blades are #15 for surgical procedures and #11 and #12 to incise and drain.

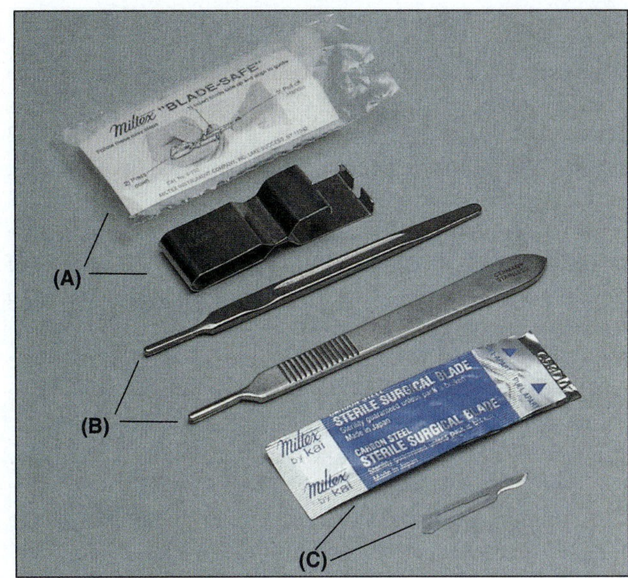

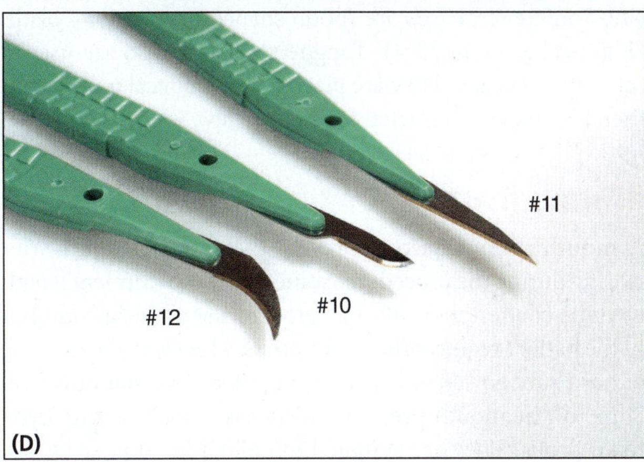

FIGURE 25-1
(A) Blade removal devices. (B) Metal scalpel handles. (C) Scalpel package and scalpel blade. (D) Scalpel blades #12, 10, and 11.

Disposable scalpels are also available. They have plastic handles with metal blades. Disposable scalpels are supplied in sterile packages and are disposed of after one use.

Use cotton pliers, a hemostat, or a blade protector to avoid injury, when removing or replacing blades on the scalpel handle. Practice placing and removing the blades to familiarize yourself with the mechanics of this skill. Disposable surgical blade removers are available. The scalpel blade is placed in the plastic cap of the remover and removed from the handle. The blade is left in the cap and discarded.

Retractor

A **retractor** is used to deflect tissue from the surgical site so that the view is unobstructed. Careful handling of retractors is necessary to avoid traumatizing the tissue. There are several types of retractors: tissue retractors, cheek and lip retractors, and tongue retractors.

A **tissue retractor** is supplied in forceps (hinged) style (**tissue forceps**) or cotton-plier style. The working ends of both types of retractors have small teeth to assist in grasping the tissue securely (Figure 25-2).

A **cheek retractor** and **lip retractor** is used to hold the patient's cheeks away from the operating site. They increase visibility by retracting the cheeks and expanding the viewing area. Cheek retractors are made of metal or plastic (Figures 25-3 and 25-4).

A **tongue retractor** is placed between the border of the tongue and the lingual surfaces of the teeth. The dental assistant gently but firmly retracts the tongue from the operating site. Tongue retractors are spoon shaped or have long blades (Figures 25-3 and 25-4). Tongue retractors also are used to retract the cheeks. They are placed on the buccal mucosa and then the tissue is retracted for a clear view.

Mouth Prop

A **mouth prop** is used to prevent the patient's mouth from closing during the procedure. Sometimes, appointment length, the type of anesthesia administered, or the physical condition of the patient requires the use of props. Mouth props are made of hard rubber, silicone, plastic, Styrofoam, or stainless steel. Some of the mouth props are disposable, such as the Styrofoam props. They are supplied in child and adult sizes. The prop is inserted into the patient's mouth with the tapered end toward the posterior teeth. This allows the muscles to relax while keeping the mouth open.

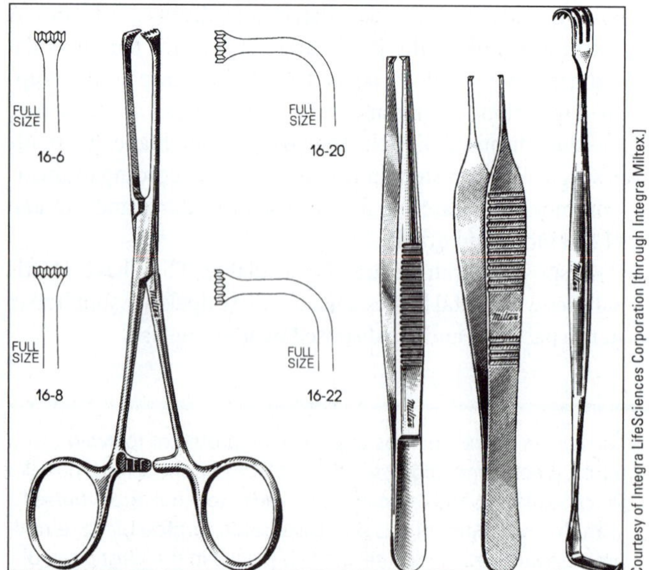

Courtesy of Integra LifeSciences Corporation [through Integra Miltex.]

FIGURE 25-2

Tissue retractors.

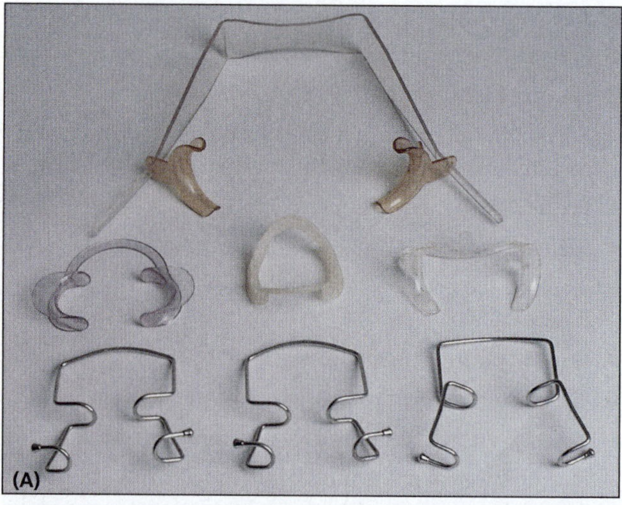

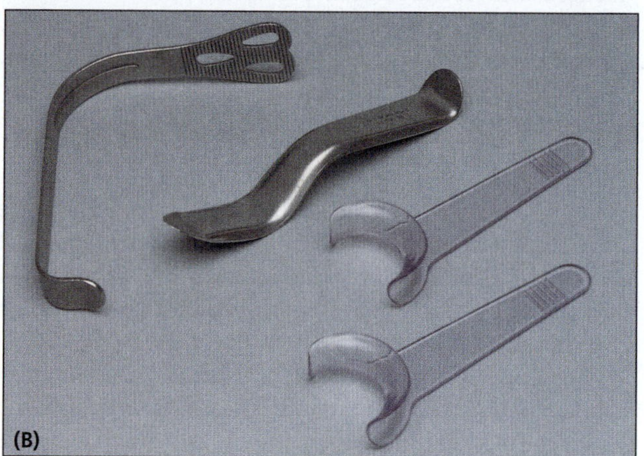

FIGURE 25-3

(A) Tongue and cheek retractors. (B) Lip, tongue, and cheek retractors.

Another type of mouth prop is the Molt mouth gag, which is hinged and has handles, a ratchet release, and beaks. Molt mouth gags are supplied in pediatric, child, and adult sizes. The beaks are closed when inserted into the patient's mouth, and the handle is gently squeezed, which opens the beaks and the patient's mouth. The forceps are locked in this position until the release is engaged (Figure 25-5).

Hemostat

A **hemostat** has multiple uses during surgical procedures. Hemostats are used to retract tissue, remove small root tips, clamp off blood vessels, and grasp loose objects. A hemostat is similar to forceps, the main differences being the working ends of the hemostat are not sharp but have long, serrated, or grooved beaks. They have locking handles that can be manipulated with one hand (Figure 25-6A).

Hemostats are supplied in various sizes to accommodate the uses of the instrument. Tissue, bone, and tooth fragments are easily grasped and removed with the hemostat. There are various types, including the Kelly and the Halstead-Mosquito. Hemostats come with straight and curved beaks.

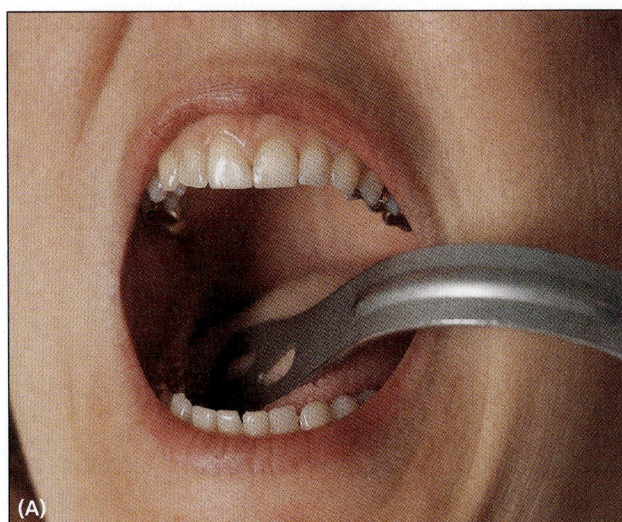

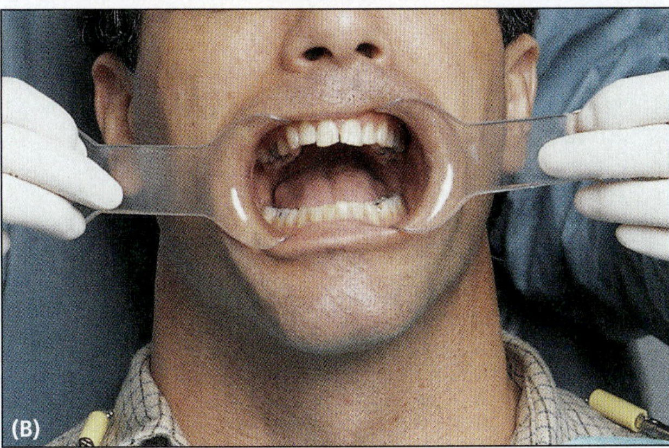

FIGURE 25-4

(A) Retracting the tongue with the University of Minnesota retractor. (B) Cheek retractor in patient's mouth.

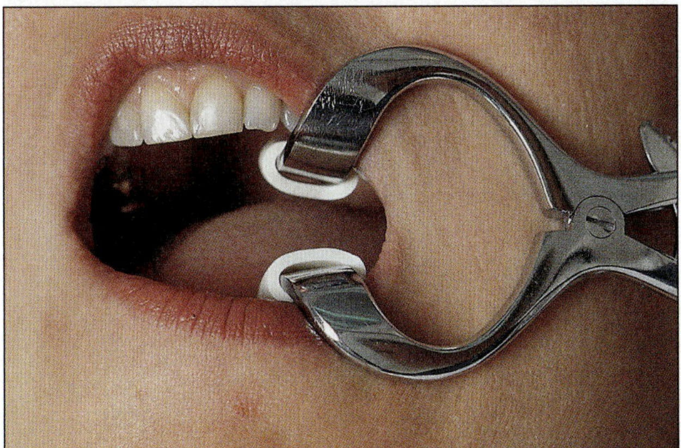

FIGURE 25-5

Molt mouth gags in patient's mouth.

Needle Holder

A **needle holder** is similar to a hemostat and functions in much the same manner. Needle holders are forceps with straight beaks, but the beaks are shorter than hemostat beaks. The needle holder has fine serrations with a groove down the center of each beak to hold the suture needle. They are supplied in various sizes (Figure 25-6B).

Surgical Scissors

The **surgical scissors** are used to cut sutures and to trim soft tissue. They are supplied in various sizes and shapes (Figure 25-7). They are made of stainless steel and should be used only for surgical procedures to maintain their sharp edges. The surgical scissors have pointed beaks with straight or angled blades.

Surgical Aspirating Tips

The **surgical aspirating tips** are made of metal or plastic. The metal tips are sterilizable, while the plastic tips are discarded after one use. The surgical aspirating tips are long tubes that are very slender or tapered to small openings. The tips are

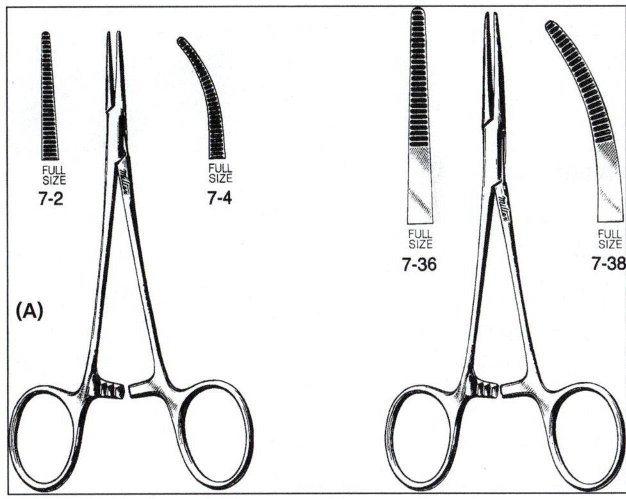

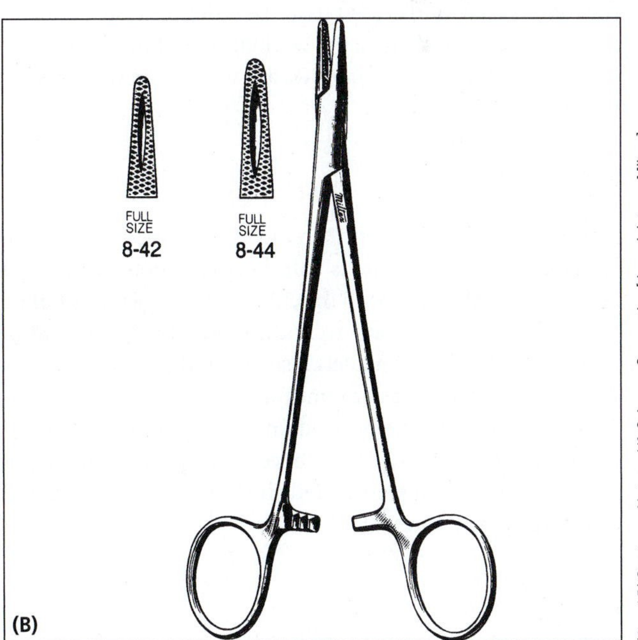

(A and B) Courtesy of Integra LifeSciences Corporation [through Integra Miltex.]

FIGURE 25-6

(A) Hemostats. (B) Needle holder.

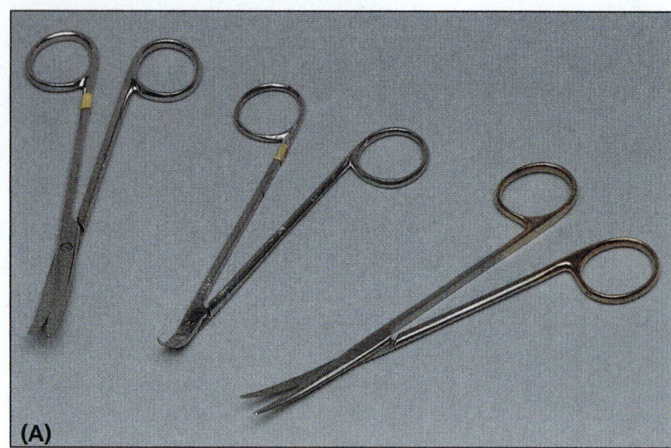

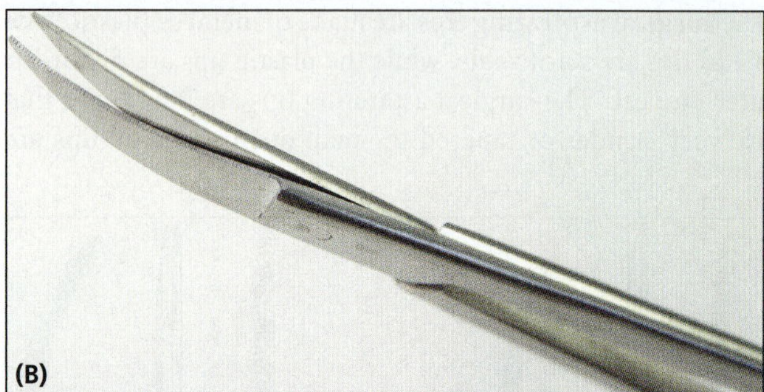

FIGURE 25-7

Surgical scissors.

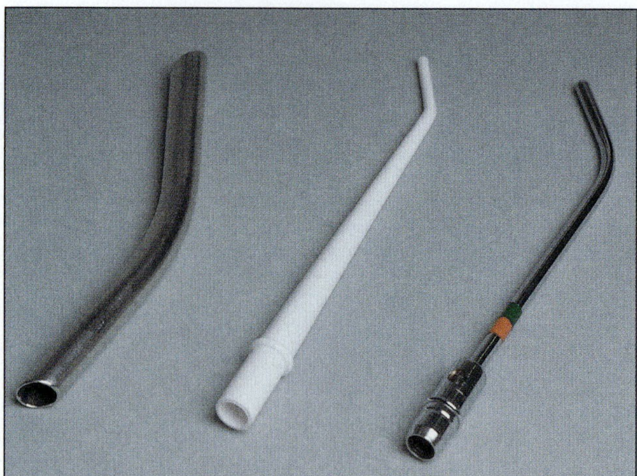

FIGURE 25-8

Surgical aspirating tips.

used to aspirate blood and debris from the surgical site and for tonsil suction for sedated patients (Figure 25-8). A **stylet** is a thin wire used to clear blood and tissue from the surgical tips.

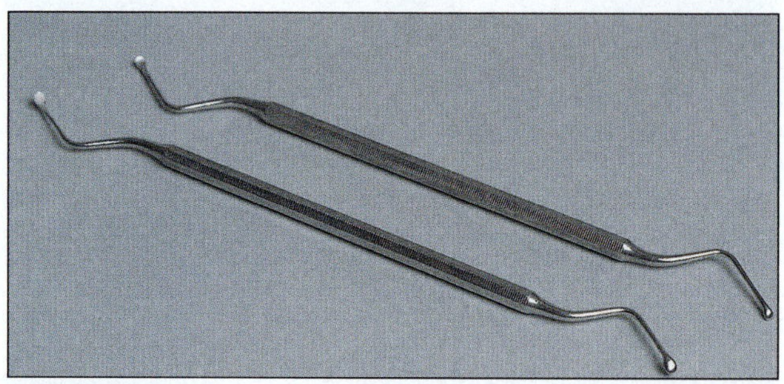

FIGURE 25-9

Surgical curettes.

Surgical Curettes

A **surgical curette** is used for curettage and debridement of the tooth socket or diseased tissue. It is double ended and has straight or curved shanks; the working end of the instrument is spoon shaped. Surgical curettes are available in various sizes (Figure 25-9).

Surgical Chisel and Mallet

A **surgical chisel** is used to remove or shape bone. It can be used alone if the bone is soft, but if the bone is dense, a **surgical mallet** is used with the chisel. The chisel is positioned on the bone, and mallets are used to gently tap the end of the chisel. Chisels and mallets also are used to split teeth into smaller portions for easier removal.

Chisels are available beveled on one surface or bi-beveled (beveled on both sides). The bi-beveled chisels are used to split a tooth, while the single-beveled chisel is used to remove and shape the bone (Figure 25-10).

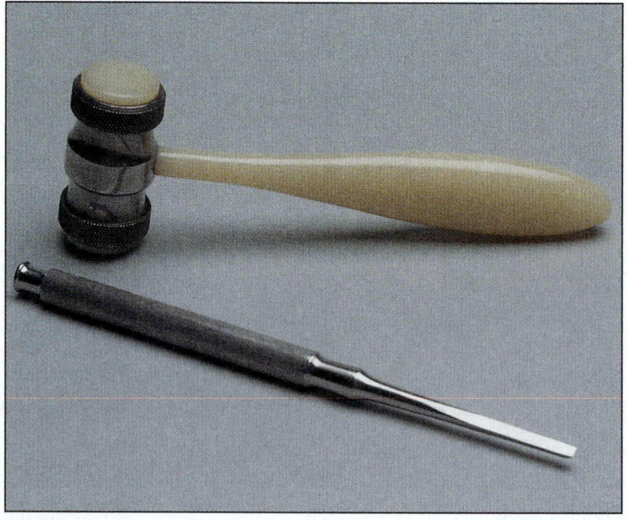

FIGURE 25-10

Surgical chisel and mallet.

Rongeurs

The **rongeurs** (**RON**-jeers) are hinged forceps with springs in the handle. They are used to trim and shape the alveolar bone after extractions. The beaks are sharp and have cutting edges, similar to fingernail trimmers. There are several sizes and shapes of rongeurs. When multiple teeth are removed and a denture is to be seated, rongeurs are necessary to contour the ridges of the alveolar bone and eliminate sharp edges (Figure 25-11).

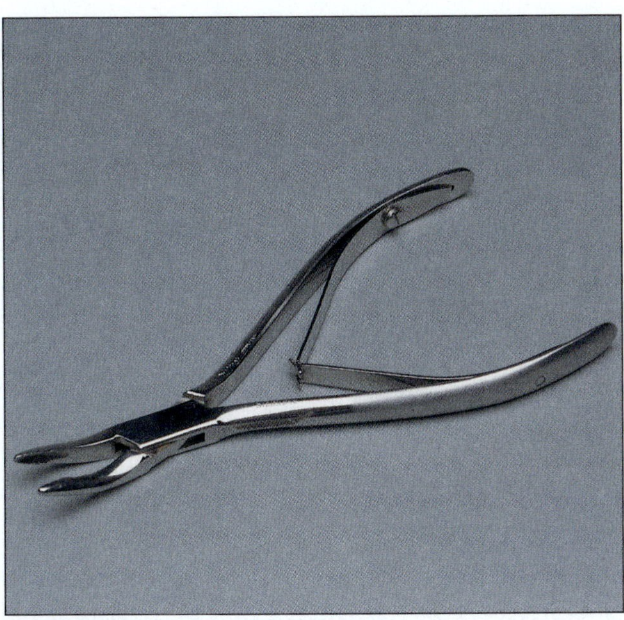

FIGURE 25-11
Surgical rongeurs.

Surgical Bone File

A **surgical bone file** is usually a double-ended instrument. It is supplied in various sizes and shapes. Bone files are used in a back-and-forth motion to smooth the edges of alveolar bone. They trim and smooth the bone after the teeth have been extracted and the rongeurs have contoured the bone (Figure 25-12).

Periosteal Elevator

The **periosteal elevator** is an instrument of many uses and is included on most surgical tray setups. It is often used to detach the periosteum (bone covering) and gingival tissues from around the tooth prior to the use of extraction forceps. The periosteal elevator is also used to reflect and lift the **mucoperiosteum** (mucosa and periosteum) from the bone.

Periosteal elevators are double-ended instruments with various working-end combinations. Often, one end is pointed and the other is rounded (Figure 25-13).

Elevator

An **elevator** is used by the surgeon to loosen and remove teeth, retained roots, and root fragments. Elevators are designed in different shapes and sizes to accommodate the variety of tasks, operating techniques, and tooth morphology. They are single-ended instruments with large, bulbous, or T-shaped handles to allow for a firm grip. Being able to firmly grip the elevator allows the surgeon to exert the necessary force. The working ends of elevators may be straight or angular and are often paired left and right. Elevators are referred to by manufacturer's number or by designer names. Two common designer elevators are Potts and Cryers (Figures 25-14B and C).

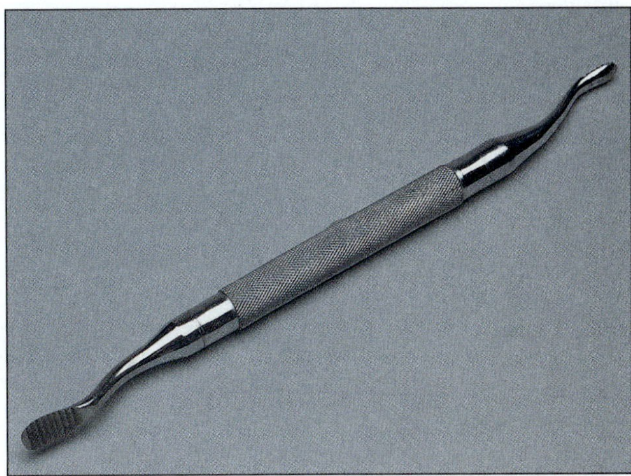

FIGURE 25-12
Surgical bone file.

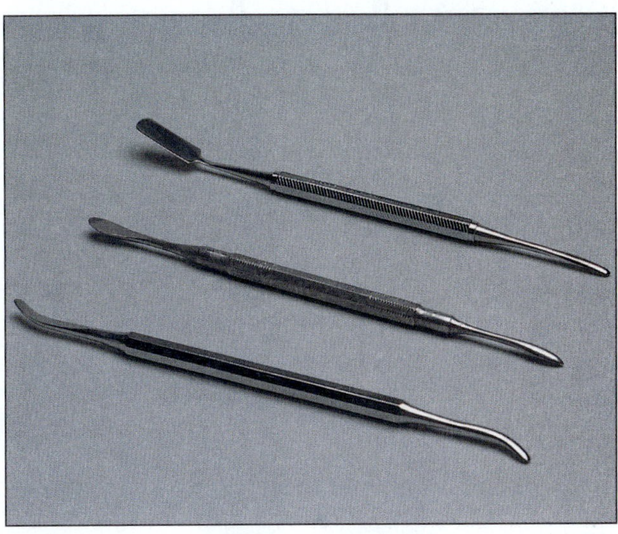

FIGURE 25-13
Periosteal elevators.

An **apical elevator** is similar to the elevators with the large handle but have smaller working ends. They are straight or angular and have longer, narrower blades to loosen and remove roots or root or bone fragments (Figure 25-14A).

A **root tip pick** or elevator is even thinner and longer than apical elevators. They are paired left and right and are also straight or angled. The root tip picks are designed to tease the root tips or fragments out of the bone socket. They are delicate instruments that break if too much force is applied (Figure 25-15).

Forceps

The **extraction forceps** are used to remove teeth from the alveolar bone. They are hinged instruments with various handles and beak styles. Specific forceps are used on certain teeth or in certain areas of the mouth. Dental assistants should be able to identify which forceps their dentists routinely use. One way to learn forceps is by manufacturer's numbers. Each instrument

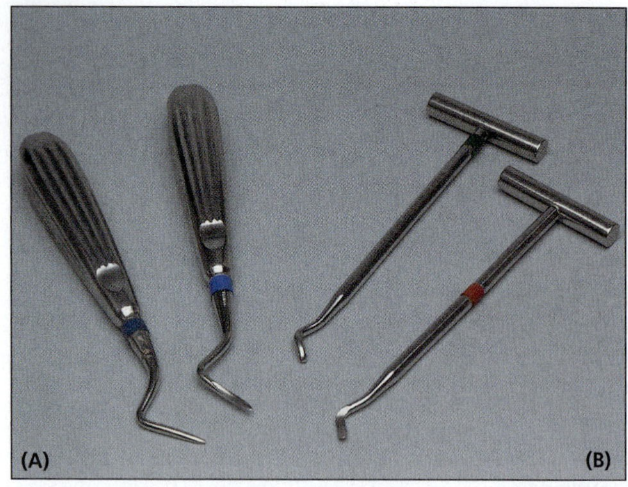

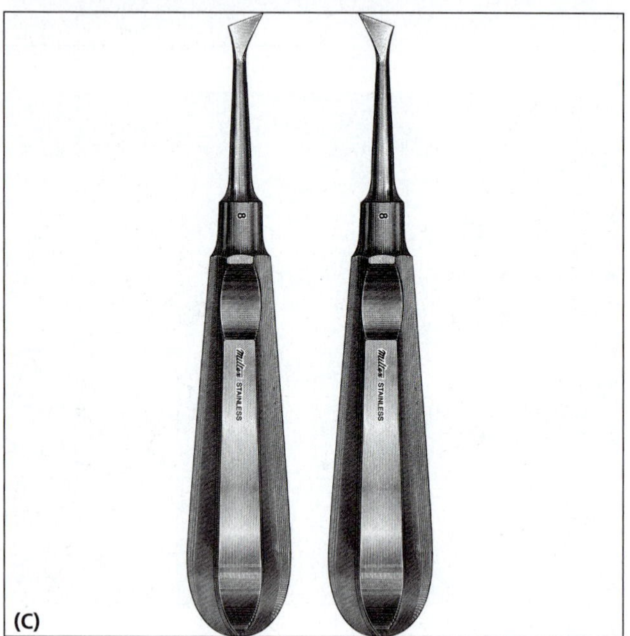

FIGURE 25-14

(A) Apical elevators. (B) Potts or T-handled elevators. (C) Cryers elevators.

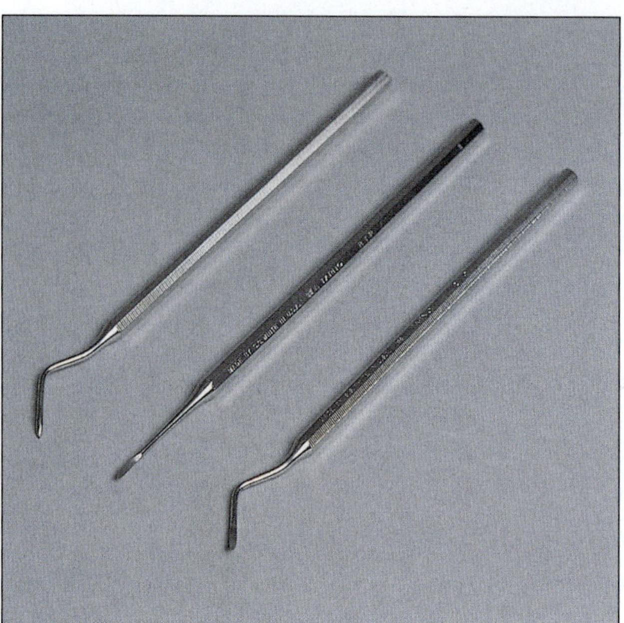

FIGURE 25-15

Root tip picks.

has a number imprinted on the handle and is labeled with an "L" or "R" for left or right. For example, #88R is used on the maxillary right first and second molars.

Another way to identify forceps is to learn how the design of the forceps applies to tooth morphology. Careful study of the various shapes of the beaks will allow determination of forceps for:

- Maxillary or mandibular teeth
- Right or left quadrant
- Anterior or posterior teeth
- Accommodation of teeth anatomy

For example, on #53R for the maxillary molars, one beak is pointed for placement in the bifurcated buccal root. On #88L for the maxillary molars, there is a pointed single beak on the buccal to be placed between the two buccal roots and a split beak on the lingual to engage the single lingual root.

The curve of the shank of the forceps indicates whether the forceps should be used on the maxillary or the mandibular. Mandibular forceps are often at more of a right angle, and the maxillary are straight, slightly curved, or have two angles (like bayonets). For example, #17 forceps are used on the mandibular first and second molars; the beaks form an angle with the handle. The forceps for the maxillary first and second molars have two angles in the working end.

Some forceps are **universal forceps** and can be used on any of the four quadrants. Another example is #101 forceps, which can be used for bicuspids and deciduous teeth in either arch. Other forceps can be used on the left or right side in the same arch. For example, the #150 forceps can be used for maxillary incisors, bicuspids, and roots on both the left and right quadrants.

Forceps used on the anterior or posterior teeth can be distinguished by beak width. For example, on mandibular forceps #151, the beaks are smaller to fit the incisors, bicuspids, and roots, while mandibular molar forceps #17 are wider to accommodate the width of the molars.

The shapes of forceps beaks are designed to accommodate the anatomy of specific teeth. For example, mandibular first and second molar forceps have narrow, pointed beaks to engage the bifurcated roots of these molars. These forceps are sometimes called the "cow horns" because of their shape.

Extraction forceps are held in a palm grasp by the operator. Some handles are straight, while others have "finger rings" or hooks on the handles. The selection is the preference of the dentist.

To better visualize and learn forceps, divide them into the arches and teeth they are used on (Figures 25-16 and 25-17).

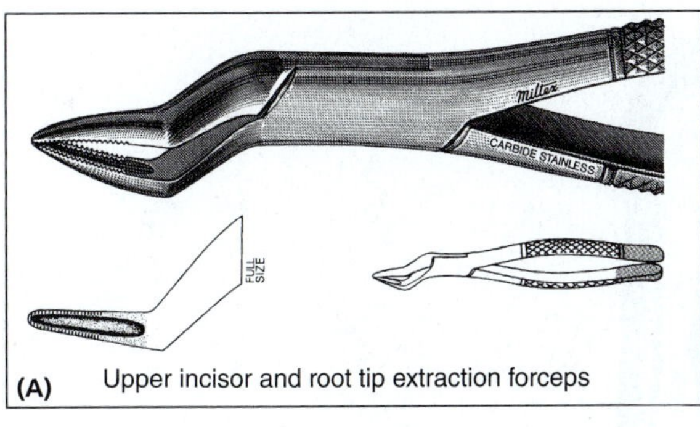

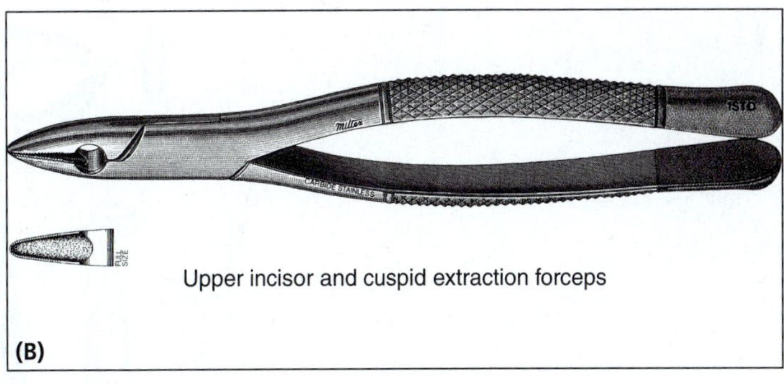

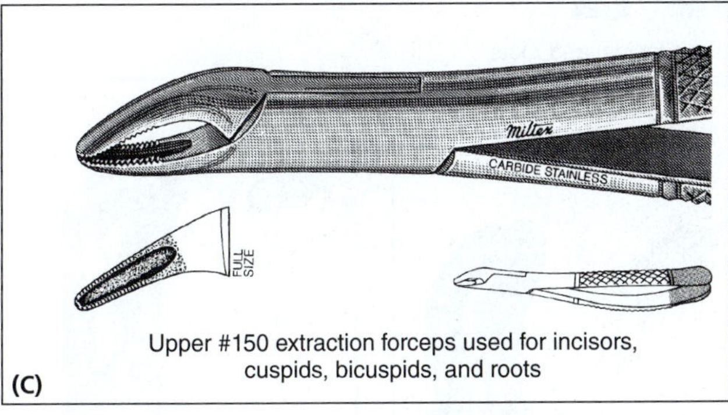

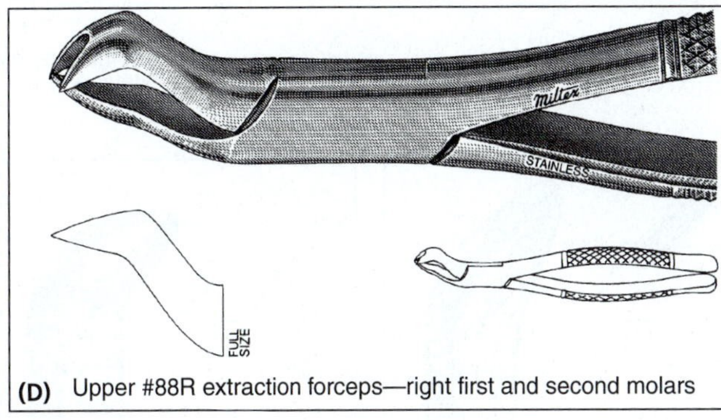

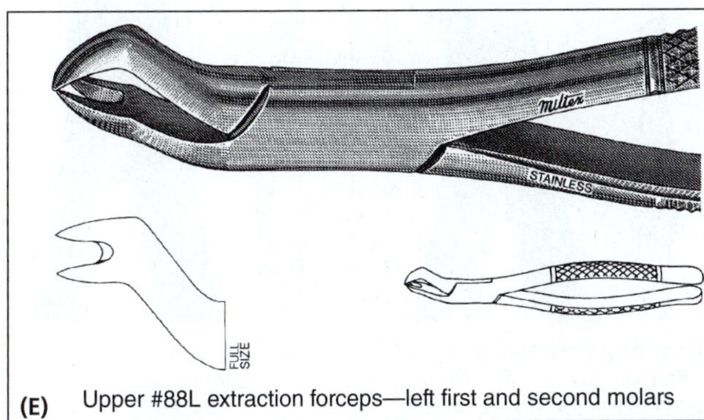

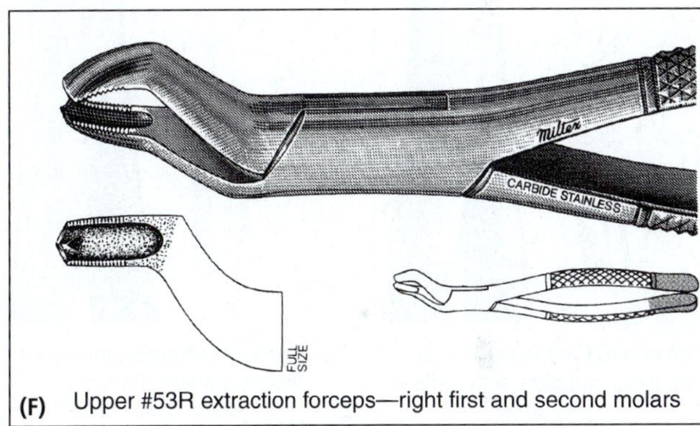

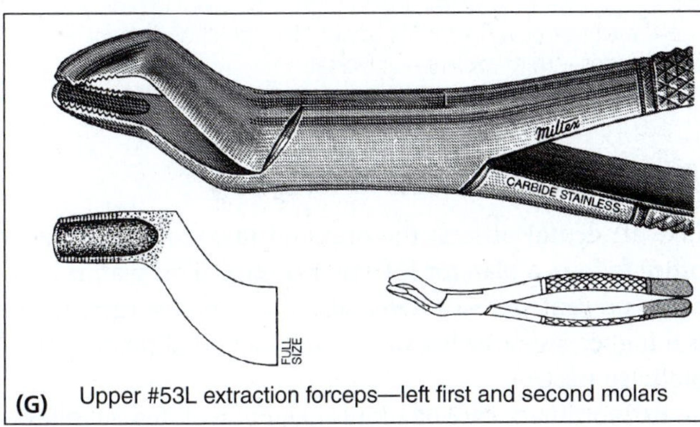

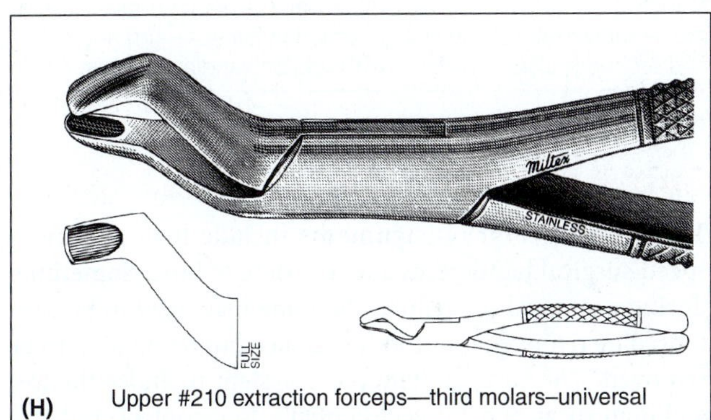

FIGURE 25-16

Maxillary extraction forceps. (A) Upper incisor and root tip extraction forceps. (B) Upper incisor and cuspid extraction forceps. (C) Upper #150 extraction forceps used for incisors, cuspids, bicuspids, and roots. (D) Upper #88L extraction forceps—left first and second molars. (E) Upper #88R extraction forceps—right first and second molars. (F) Upper #53R extraction forceps—right first and second molars. (G) Upper #53L extraction forceps—left first and second molars. (H) Upper #210 extraction forceps—third molars–universal.

(A–H) Courtesy of Integra LifeSciences Corporation [through Integra Miltex.]

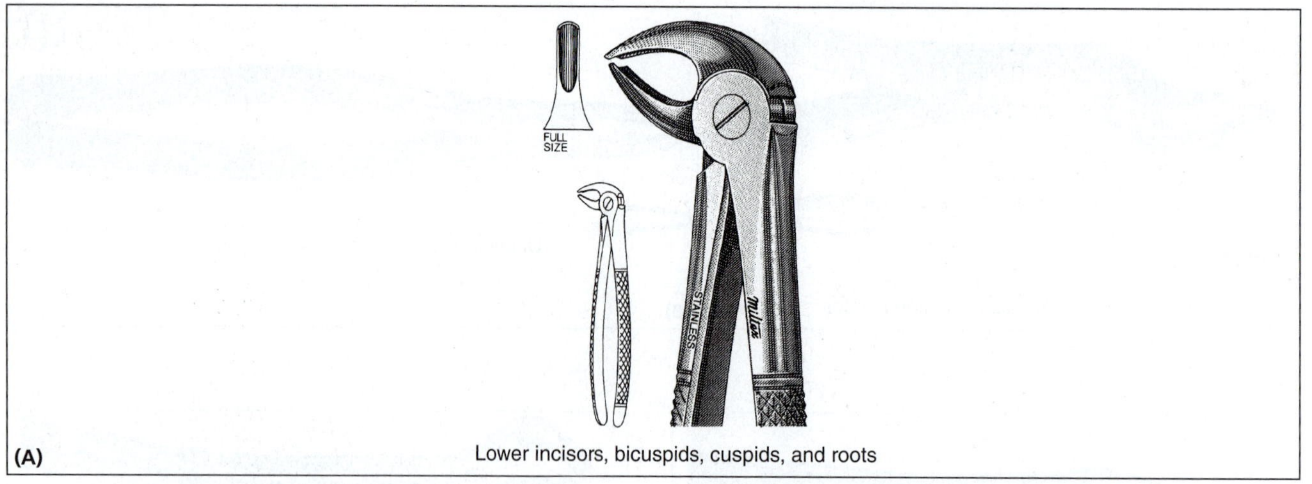

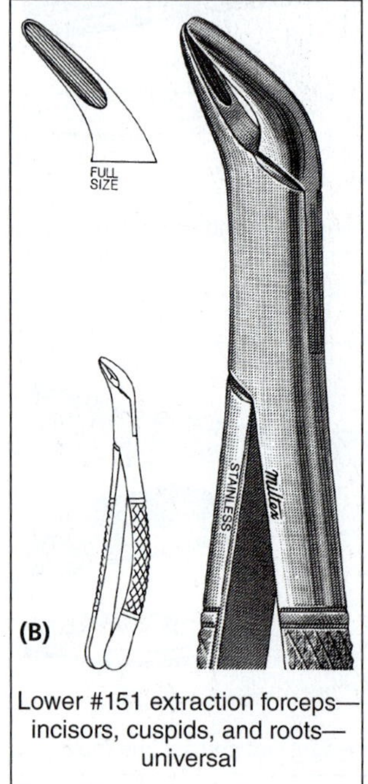

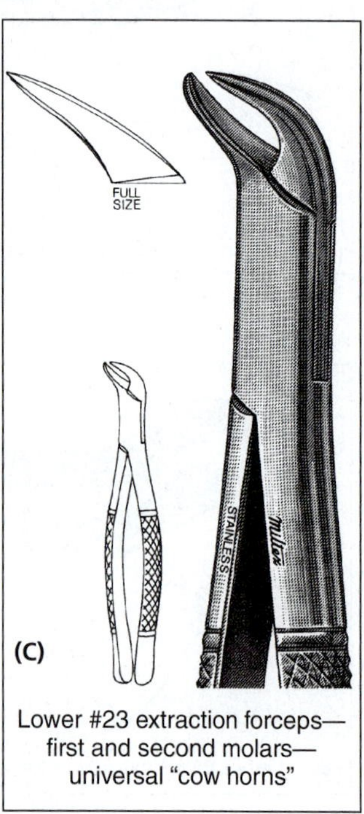

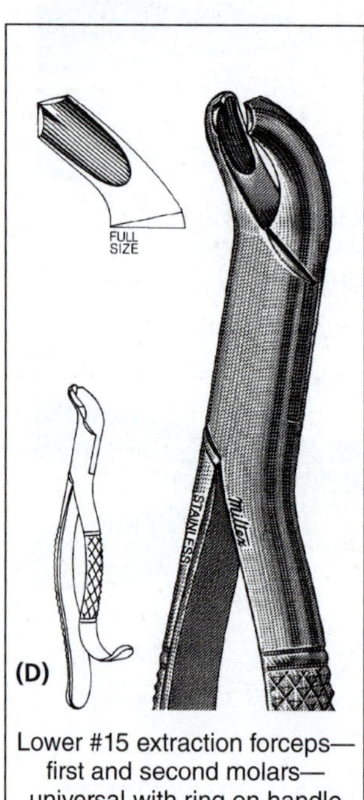

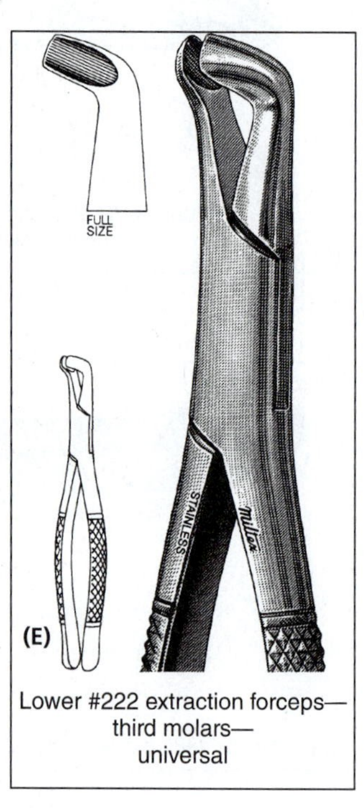

(A–E) Courtesy of Integra LifeSciences Corporation [through Integra Miltex.]

FIGURE 25-17

Mandibular extraction forceps. (A) Lower incisors, bicuspids, cuspids, and roots. (B) Lower #151 extraction forceps—incisors, cuspids, and roots—universal. (C) Lower #23 extraction forceps—first and second molars—universal "cow horns". (D) Lower #15 extraction forceps—first and second molars—universal with ring on handle. (E) Lower #222 extraction forceps—third molars—universal.

Surgical Rotary Instruments

The **surgical rotary instruments** include low- and high-speed surgical handpieces and a variety of burs. Sometimes during a surgical procedure, the bone may need to be contoured or removed or a tooth may need to be divided to be removed. The surgical handpiece system includes the low and high surgical handpiece controls, foot control, and arm to hold saline water. The surgical handpiece uses saline water as the cooling system to avoid contamination of the surgical site. There are many shapes of burs used for cutting and smoothing bone and tissue. The burs used are often longer to meet the surgical site.

Asepsis in Oral Surgery

Like all dental offices, the oral and maxillofacial surgery office follows a plan for infection control. This plan is critical to prevent cross-contamination. The oral surgery office is a higher risk area because of the increased possibility of blood contact.

Extraordinary care of surgical equipment and supplies is necessary to prevent accidental exposure. In the sterilizing room, an area should be designated for "unclean" trays where the contaminated tray is taken apart and disposable sharps are placed in a marked sharps container. Expendable items, such as gauze, cotton rolls, and so on, are placed in marked hazardous waste containers. The instruments are cleaned, and then bagged or wrapped for sterilization. The bags are carefully marked with the procedure and date. The instruments are sterilized according to various methods, such as steam autoclaving, dry heat, and chemical vapor. Current OSHA guidelines should be followed (see Chapter 11, Infection Control).

Storage of Contaminated Instruments

If contaminated instruments cannot be processed immediately, they should be presoaked to prevent blood and debris from drying on them.

The Dentist and the Dental Assistant

The dentist and the dental assistant must follow the routine requirements of personal protective equipment (PPE) for all surgical procedures. One change is in the handwashing procedure. For oral surgery, the surgical hand scrub is completed before donning sterile gloves. (See Procedure 25-1.)

Patient Considerations

During the first visit, a medical history is completed) by the patient. If surgery is anticipated, the surgeon may consult with the patient's physician about the patient's medications and physical conditions that may affect the surgical procedure.

Radiographs are sent from the general dental office to the oral surgeon's office before the patient is scheduled. Periapical radiographs are commonly used for extractions, but occlusal and extraoral radiographs such as panoramic, lateral skull, cephalometric, and computerized tomography also may be required. (Specific extraoral exposures are explained in Chapter 22, Production and Evaluation of Dental Radiographs; and Chapter 23, Extraoral and Digital Radiography.)

The oral surgeon completes a thorough examination. Once the diagnosis is made, the treatment options are explained to the patient. The patient must carefully read and sign an informed consent form prior to the procedure. The informed consent identifies and explains the surgery the patient is to receive and acknowledges any risks of the treatment.

Patient Preparation

The type of anesthetic administered will determine the preoperative instructions given to the patient. It is important for the patient to follow the instructions carefully prior to his or her appointment.

Oral Surgery Procedures

CDA

Common procedures performed in the oral surgeon's office are routine extractions, multiple extractions and alveoplasty, surgical removal of impacted third molars, biopsy procedures, and dental implant surgery.

Typical Preoperative Instructions for the Patient

1. Wear loose-fitting clothing and low-heeled shoes. Your shirt should be short sleeved or easy to roll up.
2. Remove contact lenses before surgery.
3. Notify the dentist if a cold, sore throat, fever, or other illness develops prior to surgery.
4. Do not consume alcoholic beverages 24 hours before surgery.
5. Arrange transportation to and from the office on the day of the surgery.
6. When a physical examination is requested by the oral surgeon, have the physician send written approval prior to surgery.
7. Some medical conditions, such as rheumatic heart disease or artificial heart valves, require prophylactic antibiotics to be taken prior to surgery.
8. If the surgery is in the morning, eat nothing after midnight. This includes medicines, food, and all fluids.* Food, liquids, or medications in the stomach when general anesthesia is administered may cause vomiting. The vomit may then be aspirated into the lungs.*
9. If the surgery is in the afternoon, drink only water, juice, tea, or coffee prior to 6 a.m. After 6 a.m., take absolutely nothing by mouth.*

Patient Preparation

1. The patient is escorted to the treatment room. The dental assistant checks any changes in the medical history, whether the patient followed the preoperative instructions, and whether prescribed medication was taken as directed.
2. The patient is given an antimicrobial rinse.
3. The patient is seated and a full-length drape is placed on him or her. The patient is then reclined to a routine position for the dentist.
4. A sterile towel is placed over the patient's chest.
5. Vital signs are taken and recorded. The patient is prepared for administration of the intravenous sedation.

* Food, liquids, or medications in the stomach when general anesthesia is administered may cause vomiting. The vomit may then be aspirated into the lungs.

Procedure 25-1
Surgical Scrub

This procedure is performed by the oral surgeon and the dental assistant before donning sterile gloves for a surgical procedure.

Equipment and Supplies

- Antimicrobial soap
- Sterile scrub brush or foam sponge
- Disposable sterile towels

Procedure Steps (*Follow aseptic procedures*)

1. Remove watch and rings before the scrub.
2. Use an antimicrobial soap, such as chlorhexidine gluconate.
3. Wet hands and forearms up to the elbows with warm water.
4. Dispense about 5 mL of soap into cupped hands and work into a lather.
5. Beginning with the fingernails, scrub the fingers, hands, and forearms with a surgical scrub brush.
6. Rinse thoroughly with warm water.
7. Repeat the procedure with soap but without the scrub brush.
8. Rinse with warm water, beginning at the fingertips and moving hands and forearms through the water and up so that the water drains off the forearms last (Figure 25-18). This prevents the hands from being recontaminated.
9. Dry hands and arms thoroughly with disposable sterile towels.
10. Don sterile surgical gloves.

NOTE: The surgical scrub was commonly referred to as the "5-minute scrub," but studies have indicated that scrub times of 3 to 4 minutes are as effective as 5-minute scrubs. The recommendation is to follow the scrub product manufacturer's instructions and OSHA guidelines. Do not use a brush so stiff that it creates microscopic abrasions on the skin.

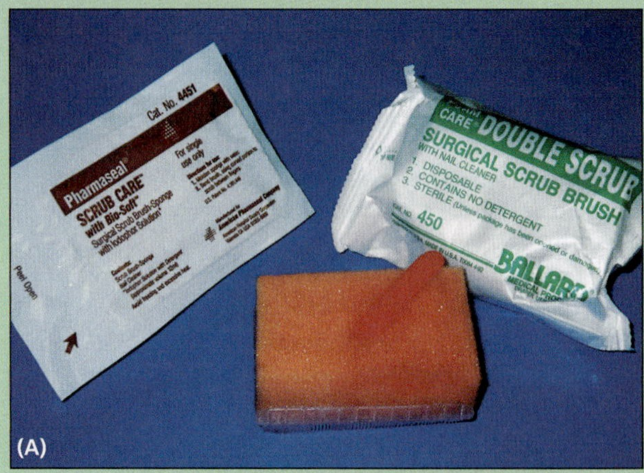

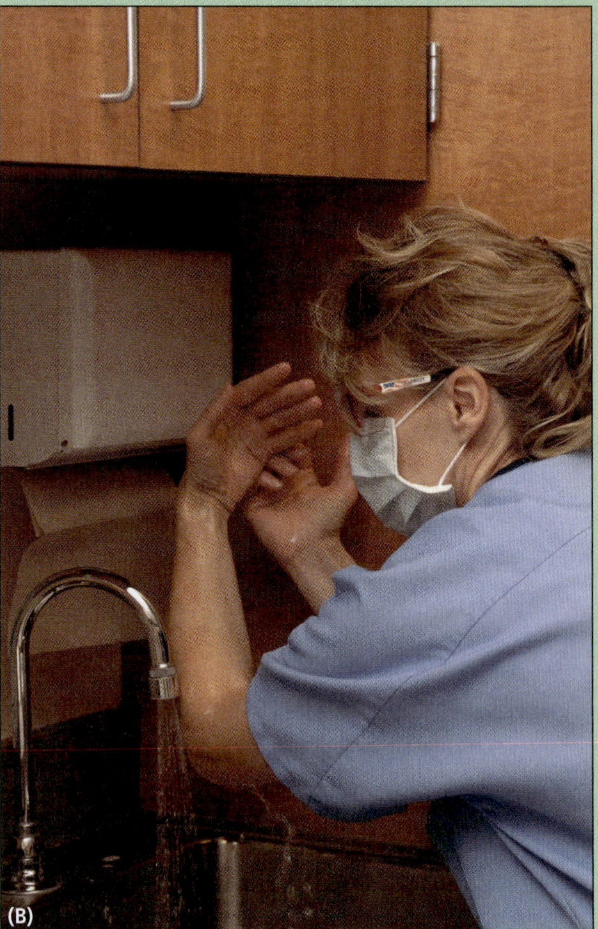

FIGURE 25-18
(A) Materials for surgical scrub. (B) Completion of surgical scrub.

Routine or Uncomplicated Extractions

Routine or uncomplicated extractions include the removal of permanent or primary teeth that are erupted into the oral cavity. These surgeries are usually less involved and performed more often than other surgeries. The dental assistant prepares the tray setup and selects forceps and elevators for the specific tooth to be extracted. (See Procedure 25-2.)

Multiple Extractions and Alveoplasty

Multiple extractions are needed when the patient is going to have a full or partial denture. The extraction process is similar for one tooth or for several teeth, but after several teeth have been removed, the bone and soft tissue must be contoured and smoothed. The contouring process is called an **alveoplasty**. The alveolar ridge must be free of any sharp edges or points in order to achieve the most comfort and function for the patient. If both the maxillary and the mandibular teeth are to be extracted at one appointment, the maxillary teeth are extracted first. This prevents hemorrhage and debris from contaminating the mandibular extraction site during surgery. Routinely, the dentist starts at the most posterior tooth and moves anteriorly.

Procedure 25-2
Routine or Uncomplicated Extraction

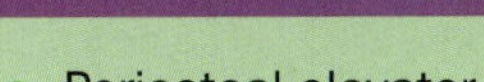

The dental assistant assists the oral surgeon throughout this procedure. The dental assistant must be prepared and thinking ahead to anticipate the surgeon's needs.

Equipment and Supplies (*Figure 25-19*)

- Mouth mirror
- Gauze sponges
- Surgical HVE tip
- University of Minnesota Retractor for the tongue and the cheek
- Local anesthetic setup
- Nitrous oxide setup (optional)

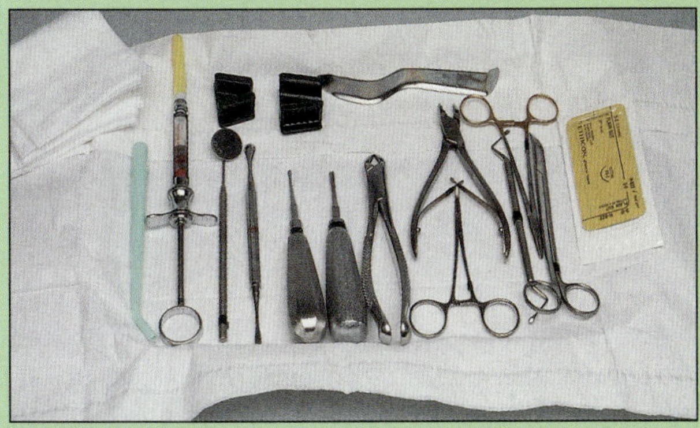

FIGURE 25-19
Tray setup for uncomplicated extraction.

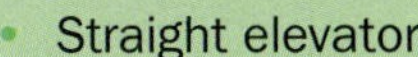

- Periosteal elevator
- Straight elevator
- Extraction forceps
- Surgical rongeurs
- Hemostat/needle holder
- Surgical curette
- Surgical scissors
- Suture setup

1. The surgeon examines the site of extraction. The patient's x-rays are mounted on the viewbox for the dentist to review. The dental assistant transfers the mouth mirror and explorer to the surgeon.
2. Topical anesthetic is placed on the mucosa, and local anesthetic is administered. The dental assistant prepares the topical anesthetic and transfers it to the surgeon (if allowed by the state practice act, the dental assistant can place the topical anesthetic). The syringe is prepared and transferred to the surgeon. The dental assistant then observes the patient.
3. Either the periosteal or a straight elevator is used by the oral surgeon to determine whether the patient is adequately numb, to separate epithelial attachment from around the tooth,

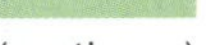

(continues)

Procedure 25-2 (continued)

and to initiate alveolar bone expansion around the neck of the tooth (to accommodate forceps placement). The dental assistant transfers and receives elevators and has gauze ready to remove blood or debris from the instruments. The dental assistant maintains the operating field, adjusts the light, and retracts tissues as needed.

4. Once the tooth is loosened in the alveolus, forceps are placed securely on the tooth and, with a firm grasp, the surgeon **luxates** (moves or dislocates) the tooth and then removes it from the socket. This may be easy, or the tooth may have to be subluxated (rocked back and forth), rotated, and lifted several times before the bone around the tooth is spread enough to lift the tooth out of the socket. During this time, the dental assistant transfers forceps and elevators as needed by the surgeon, keeps the instruments clean of debris, and retracts the cheek or tongue. The dental assistant should observe the patient for signs of anxiety or syncope. Once the tooth is extracted, the forceps beaks and tooth are received in the palm of the dental assistant's hand while transferring gauze to the surgeon (Figure 25-20). Once the forceps and tooth are placed on the tray, the tooth is examined for fractured roots.
5. The alveolus (socket) is examined for fractured root tips and debris. A surgical curette is used to remove bone chips, granulation tissue, and abscesses/cysts. The dental assistant evacuates the alveolus using the surgical HVE tip, and then transfers the surgical curette. Gauze is held close to the patient's chin to remove debris from the curette.

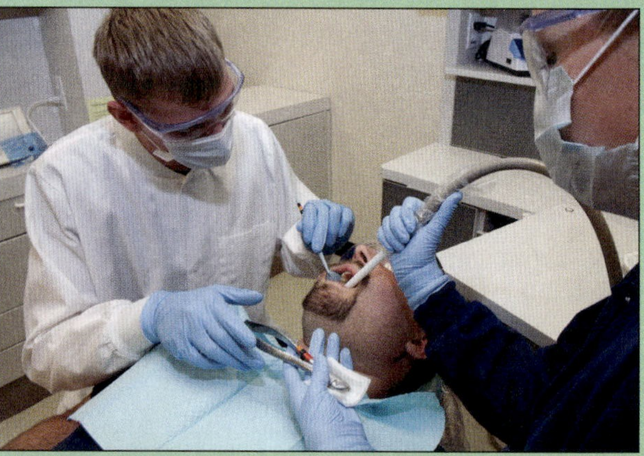

FIGURE 25-20
Dental assistant receiving extraction forceps with tooth in beaks.

6. Once the tooth and any fragments are removed, the area is debrided and the wound is covered with folded, moistened gauze as a pressure pack. The patient is instructed to bite down on the gauze to apply pressure. This aids in controlling the bleeding and in the formation of the blood clot.
7. At this point in the procedure, the dentist may place sutures. The dental assistant prepares the sutures and assists during placement. The dental assistant debrides the area with the HVE and has a moistened gauze folded and ready to place in the patient's mouth for biting on.
8. The dental assistant checks and cleans the patient's face, returns the patient to a sitting position, and allows a few minutes before giving postoperative instructions. The patient is then dismissed.

Impacted Teeth Extractions

Third molars usually erupt between the late teens and early twenties. In some cases, the patient's jaw does not grow long enough to allow the third molars or wisdom teeth to erupt or these teeth do not erupt because of blockage by other teeth. These molars then stay trapped within the jaw. Many problems can arise when this situation occurs, such as pain, inflammation, infection, destruction of neighboring teeth, destruction of the bone, or movement of the permanent teeth out of proper alignment (Figure 25-22).

Extracting impacted teeth is one of the most common procedures the oral surgeon performs, especially third molar extractions. Many factors determine the difficulty of the impacted tooth extraction, including the depth, position, or angulation of the tooth in the bone. If the third molars are partially erupted through the bone and into the soft tissues this is called a **soft tissue impaction**. A **hard tissue impaction** occurs if the teeth are impacted in bone and not through the gingival tissues. When the tooth is impacted in the bone, dental handpieces and surgical burs

Procedure 25-3
Multiple Extractions and Alveoplasty

The procedure is performed by the oral surgeon, who is assisted by the dental assistant. This sterile procedure involves the removal of several teeth and contouring the bone. Responsibilities of the dental assistant include evacuation and instrument transfer.

Equipment and Supplies (*Figure 25-21*)

- Luer-Lok syringe and sterile saline solution
- Local anesthetic setup
- Surgical HVE tip
- Mouth mirror
- Scalpel and blades
- Periosteal elevators
- Straight elevator
- Extraction forceps (selected for the teeth being extracted)
- Surgical rongeurs
- Tissue retractor
- Surgical curette
- Bone file
- Root tip picks
- Surgical scissors
- Hemostat

Across the top of the tray

- Gauze sponges
- Low-speed handpiece with surgical bur
- Retractors for tongue and cheeks
- Suture setup

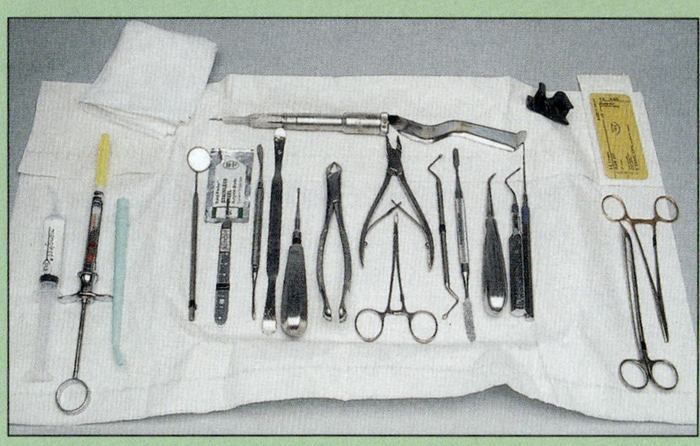

FIGURE 25-21
Tray setup for multiple extractions and alveoplasty.

Procedure Steps (*Follow aseptic procedures*)

1. The surgeon examines the teeth to be extracted.
2. When several teeth are going to be extracted, the patient may request general anesthesia. The patient will be prepared for intravenous sedation, which is followed by local anesthetic. The local anesthetic reduces bleeding at the extraction site and postoperative pain. The dental assistant prepares the materials necessary for the local and intravenous anesthetic, and then assists in the administration.
3. The teeth are removed by the same techniques described for the routine extraction.
4. After the teeth have been extracted and any root tips or debris removed, the alveoplasty procedure begins. The alveoplasty is usually accomplished one quadrant at a time. The surgeon makes an incision on the buccal and lingual surface to remove the interdental papillae and to expose the crest of the alveolar bone. The flap of tissue is reflected (folding back) for clear vision. The dental assistant transfers the scalpel and evacuates the area as necessary, receives the scalpel, and transfers the periosteal elevator to reflect the soft tissue. The dental assistant uses tissue forceps to retract the tissue and maintain the operating area.
5. Rongeurs and/or surgical burs are used for the initial trimming and contouring of the alveolar bone. The dental assistant transfers the rongeurs and/or the low-speed handpiece with surgical burs and keeps them free of debris. The dental assistant intermittently uses the HVE and the irrigation syringe with sterile saline solution to maintain the operating field.
6. Final contouring and smoothing are done with the bone file. The area is rinsed with sterile saline solution. At this point, a plastic stint (clear denture base material, molded to the same shape and size as the denture) is placed in the patient's mouth. Areas impinging on the stint can be seen by the surgeon. The surgeon continues to contour the bone until all interferences are removed. The dental

(continues)

Procedure 25-3 (continued)

assistant transfers instruments and continues to maintain the surgical site. The stint must be kept clean, so the dental assistant removes blood and debris from the stint between placements.

7. The buccal and lingual flaps are repositioned and sutured into position. The dental assistant prepares the suture materials and, once the tissue is in position, transfers the suture for placement. The dental assistant assists during the suture procedure and holds the tissue as the surgeon places the sutures.
8. A folded moist gauze pack is placed over the surgical site or the immediate denture is seated. The dental assistant prepares the gauze pack and transfers it to the surgeon. If the patient receives an immediate denture, the dental assistant readies the denture and transfers it to the surgeon for placement.
9. The patient is allowed to recover, and then postoperative instructions are given verbally and in writing.
10. The patient is scheduled for a postoperative examination and suture removal.

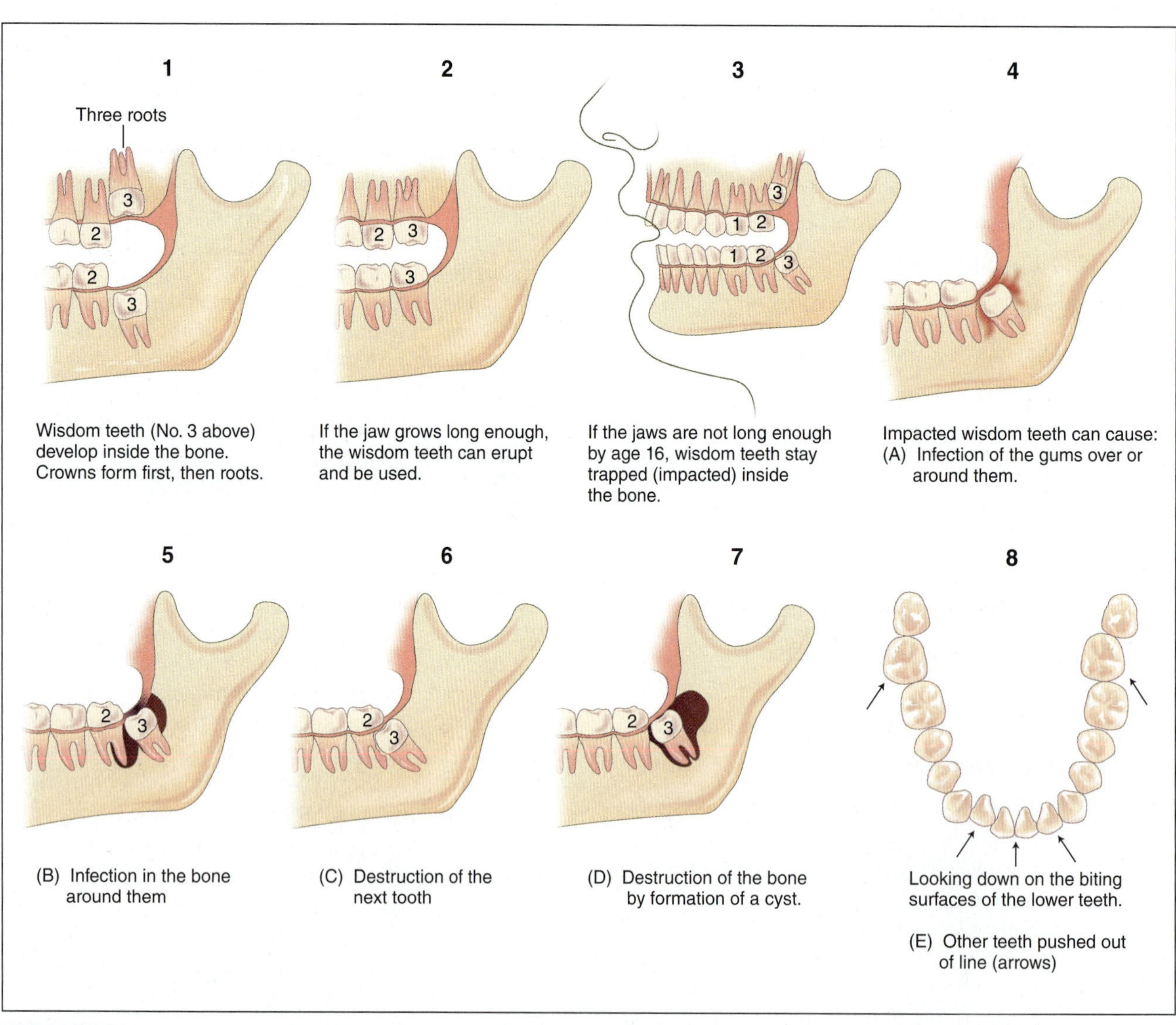

FIGURE 25-22

Problems caused by impacted wisdom teeth.

are required to gain access. Additional surgical instruments are used to facilitate the removal of the tooth from the bone such as various elevators. Often, all impacted third molars are removed at one appointment. (See Procedure 25-4 and Figure 25-23.)

Cancer and Oral Abnormalities Detection

With every patient, the dentist and staff must be aware of any abnormal tissue. Through the clinical examination, x-rays, or

Procedure 25-4
Removal of Impacted Third Molars

This procedure is performed by the oral surgeon, who is assisted by the dental assistant. This is a sterile procedure. Because the teeth are impacted, the surgeon will first have to expose the teeth by incising the tissue and removing the bone. The dental assistant transfers instruments and maintains the operating site.

Equipment and Supplies

- Basic setup: mouth mirror, explorer, and cotton pliers
- Gauze sponges
- Surgical HVE tip
- Irrigating syringe and sterile saline solution
- Retractor for the tongue and the cheek
- Local anesthetic setup
- Nitrous oxide setup (optional)
- Scalpel and blades
- Hemostat and tissue retractors
- Periosteal elevator
- Straight elevator
- Extraction forceps (if needed)
- Root tip picks
- Surgical curette
- Rongeurs
- Bone file
- Low-speed handpiece and surgical burs
- Surgical scissors
- Suture setup

Procedure Steps (*Follow aseptic procedures*)

1. The anesthetic is administered. Oral sedation may be used with local anesthetic, but the most common is intravenous (IV) anesthesia. The dental assistant prepares and transfers the anesthetic and/or assists with the IV.
2. When the patient is adequately anesthetized, an incision is made along the ridge, distal to the second molar. The scalpel incises the mucoperiosteum to the underlying bone. Depending on where the impacted tooth lies, a flap incision may be made to ensure adequate vision for the surgeon. The dental assistant transfers the scalpel and maintains the operating field with the surgical HVE (Figure 25-23A).
3. The periosteal elevator is used to retract the tissue from the alveolar bone. Once the tissue is incised, it must be reflected from the bone. The dental assistant transfers the periosteal elevator and evacuates. When the flap is completed, the dental assistant retracts the tissue (Figure 25-23B).
4. The surgeon uses a surgical bur and handpiece or a chisel and mallet to remove the bone over the tooth. The dental assistant receives the periosteal elevator and transfers the handpiece and bur or the chisel. The dental assistant continues to evacuate as needed (Figure 25-23C).
5. Once the tooth is exposed, it can often be luxated and lifted from the socket with elevators or forceps. If this is not possible, the tooth may be sectioned or divided for removal. This involves dividing the tooth into two or more parts. Burs and/or the chisel are used to separate the tooth in half to remove part or the entire crown of the tooth from the root portion. The dental assistant passes elevators and forceps. The dental assistant keeps the area clear with the HVE and periodically transfers the surgeon new gauze (Figure 25-23D).
6. When the tooth is removed, it is placed on a flat surface and examined to ensure that the entire tooth has been removed.
7. Curettes are used to remove the follicle (sac of thickened membrane) and debride the socket.

(continues)

Procedure 25-4 (continued)

The rongeurs, bone files, or burs may be used to contour the bone margins. The area is then irrigated with sterile water and evacuated. The dental assistant transfers instruments and removes debris from the working ends with gauze. The dental assistant prepares the irrigating syringe with sterile water and evacuates the area thoroughly.

8. The tissue flap is replaced to its normal position over the wound, and the operator sutures the area. The dental assistant prepares the suture and places it in the needle holder and transfers it to the oral surgeon. The cheeks are then retracted so that the surgeon can place the sutures (Figures 25-23E and F). The dental assistant has folded moist gauze ready to place when suturing is completed.
9. The patient is allowed to recover and is given postoperative instructions, an ice pack, and a prescription for pain before being dismissed. The patient will need to schedule an appointment for suture removal in 5 to 7 days. The dental assistant stays with the patient during recovery. When the patient is ready to leave, the dental assistant notifies the patient's escort and verifies that the patient has the necessary prescription(s) and postoperative instructions.

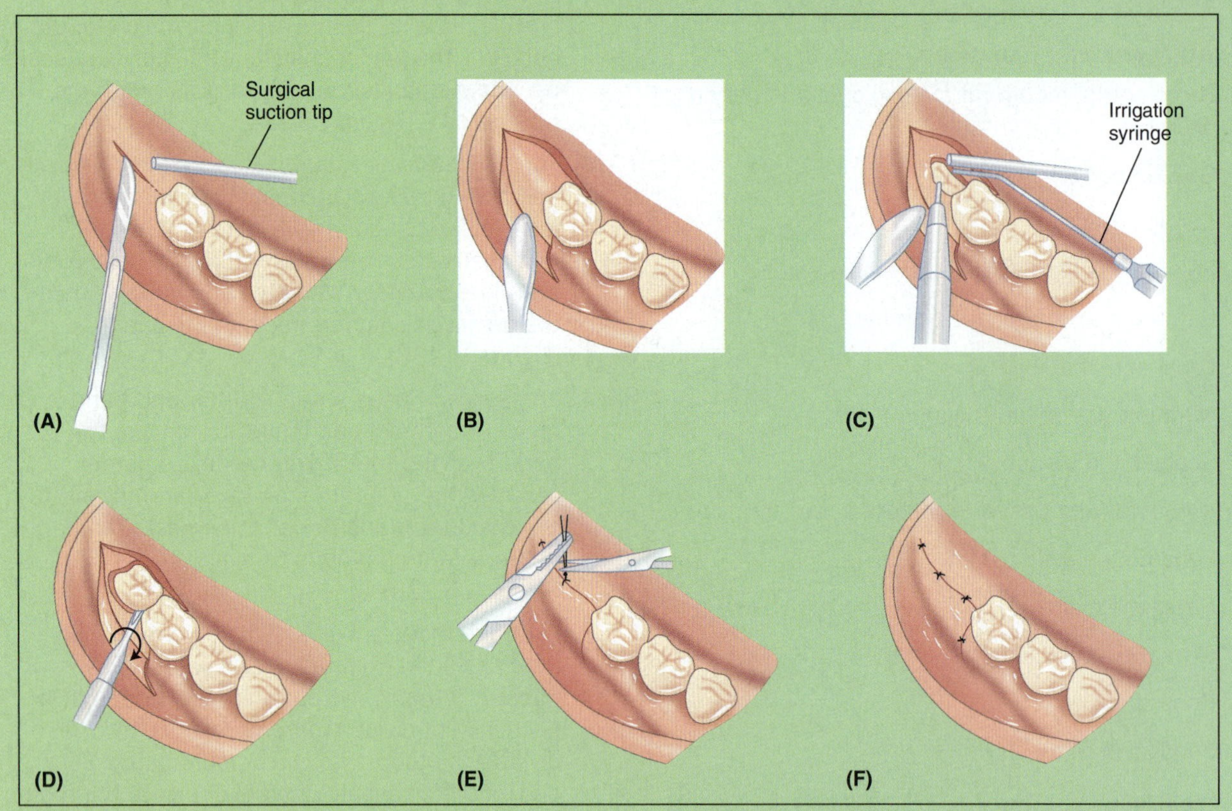

FIGURE 25-23

Steps to remove impacted third molars. (A) A flap incision is made; the assistant evacuates the area. (B) A periosteal elevator is used to retract the tissue. (C) A surgical bur is used to remove the bone over the tooth. The dental assistant evacuates and irrigates the area. (D) An elevator luxates and removes the tooth. (E) Sutures are placed. (F) The surgery is completed.

patient complaints, pathology may be discovered. Early detection of pre-malignant and/or malignant conditions can save lives. There are means to assist dental professionals in the early detection of abnormalities in the oral cavity of their patients. After the oral inspection (performed with a white light and palpation) is completed, the dental professional can use other screening techniques such as the **VELscope** and the **ViziLite** systems to inspect for disease including pre-cancerous and cancerous areas. Both of these techniques have been widely used. They are easy to use and the noninvasive examination only takes a few minutes.

The VELscope system involves a handheld, cordless handpiece with a blue-spectrum light that causes the soft tissues of the mouth to naturally fluoresce (Figure 25-24).

When healthy tissues become diseased or traumatized they fluoresce in patterns that are visibly different from healthy tissues. The VELscope assists in early detection and follow-up of abnormalities of oral soft tissues. The dentist passes the blue-spectrum light over the soft tissues, which will have a darkened appearance from the light, and looks for areas with a strong loss of fluorescence and areas of asymmetry and/or irregular shapes. In some cases, further assessment through a biopsy may be needed. To advance skills and knowledge for the dental professional, there are many avenues for further education, including the website at www.velscope.com.

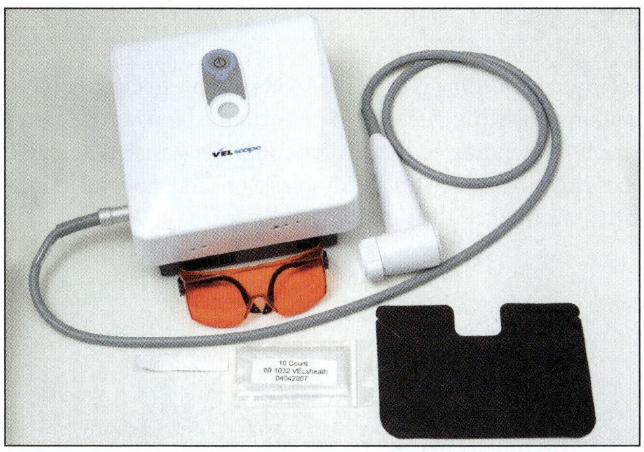

FIGURE 25-24
A VELscope is used for cancer and oral abnormalities detection.

The ViziLite system is an oral lesion identification and marking system. This system provides the dental professional with an easy, noninvasive method of identifying, evaluating, monitoring, and marking oral lesions including pre-cancerous and cancerous areas. The system includes: a pre-rinse solution, handheld disposable light stick, marking dye, disposable retractor, and single-use dose cup. With this system the patient rinses the mouth with the pre-rinse solution; the dental professional then dries the area and with dimmed overhead lights inspects the oral cavity using the light stick. Lesions will appear distinctly white; if after evaluation the lesions are considered suspicious, they are documented, possibly marked with the blue marking dye, and often a photograph of the area is taken. A biopsy of the area may be needed for further evaluation.

Biopsy Procedures

When the dentist finds a suspicious lesion or area they will want a **biopsy** performed to gain further information. The biopsy procedure, performed by an oral surgeon, involves removal of tissue from a suspicious area, either totally or partially, for microscopic examination and diagnosis. There are three types of biopsy techniques: excisional, incisional, and exfoliative. (See Procedure 25-5.)

The Incisional Biopsy. The **incisional biopsy** involves removal of a small section of the lesion, which includes a small border of normal tissue (Figure 25-25A). This technique is often performed on lesions larger than 1 cm in all dimensions,

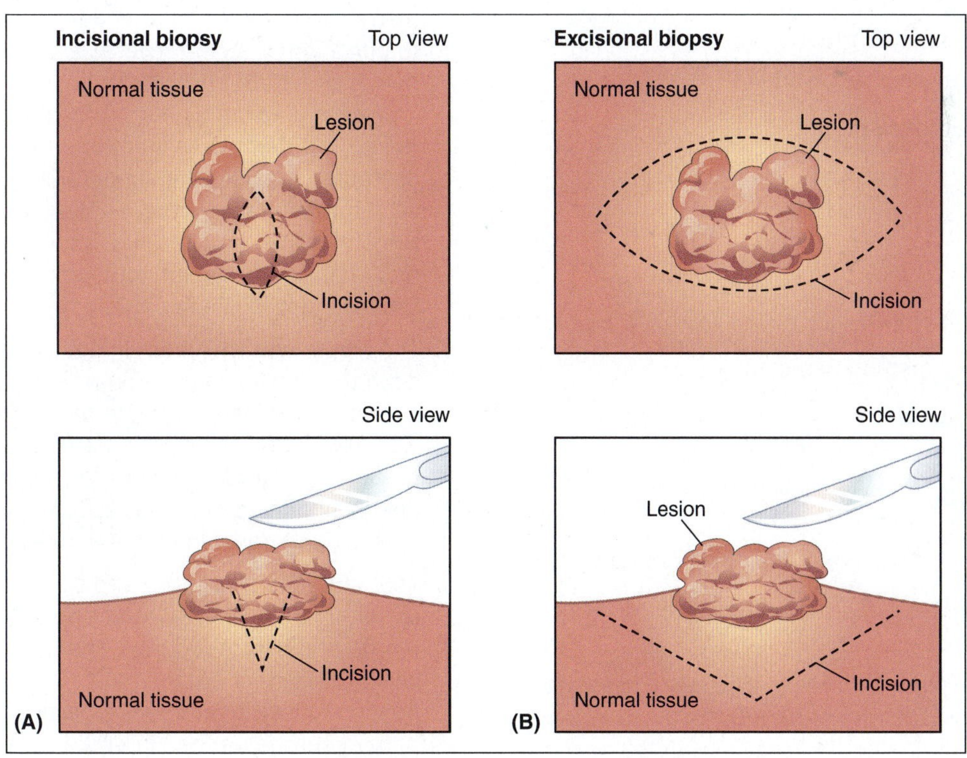

FIGURE 25-25
Biopsy techniques. (A) Incisional biopsy. (B) Excisional biopsy.

where total removal is more difficult and patient appearance and function are impaired.

The Excisional Biopsy. The **excisional biopsy** involves removal of the lesion completely, including a border of the normal tissue surrounding it (Figure 25-25B). The excisional biopsy is performed for smaller lesions, such as fibromas. Total removal of the lesions does not interfere with the patient's appearance or functioning.

The Exfoliative Cytology. The **exfoliative cytology**, or "smear biopsy," involves removal of a layer of cells from the surface of the lesion. This is a nonsurgical procedure in which the gathered cells are spread on a glass slab. This technique is used as an adjunct to the surgical biopsy techniques and is also performed by an oral surgeon.

One way this procedure is done in many dental offices is by using the **oral brush biopsy**. This technique involves using a small sterile brush to "wipe" the surface of the lesion firmly enough to remove the overlying keratin layer until pink tissue or pinpoint bleeding is evident. A kit available to dental offices contains everything needed to perform the biopsy and to prepare it for sending to the lab for computer-assisted analysis. These kits are used to test for dysplasia or cancer of oral lesions with abnormal epithelium (Figure 25-26).

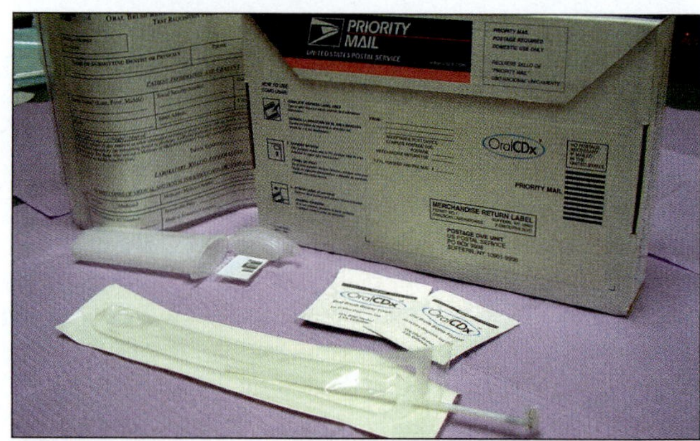

FIGURE 25-26
Oral CDX oral brush biopsy kit.

Procedure 25-5
Biopsy

This procedure is performed by the oral surgeon, who is assisted by the dental assistant. The dental assistant readies all materials that are sent to the laboratory as well as the tray setup.

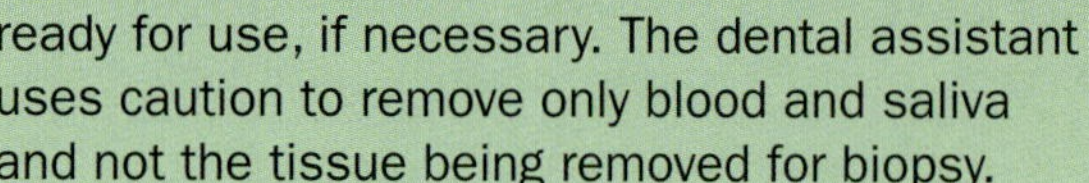

Equipment and Supplies

- Mouth mirror
- Local anesthetic setup
- Retractors (tongue, cheek, and tissue)
- Gauze sponges
- Surgical HVE tip
- Scalpel and blades
- Tissue scissors and hemostat
- Small container with a preservative solution, such as formalin
- Suture setup

Procedure Steps (*Follow aseptic procedures*)

1. The patient is anesthetized with local anesthetic.
2. A scalpel blade is used to incise or excise the lesion and a border of normal tissue. The dental assistant transfers the scalpel with the specific blade the surgeon prefers and has the HVE ready for use, if necessary. The dental assistant uses caution to remove only blood and saliva and not the tissue being removed for biopsy.
3. Tissue forceps are used to lift the biopsy specimen once freed from the underlying tissue and to place it in a small, covered container. The dental assistant retracts the cheeks and tongue, if needed, and uses gauze to control hemorrhage. The dental assistant has the specimen container ready for the surgeon. In order to prevent contamination, care is taken not to touch the outside of the specimen container. Once the tissue biopsy is placed in the container, the dental assistant replaces the cap tightly.
4. The biopsy site is closed with sutures. The surgeon then prepares the biopsy and the necessary information to be sent to the pathology laboratory. The dental assistant assists during the placement of sutures by transferring the suture needle and thread on needle forceps, retracting tissues, and transferring the suture scissors.
5. The patient is dismissed and scheduled for an appointment in 1 week for the results of the biopsy and suture removal. The dental assistant gives the patient postoperative instructions. The dental assistant gathers the pertinent information and prepares the biopsy container for pickup by the pathology laboratory.

Postoperative Care of the Patient

Following oral surgery, the patient is given postoperative home-care instructions. The instructions are given routinely by a dental assistant at the direction of the surgeon. The dental assistant gives the instructions verbally to the patient and the patient's escort. In addition, a written copy of the instructions with the office phone number is given to the patient, along with necessary prescriptions.

Postoperative Home-Care Instructions

It is important to carefully read and follow postoperative home-care instructions to prevent needless worry. Have someone with you for 24 hours following the surgery. Treatment continues until the healing process is completed.

What to expect:

1. **Discomfort** reaches a peak when the anesthetic wears off and sensation returns.
2. **Swelling** is normal following a surgical procedure. The swelling will continue up to 24 hours after surgery and can persist for 4 to 5 days. Facial discoloration may appear but will disappear in a day or so.
3. **Bleeding** or oozing may occur for the first 12 to 24 hours after surgery. The surgeon will place sterile gauze in the mouth to bite on immediately following surgery. Remove the gauze when the oozing has stopped.
4. **Difficulty opening mouth**, **a sore throat**, and **earaches** are not uncommon, especially if third molars were removed.

What to do:

1. Begin taking pain medication before the discomfort begins and the anesthetic wears off. Over-the-counter analgesics are suggested for minor discomfort, and the surgeon will prescribe a stronger medication for pain control, if necessary. Take medications as directed to avoid nausea and vomiting.
2. Use an ice pack to reduce the swelling as soon as possible. Apply the pack to the face over the extraction site for 20 minutes, and then remove for 20 minutes (20 minutes on, 20 minutes off). Continue this cycle intermittently throughout the first 12 to 24 hours. After 48 hours if the swelling has not subsided, use moist heat.
3. The best means to control bleeding is pressure. To accomplish the pressure needed, place folded gauze over the surgical site and bite down. Change the sterile gauze pads as needed. If the bleeding persists, insert a wet tea bag over the surgical site and bite down for about 20 minutes. Tea contains tannic acid, which assists in the clotting process.
4. A soft diet should be followed for 24 hours. Eat a well-balanced diet with soups, fruit juices, milk shakes, and other foods, as tolerated. Drink fluids to prevent dehydration and temperature elevation.
5. Take medications as directed to prevent infection.
6. Continue brushing and flossing areas not involved in surgery.
7. Sleep with the head elevated to reduce swelling.
8. Avoid vigorous physical exercise.
9. Rest as much as possible for the first couple of days following surgery to promote healing.

Things to avoid:

1. Avoid strenuous physical activity for 48 hours.
2. Do not suck through a straw and avoid spitting.
3. Do not smoke or chew gum.
4. Do not drive, drink alcohol, or operate machinery while taking pain medication.
5. If immediate dentures have been inserted, do not remove until your next appointment, usually within 24 hours of surgery.
6. Do not rinse vigorously for 48 hours after surgery. After this time, rinse gently with warm salt-water solution.

If you have any questions or problems, please call the office.

Dr.:______________ Telephone #:______________

Postsurgical Complications

The dental assistant should be aware of the possible complications that can arise after surgical procedures. Some of the most common include alveolitis and paresthesia.

Alveolitis

A condition called **alveolitis** (alveolar osteitis), or **dry socket**, is the most common complication following an extraction. The loss of blood clot leaves a dry socket, which is painful. Alveolitis usually develops between the third and the fifth day after surgery. In the normal process after an extraction, blood oozes into the socket and begins clotting. The clot is later replaced by connective tissue and eventually bone tissue. In some extractions, this process does not happen and the blood clot either does not form or forms and is lost. The exact etiology for this phenomenon is not clear, but insufficient blood supply to the area, infection, and trauma seem to play roles. The mandibular third molars seem to be the most frequent sites for dry socket.

The signs of dry socket are extreme pain, foul breath and taste, exposed bone, and an empty socket. Procedure 25-6 describes the treatment for alveolitis.

Paresthesia

Another postsurgical complication that sometimes occurs is **paresthesia** (see Chapter 20, Anesthesia and Sedation). In some procedures, such as hard tissue impactions, the teeth are close to the nerves. If the nerve is bruised or damaged during the surgical procedure the patient may experience numbness of the tongue, lip, or chin that may last a few days, weeks, months, or in extreme cases it may be permanent.

Procedure 25-6
Treatment for Alveolitis

This procedure is performed by the oral surgeon who is assisted by the dental assistant.

Equipment and Supplies (*Figure 25-27*)

- Local anesthetic setup (may be required)
- Mouth mirror
- Irrigating syringe and warm sterile saline solution
- Surgical HVE tip
- Surgical curettes
- Iodoform gauze or sponge material
- Cotton pliers
- Surgical scissors
- Mouth mirror
- Surgical HVE tip

Procedure Steps (*Follow aseptic procedures*)

1. Anesthetic may be administered. The sutures are removed.
2. The surgeon may gently curettage the area inside the socket to stimulate the formation of a new blood clot.
3. The alveolus (socket) is gently irrigated with the warm saline solution. The dental assistant prepares the syringe and maintains the area by retraction and evacuation.
4. The alveolus is gently packed with a medicated dressing. Narrow strips of iodoform gauze or iodoform sponge are used for packing the socket. The dental assistant prepares and transfers the materials to the surgeon for placement. In some states, such as California, a registered dental assistant can place post extraction dressings (Figure 25-28).
5. The surgeon prescribes medication for pain control, and the patient is scheduled to return in 1 to 2 days to repeat this process.

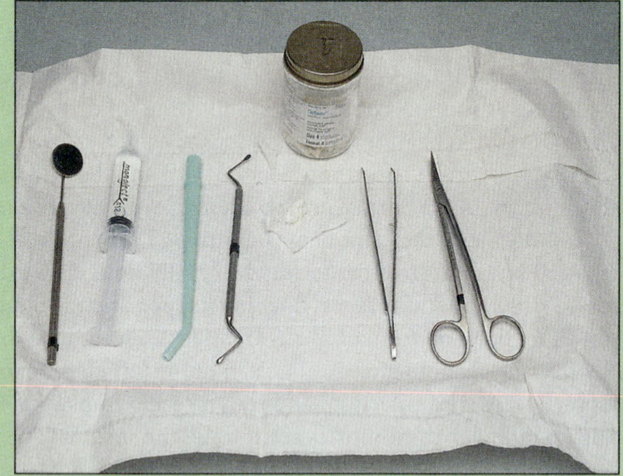

FIGURE 25-27
Tray setup for alveolitis treatment.

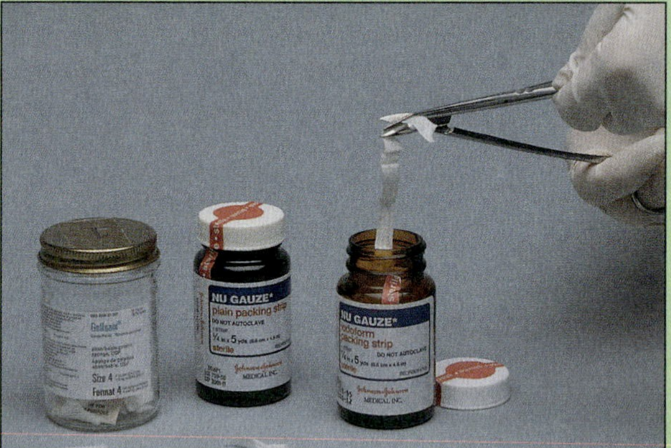

FIGURE 25-28
Examples of iodoform gauze and sponge packaging materials. The dental assistant prepares to pass the gauze packing.

Temporomandibular Joint Disease

The temporomandibular joint (TMJ) is made of muscles, bones, and joints of the jaw (refer to Chapter 7, Head and Neck Anatomy). These structures work closely together to make it possible to chew, speak, and swallow without discomfort. When these structures do not work together correctly, TMJ disease/dysfunction/disorder occurs. Other causes of TMJ problems include accidents, oral habits such as clenching or grinding the teeth (bruxism) (Figure 25-29), or diseases such as arthritis.

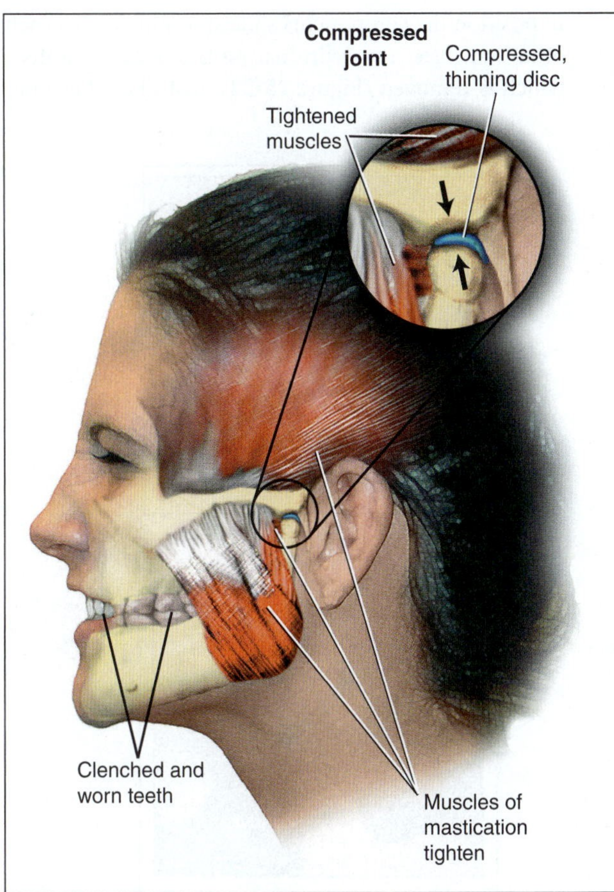

FIGURE 25-29
Clenched teeth and tightened muscles cause TMJ disc to compress.

Signs and Symptoms of TMJ Dysfunction

There are many signs and symptoms of TMJ disease/dysfunction/disorder. The most common are as follows:

- Pain around the ear, which often radiates into the face
- Tenderness of the masticatory muscles
- Popping and clicking noise when opening or closing the mouth
- **Crepitus** (crackling sound) or **tinnitus** (ringing or tinkling sound)
- Limited mandibular movement when opening
- **Trismus** (limited opening of the mouth)
- Headaches or neck aches

Diagnosing TMJ Dysfunction

Diagnosis is an important step in TMJ treatment. A medical and dental evaluation should be completed to ensure the appropriate treatment. Diagnostic procedures may include the following:

- Complete dental and medical history to gather information about the patient's symptoms, overall health, and family history. The patient may be asked about stress, teeth grinding or clenching, diseases that may affect joint function, bite problems, or any injuries to the joint area.
- Physical examination of the joint, including palpating (touching) the muscles and jaw, listening for sounds as the jaw opens and closes, and measuring how wide the patient can open the mouth.
- Tomographic radiographs and magnetic resonance imaging (MRI) may be taken (see Chapter 22, Production and Evaluation of Dental Radiographs; and Chapter 23, Extraoral and Digital Radiography).
- Dental study casts (models) of the teeth, which help the dentist evaluate the patient's bite and occlusion. The study casts may be articulated so jaw movements can be simulated.

Treatment Options for TMJ Dysfunction

Once the evaluation process is complete, the dentist will decide which type of treatment the patient needs. Often, treatment involves several phases. Sometimes, only minor treatment may be needed, but if discomfort and other symptoms continue, a more involved treatment may be required. If the patient is unresponsive to treatment options, surgery may be advised.

Noninvasive treatments for TMJ dysfunction include the following:

- Alternately applying ice and heat to the TMJ area.
- Learning to rest the jaw.
- Medication, such as pain reliever, muscle relaxant, antibiotics, and/or a nonsteroidal anti-inflammatory agent, or mood-elevator medications and/or anti-anxiety medication may be prescribed.
- Stress management, including relaxation techniques and biofeedback consultation.
- Physical therapy for jaw exercises, massage, good posture training, electrical stimulations, and ultrasound.
- Occlusal splint to relieve muscle spasms, balance the bite, relieve pressure on the joint, protect teeth from wear, and prevent grinding.
- Orthodontic treatment and restorative treatment may need to be completed.

Invasive treatments include the following:

- Surgery that involves the surgeon inserting a tiny instrument through a small incision to remove adhesions and place anti-inflammatory agents known as **arthroscopy**.
- The irrigation of the joint, known as **arthrocentesis**, is a minimally invasive procedure used to treat TMJ disease. With low risk and a high success rate, surgeons use this method before exploring more aggressive treatment options. Intravenous (IV) or general sedation is administered, and then the surgeon injects the joint with local anesthesia and fluid to flush out inflamed fluids around the joint. Steroids may also be injected to combat inflammation.

- Surgery to relieve pain and restore range of motion by realigning or reconstructing a joint, known as **arthroplasty**. This includes several types of surgeries for the TMJ:
  1. **Disc repositioning**—under general anesthetic the surgeon makes an incision and moves the displaced disc back to its original position and stitches it in place. Surrounding ligaments are also sometimes repaired (Figure 25-30).
  2. **Discectomy** is the surgical removal of the disc. When the disc has become deteriorated and damaged and is out of place or popping back and forth, this surgery is then performed as a last resort. The patient is given general anesthetic and the oral surgeon makes an incision and then removes the disc and some of the surrounding tissues, including the nerve tissue that may have caused the patient's pain. It may take a few weeks to several months for scar tissue to completely fill the joint and prevent bones from rubbing and grinding together.
  3. **Articular eminence recontouring** is performed when the articular eminence part of the joint is too steep or too deep and as a result too much pressure is put on the condyle. The surgeon shortens and smoothes the articular eminence to prevent or reduce the excessive forces and to improve the range of motion and lessen the pain (Figure 25-31).
  4. **TMJ replacement**—if a joint is badly damaged and cannot be repaired, it is removed and replaced. This is done only after other treatment options have been done and failed, or if this is the only course of treatment. Causes include severe degenerative disease, congenitally deformed TMJ, and advanced rheumatoid arthritis. Over the years these surgeries have become more common and the prosthetic TMJ joints have improved. The patient may need a partial joint replacement when only one component (disc, ball, or socket) of the TMJ is replaced. If the articular fossa no longer provides a smooth socket, a high-density polyethylene or metal liner is placed inside the joint to restore function and flexibility. If the end of the condyle is damaged and is not a ball shape, it is replaced with a prosthesis or bone from another part of the patient's body, such as the ribs. Total joint replacement is a procedure where both the ball and the socket are replaced with prostheses. Once in position the components slide smoothly across each other's surface, thus eliminating the need for a disc, which is removed (Figure 25-32). Just like other joint

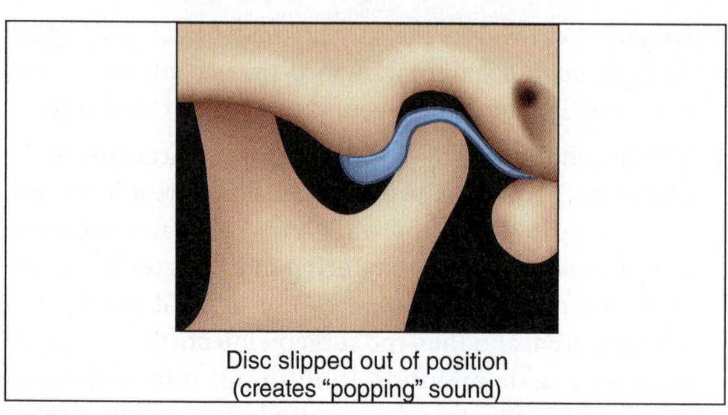

Disc slipped out of position
(creates "popping" sound)

FIGURE 25-30

Disc repositioning.

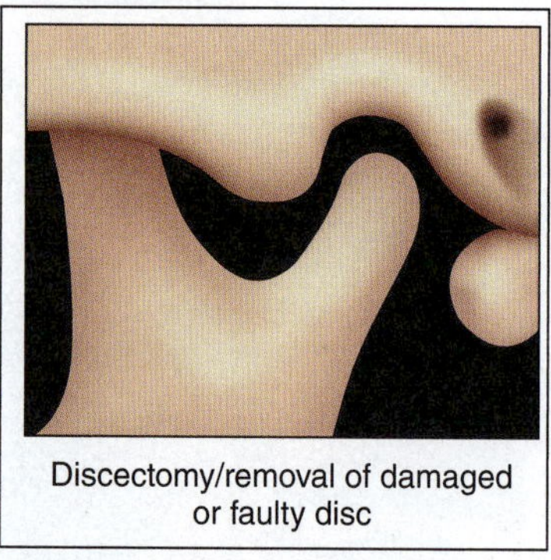

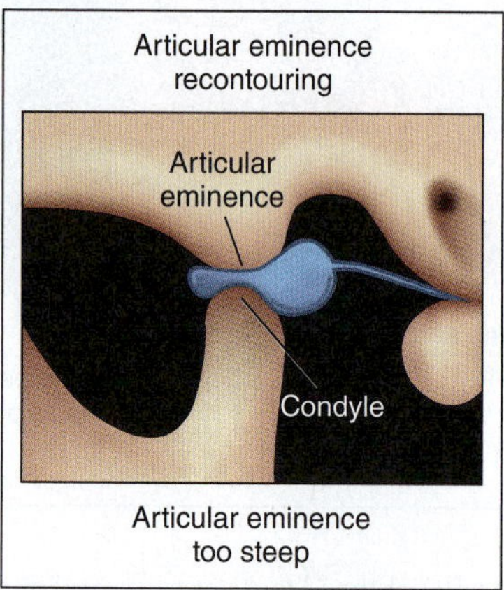

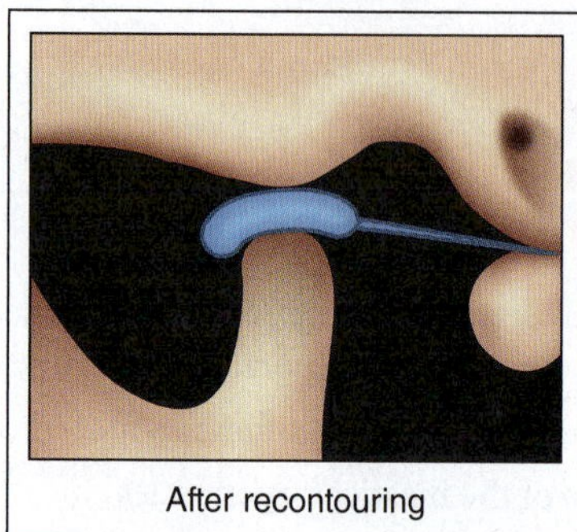

FIGURE 25-31

Articular eminence recontouring.

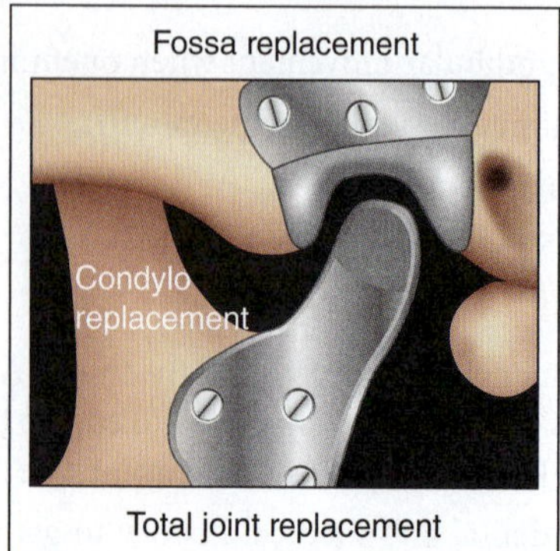

FIGURE 25-32

Temporomandibular joint replacement.

replacements (e.g., hip or knee) the patient will have some restrictions and need to make certain lifestyle and behavior changes to keep pain at a minimum and reduce the stress on the TMJ.

Hospital Dentistry

Most procedures are performed in the oral maxillofacial surgeon's office, but some cases require a hospital setting. The surgeon follows the protocol of the hospital to meet scheduling, staffing, and credentialing standards. Some hospitals allow dental assistants to assist oral surgeons, after the dental assistants meet hospital standards on asepsis and operating room protocol.

Patients who require hospitalization for dental treatment include:

- Trauma victims with facial and jaw fractures
- Patients with high-risk conditions or diseases (e.g., heart disease or diabetes)
- Patients with mental or physical disabilities who could not tolerate surgery in an office setting
- Patients who require extensive surgical procedures such as TMJ surgery or **orthognathic surgery** (surgery involving the relationships of the dental arches and/or the supporting bones of the face)

Orofacial Trauma Patients

The oral maxillofacial surgeon is called on for the treatment of orofacial trauma patients. The surgeon sees the patient in the hospital to begin treatment. At first the primary role of the surgeon is to manage any orofacial hemorrhaging, pain, and to prevent infection. With some patients treatment is given and they are sent home, however patients with major trauma are admitted to the hospital and prepared for surgery. Diagnosis is facilitated and enhanced with the advancing three-dimensional Cone Beam and CAD/CAM technologies. With this technology, the skull can be rotated and aligned to see the minutest details of the patient's anatomical structure. This allows surgical guides to be fabricated or robot-produced archwires to be placed. See Figures 25-33 and 25-34 for examples of photographs, x-rays, and skeletal views of two trauma patients and sequence of their treatment.

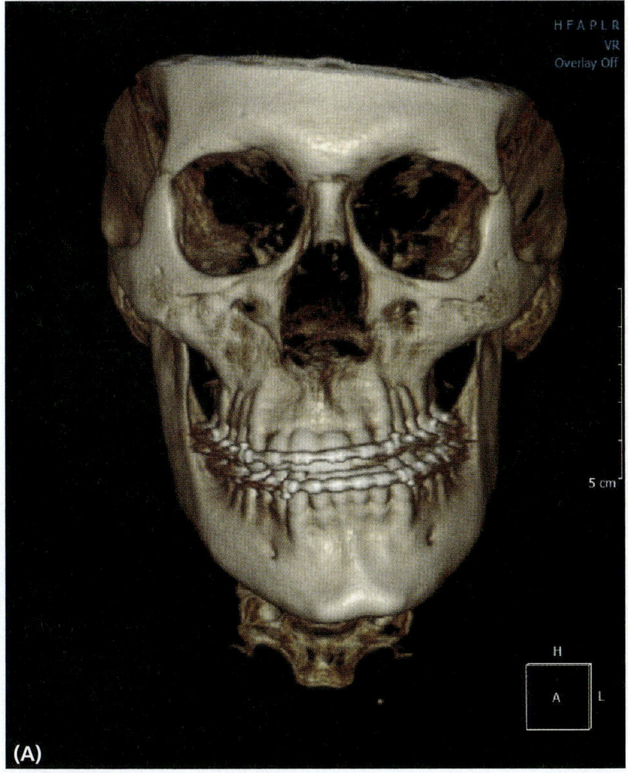

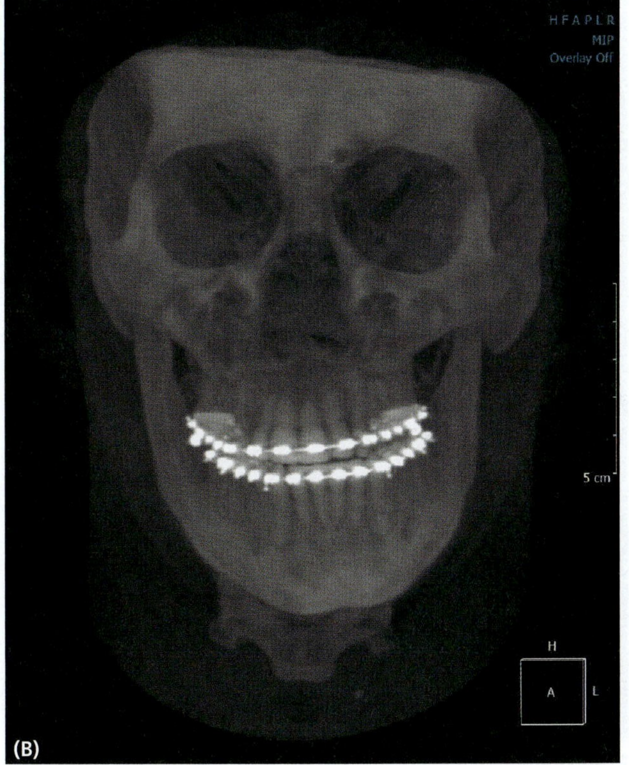

(A amd B) Courtesy of Imaging Sciences Inc.

FIGURE 25-33

Using enhanced technologies the oral surgeon has various types of views to show the before and after treatment of an orofacial trauma patient: (a) Front view showing the trauma that shifted the mandible. (B) X-ray view of the skull.

(continues)

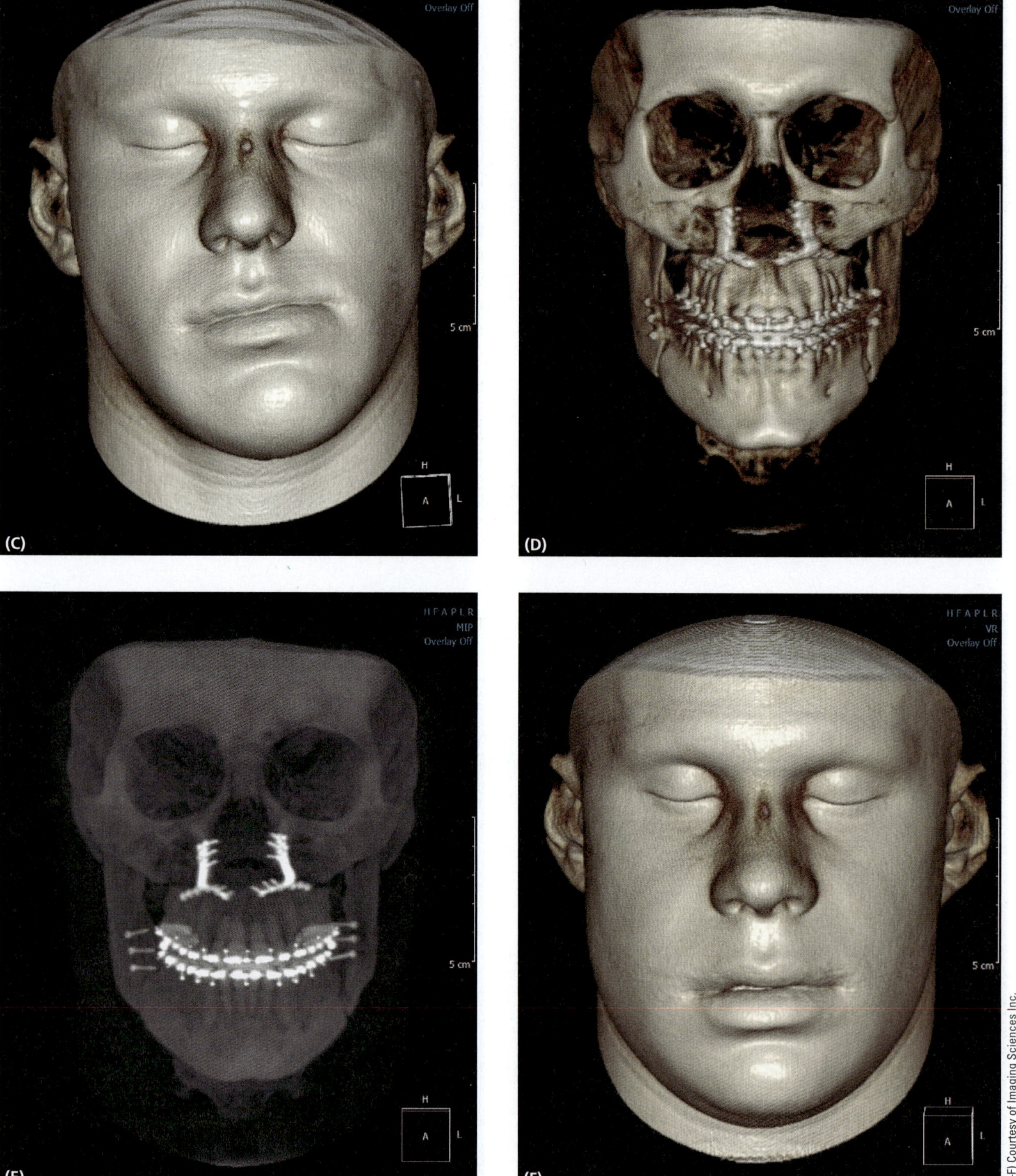

(C–F) Courtesy of Imaging Sciences Inc.

FIGURE 25-33 (continued)

(C) Photograph of a frontal view of the patient. (D) Front view showing the realignment of the maxilla and the mandible. (E) X-ray of patient after treatment. (F) Photograph of frontal view of patient after surgery.

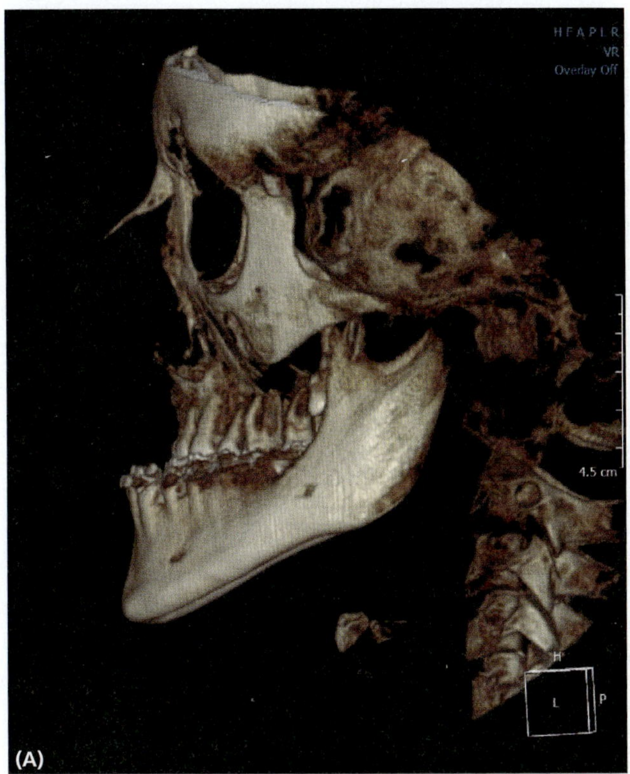

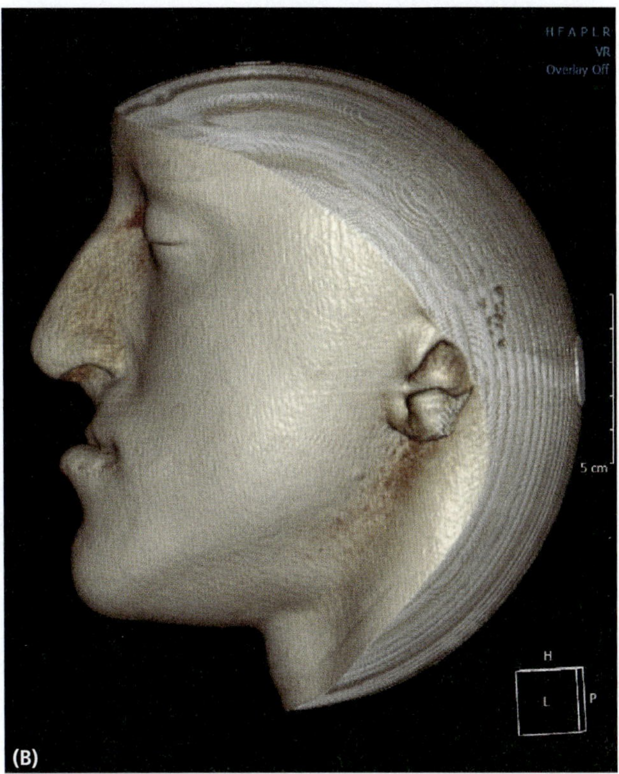

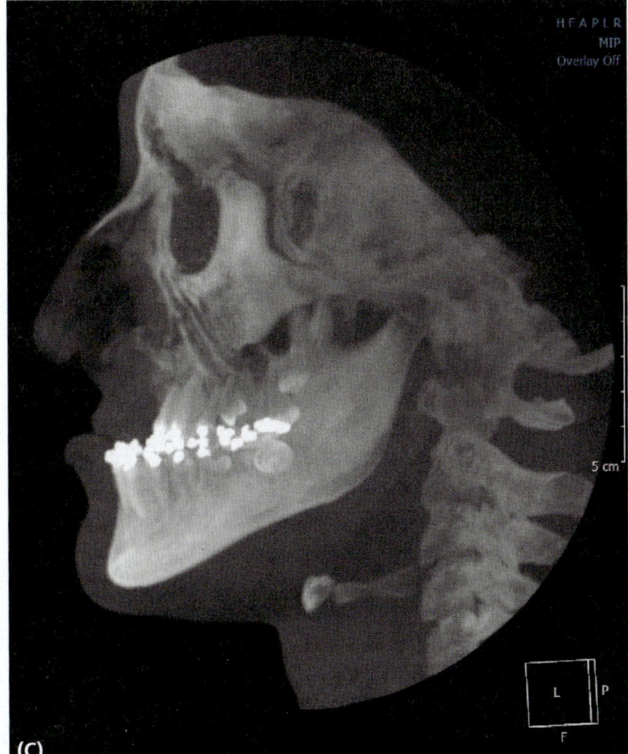

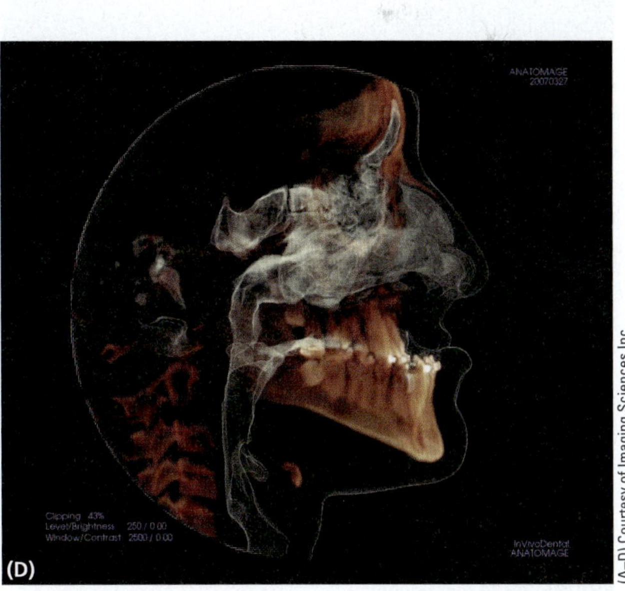

(A–D) Courtesy of Imaging Sciences Inc.

FIGURE 25-34

Advanced technology assists the oral surgeon by showing various types of views of before and after treatment of a patient in need of orofacial treatment due to trauma: (A) Lateral view of the skeleton showing the patient with a class III facial profile due to trauma. (B) Photograph of a profile view of the patient showing the collapsed maxilla. (C) X-ray of lateral view of the skull showing the trauma. (D) Enhanced view of the lateral view of the skull before surgery.

(continues)

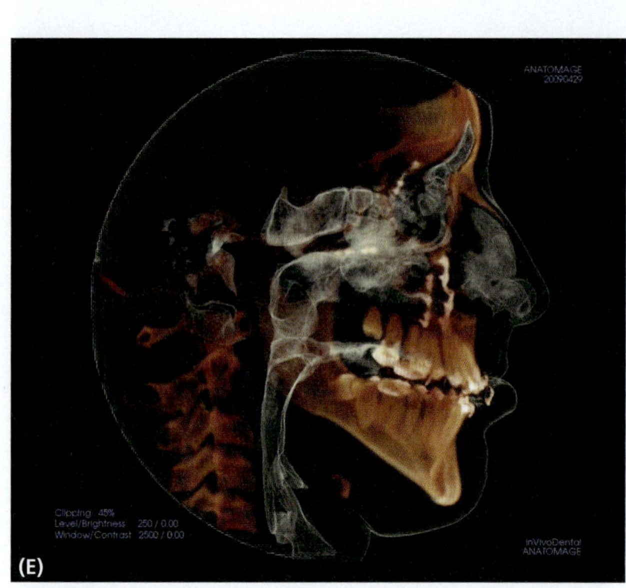

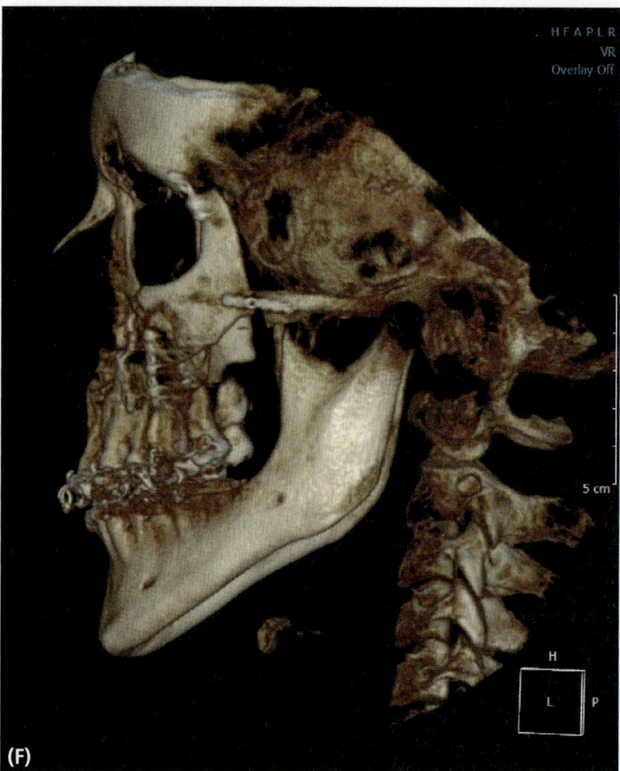

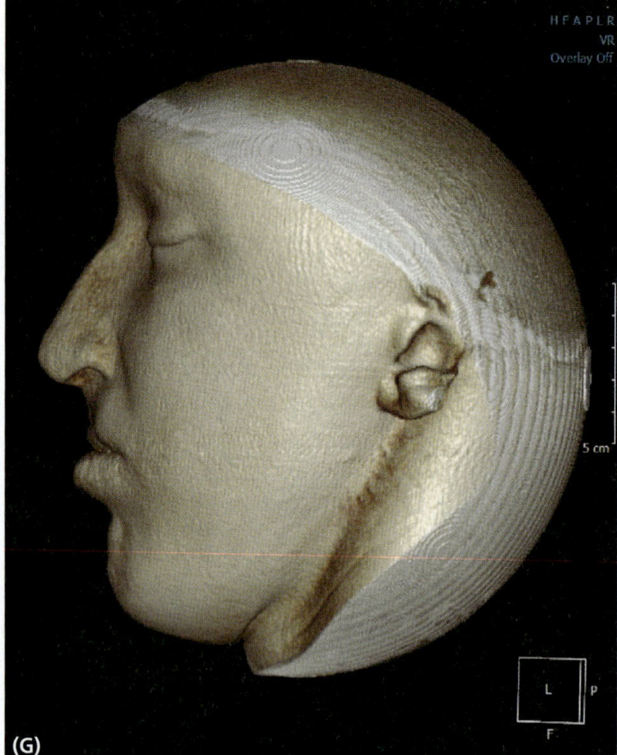

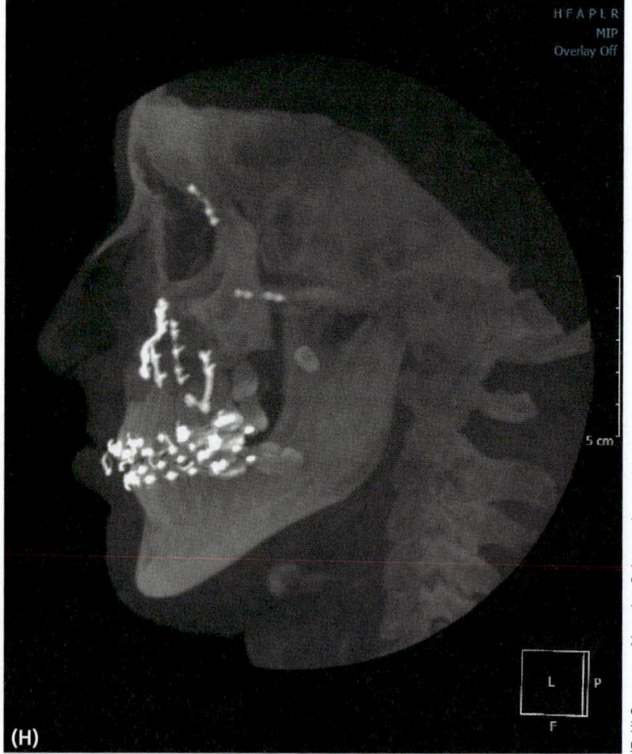

(E–H) Courtesy of Imaging Sciences Inc.

FIGURE 25-34 (continued)

(E) Enhanced view of the lateral view of the skull after treatment and the maxilla repositioned. (F) Lateral view of the skeleton showing patient positioned in a class I facial profile. (G) Photograph of profile view of the patient. (H) X-ray of the patient after surgery.

Advanced Chairside Functions

Suture Removal

Sutures hold displaced or incised tissue in its original position; they close the wound to promote healing and limit contamination by bacteria and food debris. The dental assistant assists the dentist in the placement of sutures and observes the type and number of sutures, and then records this information on the patient's chart for later reference. In 5 to 7 days, the patient returns to the office for the sutures to be removed. In some states, qualified dental assistants are allowed to remove the sutures under the supervision of the dentist. It is the responsibility of the dental assistant to gain the knowledge and the experience necessary to perform this task to the highest standard. The dentist must be aware of the patient's status and be notified immediately if diagnostic decisions are required.

Procedures Prior to Removal of Sutures

Prior to the suture removal, several steps and considerations are necessary to ensure patient comfort and safety. Included are preparing the equipment and supplies, reviewing the patient's chart, evaluating the suture site, and consulting with the dentist.

Prepare Suture Removal Equipment and Supplies. Before the patient's appointment, the tray is set up with the following items: mouth mirror, explorer, cotton pliers, suture scissors, gauze sponges, air–water syringe tip, and evacuator. This is a sterile procedure, so all aseptic guidelines are followed.

Review the Patient's Chart. Check the patient's chart for information concerning the sutures after the patient has been seated and before beginning the procedure. Ask the patient if any problems had occurred with the sutures since the last appointment.

Examine the Suture Site. Check the suture site for the following:

1. Location of the sutures
2. Number of sutures
3. Type or pattern of sutures
4. Healing of tissues in the wound area

Healing of the tissues depends on a number of factors, including the extent of the wound, the healing capabilities of the patient, whether a periodontal dressing was applied, and the amount of healing time. To evaluate the healing process, the dental assistant should **debride** (remove debris from) the suture site. Once the tissues have been cleaned, the suture site is evaluated for progress of healing and signs of infection. See Table 25-1 for descriptions of what to look for in the suture area.

Ways to Debride the Suture Site

1. Use light air and a warm water spray.
2. Use a cotton-tip applicator moistened with warm water or diluted hydrogen peroxide.
3. Use moist cotton gauze to gently dab the suture site.

Consult with the Dentist. The dental assistant should always consult with the dentist when removing sutures. After the patient has been seated, the dental assistant should check the healing of the suture site and identify the correct number of sutures to be removed. Consult with the dentist prior to suture removal for instructions, especially if there is anything unusual in the healing process or sutures cannot be located.

TABLE 25-1 Suture Site Healing Signs

Size of Wound	Appearance
Large area for flap or multiple extractions without a periodontal dressing	Area is slightly red with granulation tissue present, but no infection.
Large area for flap or multiple extractions with a periodontal dressing	Area appears slightly red with granulation tissue present. A milky film is seen where the dressing was placed.
Small area for minor surgery without a periodontal dressing placed	Area appears almost healed, with dark pink granulation tissue and no inflammation.
Any size of wound that is red and inflamed, tender, and has some bleeding	This wound is infected or irritated or has not had enough time to heal.

Advanced Chairside Functions (Continued)

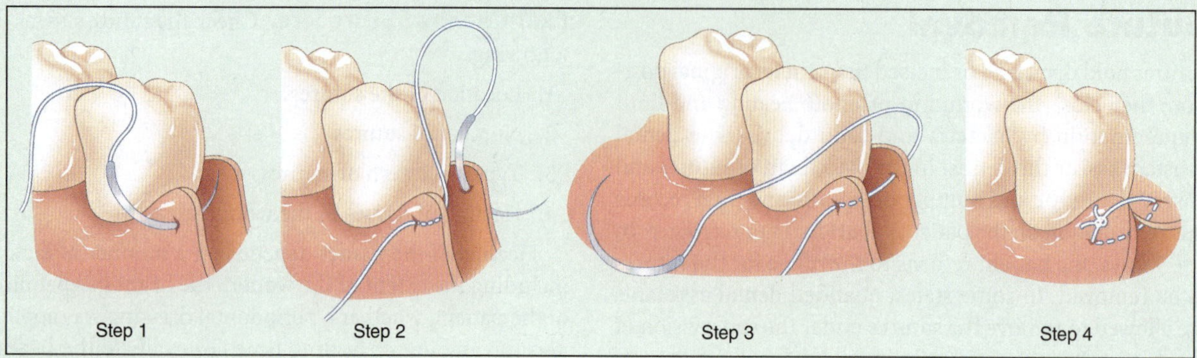

FIGURE 25-35
Simple suture pattern.

Types of Suture Patterns

To remove sutures, it is necessary to understand how the sutures are placed. There are several basic patterns, although dentists may vary their suturing techniques depending on the procedure and the patient. Detailed charting when the sutures are placed will help the dental assistant during suture removal. Most sutures are tied with simple square knots, referred to as surgeon's knots. The dental assistant should ask the dentist to place a variety of sutures in a tissue simulation, such as cotton rolls rolled into 2 × 2 inch gauze or dental dam material, to practice suture removal.

Simple Suture. The **simple suture** is the most widely used suture stitch, is very versatile, and is used in many areas of the mouth (see Figure 25-35 for steps the dentist follows to place the simple suture). Once the suture is placed, it is tied with a surgeon's knot.

Continuous Simple Suture. The **continuous simple suture** is placed when there have been multiple extractions (Figure 25-36). This series of sutures looks like hem stitching, with a surgeon's knot at either end. The number of stitches depends on the wound site.

Sling Suture. The **sling suture** is used for interproximal suturing (Figure 25-37). When a flap has been necessary, the sling suture is especially useful. An example of where a sling suture would be used is on the facial surface of the tissue. The suture needle and thread are inserted through the tissue on the facial surface (distal-facial of the tooth), and then the thread is wrapped around the lingual of the tooth, where the needle and thread are placed through the facial tissue on the opposite side of the tooth (mesial-facial). The thread is then wrapped back around the lingual of the tooth and a surgeon's knot is used to secure the suture.

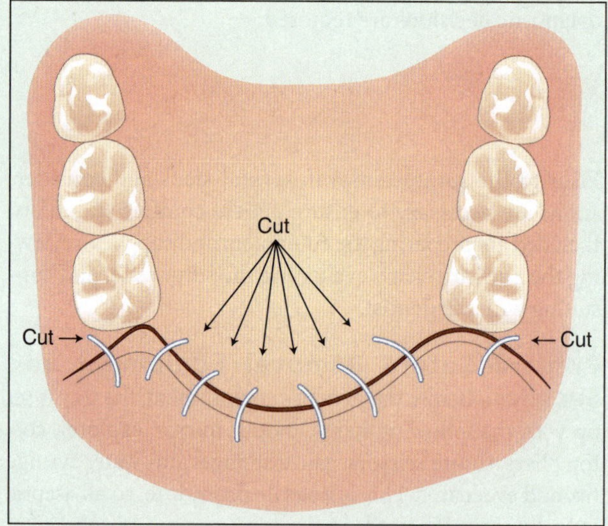

FIGURE 25-36
Continuous simple suture pattern with removable cuts.

Continuous Sling Suture. The **continuous sling suture** is placed where a large flap involving several teeth has been used (Figure 25-38). This suture involves the same steps as with the single sling, except the suture thread is wrapped around to the next tooth instead of back to the beginning side. When the tissue has been secured interproximally of each tooth involved, the suture is tied off (see Figures 25-38 and 25-39 for a continuous sling suture securing the facial tissue of several teeth).

Mattress Sutures. Mattress sutures also are used when a flap is to be sutured. The difference between the simple and the mattress sutures is that the simple suture goes into the facial surface and then emerges from the lingual surface, while the mattress sutures go in and out of the tissue on the same surface. For example, on the facial surface,

Advanced Chairside Functions

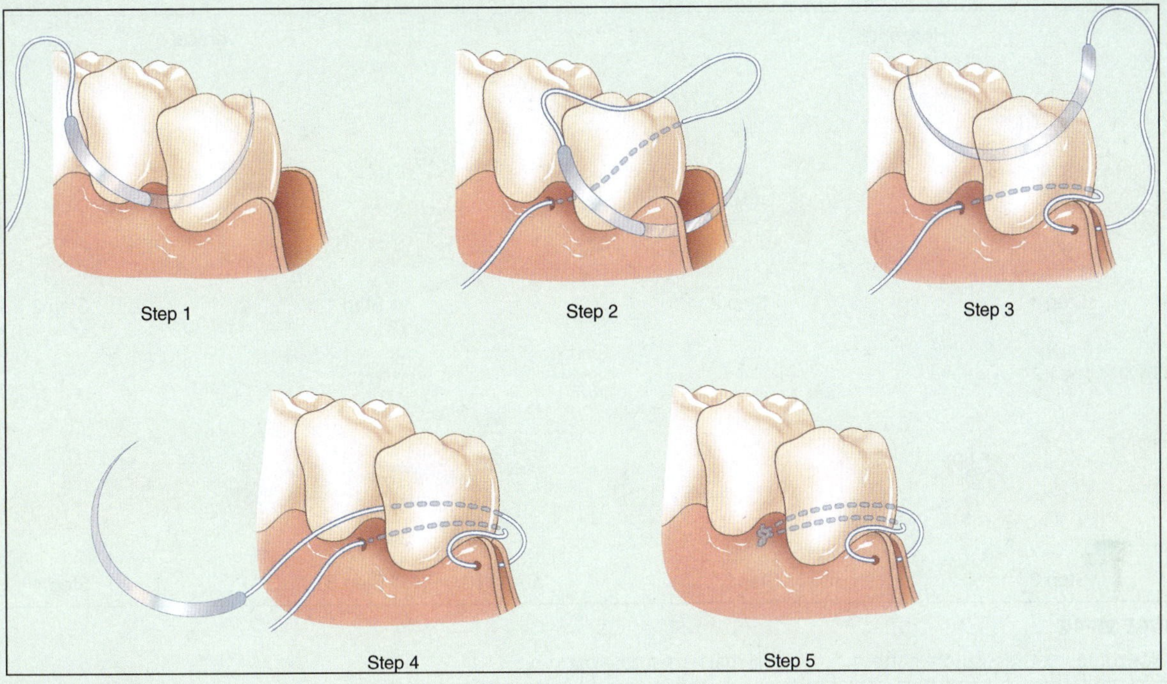

FIGURE 25-37
Sling suture pattern.

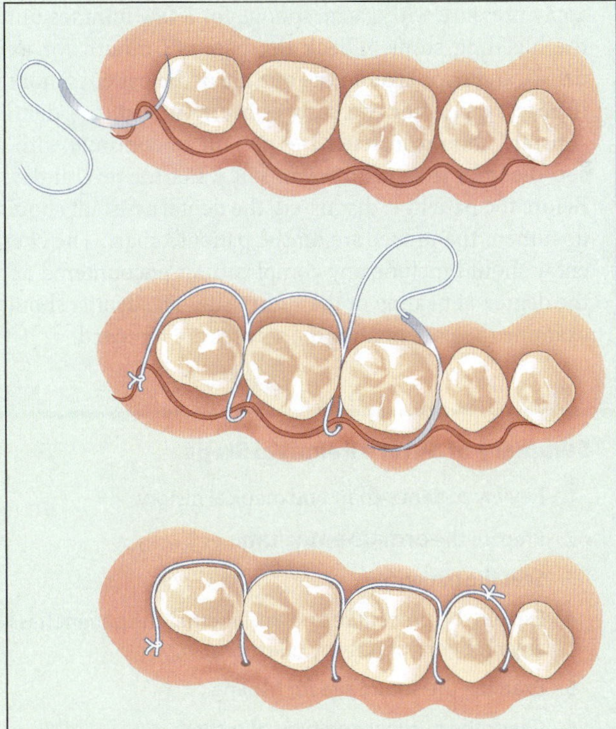

FIGURE 25-38
Continuous sling suture pattern.

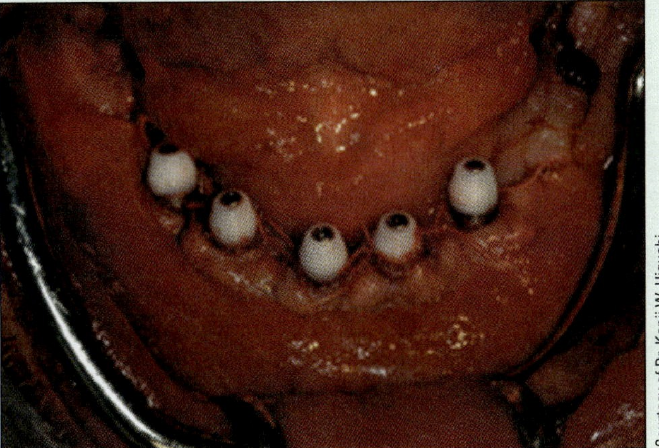

FIGURE 25-39
Patient with sutures in place.

the suture goes into and comes back out of the tissue on the same surface. If the stitch, or bite, is taken horizontally, it is a **horizontal mattress suture** (Figure 25-40A). If the stitch is taken vertically, it is a **vertical mattress suture** (Figure 25-40B). With the mattress sutures, the same stitch is taken on the facial and lingual. The mattress sutures are tied with one surgeon's knot on the surface where the suture procedure began.

Advanced Chairside Functions (Continued)

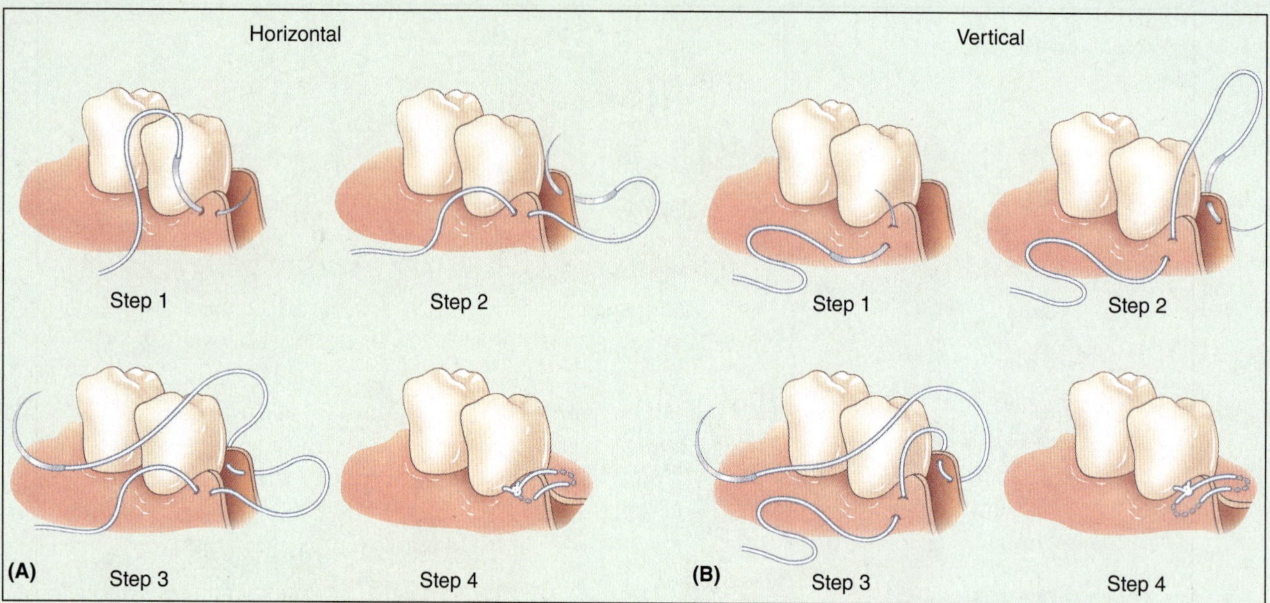

FIGURE 25-40
(A) Horizontal mattress suture pattern. (B) Vertical mattress suture pattern.

Suture Removal Criteria

The following are basic criteria to guide the dental assistant when removing sutures:

- Explain the procedure to the patient.
- The healing process should not be disturbed when removing the sutures.
- The suture is removed with the least amount of trauma to the tissues.
- All sutures are removed from the suture site.
- The knot is not cut.
- The suture is cut as closely to the tissue as possible.
- A suture that has been exposed in the mouth is not pulled through the tissue. (This suture is contaminated with saliva, food, and bacteria.)
- The knot is not pulled through the tissue.
- The hemorrhage is controlled following established procedures.
- The sutures are placed on a gauze so they can be counted.

Suture Removal

Each type of suture is placed in a specific pattern. To remove the sutures, identify the pattern and determine where the cuts are to be made. Then, follow the basic criteria and remove the sutures from the suture site. (See Procedures 25-7 through 25-9.)

Post-Suture Removal

If there was bleeding when the sutures were removed, apply pressure with gauze sponge for a few minutes until the bleeding stops. Check the patient's mouth for any debris, and wipe around the outside of the patient's mouth if necessary. After the sutures are removed, the dental assistant should instruct the patient to continue with a soft diet and rinse with warm salt water for several days. Before the patient is dismissed, the dental assistant should document the procedure on the patient's chart. The chart entry should include any complications encountered and the degree of healing of the suture site. The dentist should examine the patient after the sutures are removed.

Summary of Suture Removal Steps

1. Review patient's chart and medical history.
2. Prepare the **armamentarium**.
3. Seat the patient.
4. Explain the procedure and ask whether the patient has had any problems or has any questions.
5. Examine the suture site for healing.
6. Check the number and type of sutures.
7. Consult with the dentist.
8. Debride the suture site to prepare for suture removal.

Advanced Chairside Functions

9. Evaluate the sutures to determine where to make the cuts.
10. Gently secure and lift the sutures to position for cutting.
11. Using suture scissors or sharp, pointed surgical scissors, cut the sutures.
12. Remove the sutures and place on a gauze.
13. Blot the suture area if there is blood.
14. Count the sutures on the gauze.
15. Instruct the patient regarding care of the suture area.
16. Document the procedure on the patient's chart.
17. Call the dentist to check the patient.
18. Dismiss the patient.

Procedure 25-7
Removal of Simple Sutures and Continuous Simple Sutures

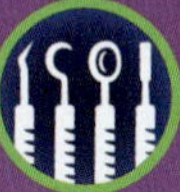

This procedure is performed by the dentist or the expanded-function dental assistant. The patient returns to the office for suture removal. The dental assistant prepares the materials needed and the patient before beginning the procedure.

Equipment and Supplies

- Basic setup: mouth mirror, explorer, and cotton pliers
- Suture scissors
- Hemostat
- Gauze sponges
- Air–water syringe tip, HVE tip

Procedure Steps (*Follow aseptic procedures*)

1. Using cotton pliers, gently lift the suture away from the tissues.
2. Take the suture scissors and cut the thread below the knot, close to the tissue.
3. Secure the knot with the cotton pliers and gently pull, lifting the suture out of the tissues.
4. Place the suture on a gauze sponge.
5. For continuous simple sutures, cut each suture and remove individually. Begin with one end and then proceed with each suture stitch.
6. Loosen the suture with the cotton pliers and, while still holding the suture thread with the cotton pliers, cut the thread close to the tissue (Figure 25-41).
7. As each suture is removed, place it on a gauze sponge so it can be counted when finished with the procedure.

Always carefully evaluate the sutures before cutting them to be sure sutures exposed in the oral cavity are not pulled through the tissue during removal.

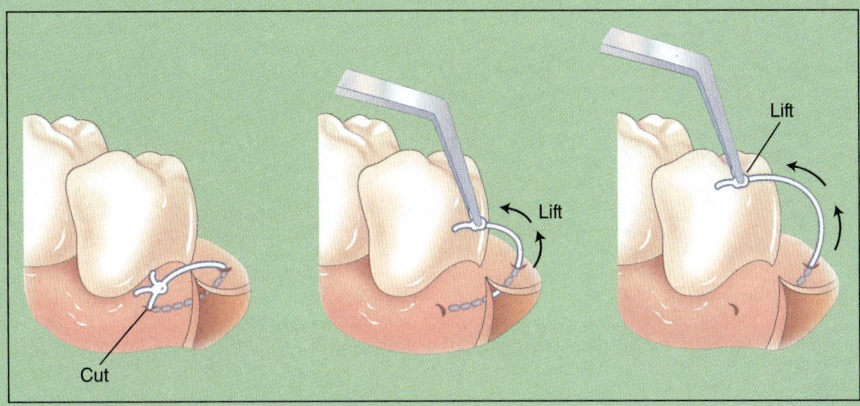

FIGURE 25-41
Removal of simple and continuous simple sutures.

Advanced Chairside Functions (Continued)

Procedure 25-8
Removal of Sling and Continuous Silng Sutures

This procedure is performed by the dentist or the expanded-function dental assistant. The patient returns to the office for suture removal. The dental assistant prepares the materials needed and the patient before beginning the procedure.

Procedure Steps (*Follow aseptic procedures*)

1. The sling suture is cut in two places. With cotton pliers, lift the suture gently on each side of the tooth to loosen the suture from the tissue (Figures 25-42A and B).

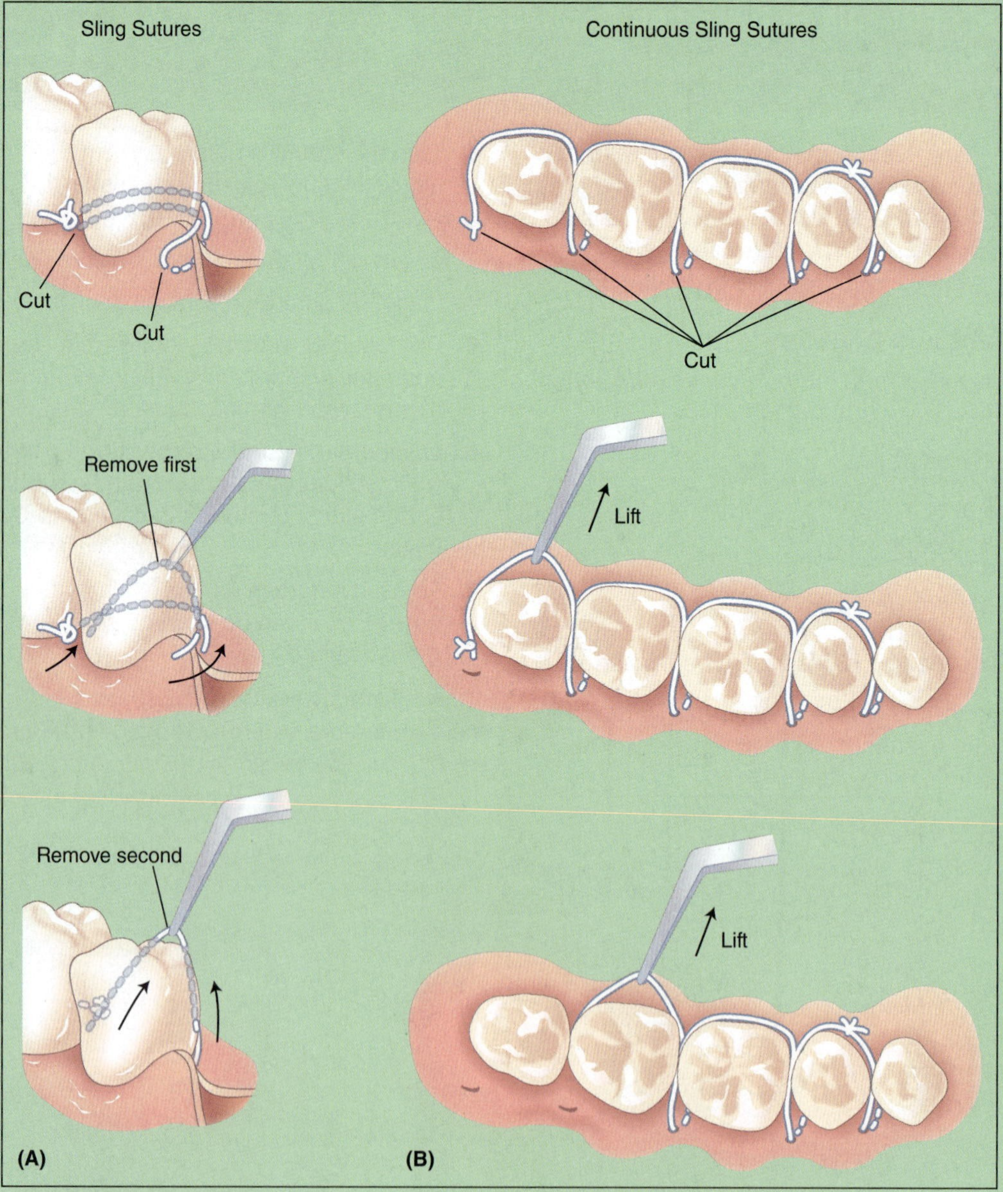

FIGURE 25-42
Removal of (A) sling sutures and (B) continuous sling sutures.

(continues)

Advanced Chairside Functions

Procedure 25-8 (continued)

2. Lift the knot gently and cut below the knot, near the tissue.
3. Lift the suture thread on the other side of the tooth, near the tissue, and cut it as close to the tissue as possible without cutting the tissue.

NOTE: When removing a continuous sling suture, this process is repeated, cutting on each side of the tooth until all sutures have been removed.

4. Using cotton pliers, remove each thread carefully, pulling toward the opposite surface, away from the flap. For example, if the suture is taken on the facial and wrapped around the lingual, pull toward the lingual to remove the sutures.
5. Place each thread of the suture on a gauze sponge to be counted.
6. Examine the suture site.

Procedure 25-9
Removal of Horizontal and Vertical Mattress Sutures

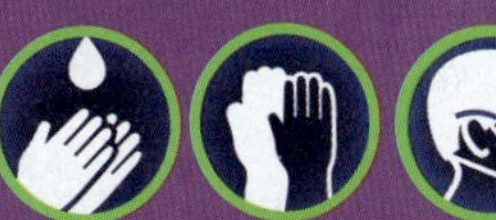

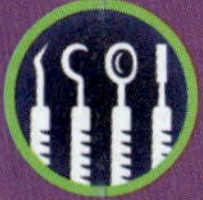

This procedure is performed by the dentist or the expanded-function dental assistant. The patient returns to the office for suture removal. The dental assistant prepares the materials needed and the patient before beginning the procedure.

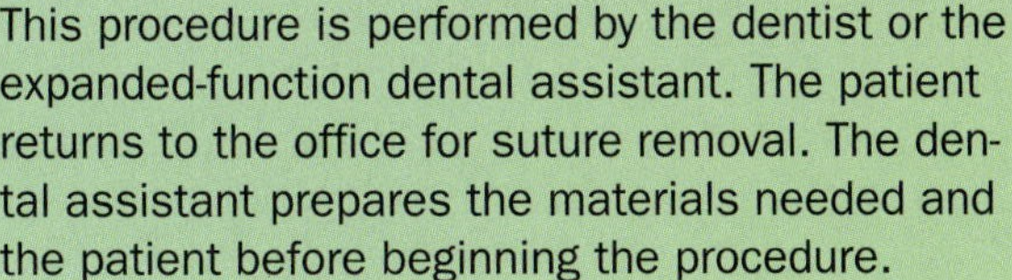

Procedure Steps (*Follow aseptic procedures*)

Although the horizontal and vertical mattress sutures are placed differently, the basic placement steps are the same. This also holds true for their removal. Two cuts are made with each mattress suture, one on each side of the suture stitch (see Figure 25-43A for the horizontal mattress and Figure 25-43B for the vertical mattress).

1. Gently lift the knot with cotton pliers.
2. Cut the suture below the knot, close to the tissue.
3. Make the second cut on the opposite surface, close to the tissue.
4. Remove one piece of the suture by holding the knot with the cotton pliers and lifting gently. Place it on a gauze sponge.
5. Remove the remaining suture thread.
6. Count pieces of the suture.
7. Examine the suture site.

(continues)

Advanced Chairside Functions (Continued)

Procedure 25-9 (continued)

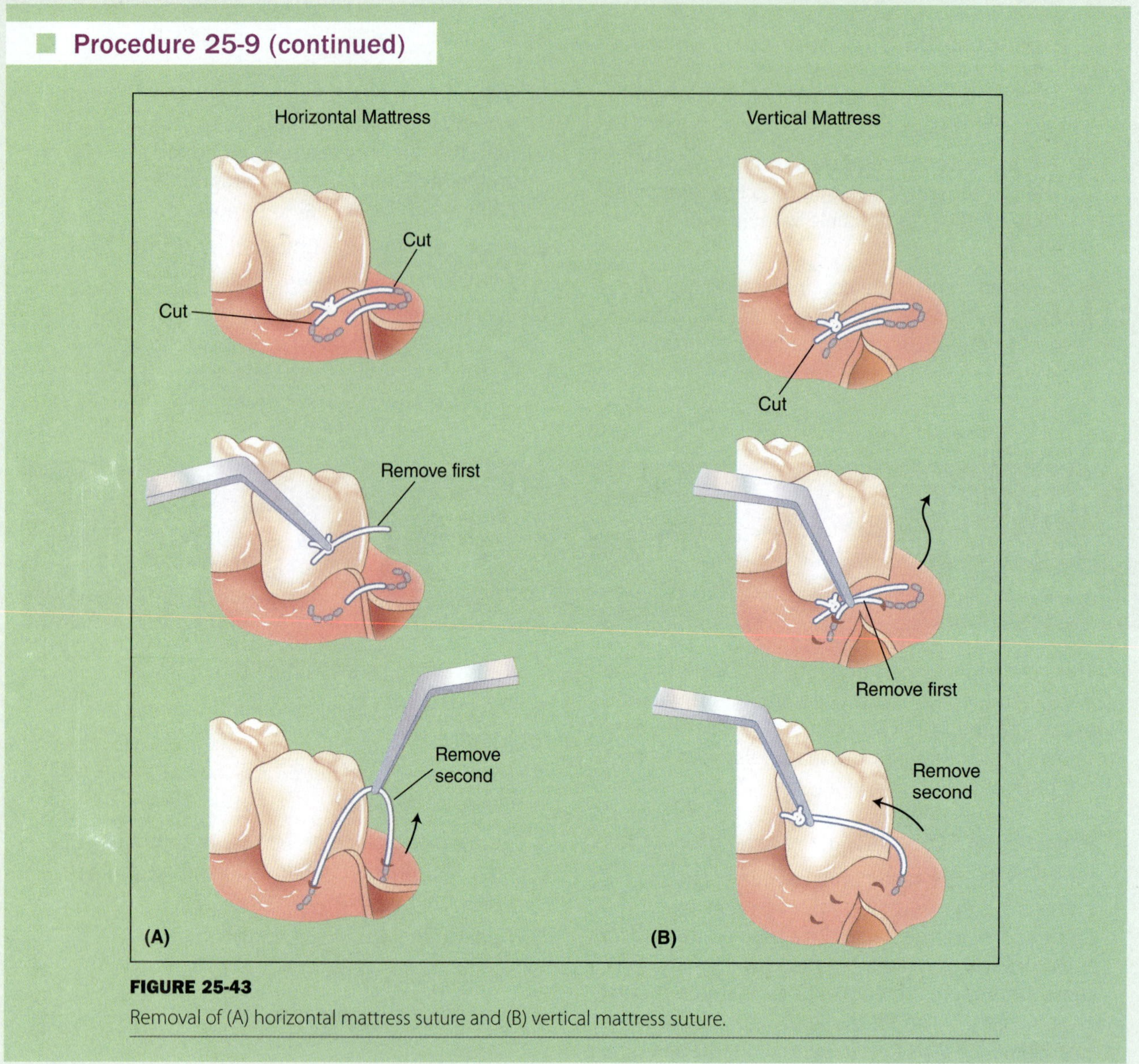

FIGURE 25-43

Removal of (A) horizontal mattress suture and (B) vertical mattress suture.

Chapter Summary

The dental surgery team may vary according to the surgeon's goals for the practice. In addition to the oral and maxillofacial surgeon, the team usually consists of the receptionist, the business office staff, the dental assistants, and, in some offices, a nurse or an anesthesiologist. The surgical dental assistant's responsibilities often vary depending on the size of the practice. Asepsis, patient preparation for oral surgery and postoperative care are discussed in this chapter. Instruments and equipment and the procedures used in oral surgery are explained. Suture removal, which is considered to be an expanded/advanced function is explained and demonstrated.

CASE STUDY

Josiah Scott, 45 years old, had his maxillary first molar removed a few years ago. The patient is experiencing no pain but has noticed that his teeth seem to be shifting. The adjacent teeth are rotating into the space left by the first molar, and the opposing first molar is supererupting. Mr. Scott is scheduled for an examination by Dr. Manwell, who is an oral surgeon.

Case Study Review

1. Why would Mr. Scott make an appointment with an oral surgeon?
2. Which procedure would correct Mr. Scott's problem?
3. What would the dental assistant need to prepare for the examination appointment?
4. Which other dental professionals would be involved in Mr. Scott's treatment?

Review Questions

Multiple Choice

1. Which of the following instruments is used to retract tissue, remove small root tips, and clamp off blood vessels?
   a. Needle holder
   b. Hemostat
   c. Tissue retractor
   d. Surgical curette
2. During surgical handwashing, the dental assistant scrubs with a scrub brush and then repeats the process with soap but without the scrub brush. This process is completed in
   a. 15 minutes.
   b. 10 minutes.
   c. 5 minutes.
   d. 1 minute.
3. Before the surgery is scheduled but after the patient's records and examination are completed, the patient must
   a. sign an informed consent.
   b. sign a waiver from the patient's general dentist.
   c. register with the oral surgeon's office.
   d. bring proof of identification to the oral surgeon's office.
4. An alveoplasty is
   a. a surgical procedure to remove teeth from the alveolar bone.
   b. a surgical procedure to remove impacted teeth from the alveolar bone.
   c. a surgical procedure to contour and smooth the alveolar bone after several teeth have been extracted.
   d. a surgical procedure to remove tissue from a suspicious area, either totally or partially, for microscopic examination and diagnosis.
5. The "rongeurs" are used in which of the following surgical procedures?
   a. Removal of impacted third molars
   b. Multiple extractions
   c. Alveoplasty
   d. All of the above
6. All of the following are included in postoperative home-care instructions *except*:
   a. Procedure for controlling swelling
   b. Patient is given a fluoride rinse
   c. Patient is given instructions to control bleeding
   d. Patient is given dietary guidelines
7. Which of the following biopsy techniques is nonsurgical and is used as an adjunct to the other surgical techniques?
   a. Incisional biopsy
   b. Excisional biopsy
   c. Exfoliative cytology
   d. None of the above
8. The diagnosing of TMJ dysfunction may include all of the following *except*:
   a. Full mouth set of radiograph will be taken
   b. Complete dental and medical history
   c. Tomographic radiographs and magnetic resonance imaging (MRI)
   d. Dental study case (models) of the teeth
9. The ________ pattern is placed where a large flap has been incised and several teeth are involved.
   a. simple suture
   b. sling suture
   c. continuous sling suture
   d. vertical mattress suture
10. When removing sutures, all of these statements are followed *except*:
    a. Do not cut the suture knot.
    b. Do not pull the suture thread that was exposed in the oral cavity through the tissues.
    c. Cut the suture thread away from the tissues as far as possible.
    d. As the sutures are removed, place them on gauze.

Critical Thinking

1. Why are the maxillary forceps designed for the left or the right quadrant and the mandibular forceps are not?
2. If a patient has had multiple extractions in preparation for a full denture, how long does the patient have to be without teeth? Does the patient have any options?

3. Explain the dental assistant's basic responsibilities during surgical procedures. Would these responsibilities ever change?
4. During a suture removal procedure, does the dentist need to examine the patient before the dental assistant removes the sutures? If so, explain the situations when the dentist would need to see the patient.
5. List several questions the dental assistant may ask the patient who is experiencing pain or discomfort in the temporomandibular joint (TMJ) area.
6. Discuss which patients might require hospitalization for dental treatment.

Web Activities

1. Visit http://www.VELscope.com and learn more about cancer screening techniques.
2. Find patient information on various oral maxillofacial treatments at http://aaoms.org.
3. Go to http://ada.org and look under *Public Resources* and then "Oral Health Topics" to find information about temporomandibular joint (TMJ) disease.

CHAPTER 26

Dental Implants

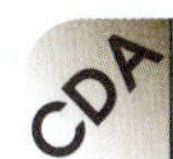

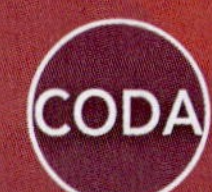

Specific Instructional Objectives

The student should strive to meet the following objectives and demonstrate an understanding of the facts and principles presented in this chapter:

1. Explain the considerations for dental implants, including patient preparedness.
2. List the indications and contraindications for dental implants.
3. List and describe the types of dental implants and explain the surgical procedures for placing the implants.
4. Describe the dental implant surgery and identify the instruments and equipment.
5. Explain the steps in the treatment sequence for dental implants.
6. Discuss postoperative homecare and maintenance for the patient with dental implants.

Key Terms

abutment post (627)
dental implant (626)
endosteal implants (628)
healing cap (627)
load (626)
mini dental implant (MDI) (629)
one-stage implant technique (626)
osseointegration (626)
subperiosteal implant (628)
surgical stent (626)
transosteal implant (630)
two-stage implant technique (627)

Introduction

Dental implants are one of the biggest advancements in dental treatment over the past 40 years. The insertion of dental implants provides a long-term option to the replacement of teeth with more traditional choices, such as bridges or partial dentures. Implants have become an effective and popular treatment for people who are missing teeth or who have lost a tooth or teeth due to advanced dental decay, periodontal disease, or injury. A **dental implant** is an artificial tooth root that is surgically placed within the alveolar bone. Once the implant is secure and stable it then holds the replacement crown, bridge, partial, or denture.

Dental Implants

Dental implants have a great success rate, with variances in success rates coming from where the implants are placed and what they do. For example, the anterior teeth success rate ranges from 90 percent to 100 percent, while the posterior teeth success rate ranges from 85 percent to 95 percent. Success also depends on the load that the implant carries; for example, with a denture the stress might be greater.

Implant failures are rare, and usually can be corrected. Reasons why implants may fail include the following:

- The soft and/or hard tissues may have infections or inflammation that did not heal.
- The implant fails to integrate.
- The implant fractures or breaks.
- There is damage to the nerve in the mandible.
- There is damage to the maxillary sinus or nasal cavity.

Dental implants often come in systems. These systems include various styles and sizes of implants, burs, instruments, and materials needed to measure and place the implants. See Figure 26-1 for models of dental implants and the parts of a dental implant. There are many different styles of implants used as prosthetic abutments, including a metal screw, cylinder, blade, or metal framework. These varieties of styles are used for many different anatomic and prosthodontic needs. Most often, the metal used to fabricate the dental implant is titanium because it is compatible with human tissue. The implant fuses with the bone tissue through a biologic bonding process. This process is called **osseointegration**. Osseointegration usually takes 3 to 6 months following surgery.

Once the implant has begun to integrate and become stable in the bone, a fixed or removable prosthesis is fabricated. The prosthesis (artificial part) may be a single crown, a bridge, a partial, or a denture (Figure 26-2).

Considerations for Dental Implants

Dental implants give the option for a fixed restoration or removable appliance that provides function and esthetics. For patients with little bone to support a denture or a partial, many times the stability of the dental implants restores the patient's confidence and comfort, and improves his or her social interactions.

Patients considering dental implants should be in reasonably good overall health, have an adequate jawbone that is healthy and strong, and have ample healing ability. A radiographic image, which includes a measure of the density of the jawbone, is evaluated to determine the quality and quantity of the jawbone, and where the implant will be placed. Sometimes patients require bone grafting to build up the bone in order to ensure a successful dental implant. See Chapter 31, Periodontics, for information on bone grafting.

The patient should also have a positive and cooperative attitude toward the implant treatment, be willing to follow all preoperative and postoperative recommendations, and be dedicated to the care of the implants once they are in place.

Treatment Sequence

The success of dental implants depends on a coordinated team approach (surgical and restorative), and good patient cooperation. At present, it can take 2 to 6 months to complete all phases of the dental implant process. The process begins with the patient meeting with the restorative dentist. After a preliminary consultation, the restorative dentist refers the patient to the oral surgeon or periodontist. Some general dentists take additional specialized training to be able to do dental implants in their office. A diagnostic consultation is scheduled. Included in this appointment are panoramic and cephalometric radiographs, a medical and dental history review, an oral examination, and study casts. Study casts may also be used to fabricate a **surgical stent**. This stent is placed over the tissues during surgery to guide the dentist in placing the implant. The stent is made of clear acrylic and is sometimes called a template (refer to Chapter 39, Laboratory Materials and Techniques). At this time, the patient must also consider the time commitment, the expense of the procedures, as implants are usually a little more expensive than traditional treatment, and the risks of a surgical procedure.

After the diagnosis is complete and the patient accepts the treatment plan, the necessary consent forms are completed by the patient, the financial arrangements are completed, and treatment appointments are scheduled.

There are several techniques used today to place dental implants. Often, one of the factors in selecting the technique is the amount of **load** the implant can tolerate and still be successful. The load is the amount of pressure or strain put on the implant once placed in the bone. Other factors include the dentist's preference and skill level.

There are usually two phases of treatment: surgical and restorative. The surgical phase can be accomplished with either a one-stage or a two-stage technique. The restorative phase is discussed in Chapter 33, Fixed Prosthodontics and Gingival Retraction and Chapter 36, Removable Prosthodontics.

In the **one-stage implant technique**, the implant is inserted into the bone, but the extruding end is not covered with gingival tissue. The implant protrudes through

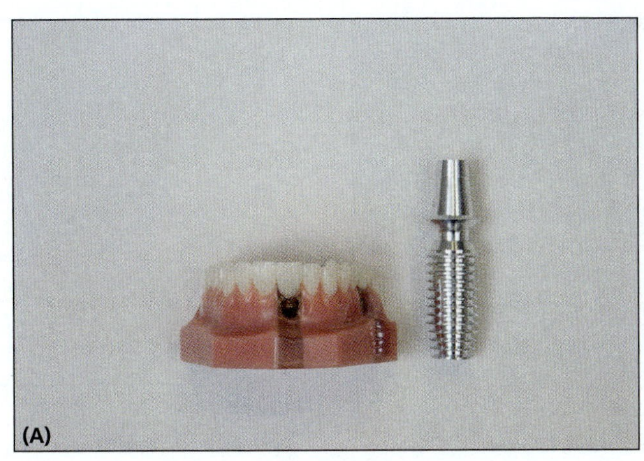

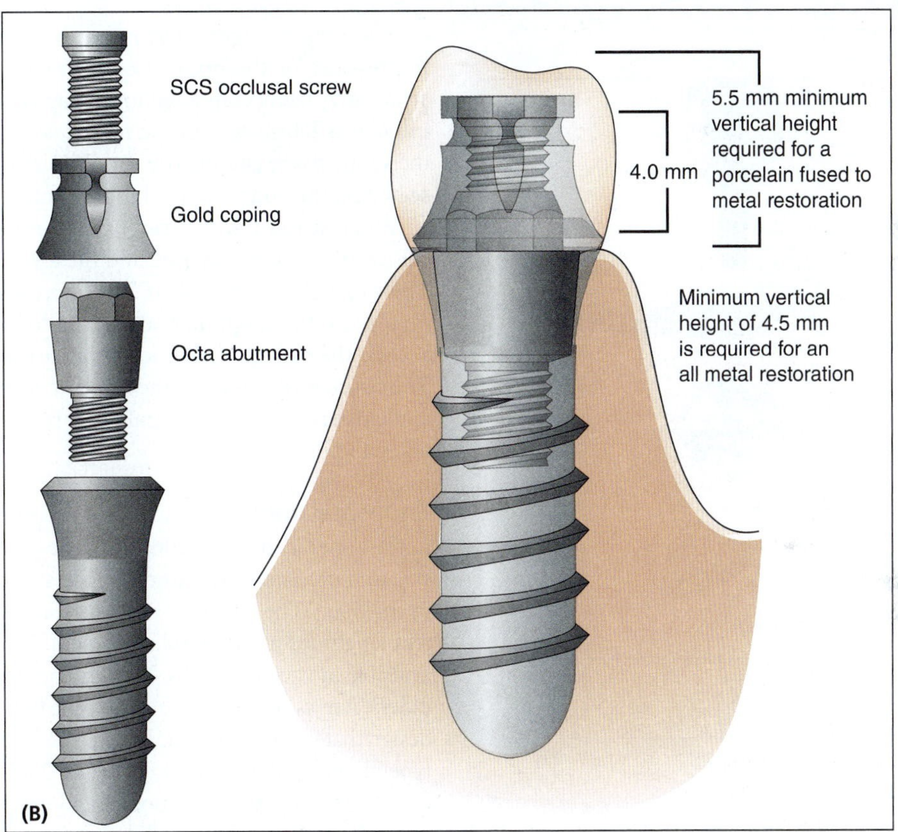

FIGURE 26-1

(A) Actual implant and model of the implant used to educate patients. (B) Components of the dental implant.

the tissue and a healing cap is placed. The **healing cap** is a metal cap or screw that fits on the dental implant and keeps tissue and debris from getting into the implant (Figure 26-3). When the healing cap is removed the **abutment post** is placed. The abutment post is screwed into the implant, and will later attach to the artificial tooth or denture. There is no load on this implant during the healing time. The healing time is 3 to 4 months, during which the osseointegration process takes place.

In the **two-stage implant technique**, the implant is placed into the bone and gingival tissue is sutured into place to cover the implant. Sutures are removed in 7 to 10 days. If there is an old prosthesis (denture), it can be modified or relined by the restorative dentist so that the patient will not be without teeth during the 3 to 4 months of healing time. After the healing time, a second surgery is scheduled. During this surgery the implant is uncovered and checked for stability. If the implant is stable, a cap or abutment is placed. The cap protrudes out of the tissue. Once the soft tissues have healed, the crown, bridge, or other prosthesis can be fabricated and placed by the general or prosthetic dentist.

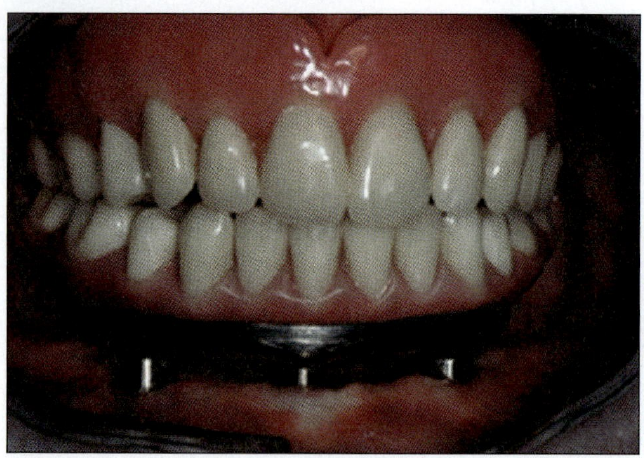

FIGURE 26-2
Subperiosteal implants in place.

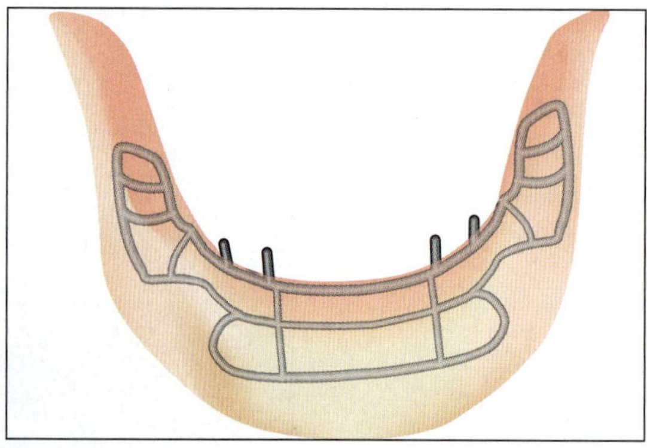

FIGURE 26-4
Subperiosteal implant.

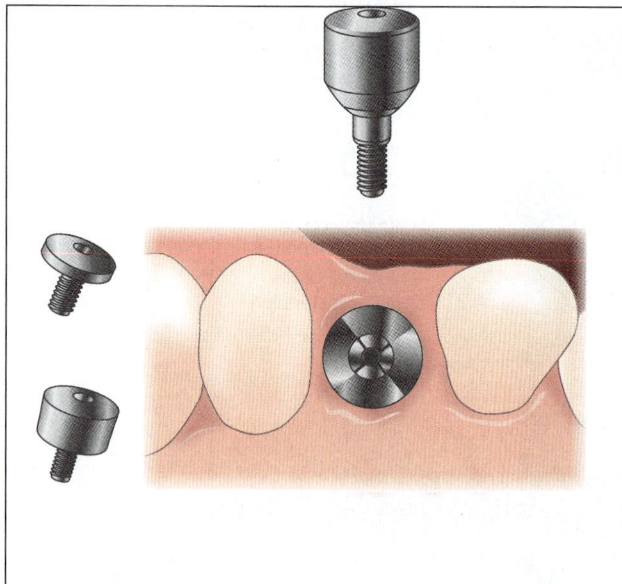

FIGURE 26-3
Healing cap on the dental implant.

Types of Implants

The two most common types of dental implants include the subperiosteal and endosteal. A third type of implant, called a mini dental implant (MDI), is also becoming very popular. A fourth type of implant is the transosteal, which is not used very often.

Subperiosteal Implant. The **subperiosteal implant** is often used on patients whose dentures have failed because the alveolar bone has atrophied (wasted away). Subperiosteal implants are most commonly placed on the mandible. The titanium implant rests on top of the alveolar bone with abutment posts or bars above the mucoperiosteum in the cuspid and first molar area. The denture connects to this structure for support and retention (Figure 26-4). The subperiosteal implant requires one or two surgeries, depending on the technique.

The *single-surgery technique* involves fabricating the impression for the implant on a model. The model is constructed by using computed tomography (CT) scans. After the implant is fabricated on the model, surgery is performed to incise the tissue and expose the alveolar bone. The implant is seated on the bone and the tissue is sutured back into place.

When using the *two-surgery technique*, during the first surgery the tissue is incised and the alveolar bone is exposed. Then an impression is taken. The impression is sent to the laboratory for the subperiosteal implant to be fabricated. Within a week, the patient returns to the office for the second surgery. The tissue is opened and the implant is seated. A transitional appliance is used while a final denture is made, which usually takes 4 to 6 weeks.

Endosteal Implant. The **endosteal implant** (endosseous, or in the bone) is the most common type of implant placed. With skill and precision these implants are surgically placed directly in the bone. The jaw bone must be sufficient in height, width, and length for a successful placement. Endosteal implants are available in various widths, lengths, and designs, including cylinders, screws, and combinations of the two. There is also a blade design that is used when the bone is too thin to support a screw-type implant without grafting (Figure 26-5). The implants may be used in any area of the mouth, and may replace one or more teeth. After the implant is placed the jawbone attaches itself to the dental implant during the osseointegration state, which lasts anywhere from 3 to 8 months. Once this stage is complete, the crown can be fabricated to be placed on the dental implant.

There are one-, two-, and three-piece systems for endosteal implants that have been approved by the American Dental Association. The components of endosteal implants include: the titanium implant, which is surgically placed in the alveolar bone; the abutment screw, which is placed in the implant once osseointegration has taken place; and the abutment post or cylinder, which is the part of the implant that attaches to the prostheses (refer to Figure 26-1).

The techniques for endosteal implants include either a one- or two-stage insertion (see Procedure 26-1). The endosteal implants are consistent, and take into consideration the bone and soft tissues. Hundreds of thousands of implants have been placed, and the techniques and materials continually advance.

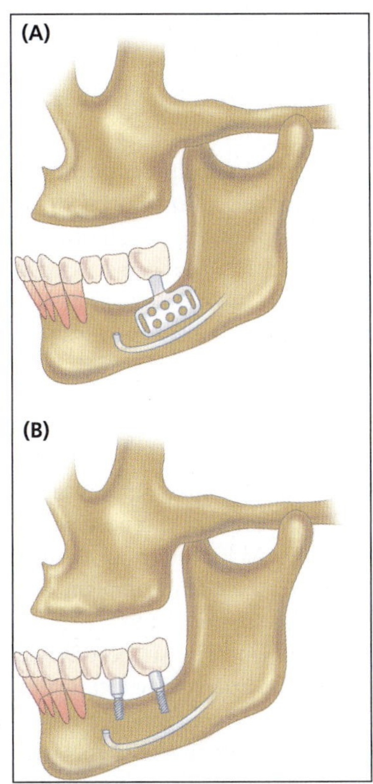

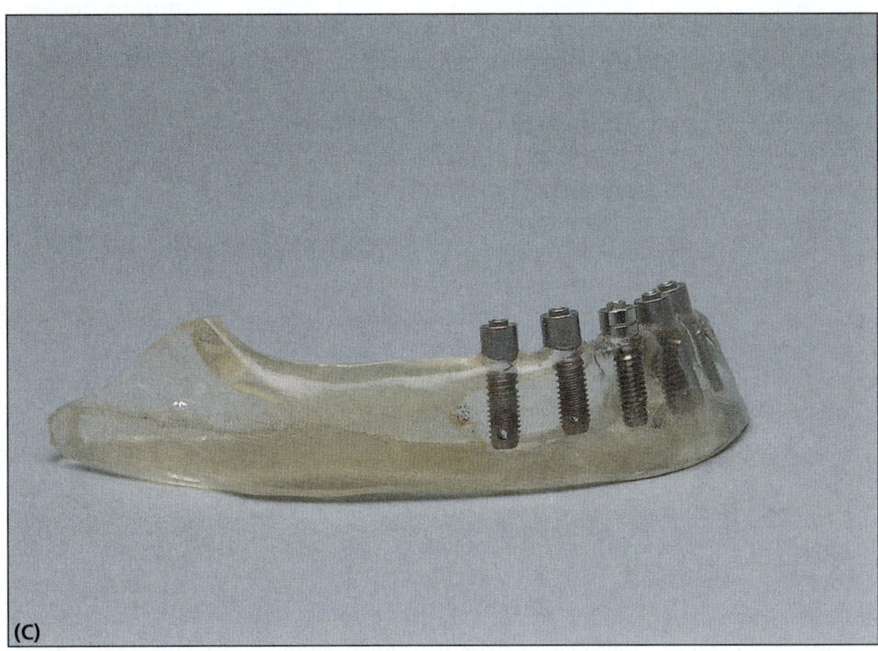

FIGURE 26-5
Sample of endosteal implants. (A) The blade implant. (B) The screw or cylinder implant. (C) A model showing the screw or cylinder implant.

Mini Dental Implants. The **mini dental implant (MDI)** is smaller in diameter (less than 3 mm) and narrower than other dental implants. It is made of biocompatible titanium alloy and can be placed directly through the mucosal tissue and into the bone. The MDIs are used for fixation of full and partial dentures, especially in the mandible; crowns in small spaces; and for retention in orthodontic procedures.

MDIs consist of various designed heads, a threaded body with various styled tips that are sharp or slightly blunted, and the metal housing (Figure 26-6). In some cases, an O-ring is placed between the MDI and the metal housing. These O-rings can be changed to keep the original retention of the full or partial denture.

Some of the benefits of MDIs include the following:

- A minimally invasive procedure
- Can be used immediately
- Less time for the procedure than traditional dental implants
- Lower cost for the patient
- Designed for stability in both soft and dense bone
- Available training programs for MDI technology

With the procedure for placing the MDIs, the dentist does not incise the tissue and lay a flap; instead, the dentist uses specially designed burs, and drills a small pilot hole through the tissue and into the bone. The dentist places the MDI in the pilot hole, and then uses a handheld driving device and a torque wrench to seat the implant. Post insertion pain and irritation are much less than with standard dental implants.

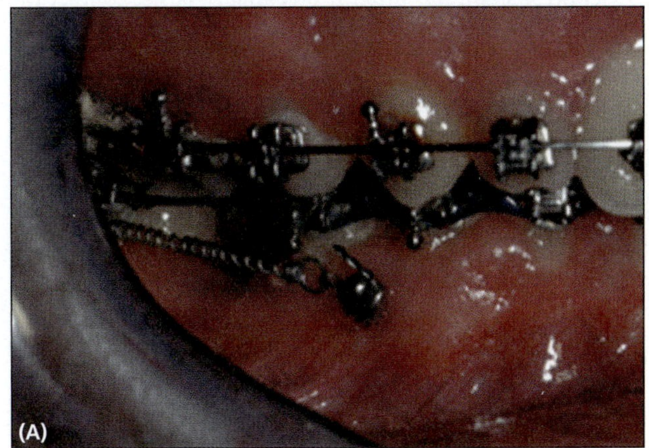

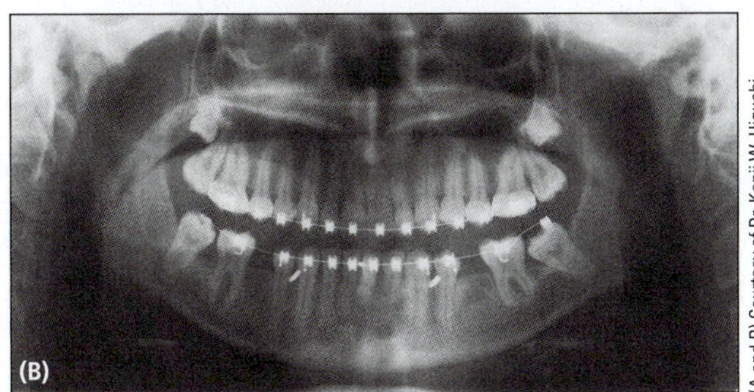

(A and B) Courtesy of Dr. Kenji W. Higuchi

FIGURE 26-6
(A) The mini dental implant (MDI) placed during orthodontic treatment. (B) Panoramic radiograph showing the mini implants in place.

MDIs systems are successfully used for retention in specific cases, but are not designed to replace osseointegrated dental implants.

Transosteal Implant. The **transosteal implant** is used in an edentulous area of the mandible, and passes through the cortical plate and the alveolar bone. Usually this type of implant is only used with patients who have severely resorbed alveolar ridges that will not support the other types of implants. These implants are also known as *staple* or *transosseous implants*. They consist of screws, nuts, and a pressure plate. The screws are inserted through the bone, penetrating the entire jaw and attaching at the bottom to the pressure plate. The denture is secured to the screws that protrude through the gingival tissue (Figure 26-7). These implants are also made of titanium and will fuse to the bone through osseointegration.

Postoperative Care and Home Care Instructions

After implant surgery, the patient should follow these postoperative care instructions:

1. Only clear liquids should be taken during the first 2 days after surgery. Milk may be taken with medication. Blended/mashed food may be added after the second day. Smoking and alcoholic beverages should be avoided.
2. Softly biting on a gauze pad for 15 to 30 minutes may control slight bleeding. If bleeding persists, contact the office.
3. Use extra pillows to elevate the head slightly during the first two nights after surgery.
4. Gently rinse the mouth with saline solution after each meal. Use no commercial mouth rinses.
5. Take daily requirements of vitamin C, D, B complex, and calcium.
6. If there are any questions or concerns about the healing process, contact the office.

Once the second surgery is completed, the exposed portion of the dental implant must be kept clean. The patient must perform daily hygiene maintenance on the implant and prosthesis. The instruments and techniques for implant hygiene are discussed in Chapter 33, Fixed Prosthodontics and Gingival Retraction. The patient should also have routine dental examinations to evaluate the implants along with the rest of the mouth.

Dental Implant Maintenance

Dental implants require maintenance just like natural teeth. Plaque and calculus builds up on the implant and needs to be removed routinely. The patient should be informed of their role and responsibility in maintaining their dental implant, and should be scheduled for continuous support and care of the peri-implant tissues as well as the implant. This support should include a clinical assessment of the condition of the soft tissues, a plaque index, depth and bleeding on probing, and a check of mobility and occlusion. Radiographs are also often taken. Some patients are at a higher risk for peri-implantitis (inflammation of the tissues surrounding the implant) due to chronic periodontitis, diabetes, poor oral hygiene, or smoking. The patient should be advised of the aids available, and a homecare regimen should be recommended. The toothbrushes selected, either automatic or manual, should be a soft, multitufted nylon brush. There are also numerous aids for use as adjuncts to the toothbrush, including:

- Threading systems
- Dental floss, including dental implant floss
- Interproximal brushes, end-tufted brushes

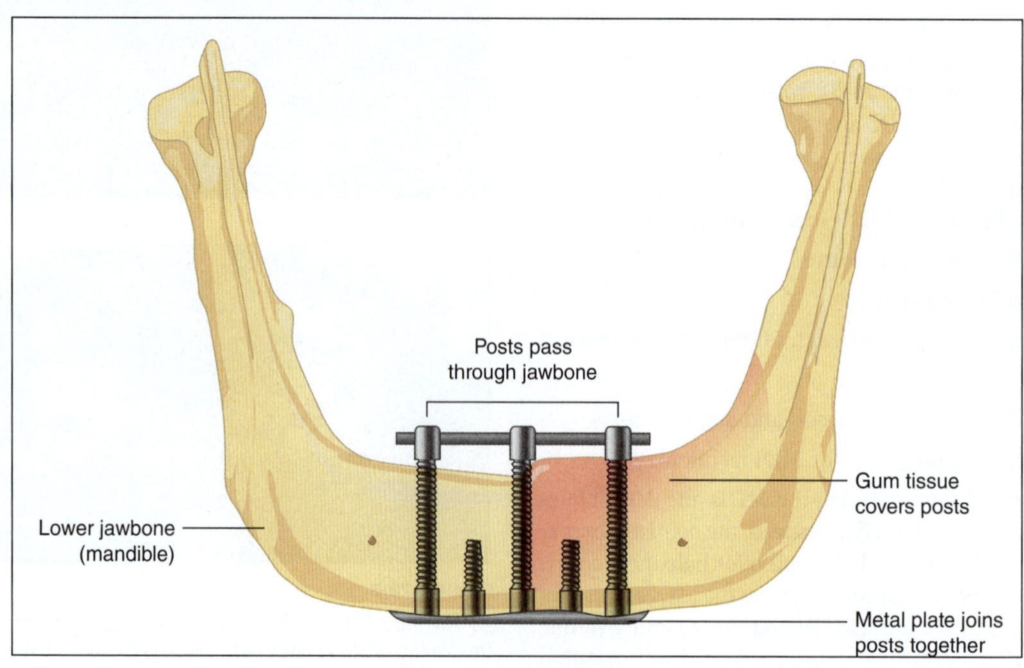

FIGURE 26-7

Placement of a transosteal dental implant.

- Water irrigators
- Antimicrobial rinses

Some dental flosses work well on dental implants, or are designed specifically for implants. The floss for dental implants is a wider band of ribbon that wraps around the implant and is moved in a back-and-forth motion (shoe-shine motion) (Figure 26-8).

Interproximal brushes and instruments provide easy access around the implant due to their small heads (Figures 26-9 and 26-10). The instruments are available in plastic, nylon, or graphite, and prevent the damaging of the titanium surface of the implant. The brushes and instruments remove plaque and stimulate the gingival tissues to increase the blood flow in the surrounding areas. The interproximal brush and instruments are inserted interdentally, and are angled toward the occlusal or incisal surface. A gently rotating motion of the brush is suggested for around the implant near the gingival margin.

During scaling and root planning procedures, plastic or plastic-coated scalers and curettes, and a soft polishing agent are used to prevent the scratching or damaging of the implant.

Water irrigators are available to remove debris and plaque from around the dental implant. The patient should be advised, however, to use the irrigators at the lowest pressure setting in order to prevent damage to the tissues. The gentle spray should be directed interproximally and kept at a horizontal level along the gingival margin. The spray should not be directed into the gingival sulcus.

Antimicrobial rinses, such as chlorhexidine gluconate and phenolic compounds, are recommended for many dental implant patients. The rinses are used once or twice daily

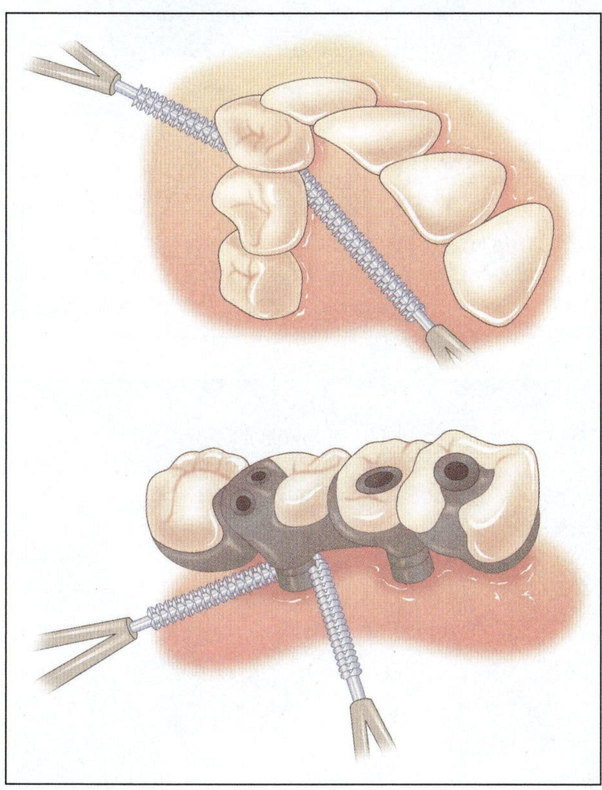

FIGURE 26-8
Dental floss used for dental implants.

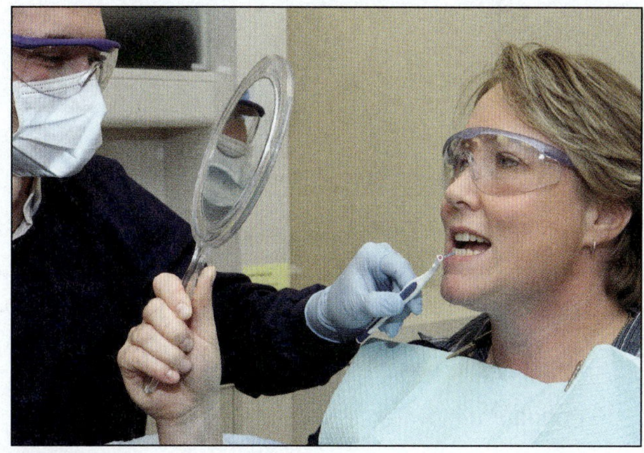

FIGURE 26-9
An interproximal brush: one piece and handle with disposable brush.

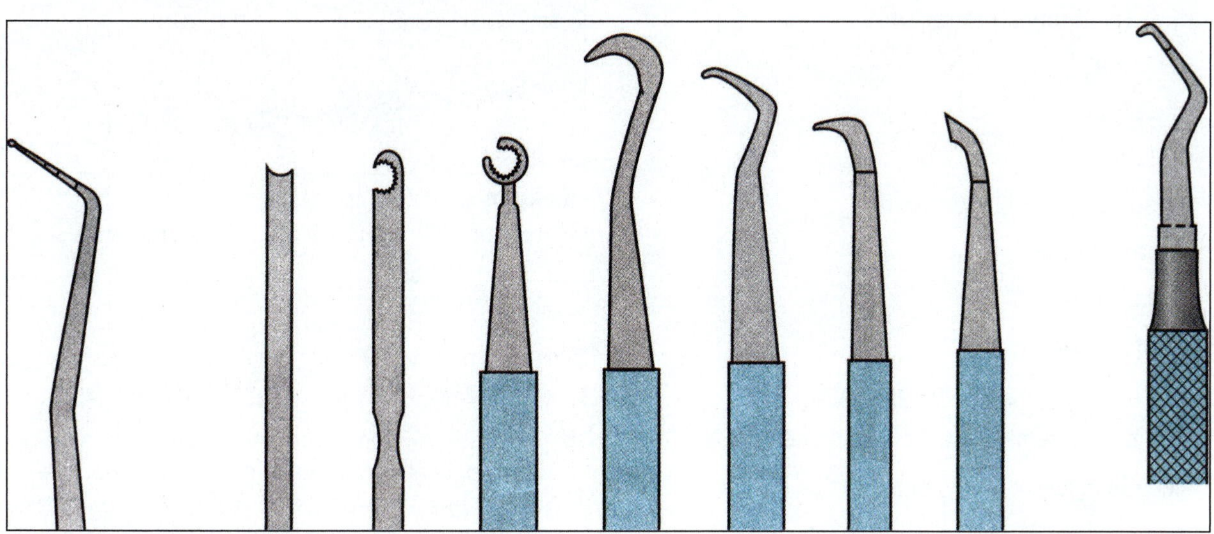

FIGURE 26-10
Plastic instruments used to clean and maintain dental implants.

Procedure 26-1
Dental Implant Surgery

The following procedure is for the placement of an endosteal implant to replace a single tooth. This is a two-stage procedure in which appointments are scheduled 3 to 4 months apart. During the presurgery appointment, the treatment is explained in detail and the patient signs a written consent for the implant surgery. Radiographs are taken, impressions for diagnostic casts are made, surgical stent templates are fabricated, and financial arrangements are completed. The patient is given intravenous sedation for this procedure.

Equipment and Supplies (*Figures 26-11A and B*)

For the first surgical procedure:

- Intravenous sedation and local anesthetic setup
- Mouth mirror
- Surgical HVE tip
- Sterile gauze and cotton pellets
- Irrigation syringe and sterile saline solution
- Low-speed handpiece
- Sterile template
- Sterile surgical drilling unit
- Scalpel and blades
- Periosteal elevator
- Rongeurs
- Surgical curette
- Tissue forceps and scissors
- Cheek and tongue retractors
- Hemostat
- Bite block
- Oral rinse
- Betadine
- Implant instrument kit
- Implant kit
- Suture setup

For the second surgical procedure:

- First seven items from the first procedure
- Electrosurgical (cautery) unit and tips (Figure 26-12)
- Hydrogen peroxide

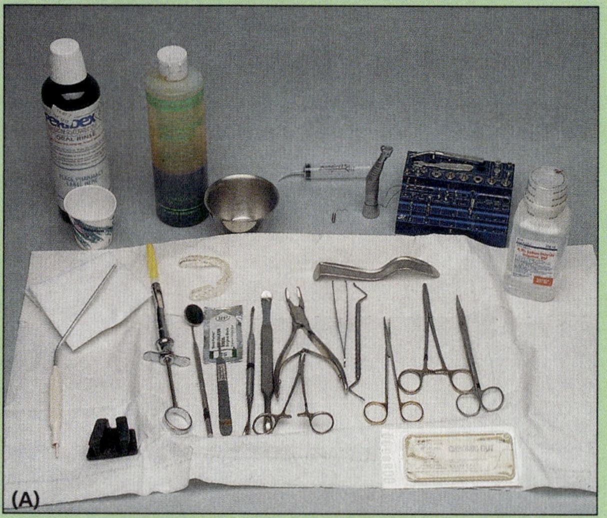
(A)

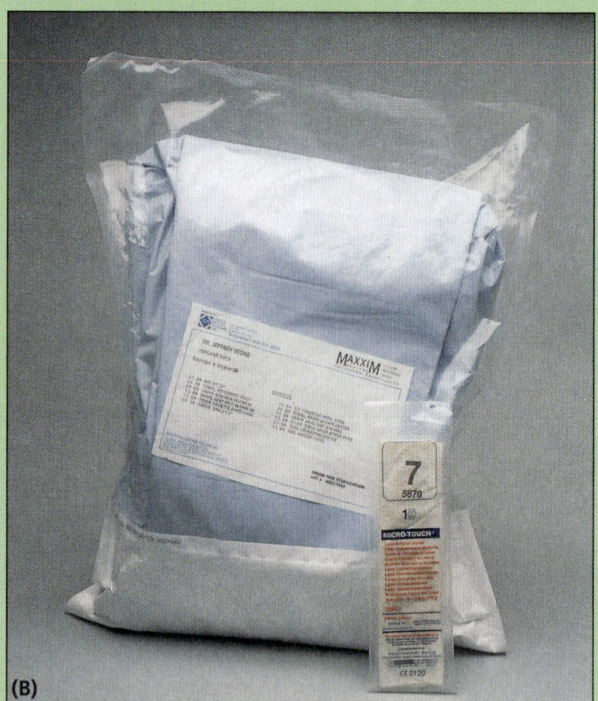

(B)

FIGURE 26-11
(A) Tray setup for implant surgery. (B) Surgical barrier kit.

Procedure Steps

First Surgery for Endosteal Implants

1. The patient is prepared and IV sedation is administered. Local anesthetic is administered. The dental assistant prepares and assists during the administration of sedation and anesthetic.

(continues)

Procedure 26-1 (continued)

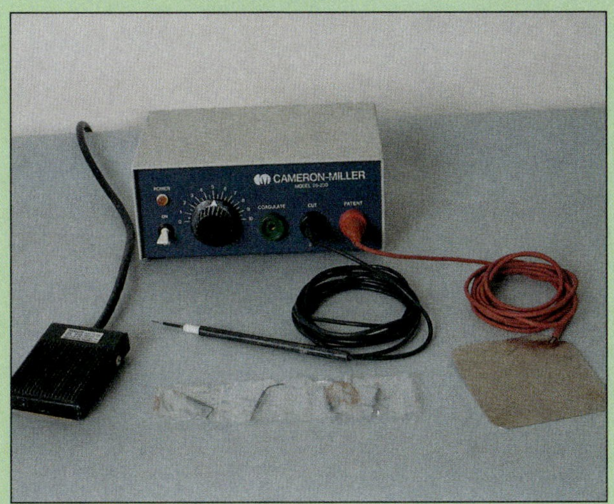

FIGURE 26-12

An electrosurge cauterizing unit used to remove and contour the tissues.

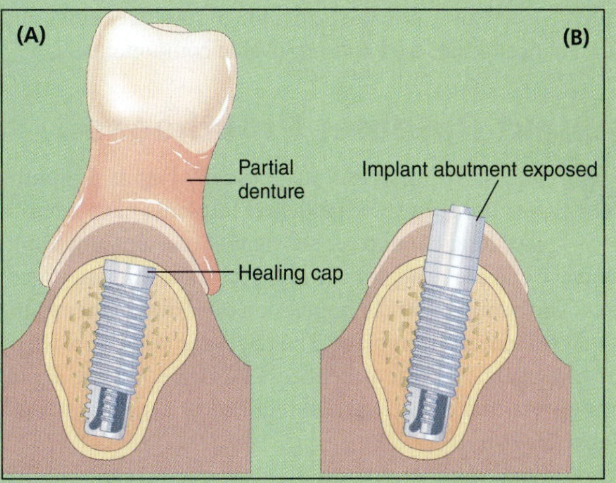

FIGURE 26-13

Implant placement procedures for (A) first-stage and (B) second-stage surgery for an endosteal implant.

2. The surgical template (stent) is seated in the patient's mouth. The target is marked through the template into the soft tissues.
3. The template is removed and the surgeon incises the tissue to expose the ridge of bone. The dental assistant prepares and transfers the scalpel and blade while maintaining the operating site.
4. A periosteal elevator is used to reflect the overlying tissues. Special spiral burs are used to prepare for the implant. The dental assistant changes the burs as size increases, and irrigates with a sterile saline solution.
5. The implant is partially placed, and then tapped or threaded into position. The dental assistant opens the sterile implant and transfers it to the surgeon. A special inserting mallet or ratchet wrench is transferred, and the dental assistant readies the healing cap and contra-angle screwdriver.
6. A healing cap is screwed into the implant. The dental assistant passes the healing cap and the contra-angle screwdriver (Figure 26-13). At this point, in the one-stage implant technique, the healing cap is left exposed in the mouth. The patient does not see the dentist for 3 to 4 months while the osseointegration takes place. Then the patient sees the oral surgeon or periodontist for a final examination. If the implant is stable, the patient returns to the dentist and final impressions are taken for the restoration to be fabricated.
7. Once the implant and healing cap are positioned, the flap is repositioned and sutured.
8. The patient is allowed to recover and given postoperative instructions.

Second Surgical Procedure

1. Local anesthetic is administered.
2. The template is positioned over the osseointegrated implant and a sharp-pointed instrument is used to mark the site. The dental assistant transfers the sterile template and the sharp-pointed instrument.
3. The template is removed and the soft tissue is excised with an electrosurgical loop. Once the healing screw is exposed, it is removed. The dental assistant receives the template and evacuates as the electrosurgical loop is used. Once the tissue is excised, the dental assistant receives the healing screw in a gauze sponge.
4. The inside of the implant is cleaned with hydrogen peroxide on a sterile cotton pellet. The dental assistant prepares the cotton pellet and transfers it to the surgeon.
5. The implant abutment is placed so that it extends slightly beyond the mucosa. The mucosa is then sutured around the abutment. The abutment is transferred to the surgeon, and then the dental assistant prepares the suture material and assists during the suturing.
6. The patient is given postoperative instructions and is then dismissed.

depending on the type. The chlorhexidine gluconate rinses are safe, and aid in fibroblast attachment to the implant surface.

Routine dental exams are also vital to the success of the implant. The exam may also include x-rays, cleaning, and maintenance to the fixed and removable components.

Implant Retainer Prostheses

CDA The fixed prosthesis stage usually begins 6 months after the surgery. The dental implants have been in place long enough for substantial osseointegration to take place and are ready for the last step of the implant procedures. The dentist will take impressions and design the retainers that will cover the implant. The retainer may be a crown or part of a bridge. The abutments are fabricated in the dental laboratory and are either screw retained or cement retained (Figure 26-14).

The screw-retained prosthesis uses one screw to attach the abutment to the implant and a second screw to attach the abutment to the prosthesis. Sometimes, a composite restoration is placed over the screw for esthetic purposes.

The cement-retained prosthesis uses transitional cement to attach the prosthesis to the abutment. Transitional cement is used so that, in case of problems with the implant, the entire system can be retrieved. The abutment is screwed into the implant like the screw-retained prosthesis (Figure 26-15).

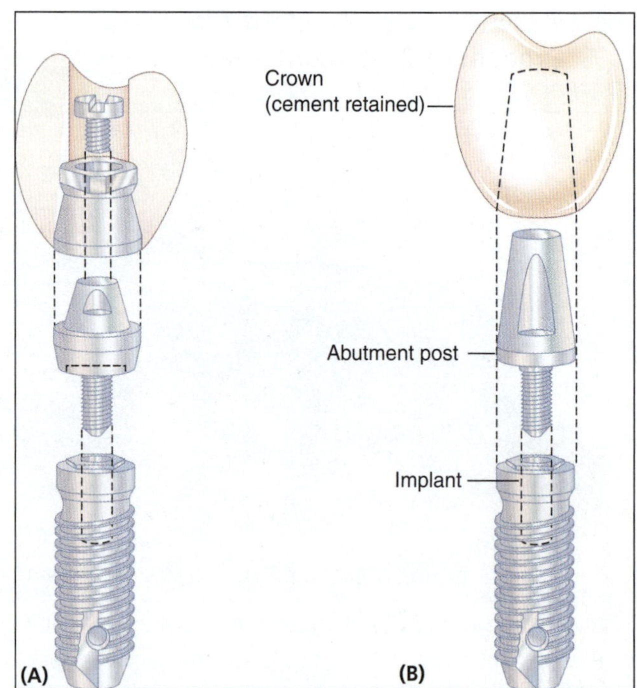

FIGURE 26-14

(A) Screw-retained implant prosthesis. (B) Cement-retained implant prosthesis.

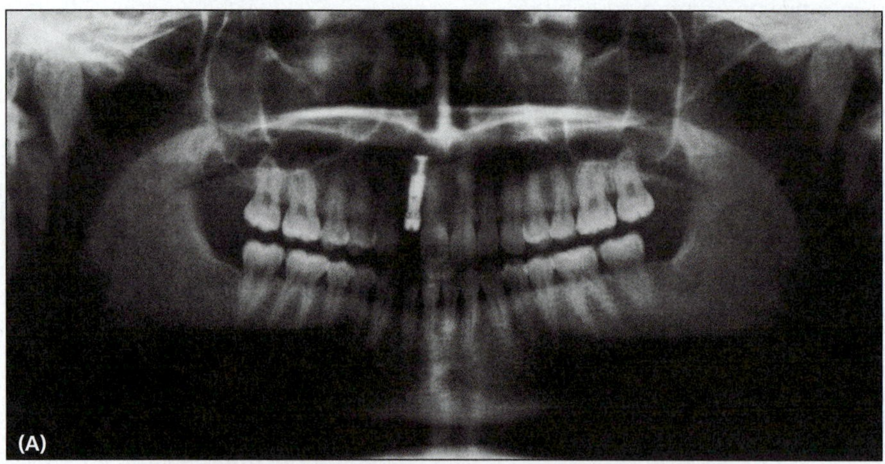

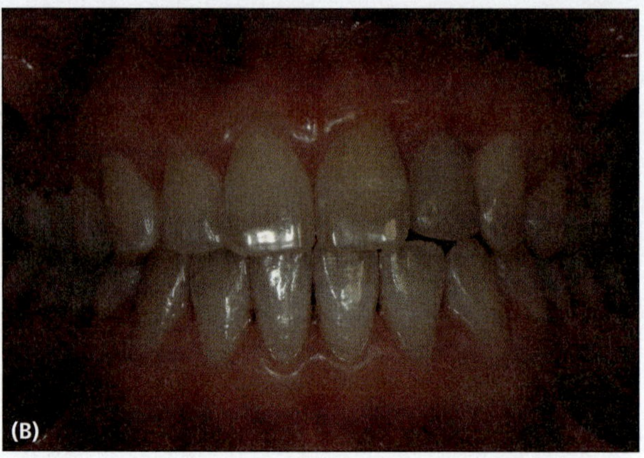

FIGURE 26-15

(A) A panoramic radiograph of the dental implant. (B) A patient's smile after the crown has been seated on the dental implant.

Chapter Summary

This chapter covers dental implants, which have become the standard of treatment for replacing missing teeth. The considerations for the patient are discussed, including preparation of the patient, number of appointments, types of implants, and steps of the procedure. Postoperative instructions as well as what is involved in the maintenance of the dental implant are covered. This chapter gives the dental assistants the information they will need to work with the patients and assist the dentist during the dental implant procedure.

CASE STUDY

Lucas Smart, 46 years old, had a retained primary (baby) tooth that was becoming loose. Over the years the roots had resorbed, and now the tooth needs to be removed. Either a bridge or an implant needs to be put into its place.

Case Study Review

1. What information would Lucas need to know about both options?
2. How many appointments would be needed for the dental implant?
3. Discuss which dental professionals would be involved with this procedure.
4. What does the maintenance of dental implants include?

Review Questions

1. When a dental implant fuses with the bone tissue through a biologic bonding process, it is called an
   a. osseointegration.
   b. alveolectomy.
   c. alveolitis.
   d. ostectomy.
2. Patients considering dental implants should
   a. be in good overall health.
   b. have a positive and cooperative attitude.
   c. have adequate jawbone that is healthy and strong.
   d. all of the above.
3. The following are all types of dental implants *except*:
   a. subperiosteal implants.
   b. mini dental implants.
   c. supraperiosteal implants.
   d. endosteal implants.
4. What is placed over the tissues during surgery and guides the dentist in placing the implant?
   a. A healing cap
   b. A surgical stent
   c. The abutment
   d. The center screw
5. The endosteal implants
   a. are used because the alveolar bone has atrophied.
   b. are most commonly placed on top of the alveolar bone.
   c. are available in a variety of widths, lengths, and designs.
   d. are smaller and narrower than other dental implants.
6. The ________ are smaller in diameter and are used for the fixation of full and partial dentures and for retention in orthodontic procedures.
   a. subperiosteal implants
   b. endosteal implants
   c. mini dental implants
   d. transosteal implants
7. In the two-stage technique the implant is inserted into the bone with the implant protruding through the tissues, and a healing cap is placed.
   a. This is a true statement.
   b. This is a false statement.
8. The three main parts of the implant include
   a. the implant, abutment screw, and the abutment post or cylinder.
   b. the implant, abutment cap, and prostheses.
   c. the abutment screw, abutment cap, and prostheses.
   d. the implant, stent, and abutment cap.
9. Postoperative care includes all of the following *except*:
   a. Take only clear liquids for the first 2 days.
   b. Softly bite on a gauze pad for 15 to 30 minutes.
   c. Gently rinse the mouth with saline solution after each meal.
   d. Do not drink milk or take vitamin C, D, B complex, or calcium.
10. Which of the following is a TRUE STATEMENT concerning homecare of dental implants?
    a. During scaling and root planning procedures, plastic or plastic-coated scalers and curettes are used to prevent scratching and damaging the implant.
    b. Water irrigators are used to remove debris, but the spray should not be directed into the sulcus.

c. Antimicrobial rinses, such as chlorhexidine gluconate and phenolic compounds, are recommended for many dental implant patients.
d. All of the above.

Critical Thinking

1. Why would a patient choose dental implants over other possible treatments?
2. List several reasons why a dental implant may fail and discuss the importance of osseointegration.
3. Explain what information needs to be gathered for the consultation appointment when a patient decides on an implant as a possible treatment.
4. What type of dental implant would assist in the retention of orthodontic appliances, and why is it the best choice?
5. What is the role of the dental assistant during a dental implant surgery?
6. Explain how dental implants are maintained both at home and in the dental office during routine examinations.

Web Activities

1. Visit http://www.straumann.us and learn more about patient information, products, and solutions concerning implants.
2. Go to www.ADA.org to find the father of dental implants, where he was from, and about the implant system he developed.
3. At http://www.Bicon.com, learn more about dental implants, types, and procedures.

CHAPTER 27

Oral Pathology 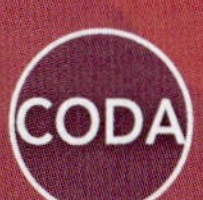

CODA

Specific Instructional Objectives

The student should strive to meet the following objectives and demonstrate an understanding of the facts and principles presented in this chapter:

1. Define oral pathology and identify the dental assistant's role in this specialty.
2. Characterize the process of inflammation including acute and chronic inflammation.
3. Identify oral lesions according to placement.
4. Identify oral diseases and lesions related to biological agents.
5. Describe oral diseases and lesions related to physical agents.
6. Identify oral diseases and lesions related to chemical agents.
7. Identify oral conditions related to hormonal disturbances.
8. Identify oral conditions related to developmental disturbances.
9. Distinguish among oral conditions related to nutritional disturbances.
10. Discuss oral cancer and its warning signs.
11. Identify the conditions and lesions of oral neoplasms.
12. Identify oral lesions related to HIV and AIDS.
13. Describe the conditions related to miscellaneous disorders affecting the oral cavity.

Key Terms

abscess (639)
actinomycosis (640)
acute inflammation (638)
amalgam tattoo (643)
amelogenesis imperfecta (647)
angular cheilitis (649)
ankyloglossia (649)
ankylosis (647)
anodontia (647)
antigenic (638)
aphthous ulcers (640)
atypical (638)
basal cell carcinoma (652)
Bell's palsy (656)
bifid tongue (649)
biopsy (638)
blister (639)
bulla (639)
Candida albicans (642)
canker sores (640)
carcinoma (650)
cellulitis (642)
Chronic inflammation (638)
congenital (647)
cyst (639)
dentinogenesis imperfecta (647)
dysplastic cells (651)
ecchymosis (639)
erosion (639)
erythroplakia (652)
etiology (638)
exostosis (648)
fibroma (653)
fissured tongue (648)
Fordyce's spots (648)
fusion (647)
gemination (647)
gingival hyperplasia (646)
glossitis (650)
granuloma (640)
gumma (641)
hairy leukoplakia (654)
hairy tongue (645)
hematoma (639)
herpes labialis (640)
herpes zoster (641)
herpetic gingivostomatitis (640)

(continues)

Key Terms (continued)

herpetic whitlow (640)
histamines (638)
human immunodeficiency virus (HIV) (653)
Hutchinson's incisors (641)
hyperkeratinized (645)
hyperplasia (643)
idiopathic (639)
inflammation (638)
innocuous (647)
Kaposi's sarcoma (654)
lesions (639)
leukemia (652)
leukoplakia (651)
lichen planus (651)
macrodontia (647)
macule (639)
malignant (651)
metastasize (652)
microdontia (648)
mucocele (655)
mulberry molars (641)
necrosis (643)
neonatal teeth (648)
neoplasm (640)
nicotine stomatitis (644)
nodule (640)
opportunistic infections (649)
oral pathology (638)
orifices (645)
palpate (638)
papilloma (653)
papule (639)
patch (639)
petechiae (639)
plaque (639)
purpura (640)
pustule (639)
pyogenic granuloma (647)
sarcoma (650)
squamous cell carcinoma (652)
supernumerary teeth (648)
syphilis (641)
thrush (642)
tori (648)
twinning (648)
ulcer (639)
varix (655)
vesicle (639)
Wickham's striae (651)

Introduction

The field of **oral pathology** is defined as the study of oral diseases, their causes (if known), and their effects on the body. A dental assistant does not diagnose oral pathological diseases but may alert the dentist to abnormal conditions in the mouth. The dental assistant must recognize abnormal conditions and must know how to prevent disease transmission, how the identified pathological condition may interfere with planned treatment, and what effect the condition will have on the overall health of the patient.

Oral pathology can originate from a number of different agents or disturbances. Biological, physical, and chemical agents may bring on a disease condition that exhibits signs in the oral cavity. Hormonal, developmental, and nutritional disturbances will also show disease signs in the mouth. In addition oral pathology can include other disorders, reactions to stress and **antigenic** (capable of causing the production of an antibody) substances, as well as neoplasms and cysts, that can develop in the oral cavity. The dental assistant has a different viewpoint of the patient's oral cavity because she or he sits on the opposite side of the patient. Anything that appears to be **atypical** (irregular or abnormal) should be brought to the attention of the dentist for further investigation, without alarming the patient. Any unusual oral *lesions*—an all-encompassing term for abnormal structures in the oral cavity—must be closely observed by the dentist. The dentist may **palpate** (feel with fingers) or perform a procedure called a biopsy on the suspicious lesion. A **biopsy** (a surgical removal of a small amount of tissue) is an accurate method for diagnosing many illnesses. After the diagnosis is made, further study is done to identify the **etiology** (cause of the disease). This biopsy is normally sent to a pathologist for examination under a microscope and further diagnosis. Dentists include any information they observe clinically or through palpation, such as size, location, color, and texture. Other information about the lesion may include how long it has been present, if it is painful to the touch, whether the area seems hot, and what the patient believes caused the situation. All this information obtained from the patient should be documented. Any additional information the doctor thinks is pertinent should be sent to the laboratory with the biopsy.

Inflammation

The body responds to disease and injury with a process known as **inflammation**. The body's response to injury or irritation can be either acute or chronic. With **acute inflammation**, the injury or irritation is minor and doesn't last long, with the tissues healing quickly. **Chronic inflammation** occurs when the tissues do not heal quickly and the inflammation process continues. Specialized cells in the area release a number of chemicals, some of which are called **histamines**. Histamines are said to bring about inflammation by increasing blood flow to the involved area and causing redness and heat. They also make the blood capillaries more hyperemic (increased amount of blood), and fluid oozes from them into the tissues, causing swelling. When the nerve endings in the area are stimulated by these chemicals, pain occurs. Four conditions are an essential part of the body's response to injury or disease: redness (erythema), heat, swelling (edema), and pain. These symptoms were first defined as the clinical features of inflammation by Cornelius Celsus (c. 25 BC–c. 50 AD), a Roman physician and medical writer. Often referred to as the *cardinal signs of inflammation*, they were known in Latin as *rubor* (redness), *calor* (warmth), *tumor* (swelling), and *dolor* (pain).

White blood cells, which are attracted to inflammation, help destroy the invading microorganisms and aid in healing. The area is encircled by a fibrous connective tissue to prevent the spread of the condition to any other area.

Inflammatory Process

- Redness
- Heat
- Swelling
- Pain

Diagnosing Oral Pathology

The dentist uses information from many sources to make a diagnosis for any oral pathology. She or he may use several diagnostic tools to identify the lesion or disease, or use a process of elimination to reach a conclusion. These diagnostic tools are radiographic, clinical, personal medical/dental and family (genetic) history, microscopic biopsy, laboratory diagnosis, surgical, and therapeutic and differential diagnosis. The dentist most often reads the radiographs and completes a clinical evaluation first. Radiographs provide views of the apical area, and the dentist can determine whether any areas of absorption have occurred. They also indicate whether cysts or abscesses are present. The dentist performs a clinical diagnosis to assess the location, size, shape, color, and texture of the lesion. The patient's genetic and medical/dental histories are often useful in making the diagnosis. There are a number of genetic disorders that may need to be illuminated. If these tools do not permit the dentist to reach a conclusion on which oral pathologic lesion is present, then further diagnostic information will be required.

The dentist can then determine that a surgery is needed to help determine the diagnosis. If the diagnosis is still not clear via visual examination during surgery, the dentist may decide to send a tissue sample to a laboratory for a biopsy analysis, blood chemistry analysis, and/or other analyses.

The therapeutic/differential diagnosis is a commonly used tool. Once an evaluation of clinical data leads to a likely diagnosis, the dentist chooses a particular therapy. If this has no effect on the condition, they will move on to the next likely diagnosis or related therapy. In contrast, when the cause of a disease or disorder is unknown, it is said to be **idiopathic**.

Oral Lesions

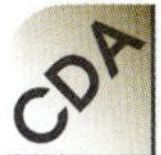

Abnormal tissues in the oral cavity, called **lesions**, are further classified according to their placement in the surface of the mucosa. They can be classified as above the surface, below the surface, or flat or even with the surface of the oral mucosa.

Above-Surface Lesions

- A **blister** is a raised area, usually oval or circular, filled with fluid that protects the damaged tissue. This fluid leaks from the blood vessels into underlying layers of skin following some type of trauma, such as a burn, friction, or disease.
- A **bulla** (BULL-ah) is a large (over one-half inch in diameter), fluid-filled blister.
- A **hematoma** is a lesion caused by bleeding from a ruptured blood vessel, which appears as a raised bruised area due to the collection of localized clotted blood. Dental assistants should watch for a hematoma after oral anesthetic. Even the best clinicians may nick a blood vessel during an injection, resulting in a hematoma. The dental assistant alerts the dentist about the condition, and then applies pressure to the area to disperse the blood in the tissue, which alleviates pressure in the area.
- A **papule** is a small (less than one-half inch in diameter), solid, raised area of skin. The surface of the papule may be pigmented in color and either smooth or bumpy.
- A **plaque** is any raised or flat patch in the oral mucosa. This term is not to be confused with dental plaque, which causes dental caries (see Chapter 4, Oral Health and Preventive Techniques).
- A **pustule** is a small, pus-containing blister.
- A **vesicle** is a small, fluid-filled blister.

Below-Surface Lesions

- An **abscess** is a concentrated area of pus formed as a result of an infection of microorganisms. Dental abscesses are periapical (at the apex of the tooth) or periodontal, and are caused by microorganisms invading the periodontal membrane of the tooth (see Chapter 31, Periodontics).
- A **cyst** is a fluid or semi-solid, fluid-filled sac. The causes of cysts are numerous. In dentistry, cysts normally occur due to the blockage of a duct leading from a fluid-forming gland. Cysts can develop around the crown of an undeveloped tooth before eruption.
- An **erosion** is the defect left from a trauma or an injury. It may arise from biting the cheek. The margins of cheek erosion are red and painful.
- An **ulcer** is due to destruction of the mucous membrane and appears as an open sore on the tissue. The ulcer may appear shallow or deeply cratered and is normally inflamed and painful.

Even or Flat with Surface Lesions

- An **ecchymosis** (eck-ih-**MOH**-sis) is a medical term for tissue bruising.
- A **macule** (**MACK**-youl) is a spot with a different texture or color than the surrounding skin.
- A **patch** is an area of skin that is different in color and/or texture from the surrounding skin.
- The **petechia (plural petechiae)** (pee-**TEE**-kee-ee) are small spots, red or purple in color, that occur in the skin or mucosal tissue. They are caused by a localized hemorrhage.

- A **purpura** (**PUR**-pew-rah) is caused by bleeding within underlying tissues. These purplish or reddish-brown areas, or spots of discoloration, can range in size from the diameter of a pin's head up to 1 inch. Small purpuras are normally called petechiae, and the larger ones are called ecchymoses or bruises.

Flat or Above-Surface Lesions

- A **granuloma**, associated with chronic inflammation, appears as a neoplasm filled with granulation tissue. The suffix "oma" refers to a neoplasm.
- A **neoplasm** is the medical term for tumor. This new, abnormal growth serves no purpose and can be either malignant (life threatening) or benign (not life threatening).
- A **nodule** is a small lump of tissue, hard or soft, that is usually more than one-quarter inch in diameter. A nodule may protrude from the tissue or form beneath the surface of the tissue.

Biological Agents

A number of microorganisms cause oral diseases that are manifested through lesions in the head and neck.

Actinomycosis

The disorder, **actinomycosis**, is an infection caused by bacteria. At first, a painful swelling appears, and then pus and yellow granules discharge from the area. Poor oral hygiene or microorganisms obtaining access to the bone through the dental socket after tooth removal are thought to be contributing factors.

Herpes Simplex

Type I herpes simplex typically occurs above the waist (normally around the mouth); Type II may appear in the oral cavity, but normally appears below the waist and is commonly called genital herpes. The Type I infection occurs in about three-fourths of middle-aged adults. Forms of the virus are responsible for cold sores (painful blisters around the mouth). These blisters, commonly called fever blisters, can appear solitary or in a cluster of small blisters on the lips, called **herpes labialis** (Figure 27-1). Normal inflammation encompasses the area.

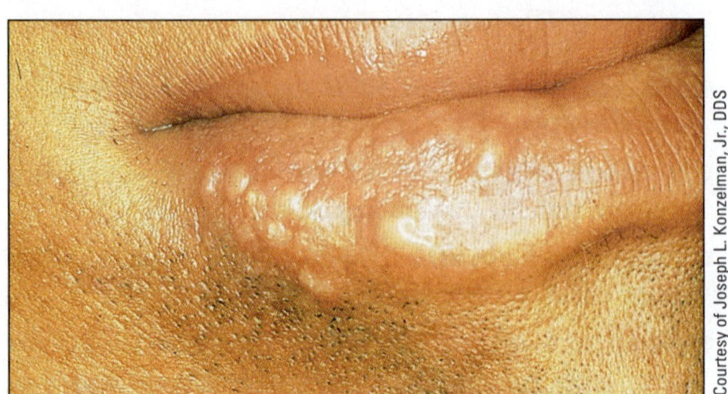

Courtesy of Joseph L. Konzelman, Jr., DDS

FIGURE 27-1
Herpes lesions on the lips, called herpes labialis.

The virus responsible for the disease is transmitted through physical contact and is seen normally in children around the age of 6 as **herpetic gingivostomatitis** (the initial infection). The virus, which is infectious both during the onset of the vesicular stage and throughout the crusted stage, is often unknowingly passed by adults to children during kissing. It exhibits symptoms much like the flu. Fever, along with body aches, is apparent, followed by scattered ulcers in the oral mucosa or on the lips. The lesions appear as nicks in the tissue and are extremely sore. These vesicle ulcerations vary in size from a pin's head to one-quarter inch in size. The symptoms reappear throughout life and usually last from 7 to 14 days. If the condition is caught early, medication is available to alleviate discomfort (see Chapter 10, Microbiology).

Dental assistants must exert extreme care while working with patients who have herpes. Stretching and pulling of the lesion causes the patient significant discomfort. Dentists may choose to reschedule the patient until after recovery from the herpes outbreak. The dental assistant must pay special attention to eliminating cross-contamination by maintaining asepsis. The herpetic virus lasts on a countertop or work surface for up to 4 hours. Health care workers are known to develop the infection if barriers are not used. If exposure is significant, gloves are not worn, and a break in the skin is accessible to the virus, **herpetic whitlow** may occur. This is a crusting ulceration on the fingers or hands that is extremely painful.

Any patient with apparent ulcers from the herpes virus that last longer than a month should be tested for immunodeficient diseases, such as HIV.

Aphthous Ulcers

Common ulcerations that recur in the oral cavity are **aphthous ulcers** (AF-thus). These painful ulcers appear as circular with yellow centers and erythematous (red) halos surrounding the lesions (Figure 27-2). The yellow necrotic center is due to dead or dying epithelial cells. The cause of this ulcer is unknown, but streptococci bacteria have been identified in numerous cases. Recurrent aphthous ulcers (RAU) are referred to by patients as **canker sores**, and they are not contagious. A patient may have as few as one or as many as six sores at one

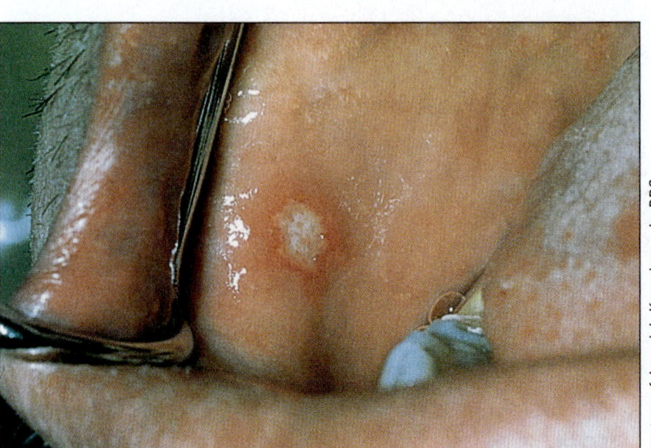

Courtesy of Joseph L. Konzelman, Jr., DDS.

FIGURE 27-2
Recurrent aphthous ulcer on buccal mucosa.

time. Heredity, trauma, stress, food allergens, and hormonal changes are associated with the recurrence of this ulceration.

Recurrent aphthous ulcers start out as small bumps that begin with a sting. These ulcers develop on an area of unattached gingiva or mucosa inside the cheeks, and present as a whitish dished-out area that is surrounded with a red ring. Nerve endings are exposed. Bacteria can invade the area, resulting in inflammation, and the area becomes even more uncomfortable.

Aphthous ulcers last from 10 to 14 days, and topical anesthetics are used to treat the painful symptoms. Patients may have to be rescheduled for dental treatment, because these sores cause significant discomfort if they are touched or stretched.

Herpes Zoster

The disorder, **herpes zoster** (shingles), appears as unilateral, painful lesions that can last up to 5 weeks. This virus, which causes varicella in children, may be latent and then activate at a time when the person is immunodeficient. Patients with human immunodeficiency virus (HIV) or advanced cancers are predisposed to herpes zoster. Acyclovir™ has been used successfully to treat the symptoms of these painful ulcers in some cases.

Syphilis

A venereal disease caused by bacteria, called **syphilis**, may be treated with antibiotics, and has three primary stages. The first stage presents with a primary lesion about one-half inch in diameter that is hard and raised (Figure 27-3). This lesion, called a chancre, appears normally on the lip. The chancre first ulcerates and then becomes crusted over. It appears much like a herpetic lesion. The chancre disappears within 5 weeks, and no clinical manifestations of the disease appear in the oral cavity until 2 months to 1 year later.

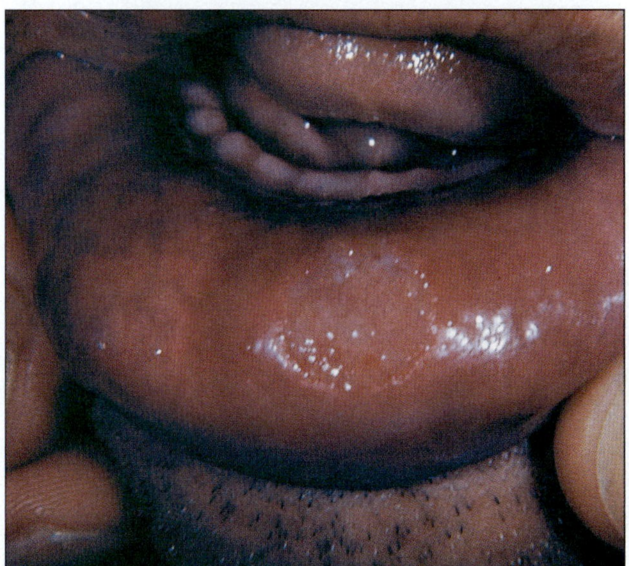

FIGURE 27-3
Lip chancre from primary syphilis.

The second stage begins with flu-like symptoms, followed by one of two types of lesions. These lesions, a mucous patch or a split papule, are both extremely infectious. In the tertiary, or third, and final stage of syphilis, a **gumma** or localized lesion appears. The final stage of syphilis may occur many years after non-treatment of secondary syphilis. This lesion destroys bone and cartilage.

Children born to mothers with syphilis may have teeth with enamel hypoplasia, or teeth that have been altered because of the infection, during the morphodifferentiation and dentinogenesis cycles of tooth development. The anterior dentition appears to be dented on the incisal edges, called **Hutchinson's incisors** (Figure 27-4). The permanent molars may appear more rounded with the occlusal surface, resembling a mulberry. Due to their appearance, they are called **mulberry molars** (Figure 27-5).

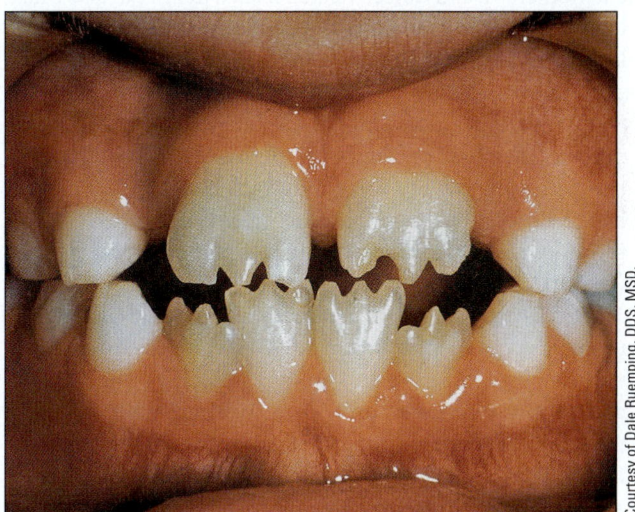

Courtesy of Dale Ruemping, DDS, MSD.

FIGURE 27-4
Hutchinson's incisors from prenatal syphilis.

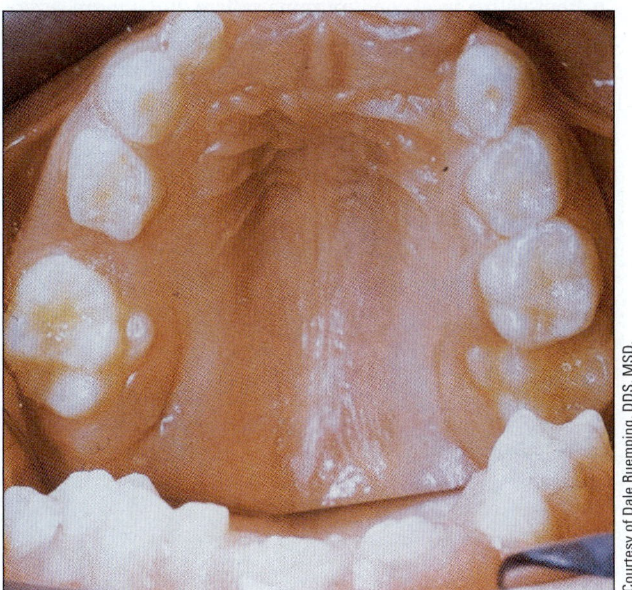

Courtesy of Dale Ruemping, DDS, MSD.

FIGURE 27-5
Mulberry molars from prenatal syphilis.

Thrush

Candidiasis is a fungal infection caused by any type of *Candida*, a type of yeast normally found in the mouth, digestive track, and skin of healthy people. The body's immune system and normal bacteria usually keep the *candida* in balance, but if the balance is interrupted the results will be an overgrowth of *candida*. When it affects the oral tissues it is called **thrush** or oral thrush. Thrush is most often caused by the yeast ***Candida albicans***, which is one of many types of yeast. Thrush infections are found in babies, toddlers, children, and the elderly, as well as in people with suppressed immune systems, with certain health conditions (such as diabetes), and in people taking some medication (such as antibiotic therapy). Risk factors include a weakened immune system due to diabetes, HIV, AIDS (see later discussion in this chapter), cancer, and dry mouth (xeostomia). Medications such as corticosteroids, chemotherapy, and cancer-related related drugs can also cause thrush. Smoking, poorly fitting dentures, and stress can also lead to the development of oral thrush. Thrush is possible to prevent in most cases by modifying the risk factors.

Thrush appears as white, thick patches covering the oral mucous membranes (Figure 27-6). Tissues can be red and raw with soreness and some mouth pain. The patient might have halitosis (bad or unpleasant breath) and a bad taste in the mouth with cracking at the corners of the mouth (chelosis, Refer to Chapter 5, Nutrition).

Most infants, toddlers, and children who develop thrush usually do not require treatment. The white covering can be removed by wiping it with two-by-two inch gauze. The fungal microorganism can grow in increasing numbers in this warm, moist environment, and causes very little discomfort to the child. In a few cases, the child's pediatrician may prescribe antifungal nystatin drops (Mycostatin, Nilstat, and Nystex), or a topical antifungal drug to be applied to the area. In adult patients with a mild case of thrush, the doctor may prescribe an antifungal mouthwash (nystatin) or lozenges for short-term use. For a patient with a weakened immune system and a more severe case of thrush, a stronger systemic medication, such as fluconazole (Diflucan) or itraconazole (Sporanox) is administered. In some severe or resistant cases of thrush, amphotericin B, an antifungal drug that is administered intravenously, may be prescribed.

Thrush is generally not contagious but can be transmitted to the mother of a nursing baby with oral thrush or from person to person through the use of dentures.

Other types of candidiasis include vaginal yeast infections and diaper rash.

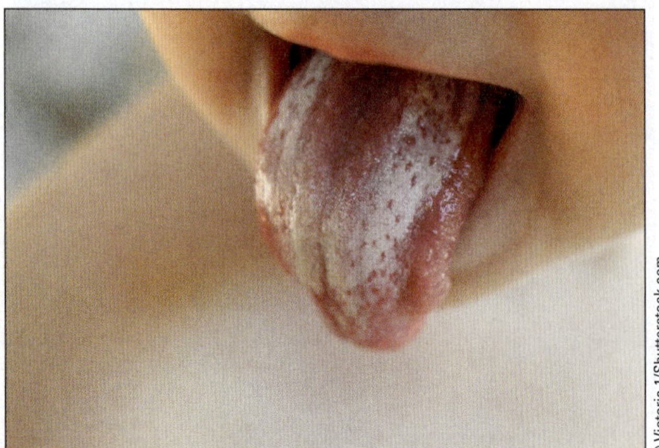
© Victoria 1/Shutterstock.com

FIGURE 27-6

A baby with thrush on lips and tongue.

Cellulitis

The condition, **cellulitis**, is a bacterial infection that spreads quickly if the inflammation is left uncontrolled. It is associated with the skin and soft tissues. Symptoms include swelling, redness of the infected area, heat, and tenderness. In the oral cavity cellulitis is often associated with an abscess tooth or other oral infections (Figure 27-7). As the infection advances, swelling develops along with redness and pain in the localized area. The dentist will examine the area and take x-rays to diagnose cellulitis. Treatment includes antibiotics and treatment of the abscessed tooth.

Physical Agents

Several physical agents can cause oral, clinical manifestations. These trauma-induced ulcerations are most often caused by accident. The patient may bite the inside of the cheek, fall on a blunt object, or wear an ill-fitting dental appliance, such as

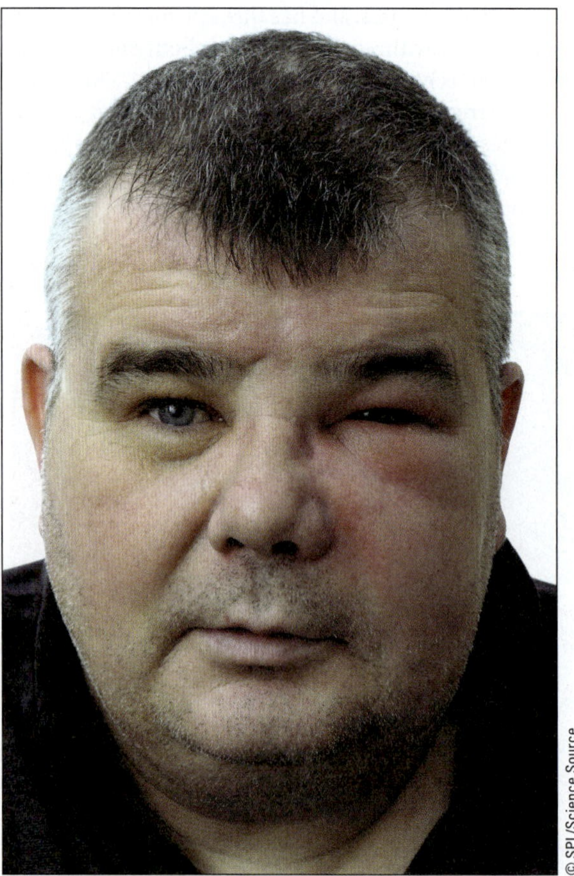
© SPL/Science Source

FIGURE 27-7

Patient with cellulitis from wisdom tooth infection.

a denture. The dental team must use great care not to induce additional trauma during dental care. The HVE has a rough edge that can cut or lacerate the patient's tissue if not handled properly. Other physical agents, such as instruments, can cause trauma by tearing or bruising the tissue if not used carefully. The dental assistant must constantly watch as instruments and materials are transferred to and from the mouth.

Overly dry cotton rolls that are removed too quickly can cause a gingival ulcer. The tissue adheres to the cotton roll so that, when it is removed, the top layer of gingival tissue is also removed. To avoid this, the dental assistant can moisten the cotton roll prior to removing it.

Denture Irritation Causing Hyperplasia

An ill-fitting denture can cause small ulcers that, after continued irritation, become folds of excess tissue called **hyperplasia** (Figure 27-8). In the palatal area, the ruga(e) palatine become inflamed and swollen. Swelling is reduced and the redness disappears if the patient does not wear the denture for several days. Soft, tissue-lining material can be placed in the denture by the dentist to allow the palate to heal prior to relining or remaking the denture.

Amalgam Tattoo

An **amalgam tattoo** can occur when amalgam particles become trapped in the tissue, either during oral surgery or during an amalgam or crown preparation procedure (Figure 27-9). The gingival tissue in the immediate area appears blue to gray. No treatment is necessary because the tattoo is asymptomatic and harmless. To prevent this condition from occurring, the dental assistant should flush the area with water to remove any amalgam particles after treatment, especially when the tissue is severely abraded. Use of a dental dam also aids in preventing amalgam tattoos.

Radiation Injury

Patients receiving excess radiation due to cancer treatment around the oral cavity may experience a number of side effects. One such side effect may be **necrosis**, which is the death of body tissue in the area that was radiated. It occurs

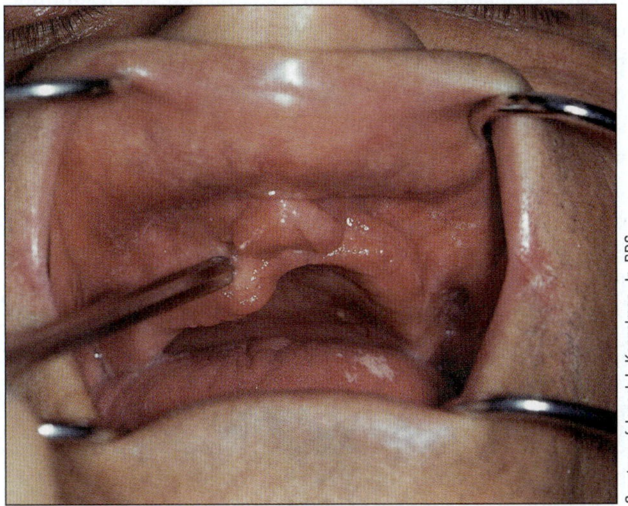

Courtesy of Joseph L. Konzelman, Jr., DDS

FIGURE 27-8

Hyperplasia from denture irritation.

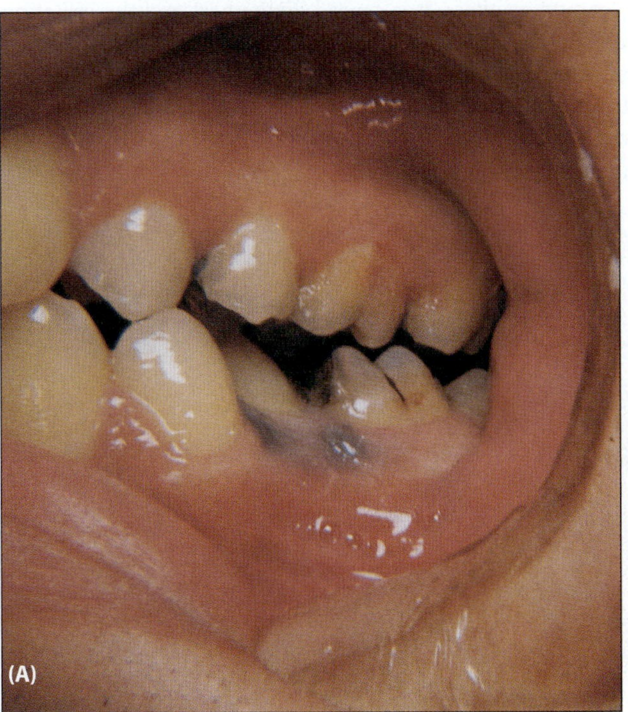

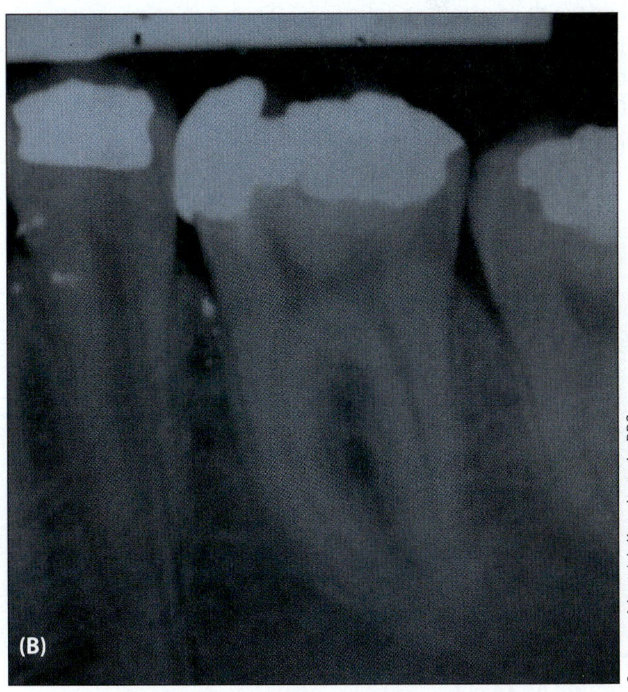

Courtesy of Joseph L. Konzelman, Jr., DDS

FIGURE 27-9

An amalgam tattoo (A) in the oral cavity, and (B) on a periapical x-ray.

when there is not enough blood flowing to the tissue. Necrosis is not reversible. Excess radiation may cause developing teeth to be malformed, dwarfed, or without roots. The deformity depends on the stage of tooth development. The soft tissue may show reddening, with apparent ulcers due to excess radiation. After the area has healed, the tissue within the area may appear pigmented. Spider-like vessels may appear in the skin that appears to be atrophied.

Oral Piercing

Oral piercings (Figure 27-10) are a means of self-expression and body art, and the majority of them involve the tongue. A barbell-shaped piece of jewelry is placed in the midline of the tongue after a needle pierces the area. Often, a temporary device is placed so that it can be adjusted if swelling occurs. When the barbell is placed through the tongue a ball is screwed on the lower side of the tongue to secure it. If a blood vessel is punctured during the piercing, severe bleeding may occur. In some instances, blood poisoning or blood clots will develop. Other sites include cheeks, lips, uvula, and the side of the tongue; sometimes multiple sites are pierced. Healing in any of these areas takes a month or more.

Before a person chooses oral piercing, possible outcomes and related symptoms should be investigated. Tongue piercings are most commonly placed in the center of the tongue to minimize vesicle and neural damage. Keeping the site clean is essential. In dentistry this is another concern because, often, the piercing affects treatments such as radiographs. Side effects are common. The most serious side effect is tongue swelling, which can actually close off the airway and, thus, hamper breathing. Other symptoms include pain, infection, swelling, increased saliva flow, teeth and tissue damage (Figure 27-11), metal hypersensitivity, scar tissue development, and problems with mastication (chewing). Speech is often affected as well. Piercing has been identified by the National Institutes of Health as a possible factor in transmission of hepatitis B, C, D, and G. (For more information see the American Dental Association's policies on oral piercing.)

Tongue Splitting

Another form of self-expression is tongue splitting, or separating the end of the tongue, resulting in a reptilian appearance. Reversing this procedure requires surgery. Compared to oral piercing, damage to teeth and tissue is less severe, speech problems are exaggerated, and the potential for infection is greater. Finally, swallowing may become more difficult.

Chemical Agents

A number of chemical agents can cause oral lesions. Some of the materials used in dentistry are caustic and may cause chemical burns. These agents include phenol, sodium hypochlorate, zinc chloride, phosphoric acid, and aspirin. The chemicals in tobacco also cause oral lesions. Certain drugs will also induce oral lesions. In the dental office, the most common effects of chemical agents seen in patients' oral cavities are aspirin burns, nicotine stomatitis, and chewing tobacco lesions.

Aspirin Burn

Some people place aspirin over the root area of a tooth to alleviate discomfort before seeking dental treatment. The placement of the aspirin causes a lesion that is white in color and rough in texture (Figure 27-12). Soreness is apparent after the aspirin is removed or dissolved.

Nicotine Stomatitis

Another condition that the dental assistant is likely to see in the dental office is **nicotine stomatitis** (Figure 27-13). Pipe smokers are more likely to develop nicotine stomatitis than cigarette smokers. It is caused by the heat and the irritating effect of the chemicals in the tobacco. The reason for more frequent occurrence in pipe smokers is that they typically place the pipe in the same area. The pipe stem then delivers a great deal of heat and tobacco to the same tissue every time the person smokes.

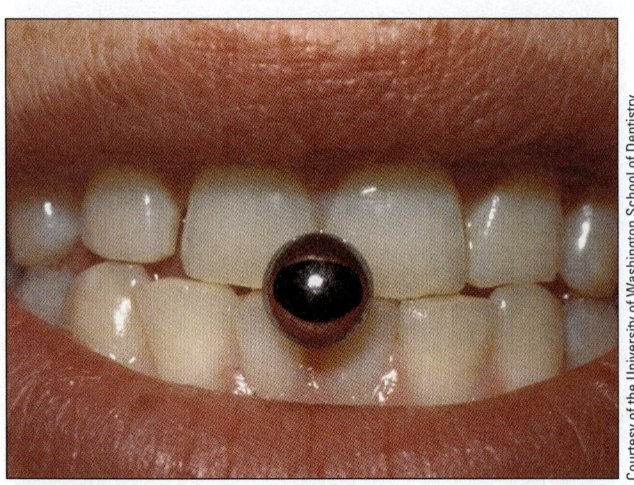
Courtesy of the University of Washington School of Dentistry

FIGURE 27-10
Oral piercing.

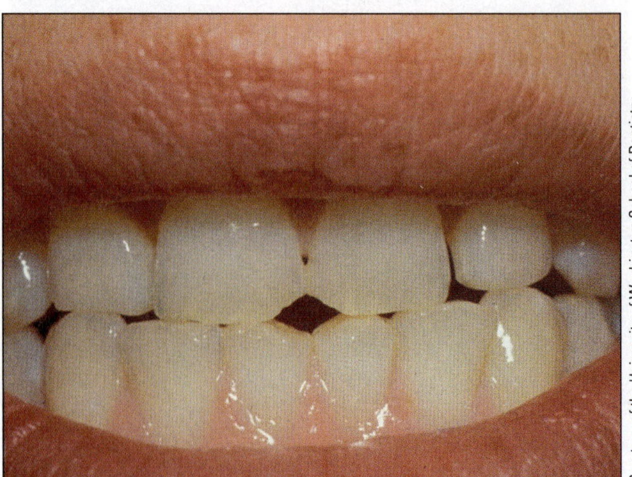
Courtesy of the University of Washington School of Dentistry

FIGURE 27-11
Oral piercing with damage to the teeth and tissues.

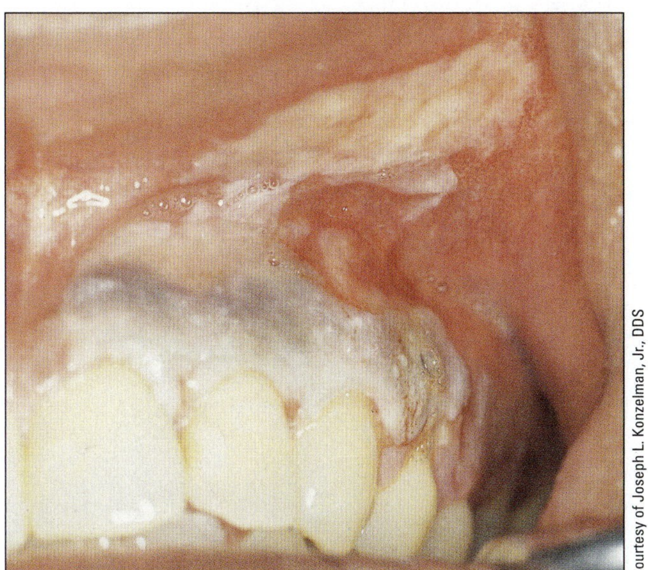

FIGURE 27-12
Aspirin burn.

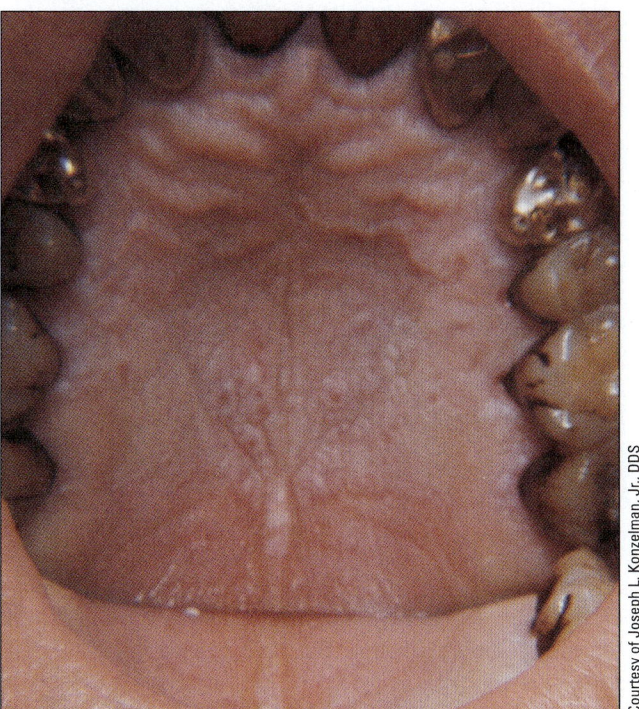

FIGURE 27-13
Nicotine stomatitis.

The affected area of tissue first turns red in response to the irritation. If the irritation continues, the tissue presents as whitened and red, **hyperkeratinized** nodules. Hyperkeratinized tissue occurs where the epithelial tissue builds up a layer of keratin as a protective coating. The **orifices** (openings) of the salivary glands appear to be inflamed. The patient should be made aware of this condition and be encouraged to stop smoking. Normally, the condition disappears if the patient ceases to smoke.

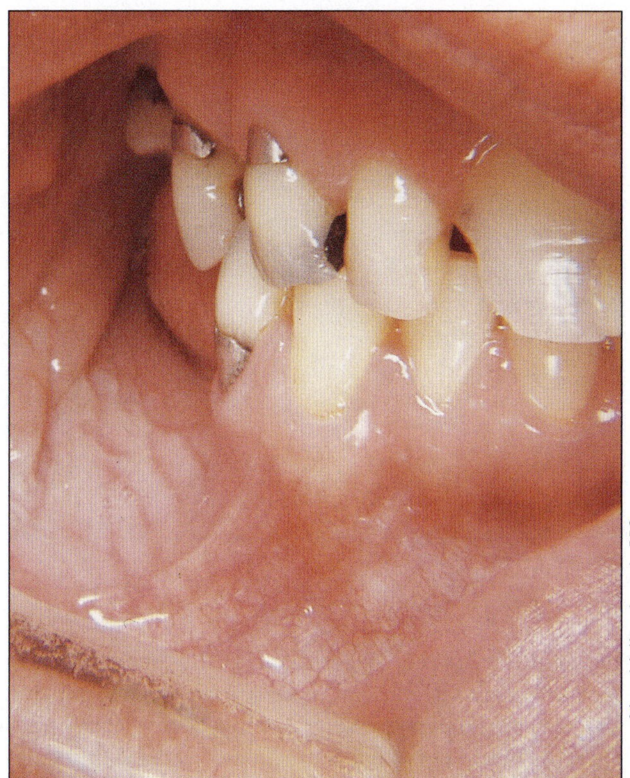

FIGURE 27-14
Chewing tobacco (snuff) lesion.

Chewing Tobacco (Snuff) Lesion

Snuff is a preparation of powdered tobacco (often mixed with other substances) for inhalation into the nose. It is also formed into a wad for chewing. It contains nicotine and is addictive. In this chapter, snuff is referred to as chewing tobacco. Lesions caused by this form of tobacco appear in the oral vestibule, normally the lower anterior area between the lip and the teeth, as wrinkled, white, thickened tissue. Like nicotine stomatitis lesions, the severity of a snuff lesion depends on how often the smokeless tobacco is used and how sensitive the individual is to the product (Figure 27-14).

Smoking Other Drugs

Individuals smoking other drugs, such as marijuana, may exhibit the clinical signs of tobacco irritation. Marijuana irritations normally are apparent in the middle anterior section of the lips, both maxillary and mandibular. This tissue appears red in the early stages, and white with thick, wrinkled tissue in the later stages. This occurs primarily because a device, such as a "roach clip," is used to hold the drug as it is smoked down to a very small piece; therefore, the heat and the drug are concentrated on the lips.

Hairy Tongue

A condition in which the filiform papillae of the tongue become elongated and appear like hairs is called **hairy tongue** (also called the black hairy tongue, lingua nigra, melanoglossia,

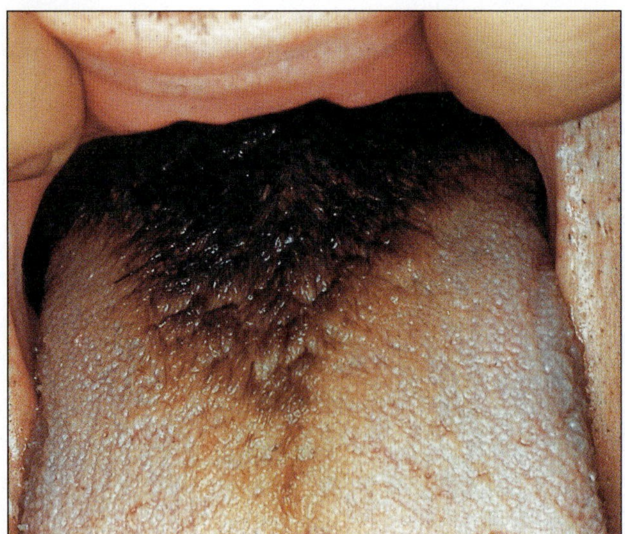

FIGURE 27-15
Hairy tongue.

and migrities linguae) (Figure 27-15). This "hair" normally becomes stained by tobacco, food, or other microorganisms, making it appear dark in color. Hairy tongue may appear without a known cause, but it is normally associated with chemotherapeutic agents such as drugs, hydrogen peroxide mouth rinses, and antibiotics. Treatment of this condition is to stop the known cause, if applicable, and use good oral hygiene, including brushing the tongue. In extreme cases, the filiform papillae grow so long that they cause the person to gag. If this happens, the papillae can be trimmed to alleviate gagging.

Gingival Hyperplasia

A condition known as **gingival hyperplasia** occurs when the connective tissue grows over the teeth (Figure 27-16). This fibrous mass is not uncomfortable to the patient but can inhibit eating and alter the patient's appearance. There are numerous causes of this condition: plaque, orthodontic braces, and various drugs. Phenytoin (Dilantin™) causes this symptom in about one-half of patients being treated with this medication. The condition is referred to as Dilantin hyperplasia.

The condition is normally reduced after the irritant is removed or the patient stops taking the drugs, but that solution is not always preferable. If ongoing drug therapy is necessary, the tissue can be removed surgically and recurrence is probable.

Meth Mouth

Methamphetamines have become an often used illegal drug in part because the drug is easily made with inexpensive ingredients, and the high from these drugs lasts up to 12 hours. Street names include ice, crank, crystal, meth, speed, fire, glass, and chalk, and the pills are called yaba. Meth is consumed via injecting, smoking, snorting, or swallowing. Effects on the oral cavity may be devastating. The acid in the drug causes cravings for high-calorie carbonated drinks. Rampant decay is common in cases of "meth mouth" (Figure 27-17),

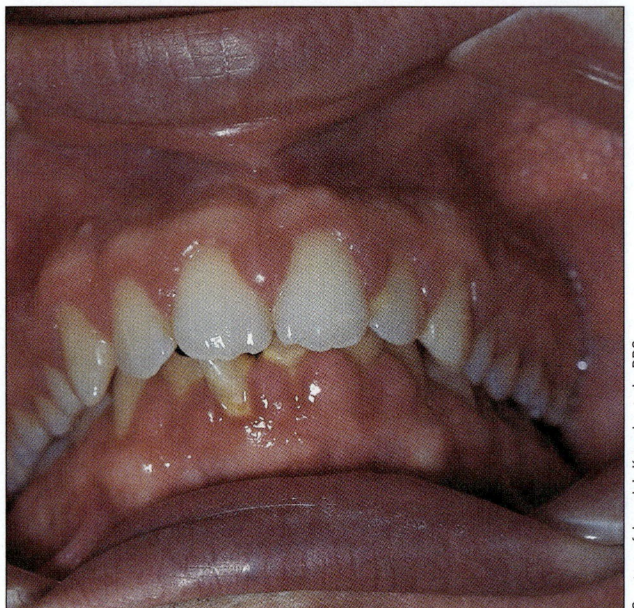

Courtesy of Joseph L. Konzelman, Jr., DDS

FIGURE 27-16
Gingival hyperplasia.

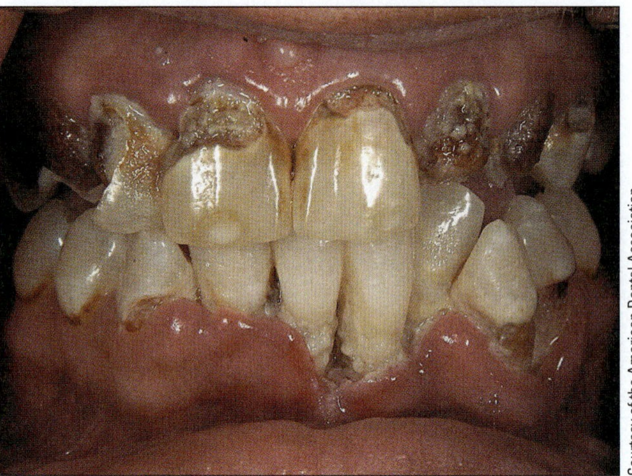

Courtesy of the American Dental Association

FIGURE 27-17
Meth mouth.

and, often, teeth seem to have exploded. Dental treatment is typically complicated, long term, and expensive.

Hormonal Disturbances

Oral conditions can be caused by a change in hormonal balance. Puberty and pregnancy cause hormonal changes that affect the oral tissues. An individual who notices soreness in the gingival tissue must pay close attention to oral hygiene so that the condition does not progress.

Pregnancy Gingivitis

Pregnancy gingivitis occurs in about 5 percent of pregnant women. The gingival tissues appear enlarged and inflamed. A few pregnant women with this condition also develop tumors (see next section). Both of these conditions clear up

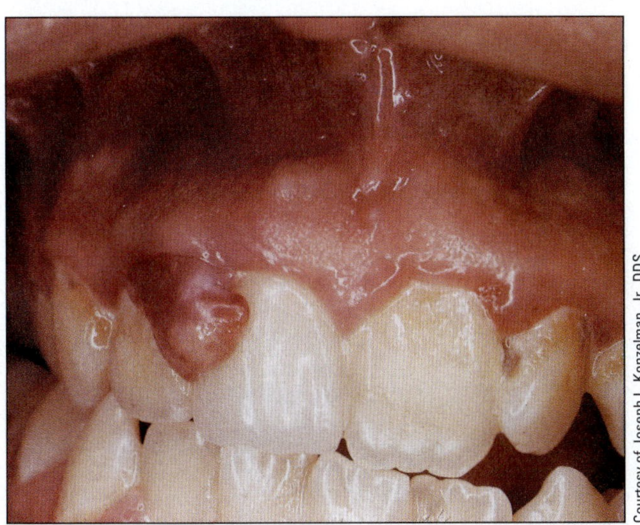

FIGURE 27-18
Pyogenic granuloma.

once the hormonal balance returns to normal, but good oral hygiene practices must be followed to control gingivitis and bleeding.

Pyogenic Granuloma

Often called a pregnancy tumor, **pyogenic granuloma** (pie-oh-**JEN**-ick) is also found in males and non-pregnant females (Figure 27-18). It may be seen in orthodontic patients where poor oral hygiene is a factor, or in patients who have extremely poor oral hygiene. This overgrowth of granulation tissue occurs as a result of local irritation. The tumor is a red, vascular mass ranging in size from a few millimeters to several centimeters, and grows rapidly. Normally, it is not painful and can be excised. The cause is hormonal disturbances, and the lesion may grow back if the situation continues. Therefore, it is not prudent to remove the lesion during the pregnancy unless the patient is uncomfortable. Other factors, such as calculus on the teeth, should be removed to eliminate irritation to the area.

Puberty Gingival Enlargement

Adolescents going through puberty can experience gingival enlargement due to hormonal changes. The condition appears much like pregnancy gingivitis as the gingival tissue is enlarged, bleeds easily, and appears soft and swollen. This condition is more common in girls than in boys. It corrects itself after hormonal balance is stabilized, and good oral hygiene practices are maintained.

Developmental Disturbances

A wide range of anomalies can take place if any stage of embryo development is disturbed. In the oral cavity, anomalies occur in about one in every 800 children born. Some of these **congenital** (present at birth) conditions are genetic (inherited). Other anomalies are caused by outside agents, such as alcohol, drugs, or a mother's illness during pregnancy such as syphilis (refer to biological agents).

One such developmental disturbance is clefting in the oral cavity, such as a cleft lip or cleft palate (see Chapter 8, Embryology and Histology). The majority of these conditions are **innocuous** (harmless); however, some conditions cause eating, speaking, and esthetic difficulties. The construction of an obturator (an appliance that aids in swallowing) for the cleft palate may be necessary to treat the condition.

Disturbances in Tooth Development

As the teeth are developing, a number of disturbances can occur.

Amelogenesis Imperfecta. One developmental disturbance, **amelogenesis imperfecta**, is a genetic (inherited) condition of the teeth in which the enamel is discolored, partially missing, or extremely thin. These teeth can be more susceptible to dental caries. Treatment may consist of composite restorations that cover the entire surface of the teeth.

Ankylosis. In the condition of **ankylosis**, the tooth, cementum, or dentin fuses with the alveolar bone, restricting the movement of the tooth as well as its eruption. An ankylosed tooth appears below the normal occlusal plane of the adjacent teeth. If this condition affects a third molar, removing the tooth becomes quite difficult. The dentist may have to use a handpiece and a bur to separate the tooth from the bone to remove it from the socket.

Anodontia. When teeth are congenitally missing this is called **anodontia**. This condition can affect primary or permanent teeth, or both. It is most often seen in permanent third molars. Many individuals only develop one or two of their third molars, or wisdom teeth. Some individuals develop no third molars.

Dentinogenesis Imperfecta. The condition of **dentinogenesis imperfecta** is characterized by enamel that appears to be opalescent, blue grey, or yellow brown in color and chips away from the dentin soon after eruption of the tooth. This hereditary condition normally appears in both deciduous and permanent teeth. The pulp chambers are missing, as are the root canals. Normally, these patients present with attrition (wearing away) due to a lack of enamel.

Fusion. A condition in which the enamel and dentin of two or more individual teeth join together is **fusion**. The incisal or occlusal surface may show an indentation between the two teeth, and they normally are much broader in appearance. This condition most often is seen in mandibular anterior deciduous teeth.

Gemination. The condition of **gemination** may appear much like a fusion, but, in this case, one tooth bud attempts to divide. The indentation on the incisal or occlusal surface is apparent.

Macrodontia. The term **macrodontia** describes teeth that are abnormally large. The entire dentition may manifest itself in macrodontia teeth, or only one or two teeth may develop in this manner.

Microdontia. The term **microdontia** describes teeth that are abnormally small. This condition is often seen in individuals with Down's syndrome and those born with congenital heart disease. Small teeth can be apparent in the entire dentition or only show up in one or two teeth. Commonly, the maxillary laterals show as microdontia teeth. In this area, the teeth are often peg shaped and small.

Neonatal Teeth. Teeth that are present at the time of birth or within the first month after birth are called **neonatal teeth** (natal teeth). Normally, the baby sheds these teeth very quickly, because the roots are not formed yet.

Supernumerary Teeth. Extra teeth are called **supernumerary teeth**. They appear dwarfed in size and shape, but normal in all other aspects. Supernumerary teeth are seen most frequently in the maxillary anterior (mesiodens) or third molar area (paramolar), both maxillary and mandibular.

Twinning. The condition of **twinning** occurs when the germination process has been successful and two separate teeth are made from a single tooth bud. The tooth appears as a clone of the original tooth in both shape and size.

Oral Tori

Bony outgrowths of tissue in the oral cavity that are benign (nonmalignant) in nature are called **tori**. In the maxillary hard palate, they are termed torus palatinus. In the mandibular canine or premolar region, they are called torus mandibularis.

Tori palatinus are normally seen close to the midline but can occur on the lateral borders (Figure 27-19). Approximately one in every five adults has a maxillary torus, and about one in every twenty has a mandibular torus. Tori mandibulares are more annoying, because food debris can collect under them (Figure 27-20). Both tori conditions present with surfaces of hard bone covered with thin coverings of tissue. The dental assistant must be careful while taking oral radiographs. He or she should examine the oral cavity carefully before placing the film or sensor into position. The radiographs can abrade the tissue and cause the patient discomfort if placed directly on the tissue covering the bony growths.

These growths are not removed unless the patient needs a prosthetic appliance, such as a denture or a lower partial. The growths are then surgically removed to allow room for the dental appliance.

Exostoses

An enlargement or nodular outgrowth of dense lamella bone (a thin structure extending from the facial surface) that appears on the facial surfaces of the mandibular and maxillary palates is called **exostosis**. These enlargements, which appear much like tori, may be variations of the same developmental disturbance. There is no treatment, unless a dental appliance is necessary, or the enlargements hamper mastication (chewing) for the patient.

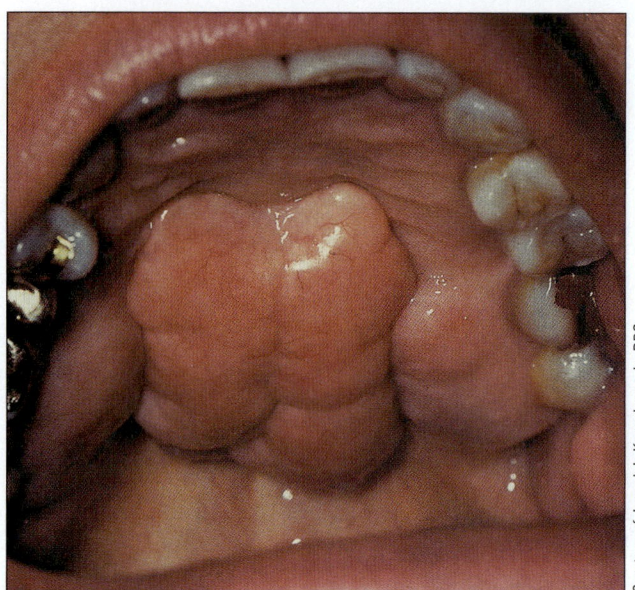

Courtesy of Joseph L. Konzelman, Jr., DDS

FIGURE 27-19
Torus palatinus.

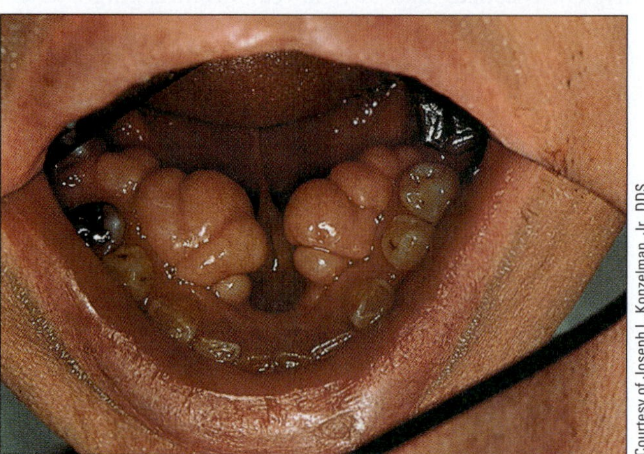

Courtesy of Joseph L. Konzelman, Jr., DDS

FIGURE 27-20
Torus mandibularis.

Fordyce's Spots (Granules)

In about 80 percent of the population, numerous light-yellow spots in the oral cavity are present. These round lesions, called **Fordyce's spots**, are sebaceous oil glands near the surface of the epithelium (Figure 27-21). They can be found anywhere in the oral cavity, but most often are on the buccal mucosa. No identified causes are known, and no treatment is necessary.

Fissured Tongue

A **fissured tongue** occurs in about 5 percent of the population (Figure 27-22). It appears as a wrinkled, deeply grooved surface on the tongue. Fissured tongue may be symmetrical or irregular in pattern. The patient may experience discomfort due to retention of debris in the deep fissures. No treatment is necessary, although the patient may use a home irrigating device to clean the fissures occasionally.

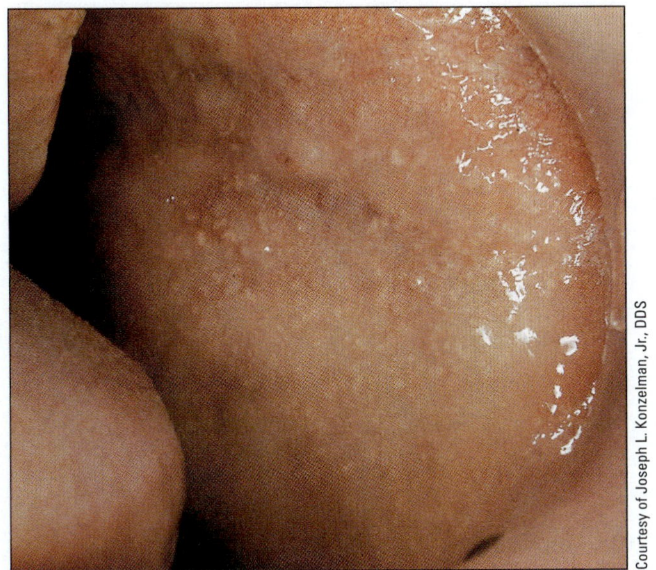

FIGURE 27-21
Fordyce's spots.

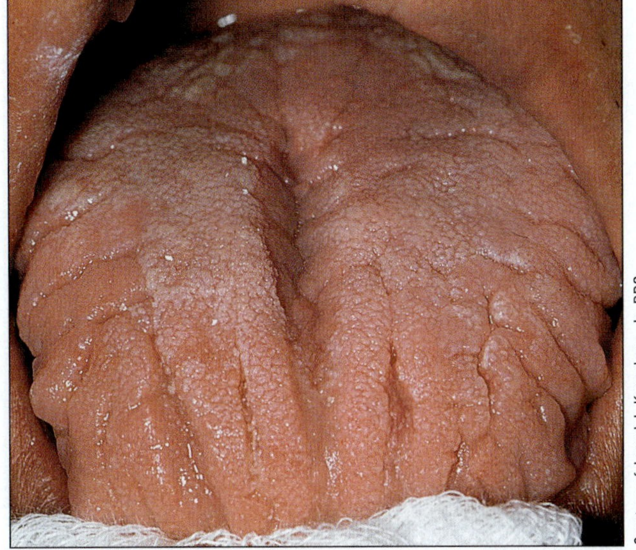

FIGURE 27-22
Fissured tongue.

Bifid Tongue

If the two lateral halves of the anterior two-thirds of the tongue fail to fuse completely, a condition known as **bifid tongue** occurs. It appears as an extra tag of muscle at the end of the tongue. No treatment is necessary, unless the extra tag of tongue is annoying; then, it is surgically removed.

Ankyloglossia

The term commonly used for **ankyloglossia** is "tongue tied" (Figure 27-23). The lingual frenulum is attached near the tip of the tongue, which limits movement of the tongue and may interfere with the enunciation of specific sounds and eating. This condition can be corrected with a simple surgical procedure, which enables the individual to overcome related speech problems. A dental assistant should watch for this condition in children. Under direction of the dentist, while waiting for local anesthetic to take effect, ask the child to stick the tongue out and move it across the upper lip from side to side. Note if a restriction is present, and bring this information to the attention of the dentist for further evaluation.

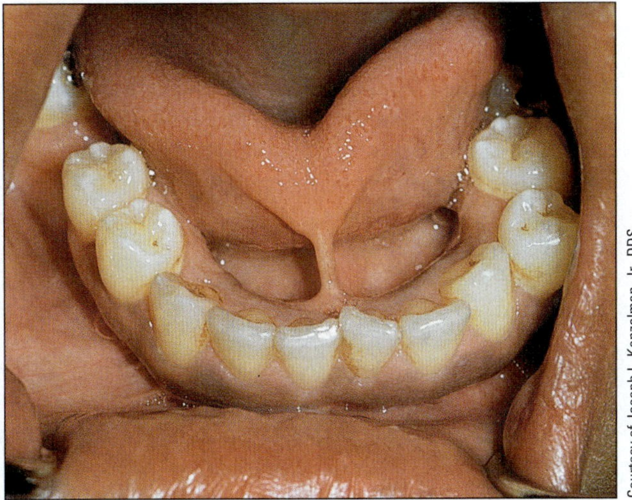

FIGURE 27-23
Ankyloglossia.

Nutritional Disturbances

The oral cavity can reveal a number of conditions resulting from inadequate diet. It is important to consult with all patients about eating a well-balanced diet (see Chapter 5, Nutrition).

Angular Cheilitis

Vitamin B complex deficiency results in a condition known as **angular cheilitis**. A lesion forms in the corner of the mouth, involving both the mucous membrane and the skin (Figure 27-24). This condition may also occur if the patient constantly licks the corners of the mouth (commissures), or if the patient loses vertical dimension of the face. A loss of vertical dimension occurs when a person overcloses the mouth because the occlusal plane is worn down or the bone structure beneath a denture is deteriorated. The end of the chin is closer to the tip of the nose, and the corners of the mouth cave in, which allows saliva to pool in the corners. This condition permits the growth of microorganisms; as a result, fungal **opportunistic infections** such as *candidiasis* are often found in this area.

This condition is treated via correction of vitamin B deficiency or the use of antifungal drugs. Dentures can be remade or the teeth crowned and extended in length to correct the loss of vertical dimension.

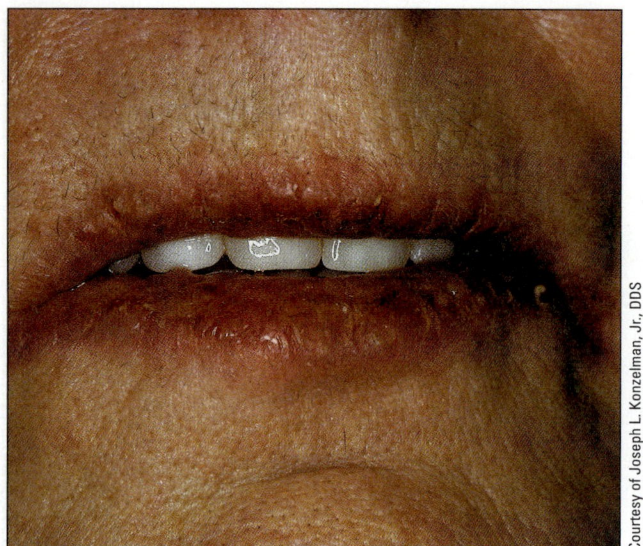
Courtesy of Joseph L. Konzelman, Jr., DDS

FIGURE 27-24
Angular cheilitis.

Glossitis (Bald Tongue)

Another condition reportedly caused by the lack of the vitamin B complex is **glossitis**. Glossitis literally means "inflammation of the tongue." The filiform papillae on the tongue are absent, and the tongue appears to be smooth, hence the name bald tongue. The tongue may be sore and the patient may experience difficulty while eating. A well-balanced diet aids in correcting this condition.

Oral Cancer

Cancer is a disease involving abnormal cell growth that has the potential to invade or spread into all areas of the body. There are over 100 types of cancer. Oral cancer is one of the most common forms of cancer. It appears as a sore or growth in the mouth and the lips, and does not go away. It is not usually painful so it can go undetected, but if it is not diagnosed and treated early, it can be life threatening. Oral cancer includes cancers of the lips, tongue, cheeks, floor of the mouth, hard and soft palate, sinuses, and pharynx (throat) (Figure 27-25). More men get oral cancer than women in the United States, according to the American Cancer Society, and men over age 50 are at the greatest risk. Smokers are six times more likely to develop oral cancers than nonsmokers, and smokeless tobacco users are 50 times more likely to develop cancers of the lips and cheek.

The signs and symptoms of oral cancer are listed in the box, Oral Cancer Warning Signs. If any of these symptoms are noticed, a dentist or health care provider should be seen immediately. The risk factors for the development of oral cancer include the following:

- Smoking cigarettes, cigars, or pipes
- People who use smokeless tobacco including dip, snuff, or chewing products
- Alcohol use in excess

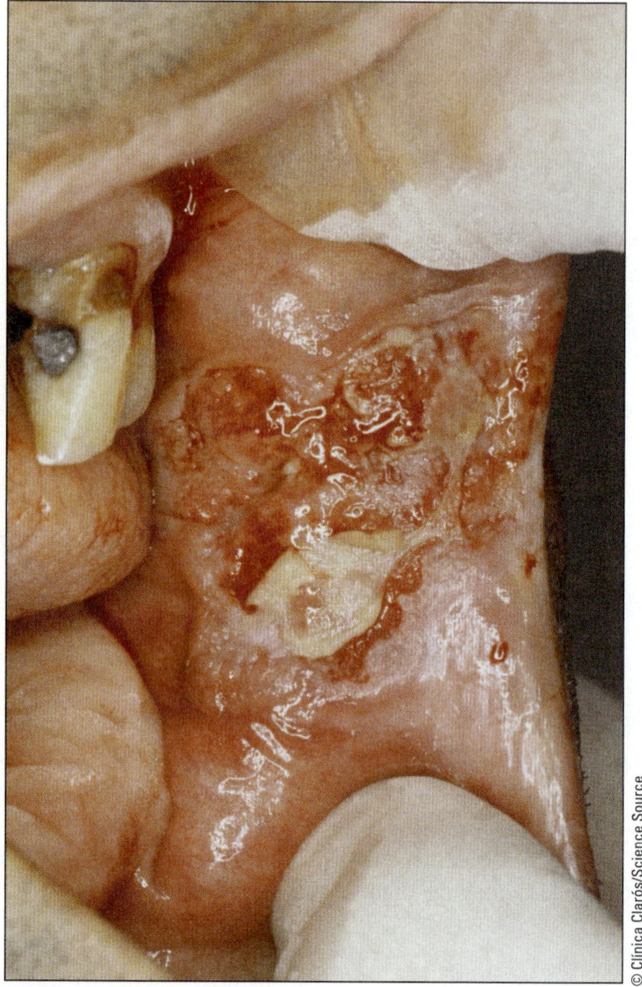
© Clínica Claros/Science Source

FIGURE 27-25
Oral cancer on the cheek.

- Family history of cancer
- Excessive exposure to the sun, especially at a young age
- Infections such as hepatitis B, hepatitis C, and human papillomavirus (HPV)

A **carcinoma** is one of the most common types of cancer. They are formed by epithelial cells, which are cells that cover the inside (lining) and outside (skin) surfaces of the body. Carcinomas are abnormal cells that spread (*metastasize*) to other parts of the body. This cancer is found on the lips, cheeks, and the floor of the mouth.

A **sarcoma** is a type of cancer cell that occurs in connective tissue cells. These tissues support the body and include cartilage, tendons, bones, muscles, and the fibrous tissue in organs. There are two main types of sarcomas: *osteosarcoma*, which develop in the bones, such as the jaw bone; and soft tissue sarcoma, which occurs in all other types of connective tissue.

Cancer is detected by specific signs and symptoms, or by screening tests. Tissues are then evaluated through medical imaging and biopsy. Once the cancer has been diagnosed it is often treated with surgery, chemotherapy, radiation therapy, targeted therapy, or a combination of these. Pain, nausea, and symptom management are part of the care.

The different treatments often have effects on tissues in the oral cavity. Examples of the effects of radiation therapy includes xerostomia (dry mouth), which occurs when radiation reduces the production of saliva or makes it so the salvia glands are no longer able to produce saliva; and dental caries which may appear with the lack of salvia. There may also be a decreased supply of blood to the jaw bone, which may cause a weakening of the bones, and may lessen any healing. Chemotherapy drugs are powerful drugs that may also affect the oral tissues.

Neoplasms

As stated earlier, *neoplasm* is a medical term for tumor. This group of lesions has great potential for becoming **malignant** (cancerous). The dental assistant should be knowledgeable about the causes of these diseases and should perform careful clinical examinations for premalignant lesions. Even if it is known that a tumor is benign (harmless), it is important that all lesions are brought to the attention of the dentist, without alarming the patient. Early recognition of the tumor could save the patient's life.

Oral Cancer Warning Signs

- A sore in the oral cavity, face, or mouth that bleeds easily and does not heal within 2 weeks
- Lumps or bumps, rough spots, or swelling in the oral cavity, on the lips, or on the neck
- White, red, or rash-like lesions in the mouth or on the lips
- Dryness in the mouth over a period of time for no apparent reason
- Hoarseness, chronic sore throat, change in the voice for no apparent reason
- Numbness, pain, tenderness in or around the oral cavity, ear, and neck
- Soreness or burning sensation in or around the oral cavity
- Feeling that something is caught in the back of the throat
- Difficulty speaking, chewing, or swallowing, or moving the jaw or the tongue
- Change in the way the teeth fit together or the way dentures fit
- Repeated bleeding in a specific area of the mouth for no apparent reason
- Significant weight lost for no known reason

Leukoplakia

A white, leathery patch that cannot be identified as any other type of lesion is termed **leukoplakia** (**loo**-koh-**PLAY**-kee-ah) (Figure 27-26). A biopsy is required to further identify the lesion. The dentist normally views these lesions with concern, because they may be precipitating factors to cancer. They are found throughout the oral mucosa and can be very dense or very diffuse. The operator is not able to wipe the lesion off with two-by-two gauze as he or she could with thrush. Leukoplakia is often seen in the lower lip of a person who uses chewing tobacco. Normally, excessive alcohol and tobacco usage, vitamin A deficiency, or trauma are associated with the lesion.

Biopsy results normally show hyperkeratinization, a thickening of the outer layer of the skin due to an excess of keratin. This condition is similar to developing corns on the feet due to constant irritation. Biopsies also could reveal **dysplastic cells**, that is, abnormal cell features such as size, shape, and rate of multiplication. Dysplasic cells often become malignant.

Lichen Planus

The initial skin lesion of **lichen planus** usually appears on the lower leg or ankle. This lesion is a flat-topped papule, dark red or violet in color. The oral lesions (reticular lichen planus) begin as small, white papules that group and form interlacing white lines known as **Wickham's striae** (Figure 27-27). In most cases, they are on the buccal mucosa. An erosive form of the lesion (erosive lichen planus) causes the loss of oral epithelium in the infected area. Both types are fairly common, with reticular lichen planus being asymptomatic

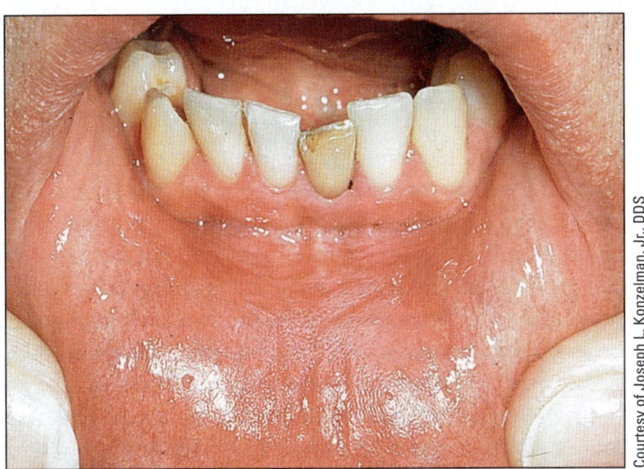

Courtesy of Joseph L. Konzelman, Jr., DDS

FIGURE 27-26
Leukoplakia.

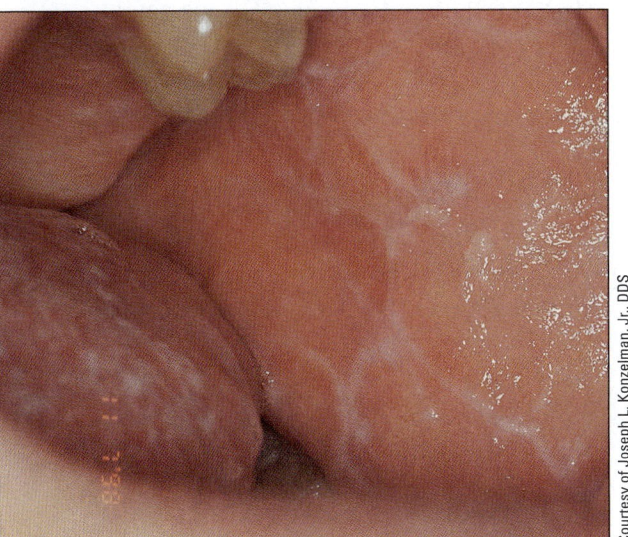

Courtesy of Joseph L. Konzelman, Jr., DDS

FIGURE 27-27
Lichen planus.

and erosive lichen planus usually being more tender and painful. A patient may exhibit pain while eating, and some foods may aggravate the condition. The treatment is topical steroid therapy.

It is unknown whether lichen planus is a premalignant condition. Patients should be examined periodically for any changes in this condition.

Erythroplakia

Any red patch of tissue in the oral cavity that cannot be associated with inflammation is termed **erythroplakia** (eh-rith-roh-**PLAY**-kee-ah). Most commonly, this condition appears in the soft palate, retromolar pad area, or the floor of the mouth. It is usually seen in patients over 60 who have used tobacco and alcoholic beverages on a regular basis.

This lesion is of great concern, because almost 100 percent of biopsies indicate premalignant or malignant tissue. Treatment depends on the extent of the lesion. In early stages, it can be removed surgically; however, in later stages, it is necessary to treat the lesion with radiation and chemotherapy.

Leukemia

The condition, **leukemia**, is a cancer of the blood cells. It starts in the bone marrow, where the blood cells are made. A person who has leukemia will make a lot of abnormal white blood cells (leukocytes) that do not work like normal cells and grow faster. The symptoms include painless lumps in the neck, underarm, stomach or groin and swollen lymph nodes, enlarged liver or spleen, bleeding, bruising, infections, night sweats, pain, weight loss, and unexplained tiredness.

The leukemia may be acute or chronic. Acute leukemia moves very fast and a person may feel sick and show signs immediately. Chronic leukemia may not show symptoms for years, and then the disease appears gradually.

Oral symptoms of leukemia include gingivitis, swelling of the tissues, and bleeding of the gums. For some, the first signs of leukemia show in the mouth (Figure 27-28).

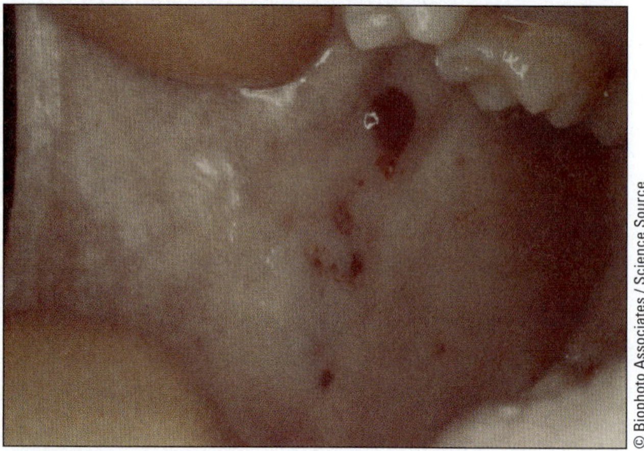

FIGURE 27-28

Leukemia.

Squamous Cell Carcinoma

A **carcinoma** is a malignant neoplasm (tumor) that can spread, or **metastasize**, into the surrounding tissue and lymph nodes. Typically, it first appears as an ulcerated area in the soft tissues of the mouth. A **squamous cell carcinoma** is cancer of the squamous epithelium (Figure 27-29). Nine out of ten oral cancers are of this type.

Factors associated with causing carcinomas are sunlight exposure and long-term use of tobacco or alcohol. Normally, squamous cell carcinomas are seen in adults over 40, but have also been found in younger patients. More cases have been documented in males than females. Squamous cell carcinoma is found primarily on the floor of the oral cavity under the tongue, on the sides or borders of the tongue, and on the soft palate tonsil area.

The lesion may first appear as a thickened, white plaque that develops into an ulcer. As it grows, this ulcer seems to encompass other tissues. Soon, a rolled border appears with the center tissue. The mass continues to grow, rising above the normal tissue level.

Treatment for squamous cell carcinoma depends on the size, site, and spread of the tumor. Early detection is essential, because if the carcinoma metastasizes into the lymph nodes, the survival rate is greatly diminished.

Basal Cell Carcinoma

The most common form of skin cancer is **basal cell carcinoma** (Figure 27-30). Lesions normally appear on the neck, ear, face, lip, and head. Because it is the area primarily exposed to the sun, the face is the principal site. Fair-skinned individuals are more susceptible to this carcinoma, as are men over 40.

Unlike squamous cells, these cells typically do not metastasize. They invade the area around them as they grow. The lesion first appears as a nodule and then ulcerates, the borders rise, and the center develops into a crater.

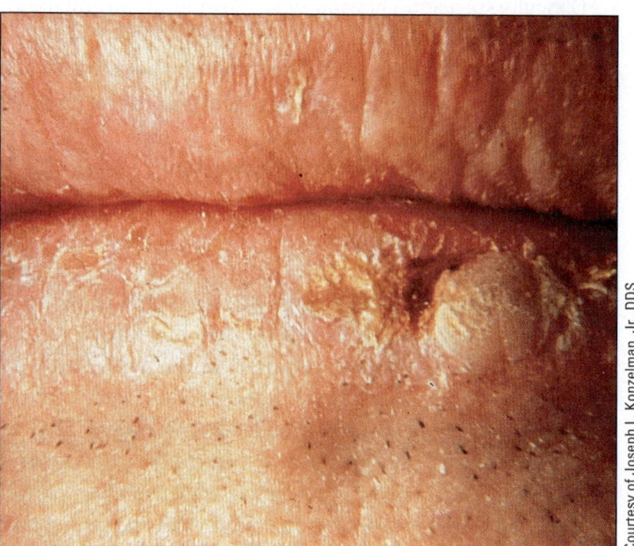

FIGURE 27-29

Squamous cell carcinoma.

Surgical removal of the lesion is the principal treatment. Patients commonly develop more than one lesion. Careful clinical examinations of the head and neck can be performed during 6-month recall appointments to identify other lesions at an early stage.

Papilloma. A lesion of squamous epithelial tissue that is benign is called a **papilloma**. A papilloma resembles a cauliflower in appearance because it seems to have a number of projections deriving from a single origin (Figure 27-31). It is not caused by continued irritation, like many of the neoplasms, but rather occurs after the individual has been infected by a virus. A number of viruses have resulted in a similar type of lesion. This lesion ranges in color from white to red, and is normally 1 to 3 cm in size.

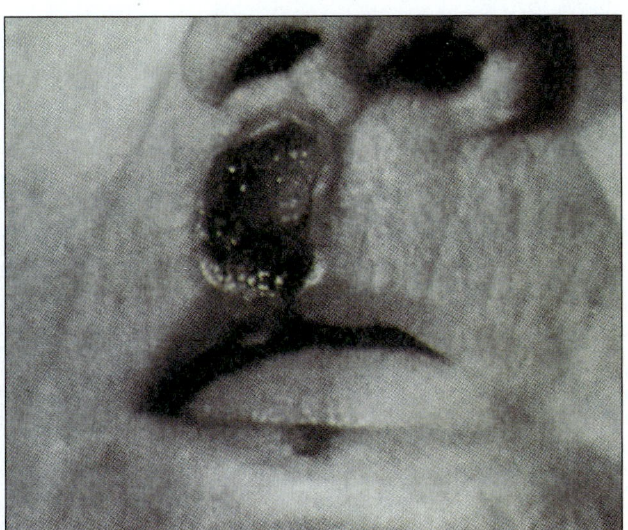

FIGURE 27-30
Basal cell carcinoma.

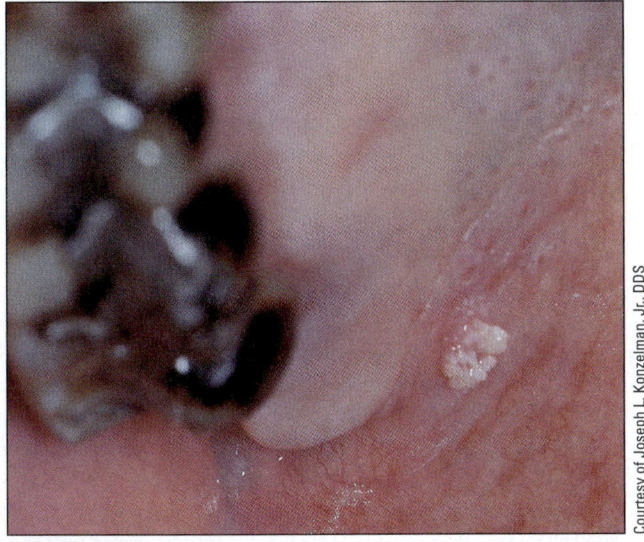

Courtesy of Joseph L. Konzelman, Jr., DDS

FIGURE 27-31
Papilloma.

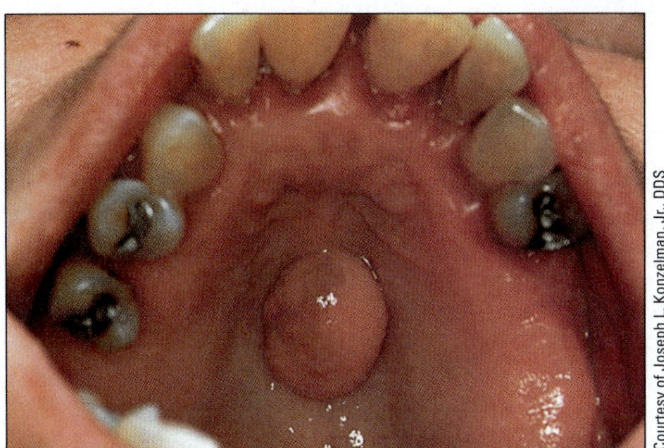

Courtesy of Joseph L. Konzelman, Jr., DDS

FIGURE 27-32
Fibroma.

Treatment of the papilloma is to surgically remove it along with a small amount of normal epithelial cells at the base of the lesion.

Fibroma

A **fibroma** is a benign tumor of connective tissue cells (cells that surround and support structures) (Figure 27-32). A fibroma is a reactive hyperplasia, rather than a true neoplasm. It presents in the oral cavity as a dome-shaped, pink-colored, smooth-surfaced lesion less than 2 cm in diameter. Normally, it is found on the buccal (cheek) surface, proximal to where the teeth occlude. The fibroma forms because of continued irritation of the teeth biting together. Continued trauma causes the connective tissue to grow. This benign tumor may be surgically excised or left without treatment. Recurrence of a fibroma is rare.

Oral Lesions Related to AIDS and HIV

AIDS is an immune system disorder that follows infection by the **human immunodeficiency virus (HIV)**. Healthy individuals can combat most microorganisms that cause disease, but individuals with suppressed immune systems do not fare as well. Opportunistic infections such as the herpes virus, hepatitis, tuberculosis, candidiasis, and pneumonia are common. There is no cure for AIDS, and treatment is focused on the complications associated with it. Patients who are infected with HIV have specific oral manifestations related to the disease.

Patients with AIDS are much more susceptible to periodontal lesions than healthy individuals. The gingival tissue becomes inflamed, red, and bulbous, and bone loss occurs. Bacteria and yeast are found in the infected area. This condition is extremely painful and the tissue bleeds readily when touched. Normal oral hygiene techniques are not as effective as they are in a healthy individual.

Treatment consists of extremely good oral hygiene, root planing and curettage, rinses, and antibiotic therapy.

Hairy Leukoplakia

In the early 1980s, a raised, white-patched lesion called **hairy leukoplakia** was identified in patients known to be infected with HIV (Figure 27-33). It appears much like the candidiasis lesion but cannot be removed by wiping with gauze. Hairy leukoplakia is a white, patterned lesion normally found on the borders of the tongue. This lesion is not painful, and no treatment is available. If the patient has not been tested for HIV, the dentist may suggest testing.

HIV/AIDS Patients, and patients who have had cancer treatment, such as chemotherapy, and are immunodepressed, are likely to develop an infection called *candidiasis*. This fungal infection is much like thrush, and is the first oral lesion manifesting from the HIV infection. The membrane presents as a white, thick, plaque-like covering in linear patterns on top of a red, inflamed surface (Figure 27-34). It can be present on numerous oral membranes, but normally appears on the tongue and buccal mucosa. Patients often report a burning sensation in the area of the infection. Treatment consists of antifungal medications such as Nystatin™ (see Chapter 15, Pharmacology).

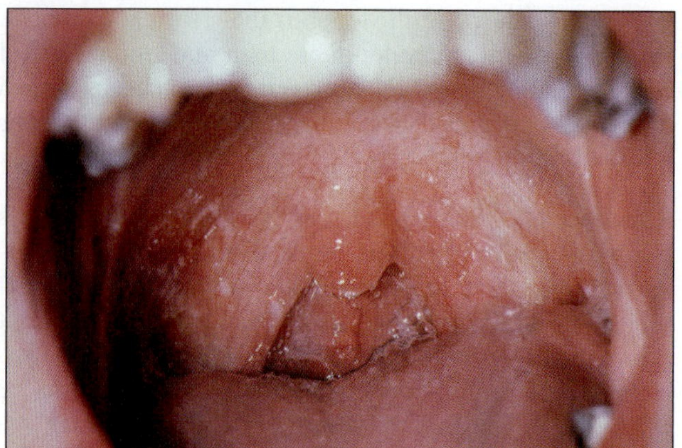

FIGURE 27-34
Candidiasis in an HIV patient.

Kaposi's Sarcoma

A number of AIDS patients present with an unusual malignant vascular tumor called **Kaposi's sarcoma** (Figure 27-35). AIDS patients are susceptible to other malignant tumors, such as squamous cell carcinoma and lymphoma; but until the 1980s and the spread of AIDS, Kaposi's sarcoma was quite rare. In patients with AIDS, Kaposi's sarcoma is aggressive and spreads rapidly.

The lesions, a diffuse blue-purple, appear all over the body, especially on the face, arms, and the palate. They are flat or nodular and, as the tumor enlarges, it becomes a hemorrhagic neoplasm. Bleeding and pain occur in the more advanced stages.

Treatment consists of low-dose radiation and/or chemotherapeutic drugs. The prognosis (outcome) is poor at this stage, and a number of people die from the lymphoreticular neoplasms related to this disease.

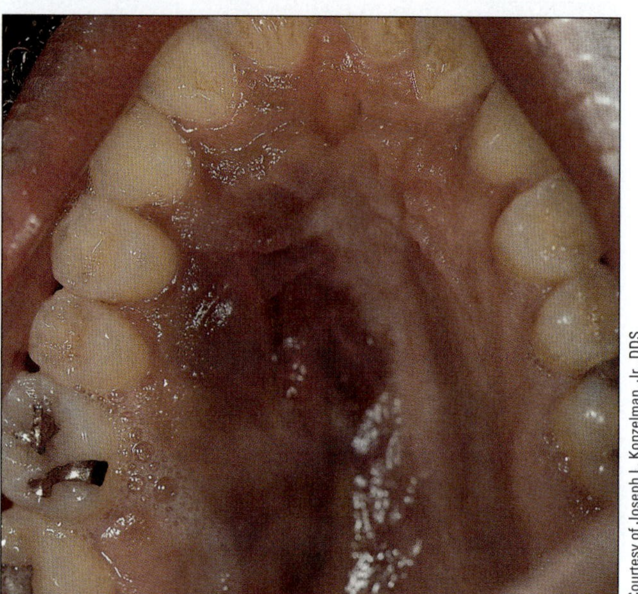

FIGURE 27-35
Kaposi's sarcoma.

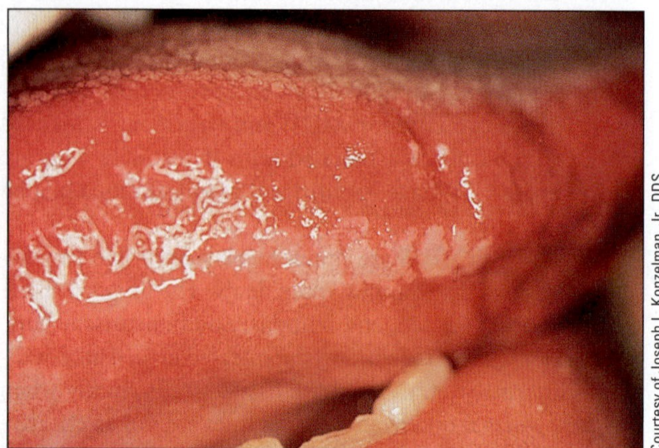

FIGURE 27-33
Hairy leukoplakia.

Miscellaneous Disorders

The dental assistant may see other disorders in the oral cavity. Any lesion appearing to be abnormal should be brought to the dentist's attention.

Acute Necrotizing Ulcerative Gingivitis

The tissues present with bleeding, infection, pain, and a foul odor in a condition known as acute necrotizing ulcerative gingivitis (ANUG) (Figure 27-36). This infectious disease is seen primarily in young adults and adolescents. Poor hygiene, lack of sleep, poor nutrition, and stress are precipitating factors. It was referred to as trench mouth years ago due to the fact that many soldiers who fought in the trenches developed ANUG. It is also seen on college campuses around final exam time.

ANUG is very painful and must be treated with thorough debridement and cleaning. Antibiotics may be prescribed along with oral rinses of warm water. Immaculate oral hygiene is also necessary to treat ANUG. After the condition resolves, the tips of the papilla will, from that time forward, appear to be blunted or flat.

Mucocele

When trauma affects a minor salivary gland, a **mucocele** (**MYOO**-ko-seal) can result (Figure 27-37). This normally takes place on the mandibular anterior lip where a patient accidentally bites into the tissue. If this is at the place of a minor salivary gland, a duct may be closed off. The mucocele may appear like a bubble on the inside of the lip.

Occasionally, a stone-like particle may block the saliva duct opening. If this happens, the gland fills with fluid and enlarges. The gland may be opened and the fluid expressed from the area. Recurrence may necessitate total removal of the duct and gland.

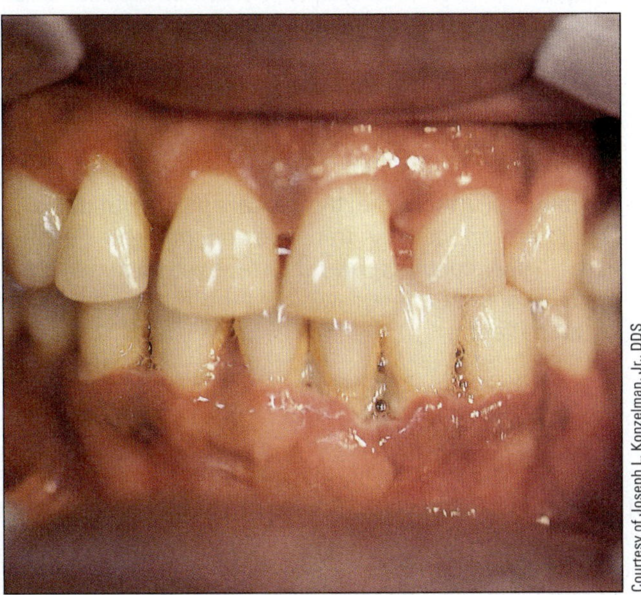

Courtesy of Joseph L. Konzelman, Jr., DDS

FIGURE 27-36

Acute necrotizing ulcerative gingivitis.

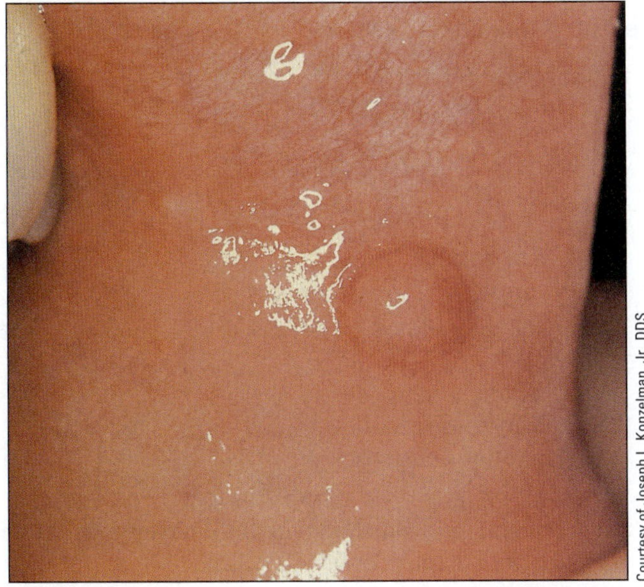

Courtesy of Joseph L. Konzelman, Jr., DDS

FIGURE 27-37

Mucocele.

Varix

A **varix** is a condition primarily seen in the elderly. The blood vessels become weakened and extended. Normally, this condition occurs in the oral cavity beneath the tongue or on the buccal mucosa. These dark-purple, extended vessels in the oral cavity are related to the varicose veins in other parts of the body. They should be noted on the patient's chart, but no treatment is necessary.

Geographic Tongue

Less than 2 percent of the population has an inflammatory condition that affects the tongue, called geographic tongue or benign migratory glossitis (Figure 27-38). It affects the dorsal and lateral surfaces of the tongue and presents as red, smooth patches absent of filiform papillae. Geographic tongue presents with patches that are normally surrounded by an elevated white or yellow border. The area of the patches makes up an ever-changing pattern on the tongue that resembles a map of the world. The condition may have periods of remission. The condition is not painful, and treatment is unnecessary.

Anorexia Nervosa and Bulimia

The diseases of anorexia nervosa (the loss of at least 15 percent body weight, and an intense fear of gaining weight) and bulimia (episodes of out-of-control eating followed by purging) have several implications in oral pathology. Anorexia nervosa is a disease in which extreme aversion to food is present. These patients may be suffering from malnutrition, with symptoms

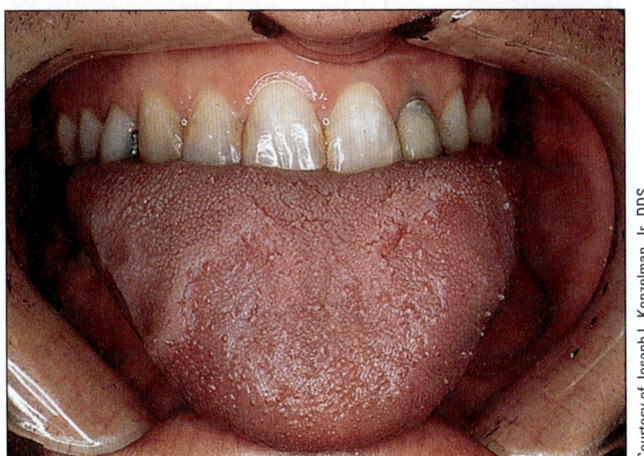

Courtesy of Joseph L. Konzelman, Jr., DDS

FIGURE 27-38

Geographic tongue.

including sore and inflamed tissues from poor periodontal health, The patient suffering from bulimia has symptoms of induced vomiting that have a direct impact on oral health.

Due to constant vomiting/purging, the lingual surfaces of the anterior teeth become decalcified and the enamel is eroded. The occlusal surfaces of the posterior teeth become eroded, causing existing restorations to deteriorate. Rampant caries and enlargement of the parotid glands are also problems, along with the other symptoms of the disease, which are life threatening.

Treatment focuses on symptoms and maintaining comfort until the eating disorder can be reversed. The patient is encouraged to practice immaculate oral hygiene, and to rinse the mouth after purging to decrease acidity and the number of microorganisms. The teeth may be sensitive where the enamel has eroded. Toothpaste for sensitive teeth is suggested as treatment. See Chapter 5, Nutrition, for more information on Anorexia Nervosa and Bulimia.

Bell's Palsy

Bell's palsy (named for Scottish surgeon Sir Charles Bell) is a temporary paralysis of the muscles on one side of the face. The cause is unknown but is thought to be related to herpes zoster (shingles). One side of the face droops down, and the patient cannot close the eye or smile. Some individuals have pain in the ear on the affected side. Taste is diminished, and sounds seem unnaturally loud. Most cases clear up without treatment, but analgesics can be given for symptoms of discomfort, and corticosteroid drugs can be given to reduce inflammation in the nerves.

Chapter Summary

The dental assistant, who sits opposite the dentist, has a different view of the patient's oral cavity. Anything that appears atypical should be brought to the dentist's attention, without alarming the patient.

The dental assistant does not diagnose oral pathological diseases but identifies abnormal conditions in the mouth. Furthermore, the dental assistant must know how to prevent disease transmission, how the identified pathological condition may interfere with planned treatment, and what effect it will have on the overall health of the patient.

CASE STUDY

Josiah Toby Edward, 20 years old, was just given an injection by Dr. Smile. The dental assistant notices that the area where the injection was given is swelling and appears to be raised and bruised. The patient feels no discomfort because the anesthetic has taken effect. Even though the dental assistant does not diagnose the condition, he or she may have some general idea about what is occurring in Toby Edward's mouth. Answer the following review questions with that in mind.

Case Study Review

1. What pathologic condition may be present in Toby Edward's mouth?
2. What should the dental assistant do to treat this condition?
3. What is the prognosis of this condition?

Review Questions

Multiple Choice

1. The first stage of syphilis manifests in a lesion called a
   a. gumma.
   b. chancre.
   c. mucous patch.
   d. split papule.
2. An oral condition that is common in children and appears as a white, thick covering over the oral mucous membranes is called
   a. a papule.
   b. a bulla.
   c. a hematoma.
   d. thrush.
3. All of the following are caused by chemical agents *except*
   a. aspirin burn.
   b. hairy tongue.
   c. nicotine stomatitis.
   d. pustule.
4. A condition in which the tooth, cementum, or dentin fuses with the alveolar bone is called
   a. amelogenesis imperfecta.
   b. ankylosis.
   c. anodontia.
   d. fusion.

5. A vitamin B complex deficiency results in a condition known as
   a. *Candida albicans.*
   b. Fordyce's spots.
   c. glossitis.
   d. angular cheilitis.
6. All but one is involved in the inflammatory process. Identify the one that is not.
   a. Redness
   b. Swelling
   c. Pain
   d. Erosion
7. ________ or shingles appears as unilateral, painful lesions that can last up to 5 weeks.
   a. Syphilis
   b. Herpes zoster
   c. Herpes simplex
   d. Actinomycosis
8. The common name for the fungal infection, candidiasis, in children is ________.
   a. hyperplasia
   b. chickenpox
   c. measles
   d. thrush
9. When connective tissue grows over the teeth, this condition is known as ________.
   a. gingival hyperplasia
   b. Dilantin hyperplasia
   c. pyogenic granuloma
   d. anodontia
10. Extra teeth are ________.
    a. gemination
    b. supernumerary teeth
    c. neonatal teeth
    d. anodontia

Critical Thinking

1. If a dental assistant is taking radiographs on a patient who presents with tori mandibulares, what should be done?
2. A patient presents with a bald tongue. What causes this condition? Is it uncomfortable for the patient? What will help correct the condition?
3. What are the warning signs of oral cancer?

Web Activities

1. Go to http://www.oralcancer.org and find the number of individuals who will develop oral cancer this year.
2. Go to http://www.HIV.org and identify the number of people currently living with AIDS, and look at the data to find the number of AIDS related deaths most recently recorded.
3. Go to http://www.anad.org and identify the physical repercussions of anorexia nervosa and bulimia nervosa. Which of these physical repercussions are related specifically to dentistry?

CHAPTER 28

Orthodontics

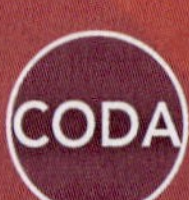

Specific Instructional Objectives

The student should strive to meet the following objectives and demonstrate an understanding of the facts and principles presented in this chapter:

1. Define orthodontics and describe the orthodontic setting.
2. Define the role of the dental assistant in an orthodontic setting.
3. Define and describe occlusion and malocclusion.
4. Identify the causes of malocclusion.
5. Describe preventive, interceptive, and corrective orthodontics.
6. Explain the process of tooth movement.
7. Describe the preorthodontic appointment for diagnostic records.
8. Describe the consultation appointment and the roles of the assistant, patient, and orthodontist.
9. Differentiate between fixed and removable appliances.
10. Identify and describe the function of basic orthodontic instruments.
11. Describe the stages of orthodontic treatment.
12. Explain the procedure for removing orthodontic appliances and how the teeth are kept in position after appliance removal.

Key Terms

activator (671)
Angle's classification (661)
arch wire (667)
Bionator appliance (671)
brackets (667)
buccal tubes (669)
buccoversion (661)
corrective orthodontics (664)
deposition (664)
distoversion (661)
elastics (669)
fixed appliance (664)
Frankel appliance (672)
Hawley retainer (673)
headgear (671)
Herbst appliance (671)
infraversion (661)
interceptive (664)
labioversion (661)
ligature wire (669)
linguoversion (661)
malocclusion (661)
mesioversion (661)
normal occlusion (661)
orthodontic bands (667)
osteoblasts (664)
osteoclasts (664)
overbite (671)
palatal expanding appliance (670)
plastic rings (669)
preventive (664)
removable appliance (664)
resorption (664)
self-ligating bracket (683)
separators (677)
space maintainer (670)
springs (669)
supraversion (661)
tooth positioner (673)
torsoversion (661)
transposition (661)
transversion (661)

Introduction

Orthodontics is the dental specialty that is focused on the recognition, prevention, and treatment of malalignment and irregularities of the teeth, jaws, and facial profile. Patients are of all ages, ranging from children to teenagers, adults, and seniors. Orthodontic treatment provides a beautiful smile that brings teeth, lips, and jaws into proper alignment. Improved teeth and jaw alignment provides better function and easier cleaning, with long-lasting results.

The Orthodontic Practice

The orthodontist spends an additional 2 to 3 academic years of education in an orthodontic residency program after graduating from dental school. Orthodontists continue their education with ongoing courses/seminars in new and advanced technologies and practices. Although the general dentist may perform limited orthodontic treatment, most patients requiring tooth alignment are referred to an orthodontist. Working together the general dentist and orthodontist provide the best treatment for patients. Treatment may extend over several years as the child patient grows and develops and the adult patient's teeth move into the desired position.

Although the orthodontic practice treats mainly children and young adults, the number of adult patients who see an orthodontist is increasing. Adults seek orthodontic treatment for both cosmetic and functional reasons.

Office

The orthodontic office is designed to facilitate a number of patients at different stages of treatment. Specific rooms or areas are used for examination, diagnostic records, and treatment consultations before treatment begins. The treatment area contains several dental chairs and units.

This area is an "open bay," meaning there are no walls separating the dental units (Figure 28-1). The laboratory in the orthodontic office is where appliances and models are fabricated. This area contains equipment and materials necessary to pour impressions, trim study models, and construct orthodontic appliances.

Team

The orthodontic team consists of the orthodontist, reception and business office staff, office coordinator, orthodontic/dental assistants, and laboratory technician(s).

Orthodontist. Orthodontists examine patients, make diagnoses for treatment, and perform orthodontic procedures. They check and evaluate the progress of patients throughout treatment.

Reception and Business Office Staff. The receptionist greets patients and schedules appointments. The business staff takes care of financial arrangements and manages the business administration of the office. They maintain communication with the patients, parents, and the general dentist during the course of treatment.

Office Coordinator. The office coordinator makes sure that the office is run smoothly and efficiently. The coordinator provides information to families considering orthodontic treatment and coordinates the orthodontic assistant's responsibilities during the various phases of patient treatment.

Laboratory Technician. The laboratory technician may pour and trim diagnostic models and working casts. The technician constructs orthodontic appliances and retainers to the specifications of the orthodontist.

Orthodontic Assistant. The orthodontic assistant has a variety of responsibilities depending on the size of the practice and the number of assistants in the practice. *More important, functions allowed also vary with each state's Dental Practice Act.* The orthodontic assistant works with the orthodontist but also functions independently to complete many orthodontic tasks. Examine the state Dental Practice Act to become familiar with which skills are allowed to be used. Several states have different skill levels that coordinate with the levels of education the dental assistant has received.

Generally, the orthodontic assistant is allowed to perform the following tasks:

- Take study model impressions and/or digital intraoral impression
- Take and process intraoral radiographs
- Take and process extraoral radiographs (panoramic and cephalometric)
- Take intraoral measurements and do the tracings on cephalometric radiographs or computer imaging

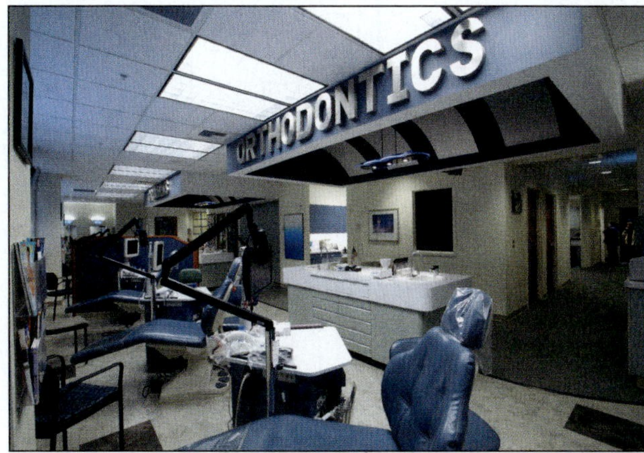

FIGURE 28-1

(A) Treatment area in orthodontic office. The chairs are arranged in an "open bay" concept.

(continues)

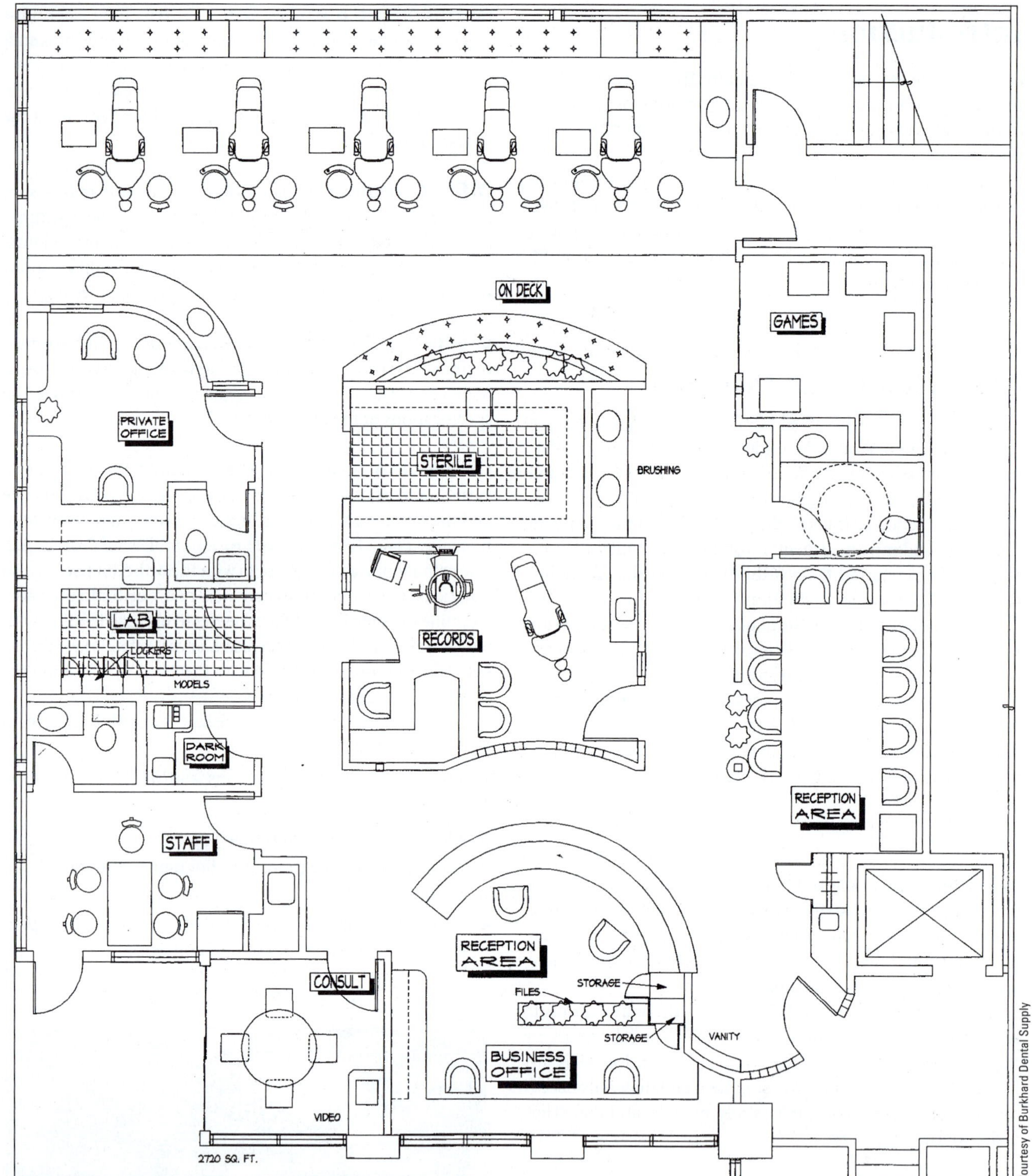

Courtesy of Burkhard Dental Supply

FIGURE 28-1 (continued)
(B) Blueprint of an orthodontic office.

- Take intraoral and extraoral photographs
- Assist the orthodontist during the consultation appointment
- Perform general chairside assisting responsibilities during treatment appointments
- Polish the patient's teeth at various stages of treatment
- Give oral hygiene instructions
- Apply enamel sealants to teeth to be bonded
- Place and remove orthodontic separators*
- Pre-fit bands before cementation*

- Prepare brackets for placement by the orthodontist*
- Prepare and assist with application of bonding agents/cements*
- Remove excess cement from bands and brackets*
- Place and remove arch wires and ligatures*
- Place adjusted retainers and/or headgear*
- Check for loose and broken appliances at each appointment*
- Give instructions on appliance wear and care
- Prep teeth for bonding*
- Select, pre-position, and light cure brackets after positioned by orthodontist*
- Size, fit, and cement bands after positioned by orthodontist*
- Maintain and sterilize instruments
- Maintain inventory and supplies

**With additional training and if allowed by the state Dental Practice Act*

Credentialed Orthodontic Assistant

To become a credentialed orthodontic assistant, a specialty examination must be passed. The examinations are administered by the Dental Assisting National Board (DANB) and/or the individual state board of dentistry. DANB administers an examination and, upon successful completion, the candidate is awarded the title of Certified Orthodontic Assistant (COA).

Occlusion and Malocclusion

The dental assistant must understand the terminology related to occlusion to effectively assist the dentist during orthodontic treatment as well as to educate and motivate the patient during treatment.

Normal Occlusion

A **normal** (or ideal) **occlusion** describes the contact relationship of the mandibular arch with the maxillary arch. This usually focuses on occlusal contacts, alignment of teeth, and arrangement and relationship of the teeth within and between the arches.

Characteristics of normal occlusion are as follows:

- The mandibular teeth are in maximum contact with the maxillary teeth and the teeth are not rotated or spaced abnormally.
- The maxillary anterior teeth overlap the incisal edge of the mandibular anterior teeth by 2 mm.
- The maxillary posterior teeth are one cusp distal to the mandibular posterior teeth.
- The mesial buccal cusp of the maxillary first permanent molar occludes in the buccal groove of the mandibular first molar (Figure 28-2).

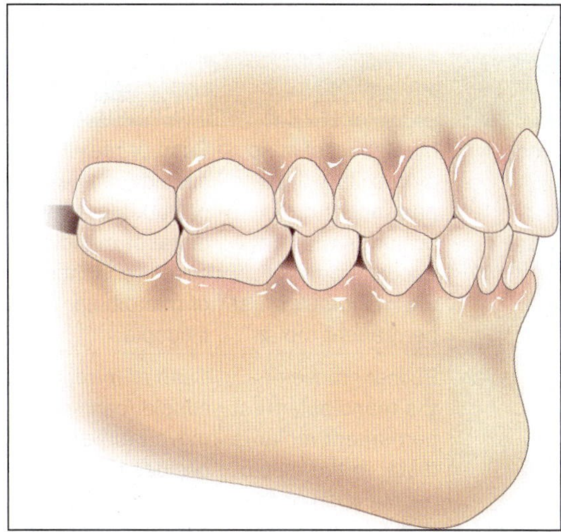

FIGURE 28-2

Example of normal occlusion.

Malocclusion

A **malocclusion** is any deviation from normal occlusion, including misalignment of a single tooth, a group of teeth, or an entire arch. Table 28-1 shows the most common method of classification, called **Angle's classification**. Also included in the table are the matching facial profiles.

In 1899, Edward Angle established a system to classify malocclusion. It is still commonly used today.

Malpositions of Individual Teeth and Groups of Teeth

There are numerous variations in the position of individual teeth in the alveolar bone. The following terms describe these deviations:

- **Torsoversion**—Tooth is rotated or turned.
- **Mesioversion**—Tooth is mesial to normal position.
- **Distoversion**—Tooth is distal to normal position.
- **Linguoversion**—Tooth is lingual to normal position.
- **Labioversion** or **buccoversion**—Tooth is tipped toward the lip or cheek.
- **Supraversion**—Tooth extends above the normal line of occlusion.
- **Infraversion**—Tooth is positioned below the normal line of occlusion.
- **Transversion** or **transposition**—Tooth is in the wrong order in the arch.

Groups of teeth sometimes deviate from the normal tooth positions. Table 28-2 lists the terms, provides a description of the variations, and shows illustrations.

TABLE 28-1 Angle's Classifications of Malocclusion and Facial Profiles

Class Name	Molar Relationship	Cuspid Relationship	Description	Illustration	Facial Profile
Neutrocclusion	Mesiobuccal cusp of maxillary first permanent molar occludes with the buccal groove of the mandibular first permanent molar.	Cusp of maxillary cuspid (canine) occludes between distal of mandibular cuspid and mesial of mandibular first bicuspid.	Similar to normal occlusion with individual teeth or groups of teeth out of position.	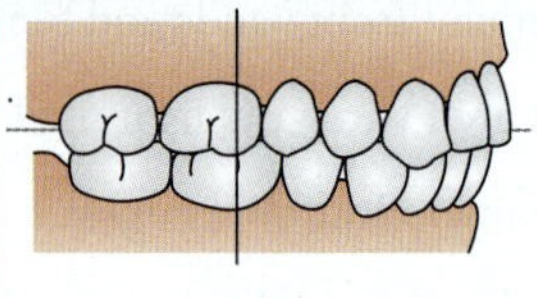 Class I	Mesognathic 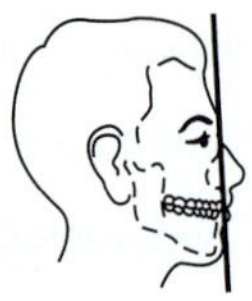
Distocclusion	Buccal groove of the mandibular first permanent molar is distal to the mesiobuccal cusp of the maxillary first permanent molar.	Cusp of maxillary cuspid (canine) is moved forward and occludes between distal of mandibular lateral incisor and mesial of mandibular cuspid.	Division 1—Maxillary teeth in labioversion (teeth protrude outward, toward lips). Division 2—Linguoversion of mandibular teeth (teeth tilt backward toward the tongue).	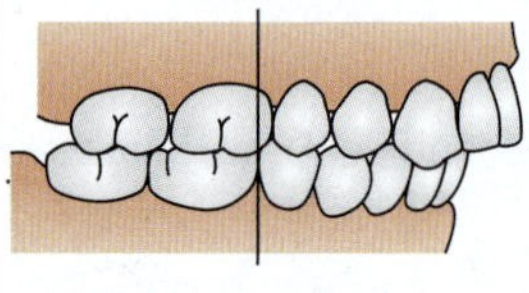 Class II, Division 1 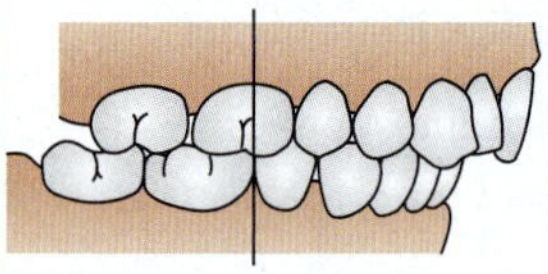 Class II, Division 2	Retrognathic 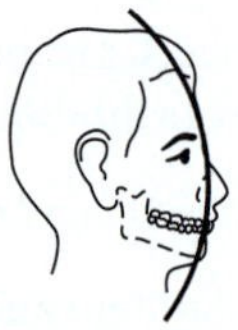 Retrognathic
Mesioclusion	Buccal groove of the mandibular first permanent molar is mesial to the mesiobuccal cusp of the maxillary first permanent molar.	Cusp of maxillary cuspid (canine) is moved back and occludes behind mandibular cuspid and in the middle of mandibular first molar.	Mandibular teeth mesial to normal position.	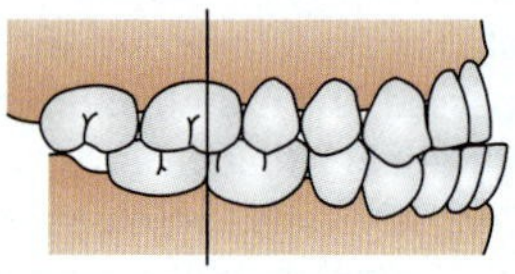 Class III	Prognathic 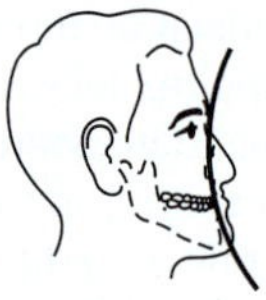

TABLE 28-2 Malpositions of Groups of Teeth

Term	Description	Illustration
Anterior cross-bite	Abnormal relationship of a tooth or a group of teeth in one arch to the opposing teeth in the other arch. In anterior cross-bite, the maxillary incisors are lingual to the opposing mandibular incisors.	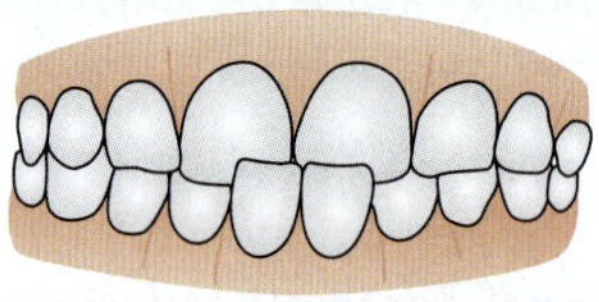
Posterior cross-bite	Abnormal relationship of teeth in one arch to the opposing teeth in the other arch. In posterior cross-bite, the primary or permanent maxillary posterior teeth are lingual to the mandibular teeth.	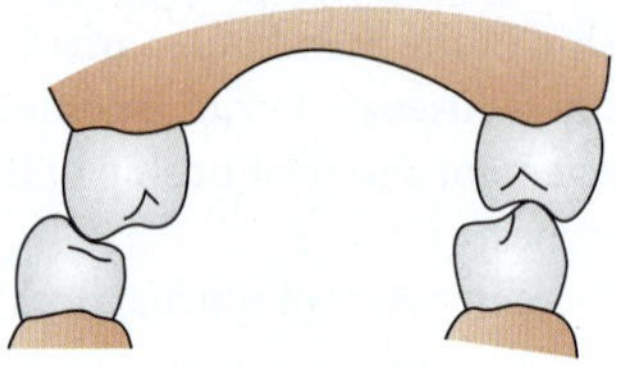
Edge-to-edge bite	Incisal surfaces of the maxillary anterior teeth meet the incisal surfaces of the mandibular anterior teeth.	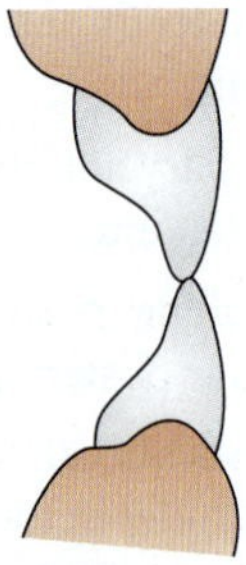

(continues)

TABLE 28-2 Malpositions of Groups of Teeth (continued)

Term	Description	Illustration
End-to-end bite	Maxillary posterior teeth meet the mandibular posterior teeth cusp-to-cusp instead of in normal fashion.	
Open bite	Failure of the maxillary and mandibular to occlude (meet).	
Overjet (horizontal overlap)	An abnormal horizontal distance between the labial surface of the mandibular anterior teeth and the lingual surface of the maxillary anterior teeth.	
Overbite (vertical overlap)	Normally, the maxillary teeth extend vertically over the incisal one-third of the mandibular anterior teeth. When the vertical overlap is greater than this, the person is said to have an overbite.	
Underjet	Maxillary anteriors positioned lingually to the mandibular anteriors with excessive space between the labial of the maxillary anteriors and the lingual of the mandibular anteriors.	

Etiology of Malocclusion

The etiology or cause of malocclusion falls into one of three categories:

1. **Genetic or heredity** factors may be responsible for deviations such as supernumerary teeth, facial and palatal clefts, abnormal jaw relationships, abnormal teeth-to-jaw relationships, and congenitally missing teeth.
2. **Systemic** factors include systemic diseases and nutritional disturbances that upset the normal schedule of dentition development during infancy and early childhood.
3. **Local** factors include trauma and habits such as thumb sucking, tongue thrusting, tongue sucking, mouth breathing, bruxism (involuntary grinding or clenching of teeth), and nail biting.

Types of Orthodontic Treatments

Orthodontic treatment involves much more than straightening teeth. The scope of treatments in orthodontics includes:

- Maintaining or establishing a normal or functional occlusion
- Improving the esthetic appearance of the face
- Eliminating problems that may disrupt normal development of the teeth and facial structures
- Correcting several facial and oral deformities through cooperative work with the oral and maxillofacial surgeon

Orthodontic treatments are divided into cases where malocclusion may be prevented or intercepted and cases where malocclusion already exists and correction is needed.

Preventive and Interceptive Orthodontics

Orthodontic treatment may be **preventive** and **interceptive**. Often, the general dentist and the pediatric dentist work with the orthodontist on a treatment plan for the patient.

Common treatments that are considered preventive and interceptive include:

- Placing restorations to prevent premature loss of teeth
- Placing space maintainers to hold space for a missing tooth
- Recognizing any deviation from the normal
- Observing growth patterns and development of teeth and bones
- Correcting bad habits affecting the oral cavity as early as possible
- Extracting teeth to prevent overcrowding
- Removing deciduous teeth to provide space for permanent teeth

Corrective Orthodontics

The area of **corrective orthodontics** involves improving existing problems. This type of orthodontics is primarily accomplished on children in the last stage of mixed dentition entering full permanent dentition. Treatment of adults may also fall into corrective orthodontics.

Common treatments that are considered corrective orthodontics include the following:

- Placement of fixed or removable appliances. A **fixed appliance**, which is attached to the teeth and cannot be removed by the patient, includes "braces," bands, brackets, arch wires, and ties. A **removable appliance**, which is inserted into the mouth and removed by the patient, include functional retainers.
- Orthognathic surgery for severe cases.

Process of Tooth Movement

Orthodontic appliances are devices that move teeth by applying force. They also hold teeth in position. The appliances are carefully designed to achieve the desired movement and position of the teeth. The teeth are allowed to be moved through the process of **resorption**, which eliminates tissues no longer needed by the body. The teeth are retained in position through the process of **deposition**, which creates and deposits new cells.

The force of the orthodontic appliance compresses the periodontal ligament and reduces the blood supply to one side of the tooth. Specialized bone cells called **osteoclasts** cause the bone to resorb, or break down. As the tooth moves into the new space, the periodontal ligaments on the other side of the tooth are stretched, causing tension. As the tension increases, bone cells called **osteoblasts** deposit new bone to hold the tooth in its new position.

The principles of tooth movement are the same for all patients regardless of age; however, the rate of movement may be slower in the adult patient. Redeposited bone tissue takes 6 to 12 months for osteogenesis to take place. Thus, appliances such as retainers are required to hold the teeth in position. Overall, tooth movement depends on the:

- Magnitude of force
- Duration of application of force
- Direction of force
- Distribution of force

Preorthodontic Treatment

The purpose of a patient's first visit to the orthodontist is often a preliminary examination. This enables the orthodontist to make an initial recommendation as to whether treatment is advisable at that time or should be delayed until there is further dental development. If treatment is delayed, follow-up appointments may be scheduled periodically to evaluate the patient's growth patterns. If treatment is advised, an appointment is scheduled for diagnostic records.

To ensure successful treatment, the orthodontist must have the cooperation of the patient and the support of the patient's family. This is an important aspect, because orthodontic treatment may take several years to complete. The patient must be willing to follow the directions of the orthodontist concerning appliances and must also be willing to maintain good oral hygiene.

Diagnostic Records

Orthodontic offices are now using computer software programs for retaining all records that make up the patient treatment, including the chart, treatment plan and notes, information on the patient's teeth, and a chart of the teeth and face. Digital images that are transferred into electronic software programs include photographs as well as panoramic and cephalometric radiographs. Some programs allow three-dimensional (3D) digital models to be stored as part of the patient record, thus making a paperless practice without the additional need of storage of study models. Diagnostic records for orthodontic treatment include a medical and dental history, clinical examination, panoramic x-rays, cephalometric (**SEF**-ah-loh-meh-trick) x-rays, intraoral and facial photographs, and plaster study models of the teeth or using a digital imaging system.

Medical–Dental History

Treatment begins with a complete medical history to evaluate the general health of the patient. Some conditions and medications have an effect on the patient's response to treatment or may require that the process proceed at a slower pace. Treatment may last for several years, so the medical history must be reviewed periodically.

The dental history provides information about the patient's past exposure to dental treatment. For example, caries incidence, missing teeth, and whether the patient has received routine dental care or only emergency dental care impact the outcome of orthodontic treatment. The dental history gives the orthodontist a guideline when designing the overall treatment plan to facilitate specific needs of the patient.

Clinical Examination

The dentist evaluates the results of an extensive examination of the face, jaws, and teeth, looking for symmetry between them. The teeth are evaluated for size, shape, color, and position. The jaws are examined for size, shape, and relationship to one another. The Angle classification of occlusion is often used to determine the classification on both sides of the mouth.

The oral cavity is also examined for abnormal functional and neuromuscular patterns, such as tongue sucking, tongue thrusting, mouth breathing, and bruxism. The orthodontist commonly uses the Palmer method of charting (refer to Chapter 14, Dental Charting), and measurements.

Radiographs

The orthodontist takes radiographs as part of the diagnostic procedure. The most common types of radiographs for orthodontics are panoramic and cephalometric. Some intraoral films such as full-mouth x-rays and occlusals are also taken for more detail of particular areas.

Panoramic x-rays are taken for an overall view of the dentition and surrounding area. Impacted teeth, abscesses, supernumerary teeth, or disorders of the temporomandibular joint can be determined from the panoramic film (Figure 28-3).

Cephalometric films are taken to evaluate the growth patterns and to determine the course of treatment. The cephalometric radiograph is a lateral view of the patient's head that shows the jaw and the teeth. Cephalometric radiograph tracings are performed to determine the relationship of certain landmarks.

Once the measurements are obtained, they are used for diagnosis, treatment planning, and/or assessment of treatment effects. Cephalometric analyses help the orthodontist determine the shape of the face currently, how the face has grown, what the expected growth will be, and the changes that need to be made. These cephalometric tracings are done either manually, using tracing paper and a special pen, or by computer (Figure 28-4). Cephalometric radiographs are taken periodically during treatment to monitor the patient's oral and facial growth.

Photographs

Intraoral and extraoral photographs are taken as part of the patient's records before and after treatment. Facial photographs include a full frontal view and a profile view

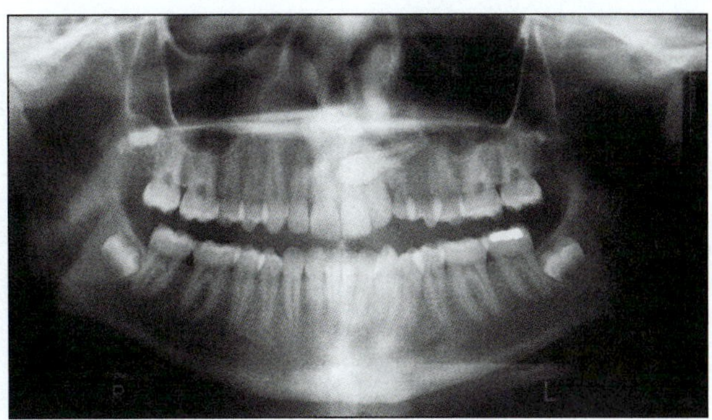

FIGURE 28-3

Panoramic radiograph needed for diagnosis.

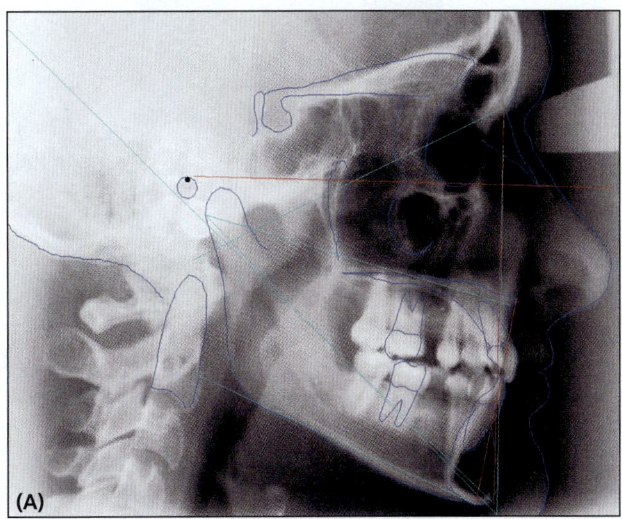

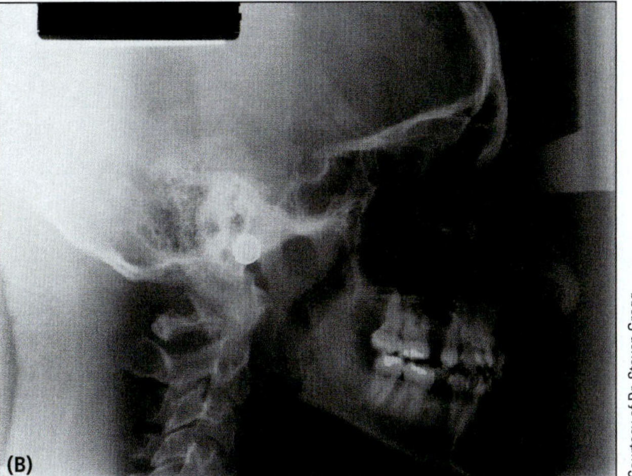

FIGURE 28-4

(A) Cephalometric radiograph. (B) Cephalometric tracing on a radiograph.

(Figure 28-5A). These are used to evaluate the symmetry and balance of the face.

Cheek retractors and mirrors are used when exposing intraoral photographs (Figure 28-5B). Intraoral photos are a visual record of the teeth and are used for planning treatment.

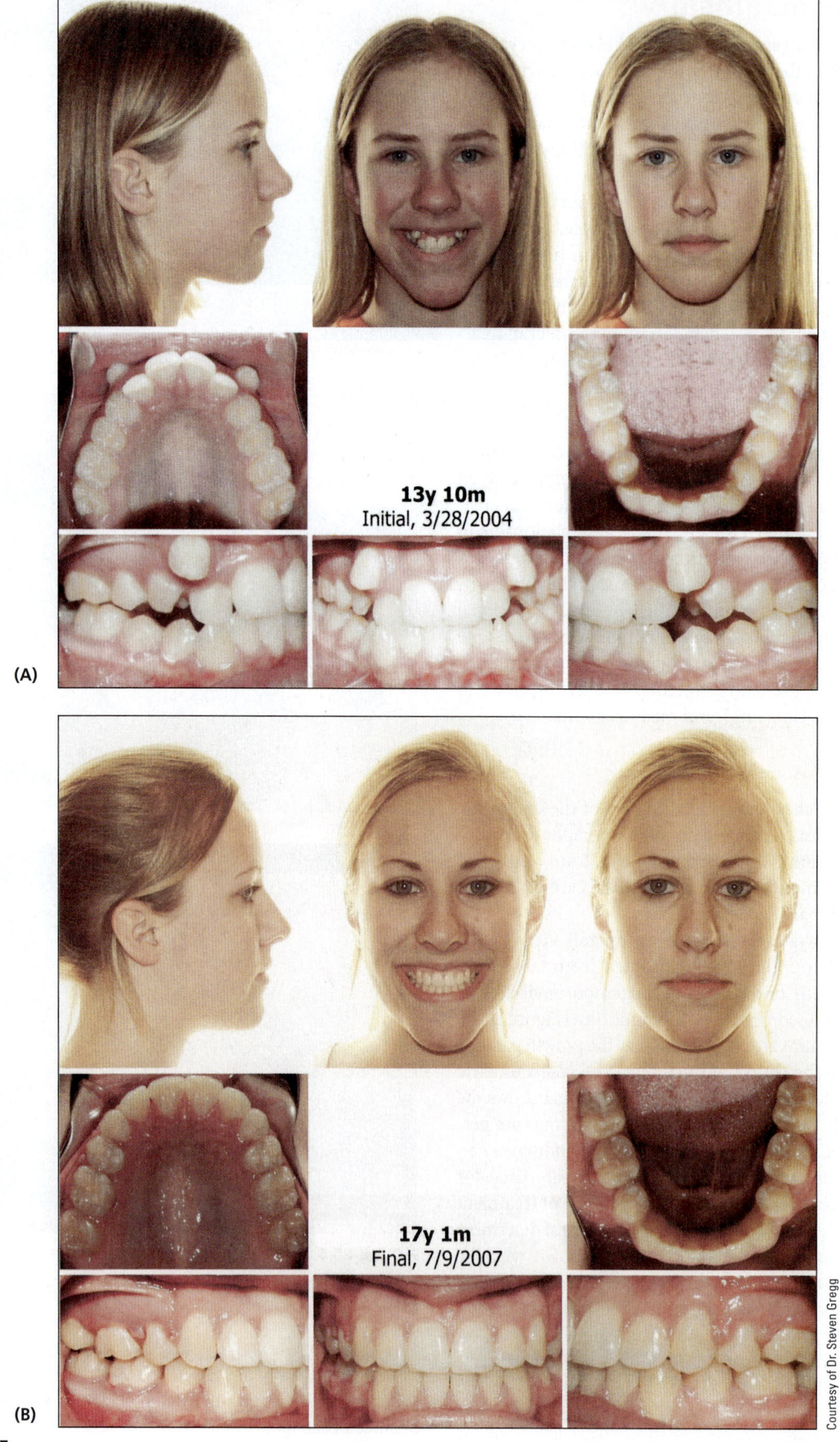

FIGURE 28-5

Top row: Patient profile view and frontal views. Middle row: Intraoral photographs of the maxillary and mandibular arches using mirrors. Bottom row: Dentition from various angles using mirrors and cheek retractors.

Study Models

Study models or diagnostic casts are used as part of the patient's record. They show how the teeth, mouth, and arches relate to one another. The study casts allow the study of the sizes and positions of the teeth along with the widths and lengths of the arches.

The first step is to take an alginate impression of the patient's teeth. The impression is then poured in stone or orthodontic plaster, trimmed, and finished. Orthodontic models are very detailed and symmetrical (Figure 28-6). The finished study models are used in the case presentation as visual aids and are kept as a reference throughout the patient's treatment. (Refer to Chapter 35, Laboratory Materials and Techniques.) Orthodontist are increasingly implementing the digital scanning systems for impressions.

Consultation Appointment

After the diagnostic appointment, the patient (and a parent if the patient is under age 18) is scheduled for a consultation appointment. The orthodontist studies the information gathered, makes a diagnosis, and prepares a treatment plan before the patient's appointment. Sufficient time must be allowed to present all the information to the patient (and parents). Radiographs, photographs, study models, and other visual aids are used in the presentation. During the consultation, the treatment, duration of treatment, involvement, and costs are explained. The responsibility of the patient is reviewed at this time so that it is understood what he or she must do to facilitate treatment progress as planned. If the patient accepts the treatment plan, consent papers are signed and financial arrangements are made.

Sometimes, the age and development of the individual patient indicate that treatment be divided into several phases. The first phase may involve the patient wearing removable appliances and/or headgear. The patient often has mixed dentition, and treatment may last several months to 2 years. Next is the fixed appliance phase, which is started when the patient is in full permanent dentition.

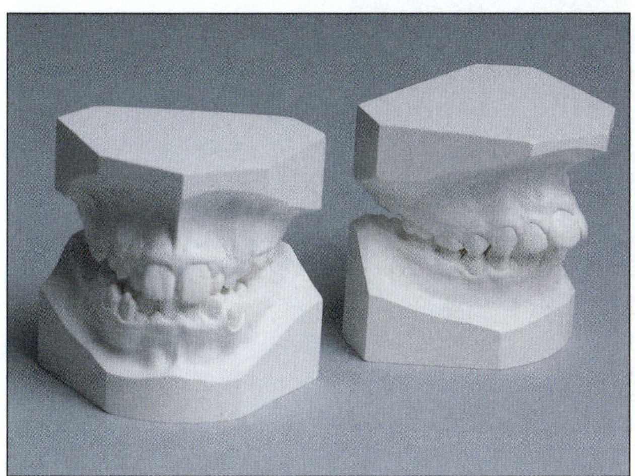

FIGURE 28-6

Orthodontic study model trimmed symmetrically.

Orthodontic Appliances

Orthodontic appliances are classified into two categories: fixed appliances and removable appliances.

Fixed Appliances

Fixed appliances are attached to the teeth and cannot be removed by the patient. The appliances are directly bonded onto the tooth or cemented into place with dental cement. The treatment is more controlled with fixed appliances, because the patient cannot remove them. Fixed appliances are commonly known as braces (Figure 28-7).

Orthodontic Bands. The **orthodontic bands** are thin bands of stainless steel that are carefully fitted around each tooth. Bands are supplied in a variety of sizes, and are presized on the patient's model before cementation. Glass ionomer, polycarboxylate, or zinc phosphate cement is commonly used for cementing orthodontic bands. Bands are used on the posterior teeth because they provide the means to hold and control tooth movement. Depending on the individual case, various attachments such as brackets or buccal tubes are placed on the bands (Figures 28-8A and B).

Brackets. Brackets are attachments that are either welded to the bands or bonded directly to the teeth. The function of **brackets** is to hold the arch wire in place and to transmit the force of the arch wire to move the tooth. Brackets for the posterior teeth are made of stainless steel and are either cemented on the tooth or welded directly to the band. Brackets for the anterior teeth are made of stainless steel, ceramic, or acrylic, and are cemented or directly bonded to the teeth (Figures 28-8B through E). Tooth-colored ceramic and acrylic brackets are popular because they are barely noticeable on the anterior teeth.

Arch Wires. An **arch wire** is a wire that conforms to the shape of the dental arch. The arch wire is placed in the brackets and

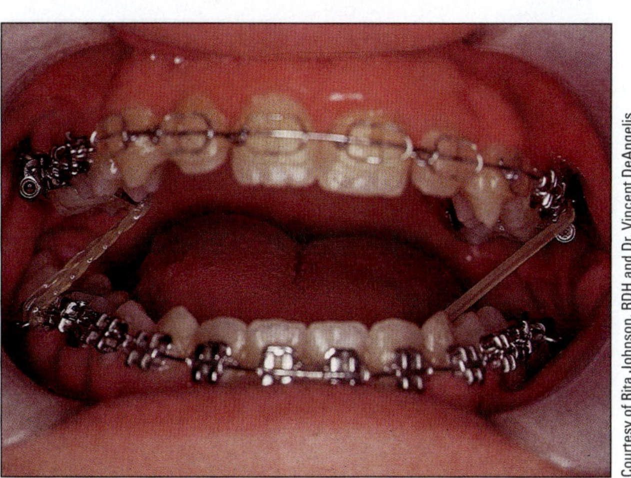

Courtesy of Rita Johnson, RDH and Dr. Vincent DeAngelis

FIGURE 28-7

Patient in full braces. The posterior teeth are banded; the anterior teeth have brackets only.

through a buccal tube on a posterior molar. At each bracket, ligature wire or elastics are wrapped around the bracket to secure the arch wire in place. The arch wire is the force used to correct the position of teeth. They can also be used to maintain the teeth in position upon completion of orthodontic treatment.

Arch wires are made of several different types of material, most commonly stainless steel, nickel-titanium alloy, and beta-titanium alloy.

- Stainless steel wires are high strength and not very elastic, thus if they are bent too much they will not return to their original shape. These wires are used in the middle-to-end stages of orthodontic treatment where the dentist needs more control of tooth movement.
- Nickel-titanium alloy (Ni-Ti) arch wires are very resistant to deformation. The elasticity of this wire allows it to return to its original shape while gently applying force to move

Orthodontic band
Buccal tube
(A)

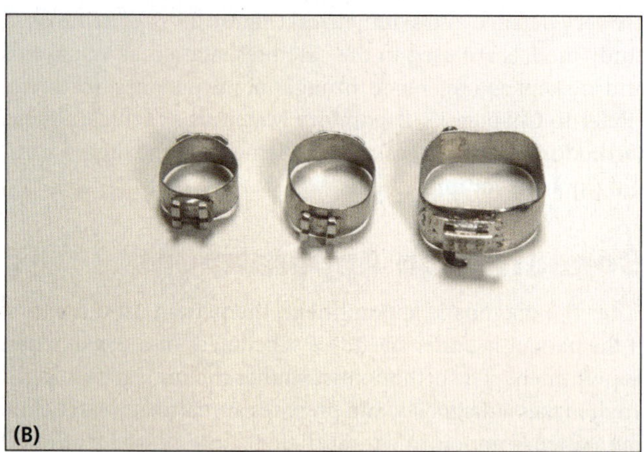

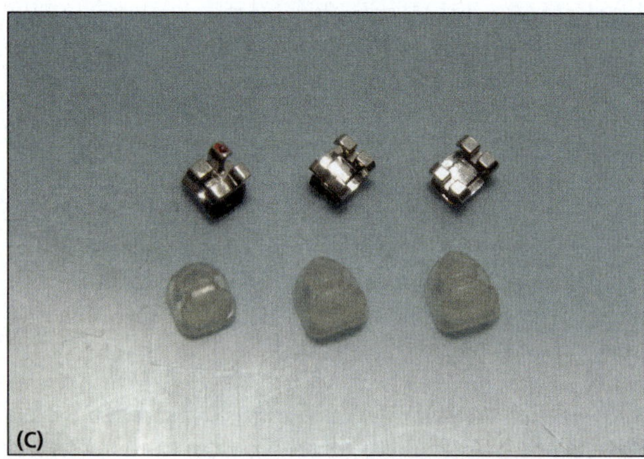

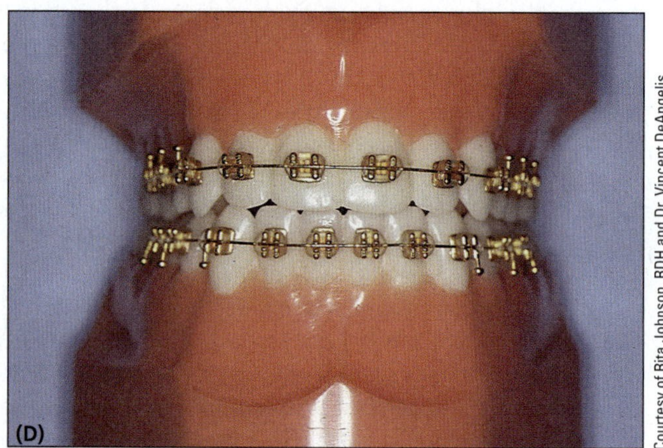

Courtesy of Rita Johnson, RDH and Dr. Vincent DeAngelis

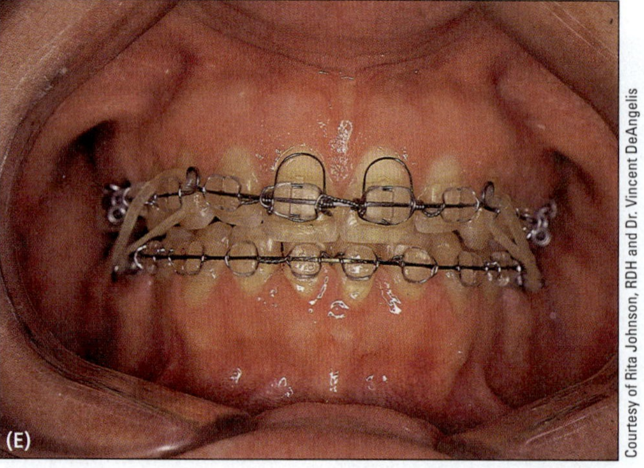

Courtesy of Rita Johnson, RDH and Dr. Vincent DeAngelis

FIGURE 28-8

(A) Orthodontic band with buccal tube. (B) Various orthodontic bands with bracket or tube attached. (C) Metal and plastic/porcelain brackets. (D) Metal brackets on a model. (E) Tooth-colored brackets.

the teeth with it at the same time. Some of the Ni-Ti wires are heat-activated (Copper Ni-Ti) wires. These wires can hold the deformed shape at room temperature so they can be secured in the brackets, but when the wire reaches the temperature of the patient's mouth, the wire will move to return to its original U shape carrying the teeth with it.

- Beta-titanium wires are made of titanium and molybdenum and were developed after the Ni-Ti wires. They have a medium range of elasticity and strength so they are a good intermediary wire between NI-Ti and stainless steel.

The arch wires come in different "sizes," which refers to the cross-section or the thickness of the wire. The wires are also supplied in several shapes: square, rectangular, and round. Considering that arch wires are made from identical materials, the smaller the wire, the more elastic and less stiff the wire will be. As the wires progress in size, they become stiffer and less elastic (Figure 28-9A).

All patients are different and each orthodontist has his or her own techniques, but most orthodontists use small Ni-Ti arch wires at the beginning of the treatment to align the teeth and then progress to larger stainless steel or beta-titanium wires. Wires are not usually changed at every visit, but depending on the case, they are changed three to five times during treatment with different types of wires at different stages of treatment.

Ligature Wire and Plastic Chains/Ties. A **ligature wire** and **plastic rings** are used to hold the arch wire to the brackets. Ligature wire is a very thin, flexible wire that usually comes in precut lengths or on spools (Figure 28-9B). The wire wraps around the bracket and then is tightened by twisting the wire, which ties or "ligates" the arch wire to the bracket. Plastic rings, also called elastic ties, are small bands that are supplied in a variety of colors. The elastic bands slip over the bracket to secure the arch wire. Also commonly used are elastic chains. The chain is a continuous chain of "Os." The elastic chain attaches several adjacent teeth together. This continuous pressure brings the teeth together (Figure 28-9C).

Buccal Tubes. The **buccal tubes** are small cylinders of metal welded to the molar bands, usually on the buccal surface. Their function is to provide a means of attachment for the arch wire to the band in the posterior area (Figures 28-8 and 28-10).

Springs. The **springs** are specially bent or shaped wires that are attached to the main arch wire. There are two main kinds of springs: the finger spring and the coil spring. The finger spring provides gentle pressure on individual teeth (Figure 28-11A). Coil springs are designed for space closure and maintenance application or to effectively open and maintain a space (Figure 28-11B).

Elastics. The **elastics** are rubber bands that are available in a variety of sizes. Elastics provide force for movement. They are often used between the upper and lower arches. Elastics are attached to hooks or buttons that are secured on the band or brackets (Figure 28-12).

New developments in ligature ties include fluoride-releasing ties that aid in reducing decalcification of the tooth.

Special Fixed Appliances

There are several fixed orthodontic appliances that are not part of routine braces. These appliances are cemented in place and have a specific function for a specific treatment or phases of treatment. They include lingual braces, lingual arch wire, space maintainers, and the palatal expansion appliance.

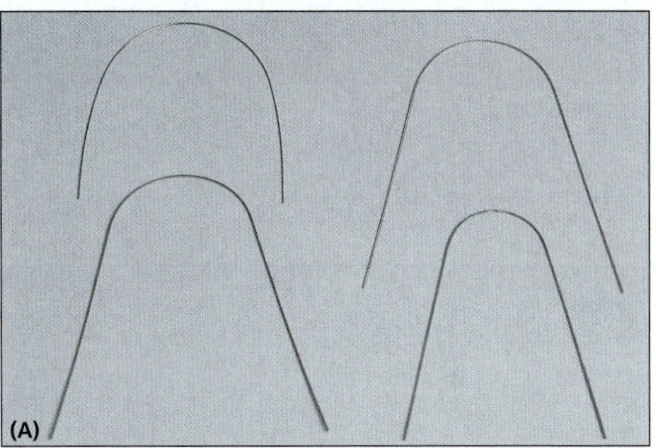
(A)

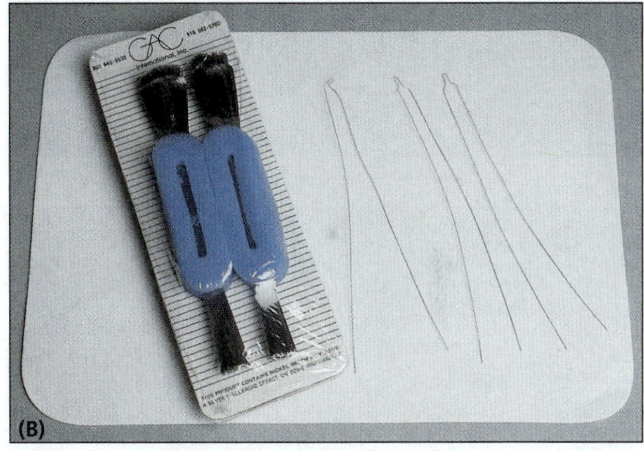

(B)

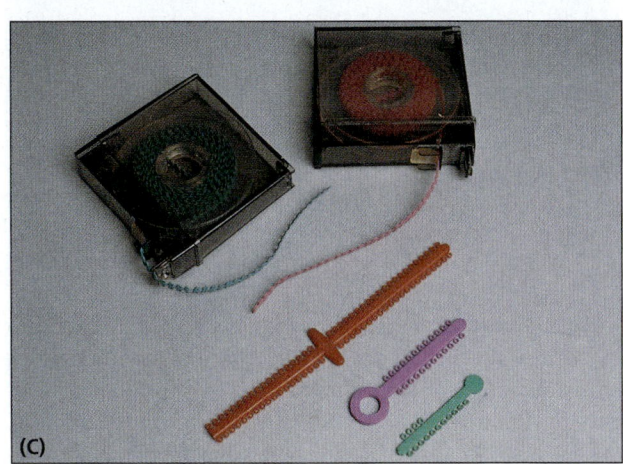
(C)

FIGURE 28-9

(A) Various arch wires. (B) Ligature wire used to secure the arch wire to the brackets. (C) Elastic bands, "Os," and chain elastics are also used to secure the arch wire to the brackets.

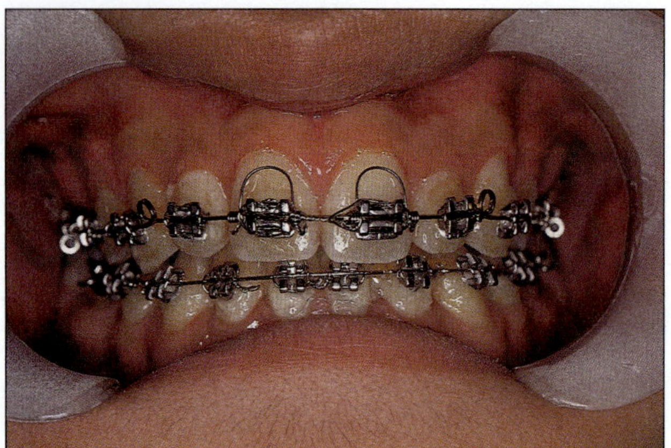

FIGURE 28-10

Patient with full braces: bands with buccal tubes, brackets, arch wire, ligature wire, elastics, and finger springs.

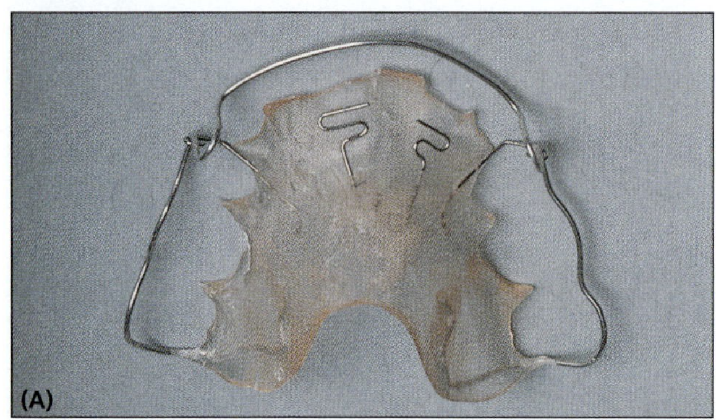

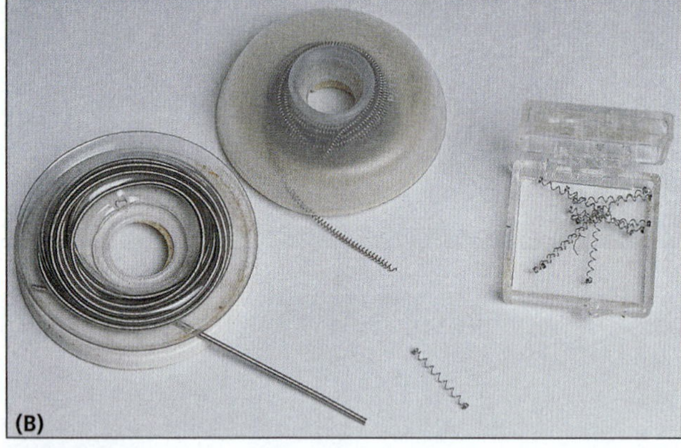

FIGURE 28-11

(A) Finger spring on palate of retainer. (B) Coil springs.

Lingual Braces. Lingual braces, sometimes called invisible braces, are attached to the lingual surface of the teeth. These braces allow patients who are apprehensive about their appearance during treatment an alternative to conventional braces. When the braces are placed on the lingual surfaces they are much less noticeable. The disadvantages to lingual braces include placement and maintenance. It is difficult to keep the areas dry during cementation, and they are troublesome for the patient to maintain.

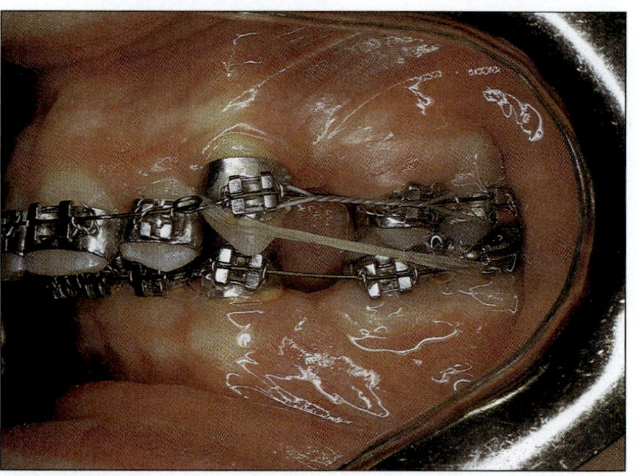

Courtesy of Rita Johnson, RDH and Dr. Vincent DeAngelis

FIGURE 28-12

Patient in full braces with rubber elastic from one arch to the other. The rubber bands provide the force for movement.

Lingual Arch Wire. The lingual arch wire is placed on the lingual surface instead of the facial. Orthodontic bands are placed on the first permanent molars, and the arch wire is closely adapted to the lingual surfaces of the teeth. The function of the lingual arch wire is to maintain the arch by holding the teeth in position until the permanent teeth erupt (Figures 28-13A and B).

Space Maintainer. The **space maintainer** is composed of a band and a wire loop soldered together (Figure 28-14). Its function is to maintain space for the permanent tooth to erupt after premature loss of the primary tooth. There are several varieties of space maintainers that can be adapted to the patient's teeth.

Maintaining this space until the permanent tooth begins to erupt is important. If the space is not held open, the adjacent teeth will drift in and begin to fill the space, which makes it more difficult for the permanent tooth to erupt as well as to come in straight.

The space maintainer must be cemented in place to hold the teeth in position; if the maintainer loosens or comes out, it should be replaced as soon as possible to prevent the teeth from moving. If it is left out too long, a new impression must be taken and a new space maintainer must be fabricated.

Palatal Expander Appliance. The **palatal expanding appliance** is composed of an acrylic palatal portion that is split along the midline. The acrylic palatal portion is attached to bands, and the bands are cemented to the posterior teeth for stability. In the middle of the acrylic is a screw-like device called the rapid palatal expander (RPE) that can be adjusted to expand the arch. The function of the palatal separating appliance is to spread the mid-palatal suture (see Chapter 7, Head and Neck Anatomy). This process takes about 2 to 3 weeks. Bone tissue fills in the opening and closes the space (Figure 28-15).

The screw must be turned twice each day once the device is cemented in place. A "key" is inserted into one of the holes on the screw and pushed toward the throat. The next hole

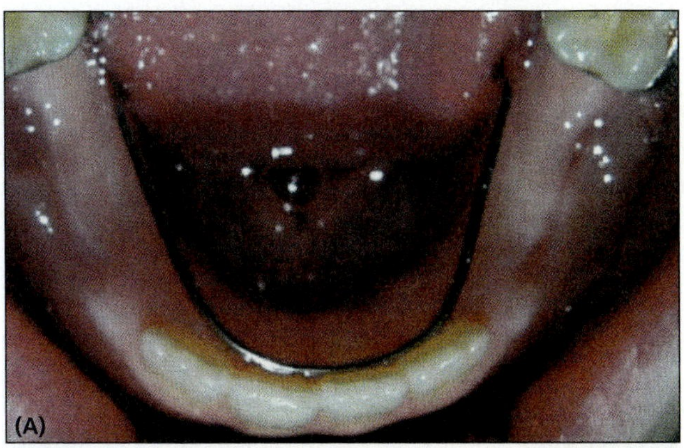

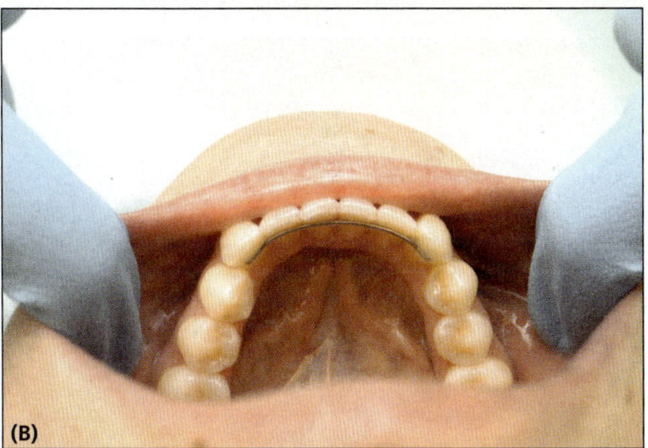

FIGURE 28-13

(A) Patient with a lingual arch wire. (B) Patient with a lingual arch bar from cuspid to cuspid.

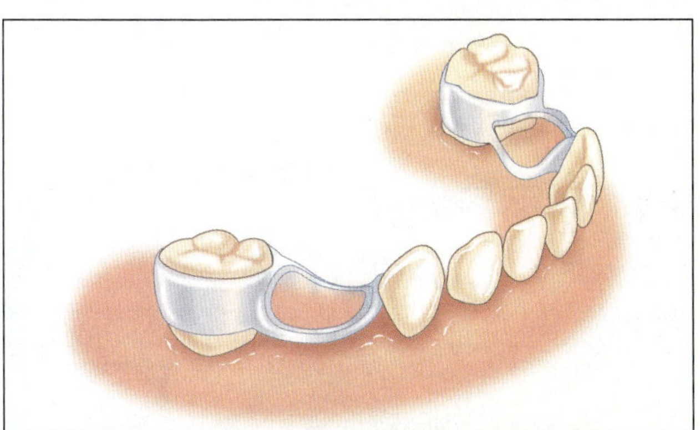

FIGURE 28-14

Space maintainer to hold space when a tooth is lost prematurely.

will then be exposed for the next turn. The key should always be secured by wrapping the string that is attached to the key around the wrist to prevent the possibility of swallowing the key. The tightening process may be a little uncomfortable until the palate separates to the desired space; subsequently, the patient may feel as if the roof of the mouth itches. The space between the maxillary central incisors may widen during the first 2 weeks as the appliance spreads the arch. The space will disappear soon when it is no longer necessary to turn the screw on the separator.

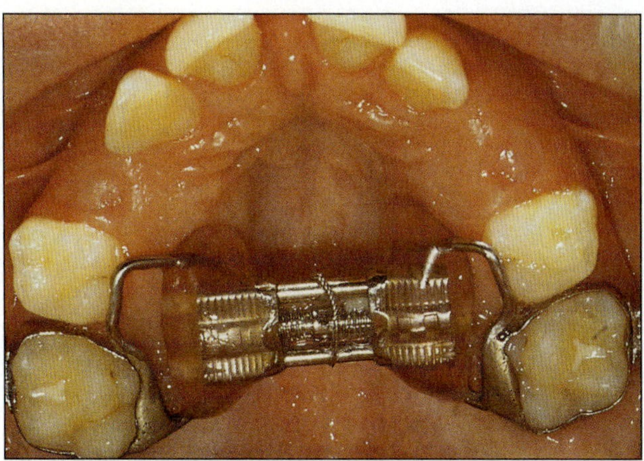

Courtesy of Rita Johnson, RDH and Dr. Vincent DeAngelis

FIGURE 28-15

palatal expanding appliance.

Removable Appliances

Removable appliances are designed to be inserted into the mouth and removed by the patient. There are numerous varieties of removable appliances and many ways to categorize them. The more commonly used removable appliances include headgear, functional appliances, retainers, and positioners. Also in this category of removable appliances is the invisible straightening of fully erupted permanent teeth with a series of removable custom plastic "aligners."

Headgear. The **headgear** consists of a strap that goes behind the patient's head or neck and a facebow that attaches to buccal tubes on molar bands. There are many designs to meet the individual patient's needs. Headgear is used to apply force to move teeth, to restrain or alter cranial-facial bone growth, and to reinforce stability of intraoral appliances. Usually, patients wear headgear for a specific number of hours per day (Figure 28-16).

Functional Appliances. Functional appliances are removable appliances that are routinely used before fixed appliances are placed. Functional appliances are used while the teeth and cranial-facial skeleton are still developing. There are a wide variety of functional appliances. Some guide newly erupting teeth into position, others change the direction of cranial-facial skeletal growth, and still others inhibit the growth rate of one arch. The **activator** is the original functional jaw orthopedic appliance, and it has been modified many times. The activator is used to expand the width of the maxillary arch, for minor tooth movement, to make changes in skeletal growth patterns, and to reduce **overbite** (projection of upper teeth over the lower). The most common activators are the Bionator, the Herbst, and the Frankel (Figure 28-17). The **Bionator appliance** is an acrylic appliance which fits on the upper and lower teeth, and positions the lower jaw forward. It is used to encourage lower jaw growth.

The **Herbst appliance** is a fixed appliance that improves the overbite by encouraging lower jaw growth. The

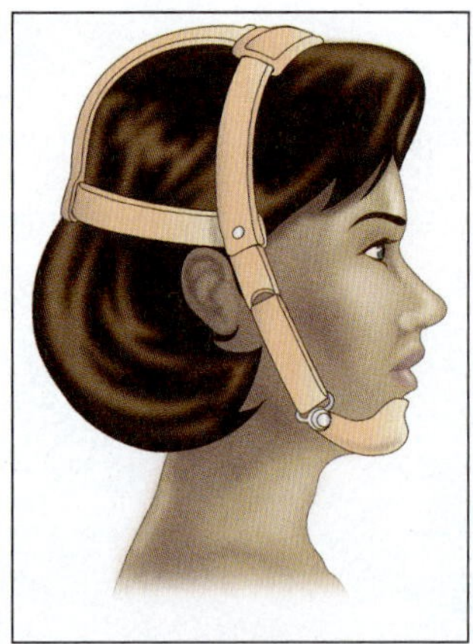

FIGURE 28-16

Headgear with adjustable straps used to apply force to move teeth.

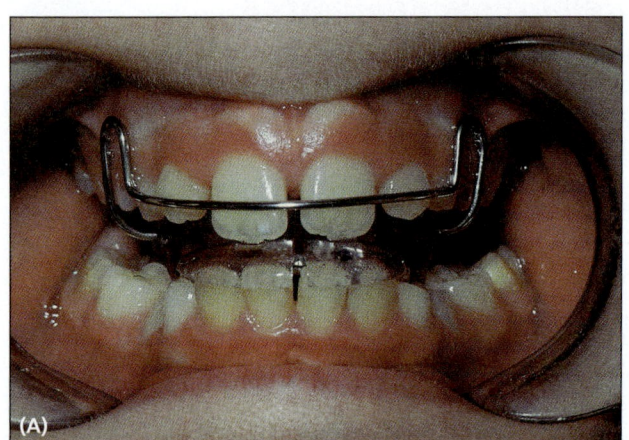

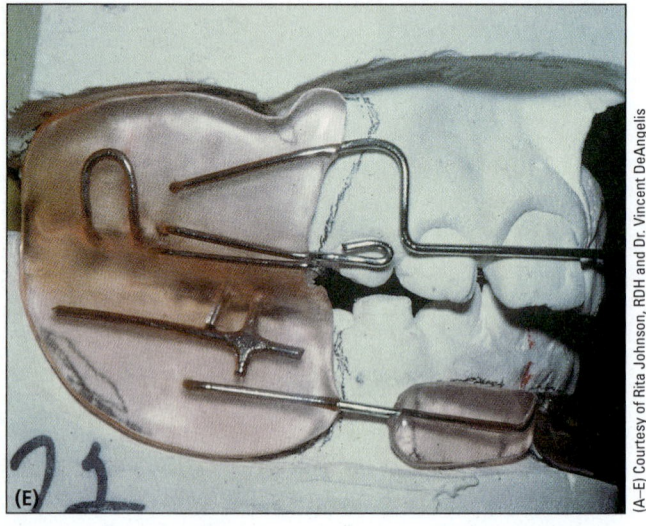

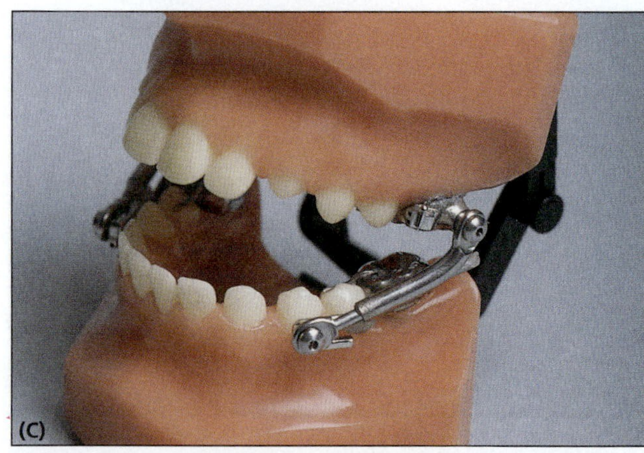

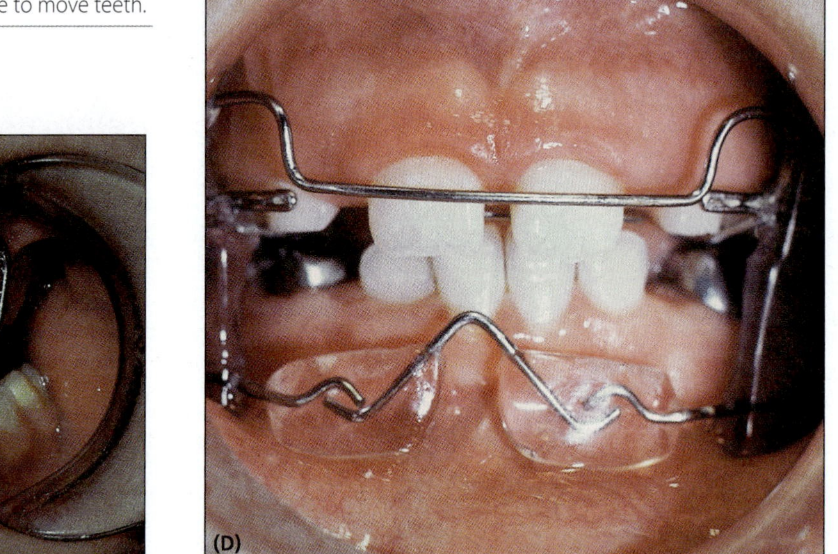

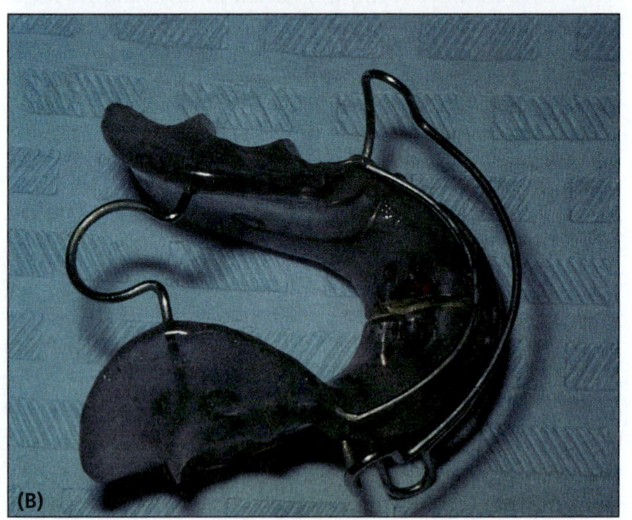

(A–E) Courtesy of Rita Johnson, RDH and Dr. Vincent DeAngelis

FIGURE 28-17

(A) Patient with Bionator appliance. (B) Bionator appliance. (C) Herbst appliance. (D) Patient with Frankel appliance. (E) Frankel appliance.

Frankel appliance uses headgear to assist the mandible to advance and grow forward while stopping the maxilla from growing. The front teeth are pulled back, which results in flattening the open bite.

Retainers. Retainers are custom-made appliances fitted to the patient's arch. They are made of acrylic, or metal wire and acrylic, and are secured in the patient's mouth by wires braced against and/or around the teeth. They are used to retain the teeth in position after the fixed appliances have been removed. The **Hawley retainer** is an example of a retainer (Figure 28-18).

Tooth Positioner. The **tooth positioner** is a flexible rubber or soft-plastic appliance that surrounds the crowns of all teeth in both arches when positioned in the patient's mouth. Positioners are custom made for the patient after the removal of fixed appliances. Their function is to maintain the ideal position of the teeth upon completion of fixed treatment (Figure 28-19). The positioners are worn by the patient until the teeth are set in their new location.

Esthetic Orthodontic Aligners. The *aligner* is an esthetic orthodontic appliance that, in conjunction with a dentist's diagnosis, treatment plan, and advances in medical imaging technology, corrects malocclusion using a series of custom-made, nearly invisible, removable aligners.

Patients wear each aligner for a minimum of 2 weeks, for about 22 hours per day. Treatment generally can last from 6 months to 1 year. Aligners are only removed for eating, brushing, and flossing. Teeth are moved gradually as each aligner is replaced with the next, until the desired results are achieved (Figure 28-20).

The aligners are similar to whitening or fluoride trays in that they are custom made, but are thinner, even more precise, and fabricated from a more rigid, proprietary material. The number of aligners and length of treatment depend on the complexity of the case. As with traditional braces, patients experience a brief period of adjustment as they transition to each new set of aligners. Since the aligners are removable, oral hygiene is easy to maintain while patients eat, brush, and floss as they normally would.

Orthodontists or dentist must complete a training/certification program offered through the manufacturer in order to treat patients with their product. Dental auxiliaries attending the certification program will learn the submission process, which includes PVS impressions or digital scanning impressions and bite, x-rays, intra- and extraoral photographs, and the dentist's treatment plan. Additionally, modules on case management and practice building are presented. See Table 28-3 for an example of a sequence of treatment.

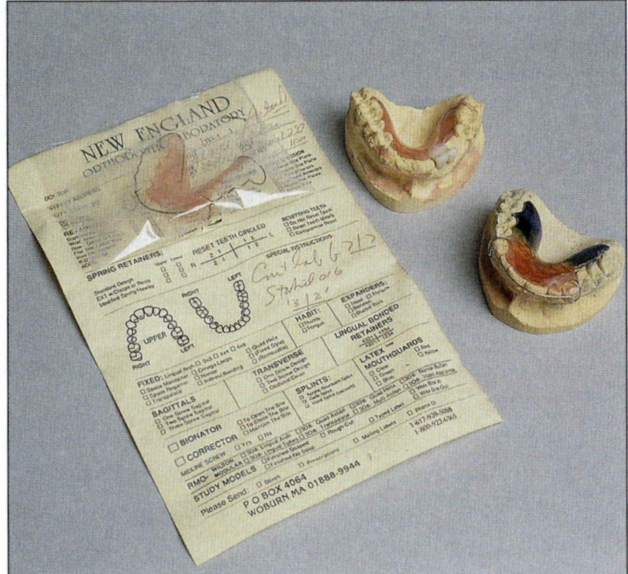

FIGURE 28-18

Various Hawley appliances with lab prescription.

Aesthetic Short-Term Orthodontic Treatment

Cosmetic orthodontic systems are on the rise with the adult population looking for quick results. Systems focusing on the anterior six teeth on both the maxillary and the mandibular arch use one of three techniques and are cosmetic in nature.

- Clear brackets and wires
- Clear aligner
- Invisible braces (brackets and wires placed on the lingual side of the teeth)

These techniques are focused on aesthetics of the anterior teeth only.

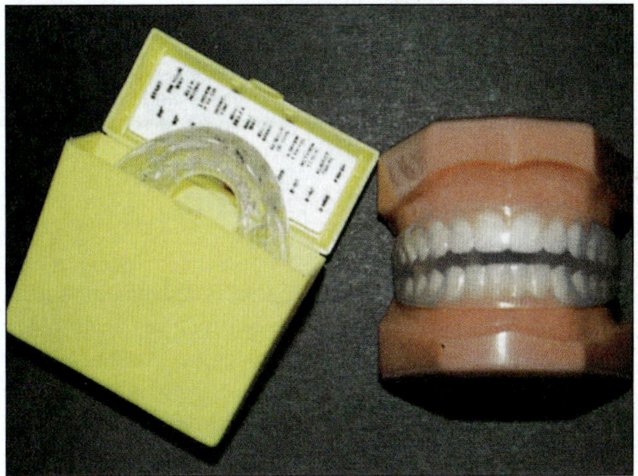

FIGURE 28-19

Tooth positioner in storage container and in mouth.

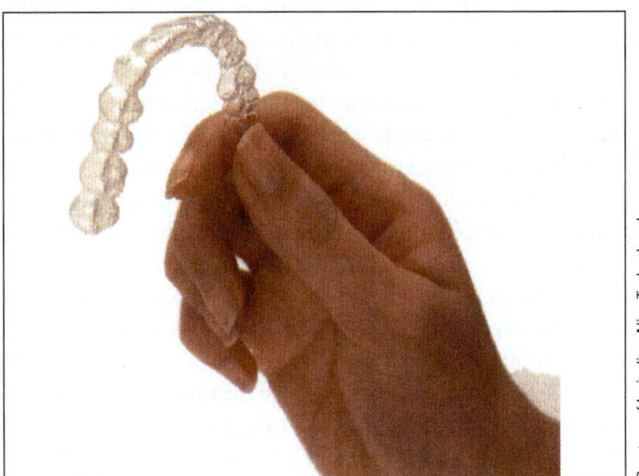

Courtesy of Invisalign-Align Technology Inc.

FIGURE 28-20

Invisalign® esthetic orthodontic appliance.

TABLE 28-3 Sequence of Treatment for Invisalign® Aligners

Dental office evaluation	Complete examination and discussion of patient's chief complaint.
	Complete records: • FMX or panorex (cephalometric optional) • PVS impressions (full maxillary and mandibular) • PVS bite • Series of intraoral and extraoral photographs • Prescription and diagnosis forms completed
Submit case to Align Technology	Align receives records (x-rays, impressions, and photos). Impressions are scanned to create a highly accurate 3D model of the patient's teeth. A computerized movie called ClinCheck® is then made depicting the movement of teeth from the beginning of treatment to the projected final result. This software allows the dentist to take an online virtual tour of the patient's teeth. You will see the patient's teeth the way they are at the beginning of treatment, the way they will look at the end, and each stage in between. Aligners are not manufactured until the treating dentist approves this ClinCheck file.
Dental office	Dentist reviews ClinCheck file, makes any necessary modifications, and accepts the case to authorize fabrication of Aligners.
Manufacturing of aligners	From the approved ClinCheck file, Align uses lasers to build a set of resin models for each stage/set of Aligners to be fabricated for the patient. From the resin models, Align Technology manufactures a series of clear Aligners with the specified movements built into the shape of each one sequentially. All Aligners are shipped to the treating dentist.
Dental office	Dentist dispenses first set of Aligners to patient and schedules next appointment for 2 weeks to evaluate and deliver subsequent sets of Aligners. Normally after the second appointment, patients can be given two to three sets of Aligners at one time, with future visits scheduled 6 weeks apart.

3D Orthodontic Imaging Treatment

3D technology has advanced many aspects of dental treatment, including orthodontic treatment. 3D imaging technology provides interaction between the machine (hardware) and the software programs. They integrate technology to provide diagnoses, treatment planning, and orthodontic treatment. With 3D orthodontic imaging technology, orthodontists are providing treatment through nontraditional means without the need for plaster study models, x-rays, and hand bending of wires.

To create a 3D model, this advanced system uses a specially designed handheld scanner to take pictures of the teeth. The orthodontist may also use cone and beam computer tomography along with the scanner to better analyze the orientation and position of the teeth. This is done by showing more detail between the bone, teeth, nerves, and soft tissues.

Once the 3D model is finished, the orthodontist uses special treatment planning software that includes virtual simulation tools to see the teeth and how they occlude from any angle. The dentist then determines the final position of the teeth and creates an effective treatment plan to be presented to the patient.

Once the patient has accepted the treatment plan, the information that was gathered is sent to a center where robots are used to bend a shape-memory alloy arch wire according to the orthodontist's specifications. The arch wire is then sent to the office, where it is ready to be placed once the brackets are bonded on the patient.

Orthodontic treatment designed with 3D imaging technology may be shorter due to the accuracy of the computerized treatment plan, but like traditional treatment, each case is individual and may vary. Overall patients may experience less pain due to the need of fewer wire changes and adjustments. This state-of-the-art orthodontic treatment is changing the way orthodontic treatment has been done for many years. The 3D imaging, virtual simulations, and use of robotics add a new dimension to orthodontic treatment. The dental assistant has the opportunity to learn new technology and skills, and to be part of the change in orthodontic treatment (Figure 28-21).

Orthodontic Instruments

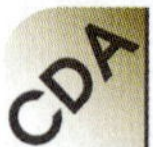

Listed below are commonly used instruments and their functions:

- Coon ligature tying pliers—Manipulates ligature wire (Figure 28-22)
- Mathieu needle holder—Ties ligature wire and places elastic ligatures (Figure 28-23)
- Ligature director—Tucks twisted ligature wire ends into interproximal spaces (a small condenser may also be used) (Figure 28-24)
- Pin and ligature cutter or light wire cutter—Cuts thin ligature wire (Figure 28-25)
- Howe pliers—Utility pliers to manipulate ligature wire (Figure 28-26)

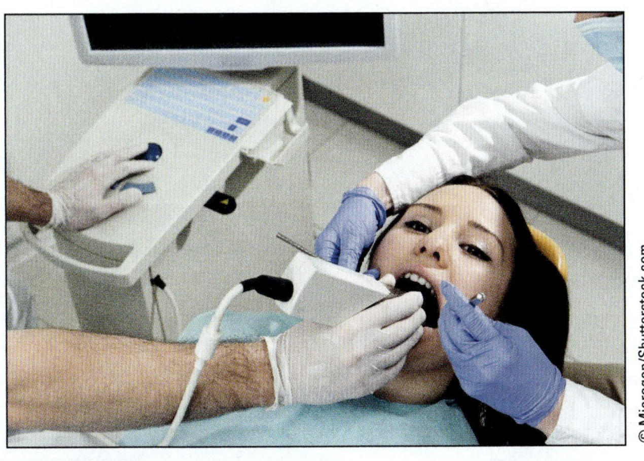

FIGURE 28-21

3D Imaging of an Orthodontic Patient

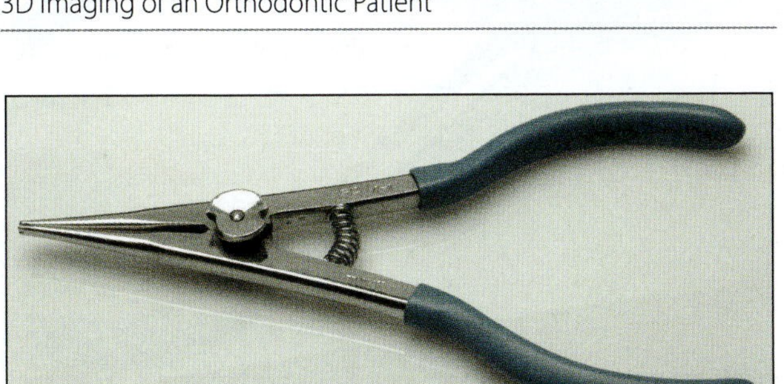

FIGURE 28-22

Coon ligature-typing pliers.

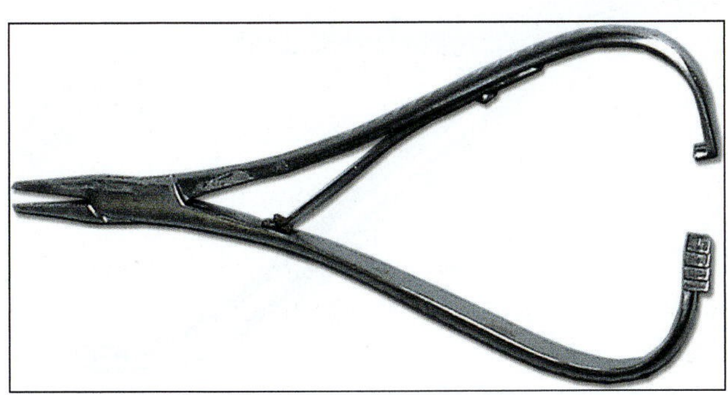

FIGURE 28-23

Mathieu needle holder.

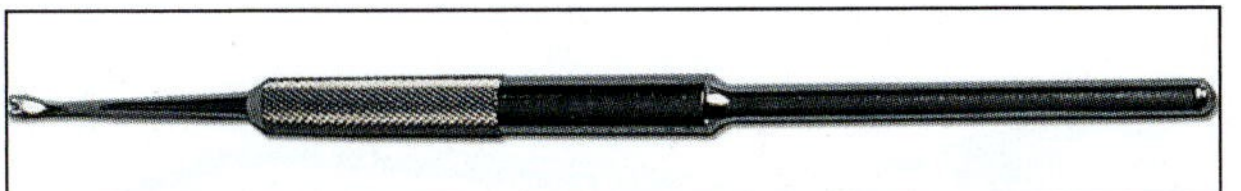

FIGURE 28-24

Ligature director.

- Band seater—Seats posterior metal bands (Figure 28-27A)
- Scaler—Removes excess cement and used to remove elastic ties (Figure 28-27B)
- Bite stick band seater—Uses force of occlusion to seat the band (Figure 28-28)

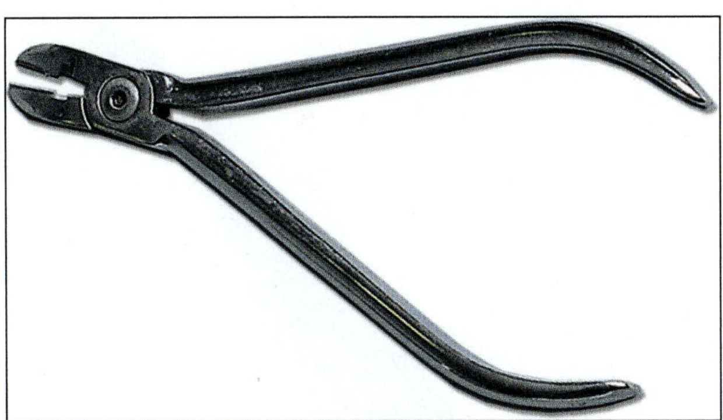

FIGURE 28-25

Pin and ligature cutter.

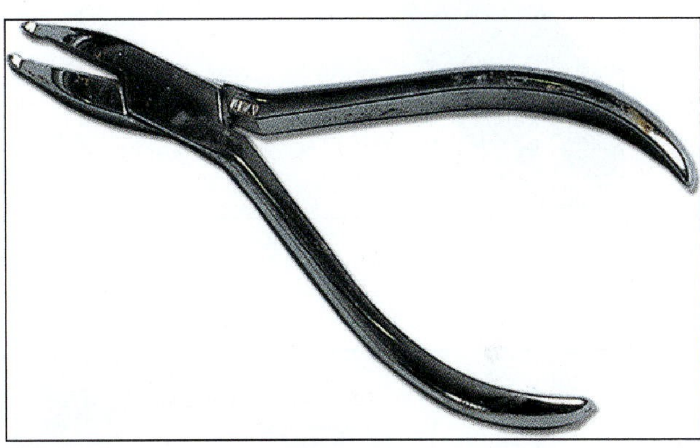

FIGURE 28-26

Howe pliers.

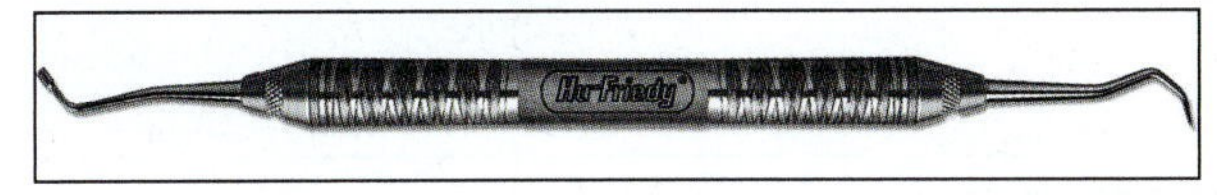

FIGURE 28-27

(A) Band seater. (B) Scaler.

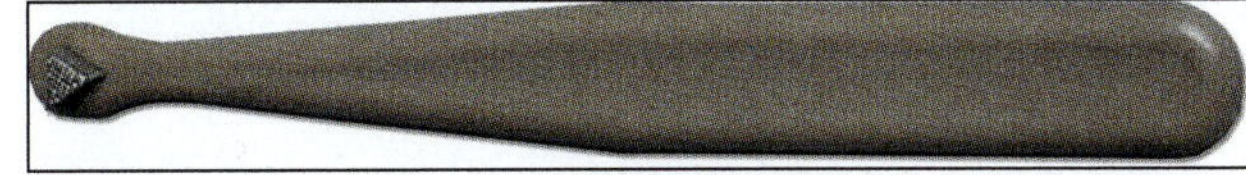

FIGURE 28-28

Bite stick with band seater.

- Band driver—Pushes the band into place (Figure 28-29)
- Posterior band-removing pliers—Removes posterior bands (Figure 28-30)
- Band-contouring pliers—Stretches and shapes the posterior bands to adapt to the tooth (Figure 28-31)
- Bracket forceps—Holds brackets for placement and positioning (Figure 28-32)
- Wire-bending pliers (sometimes called "Bird-beak" pliers)—Contours wire and forms springs (Figure 28-33)
- Elastic-separating pliers—Places elastic on brackets
- Three-prong pliers—Adjusts and bends wire and clasps (Figure 28-34)

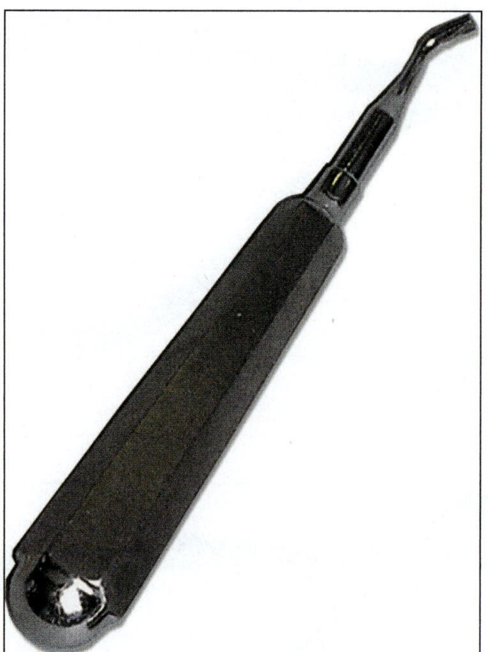

FIGURE 28-29
Band driver (pusher).

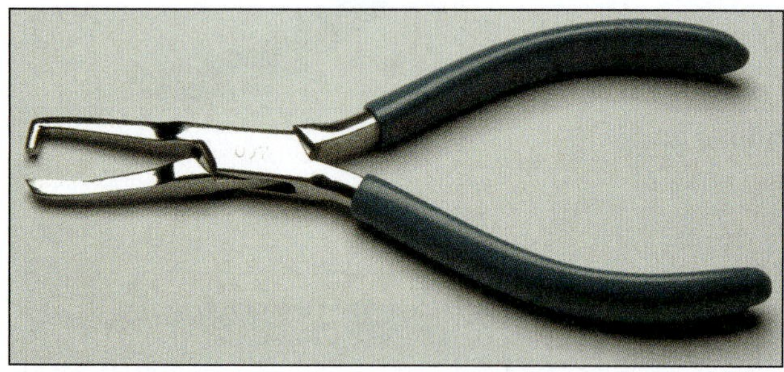

FIGURE 28-30
Posterior band–removing pliers.

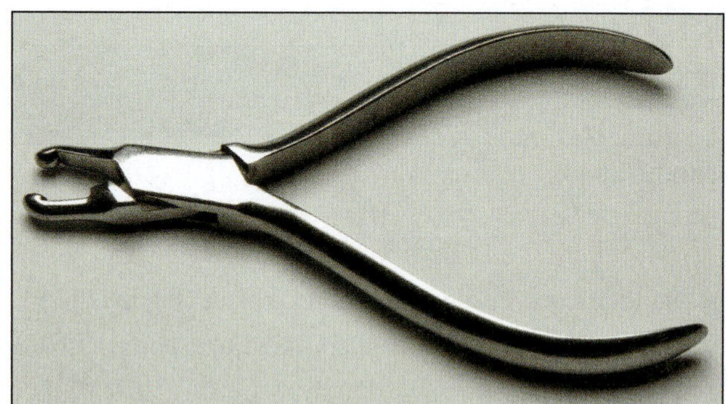

FIGURE 28-31
Band-contouring pliers.

- Weingart utility pliers—Places the arch wire (Figure 28-35)
- Tweed loop pliers—Forms loops and springs in wire (Figure 28-36)
- Distal end–cutting pliers—Used intraorally, these pliers cut the distal ends of the arch wire and have a mechanism that grasps the cut piece of the arch wire so it does not drop down the patient's throat (Figure 28-37)

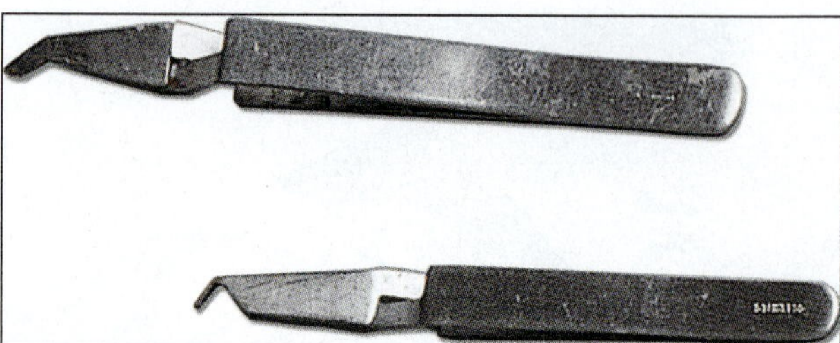

FIGURE 28-32
Bracket forceps.

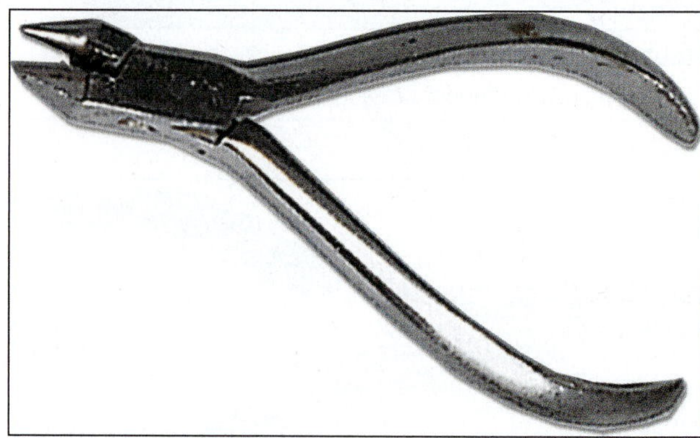

FIGURE 28-33
Wire-bending pliers, sometimes called "bird-beak" pliers.

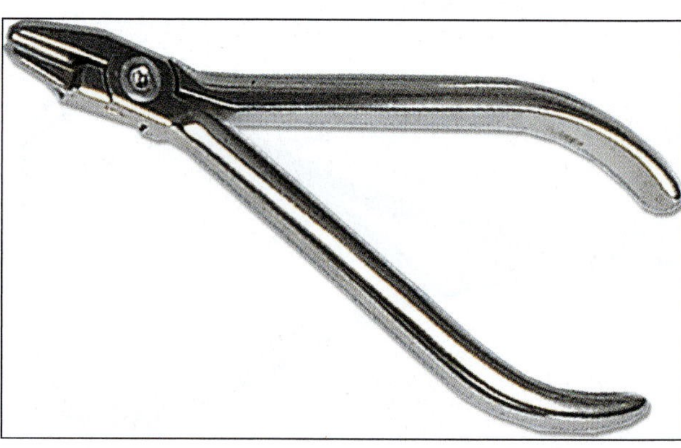

FIGURE 28-34
Three-prong pliers.

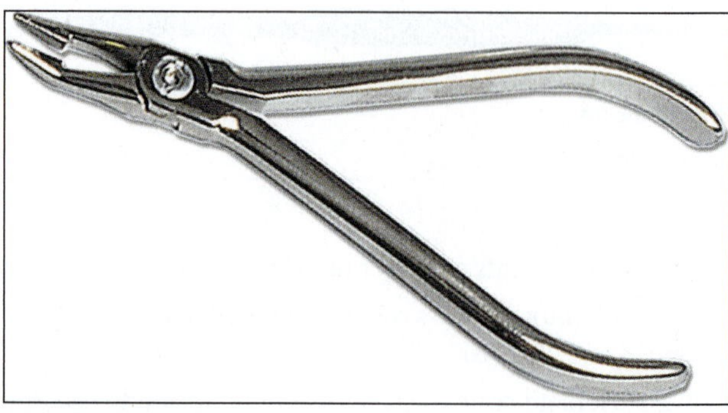

FIGURE 28-35
Weingart utility pliers.

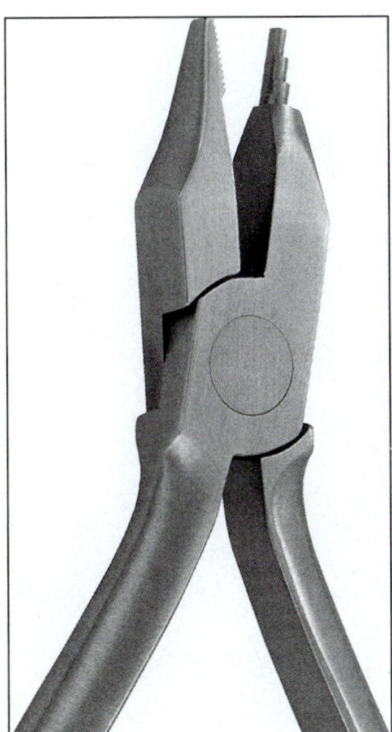

FIGURE 28-36
Tweed loop pliers.

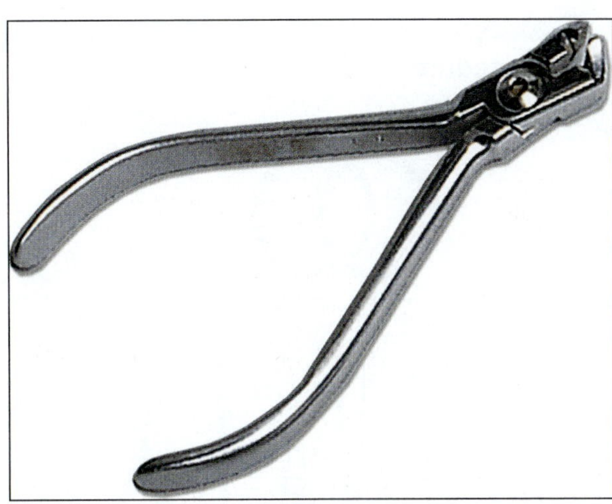

FIGURE 28-37
Distal end–cutting pliers.

Orthodontic Treatment

Orthodontic treatment begins after the patient has finished the consultation appointment, the general dentist has restored all areas of decay, and the patient has been given a prophylaxis and fluoride treatment.

The orthodontic treatment sequence follows:

1. Application of separators
2. Placement of posterior bands
3. Placement of anterior brackets
4. Placement of arch wire
5. Interval checkups
6. Completion appointment

Separators

A few days before the bands are placed on the posterior teeth, the patient is scheduled for placement of **separators**. Separators are placed in the contact areas between the teeth, forcing the teeth to spread apart to accommodate the orthodontic bands. Types of separators include elastics, steel spring, and brass wire.

Elastic separators are used because they provide a constant force as the teeth move, are easy to apply, and are more comfortable for the patient. The elastic separators are small circles that are stretched for placement. They fit around the contact area and, when released, apply a constant pressure until the teeth move apart, usually within a couple of days. The dental assistant may be permitted, in some states, to place and remove these separators (Procedures 28-1, 28-2, and 28-3).

Procedure 28-1
Placement and Removal of Elastic Separators

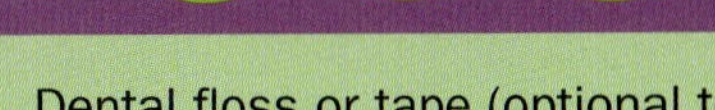

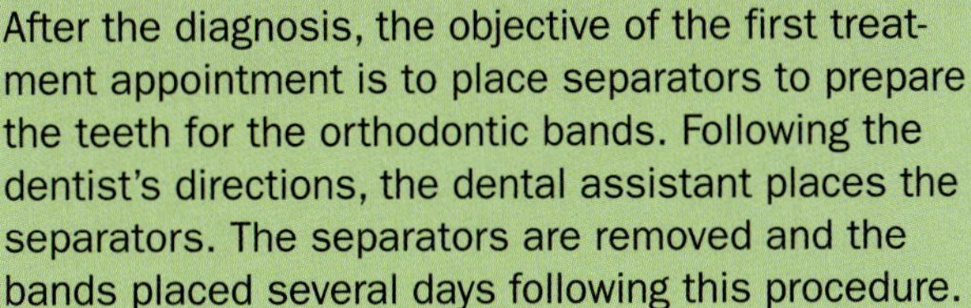

After the diagnosis, the objective of the first treatment appointment is to place separators to prepare the teeth for the orthodontic bands. Following the dentist's directions, the dental assistant places the separators. The separators are removed and the bands placed several days following this procedure.

Equipment and Supplies (*Figure 28-38*)

- Basic setup: mouth mirror, explorer, and cotton pliers
- Separation pliers
- Separators (wire or elastic)
- Dental floss or tape (optional technique)
- Scaler
- Mathieu needle holder

Procedure Steps (*Follow aseptic procedures*)

Placement of Elastic Separators with Separating Pliers

1. Examine the patient's mouth using the mouth mirror.
2. Place elastic separator over the beaks of the separating pliers. Squeeze the pliers to secure the elastic on the pliers.

(continues)

Procedure 28-1 (continued)

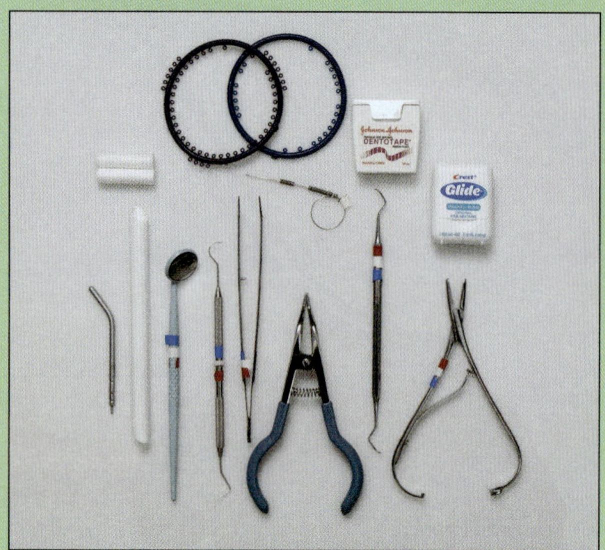

FIGURE 28-38
Tray setup for placement and removal of elastic separators.

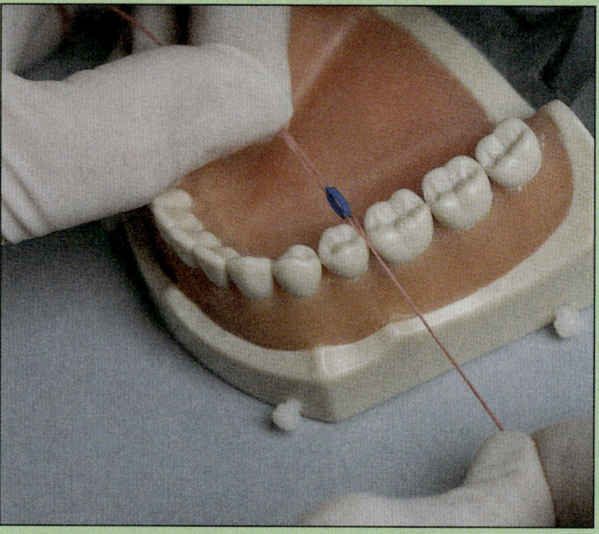

FIGURE 28-39
Placement of separators. Dental floss stretches elastic separator for placement.

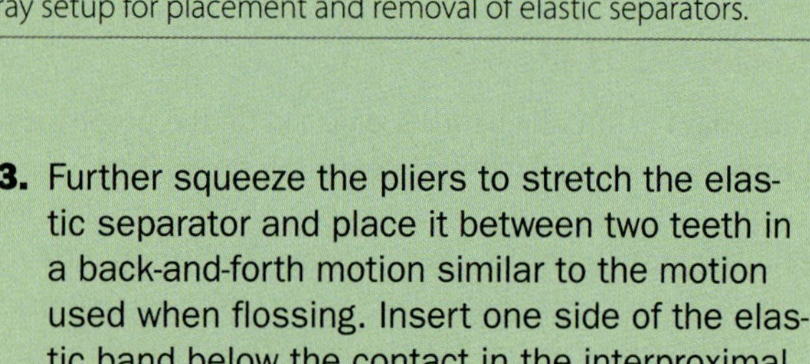

3. Further squeeze the pliers to stretch the elastic separator and place it between two teeth in a back-and-forth motion similar to the motion used when flossing. Insert one side of the elastic band below the contact in the interproximal space.
4. Release the tension on the separating pliers and remove the pliers. Repeat this process on all interproximal spaces around the teeth that will receive metal bands.

Placement of Separators with Dental Floss (*Figure 28-39*)

1. Place two lengths of dental floss through an elastic separator.
2. Fold over each floss length until the ends meet. Pull each piece of floss by the ends to stretch the elastic.
3. Using a back-and-forth motion, insert the separator into place.
4. Once the separator is in place, release the floss and pull free.

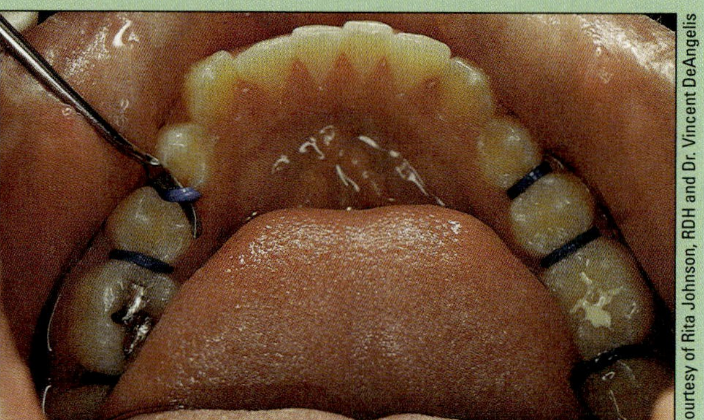

FIGURE 28-40
Removal of elastic separators.

Courtesy of Rita Johnson, RDH and Dr. Vincent DeAngelis

Removal of Elastic Separators (*Figure 28-40*)

1. Using a scaler or an explorer, insert one end into the ring of the elastic separator.
2. Place a finger over the top of the separator to prevent the separator from snapping and injuring the patient.
3. Pull gently on the instrument toward the occlusal until the elastic is free of the contact.

Selection of Orthodontic Bands

The patient returns to the office in a few days to have the separators removed and orthodontic bands placed. The bands may be selected and sized on the patient's study model before the appointment, or the selection may take place directly on the patient during the appointment. Bands are supplied in a wide variety of sizes for each tooth in the arch. They often have an identifying code printed on one surface. The code is helpful when selecting bands and replacing unused, sterilized bands.

Procedure 28-2
Placement and Removal of Steel Spring Separators

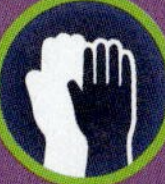

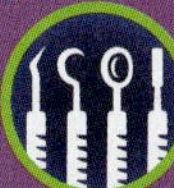

This technique involves placing and removing steel spring separators.

Equipment and Supplies

- Basic setup: mouth mirror, explorer, and cotton pliers
- Dental floss
- Bird-beak or #139 pliers
- Steel spring separators

Procedure Steps (*Follow aseptic procedures*)

Placing Steel Spring Separators (*Figure 28-41*)

1. Using the selected pliers or a hemostat, grasp the short end of the steel spring close to the coiled end.
2. Hook and engage the long arm of the separator over the occlusal surface of the tooth, engaging the hook into the lingual contact.
3. Place your finger over the occlusal arm (long) while stretching the gingival (short) arm out and then release the short side of the spring separator and slide it in under the contact.
4. The coil should be on the buccal/facial side; the long arm resting over the contact on the occlusal surface, the short arm under the contact on the gingival side and the spring should be close to the tooth.
5. Gently press the spring separator to test that it is securely in place.

Removing Steel Spring Separators

1. Place the finger of one hand over the spring to prevent injury to the patient.
2. Place one end of a scaler in the coil and lift upward.
3. Once the longest side of the spring is free of the lingual embrasure, pull the coil toward the facial aspect.

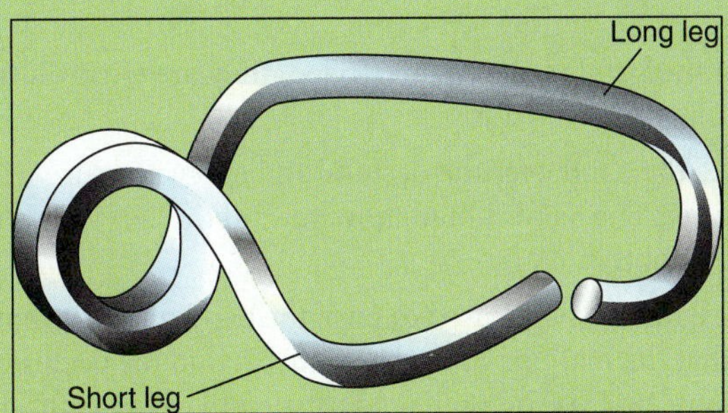

FIGURE 28-41
Steel spring separator.

Procedure 28-3
Placement and Removal of Brass Wire

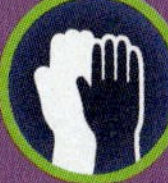

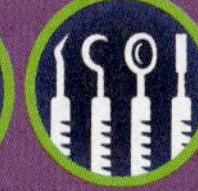

This procedure involves placing and removing brass wire separators.

Equipment and Supplies

- Basic setup: mouth mirror, explorer, and cotton pliers
- Spool of brass wire (*Figure 28-42*)
- Hemostat
- Ligature wire cutter
- Condenser

Placing Brass Wire Separators

1. Bend brass wire into C-shape, leaving a “tail” portion.
2. Starting from the lingual surface, place one part of the wire under the contact using a hemostat.
3. Fold the other part of the wire over the contact and pull toward the facial. Bring the ends of the wire together and twist.
4. Cut the twisted ends with the ligature cutting pliers and tuck them into the gingival embrasure.

(continues)

Procedure 28-3 (continued)

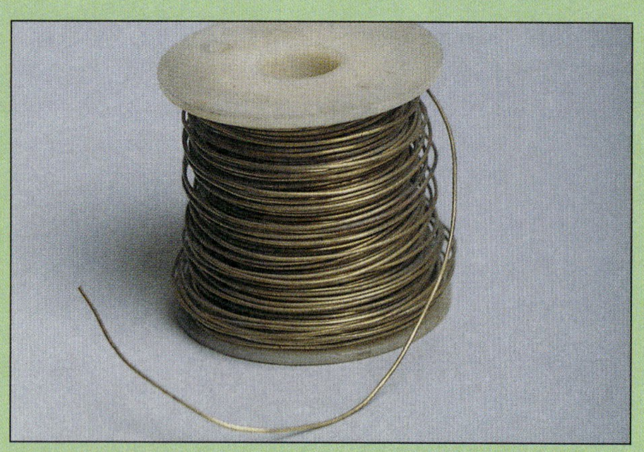

FIGURE 28-42

Spool of brass wire used to separate the teeth.

Removing Brass Wire Separators

1. Lift the brass wire carefully near the occlusal surface on the lingual side. Cut the wire using ligature cutting pliers.
2. Use the hemostat to remove both sections of the wire from under the contact on the facial side.

Once the bands have been selected, they are tried on the teeth in the following way:

1. Place the band over the occlusal and apply pressure with a finger. The band should move toward the cervical third of the tooth.
2. The band pusher is used to push the band onto the tooth so that the margins of the band are beyond the occlusion (Figure 28-43). The band is adjusted until it closely fits the tooth contours.
3. After all bands have been sized, they are removed with band removal pliers and placed on a model.
4. The orthodontist or lab technician then prepares the bands for final cementation by smoothing the margins of the bands with a handpiece and bur. If the bands have brackets or buccal tubes, the bands are fitted with pins or wax in the openings to prevent cement from filling the bracket holes and the buccal tubes.

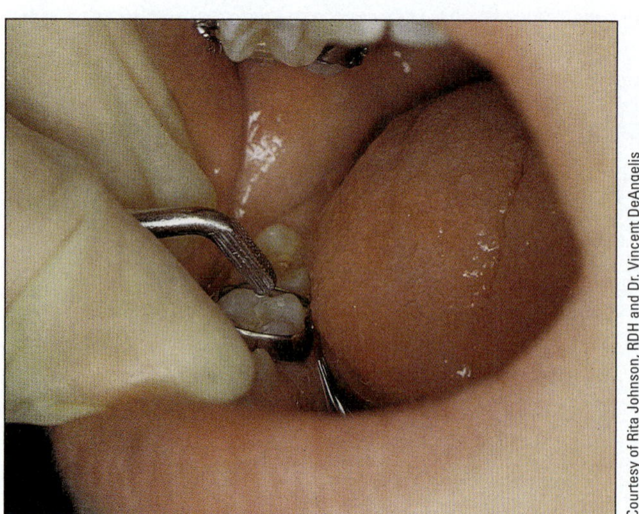

Courtesy of Rita Johnson, RDH and Dr. Vincent DeAngelis

FIGURE 28-43

Band pusher is used to seat the band on the tooth.

Band Cementation

Orthodontic bands are cemented using a variety of cements, including glass ionomer, polycarboxylate, and zinc phosphate. Although zinc phosphate cement has been used for many years, glass ionomer cement is becoming the preferred cement because it releases fluoride, which helps prevent decay under the bands during treatment.

Generally, the cement is thick for orthodontic band cementation and has a long setting time to permit final seating and adaptation. Follow manufacturer's instructions and technique suggestions (Procedure 28-4).

Direct Bonding Brackets

The placement of brackets directly on the anterior teeth is a popular choice of treatment. Patients like the brackets because they are more esthetic than the full bands and it is easier to maintain good oral hygiene. The brackets are often purchased in kits or sets. The kit includes brackets from the left second bicuspid to right second bicuspid on both arches.

The brackets are bonded to the tooth surface with a similar material and technique used to restore anterior teeth composite resin (Refer to Chapter 38, Restorative Materials, Matrix, and Wedge) (Procedure 28-5).

Procedure 28-4
Cementation of Orthodontic Bands

Orthodontic bands are prepared for the individual patient. The orthodontist places the bands on the teeth to accomplish the task needed to correct the patient's malocclusion. The dental assistant mixes the cement and prepares the band for seating.

Equipment and Supplies (*Figure 28-44*)

- Basic setup: mouth mirror, explorer, and cotton pliers
- Cotton rolls and gauze
- Saliva ejector and HVE
- Low-speed handpiece with rubber cup and prophy paste
- Selected and prepared bands
- Band pusher
- Bite stick
- Scaler
- Cement of choice
- Paper pad or glass slab
- Cement spatula
- Plastic filling instrument (PFI)

Procedure Steps (*Follow aseptic procedures*)

1. Once the separators are removed, the teeth are given a rubber cup polish.
2. The patient's mouth is rinsed thoroughly. The teeth are dried and cotton rolls are placed for isolation in the areas where the bands are to be placed.
3. Mix the cement according to manufacturer's directions and load the first band. Place cement from the gingival edge, covering the inside of the band. Once the band is ready, transfer it to the orthodontist. There are many methods to transfer the bands. Some orthodontists prefer placement on the mixing slab or pad in order. Others like the bands passed on the end of the spatula or on a piece of wax or masking tape. Transferring the band needs to be made as easy as possible. Position the bands so that the orthodontist can pick them up in order of placement sequence (Figure 28-45A).
4. The orthodontist seats the band on the tooth. Transfer the band driver and any other instrument the orthodontist requests until the band is properly seated.
5. The banding procedure is repeated. Continue to fill the bands and transfer them to the operator until all bands have been cemented or until the cement becomes too thick and a new mix is required. If a new mix is required, clean the instruments with wet gauze or an alcohol wipe and mix additional cement.
6. Once all bands are in place, the cement is allowed to set. During this time, clean the cement off all used instruments.
7. After the cement is set, remove the excess cement with a scaler. When all the cement has been removed, the protective pins or wax are removed from the brackets and the patient's mouth is rinsed (Figure 28-45B).

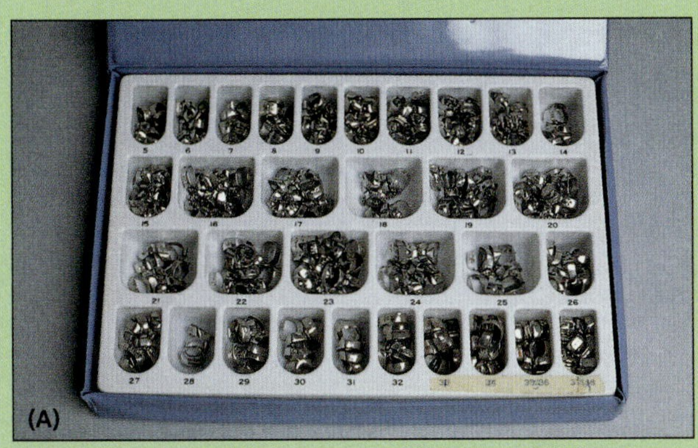

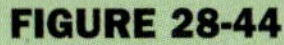

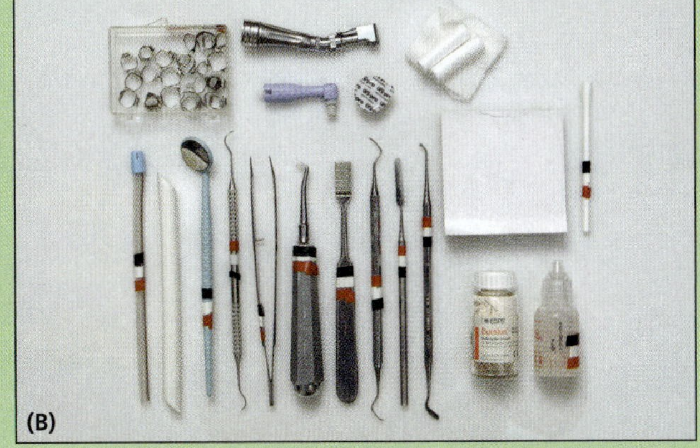

FIGURE 28-44

(A) Selection of bands. (B) Tray setup for cementation of orthodontic bands.

(continues)

Procedure 28-4 (continued)

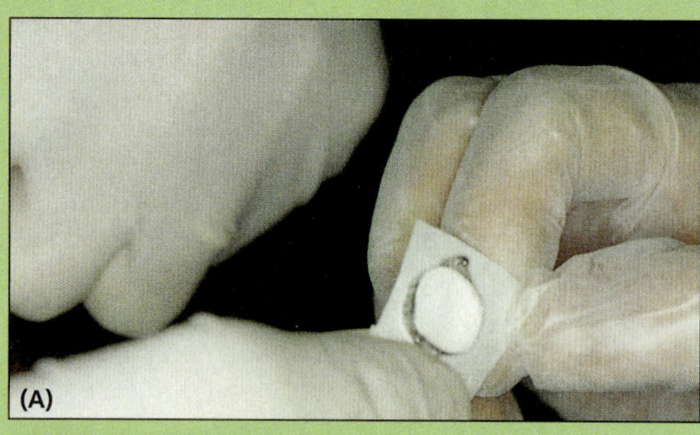

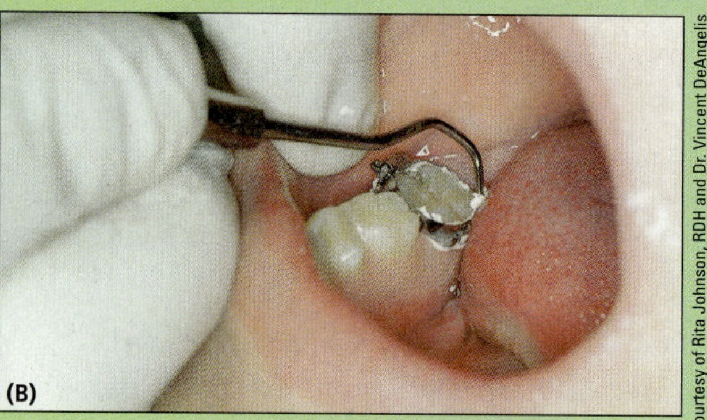

FIGURE 28-45

(A) Assistant passes the band filled with cement to operator. (The band is held on a piece of tape.) (B) Excess cement is removed from the tooth around the band.

(A and B) Courtesy of Rita Johnson, RDH and Dr. Vincent DeAngelis

Procedure 28-5

Direct Bonding of Brackets

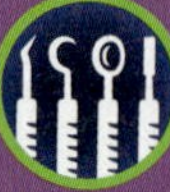

This procedure involves bonding the brackets to the teeth.

Equipment and Supplies (*Figure 28-46*)

- Basic setup: mouth mirror, explorer, and cotton pliers
- Cotton rolls and gauze
- Saliva ejector and HVE
- Low-speed handpiece with rubber cup and pumice
- Bracket kit
- Retractors for cheeks and lips

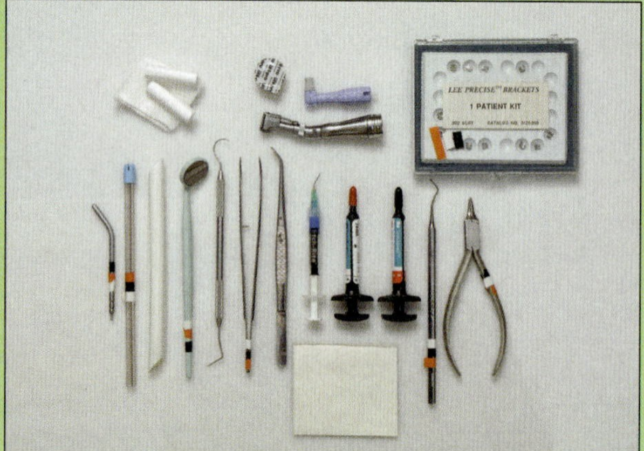

FIGURE 28-46

Tray setup for direct bonding of brackets.

- Bracket forceps
- Acid etchant
- Bonding agent
- Scaler

Procedure Steps (*Follow aseptic procedures*)

1. Polish the teeth that are to receive brackets with a rubber cup and pumice (Figure 28-47A). (Polishing paste with fluoride is not used because some of the ingredients will interfere with the bonding process.)
2. The patient's mouth is rinsed and dried. Cotton rolls are placed in the area where brackets are to be bonded and retractors are positioned.
3. The acid etchant is placed on the enamel surface. The etchant remains on the tooth for a specific amount of time, as per the manufacturer's directions. Prepare the etchant and transfer it to the operator. Maintain the operating field to be sure it stays dry.
4. Rinse the patient's mouth long enough to ensure that all the etchant is removed from the tooth surface (approximately 30 seconds) and then dry the tooth/teeth. The teeth will have a chalky appearance.
5. Prepare the bonding agent according to the manufacturer's directions and apply it to the

(continues)

Procedure 28-5 (continued)

back of the bracket (Figure 28-47B). Transfer the agent to the dentist for placement on the tooth. Then pass the bracket. The orthodontist positions it on the tooth. Any excess bonding agent is removed from around the bracket with a scaler or similar instrument. Care is used not to remove any bonding agent from between the bracket and the tooth; this would weaken the seal and could lead to decalcification and decay.

6. The brackets are then held in position on the tooth until the bonding material is set chemically or with a curing light (Figure 28-47C).
7. Remove the cotton rolls and retractors from the patient's mouth.

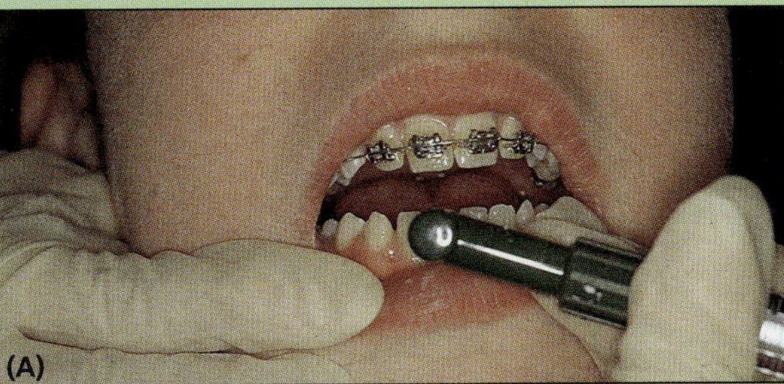

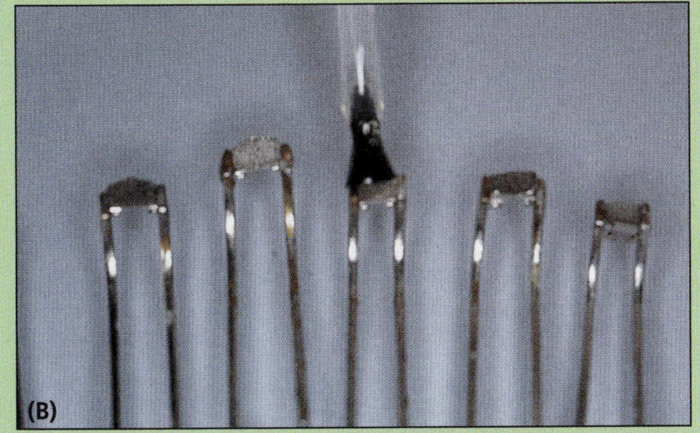

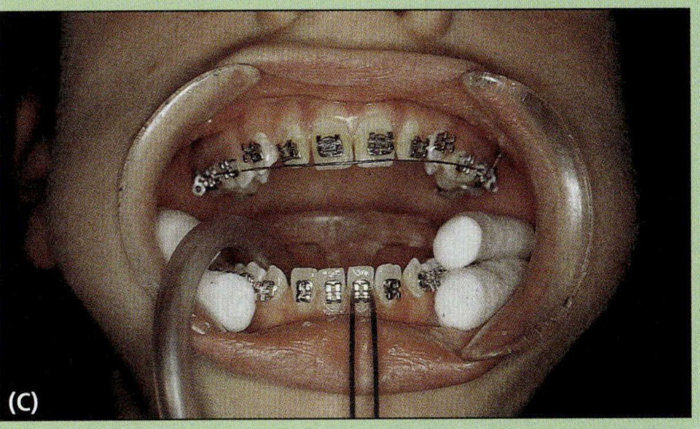

(A–C) Courtesy of Rita Johnson, RDH and Dr. Vincent DeAngelis

FIGURE 28-47
Steps in placement of direct-bonded brackets. (A) Clean tooth surface. (B) Apply bonding agent. (C) Place bracket on tooth and light cure.

Placement of Arch Wire

The orthodontist selects and shapes the arch wire, so once the bands and brackets are placed, the arch wire can be positioned and secured in place (Procedure 28-6). The arch wire is commonly secured into the brackets with elastic or stainless steel ligatures (ties). There is also a bracket that does not require ligature ties; instead, the bracket has a slot that opens for placement and removal of the arch wire. It is called the "Damon SL" **self-ligating bracket** (Figure 28-48).

Oral Hygiene Instructions

Oral hygiene instructions are given to the patient once the braces are in place. With fixed braces, food and debris have many places to hide in and attach to, making the patient more caries susceptible. Good oral hygiene is necessary to prevent plaque buildup in these areas. The dental assistant educates and motivates the patient. This process is continued throughout the treatment. Keeping some patients motivated can be a challenge, and

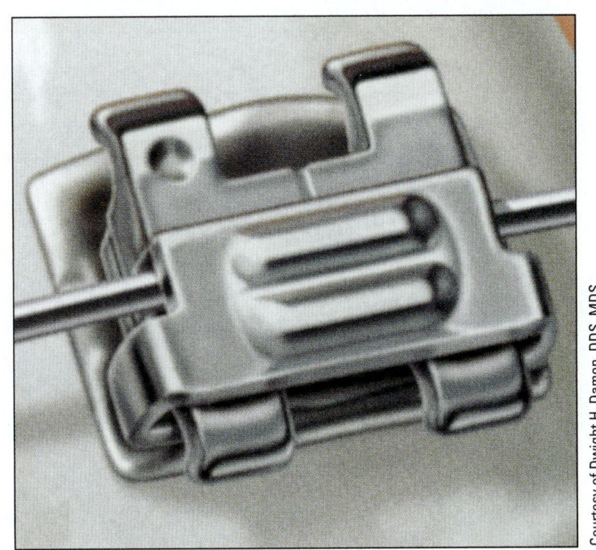

Courtesy of Dwight H. Damon, DDS, MDS.

FIGURE 28-48
Damon self-ligating brackets.

Procedure 28-6
Placement of Arch Wire and Ligature Ties

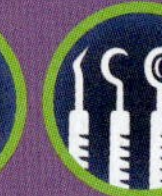
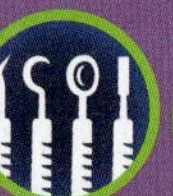

This procedure involves placing the arch wire and ligature ties.

Equipment and Supplies (*Figure 28-49*)

- Basic setup: mouth mirror, explorer, and cotton pliers
- Cotton rolls and gauze
- Saliva ejector and HVE
- Selected arch wire
- Weingart pliers
- Bird-beak pliers
- Elastics or ligature wire
- Ligature-cutting pliers
- Ligature-tying pliers
- Distal end–cutting pliers
- Condenser

Procedure Steps

1. Insert the arch wire into the buccal tubes on the molar bands using the Weingart pliers. If the wire is too long, cut off the ends with the distal-end cutting pliers.
2. The arch wire is placed in the horizontal slot of each bracket and held in place with plastic rings/elastic ties, ligature wire, or with the self-ligating bracket (Figure 28-50).

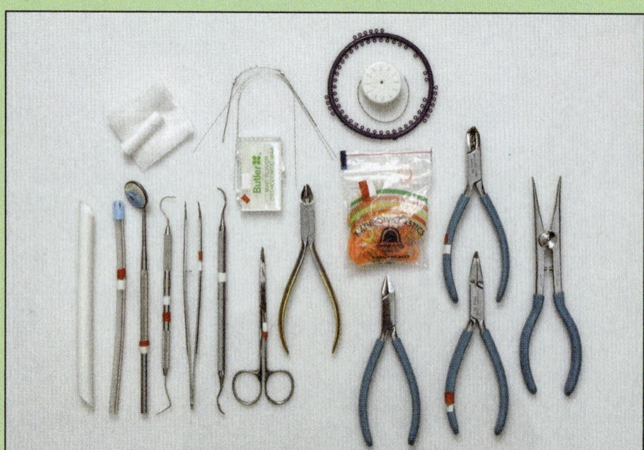

FIGURE 28-49

Tray setup for placement of arch wire and ligature ties or elastics to secure the arch wire.

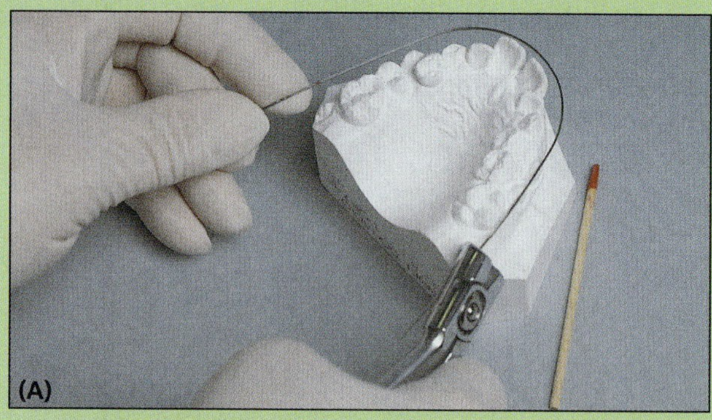

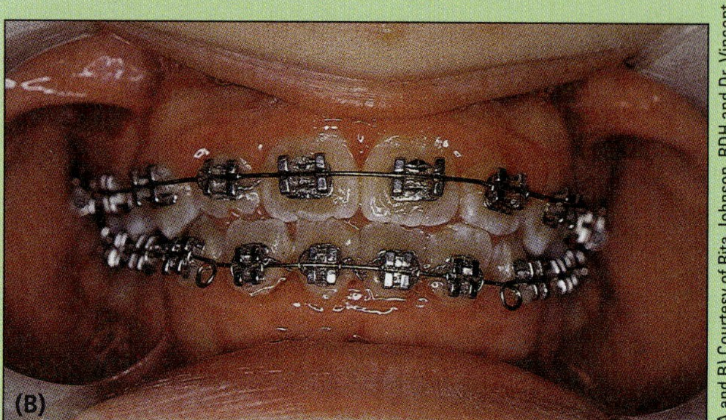

(A and B) Courtesy of Rita Johnson, RDH and Dr. Vincent DeAngelis

FIGURE 28-50

(A) Arch wire is cut to size with distal end–cutting pliers.
(B) Place arch wire in buccal tubes.

Elastic Ties Placement

3. The elastic ties are slipped over the brackets using ligature-tying pliers or a hemostat. The ring ties are spread and placed on the gingival extensions of the brackets, pulled over the arch wire, and then wrapped around the occlusal extensions of the brackets (Figure 28-51).

Ligature Wire Ties placement

4. Hold the ligature wire between the thumb and the index finger. Wrap the wire around the occlusal and gingival wings of the bracket in a distal-mesial direction. Cross the ends of the wire together. Using a hemostat or ligature-tying pliers, twist the ends of the wire together for several rotations. Repeat the process to secure the arch wire (Figure 28-52A).

(continues)

Procedure 28-6 (continued)

5. The twisted ends of the ligature wire, called the "pigtail," are cut with ligature-wire cutting pliers to a length of 3 to 4 mm (Figures 28-52B and C).
6. The pigtail is bent into the embrasure space with a condenser (Figure 28-52D).

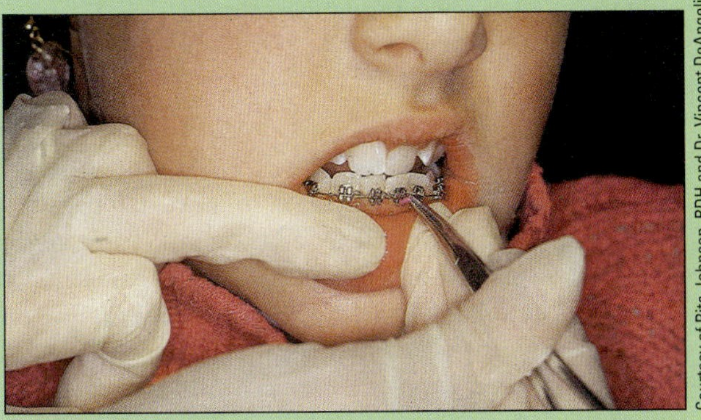

Courtesy of Rita Johnson, RDH and Dr. Vincent DeAngelis

FIGURE 28-51

Elastic rings being placed on anterior brackets, using a hemostat.

7. After all the pigtail ends have been tucked into place, run a finger over the area to check for sharp ends.
8. Check the distal ends of the arch wire. Cut any excess with distal end–cutting pliers.
9. If the patient's treatment requires rubber elastic bands, they are placed at this appointment. The patient is shown how to place and remove them.

The rubber bands stretch over time, so the orthodontist will give instructions on how often to change the rubber bands. The patient is given a sufficient number of elastics with instructions to call the office for more, if needed.

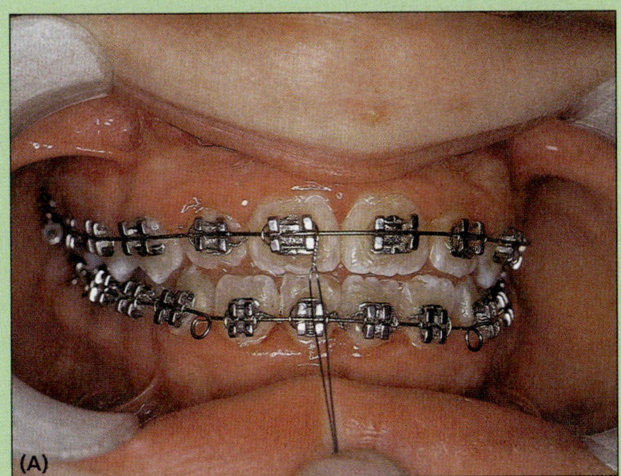

(A)

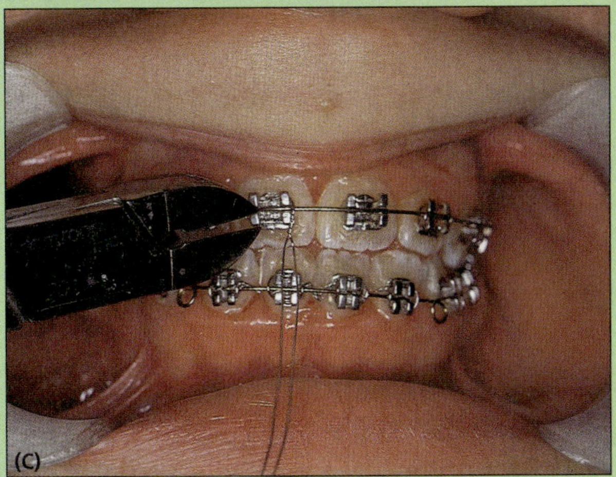

(C)

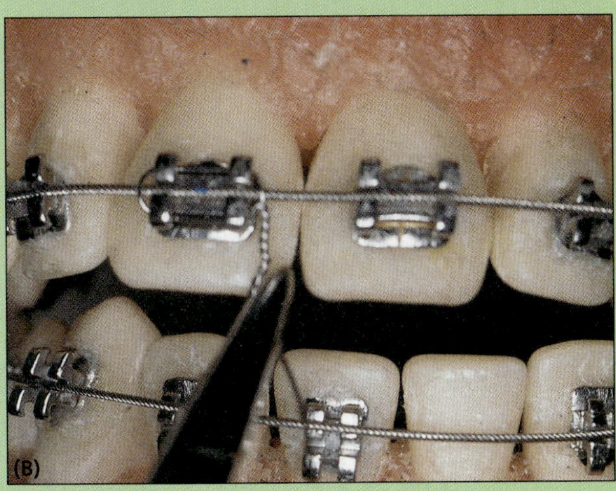

(B)

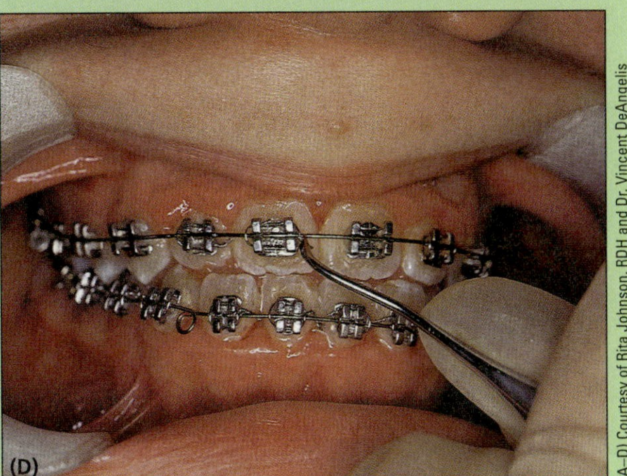

(D)

(A–D) Courtesy of Rita Johnson, RDH and Dr. Vincent DeAngelis

FIGURE 28-52

(A) Ligature wire being looped around brackets. (B) Ligature wire is twisted. (C) Ligature wire is cut with cutting pliers. (D) Ligature wire is tucked into embrasure space.

numerous approaches must be used. Instructions include the following:

- Brushing—The patient is given an orthodontic toothbrush and shown how to brush around the fixed appliances in order to remove plaque. The toothbrush is contoured to fit around the brackets and into the space between the band and the gingival margin. The patient will need to spend more time after meals and at bedtime to keep the teeth clean (Figures 28-53A and B).
- Flossing—Supply the patient with a floss threader to thread the floss under the arch wire and through the interproximal area. Motivating the patient to take the time to floss routinely may be a challenge (Figure 28-54). Patients may use interproximal brushes to help with hygiene compliance.
- Diet—The patient should avoid certain foods that may damage the bands, arch wire, or brackets. Foods that are sticky, crunchy, and hard should be avoided. Examples include caramels, chewing gum, popcorn, and raw vegetables (unless they are cut into small pieces).
- Fluoride rinses—These may be prescribed for the patient's home use during orthodontic treatment.

Periodic Office Visits for Adjustments

As time passes and the teeth begin to move, the patient will need to see the orthodontist for adjustments. These appointments are usually short, unless the arch wire needs to be changed. The orthodontist reviews the patient's progress, checks the appliances, and makes any adjustments. The dental assistant performs some of these tasks under direct supervision of the dentist.

These appointments are also used for oral hygiene checks. If the patient is not doing an adequate job, the dental assistant reviews brushing and flossing and talks with the patient to motivate and encourage the patient. Helping some patients stay motivated to maintain their oral hygiene can be a challenge. Educating the patient is the first step, followed by demonstrating various techniques to improve brushing and flossing with their braces in place. Each orthodontic office has different ways to encourage, motivate, and reward patients who maintain their oral hygiene effectively. Verbal and written encouragement, prizes, gift cards, passes to movies, and placing the patient's name in a drawing for a larger prize are just a few ways to motivate and reward the patient for good oral hygiene and for following instructions.

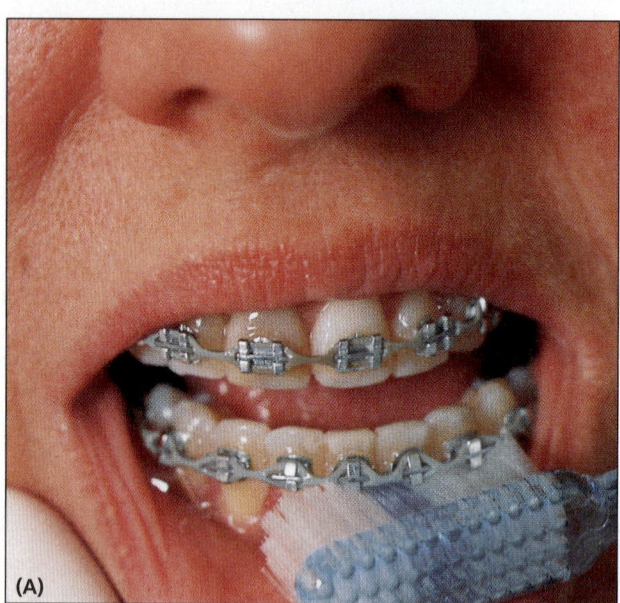
(A)

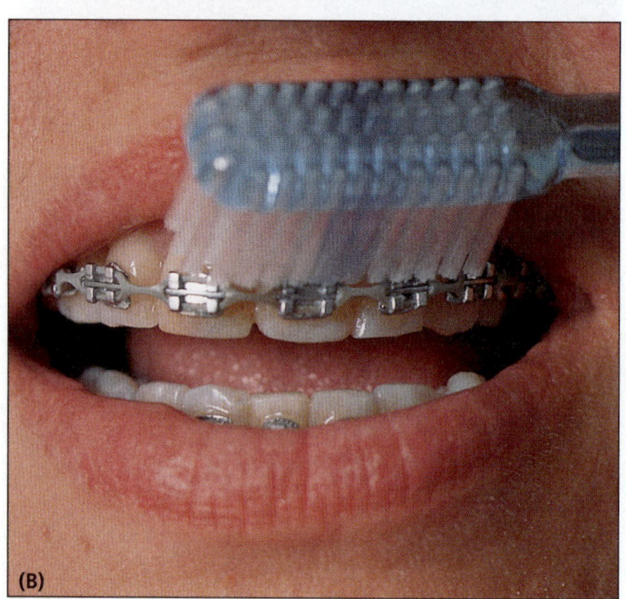
(B)

FIGURE 28-53

Tooth brushing techniques on a patient with fixed orthodontic appliances. Toothbrush positioned properly on (A) maxillary teeth and (B) mandibular teeth.

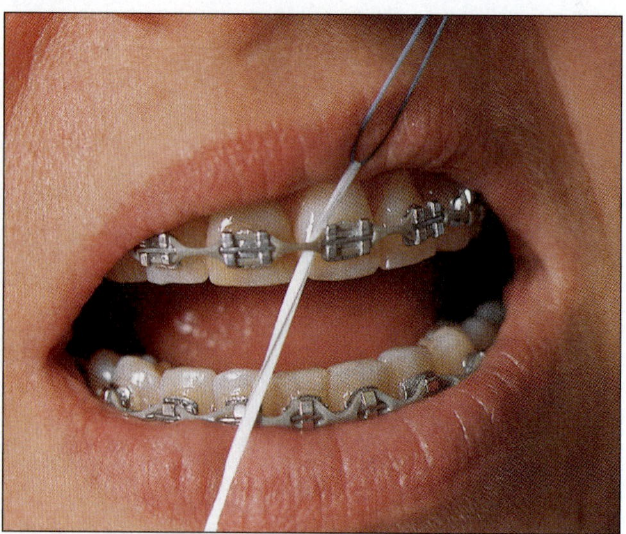

FIGURE 28-54

Floss being threaded under arch wire.

Completion Appointment

Once the teeth have moved into position and the orthodontist is satisfied with the treatment, the braces are removed. The patient receives a coronal polish and an impression is taken for construction of a retainer (Procedure 28-7) or positioner to hold the teeth in position for the alveolar bone to stabilize the new positions of the teeth.

Procedure 28-7
Completion Appointment

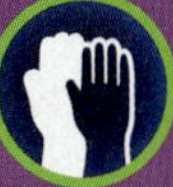

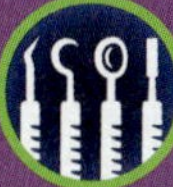

When the orthodontist determines that the patient's teeth have moved to the desired positions, the appliances are removed.

Equipment and Supplies (*Figure 28-55*)

- Basic setup: mouth mirror, explorer, and cotton pliers
- Cotton rolls and gauze
- Scaler
- Ligature-wire cutting pliers Hemostat
- Bracket- and adhesive-removing pliers
- Posterior band remover
- Ultrasonic scaler (optional)
- Prophy angle, cups, and prophy paste
- Alginate impression material and selected tray

Procedure Steps (*Follow aseptic procedures*)

Ligature Wire Ties

1. The ligature ties are removed first. They are loosened with a scaler or an explorer and then cut with the ligature-wire cutting pliers.

Elastic Bands

2. Place the beaks of ligature-wire cutting pliers where the wire is exposed and cut the wire.
3. Carefully remove the wire from the wings of the bracket. Repeat on each tooth until all ligature wires are removed.
4. Elastic ties are removed with a scaler.
5. The tip of the scaler explorer is placed under the elastic and rolled over the bracket wings until the elastic is released (Figure 28-56).

Removal of Arch Wire

6. Using a hemostat, remove the arch wire from the brackets (Figure 28-57). Pull the arch wire from the buccal tube on one side. Then hold it securely to prevent injury to the patient while removing the opposite end.
7. To remove the anterior brackets, use a bracket and adhesive-removing pliers. The lower beak of the pliers, with a very sharp edge, is placed on the gingival edge of the bracket; the upper beak, with a nylon tip, is placed on the occlusal edge of the bracket. When the pliers are squeezed together, the sharp lower beak breaks the bond and removes some cement (Figure 28-58).

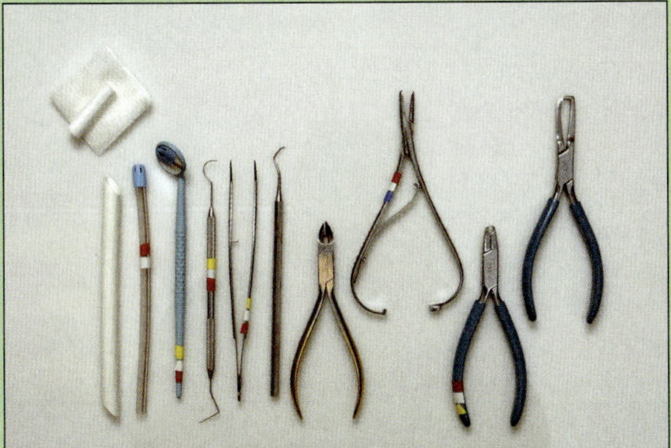

FIGURE 28-55
Completion appointment tray setup.

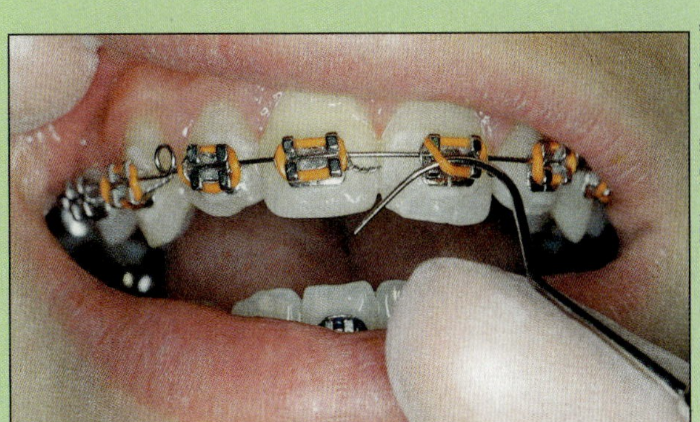

Courtesy of Rita Johnson, RDH and Dr. Vincent DeAngelis

FIGURE 28-56
Removal of elastic rings. Insert end of scaler or explorer under elastic, and roll elastic rings over wings of bracket.

(continues)

Procedure 28-7 (continued)

8. To remove the posterior bands, band-removing pliers are placed with the cushioned end on the buccal cusp. The end with the blade is placed against the gingival edge of the band. The band is gently lifted toward the occlusal surface (Figure 28-59).
9. This process is repeated on the lingual surfaces until the band is free.
10. Cement and direct bonding materials are removed from the tooth surface with a hand scaler, an ultrasonic scaler, and/or a finishing bur.
11. A rubber cup polish is completed. Photographs may be taken.
12. An alginate impression is taken of both arches. The impressions are sent to the lab to be used in construction of the retainer.
13. The patient is reappointed for later that day or for the next day. The retainer or positioner is then placed.
14. The patient is given instructions on placement and removal of the retainer and the wearing schedule.

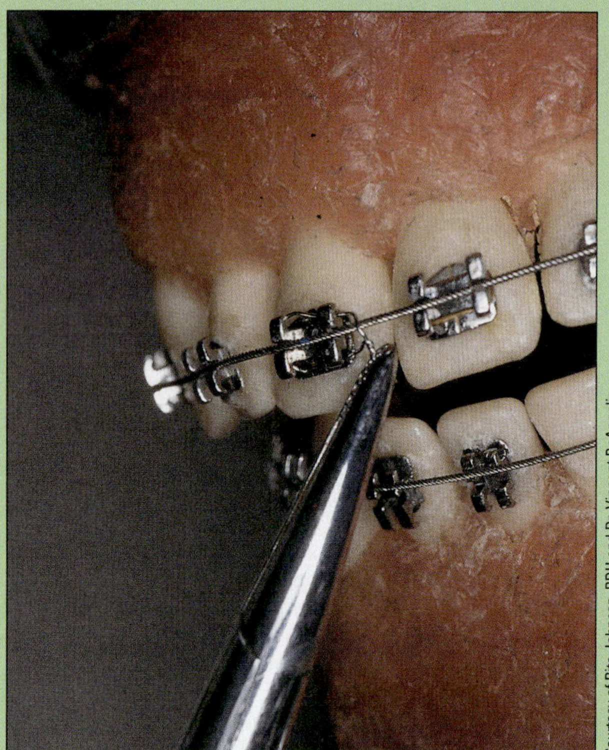

FIGURE 28-57

Removal of ligature wire. Pull twisted "pigtail" wire from embrasure. Cut wire. Unwind from wings of bracket in an occlusal direction.

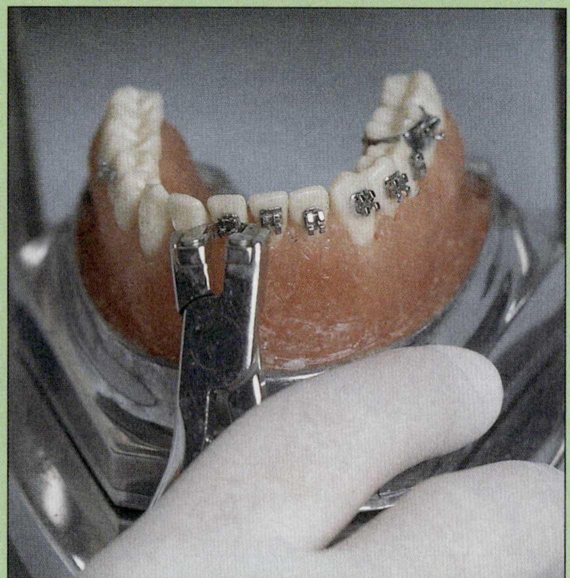

FIGURE 28-58

Bracket removal.

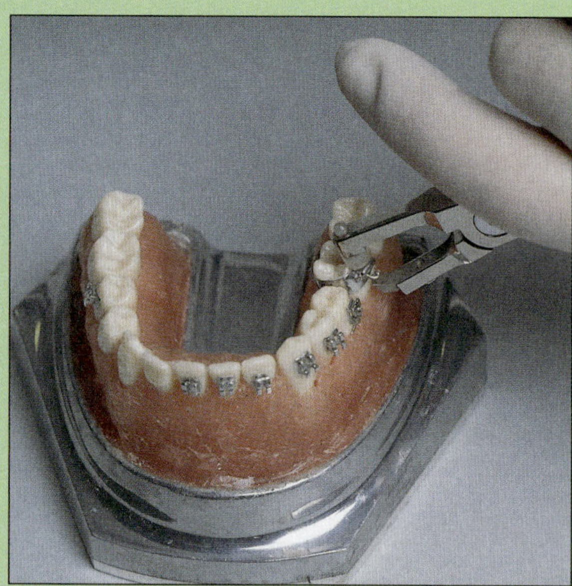

FIGURE 28-59

Band removal with band-removal pliers.

Chapter Summary

Orthodontics is an exciting specialty that provides many opportunities for the dental assistant. Depending on the size of the practice and the number of auxiliaries, the assistant assists the dentist, performs many chairside skills independently, motivates patients, provides oral hygiene instruction, does laboratory tasks, and may work with the orthodontist during case presentations/consultations.

This chapter covers the various appointments needed for orthodontic treatment, the materials and instruments used, and types of orthodontic appliances most commonly used. Each state regulates the education and the skills the dental assistant may perform directly and indirectly on the orthodontic patient. To become a certified orthodontic assistant, the assistant must pass a specialty examination administered by the Dental Assistant National Board and/or the individual state board of dentistry.

CASE STUDY

Chaz Danton, 12 years old, had an appointment with the orthodontist, Dr. Snyder. Chaz has an overbite and a receded mandible. When eating crunchy foods, such as toast and pizza crust, his palate becomes inflamed and irritated. Chaz is missing his permanent bicuspids.

Review

1. What should the dental assistant prepare for Chaz's appointment?
2. Is Chaz's age a factor in the orthodontist's diagnosis?
3. What stage of tooth eruption should the dental assistant expect Chaz to be in? Which primary teeth are normally present?
4. Which of Dr. Angle's classes of malocclusion do you expect to see and record?

Review Questions

Multiple Choice

1. When individual teeth are turned or rotated in the socket, they are said to be
   a. infraverted.
   b. linguoverted.
   c. transposed.
   d. torsoverted.
2. Which of the following types of orthodontic treatments involve fixing an existing problem?
   a. Preventive treatment
   b. Interceptive treatment
   c. Corrective treatment
3. Orthodontic tracings are made using which of the following types of radiographs?
   a. Bite-wing
   b. Periapical
   c. Cephalometric
   d. Panoramic
4. To secure the arch wire in position on the posterior bands, use
   a. buccal tubes.
   b. brackets.
   c. springs.
   d. plastic rings.
5. All of the following are true statements about orthodontic brackets *except*
   a. brackets are welded onto orthodontic bands or bonded directly to the teeth.
   b. brackets are made of stainless steel, ceramic, or acrylic.
   c. brackets hold the bands in place on the teeth.
   d. brackets hold the arch wire in place.
6. An abnormal horizontal distance between the labial surface of the mandibular anterior teeth and the lingual surface of maxillary teeth is a(an)
   a. open bite.
   b. overjet.
   c. underbite.
   d. overbite.

7. Specialized bone cells that cause the bone to resorb or break down are
   a. osteoclasts.
   b. osteoblasts.
   c. odontoclasts.
   d. odontoblasts.
8. During the consultation appointment, which of the following is discussed?
   a. Cost of treatment
   b. Patient's responsibility
   c. Duration of treatment
   d. All of the above
9. Which of the following instruments is used to tie ligature wire and/or place elastic ligatures?
   a. Coons pliers
   b. Ligature director
   c. Mathieu pliers
   d. ligature-wire cutting pliers
10. Elastic ties are removed with which of the following?
   a. Bird-beak pliers
   b. Weingart utility pliers
   c. Scaler
   d. Howe pliers

Critical Thinking

1. Do you have teeth that are out of alignment? Using orthodontic terms, describe the deviations and identify the malpositioned teeth.
2. Which foods should the orthodontic patient avoid? What are some alternatives?
3. Name the three categories of causes of malocclusion. Give three examples in each category. Have you or anyone in your family had an orthodontic condition? Trace the etiology to one of the categories.
4. Discuss the importance of using a space maintainer and why it should stay in the patient's mouth until the permanent tooth erupts.
5. List ways to motivate the orthodontic patient to brush and floss during orthodontic treatment.

Web Activities

1. Go to http://www.invisalign.com and find out if this treatment would work for you.
2. Go to http://www.ormco.com and watch the video on the Damon bracket system.
3. Go to http://www.www1.mylifemysmile.org and find out which month is orthodontic health month. Learn about the history of orthodontics.
4. Go to http://www.cfastresults.com and http://www.*6monthsmiles*.com to learn more about treatments that general dentist are incorporating into their practices.

CHAPTER

29

Pediatric Dentistry

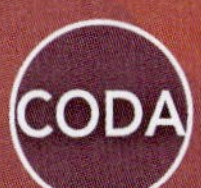

CODA

Specific Instructional Objectives

The student should strive to meet the following objectives and demonstrate an understanding of the facts and principles presented in this chapter:

1. Define pediatric dentistry as a specialty.
2. Describe the pediatric office and team members.
3. Explain the common behavioral characteristics of children of various ages.
4. Describe child behavior management techniques.
5. Explain the role of the parent or guardian in pediatric dentistry.
6. Identify common procedures in pediatric dentistry, including preventive procedures, diet, restorative procedures, preventive and interceptive orthodontic treatment, and restorative procedures.
7. Identify the equipment unique to pediatric dentistry.
8. Explain common emergencies in pediatric dentistry and the treatment for these emergencies.
9. Identify the signs of child abuse and the procedure for reporting suspected child abuse cases.

Key Terms

apexogenesis (704)
avulsed tooth (708)
behavior management (695)
direct pulp capping (DPC) (701)
fluoride application (698)
fluoride varnish (698)
Formocresol (704)
hand-over-mouth (HOM) technique (696)
indirect pulp treatment (IPT) (701)
maturation (693)
modeling technique (695)
mouth guard (698)
objective fears (694)
papoose board (696)
pedodontics (692)
pulpectomy (704)
pulpotomy (701)
space maintainer (699)
spot-welded matrix band (700)
stainless steel crown (704)
subjective fears (694)
T-band matrix (700)
tell, show, and do technique (695)
tongue thrusting (699)
traumatic intrusion (707)

Introduction

The pediatric dental practice provides dental care for children and is often referred to as **pedodontics**. The pediatric specialist treats children from birth through the eruption of their second permanent molars. The pediatric practice sometimes treats medically, mentally, or emotionally compromised adults as well. The scope of pediatric treatment for children includes restoring and maintaining the primary, mixed, and permanent dentition, and applying preventive measures for dental caries, periodontal disease, and malocclusion. The restorative aspect is a large part of the practice, but the primary focus of the pediatric dental practice is preventive treatment.

The pediatric specialist is concerned with the basic needs and special requirements for treatment of the young patient. The pediatric dentist has 2 to 3 years of additional training after dental school. This advanced education includes study in pediatric growth patterns, development, and behavior management. This training enables the pediatric dentist to successfully treat the emotionally and physically developing child as well as the patient with special needs.

American Academy of Pediatrics (AAP)

The AAP is the guiding organization of the pediatric dentist. "The mission of the AAP is to attain optimal physical, mental, and social health and well-being for all infants, children, adolescents and young adults." The AAP works with the community, government, and other national organizations as an advocate for health care and an educator about safety issues for children from infancy to young adulthood, as well as for patients with special needs. The AAP provides the means for research programs and publications for consumers, physicians, and other health care professionals. Along with brochures and books, there is also a parent-oriented website, HealthyChildren.org, which offers up-to-date dental health care advice.

The general dentist, other specialists, and physicians refer patients to the pediatric specialist for treatment. The general dentist, orthodontist, and pediatric dentist work closely together to ensure that the child patient receives the best overall dental care and education. Pediatric dentists as a group have been very instrumental in improving dental care for children, and in educating children and parents/guardians. Many programs are available, but the need to provide these services is still great. Some areas have federal, state, or local programs to provide dental care for children, while others have little, if any, assistance. There is a great deal that can be done to prevent tooth decay and early loss of primary teeth. Dentists, dental assistants, and dental hygienists are working with communities to provide education and various services for children. The Surgeon General of the United States, along with the ADA and the American Association of Pediatrics (AAP), has expressed such concerns, and continually seeks means and ways to meet this need. One such example is the ABCD Program, which is recognized by the ADA and the AAP. This program provides dental access to high-risk preschool children. The program was developed in the state of Washington by concerned dentists, dental educators, public health agencies, the state dental association, and state Medicaid representatives. The focus is on prevention and restorative dental care for Medicaid-eligible children from birth to age six. The goal is to start dental visits early in order to produce positive behaviors from both parents and children, and reducing the need for costly dental work as the child ages by controlling the dental decay process. Go to http://www.abcd-dental.org for more information.

The Pediatric Dental Office

The pediatric office is open and friendly to make the child patient feel comfortable and secure. Pediatric office settings are creative and imaginative. The decor is often brightly designed with things children are attracted to. The reception room usually has an area for coloring or reading, a cage for small animals or a fish tank, toys for various age groups, and a display area with pictures of patients (Figure 29-1).

In some pediatric offices, the treatment areas are designed with several dental chairs arranged in an open area. This open bay concept allows children to see one another. It is reassuring for the child patient to know that other children are there and receiving treatment. Many offices have headphones with a variety of programs or music available, or televisions with either movies or patient education programs running.

Often the pediatric office will include a quiet room for patients who are difficult to manage. This room is separate and closed off from the others so that if patient management problems occur, they will not upset the other children in the office.

The Pediatric Dental Team

The composition of the pediatric dental team is similar to the general dental office team, including the pediatric dentist, dental assistants, expanded function dental assistants, hygienist, and the reception and business office auxiliary. The difference may be the personalities of the team members, and their desire to work with children. The entire staff needs to enjoy children, and be sincere and honest in their actions and feelings. To be effective in managing children, the dental team must be upbeat, motivated, and aware.

The pediatric staff often wears bright colors and designs. Safety glasses, masks, and gloves are routinely worn. To make the mask look less threatening, some masks can be purchased that have designs printed on them.

Dental Assistant's Role in Pediatric Dentistry

The role of the dental assistant in the pediatric practice varies depending on areas of responsibility. One aspect is management of the child, and another is working at chairside. Skills

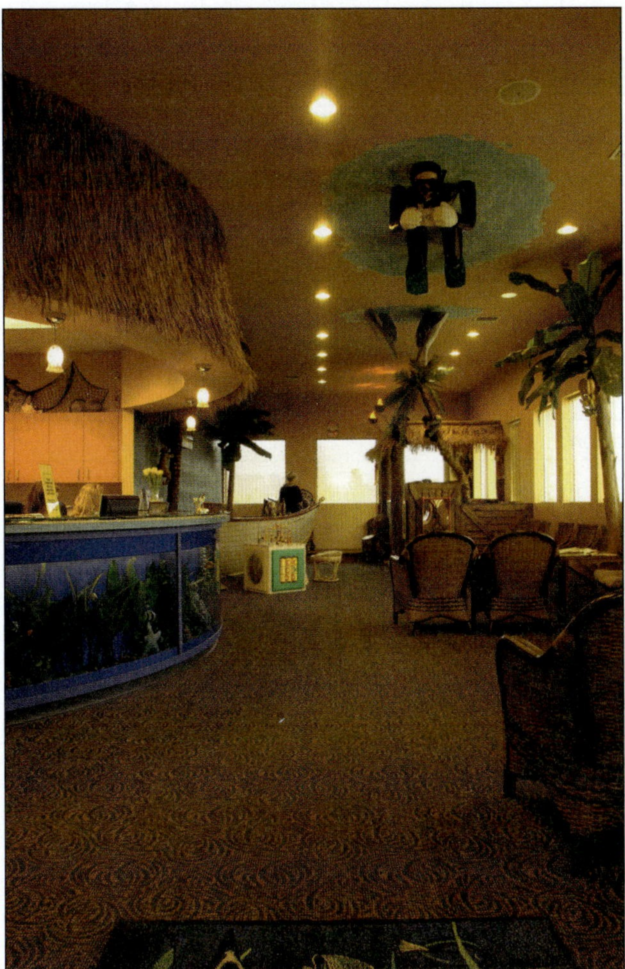

FIGURE 29-1

Reception areas in pediatric practices often include various toys, activities, books, television, and video games. The practice of Dr. Jay Enzler has adopted an under-the-sea theme to make the experience less threatening and more enjoyable for young patients.

that the assistant performs at chairside vary in every office and from state to state depending on the state's Dental Practice Act. In the pediatric practice the dental assistant may be registered or licensed to perform expanded or advanced duties. The expanded function assistant may perform legal preventive procedures such as a coronal polish, the application of dental sealants, and taking preliminary impressions. Some states have additional expanded functions in restorative dentistry. In these states the dental assistant completes advanced training and licensing to place amalgam and composite restoration after the dentist has prepped the tooth. When the assistant works independently, he or she assumes the authority role and must maintain control of the child.

In many offices, the assistant plays the primary role in greeting the child, escorting him or her to the treatment area, and preparing him or her for treatment. The assistant transfers attention and control to the dentist when the dentist comes into the room. The assistant's role during treatment is to support the dentist in a manner that the assistant and the dentist have discussed. Usually, this is office policy and a good topic for staff meeting discussions.

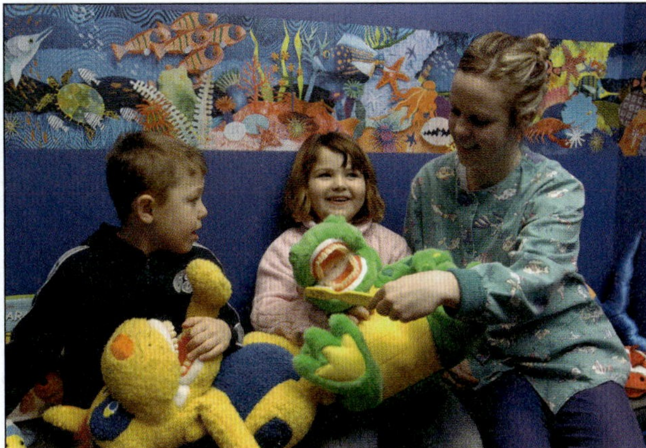

FIGURE 29-2

A dental assistant showing children how to brush their teeth by demonstrating on a puppet.

The dental assistant is also an educator of both the child and the parents. The assistant answers questions or refers them to the pediatric dentist. Topics that might be discussed include oral hygiene techniques, dental nutrition, tooth eruption, and the application of fluoride (Figure 29-2).

Behavioral Characteristics of Children at Various Ages

Each child develops on his or her own special time schedule, but there are some common levels of psychological and physical growth. The term, **maturation**, means growth to a certain level, and then learning on that level. The *chronological age* of a child may be 7 years old, but that child may not be mature enough to learn on this level. The *mental age* (level of intellectual development) and the *emotional age* (emotional maturity) may be at different levels. Development takes longer for some than for others, and environment, age, experiences, and other people all influence this psychological growth. Table 29-1 provides general characteristics of behavior in children at various ages. These are generalizations and are not meant to be comprehensive.

Understanding the behavior of children at various ages will give the dental assistant a better way to establish a relationship with children. Having some idea of their learning levels, communication abilities, and interests enables the assistant to understand the patient, and effectively manage the child to make his or her experience with dentistry a positive one. It is believed that early dental care can promote a lifetime of good oral health for the child. The best ages to introduce a child to dental care in the dental office is between 2 and 6 years, but some offices encourage parents to bring the child in by their first birthday in order to familiarize the child with the dental office and the examination process. By the age of 2 some children will sit for the exam and polish procedures and are learning to brush and floss with parents' guidance.

(To review the stages of tooth eruption, refer to Appendix B in the back of the textbook.)

TABLE 29-1 General Behavioral Characteristics of Children at Various Ages

Age	Behavior
2 to 6 years overall	Likes to be with parents and siblings
	Likes to play (e.g., having a "ride" in the dental chair, seeing the "squirt gun")
	Can respond to dentist's instructions and understands simple explanations
	Transitional time from infantile behavior patterns to the more independent preschool child
2 to 4 years	Short attention span
	Wide variety of interests
	Parallel play without bothering other children
	Responds to fantasy
4 to 6 years	Shows feelings with facial expression
	Parents are very influential
	Greatest number of management problems
	Needs constant reassurance
	Moves toward integrated play
	Shows some tolerance with dislikes
6 to 12 years overall	Period of socializing
	Asserts independence
	Differences between boys and girls are more noticeable
6 to 9 years	Learning to get along with people and the regulations of society
	Friendships are important
	Usually prefers to come in for treatment without a parent
	Likes to collect things
	Aware of his or her place in society and likes to belong to a group
	Likes to be spoken to directly
9 to 12 years	Usually not difficult to manage
	May respond passively
	Girls are more mature
	Will respond when things are explained
	Boys sometimes act like they know it all
	Likes to be treated as an adult

Patient Management

Patient management is a team effort. Successful treatment is the result of how well the patient is managed. The dental team must work together and know each other's responsibilities and roles. A positive, trusting relationship with some children takes time and effort. The dental team must have consistent management policies and procedure sequences, and must consistently use the same terminology when speaking with patients.

Longevity of staff members provides the opportunity to better respond as a unit. Over time, the team will encounter various management problems; once the problems have occurred, discuss them and decide how they will be handled in the future.

Fear is a large factor in behavior problems with children. Some of the fears are based on feelings, attitudes, and concerns that have developed from suggestions of others, including parents, siblings, and friends. These are called **subjective fears**. Other fears that are based on the child's own experiences, are known as **objective fears**.

When a child has questions, the dental team should give honest, brief, and simple answers. Try to relate the answer to something the child already knows about or has experienced. For example, relate the pinch of an injection to the pinch of a mosquito.

Behavioral Assessment

One main aspect of child management during dental treatment is managing dental anxiety. The pediatric dentist is trained to assess and manage the child's behavior during dental treatment. The dentist treating a child patient almost always assesses the child's ability to cooperate first. Cooperative behavior is the key to delivering treatment; therefore, to begin the assessment process during the initial exam, the dentist evaluates and classifies the child's behavior and estimates the child's ability to cooperate. This will assist the dentist in deciding whether the patient will need nonpharmacologic intervention, oral conscious sedation, IV sedation, or general anesthesia. There are many patient behavior management assessment scales used in pediatric dentistry to accomplish this task. Two prominent examples are the Frankl's Behavior Rating Scale (Table 29-2) and the Wright's Classification Scale (Table 29-3).

Children who demonstrate management problems can affect the office by causing a loss of treatment time, making it difficult to get things done, and sometimes presenting unsatisfactory results. To decrease the child's fear and anxiety, the office should provide a safe, controlled environment and use different communication and management techniques.

Behavior Management Techniques

There are many **behavior management** techniques, a few are covered here to provide the dental assistant with some ideas. In the management of a child's behavior it is important not to lie to the child, but answer questions and make explanations in such a manner that the child can relate to it on their level of understanding. Consider words the child can relate to, such as "rain coat" instead of dental dam, or "pinch" for the feeling of an anesthetic needle.

The following techniques are taken from the American Academy of Pediatric Dentistry's published *Standards of Care for Behavior Management.*

Tell, Show, and Do. With the **tell, show, and do technique,** the assistant names a dental instrument and demonstrates its use, often using either his or her own hand or fingers, or the child's hand. Once the child is comfortable, the instrument is used.

Voice Control. Speaking calmly but firmly lets the child know the dentist is in control and is serious about the treatment and the child's behavior.

Distraction. Distract the child's attention from perceived unpleasant procedures. Watching videos, listening to tapes, or getting the child to think of something pleasant are methods of distraction (Figure 29-3).

Nonverbal Communication. Nonverbal communication gains the attention of the child and guides his or her behavior. The dental team's facial expressions, postures, and contact with the child reinforce positive behavior.

Modeling. The **modeling technique** pairs a timid child in the dental care setting with a cooperative child of a similar age. The open bay treatment areas provide the opportunity for the modeling process.

Positive Reinforcement. Give the patient positive reinforcement at the appropriate time. Every child does something right during the dental visit. Praise him or her in order to reinforce the positive behavior. Be sure the praise or positive reinforcement is honest, sincere, and for worthy behavior.

Gentle Restraints. Sometimes a child's behavior during treatment requires management for his or her own protection from possible injury. Some children

TABLE 29-2 Frankl's Behavior Scale

Rating	Attitude	Definition
1	Definitely Negative	Completely uncooperative, refusal of treatment, crying, very difficult to make progress
2	Negative	Reluctant to listen or accept treatment, uncooperative, sullen, withdrawn
3	Positive	Acceptance of treatment and cooperative, but somewhat shy and reluctant; follows directions
4	Definitely Positive	Completely cooperative, has good rapport with the dentist and is interested in and enjoys the experience

Source: McDonald and Avery, Eds. *Dentistry for child and adolescent,* 9th ed. 2010 Philadelphia: CV Mosby.

TABLE 29-3 Wright's Classification of Behavior Scale

Classification	Attitude	Description
1	Cooperative	Understands the procedure, follows directions, and engages in conversations
2	Lacking Cooperation	Lacking in cooperation ability, the patient is usually very young, or mentally or physically disabled. Manage with the use of sedation or general anesthetic.
3	Potentially Cooperative	Patients are potentially cooperative and are usually 3 to 12 years old. Outstanding features are subjective and objective fears.

Source: McDonald and Avery, Eds. *Dentistry for child and adolescent,* 9th ed. 2010 Philadelphia: CV Mosby.

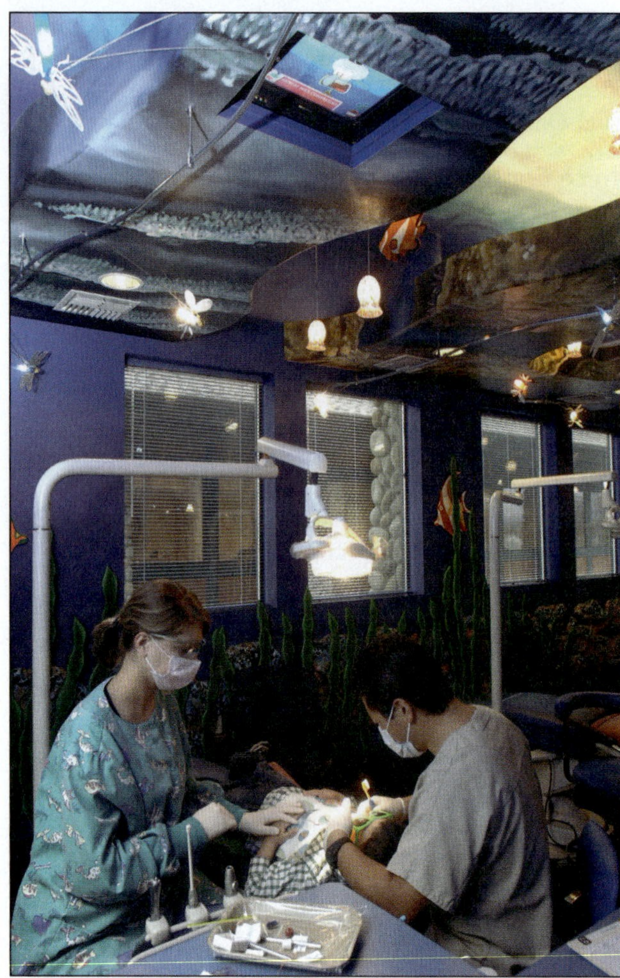

FIGURE 29-3
A child being distracted while receiving dental treatment with a ceiling monitor showing a movie.

need gentle restraint of the arms and legs to reduce or eliminate movement. This is for the safety of the patient and the operator. With the informed consent of the parent/guardian a **papoose board** and pedi-wrap are used for this kind of restraint (Figure 29-4).

Hand Over Mouth. The **hand-over-mouth (HOM) technique** works to gain the child's attention for establishing communication, eliminates inappropriate avoidance responses, enhances the child's self-confidence for coping during treatment, and ensures safety during delivery of care. The dentist places his or her hand over the patient's mouth and, in a very calm voice, explains behavior expectations. The hand is removed when behavior is appropriate. The process is reapplied, if necessary.

HOM requires informed consent and, although effective, this technique is not used often.

Mild Sedation. An anxious child may benefit from sedation. Conscious sedation and nitrous oxide inhalation are two forms used in the pediatric office. Both require informed consent before being administered. Conscious sedation and nitrous oxide inhalation are preoperative or intraoperative.

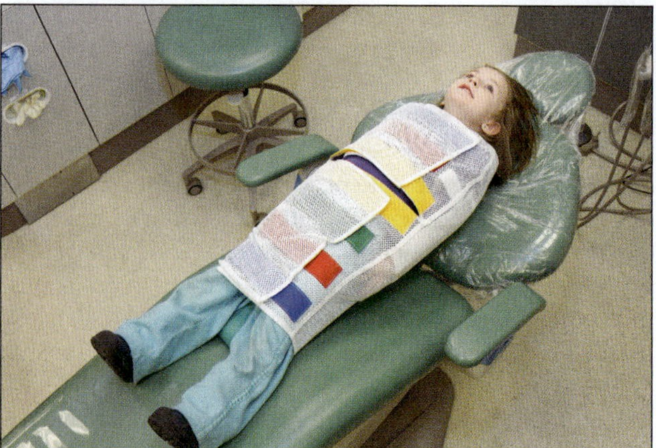

FIGURE 29-4
A child positioned in a papoose board with pedi-wrap.

Both reduce anxiety and movement by the patient, increase tolerance for longer periods, and enhance communication. Sedation also aids in the treatment of mentally, physically, or medically compromised patients.

General Anesthesia. General anesthesia is administered for treatment if a child is extremely fearful or uncooperative, or if the patient has certain physical, mental, or medical conditions. This provides a safe, efficient, and effective means for dental care.

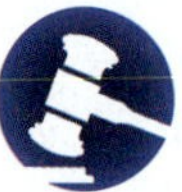

General anesthesia requires informed consent from the child's parent or guardian and is usually administered in a hospital setting.

Patients with Special Health Care Needs

Providing preventive and therapeutic oral health care to individuals with *special health care needs* (SHCN) is a part of the practice of pediatric dentistry. Guidelines on Management of Dental Patients with Special Health Care Needs from the American Academy of Pediatric Dentistry (AAPD) states that: SHCN patients include "any physical, developmental, mental, sensory, behavioral, cognitive, or emotional impairment of limiting condition that requires medical management, health care intervention, and/or use of specialized services or programs. The condition may be congenital, developmental, or acquired through disease, trauma, or environmental cause and may impose limitation in performing daily self-maintenance activities or substantial limitations in a major life activity. Health care for individuals with special needs requires specialized knowledge acquired by additional training, as well as increased awareness and attention, adaptation, and accommodative measures beyond what are considered routine." Individuals with special needs who are treated in the pediatric office include the following:

- Patients with orofacial disorders or conditions, such as cleft lip/palate, amelogenesis, or dentinogenesis imperfecta (see Chapter 8, Embryology and Histology and Chapter 27, Oral Pathology).

- Some SHCN patients with systemic health conditions, such as leukemia or cardiac problems, that may be at a greater risk for oral diseases.
- Patients with mental, developmental, or physical disabilities, including children with autism, Down syndrome, anxiety, cerebral palsy, and spinal cord injuries. These patients may not have the ability to understand or perform daily preventive oral health care.

The pediatric practice successfully treats patients (children and adults) who have been diagnosed with special needs. Depending on the severity of their condition they may be treated in the pediatric office or in the hospital setting. Some offices have a quiet or special care room that is customized and adapted, where safe treatment can be provided. The pediatric dentist is often board certified at a nearby hospital so they can provide treatment there when necessary.

The pediatric dentist will take a medical and dental history, and sometimes confer with the patient's medical care provider(s) to determine the best means for treatment. It is important to make patients comfortable and feel safe whatever their needs. Several things are considered before treatment begins, including the length of the appointments, the need for additional auxiliary staff to accommodate the patient needs effectively, and any additional aids to accommodate the patients' unique circumstances. To create a nonthreatening environment the dentist and staff will spend a lot of time at the beginning of treatment establishing a relationship with the patient. An example is to use a lot of tell-show-do to introduce many aspects of the treatment, like showing the air–water syringe and how it works on their hand before using it in their mouth.

Interacting with the child on a level they are comfortable with makes them more cooperative and reduces anxiety. Sometimes the parents are welcomed back into the operatory and are involved in the process. With the assistance of the parent or caregiver, most of the patient's physical and mental disabilities can be managed. Protective stabilization, nitrous oxide sedation, or general anesthesia are some additional means to work with the anxiety and resistant behaviors of these children.

The Role of the Parent or Guardian

Parents or guardians often require assistance to best prepare the child for dental care. Sometimes, the parents' or guardians' past experiences influence how they feel about dental treatment, and this is transmitted to the child. Then the child may become apprehensive and hesitant.

Many offices have suggestions for parents to help prepare the child for treatment. There are pamphlets, books, and videos to instruct the parents on how to explain what the child is going to experience in the dental office. It is important that the child's questions be answered truthfully but in terms they understand and with minimal explanation. If the parents are not sure of the treatment or how to answer the questions, they should tell the child to ask the dentist.

When the first appointment is made, the parent should be informed of what to expect. This usually means examining the child's teeth and taking x-rays. A treatment plan may include restorations and preventive treatment. The parents are encouraged to discuss concerns they might have with the dentist, away from the child.

Each office has a policy on parents coming into the treatment room with the child during the appointment. The dental assistants must know how the dentist feels about having the parents with the child during treatment. Some dentists feel that they can manage the child better if the parents are not in the treatment room. Others feel that as long as the parents do not interfere, they can remain. The parents usually are eager to cooperate with the office policies. If the child wants the parent to come into the treatment area, offer the parent a chair near the foot of the patient's chair so that he or she is not in the direct view of the child when the child is reclined and the dentist and dental assistant are seated. The dental team remains focused on establishing a relationship with the child. On occasion, the dentist may use the presence of the parents to control behavior. For example, the dentist might say that if the child cooperates, the parent can stay in the treatment area, but if the child does not cooperate, the parent will be asked to leave. Some dentists feel that if the child does not behave, it is the parent's responsibility to manage the child in order for dental care to be completed.

Parents are generally very supportive if they are informed, know what is happening, and know what is expected of them.

Procedures in Pediatric Dentistry

The first appointment with the pediatric dentist may be for a routine examination followed by treatment, or it may be an emergency appointment due to an injury. Dental care for children involves both the primary and permanent dentition. Sometimes the parents may question the need to restore primary teeth because they are not permanent and will be replaced. The primary dentition is restored for the following reasons:

- The primary teeth are needed to hold space for the permanent teeth.
- They maintain the functions of the teeth in chewing, speech, and esthetics.
- They act as guides for the permanent dentition during eruption.

Educating the parents so that they understand the importance of the primary teeth is necessary with all types of pediatric dental treatments (see Appendix B, Stages of Tooth Eruption).

The Examination

The examination of a child patient is similar to that of an adult. The gingiva, supporting tissues, and oral mucosa are checked. The surfaces of the teeth are examined with a mouth mirror and an explorer. Radiographs are exposed to show the conditions of the primary teeth and the positions and development of the permanent teeth (refer to Chapter 22, Production and Evaluation of Dental Radiographs, for suggestions and types of pediatric x-ray exposures).

The patient's medical and dental history is recorded by the parent or guardian. The medical history provides information about past dental experiences, any allergies, facial habits, illnesses, and general development of the child.

Preventive Procedures

Preventive procedures in pediatric dentistry include educating both the child and the parent regarding diet suggestions, oral hygiene techniques, use of fluorides, pit and fissure sealants, use of mouth guards for sports activities, and preventive orthodontic treatment.

Oral Hygiene Techniques. Oral hygiene techniques are coordinated with the child's age and physical ability (see Chapter 4, Oral Health and Preventive Techniques, for oral hygiene techniques for children). The parent is given information on toothbrushing and flossing techniques in order to assist the child.

Coronal Polishing. The coronal polish is a rubber cup polish of the crowns of the teeth. Polishing paste is applied to the teeth with the rubber cup to remove plaque and some stains (see Chapter 32, Coronal Polish). This is routinely performed by the dental hygienist, but in many states dental assistants can also perform the coronal polish.

Pit and Fissure Sealants. Pit and fissure sealants are routinely placed to protect newly erupted teeth and teeth where sealants are indicated. The sealants protect the deep pits and fissure areas of the primary molars, and the premolars and molars of the permanent teeth. Sealants have successfully reduced the number of cavities in children (refer to Chapter 30, Dental Sealants).

Fluoride Applications and Fluoride Varnishes. A **fluoride application** and **fluoride varnish** is routinely applied after the coronal polish and pit and fissure sealants have been placed. Periodically the dentist will determine a fluoride therapy plan with the parents. How and when fluoride is given to a child often depends on if the water supply is fluoridated, the patient's oral hygiene techniques, and how often the patient visits the dentist. Fluoride is administered in the office as a gel or foam solution, and is placed in the child's mouth in trays, or as a rinse (see Chapter 4, Oral Health and Preventive Techniques). Fluoride varnish usually contains 5 percent sodium fluoride in an alcohol solution with natural resins. The resins make the solution sticky allowing the varnish to adhere to the teeth as the alcohol evaporates. The varnish is painted on the surfaces of the teeth setting on contact with saliva, and then it dries to a natural tooth color. Fluoride varnish comes in various forms including premeasured unit doses, individual applications with applicator brushes, and tubes.

Diet. In the pediatric office the child's diet should be discussed with the child and the parent. Usually there is information to give the parents, such as brochures and websites, to assist them with diet recommendations. The dental team will suggest a good diet built on nutritious foods from each of the main food groups (refer to Chapter 5, Nutrition). The AAP recommends the following:

- Selecting a mix of foods from the five food groups: vegetables, fruits, grains, low-fat dairy, and quality protein sources, including lean meats, fish, nuts, seeds and eggs.
- Avoid highly processed foods.
- Offer a variety of food choices.
- Use small amounts of sugar, salt, fats, and oils with highly nutritious foods to enhance enjoyment and consumption, for example, placing brown sugar on oatmeal.
- Offer appropriate portions.

Discussions many include: limiting snacks and snacking time, choosing sugarless gum and diet sodas instead of the high sugar types of gum and soda; including orange juice with calcium; not putting the child to bed with a bottle of milk, formula, or juice; encouraging the child to rinse their mouth after eating or snacking; and limiting fun foods to special occasions.

Mouth Guards. When children are active in any recreational activity that poses a risk of injury to the mouth, they should be wearing a **mouth guard**. A properly fitted mouth guard offers protection from a premature loss of teeth; can prevent broken or fractured teeth; and can prevent injuries to the lips, tongue, face, and jaw. Mouth guards are mainly worn on the maxillary teeth, and are designed to stay in place while allowing the child to talk and breathe normally.

There are various types of mouth guards, including the following:

- Custom-fitted mouth guards are made by the dentist specifically for the patient. They involve taking impressions of the patient for a study model. The impressions are poured to make study models that are then used to fabricate a mouth guard. Once the mouth guard material is vacuum formed over the model, it is trimmed and finished for the patient (see Chapter 35, Laboratory Materials and Techniques) (Figure 29-5A). These mouth guards are more expensive, but offer a better fit and the most protection to the mouth.
- Mouth-formed, or "boil and bite," mouth guards are mouth protectors that are usually purchased in sporting goods or athletic stores. These mouth guards are softened in heated water, inserted into the mouth, and then molded to fit the individual's arch (Figure 29-5B). With this type of mouth guard, directions must be followed carefully to ensure that the mouth guard fits properly.
- Stock or ready-made mouth guards are pre-formed and ready to wear. They are inexpensive and do not fit as well as the other two types of mouth guards.

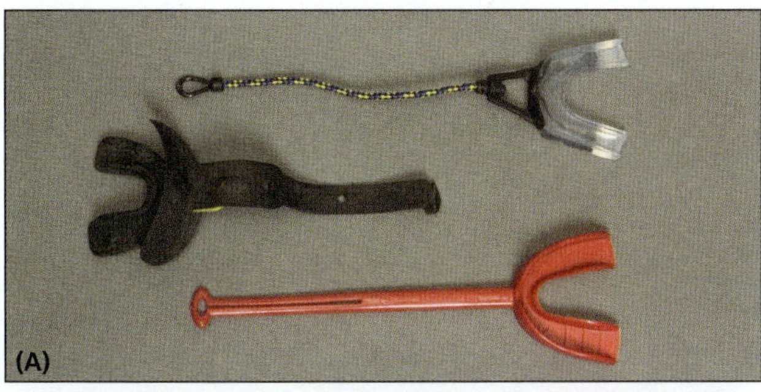

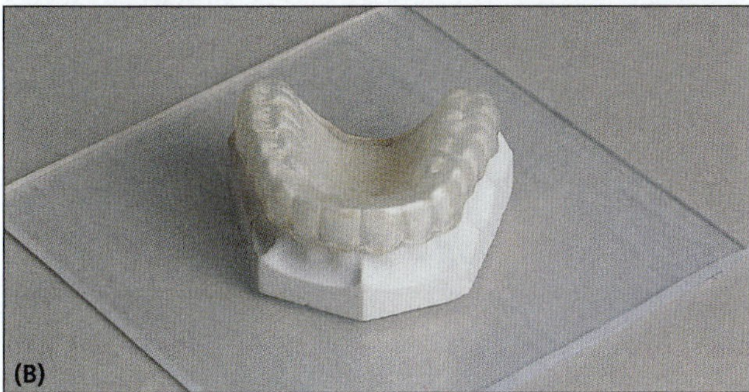

FIGURE 29-5

(A) Various mouth guards used in athletics. (B) An example of mouth guard material and a formed mouth guard.

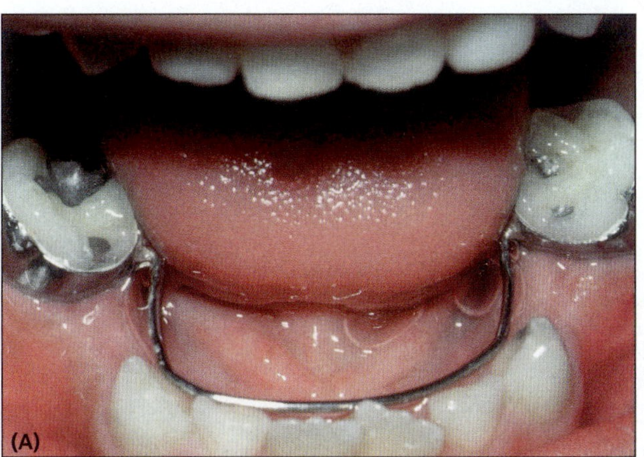

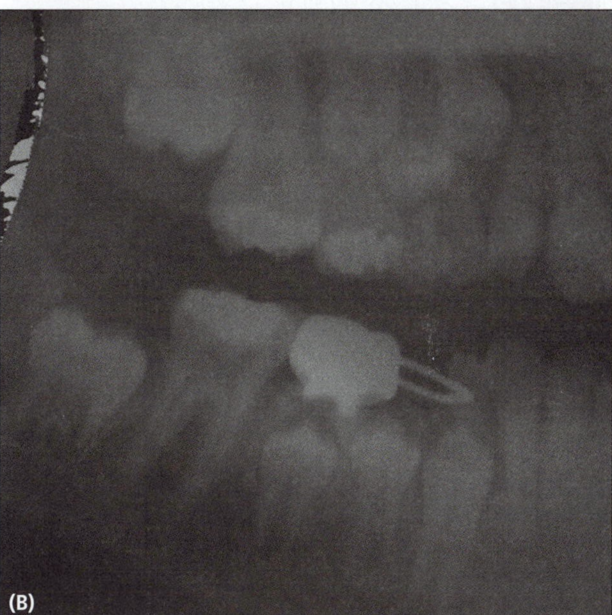

FIGURE 29-6

(A) Fixed bilateral space maintainer. (B) An x-ray of a patient with a fixed unilateral space maintainer.

Preventive and Interceptive Orthodontic Treatment. Preventive and interceptive orthodontic treatment includes a variety of orthodontic treatments. Two common procedures are placing space maintainers and correcting oral habits.

A **space maintainer** is designed to maintain a space until the permanent tooth erupts. The space is the result of the premature loss of a primary tooth. A space maintainer may be a fixed or removable appliance. The appliance is designed to meet the needs of the child patient.

There are different types of space maintainers, including the fixed unilateral appliance, the fixed bilateral space maintainer, and the Nance appliance (Figure 29-6). Most space maintainers are fixed (cemented) in place so that the patient cannot remove them, but if the child is responsible enough to care for the appliance, a removable space maintainer, such as a dental crown or fake tooth, can be fabricated by the lab to hold open the space. This type of space maintainer is more aesthetic, but must be kept cleaned.

If more than one tooth is missing, a child denture or partial can also be made to hold the spaces open until the permanent teeth can erupt, or the child is ready for a permanent fixed prosthesis, such as a bridge or implant (refer to Chapter 28, Orthodontics, for more information on space maintainers).

Oral habits such as thumb sucking and tongue thrusting may need intervention because they can lead to abnormal muscle function, distorted growth of the jaw, malocclusion, changed facial contour, and problems with speech.

Thumb sucking is a controversial subject with many opinions on whether the habit should be treated. Most orthodontists leave the thumb sucking of a child alone until the child's maxillary anterior teeth erupt; hopefully, by then, the habit will have disappeared. Most dentists begin some form of treatment if the child continues to suck his or her thumb at age 5. Treatment includes counseling with the child and the parents, gentle persuasion, and behavior modification techniques. Fixed appliances, such as cribs and rakes, are also used if the habit continues (Figure 29-7).

The habit of **tongue thrusting**, in which a child's tongue pushes against the anterior teeth during swallowing, causes an anterior open bite. Treatment for this habit includes myofunctional exercises (therapy) or the use of appliances.

Restorative Procedures

Restorative procedures are similar to those performed on adult patients. The materials used in pediatric dentistry are the same as those used in the restoration of permanent teeth. Amalgam is used most frequently for posterior teeth, and it is approved by the ADA. Some dentists are placing more tooth-colored restorations because of their more natural appearance. These

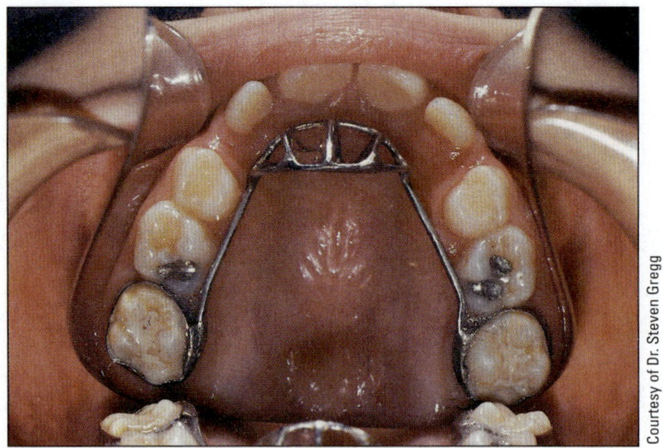
Courtesy of Dr. Steven Gregg

FIGURE 29-7
A crib appliance that stops a child from sucking his or her thumb.

are placed in both the anterior and posterior regions of the child's mouth. Esthetic restorations include composites, glass ionomers, resin-modified glass ionomers, and compomers—a combination of composite resins and glass ionomers (see Chapter 38, Restorative Materials and Matrix and Wedge). Badly decayed teeth are protected with stainless steel crowns that are permanently cemented in place. In very rare cases, partials and dentures are made for pediatric patients.

The difference between pediatric and adult restorative procedures is the size of the instruments. Examples of instruments and materials that are reduced in size include the dental high-speed handpiece and burs, dental dam material, and dental dam clamps. The dental dam material is smaller in size and the width of the jaws of the clamps is smaller to accommodate the primary teeth. The high-speed handpiece has a compact head to allow for better access in the child's mouth, and the burs have shorter shanks.

Pedodontic Matrices. The dental matrices used in restorative procedures are adapted to the sizes and shapes of the teeth. The Tofflemire matrix is used in pediatrics, but custom matrices are more common (see Chapter 34). Two custom matrices are the **T-band matrix** and the **spot-welded matrix band**.

T-bands are designed for, and used on, primary teeth. Often made of brass strips that are crossed at one end, they are available in various designs and sizes. The T-bands do not require retainers, are adjustable, and can be secured on the tooth (Figure 29-8; and see Procedure 29-1).

Spot-welded matrix bands are also used for primary teeth (Procedure 29-2). The custom-made bands are used for Class II restorations. The matrix material comes in rolls of various width and thickness. This custom matrix does not require a retainer to be secure on the tooth, but a spot-welding machine is required. The band is quickly made at chairside.

Dental Dam Procedure

Using a dental dam during pediatric procedures protects the patient's busy and curious tongue and prevents materials from being aspirated into the throat. It also provides a dry area while also improving visibility. It often reduces the procedure time by restricting patient talking and providing an isolated treatment area in the oral cavity.

Pediatric dental dams are smaller than dams for adults, typically comprised of 5 × 5 inch pieces of material. The dental dam punch is the same one used for adults, but holes are smaller and the distance between holes is shorter. To cover the area, usually three or four holes are punched in a quadrant. The dental dam clamps are smaller and sometimes have projections for better retention. (For more information and the procedure sequence, see Chapter 38, Restorative Materials and Matrix, and Wedge).

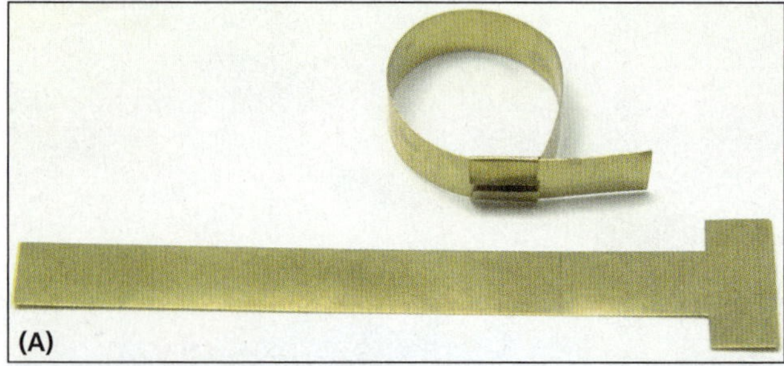
(A)

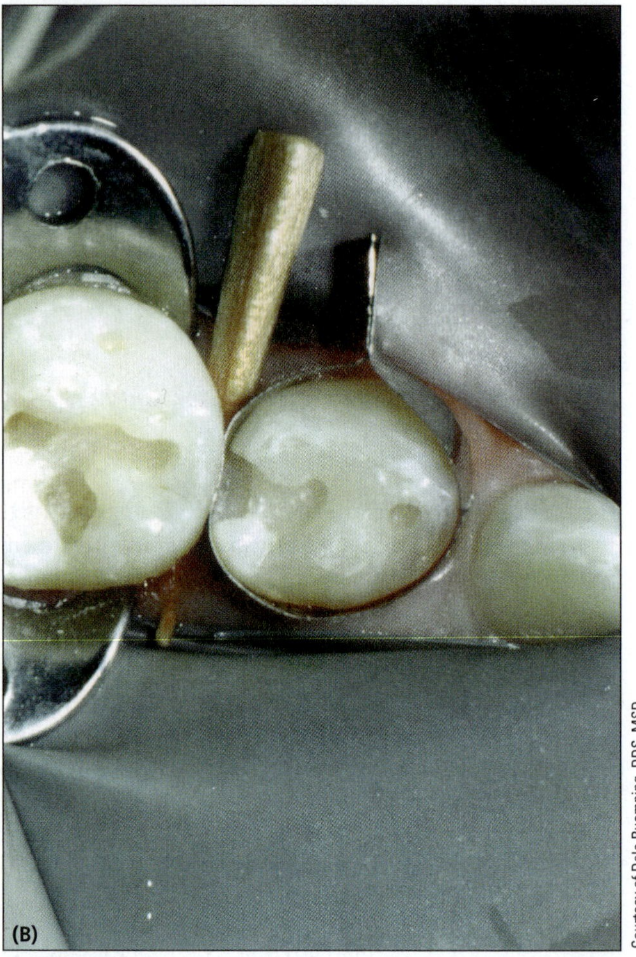
(B)
Courtesy of Dale Ruemping, DDS, MSD

FIGURE 29-8
(A) T-bands. (B) T-band correctly assembled on a tooth.

Procedure 29-1
T-Band Placement

For this procedure, the tooth has been prepared and a matrix is assembled and placed on the tooth. The dentist places the T-band unless the state's Dental Practice Act allows the dental assistant to perform this skill.

Equipment and Supplies (*Figure 29-9*)

- T-band assortment
- Burnisher
- Cotton pliers or hemostat
- Crown and collar scissors

Procedure Steps (*Follow aseptic procedures*)

1. Prepare the T-band ahead of time by selecting the appropriate band size.
2. Loop the band to shape the approximate diameter of the tooth.
3. Fold the "T" ends over the band loop, leaving a circle with a long tail or end.
4. Place the band on the tooth in the interproximal space covering the margins of the preparation.
5. Place the portion of the band where the "T" is folded on the buccal surface, away from the margins of the preparation.
6. Tighten the band by pulling on the free end (tail) until the band is tight around the tooth.
7. Bend the free end back toward the "T" to secure the band. Remove any excess band with scissors.
8. Burnish the band and place a wedge as needed.
9. To remove the T-band, fold back the overlapping section of the band to loosen the band. Use cotton pliers to remove the band from the tooth.

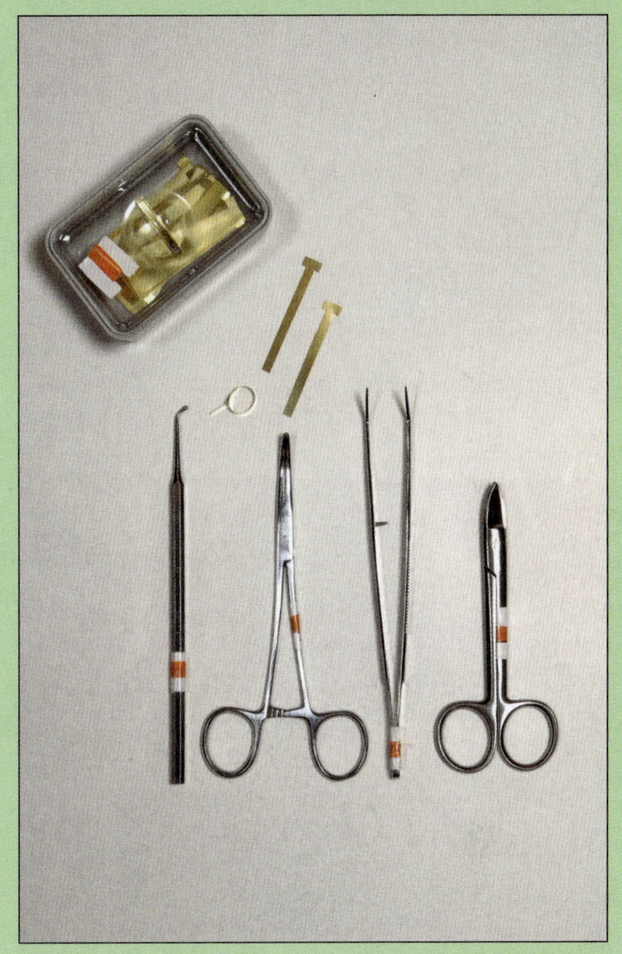

FIGURE 29-9
A Tray setup for T-band placement.

Pulp Therapy in Primary and Young Permanent Teeth

Caries or traumatic injuries can damage both primary and permanent teeth. The teeth are assessed to determine the status of the pulp. The duration, frequency, and location of pain are recorded. The clinical assessment includes a visual examination and radiographs. The extent of a lesion is determined by the following: presence of fistula (pathway from abscess to mucosa), whether the tooth is mobile, presence of swelling, and/or sensitivity to heat or percussion.

Vital Pulp Therapy. Vital pulp therapy involves the removal of tissue that is potentially infected and focuses on the reparative ability of the pulp. This procedure will maintain the tooth in a healthy state so that the tooth is not lost. There are three choices in treatment depending on the status of the pulp: **indirect pulp treatment (IPT)**, **direct pulp capping (DPC)**, or a **pulpotomy** (Procedure 29-3).

If the pulp is not yet exposed, indirect pulp treatment (IPT), also known as indirect pulp capping, is indicated (Figure 29-12A). In this case, the pulp has not yet been exposed, but there is a chance that the pulp will be exposed while removing the caries. The technique involves the following:

1. Leaving a thin layer of sound or carious dentin with no evidence of pulp exposure
2. Placing a medicament and a temporary restoration that seals completely

Procedure 29-2
Spot-Welded Matrix Band Placement

For this procedure, the tooth has been prepared for restoration and the spot-welded matrix band is prepared by the dental assistant at chairside.

Equipment and Supplies

- Spot-welded matrix band material
- Crown and collar scissors
- Cotton pliers, hemostat, or Howe pliers
- Burnisher
- Spot-welding unit (Figure 29-10)

Procedure Steps (*Follow aseptic procedures*)

1. Cut an approximate length of matrix band material. Turn on the spot-welding unit to warm it up.

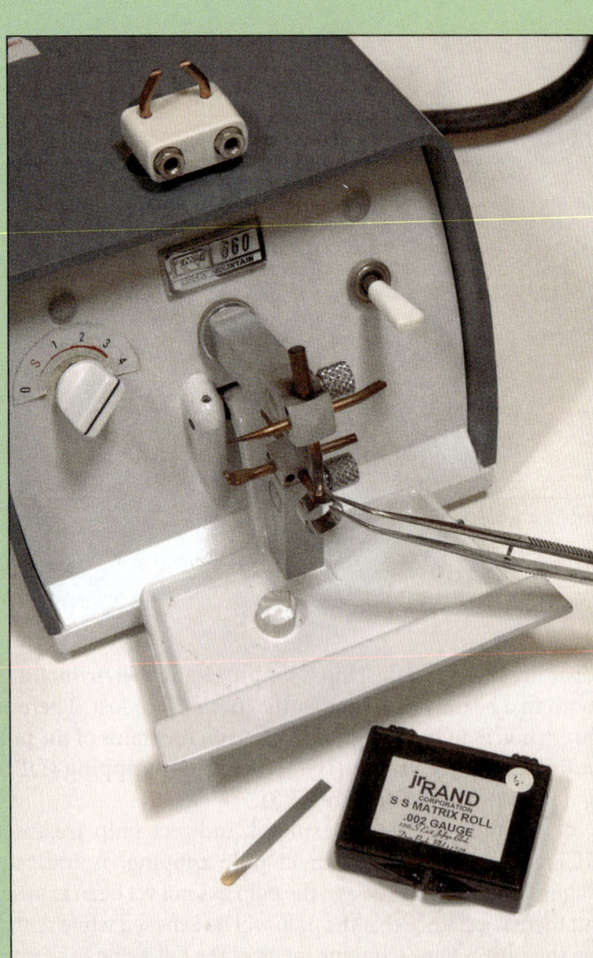

FIGURE 29-10
A spot-welding machine with matrix band material.

2. Loop the matrix material around the tooth, bringing the ends of the material together on the buccal surface.
3. Pinch the band tightly together with a hemostat, cotton pliers, or Howe pliers.
4. Bend the excess material to one side.
5. Take the band to the spot-welding unit and spot-weld the band together to form a circle the diameter of the tooth (Figure 29-11).
6. Trim off the excess and sharp edges of the band.
7. Replace the band on the tooth with the welded area on the buccal surface. Place the wedges into the interproximal space and along the contour of the tooth.
8. To remove the band after the amalgam has been placed, cut the lingual aspect of the band and pull it in an occlusal or buccal direction with cotton pliers.

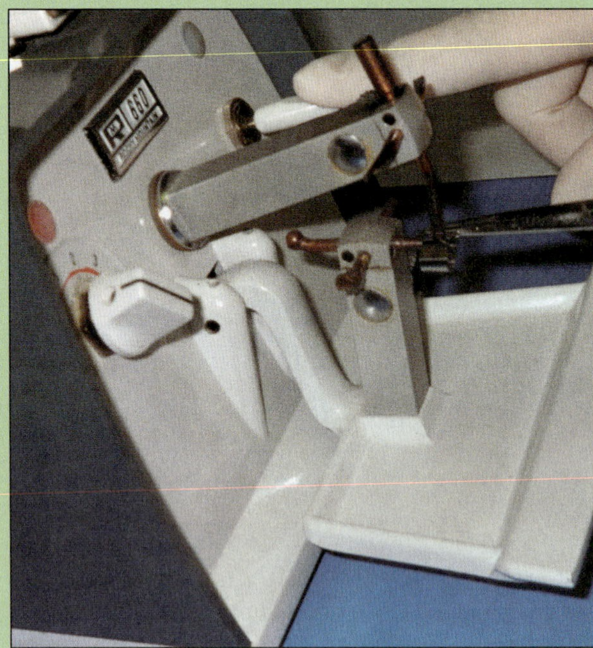

FIGURE 29-11
Spot-welding a matrix band.

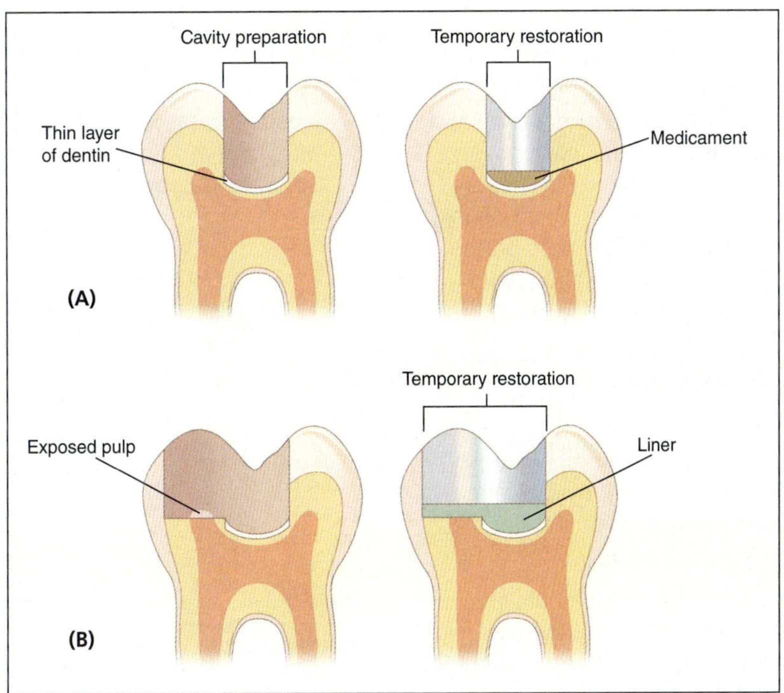

FIGURE 29-12
(A) Indirect pulp treatment or capping. (B) Direct pulp treatment or capping.

Procedure 29-3
Pulpotomy

This procedure is performed by the dentist with the help of a dental assistant. The dental assistant prepares the treatment room, patient, equipment, and supplies. The tooth is opened and treated before a temporary restoration is placed.

Equipment and Supplies (*Figure 29-13*)

- Amalgam setup
- Formocresol
- Sterile round burs
- Zinc oxide-eugenol cement (ZOE or IRM)

Procedure Steps (*Follow aseptic procedures*)

1. Anesthetic is administered.
2. Place the dental dam.
3. Using the high-speed handpiece, a large opening is made in the occlusal surface of the tooth, exposing the coronal portion of the pulp (Figure 29-14A).
4. The coronal portion of the pulp is then removed with a spoon excavator or round bur (Figure 29-14B).

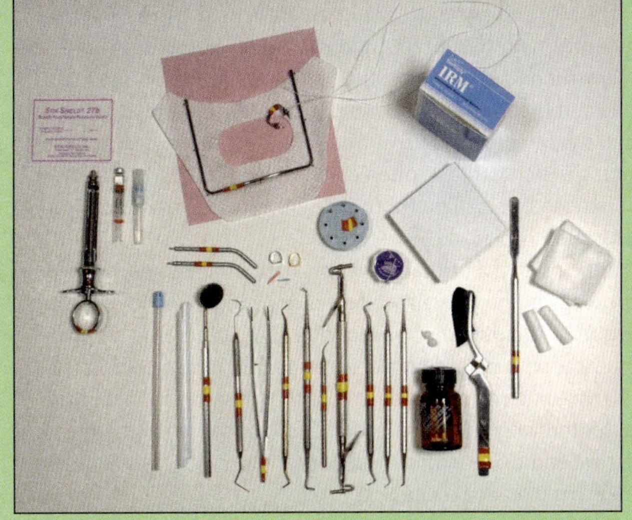

FIGURE 29-13
Pulpotomy tray setup.

5. Prepare a sterile cotton pellet by wetting it in formocresol solution. The dentist places the pellet in the chamber for 5 minutes (Figure 29-14C). Formocresol is bactericidal—it preserves a thin layer of the remaining pulp

(continues)

Procedure 29-3 (continued)

tissue to control hemorrhage. **Formocresol** is a solution of formaldehyde, cresol, glycerin, and water. It is used in vital pulpotomy and as a temporary intracanal medicament used during root canal therapy. If formocresol gets on the skin, it will cause a burning sensation. Wash with soap and water, and treat as a burn.

6. After the hemorrhage is controlled, the cotton pellet is removed and the pulp chamber is rinsed and dried.
7. Mix zinc oxide eugenol to a base consistency and transfer it to the dentist. A layer of the zinc oxide base is placed in the chamber over the remaining pulp (Figure 29-14D).
8. Place the restoration, such as an amalgam, remove the dental dam, and check the occlusion. Stainless steel crowns are also used if little tooth structure remains. Sometimes, the dentist will choose to place a temporary restoration instead of a final restoration. This delays final treatment until the outcome of the injured pulp is known.

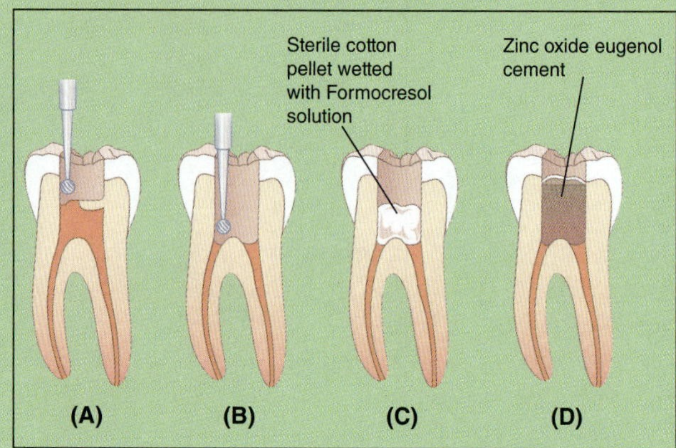

FIGURE 29-14
A pulpotomy procedure, showing direct pulp exposure.

3. Leaving the medicament and restoration for 6 to 8 weeks
4. Opening the tooth and removing the remaining caries
5. Placing restoration

If the pulp has been exposed through mechanical or traumatic means, but there is a chance for a favorable response, a direct pulp capping (DPC) (Figure 29-12B) procedure is indicated. The patient should be informed of the possible outcomes with the direct pulp capping treatment. It may be successful and the pulp will heal, or the infection may continue and the tooth will abscess. In the case of an abscess, root canal treatment may be required. The DPC procedure involves placing a medicament, often calcium hydroxide, directly over the exposed pulp. The tooth is then restored or a temporary restoration is placed.

If the pulp of a primary or young permanent tooth has been exposed, a pulpotomy procedure may be indicated to remove a portion of the pulp. For primary teeth, a pulpotomy keeps the pulp vital, with no prolonged adverse signs, internal resorption, or harm to succedaneous teeth. For the young permanent teeth, a pulpotomy maintains pulp vitality and allows enough time for the root end to develop and close (in these cases, the treatment is referred to as **apexogenesis**).

Nonvital Pulp Therapy. Nonvital pulp therapy may be indicated for both primary and newly erupted permanent teeth. The tooth is extracted or a **pulpectomy** is indicated. This procedure involves the complete removal of the dental pulp (see Chapter 24, Endodontics).

Stainless Steel Crowns

A **stainless steel crown** is used on both primary and permanent teeth. On primary teeth, they are placed until permanent dentition erupts. On permanent teeth, these crowns are placed until the patient can have them replaced with cast gold or porcelain fused to metal crowns. Indications for use of a stainless steel crown include the following:

- Extensive carious lesions
- Hypoplastic or hypocalcified teeth
- Treatment following a pulpotomy or pulpectomy procedure
- A primary tooth is used as an abutment tooth for a space maintainer
- Temporary restoration of fractured teeth

Stainless steel crowns are available in various sizes, and can be purchased individually or in complete kits (Figure 29-15A and B). See Procedure 29-4 for an overview of the steps involved in placing a crown.

Emergency Treatment for Traumatic Injuries

Children are prone to accidents as their bodies and coordination skills grow and develop. Traumatic injuries to children's teeth are not uncommon, resulting in fractured, displaced, or avulsed teeth. Another injury seen in the pediatric population is traumatic intrusion.

Fractured Teeth

Fractured teeth are a common emergency in the pediatric practice (Figure 29-18). The anterior teeth are most often involved. The child should be seen by the dentist as soon as possible after the accident. The dentist examines the teeth, documents the history of the accident, performs vitality tests, and takes radiographs. Treatment is determined by the extent

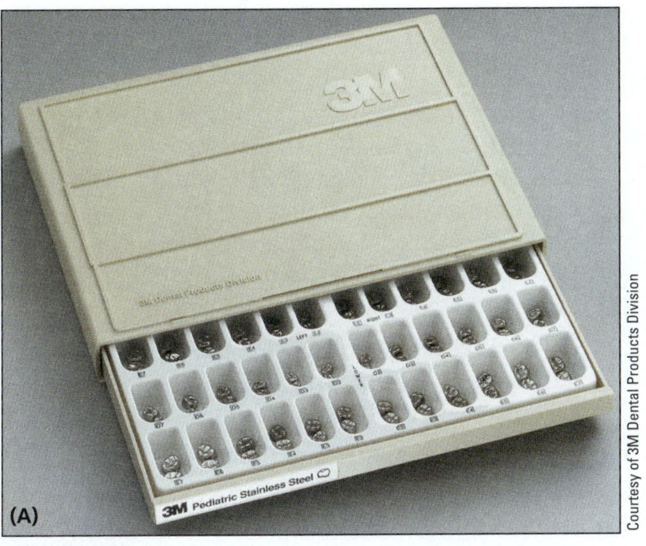

Courtesy of 3M Dental Products Division

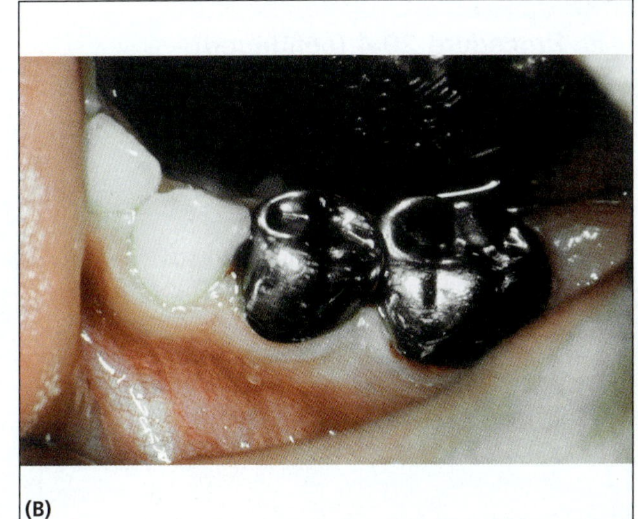

Courtesy of Dale Ruemping, DDS, MSD

FIGURE 29-15
(A) Stainless steel crown kit. (B) Stainless steel crown placed on a tooth.

Procedure 29-4
Stainless Steel Crown Placement

This procedure is performed by the dentist with the help of the dental assistant. The assistant maintains the operating field, mixes materials, and assists in preparation of the stainless steel crown.

Equipment and Supplies (*Figure 29-16*)

- Basic setup: mouth mirror, explorer, and cotton pliers
- Cotton rolls and gauze
- HVE and saliva ejector
- High-speed handpiece with selected burs
- Low-speed handpiece with green stone and rubber abrasive wheel
- Spoon excavator
- Selection of stainless steel crowns
- Crown and collar scissors
- Contouring and crimping pliers
- Mixing spatula, paper pad, and permanent cement
- Articulating forceps and paper
- Dental floss

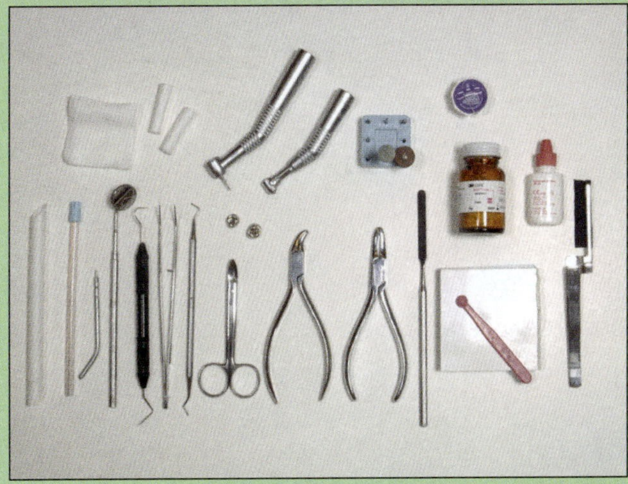

FIGURE 29-16
Stainless steel crown tray setup.

Procedure Steps (*Follow aseptic procedures*)

1. Local anesthetic is administered and the tooth is prepared, similar to the preparation for a cast gold crown. The high-speed handpiece with tapered diamonds is commonly used. Transfer instruments and evacuate during the preparation of the tooth.

(continues)

Procedure 29-4 (continued)

2. The circumference and height of the tooth are reduced.
3. Decay is removed using conventional methods and cavity medications are placed.
4. A stainless steel crown is selected from the kit, and it is tried on the tooth. The crown must fit around the circumference of the prepared tooth and contact the adjacent teeth, mesially and distally. Assist the dentist in the selection of the crown. Some states do not allow dental assistants to perform the function of fitting the crown.
5. Once the crown is selected, the crown and collar scissors are used to adjust the occlusal-gingival height (Figure 29-17A). The gingival margin of the crown should extend 1 millimeter beyond the margin of the tooth preparation.
6. A green stone is used to smooth the rough edges of the crown. This area is polished with a rubber abrasive wheel (Figure 29-17B).
7. Place the crown on the tooth and check the patient's occlusion with articulating paper. Make adjustments, if necessary. Use dental floss to check the contacts. Prepare the articulating paper, dry the tooth, and transfer the paper. Receive the articulating forceps and paper and prepare the handpiece, if necessary.
8. Using contouring and crimping pliers, contour the crown, and then crimp the cervical margins of the crown in toward the tooth (Figure 29-17C).
9. The crown is removed and the tooth is dried thoroughly.
10. The cement is mixed and placed in the crown and on the tooth (Figure 29-17D). Mix the cement and place it in the crown. Transfer the crown to the dentist for placement.
11. Remove the excess cement from around the crown.
12. Rinse the patient's mouth and then dismiss the patient.

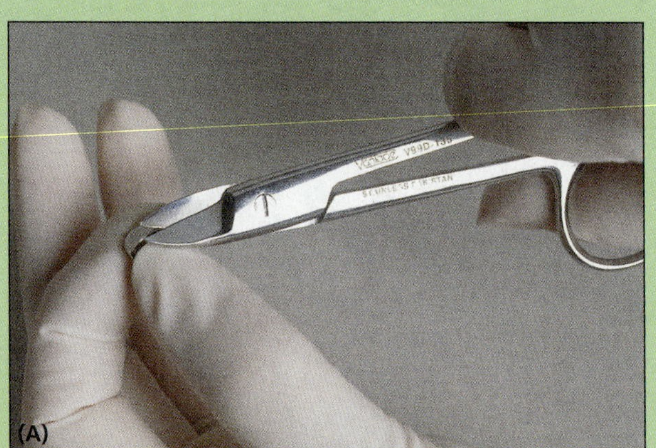
(A)

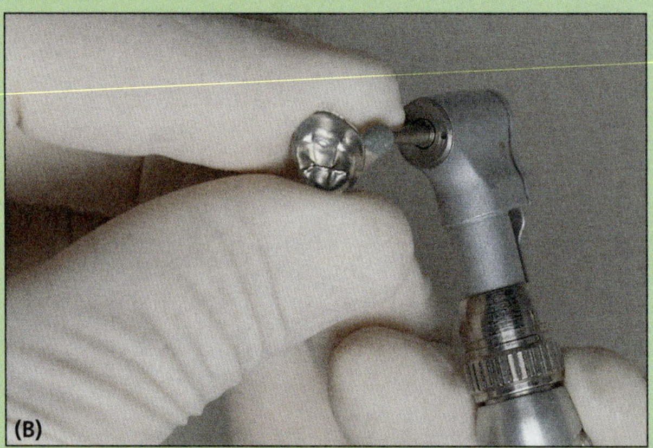
(B)

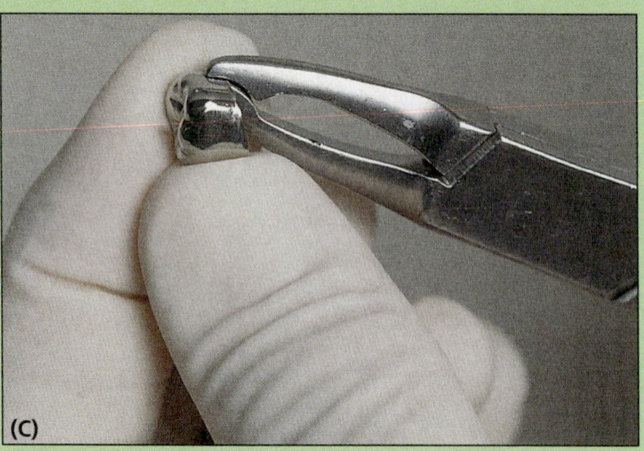
(C)

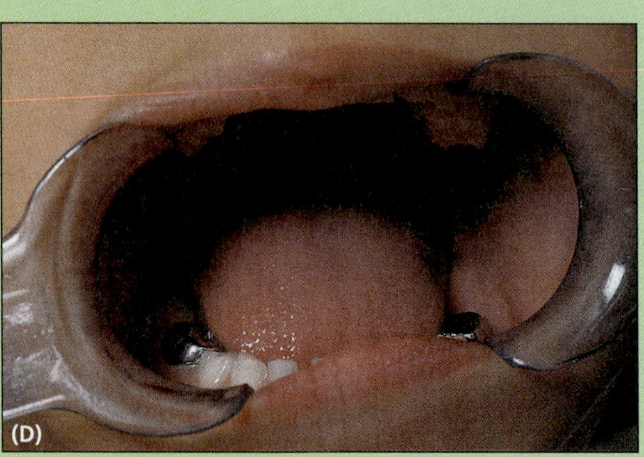
(D)

FIGURE 29-17

(A) Stainless steel crown selected and trimmed with crown and collar scissors. (B) Crown margins smoothed with the green stone. (C) Crown contoured with contouring pliers; margins are then crimped with crimping pliers. (D) Crown cemented on the tooth.

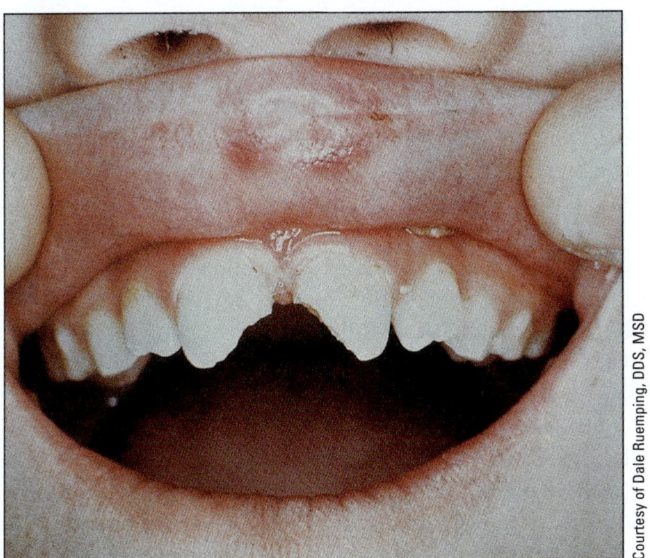

Courtesy of Dale Ruemping, DDS, MSD

FIGURE 29-18

Fractured anterior central incisors.

of the injury and the vitality of the pulp (see Table 29-4 for classifications of fractures and suggested treatment).

At this initial appointment, the pulp is treated and a temporary restoration is placed if needed for protection. Generally, the dentist will wait 3 to 6 months for further treatment. This gives the pulp a chance to recover without additional injury. If the tooth recovers in 6 months, a permanent restoration is placed.

Traumatic Intrusion

A **traumatic intrusion** occurs when the teeth are forcibly driven into the alveolus so that only a portion of the crown is visible. The treatment for intrusion is to either allow the teeth to re-erupt on their own, or see the dentist for repositioning the teeth and splinting adjacent teeth to hold the position. These teeth may become nonvital and later require endodontic treatment.

Traumatic intrusion of the primary teeth may cause damage to the underlying developing permanent teeth (Figure 29-19). The damage can result from physical trauma or from infection of the traumatized teeth. The damage is determined when the permanent teeth erupt.

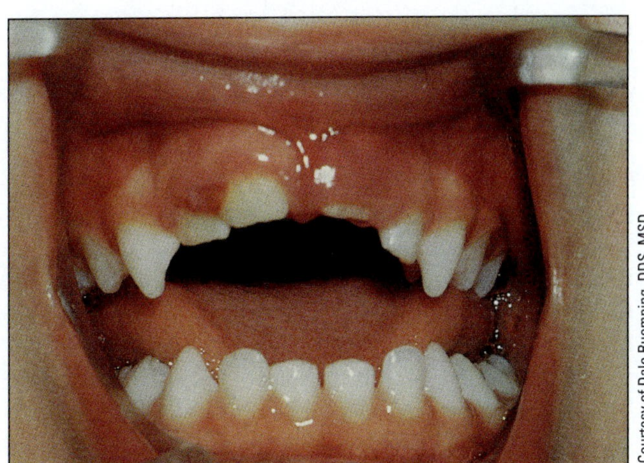

Courtesy of Dale Ruemping, DDS, MSD

FIGURE 29-19

A traumatic intrusion.

Displaced Teeth

Lateral or extrusive displacement, or luxation (when a tooth is moved from its original position), of primary teeth should be repositioned by the dentist as soon as possible. The roots of primary teeth go through resorption faster after an injury and if the teeth are mobile. If infection occurs, the teeth are removed.

After the teeth are repositioned, they are held in place with a splint (Figure 29-20). The splint is left in place for 2 to 4 weeks in order to stabilize the teeth. Often with these

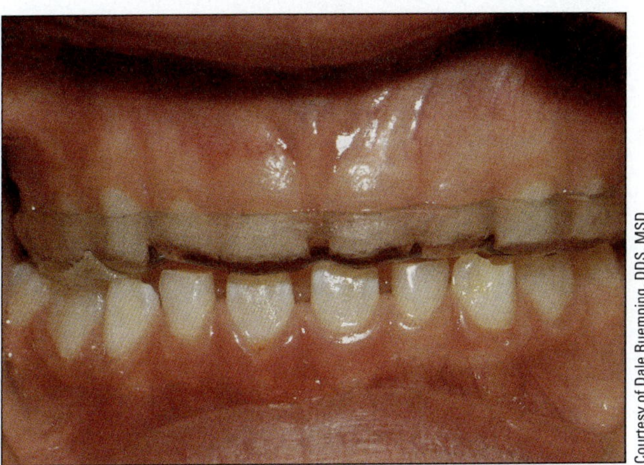

Courtesy of Dale Ruemping, DDS, MSD

FIGURE 29-20

A child with teeth in a splint.

TABLE 29-4 Classifications of Tooth Fractures and Treatment

Classification	Treatment
Enamel	Smooth the rough edges.
Enamel and dentin are involved in fracture	Exposed dentin is protected with glass ionomer, calcium hydroxide, and a bonding agent with composite restoration.
Enamel, dentin, and pulp are involved	Depending on the clinical examination, a direct pulp capping, pulpotomy, or pulpectomy may be indicated.
Crown is fractured with pulp exposure	Root canal treatment, if indicated, and a post and cast crown are completed to stabilize and protect the tooth.

injuries, the periodontal ligament is damaged extensively. The teeth are monitored for vitality and assessed for endodontic treatment.

Avulsed Teeth

An **avulsed tooth** has been completely removed from the mouth. Primary avulsed teeth are not replaced because infection or ankylosis (**ANG**-kill-loh-sis) may occur. Ankylosis is the fusion of bone and cementum. Permanent teeth that have been avulsed should be replaced as soon as possible after the injury. Instruct the parents to replant the tooth immediately. The success rate is relatively high if this is done. If the tooth cannot be replanted, instruct the parent to place the tooth in milk, saliva, saline, or water and transport the patient and tooth to the dental office immediately. Caution should be taken with the avulsed tooth to place it carefully in liquid and not rinse it off.

Time is important if the tooth is to be saved. The patient should see the dentist as soon as possible, and the dentist should be called immediately for instructions.

Replacing an Avulsed Tooth

1. The tooth is kept moist and the site in the mouth is examined.
2. Local anesthetic is administered.
3. X-rays are taken.
4. The blood clot is removed from the alveolus.
5. The avulsed tooth is cleaned off in a saline solution and then inserted into the alveolus.
6. A splint is placed to retain the tooth in position.
7. Antibiotics, analgesics, and chlorhexidine rinses are prescribed.
8. Endodontic treatment may be required later.

Child Abuse

Child abuse and neglect is a serious problem that all health professionals encounter. The dental office provides an opportunity for children who are abused to be observed and for the abuse to be reported. The entire dental team needs to be aware of the types of child abuse and the signs of child abuse.

Types of child abuse can be physical, sexual, neglectful, and emotional. Injuries associated with child abuse that might be evident in the dental office include fractured teeth and jaw bones, lacerations around the labial frenulum, missing teeth with no explanation, and bruises or scars on the lips. Marks on the child's arms, legs, and neck may also be noticed by the dental team. Lack of personal hygiene or appropriate clothing for the season, extensive caries, and a lack of response toward the need of the child to receive dental treatment are concerns of the dental team, and should be noted and followed if the child's health and welfare are continually compromised.

The Law and Reporting Child Abuse

Laws regarding reporting child abuse may differ from state to state, but most require the dentist to report signs of abuse. The laws are designed to protect children and provide help for families.

Reports should include the following:

- The nature of the concern
- Description of the injury, including type, color, size, characteristics, and location
- X-rays and color photographs
- Child's name, age, address, sex, and date of birth
- Parent or caregiver names
- Physician's name
- Explanations by the child and caregiver for the injury

The dentist is required to report the findings to a social service agency, the local police department, or a child protective service. The dentist may be asked to appear in court and/or file a report.

Chapter Summary

The scope of pediatric treatment includes restoring and maintaining the primary, mixed, and permanent dentition, and applying preventive measures for dental caries, periodontal disease, and malocclusion. The primary focus of the pediatric dental practice is preventive treatment and dealing with the compromised child patient. The whole staff needs to enjoy working with children and be sincere and honest in their actions and feelings. To be effective in the management of children, the dental team must be upbeat, motivated, and aware.

The role of the dental assistant in the pediatric practice will vary according to areas of responsibility. One part that the assistant is involved in is managing the child. Another part is the tasks that the assistant performs at chairside. Depending on the state, when assistants work independently, they assume the authority role and must maintain control of the child. The dental assistant is also an educator of the child and parents.

CASE STUDY

On Friday afternoon, Mrs. Anderson brought her 4-year-old daughter, Noelle, to Dr. Bryan's office for emergency treatment. Noelle had fallen and hit her face. Her maxillary left central incisor was pushed into the alveolus so that only the incisal third of the tooth was exposed. Noelle had seen Dr. Bryan for an exam when she was 3 years old.

Case Study Review

1. What is the condition of Noelle's teeth called?
2. At what stage of tooth eruption is Noelle likely to be? What could happen to Noelle's teeth as a result of the physical trauma? Are the permanent teeth affected?
3. Because Noelle had only been in the office for one visit when she was 3 years, would behavior management be a consideration?

Review Questions

Multiple Choice

1. The best age range for introducing dental care in the dental office is
   a. 2 to 6 years old.
   b. 4 to 8 years old.
   c. 6 to 10 years old.
   d. 10 to 12 years old.
2. Fear that is based on a person's own personal experiences is called
   a. objective.
   b. subjective.
   c. intraverted.
   d. extraverted.
3. If the pulp of a primary tooth has been exposed, which of the following procedures would be indicated?
   a. Pulpectomy
   b. Pulpotomy
   c. Apexification
   d. Root canal
4. Stainless steel crowns are indicated for all of the following *except:*
   a. Following a pulpotomy procedure
   b. Hypoplastic or hypocalcified teeth
   c. Incipient decay
   d. Extensive carious decay
5. Tongue thrusting
   a. pushes the tongue against the posterior teeth.
   b. pushes the tongue against the anterior teeth when swallowing.
   c. pushes the tongue against the palate when swallowing.
   d. pushes the tongue against the floor of the mouth.
6. Behavior management techniques used in the pediatric practice include
   a. voice control.
   b. positive reinforcement.
   c. distraction.
   d. all of the above.
7. The most common pedodontic matrices are:
   a. the tofflemire matrix
   b. the T-band matrix
   c. the spot-welded matrix
   d. both b and c
8. Which of the following is not a preventive procedure?
   a. Coronal polish
   b. Fluoride varnish
   c. Amalgam restoration
   d. Enamel sealants
9. All of the following patients are treated in the pediatric office *except*:
   a. autistic children.
   b. down's syndrome patients.
   c. cleft lip/palate patients.
   d. normal adult patients.
10. A child with mixed dentition has
   a. deciduous and permanent teeth existing simultaneously in the mouth.
   b. deciduous teeth only.
   c. permanent teeth only.
   d. deciduous teeth with decay.

Critical Thinking

1. Think of an office theme or design that would be attractive to children. Would the assistant be responsible for any maintenance?
2. List three behavior management techniques that would be effective with a young patient who is visiting the dental office for the first time.
3. A 5-year-old child arrives at the dental office with bruising on the upper arms and cuts around and inside the mouth. List some steps that may be taken in a pediatric dental office with a suspected child abuse case.
4. Discuss why primary teeth are not replaced in the socket once they have been avulsed. List several considerations when replacing a permanent avulsed tooth.

5. What steps should the dental team take when working with special needs patients?

Web Activities

1. The American Academy of Pediatrics is a wonderful resource. Go to http://www.aapd.org and identify Children's Dental Health month. Also, examine the brochures available for parent and patient information.
2. Return to http://www.aapd.org to locate the questions parents most frequently ask about their children's teeth.
3. Go to the Web site, HealthyChildren.org and look at "Ages & Stages." Review the physical and social characteristics of the toddler, preschooler, grade school child, teenager, and young adult.

CHAPTER

30

Enamel Sealants 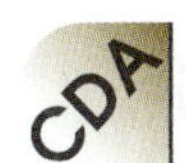

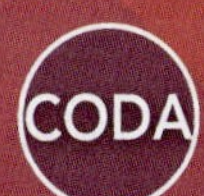

Specific Instructional Objectives

The student should strive to meet the following objectives and demonstrate an understanding of the facts and principles presented in this chapter:

1. Explain the purpose of using dental sealants and where they are placed.
2. List the indications and contraindications of placing sealants.
3. Explain how the dentist decides where and when to place the dental sealant.
4. Discuss the role of the dental assistant in the placement of dental sealants.
5. Describe the process of dental decay and how the sealants work.
6. Describe the types of sealant materials, including composite, glass ionomer, and filled and unfilled sealants.
7. Explain the two methods of polymerization.
8. Discuss the problems with placement of dental sealants.
9. List and describe the steps of the application procedure.

Key Terms

bonding (715)
cannula (714)
Chemically cured (716)
coalesced (713)
color-changing sealants (714)
dental composite resins (BIS-GMA) (714)
etched (715)
glass ionomers (714)
Light cured (716)
mechanical bond (715)
photopolymerized sealant (714)
pit and fissure sealant (712)
polymerization (716)
sealants (712)

Introduction

Dental **sealants** (also known as "**pit and fissure sealants**") are recognized as an effective means to prevent cavities and to prevent the initiation and progression of early carious lesions. They provide a plastic coating over the chewing surfaces of the premolars and molars where decay most often occurs. Tooth brushing and flossing remove plaque and food debris from the smooth surfaces of the teeth, but the toothbrush bristles cannot get into the pits and fissures to remove the debris there (Figure 30-1). The sealants act as a barrier that protects these vulnerable areas on the enamel from accumulation of plaque and food debris. The sealants hold up under the normal stresses of chewing, and, as long as the sealant remains intact, the tooth will be protected from decay. The dentist will check the sealants at routine checkup appointments and will evaluate the effectiveness of the sealant to determine if it needs to be replaced.

Sealants are placed on children and teenagers, but adults can also benefit. The possibility of dental decay begins early in life, and so it is best if sealants are placed as the molars and premolars erupt into the mouth. The pits and fissures on the occlusal surface of the tooth are cleaned thoroughly with a toothbrush, periodontal probe, explorer, or a prophy brush prior to placing the sealant material. The sealant is painted onto the tooth enamel where it bonds to the tooth and hardens.

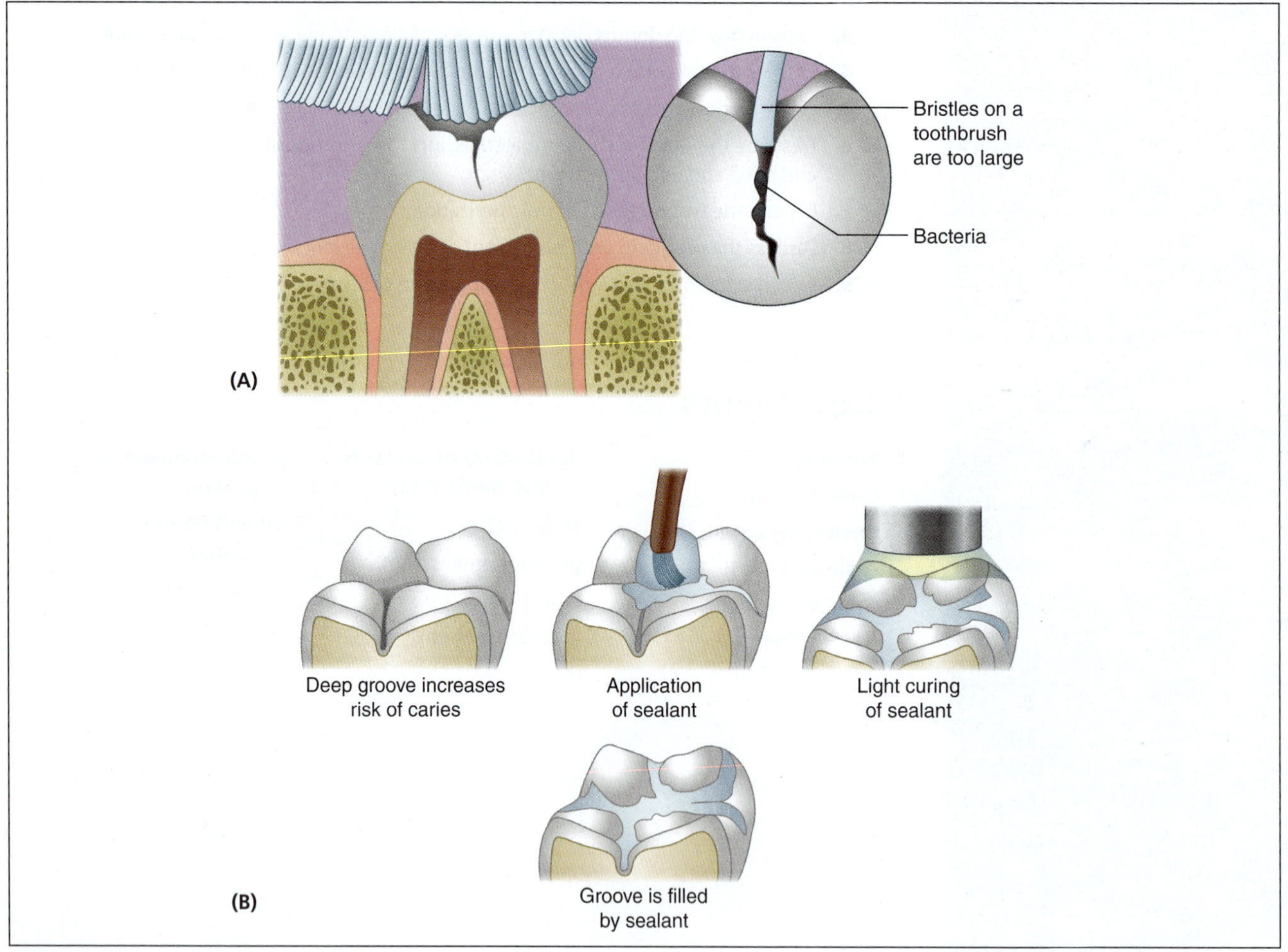

FIGURE 30-1
(A) Toothbrush bristle that is too large to get into the pits and fissures of the tooth. (B) Application of a sealant.

Advanced Chairside Functions

Dental Sealants

Dental sealants are hard resin materials that are applied to the caries-free occlusal surfaces of the premolars and molars. These pit and fissure teeth are particularly susceptible to caries because of the deep pits and fissures in the enamel on the occlusal surface. Tooth brushing is not always an adequate means of removing the bacteria and debris that are lodged into the pits and fissures. Fluoride is very effective at preventing decay on the smooth enamel surfaces of the teeth but is less effective in the pits and fissures. Sealants bond to the tooth to seal the pits and fissures, thereby preventing the decay process from starting. The barrier costs less than a restoration, but does not last as long. On average, sealants remain in place for 5 to 10 years. The combined use of pit and fissure sealants and fluoride has proven to be an effective measure that greatly reduces dental caries in patients through age 16.

Under the *Healthy People 2010* initiative, the U.S. government set a goal that 50 percent of all children will have sealants by 2010. For children aged 8, 33 percent of this target was achieved. For children aged 14, 17 percent of this goal was achieved. The number of school-based health centers providing oral health care and sealants has doubled. The new *Healthy People 2020* initiative has modified the 2010 goal by tracking treatment of dental sealants in children aged 6 through 9 and 13 through 15. (The *Healthy People* initiatives, which challenge private and public sectors at all levels, are managed by the U.S. Department of Health and Human Services.)

Indications and Contraindications for Sealants

Dental sealants are *indicated* when the patient

- has low-to-moderate caries activity;
- practices good oral hygiene techniques;
- teeth are erupted into the mouth enough for the occlusal surface to be accessible;
- eats a balanced diet, preferably low in sugar;
- has a good quantity and quality of saliva; and
- has fluoridated water or takes a fluoride supplement.

Sealants are most beneficial if applied

- on occlusal pits and fissures of non-carious primary and permanent teeth;
- on deep pits on the maxillary central and lateral incisors;
- on recently erupted teeth;
- on patients with a high number of occlusal caries and deep fissures; and
- along with preventive treatment.

Contraindications to placing dental sealants include

- teeth that have been caries free for 4 or more years (because the chances are minimal that occlusal decay will occur);
- teeth with shallow open grooves, because, usually, these teeth are easy to keep clean, making them more resistant to decay, and sealants are not well retained in these areas;
- teeth with well **coalesced** (blended) pits and fissures;
- patients with occlusal decay or who have occlusal restorations; and
- the patient who is allergic to methacrylate, which is contained in the sealant material, because oral tissues may come in contact with it during sealant placement.

Determination to Place Dental Sealants

Dentists use their professional judgment, ADA and CDC guidelines, as well as the patient's needs and preference to determine where and when dental sealants are placed. The dentist will perform a caries risk assessment to assist them in this decision process, and it is important that they reevaluate a patient's caries-risk status periodically.

During the examination the dentist may use a periodontal probe or explorer to examine the pits and fissures on the molars and premolars, and take x-rays of the teeth to determine the need for sealants (Figure 30-2). A caries detection device or dye may also be used as an aid in the decision-making process.

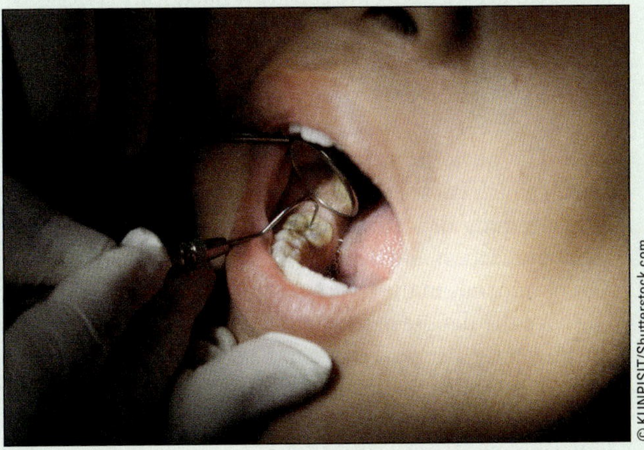

FIGURE 30-2
A dentist checking pits and fissures.

Advanced Chairside Functions (Continued)

Refer to Chapter 37, Dental Cements, Bases, Liners, and Bonding Agents for more information on caries detection.

Some children are at a higher risk for dental decay due to genetics, tooth anatomy (occlusal anatomy with deep pits and fissures), poor oral hygiene, and high-sugar diets. These patients would greatly benefit from the placement of dental sealants.

Role of the Dental Assistant

Applying dental sealants is an expanded duty delegated to the dental hygienist or the dental assistant in some states. The laws governing the dental assistant's responsibilities vary greatly with each state, so become familiar with state practice acts. In some states, the dental assistant can assist the dentist in this procedure by helping in the isolation of the teeth and keeping them dry and free of debris until the sealant is placed. In other states, the dental assistant can place the sealants with education and training. The dental assistant can then follow through with the total preventive program, and apply both the fluoride and the pit and fissure sealants.

It is important for the dental assistant to stay informed and current on enamel sealants. Research on sealant effectiveness, chemical properties, and potential is ongoing, so reading, and attending seminars keeps the dental assistant well informed. Refer to the American Dental Association and the CDC for recommendations and updates on sealant materials, technique changes, and when to place sealants.

Dental Caries and How Dental Sealants Work

Dental sealants are placed, first, to prevent decay in teeth with deep pits and fissures, and second, as a preventive approach to areas that have early (cavitated) carious lesions. A cavitation is a cavity that goes untreated. The cavitation can harbor bacteria and lead to dental decay.

The dental caries process occurs over time with the interaction between the dental plaque and the tooth structure. The bacteria in the plaque become metabolically active, which causes changes in the pH level of the tooth, either gaining or losing minerals. This imbalance in the remineralization and demineralization process leads to a loss of minerals in the tooth structures.

Once the dentist determines that dental decay is present they must also look to see if the decay process is active, and if it is progressing rapidly or slowly. Caries can be prevented, and secondary prevention can occur by intervening in the progression of early caries, before cavitation, with the placement of dental sealant.

Dental Sealant Materials

Several materials have been used as sealants for occlusal pits and fissures, with no single material being superior to the others. The most commonly used are **dental composite resins (BIS-GMA)** or resin based in order to enhance the flow that is typically required for sealants, and these composites have been diluted and are, thus, less viscous. Composites used as sealants are either *unfilled* or *filled*. The filled composite sealant contains a small amount of quartz and silica particles. The unfilled sealant materials do not usually require an occlusal adjustment after the sealant placement is complete. It will wear down naturally with normal chewing. The more filler that is added, the more the sealant material will need to be adjusted. Usually a disc, stone, or bur is used to reduce the occlusion.

Dental composites, which will last up to 10 years, are inexpensive and come in kits with everything you need for application. They are quick and easy to use, which is important when working on active children. Composite sealants require no mixing because they usually come in syringes with disposable applicator tips, cartridges with a **cannula** (small hollow tube) for application, or single-use dispensing tips.

Also available are dental-composite sealant materials containing *fluoride* for the added benefit of fluoride release under the sealant. The fluoride is released after the polymerization of the sealant and creates a fluoride layer. This layer may help with the remineralization process and makes the tooth more resistant to decay. Fluoride may also be in the polishing pastes used to clean the tooth prior to the sealant procedure. Some sealant manufacturer's directions recommend not using this type of paste, and others do not consider the fluoride in the polishing pastes to be a problem. Be sure to check the manufacturer's directions with each material used.

Composite materials come in clear, opaque, or lightly tinted colors. The advantage to the opaque and tinted composites is visibility, which makes placement less difficult, and identification of the sealants at follow-up exams easier. Patients, however, prefer the clear or opaque options because of esthetic appeal. The use of **color-changing sealants**, or **photopolymerized sealant** material, is a relatively new and popular option. These sealants contain a photoactive color additive; they are tinted (usually pink or green) on the initial application, and then change to opaque white after being light cured. This is an improvement that allows for better visibility during sealant placement (Figure 30-3).

The use of **glass ionomers**, another choice for pit and fissure sealant material, is popular in some offices because

Advanced Chairside Functions

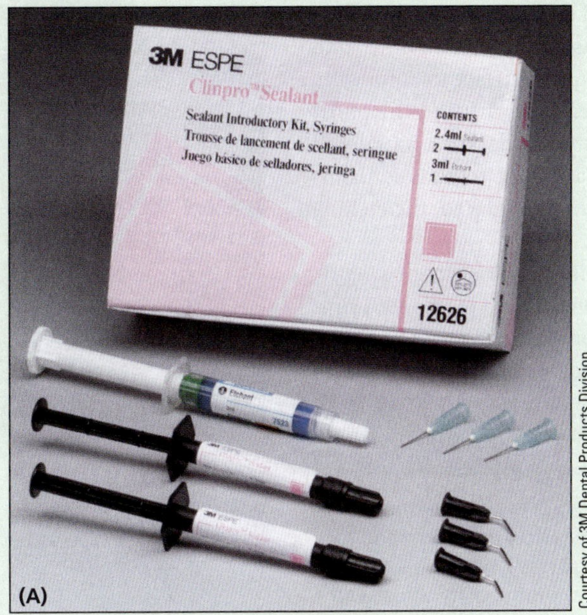

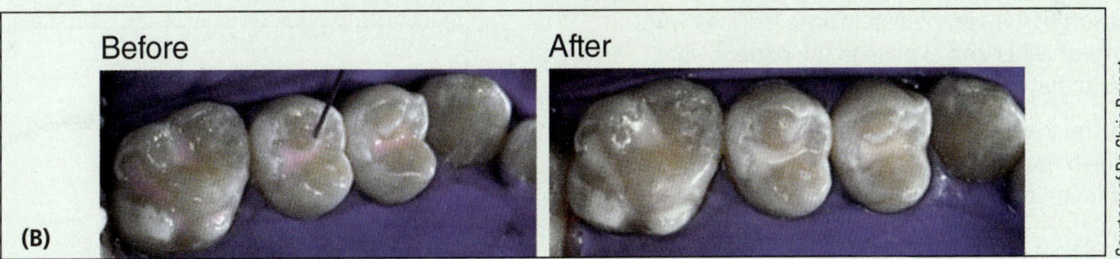

FIGURE 30-3

(A) Color-changing composite resin sealant. (B) The sealant being placed on several etched teeth (Before); and the teeth after the sealant has been light cured (After).

they need not purchase separate material for sealant procedures. In addition, they

- contain fluoride,
- are generally easier to place than resin-based sealants,
- require no etching or bonding agent,
- can be used on smooth surfaces of the tooth because they are less fluid than composites,
- do not require that the area be completely dry for placement because they are not moisture sensitive, and
- bond directly with the enamel.

The fluoride in the glass ionomer material is released continually for about 2 years, which is why glass ionomers are used if the patient has a high rate of caries or xerostomia (dryness of mouth caused by reduced saliva). Glass ionomers are available in powder or liquid form, in capsules with cannula for dispensing the material, and in a syringe with disposable applicator tips.

Bonding, Etching, and Conditioning

Bonding agents, also known as adhesives, may be used in the pit and fissure sealant application. Attachment to the tooth surface, or **bonding**, occurs differently for the composite sealants than for the glass ionomer sealants.

Composite sealants bond to the tooth mechanically. The **mechanical bond** is accomplished when the sealant flows into the irregularities of the treated enamel and locks into place. The enamel surface is **etched**, or conditioned, by a phosphoric acid (or another type of acid) solution that is applied to a clean tooth with a brush, syringe, or small cotton-tipped applicator. The etchant comes in a gel or liquid, and is applied for a specified amount of time, usually 15 to 30 seconds. During the application time, the etchant is dabbed or flowed over the area, but never rubbed. The phosphoric acid removes some of the matrix of the enamel, leaving the enamel rods intact for the sealant material to

Advanced Chairside Functions (Continued)

bond to once it is light cured. If the etchant is rubbed during application, the enamel rods will be broken down and the sealant will not have an adequate surface to bond with. It is very important for the area to be dry and the phosphoric acid to be placed correctly in order for a good bond to occur and for the sealant to last. If the tooth is contaminated with saliva before the sealant is placed, the etching procedure must also be redone.

One-step etching and bonding materials are currently available. These materials combine the acid etchants, primers, and adhesives in an all-in-one system. These materials are placed on the tooth and dried, but not rinsed; the tooth is then ready for sealant placement.

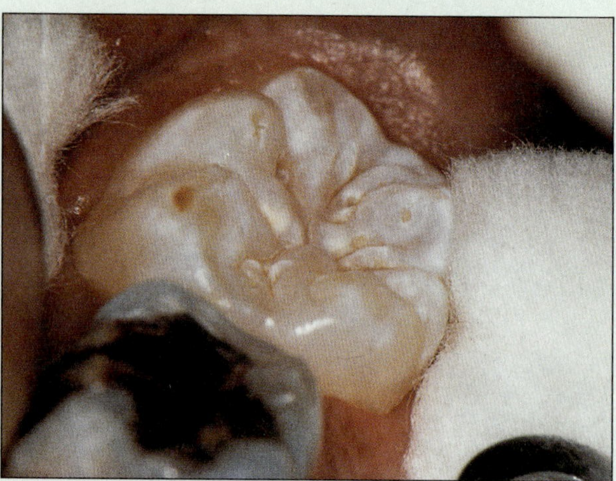

FIGURE 30-4
White chalky area on the occlusal surface of the tooth is where the acid etchant was placed.

Care must be given to the etching process because most etching agents contain phosphoric acid. The patient and the assistant should wear protective glasses when etchants are used. If the etchant gets into the eye, immediately flush with water and check with a doctor. If the etching agent accidently contacts the soft tissues, immediately rinse the area with large amounts of water and explain to the patient what happened, and that the area may be sensitive.

As noted, the tooth must be etched beyond the sealant, it has been shown that this etched area of the tooth surface will begin to remineralize after it is covered with salvia again.

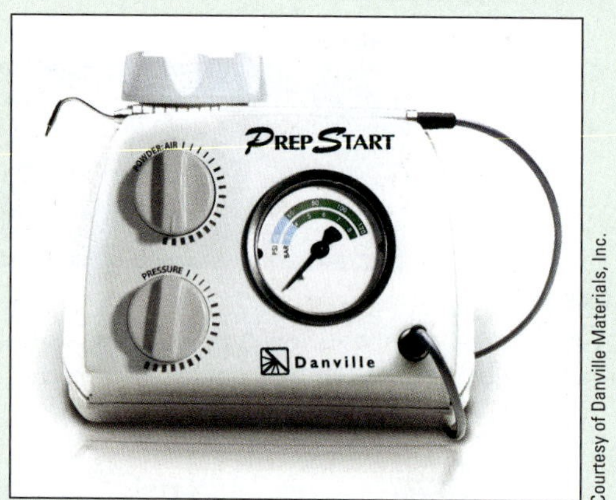

Courtesy of Danville Materials, Inc.

FIGURE 30-5
An air abrasion unit.

When the *time* specified for application has passed, the tooth is rinsed thoroughly for the specified amount of time, usually 30 to 60 seconds. After the tooth has been etched, the surface looks frosted or chalky and appears dull (Figure 30-4). If the enamel does not appear chalky and white, the procedure must be repeated. The etchant or conditioner is applied on the occlusal surface 2 to 3 mm beyond the area to be sealed. The tooth must be etched beyond the sealant to prevent fracture of the sealant and possible *microleakage*.

The glass ionomer sealant materials bond to the tooth chemically. An acid in the glass ionomer material breaks down the enamel and then fuses with it. This is a very strong bond with less chance of marginal chipping or poor bonding.

Other methods used to prepare the tooth by opening the fissures before placing sealants include air abrasion etchers and micro etchers (Figure 30-5). Both the air abrasion and the micro-etching units can be controlled to remove small amounts of decay and tooth structure. When using the air abrasion unit or micro etchers, all debris from the tooth surface must be removed before placing the sealant. Refer to Chapter 18, Basic Chairside Instruments, Tray Systems, and Instrument Transfer.

Another etching method is by modification with a bur (enameloplasty). The dentist will use a fissurotomy bur to open the pits and fissures for better retention of the sealant material (Figure 30-6).

Curing Process

Another difference in the types of sealant materials is the curing or hardening process. The two methods of **polymerization** (hardening) follow:

1. **Chemically cured**, also known as self-curing or auto polymerization.
2. **Light cured**, in which a curing light is used to harden materials.

Advanced Chairside Functions

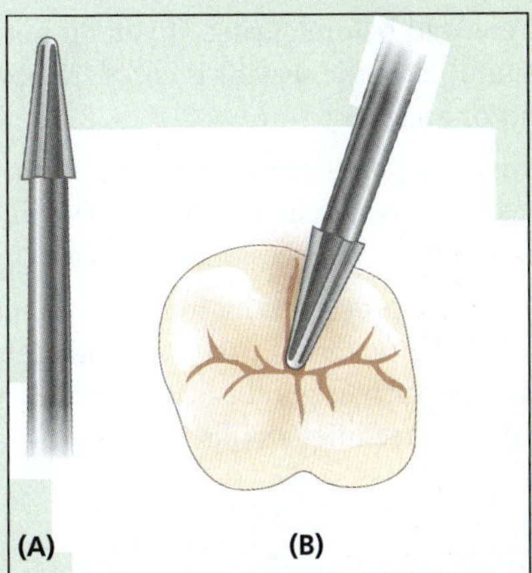

FIGURE 30-6

(A) Fissurotomy Bur. (B) A fissurotomy bur being used to open up a deep pit.

Chemically cured materials consist of a catalyst and a base. When the two are mixed together, they chemically react to polymerize in about 1 minute.

Light-cured sealants are packaged as single-component systems that are activated by a curing light. The advantages of light-curing systems include increased working time, the operator has control of the setting time, and no mixing is required.

Placement of Dental Sealants

The dentist diagnoses which teeth need dental sealants after a thorough examination that includes radiographs. Some dentists also use a caries detection dye, magnified visual inspection, or the new, nondestructive qualitative laser fluorescence. Children with newly erupted molars and premolars that are caries free benefit the most from sealants. Partially erupted teeth may be sealed provided there is no flap over the occlusal surface that might interfere with sealant application.

Isolation is a very important step during sealant placement, because the tooth must be kept dry and free from contamination after the etchant is placed. Using the dental dam is the best method for isolating the tooth or teeth. If placed correctly, the tooth is easier to see and the area is kept dry. The main disadvantage to using the dental dam is that placing it is time consuming. The rubber dam will help control saliva and tongue movement during the procedure. It is usually used when more than one tooth is sealed.

Other means of isolating the tooth include cotton rolls or Garmer® clamps with cotton rolls. Dri-Angles® or Dry-Tips® can also be used to block the Stensen's duct on the buccal mucosa and assist in keeping the mouth open. It is the operator's preference as to when to isolate the teeth: before or after the polish. Usually, sealants are placed on one or two quadrants at a time to ensure adequate isolation of the teeth.

Typically, the tooth is cleaned before it is etched and sealed. The occlusal surface must be free of debris so that the etchant can attach to the enamel surface. Prophy pastes, which are normally used for coronal polishing, should only be used when the manufacturer's directions permit them for use with that type of sealant material. The prophy pastes may not be able to be used because they contain flavoring oils and fluoride that may interfere with the mechanical bonding of the sealant. Another material used for cleaning is flour of pumice with a rubber cup or bristle brush. Other means of cleaning the tooth include using an air abrasion unit (micro abrasion), port polisher, or fissurotomy burs. These will clean the pits and fissures and remove any incipient decay so that the tooth is prepared for the sealant. After cleaning the tooth to remove any debris that might be deep in the pit or fissure, the tooth is rinsed thoroughly and then dried.

Always follow the manufacturer's instructions for preparing the tooth and placing the sealant. Procedure 30-1 demonstrates the steps used in the placement of dental sealants.

Helpful Hints

- The most likely cause of sealant failure is lack of moisture control. Be sure to isolate the area well and maintain isolation throughout the procedure.
- Ask the patient to keep the tongue still to prevent contamination.
- Dri-Angles® can be placed to reduce saliva flow. Place on the buccal mucosa with the widest end toward the anterior of the mouth.
- Sealant patients can sometimes be a challenge, so be prepared and work quickly and efficiently in order to finish as soon as possible.
- Read the manufacturer's instructions to check for any changes in technique or product.

Problems with Sealants

The following are problems that may occur during and after the placement of sealants.

- The tooth may not be etched completely, leaving voids on the surface. After the tooth is etched, carefully examine it, and if there are any voids or air bubbles, the tooth needs to be re-etched.
- Sealant retention is most often compromised if there is moisture contamination during the placement. Practice good isolation techniques to prevent this problem. If

Advanced Chairside Functions (Continued)

the sealant is lost, clean, re-etch, and apply the sealant. Sealants should always be examined carefully at routine checkups.

- Sealant interferes with the bite because too much sealant material was placed on the tooth. After the sealant placement check the patients bite, if the sealant is too high, use a bur to reduce the height of the sealant and clear the bite. Be careful to place the sealant with just enough material to extend just beyond the pits and fissures. This is the same for sealants that block the contact areas. Too much sealant has been applied and needs to be removed before curing. If you do not notice the excess until after the sealant is cured, remove it with a bur and/or a scaler.
- Sometimes sealants remain intact but have chipped margins or areas that leak. This is where microleakage occurs, and there is a possibility of decay.

Problems can be prevented by following manufacturer's directions on the materials used and with detailed technique practices, such as good isolation, knowledge on use of materials, and technique skills.

Procedure 30-1
Procedure for Placing Dental Sealants

This procedure is performed by the dental assistant, hygienist, or dentist depending on the state's Dental Practice Act. Before the sealant is placed, the teeth are evaluated for caries, and then the tooth or teeth are polished with a rubber cup. Equipment for preparation of the tooth or teeth and the sealant placement procedure steps are listed below.

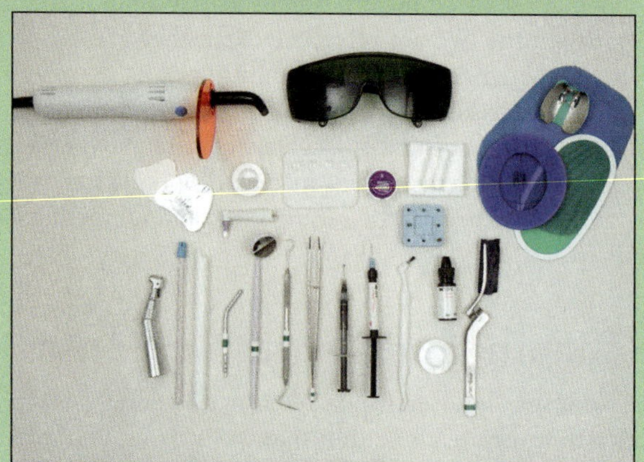

FIGURE 30-7
The tray setup for the placement of dental sealants.

Equipment and Supplies (*Figure 30-7*)

- Basic setup: mouth mirror, explorer, and cotton pliers
- Air–water syringe tip, HVE tips, and saliva ejector
- Rubber cup or brush
- Dri-Angles®
- Low-speed handpiece with right angle (prophy angle) attachment
- Flour of pumice or prophy paste (without fluoride), air polisher, dry toothbrush, or fissurotomy burs
- Dental dam setup, cotton rolls, or Garmers cotton roll holders and short and long cotton rolls
- Etchant or conditioner
- Sealant material: base material and catalyst (for self-cure), or syringe or capsule (for light cure)
- Applicators (microbrush, small cotton-tipped applicator, or syringe) for etchant
- Bonding agent
- Light-curing unit
- Articulating paper and forceps
- Assorted burs and/or stones for reducing high spots

Procedure Steps (*Follow aseptic procedures*)

Prepare the Teeth

1. Check tooth or teeth with explorer. Polish the occlusal surface of the teeth to receive sealants.
2. Use flour of pumice or a non-fluoride prophy paste with a rubber cup or bristle brush to clean the occlusal surfaces. An air polisher, a dry toothbrush, or fissurotomy burs can also

(continues)

Advanced Chairside Functions

Procedure 30-1 (continued)

be used. Once polished, rinse the teeth and dry thoroughly. If the pits and fissures are deep, check them with an explorer, and then rinse and dry again.

Isolate the Teeth

3. Dental dam isolation is ideal because it keeps the teeth dry and protects the tissues from the etchant. Depending on the skill of the operator, the dental dam may be placed on more than one quadrant at a time. (Refer to information on dental dams in Chapter 19, Instrument Transfer and Maintaining the Operating Field.) Cotton roll isolation is commonly used, but care must be given to ensure that the teeth are kept isolated. Garmers clamps used with long and short cotton rolls are very effective. Place cotton rolls on both buccal and lingual areas for the mandibular teeth, and only on the buccal for the maxillary teeth. Place a Dri-Angle on the buccal mucosa.

Dry Surfaces and Etch

4. After the tooth is isolated, completely dry the tooth. Following manufacturer's directions, apply the etchant. Using an applicator, apply etchant to the occlusal surface, into the pits and fissures, and two-thirds up the cuspid incline. Use a gentle dabbing motion while applying the sealant for the designated amount of time (usually 15 to 30 seconds).

Rinsing and Drying the Teeth

5. Rinse the tooth with water, and use the evacuator tip to remove the remaining acid and water. Rinse for 20 to 30 seconds. Re-isolate with dry cotton rolls if this method was used.
6. Dry the tooth with the air and examine the etched surface. It should appear dull and chalky white. If the tooth does not have this appearance, etch again for 15 to 30 seconds (Figure 30-8).

Application of Sealant Material

7. Follow manufacturer's directions to prepare and apply the sealant material. With the applicator selected, place the sealant so that

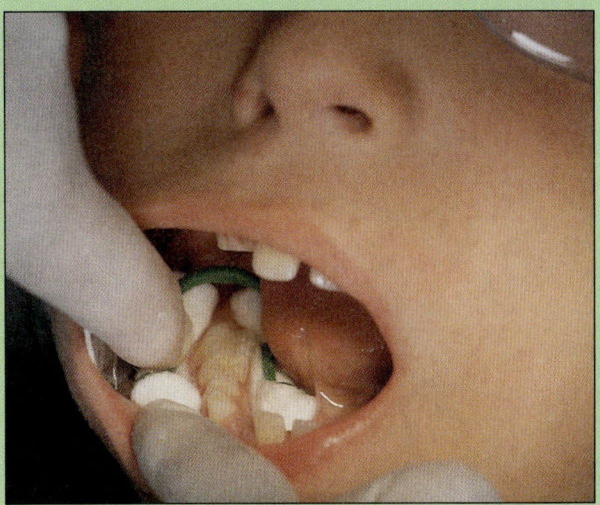

FIGURE 30-8
An isolated tooth with etched enamel. Its appearance is white and chalky where the etchant was placed.

it flows into the pits and fissures and reaches the desired thickness. Place the sealant on the mesial side of the tooth and allow it to flow toward the distal side of the tooth. The applicator tip or a microbrush can be used to carefully move the sealant and prevent air bubbles.

8. Allow the self-curing sealants to set (polymerize) for the time recommended by the manufacturer. For light-cured sealants, hold the curing light 2 mm directly above the occlusal surface and expose for the appropriate time (materials differ, so the curing time can range from 20 to 60 seconds).

NOTE: Use tinted protective eyewear during the curing process.

9. Evaluate the sealant (Figure 30-9). With an explorer, carefully check to see whether the sealant is hardened and smooth. If there are irregularities or voids, repeat the process to properly seal those areas. If the surface has been free of saliva, then additional sealant can be added without etching the tooth first. However, if saliva has contacted the tooth, then the process must be repeated.
10. After the sealant has set, rinse or wipe the surface with a moist cotton roll or pellet to remove the air-inhibited layer.

Advanced Chairside Functions (Continued)

Procedure 30-1 (continued)

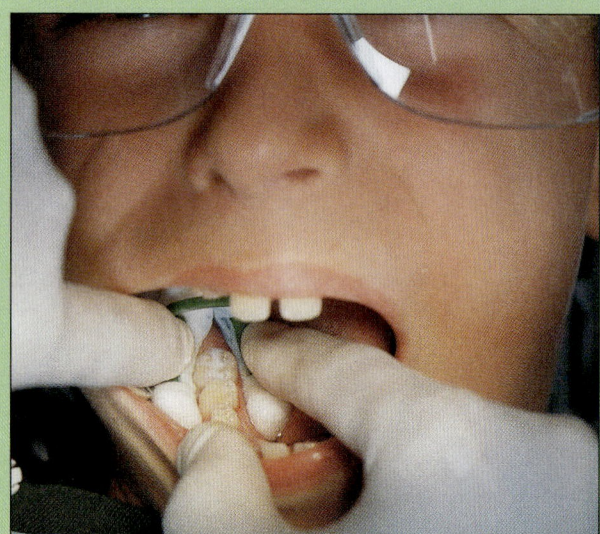

FIGURE 30-9
A tooth with sealant in place.

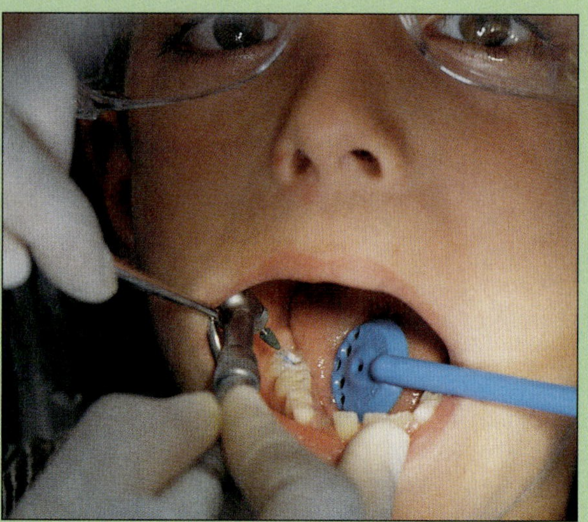

FIGURE 30-10
Articulating paper has marked high spots on the sealant. Before the patient is dismissed, the sealant is reduced with assorted burs and stones.

Occlusal Evaluation

11. Remove the cotton rolls or the dental dam. Check the contacts with dental floss, and look for any excess materials. Dry the teeth and, with articulating paper, evaluate for any high spots (Figure 30-10). If the markings are dark, use a bur or stone to reduce them. It does not take much to reduce the sealant, and areas just a little high will wear down in 2 to 3 days with very little patient awareness.

Finish and Set Evaluation Sequence

12. Apply fluoride to the sealed tooth to cover any areas that were etched but not sealed. Sealants are recorded on the patient's chart. Instruct the patient to have the sealants checked every 6 months to a year to ensure that they have been completely retained.

Chapter Summary

Dental sealants are an excellent means of preventing and reducing tooth decay. Sealants are placed mainly on permanent teeth, preferably just after they erupt in the mouth. There are several types of sealants, including composite resins and glass ionomers. There is discussion on how the tooth is prepared, how the sealant is retained on the tooth, and the curing process of the materials. Depending on individual state's Dental Practice Acts, the dental assistant may or may not place sealants. If dental assistants are allowed to place sealants, they must obtain the needed additional education and skills. The technique for placing sealants requires practice to become proficient.

CASE STUDY

Emery Ann Jones has four newly erupted permanent teeth in her mouth. On her recent visit to the pediatric dentist, they suggested Emery have sealants placed on two of her teeth. Of the other two teeth, one has shallow open grooves and the other has occlusal decay.

Case Study Review

1. List the advantages of placing dental sealants on newly erupted teeth.
2. Discuss placing dental sealants on teeth that have shallow open grooves or occlusal decay.
3. What are the other contraindications to placing sealants?

Review Questions

Multiple Choice

1. Dental sealants are indicated for all of the following *except*
   a. recently erupted teeth.
   b. teeth that have been caries free for 4 or more years.
   c. on occlusal pits and fissures of noncarious primary teeth.
   d. on deep occlusal fissures.
2. All of the following statements are true about dental sealants *except*:
   a. Sealants bond mechanically to the tooth surface.
   b. The teeth are etched before sealants are placed.
   c. Sealants are light cured only.
   d. Sealants are placed on caries-free occlusal surfaces.
3. What are the two methods of polymerization?
   a. Chemically cured and light cured
   b. Water cured and chemically cured
   c. Light cured and heat cured
   d. Heat cured and water cured
4. All the following statements are true about the opaque or tinted sealants *except*:
   a. The advantage is visibility.
   b. The placement is easier because of good visibility.
   c. These sealants are less difficult to identify.
   d. Patients prefer the tinted sealants.
5. What type of material is used for sealants?
   a. Glass ionomers
   b. Composite resins (BIS-GMA)
   c. Both a and b
   d. Only b
6. All of the following statements about fluoride are true, *except*:
   a. Fluoride is released after polymerization and creates a fluoride layer.
   b. There is no fluoride in any dental sealant materials.
   c. The fluoride in the glass ionomer material is released for about 2 years.
   d. Check with the manufacturer's directions to see if fluoride prophy pastes are compatible with the sealant materials.
7. These composite resins may contain small amounts of quartz and silica particles.
   a. Filled composite resins
   b. Unfilled composite resins
   c. Glass ionomers
   d. Etchants
8. The air abrasion units and the fissurotomy burs are
   a. used to prepare the tooth for sealants.
   b. used to finish the sealant material.
   c. used to begin the polymerization of the sealant.
   d. not used in the sealant procedure.
9. All the following statements are true *except*:
   a. Most etchants contain phosphoric acid.
   b. The patient and the assistant should wear protective glasses during the placement of the sealant.
   c. The etched area of the tooth surface will never remineralize.
   d. If the etchant contacts soft tissues, rinse with a large amount of water.
10. Where do you find out whether dental assistants can legally place dental sealants in your state?
    a. American Dental Association
    b. American Academy of Pediatric Dentistry
    c. The state's Dental Practice Act
    d. Dental assistants can place sealants in all states.

Critical Thinking

1. On a 6-month recall appointment for a child patient, you notice that a sealant is missing on tooth #30. Should the sealant be replaced? If so, can the sealant be replaced without etching the tooth first?
2. Discuss the various methods for keeping the area dry when placing a sealant.

3. When should dental sealants be placed on a patient? Are sealants only placed on children?

Web Activities

1. Sealants are a very important part of preventive treatment for children. To find out more about sealants go to the ADA Web site.
2. Go to https://www.aap.org to read recent articles on dental sealant materials and techniques.
3. To find out what dental sealants are, why they are needed, and more health-related information go to http://www.nidcr.nih.gov/OralHealth/Topics/Sealants

CHAPTER 31

Periodontics

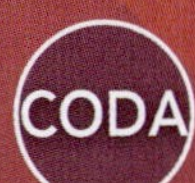

Specific Instructional Objectives

The student should strive to meet the following objectives and demonstrate an understanding of the facts and principles presented in this chapter:

1. Describe the scope of periodontics.
2. Identify members of the periodontal team and their roles.
3. Describe the stages of periodontal disease.
4. Explain the diagnostic procedures involved in the patient's first visit to the periodontal office.
5. Identify and describe periodontal instruments and their uses.
6. Describe the use and the benefits of lasers in dentistry.
7. Explain the safety precautions when using dental lasers.
8. Describe nonsurgical procedures and the dental assistant's role in each procedure.
9. Explain surgical procedures and dental assisting responsibilities.
10. Describe plastic (esthetic) periodontal surgery and list the types of surgeries.
11. Explain the purpose of periodontal dressing.
12. Identify the types of periodontal dressings and how they are prepared, placed, and removed.
13. Describe periodontal maintenance procedures and the patient's role relating to each.

Key Terms

air polishing systems (736)
bacterial plaque (725)
bleeding index (732)
bone grafting (746)
bruxism (725)
calculus (725)
chisel scaler (735)
coronal polish (742)
curette (734)
electrosurgery (737)
frenectomy (747)
furcation (728)
gingival cleft (732)
gingival grafting (747)
gingivectomy (743)
gingivitis (725)
gingivoplasty (743)
Gracey curette (735)
guided tissue regeneration (GTR) (748)
hoe scaler (735)
horizontal bone resorption (732)
interdental knife (736)
laser (739)
mucogingival surgery (747)
necrotizing ulcerative gingivitis (NUG) (728)
necrotizing ulcerative periodontitis (NUP) (729)
occlusal equilibration (732)
osseous surgery (746)
ostectomy (746)
osteoplasty (746)
periodontal dressing (745)
periodontal flap surgery (745)
periodontal knife (736)
periodontal pocket (730)
periodontal probe (734)
periodontal probing (730)
periodontal scissors (738)
periodontal screening and recording (PSR) (732)
periodontitis (725)

(continues)

Key Terms (continued)

Introduction

The periodontist specializes in diseases of the tissue around the root of the tooth. This specialty deals with symptoms, probable causes, diagnosis, and treatment of periodontal disease.

Periodontal Team

The team in a periodontal office includes the periodontist, dental assistants, dental hygienists, and business office staff.

- The periodontist coordinates treatment with the general dentist in the overall care of the patient. The periodontist screens the patient, performs the surgical care, and provides continual care according to the patient's needs.
- The dental assistant performs chairside assisting duties and expanded functions allowed by state Dental Practice Acts, including placing and removing periodontal dressing, removing sutures, and performing coronal polishes. The dental assistant takes radiographs, takes impressions for study models, places sealants, and administers fluoride treatments. The dental assistant also gives pre- and postoperative instructions and prepares the treatment room for surgery. These functions are in addition to treatment room preparation and maintenance and sterilization procedures. The dental assistant is involved in educating and motivating the patient throughout the treatment. In some offices, the dental assistant may also perform laboratory tasks, such as pouring study models or making periodontal splints.
- The dental hygienist performs traditional hygiene procedures and, depending on the state Dental Practice Act, may also administer local anesthetic. In a periodontal practice, the hygienist often sees patients who have more advanced periodontal disease; therefore, responsibilities include curettage, root planing, and clinical examination procedures.

Periodontal Disease

Ancient human skulls demonstrate evidence of bone destruction associated with periodontal disease, and early civilizations had treatment methods such as using wire to tie loose teeth together. According to the American Academy of Periodontology, three out of four adults will experience, to some degree, periodontal problems at some time in their lives. Periodontal disease occurs in children and adolescents with marginal gingivitis and gingival recession, which are the most prevalent conditions (Figure 31-1).

Periodontal disease involves the **periodontium**, which represents the tissues that support the teeth and includes the following (see Chapter 8, Embryology and Histology, to review the tissues that support the tooth):

- **Gingiva**—Tissues that surround the teeth.
- **Epithelial attachment**—Area at the bottom of the sulcus where the gingiva attaches to the tooth.
- **Periodontal ligaments or membranes**—Fibers of connective tissue that surround the root of the tooth and attach the cementum to the bone.
- **Cementum**—Hard surface that covers the dentin on the root of the tooth.
- **Alveolar bone**—Bone that forms the socket that encases the root of the tooth.
- **Sulcus**—Space between the tooth and the free gingiva. In healthy mouths, the sulcus is 1 to 3 mm deep.

Symptoms of Periodontal Disease

The symptoms of periodontal disease include bleeding gums, loose teeth (mobility), inflamed gingiva, abnormal contour of the gingiva, periodontal pocket formation, malocclusion, halitosis, pain and tenderness, and recession and discoloration. All of these symptoms may be present or the symptoms may vary (Figure 31-2A).

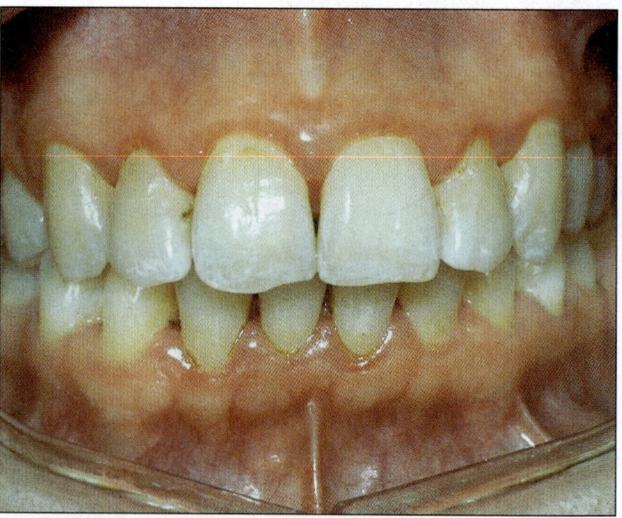

FIGURE 31-1
View of patient with mild gingivitis.

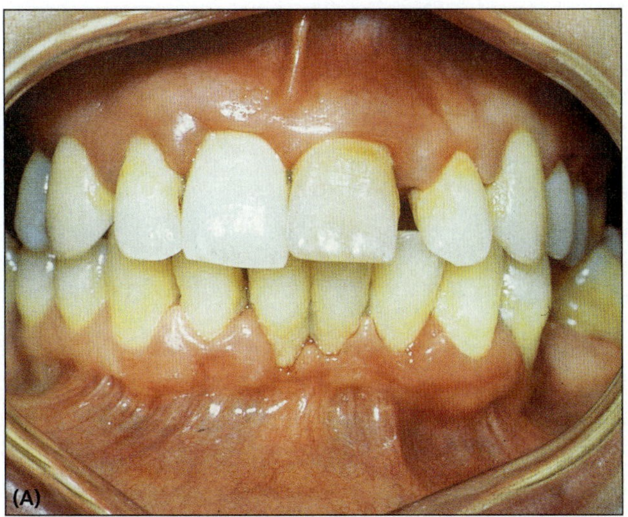
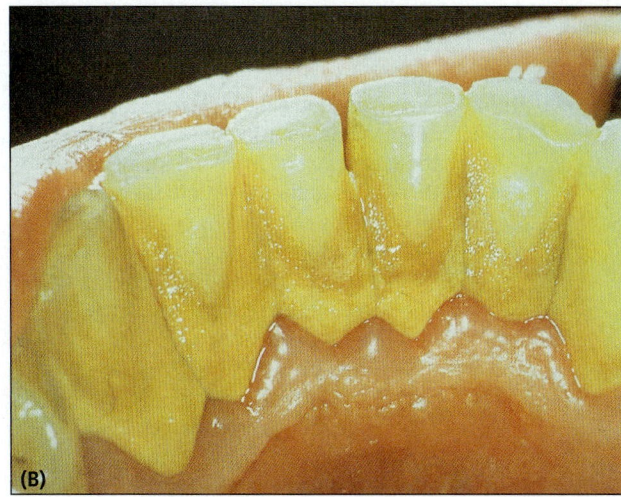

FIGURE 31-2
(A) View of patient with unhealthy gingival tissues—advanced gingival inflammation. (B) Unhealthy gingival tissues and lingual calculus.

Causes of Periodontal Disease

Local irritants are a significant cause of periodontal disease. One irritant, **bacterial plaque**, is a common cause of the inflammation of the gingival tissues. The bacterial plaque forms around the margin of the gingiva and, if left undisturbed, mineralizes and appears as a yellow or brown deposit on the teeth. This hard deposit is called **calculus** (tartar) (Figure 31-2B). If plaque and calculus are not removed, they continue to develop and grow on both supragingival and subgingival surfaces.

Poor oral hygiene results in the buildup of plaque and calculus. When we do not brush and floss daily this can lead to plaque formation and debris buildup on the teeth and appliances. (Proper brushing and flossing techniques are discussed in Chapter 4, Oral Health and Preventive Techniques.)

Improper nutrition leads to overall poor health, which often is evident in the gingival tissues. When we eat a balanced diet, including foods that keep teeth strong and the tissues free of disease, this can aid in maintaining a healthy mouth.

Malocclusion can be a factor in periodontal disease. Improper tooth alignment and occlusion can lead to plaque and calculus formation in areas where food and debris are not removed easily. Also, patients with sensitive teeth or who need dental restorations will favor these areas and alter chewing patterns, putting additional pressure on periodontal structures.

Stress can lead to **bruxism** (grinding of the teeth), which puts pressure on the teeth and surrounding tissues. Problems with the periodontium during times of stress may be evident because the patient may not eat healthy foods or maintain proper oral hygiene.

Systemic factors, including hormonal imbalances, hereditary predisposition, and certain diseases and medications, are often reflected in the gingival tissues. Examples include hormonal changes due to pregnancy, diabetes, cardiovascular disease such as hypertension, blood diseases such as leukemia, HIV infection, genetic conditions such as Down syndrome, emotional disorders, systemic drugs such as Dilantin or immunosuppressants, and thyroid deficiencies.

Classifications of Periodontal Disease

There are two main classifications of periodontal disease: **gingivitis** and **periodontitis**. Through clinical research and improved technology, the understanding of periodontal disease has broadened in scope. Considering the course and characteristics of the disease, more classifications have been added. In 1999 at the International Workshop for a Classification of Periodontal Diseases and Conditions, the American Academy of Periodontology proposed a new classification system (Table 31-1). The revisions are inclusive and describe distinct types of periodontal diseases. The classifications are based on clinical (extent and severity of disease), radiographic, and historical data. Stages of periodontal disease have also been refined (Table 31-2).

Gingivitis. Gingivitis is inflammation of the gingival tissues. It is common in all ages. Causes may include buildup of plaque and calculus, poor-fitting appliances, and poor occlusion, and the condition may occur in association with certain systemic diseases (scurvy), hormonal changes (pregnancy), or prolonged drug therapy (phenytoin, which is an anticonvulsant drug). The tissues become reddish in color, interdental papilla may be swollen and bulbous, and tissues may bleed after brushing and flossing. Gingivitis precedes periodontitis but does not always progress to it. Proper brushing and flossing can reverse this condition in some cases by removing the plaque.

In the classification system, the section on gingival diseases is divided into plaque-induced gingivitis and non-plaque-induced diseases. Each section covers types of gingival conditions that are seen in periodontal and general dental practice. According to the section on plaque-induced diseases, gingivitis can be modified by systemic factors, medications, or malnutrition. The section on non-plaque-induced gingivitis includes a wide range of gingival diseases that are specific according to bacteria. This section also includes wide-ranging manifestations of system conditions and allergic reactions.

TABLE 31-1 Classification of Periodontal Diseases and Conditions

- I. Gingival diseases
  - A. Dental plaque–induced gingival diseases*
    - 1. Gingivitis associated with dental plaque only
      - a. Without other local contributing factors
      - b. With local contributing factors (see VIIIA)
    - 2. Gingival diseases modified by systemic factors
      - a. Associated with the endocrine system
        - (1) Puberty-associated gingivitis
        - (2) Menstrual cycle–associated gingivitis
        - (3) Pregnancy-associated
          - (a) Gingivitis
          - (b) Pyogenic granuloma
        - (4) Diabetes mellitus–associated gingivitis
      - b. Associated with blood dyscrasias
        - (1) Leukemia-associated gingivitis
        - (2) Other
    - 3. Gingival diseases modified by medications
      - a. Drug-influenced gingival diseases
        - (1) Drug-influenced gingival enlargements
        - (2) Drug-influenced gingivitis
          - (a) Oral contraceptive–associated gingivitis
          - (b) Other
    - 4. Gingival diseases modified by malnutrition
      - a. Ascorbic acid–deficiency gingivitis
      - b. Other
  - B. Non–plaque-induced gingival lesions
    - 1. Gingival diseases of specific bacterial origin
      - a. *Neisseria gonorrhoeae–associated* lesions
      - b. *Treponema pallidum*–associated lesions
      - c. Streptococcal species–associated lesions
      - d. Other
    - 2. Gingival diseases of viral origin
      - a. Herpes virus infections
        - (1) Primary herpetic gingivostomatitis
        - (2) Recurrent oral herpes
        - (3) Varicella-zoster infections
      - b. Other
    - 3. Gingival diseases of fungal origin
      - a. *Candida* species infections
        - (1) Generalized gingival candidiasis
      - b. Linear gingival erythema
      - c. Histoplasmosis
      - d. Other
    - 4. Gingival lesions of genetic origin
      - a. Hereditary gingival fibromatosis
      - b. Other
    - 5. Gingival manifestations of systemic conditions
      - a. Mucocutaneous disorders
        - (1) Lichen planus
        - (2) Pemphigoid
        - (3) Pemphigus vulgaris
        - (4) Erythema multiforme
        - (5) Lupus erythematosus
        - (6) Drug-induced
        - (7) Other
      - b. Allergic reactions
        - (1) Dental restorative materials
          - (a) Mercury
          - (b) Nickel

(continues)

TABLE 31-1 Classification of Periodontal Diseases and Conditions (continued)

(c) Acrylic
(d) Other
(2) Reactions attributable to
(a) Toothpastes/dentifrices
(b) Mouthrinses/mouthwashes
(c) Chewing gum additives
(d) Foods and additives
(3) Other
6. Traumatic lesions (factitious, iatrogenic, accidental)
(a) Chemical injury
(b) Physical injury
(c) Thermal injury
7. Foreign-body reactions
8. Not otherwise specified
II. Chronic periodontitis†
A. Localized
B. Generalized
III. Aggressive periodontitis†
A. Localized
B. Generalized
IV. Periodontitis as a manifestation of systemic diseases
A. Associated with hematologic disorders
1. Acquired neutropenia
2. Leukemias
3. Other
B. Associated with genetic disorders
1. Familial and cyclic neutropenia
2. Down syndrome
3. Leukocyte adhesion deficiency syndromes
4. Papillon-Lefévre syndrome
5. Chediak-Higashi syndromes
6. Histiocytosis syndromes
7. Glycogen storage disease
8. Infantile genetic agranulocytosis
9. Cohen syndrome
10. Ehlers-Danlos syndrome (Types IV and VIIIAD)
11. Hypophosphatasia
12. Other
C. Not otherwise specified (NOS)
V. Necrotizing periodontal diseases
A. Necrotizing ulcerative gingivitis (NUG)
B. Necrotizing ulcerative periodontitis (NUP)
VI. Abscesses of the periodontium
A. Gingival abscess
B. Periodontal abscess
C. Pericoronal abscess
VII. Periodontitis associated with endodontic lesions
A. Combined periodontal–endodontic lesions
VIII. Developmental or acquired deformities and conditions
A. Localized tooth-related factors that modify or predispose to plaque-induced gingival diseases/periodontitis
1. Tooth anatomic factors
2. Dental restorations/appliances
3. Root fractures
4. Cervical root resorption and cemental tears
B. Mucogingival deformities and conditions around teeth
1. Gingival/soft tissue recession
a. Facial or lingual surfaces
b. Interproximal (papillary)

(continues)

TABLE 31-1 Classification of Periodontal Diseases and Conditions (continued)

2. Lack of keratinized gingiva
3. Decreased vestibular depth
4. Aberrant frenum/muscle position
5. Gingival excess
   a. Pseudopocket
   b. Inconsistent gingival margin
   c. Excessive gingival display
   d. Gingival enlargement (see IA3 and IB4)
6. Abnormal color

C. Mucogingival deformities and conditions on edentulous ridges
   1. Vertical and/or horizontal ridge deficiency
   2. Lack of gingiva/keratinized tissue
   3. Gingival/soft tissue enlargement
   4. Aberrant frenum/muscle position
   5. Decreased vestibular depth
   6. Abnormal color

D. Occlusal trauma
   1. Primary occlusal trauma
   2. Secondary occlusal trauma

*Can occur on a periodontium with no attachment loss or on a periodontium with attachment loss that is not progressing.
†Can be further classified on the basis of extent and severity. As a general guide, extent can be characterized as localized if ≤30% and generalized if ≥30% of sites involved. Severity can be characterized on the basis of the amount of clinical attachment loss (CAL) as follows: slight, 1–2 mm CAL; moderate, 3–4 mm CAL; and severe, ≥5 mm CAL.

Source: Armitage, G.C. 1999. Development of a classification system for periodontal diseases and conditions. *Ann Periodontal* 4: 1–6.

TABLE 31-2 Periodontal Disease Stages

Periodontal disease is caused by plaque, the colorless, sticky bacterial film that forms constantly on the teeth. The bacteria in plaque produce by-products that can irritate the gums and, over time, seriously damage the structures that support the teeth.

Healthy Tissues	Gingivitis	Early Periodontitis	Moderate Periodontitis	Advanced Periodontitis
Gum is firm, fits tightly to the teeth, and does not bleed.	Gum tissue may be inflamed, swollen, and bleeds easily during brushing, flossing, or examination by your dental professional.	Continued inflammation, loss of gum attachment and bone support.	Supporting gum and bone tissue have deteriorated, tooth loosens.	Severe destruction of tissue and bone, causing tooth loss.

Periodontitis. Periodontitis involves the formation of periodontal pockets. This occurs when margins of the gingiva and periodontal fibers recede and the supporting bone becomes inflamed and destroyed (Figure 31-3). There is an increase in tooth mobility as the pockets become deeper, and there may be **furcation** (area where the roots divide) involvement in multirooted teeth.

The classification system now refers to "chronic periodontitis" instead of "adult periodontitis" because adolescents as well as adults can develop periodontitis. Chronic periodontitis is a progressive disease process with the patient experiencing loss of tissue attachment and bone. Periodontitis can also be evaluated on the basis of extent and severity. Extent is characterized using the following guideline: extent is localized if less than 30 percent of sites are involved, and generalized if more than 30 percent are involved. Severity is characterized by the amount of clinical attachment loss (CAL): slight = 1–2 mm CAL, moderate = 3–4 mm CAL, and severe = ≥5 mm CAL.

Aggressive periodontitis is a form of periodontitis that acts rapidly and aggressively destroys the tissue attachment and bone. Extent of the disease determines whether it falls under the localized or generalized classification.

Patients with periodontitis that is associated with complicated systemic involvement, such as diabetes, are addressed in the "Periodontitis as a Manifestation of Systemic Diseases" section (see Table 31-1, section IV).

Necrotizing Ulcerative Gingivitis and Necrotizing Ulcerative Periodontitis. A **necrotizing ulcerative gingivitis (NUG)** occurs most frequently in young adults 16 to 30 years old. Causes include stress, smoking, inadequate diet,

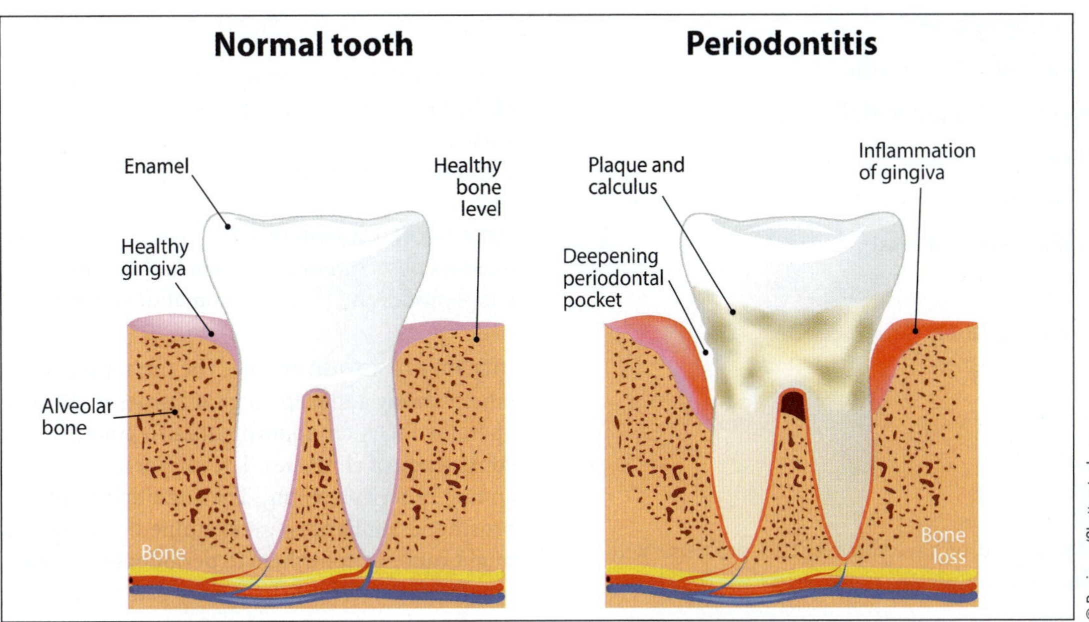

FIGURE 31-3
Periodontitis.

and poor oral hygiene. Characteristics of this form of gingivitis are inflamed gingiva, metallic taste, bad breath, pain, and hemorrhage of the tissues. This condition is also known as Vincent's disease and trench mouth. It appears in individuals in the same unhealthy state and frequently occurs in college students around the time of final examinations (because of stress).

HIV periodontitis is now known as **necrotizing ulcerative periodontitis (NUP)**. NUP is not limited to patients with HIV infections, but is also seen in patients who are severely malnourished and immunosuppressed. Patients with NUP are often in severe pain, the sites bleed easily, and tissue and bone destruction is extensive.

Periodontal Diagnostic Procedures

CDA The first appointment with the periodontist is often an information-gathering appointment. After completing the medical dental history, the patient is seated in the treatment room for an extraoral and intraoral examination. Radiographs and impressions are taken and a periodontal screening is completed. Developing rapport with the patient is essential for successful treatment. The patient must have confidence in the dentist and the staff. The patient has responsibility in the treatment of periodontal disease and should be educated and motivated. Information to share with each patient includes the importance of following oral hygiene instructions, diet suggestions and modifications, personal habit changes, and routine office visits.

Medical Dental History

The medical dental history gives the operator and the patient the opportunity to learn about each other. The operator gains information about why the patient is seeking treatment; if there is a systemic condition such as tuberculosis, HIV, AIDS, or diabetes; how the patient feels about his or her teeth; previous dental treatment; and if the patient has any oral habits that have contributed to the present condition. The patient has the opportunity to ask questions to the dentist and gain an understanding of what is involved with periodontal treatment. The patient's history must be accurate and complete. A history checklist should open the way for significant conversation between the patient, the dental assistant, and/or the dentist.

Sample Medical History Form. The following types of questions should be answered by the patient.

1. Chief complaints:
   - Why did you come to the periodontist?
   - Specifically, what area(s) of your mouth is (are) causing you concern?
   - Do you currently have pain in or near your ears?
   - Does any part of your mouth hurt when clenched?
   - Are there any areas in your mouth that have unhealed or inflamed sores?
2. Medical history:
   - Are you ill at this time? If so, what is (are) your ailment(s)?
   - Are you currently undergoing any medical treatment(s)? If so, what kind(s)?
   - Are you taking any medication(s)? If so, what kind(s)?
   - Have you ever had adverse responses to any type(s) of antibiotic? If so, what type(s)?
   - Have you ever had adverse responses to any type(s) of anesthetic? If so, what type(s)?

- Are you pregnant?
- Are you allergic to anything?
- Do you have any of the following?

  Rheumatic fever

  Heart murmur

  Cardiovascular disease

  Hepatitis

  Kidney infection

  Tuberculosis

  Diabetes

  AIDS

  HIV
- Do you have, or have you ever had, problems with any of the following?

  Prolonged bleeding

  Allergies

  Oral symptoms related to pregnancy, menstruation, or menopause
- Do you have any oral conditions present? If so, how long have they been present and has there been any treatment for them?

3. Oral history:
   - Have you had any extractions? Have you had any restorations?
   - Do you have any problems after dental treatment, such as bleeding, pain, or swelling?
   - Do you have any problems with your teeth, such as bleeding gums, pain, mobility, or sensitivity?
   - Do you have difficulty with your joints when eating or opening and closing your mouth?
4. Oral habits:
   - Do you have any habits such as grinding, clenching, or mouth breathing?
   - Do you smoke?
   - Do you use alcohol or drugs?
5. Family history:
   - Does anyone in your family have a history of periodontal disease?
6. Oral hygiene:
   - Which brushing technique do you use?
   - Do you floss? If so, how often?
   - What type of toothbrush and toothpaste do you use?
   - Do you use any other oral hygiene aids? If so, what kinds?

Clinical Examination

The clinical examination includes an extraoral examination of the face and neck; an intraoral examination of the tongue, palate, buccal mucosa, the teeth, and the oropharynx area; and the periodontal examination.

Extraoral Examination. The extraoral examination includes observation of the skin and lips and palpation of the lymph nodes and the temporomandibular joint.

Intraoral Examination. The intraoral examination combines viewing and palpating the tissues in the oral cavity. The operator looks for abnormalities in color, size, texture, and consistency of all tissues. The intraoral examination includes an oral cancer screening. The condition of the teeth and any prosthetic appliances are examined, noting any areas that might cause or contribute to periodontal disease. Any necessary treatment is recorded on the patient's chart.

Periodontal Examination. The periodontal examination is a thorough examination of the periodontium using periodontal charts. The periodontal charts depict the condition of the patient's periodontal tissues. The charting is completed either manually or on a computer. The oral cavity is examined, and information is gathered by the dentist or hygienist while the dental assistant records the information on the periodontal chart (Figure 31-4).

- Patient's oral hygiene is evaluated and the amount of **plaque** and calculus present is determined. This evaluation includes both supragingival and subgingival deposits.
- The process of **periodontal probing** measures the depth of the **periodontal pocket** with a periodontal probe (refer to the Periodontal Instruments—Periodontal Probes section). A normal sulcus is 3 mm deep or less. When the depth is greater than 3 mm, it is termed a periodontal pocket. To determine the sulcus depth, six sites are probed and recorded on each tooth. There are three sites on the facial, including mesiofacial, midfacial, and distofacial, and three sites on the lingual, including mesiolingual, midlingual, and distolingual. The periodontal probe is inserted into the sulcus until the operator feels resistance (Figure 31-5). Tactile sensation indicates the level of the epithelium attachment. The calibrations on the probe measure the depth of the pocket. These are recorded on the chart.
- The **tooth mobility** measures the movement of the tooth within the socket. The mobility test is accomplished by pushing the tooth in a buccolingual direction using the handle ends of two instruments or by using the automatic device for assessing mobility. Mobility is usually recorded using a scale of 0 to 3: 0 = normal, 1 = slight or 1 mm, 2 = moderate or 2 mm, and 3 = severe or 3 mm.
- Furcation involvement measures destruction of interradicular bone in the furcation area of multi rooted teeth. A curved instrument is inserted in the furcation to determine the amount of involvement.

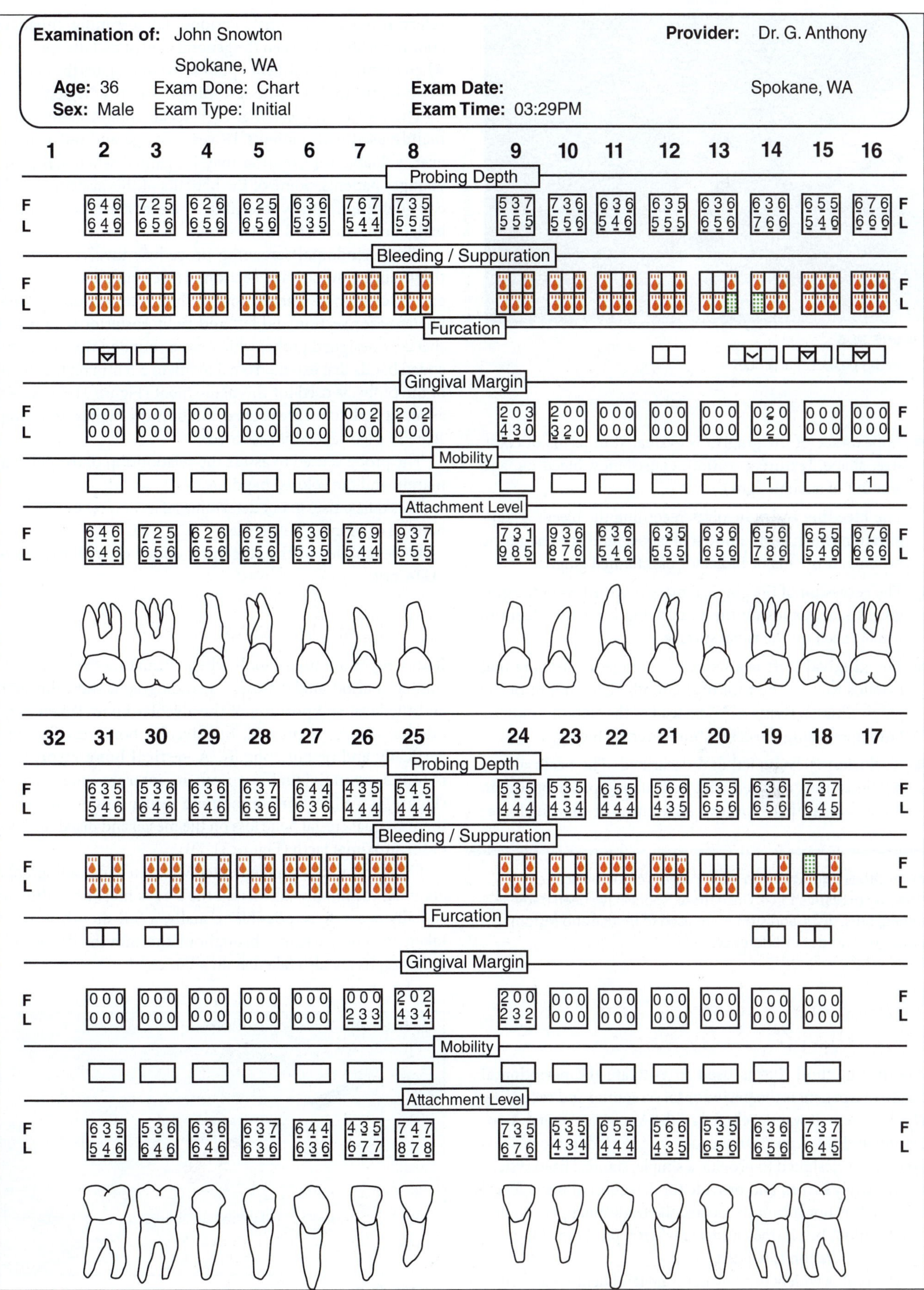

FIGURE 31-4

Periodontal chart includes probing depth, bleeding index, notation for any furcation involvement, level of gingival margin, tooth mobility, and the attachment level for both arches.

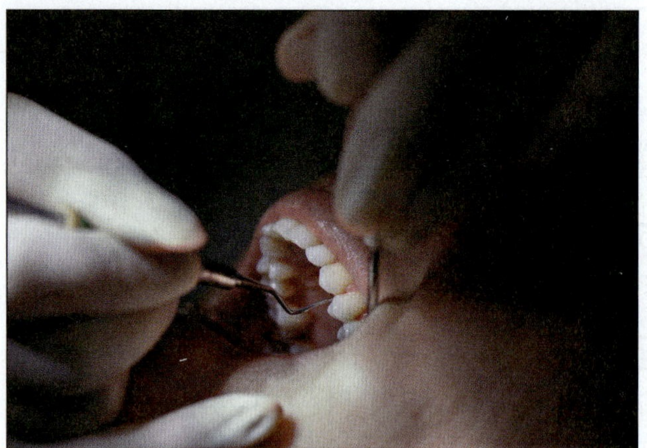

FIGURE 31-5
Using the periodontal probe.

- Appearance of the gingiva is evaluated in terms of color, size, shape, texture, position, consistency, bleeding, and amount of exudate (pus).
- The **bleeding index** involves recording the bleeding/suppuration which is the amount of blood/fluid present during probing. It is a major indicator of inflamed gingiva.
- The **recession** of the gingival margin is the loss of the gingival tissue, exposing the underlying cementum/dentin, usually seen on the facial surface.
- The **gingival cleft** is a fissure or elongated opening that extends toward the root of the tooth. The margin of the gingival tissue forms a "V" instead of the smooth rounded border exposing the cementum covering the root.
- Occlusion is evaluated and described. The occlusal bite relationship is checked with articulating paper or wax to identify areas that show excessive biting or chewing force.

An **occlusal equilibration** is the process of removing areas showing excessive force. Once these "spots" have been determined, burs, discs, and stones are used to reduce and restore occlusion without interference.

Periodontal Screening and Recording (PSR) System

Another method that is used to evaluate the periodontal health of a patient is the **periodontal screening and recording (PSR)** system. It was developed by the American Dental Association and the American Academy of Periodontology. This system was designed to provide a simple, standardized system to effectively screen and provide for detection of periodontal disease. It is not meant to replace the traditional periodontal examination, but it does indicate when a partial or full periodontal evaluation is needed.

The PSR is widely used by many general dentists as well as the periodontist. This system assists the dentist to determine the best treatment plan for a patient, which might involve the referral to a periodontist. Periodontal screening enhances communication between the general dentist and the specialist when discussing treatment options. In some states the dentist/periodontist may delegate screening duties to a hygienist.

The PSR is completed at each recall appointment and is mainly used with patients 18 years of age and older; however, valuable information may be gained when screening younger patients. Some of the benefits of this system include early detection, timely screening, and that it can be helpful in patient education and motivation.

The periodontal screening procedure involves dividing the mouth into sextant sections (three maxillary sections and three mandibular sections). The three sections include one anterior section and left and right posterior sections. A specially designed probe, which has a rounded tip and color-coded bands that extend from 3.5 mm to 5.5 mm on the shank of the probe, is used for this assessment (Figure 31-6). All six areas on each tooth are probed, but only the highest screening score in each sextant is recorded.

The probe is used to assess the relationship of the gingival margin and the colored band.

This quick assessment determines if a comprehensive periodontal examination is needed.

For examples of the screening codes go to http://www.ADA.org.

Radiographic Interpretation

Radiographs are useful tools when evaluating the periodontium for periodontal disease. The radiographs show the teeth and the level and position of the alveolar bone. When periodontal disease is present, the alveolar bone recedes both vertically and/or horizontally. A **vertical bone resorption** is found on individual teeth on the interproximal surface (Figure 31-7A). A **horizontal bone resorption** occurs when there is equal crestal bone loss on the mesial and distal surfaces of the proximal teeth (Figure 31-7B).

Periapical x-rays supplemented with bitewing radiographs are most commonly taken, and the x-rays must be as dimensionally accurate as possible. Usually, a full-mouth series is taken for comparisons throughout the mouth. Panoramic radiographs are also taken as an adjunct.

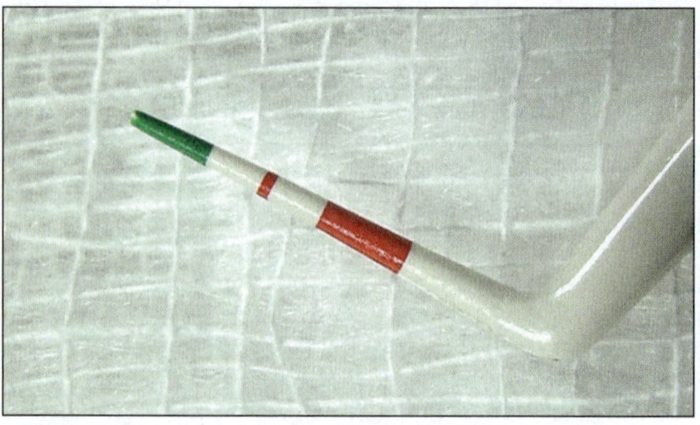

FIGURE 31-6
PSR color-coded probe.

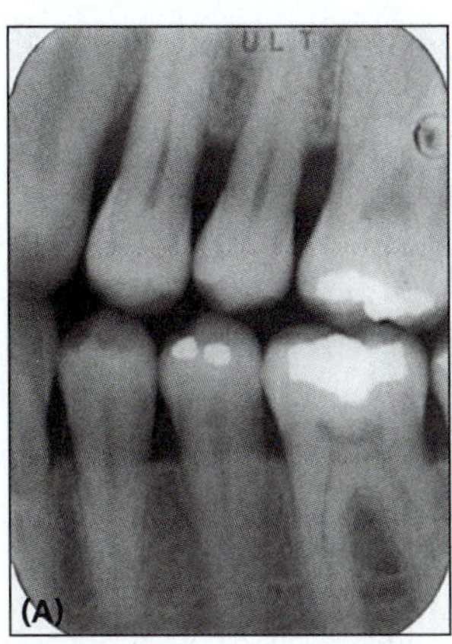

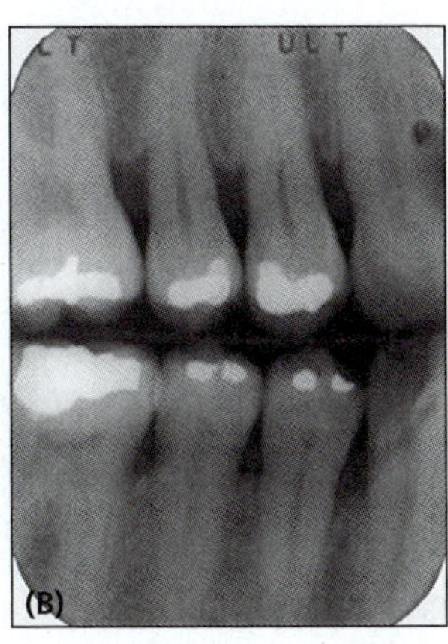

FIGURE 31-7

(A) Vertical bone loss shown on x-ray, on the mesial of the maxillary left first bicuspid (#12). (B) Horizontal bone loss shown on x-ray between the maxillary right molar, bicuspids, and cuspid (# 3, 4, 5, and 6).

Presentation of Treatment Plan

After gathering all the periodontal diagnostic information, the periodontist determines the appropriate treatment plan for the patient. The patient is scheduled for a consultation appointment. During this appointment, the prognosis (anticipated outcome) of the patient's condition and the treatment sequence are explained. Charts, radiographs, study models, and photographs are used to educate the patient. The patient's role in the treatment is discussed. The patient must be actively involved in the treatment and motivated to follow the home care plan and keep treatment appointments. Once all questions are answered and the treatment plan is understood, appointments and financial arrangements are completed.

Chemotherapeutic Agents

In the treatment of periodontal disease, the periodontist mechanically removes dental plaque and calculus from the tooth root surface. Most patients have an excellent response to this treatment but for those patients who do not respond to the removal of dental deposits, and/or for those patients who have aggressive forms of periodontitis, the periodontist may also prescribe therapeutic agents, including antibiotics and nonsteroidal anti-inflammatory agents.

Some of the antibiotics commonly prescribed are penicillin or amoxicillin, tetracycline, erythromycin, and clindamycin. These are commonly administered between 5 and 14 days prior to surgical procedures. In nonsurgical periodontal therapy, which is normally from two to four appointments, at 1- or 2-week intervals, antibiotic therapy is provided during and after the periodontal treatments.

The anti-inflammatory drugs reduce the level of inflammation and are effective adjuncts in periodontal therapy. A few examples of the drugs administered include ibuprofen and acetylsalicylic acid (aspirin).

Periodontal Instruments

Periodontal instruments are designed to probe, scrape, file, and cut the hard surfaces of the teeth, alveolar bone, and soft tissues of the gingiva. These instruments must be kept sharp. Usually, the hygienist or a specially trained assistant is responsible for maintaining periodontal hand instruments.

Instrument Sharpening

There are many benefits of using properly sharpened instruments. Sharp edges make the operator's work easier and faster, improve the quality of procedures, and enhance patient comfort. After repeated use, the cutting edges of instruments become dull and rounded, making the blades less effective and more difficult to use. At this point, the operator applies more pressure and becomes fatigued more easily. The patient may feel the added pressure and discomfort.

There are manual and mechanical methods for sharpening periodontal instruments. Mechanical devices are more expensive, but they are effective and easy to use, and provide consistent, precision sharpening. These devices usually have sharpening guides that adjust for various instruments and mechanically rotating discs (Figure 31-8). Manually sharpening instruments involves using handheld sharpening stones (Figures 31-9A and B). Sharpening stones are frequently used and are available in various shapes, sizes, and hardness (grits). Finer grits are often used to sharpen dental instruments because the finer grit (smaller particles) abrades metal slowly. There are several types of stones, including Arkansas stone, India oilstone, and ceramic stones.

Water is used with some of the stones as a lubricant; with some others, honing oil is used. Other types of oil are not used, because they may leave a residue that cannot be removed. The lubricant serves as a means for moving the metal particles of the instrument

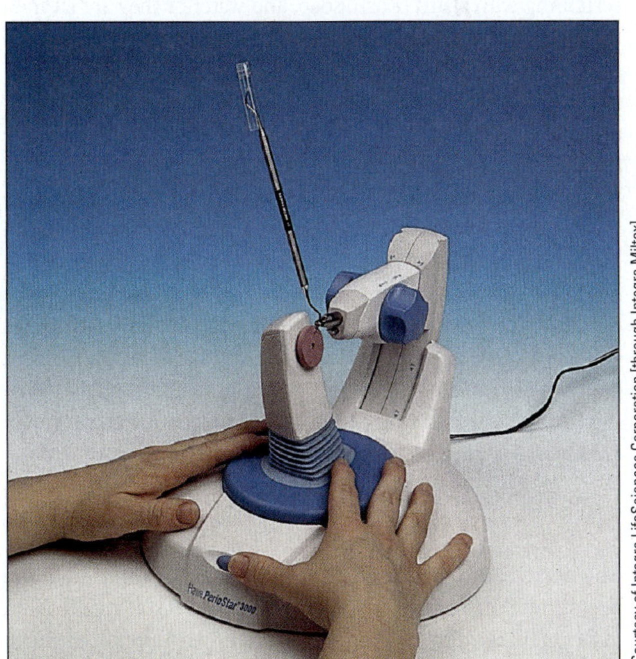

FIGURE 31-8

Mechanical sharpening device.

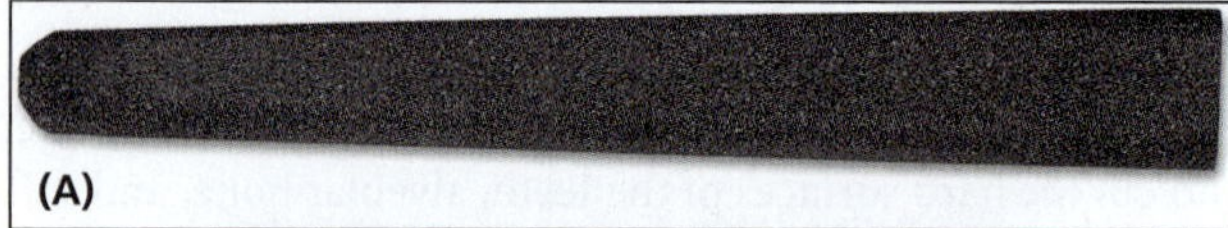

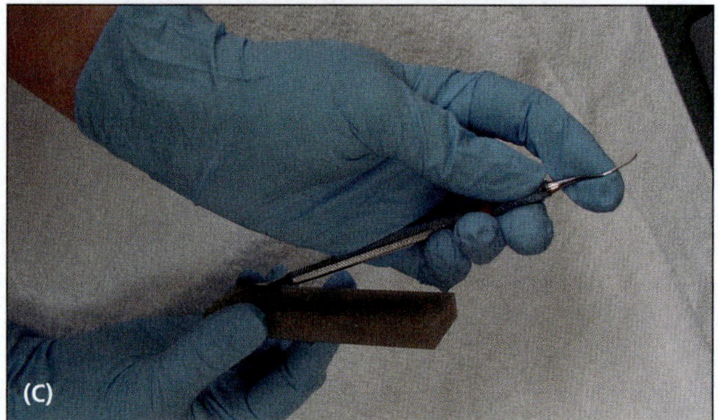

FIGURE 31-9

(A) Arkansas cylindrical dental instrument sharpening stone.
(B) Arkansas thick wedge dental instrument sharpening stone.
(C) Correct grasp and position when sharpening a dental instrument using the Arkansas stone.

away from the blade and preventing them from becoming embedded in the stone. After use, the stones are thoroughly cleaned by scrubbing with a stiff brush, soap, and water or they are cleaned ultrasonically. The stones are then sterilized properly.

There are many techniques for sharpening dental instruments; some use geometric concepts and terms while others use the "telling time" approach. The latter technique uses the face of a clock for orientation and positioning. With this method, the instrument is held stationary and the stone moves. The elbow is positioned on a stable surface with the hand upright. The end of the instrument to be sharpened is held downward in one hand, toward the wrist; the other hand holds and moves the sharpening stone against the instrument (Figure 31-9C). The positioning and technique of sharpening dental instruments requires additional information and training. It is a skill that takes time and practice, but is extremely valuable to dentists and hygienists using these instruments.

Periodontal Probes

The **periodontal probe** is the primary instrument used in the periodontal examination (Figure 31-10). This is a calibrated instrument used to measure the depth of periodontal pockets. The probe is also used to measure areas of recession, bleeding, or exudate. The calibrations on the periodontal probe are in millimeters and vary depending on the manufacturer and the

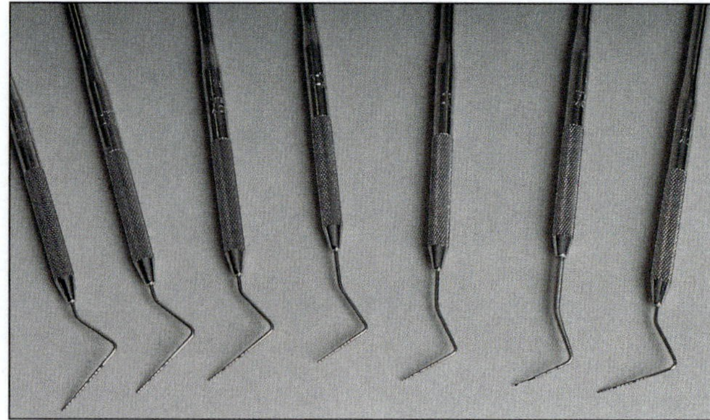

FIGURE 31-10

Varied periodontal probes.

operator's preference. These markings may be indentations or color coded for easy reading. The probe may be flat, oval, or round in cross section but must be thin enough to fit easily into the gingival sulcus.

A computerized probe system detects and stores information on pocket depth, recession, furcation involvement, and mobility. The information is shown on a computer screen and can be printed out.

Explorers

Explorers are used to detect and locate calculus, tooth irregularities, faulty margins on restorations, and furcation involvement. The explorer gives the operator the best tactile information for assessment.

The explorers used in periodontics are supplied in a variety of shapes, similar to those also used in general dental procedures. The working ends are thin and sharp. They may be curved or at near right angles to adapt to the curves of the tooth surfaces.

Curettes

The **curette** is a hand instrument used for removing subgingival calculus, smoothing the root surface, and removing the soft tissue lining of the periodontal pocket. The working end has a cutting edge on one or both sides of the blade and the end is rounded, not pointed like the scaler (Figure 31-11). The curette is an instrument that is designed to adapt to the curves of the root surfaces. There are two basic curettes: **universal curettes**,

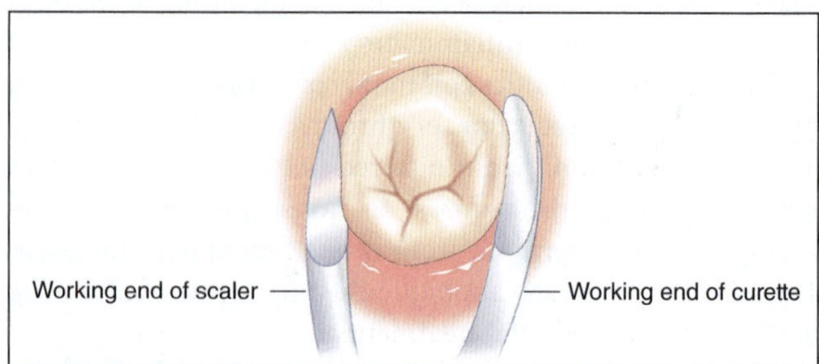

FIGURE 31-11

The working ends of a scaler and a curette showing how they are positioned on a tooth.

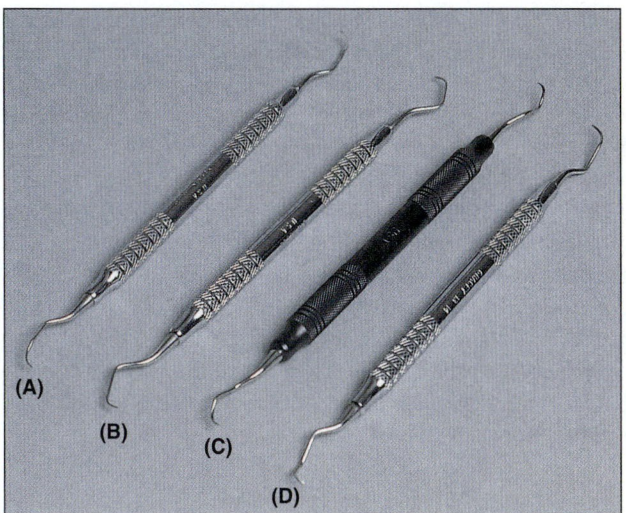

FIGURE 31-12

Gracey periodontal curettes. (A) No. 5-6. (B) No. 7-8. (C) No. 9-10. (D)No. 13-14.

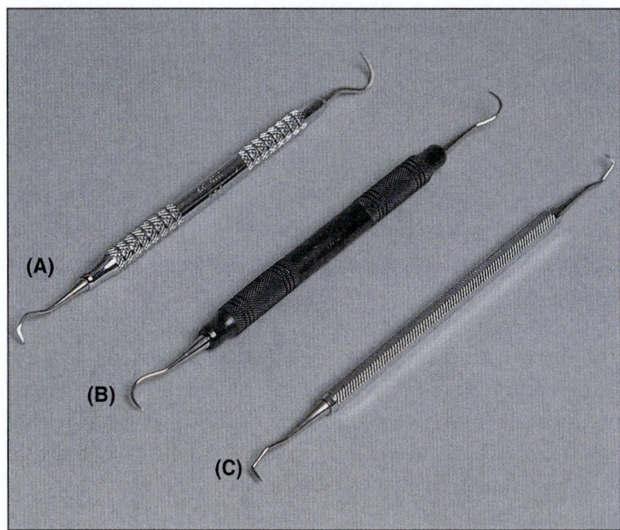

FIGURE 31-13

Types of periodontal scalers. (A) Combination instrument with a sickle scaler on one end and a Jacquette scaler on the other. (B) Sickle scaler. (C) Jacquette scaler.

which are used throughout the mouth, and **Gracey curettes**, which are supplied in a set of several instruments that are designed and angled to be used in specific areas (Figure 31-12). The curette handles are similar to those on the scalers.

Scalers

A **scaler** is a sharp hand instrument that is used to remove hard deposits such as **supragingival** (above the gingiva) and **subgingival** (below the gingiva) calculus from the teeth. Scalers are supplied in a variety of shapes and angulations to access all surfaces of the teeth. The working end of a scaler has two sharp edges that come to a point (Figure 31-11). The handles are often large and are ribbed, serrated, or knurled. Sometimes, the metal handles are covered with color-coded rubber grips to prevent muscle fatigue and for better control of the instrument.

Sickle Scalers. Sickle scalers are designed to remove supragingival calculus. The sickle scaler is also called the Shepherd's hook. These scalers have two cutting edges along the margins of the curved blade (Figures 31-13A and B).

Jacquette Scalers. Jacquette scalers, like sickle scalers, are designed to remove supragingival deposits. They have straight blades with cutting edges on both the sides. The Jacquette scaler has three angles in the shank of the instrument (Figures 31-13A and C).

Chisel Scalers. A **chisel scaler** is used most often in the anterior of the mouth. The blade of the chisel is slightly curved and the cutting edge is beveled (Figure 31-14A).

Hoe Scalers. The **hoe scaler** has a blade bent at a 90-degree-angle at the end of the working end. This cutting edge is beveled and sharp. The hoe scaler is placed in the periodontal pocket to the base and then pulled toward the crown of the

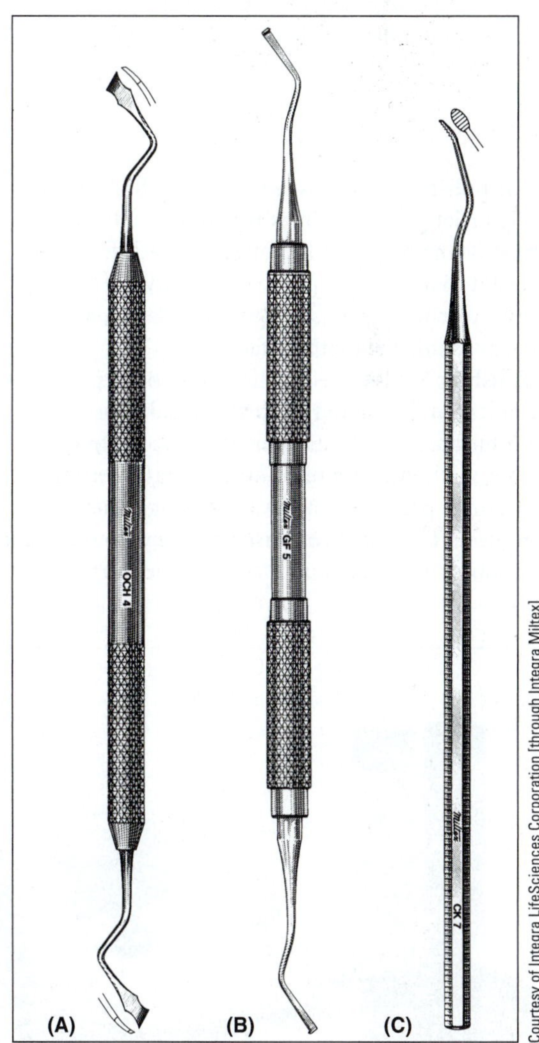

Courtesy of Integra LifeSciences Corporation [through Integra Miltex]

FIGURE 31-14

Periodontal (A) chisel, (B) hoe, and (C) file.

tooth with even pressure to plane and smooth the root surface (Figure 31-14B).

Files

Periodontal files are supplied in a variety of blade shapes and shank angulations (Figure 31-14C). They are used in a pulling motion interproximally to remove calculus and for root planing. Files are also used to remove overhanging margins of dental restorations.

Ultrasonic Instruments. The **ultrasonic instruments** are used to remove hard deposits, stains, and debris during scaling, curettage, and root-planing procedures. Typically, they are used as an adjunct to manual scaling procedures. Ultrasonic units generate high-power vibrations to a handpiece with a variety of tips. These vibrations cause the calculus to fracture and be dislodged. Because ultrasonic vibrations cause heat, the units have cooling systems that circulate water through the handpieces and out openings near the tips (Figure 31-15B). The water spray cools and also flushes the area. It is beneficial for a dental assistant to be present to evacuate the volume of water and debris. Although the ultrasonic units are effective and fast, care must be taken to prevent injury to the tissues and the teeth.

Air Polishing Systems

An **air polishing system** is sometimes called air-powder polishing or jet polishing. This is another method used by the dentist or the hygienist to polish the teeth following scaling and root planing. The primary objective of polishing is to remove extrinsic stain, supragingival plaque, and soft debris while polishing the tooth surface.

Polishing is also used to clean the tooth prior to sealant placement and bonding procedures and is used on exposed tooth surfaces of patients in orthodontic treatment.

This method uses a fine powder abrasive, air that is delivered under pressure, and water through the nozzle of the handpiece. The abrasive is usually finely powdered sodium bicarbonate or nonsodium powder as the slurry.

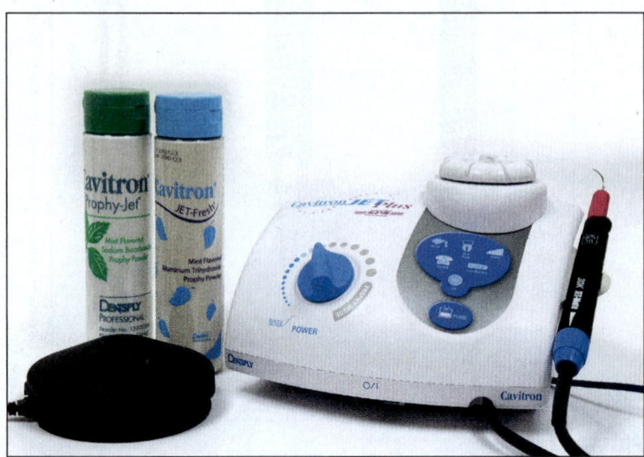

FIGURE 31-15
Ultrasonic Unit.

The removal of plaque and extrinsic stain is accomplished in a reasonable amount of time and there is minimal loss of tooth structure when the air polishing system is used as directed by the manufacturer. This system is used to polish both the crown and the root surface.

Some disadvantages of the air polishing systems include: significant aerosol spray; may cause mild stinging in other areas of the mouth due to the deflected spray; contraindicated for patients with respiratory illness; and they are not used on composite restorations, demineralized enamel, or on the margins of porcelain or cast restorations.

When using the air-powder polisher, the handpiece tip is held 4–5 mm away from the tooth surface and is kept in constant motion.

Periodontal Knives

A **periodontal knife** or gingivectomy knife is used to remove gingival tissue during periodontal surgery. The knives most commonly used are the broad-bladed Kirkland knives (Figure 31-16A). These knives are kidney shaped and sharp around the entire periphery of the blade. They are supplied as either single- or double-ended instruments.

Interdental Knives

A periodontal knife that is used to remove soft tissue interproximally is called an **interdental knife**. The Orban No. 1 and 2 are very popular interdental knives. These spear-shaped knives have long, narrow blades with cutting edges on both sides of the blade (Figure 31-16).

Periotomes

A **periotome** is a fairly new instrument that is used to sever the periodontal ligament (PDL) prior to a traumatic extraction as well as to prepare the tissue for dental implants.

These instruments are available in a variety of shapes, including narrow, angled, and wide. Some are designed for use on anterior teeth and others for posterior teeth. Periotome blades are thin, flexible, and sharp enough to cause minimal damage to periodontal ligaments. Periotomes may be single ended or double ended, and are made of stainless steel (Figure 31-17).

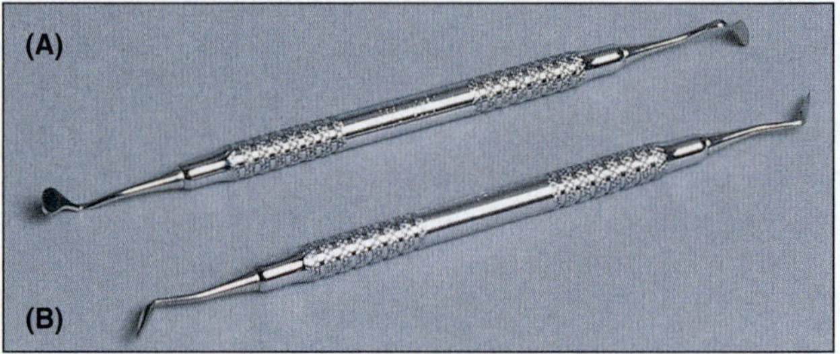

FIGURE 31-16
Gingivectomy knives. (A) Kirkland broad-blade knife. (B) Orban interdental knife.

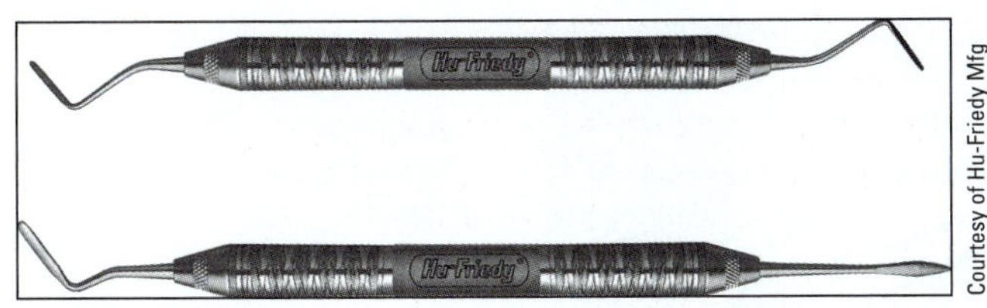
Courtesy of Hu-Friedy Mfg

FIGURE 31-17
Periotomes.

Surgical Scalpel

A **surgical scalpel** is used for periodontal surgical procedures to remove gingival tissue. The surgical scalpel is also known as the Bard-Parker scalpel. The scalpel has two components: a sterilizable metal or plastic handle and a disposable blade. The blades come in different shapes and sizes. Disposable scalpels are also available (Figure 31-18).

Electrosurgery

An **electrosurgery** cauterizes the tissues during many periodontal surgeries. The electrosurgery unit uses tiny electrical currents to remove or contour soft tissues and lesions and also coagulates (provides hemostasis) the blood during the procedure (Figure 31-19). The electrosurgery unit consists of a control box, foot-operated on-off controls, a terminal plate that is placed behind the patient's back or shoulders, and another terminal that is a probe with various cutting tips that the dentist uses for the surgery. There is also a cordless electrosurgical cauterizer that is DC battery powered which eliminates the need to ground the patient, this unit will run for 35 to 40 minutes before the batteries need to be changed. The dental assistant must keep the oral evacuator near the surgical site to remove the debris and odors.

Pocket Marking Pliers

The **pocket marking plier** is used to transfer the measurement of the pocket to the outside of the tissue so that the operator can see the depth level of the pocket. The pocket marking pliers have one straight, thin beak placed in the pocket, and another bent at a right angle at the tip. When the beaks are pinched together, the gingival tissue is perforated, leaving small, pinpoint markings (Figure 31-20).

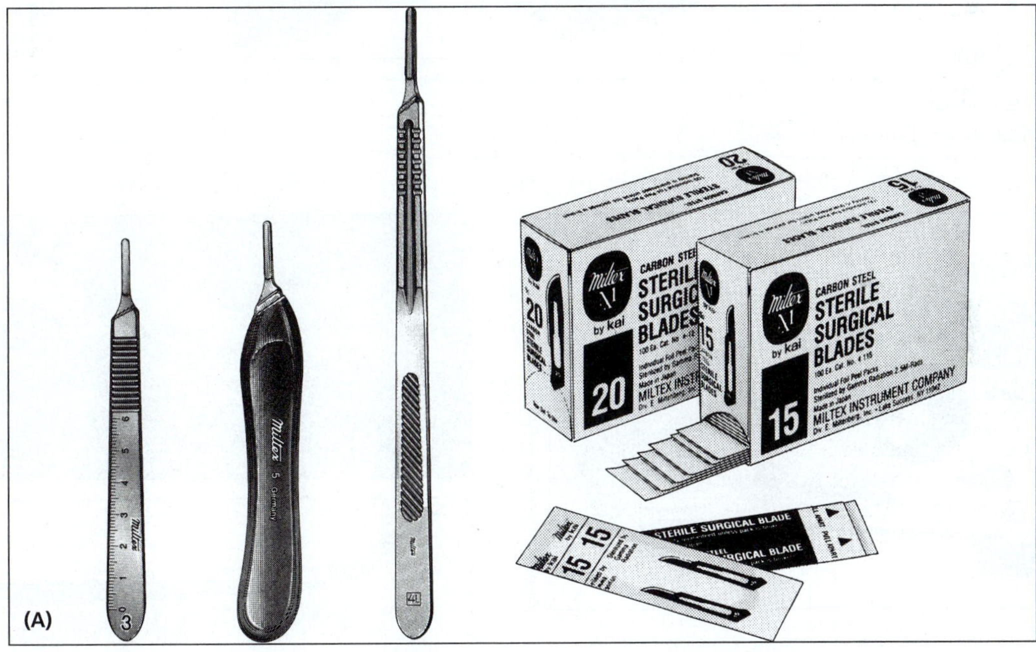

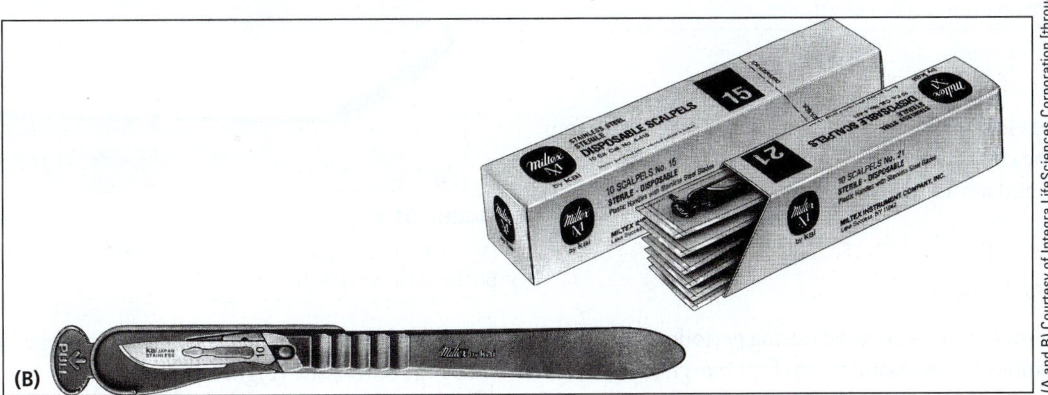

(A and B) Courtesy of Integra LifeSciences Corporation [through Integra Miltex]

FIGURE 31-18
(A) Surgical knife, Bard-parker, and blades. (B) Disposable scalpels.

(continued)

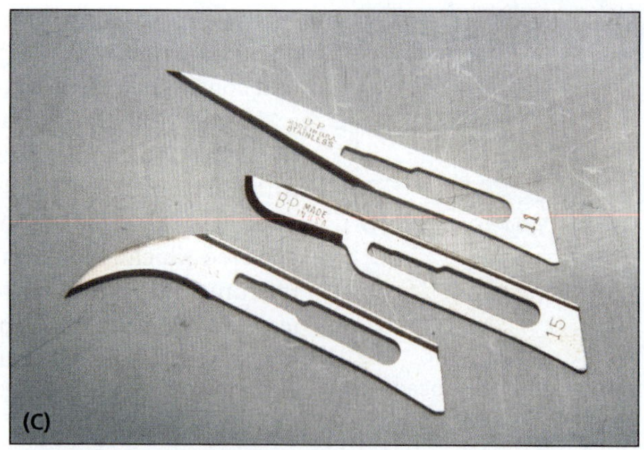
11
15

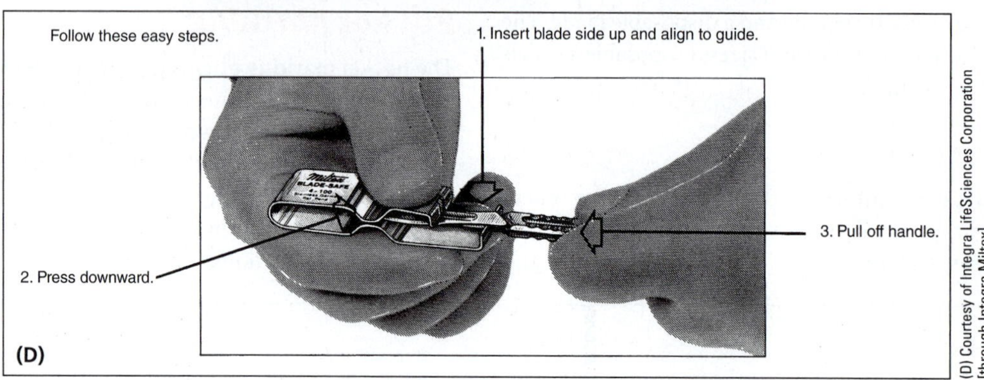
Follow these easy steps.
1. Insert blade side up and align to guide.
2. Press downward.
3. Pull off handle.

(D) Courtesy of Integra LifeSciences Corporation [through Integra Miltex]

FIGURE 31-18 (continued)
(C) Various surgical blades. (D) Blade remover.

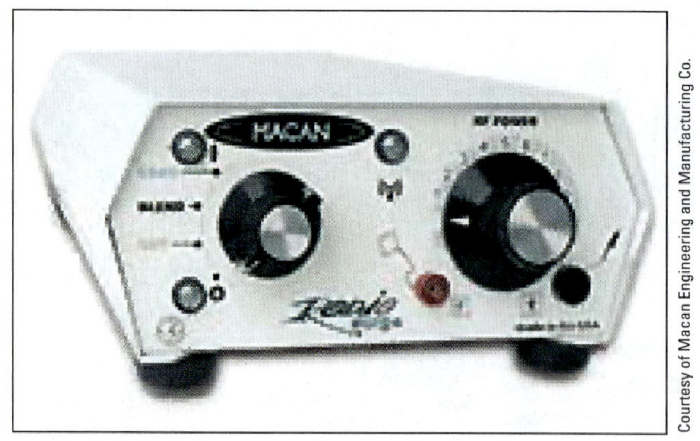
MACAN

Courtesy of Macan Engineering and Manufacturing Co.

FIGURE 31-19
Electrosurgical unit with various electrodes.

Periosteal Elevators

A **periosteal elevator** is used to reflect soft tissue away from the bone. The elevators are usually double ended, with a long, tapered end and a round, bladed end (Figure 31-21).

Periodontal Scissors, Rongeurs, and Forceps

The **periodontal scissors** are used during periodontal surgery, mainly to remove tags of tissue and to trim margins. There are other uses and many varieties, but most often the blades are long and very thin.

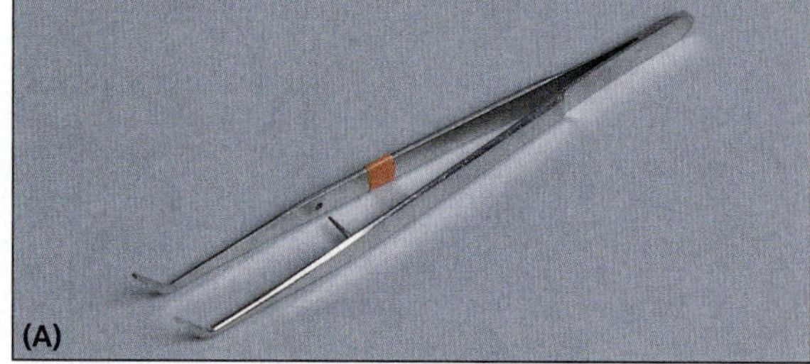

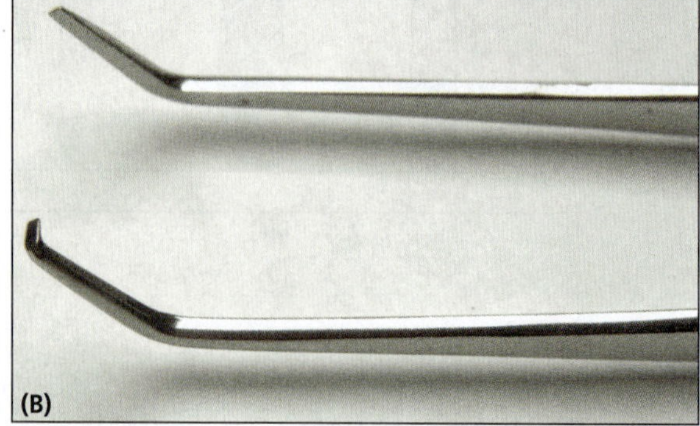

FIGURE 31-20
(A) Pocket marking pliers. (B) Close-up of the working ends of the pocket marking pliers.

A **soft tissue rongeur** or nipper is a hinged plier used to shape the soft tissue (Figure 31-22A).

Tissue forceps are used to retract tissue or to hold the tissue in place. They are designed similar to hemostats, except

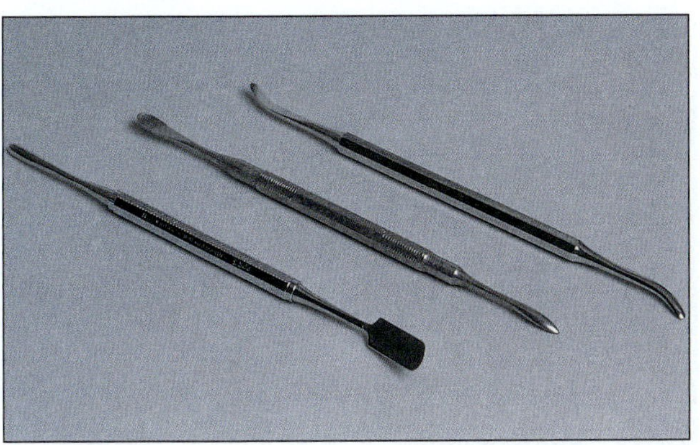

FIGURE 31-21
Various periosteal elevators.

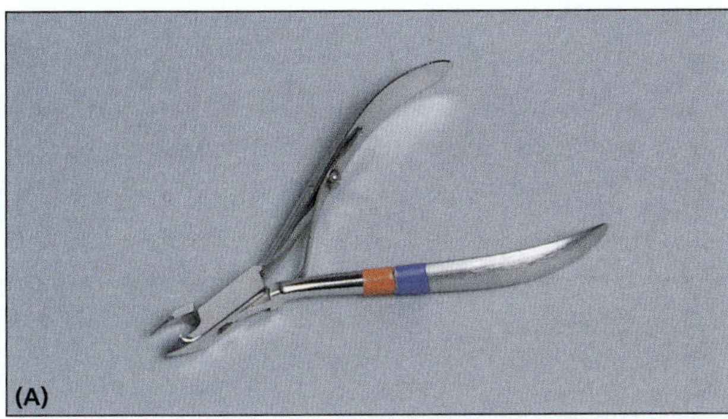

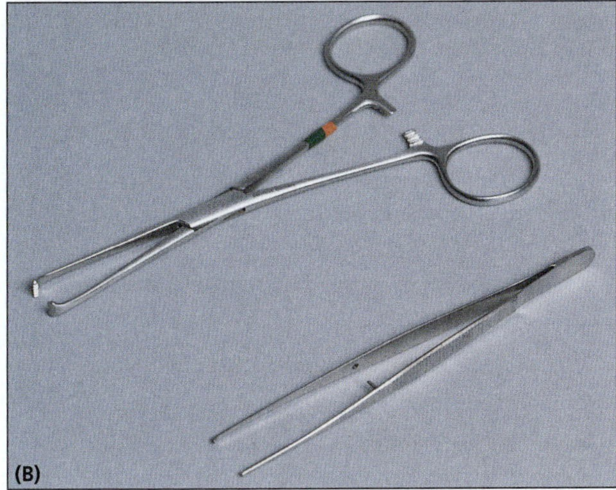

FIGURE 31-22
(A) Soft tissue rongeurs. (B) Tissue forceps.

that the beaks are curved near the end at right angles to each other (Figure 31-22B).

Lasers

A dental **laser** is a medical device that generates a precise beam of concentrated light energy. "Laser" is an acronym for **L**ight **A**ctivated by **S**timulated **E**mission of **R**adiation. The efficiency of the laser is based on the peak absorption rates of unique laser wavelengths by hard/soft tissues and other dental materials (e.g., composites or whitening solutions). There are many types of dental laser wavelengths to meet the needs of the dentist. Some standard dental laser wavelengths include the Erbium (Er:YAG), the Nd:YAG, the argon, CO_2, and the diode laser wavelengths. There is also a water-using device called the YSGG hydrokinetic system, which has very similar uses and benefits.

The dentist must complete training to become qualified to use lasers. There are many courses available, and the companies that sell dental lasers offer comprehensive training and support packages. When the dental laser is used in the office, there is training for dental assistants and hygienists as well. For more information, visit the Institute for Laser Dentistry (ILD) Web site at http://www.laserdentistry.ca.

Who Regulates Lasers in Dentistry

The Food and Drug Administration (FDA) regulates lasers as medical devices. They control the following:

- Engineering controls such as on/off key or password
- Emergency stop button
- Foot control cover guard
- Safety interlock on paneling and housing
- Software diagnostics
- Five-second delay in standby mode
- System time out
- Visible and auditory sounds when laser is being used

The American National Standards Institute (ANSI) also provides recommendations when using dental lasers. The office should have a person designated as the laser safety officer. This person would be responsible for making sure all engineering controls (these are listed under the FDA requirements) are in place. The safety officer determines the hazard zone for each laser and places a "Danger Laser Operating" sign outside the treatment area when the laser is being used (Figure 31-23). The ANSI also suggests the importance of reviewing and following the manufacturer's instructions for each laser used in the office. The safety officer selects and makes sure appropriate protective eyewear is available. They

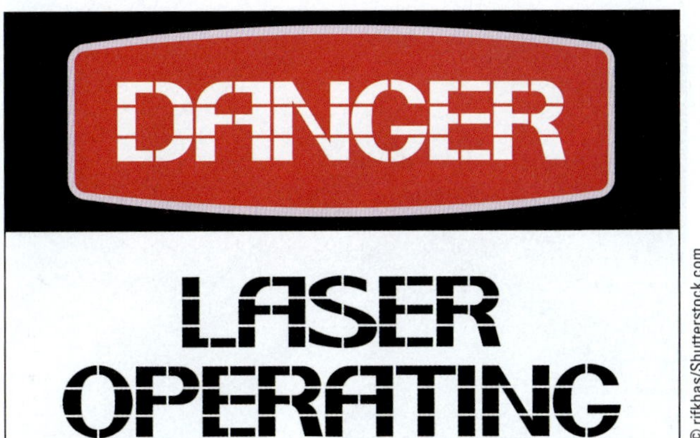

FIGURE 31-23
Warning signs must be posted in areas where lasers are being used to prevent injury to the eyes of others who may come into the area and are not wearing the filtered eyewear.

should check with the manufacturer to find the kind of specially filtered eyewear that is needed with the brand/type of laser in use.

Uses of the Dental Laser

Dental laser uses include procedures on hard and soft tissues. In periodontal practice, laser uses include the following:

- Sulcular debridement and laser curettage
- Gingivectomy, gingivoplasty, and frenectomy
- Fibroma and other tumor and lesion removal
- Excisional new attachment procedure (ENAP)
- Implant exposure
- Treatment for aphthous ulcers
- Tissue fusion, which eliminates the need for sutures
- Eliminates granulation tissue
- Biopsy
- Crown lengthening
- Control of bleeding
- Osseous procedures

Other uses of the dental laser include tissue retraction for crown impressions, some cavity preparation and caries removal, transillumination for detection of caries microfracture, laser etching, composite curing, endodontic therapy, pulpotomy treatment, and in-office whitening (bleaching) (Figure 31-24).

Safety When Using Lasers

The primary required safety measure is protective eyewear to be worn by the dentist, staff, and patient when the laser is being used (Figure 31-25). When using high-powered lasers such as diodes, Nd:YAG, or erbium special filtered protective eyewear must be worn. Also the tissues surrounding the area being worked on should be covered or shielded during the procedure with wet gauze. The dental assistant should use high-volume evacuation to draw the "cloud or plume" once the tissue is vaporized as well as other debris. Instruments that may be used when using the laser are matte coated to prevent any laser reflection during a procedure.

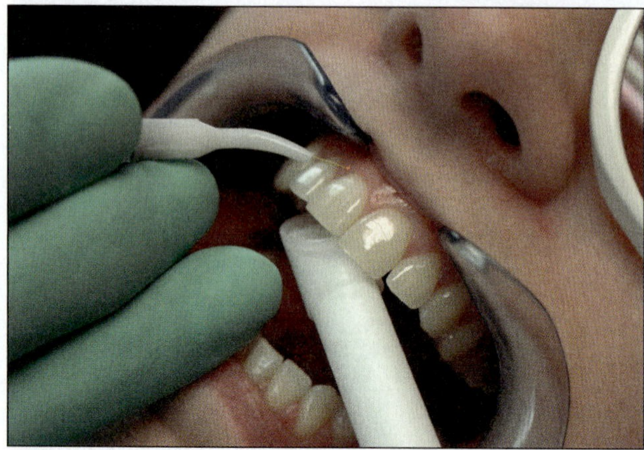

FIGURE 31-24
Dental laser in use.

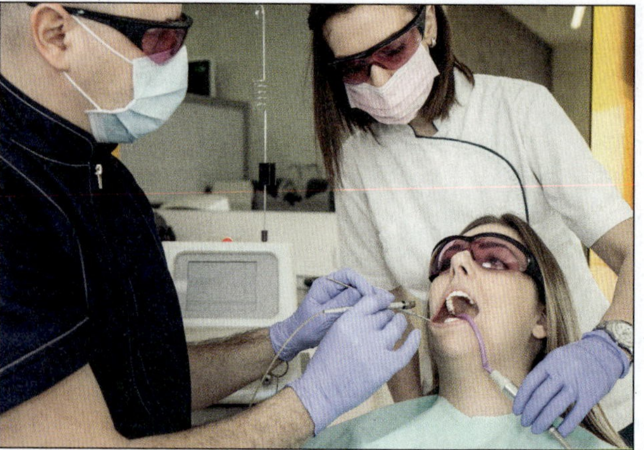

FIGURE 31-25
Dental laser safety: dentist, assistant, and patient wearing safety glasses.

The protective eyewear is expensive and care should be given when cleaning. Use soap and water and dry with a scratch-free soft cloth. This will prevent the removal of the protective film on the lens. If the lens is scratched they cannot be worn when using the laser equipment.

Benefits of Lasers in Dentistry

Laser technology is rapidly advancing as applications expand and awareness of benefits increases. Following are some of the benefits of this technology:

- A near-bloodless operating field so that vision is improved
- Minimal or no anesthesia
- Minimizes postoperative swelling and discomfort
- Enhances coagulation (hemostasis)
- Minimizes healing time
- Reduces damage to surrounding healthy tissues
- Reduces chance of infection, because areas are sterilized by the laser during procedure
- Surgical treatment sites often do not require stitches
- Increases accuracy of cutting
- Reduces chair time
- Less fear and anxiety for the patient

Nonsurgical Periodontal Procedures

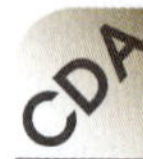

Nonsurgical treatments for periodontal diseases include occlusal adjustment, scaling and polishing, root planning, and gingival curettage.

Principles of Periodontal Procedures

For periodontal treatment that is effective and efficient with minimal discomfort to the patient or stress to the operator, the following principles are followed:

- Comfortable position for the operator and the patient
- Effective pain control for the patient
- Use of a dental assistant to maintain the operating field for clear vision, good illumination, and retraction
- Maintain instruments properly (sharp and in order for use during the procedure)
- Correct instrument grasp, fulcrum, and instrument adaptation

Occlusal Adjustment

The occlusal adjustment or equilibration procedure involves adjustment of the occlusal surface to eliminate detrimental forces and to provide functional forces for stimulation of a healthy periodontium. The adjustment procedure is performed quadrant by quadrant and may require several appointments to fully equilibrate the patient's whole mouth (Procedure 31-1).

Scaling and Polishing

The purpose of **scaling** is to remove plaque, calculus, and stains from the surfaces of the teeth. The deposits above the gingival margin, supragingival deposits, and those

Procedure 31-1
Occlusal Adjustment

The procedure is performed by the periodontist. It involves marking the patient's bite and adjusting the occlusal surfaces of the teeth. The dental assistant prepares the articulating paper or wax; maintains the operating field; and changes burs, discs, and stones in the handpiece.

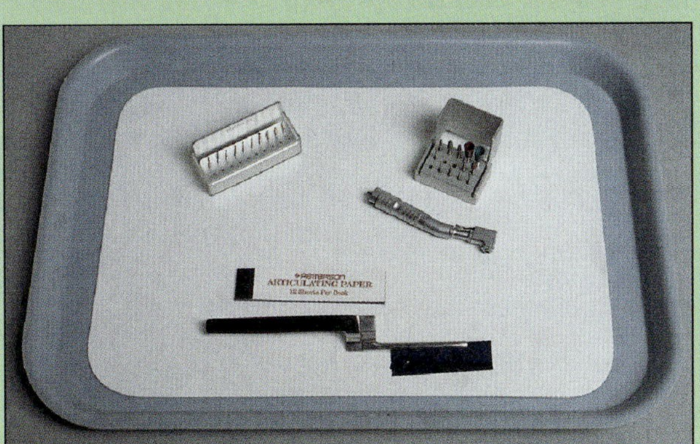

FIGURE 31-26
Occlusal equilibration armamentarium.

Equipment and Supplies (*Figure 31-26*)

- Basic setup: mouth mirror, explorer, and cotton pliers
- Cotton rolls and 2 × 2 inch gauze sponges
- Saliva ejector, HVE tip, air–water syringe tip
- Articulation forceps and articulating paper and/or occlusal wax
- Low-speed handpiece
- Diamond burs, various discs, and stones
- Polishing wheels and discs

Procedure Steps (*Follow aseptic procedures*)

1. Seat and prepare the patient for the occlusal adjustment procedure.
2. Prepare the articulating forceps with paper, or prepare to transfer the wax. Dry the quadrant with the air syringe or a gauze sponge.
3. The periodontist places the articulating paper over the occlusal surfaces and instructs the patient to bite down and grind the teeth side to side.
4. The articulating paper is removed, and the colored marks left by the paper are evaluated. The markings indicate how teeth in the maxillary and mandibular arches occlude.
5. Change burs, discs, and stones as requested by the periodontist. Transfer the handpiece to the periodontist, and use the air–water syringe and the evacuator to keep the area clean and clear during the adjustment procedure.
6. This process is repeated until the teeth occlude evenly over the quadrant.
7. Each quadrant is evaluated and adjusted.

just below the gingival margin are removed with scalers and curettes. After this, the coronal surfaces of the teeth are polished with rubber cups, brushes, an abrasive, and dental tape and floss (Procedure 31-2). This procedure is called a **prophylaxis** and can be performed by the dentist or the dental hygienist. Depending on the state Dental Practice Act, dental assistants can remove supragingival deposits and/or perform the **coronal polish** (discussed in Chapter 32).

In a routine prophylaxis, deposits from above and just slightly below the gingival margins are removed. In a periodontal scaling, the subgingival deposits are more extensive and involve removal of irritants from deep pockets and smoothing of the root surface (Figure 31-28).

Procedure 31-2
Scaling, Curettage, and Polishing

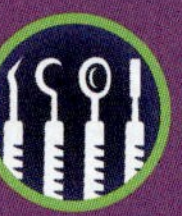

This procedure is done by the periodontist or the dental hygienist. A dental hygiene assistant assists during this procedure. Responsibilities include instrument transfer, rinsing the oral cavity, evacuation with the HVE, removing debris from instruments, retraction, and maintaining patient comfort.

Equipment and Supplies (*Figure 31-27*)

- Basic setup: mouth mirror, explorer, and cotton pliers
- Saliva ejector, HVE tip, and air–water syringe tip
- Cotton rolls and gauze sponges
- Periodontal probe
- Scalers: Jacquette and Shepherd's hook
- Curettes: Universal and Gracey
- Dental floss and dental tape
- Prophy angle—rubber cups and brushes
- Prophy paste
- Optional—disclosing solution or tablets

Procedure Steps (*Follow aseptic procedures*)

1. The operator examines the oral cavity.
2. The operator uses scalers and curettes to remove calculus and debris from around the teeth. Often, the operator cleans all surfaces of the teeth in one quadrant before moving to the next quadrant.
3. After all the calculus has been removed, the operator polishes the teeth with prophy paste, rubber cup, and brush.

NOTE: Some practices use a prophy jet (spray saltwater) as an alternative to the rubber cup polish (discussed later in this chapter).

4. The operator uses dental tape and prophy paste to clean the interproximal areas. Then the entire mouth is flossed and rinsed.

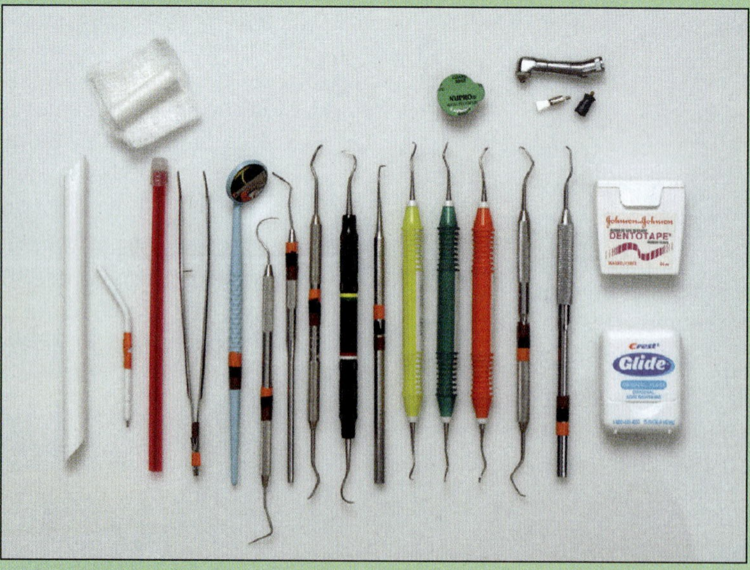

FIGURE 31-27
Scale and polish (prophylaxis) tray setup.

Root Planing

After the plaque and calculus are removed from the periodontal pocket and the root surface, the cementum is often rough and irregular. This provides a surface ideal for accumulation of plaque and calculus formation. The roughness is removed by **root planing**. This is a process of planing or shaving the root surface with curettes and other periodontal instruments to leave a smooth root surface. For the patient's comfort, anesthetic is sometimes given during this procedure.

Gingival Curettage

Gingival curettage, also known as soft tissue curettage, is a procedure that involves scraping the inner gingival walls of the periodontal pockets to remove inflamed tissue and debris. This is accomplished with curettes, and ideally performed after the scaling and root planing of the tooth. By removing diseased tissue and irritants, the edema is reduced and the gingival tissue may begin to heal itself.

Postoperative Treatment

Upon completion of this level of treatment the dental assistant, following the dentist's directions, will give the patient postoperative instructions including the following:

- **Pain control.** The periodontist will often prescribe a pain medication (analgesic) for the patient. Depending on the extent of the procedure and the tissues involved, the patient may need something to relieve any discomfort.
- **Oral hygiene.** The patient is taught good brushing and flossing techniques. Periodontal aids such as interproximal brushes, soft wooden tips, and/or bridge threaders are selected to assist the patient in cleaning large interdental spaces or around fixed appliances. Videos, pamphlets, and various other aids are used to motivate and educate the patient.
- **Antibacterial therapy.** Antimicrobial mouth rinses and antibiotic regimens are used in addition to routine treatments. Fluorides are also prescribed because they have bactericidal effects against the formation of plaque.

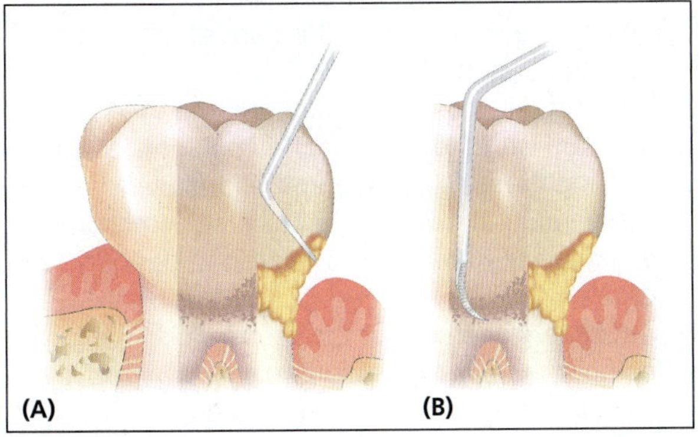

FIGURE 31-28
Placement of instruments for scaling. (A) Supragingival scaling. (B) Subgingival scaling.

- **Diet and smoking.** Patients should be advised to avoid spicy foods, citrus fruits, and alcoholic beverages and to otherwise follow a normal diet. Smoking should be stopped, because the smoke irritates the tissues and delays the healing process.

Surgical Periodontal Procedures

The accepted rationale for periodontal surgery has been to arrest the disease process, reduce the periodontium to a level that is easier for the patient to keep clean, and perform effective scaling and root-planing procedures.

Preoperative Instructions

Before the procedure the dental assistant, following the dentists instructions, should complete the following:

- Confirm that the patient understands what procedure he or she is there for that day
- Explain the procedure and answer any questions
- Confirm the patient has prepared as instructed—instructions will vary depending on the type of anesthetic the patient is receiving
- Provide instructions if the patient is to receive IV sedation

Gingivectomy

A **gingivectomy** is the surgical removal of diseased gingival tissue that forms the periodontal pocket. The pocket must be eliminated to prevent the accumulation of debris and bacteria. This surgical procedure reduces the height of the gingival tissue, which provides visibility and access in order to remove irritants and smooth the root surface. This promotes the healing process and makes it easier for the patient to access the area during cleaning.

The gingivectomy procedure involves marking the pocket depths with pocket marking pliers and then excising the gingival tissue with periodontal knives, a scalpel, surgical scissors, or electrosurgery. After the tissue is excised, calculus and necrotic root tissue are removed and smoothed with scalers and curettes. The area is rinsed gently and covered with a gauze sponge until the hemorrhage is controlled. Once the blood clots have formed, a periodontal dressing is placed to promote healing, reduce the chance of infection, and prevent disturbance to the area (Procedure 31-3).

Gingivoplasty

A **gingivoplasty** is reshaping the gingival tissue to remove deformities such as clefts, craters, and enlargements. A gingivoplasty does not involve the removal of periodontal pockets; it is completed to recontour the gingiva and often immediately follows a gingivectomy. A gingivoplasty is performed with periodontal knives, a scalpel, rongeurs, rotary diamonds, curettes, and surgical scissors. The gingival margin is tapered and thinned, creating a scalloped edge. Interdental grooves are contoured.

Procedure 31-3
Gingivectomy

This procedure is performed by the periodontist in order to remove diseased gingiva and clean the periodontal pockets. The dental assistant prepares the instruments and materials, prepares the patient, and performs assisting responsibilities during the procedure. Depending on the state Dental Practice Act, the dental assistant may place and remove the periodontal dressing.

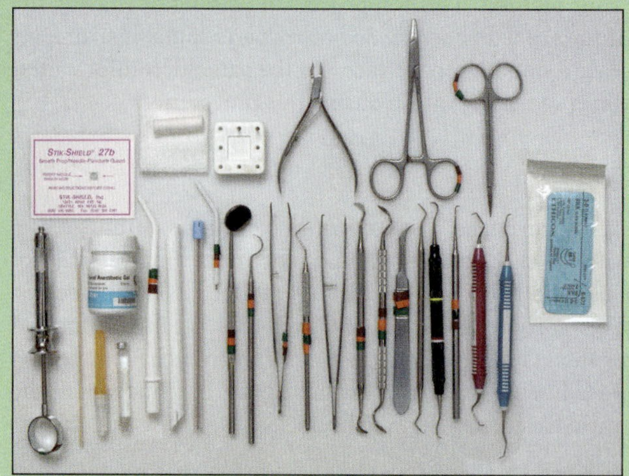

FIGURE 31-29
Gingivectomy tray setup.

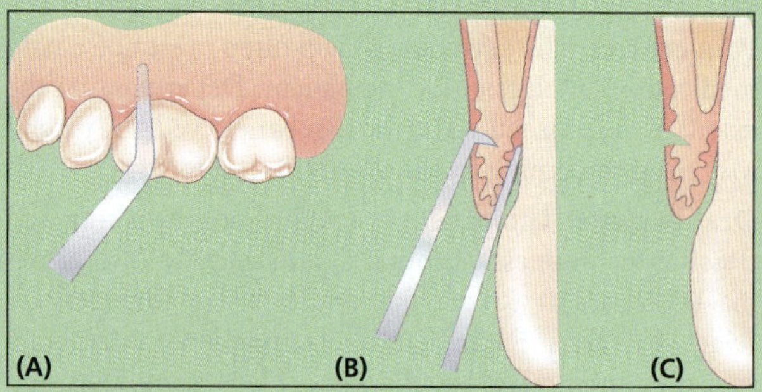

FIGURE 31-30
Gingivectomy procedure. (A, B) Marking pocket depth with pocket marker. (C) Incising marked tissues with periodontal knives.

Equipment and Supplies (*Figure 31-29*)

- Basic setup: mouth mirror, explorer, cotton pliers
- Periodontal probe
- Cotton rolls and gauze sponges
- Saliva ejector, HVE tip, air-water syringe tip, and surgical aspirator tip
- Anesthetic setup
- Pocket marker
- Periodontal knives—broad bladed and interproximal
- Scalpel, blades, and diamond burs
- Scalers and curettes
- Soft tissue rongeurs and surgical scissors
- Hemostat
- Suture needle and thread
- Periodontal dressing materials

Procedure Steps (*Follow aseptic procedures*)

1. The anesthetic is administered to anesthetize the tissues and reduce blood flow to the area.
2. The periodontist examines the patient's periodontal chart, and then the area is examined with a periodontal probe.
3. The depths of the pockets are marked with pocket markers (Figures 31-30A and B).
4. The broad-bladed knife or scalpel is used to incise the marked gingiva. Evacuate the area and transfer instruments (Figure 31-30C).
5. Interdental knives are used to remove interproximal tissue. Scissors, rongeurs, and burs are used to remove tissue tags. Have gauze ready to receive any tissue from instruments and to clean the area of debris.
6. After the tissue is removed, the periodontist scales and planes the root surfaces. Irritants are removed and the surfaces are smoothed to promote healing. Continue to pass instruments and evacuate the area. A sterile saline solution may be used to irrigate the area.
7. If sutures are needed, they are placed at this time. Prepare the suture needle and thread and have them positioned in a hemostat or needle holder, ready to pass to the dentist. Retract tissue as needed.
8. After the sutures are placed and the area is irrigated with the sterile saline solution, a periodontal dressing is prepared and placed. Assist the periodontist with the suture placement, evacuate the area, and prepare the periodontal dressing.
9. After the placement of the dressing is completed, the patient is given postoperative instructions and dismissed. Make sure the patient does not have any debris on his or her face.

Postoperative Treatment Following Surgery

Upon completion of a surgical procedure the dental assistant, following the dentists directions, will give the patient postoperative instructions. These instructions are given to the patient (and also to the support person) both verbally and in written form to take home with them. The instructions include office phone numbers in case the patient has questions or problems with the surgery, and also include the following information:

- **Medications and pain management.** The patient can expect mild to moderate discomfort after surgery. Analgesic tablets (i.e., Tylenol, Motrin, or nonaspirin analgesics) can be taken as needed or as directed by the periodontist. Prescription medications should be taken for 2 to 3 days after surgery or as directed. Antibiotics may also be prescribed; the patient should carefully follow the instructions and take the antibiotics as directed until they are completely gone.
- **Activity.** The patient should limit their activity for 24 hours following surgery because increased activity can lead to increased bleeding.
- **Smoking.** The patient should not smoke or chew tobacco for 12 to 72 hours depending on the surgery and the periodontist instructions. Tobacco interferes with and slows the healing process.
- **Oral hygiene.** Normal brushing and flossing should be completed by the patient in areas not involved in the surgery. Brush only the biting surfaces of the teeth involved in surgery. Gently rinse the mouth with warm salt water after 24 hours.
- **Diet.** The patient should avoid hot, spicy foods and citrus foods; eat soft foods; and chew on the healthy side of the mouth so that the periodontal dressing is not disturbed.
- **Swelling and bleeding.** Some swelling may occur. The patient should place an ice pack over the area for 10 minutes and then remove for 10 minutes, repeating as needed. Some seepage and bleeding may occur and is normal; however, if it persists, the patient should call the dentist.

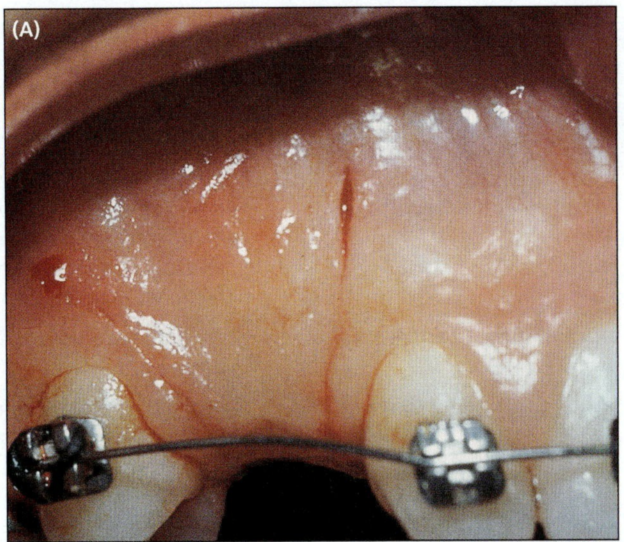

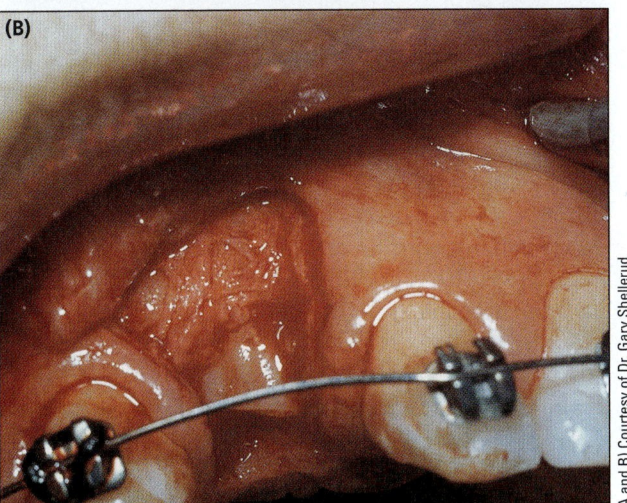

(A and B) Courtesy of Dr. Gary Shellerud

FIGURE 31-31

Flap surgery to expose an impacted tooth. (A) Making incision. (B) Retracting tissue.

Periodontal Flap Surgery

A **periodontal flap surgery** involves surgically separating the gingiva from the underlying tissue. The gingiva is incised with a scalpel and then separated with a periosteal elevator. Once the tissue is retracted, the periodontist has good visibility and access to bone, tooth, and the tooth roots (Figures 31-31 and 31-32).

The design of the flap depends on the objectives of the surgery and the periodontist. The amount of exposure necessary for the surgery and the repositioning of the flap are important considerations. The periodontist exposes an area large enough to remove the irritants completely with the periodontal instruments. The appearance of the gingiva after the surgery depends on the proper repositioning of the flap. The tissue is positioned to heal in a manner that leaves as little evidence of the surgery as possible.

When the flap is retracted, the diseased tissue and debris are removed, the roots are planed, and the alveolar bone is trimmed and contoured. The area is rinsed with a saline solution and the flap is repositioned and sutured. A **periodontal dressing** may be applied to protect the surgical site.

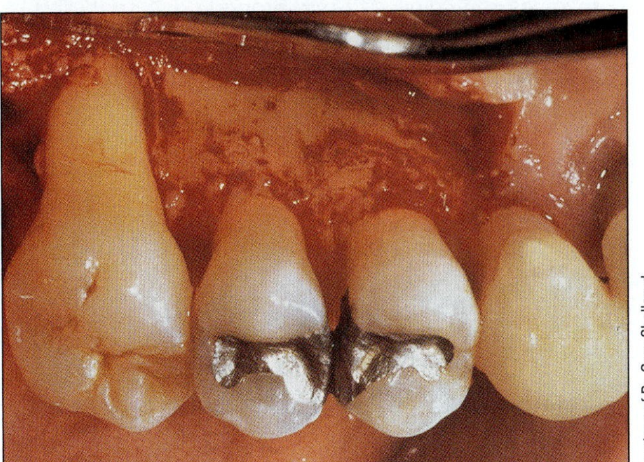

Courtesy of Dr. Gary Shellerud

FIGURE 31-32

Periodontal flap and osseous surgery. A flap is laid and alveolar bone exposed.

TABLE 31-3 Descriptions of Bone Replacement Grafts

Autogenous (autografts)	Cortical and cancellous bone extracted from intraoral and extraoral sites. Examples are bone removed during an osteoplasty or an ostectomy, bone harvested from a healing socket after an extraction, and donor bone from maxillary tuberosities, edentulous ridges, or retromolar areas.
Allogeneic (allografts)	An allograft is tissue transplanted between people of the same species. Bone tissue is carefully selected from donor cadavers; tested to ensure it is free of any transmissible pathologic condition; freeze dried; ground to average bone particle size; and placed in sterile, vacuum-sealed bottles with an indefinite shelf life.
Xenogeneic (xenografts)	Xenografts are tissues from different species. Cows and pigs are used most often for humans.
Allogeneic (alloplastic grafts)	Alloplastic grafts are various synthetic materials, including hydroxyapatite, calcium carbonate, polymers, bioactive glasses, and tricalcium phosphate.

Osseous Surgery

An **osseous surgery** removes defects/deformities in the bone caused by periodontal disease and other related conditions (Procedure 31-4). Two types of bone surgeries that correct the deformities are **osteoplasty**, reshaping the bone, and **ostectomy**, removal of bone.

Osseous surgery can be either additive or subtractive. During additive osseous surgery (sometimes called *bone augmentation*), bone or bone substitute is added to fill in areas. This is a **bone grafting** (moving tissue from one area to another) procedure.

Bone Grafting. Bone grafting offers some hope to restore lost bone and regeneration of a functional attachment of the periodontium. After careful patient evaluation, this procedure may be selected to improve the patient's condition. There are several types of bone replacement grafts: autogenous, allogeneic, xenogeneic, and alloplastic (see Table 31-3). Autogenous grafts have the best results; but because often only a limited amount of host bone is conveniently available in the oral cavity, other grafts may be indicated. Research reports that all bone replacement grafts fill the original intrabony defects about 60 to 70 percent.

During subtractive osseous surgery, the bone is removed with chisels, rongeurs, files, diamond burs, and stones.

After the bone has been grafted or removed and contoured, the flap is repositioned and sutures are placed. The area is rinsed gently and blotted dry before a periodontal dressing is placed.

Procedure 31-4
Osseous Surgery

This procedure is performed by the periodontist. It involves removing and recontouring diseased and defective bone tissue. The extent of the periodontal disease process determines the amount and type of surgery performed.

Equipment and Supplies (*Figure 31-33*)

- Basic setup: mouth mirror, explorer, and cotton pliers
- Periodontal probe
- Cotton rolls and gauze sponges
- Saliva ejector, HVE tip, air–water syringe tip, and surgical aspirator tip
- Anesthetic setup
- Scalpel and blades

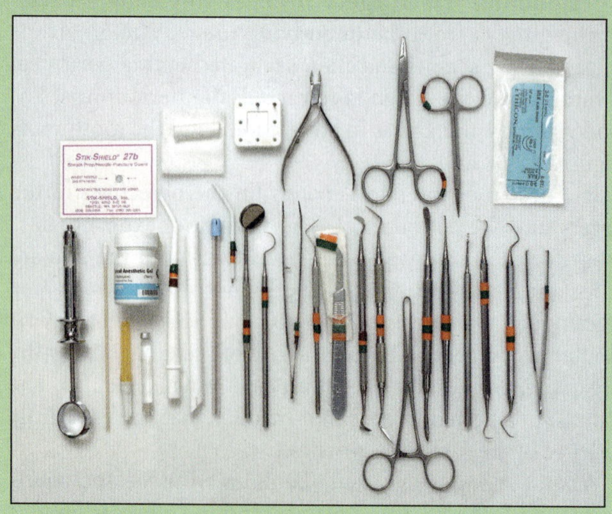

FIGURE 31-33
Osseous surgery tray setup.

(continues)

Procedure 31-4 (continued)

- Periodontal knives—broad bladed and interproximal
- Tissue retractor
- Periosteal elevator
- Diamond burs and stones
- Rongeurs, chisels, and files
- Scalers and curettes
- Hemostat and surgical scissors
- Suture setup
- Periodontal dressing materials

Procedure Steps (*Follow aseptic procedures*)

In osseous surgery, a flap of soft tissue is incised and reflected to expose the bone for reshaping and/or removal. This procedure is performed by the periodontist.

1. After the anesthetic is administered, the soft tissue is incised and loosened from the underlying bone. Transfer instruments and maintain good visibility for the operator.
2. The tissue flap is reflected and stabilized with tissue retractors. Retract and hold the tissue.
3. Once the bone is exposed, the diseased bone tissue is excised. Scalers and curettes are used to remove calculus and diseased tissue, and the roots are planed. Transfer instruments, rinse the area with a sterile saline solution as needed, evacuate, and keep the instruments clean by removing debris from instruments with the gauze sponge.
4. The bone is shaped and contoured using diamond burs and stones, rongeurs, chisels, and files.
5. The tissue flap is replaced and positioned over the alveolar bone and then sutured in place. Prepare the suture and stabilize the tissue with tissue forceps during the suturing procedure.
6. Prepare the periodontal dressing materials and assist the operator in the placement. In some states, the dental assistant is allowed to place and remove the periodontal dressing.
7. Remove any debris from the patient's face, give postoperative instructions, and dismiss the patient.

Mucogingival Surgery

A **mucogingival surgery** is reconstructive surgery on the gingiva and/or mucosa tissues. The surgeries may involve covering exposed roots, increasing the width of the gingival tissue, and reducing frenum or muscle attachments. Periodontal disease can cause negative changes in the gingiva, and mucogingival surgery improves these areas. Two common examples of mucogingival surgery are gingival grafting and the frenectomy.

Gingival Grafting/Connective Tissue Grafting

During a **gingival grafting** procedure, tissue is taken from one site and placed on another. The procedure involves preparation of the site of the graft by eliminating any periodontal pockets and exposing a bed of connective tissue. Then, a graft (section of tissue) is obtained from the donor site, often the palate area. This graft is positioned carefully and sutured securely in place. The donor site is covered with a periodontal dressing or another protective material until it is healed, which usually takes 1 to 2 weeks (Figure 31-34).

Other types of soft tissue grafts include *free gingival grafts* and *pedicle grafts*. Free gingival grafts are similar to connective tissue grafts in that the free gingival grafts involve the use of palatal tissues and the blood supply is not part of the graft. A flap of tissue is removed from the roof of the mouth or edentulous area and tissues from under the flap, called subepithelial connective tissue, are removed from the flap and sutured to the gingival tissue surrounding the exposed root. The palatal flap is then sutured back down.

The pedicle graft procedure involves taking tissue from near the tooth needing repair. The flap is cut away on three sides leaving one edge attached, keeping the blood supply. The tissue is pulled to cover the exposed root and then is sutured in place.

Some dentists prefer to use graft material from a tissue bank instead of the roof of the mouth. There are also the tissue-stimulating proteins that are used to encourage the body's natural ability to grow bone and tissue.

Frenectomy

The **frenectomy** is a complete removal of the frenum, including the attachment to the underlying bone. The frenum may be removed if it is attached too close to the marginal gingiva. The procedure involves incising the frenum and removing a triangular section. The periodontal fibers are separated and cut to the bone. The labial mucosa is then sutured to the apical periosteum. The periodontal dressing is prepared and placed over the suture site.

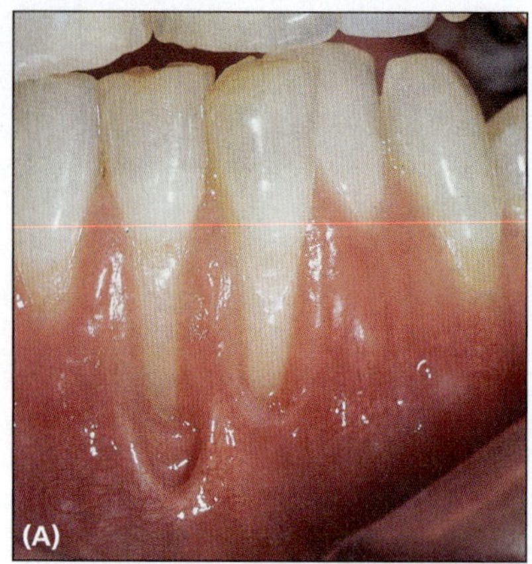

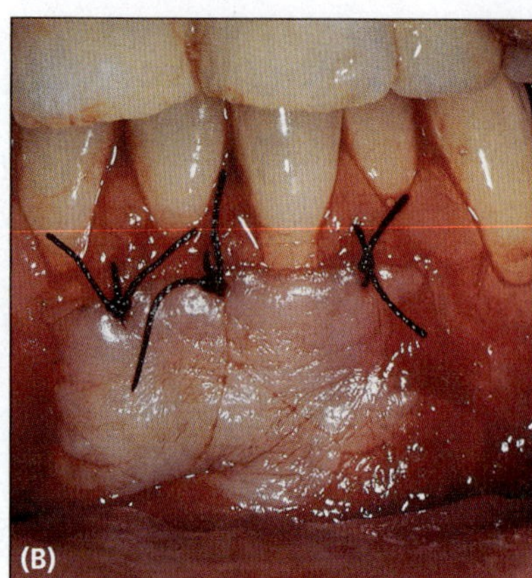

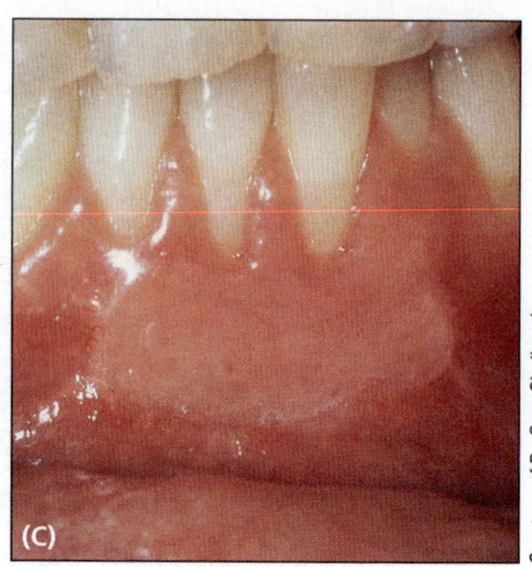

Courtesy of Dr. Gary Shellerud

FIGURE 31-34

Gingival graft. (A) Gingival recession shows need for graft. (B) Palatal tissue graft is positioned over area of recession and then sutured in place. (C) Graft after healing period.

Guided Tissue Regeneration

A **guided tissue regeneration (GTR)**, or selective cell reproduction, uses barrier membranes to maintain a space between the gingival flap and the root surface of the tooth in order for tissues to regenerate in a periodontal defect. Cells capable of forming new cementum, periodontal ligament, and supporting alveolar bone must move into the surgical site to produce these tissues, but they must not be interfered with. Therefore, apical epithelial migration must be delayed and gingival connective tissue from the flap must be kept away from the surgical area for regeneration to take place.

The membranes used as a barrier are classified as nonabsorbable or absorbable. Both have proven to be successful techniques. The technique involving nonabsorbablemembranes has been on the market longer and requires a second appointment in about 3 to 4 weeks to remove the barrier. Selection of the type of membrane to be used is determined by the dentist's preference and the type of periodontal defect.

Periodontal Plastic Surgery

Periodontal plastic surgery is a generic name for any number of periodontal surgical procedures. Periodontal plastic surgery involves the gingival tissues and defects in these tissues. These procedures are often performed when a patient is unhappy with the appearance his or her teeth and seeks cosmetic dental treatment. The periodontist works with the cosmetic dentist or general dentist to provide optimum periodontal health and the esthetics the patient is looking for. Some surgeries involve removing gingival tissue such as with crown lengthening while others involve adding gingival tissues such as covering exposed root surfaces or adding tissue around dental implants. (See more information in Chapter 35, Cosmetic Dentistry and Teeth Whitening.)

Periodontal Dressing

Periodontal dressings or packs are placed after periodontal surgical procedures. The dressings do not have any medicinal qualities; they are bandages used to protect the tissue during the healing process.

The following are objectives of the periodontal dressing:

- Minimizing postoperative infection and hemorrhage
- Protecting the tissues during mastication
- Covering the surgical site in order to reduce pain due to trauma or irritation
- Providing support for teeth that are mobile
- Helping to hold flaps in position

Types of Periodontal Dressings

The most common types of materials used as periodontal dressings are zinc oxide–eugenol materials, noneugenol materials, the light-cured dressings, and gelatin-based materials.

Zinc Oxide–Eugenol Materials. Zinc oxide–eugenol materials are supplied in a powder (zinc oxide) or liquid (eugenol) form that can be mixed before the procedure and stored for later use. In some offices the material is mixed, wrapped in wax paper, and then frozen until needed.

The presence of eugenol in this dressing can cause an allergic reaction. The area becomes red and a burning sensation is experienced by the patient.

Noneugenol Materials. The noneugenol materials come in a two-paste system: one tube of base material and one tube of accelerator. The two pastes are dispensed in equal portions on a paper pad and mixed together prior to placement (Procedures 31-5 and 31-6).

The noneugenol dressings do not cause sensitivity problems, and some noneugenol dressing materials have bacteriostatic agents added.

Light-Cured Periodontal Dressing. Light-cured periodontal dressing material comes in syringes. It can be placed directly on the surgical site or placed on a mixing pad. If it

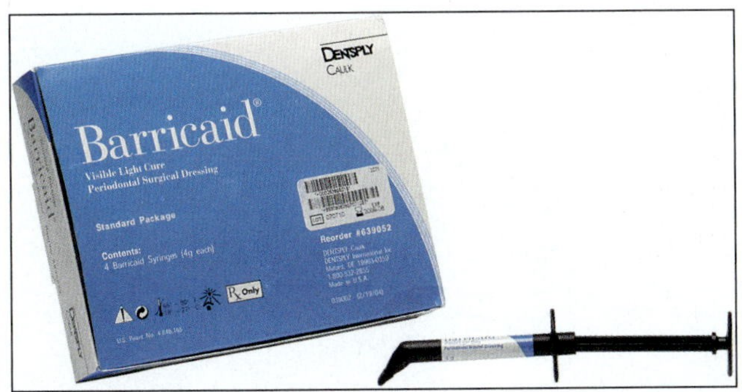

FIGURE 31-35
Light-cured periodontal dressing.

is placed directly on the tissues it can be contoured into the desired position, and then light cured. The material may also be dispensed onto a paper pad, manipulated to the required shape and size, placed over the tissues, and then light cured (Figure 31-35).

Gelatin-Base Dressings. Gelatin-base dressings offer good stability and dissolve in 24 to 48 hours. They are excellent for use after soft-tissue augmentation.

Procedure 31-5
Preparation and Placement of Noneugenol Periodontal Dressing

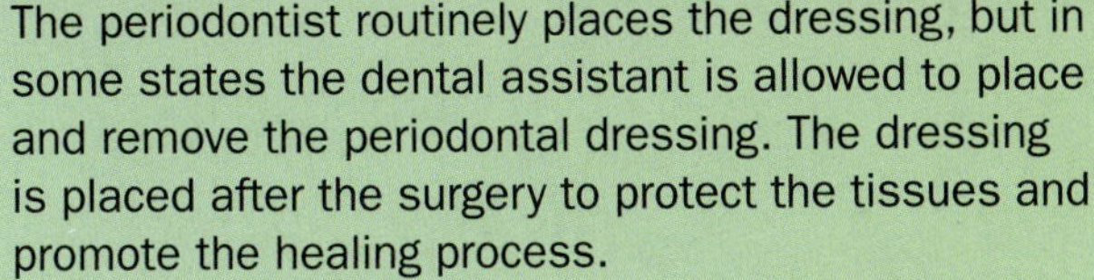

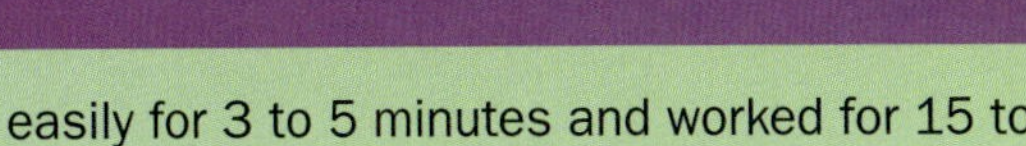

The periodontist routinely places the dressing, but in some states the dental assistant is allowed to place and remove the periodontal dressing. The dressing is placed after the surgery to protect the tissues and promote the healing process.

Equipment and Supplies

- Basic setup: mouth mirror, explorer, and cotton pliers
- Gauze sponges
- Noneugenol periodontal dressing material (base and accelerator)
- Paper pad and tongue depressor
- Approved lubricant
- Instrument to contour dressing (spoon excavator and, sickle scaler)

Procedure Steps (*Follow aseptic procedures*)

1. After the hemorrhaging is controlled, the patient's lips are coated lightly with approved lubricant.
2. The dressing materials are dispensed into equal lengths and mixed with a tongue blade until homogeneous. (Cleanup is made easier by using a paper pad and a tongue blade.) The material is allowed to set for 2 to 3 minutes until the tackiness is gone (Figure 31-36A).
3. Lubricate gloved fingers with approved lubricant so the putty-like material can be handled easily.
4. The dressing comes with a retardant to slow the setting time, if necessary; it can be molded easily for 3 to 5 minutes and worked for 15 to 20 minutes.
5. The dressing is molded into a thin strip slightly longer than the length of the surgical site. Divide the strip into two equal lengths, one for the facial surface and one for the lingual surface (Figure 31-36B).
6. To begin the placement, form the end of one strip into a hook shape. Wrap this hook around the distal of the most posterior tooth (Figure 31-36C).
7. Adapt the rest of the strip along the facial surface, gently pressing the pack into the interproximal areas (Figure 31-36D).
8. The second strip is applied to the lingual surface in the same manner. The pack is wrapped around the last posterior tooth and then adapted to the lingual surface, moving toward the midline.
9. The pack should cover the gingiva evenly without interfering with occlusion, tongue movements, or frenum attachments.
10. Check the dressing for overextensions. These areas are removed with a spoon excavator or scaler. Gently press the instrument into the dressing to detach the extra material. Smooth the pack and evaluate it for even thickness.
11. Ask the patient how the pack feels. Instruct the patient to move his or her tongue, cheeks, and lips to mold the pack. Make any adjustments to ensure that the dressing is securely in place, trimmed, and contoured.

(continues)

Procedure 31-5 (continued)

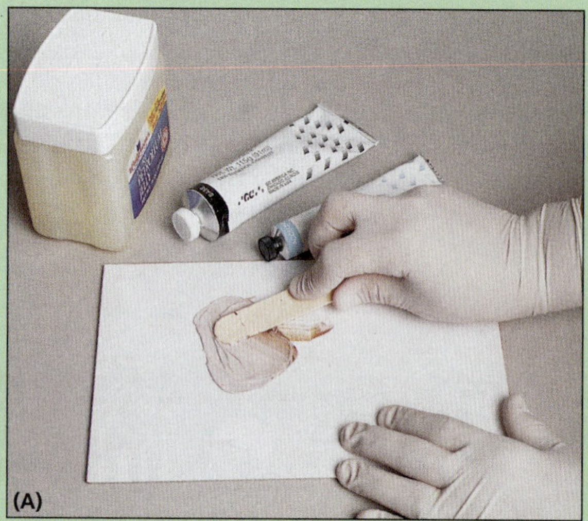

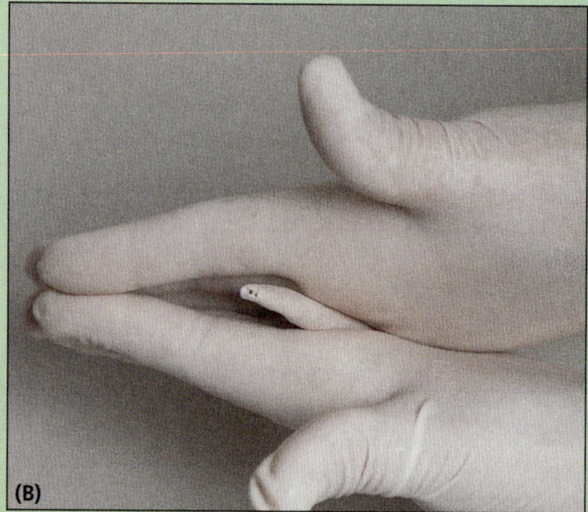

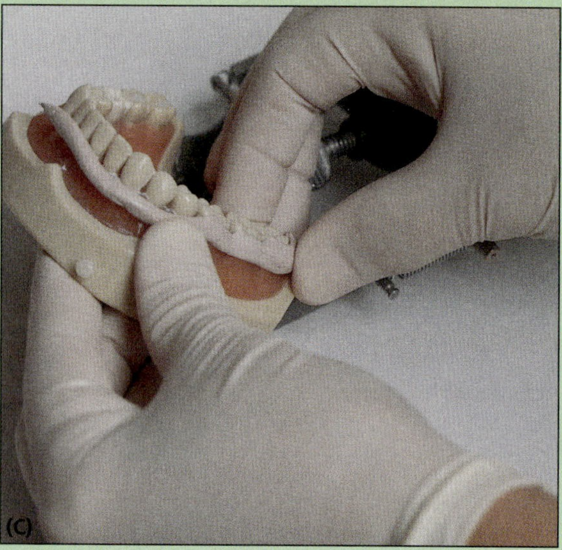

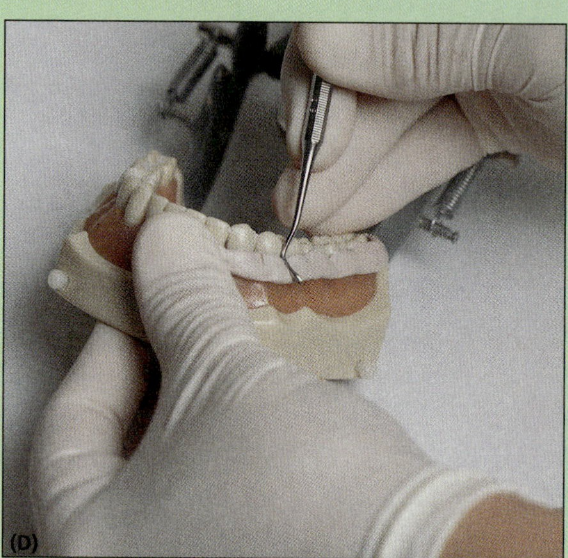

FIGURE 31-36

Preparation and placement of periodontal dressing. (A) Mixing the materials. (B) Preparing the materials for placement. (C) Placing the dressing on tissue. (D) Contouring dressing.

12. Give the patient instructions about the periodontal dressing, including:

- The pack is kept on for 1 week after surgery.
- The pack will harden in a few hours and then withstand normal chewing stresses.
- The pack may chip and break off during the week but should remain intact as long as possible. If there is pain when pieces of the pack come off or the pack becomes rough, the patient should call the office.
- The patient should brush the occlusal surface of the teeth involved in the surgery and continue to brush and floss the rest of the teeth as normal.

Procedure 31-6
Removal of Periodontal Dressing

This procedure is performed by the periodontist or the dental assistant depending on the expanded functions. The patient has worn the dressing for a week to 10 days. The patient's mouth is examined before removing the dressing to check for areas where the dressing may have loosened or come off completely.

Equipment

- Basic setup: mouth mirror, explorer, and cotton pliers
- Saliva ejector, HVE tip, and air–water syringe tip
- Gauze sponges and tissue
- Instruments to remove the dressing (spoon excavator, sickle explorer, and surgical hoe)

Procedure Steps (*Follow aseptic procedures*)

1. After seating the patient, the surgical site is evaluated and the dressing is removed.
2. A surgical hoe or a spoon excavator is inserted along the margin. Lateral pressure is applied to pry the dressing away from the tissue (Figure 31-37).
3. The pack may come off in large pieces and then scalers and floss can be used to remove any particles from the interproximal areas and tooth surfaces. Cotton pliers are used to remove particles of dressing embedded in the surgical site.
4. Gently rinse the entire area with warm water to remove any debris. The air–water syringe can be used carefully.

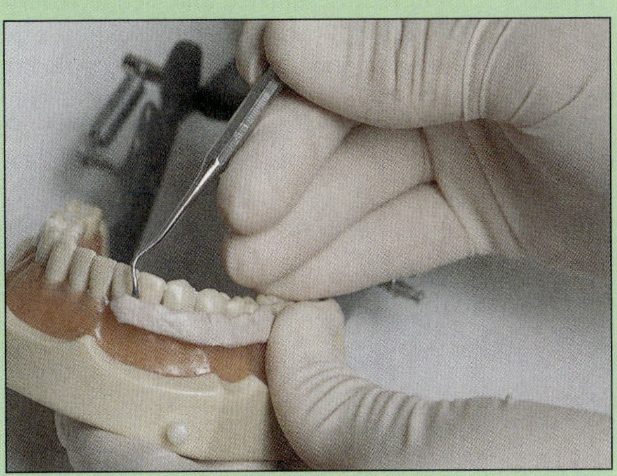

FIGURE 31-37
Removing periodontal dressing.

Periodontal Maintenance Procedures

Periodontal surgery does not end the need for periodontal treatment. The patient determines the success of the treatment by being committed and following the designed therapy. Periodontal disease is an ongoing process, but continual care maintains the status of periodontal health after surgery. Dedicated home oral-hygiene routines and periodic visits to the dentist are necessary for successful periodontal care.

Once the patient has accepted the treatment plan, plaque-control techniques are taught by the dental assistant and/or the hygienist. As the patient continues through treatment, the patient's hygiene skills and personalized intraoral aids are evaluated and adjusted according to the patient's individual needs. After surgery, the patient is instructed to keep the area as clean as possible to enhance the healing process. After the periodontal dressing is removed, interdental cleaners, floss, and water irrigators may be used to remove plaque and debris. When the tissues have healed sufficiently, the patient can begin the oral hygiene regimen prescribed.

Chapter Summary

Periodontal disease is as old as the human race. According to the American Academy of Periodontology, three out of four adults will experience, to some degree, periodontal problems at some time in their lives. In children and adolescents, marginal gingivitis and gingival recession are the most prevalent conditions.

In this chapter the dental assistant student will learn the symptoms, causes, and classifications of periodontal disease. Diagnostic procedures including the medical/dental history, the clinical examination, periodontal screening and recording system, types of x-rays taken, and how the treatment plan is put together and presented to the patient are described. The student will learn the instruments and equipment used as well as the nonsurgical and surgical procedures routinely completed in a periodontal office. There is also information on the use, benefits, and safety of dental lasers. The dental assistant performs chairside assisting duties and the expanded functions allowed by the state Dental Practice Act, including placing and removing periodontal dressing, removing sutures, and performing coronal polishes. The dental assistant takes radiographs, takes impressions for study models, and administers fluoride treatments. The assistant also gives pre- and postoperative instructions and prepares the treatment room for surgery. These functions are in addition to treatment room preparation and maintenance and sterilization procedures. The dental assistant is involved in educating and motivating the patient throughout the treatment. In some offices, the dental assistant may also perform laboratory tasks, such as pouring study models or making periodontal splints.

CASE STUDY

Melissa Moore is 42 years old. She has been Dr. Sanchez's patient for 14 years. Melissa has her teeth examined and cleaned every 6 months. Over the years, she has developed several teeth with pocket readings of between six and eight. At Melissa's last cleaning appointment, the hygienist explained that she found over 10 areas with periodontal probing readings of over six and areas where the tissues bleed easily. Melissa is in good general health but has been taking medication to reduce anxiety for the past 6 months.

Case Study Review

1. Are Melissa's periodontal readings within the normal range?
2. What questions should be asked in reference to the change in her condition over such a short period of time?
3. Explain how stress could affect Melissa's periodontal health.

Review Questions

Multiple Choice

1. The periodontium includes
   a. gingiva, epithelial attachment, cementum, sulcus, enamel, and pulp chamber.
   b. gingiva, enamel, cementum, dentin, sulcus, and periodontal ligaments.
   c. gingiva, epithelial attachment, periodontal ligaments, cementum, and alveolar bone.
   d. periodontal ligaments, sulcus, gingiva, salivary glands, and mucous membrane.
2. Periodontal disease is a virus that can be transmitted from one individual to another.
   a. True
   b. False
3. The working end of the periodontal instrument used to remove subgingival calculus and smooth the root surface is rounded and has cutting edges on both sides of the blade. This instrument is a
   a. hoe.
   b. file.
   c. scaler.
   d. curette.
4. The procedure to remove calculus and debris from the tooth and periodontal pocket is known as
   a. root planing.
   b. scaling and curettage.
   c. polishing procedure.
   d. occlusal adjustment.
5. Periodontal surgery that involves recontouring of the alveolar bone is called
   a. mucogingival surgery.
   b. gingival grafting.
   c. osteoplasty.
   d. ostectomy.
6. All of the following are safety measures to be in place when using dental lasers *except*:
   a. Special protective eyewear should be worn by the dentist only.
   b. A warning sign should be posted by the treatment room when lasers are in use.
   c. A moist gauze should cover tissues not being treated with the laser.
   d. Matte-coated instruments should be used.
7. ________ are hinged instruments used to shape soft tissue.
   a. Pocket marking pliers
   b. Periosteal elevators

c. Soft tissue rongeurs
d. Tissue forceps

8. How many sites are probed to determine the sulcus depth?
   a. 5
   b. 6
   c. 10
   d. 12
9. When placing the periodontal dressing the assistant should
   a. use lubricated gloved fingers to mold the dressing into a thin strip.
   b. divide the dressing into two equal lengths, one for facial/buccal surface and one for lingual surface.
   c. place the first strip on the facial/buccal surface and the second on the lingual surface.
   d. All of the answers are correct
10. All of the following are types of periodontal dressing *except*:
   a. zinc oxide-eugenol.
   b. adhesive surgical dressing.
   c. noneugenol dressing.
   d. light-cured periodontal dressing.

Critical Thinking

1. What are the signs and symptoms of periodontal disease?
2. Name the periodontal disease that occurs in young adults and discuss why this occurs in this age group.
3. Patients must take an active part in the treatment of periodontal disease. List several means the dental assistant uses to aid the patient.
4. Lasers are being used more and more for dental treatments. Discuss the benefits of using lasers in the periodontal office.
5. Discuss the purpose of placing periodontal dressing and which type of periodontal dressing might cause an allergic reaction to the patient.

Web Activities

1. Go to http://www.perio.org for consumer information and the frequently asked questions about periodontal disease and treatments.
2. To learn about the academy of laser dentistry, patient overview, and dental lasers, visit http://www.laserdentistry.org.
3. Take the quiz at http://www.perio.org to see if you have periodontal disease.

CHAPTER

32 Coronal Polish

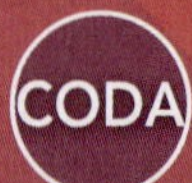

Specific Instructional Objectives

The student should strive to meet the following objectives and demonstrate an understanding of the facts and principles presented in this chapter:

1. Define coronal polish.
2. Describe and explain the rational for each step in the coronal polish procedure.
3. Explain the indications and contraindications for coronal polish.
4. Describe and identify the dental deposits and stains.
5. List the types of abrasives and explain the characteristics of each type.
6. List and explain the types of equipment and materials used to perform a coronal polish.
7. Explain how to maintain the oral cavity during a coronal polish.
8. List the auxiliary polishing aids and explain their functions.
9. Describe the steps in the coronal polish procedure.

Key Terms

abrasive (759)
abrasive polishing strip (768)
auxiliary polishing aid (768)
black line stain (759)
bridge threader (768)
brown stain (758)
chalk (760)
coronal polish (755)
dental floss (762)
dental fluorosis (758)
dental tape (762)
endogenous (757)
exogenous (756)
extrinsic (756)
flour of pumice (760)
fluoride prophylaxis paste (760)
green stain (759)
hard deposits (755)
humectant (760)
interproximal brush (769)
intrinsic (756)
metallic stain (758)
oral prophylaxis (755)
pellicle (756)
polishing (759)
prophy brush (762)
soft deposit (756)
soft wood points (769)
tetracycline stain (758)
tin oxide (760)
tobacco stain (758)
yellow stain (758)
zirconium silicate (760)

Introduction

The **oral prophylaxis** procedure is actually twofold. First, the **hard deposits** (scaling) are removed by the dentist or dental hygienist. Second, the teeth are polished with a rubber cup. In some states, a registered or an expanded-function dental assistant can perform this part of the prophylaxis, in addition to the dentist and the hygienist.

The **coronal polish** procedure involves removing soft deposits and extrinsic stains (i.e., stains removed by polishing) from the surfaces of the teeth and restorations. This is accomplished with an abrasive, dental handpiece, rubber cup (sometimes this procedure is called a "rubber cup" polish), brush, dental tape, and floss. The coronal polish is the polishing of the clinical crown of the tooth. The clinical crown on a newly erupted tooth would involve polishing the enamel surface, while the clinical crown on a tooth with some gingival recession may involve the enamel and the dentin (Figure 32-1). Often, exposed dentin is not polished because of the possibility of increased sensitivity. Composite restorations, acrylic veneers, and porcelain-filled surfaces are also not polished or carefully polished because of the possibility of removing the finish and decreasing surface hardness. Different abrasives are used on each surface.

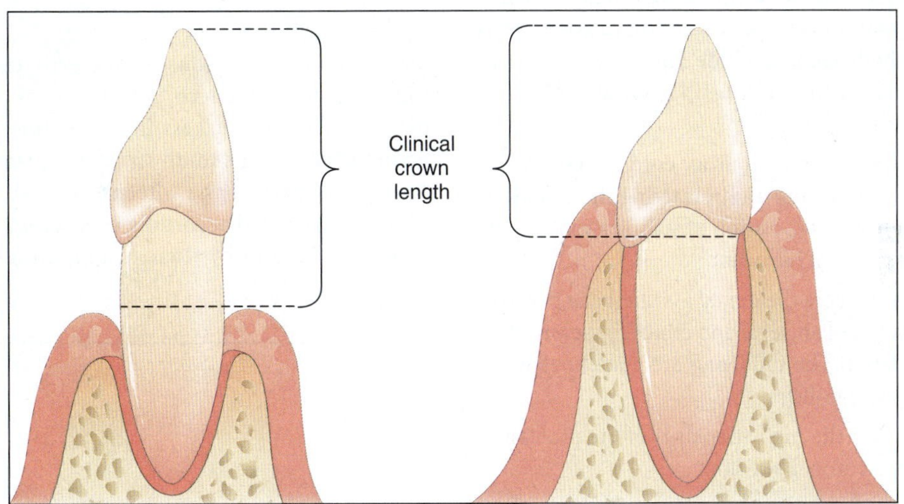

FIGURE 32-1
Varying length of clinical crown of tooth.

Advanced Chairside Functions

Rationale for Performing Coronal Polish

After the teeth have been scaled to remove the hard deposits, the polish is done to provide a smooth, polished surface. Additional benefits and indications include the following:

- A polish makes it easier for the patient to keep the teeth clean.
- The tooth surface absorbs fluoride better.
- The process of accumulation of new deposits is slowed.
- A clean tooth surface motivates the patient to maintain good oral hygiene habits.
- The teeth are prepared for placement of enamel sealant.
- The teeth are prepared for orthodontic bracket and band placement.

Contraindications and Modifications

Conditions that contraindicate a coronal polish involve the gingival tissues. The abrasive agents used in the coronal polish may cause problems, and the polish technique could traumatize the already irritated tissues. Whether the cause of the gingival irritation is systemic or local, whenever the gingival tissues are irritated, inflamed, sensitive, or hemorrhage easily, it is best to evaluate the necessity of the coronal polish. For some patients, the polish should be postponed until the condition of the tissue improves. For other patients, the polish removes the source of irritation. The dentist makes the decision on an individual patient basis.

Advanced Chairside Functions (Continued)

The following conditions may require modification of coronal polish techniques:

- **Orthodontic appliances**—Use of a small rubber cup and a pointed or tapered brush, especially around the brackets.
- **Hypersensitive teeth**—Use a very wet abrasive agent with a light, intermittent stroke. Use a cotton roll or cotton swab to dry the area.
- **Green chromogenic bacterial stain**—Before beginning the coronal polish, use a solution of equal parts of 3 percent hydrogen peroxide and water. Apply to the stained areas with a cotton-tip applicator for a few seconds, and then rinse.
- **Minor oral irritations, such as cold sores**—Avoid the areas when polishing and retracting the tissues or establishing a *fulcrum* (position of stabilization). Apply a protective coating of lubricant.

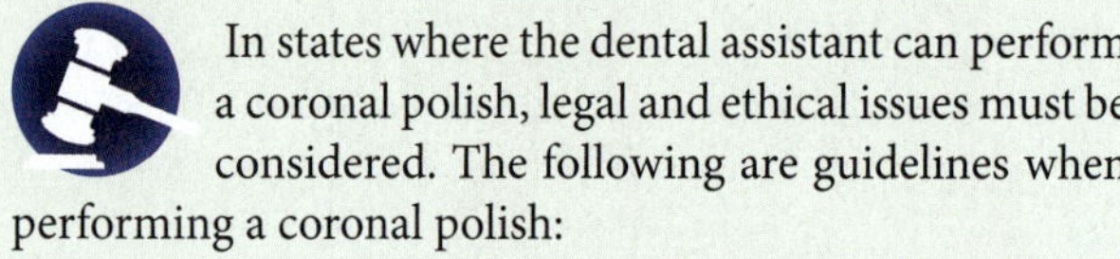

In states where the dental assistant can perform a coronal polish, legal and ethical issues must be considered. The following are guidelines when performing a coronal polish:

- Consistently meet the high standards of the profession in performing a coronal polish.
- Follow aseptic techniques and OSHA guidelines.
- Request assistance when needed to best serve the patient.
- Refer all diagnosing to the dentist.

Dental Deposits

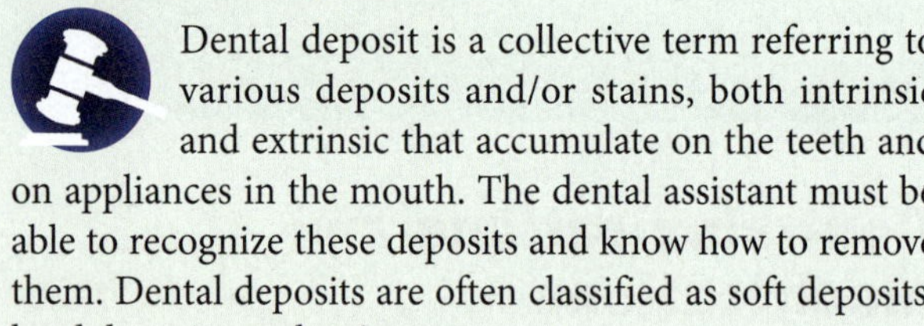

Dental deposit is a collective term referring to various deposits and/or stains, both intrinsic and extrinsic that accumulate on the teeth and on appliances in the mouth. The dental assistant must be able to recognize these deposits and know how to remove them. Dental deposits are often classified as soft deposits, hard deposits, and stains.

Soft Deposits

The **soft deposits** include the acquired dental **pellicle**, materia alba, food debris, and plaque. The dental assistant can remove these soft deposits while performing a coronal polish (Table 32-1). To aid in identifying the soft deposits the dental assistant can apply a red disclosing solution to the teeth (Figure 32-2).

Calculus

Dental calculus is a hard, calcified deposit that forms on the teeth, restorations, and dental appliances. Another name for calculus is "tartar." Calculus is mineralized plaque with few, if any, living organisms in its structure. It is often covered with a layer of plaque and is attached firmly to the tooth.

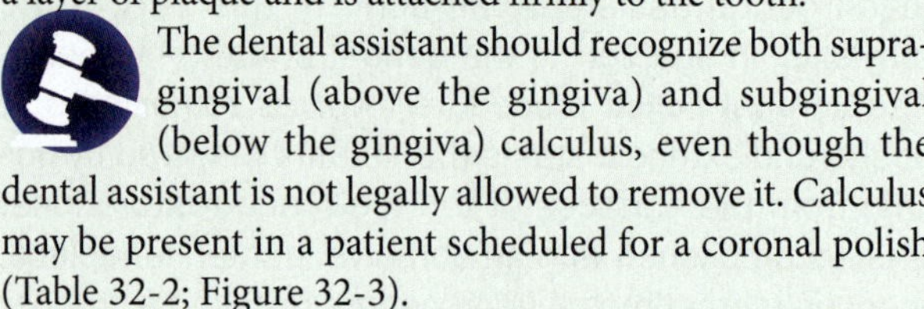

The dental assistant should recognize both supragingival (above the gingiva) and subgingival (below the gingiva) calculus, even though the dental assistant is not legally allowed to remove it. Calculus may be present in a patient scheduled for a coronal polish (Table 32-2; Figure 32-3).

Stains

Stains are discolorations of the teeth and are caused by foods, bacteria, tobacco, metals, drugs, imperfect tooth development, and excess fluoride, among other things. Stains adhere to the tooth structure, plaque, and calculus or may be part of the internal structure of the tooth. They are classified according to location, either **intrinsic** or **extrinsic**, and by their origin, either **exogenous** or

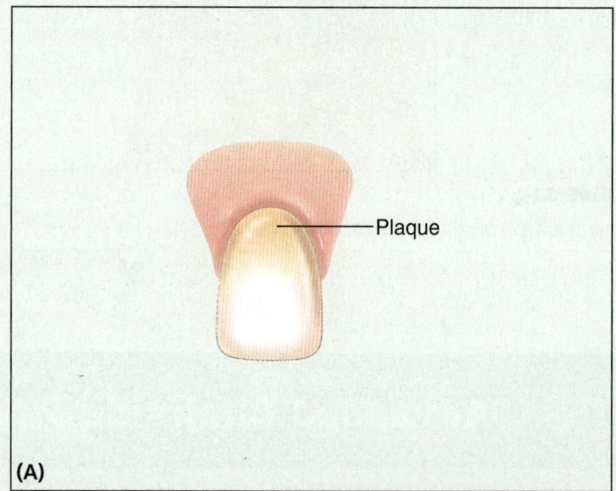

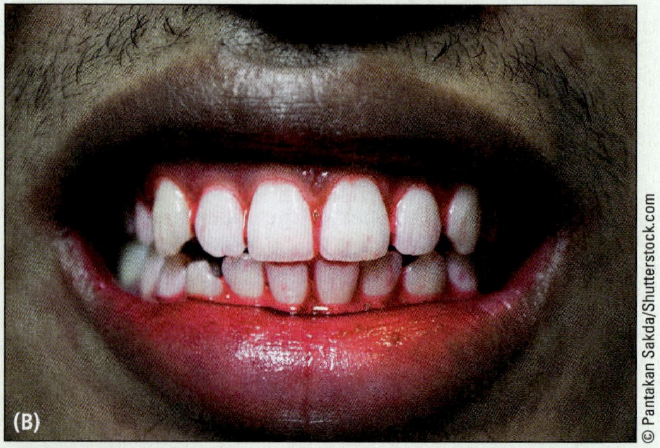

FIGURE 32-2
(A) Soft deposits on teeth. (B) Plaque is shown after application of red disclosing solution.

Advanced Chairside Functions

TABLE 32-1 Soft Deposits

	Pellicle	Materia Alba	Food Debris	Plaque
Appearance	Thin, clear film, sometimes stained	Soft, bulky mass, cottage cheese-like, white to yellow	Small particles of food	Soft, dense, furry-like deposit
Composition	A cellular, insoluble proteins, fats, and other materials	Unstructured, living and dead microorganisms. Food debris, desquamated epithelial cells, disintegrating leukocytes, and proteins	Food particles	Organized mass of many types of microorganisms in a sticky matrix. Approximately 80 percent water and 20 percent organic and inorganic solids, with most of the solids being microorganisms
Source	Saliva and sulcular fluids	Accumulation of materials and bacterial growth	Diet	Microorganisms
Formation	Forms within minutes of removal	Time varies	Forms while eating	Forms within 12–24 hours of removal
Attachment	Tooth surface, restorations, and appliances	Loosely attached, collects in grooves and spaces on and between teeth, gingiva, and appliances	Loosely attached, collects in spaces and grooves in and around teeth and appliances	Gingival areas in difficult areas to clean and lingual and occlusal grooves
Classification	Unstained and stained surface	None	None	Location on tooth with pathogenic effect
Significance	May protect enamel or may provide attachment and breeding ground for plaque and calculus	Provides source for plaque development	Provides nutrients	Dental caries, gingivitis, and periodontal disease
Methods of removal	Polishing with an abrasive	Rinsing, toothbrushing, and flossing	Rinsing, toothbrushing, and flossing	Toothbrushing, flossing, and coronal polish

TABLE 32-2 Calculus

	Supragingival Calculus	Subgingival Calculus
Appearance	Chalky white, yellow, gray, or stained by food	Black, brown, or dark green
Formation	Surfaces above the gingival margin. Most common on lingual of mandibular incisors and buccal of maxillary molars	Surfaces below the gingival margin
Removal	Mechanical methods	Mechanical methods
Age of patient	Uncommon in children under age 9	Very rare in children under age 9

endogenous. Intrinsic stains are inside the tooth structure and are mostly permanent (in some cases, bleaching is successful). The origin of intrinsic stains can be both endogenous (originating from inside the tooth) and exogenous (originating from outside the tooth). Extrinsic stains are on the outside of the tooth structure and can be removed by scaling and polishing. Extrinsic stains are exogenous only.

Dental stains are significant because of their unattractive appearance. They also may provide rough surfaces for deposits to adhere to. Stains may indicate past or present physical habits or conditions, which aid the dental assistant

Advanced Chairside Functions (Continued)

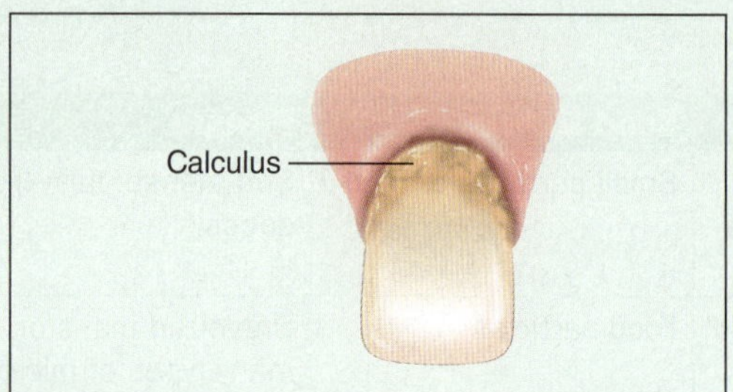

FIGURE 32-3
Calculus on teeth.

in determining oral hygiene information and instructions to be given to the patient.

It is important for the dental assistant to be able to distinguish between intrinsic and extrinsic stains and to know what stains can and cannot be removed. The dental assistant can explain to the patient the cause of the stains and what their options are for removal if possible or for further treatment if they are not removable. These options may include professional whitening, enamel micro abrasion, and cosmetic restorative procedures.

Intrinsic Stains. Categories of these stains are described below.

Dental Fluorosis. A **dental fluorosis** occurs as a result of high concentrations of fluoride received systemically during tooth development. The color of the stain varies from white to yellow-brown or gray-brown. The outer surface may be pitted and rough depending on severity. The stain is distributed relative to the stage of development of the teeth. Other names include brown stain and mottled enamel (Figure 32-4).

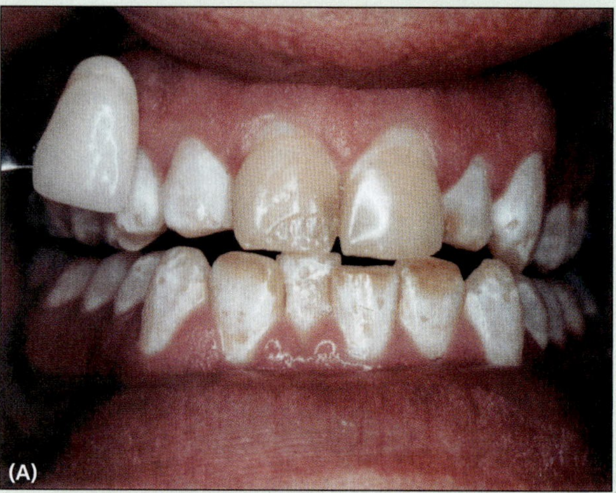

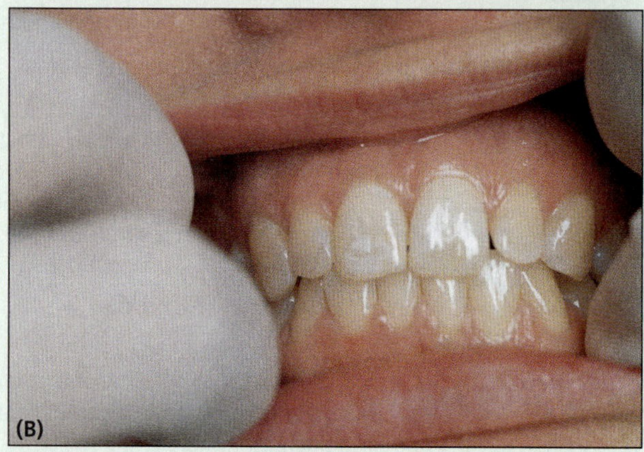

FIGURE 32-4
(A) Severe dental fluorosis. (B) Mild dental fluorosis.

Pulp Damaged or Nonvital Tooth Stain. This type of intrinsic stain occurs when the pulp is damaged or removed. This stain can vary in color from light yellow to black to green to magenta and is caused by blood and pulp tissues seeping into the dentin tubules.

Tetracycline Stain. A **tetracycline stain** is the result of high concentrations of tetracycline antibiotics taken during the time the tooth was developing. The stain varies in color from light green or yellow to dark gray-brown.

Metallic Stain. A **metallic stain** can be intrinsic and/or extrinsic. Metals and metallic salts may be inhaled in industrial settings or taken orally in certain drugs, or may comprise part of the materials used to restore teeth. The metals adhere to the pellicle and other soft deposits, or they penetrate the tooth surface to become part of the tooth structure. Several metals that can cause permanent stains are copper dust, which causes a green to greenish-blue stain; amalgam deposits that cause a gray to black or bluish-black stain; iron dust that causes a brown stain; and iron drugs, which cause a black stain.

Extrinsic Stains. Extrinsic stains also have several classifications.

Yellow and Brown Stains. A **yellow stain** and a **brown stain** are usually associated with poor oral hygiene and are dull yellow to a light brownish color. They are generally associated with plaque and most commonly found on the buccal surface of the maxillary molars and lingual surface of the mandibular incisors.

Tobacco Stain. A **tobacco stain** is the result of coal tar combustion in cigarettes and pigments from chewing tobacco penetrating the pits and fissures on the enamel and dentin surfaces. The stain is light brown to black in color,

Advanced Chairside Functions

and the amount of stain depends on the individual's oral hygiene habits and how often the person smokes.

Green Stain. A **green stain** varies in color from light to dark green or a yellowish green and is found most frequently in children. It is found on the facial surface of the maxillary anterior teeth at the cervical third and contains chromogenic bacteria and fungi.

Black Line Stain. A **black line stain** forms a thin black to dark-brown line slightly above the gingiva and follows the contour of the gingival margin. It is found primarily in women and often where there is excellent oral hygiene. The black line stain forms on the facial and lingual surfaces of the teeth and tends to reform after removal.

Orange Stain. This extrinsic stain is believed to be caused by chromogenic bacteria often related to drug therapy, such as antibiotics. It is uncommon, but if it does occur, it can be found on the lingual and facial surfaces of the anterior teeth near the gingival margin.

Chlorhexidine Stain. This stain occurs with prolonged use of chlorhexidine, which is found in chewing gum and mouth rinse. It is yellowish to green to brown in color and appears on restorations, the tongue, in plaque, and in the cervical and interproximal surfaces of the teeth. This is not a permanent stain and can be removed with tooth brushing and/or a coronal polish.

Abrasives and Polishing Agents

An **abrasive** is a material that cuts or grinds the surface, leaving grooves and a rough surface, while **polishing** produces a smooth, glossy surface with fine abrasive materials. It is important to understand abrasives and their characteristics and their actions to select the best materials for the patient without damaging the tooth. Abrasives remove small amounts of enamel during the polishing procedure; therefore, it is best to follow the coronal polish procedure with a fluoride treatment and/or to use a fluoride prophy agent.

Abrasives

Abrasives are materials composed of particles that come in powders or pastes. They are selected according to the amount of stain and soft deposits that are to be removed. Abrasives should always be as moist as possible yet easy to use without dripping or spattering. These particles have characteristics that affect their abrasiveness (Table 32-3).

Rate of Abrasion. The rate of abrasion is the time it takes to remove stains and deposits from a surface. This depends on several factors:

- By *increasing the speed of the handpiece*, the rate of abrasion is increased accordingly. This also increases the heat production.
- The *pressure* can control the rate of abrasion. The firmer the pressure, the more abrasive. Also, frictional heat increases.
- The *amount of abrasive* material used affects the rate of abrasion. The more material that is used, the faster the abrasive works.
- The *type of abrasive* used determines the rate of abrasion. The larger and harder the particles, the faster the abrasion. Also, the rate of heat production increases.
- The *dryer the abrasive* materials, the more abrasive they are.

TABLE 32-3 Characteristics of Abrasives

Characteristic	Effect on Abrasive
Particle shape	Sharp-edged particles are more abrasive than dull, rounded particles.
Particle hardness	Harder particles abrade faster. Particles must be harder than the surfaces they are used on.
Particle strength	Resistance of particles to break up during the polish; therefore, less material is used.
Particle size	The larger the particle, the more abrasive it is.
Grit or grade of abrasive particles	Materials are sifted through standardized sieves to grade fineness. Fine abrasives are called powders or flours and are graded F, FF, and FFF for increasing fineness.
Particle attrition resistance	Particles that do not dull or become embedded in the surface being polished are the most effective.

Advanced Chairside Functions (Continued)

Select an abrasive material that is coarse enough to cut through the deposits and stains and polish until the surfaces are as smooth as possible. Then, select a finer material, if needed, to polish the surface until it is smooth and free of deposits and stains. Usually, one abrasive is enough to complete the task, but if the patient has a lot of stain, a more coarse abrasive should be used. In the case of gingival recession, a finer abrasive is used on these areas after finishing all other areas with a coarser abrasive. When using two types of abrasives, completely finish with one abrasive, and then rinse the patient's mouth thoroughly before beginning with another abrasive. Also, use separate dappen dishes, rubber cups, and brushes for each abrasive.

Types of Abrasives. The abrasives come in powders and pastes and in bulk form or individually packaged. Besides the abrasive, most commercial preparations contain water, a binder, **humectant** (retains moisture), color, and a flavoring. Prophy pastes can contain materials that stimulate the remineralization of tooth enamel, prevent the loss of enamel, have desensitizing agents, remove stains, and polish the tooth surface. The pastes come in a variety of grits including super fine, fine, medium, and coarse. They also come in many flavors and some are non-splattering formulas. The prophy pastes come with a finger holder for easy access of the paste during the polishing procedure (Figure 32-5).

- **Zirconium silicate**—Used for stain removal and polishing. This material may be used on gold restorations, exposed dentin, and tooth-colored restorations, as well as enamel.
- **Silica/fine silica**—Used to remove stains, as a high-powered cleaning agent and a fine polishing agent. Course silica particles break down during the application and become a fine grit to polish.
- **Tin oxide**—A very fine polishing agent used on enamel and metallic restorations. Used in a paste form, it is mixed with water, alcohol, or glycerin.
- **Flour of pumice**—Used to remove stains from the enamel. It is relatively coarse and should be followed by a fine polishing agent. It is not used on exposed dentin, tooth-colored restorations, or gold restorations because of its high abrasiveness.
- **Chalk** (also known as whiting)—A mild abrasive, it is used in some prophylactic pastes.
- **Fluoride prophylaxis pastes**—Available and very popular. Fluoride is added to commercially prepared prophylaxis pastes to replace the fluoride lost in the enamel surface during the polishing procedure due to abrasion. Fluoride prophylaxis pastes should not be used if the teeth are to receive enamel sealants after the coronal polish.

Equipment and Supplies

The tray setup for the coronal polish includes patient safety glasses, hand mirror, mouth mirror, explorer, cotton pliers, cotton swabs (Q-Tips), 2 × 2 gauze, cotton rolls, saliva ejector, evacuator, air–water syringe tip, low-speed handpiece, rubber cups, brushes, prophy paste, tongue depressor, dental floss, dental tape, disclosing solution, and dappen dish for disclosing solution (see Figure 32-10). Barriers are placed on the dental unit, and the dental assistant follows OSHA guidelines and wears PPE.

Use of Dental Handpiece for Coronal Polish

For the coronal polish procedure, a low-speed dental handpiece is used with a prophy angle attachment (right angle). The handpiece is held in a modified pen grasp. The

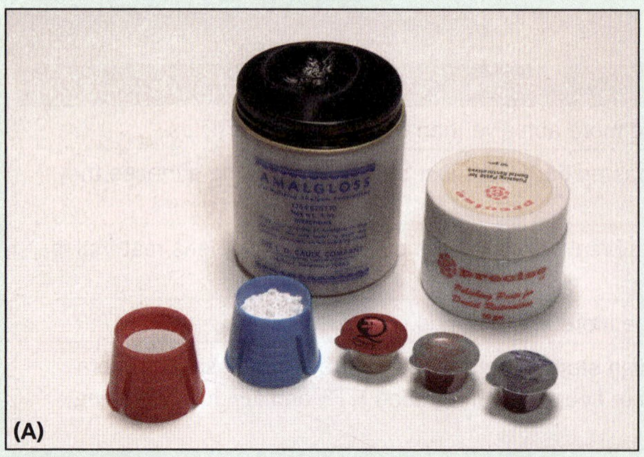

(A)

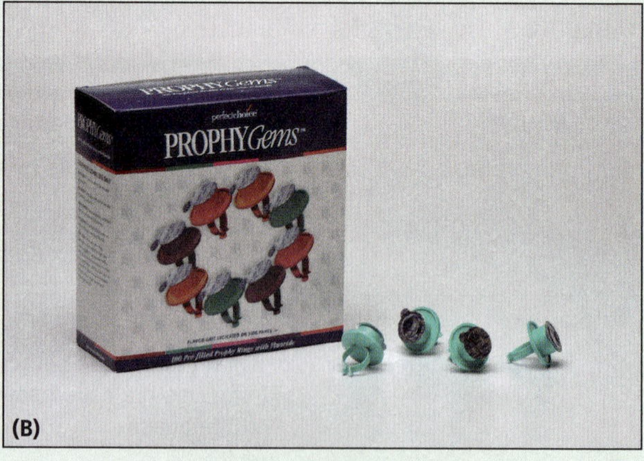

(B)

FIGURE 32-5
(A) Various types of abrasives, including powders and pastes. (B) Polishing agent in finger holder for easier application.

Advanced Chairside Functions

fingers should close up on the prophy angle attachment, and the body of the handpiece should rest in the "V" of the hand. This gives the operator control and prevents fatigue (Figure 32-6).

When the correct grasp is used, the procedure is performed efficiently and effectively. The speed of the handpiece is controlled by steady foot pressure on the rheostat. Keeping the speed even takes practice. An even, slow speed is desired, with just enough pressure to keep the cups and brushes rotating. Apply the handpiece to the tooth with light-to-moderate pressure. The handpiece should be started when it is in the mouth, near the tooth to be polished. This establishes the speed of the handpiece before placing the cup/brush on the tooth. When the handpiece is removed from the tooth for more than a moment, release the pressure on the rheostat so that the handpiece stops before being removed from the mouth. This prevents debris from splattering.

When the modified pen grasp is used, the ring finger is the fulcrum finger. The little finger is also used to supplement the ring finger as a fulcrum. During the procedure, *tooth structure provides the most stable fulcrum*. However, the soft tissue is used as a fulcrum. Cover the tissue with a 2 × 2 gauze first to prevent slipping. Using a fulcrum provides stability and control of the handpiece and patient comfort, and helps reduce fatigue of the dental assistant.

Points for Using a Dental Handpiece

- Use a slow, even speed.
- Use light-to-moderate pressure.
- Always use a fulcrum.
- Start and stop handpiece inside patient's mouth.

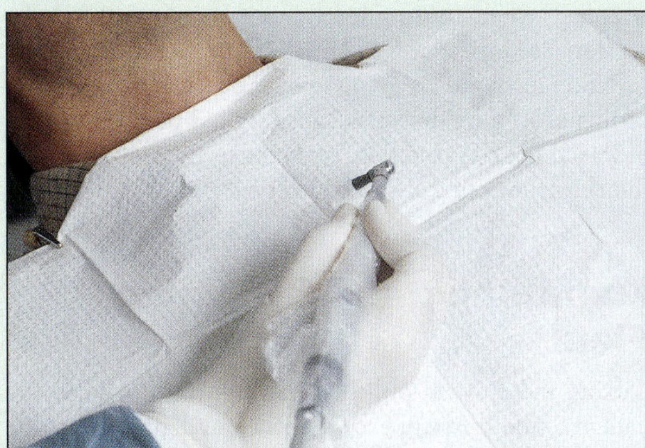

FIGURE 32-6

Modified pen grasp and dental handpiece.

Use of Rubber Prophy Cup

The rubber prophy cup is used with an abrasive agent to polish the teeth and dental appliances (Procedure 32-1). Rubber prophy cups are available in several designs to fit the prophy angles. On the back of the prophy cup there may be a small metal screw attachment that is screwed into the corresponding prophy angle or a small hole that slips over a knob on the prophy angle. Disposable prophy angles with attached prophy cups and brushes are also available (Figure 32-7).

Rubber prophy cups are made of either natural or synthetic rubber. Natural rubber cups are resilient and will not stain the teeth. Synthetic rubber cups are stiffer than the natural rubber, and the black cups may stain the teeth during the polish.

The rubber cup should be soft and flexible to adapt to the contours of the teeth. Edges should not be rough or frayed, which could irritate the tissues. The number of cups needed for the polishing depends on the number of abrasives used. One cup is used for each polishing agent. The edge of the cup is the part that actually does the polishing. The center of the cup holds and transports the abrasive agent. The cup is flexed to adapt to the tooth surface by applying slight pressure to one edge (Figure 32-8). The cup is most efficient on the facial and lingual surfaces of the teeth and fixed appliances, along the gingival margin, and 1 to 2 mm into the sulcus.

The hand and wrist are used to move the handpiece to adapt the cup to the tooth surface. When working on the lingual or facial surfaces move the edge of the rubber cup as far as possible into the proximal and manipulate the cup into the sulcus, *not* on the gingival margin. The next step

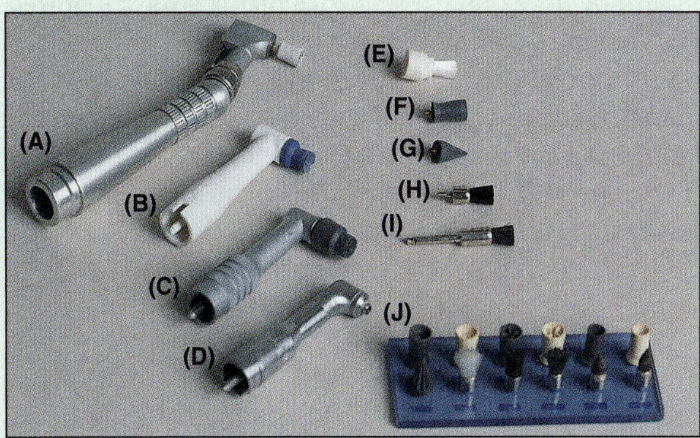

FIGURE 32-7

(A) Contra-angle with latch prophy cup. (B) Disposable prophy angle cup. (C) Right angle with snap-on prophy cup. (D) Right angle (prophy angle) for screw cup or brush. (E) Snap-on prophy brush. (F) Screw-on prophy cup. (G) Rubber point. (H) Screw-on prophy brush. (I) Latch brush. (J) Assortment of cups, brushes, and points.

Advanced Chairside Functions (Continued)

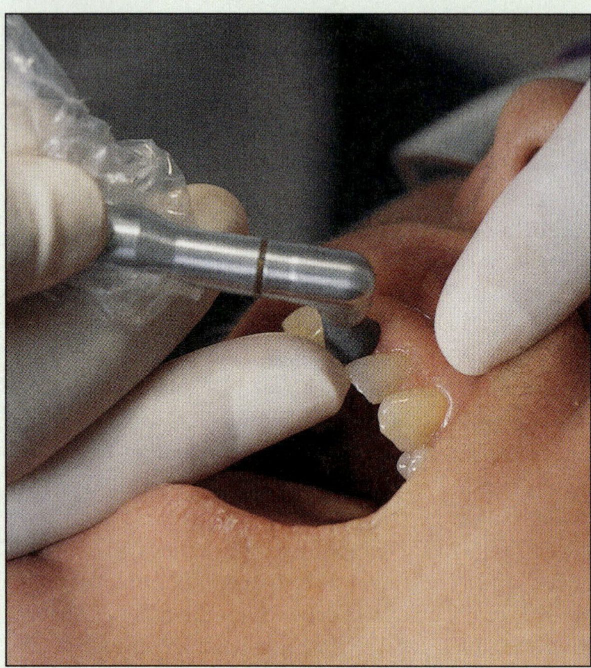

FIGURE 32-8
Adapting rubber cup to tooth surface.

in learning to use the prophy cup is to learn the stroke. A short, intermittent, overlapping stroke is used with a slow-revolving rubber cup. This stroke covers the tooth, leaves no unpolished surfaces, and minimizes the frictional heat produced (Figure 32-9).

Systematic Procedure

Follow a systematic procedure when polishing the entire mouth by developing a sequence that is always followed. For example, always start in the same quadrant or begin on the buccal surface of the most posterior tooth in the mandibular right quadrant and polish each tooth, moving around the entire arch; then make a loop around the most posterior tooth on the mandibular left quadrant and polish the lingual surface, ending on the right side.

Prophy Brush

The **prophy brush** that is used for the coronal polish procedure comes in several styles. Like the rubber cup, prophy brushes are "snap on" or "screw on," depending on which prophy angle they are used (see Figure 32-7). Brushes are available with nylon or natural bristles. Some brushes are tapered, while others are flat on the end. For the coronal polishes, a soft and flexible brush is used. Softening can be accomplished by soaking the brush in hot water before using it.

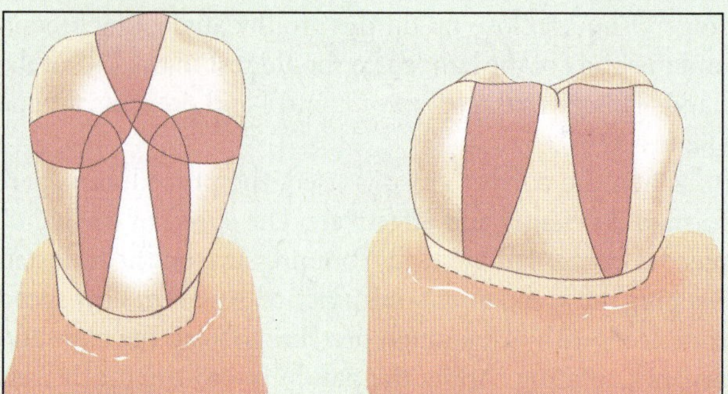

FIGURE 32-9
Examples of the overlapping polishing stroke.

Prophy brushes are used on the occlusal surfaces to effectively clean the deep pits and fissures and also on the lingual of the anterior teeth, but the bristles should *never* contact the gingival tissues and should be positioned only above the gingival third of the tooth. This brush is used only on the enamel surface. Used in the same manner as the cup, the brush is flexed in the central fossa with a light, intermittent, and overlapping stroke. On lingual surfaces, the brush is placed in the lingual pit and moved toward the incisal edge. Procedure 32-1 outlines the use of the prophy brush for polishing.

Dental Tape and Dental Floss

A **dental tape** is used on the interproximal surfaces of the teeth with an abrasive agent. Care must be used not to damage the interdental papilla and free gingival margins when using the tape. After all the interproximal surfaces have been polished with dental tape and abrasive, the teeth must be flossed to remove any particles of abrasive that were left after rinsing. The **dental floss** is placed interproximally, wrapped around the tooth, and moved in an up-and-down motion (see Procedure 32-2).

Note: If fluoride is going to be applied as the next step of this procedure, unwaxed floss should be used instead of waxed floss. Waxed floss coats the teeth, preventing the fluoride from being absorbed by the teeth.

Maintaining the Operating Field

During the coronal polish, it is important to keep the patient's mouth free of excess saliva and debris, direct the dental light for maximum light for the operator (dental assistant), keep the patient comfortable, and maintain correct positioning of the dental assistant and patient.

Advanced Chairside Functions

Procedure 32-1
Polishing with the Rubber Cup

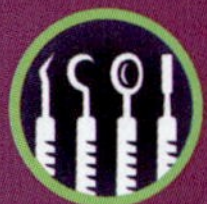

This procedure is performed by the dental assistant, hygienist, or dentist. The following procedure for polishing with the rubber cup explains positioning techniques and action of the rubber cup. Examine rubber cup placement on both arches and each quadrant on the facial and lingual surfaces.

Equipment and Supplies (*Figure 32-10*)

- Basic setup: mouth mirror, explorer/periodontal probe, and cotton pliers
- Saliva ejector, HVE tip, and air–water syringe tip
- 2 × 2 inch gauze sponges and cotton-tip applicator
- Dappen dish
- Lip lubricant
- Disclosing solution (optional)
- Low-speed handpiece
- Prophy angle attachment
- Assortment of rubber cups and brushes
- Prophy paste in different grits
- Finger rings to hold prophy paste cup
- Dental tape and dental floss

Procedure Steps (*Follow aseptic procedures*)

1. The patient is seated and prepared for the coronal polish procedure. Lip lubricant is sometimes offered for the patient's comfort. The dental assistant reviews the patient's medical history and inspects the oral cavity. The amount of extrinsic stain determines the grit of the abrasive to be used.
2. The dental assistant may dry the teeth and place disclosing solution on the teeth for easier detection of plaque.
3. After the teeth are dry, a cotton-tip applicator is used to place the solution on all surfaces of the teeth. This is accomplished one quadrant, one arch, or one side at a time.
4. After placing abrasive polishing agent in the cup, place the handpiece in the patient's mouth and start it. Then place the cup near the gingival sulcus and as far into the mesial or distal surface as possible. Establish a fulcrum as close to the tooth being polished as possible.

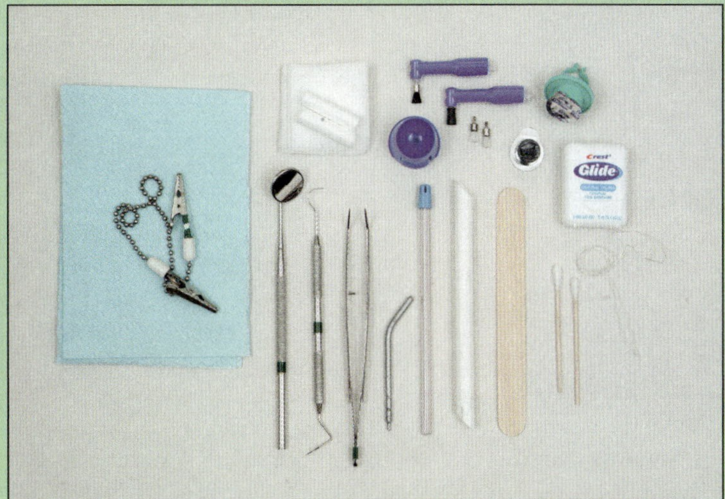

FIGURE 32-10
Tray setup for coronal polish procedure.

(continues)

Advanced Chairside Functions (Continued)

Procedure 32-1 (continued)

5. Apply light pressure to flex the cup and flare it into the sulcus 1 to 2 mm.
6. Sweep the rubber cup toward the incisal or occlusal edge. If the crown of the tooth is long, lift the cup halfway up the tooth and make a second stroke toward the occlusal.
7. At the incisal or occlusal edge, lift the cup slightly off the tooth and reposition it near the gingival to repeat the stroke, moving toward the opposite side of the tooth.
8. Repeat the stroke, overlapping each time, until the entire tooth surface is polished.
9. When finished with one tooth, move to the adjacent tooth using the same steps until the surfaces of all teeth have been polished.
10. For the patient's comfort, rinse the mouth frequently, at least after polishing each quadrant.
11. When all teeth have been polished, rinse and evacuate the patient's mouth thoroughly, removing all debris (Figures 32-11A through F).

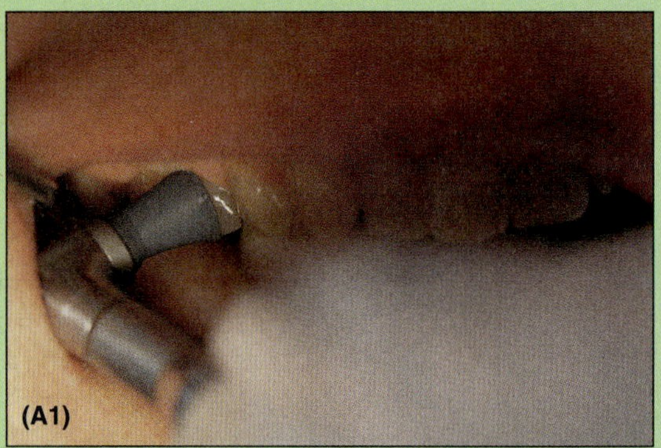
(A1)

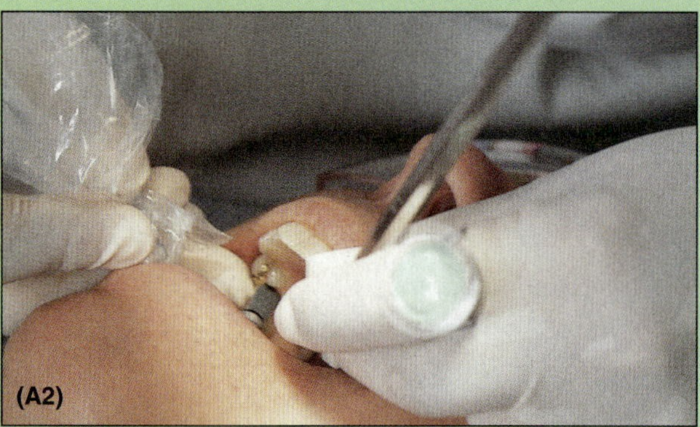
(A2)

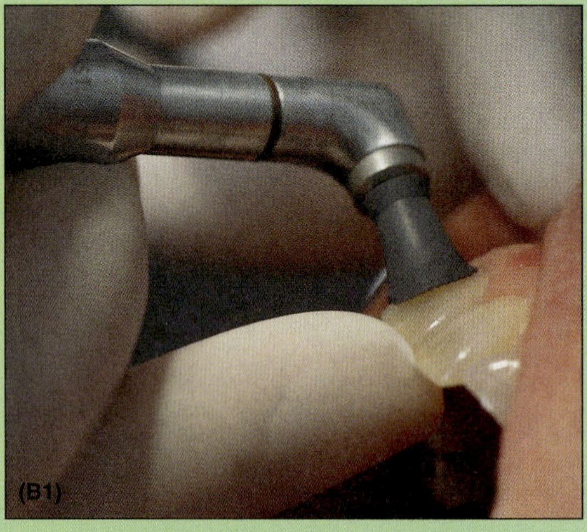
(B1)

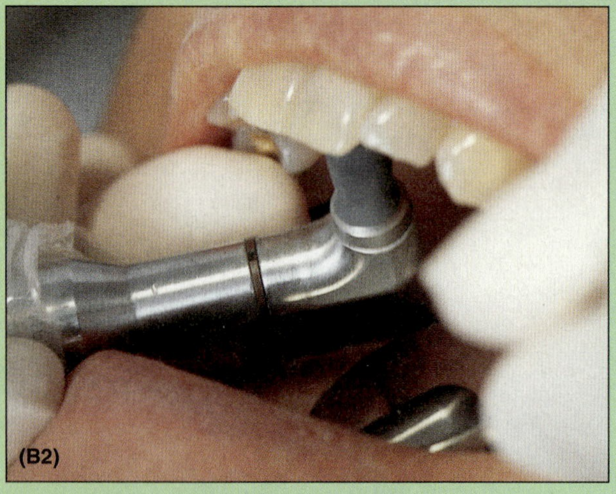
(B2)

FIGURE 32-11

Correct cup placement and fulcrum. (A) Maxillary right posterior, buccal surface and lingual surface. (A1) Cheek is retracted to position cup on tooth. Fulcrum on same arch. (A2) Use indirect vision and fulcrum on same arch. (B) Maxillary anteriors, facial surface and lingual surface. (B1) Retract lip and fulcrum on incisal edge. (B2) Use a mouth mirror for indirect vision.

(continues)

Advanced Chairside Functions

Procedure 32-1 (continued)

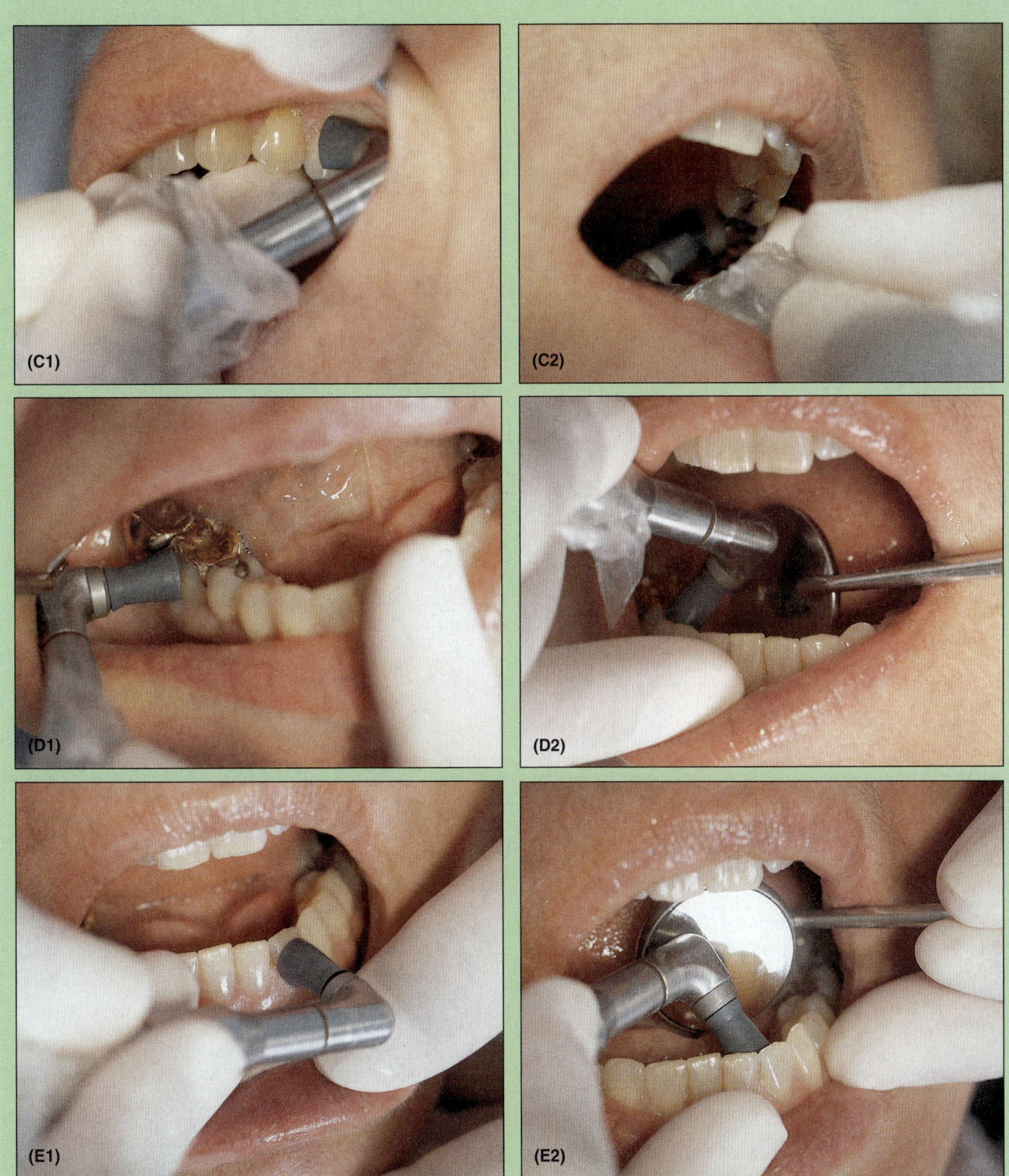

FIGURE 32-11 (continued)
(C) Maxillary left posterior, buccal and lingual surface. (C1) Retract cheek to position prophy angle and have patient close slightly. Fulcrum on same arch. (C2) Adapt cup to lingual surface. (D) Mandibular right posterior, buccal surface and lingual surface. (D1) Retract tissue to place prophy angle and have patient close slightly. (D2) Retract tongue with mouth mirror. (E) Mandibular anteriors, facial and lingual surface. (E1) Retract lip with a finger. (E2) Use mouth mirror for indirect vision and retraction of the tongue.

(continues)

Advanced Chairside Functions (Continued)

Procedure 32-1 (continued)

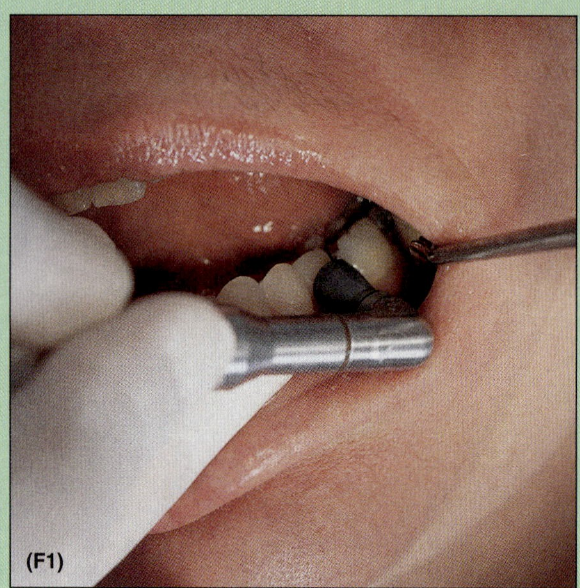

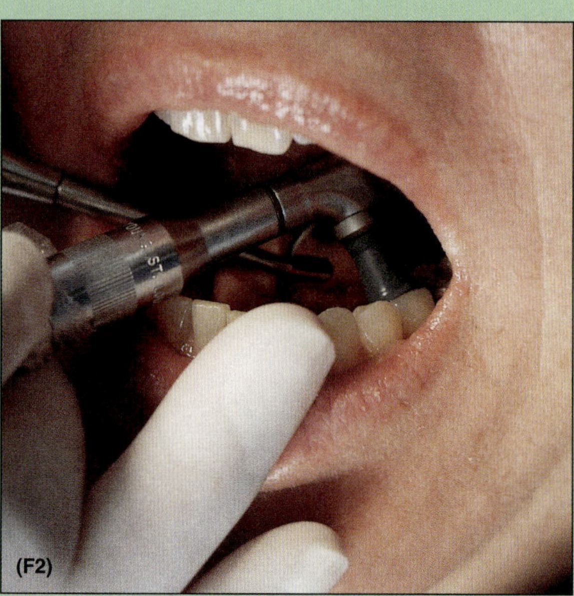

FIGURE 32-11 (continued)

(F) Mandibular left posterior, buccal and lingual surface. (F1) Retract cheek and position prophy cup. (F2) Retract tongue with mouth mirror to position prophy cup.

Procedure 32-2
Using the Prophy Brush

This procedure is performed by the dental assistant, hygienist, or dentist. The prophy brush procedure follows the rubber cup polish, and includes the techniques used to manipulate and position the brush (Figure 32-12).

Equipment and Supplies

- See Procedure 32-1, Polishing with the Rubber Cup.

Procedure Steps (*Follow aseptic procedures*)

1. Place the softened brush on the prophy angle and apply prophy paste to the brush.
2. Establish a fulcrum close to the posterior tooth to be polished.
3. Move the brush bristles toward the mesial buccal cusp tip and continue until the brush comes off the occlusal surface.
4. Replace the brush bristles in the central fossa.
5. Apply slight pressure again, and move the brush up toward the distal buccal cusp until the brush comes off the occlusal surface.
6. Repeat this procedure on the occlusal surface of each posterior tooth until all of the occlusal surfaces are cleaned.
7. Repeat this process on the occlusal surfaces of all teeth.

(continues)

Advanced Chairside Functions

Procedure 32-2 (continued)

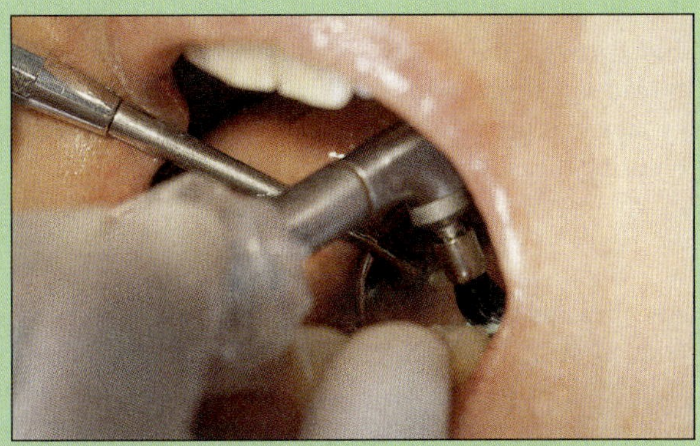

FIGURE 32-12
Prophy brush on occlusal surface.

8. For the lingual surfaces of the anterior teeth, place the prophy brush in the lingual pit, above the cingulum.
9. Apply light pressure to flex and spread the brush bristles.
10. Move the brush toward the incisal edge to polish the lingual surface.
11. Repeat on all lingual surfaces that have deep pits and grooves.
12. When finished with the brush, rinse and evacuate the oral cavity thoroughly.

Procedure 32-3
Polishing with Dental Tape and Dental Floss

    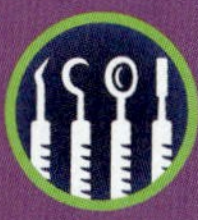

This procedure is part of the coronal polish. After the rubber cup and brush have been used, the interproximal surfaces of the teeth are cleaned with dental tape and then dental floss is used.

Equipment and Supplies

- See Procedure 32-1, Polishing with the Rubber Cup.

Procedure Steps (*Follow aseptic procedures*)

1. Cut off a piece of dental tape 12 to 18 inches long.
2. Wipe some abrasive agent into the interproximal contact areas of the teeth in a quadrant, with a cotton tip or finger.
3. Wrap the tape around the middle fingers of both hands, leaving a length of tape just long enough to wrap around the tooth while maintaining control.
4. Take the tape through the contact at an oblique (slanting or diagonal) angle (\) in a back-and-forth motion, using gentle pressure and holding the tape against the tooth. This assists in preventing the tape from snapping through the contact and damaging the gingiva.
5. Wrap the tape around the tooth to cover the line angles of the tooth on both the buccal and the lingual.
6. When the proximal surface of one tooth is complete, lift the tape up and over the interdental papilla without removing the tape through the contact and readapt the tape on the proximal surface of the adjacent tooth.
7. Polish this surface with the tape and abrasive and then remove the tape up through the contact. If the tape is pulled through the embrasure area, be careful not to injure the gingival tissues.
8. Continue around each tooth in both arches until all proximal surfaces have been polished, including the most distal surface of each quadrant. Use different areas of the tape as needed, and rinse areas thoroughly and evacuate all debris.
9. Follow the taping by using dental floss to remove any remaining debris. Floss all areas and rinse thoroughly.

Advanced Chairside Functions (Continued)

Dental Assistant Guidelines

The dental assistant should follow the guidelines for positioning discussed in previous chapters. When dental assistants become operators, they should sit on the side of the patient where they are most comfortable. For example, a right-handed dental assistant usually finds being on the right side of the patient more convenient. Dental assistants should adjust the operator's chair so that their feet are flat on the floor and movement around the patient's head is unrestricted. The dental assistant usually sits between the 8 and 9 o'clock positions when performing the polish if right-handed and between 3 and 4 o'clock if left-handed.

Patient Considerations

The patient is seated and reclined to the correct height for the dental assistant. During the coronal polish procedure, the patient's head may be positioned up and down and left and right depending on the arch and the quadrant that the dental assistant is working on.

Dental Light Use

The dental light needs to be adjusted for good direct and indirect vision. The dental assistant can maintain good illumination of the mouth by remembering to adjust the light whenever the patient's head position is changed.

Oral Cavity Maintenance

The oral cavity should be rinsed frequently during the polish using the air–water syringe and evacuator. The saliva ejector helps to keep saliva to a minimum if placed in the patient's mouth during use of the prophy cup and brush. This also reduces splattering of the polishing agent. Another way to reduce splattering is to wipe the debris from the cup and the brush with a 2 × 2 inch gauze when removing the cup and brush from the mouth.

Auxiliary Polishing Aids

Several **auxiliary polishing aids** may be needed during a coronal polish. These aids include bridge threaders, abrasive polishing strips, soft wooden points, and small interproximal brushes (Figure 32-13).

Bridge Threaders

The **bridge threader** is used to pull the dental tape and floss under fixed appliances, around orthodontic appliances, and around splints so that all proximal surfaces can be cleaned and polished. There are several types of bridge threaders. Usually, they are made of plastic with loops or eyes for the tape or floss to slide through and pointed ends (Figure 32-14). After the floss or tape is threaded through the eye of the threader on the facial side, slip the pointed end through the gingival embrasure. Once the bridge threader is through the embrasure, take hold of the floss or tape and proceed as described in the previous section on using the dental tape and floss.

Abrasive Polishing Strips

An **abrasive polishing strip** is used occasionally when a small stain is difficult to remove. Polishing strips or "finishing strips" are used only on enamel surfaces. They

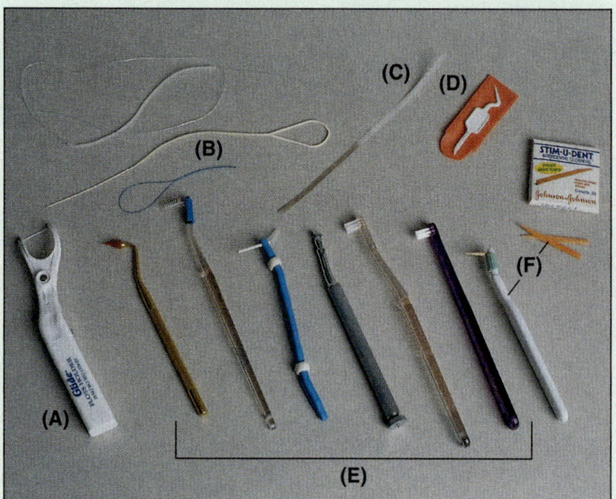

FIGURE 32-13

Various auxiliary polishing aids. (A) Flossing aid. (B) Bridge threaders. (C) Abrasive polishing strip. (D) Disposable interproximal pick. (E) Various small interproximal brushes. (F) Soft wooden points.

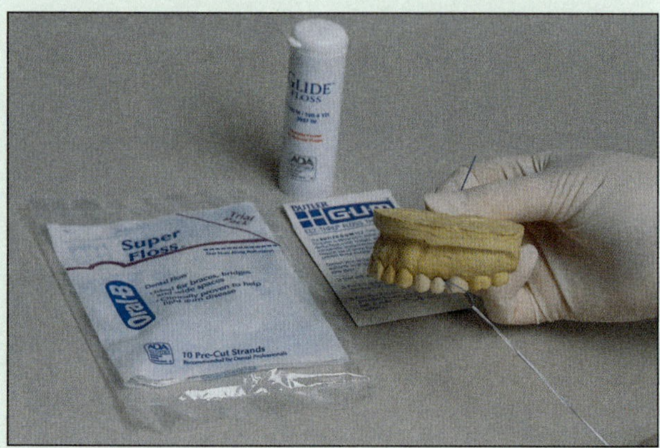

FIGURE 32-14

Bridge threader going under fixed bridge near abutment tooth.

Advanced Chairside Functions

come in various grits and widths. The polishing strip is worked interproximally, pulled tight against the proximal surface of the tooth, and then moved in a back-and-forth motion until the stain is gone. Care must be taken not to cut surrounding soft tissues, because the edges of the strip are sharp.

Soft Wood Points

The **soft wood points** are sometimes used with polishing agents to polish occlusal grooves and pits, proximal surfaces of sensitive teeth, and areas other polishing instruments cannot reach. Soft wood points are made of balsa wood; orangewood sticks; round, wooden toothpicks; and several other types of soft wood. The soft wood points can be used alone or with handles. The points are narrow and come in either wedge shapes for the proximal surfaces or cone shapes for the pits and grooves.

Interproximal Brushes

An **interproximal brush** is a small, soft-bristled brush that comes in a variety of shapes and sizes. The brushes come in packages of three or four and are used by attaching them to metal or plastic handles. After selecting the best shape of brush to clean a specific area, attach the brush to the handle and insert the brush with light pressure. Use a back-and-forth motion to work the brush (Figure 32-15).

Interproximal brushes are useful in the following conditions:

- Open contact areas
- Around orthodontic braces and wires
- Around exposed bifurcation or trifurcation of the roots
- On abutment teeth of a hygienic bridge

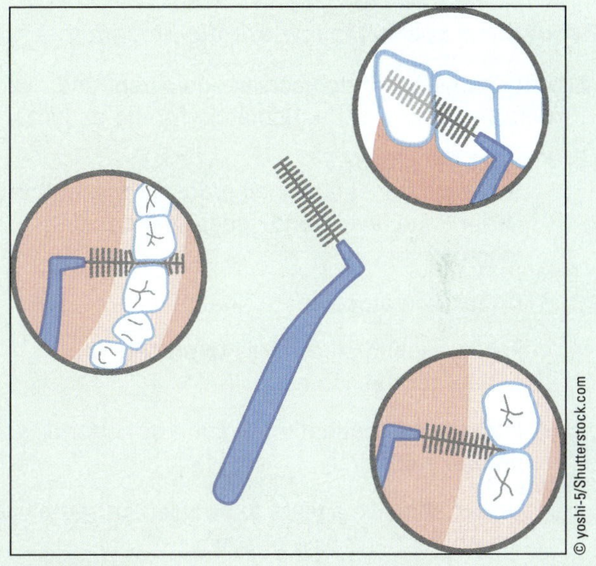

FIGURE 32-15
Interproximal brush

Procedure 32-4
Coronal Polish

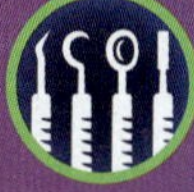

This procedure is performed routinely by the dental assistant and dental hygienist. The protocol for performing a coronal polish is described, including preparation of materials and the patient, positioning of the operator and the patient, sequence of procedure, and evaluating the procedure.

Equipment and Supplies
(*see Figure 32-10*)

- Basic three setup: mouth mirror, explorer, and cotton pliers
- Saliva ejector, HVE tip, and air–water syringe tip
- 2 × 2 inch gauze sponges, cotton-tip applicators, tongue blade, and cotton rolls
- Lip lubricant and disclosing solution in dappen dish
- Low-speed handpiece with prophy angle attachment
- Prophy cups and brushes (dappen dish with warm water to soak brushes in)
- Prophy pastes, with a variety of grits and finger ring holder
- Dental tape and dental floss
- Auxiliary aids as needed

The following items are needed off the tray:

- Patient's chart
- Red/blue pencil, lead pencil, and pen

(continues)

Advanced Chairside Functions (Continued)

Procedure 32-4 (continued)

- Barriers for the dental unit
- Patient napkin and napkin chain
- Patient safety glasses
- Patient hand mirror

Procedure Steps (*Follow aseptic procedures*)

1. After gathering the preceding equipment and materials, prepare the operatory for the patient.
2. Prepare the patient.
   - Following the established procedure, seat the patient and review and update the patient's records.
   - Explain the procedure to the patient.
   - Follow aseptic procedures to prepare the patient for the coronal polish.
   - Evaluate the patient's condition by performing an oral inspection.
   - Select abrasive agents to be used, based on the amount and type of stain.
   - Lubricate the patient's lips, dry the teeth, and apply the disclosing agent with the cotton-tip applicator.
   - Adjust the dental unit light for good vision.
3. Position the operator and the patient. When the operator is polishing the maxillary and mandibular right facial and the maxillary and mandibular left lingual, the patient's head is turned away from the operator (Figure 32-16). When the operator is polishing the maxillary and mandibular right lingual and the maxillary and mandibular left facial, the patient's head is turned toward the operator (Figure 32-17).
4. Initiate the procedure sequence.
   - Begin the polish on the quadrant or arch according to the predetermined, established routine.
   - Follow criteria previously discussed regarding the use of abrasives and the rubber cup, prophy brush, tape, and floss.
   - Rinse the patient's mouth after each quadrant is polished or as needed.

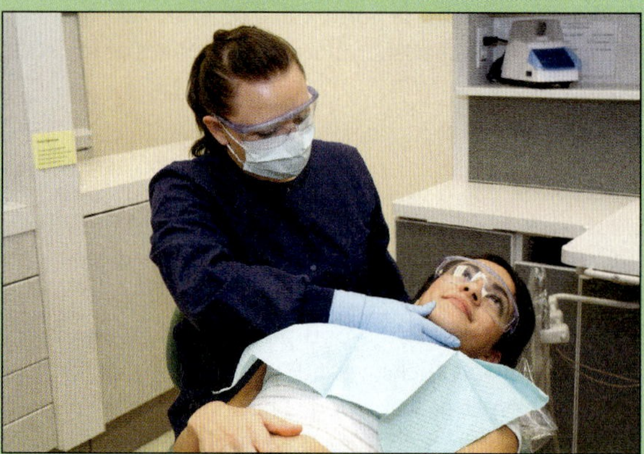

FIGURE 32-16
Positioning patient's head away from dental assistant.

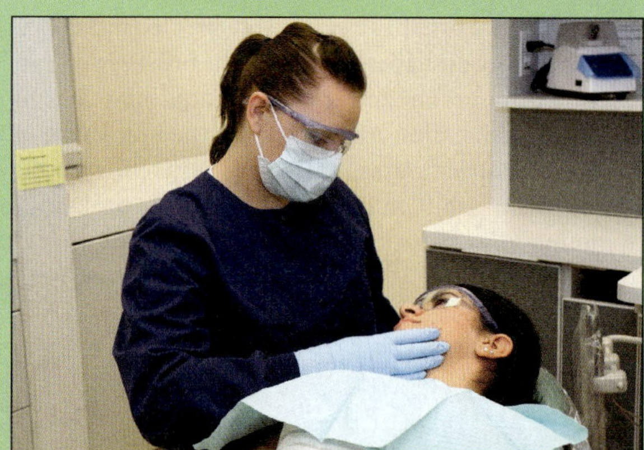

FIGURE 32-17
Positioning patient's head toward the dental assistant.

5. Evaluate coronal polish.
   - Once all steps of the coronal polish have been completed, rinse the patient's mouth thoroughly with spray from the air–water syringe and evacuator.
   - Apply disclosing solution to detect any areas of plaque or stain that were missed.
   - Using the mouth mirror and the air syringe, inspect each surface for any remaining soft deposits and/or stains. Note these areas on the patient's chart or paper for future reference.

(continues)

Advanced Chairside Functions

Procedure 32-4 (continued)

- Polish the areas missed with a prophy cup and/or brush.
- Rinse the patient's mouth to remove all of the abrasive agent.
- Inspect the teeth for a lustrous shine showing no debris or extrinsic stains. The soft tissues should be free of abrasion or trauma. The patient is ready for a fluoride treatment. The dentist may want to see the patient before he or she is dismissed.

6. Chart the coronal polish. It is the dental assistant's responsibility to record the coronal polish completely and accurately on the patient's dental chart. The entry is recorded in ink, dated, and signed or entered into the computer system. Include any comments about the condition of the patient's mouth and type(s) of material(s) used.

Chapter Summary

In the coronal polish chapter there is discussion on the rational for and against performing the coronal polish. Learning about dental deposits and stains aids the dental assistant when trying to remove them and in educating the patient in home care techniques. Materials and equipment required to complete a coronal polish are discussed as well as the techniques. Performing a coronal polish, an expanded function, requires increased skill and responsibility. This task is delegated by the dentist according to the state Dental Practice Act. Some states require additional education, certification, or registration to perform this function.

CASE STUDY

Emery Smith is 15 years old. She was scheduled for a coronal polish procedure. When the dental assistant examined her teeth before beginning the polish, she noticed Emery had orthodontic bands on her molars. She also had yellow/brown stains on the buccal surface of the maxillary molars and the lingual surface of the mandibular incisors.

Case Study Review

1. Would a coronal polish procedure be contraindicated because Emery still had orthodontic bands on her molars? Explain.
2. Are Emery's stains intrinsic or extrinsic? What are the stains likely to be caused by?
3. How would the assistant remove the stains? What materials would work best with the yellow/brown stains?

Review Questions

Multiple Choice

1. The clinical crown on the tooth
   a. may involve the enamel and exposed cementum/dentin.
   b. is the part of the tooth that is visible in the mouth.
   c. is polished during the coronal polish.
   d. All of the above.
2. All of the following are conditions that may require modification of the coronal polish techniques *except*
   a. orthodontic appliances.
   b. hypersensitive teeth.
   c. mixed dentition.
   d. minor oral irritations, such as cold sores.
3. ________ is the soft, bulky mass, white to yellow in color that accumulates on the tooth surface near the gingival tissue.
   a. Pellicle
   b. Plaque
   c. Materia Alba
   d. Food debris
4. A hard, calcified deposit that forms on the teeth, restorations, and dental appliances is called
   a. plaque.
   b. calculus.
   c. materia Alba.
   d. intrinsic stain.
5. All of the following statements are true about dental stains on the teeth *except:*
   a. Stains are found only in mineralized plaque.
   b. Stains are caused by imperfect tooth development and excess fluoride.
   c. Stains are caused by foods, bacteria, tobacco, metals, and drugs.
   d. Stains adhere to the tooth structure, plaque, or calculus .
6. Dental fluorosis is classified as an
   a. intrinsic stain.
   b. extrinsic stain.
7. The abrasive material zirconium silicate is
   a. a mild abrasive, also known as whiting.
   b. a very fine polishing agent used on metallic restorations.
   c. a relatively coarse material and is not used on exposed dentin.
   d. used as a stain removal and polishing agent.
8. All of the following are true statements about the rubber prophy cup *except:*
   a. The prophy cup is used to carry the abrasive agent to polish the teeth.
   b. The prophy cup should be hard and stiff to remove the soft deposits from the teeth.
   c. The rubber prophy cup is made of natural or synthetic rubber materials.
   d. The prophy cup should be soft and flexible to adapt to the contours of the teeth.
9. Apply light pressure to flex the cup and flare it into the sulcus 1 to 2 mm.
   a. This is a *true statement.*
   b. This is a *false statement.*
10. When performing a rubber cup polish, all of the following statements are true *except:*
    a. Use a slow, even speed.
    b. Always use a fulcrum.
    c. Use the edge of the rubber prophy cup to polish.
    d. Start and stop the low-speed handpiece outside the patient's mouth.

Critical Thinking

1. Review auxiliary polishing aids that are available, and then select the polishing aids that you would suggest to a patient who has a fixed bridge.
2. Discuss various ways to ensure that a fulcrum is always used when performing a coronal polish.
3. The coronal polish is the polishing of the "clinical crown," Discuss the clinical crown and what tooth surfaces are polished.
4. Discuss the indications and the contraindications to performing a coronal polish.
5. Discuss how stains are classified and how they are removed.

Web Activities

1. Go to http://www.ada.org/, type in "dental stains" in the search box. Read the articles relating to dental stains.
2. To learn about the many types of fluoride prophy pastes, search the various manufacturers on the web. Find their fluoride prophy pastes and look for the grit, flavors, etc. Suggestions include: Dentsply, Patterson Dental, Henry Schein Dental, and WaterPik.
3. Research your state Dental Practice Act to see if the coronal polish is listed as an expanded function and if a license or registration is required.

CHAPTER

33

Fixed Prosthodontics and Gingival Retraction

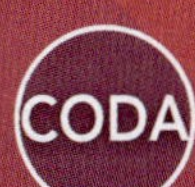

Specific Instructional Objectives

The student should strive to meet the following objectives and demonstrate an understanding of the facts and principles presented in this chapter:

1. Define the scope of fixed prosthodontics.
2. Describe the role of the dental assistant in all phases of fixed prosthodontic treatment.
3. Explain the dentist's considerations when recommending various prostheses to a patient.
4. Describe various types of fixed prostheses and their functions.
5. Describe dental materials used in fixed prostheses.
6. Identify the general steps for the procedure for fixed prostheses.
7. Explain the involvement of the laboratory technician in the fabrication of fixed prostheses.
8. Explain the techniques for retaining the prosthesis when there is little or no crown on the tooth, including core buildups, pins, and posts.
9. Explain the techniques for maintaining fixed prostheses.

Advanced Chairside Functions

10. Explain the function of gingival retraction.
11. Describe the different types of gingival retraction.
12. Explain the steps for placing and removing the gingival retraction cord.

Key Terms

abutments (776)
bevel (783)
bite registration (785)
cantilever bridge (776)
cast restoration (775)
chamfer (783)
core buildup (789)
dental casting alloy (781)
die (788)
direct resin veneer (777)
full-cast crown (775)
gingival retraction (792)
indirect resin veneer (777)
indirect restoration (775)
inlay (775)
ischemia (795)
Maryland bridge (776)
onlay (776)
partial crown (775)
pontic (776)
porcelain veneer (778)
porcelain-fused-to-metal crowns (781)
post-retained core (790)
prostheses (774)
prosthodontist (774)
retention core (789)
retention pin (789)
shade guide (783)
shoulder (783)
silane coupling agent (781)
three-quarter crown (775)
units (776)
veneer (777)

Introduction

Fixed prosthodontics is the specialty that deals with replacement of missing teeth or parts of teeth with extensive restorations. The restorations or **prostheses** (artificial parts for missing tissues) are fabricated in a dental laboratory from detailed impressions taken in the dental office. When finished, the prostheses are cemented permanently in the patient's mouth.

Fixed prostheses replace missing teeth and tooth structures in order to

- restore masticatory function;
- improve esthetics, and often self-esteem;
- improve speech;
- promote good oral hygiene; and
- prevent further movement of the teeth because of support of the prostheses.

The fixed prosthesis becomes part of the natural dentition and is maintained with routine brushing and flossing techniques. The main disadvantages are the expense of the prosthesis and the time involved in preparing the tooth, taking the impression, fabricating the restoration, and permanently cementing it in place. Restorations routinely take at least two appointments to complete. Dental insurance may cover some of the expense of prosthetic restorations.

There are several advantages of having a permanent restoration. The restoration is secure in the mouth, it is esthetic, and it restores function for many years. These advantages outweigh the initial monetary expense and time commitment.

General dentists normally include fixed prosthodontic procedures in their practice; however, cases that are beyond their level of expertise are referred to a specialist. The **prosthodontist** receives additional education and clinical practice to specialize in fixed and removable prosthodontic procedures. Patient cases may include fixed prosthetic procedures that are difficult, involved, and extensive. Such cases might include patients who have had extensive surgery due to cancer of the mouth, or patients who need full mouth reconstruction. The patients are referred by general dentists and other specialists to the prosthodontist.

There are many types of fixed prostheses and a variety of materials are used for their preparation, fabrication, and cementation.

Role of the Dental Assistant

The dental assistant is involved in all stages of fixed prosthodontic treatment. It is important to understand the sequence of the procedure, and the various types of restorations when assisting the dentist. The dental assistant explains the steps of the procedure to the patient, answers questions, and gives postoperative and home care instructions.

Responsibilities include the preparation of equipment and supplies needed for both appointments. Each tray setup is arranged according to the sequence of the procedure, with auxiliary instruments and materials close at hand. The procedures require many different types of dental materials, including alginate, bite registration materials, final impression materials, a retraction cord, temporization materials, and final cements. The dental assistant prepares and utilizes these materials throughout the procedure.

The dental assistant assists the dentist in all aspects of the procedure, from selecting the shade of the tooth to general chairside assisting. In some states, the qualified dental assistant can perform some of the procedures, such as placing the retraction cord, placing and removing temporaries, taking preliminary impressions, and removing excess cement. The dental assistant also coordinates the patient's appointments and the laboratory schedule. In some offices, the dental assistant may perform selected laboratory functions, such as making custom trays and pouring study models.

Dental assistants are also learning new CAD/CAM restorative techniques (refer to Chapter 26, Dental Implants). This involves working with specially designed software and operating the milling chamber. Continued education and training is required to keep up with the latest technology.

Patient Considerations

When a patient needs fixed prosthodontic treatment, the dentist performs an examination that includes the following:

- Medical and dental history
- Examination of the intraoral and extraoral tissues
- Radiographs
- Impressions for study models (diagnostic casts)
- Intraoral photographs taken with an intraoral camera
- Extraoral photographs

Patients who are candidates for fixed prostheses should be in good general health, have healthy supportive tissues, and be motivated to maintain the prostheses. Sometimes, patients need to have periodontal or orthodontic treatment prior to the fixed prosthodontic treatment.

Case Presentation

With less complicated cases, the dentist presents the treatment to the patient at the time of the examination. Other cases require time for the dentist to make the diagnosis and treatment plan before the patient is scheduled for the case presentation.

At the case presentation, the dentist recommends the type of prosthesis and explains what is involved in treatment, including the number of appointments and what the patient can expect. The dentist uses study models, radiographs, pictures of completed cases, samples of various dental prostheses on models, pamphlets, educational videos, and computer images in the presentation. The computer-imaging component shows the patient's before and after images.

When presenting the treatment choices to the patient, the dentist or the office manager explains the cost of the prosthesis, whether insurance will cover any of the treatment, and the number of appointments required. The dentist's business manager works with the patient to meet the cost and time commitments for this treatment. Sometimes the procedure is scheduled over a 2-year time span to take advantage of insurance coverage.

Types of Fixed Prostheses

Fixed prostheses are designed to replace the missing tooth structure in a variety of ways, including full crowns, partial crowns, inlays, onlays, bridges, and veneers. They can be completed using the indirect technique. The indirect technique means the restoration is not placed directly in the tooth preparation as it is with composite and amalgam fillings. The **indirect restoration** involves preparing the tooth, taking impressions, and placing a provisional restoration. The impressions are sent to a commercial laboratory, which then fabricates the permanent prostheses. The patient comes back for a second appointment to have the restoration cemented or bonded in place. This restoration is also known as a **cast restoration**.

Indirect restorations can also be created with the use of the CAD/CAM (computer-aided design/computer-aided manufacturing) technologies (see Chapter 34, Computerized Impressions and Restorative Systems). With a CAD/CAM system the tooth is prepared and the restoration is fabricated right in the office. After the tooth is prepped a computer program is used to design a crown, inlay, and so on. This information is sent to the milling machine, which is right in the office, for fabrication. Once completed the finished restoration is ready to be cemented or bonded in place. The patient only needs one appointment and never has to wear a provisional restoration.

Crowns

Crowns cover teeth that have extensive decay or breakdown. The prepared tooth is covered with an anatomically shaped and fitted crown. Crowns are constructed of various materials including full gold crowns, porcelain-fused-to-metal crowns, or full porcelain crowns. The tooth may require a full crown, which is often referred to as a **full-cast crown** (Figures 33-1A and B). A full crown covers the entire coronal surface of the tooth. Sometimes, the tooth is broken down so badly that means to retain the full crown on the tooth are required. (Retention is discussed later in this chapter.)

A **partial crown** is a cast restoration that covers three or more, but not all, surfaces of a tooth. A **three-quarter crown** is normally prepared so that the mesial, distal, and lingual surfaces are reduced but the facial surface is left intact (Figure 33-2). The incisal or occlusal surface of the tooth is also reduced.

Inlays and Onlays

Inlays and onlays are restorations that replace the missing tooth structure within the tooth. An **inlay** covers the area between the cusps in the middle of the tooth, and the proximal

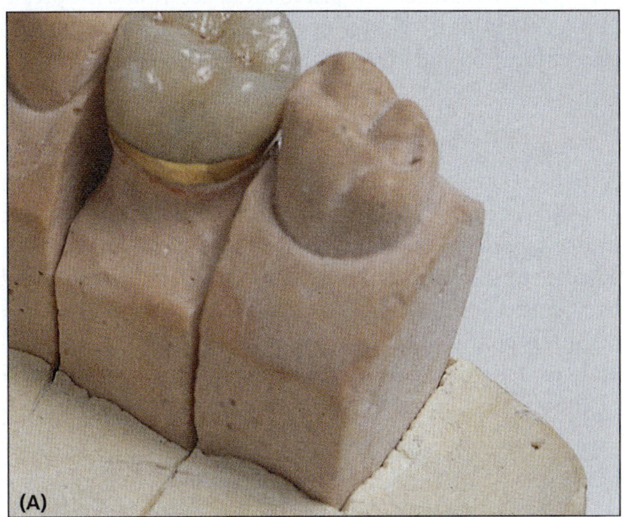

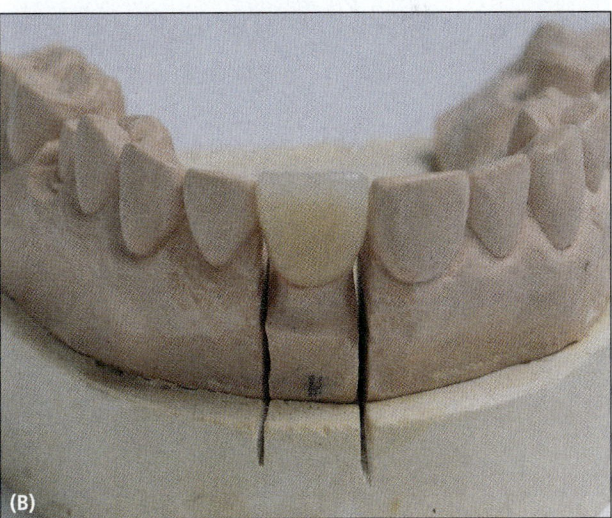

FIGURE 33-1
(A) Porcelain-fused-to-metal crown. (B) Full porcelain crown.

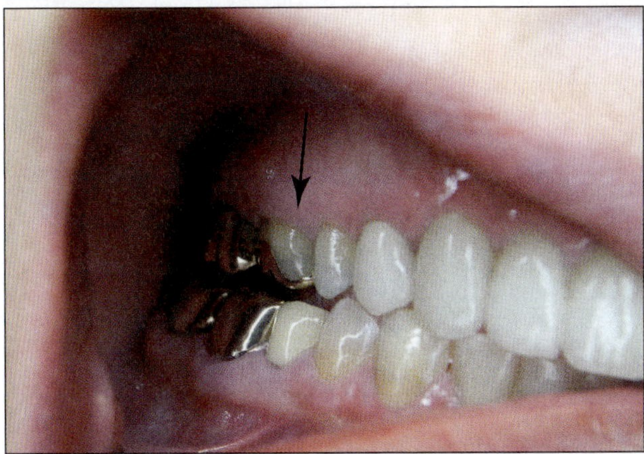

FIGURE 33-2
Three-quarter crown.

surfaces that are involved (Figure 33-3A). Inlays are MOD (mesio-occluso-distal), MO (mesio-occlusal), DO (disto-occlusal), or O (occlusal). An **onlay** is like an inlay except it includes the cusp ridges of the tooth (Figure 33-3B). Inlays and onlays are also cast restorations that are made of a variety of materials. The extent of the lost tooth structure and the preparation determine which type of cast restoration is best suited to restore function and preserve the strength of the tooth.

Bridges

A bridge is a restoration that spans the space of a missing tooth or teeth. The bridge is divided into **units**, and each unit of a bridge represents a tooth. A bridge may replace one or more adjacent teeth in the same arch. The missing tooth is replaced by a **pontic**, which can be designed in a variety of forms. Two common pontics are the hygienic (free cleansing/sanitary) and cosmetic (ovate). The hygienic pontics allow for space between the tissue and pontic, usually seen in the posterior area. The cosmetic pontics are tooth colored and fill in the entire space to the gingival tissue.

The teeth adjacent to the pontic are called **abutments**. Crowns, inlays, or onlays may be placed on the abutment teeth to support and stabilize the pontic (Figures 33-4A and B).

Bridges are made of a variety of materials to meet the patient's esthetic and functional needs. After the bridges have been fabricated, they are permanently cemented in the patient's mouth. Bridges can also be retained by one or two teeth on the same side. This type of bridge is known as a **cantilever bridge**. The cantilever bridge is used in areas of the mouth that are under less stress, such as the front teeth. This procedure involves anchoring the false tooth to one side over one or more natural and adjacent teeth.

A **Maryland bridge**, or resin-retained fixed bridge, is used to replace one tooth. Abutment teeth have very little tooth structure removed during preparation. The bridge consists of a pontic with extensions (retainers) of varying shapes. The

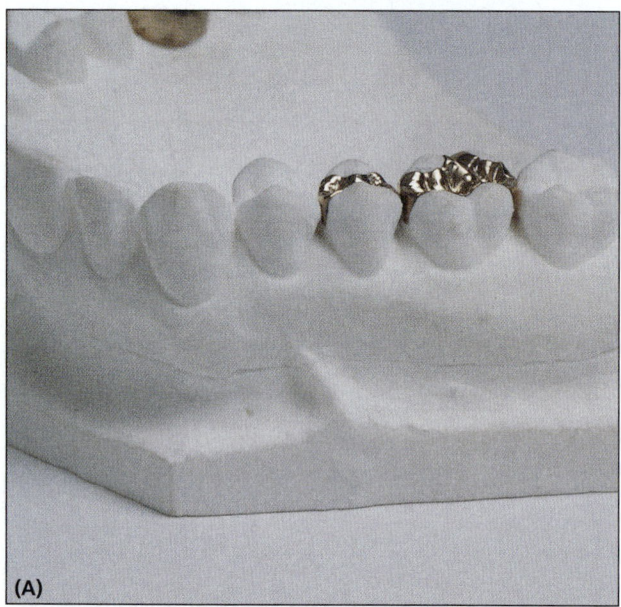

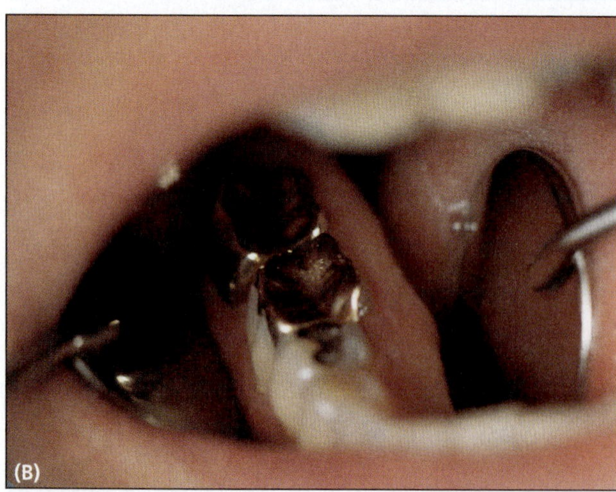

FIGURE 33-3

(A) Gold inlay restorations. (B) Gold onlay restoration on a mandibular first molar.

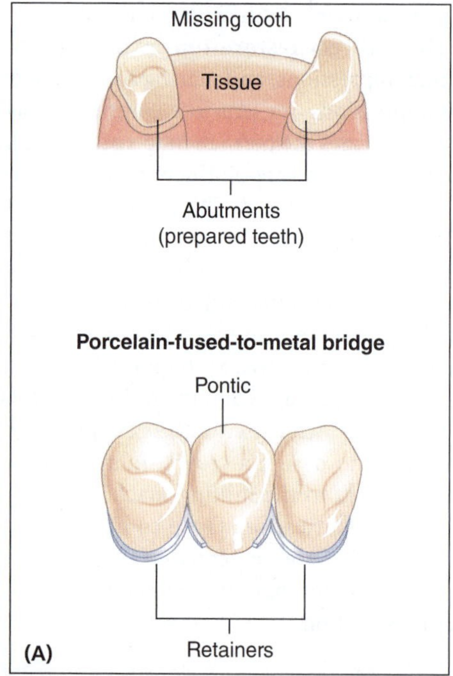

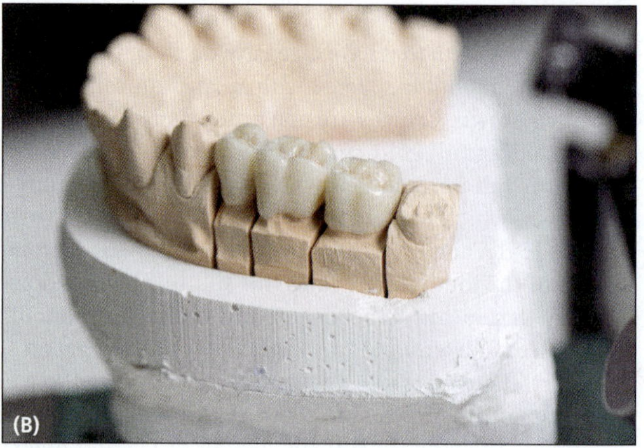

FIGURE 33-4

Three-unit bridge abutments, pontics, and retainers.

extensions are designed to attach to the abutment teeth, on or toward the lingual surface. The retainers of the Maryland bridge are roughened by electrolytic etching to increase their bonding to the natural tooth structure (Figure 33-5).

Preparation of the teeth for the Maryland Bridge is usually minimal. The impressions are taken and temporaries may be placed. The laboratory procedures are the same for all cases except the electrolytic etching of the inside of the bridge retainers. Cementation steps are as follows:

1. A dental dam is placed to protect the tissues from the acid etching.
2. The abutment teeth are cleaned with pumice and water, and then rinsed and dried thoroughly.
3. The prepared surfaces of the teeth are acid etched for 30 to 60 seconds, rinsed thoroughly, and dried.
4. A dual-cured composite cementing material is applied to the etched surfaces of the bridge retainers and the etched tooth surface.
5. The bridge is positioned on the abutment teeth.
6. Once the material has set, excess cement material is removed.

Veneers

A **veneer** is a thin layer of tooth-colored material that covers much of the facial surface. Veneers are used to cover teeth stained intrinsically; teeth affected by abrasion, erosion, and enamel hypoplasia; or to reshape the anatomy of the teeth. Veneers improve appearance with very little removal of the tooth structure. Examples include the following:

- Full facial coverage on anterior maxillary teeth—covered with veneers for a natural appearance (Figures 33-6A and B).
- Tetracycline stains on the maxillary anterior teeth—veneers cover the stain for improved appearance (Figures 33-7A and B).
- Diastema (an abnormal space between two adjacent teeth in the same arch) on maxillary central incisors—veneers close the space (Figures 33-8A and B).

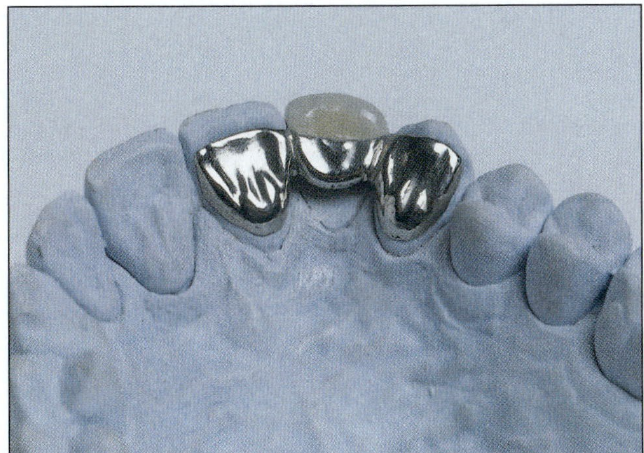

FIGURE 33-5
Maryland bridge.

Veneer procedures are changing constantly as technology progresses. There are many types of veneers, materials used, and techniques. Direct resin veneers, indirect resin veneers, and porcelain veneers are the three types that are discussed in the following sections.

Direct Resin Veneers. A **direct resin veneer** is made in the dental office directly on the patient's tooth. This procedure requires one appointment. In preparation for the veneer procedure, little, if any, tooth structure is removed. The tooth is etched, adhesive is applied, and opaquers and body shade are placed. The incisal shade follows. The shade can be varied between the incisal edge and body of the veneer. The veneers are contoured and finished. Generally, these materials are light cured and require routine polishing and periodic maintenance.

Indirect Resin Veneers. An **indirect resin veneer** requires two appointments. At the first appointment, the tooth is prepared and an impression is taken. The impression is sent to the laboratory for fabrication of the veneer. During the second appointment, the veneer is bonded in place. These veneers do not bond well to resin cement. They lack strength and wear at a faster rate than porcelain veneers.

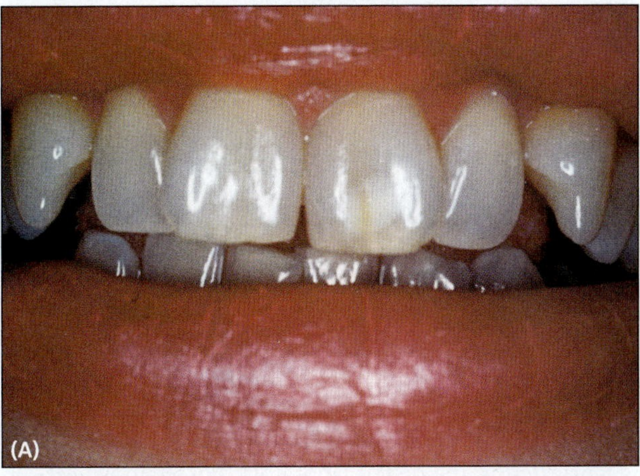

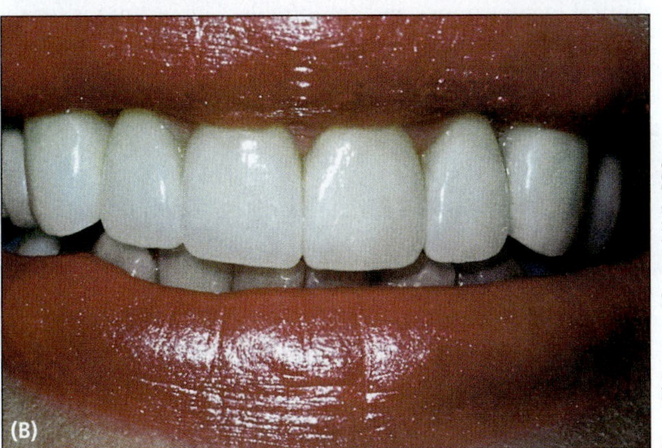

(A and B) Courtesy of George J. Velis, DDS

FIGURE 33-6
Veneers on anterior teeth. (A) Before placement. (B) After placement of veneers.

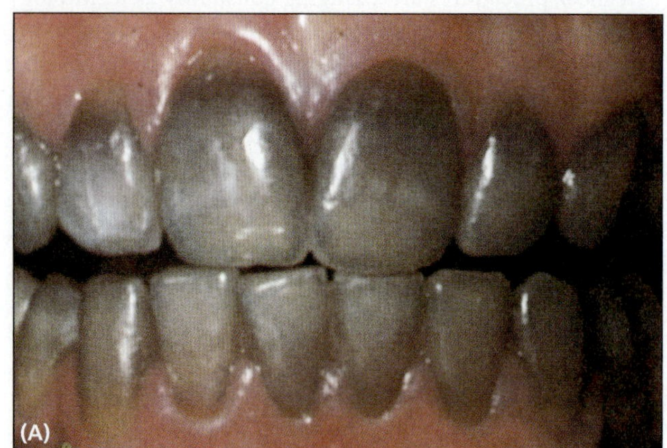

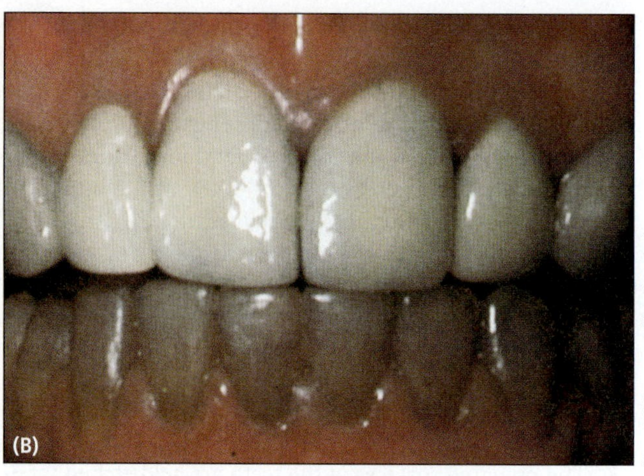

(A and B) Courtesy of Kerr Corporation

FIGURE 33-7

(A) Patient with tetracycline staining. (B) Patient with tetracycline staining after direct resin veneers have been placed.

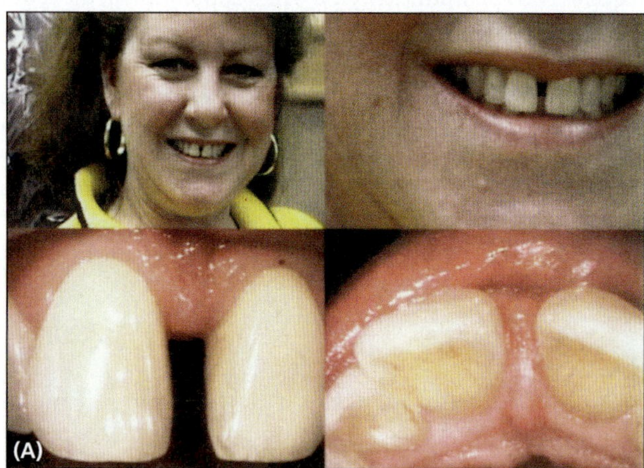

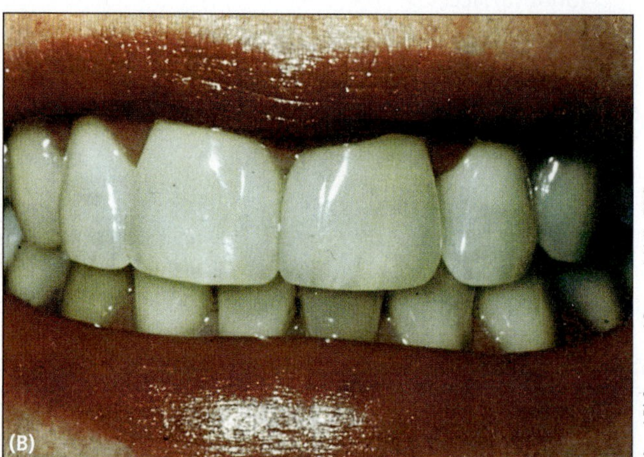

(A and B) Courtesy of George J. Velis, DDS

FIGURE 33-8

(A) Patient with diastema between two central incisors. (B) Same patient with diastema after indirect resin veneers have been placed.

Porcelain Veneers. A **porcelain veneer** is similar to an indirect resin veneer in that it requires two appointments and is fabricated in the dental laboratory. Porcelain veneers are natural in appearance and are durable. The technique for the porcelain veneer is sensitive to shade selection and gingival margin adaptation if the veneer is to look natural and adapt well. Procedure 33-1 outlines the steps involved in placing porcelain veneers.

Procedure 33-1
Porcelain Veneers

This procedure is performed by the prosthodontist and is completed in two appointments. During the first appointment, the tooth is prepared and impressions are taken; at the second appointment, the porcelain veneer is applied. Between appointments, the impressions are sent to a dental laboratory, where the porcelain veneer is fabricated.

Equipment *(For the preparation appointment) (Figure 33-9)*

- Basic setup: mouth mirror, explorer, and cotton pliers
- Cotton rolls and 2 × 2 inch gauze
- HVE tip and air–water syringe tip

(continues)

Procedure 33-1 (continued)

- Anesthetic setup
- High-speed handpiece and assorted burs
- Shade guide
- Spoon excavator
- Low-speed handpiece with prophy angle, rubber cup, and pumice
- Retraction cord and placement instrument
- Bite registration materials
- Alginate impression materials for model of opposing arch
- Final impression materials (polysiloxane or polyether)
- Provisional veneer (optional)
- Laboratory prescription form

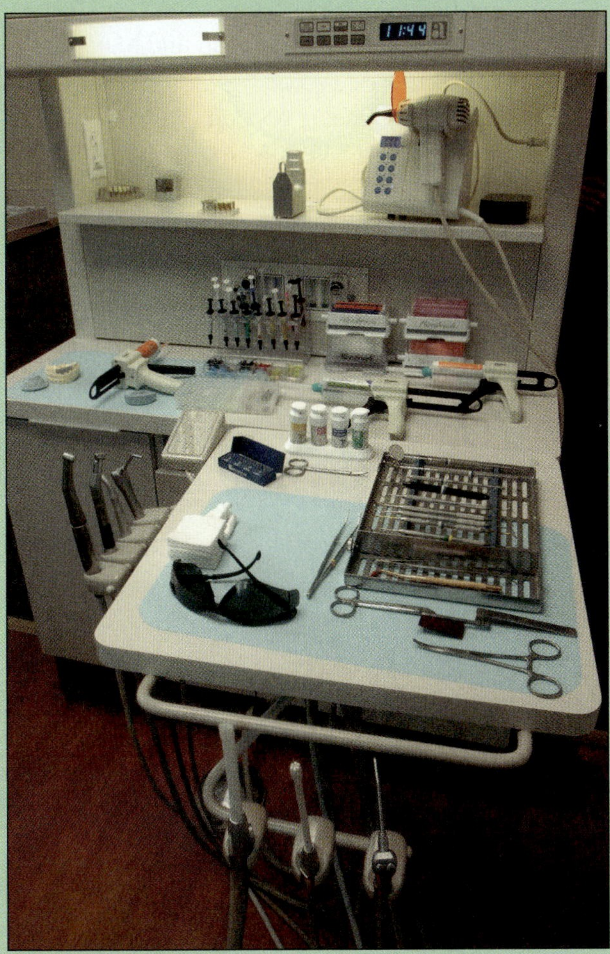

FIGURE 33-9

Porcelain veneers tray set up for preparation appointment, including the impression materials, bite registration materials, curing light, shade guide, and provisional materials.

Procedure Steps (*Follow aseptic procedures*)

Preparation Appointment (First Appointment)

1. Bite registration and opposing arch impression are taken.
2. The teeth are cleaned with a rubber cup and pumice to remove extrinsic stains. A shade is selected by the dentist to determine how light the patient wants the veneers and to estimate how light the finished shade will be.
3. The teeth are prepared according to the design of the veneer. The incisal edge and the cervical margin are prepared carefully so that the finished veneer is even with the gingival crest, or just slightly subgingival.
4. The retraction cord is placed to achieve hemostasis and ensure visualization of the margins.
5. A final impression is taken with a dimensionally stable material such as polysiloxane or polyether.
6. Provisional veneers are placed if necessary, although most patients do not require provisional veneers.
7. The retraction cord is removed after the provisional veneers are placed.
8. The patient is informed that the gums will be tender for several days because of the retraction cord placement.
9. The patient is dismissed.

Laboratory Fabrication

1. The impressions are disinfected and sent to the dental laboratory with a laboratory prescription.
2. The laboratory follows the dentist's prescription regarding length of veneer, shade, thickness, and texture. Color photos of the patient are helpful in the designing and shading process.
3. The laboratory fabricates the veneers and returns them to the office.

Equipment (*For the cementation appointment*) (*Figure 33-10*)

- Basic setup: mouth mirror, explorer, and cotton pliers
- Cotton rolls, 2 × 2 inch gauze, and cheek and lip retractors
- Saliva ejector, HVE tip, and air–water syringe tip
- Porcelain veneers from the laboratory

(continues)

Procedure 33-1 (continued)

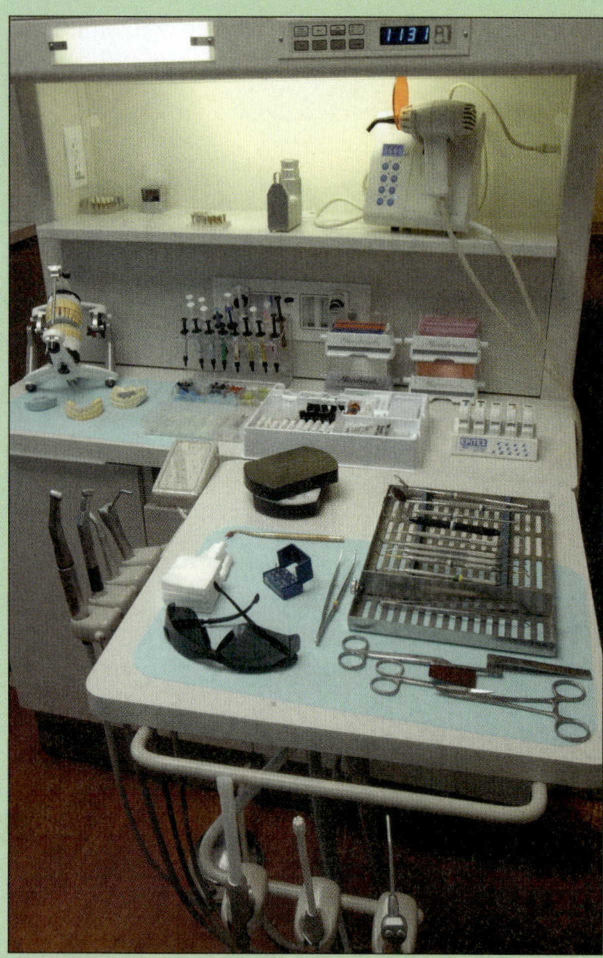

FIGURE 33-10
Porcelain veneers tray setup for cementation appointment, including veneers back from the lab, curing light, and permanent cement/bonding agent.

- Low-speed handpiece with prophy angle, rubber cup, and pumice
- Silane coupling agent and small applicator (brush)
- Retraction cord and placement instrument
- Chlorhexidine soap
- Plastic or ultrathin metal strips
- Etchant and applicator
- Bonding agent and curing light

Cementation Appointment (Second Appointment)

1. The second appointment should be scheduled as soon as possible after the first appointment because the patient is often without provisional coverage. The laboratory should be scheduled ahead of time so the turnaround time is minimal.
2. Complete a preliminary cleaning of the teeth with pumice to remove plaque and stains.
3. The veneers are tried on the tooth and adjustments are made with finishing diamonds. The veneers are very fragile and require careful handling.
4. Once all adjustments are complete, clean and dry the inside of the veneers thoroughly. Acid etchant is used to clean and decontaminate the inside surface of the veneer.
5. Apply a thin layer of silane coupling agent (this material allows bonding to porcelain).
6. Place the light-cured bonding agent in the veneers. Make sure there are no air bubbles. The material fills the veneer and is spread evenly. The veneers are then placed in a light-protected area or box until the teeth are prepared.
7. Prepare the teeth for bonding by placing a retraction cord on the facial surface. Clean the facial surface with chlorhexidine soap and a prophy cup or brush.
8. Isolate the teeth being bonded with cotton rolls, cheek and lip retractors, a saliva ejector, and plastic or ultrathin metal strips.
9. Etch the teeth to be bonded, following the directions of the adhesive system's manufacturer.
10. Apply the adhesive to the teeth being bonded.
11. Seat each veneer in the correct position.
12. In some cases, the veneer is spot cured and excess cement is removed.
13. Light cure each veneer in place.
14. Remove excess cement with a scalpel.
15. Contour and refine the margins with finishing diamonds or burs (Figure 33-11).
16. Polish the veneers with rubber wheels, cups, and polishing paste.

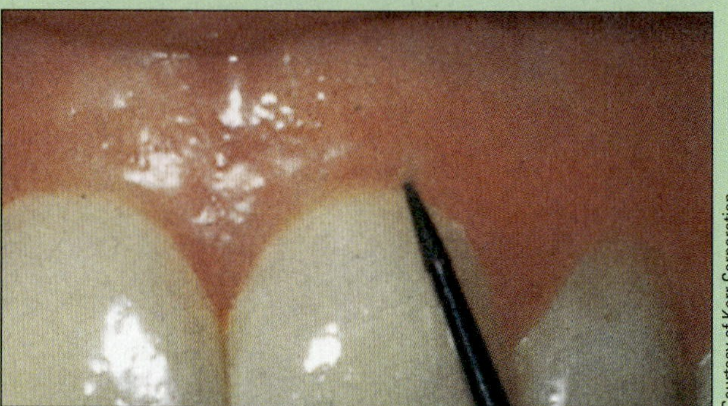

Courtesy of Kerr Corporation

FIGURE 33-11
Finishing porcelain veneer margins with diamond bur.

Types of Materials Used for Fixed Prostheses

CDA The materials used for the construction of fixed crowns, bridges, inlays, onlays, and veneers depend, among other considerations, on their locations in the mouth, required strength, amount of tooth structure, and esthetics—although at one time having gold showing was desirable, natural-looking teeth are the current trend. Because patients want tooth-colored restorations, porcelain and composite materials are commonly used today.

Before discussing the types of materials used to construct fixed prostheses, many materials used during the various procedures should also be mentioned. In the initial preparation appointment and final cementation appointment, the following materials are used:

- Shade guide—a holder with a number of different shades that usually has a variety of light and dark shades in yellow, brown, white, and black tones. The shade guide is used to determine the finished shade of the prostheses. The shade guide is held next to the tooth and the shade is taken under natural light with the teeth slightly moist.

Digital Shade Guide

The new digital shade guide will measure tooth shades under any lighting condition. It is used to measure natural teeth, evaluate bleaching progress, and check restoration for shade accuracy. This shade guide measures a number of shades to meet the accuracy needed to achieve the closest match possible. The digital shade guide is used to take measurements at the cervical (neck) surface of the tooth, the middle or central portion of the tooth, and at the incisal edge. Up to 25 measurements are stored within the machine, and the information is integrated with the accompanying software for the precise shade solution.

- Alginate impression material—used to take an opposing arch impression and to make a provisional restoration.
- Bite registration materials—used to take an impression of how the patient bites. Materials used for bite registration include wax and polysiloxane.
- Retraction cord—used to retract the gingival tissue around the prepped tooth.
- Final impression material—used to take a final impression of the prepped tooth. Various types of final impression materials are used including silicone (modified polysiloxane and polyvinyl), polysulfide, polyether, and hydrocolloid. The final impression is poured in stone (a high-strength die stone, see Chapter 39, Laboratory Materials and Techniques) to make the *master cast*, which is used to construct the prosthesis.
- Provisional cement—used to cement provisional restorations.
- Bonding agent—used to assist in the bonding of permanent restorations. The bonding agent is placed before the permanent cement.
- Permanent cement—used to cement permanent restorations. Permanent cements include polycarboxylate, glass ionomer, resins, or a combination of these materials.
- **Silane coupling agent**—allows bonding between ceramic materials (i.e., composite fillers and porcelain) to polymer resins.

To learn more about these materials or to review them, see Chapter 37, Dental Cements, Bases, Liners, and Bonding Agents, and Chapter 39, Laboratory Materials and Techniques.

Gold Casting Alloys

Gold used in crowns, inlays, and onlays is not pure gold but a combination of metals. When two or more metals are combined, they form an alloy. Pure gold is too soft for use in cast restorations; therefore, other metals, such as platinum and palladium, are added, along with iron, tin, or zinc, to form a **dental casting alloy**.

Restorations made of gold alloy include full gold crowns, inlays, and onlays. These are fabricated mainly for the posterior teeth where they are less visible. Gold crowns are also fabricated with tooth-colored veneers. The veneers may cover the entire crown or just the facial surface. Crowns that have veneers are known as **porcelain-fused-to-metal crowns**, or ceramometal crowns (Figures 30-12A and B).

Porcelain-fused-to-metal crowns are very popular and are commonly used where strength and esthetics are needed. These crowns resist fracture, abrasion, and discoloration, and are used in all areas of the mouth for single-tooth restorations or bridges. The disadvantages are that the tooth requires more reduction to allow for the thickness of the porcelain, and that the porcelain is abrasive and can wear down natural teeth or metal restorations.

Tooth-Colored Cast Restorations

Tooth-colored cast restorations are made either of porcelain or composite resin. Use of these materials is increasing for esthetic reasons. Porcelain is used for inlays, bonded veneers, porcelain-fused-to-metal crowns, and bridges. Porcelain cast restorations require at least two appointments and are more expensive than gold cast restorations. Porcelain, a type of ceramic, resembles the natural tooth structure but is not as strong when used alone. Porcelain is susceptible to fracture under occlusal stresses, but resin-bonding techniques have reduced this concern. Restorations that are solely porcelain are used mainly on single teeth, and rarely for fixed bridges.

Composite-resin indirect technique restorations are fabricated in a dental laboratory. Inlays, onlays, and veneers are made from impressions taken at the first appointment; then

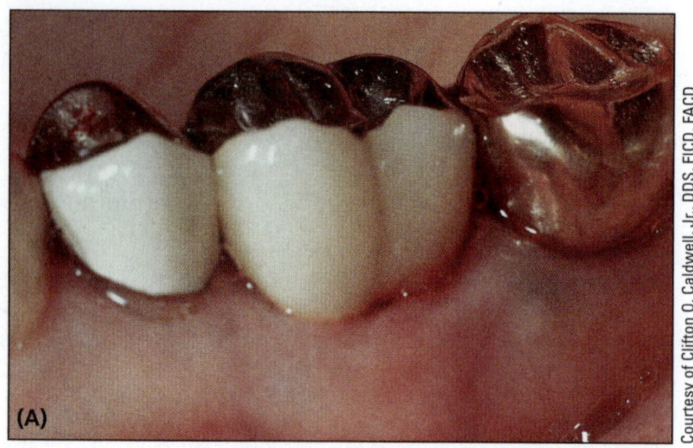

Courtesy of Clifton O. Caldwell, Jr., DDS, FICD, FACD

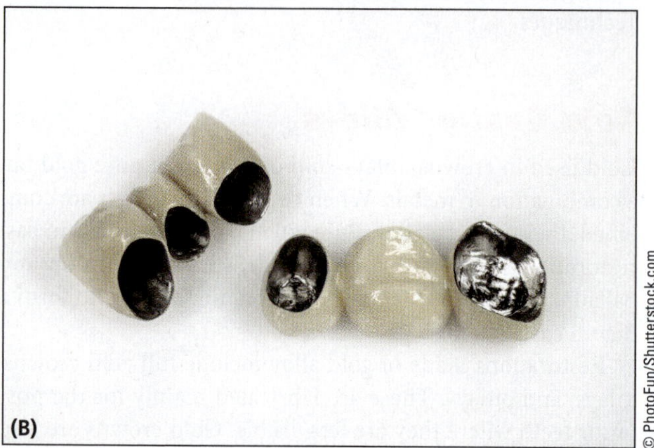

© PhotoFun/Shutterstock.com

FIGURE 33-12

(A) Bridge with a full gold crown on the second molar, and two metal crowns with porcelain facings on the first molar and the second bicuspid. (B) Porcelain-fused-to-metal bridges.

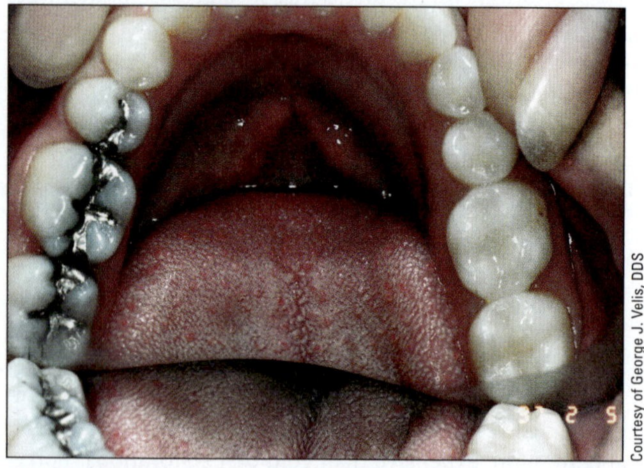

Courtesy of George J. Velis, DDS

FIGURE 33-13

Mirror view of composite resin inlays on patient's left mandibular.

the dental laboratory creates the restorations from composite resin material. This material is heated and placed under pressure. These restorations are stronger than direct composite resin restorations and are bonded in place during the second appointment (Figure 33-13).

General Steps in Fixed Prosthesis Procedures

After the initial appointment, and once the patient has agreed to the treatment, there are general steps followed in all fixed prosthesis procedures, which are usually completed in two appointments. These steps may vary depending upon the type of prostheses and the impression materials used. The appointments are scheduled with the lab to determine the amount of time they need to complete the crown, bridge, inlay, onlay, or veneer (usually about 2 weeks). The CAD/CAM computerized systems allow all the steps to be completed in 1 day (see Chapter 34, Computerize Impressions and Restorative Systems).

The steps for the prosthesis procedures include the following:

1. Patient is given a local anesthetic.
2. The dental assistant takes an alginate impression for fabrication of the provisional, and for use as a model of the opposing arch.
3. A shade is taken with the shade guide and recorded on the patient chart and lab prescription.
4. The tooth is then prepared by the dentist.
5. A retraction cord is placed around the prepared tooth to clearly see the preparation margins.
6. The retraction cord is removed, and the final impression is taken. This is usually a two-step process: the syringe material is placed first, and then the tray material.
7. The dental assistant then takes the bite registration. Note that the bite registration may be taken with the alginate impression at the beginning of the procedure.
8. The dental assistant fabricates, places, and adjusts the provisional coverage.
9. The patient is dismissed.
10. At the second appointment, the patient is given a local anesthetic.
11. The provisional is removed and debris is rinsed off.
12. The dentist tries the crown on the patient, checks the patient's occlusion, and adjusts with burs, discs, and stones.
13. Permanent cement is prepared and placed into the prosthesis.
14. The prosthesis is given to the dentist to seat.
15. Once the cement has dried the patient's bite is sometimes checked one more time.
16. The patient is dismissed.
17. The dental assistant gathers and disinfects the alginate impressions, the bite registration, and the final impression. The dental assistant then prepares the lab prescription for lab delivery.

Procedures 33-2 and 33-3 present the steps and techniques for the preparation and cementation of porcelain-fused-to-metal crowns.

Procedure 33-2
Preparation for a Porcelain-Fused-to-Metal Crown

This procedure is performed by the prosthodontist and dental assistant. Like the porcelain veneer procedure, this process involves two appointments. The following procedure includes the steps in the preparation appointment, including retention procedures, and steps in the cementation appointment.

Equipment (*Figure 33-14*)

- Basic setup: mouth mirror, explorer, and cotton pliers
- Cotton rolls, gauze, dental floss, articulating paper, and forceps
- HVE tip, saliva ejector, and three-way syringe tip
- Anesthetic setup
- Dental dam setup
- High-speed handpiece with a selection of diamonds, discs, and burs
- Irreversible hydrocolloid (alginate) impression materials
- Spoon excavator, scaler, plastic filling instrument, and cement spatula
- Tooth shade guide (optional)
- Retention materials depending on the amount of tooth structure retained—core buildup materials and post-retention pins (optional)
- Gingival retraction cord and placement instrument
- Final impression materials and tray (stock or custom tray)
- Bite registration materials

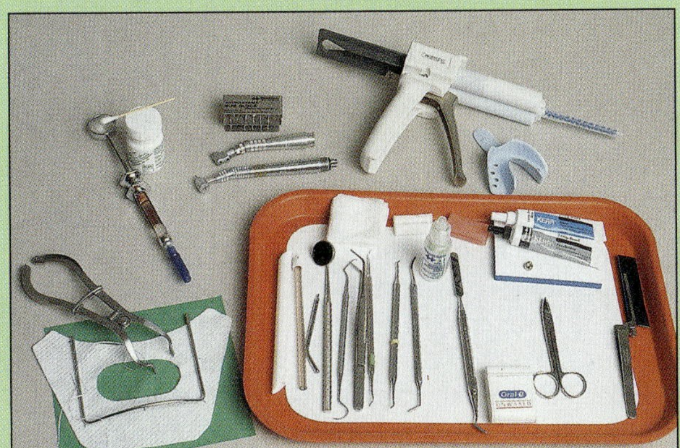

FIGURE 33-14
Tray setup for the preparation appointment.

- Crown and collar scissors
- Provisional coverage materials
- Low-speed handpiece with burs, discs, and stones
- Laboratory prescription and container for impressions (off-tray item)

Procedure Steps (*Follow aseptic procedures*)

1. The patient is given a local anesthetic. Prepare the syringe, transfer the syringe to the prosthodontist, and, during the administration of the anesthetic, observe the patient.
2. Alginate impressions are taken for fabrication of certain types of temporaries, and also for a model of the opposing arch. Select the trays, mix the irreversible hydrocolloid, and take the impressions. The impressions are stored properly until needed and/or poured in plaster or stone. See Chapter 39, Laboratory Materials and Techniques.
3. While waiting for the anesthetic to be effective before the tooth is prepared, the tooth shade is selected. A **shade guide** is used to match the natural teeth.

NOTE: This is a very important step for the esthetics of the crown and the appearance of the patient. The shade guide includes a variety of shades, and the shades can be variegated to match the varying shading of the patient's natural teeth (Figure 33-15A).

Moisten the shade guide and hold it close to the natural teeth under natural light (Figure 33-15B). The patient's teeth should be wet also. Record the information on the patient's chart and on the laboratory prescription.

4. Crowns are prepared with the high-speed handpiece with various diamonds and burs. The tooth must be reduced to accommodate the thickness of the metal and porcelain materials, and to have enough strength.
5. The margins of the preparation are either finished in a **chamfer** or **shoulder** preparation. The chamfer provides adequate bulk and extends easily into the gingival sulcus. The shoulder provides a ledge that is sometimes beveled (Figure 33-16). A **bevel** is an angled or slanted, instead of horizontal, surface. Prepare and

(continues)

Procedure 33-2 (continued)

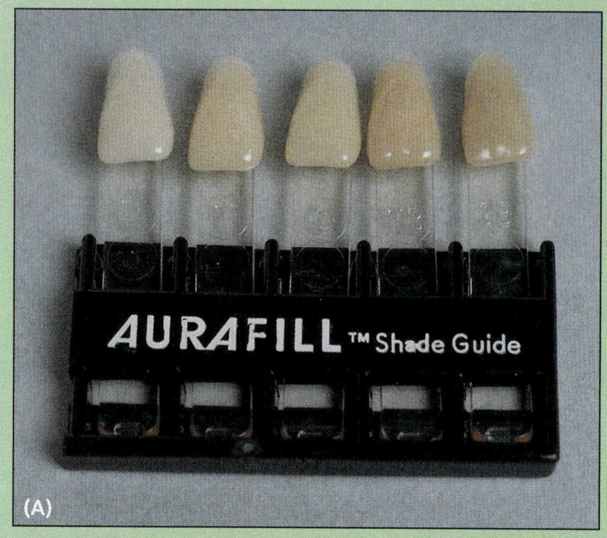

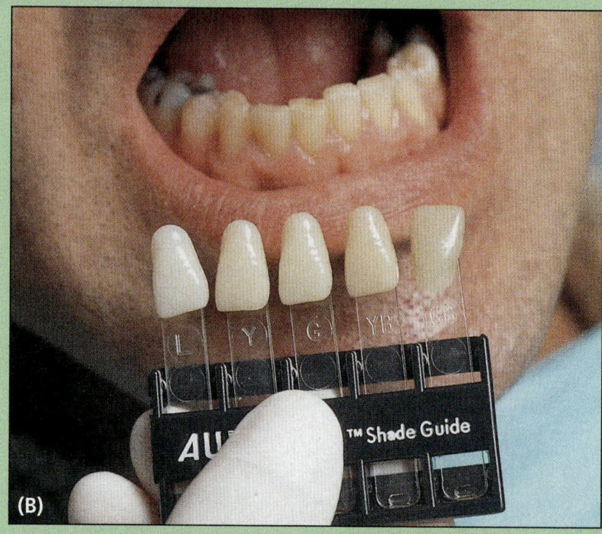

FIGURE 33-15

(A) Shade guide. (B) Matching the shade guide to a patient's natural teeth.

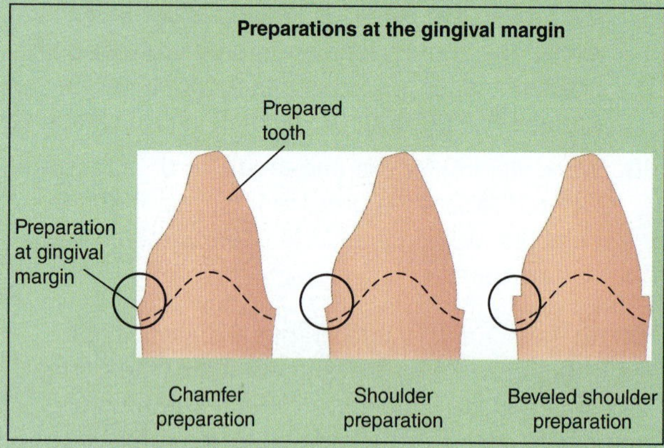

FIGURE 33-16

Examples of how the dentist prepares the margin of the tooth for a crown restoration.

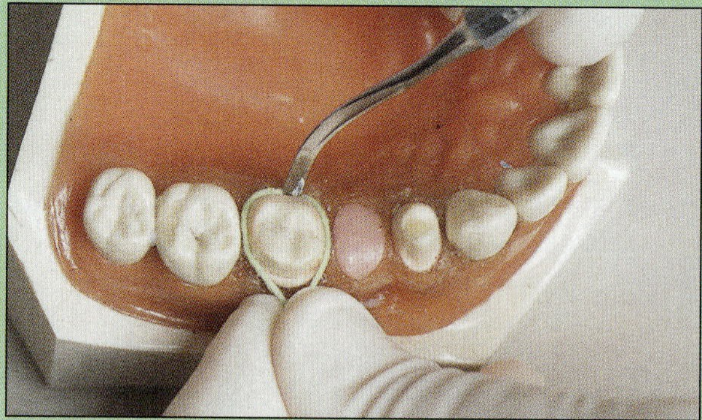

FIGURE 33-17

Placing the retraction cord around a prepared tooth.

transfer the high-speed handpiece, and then evacuate and maintain the operating field with the air–water syringe. Retract and exchange instruments as needed.

Tooth Preparation for Crowns

The abutment teeth are prepared for full crowns by tapering margins of the preparation to the crown of the tooth. This preparation design allows for the placement and withdrawal of the finished restoration.

6. Once the tooth is prepared, the gingival tissue is retracted from the preparation so that a detailed impression can be made of the margins. The margins of the preparation must be detailed in the impressions so that the finished crown fits snugly and securely on the tooth. The retraction cord is placed around the prepared tooth and pushed into the sulcus with a plastic filling instrument or a retraction cord-condensing instrument (Figure 33-17). (Gingival retraction techniques are discussed in detail later in this chapter.) In some states, the dental assistant is permitted to place the gingival retraction cord. Transfer a piece of retraction cord in cotton pliers to the prosthodontist. Then transfer the appropriate cord-condensing instrument. The retraction cord remains in place for 5 minutes.

(continues)

Procedure 33-2 (continued)

7. The prosthodontist selects the tray and impression material to be used. There are a variety of materials that are suitable for final impressions (see Chapter 39, Laboratory Materials and Techniques). The tray and syringe are selected and prepared, and the materials are mixed.

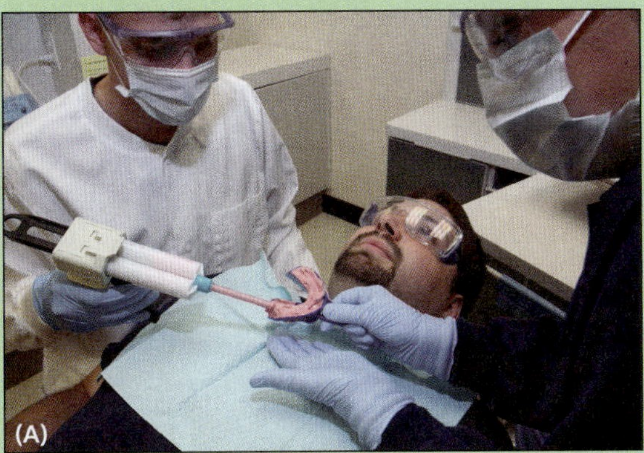

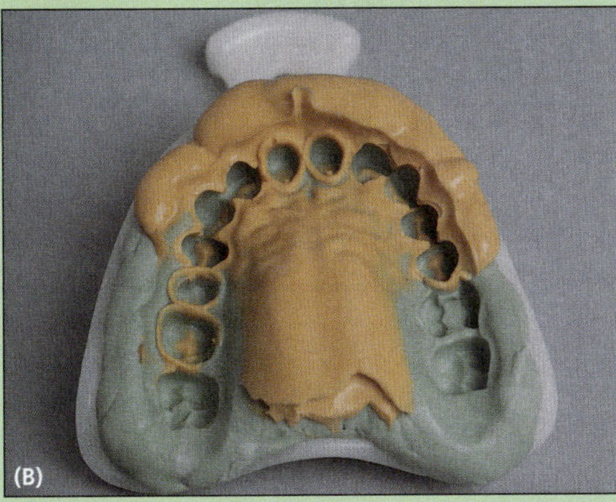

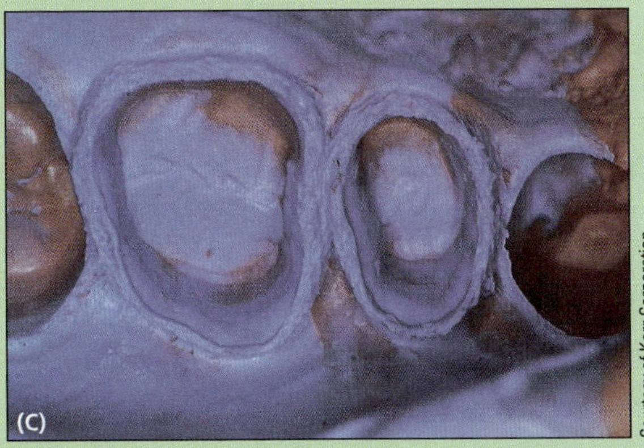

Courtesy of Kerr Corporation

FIGURE 33-18

(A) A dental assistant receives a syringe with light-body impression material and transfers the tray with medium-to heavy-bodied impression material to the dentist. (B) Final impression. (C) A close-up of the preparation margins in the final impression.

8. Transfer cotton pliers to remove the retraction cord. Transfer the syringe material and receive the cotton pliers and cord. The prosthodontist removes the retraction cord, receives the syringe, and dispenses the material around the margins of the preparation (Figure 33-18A). During this time, mix and load the heavier material into the tray. The prosthodontist places and holds the tray with the impression material in the patient's mouth. Once the prosthodontist has seated the tray, move the light from the patient's face and clean up the impression materials. The final impression is rinsed, disinfected, and placed in a plastic laboratory container (Figures 33-18B and C).

9. The **bite registration**, also called the occlusal registration, is taken after the final impression is completed. The purpose of the bite registration is to record the way the patient occludes the maxillary and mandibular teeth. There are many types of materials that can be used to record the bite of the patient, including wax and vinyl polysiloxane materials (Figure 33-19). Prepare the materials and transfer them to the prosthodontist, who places the tray and takes the bite impression. In some states, the dental assistant can take the bite impression. After the bite registration is taken, rinse the patient's mouth. The materials are rinsed, disinfected, and placed in a plastic laboratory container.

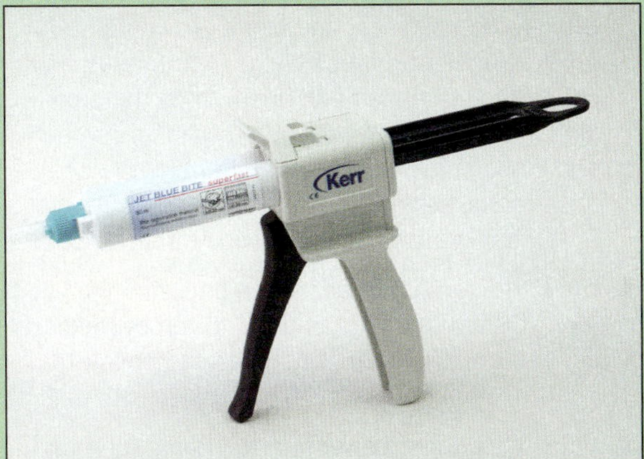

FIGURE 33-19

Dispensing gun with materials for taking a bite registration.

(continues)

Procedure 33-2 (continued)

Provisionals

The provisional restoration is very important in crown and bridge construction. The provisional retains the teeth in the same position so that the adjacent and opposing teeth do not shift position. The provisional protects the prepared tooth so that the patient can function normally. Between appointments, the provisional should look natural and be acceptable to the patient. Usually, the patient wears the provisional for 7 to 10 days, sometimes longer, depending on the extent of the prosthetics.

There are many types of provisional techniques and materials available (see Chapter 39, Laboratory Materials and Techniques). Some provisional crown forms are preformed, while others are custom made for each patient (Figure 33-20). The provisional must be fitted to the tooth in order to protect the margins, maintain the space, and be esthetically pleasing.

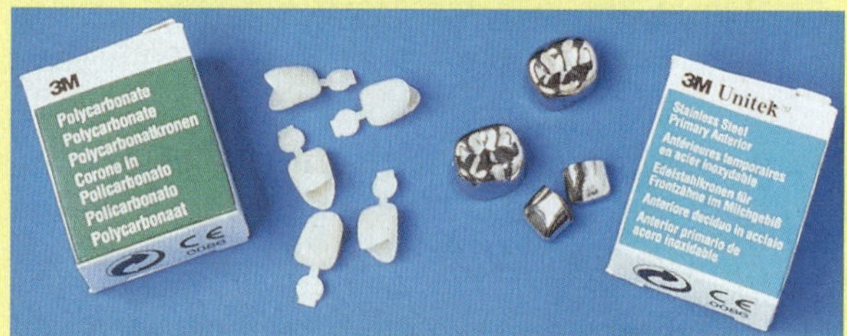

FIGURE 33-20
Anterior and posterior preformed temporaries.

10. After trimming and contouring the provisional, it is polished and cemented with provisional cement. The dental assistant either assists the prosthodontist or makes the provisional restoration, depending on the expanded functions laws. When assisting with the provisional, prepare the materials and trays as dictated by the technique. Some temporaries require crown and bridge scissors, and crimping and contour pliers, while others need burs, discs, and stones to contour and finish. Transfer and receive the instruments and keep the area rinsed and dried. Once the provisional is completed, mix the provisional cement and place some in the crown. Transfer the bite stick for the patient to bite on, and then transfer a 2 × 2 inch gauze sponge to wipe off any excess.

11. Once the cement is dried, the bite stick is removed and a scaler is used to remove excess dry cement. Transfer dental floss to check the interproximal contacts.

12. Hold articulating paper in articulating forceps for the patient to bite on to test the bite. If adjustments are needed, transfer the low-speed handpiece with finishing burs. The patient's mouth is rinsed and evacuated before the patient is dismissed.

13. After the patient has been dismissed, the patient's impressions and models are disinfected and readied, along with the laboratory prescription, for laboratory pickup (Figure 33-21). The following information is usually included on the laboratory prescription:

- Patient's name
- Description of the prosthesis
- Types of materials the prosthodontist wants the prosthesis to be constructed from
- Shade or shading desired
- Prosthodontist's name, license number, address, telephone number, fax number, and signature
- Date when the case will be back in the dental office

LAB COPY
CASE NO. 1972 Date March 18 20__
To M.P. Lab (NAME OF LABORATORY)
Address 5511 N. Walton Ave.
Patient's Name Sarah Grant
Patient's Address 3404 W. Greenwood
City Spokane State WA
℞
#14 Porcelain Crown fused to high noble metal – porcelain occlusion

FOR ADDITIONAL INSTRUCTIONS USE BACK
SHADE A-2 GINGIVAL INCISAL
MAKE OF TEETH ANT. POST. N/A
Age 27 Sex F ☒ DELICATE– ☐ –MEDIUM VIGOROUS– ☐

	DATE	HOUR
TRAYS	N/A	
BITE	N/A	
TRYIN	4/1	1 pm

FINISH DAY APRIL 1st HOUR 1 AM PM
UPPER LOWER RIGHT LEFT LEFT RIGHT
GOLD - dwt. gr. TOTAL INVOICE $ 104.00
DR. SIGNATURE Randy Stephens LICENSE NO. 7013
DR. ADDRESS 9146 N. Monroe PHONE NO. 3279533
DENTAL WORK AUTHORIZATION

Courtesy of Dr. Randall Stephens

FIGURE 33-21
Laboratory prescription.

Procedure 33-3
Cementation of Porcelain-Fused-to-Metal Crown

The following procedure is performed by the prosthodontist and the dental assistant. The provisional is removed, the permanent prosthesis is evaluated, and the final cementation is completed.

Equipment (*Figure 33-22*)

- Basic setup: mouth mirror, explorer, and cotton pliers
- Cotton rolls, gauze, dental floss, articulating paper, and forceps
- HVE tip, saliva ejector, and air–water syringe tip
- Low-speed handpiece with finishing burs, discs, and stones
- Anesthetic setup
- Spoon excavator and scaler
- Plastic filling instrument (PFI) and cement spatula
- Orangewood bite stick (crown remover, crown seater, and mallet are optional)
- Final cementation materials (glass ionomer cement, polycarboxylate cement, resin cements, or zinc phosphate cement)
- Porcelain-fused-to-metal crown from laboratory

Procedure Steps (*Follow aseptic procedures*)

1. The day before the patient's appointment, make sure the laboratory has completed the crown and that it is in the office.
2. Once the patient arrives for the appointment, prepare him or her and explain the treatment. Prepare the topical and local anesthetic, and then transfer the syringe and observe the patient. Once the anesthetic is placed, rinse and evacuate the mouth.
3. The provisional coverage is removed with a crown remover, scaler, and other instruments that fit under the margin of the provisional.
4. Remove the provisional, and then the excess cement. The dental assistant either assists during this stage of the procedure by transferring instruments and keeping the area clean and free of debris, or removes the provisional and excess cement as part of the expanded functions. Once the provisional is removed, rinse and dry the area and prepare the crown.
5. The cast crown is positioned on the preparation. If there is difficulty in seating the crown, a bite stick and/or mallet may be used. The occlusion, margins, and contacts are evaluated and adjustments are made, if necessary. If the porcelain is adjusted, it is sent back to the laboratory to be refinished. Transfer instruments, dental floss, and articulating paper and forceps. Keep the area clean and dry and transfer the low-speed handpiece with finishing burs, discs, and stones. If the casting has to be returned to the laboratory, disinfect the crown and prepare it for return to the laboratory.
6. Before cementing the crown, the area is isolated with cotton rolls and protective liners, and/or a cavity varnish is placed.
7. The permanent cement is mixed according to the manufacturer's directions and placed in the crown and on the prepared tooth (Figure 33-23).

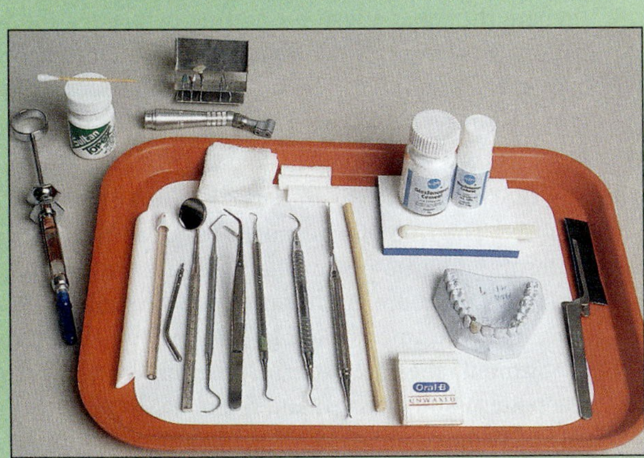

FIGURE 33-22
Tray setup for cementation appointment.

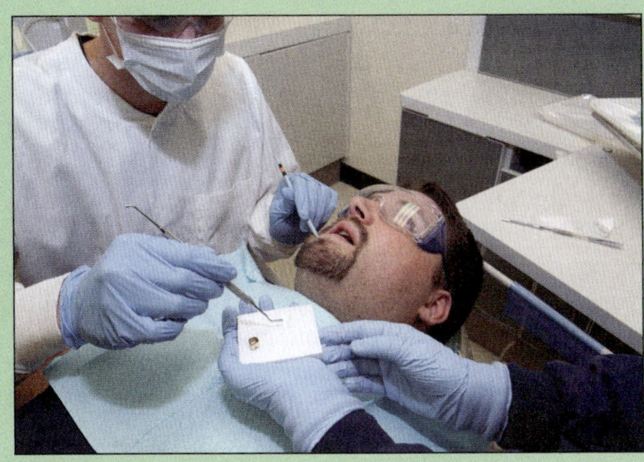

FIGURE 33-23
The dental assistant passes the final cement and crown for cementation.

(continues)

Procedure 33-3 (continued)

8. Prepare the permanent cement when the prosthodontist is ready, and place some cement in the crown. Pass the plastic filling instrument, so that the dentist can place cement on the preparation. Receive the PFI, and transfer the crown and the bite stick for the patient to bite down on. Once the crown is seated on the tooth, the patient bites on a bite stick or crown seater until the cement hardens.
9. After the cement has hardened, remove it with a scaler, excavator, or explorer (Figure 33-24). The patient's mouth is rinsed and evacuated. Use dental floss to remove excess cement interproximally.
10. The patient is given instructions for brushing and flossing the area, and is told to call the office if questions or problems develop. Document the procedure and dismiss the patient.

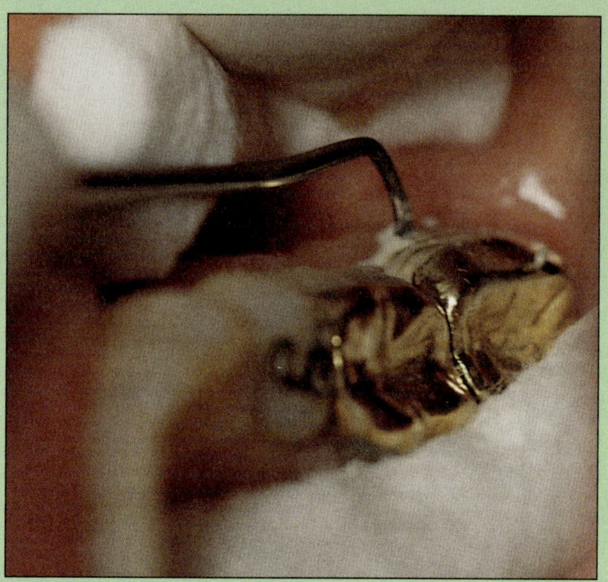

FIGURE 33-24
After the crown is cemented permanently, excess cement is removed from the margins of the crown.

CAD/CAM Restorative Systems

In-office CAD/CAM (Computer-Aided Design/Computer Controlled Manufacturing) restorative systems are also used to complete prostheses procedures. They are used after the tooth is prepped to take the impression, and for fabricating the inlays, onlays, posterior and anterior crowns, and veneers in the office. These systems allow the whole procedure to be completed in 1 day. See Chapter 34, Computerized Impression and Restorative Systems, for more information.

Role of the Laboratory Technician

The dental laboratory technician and dentist work closely together in order to give the patient quality restorations. The relationship between the laboratory and the dental office is critical. Good communication and clearly defined expectations are essential.

The laboratory technician performs the following procedures in fixed prosthesis construction: making custom trays, pouring impressions, articulating stone casts (models), preparing wax patterns, investing, and casting gold alloy restorations. The laboratory technician also constructs porcelain and porcelain-fused-to-metal restorations, and fabricates the prosthesis according to the dentist's prescription and the impressions sent from the dental office.

It is important that the impression materials be handled properly and that everything needed is sent to the laboratory. The dental assistant is often responsible for having everything ready for the laboratory pickup.

Fabrication of a Prosthesis in the Dental Laboratory

Once the case is in the dental laboratory, several steps are involved in fabricating the prosthesis, depending on the number of units and types of materials used.

Laboratory steps include the following:

1. Pour the alginate impression of the opposing arch in plaster (a low-strength material to make a model, see Chapter 39, Laboratory Materials and Techniques).
2. Pour the final impression to make the master model and **die** (replica of prepared tooth) (Figure 33-25).
3. Create a wax pattern on the die, which is then removed from the master model.
4. Prepare the wax pattern for casting by placing the wax pattern on a sprue pin and placing the pin on the mold base in the ring mold. The sprue pin will later provide a passage for the molten metal to flow into the investment mold.
5. Mix the *investment material*, pour it into the mold, and let it set. The ring of investment material, with the wax pattern and sprue pin in the middle, is heated to the desired temperature. At the same time the metal is heated. Once the investment material has been heated enough to "burnout" the wax pattern/sprue pin, leaving a negative pattern and passage, and the metal has reached the desired temperature, a centrifuge-casting machine is used to complete the casting procedure.
6. The casting ring is then cooled by placing it in water to aid in the removal of the investment material. The excess

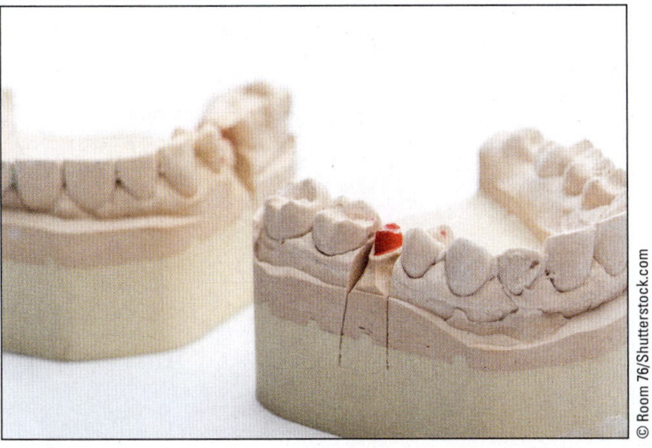

FIGURE 33-25

(A) Die prepared for wax-up. (B) A drawing of the wax pattern placed on a sprue pin, and placed on a mold base in a casting ring ready for investment material to be poured into the ring.

casting metal from the sprue channel and base is removed from the casting with laboratory burs and discs. The casting is then polished.

7. Prepare the gold casting for making the porcelain veneer.
8. Paint the porcelain on the crown in layers, and then cure it in an oven at high temperatures.
9. Finish and polish the porcelain-fused-to-metal crown.

Retention Techniques

Often, the teeth being restored with a fixed prosthesis have substantial loss of tooth structure due to decay, fractures, or large deteriorated restorations. Also, root canal therapy may be required before crowns and bridges are made.

The dentist improves the retentive capability of the tooth if the tooth being restored cannot retain the restoration alone. There are several options for building up the tooth, including core buildups, retention pins, and post-retained cores.

Core Buildups

A **core buildup** is a treatment performed for vital teeth, and nonvital teeth that have very little crown structure. For this procedure, the dentist removes any decay and defective restoration, and then builds a core that supports and provides more retention for the cast restoration.

The core buildup, or **retention core**, is made of amalgam, composite, or a silver alloy/glass ionomer combination (Figure 33-26). These materials come in a powder or liquid, syringe, or capsule form and are either set chemically or light cured.

Retention Pins

The dentist often places a **retention pin** for additional retention of the core buildup. The pins are placed strategically, depending on the amount of buildup needed and the type of restoration. They are placed before the core material; and the core buildup material surrounds the pins (Figure 33-27).

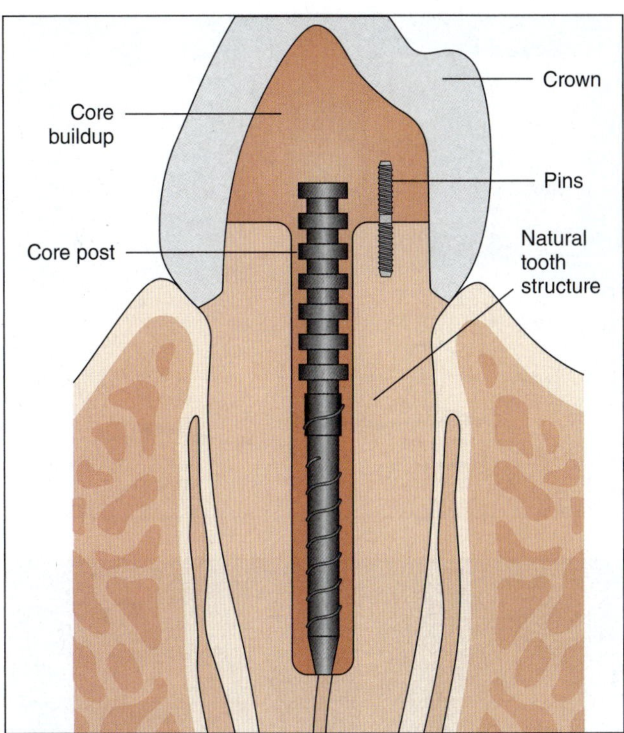

FIGURE 33-26

Tooth with core post, core buildup, and pins.

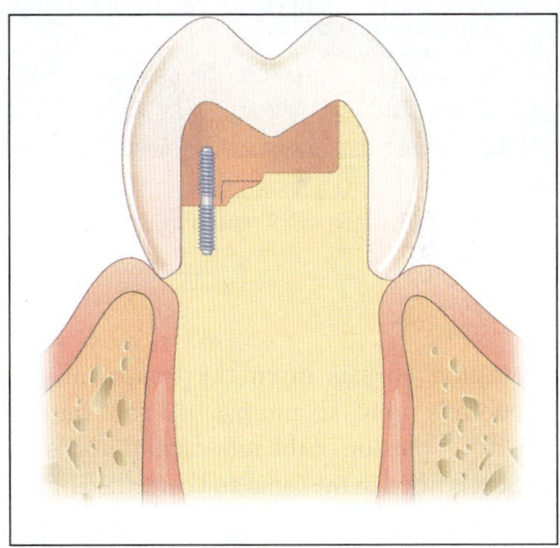

FIGURE 33-27

Pins placed in a prepared tooth for support and retention.

Pins often come in kits with various sized pins, drills, and a hand driver or mechanical placement device (Figures 33-28A and B). The drills are used in a low-speed handpiece to drill holes for the pins, which are retained in the holes.

Retention Pins in Amalgam

Retention pins are also used in an amalgam restoration for retention and support when a large surface of the tooth is being replaced. One example of this is replacing the distal-buccal cusp with amalgam.

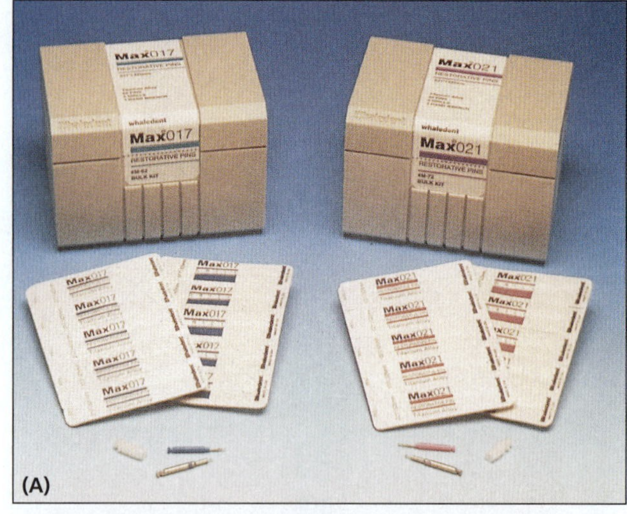

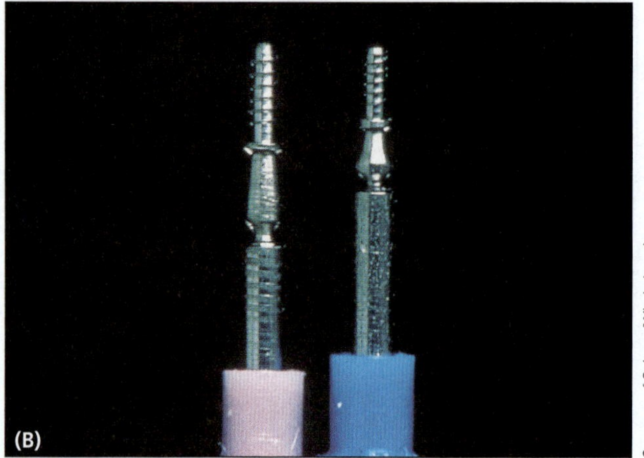

FIGURE 33-28

(A) Retention pin kit. (B) Close-up of pins (maxillary restorative pins).

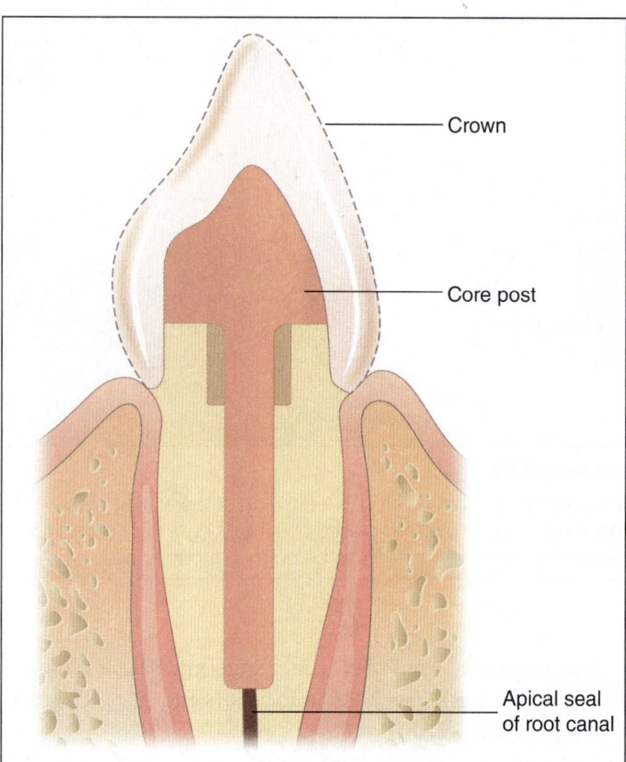

FIGURE 33-29

Core post in a nonvital tooth.

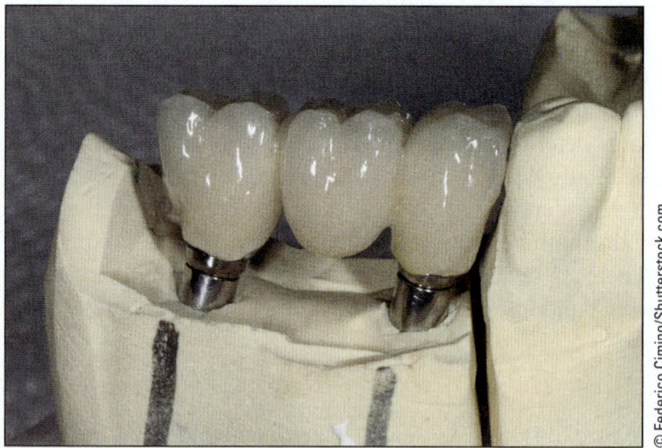

FIGURE 33-30

A three-unit bridge with two full crowns and a pontic on two implants.

Post-Retained Cores

A **post-retained core** is often the treatment of choice when the tooth is nonvital, and has had root canal therapy (Figure 33-29). A portion of the root canal filling is removed, and a cast post is fitted in the canal and cemented in place. The posts are made of materials such as titanium, titanium alloy, gold-plated metal, and stainless steel. They come in different sizes and are often purchased in a kit. The kits contain various sized posts, drills, reamers used to prepare the tooth, and wrenches or keys for hand placement.

Once the post is fitted in the root canal, it is cemented in place. Core buildup materials are then placed around the post. The tooth is then ready for the preparation of the prosthesis.

Implant Retainer Prostheses

Implants are also used as retainers for crowns and bridges (Figure 33-30). The steps for fabrication of the prostheses are basically the same as with natural teeth. For more information on dental implants refer to Chapter 26, Dental Implants.

Maintenance of the Fixed Prosthodontics

The patient is given home care instructions on how to properly maintain the new crown or bridge and is instructed to call the office if the restoration comes loose or falls out.

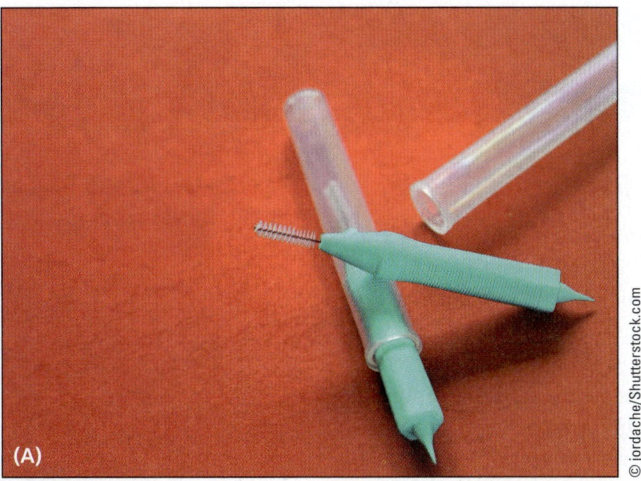
(A)
© jordache/Shutterstock.com

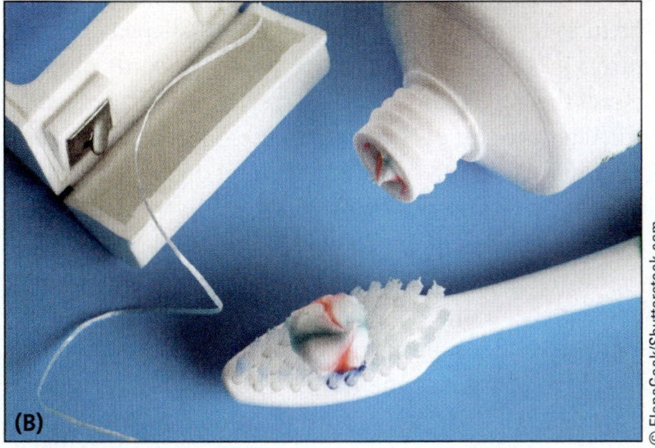
(B)
© ElenaGaak/Shutterstock.com

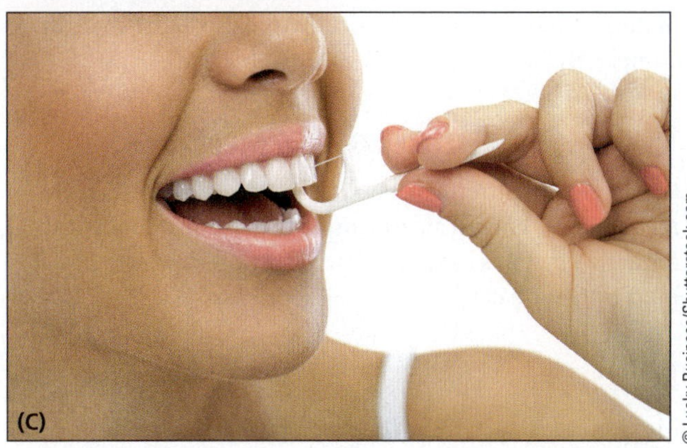
(C)
© Lucky Business/Shutterstock.com

FIGURE 33-31
The following are aids for maintaining dental prostheses: (A) Interproximal brush. (B) Floss and toothbrush. (C) Dental floss and pick.

Fixed Prostheses Maintenance

Maintenance of the fixed prosthesis should become part of the patient's daily regimen. Brushing and flossing are continued. Depending on the patient's individual needs, various aids can assist in cleaning hard-to-reach areas. Toothbrushes should be soft and multitufted, and have heads small enough to reach all areas in each quadrant. Dental floss works well under bridgework. A bridge threader can be used with the floss to clean under the pontic and along the abutment teeth. Interproximal brushes and tips are designed for removal of plaque around the fixed prosthesis (Figures 33-31A–C and 33-32).

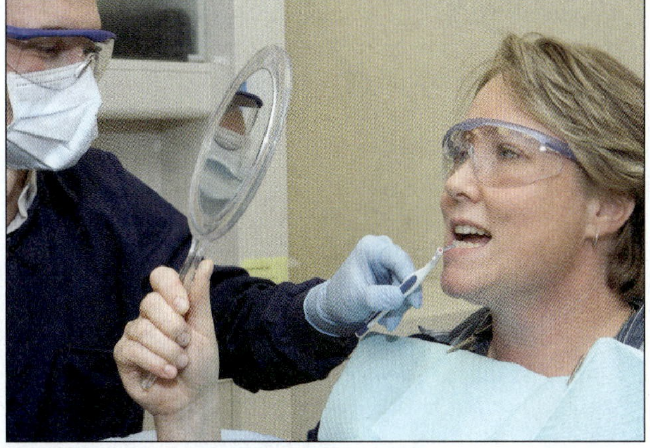

FIGURE 33-32
A dental assistant showing a patient how to use an interproximal brush.

Advanced Chairside Functions

Gingival Retraction

After a tooth is prepared for a crown, **gingival retraction** is done to ensure that an impression with clear margins can be obtained (Procedure 33-4). During this process, all hemorrhaging must be arrested, and all hard and soft tissue the operator wants to reproduce must be clean and dry. The margins are ideally supragingival, or above the gingiva, but many may be subgingival, or below the gingiva. The tissue must be retracted horizontally to allow room for a sufficient amount of impression material, and displaced vertically to expose the margin completely.

Types of Gingival Retraction

Gingival retraction can be effectively accomplished by mechanical, chemical, or surgical methods. Recently, retraction systems have been used as an alternative to placing a retraction cord.

Mechanical Retraction

Mechanical retraction can be accomplished in a number of ways. Without the use of drugs, tissue shrinkage or hemostasis will not be accomplished; however, the tissue can be displaced to allow access to the margin. A retraction cord is placed in the sulcus of a healthy and inflammation-free gingiva. The cotton cord is left in place for 10 to 15 minutes (instead of 5 minutes that it would take with a chemical retraction cord). Retraction cords are available in a variety of sizes, configurations, and chemical treatments (Figures 33-33A and B). The cord comes in a dispensing package for easy use, and may be twisted, braided, or woven to hold its shape.

If any of the cords is placed too deep, the crevice opens at the bottom but is narrow at the top (Figure 33-34A). The operator may be able to get the impression material into the crevice after the cord is removed, but the material has a tendency to fracture near the edge of the preparation. If the cord is placed too shallow in the crevice, the space is inadequate to allow an accurate reproduction of the margin of the preparation (Figure 33-34B). The proper position of the tucked cord is 1 to 3 mm into the V-shaped crevice (Figure 33-34C). The dentist may want two cords placed to retract the gingival tissues. The crevice is V-shaped, and this dictates the size of the cords to use. The smaller cords are placed at the depth of the crevice, and the larger cord is placed on top (Figure 33-34D).

Another means of mechanical retraction is accomplished by lengthening a provisional crown form to cause tissue displacement, and then taking the impression at a later date. Another method uses a dental dam clamp and a rubber dam to displace the tissue. The clamp and rubber dam are placed, and then removed just before taking the final impression. Both of these techniques may cause the tissue to bleed and the impression to be distorted.

Retraction Systems

Gingival retraction systems are now available that offer alternatives to placing a retraction cord. These systems use a silicone material that retracts the gingival tissues;

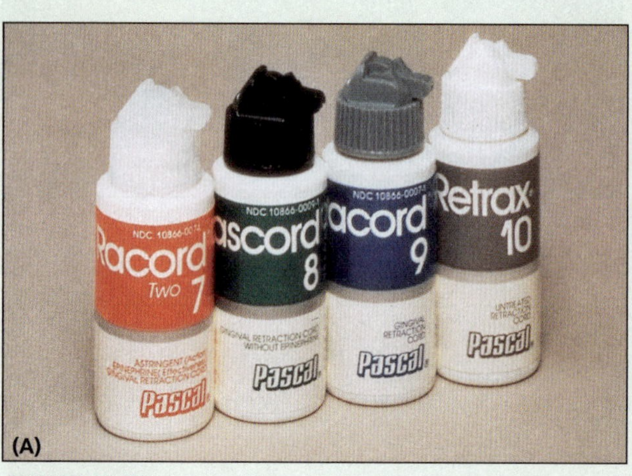

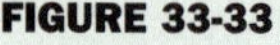
(A)

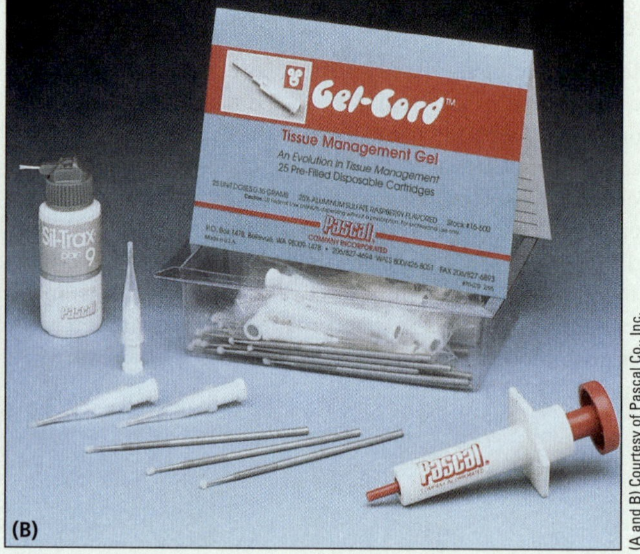

(B)

(A and B) Courtesy of Pascal Co., Inc.

FIGURE 33-33
(A) Various types of retraction cords. (B) Tissue management gel kit.

Advanced Chairside Functions

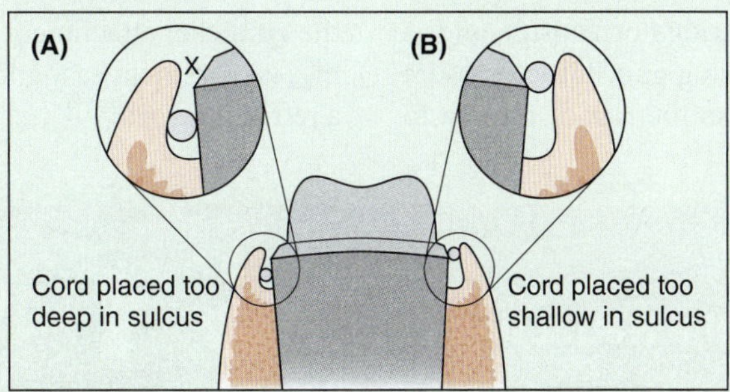

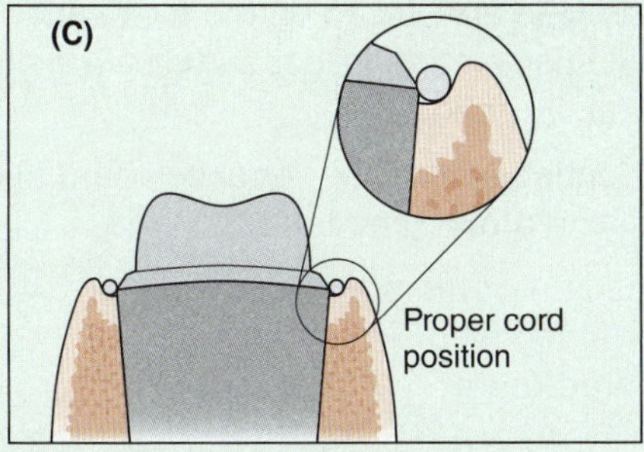

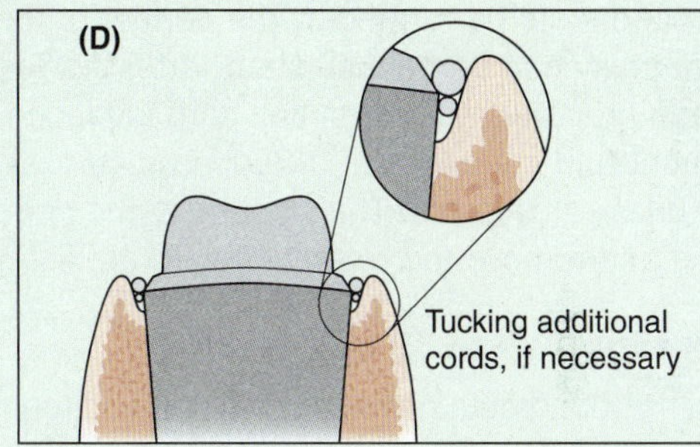

FIGURE 33-34

(A) Retraction cord placement at root depth. (B) Retraction cord placed too shallow. (C) Retraction cord placed correctly. (D) Double retraction cords placed correctly.

aluminum chloride (hemostatic agent) has been added to the material to prevent bleeding and crevicular seepage. The material is rigid enough to create a space between the tooth and tissue, and to expose the subgingival margins and keep the area dry. The paste is dispensed into the sulcus with enough material to fill it. It is left in place for 1 to 2 minutes, and then is rinsed before the final impression is taken (Figures 33-35A–F).

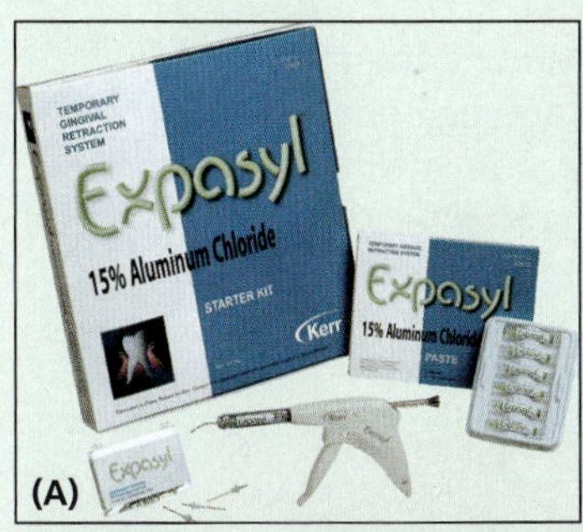

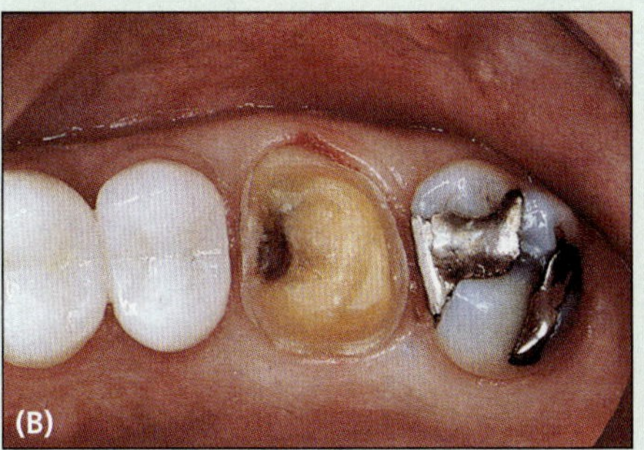

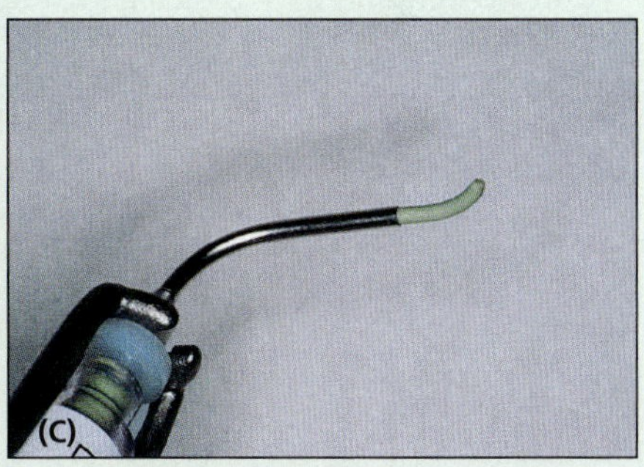

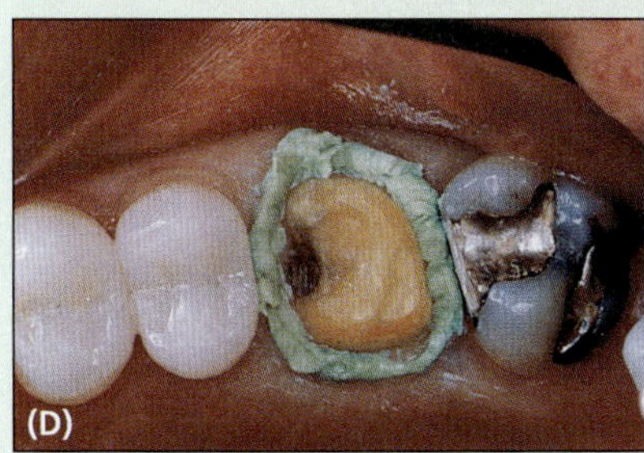

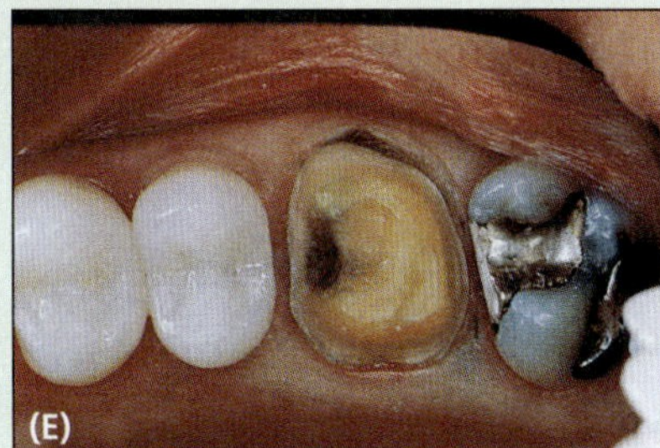

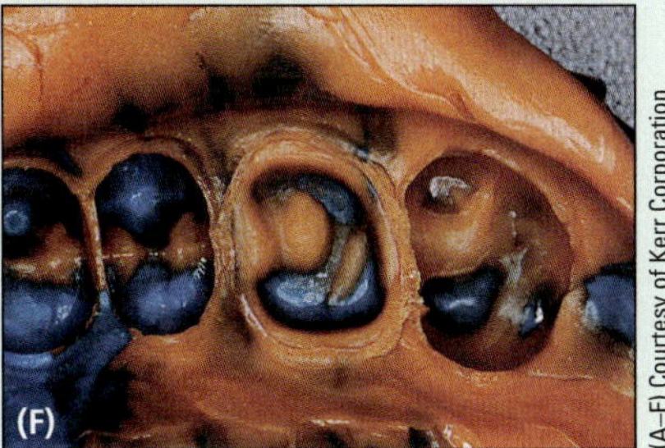

FIGURE 33-35

(A) An expasyl gingival retraction material kit. (B–F) Steps for placing a syringe-type gingival retraction cord. (B) Preparation ready for the gingival retraction material. (C) Making sure material is dispensing correctly. (D) Retraction material placed around the prepared tooth. (E) Retraction material removed and ready for impression. (F) Final impression with clear margins around the prep.

Advanced Chairside Functions (Continued)

The material comes in a cartridge or capsule and is dispensed with a mixing dispensing gun. Little pressure is needed to place the material, so the risk of trauma to the epithelial attachment is reduced. The dispensing gun makes placement easy and saves time compared to placing a retraction cord.

Procedure 33-4
Placing and Removing the Retraction Cord

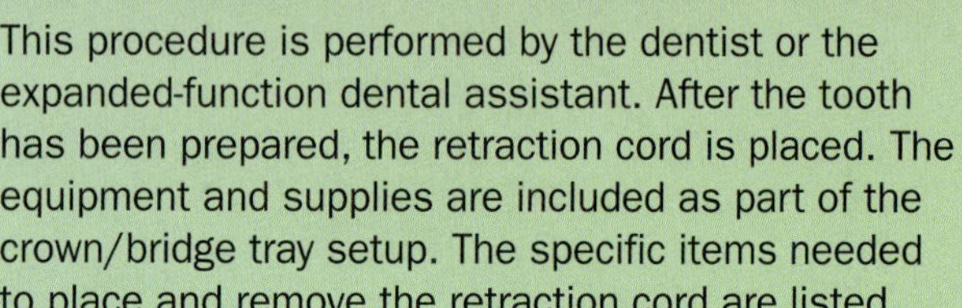

This procedure is performed by the dentist or the expanded-function dental assistant. After the tooth has been prepared, the retraction cord is placed. The equipment and supplies are included as part of the crown/bridge tray setup. The specific items needed to place and remove the retraction cord are listed.

Equipment (*Figure 33-36*)

- Basic setup: mouth mirror, explorer, and cotton pliers
- HVE tip and air–water syringe tip
- Scissors
- Hemostat
- Retraction cord(s)
- Retraction cord placement instrument or plastic instrument
- Cotton rolls and 2 × 2 inch gauze sponges

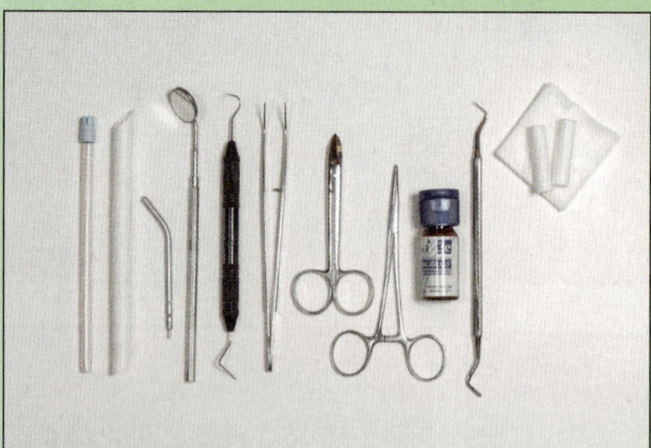

FIGURE 33-36
Placing and removing the retraction cord tray setup.

Procedure Steps (*Follow aseptic procedures*)

1. The dentist prepares the tooth for the crown.
2. Rinse and dry the area in preparation for the placement of the retraction cord.
3. Cotton rolls are placed on the facial and, if mandibular, on the lingual surface. The area is carefully dried.
4. The dentist selects the retraction cord(s) to be placed around the tooth.
5. The length of the cord needed is determined by the circumference of the prepared tooth.

Note: The desired length is determined by wrapping the cord around the small finger for an anterior tooth and around a larger finger for a molar.

6. The cord is cut to the appropriate length.
7. Twist the cord ends to compress the fibers together.
8. The cord is looped and placed in a hemostat or cotton pliers.
9. The cord is looped around the margin of the prepared tooth and tightened slightly (Figure 33-37). This aids in slipping the cord into the sulcus area. Normally, the ends of the cord are toward the buccal surface for easy access.

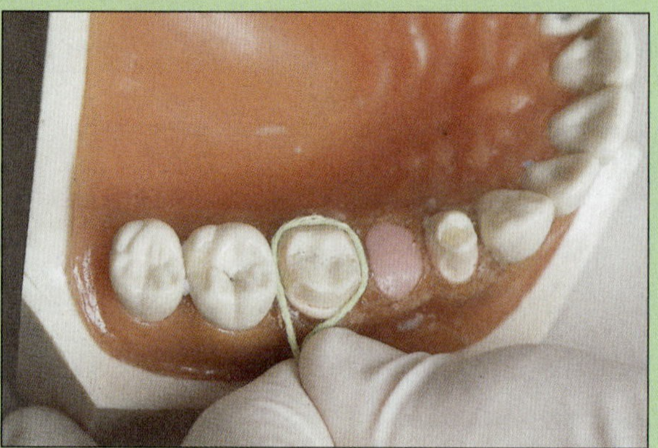

FIGURE 33-37
A retraction cord looped around a prepared tooth for placement in the gingival sulcus.

(continues)

Advanced Chairside Functions

Procedure 33-4 (continued)

10. The hemostat or cotton pliers are released, leaving the cord in the sulcus.

11. The retraction cord is packed into position with a packing instrument or a plastic instrument.

12. The cord is gently packed around the cervical area, apical to the preparation.

13. The cord is packed around the tooth, and overlaps, usually on the facial surface.

14. A tip of the cord is left showing out of the sulcus for easy removal just before taking the impression (Figure 33-38).

15. The retraction cord is left in place for 5 minutes when a chemical retraction cord is used, and for 10 to 15 minutes for mechanical retraction.

16. The end of the retraction cord is grasped and removed in a circular motion just before the impression material is placed.

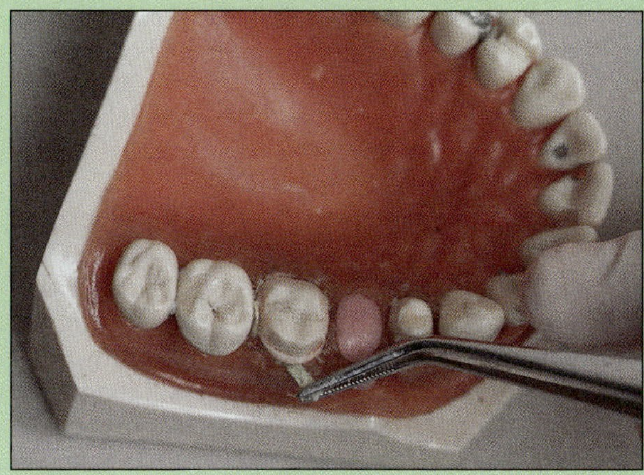

FIGURE 33-38
A retraction cord around a prepared tooth with a tag left out for easy removal.

Chemical Retraction

Chemical retraction may be performed prior to placement of the cord, by impregnating the cord and then placing it, or both. One of the newer ways is to use a topical hemostatic solution, an astringent with dentoinfusion tubes, and a plastic Luer-Lok syringe. The solution is placed using a disposable metal tip bent to the desired area. As the solution is placed, the blood and the solution merge together and are washed away with the air–water syringe. What is left in the tissue is a provisional coagulum seal that does not allow any seepage. The tissue may appear slightly darkened, but this technique allows for hemorrhaging to be arrested. A retraction cord of interwoven cotton, with or without solution, is packed vertically to expose the prepared margin. This packing of the cord provides horizontal retraction, which allows for a sufficient bulk of the impression material to flow around the margin.

The retraction cord could also be impregnated with aluminum chloride or an astringent of aluminum salts for chemical retraction. This technique causes a shrinking of the tissues, or **ischemia**, and obtains clear access to the margin of the preparation. A substance used to obtain this result is epinephrine, which is an astringent and a vasoconstrictor. It provides hemostasis and shrinks the tissues by constricting the blood vessels. Epinephrine causes an increased heartbeat, or tachycardia, for the patient. Epinephrine is definitely contraindicated for a patient with heart disease, diabetes, or hyperthyroidism, or if taking certain drugs.

Note: The dental assistant should watch for patients who exhibit hypertension, knowing that most hyperthyroid and diabetic patients are usually hypertensive. Normally, the dentist prefers to use a chemical retraction cord, so the patient's medical history should be reviewed carefully.

Surgical Retraction

Instead of retraction, the dentist may choose to remove the tissue around the preparation. This approach is accomplished by using a surgical knife or by performing electrosurgery. With the surgical knife, the dentist excises the tissue and exposes the margin of the preparation. The area where the tissue has been removed may bleed and require additional treatment in order to get a good impression of the area.

The dentist may decide to use an electrosurgery unit, which cauterizes the tissues as it removes them. Therefore, the tissue is removed without bleeding. The unit passes a high-frequency current into a small electrode, which passes through the tissue. The tip of the unit is a metal wire or loop. As the tip touches the tissue, the unit is activated to remove the tissue. It is especially important with this treatment that soft tissue anesthesia is maintained.

Advanced Chairside Functions (Continued)

Electrosurgery is not used with patients who are receiving radiation therapy, have cardiac pacemakers, or have any diseases that slow healing.

Constant use of a nonmetal HVE tip during the surgery is important due to the odor given off as the tissues are cauterized. The evacuator reduces the odor if it is placed near the surgical site. After the tissue is removed, the sulcus is cleaned with a hydrogen peroxide rinse. Immediately following the procedure, the final impression is taken.

Chapter Summary

Fixed prosthodontics encompasses replacement of missing teeth or parts of teeth with extensive restorations. There are many types of fixed prostheses and a variety of materials used for preparation, fabrication, and cementation. The dental assistant is involved in all stages of fixed prosthodontic treatment. It is important to understand the sequence of the procedure and the various types of restorations when assisting the dentist.

The goal of this chapter was to assess the more common procedures in order to give the dental assistant the background needed to assist the dentist. Restorations routinely take at least two appointments to complete. The assistant explains the steps of the procedure to the patient, answers questions, and provides postoperative and home care instructions.

Gingival retraction is an important step when preparing the tooth for the final impression. Margins of the preparations must be exposed so that the impression will reflect an accurate image of the tooth and preparation, and, thus, ensure that the fixed prosthesis will fit perfectly. Learning about the various materials and techniques helps the dental assistant become more skilled when working with the dentist.

CASE STUDY

Ann Arthur is unhappy with the appearance of her anterior teeth. The maxillary and mandibular incisors are a dull, medium-yellow shade. There is a slight diastema (space) between the maxillary central incisors. Ann has considered treatment for several years and has scheduled an appointment for next week. She has dental insurance through her husband's insurance plan.

Case Study Review

1. What are the two concerns Ann has about her anterior teeth?
2. What treatment options are available?
3. Once a treatment plan is in place, how might financial information, such as insurance, be considered by the business staff?

Review Questions

Multiple Choice

1. Which of the following prosthetic restorations covers only the area between the cusps on the occlusal surface of the tooth?
   a. Three-quarter crown
   b. Inlay restoration
   c. Onlay restoration
   d. Veneer restoration
2. The dental bridge part that replaces the missing tooth is called the
   a. abutment.
   b. pontic.
   c. connector.
   d. retainer.
3. Materials used to fabricate crowns and bridges include all of the following *except*
   a. gold alloy.
   b. porcelain.

c. composite resin.
d. amalgam.

4. During the preparation appointment, the retraction cord is
   a. placed after the tooth is prepared, but before the final impressions are taken.
   b. placed after the final impressions are taken.
   c. placed before the tooth is prepared.
   d. placed with the provisional restoration.
5. All of the following materials are needed during the preparation appointment *except*
   a. alginate.
   b. gingival retraction cord.
   c. bonding agent.
   d. provisional cement.
6. If a tooth is badly broken down, all of the following methods are used to add the needed support *except*
   a. glass ionomer cement base.
   b. core buildup.
   c. retention pins.
   d. post-retained cores.
7. All of the following are types of veneers *except*
   a. direct resin veneers.
   b. indirect resin veneers.
   c. direct glass ionomer veneers.
   d. porcelain veneers.
8. Which of the following materials is *not* used to take the final impression after the tooth is prepared?
   a. Polysiloxane
   b. Alginate
   c. Hydrocolloid
   d. Silicone impression materials
9. How many types of gingival retraction are used in fixed prosthodontic procedures?
   a. Two
   b. Three
   c. Five
   d. Six
10. Which type of gingival retraction is accomplished by placement of a retraction cord?
   a. Mechanical
   b. Chemical
   c. Surgical
   d. None of the above

Critical Thinking

1. Which expanded functions in your state relate to fixed prosthodontic procedures?
2. Name the restoration types that are fabricated of gold alloy, porcelain-fused-to-metal, or porcelain.
3. Name possible techniques for building up a crown that is badly broken down.
4. Discuss what happens if the retraction cord is placed too deep in the sulcus.
5. Explain why the dentist may place additional retraction cords in the sulcus before the final impression is taken.

Web Activities

1. Go to http://vitanorthamerica.com and search under products for information on the new digital shade guide.
2. Go to www.academyofprosthodontics.org and click on View Glossary, and review common terms covered in Chapter 33, Fixed Prosthodontics.
3. To find more information on home care products that can assist patients with fixed prostheses go to http://www.gumbrand.com/. Look under Products and Oral Care Topics.
4. Go to http://www.gingi-pak.com and continue to the area on Training and Support. Locate retraction techniques in this area. List three techniques for various cord-packing materials that are identified on this Web site.

CHAPTER

34

Computerized Impression and Restorative Systems

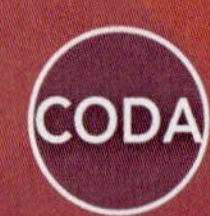

Specific Instructional Objectives

The student should strive to meet the following objectives and demonstrate an understanding of the facts and principles presented in this chapter:

1. Identify and explain the computer-aided design (CAD) and the computer-aided manufacturing (CAM) restorative systems.
2. List the advantages and disadvantages of the CAD/CAM technology.
3. Explain the role of the dental assistant during cavity preparation, and while using the CAD/CAM systems to design and manufacture an indirect restoration.
4. Describe the considerations the patient should be made aware of when using CAD/CAM technology.
5. Gain an understanding of the CAD equipment, and the CAM systems.
6. Discuss how the CAD/CAM systems are used in the dental office and in the dental laboratory.
7. List and describe the steps for preparing the tooth, designing the restoration, and manufacturing the final restoration.

Key Terms

CAD/CAM restorative systems (799)

CEREC (799)

computer-aided design (CAD) (799)

computer-aided manufacturing (CAM) (799)

computer surface digitization (CSD) (802)

digital impression (802)

Introduction

Over the last 30 years, **computer-aided design (CAD)** and **computer-aided manufacturing (CAM)** technology has become increasingly popular for the fields of dentistry and prosthodontics. Techniques, software, and materials have improved, becoming easier to use and incorporate into dental practice; and this technology continues to advance. CAD/CAM technology is used in both the dental office and in the dental laboratory. This technology is capable of many procedures from digital impressions and design, to the production of complete restorations, surgical guides, fixed partial and full dentures, implant abutments, and orthodontic appliances.

With a CAD/CAM system, the tooth can be prepared and the restoration fabricated right in the office. After the tooth is prepped a computer program is used to design the crown, inlay, and so on. This information is sent to the milling machine for fabrication. Once completed the finished restoration is ready to be cemented or bonded in place. The patient only needs one appointment and never has to wear a provisional restoration.

The advantages of the CAD/CAM system include the following:

- The procedure is completed in 1 day.
- No impressions are taken.
- The patient does not need to have provisional restorations.
- Without the provisional restoration, tooth sensitivity may be reduced.
- Saves time for the patient.
- The dental laboratory is not involved.

The disadvantages of the CAD/CAM system include the following:

- The cost may be greater than traditional restoration procedures.
- Involves extra time for the dentist or dental assistant.
- May involve a long appointment for the patient.

The Role of the Dental Assistant

The dental assistant's role in CAD/CAM procedures will vary from office to office following the dentist's directions and preferences. In some offices the dental assistant sets up the scanner, gets the computer software open and ready, and prepares the milling machine. During the procedure the assistant will assist the dentist, and make sure they have what they need to complete the procedure. In other offices the dental assistant may assist the dentist during cavity preparation and then, depending on his or her training and skills, he or she may scan the preparation to create the digital impression. The digitized impression can be modified to enhance the gingival margins of the preparation with CAD/CAM software.

Once the impression is approved by the dentist, a virtual restoration is designed for the dentist to evaluate and double-check, especially along the margins.

When the dentist has approved the virtual restoration, the assistant sends this information to the CAM equipment for the milling of the restoration.

Upon completion of the restoration, the dental assistant will assist the dentist as the restoration is tried on the tooth to ensure the margins, contacts, and occlusion are where the dentist wants them to be. The assistant may then polish and glaze the restoration before assisting the dentist with the final cementation.

It takes training for the dental assistant to become proficient in using these systems. Many of the manufacturers will provide training to the dentist and his or her team members when the units are purchased. Many schools and consultants are also training dental team members and dentists on how to integrate CAD/CAM into their offices. Continued education and training is required to keep up with the latest technology. Learning this new technology advances the dental assistant's knowledge and skills, making the dental assistant a more valued member of the dental team. Learning new technologies can also be motivating and rewarding for the dental assistant's career.

Patient Considerations

Patient considerations include providing the patient with the information he or she needs to understand the treatment, the time commitment involved, and the cost of the procedure. Once the patient understands the need for a crown, bridge, inlay, or onlay, the treatment options are explained. Some offices have videos, pictures, or brochures for the patient to look at. When CAD/CAM technology is used for prosthetic restoration, the procedure is completed in one appointment. Although this treatment only requires one appointment, it is usually a much longer appointment. The patient should be aware of the cost differences between the routine treatment and the CAD/CAM system. Once the patient understands this option, the dentist will determine if this treatment is best for them. The CAD/CAM restoration will be similar to routine fixed prosthodontic treatments, providing quality work, materials, and results.

CAD/CAM Restorative Systems for the Dental Office

In-office **CAD/CAM restorative systems** are becoming increasingly common. These systems allow for metal-free, tooth-colored restorations to be fabricated within a single appointment. All types of restorations including inlays, onlays, posterior and anterior crowns, and veneers can be designed and milled at the chairside. With this type of system, there are no unpleasant impressions, no need for provisionals, and more of the healthy tooth structure may be maintained.

The first CAD/CAM restorative system, called **CEREC** (chairside economical restorations of esthetic ceramics), was developed in Switzerland in 1980 (Figure 34-1). The CEREC 3 has the ADA Seal of Acceptance. Since then there have been a number of systems on the market, each with their own technology and computer programs.

Several factors should be addressed before the dentist decides to add this technology to the practice. First, a time investment is required to integrate the system into the office

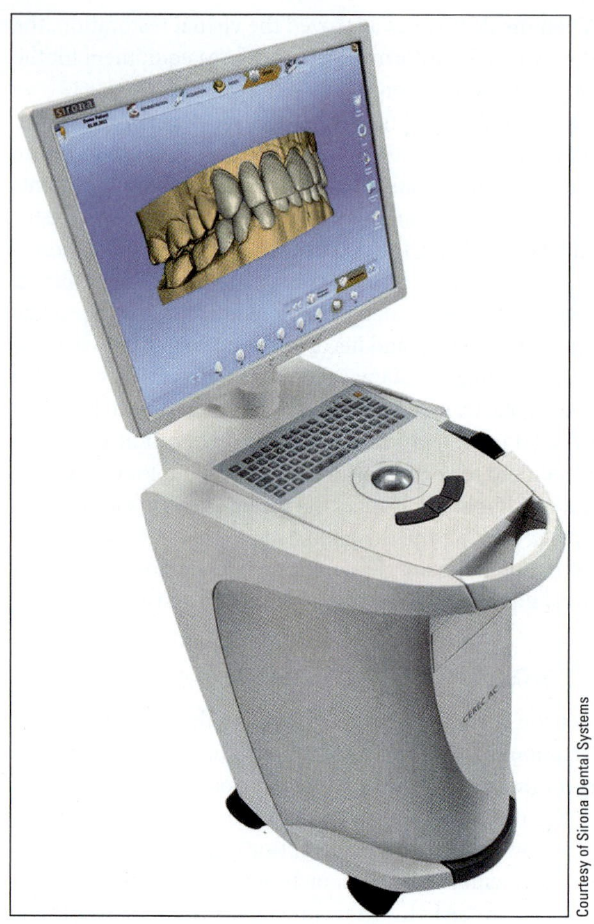

Courtesy of Sirona Dental Systems

FIGURE 34-1

The CEREC CAD machine.

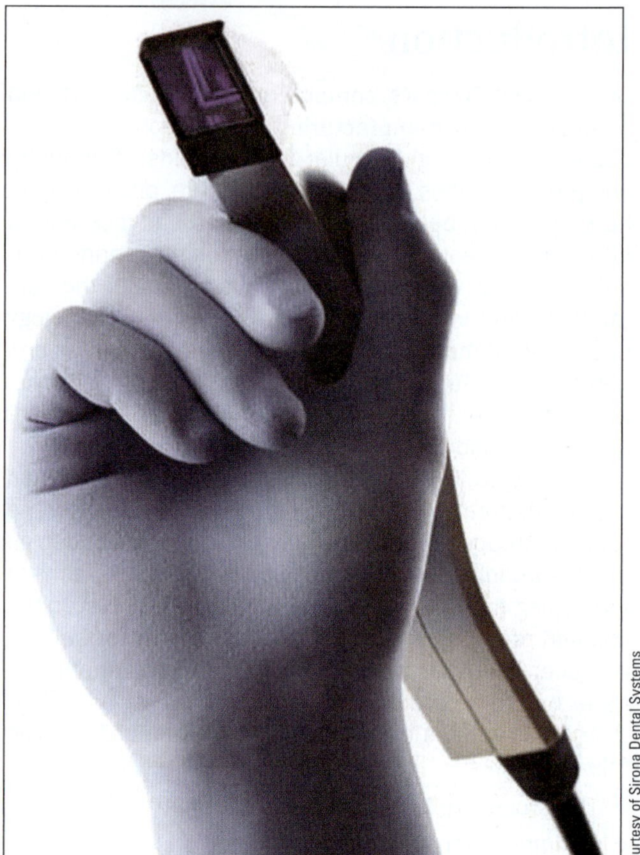

Courtesy of Sirona Dental Systems

FIGURE 34-2

CAD/CAM scanner used to scan an image of the teeth into the computer.

scheduling and routines. The dentist and staff must be trained, and they need time to practice using both the hardware and software in order to become proficient. Training programs are available when the CAD/CAM system is purchased and for continued education. Second, a large financial investment is required for purchasing the system and for training. The learning curve may affect patient scheduling and production until the technique is mastered by the dental team. Third, the dentist and staff should be familiar with computers, be committed to learning the system, and be dedicated and enthusiastic about understanding and becoming skilled in this technology.

Taking Virtual Impressions in the Dental Office

The first segment of the CAD/CAM system contains the intraoral camera (scanner) that takes the digital impression (Figure 34-2). After the tooth is prepared, the dentist may use a gingival retraction cord to retract the tissues from around the margins of the preparation, ensuring that an impression with clear margins can be obtained. Before the cavity preparation is scanned, the retraction cord is removed, and, sometimes, the tooth and surrounding tissues are coated with a reflective powder to enhance the scanning process. The images can be captured in different ways with different technology. One system may use a laser and manual capture, another may use an LED camera with automatic capture, and still another may use a video and manual capture to obtain the image. Table 34-1 lists four CAD/CAM systems and what they offer. Each system has specially designed software that receives the impression data, and then displays a three-dimensional (3D) image of the preparation and the surrounding teeth and tissues on the computer monitor (Figure 34-3).

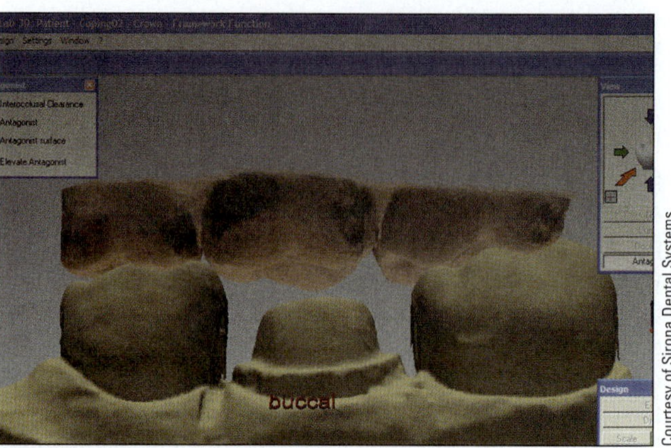

Courtesy of Sirona Dental Systems

FIGURE 34-3

A computerized image of a prepared tooth that is ready for a crown to be designed.

TABLE 34-1 Digital Impressions and CAD/CAM Systems

CAD/CAM Systems	CEREC AC	E4D	iTero	Lava COS
Powdering Required?	Yes, spray with a light coat of opaquing medium	Powder obtains a better image but is not required	No	A small amount
Image Capture	Blue light LED camera	Red light laser camera	Video camera	Laser camera
Full Arch Digital Impression?	Yes	No	Yes	Yes
Can Be Sent to a Dental Laboratory?	Yes	No	Yes	Yes
Software for Designing Restorations?	Yes	Yes	No	No
In Office Milling?	Yes	Yes	No	No
Time to Mill Most Restorations	3–8 minutes	10–20 minutes	N/A	N/A
Mills Bridges?	Yes	No	No	No

Fabricating and Milling the Restoration

Once the digital impression has been scanned into the computer, the software allows the dentist or dental assistant to create the missing areas of the tooth, creating a virtual restoration. This is called reverse engineering.

The second segment of the system is the milling machine, which is usually located in the lab area of the office (Figure 34-4). After the dentist designs the digital restoration with the CAD software, it is transferred to the milling machine. The milling chamber contains an attachment for a block of ceramic material, two diamond burs, and water (Figure 34-5). A block of ceramic material matching the patient's tooth color is selected and placed in the milling chamber. The CAM software uses the transferred information on the restoration, and begins the milling process. Within a determined amount of time, the restoration is milled.

Several ceramic materials are available for the dentist to choose from including leucite-reinforced glass ceramic; fine grained, feldspathic porcelain; and a polymer ceramic based on MZ100 composite restorative material (Figure 34-6).

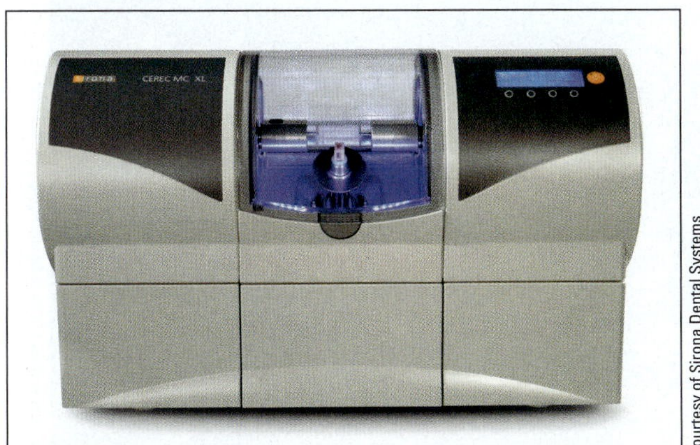

Courtesy of Sirona Dental Systems

FIGURE 34-4

A CAM system unit, which mills ceramic blocks into restorations, such as crowns.

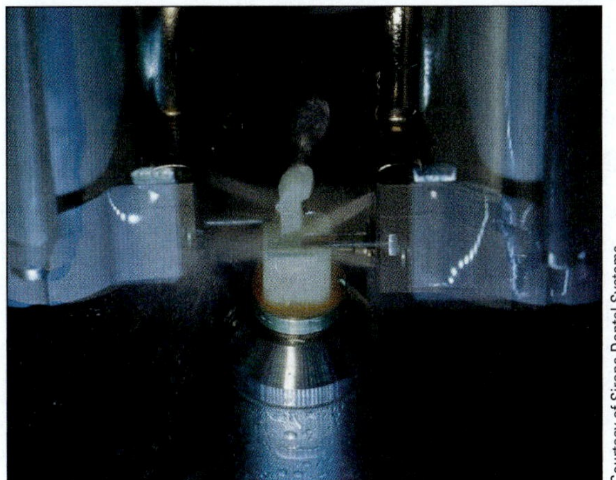

Courtesy of Sirona Dental Systems

FIGURE 34-5

A close up of the milling process.

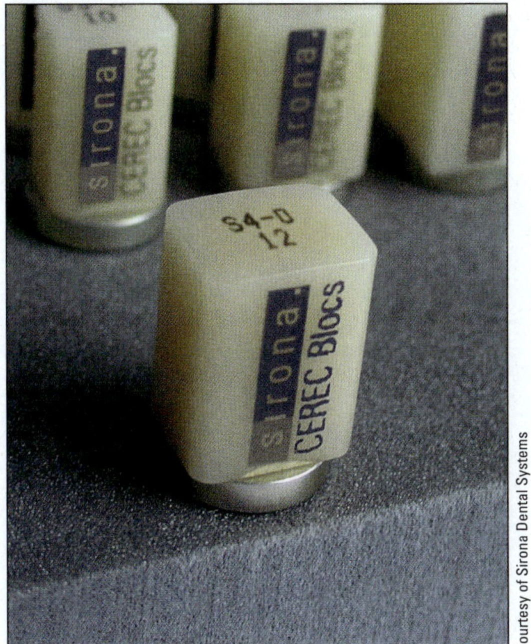

Courtesy of Sirona Dental Systems

FIGURE 34-6

Ceramic blocks for the CAM.

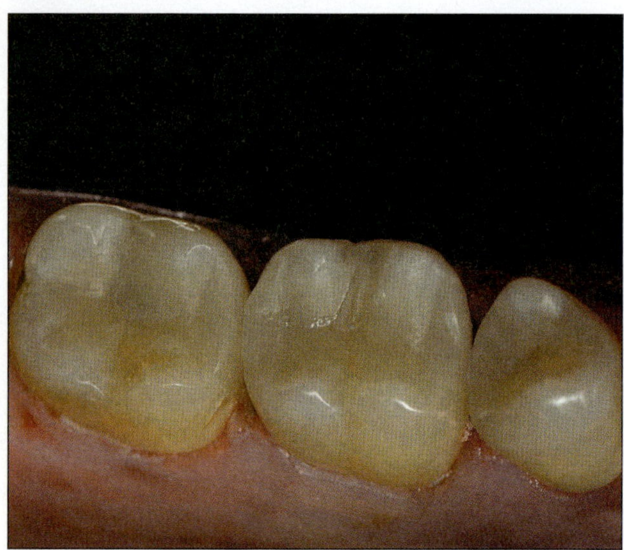

FIGURE 34-7
Teeth restored with a ceramic restoration designed and fabricated by the CEREC system.

Completion of the Restoration

Once the restoration is completed it is tried in the patient's mouth. The gingival margins and occlusions are evaluated, and then adjusted using discs and burs. The restoration is then ready to be cemented. Sometimes the restoration is glazed before cementation. Once cemented, the restoration is then polished (Figure 34-7).

Millions of restorations have been fabricated and placed since the introduction of the CAD/CAM technology. Patient satisfaction with the restorations from these systems has been very high because the restoration is esthetically pleasing, comfortable, and only takes a single appointment to complete. Impressions and provisionals are nonexistent, and there are fewer injections. The CAD/CAM system provides the dentist with precision technology for creating dental restorations in the dental office.

There is an exception, however; if the dentist prefers to dedicate more time to the design process, then the patient would be scheduled for a second appointment, and the patient would have to wear provisionals during that time.

CAD/CAM Systems for Dental Laboratories

Another option for the dentist with a CAD system is to take a **digital impression** in the office, and have the restoration designed and made in a dental lab. This eliminates the need for the dentist to purchase the milling unit and to learn the necessary skills to fabricate the restoration. With this system the dentist prepares the tooth and then uses a specially designed scanner and software to capture a digital impression of the prepared tooth, the adjacent teeth, and the opposing arch (Figure 34-8). The digital impressions are then sent electronically to a designated lab that has shared software. The impressions are received immediately by the lab, giving the dentist a chance to discuss the details of the case with the lab technician, if necessary, before the patient leaves the office.

Many dental laboratories have a CAD/CAM system that is designed to interface with dental offices. The system technology is often standardized to provide a smooth transition when exchanging information and data between the dental office and the dental lab. The construction of crowns and bridges is done in dental laboratories, where they use **computer surface digitization (CSD)** to acquire a 3D record of the geometry of a preparation. Once the lab technician receives the information the dentist scanned, a digital restoration is designed. The dentist sends the shade and type of ceramic material to be used. A ceramic block is selected and placed in the chamber and milled according to the dentist's directions (Figure 34-9). The restoration and models are then sent to the dental office for the patient's next appointment.

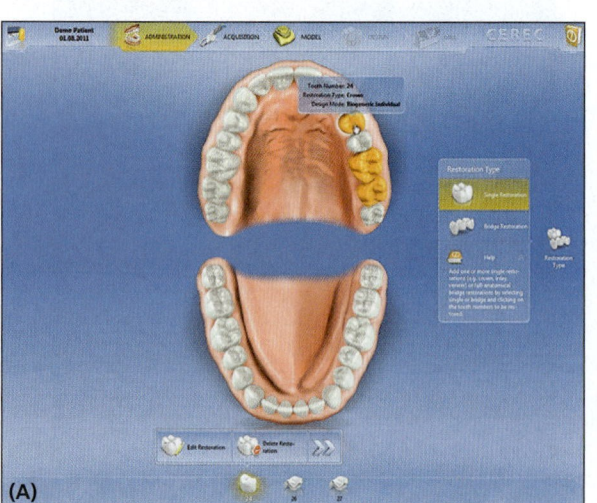

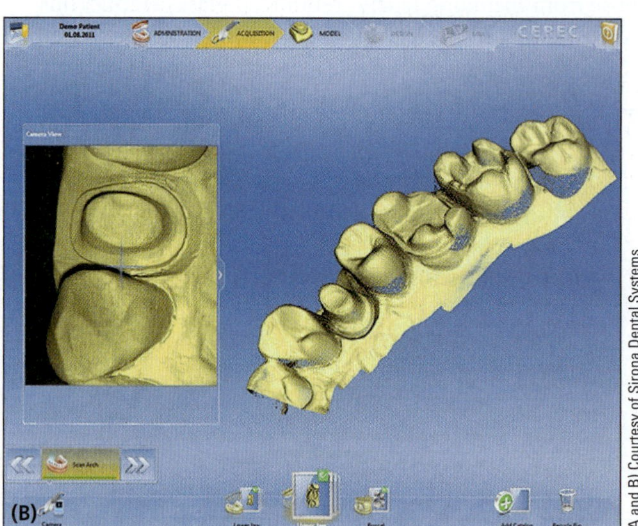

(A and B) Courtesy of Sirona Dental Systems

FIGURE 34-8
(A and B) CAD digital impressions.

(continued)

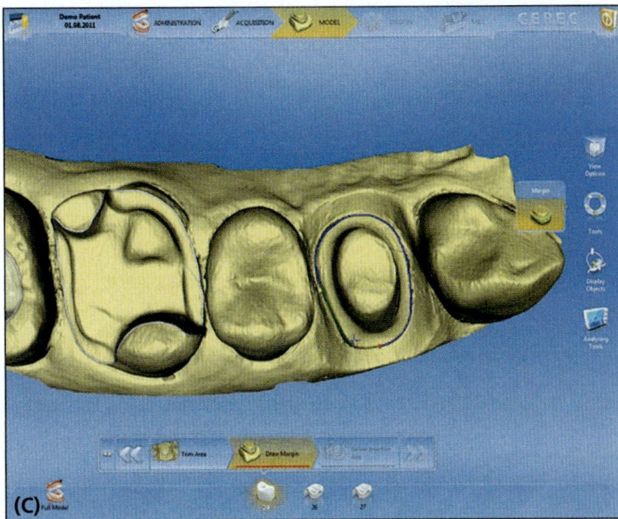
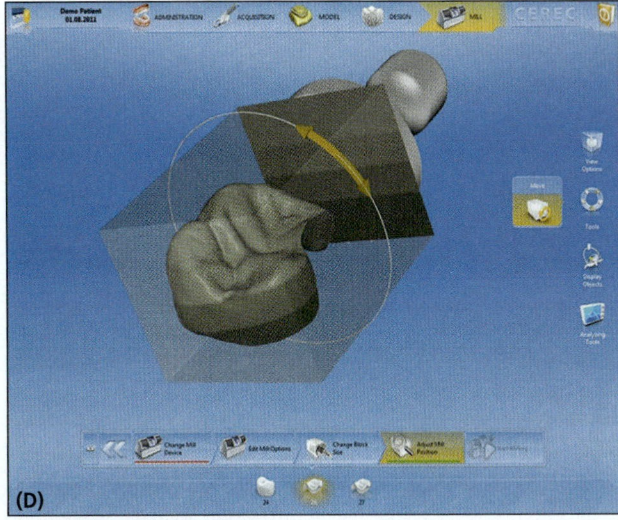
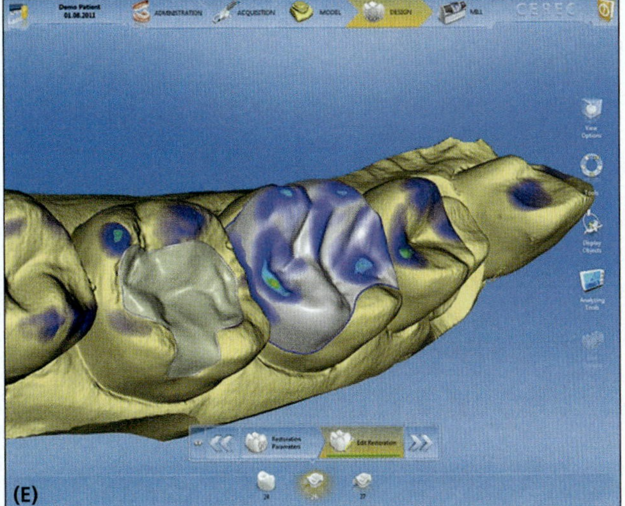

(C–E) Courtesy of Sirona Dental Systems

FIGURE 34-8 (continued)
(C) CAD digital impressions. (D) A restoration milled from a ceramic block. (E) A virtually designed restoration.

Digital impressions are very accurate and can be transferred to the dental laboratory or CAM system rapidly. Routine dental impression materials have to be set up and sometimes need to be retaken because of a bubble in the material or a problem during the loading of the material in the tray. The materials then need to be disinfected and taken to the dental laboratory, and the patient needs to return to seat the crown after it has been fabricated. CAD impressions can be seen on the screen to ensure that accuracy has been achieved prior to sending them to the laboratory. If inaccurate or if the margins aren't clear, the scan can be repeated immediately, much like a photo on a digital camera or phone, and the prior one is deleted. The CAD impression re-scanning may take more time but there are no additional material expenses.

This technique can be used for inlays, onlays, veneers, full crowns, copings, bridge frameworks, provisionals, wax-ups, and abutments for implants. Materials used to fabricate the restoration include all ceramics, polymers, and metals. With this technique the patient will need two appointments to complete the procedure, just like the traditional procedure, but this eliminates the need for in-office impressions.

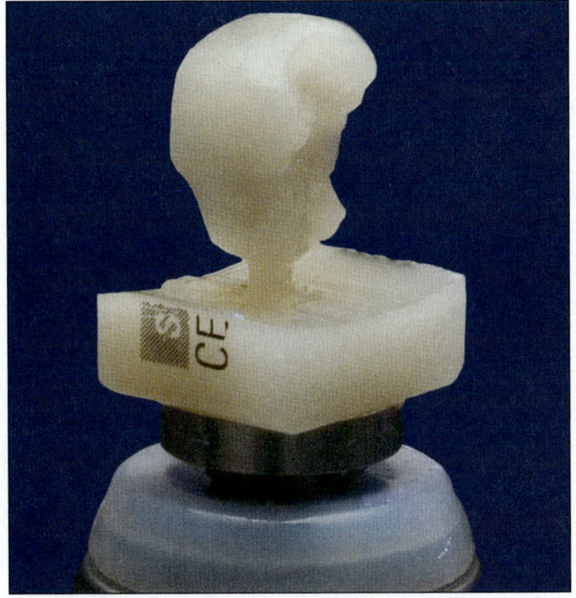

FIGURE 34-9
A finished restoration after the completion of the milling process, before being cut from the ceramic block.

Procedure 34-1
CAD/CAM Restoration

This procedure is performed by the dentist and the dental assistant, and is completed in one appointment. In the first step the tooth is prepared. The next step is to scan the tooth preparation and the surrounding tissues for the impression using the CAD system. The CAD system then designs the restoration and sends the information to the CAM system. The CAM system then mills the restoration. After trying the restoration on the patient, and making any necessary adjustments, it is ready for cementation.

Equipment and Supplies

- Basic setup: mouth mirror, explorer, and cotton pliers
- Anesthetic setup
- Cotton rolls, dry angles, gauze, dental floss, articulating paper, and forceps
- HVE tip, saliva ejector, and three-way syringe tip
- Isolation setup (dental dam or an isolation system)
- High-speed handpiece with selection of diamond burs, discs, and burs
- Spoon excavator, scaler, and plastic filling instrument
- Ceramic shade guide
- Gingival retraction setup (preference of dentist)
- Opti spray (reflective powder that assists the scanner in picking up details of the preparation)
- Ceramic block selection
- Cementation setup (including etching materials)

Preparation Steps

1. Turn on and prepare the CAD system.
2. Have the ceramic blocks ready for selection.
3. Turn on and prepare the CAM system for the milling process.

Procedure Steps (*Follow aseptic procedures*)

1. The patient is seated and given local anesthetic.
2. While waiting for the anesthetic to be effective, the shade of the ceramic material block is selected using a ceramic shade guide (Figure 34-10).
3. The ceramic block is placed in the milling machine.
4. The teeth and surrounding tissues are sprayed with the Opti spray to enhance the occlusion and bite registration on the images before the tooth is prepared.
5. The images are scanned into the computer.
6. The tooth is prepared removing any existing restorations and decay. The dentist will use the high-speed handpiece with diamond burs and hand-cutting instruments.
7. After the dentist prepares the tooth for the ceramic restoration, if needed, the gingival tissue is retracted from the preparation with gingival retraction cord.
8. The tooth preparation and surrounding tissues are coated with reflective powder for the scanning of the three-dimensional impression.
9. An instant digital impression is obtained by positioning the camera over the preparation.
10. The dentist designs the replacement part for the missing areas of the tooth, creating a virtual restoration using data from the proprietary software.
11. The software transfers this virtual data to the milling machine, where diamond burs will work simultaneously under water coolant to mill the restoration from the ceramic block (Figure 34-11).

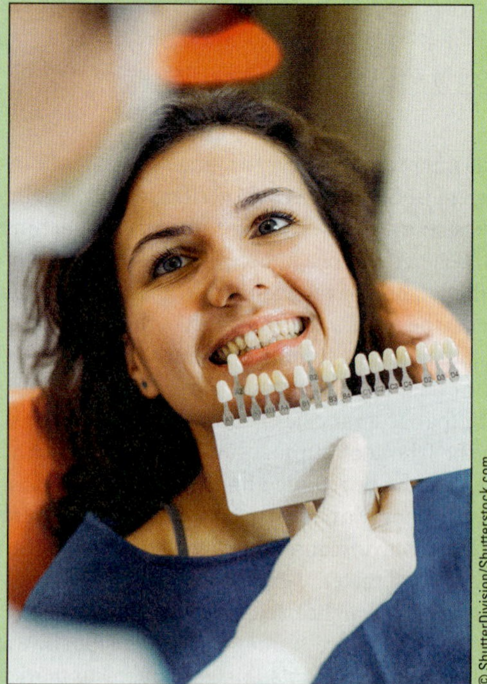

FIGURE 34-10
Selecting a shade with a ceramic shade guide.

(continues)

Procedure 34-1 (continued)

12. The finished model from the milling process is removed from the ceramic block with a bur, and is ready for the finishing process (Figure 34-12).

13. The milled restoration is placed in the patient's mouth and any adjustments are made, if needed.

14. The tooth preparation is etched, rinsed, and the bonding agent is placed to prepare for cementation.

15. The restoration is cemented in place. The occlusion and contacts are checked.

16. The patient is given home care instructions and told to call the office if questions or problems develop.

17. Document the procedure and dismiss the patient.

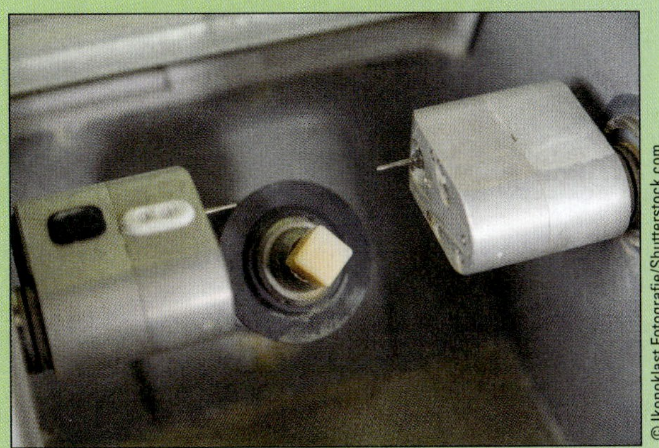

© Ikonoklast Fotografie/Shutterstock.com

FIGURE 34-11
A ceramic block ready for milling by the CAM system.

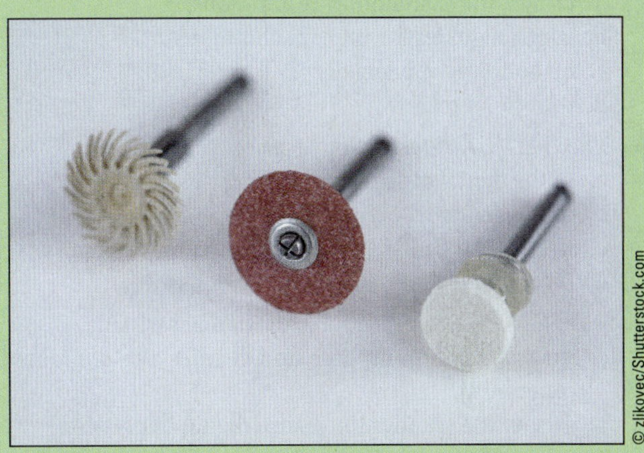

© zlikovec/Shutterstock.com

FIGURE 34-12
Discs, a rubber-polishing wheel, and ceramic stones are used to adjust and polish the restoration.

Chapter Summary

This chapter covers information on the ever-growing and advancing CAD/CAM technology. CAD/CAM systems are used by the dentist in the dental office and in the dental laboratory. As the software developed, the use of these systems has expanded into orthodontics and oral maxillofacial surgery. After reading this chapter, the student will have gained an understanding of computer-aided design (CAD) equipment and computer-aided manufacturing (CAM) systems. The components of the CAD/CAM systems are identified and explained. The steps for preparing the tooth, taking the digitized impression, designing the virtual restoration, and manufacturing the final restoration are described in detail. The technology is discussed including patient considerations and the role of the dental assistant. Also explained is how CAD/CAM systems are used with dental laboratories.

CASE STUDY

Kendra James was in for her routine dental examination and Dr. Mendes has found decay under an MOD restoration on tooth #5. After taking x-rays and completing the examination, Dr. Mendes has recommended that the MOD restoration be replaced with a crown. Kendra was concerned about the time involved and the cost of the crown. Dr. Mendes has included the CAD/CAM technology in his office since Kendra's last appointment. After talking with Kendra the dental assistant found out that Kendra was also concerned about the impressions because she has a gagging problem.

Case Study Review

1. What can be explained to Kendra about the time and expense of a crown procedure?
2. Discuss the steps involved with the CAD/CAM technology.
3. What can the dental assistant do to help Kendra with her gagging concerns?

Review Questions

Multiple Choice

1. When referring to digital impressions, CAD stands for
   a. computer-assisted design.
   b. computer-aided draft.
   c. computer-aided digital.
   d. computer-aided design.
2. The CAD/CAM systems can be used in all of the following procedures *except*:
   a. crown, inlay, and onlay restorations.
   b. surgical guides for implant abutments.
   c. orthodontic appliances.
   d. root canal therapy.
3. The CAD/CAM technology is used
   a. in the dental office only.
   b. in the dental laboratory only.
   c. in both the dental office and the dental laboratory.
   d. none of the above.
4. With CAD/CAM procedures the dental assistant
   a. turns on the computer and readies the computer programs.
   b. sets up the scanner to create a digital impression.
   c. prepares the ceramic block to be milled.
   d. all of the above.
5. With CAD/CAM training the dental assistant can complete all of the following *except*:
   a. Scan the cavity preparation to create a digital impression.
   b. Create the digital restoration using the CAD system.
   c. Send the digitized restoration to the CAM for milling *without* the dentist's evaluation and consent.
   d. Place the ceramic block in the milling machine.
6. The advantages of the CAD/CAM system used in the dental office include all of the following *except*:
   a. The fee is reduced because there is no dental laboratory involvement.
   b. No impressions are taken with routine materials and trays.
   c. The patient does not need to have provisional restorations.
   d. Saves time for the patient.
7. All of the following are components of the CAD/CAM system *except*:
   a. intraoral camera (scanner).
   b. cAD/CAM software.
   c. milling machine.
   d. gold or gold alloy blocks.
8. With the CAD/CAM technology all of the following statements are true *except*:
   a. Images of the occlusion or bite registration are scanned before the tooth is prepared.
   b. No shade needs to be taken; the computer selects the shade to match the patient's teeth.
   c. The digitized impression can be modified to enhance the gingival margins of the preparation.
   d. Diamond burs and water are used during the milling process of the ceramic block.
9. Restorations using CAD/CAM technology in the dental office and laboratory are
   a. completed in one appointment.
   b. completed in two appointments.
   c. a and b are both correct.
   d. only a is correct.
10. CAD/CAM systems sometimes use a ________ to obtain an enhanced digital image.
    a. reflective powder
    b. polishing agent
    c. desensitizing agent
    d. water solution

Critical Thinking

1. What are the advantages of using CAD/CAM technology in the office?
2. What is the importance of CAD/CAM technology to the dental assistant?
3. Name the types of materials that are used to mill the restoration.
4. Explain why the dentist may choose to place a gingival retraction cord before the preparation is scanned.
5. List the types of cameras used to capture the image.

Web Activities

1. Find the latest updates on the CEREC CAD/CAM system at http://www.cerec.net or http://www.sirona.com.
2. Go to http://www.ada.org/ and search for CAD/CAM systems to find out the ADA information on CAD/CAM systems used in dentistry today.
3. For more information on the four systems listed in Table 34-1 go to the individual Web sites. CERAC https://www.cereconline.com; E4D https://e4d.com; iTero, www.itero.com; and Lava COS www.3m.com.

CHAPTER

35

Cosmetic Dentistry and Teeth Whitening

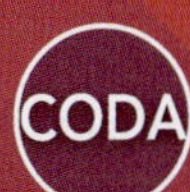

Specific Instructional Objectives

The student should strive to meet the following objectives and demonstrate an understanding of the facts and principles presented in this chapter:

1. Define cosmetic dentistry and describe what is involved in cosmetic dentistry.
2. Describe who performs cosmetic dentistry and education requirements.
3. Explain the role of the dental assistant in cosmetic dentistry.
4. Explain the scope of cosmetic dentistry.
5. Describe fundamental principles that the cosmetic dentist must learn when creating the perfect smile.
6. Discuss the basic elements of psychology and sociology that are considered for cosmetic treatment.
7. Explain what the patient should consider when selecting a dentist for cosmetic treatment.
8. Identify and describe specific procedures performed in cosmetic dentistry, including diagnosis and treatment planning, legal forms, and documentation.
9. Describe the role that oral photography has in cosmetic dentistry, the equipment needed, and how the patient is set up for the photographs to be taken.
10. Describe why soft tissue surgery may be needed in cosmetic dentistry, how it is performed, and how lasers and electrosurgery are involved.
11. Explain why the dental team needs to know about occlusion in cosmetic dentistry.
12. Describe the types of restorations that are placed and materials used for cosmetic restorations.
13. Describe the marketing techniques for cosmetic dentistry.

Advanced Chairside Functions

14. Explain how teeth are whitened, and causes of intrinsic and extrinsic tooth staining.
15. Explain the benefits of whitening techniques used in dentistry.
16. Describe the role of the dental assistant in the whitening process.
17. List and describe types of whitening techniques.
18. Describe the procedures for dental office whitening for vital and nonvital teeth, and for home whitening and over-the-counter whitening materials.
19. Explain information given to the patient about outcomes, procedures, responsibilities, and precautions related to teeth whitening.

Key Terms

American Academy of Cosmetic Dentistry (AACD) (808)
assisted whitening (827)
bleaching/whitening (823)
carbamide peroxide (824)
ceramometal restoration (821)
chroma (811)

(continues)

Key Terms (continued)

composite resin (821)
cosmetic dentistry (808)
crown lengthening (819)
documentation (817)
hue (811)
hydrogen peroxide (824)
illusion (811)
legal form (815)
mandibular occlusal view (819)
maxillary occlusal view (819)
natural light (810)
neuromuscular dentistry (820)
opacity (811)
porcelain restoration (821)
power whitening (826)
sodium perborate (824)
transitional line angles (812)
translucency (811)
value (811)
walking whitening technique (825)
white light teeth whitening systems (828)

Introduction

The search for means of enhancing the appearance of teeth dates at least to the Phoenicians around 800 BC. Animal tusks that were carved to resemble the shape, form, and hue of natural teeth were used as pontics to improve the appearance of the teeth. In the seventeenth century, gold shell crowns with enamel "veneers" were developed for improving esthetics. In the same century, a tooth powder was used to whiten teeth.

Porcelain teeth were first manufactured in the early part of the nineteenth century, while various techniques for esthetic crowns such as open-face crowns, porcelain jackets, and three-quarter crowns were developed later. In 1904, the first truly cosmetic restorative material was developed, a combination of acid-soluble glass blended with a liquid containing phosphoric acid. Shortly thereafter, a chemically activated acrylic resin was developed and acrylic veneer facings were widely used. In the 1970s, composite resins almost completely replaced acrylic resins. Since that time, numerous refinements of the basic formula of resin matrix and glass filler have been introduced, and new and improved products are continually placed on the market. With the advancement of various materials and inventive techniques, cosmetic dentistry is becoming increasingly popular.

Research continues, study groups are formed, continuing education courses/seminars are offered, and societies and journals are dedicated to cosmetic dentistry. Everyone wants a beautiful smile, and cosmetic dentistry has changed from a need-based treatment to an elective-based treatment.

In this chapter, various aspects of **cosmetic dentistry** are discussed, but details and procedures on the various types of crowns and veneers are included in Chapter 33, Fixed Prosthodontics and Gingival Retraction. Cosmetic dentistry also includes some orthodontic treatments (Chapter 28, Orthodontics) and oral surgery procedures (Chapter 25, Oral and Maxillofacial Surgery). If a patient requires either orthodontics or oral surgery, these become part of the treatment plan and are completed before cosmetic dentistry procedures are performed. Many dental patients want teeth that are caries free and esthetically pleasing. Because of this more periodontal plastic surgery is also involved in treatment planning. See Chapter 31, Periodontics, for more information on plastic surgery involving the periodontal tissues.

Cosmetic Dentist and Staff

The general dentist and prosthodontist perform many procedures that are part of cosmetic dentistry. Courses, seminars, and institutes on "smile designs or enhancements" provide extended training, both through lecture and clinical practice. Upon completing this training, dentists and staff members receive a certificate.

Established in 1984, the **American Academy of Cosmetic Dentistry (AACD)** is the largest international dental organization dedicated to the art and science of cosmetic dentistry. Members from all over the world include cosmetic and reconstructive dentists, dental laboratory technicians, educators, researchers, dental students, hygienists, corporations, and dental auxiliaries. To keep up-to-date with ongoing advancements in cosmetic dentistry, the AACD offers continued education through workshops, lectures, and publications. Dentists and their staff may also belong to local study clubs that provide support and updated information on products and techniques.

Two advanced credentialing programs are offered through the American Academy of Cosmetic Dentistry: Accreditation and Fellowship. To become an accredited member, the dentist must take continuing education courses and pass an examination process. This process includes a written exam and a clinical exam, in which the dentist submits clinical casework. Once the dentist successfully passes the written and clinical exams and becomes an accredited member of the AACD, she or he may choose to continue the pursuit of clinical education and fellowship. Fellowship is achieved when the dentist submits 50 clinical cases that exhibit competency in cosmetic dentistry.

Dental Staff

The staff of the dentist who performs cosmetic dentistry is similar to the staff of any dental office: front office personnel, business office staff, chairside assistants, and dental hygienists. Each member of the team plays an important part in the process of enhancing the appearance of a person's smile.

Office personnel ensure that the patient is scheduled in a convenient and timely manner. They also are the first to greet the patient and the last the patient sees before leaving the office. Their contact with the patient should be friendly and reassuring so that the patient is comfortable and confident in the treatment.

The business office staff will want to be familiar with the various dental insurance plans so that they can effectively communicate with the insurance companies. These staff members are also responsible for making financial arrangement with the patient that will work for both the dentist and the patient.

Most dental offices cannot accept long-term payment plans for services rendered. Currently, dental offices are often affiliated with banks and savings and loan institutions and recommend that the patient make financial arrangements through them.

At chairside, the assistant works with the dentist during cosmetic procedures that often include many expanded functions, such as placing and removing the rubber dam, taking detailed impressions, and creating esthetic temporaries for the patient to wear between treatments. The assistant is available to answer the patient's questions and provide reassurance and positive support throughout the procedure. The dental assistant may also accompany the dentist in additional training seminars, courses, and workshops, and therefore is knowledgeable about assisting with specific techniques and preparing various materials. Because they are close to both the dentist and the patient, assistants may be involved in designing the right smile for a specific person (Figure 35-1).

Dental hygienists often provide the patient with available options for improving the appearance of their teeth. They also speak with patients during hygiene treatment and learn about their desires regarding appearance. The hygienist can educate the patient about individual oral health needs and motivate them to talk to the dentist and other staff members. The hygienist may also be involved in providing oral hygiene care with detailed prophylaxis, fluoride treatments, and home care instructions.

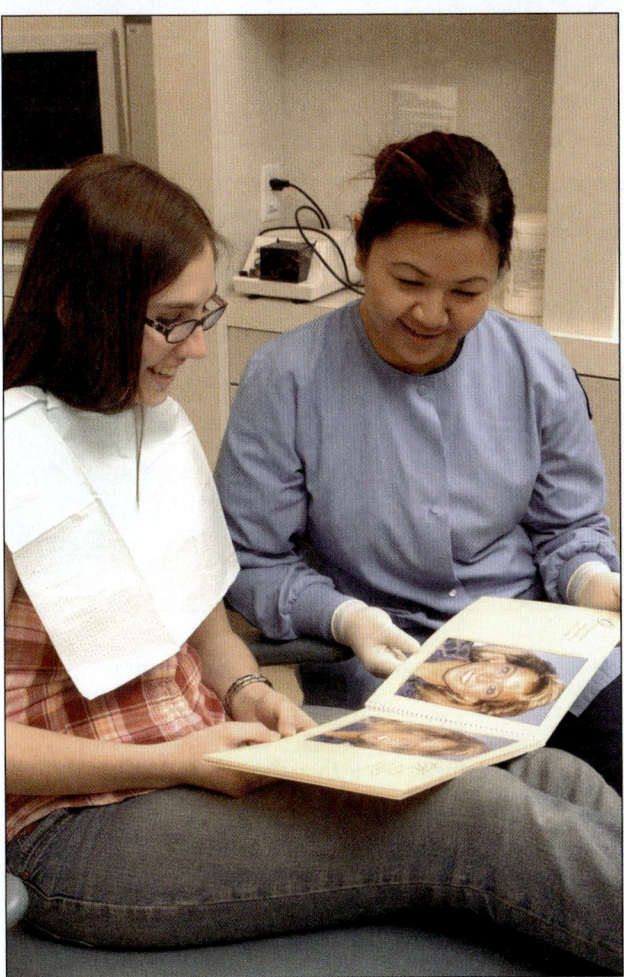

FIGURE 35-1
Dental assistant talking to a patient about cosmetic dentistry.

Scope of Cosmetic/Esthetic Dentistry

The scope of cosmetic/esthetic dentistry is very broad and diversified. General dentistry includes many aspects that we now consider to be part of "cosmetic dentistry," which sometimes makes the concept of this type of dental practice confusing. Most dentists do some cosmetic dentistry, but to be an actual "cosmetic dentist," the dentist needs continuing education at the postgraduate level and additional credentialing as mentioned previously.

Many procedures are included in cosmetic/esthetic dentistry. The cosmetic dentist performs some of these, and others are completed by various specialty dentists, including the orthodontist, periodontist, oral and maxillofacial surgeon, and prosthodontist. Selected cosmetic procedures are listed below:

- Bridges and crowns (Chapter 33, Fixed Prosthodontics and Gingival Retraction).
- Veneers (Chapter 33, Fixed Prosthodontics and Gingival Retraction).
- Tooth whitening (current chapter).
- Repositioning or straightening the teeth (orthodontics), including accelerated orthodontics (Chapter 28, Orthodontics).
- Lengthening the teeth (involves removal of gingival tissue with a laser and electrosurgery unit or scalpel). A periodontist often performs this stage of treatment (Chapter 31, Periodontics).
- Recontouring the gingival tissues (Chapter 31, Periodontics).
- Restoring length to crowns of the teeth (Chapter 31, Periodontics).
- Changing bite relationships (Chapter 28, Orthodontics).
- Closing gaps (diastema) (Chapter 33, Fixed Prosthodontics and Gingival Retraction).
- Repairing chips or fractures (Chapter 38, Restorative Materials and Matrix, and Wedge).
- Changing the shape and shade of the teeth (Chapter 33, Fixed Prosthodontics and Gingival Retraction).
- Replacing old metal restorations with cosmetic restorations (Chapter 38, Restorative Materials and Matrix, and Wedge).
- Replacing missing teeth with dental implants (Chapter 25, Oral and Maxillofacial Surgery).
- Dentures (Chapter 36, Removable Prosthodontics).
- Endodontic procedures (Chapter 24, Endodontics).

Cosmetic dentistry includes many procedures that improve patients' smiles, appearances, and how they feel about their teeth. All of the listed treatments are covered in other chapters of this book (excepting whitening)—this chapter's focus is on cosmetic dentistry as compared to general dentistry.

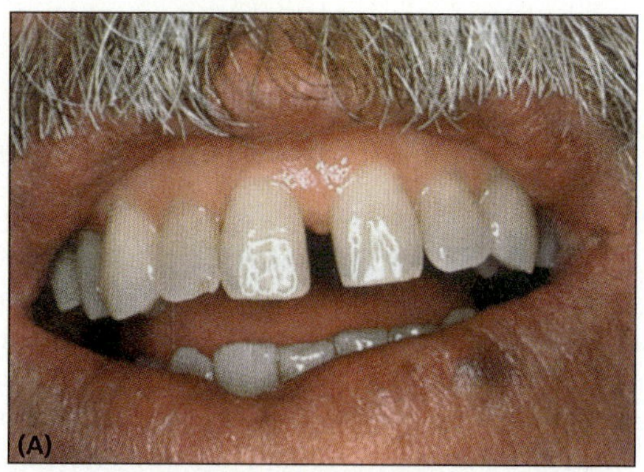
(A)

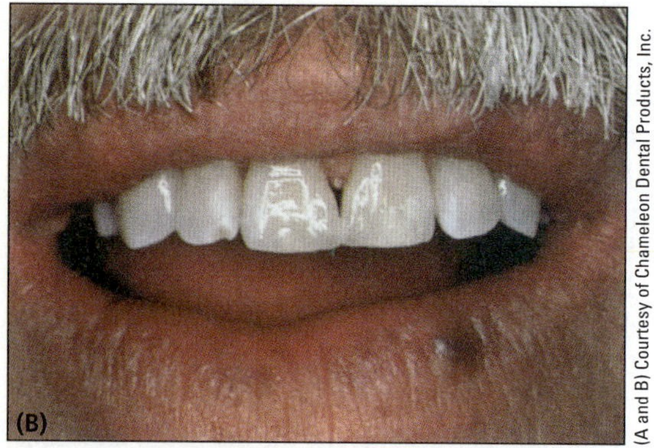
(B)

(A and B) Courtesy of Chameleon Dental Products, Inc.

FIGURE 35-2

(A) Patient with a large diastema between the central incisors. (B) Same patient after ceramic crowns have been placed to close the diastema.

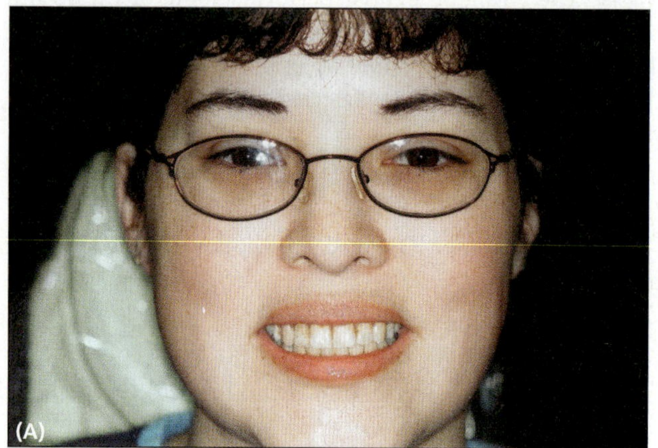
(A)

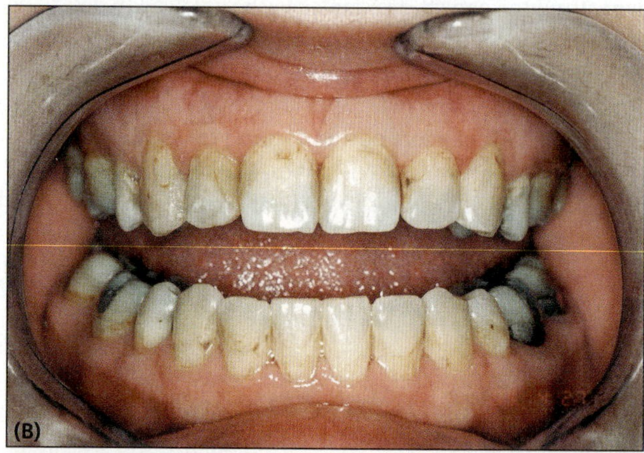
(B)

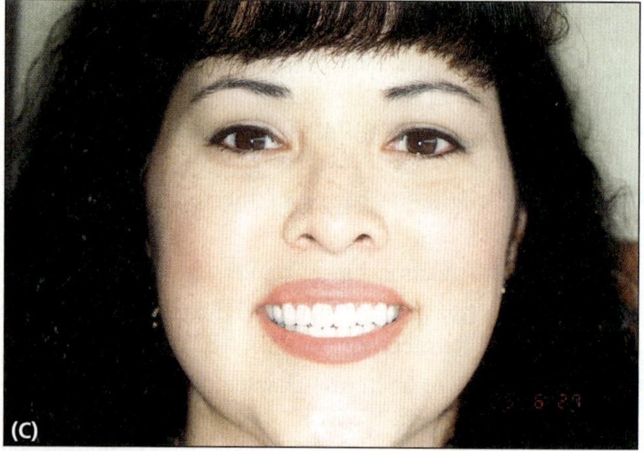
(C)

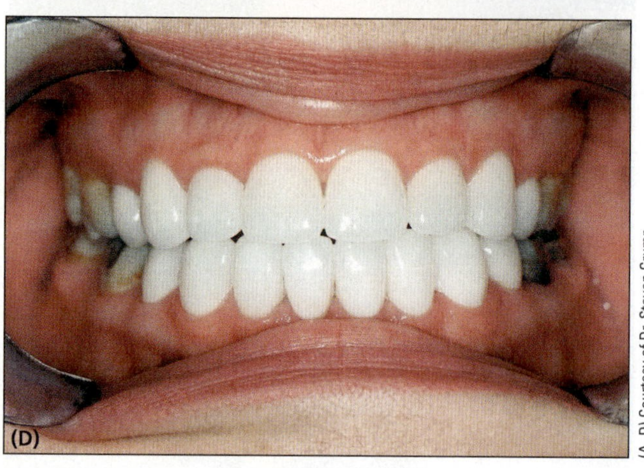
(D)

(A–D) Courtesy of Dr. Steven Crump

FIGURE 35-3

(A) Patient wanting to improve her smile. (B) The teeth are badly stained. (C) Patient after cosmetic dentistry with a beautiful smile. (D) Close-up of the cosmetic crowns.

Figures 35-2A and B and 35-3A–D illustrate before and after results of cosmetic dentistry treatment designs.

Fundamentals of Cosmetic Dentistry

The cosmetic dentist looks at the entire picture of the patient's teeth and gingival tissues. Everything is taken into consideration, including the light, color, illusion, shape, and form to create a more esthetic whole than the original. In the following sections, aspects considered by the cosmetic dentist and staff are briefly described.

Light

When selecting the shade of the teeth, **natural light** must be used. Natural light is multidirectional, casting shadows and showing texture. Dental restoration can be manipulated to cast a shadow and provide a feeling of depth to match adjacent teeth.

Color

There is much to learn about principles of color and how color is interpreted. The **hue** is the color per se (e.g., bright white, beige, and yellow). Younger permanent teeth appear to be similar in color throughout the mouth, but as the person ages and the teeth pick up intrinsic and extrinsic stains from smoking, foods, and restorative materials, hue will vary throughout the mouth. The **chroma** is the intensity or quality of the hue. Thus, to increase the chroma of a veneer, more color (hue) is added. The chroma of teeth responds to tooth whitening in both vital and nonvital teeth. The **value** corresponds to brightness, which is very important when matching shades.

The dentist and lab technician strive to match primary, secondary, and complementary hues. Often a variety of lights are used in color selection for a patient. In the dental treatment room, three lights can be used: the overhead light, usually a white fluorescent light, natural light from a window, and the dental unit light.

The dentist also must consider the **opacity** and **translucency** of a material. Opaque materials reflect light, and thus do not permit light to pass through. For instance, an extra layer of opaque porcelain is applied in a porcelain-fused-to-metal crown to prevent metal from showing through the crown. Translucent materials are the opposite—they allow light to pass through. Translucency of crowns and veneers makes them appear more natural.

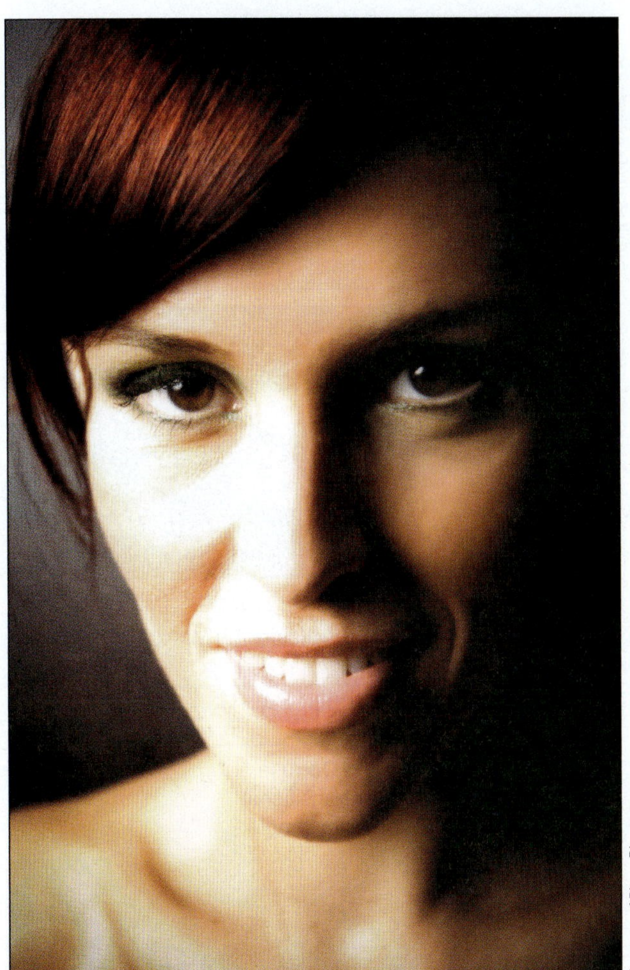

Courtesy of Photo Disc.

FIGURE 35-4
Photograph showing the principle of illumination. The light side comes forward while the dark side recedes.

Illusion

An **illusion** is the art of making something appear to be different than it actually is. Teeth can be made to appear larger or smaller and of various shapes through illusion. An artistic principle is that light areas appear to be closer or highlighted, whereas dark areas appear to recede. Manipulating light in this fashion will give the tooth dimension (depth) along with length and width (Figure 35-4).

Another aspect of illusion concerns the horizontal and vertical dimensions. Horizontal lines make the tooth appear to be wider while vertical lines make the tooth appear longer (Figure 35-5). This phenomenon is analogous to a person wearing horizontal- versus vertical-striped clothing; horizontal stripes tend to make a person appear shorter and wider, while vertical stripes make a person look taller and thinner.

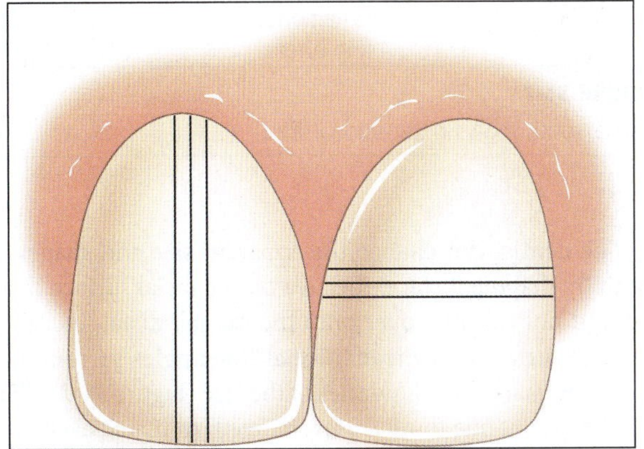

FIGURE 35-5
Drawing of tooth with horizontal lines and tooth with vertical lines, which shows illusion of length and width, respectively.

Shape and Form

In cosmetic dentistry, a tooth is viewed in an environment of other teeth. We perceive certain qualities about a tooth based on individual and cultural assumptions. For instance, many people assume that stained, heavily worn, and dark teeth belong to an older person. We have cultural and artistic biases on how we perceive a person's teeth, which include gender-based features of the teeth and how the teeth are proportioned. For example, women's teeth are often perceived as more rounded and translucent, while men's are more angled with a squared incisal edge (Figure 35-6 A and B). The cosmetic dentist can esthetically restore a person's teeth to persuade the eye of the observer that the latter, perceived qualities, conform to such biases.

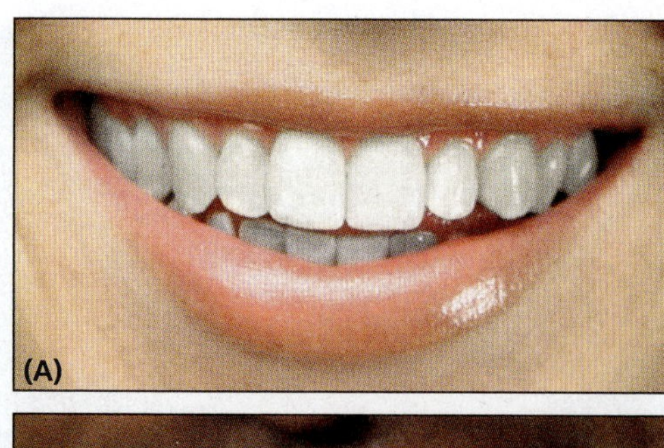

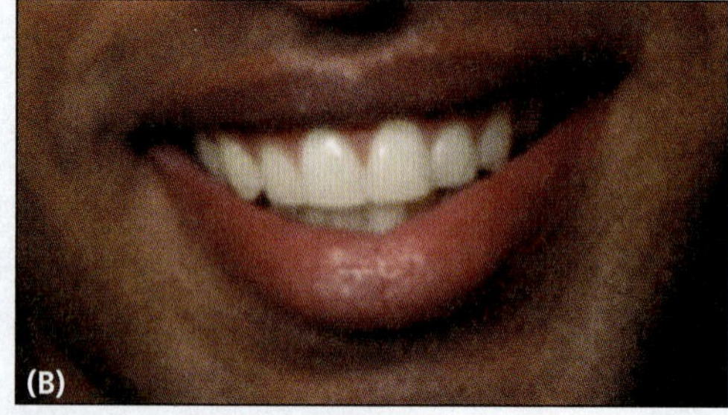

FIGURE 35-6

(A) Feminine teeth appear more rounded. (B) Masculine teeth appear squarer.

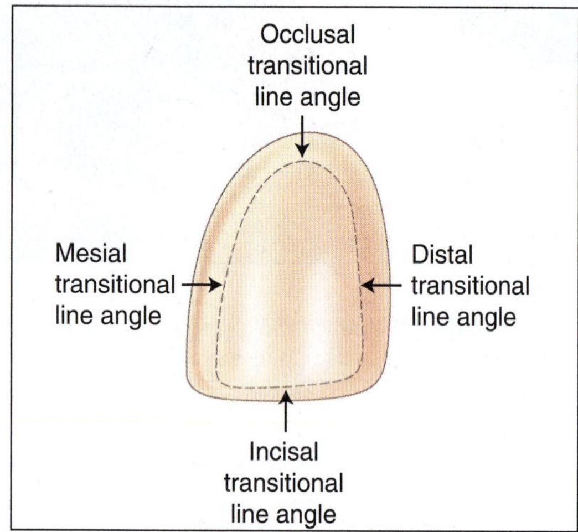

FIGURE 35-7

Face of tooth showing transitional lines.

The dentist can change the apparent size and shape of a tooth by shaping its face, the area on the facial surface that is flat and not running over onto the mesial, distal, incisal, or gingival surfaces. The **transitional line angles** surround the tooth and mark the boundaries of the face (Figure 35-7). Shaping the face of one tooth or several teeth to match each other will give the illusion that they are the same size and shape.

Cosmetic Dentistry and Psychology

Understanding a patient's feelings concerning their appearance and the appearance of their teeth is important. Knowledge of the patient's personality, motivations, desires, and expectations as well as the patient's ability to accept change

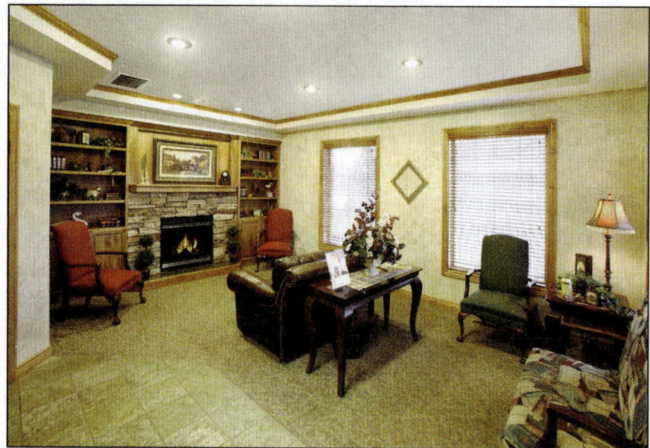

FIGURE 35-8

Open, friendly, private, and caring office reception area.

and cooperate will enhance and even determine the success of dental treatment. The dentist and dental team should be aware of Maslow's hierarchy of needs (see Chapter 2, Psychology, Communication, and Multicultural Interaction) and should have as well a general appreciation for the principles of psychology and sociology.

Psychological Influences

Psychological influences require learning about the patient's personality and his or her motivations, desires, and expectations. Establishing trust between dentist and patient requires that the dentist/dental team communicate empathetically and with a sincere desire to understand the patient and his or her dental cosmetic goals. Some dentists prefer the informal process of getting to know the patient's personality, which includes an interview and observation of the patient, while others prefer using questionnaires or personality tests.

Sometimes the dentist learns from the personality evaluation that the patient may need a family member to assist him or her in making decisions and to provide support during treatment. This person will be involved in all communications and may also come to appointments in which esthetic decisions are involved.

Psychological Environment. As it is true for all dental treatment, the need for a human touch is especially true for cosmetic treatment. Patients should feel that the entire office staff (or at least the individuals with whom he or she has contact) sincerely care about their welfare and are concerned with their dental treatment. The dentist and office staff should handle patients with respect and dignity throughout the treatment process. This is reflected in making patients comfortable, respecting their privacy, and being considerate of their time and schedules (Figure 35-8).

Sociological Influences

A number of social contemporary trends encourage individuals to seek esthetic dental treatment. The visual media (e.g., television, magazines, and advertising) exert a major influence on perceptions and attitudes about appearance. People are barraged with information on a daily basis about teeth whitening, veneers, orthodontic treatment, cosmetic surgery, and so on, and how much better they will feel and look once they partake in such services.

With escalating health care costs, many people are becoming more interested in disease prevention, and thus on maintaining health and fitness. The dental profession also endorses preventive care and clinical focus has shifted from caries to maintenance of oral health and esthetics. Meanwhile, people have become more involved in their medical/dental treatment, and they expect to participate and understand their options in order to make informed decisions.

How a Patient Selects a Cosmetic Dentist

If a patient is unhappy with the appearance or color of his or her teeth, or avoids smiling because of embarrassment about his or her teeth, he or she may be a candidate for cosmetic dentistry. A smile makeover can change a person's whole outlook on life and thus enhance self-confidence and self-esteem.

Finding a cosmetic dentist who understands the type of results a patient wishes to achieve is important. Good communication between the dentist/dental team and the patient is key to successful cosmetic treatment. The American Academy of Cosmetic Dentistry suggests that the patient look for a dentist who is skilled in cosmetic dentistry procedures. Patients are encouraged to consult with the dentist to identify the right procedures to meet their goals (Figure 35-9). Several areas that the patient should consider when selecting a cosmetic dentist are as follows:

- Get a referral—ask friends and family about the type and quality of care the dentist has provided.
- Ask the dentist for credentials on cosmetic dentistry. Has she or he completed continuing education courses to remain up-to-date on the latest techniques in clinical cosmetic dentistry?
- Examine before and after pictures—ask the dentist for such photographs of other patients who have completed cosmetic dental treatment in his or her office.

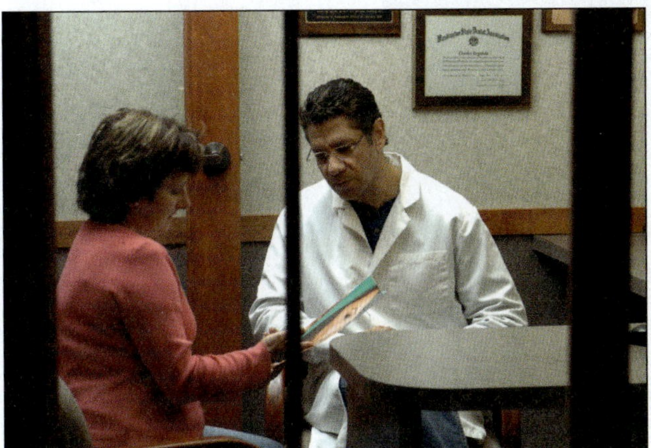

FIGURE 35-9
Patient interviewing cosmetic dentist.

The patient might also consider the availability of appointments, that is, whether the office schedule is compatible with his or her timeframe. In addition, the patient should ask about how a patient is scheduled if a problem occurs or an adjustment needs to be made.

Another consideration is the availability of financial arrangements and options for payments. The patient should determine the dental office financial policies, requirements, and communication responsibilities for working with his or her insurance company.

Procedures in Cosmetic Dentistry

Before any dental treatment begins, the dentist should thoroughly discuss with patients their expectations and esthetic desires. This discussion should include a history as well as the patient's attitude toward previous treatments. These first steps can facilitate success of the cosmetic treatment by establishing clear and open communication between the patient and the dentist and dental staff. Patients need to explain their concerns with the appearance of their teeth in as much detail as possible. The dentist may inform the patient of ways that the appearance of their teeth can be enhanced, with the use of before and after pictures, models, videos, computer programs, and pamphlets (Figures 35-10 A–C).

Diagnosis and Treatment Planning

The following items are items needed for the diagnostic records before a treatment plan can be designed for an individual patient:

- Medical and dental history
- Full-mouth x-rays
- Panoramic radiographs
- Periodontal charting
- Examination of existing restorations
- Occlusal analysis
- Study models
- Photographic series

Once all information is gathered, the dentist reviews it and designs a treatment plan. An appointment is set up with the patient for the case presentation. During the case presentation the dentist and staff members must educate the patient about oral health requirements for cosmetic dental treatment. With the use of visual aids, such as study models, photographs, and dental radiographs, the dentist can inform the patient about what needs to be done to attain his or her desired results. At this time the dentist explains to the patient everything involved in the treatment plan. Sometimes the patient needs to be referred to a specialist for treatment before cosmetic treatment actually begins. Once the patient understands what is involved in the treatment, the dentist and staff must motivate

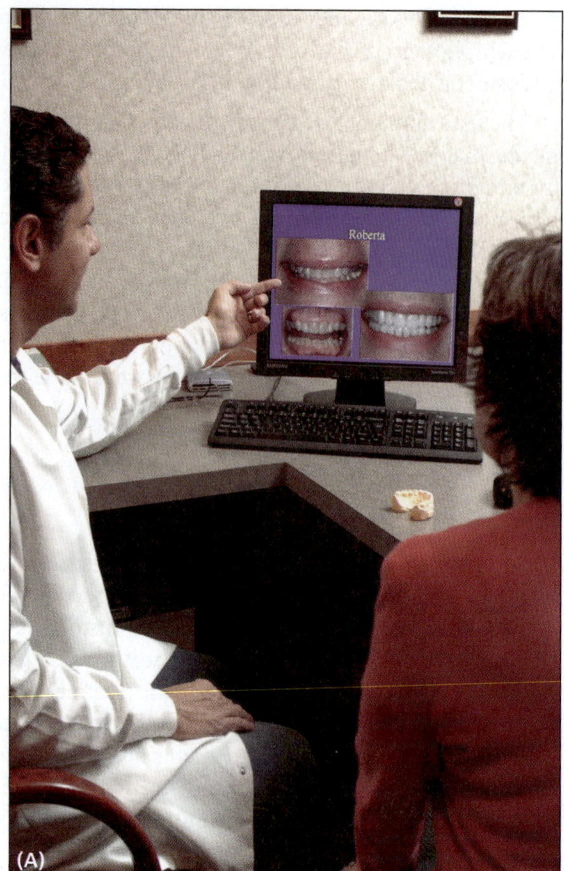

(A)

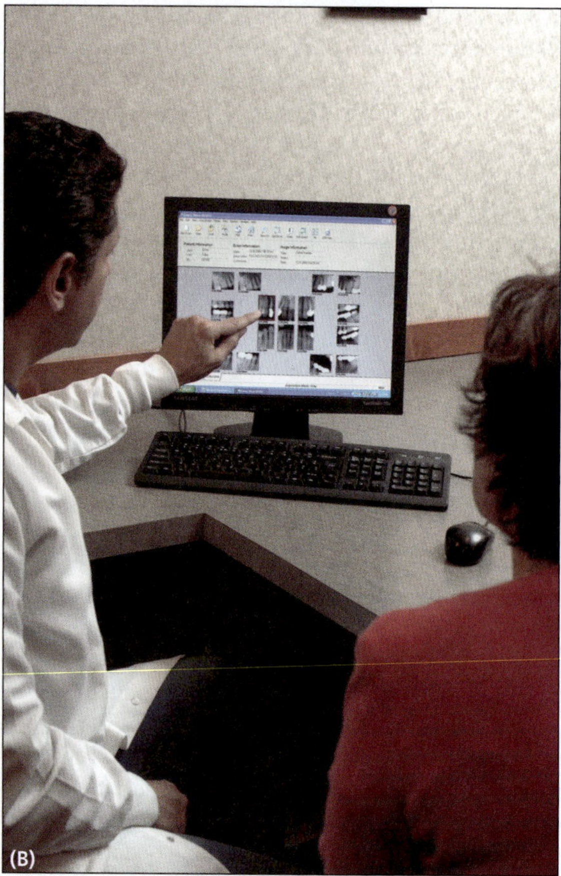
(B)

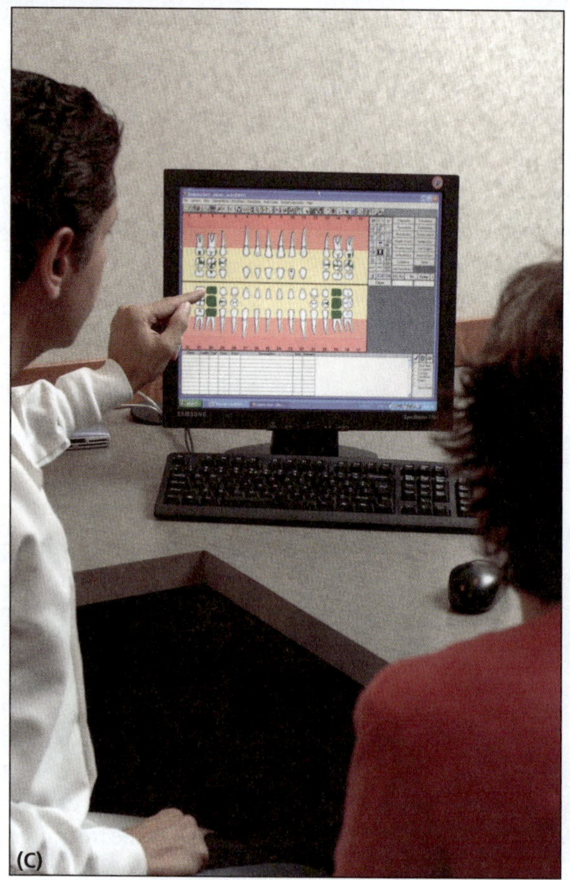
(C)

FIGURE 35-10

Everything needed for cosmetic case presentation: medical/dental history. (A) Photographs. (B) X-rays, panoramic x-ray. (C) Periodontal and restoration chart and occlusal evaluation.

the patient to accept and make financial arrangements to pay for the treatment.

Legal Forms and Documentation

Because cosmetic dentistry involves increased risk, following a specific format with every patient is important. All **legal forms** should accurately describe the treatment and the expected outcome. The patient should sign a consent form that is specifically designed for the dentist and the expected treatment (Figures 35-11 A–C).

The dentist and staff must determine whether the patient fails to realize the limitations of dentistry. Special precautions must be taken by dentists who practice primarily cosmetic dentistry because subjective opinions about treatment results may determine whether a patient files a lawsuit. See Chapter 40,

(A) Consent to Dental Treatment

I, (print name) ______________________________ have been

informed by Dr. (print name) ______________________________, of the need to

undergo dental treatment as presented to me on ______________________ .

I have been fully informed about the details of the recommended treatment and alternatives, and agree to accept the treatment as recommended by the doctor.

I understand that as the treatment proceeds there may be need to change the treatment plan. If this occurs I expect to be informed before any change is instituted.

I further understand that individual reactions to treatment cannot be predicted, and that if I experience any unanticipated reactions during or following any treatment, I agree to report them to the office as soon as possible.

I have been told that the success of the recommended treatment depends upon my cooperation in keeping scheduled appointments, following home care instruction, including oral hygiene and dietary instructions, and reporting to the office any change in my health status as soon as possible.

I have discussed all of the above with the doctor, and all my questions have been answered.

I acknowledge that no guarantees or assurances have been given by anyone as to the results that may be obtained.

Following the explanation, the discussion, and the answers to my questions, I authorize the doctor to complete the treatment as described.

______________________________ Patient's Signature

______________________________ If a Minor, Signature of Parent Or Guardian

______________________________ Witness Signature

______________________________ Doctor's Signature

______________________________ Date

FIGURE 35-11

(A) Consent to dental treatment form.

(continues)

(B)

Request for Release of Health Information

I, (print name) ______________________________, hereby grant permission to (print name of doctor or hospital) ______________________________ to release information related to my health history, status, and treatment, and copies of my health record, X-rays, and any test results to:

____

At ______________________________

____

Signature ______________________________ Date ______________

(if a minor, parent or guardian must sign)

(C)

Permission to Take Photographs, Slides, & Videos

I, (print name) ______________________________, hereby authorize Dr. (print name) ______________________________ to take photographs, slides, and/or videos of my face, jaws, and teeth.

I understand that the photographs, slides, and/or videos will be used as a record of my care, and may be used for educational purposes in lectures, demonstrations, and professional publications.

I further understand that if the photographs, slides, and/or videos are used in any publication, or as part of a demonstration, reasonable attempts will be made to conceal my identity.

____
Patient's Signature

____
If a Minor, Signature of Parent Or Guardian

____
Witness Signature

____
Doctor's Signature

____
Date

FIGURE 35-11 (continued)

(B) Request for release of health information form. (C) Permission form.

Dental Office Management for more information on consent and informed consent.

Careful and detailed **documentation** should be routine procedure for all treatments. Examples of information that should be documented are as follows:

- A detailed treatment plan was given to the patient, the patient signed a consent form before treatment began, and the patient was informed about all the risks and benefits of treatment.
- Comments made by the patient during the case presentation or course of treatment that indicate concerns or doubts.
- Adverse occurrences or problems that arose during the course of treatment.
- Requests for consultation with other health care practitioners.
- Cancellations, late arrivals, and changes of appointments.
- Evidence that the patient did not follow the treatment plan involving other dental specialists, such as orthodontic treatment or periodontal surgery required before cosmetic treatment can begin.
- Instances in which the patient did not follow home care instructions.

Oral Photography

Oral photography is a new skill that many cosmetic dentists must acquire. The digital or 35-mm camera has become an indispensable piece of equipment in the cosmetic practice. Although the use of film as a storage medium has declined (due to use of computers, digital cameras, and printers), conventional photography at present produces a clearer and higher-quality photograph.

Uses of Oral Photography

- Case presentation—Close-up photographs should be taken before any dental treatment begins. These photos are used during the case presentation to explain the proposed treatment plan to the patient. These photos can also be used with a portfolio of before and after photographs of similar, successfully treated cases. Photographs are also taken once the treatment is complete.
- Patient records—Before and after photographs are kept as part of the patient's records. The dentist should have the patient sign a release form so the photographs can be used in office displays and in case presentations.
- Laboratory communication—Oral photographs give the dental laboratory technician another means of visualizing desired treatment outcomes for the patient.
- Insurance—Treatment plans may have a better chance of acceptance if photographs accompany insurance claims. Photographs will display certain things that are not evident on radiographs. Insurance programs may reimburse the patient for the cost of the photographs just as radiographs are covered.
- Quality control—A magnified image sometimes shows things that are not evident by viewing the patient. Photographs also are used by the dentist when she or he is studying a case in the patient's absence.
- Marketing and education—Before and after photographs are a wonderful marketing tool. The photographs can be displayed in the office or in pamphlets, newsletters, and so on that advertises a particular dentist's work. Photographs can also be used when the dentist is lecturing, sharing information at study clubs, or conferring with other dentists or dental specialists.

Basic Equipment for Dental Photography

The basic equipment necessary for taking quality photographs includes a 35-mm SLR camera, digital cameras, a macro lens, a flash unit to obtain proper lighting, film that is suitable for dental exposures, a variety of shapes and sizes of frontal surface glass mirrors to produce a clear view, and lip and cheek retractors (Figures 35-12 and 35-13). Some dental offices have

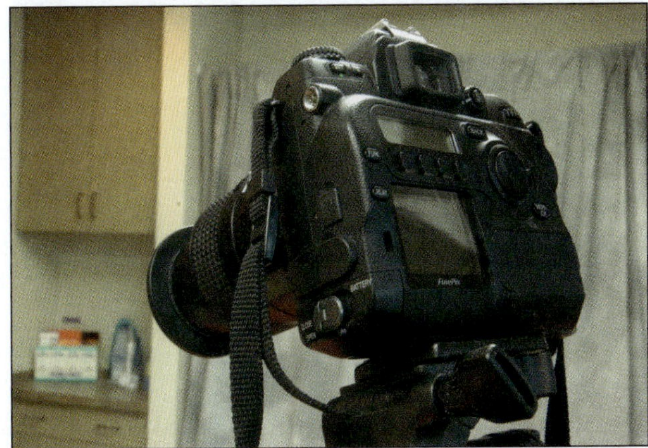

FIGURE 35-12

Camera used to take photographs in preparation for cosmetic dentistry.

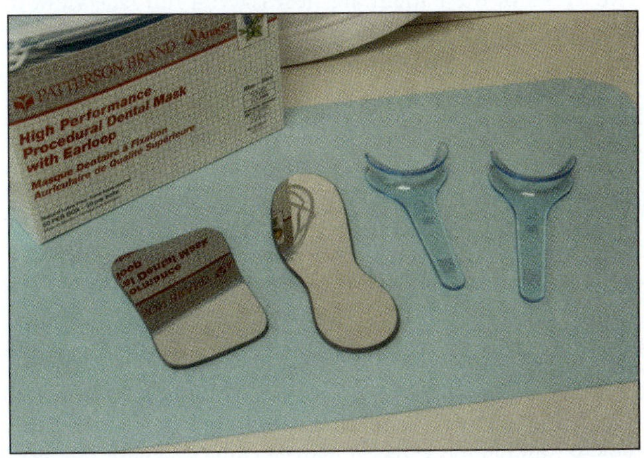

FIGURE 35-13

Various mirrors and cheek retractors used to take oral photographs of maxillary and mandibular arches.

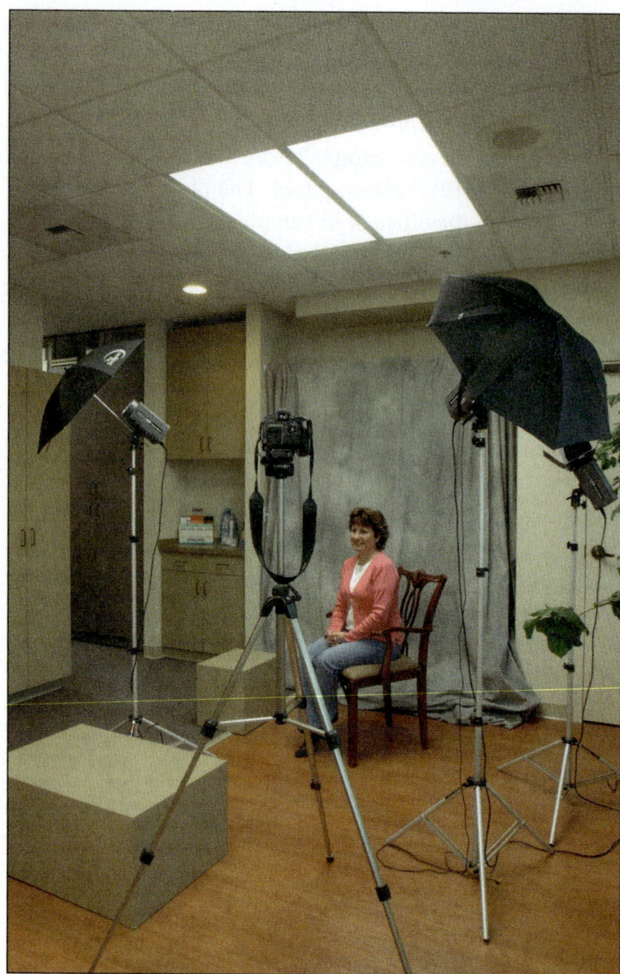

FIGURE 35-14
Area in dental office where photographs are taken.

a special area set up for photographs, while in others the photographs are taken when the patient is seated in the dental chair (Figure 35-14).

Extraoral Techniques

Two views of the patient are necessary: a full face view, in which the patient is seated with the head positioned looking straight ahead with the line from the ala of the nose to the tragus of the ear parallel to the floor (Figures 35-15 A and B); and a profile view, in which the patient's head is positioned showing one side of the face (the profile) with the ala of the nose to the tragus of the ear parallel to the floor (Figure 35-16).

Intraoral Techniques

Intraoral techniques involve using retraction means and mirrors. The anterior or frontal view, which can be taken with the use of cheek and lip retractors, shows the entire anterior dentition. Sometimes a more relaxed, casual view is also taken; this type of photograph shows a natural smile line with the teeth exposed (retractors are not used).

The maxillary occlusal and mandibular occlusal views are difficult to expose. The patient is positioned in a semi-upright

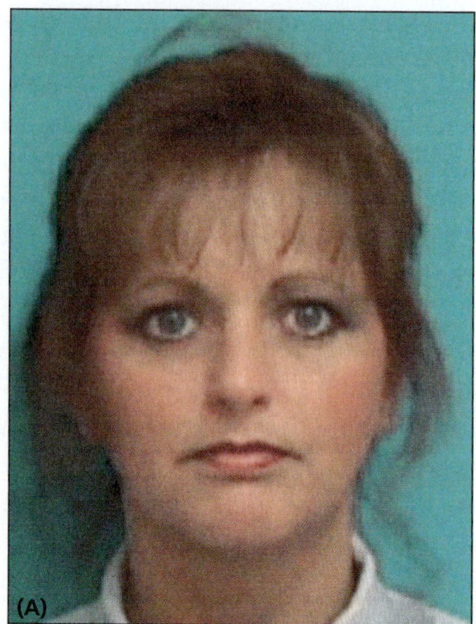

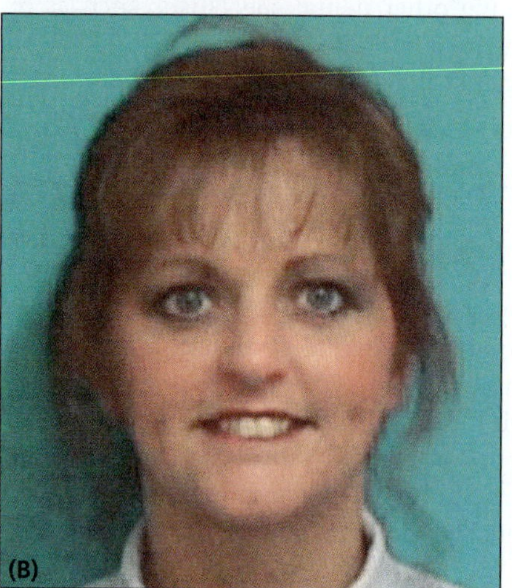

FIGURE 35-15
Photograph of full face view with (A) the lips closed (B) the patient smiling.

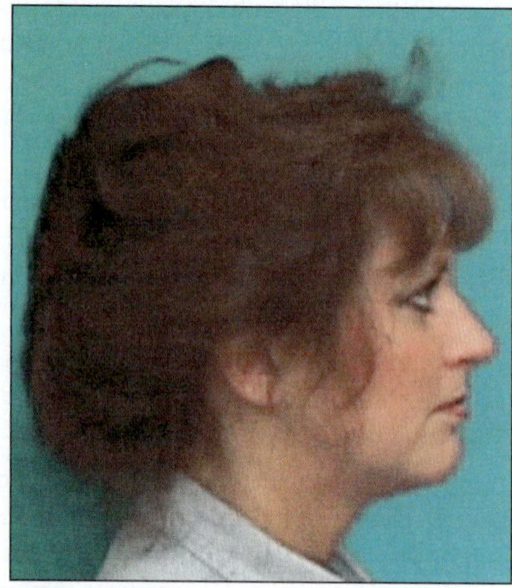

FIGURE 35-16
Photograph of side-face (profile) view.

position with his or her mouth open. Usually one assistant holds the lip and cheek retractors in the patient's mouth while another assistant positions the mirror so that it is resting on the maxillary tuberosity (Figure 35-17).

The **mandibular occlusal view** is the reverse of the **maxillary occlusal view**; the patient is positioned in the supine position parallel to the floor. The head is tilted back and the occlusal plane is parallel to the floor. One assistant places the retractors and another positions the mirror to rest on the retromolar pad (Figure 35-18).

The buccal views and lingual views are taken using mirrors and lip retractors. The buccal views are ideal for showing the patient's centric occlusion and bite relationship, while the lingual views show the lingual right or left side of the maxillary or mandibular arch (Figures 35-19 A and B).

Contouring Soft Tissues in Cosmetic Dentistry

Cosmetic dental treatment may also include contouring of the soft tissues. As part of the evaluation, the dentist will examine and probe the gingival tissues and sulcus. The appearance of the gingival tissues is just as important as other elements in the mouth for achieving a pleasing smile (Figure 35-20).

Indications for Treatment

Indications for soft tissue contouring include incomplete passive eruption of one or more teeth. With this condition, the patient appears to have very short teeth with a lot of gum tissue showing, hypertrophied or malpositioned papilla, inflamed tissues as a result of orthodontic treatment, hypertrophied gingival tissue from drug therapy (such as Dilantin), or hypertrophied gingival tissue from poor oral hygiene or pathologic conditions.

In some cases, the anterior teeth appear shorter than normal. This can be caused by gingival tissue enlargement, short clinical crowns, or altered or delayed eruption. It is important for the dentist to evaluate the cause of the problem before proceeding with treatment. For example, gingival enlargement may be caused by gingival inflammation from a systemic problem such as diabetes or pregnancy, or from a hereditary problem such as gingival fibromatosis. In some cases, the tooth fails to erupt normally and the width of the gingiva can be quite large; in others a short clinical crown may be the result of attrition due to bruxism. After the diagnosis and etiology is determined, a treatment can be selected that may include esthetic **crown lengthening** to improve the patient's appearance. Esthetic crown lengthening is indicated to establish the proper relation of the gingival margin with the lip and to increase the length of the teeth for appearance and for prosthetic crown retention.

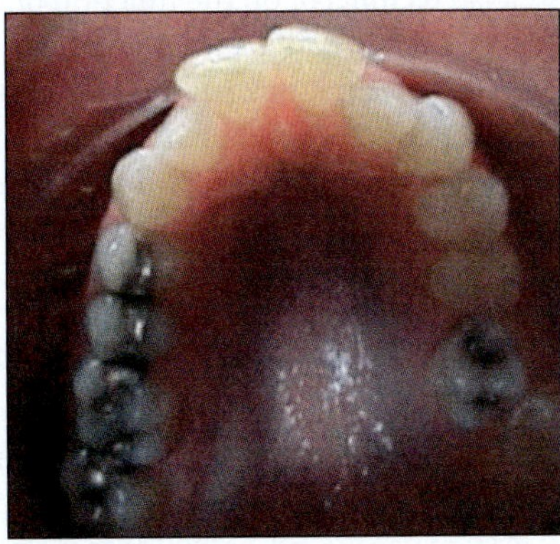

FIGURE 35-17
Photograph of maxillary occlusal view.

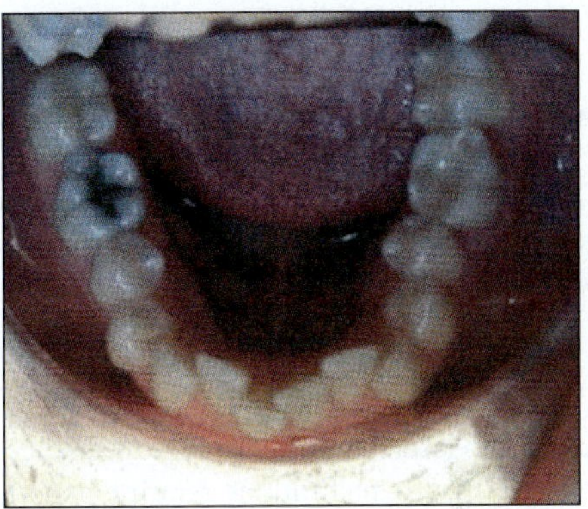

FIGURE 35-18
Photograph of mandibular occlusal view.

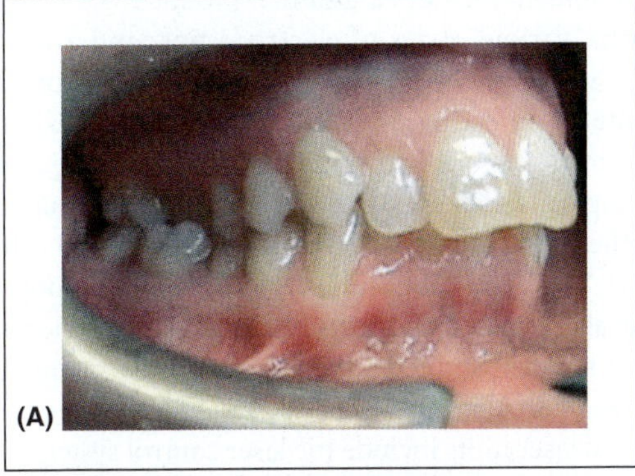

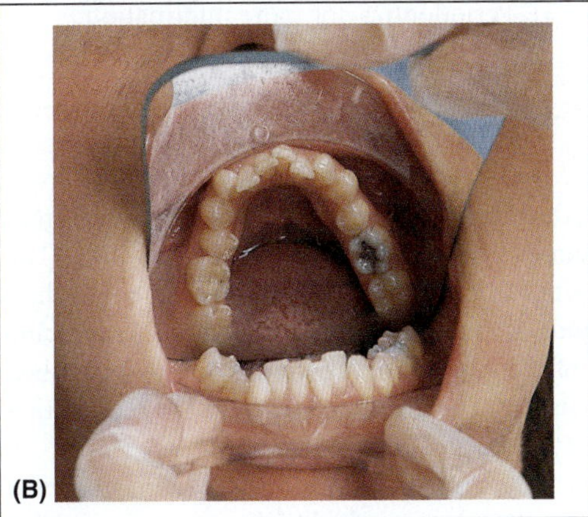

FIGURE 35-19
(A) Buccal view (B) Lingual view using a mirror.

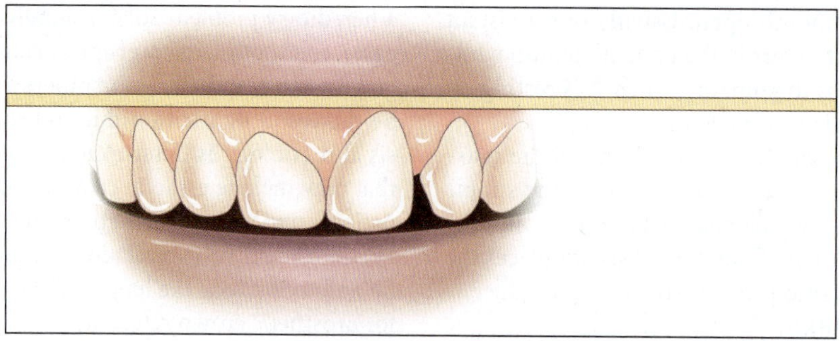

FIGURE 35-20
Evaluation of gingival tissue symmetry.

In this procedure, to determine the amount of tissue that needs to be removed, the dentist locates the Cementoenamel Junction (CEJ) (which is significantly subgingival) and determines the bone level (which is usually 1 to 2 mm apical to the CEJ) before proceeding with the crown lengthening.

Methods for Soft Tissue Contouring

Electrosurgery or lasers are used to remove and contour the gingival tissues. Both techniques require that the dentist become familiar with the equipment and skilled in the detailed application steps.

Electrosurgery equipment and techniques have been used for many years. The equipment has improved as have the precise techniques required for esthetic contouring. Electrosurgery equipment includes a unit that produces various current strengths, various styles of electrode tips, and a foot pedal control. See Chapter 31, Periodontics, for more information.

Dental lasers are becoming increasingly popular, and have proven to be an ideal technology for gum contouring and reshaping. Soft tissue lasers offer degrees of precision that surpass other techniques while minimizing pain and other discomfort. The dentist will choose a dental laser among several types available based on primary intended use. Education and training for dentist and staff are provided by manufacturers when the dentist purchases a laser system.

Dental laser units include the laser control system, a handpiece with various tips, water reservoir, and a foot pedal. See Chapter 31, Periodontics, for more information.

Basic Clinical Technique for Soft Tissue Contouring

Ideally, the height of the gingival tissues of the central incisors is the same as the height of the cuspids (canines). The height of the gingival tissues of the laterals is just below the centrals or cuspids. If the first premolars (bicuspids) are included, the height of the gingival tissue should be 1 to 2 mm below that of the cuspids. The techniques involved to achieve these goals must be precise and accurate.

After the anesthetic is administered, the sulcular areas of the involved teeth are probed to determine the depth and orientation of the sulcus. A guide tooth is selected, usually an anterior tooth that is not involved in the surgical procedure. A straightedge tangent is held to the gingival height and parallel to the pupils of the patient's eyes to determine the amount of gingival tissues to be removed for achieving symmetry. An explorer is used to penetrate the gingival tissue to mark the amount of tissue to be removed. The dentist evaluates whether sufficient gingiva exists to perform the contouring before proceeding (remember the adage "measure twice, cut once"). The tissues are then contoured and reshaped with a dental laser or electrosurgery. Typically, little bleeding occurs when either of these techniques is used. The gingival tissue height is evaluated throughout the procedure and then confirmed for accuracy using a straight line once all the tissue has been contoured.

Occlusion in Cosmetic Dentistry

Another area considered essential in successful esthetic treatment is occlusion. The cosmetic dentist will examine the patient's occlusion to determine whether any malocclusion exists. Malocclusions may result from skeletal, dental, or muscular problems. The mandible and maxilla are evaluated separately and in relationship to each other. A patient with occlusal problems involving orthodontic principles beyond the scope of the dentist should be referred to a specialist for a diagnosis. The orthodontist must consider whether restorative techniques may be a better means of treatment than extensive orthodontic therapy.

Traditionally, the dentist takes detailed, precise impressions of the patient's maxillary and mandibular arches. These impressions are poured up in stone and articulated. The dentist consults with a lab technician on the function of the patient's bite and how esthetic restorations will be affected.

Placing cosmetic restorations has a significant impact on occlusion, which is a topic in the subdiscipline of **neuromuscular dentistry**. The field of neuromuscular dentistry is defined as "the science of occlusion that objectively measures the physiologic functions affected by occlusion to achieve an optimal relationship between the skull and the mandible."

Occlusion is evaluated and treated so that the muscles that control the jaw position are optimal for ideal function and the patient's comfort. Several devices are used to assist in evaluating occlusion before cosmetic treatment begins. One such analysis system uses a grid-based sensor to provide vivid graphics for the dentist to use in determining and adjusting a patient's bite to achieve the perfect bite (Figures 35-21 A–C).

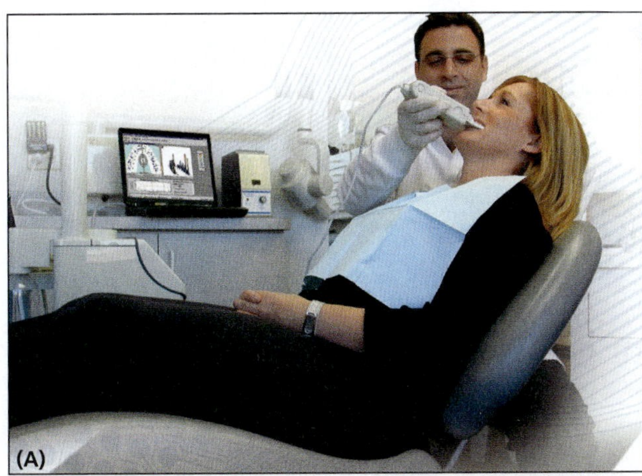

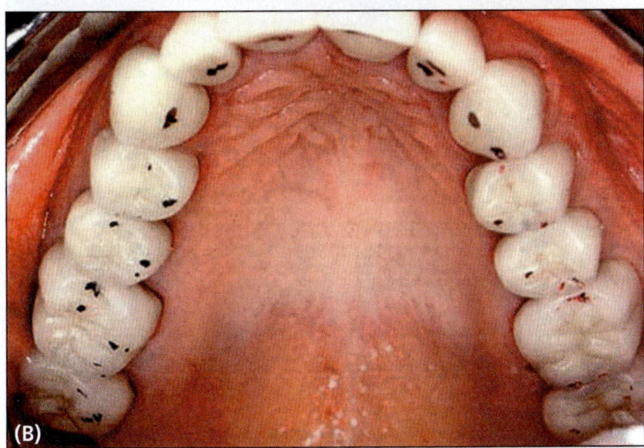

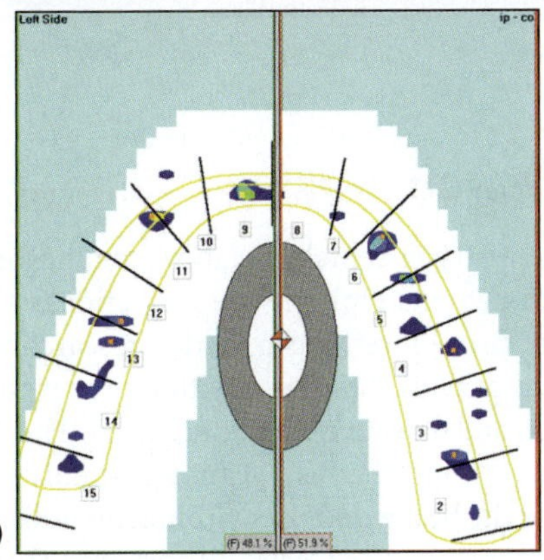

(A–C) Courtesy of Tekscan, Inc.

FIGURE 35-21

(A) Patient having occlusion scanned/evaluated. (B) Arch marked with articulating paper. (C) Graphic scan of occlusal analysis.

Types of Restorations and Materials

While most types of restorations and materials used in cosmetic dentistry have been around for awhile, they are continually being improved and updated. Some of these materials, such as dentin-bonding materials, are into respective fourth and fifth generations of development. The dentist and the dental staff must keep themselves up-to-date on new techniques and steps in a given procedure. This section provides a brief overview of selected types of restorations and materials used in cosmetic dentistry.

The **composite resin** is used in both direct and indirect techniques.

- The direct composite resin technique involves preparation of the tooth; placement of liners and bonding agents; and insertion of the composite resin into the tooth, carving, and filling completion. Many types of composite resins are available, and resin selection depends on the design and location of the cavity. Most of these materials are light cured and placed in increments or layers. Each layer is placed and then light cured before the next layer is placed. Direct composite resins are available in various shades to match the tooth and provide the patient with an esthetically pleasing restoration. More information on the various types of direct composite resins and their composition and characteristics is found in Chapter 38, Restorative Materials and Matrix, and Wedge.
- The indirect composite resin technique involves preparation of the tooth, taking a final impression and sending it to a dental laboratory, and fabrication of a restoration with a laboratory-processed composite resin. One advantage of this technique derives from rapid advances in composite resin technology. These materials have physical properties and appearance that are similar to porcelain, but without some of the problems associated with porcelain. For example, porcelain is harder than tooth enamel and can cause the opposing tooth structure to wear during normal function. In addition, if a porcelain restoration needs to be adjusted, it cannot be polished as well as a composite resin restoration.

Composite resins used for direct and indirect restorations are improving rapidly, and systems for the office and laboratory use will be available soon. These systems are expected to meet both esthetic and functional expectations.

A **ceramometal restoration** is used in conditions of heavy occlusal stress and for multiple-unit fixed prostheses. These crowns offer both strength and acceptable appearance. A ceramometal restoration is comprised of metal alloy on the inside for strength, and porcelain on the outside for esthetics. The porcelain-to-metal bond is very strong and technique sensitive. In the dental laboratory, the first step is to make the metal crown, followed by fabrication of the porcelain cap, which is painted on and then fired. See Chapter 33, Fixed Prosthodontics and Gingival Retraction, for further details.

A **porcelain restoration** can be made as full crowns/coverage or as partial veneers/coverage. These ceramic restorations are esthetically advanced compared to metaloceramic restorations. Drawbacks of porcelain restorations are their relative lack of strength and the fact that usage is limited to single teeth.

All-ceramic (porcelain) materials are used in the following restorations: jacket crowns (Figure 35-22), Dicor crowns, IPS Empress Crowns, and In-Ceram and Procera AllCeram crowns. Each of these systems has advantages and disadvantages, with

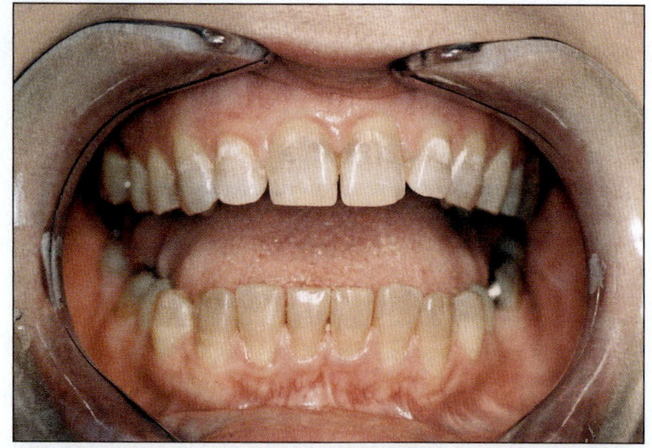

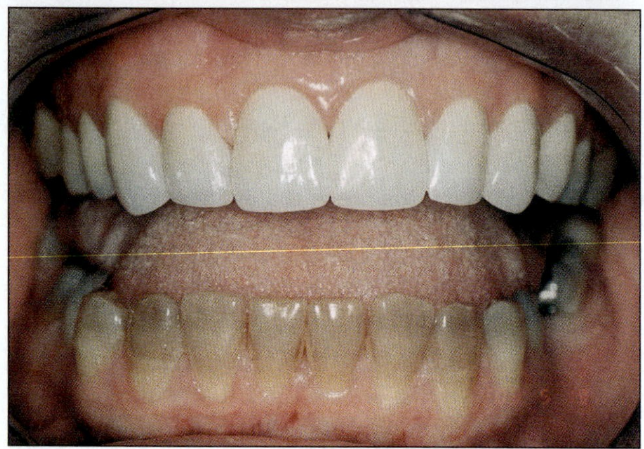

FIGURE 35-22
Before and after photographs of maxillary porcelain crowns.

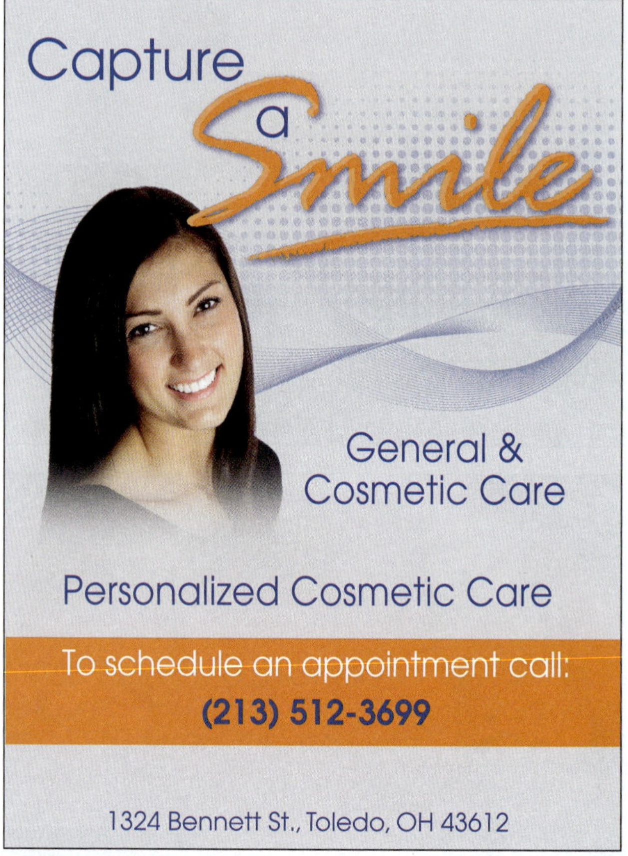

FIGURE 35-23
Advertisement for cosmetic dentistry.

the newer systems presenting improvements in the areas of strength, versatility, and natural appearance.

Veneers can be fabricated right in the office or at a dental laboratory. For more information, see Chapter 33, Fixed Prosthodontics and Gingival Retraction.

Marketing Cosmetic Dentistry

Marketing cosmetic dentistry is similar to marketing for any other product or service. Various techniques are used to motivate a particular individual to become informed on available cosmetic services that would make possible that perfect smile they have always wanted. Marketing then motivates the person to take action by finding a cosmetic dentist and going ahead with the treatment.

Marketing through advertising involves relaying a specific message by means of television, radio, magazines, and newspapers (Figure 35-23). Advertising also includes direct mailings, such as office newsletters or information on services and coupons for services. Marketing messages can be printed on pens, calendars, or cups, and then distributed to patients and prospective patients. All of these means should be considered as part of the dental practice's marketing plan.

Marketing Plan for the Dental Office

Cosmetic dentistry is dental care above and beyond routine services, and patients typically use discretionary income to pay for these procedures. Basic market research is typically carried out to provide the dentist with a clear picture of how practice goals and objectives can be achieved. The dentist and dental staff work together as a team to formulate goals and objectives for the best working environment, utilizing the talents of each team member. Goals and objectives then are those of the dentist and staff.

A marketing plan may include the following:

- Goals and objectives of practice
- Assessment of target audience
- Specific marketing tools and activities
- Timeframes and budget
- Method to evaluate results

Goals and objectives may be specific, relating to cosmetic dentistry and marketing this aspect of the practice. Some dental practices are wholly dedicated to cosmetic dentistry, while others provide both general dentistry and cosmetic dentistry services.

A profile of existing active patients and a profile of potential patients will assist the dentist and staff in determining the marketing plan direction. The practice should consider the age and income levels of their patients, and the most common types of treatments completed. Then the marketing plan can include ways to educate, motivate, and facilitate these individuals.

Specific marketing techniques should be discussed and then implemented for a predetermined time period. Marketing can be done in and out of the office. In-office marketing can be accomplished by dental team members answering patient questions and using videos, pamphlets, and other means of suggesting cosmetic options during case presentations. Opening doors for questions about cosmetic treatment is a large part of motivating the patient to act (Figure 35-24).

Marketing outside the office may include mailing a newsletter to residents in the surrounding area, and ads in the Yellow Pages, on radio and television, billboards, on buses and subway cars, and in local magazines. Search the Internet and social media for cosmetic dentists to view various styles of marketing.

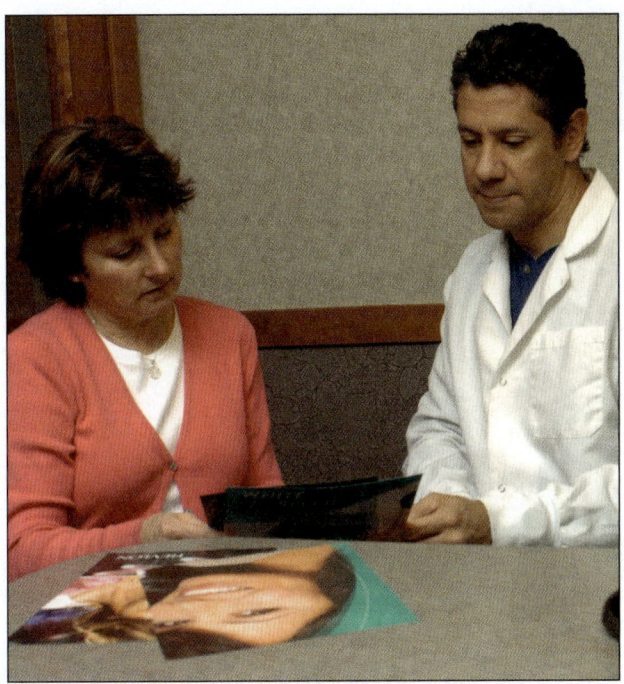

FIGURE 35-24

Here a cosmetic dentist is showing to a patient who is considering cosmetic treatment before and after photos of patients who have completed treatment.

Advanced Chairside Functions

Introduction to Tooth Whitening

Many attempts have been made to esthetically improve the shade of one's teeth. The process of **whitening/bleaching** has become one of the most requested services provided by the dental profession.

In many states the dental assistant is allowed to provide a whitening procedure. This function will be listed in the individual dental state practice act with the specific training and clinical experience necessary for the dental assistant to become confident and competent to complete a whitening procedure on patients following the dentist's instructions.

Whitening procedures have been proven safe and effective by the ADA and the Food and Drug Administration. Research is continually being done and dental professionals need to keep up-to-date on new materials and techniques.

The procedure for lightening teeth may be referred to as tooth whitening or tooth bleaching. According to the FDA, the term "whitening" refers to the restoration of a tooth's surface by removing dirt and debris. Any product that cleans (e.g., toothpaste) is considered a whitener. The FDA allows the term "bleaching" to be used only when the teeth can be whitened beyond their natural color. The term whitening is more commonly used because whitening sounds better than bleaching, even when describing procedures and products that contain bleach.

Causes of tooth stains or discolorations are varied and the whitening/bleaching techniques are selected based on the extent of the stain and its causes. In this section, we discuss the causes of stains and discolorations, the types of materials used to whiten the teeth, procedures used to whiten the teeth, and certain precautions to be exercised during procedures (Figure 35-25).

Shade Guides

Shade guides are used in the dental office to measure tooth shades before and after tooth whitening. Most shade guides are hand-held displays of a wide range of tooth shades (Figures 31-26A and B). Most manufacturers provide shade guides with their specific materials, which are generally not interchangeable. But manufacturers also cross-reference their shade guides with those of the Vitapan Classic Shade Guide. The standard shade guides usually include 16 shades. The shades are arranged on the display beginning with the light shades and progressing to the darker shades. Teeth are predominately white, with varying degrees of gray, yellow, or orange tints. The shade also varies depending on the

Advanced Chairside Functions (Continued)

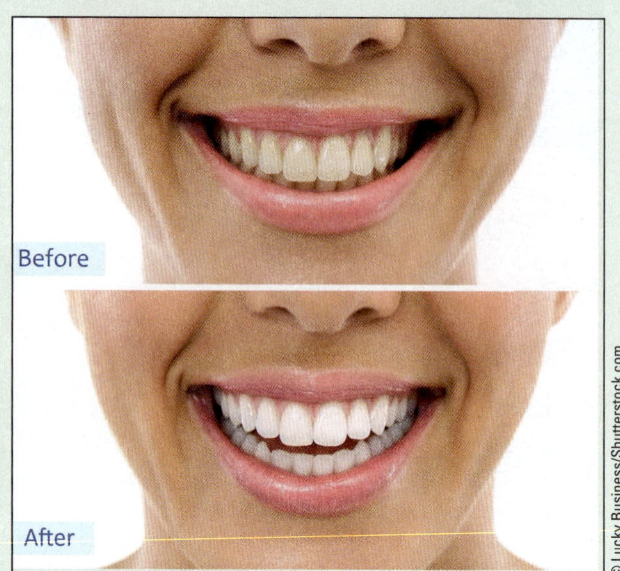

FIGURE 35-25

Patient before and after whitening procedure.

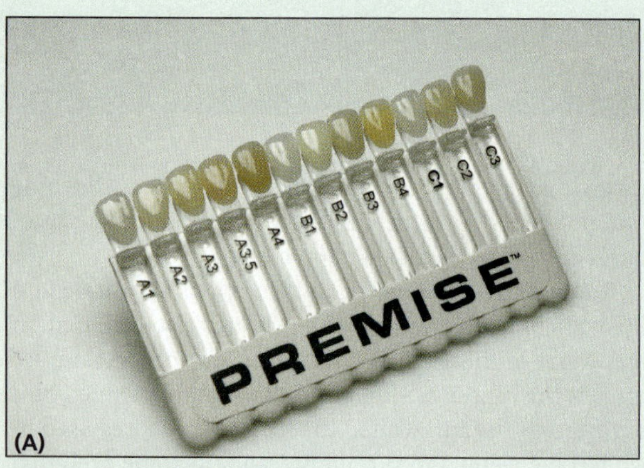

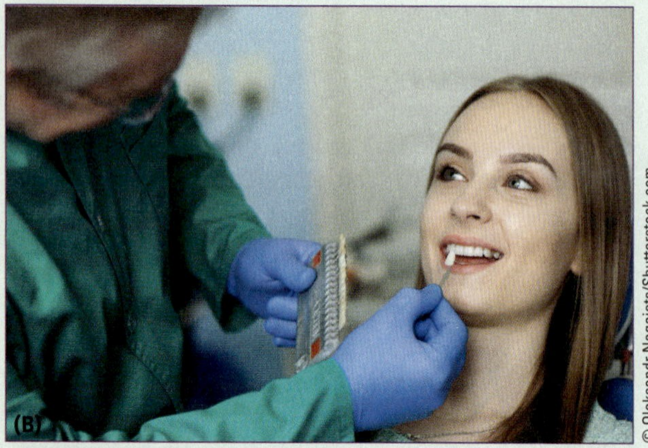

FIGURE 35-26

(A) Shade guide. (B) Checking the shade before the whitening process.

patient's age, the thickness and translucency of the teeth, and the distribution of enamel and dentin on the tooth.

The shade of the whitening material should be selected before the teeth are subjected to any prolonged drying because dehydrated teeth become lighter in shade as they lose translucency. Also good lighting is necessary when choosing the color. Natural light is preferred, but overhead/ceiling lights or the dental light may be used—however, keep them at a distance to decrease the intensity. The shade guide is held next to the teeth as close as possible. Some dentists have their dental assistants select or assist in the shade selection. The final shade selection is verified by the patient with use of a hand mirror.

How Teeth Are Whitened

The teeth turn a lighter shade when hydrogen peroxide or nonperoxide whitening material penetrates the enamel and into the dentin. The whitening process is accelerated mainly by the use of low-intensity heat or sometimes by a high-intensity curing light or a laser.

Today, the most commonly used materials are **hydrogen peroxide**, **carbamide peroxide**, and **sodium perborate**. Sodium perborate is a non-hydrogen peroxide system that contains sodium chloride, oxygen, and fluoride.

Hydrogen Peroxide

Hydrogen peroxide breaks down into water and oxygen. When this happens, free radicals of oxygen are released and they act with pigments in both intrinsic and extrinsic stains, producing a whitening effect. Available in liquid and gel forms, it varies in strength from a 5 to 35 percent solution.

Hydrogen peroxide may cause temporary sensitivity of the pulp when the solution penetrates the enamel and dentin. This is the most common side effect. Hydrogen peroxide will irritate the tissue and discolors clothing; therefore, precautions should be taken to protect the patient's eyes, face, lips, cheeks, tongue, and clothing when using hydrogen peroxide.

Carbamide Peroxide

Carbamide peroxide, a complex form of urea and hydrogen peroxide, is used in a 10 to 20 percent solution. It is weaker than hydrogen peroxide solution, but more stable. This solution is also available in liquid or gel form. A thickening agent is added to increase adhesion to the tooth and prolong exposure to the whitening agent (Figures 35-27A and B).

Sodium Perborate

Sodium perborate, another weak oxidizing agent, is sometimes mixed with hydrogen peroxide and used to whiten nonvital teeth. This compound is the ingredient used in many household bleaching agents that are safe for colors.

Advanced Chairside Functions

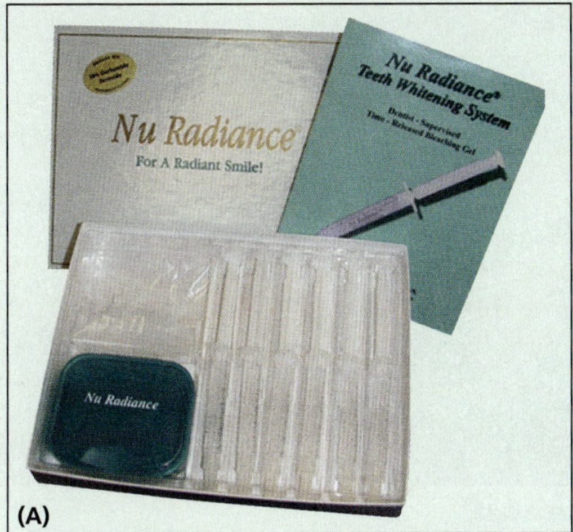

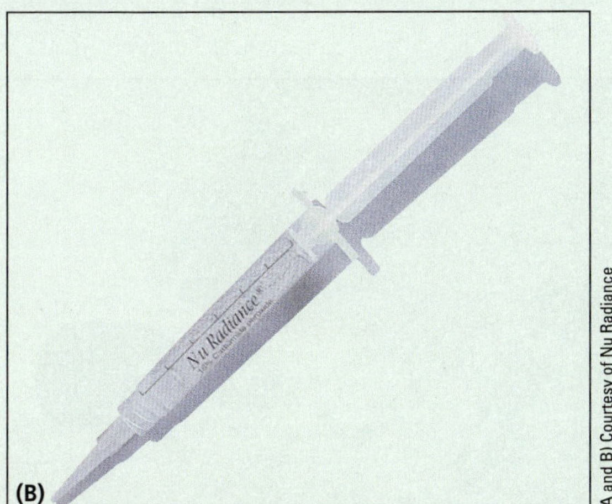

(A and B) Courtesy of Nu Radiance

FIGURE 35-27
(A) Nu Radiance whitening kit. (B) Syringe.

Causes of Tooth Stains

Examples of extrinsic stains include stains from diets and habits, such as tobacco, tea, and coffee. As teeth age they also naturally change color. The teeth develop various yellow to brown stains, and the success of the bleaching process depends on the amount of stain. Intrinsic stains include tetracycline stains, dental fluorosis, discoloration due to injury, and nonvital endodontically treated teeth. (See Chapter 32, Coronal Polish, for more information on dental stains.) Sometimes, the shade of the teeth is naturally toward yellow or gray, and these patients can esthetically enhance the color of their teeth with bleaching.

Role of the Dental Assistant

The dental assistant and the hygienist may perform some or all aspects involving whitening, such as the following:

- Providing information and answering questions the patient may have about whitening
- Obtaining the signed informed consent form from the patient
- Take and pour the impressions for the custom trays
- Fabricating custom whitening trays
- Assist in shade selection
- Chairside assisting for whitening treatments
- Providers of home whitening information, including instructions for proper use of whitening and care of trays
- Take intraoral photographs before and after treatments
- Provide posttreatment instructions to the patient
- Schedule patient for additional appointments as needed for examination and reapplication of the whitening gel

Whitening Techniques

There are two methods of whitening: one method is performed in the dental office, and the other method at home. Patients can use one or the other or a combination to meet their needs. Both vital and nonvital teeth are bleached in the office. There are advantages and disadvantages to each method, and these should be presented to the patient. Considerations include the amount of stain and its origin, number of visits to the office versus the amount of time the whitening trays are worn at home, expense of in-office whitening (which is higher than in-home whitening), and the amount of instruction and guidance the patient requires.

When patients inquire about teeth whitening, discussing available options and understanding their perceptions about their appearance are important. Factors to consider—and which determine the ultimate success of the whitening process—are summarized as follows:

- Degree of stains or discolorations
- Cause of stains or discolorations
- Whitening technique
- Whitening solution and strength of solution
- Vital versus nonvital teeth
- Presence or absence of restorations in teeth to be whitened (existing restorations will not change color with whitening techniques)

Nonvital Whitening

Endodontically treated teeth sometimes turn dark due to blood, pulpal debris, and restorative materials that are used to fill the canal. These teeth can be lightened by both internal and external bleaching. One of the most common bleaching techniques is the **walking whitening technique**. This technique calls for a thick paste of hydrogen peroxide, sodium perborate, or a combination of the two to be placed on the coronal portion of the nonvital tooth. With the bleach mixture temporarily sealed in place, the patient can leave the

Advanced Chairside Functions (Continued)

office and return for evaluation and another possible treatment as instructed by the dentist. Sometimes, heat is applied with a heated instrument/unit in order to achieve desired results.

An alternate method for whitening nonvital teeth consists of two major steps: (1) after the tooth has been treated endodontically, it is isolated with the paint on rubber dam; (2) then a whitening agent is placed in the unfilled pulp chamber of the tooth. A 30 to 35 percent hydrogen peroxide solution (Superoxol) is applied with cotton tips or cotton pellets (Figure 35-28). A heated instrument is then placed in the pulp chamber to activate the peroxide. This procedure may be repeated several times to reach the desired whitening effect.

Vital Whitening in Dental Office

Whitening vital teeth in the office involves the application of whitening liquids or gels, often with the application of heat, a curing light, or laser. This is sometimes called **power whitening** or laser whitening if a laser is used for the setting process. The patient's teeth are isolated tightly, with the dental dam or a light reflective barrier, to prevent irritation to the gingiva by any chemicals, and then they are polished with a pumice or prophy paste. The actual whitening steps depend on the types of materials used and the technique. The whitening materials are cured by the laser or light and then the excess material is removed between applications (Figure 35-29). The whitening may take several applications before the desired shade is reached. When the procedure is finished, the teeth are rinsed thoroughly, the isolation removed, and the teeth may be polished with a fluoride prophy paste (Figure 35-30).

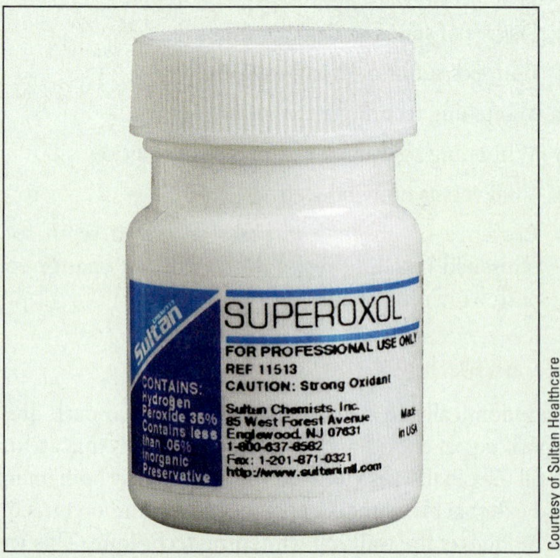

Courtesy of Sultan Healthcare

FIGURE 35-28
Superoxol (30 to 35 percent hydrogen peroxide).

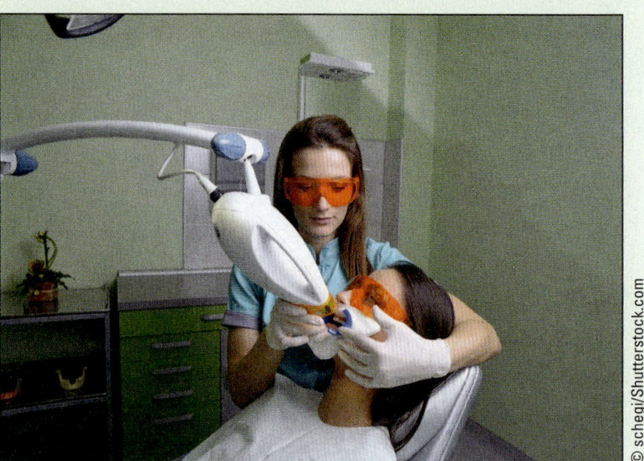

© schegi/Shutterstock.com

FIGURE 35-29
Laser whitening process.

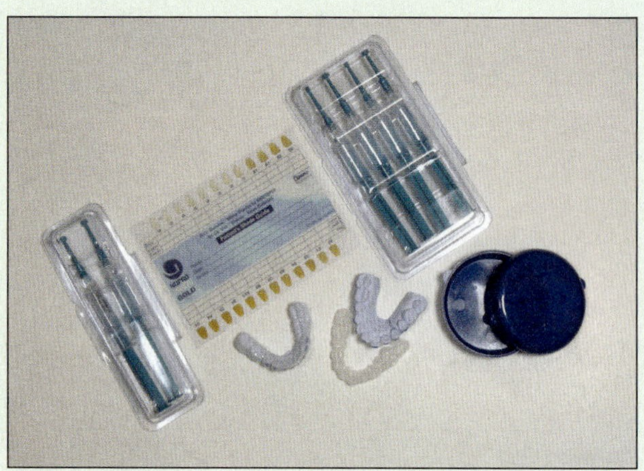

FIGURE 35-30
In-office whitening materials.

If the patient had the laser whitening, he or she will be scheduled for a checkup and possible refresh treatment. When the heat treatment procedure is used the patient is scheduled for his or her next whitening appointment within 1 to 2 weeks. The patient should be told that the teeth may be sensitive. This process usually takes three appointments.

Dehydration during Whitening Procedures

Teeth dehydrate when they are isolated for a period of time and may temporarily appear whiter after dehydrating for several hours.

Dehydration may also cause the teeth to be more sensitive during the procedure.

Advanced Chairside Functions

Home Whitening Techniques

For home whitening, the patient applies a bleaching agent, usually carbamide peroxide or diluted hydrogen peroxide, in a custom-fit tray for specific amounts of time. There are multiple materials, and the techniques vary greatly. The dental staff must become familiar with materials being prescribed for their patients. The advantages of the home bleaching techniques include fewer visits to the dental office, less expense, and convenience. The disadvantages of these techniques are that the patients must be motivated to follow the routine, the time involved for the bleaching process can take several weeks, the bleaching materials can cause nausea and sensitivity to the gingiva, and there is lack of direct monitoring by the dentist. Home bleaching is very popular with patients because of the lower cost and the positive results when done properly. As an alternative, patients can come to the office for a startup appointment, or **assisted whitening**, and then complete the process with home bleaching. Usually, the two appointments are needed to set up the patient for home bleaching. At the first appointment, the impressions for the custom trays are made. The second appointment is for delivery of the bleaching trays; instructions are also given to the patient (Figures 35-31A and B).

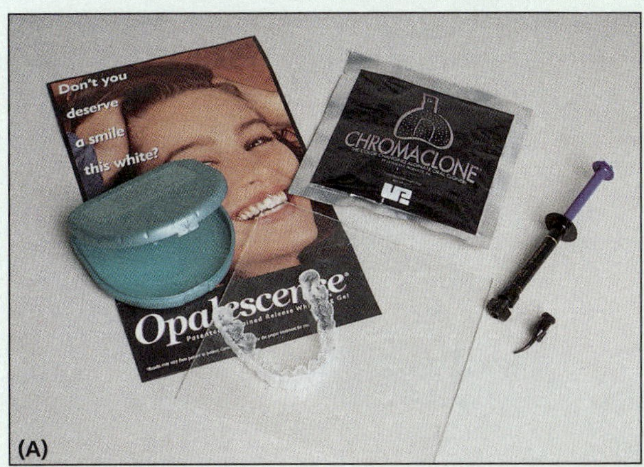

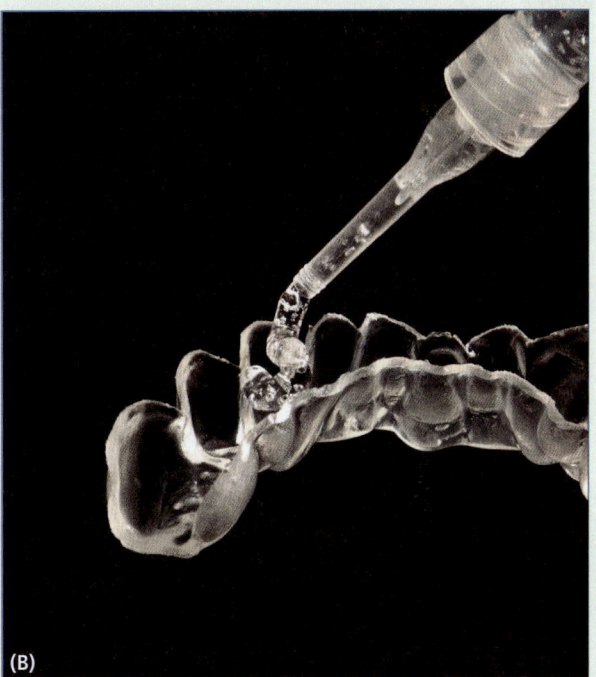

FIGURE 35-31

(A) Home whitening kit. (B) Loading custom tray with whitening gel.

Over-the-Counter Whitening Materials

Many over-the-counter (OTC) whitening products are available, including whitening strips, gels, tray systems, toothpastes, mouth rinses, and even chewing gum. Although these methods do whiten the teeth to varying degrees, there is no professional guidance or evaluation. The ADA recommends that patients consult with their dentist to determine the most appropriate means of whitening their teeth. This is especially important if the patient has many restorations, crowns, and distinctive stains. If the patient chooses an OTC method, he or she must follow the manufacturer's directions carefully and proceed with caution. The most common side effects include temporary tooth and gingival sensitivity, and on rare occasions, irreversible tooth damage. These products generally contain a less-concentrated whitening agent (compared to agents used in dental practices), usually hydrogen peroxide gel or carbamide peroxide (Figure 35-32).

Whitening Strips

Whitening strips (e.g., Crest Whitestrips) are an alternative to tray-based whitening systems. Because the strips are very thin, they do not interfere with the user's normal routine. The number of strips in a kit depends on the concentration of the whitening agent. OTC products are available in a 6 percent hydrogen peroxide solution to be worn over a 14-day period, or a 10 percent solution that is worn for 7 days. The user may achieve desired results before using all kit contents, and can stop at any time.

The strips are gently pressed on the facial surface of the anterior teeth to create maximum contact with the teeth. They are typically intended to be worn for 30 minutes two times a day. The initial whitening can be seen in a couple of days and final results will last for about 4 months.

Strip users should be aware that these products do not work on existing restorations and may cause temporary tooth and

Advanced Chairside Functions (Continued)

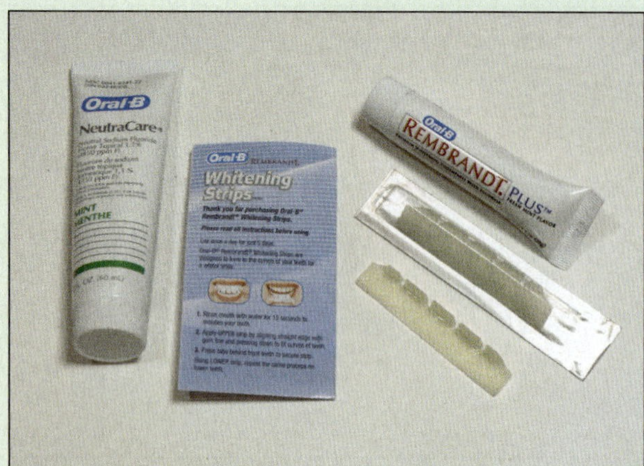

FIGURE 35-32
Over-the-counter whitening products.

gingival tissue sensitivity. Patients are encouraged to consult with their dentist when using OTC teeth-whitening products.

Whitening Gel

OTC whitening gels are painted on the facial surface of the anterior teeth. Care should be taken to keep the gel on the tooth surface and away from the gingival tissues. Some gels contain 18 percent carbamide peroxide agent and can be used on a daily basis.

Home Tray Whitening Systems

Although many tray whitening systems are delivered through the dental office, OTC systems are available as well. The trays in these systems may be preformed stock trays or thermoplastic trays that can be heated and then molded to the teeth. The trays often do not properly adapt to the teeth and they are not trimmed or contoured to prevent excess whitening agent from contacting the gingival tissues. The manufacturer's instructions should be followed carefully, and a less-aggressive approach should be taken to prevent tooth and gingival sensitivity.

The tray with the whitening solution is usually worn for a couple of hours every day to every night for up to 4 weeks or longer depending on the staining and the desired level of whitening. Several **white light teeth whitening systems** are now available that can be done at home. These systems are similar to the laser but use an advanced light transmitter to activate the whitening gel. The systems come with a tray that holds the gel when placed in the mouth. The light is then placed to cover the tray for 10 minutes. Once the desired shade is reached the procedure is repeated once a month for maintenance.

Whitening Toothpastes

Most toothpastes contain a "whitening agent," and some toothpastes are designed specifically as whitening agents. The whitening agents used in toothpaste include hydrogen peroxide, calcium peroxide, and sodium percarbonate. These agents contribute to the whitening effect, but the primary whitening is accomplished by the mild abrasive in the toothpaste. The abrasive agent (hydrated silica, dicalcium phosphate dehydrate, and calcium carbonate) rates very low on abrasive rankings. Whitening toothpastes can lighten the shade of the tooth to one shade lighter, while in dental office light-activated whitening can lighten the tooth eight shades. The ADA Seal on toothpaste packaging indicates that abrasive particles do not exceed the maximum acceptable abrasive ranking (Figure 35-33).

Mouth Rinses and Chewing Gum. Mouth rinses and even a few chewing gum products contain whitening agents. Like whitening toothpastes, the percentage of whitening agent in these products is very low. Chewing gum contains ingredients that act like stain removers and other ingredients that coat the tooth and make it harder for stains to adhere to the tooth. The minimum whitening effects of gum are temporary but tooth whitening gum can be helpful in maintaining the whitening obtained from professional or over-the-counter whitening when chewed between meals.

The whitening rinses, also freshen breath and reduce dental plaque and gum disease. It is recommended they be swished around the mouth for 60 seconds twice a day before brushing. Results should be seen in 12 weeks according to manufacturers. Because of the short exposure time whitening rinses are not as effective as other whitening

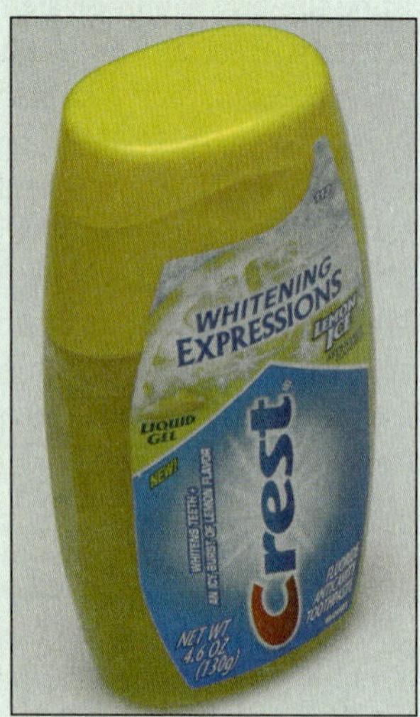

FIGURE 35-33
Whitening toothpaste.

Advanced Chairside Functions

techniques. Discontinuation of use is advised if the teeth or gingival tissues become irritated or sensitive.

Patient Information

With all bleaching procedures, the patient needs to understand the procedure steps and the outcome possibilities. The bleaching process will "lighten" most teeth; and although some teeth will never be the whitest or the brightest—they will be improved. The patient's dedication to following procedures and limiting foods and habits that stain the teeth will enhance the process and bleach the teeth faster. The health of the gingiva and surrounding tissues must be protected by adhering to technique suggestions. Ingestion of the solutions should be kept to a minimum. The patient must realize that bleaching may be an ongoing treatment, with repeated bleaching necessary every few years.

Precautions with Tooth Whitening Techniques

Whitening materials may cause tooth sensitivity to hot and cold. The patient should be advised to use a toothpaste for sensitive teeth.

Whitening may cause irritation to gingival tissues in affected areas.

Sloughing of gingival, lip, and cheek tissues may occur.

Patients should contact their dentist if any of these side effects occur.

Tooth sensitivity is sometimes treated with sodium fluoride.

Patients should be instructed to discontinue whitening procedures until sensitivity has disappeared and they have checked with their dentist.

Procedure 35-1
Nonvital Whitening

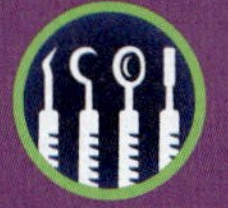

This procedure is performed by the dentist. The patient has received information on the procedure and possible outcome before the procedure begins. More than one treatment may be necessary.

Equipment and Supplies

- Basic setup: mouth mirror, explorer, and cotton pliers
- Cotton rolls, gauze sponges, cotton pellets
- HVE tip, air–water syringe tip, and saliva ejector
- Dental dam setup
- Protective gel
- Waxed dental floss
- High-speed handpiece and assorted burs
- Low-speed handpiece
- Prophy brush
- Cement base materials
- Whitening/bleaching materials
- Heat source
- Temporary coverage and cement
- Finishing burs

Procedure Steps (*Follow aseptic procedures*)

1. The dentist examines and evaluates the root canal–treated tooth.
2. Place the dental dam and ligature of waxed dental floss on the designated tooth or teeth. Once the dam is in place, apply more protective gel to further seal the dam.
3. Remove the excess restoration and any debris in the crown. With the crown of the tooth open, some dentists scrub the chamber with a soap solution and a prophy brush or cotton pellet.
4. The root canal is sealed with 2 to 3 mm of thick base cement or with a light-cured resin ionomer or bonded composite. This is a critical step, because the tooth must be sealed in order to prevent the bleach from penetrating the root. This can be done using the gel bleach in the office, the walking technique, or a combination of both techniques. If bleaching results are not achieved, heat may be also used with the office-based bleaching gel technique. Stains caused by endodontic procedures and drugs often require application of heat with the bleaching agents.
   - Gel bleaching in the office involves the chamber being filled for 30 minutes. Change the

(continues)

Advanced Chairside Functions (Continued)

Procedure 35-1 (continued)

bleaching gel every 10 minutes. Then, place a cotton pellet and temporary in the crown. The patient should be reappointed in 3 to 7 days for evaluation.

- With walking bleaching, a thick mixture of bleaching agent is placed in the crown and covered with temporary cement. Reappoint the patient in 2 to 5 days to remove the cotton pellet.

5. Desired results should be achieved in three appointments, but if the tooth remains darker than the patient prefers, a veneer should be considered. The shade can be altered slightly with the shade of the restorative materials. The temporary filling is removed, and the chamber is rinsed and evacuated. Etching is applied to the inside of the crown. Rinse. Apply the dental adhesive and then fill the chamber with restorative material and light cure.
6. Polish the restoration with finishing burs and polish.
7. Reappoint the patient in a few days to evaluate the color and whether there is the possible need of a veneer.

Procedure 35-2
In-Office Laser Whitening for Vital Teeth

This procedure is performed by the dentist or expanded-function dental assistant in the dental office. The procedure is explained to the patient with the possible outcomes.

Equipment and Supplies

- Basic set up: mouth mirror, explorer, and cotton pliers
- HVE tip, air–water syringe tip, and saliva ejector
- Lip lubricant
- Protective gel
- Rubber dam setup/lip and cheek retractor
- Cotton rolls and gauze sponges
- low-speed handpiece
- Prophy cup
- Polishing paste
- Whitening/bleaching materials
- Applicator, brush or syringe
- Laser
- Curing light
- Finishing burs

Procedure Steps (*Follow aseptic procedures*)

1. The procedure is explained and videos, photos, and pamphlets may be available for the patient. The teeth and surrounding tissues are examined. "Before" treatment photos may be taken of the patient.
2. Polish the crowns of the teeth to remove plaque and debris that may interfere with the bleaching process. Prophy paste or flour of pumice may be used.
3. Isolating with the dental dam is the safest method to protect the tissues. Place the dental dam, punching the holes as close as possible to match the tooth. If you do not use the dental dam, lip and cheek retractor will also isolate the teeth. Place protective gel on the gingival tissues, being careful not to get any of the gel on the tooth surface. Light cure material until set. The gel acts as a barrier to protect the tissues from the whitening agent.
4. Place cotton rolls in vestibule to keep the area dry.
5. Follow the manufacturer's instructions for the specific steps of the materials being used. Using a brush, applicator or syringe apply the whitening gel to the tooth surface.

(continues)

Advanced Chairside Functions

Procedure 35-2 (continued)

6. Position the laser over the teeth and turn on for 15 minutes (Figure 35-34). Repeat up to three times until the desired shade is reached. Rinse and evacuate between each application to remove the bulk of the whitening gel.
7. When whitening steps are completed, thoroughly rinse the area, cut the interseptal dental dam and remove it from the patient's mouth. Rinse again, and remove any protective gel with floss and wet gauze.
8. The patient's tissues are examined and the patient is instructed to avoid substances that may stain the teeth. The patient should also be warned that the teeth may be sensitive following the whitening procedure. The patient is scheduled for a follow-up appointment and then for an evaluation and reapplication appointment. The whitening is not permanent and will need to be refreshed periodically.

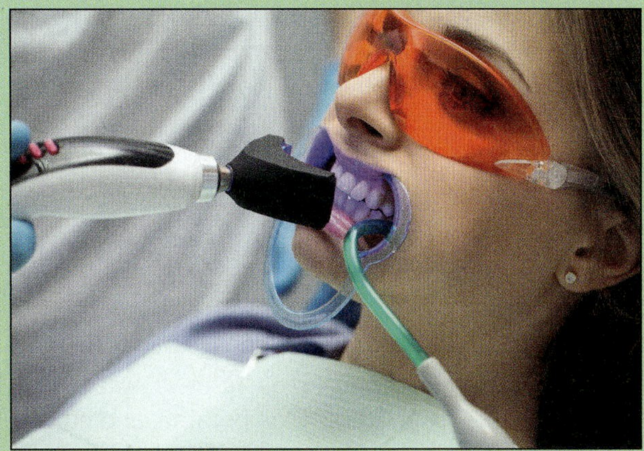

FIGURE 35-34
In-Office whitening for vital teeth.

Procedure 35-3
Home Whitening

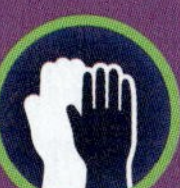

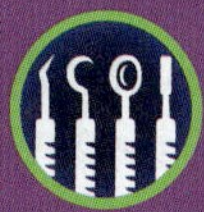

This procedure is performed by the patient at home after an examination by the dentist. The patient is given a bleaching kit and step-by-step instructions from the dentist. This procedure is divided into appointments and steps that occur between appointments.

Equipment and Supplies

- Basic setup: mouth mirror, explorer, and cotton pliers
- Alginate
- Rubber mixing bowl and spatula
- Impression trays
- Camera
- Custom-fit, vacuum-formed tray (see Chapter 39, Laboratory Materials and Techniques)
- Home bleaching kit
- Shade guide for before and after color comparisons

Procedure Steps (*Follow aseptic procedures*)

First Appointment

1. The dentist examines the teeth, considering the shade of the teeth, sensitivity, restorations, and areas of abrasion and erosion. General procedures are completed before the bleaching process begins. The bleaching techniques are explained, and the procedure that best meets the patient's needs is selected.
2. Alginate impressions are taken of the arches being bleached. "Before" photographs are taken.

Between Appointments

1. The alginate impressions are poured in stone and prepared.

(continues)

Advanced Chairside Functions (Continued)

Procedure 35-3 (continued)

2. A custom-fit, vacuum-formed tray is made. This may be done in the office lab or at a commercial lab. (Refer to Chapter 39, Laboratory Materials and Techniques.)

Second Appointment

1. With the home technique, the patient tries on the trays to ensure a good fit.
2. Instructions are given, including when and for how long to wear the trays, how to prepare the materials, how to place the custom-fit trays, what to do in case the gingiva becomes irritated, and how to handle other side effects.
3. In some cases, the patient receives one bleaching in the office, before beginning the home bleaching. The patient's teeth are polished and then the mouth is rinsed and wiped dry with tissue prior to insertion of the tray. The tray is loaded by placing small drops of gel/solution around the tray where it will contact the teeth. Do not overload the tray.
4. Place the tray firmly into position over the teeth. Wipe off any excess material with a tissue. The patient wears the tray for 1 hour this time, but may wear the tray from 1 to 4 hours per day or as recommended by the dentist. The patient should not smoke, eat, or drink while wearing the tray. Most of the bleaching takes place in the first hour. To achieve the best results, the dentist's instructions should be followed regarding how often and how long to wear the trays.
5. Some offices schedule an appointment to follow-up with the patient's progress and to examine the tissues. This appointment is usually within 2 weeks of the second appointment.

Chapter Summary

Cosmetic dentistry can be a life-changing experience for both the patient and the dental team. These procedures involve many and varied aspects of dentistry and provide esthetic services to patients. Cosmetic dentistry involves very detailed, comprehensive treatments that can involve orthodontics, oral maxillofacial surgery, occlusion adjustments, endodontic treatment, and periodontics. The fundamentals of cosmetic dentistry are discussed as well as the psychology of working with patients interested in improving their smile.

Tooth whitening may also be a part of esthetic treatments desired by patients to improve the appearance of their teeth. Various materials and techniques are discussed including nonvital and vital tooth whitening, in-office and home whitening techniques, and available OTC products.

The dental assistant plays an important role in all cosmetic and tooth-whitening procedures. The assistant must be educated and trained to assist the dentist and be actively involved in providing information to the patient.

CASE STUDY

Chance Hall works with the public, and is very concerned about the color of his teeth. He scheduled several tooth-whitening treatments with Dr. Garrett. After several appointments, Chance's teeth became very sensitive and gingival tissues were irritated. Now he wonders if he will ever have the bright smile he wants without sensitivity.

Case Study Review

1. List the potential problems of tooth whitening.
2. What should the dental assistant have explained to Chance about the side effects of tooth whitening?
3. Discuss options available to Chance to achieve his goal of having whiter teeth.

Review Questions

Multiple Choice

1. Which of the following organizations is dedicated to cosmetic dentistry?
   a. ADA
   b. ADHA
   c. AACD
   d. AAPD
2. Soft tissue contouring is accomplished with a
   a. dental laser.
   b. electrosurgery unit.
   c. both a and b.
   d. None of the above
3. All of the following procedures are included in cosmetic dentistry, *except*
   a. amalgam restorations.
   b. veneers.
   c. tooth whitening.
   d. dentures.
4. ________ surround(s) the tooth and marks the boundaries of the face of the tooth.
   a. The dental hue
   b. The chroma
   c. Opacity
   d. Transitional line angles
5. ________ is the science of occlusion that objectively measures the physiologic functions affected by occlusion to achieve an optimal relationship between the skull and the mandible.
   a. Neurological dentistry
   b. Neuromuscular dentistry
   c. Skeletal dentistry
   d. Skeletal muscular dentistry
6. Whitening procedures can remove both intrinsic and extrinsic stains to varying degrees.
   a. This is a true statement.
   b. This is a false statement.
7. Which of the following agencies/organizations has proven the safety and effectiveness of whitening procedures?
   a. American Dental Association
   b. State drug administration
   c. Food and Drug Administration
   d. Both a and c
8. When a tooth is endodontically treated and turns dark due to blood, pulpal debris, and/or restorative materials, it can be lightened by
   a. vital whitening procedures.
   b. nonvital whitening procedures.
   c. home whitening procedures.
   d. None of the above, because it cannot be lightened with any whitening procedures.
9. All of the following are true statements about in-office whitening *except*:
   a. The teeth are polished before application of the whitening materials.
   b. The actual whitening steps depend on the type of materials applied.
   c. The patient is scheduled for another appointment in 2 to 6 months.
   d. The teeth are polished with a fluoride prophy paste after the whitening materials have been placed and then the mouth is rinsed thoroughly.
10. Which of the following whitening materials is typically used in home whitening techniques?
    a. Diluted hydrogen peroxide
    b. Sodium hypochloride
    c. Sodium fluoride
    d. Phosphoric acid

Critical Thinking

1. Discuss everything that would be needed to make a case presentation to a patient who wants to have a beautiful smile.
2. Explain why formal informed consents must be part of the patient's records.
3. When patients mention that they are interested in teeth whitening, what options could the dental assistant tell them about?

Web Activities

1. Go to http://www.cosmeticdentistry.com to view specific procedures included in cosmetic dentistry and locate a cosmetic dentist in your area.
2. To learn more about cosmetic dentistry certification, go to http://www.aacd.com.
3. To find out more about tooth whitening and recommendations by the American Dental Association, go to http://www.ada.org, public information section.
4. Go to http://www.usa.philips.com to learn more about the power whitening–Zoom.

CHAPTER

36

Removable Prosthodontics

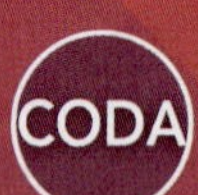

Specific Instructional Objectives

The student should strive to meet the following objectives and demonstrate an understanding of the facts and principles presented in this chapter:

1. Define removable prostheses and list the reasons for using them.
2. Describe considerations about the patient related to removable prosthetic treatment.
3. Explain the dental assistant's role in removable prosthetic treatment.
4. Outline the steps of the diagnostic appointment and list the materials needed.
5. Describe the consultation appointment and the materials required for case presentation.
6. Describe the advantages and disadvantages of the partial denture, its components, and the appointment schedule.
7. List the home care instructions for a partial denture.
8. Describe the complete denture, considerations about the patient, and the appointment schedule.
9. Discuss the appointment sequence, the advantages & disadvantages, and the construction of an immediate denture.
10. List the home care instructions for a complete denture.
11. Explain the types and steps of denture reline procedures.
12. Describe the procedure for a denture repair.
13. List the steps to polish a removable prosthetic appliance.
14. Explain the overdenture and the advantages and disadvantages related to it.

Key Terms

alveoplasty (844)
anatomical (843)
artificial teeth (836)
bar-type clasp (838)
baseplate (848)
bite rim (848)
border molding (846)
centric occlusion (847)
centric relation (847)
circumferential-type clasp (838)
connector (837)
denture base (836)
facebow (847)
facebow transfer (847)
flange (843)
framework (836)
hinge (837)
immediate denture (844)
intercuspation (847)
lateral excursion (847)
muscle trimming (846)
nonanatomical (843)
overdenture (855)
partial denture (835)
protrusion (847)
relined (852)
rest (836)
retainer (836)
retrusion (847)
vertical dimension (847)

Introduction

Removable prosthodontics, like fixed prosthodontics, refers to the replacement of missing teeth and tissues with artificial structures, or prostheses. The difference is that with removable prosthodontics, the prosthesis can be removed from the mouth by the patient for cleaning, examination, and repair. Removable prosthodontics involves two types of prostheses: **partial denture** and complete (full) dentures (Figure 36-1).

The partial denture replaces one or more teeth in one arch and is retained and supported by the underlying tissues and remaining teeth.

The complete denture replaces all the teeth in one arch. A full denture is retained and supported by the underlying tissues of the gingiva and oral mucosa, the alveolar ridges, and the hard palate. In some cases, teeth are retained in the arch or implants are placed to support the denture.

The goals of removable prosthodontics are to restore lost functions, stabilize the arch, and improve esthetics. The lost functions include the ability to masticate food properly and to have clear speech. With removable prosthodontics, the patient regains these functions, improves appearance, and, within a short adjustment period, becomes very comfortable and confident with the prosthesis.

Most patients prefer to have fixed prostheses, but in some cases it may not be the treatment of choice due to existing conditions, such as unhealthy bone structure, not having the motivation to maintain good oral hygiene, or financial restrictions. Removable prosthodontics offers an alternative that restores function and esthetics for the patient.

Prosthodontics is a specialty that requires additional training upon completion of dental school. Routine prosthodontic procedures are performed by the general dentist as well as the prosthodontist. The prosthodontist may see patients who need surgery as a result of cancer, patients who have been in accidents involving severe facial/jaw trauma, and/or patients with anomalies such as cleft lip or cleft palate.

Patient Considerations

Good communication between the patient and the prosthodontic staff is required for successful removable prosthodontics. The patient should be in good health, have a positive attitude, and be cooperative. The patient's mental and physical capabilities must be such that he or she can adapt to wearing the prosthesis and be able to maintain good oral hygiene. Impaired health may contribute to a lack of muscle coordination that is needed to place and remove the partial prosthesis or to retain a denture in place. If the patient is in poor health, it is often reflected in the oral cavity. Also, the added stress of a new appliance may lower the resistance of unhealthy tissue and complications may occur. Fluctuations in the patient's weight may alter the fit of the prosthesis, and it may need to be relined.

Patients are often very conscientious and require patience and understanding during the time they are adjusting to their new denture or partial. There are also pamphlets and videos available to inform patients about their new prostheses (Figure 36-2).

Dental Assistant's Role

The dental assistant's main functions are to prepare materials, record measurements and details for the fabrication of the denture, provide patient education and support, and perform selective laboratory procedures. Procedures in removable prosthodontics do not require many instrument exchanges, and the dental assistant does not continually maintain the oral cavity throughout the appointment with the air–water syringe and the HVE. The steps in removable prosthodontics involve as many extraoral as intraoral procedures.

Diagnosis and Treatment Planning

The first appointment for a removable prosthesis is dedicated to examining the patient. A medical history is taken or reviewed to determine the patient's state of health. The dentist may also talk with the patient to determine how the patient

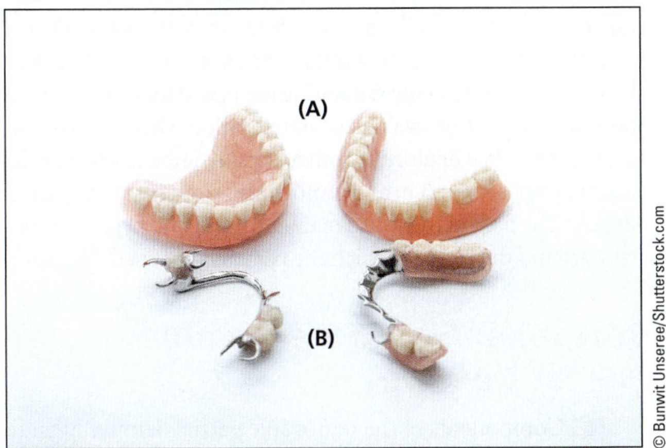

FIGURE 36-1

Example of (A) full denture and (B) partial denture.

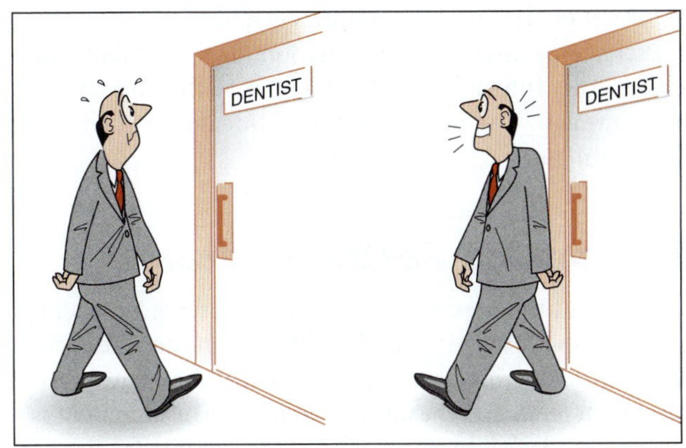

FIGURE 36-2

Nervous patient coming to dentist to have full dentures placed compared to patient that has received dentures and feels great about their appearance and the restoration of a natural appearance.

feels about his or her existing oral condition and about the prospect of having a partial or full denture. The dentist examines the patient's remaining teeth and tissues.

After a prophylaxis, preliminary impressions for study models and working casts are taken. (Review Chapter 39, Laboratory Materials and Techniques, for more information on taking alginate impressions.) Radiographic films are exposed and processed by the dental assistant as part of the diagnostic aids. Photographs are made of the patient, including a full face, frontal view, profile view, and close-up. The patient is then scheduled for a consultation appointment a few days later.

Consultation Appointment

The patient is seated in an area designed for patient consultations. The following aids are present to help the patient better understand what is involved in the treatment:

- Study models of the patient's mouth
- Radiographs mounted on a viewbox or viewed on a computer screen
- Patient's photographs
- Visual aids to explain the types of removable prostheses (this may include pamphlets, models, pictures, or video programs)
- Proposed treatment plan

The dental assistant has all of the items prepared so that the dentist can explain the diagnosis, proposed treatment plan, and prognosis to the patient. The dentist answers any questions and concerns expressed by the patient. As with other dental procedures, a cost estimate is prepared and presented to the patient, along with the number of appointments the procedure will require. The treatment plan may involve restorative dentistry, periodontal treatment, endodontic treatment, and/or surgical procedures. These procedures must be completed and the patient must be completely healed before the prosthodontic preparation can begin.

When the patient has accepted the treatment plan, a suitable financial plan is approved and insurance information collected. Often, the dental office takes insurance information at the first appointment and then contacts the insurance company for information on the patient's coverage. This information is presented at the consultation appointment. The necessary appointments are then made for treatment.

Removable Partial Denture

Partial dentures are designed to restore missing teeth and to preserve the remaining hard and soft tissues of the arches. The partial distributes the forces of mastication between the abutment teeth and the alveolar mucosa. The abutment is a natural tooth that becomes part of the support for the partial. The abutment teeth must be in good condition or be restored to withstand the stresses of chewing with a partial denture.

Advantages of a Removable Partial Denture

Reasons that a partial denture may be part of a patient's treatment plan when he or she has missing teeth are as follows:

- Partial dentures are repaired and adjusted easily. If teeth are lost in the dental arch, they can be added to the partial denture.
- When there are no teeth for a distal attachment, the removable partial denture is one treatment choice to restore function to that quadrant.
- Partial dentures require fewer intraoral procedures than fixed prostheses. This means fewer appointments and less chair time for the patient.
- Maintaining good oral hygiene of the abutments and the appliance is easier for the patient because the prosthesis is removable.
- The partial restores the mesial-distal contacts between the teeth and the anterior-posterior continuity of the arch. This provides support that teeth standing alone do not have; therefore, the arch is stabilized.
- The partial maintains a proper occlusal plane by preventing supra-eruption of the teeth on the opposing arch.
- The removable partial makes it unnecessary to reduce tooth structure. The partial appliance can be fitted to children and adolescents and is replaced easily to compensate for a child's growth.
- When several teeth are missing in both quadrants of an arch, a removable partial denture is designed to restore lost dentition in the both quadrants. The missing teeth of both quadrants are then connected in one long span appliance.
- Removable prostheses may be designed to support periodontally involved teeth.
- Compared to a fixed prosthesis, the partial prosthesis is a less expensive treatment.

Considerations for a Partial Denture

Before choosing the partial denture as the treatment, the dentist must consider several factors. There must be a number of sufficiently positioned teeth in the arch to support and stabilize a removable prosthesis. To retain the appliance, there must be adequate root structure of the remaining teeth, and the alveolar bone and mucosa must be evaluated to determine whether they can support the partial denture. Another consideration is whether the patient exhibits interest in and is motivated to adjust to the partial denture. The patient must also maintain good oral hygiene, especially around the teeth to which the partial is attached.

Components of a Removable Partial Denture

CDA Components of the removable partial denture include the metal **framework**, **rest**, connectors, **retainer**, **denture base**, and **artificial teeth** (Figure 36-3). Partial dentures are designed for individual patients without

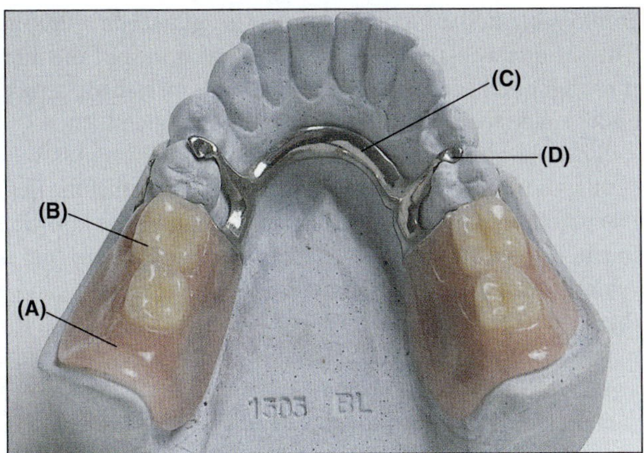

FIGURE 36-3

Mandibular partial denture. (A) Denture base. (B) Denture teeth. (C) Connectors (lingual bar). (D) Occlusal rest.

set patterns. This means the number of teeth involved, their position, and shade (color) may all be different, and the partial is designed according to the patient's needs.

Metal Framework. The metal framework is the skeleton of the removable partial (Figure 36-4A) to which the remaining units (such as the rests, connectors, and retainers) are attached. Part of the framework is a mesh or loop area designed to retain the acrylic base material. The acrylic portion of the partial denture surrounds the framework.

Rests. The rests are the part of the removable partial denture that contact a tooth to provide vertical and horizontal support. The rests control the position of the partial in relationship to the supporting structures. To provide the best support, the rests are placed as close as possible to the center of the tooth so that they can direct functional forces to the long axis of the tooth. These rests are positioned on the occlusal, incisal, or cingulum (lingual) surfaces (Figures 36-4B and C).

Connectors. A **connector** unites the various parts of the partial into a single unit, hold the working parts in the proper position, and distribute the stresses. They are divided into major and minor connectors. The *major connectors* connect the left and right quadrants of the partial. On the mandibular, the major connector is often a lingual bar or plate. On the maxillary, the major connector is a palatal bar or strap or a complete palatal plate (Figure 36-5). A stress-breaker, or **hinge**, may be built into the partial. This is a metal device that relieves pressure on the abutment teeth. The stress-breaker is like a hinge that gives some release to the occlusal stresses during mastication.

The *minor connectors* connect the major connectors with the other units of the partial, such as the clasps and rests. They maintain the integrity of the arch by an anterior-posterior bracing action. The minor connectors protect against food impaction by filling the tooth–tissue junctions.

Retainer. Sometimes called a clasp; the retainer contacts the abutment teeth and prevents the partial from moving. The position of the prosthesis is controlled by the retainer and its

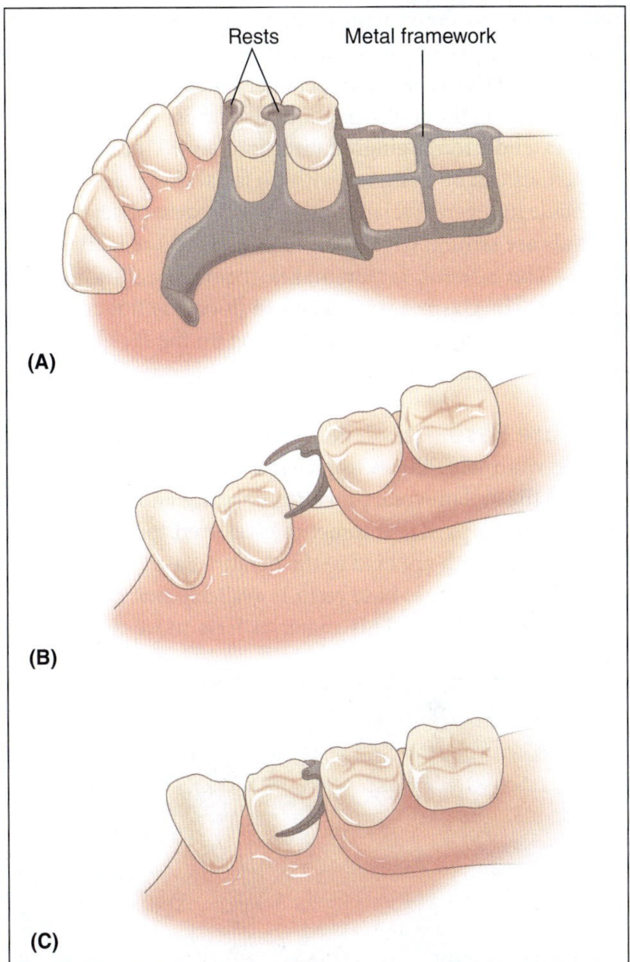

FIGURE 36-4

(A) Partial denture with metal framework. (B) Placement of clasp with rest on tooth. (C) Partial in place.

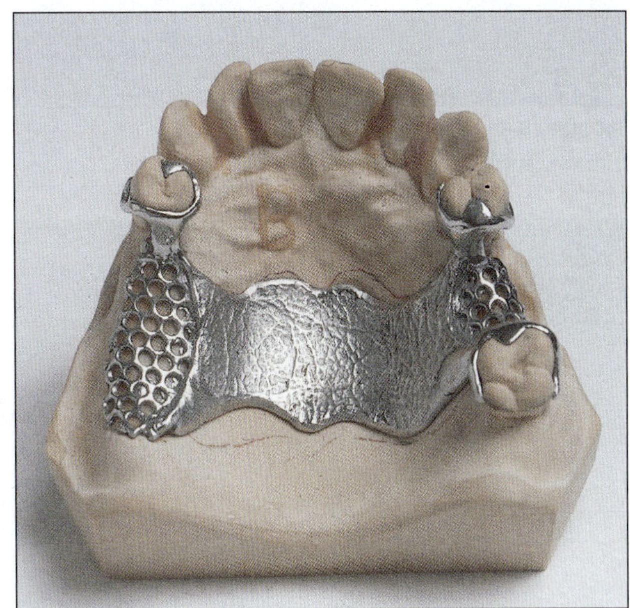

FIGURE 36-5

Major connector for maxillary palatal strap.

relationship to the remaining teeth and support structures. Retainer designs are usually circumferential or bar type. The **circumferential-type clasp** (retainer) encircles and adapts to the contours of the abutment tooth (Figure 36-6). The **bar-type clasp** extends from a gingival direction toward the occlusal.

Partials can be designed with no facial clasp showing, and are made in several variations that will fit most patients. These partials are strong, have good retention, and reliably stay in place. The esthetic factor makes them appealing to most patients. The clasps are designed to fit on the lingual, wrapping interproximally without showing on the facial. In some designs the metal also extends onto the occlusal (Figure 36-7).

Denture Base. The denture base is most often made of acrylic resin with fibers to provide a natural appearance. It rests on the oral mucosa, providing coverage and stability. This portion of the partial is sometimes referred to as the saddle. The denture teeth are held in the denture base.

A flexible denture base resin is available that can be used for partial dentures. This material feels more natural and comfortable in the mouth because it is lightweight and thin. The resin is available in basic shade categories of medium pink, light pink, and ethnic. This partial is an esthetic choice, and is suggested by some dentists for their patients.

The technique for the flexible resin base partial is very similar to the regular hard resin material, except that the flexible partial is immersed in very hot tap water before insertion in the patient's mouth. After about a minute, the partial is removed from the water and allowed to cool until it can be tolerated by the patient. The partial then adapts well with the natural tissues in the mouth. If adjustments need to be made, a green mounted stone is suggested followed by using a brown rubber wheel to smooth rough surfaces (Figure 36-8).

Artificial Teeth. The artificial teeth are made of acrylic resin or porcelain, and are available in a variety of shapes (molds), sizes, and shades. The artificial teeth are secured to the denture base by pins or holes on the undersides of the teeth (see Denture Teeth under the Components of a Complete Dentures section in this chapter).

Partial Denture Procedure

The abutment teeth where the metal framework of the partial rests must be prepared before the final impressions are taken. The occlusal surfaces of the teeth are reduced to allow for clearance of the metal framework of the partial between the arches. This surface must be contoured so that the partial denture will be held firmly in place. The buccal and lingual surfaces are prepared to allow the partial to be inserted and removed without binding. If the teeth cannot be contoured adequately with burs, discs, and stones, they are prepared for fixed crowns before the partial denture is fabricated.

After the abutment teeth have been prepared, the dentist takes final impressions and a bite registration (Procedure 36-1). These

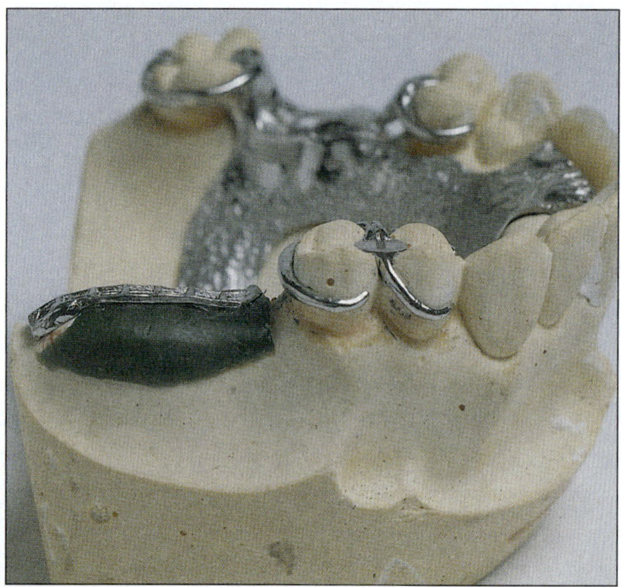

FIGURE 36-6
Circumferential clasp.

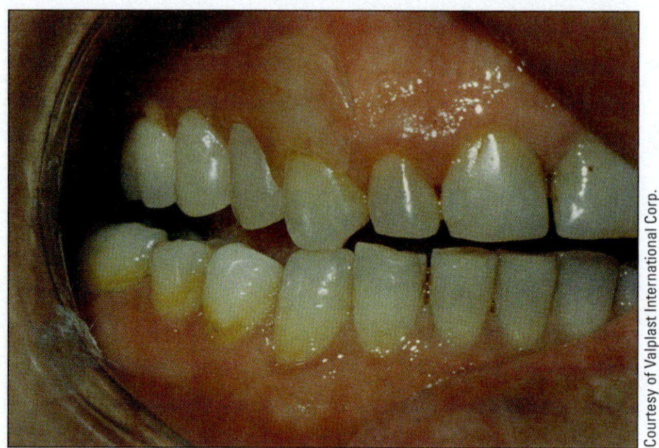

Courtesy of Valplast International Corp.

FIGURE 36-7
Esthetic clasp on removable partial denture.

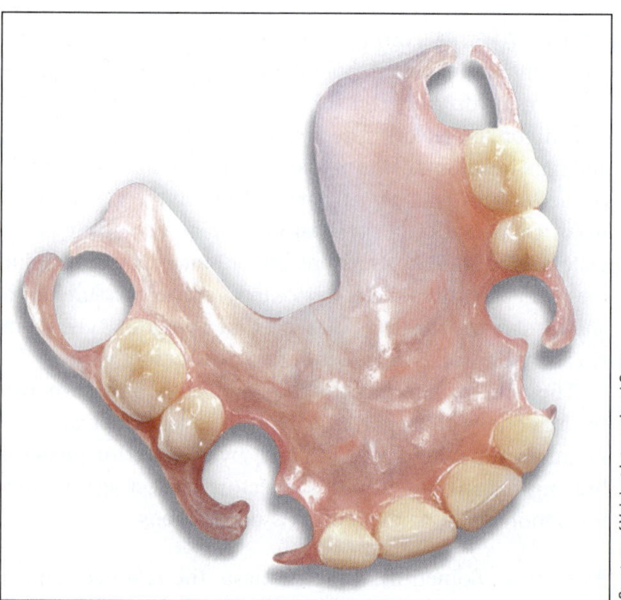

Courtesy of Valplast International Corp

FIGURE 36-8
Flexible denture base resin for partial dentures.

are sent to the dental laboratory with a laboratory prescription form. The dental laboratory follows the dentist's instructions and constructs an appliance that consists of the cast framework and denture teeth set in the wax bite rim (Figures 36-9 A–C). The partial denture is articulated on the models to simulate how the appliance will occlude and mesh in various jaw positions. The laboratory then sends the partial to the dental office for the try-in and any adjustments (Procedure 36-2). The delivery appointment is outlined in Procedure 36-3. See Table 36-1 for the appointments for a partial denture.

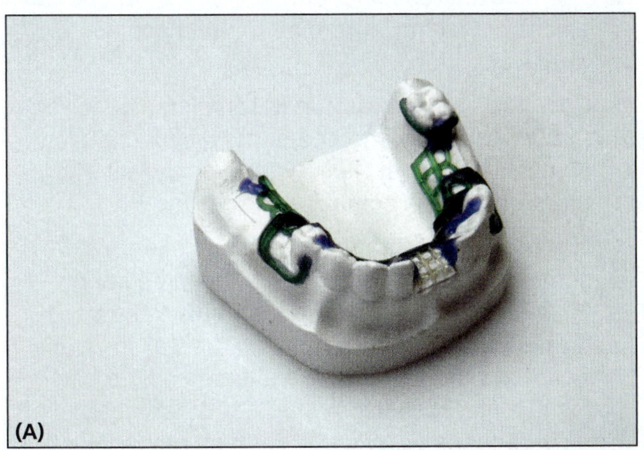

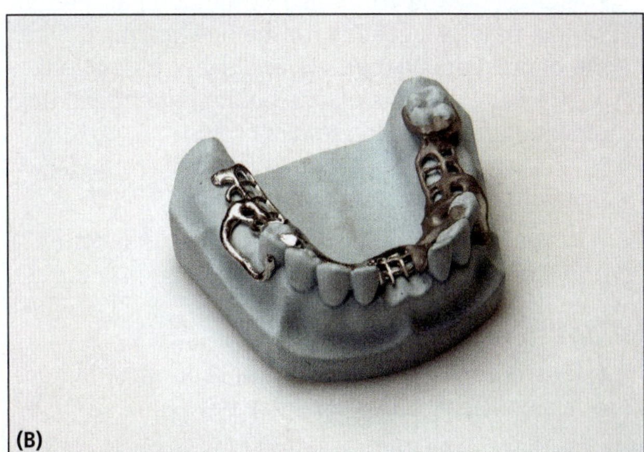

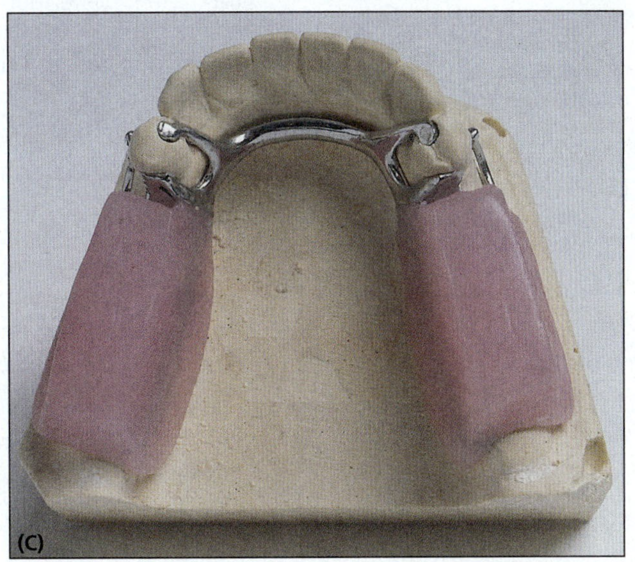

FIGURE 36-9

(A) Wax-up of a partial denture. (B) Metal framework made from wax-up of partial. (C) Metal framework with wax bite rims ready for placement of the denture teeth.

TABLE 36-1 Appointments for Partial Denture

Appointment	Procedure
Examination	Prophylaxis is completed, preliminary impressions are taken, and radiographs and photographs are taken.
Consultation	Treatment is explained to the patient and treatment is chosen.
Final impressions	Abutment teeth are prepared, final impressions are taken, bite or occlusal registration is taken, and the shade and mold of artificial teeth are selected. **Note:** Sometimes restorative, periodontal, endodontic, or surgical procedures must be completed before the final impressions can be completed.
Try-in and adjustment	The framework is placed in the patient's mouth and adjustments are made accordingly.
Delivery	The partial is seated in the patient's mouth and instructions are given regarding how to place and remove the partial and about oral hygiene techniques.
Adjustment	As needed, adjustments are made at regular intervals to ensure proper fit.

Procedure 36-1
Final Impressions for Partial Denture

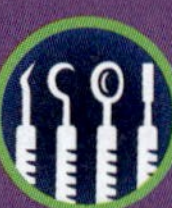

This procedure is performed by the dentist. After preparing materials needed for the final impressions, the dental assistant greets and seats the patient. A protective drape is placed on the patient and the procedure is explained to him or her.

Equipment and Supplies (*Figure 36-10*)

- Basic setup: mouth mirror, explorer, and cotton pliers
- Mouthwash
- Custom tray (see Chapter 39, Laboratory Materials and Techniques) or stock tray
- Contouring wax for the impression trays
- Impression materials—spatula and mixing pad or dispensing gun and tips
- Wax or silicone bite registration materials
- Tooth shade and mold guides
- Laboratory prescription form
- Disinfectant and container for impressions and bite registration

Procedure Steps (*Follow aseptic procedures*)

1. The dentist examines the oral cavity and tries the custom or stock tray in the patient's mouth. Sometimes, wax is placed on the borders of the tray to secure a contoured fit. Once the tray is prepared, an adhesive is painted on the inside of the tray.
2. The final impression material is prepared and placed in the tray according to the manufacturer's directions.
3. Once the final impression is completed, receive the final impressions and either disinfect them immediately or set them aside to disinfect after the procedure is completed.
4. The occlusal or bite registration is taken. When completed, it is also disinfected in preparation for the laboratory. Prepare materials to be used for the bite registration. Soften the wax in warm water and then fold it several times before placing it in the patient's mouth. Mix other materials on a paper pad and place them on a quadrant tray. Then, place them in the patient's mouth or dispense them directly into the oral cavity with a dispensing gun and tip. After the bite materials set and are removed from the mouth, disinfect them and put them with the final impressions.
5. The shade of the artificial teeth is taken with a moistened shade guide under natural light. This can be completed at any point in the appointment sequence. Once the shade is determined, record it on the laboratory prescription and the patient's chart. Assist the dentist in shade determination and recording.
6. The dentist completes the laboratory prescription with details of the partial denture design. Make sure that the patient's face is clean of impression materials and debris and then dismiss the patient.

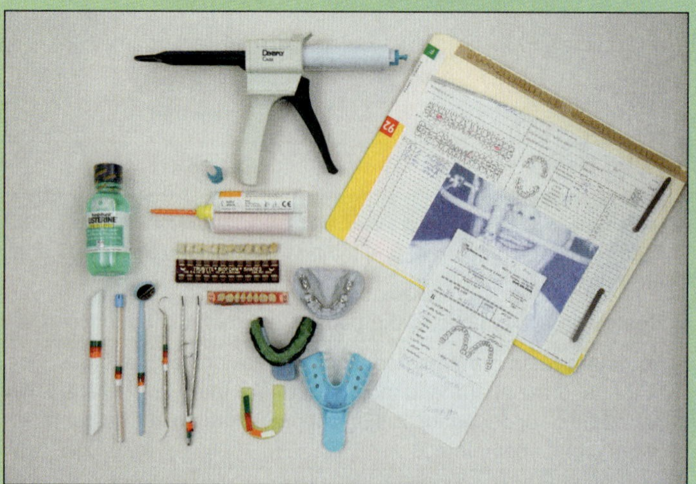

FIGURE 36-10
Tray setup for final impression of partial denture.

Procedure 36-2
Try-In Appointment for Partial Denture

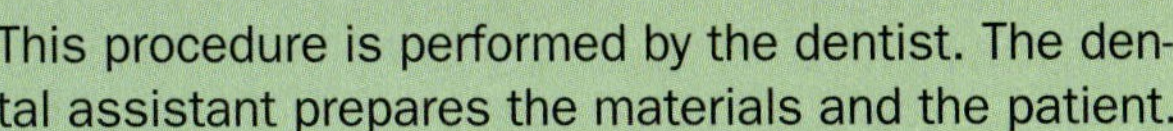

This procedure is performed by the dentist. The dental assistant prepares the materials and the patient.

Equipment and Supplies (*Figure 36-11*)

- Basic setup: mouth mirror, explorer, and cotton pliers
- Evacuating tip
- Hand mirror for patient viewing
- Articulating paper and forceps
- Adjusting instruments, including wax spatula, pliers, and a heat source
- Low-speed handpiece with burs, discs, and stones
- Contour pliers
- Partial denture from the laboratory

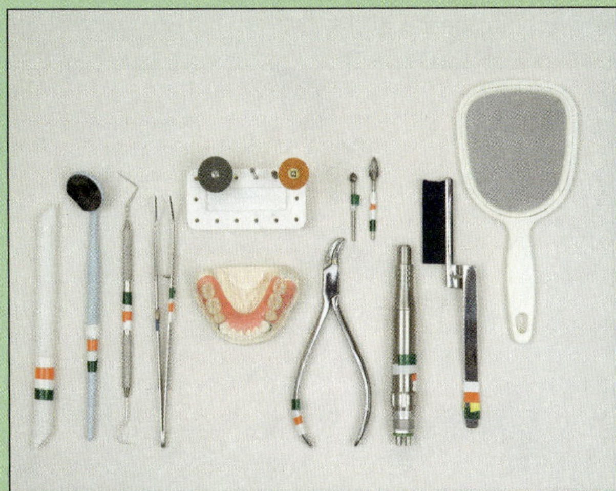

FIGURE 36-11
Tray setup for partial denture try-in appointment.

Procedure Steps (*Follow aseptic procedures*)

1. The appliance is placed in the patient's mouth and adjustments are made accordingly. If adjustments are made to the denture base and/or the position of the teeth, prepare the spatula by warming it in the heat source (alcohol torch or Bunsen burner) and transfer it to the dentist. Transfer the articulating paper and evaluate the occlusion. If adjustments are needed, transfer the handpiece and burs.
2. The patient is given a hand mirror for viewing. Dismiss the patient and disinfect the partial to prepare it for the laboratory.

Procedure 36-3
Delivery Appointment for Partial Denture

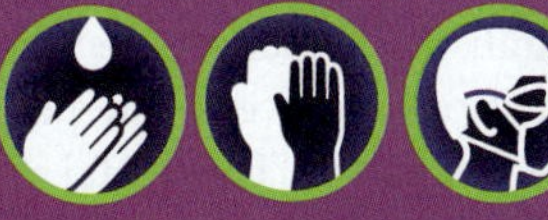

This procedure is performed by the dentist with assistance by the dental assistant. The partial denture is returned from the laboratory in a sealed container.

Equipment and Supplies

- Basic setup: mouth mirror, explorer, and cotton pliers
- Partial denture (Figure 36-12)
- Articulating paper and forceps
- Low-speed handpiece and acrylic burs and finishing burs

Procedure Steps (*Follow aseptic procedures*)

1. Preparations for the patient are completed.
2. The materials and equipment are similar to the try-in appointment with the exception of the wax adjustment instruments.

(continues)

Procedure 36-3 (continued)

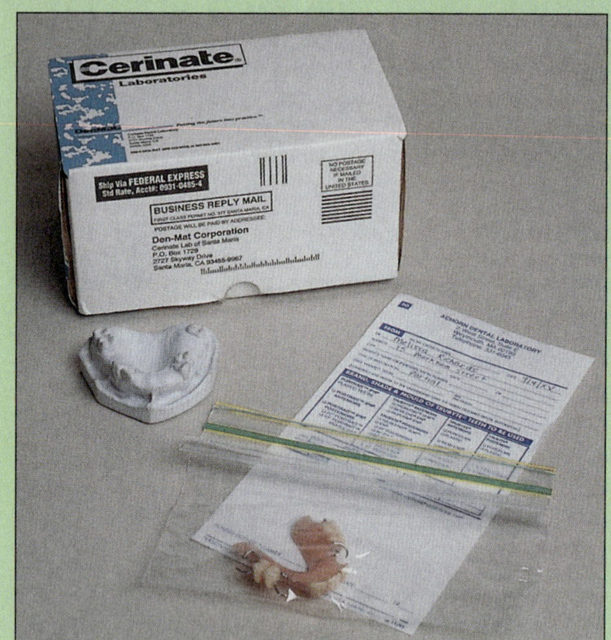

FIGURE 36-12
Complete partial denture returned from denture laboratory.

3. The patient is seated. If the patient has an old appliance, it is removed and placed in a cup with water.
4. The dentist seats the new partial denture and makes any necessary adjustments (Figure 36-13). Rinse the partial denture and hand it to the dentist for insertion. Articulating paper is used to check the patient's occlusion. If adjustments are needed, transfer the low-speed handpiece with finishing or acrylic burs. Transfer contouring pliers for adjustments to the metal clasps.
5. Provide postoperative instructions. The dentist instructs the patient on how to insert and remove the partial denture. Explain care of the partial and supporting teeth. Also explain that it may take several days to adjust to the partial and sore spots may appear. If the patient has any problems or questions, instruct him or her to call the office for an appointment right away.

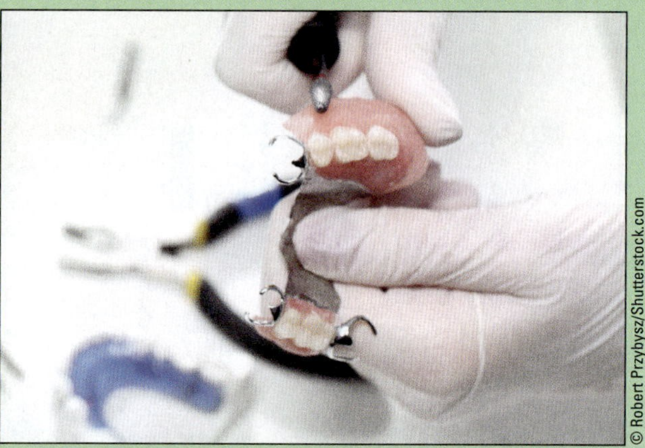

FIGURE 36-13
Partial denture being adjusted with acrylic bur.

Home Care Instructions for a Partial Denture

Patients with removable partial dentures should be given instructions on the care of their partial denture and maintaining good overall oral hygiene. Often the office has a guide or written instructions to give to the patient to take home when they receive the partial. The dental assistant will go over the instructions with the patient and address any questions the patient may have. The dental assistant will also work with the patient in placing and removing their partial until comfortable with the process.

Removable partial dentures, just like natural teeth, require proper care to keep them clean. Home care instructions for a partial denture include the following:

- Remove and rinse the partial denture after eating. Run water over the partial to remove food debris or brush.
- Handle the partial denture carefully. Place a towel on the counter/sink or put some water in the sink to prevent damage if dropped. Do not bend the plastic or clasp portion of the partial.
- Do not try to adjust the clasps, if you are having problems with the partial contact the dentist.
- Brush your partial denture at least once a day. Clean the partial by brushing or soaking to remove food, plaque, and other debris. Use a soft toothbrush to clean the artificial teeth and tissues and also clean in and around the clasps portion of the partial.
- Brush and floss the rest of your mouth especially the abutment teeth as part of your daily oral hygiene care.
- Schedule regular dental checkups. The dentist will evaluate the partial denture routinely to ensure it is comfortable and has a proper fit.

Complete Denture

The complete denture is also called the full denture. When all natural teeth are lost, a denture is fabricated to restore function and improve esthetics for the patient. (A person is said to be *edentulous* when he or she has no teeth remaining.) The denture is supported by the alveolar bone and oral mucosa.

The shape and condition of the tissues determine how much support the denture will have.

Considerations for a Complete Denture

- There is extensive bone loss and lack of support for remaining teeth in the arch.
- The patient has exhibited lack of motivation and/or ability to maintain the remaining teeth.
- The remaining teeth have gross decay, periodontal disease, or abscesses.
- The patient is edentulous.
- The patient lacks the financial means to have alternative treatments, including dental implants and fixed prostheses.

Necessities for Successful Denture Treatment

Dentures are not like natural teeth. They are prosthetic appliances that the patient must adjust to. For the patient to have success with dentures, he or she should have a positive attitude about the procedure and about wearing dentures. Dentures take time and patience to adjust to, and the patient who understands this will be more successful wearing them. Educate the patient so that he or she can prepare mentally. There are many pamphlets and videos available to explain to the patient what he or she can expect and how to function when wearing a denture.

The patient should be in good health. When a patient is in poor health, it is often reflected in the oral cavity. The added stress of a denture may lower the resistance of unhealthy tissues. Also, if there is weight loss or gain, the way the denture fits may change and a reline of the denture may be required. Impaired health may contribute to a lack of muscle coordination, which is needed to keep the denture in place.

The patient should have healthy alveolar ridges and oral mucosa. These tissues will be under stress from the denture and, if the denture does not fit properly, degeneration can occur at a much faster rate.

Components of a Complete Denture

The denture has two basic components: base and denture teeth (Figure 36-14). The external surface of the denture resembles natural tissues and extends over the retromolar pad on the mandible or the maxillary tuberosity area on the maxilla. The external surface is smooth and polished, while the internal surface matches the contours of the oral mucosa and the alveolar bone. The denture teeth are articulated to occlude with the natural or artificial teeth of the opposing arch.

Denture Base. The base is made of denture acrylic and may have a metal mesh embedded in the acrylic for additional strength. The acrylic is pigmented to resemble the normal gingiva; often, fibers are added to the acrylic to give the denture a natural appearance. The **flange** part of the base covers the alveolar ridge and gingival tissues. On the maxillary, the flange base extends beyond the ridge to the attached mucosa, back to cover the tuberosities and the junction of the hard and soft palate. On the mandibular, the flange base extends to the attached mucosa covering the oblique and mylohyoid ridges and back to cover the retromolar pad areas. Refer to Chapter 7, Head and Neck Anatomy, for more information. The denture teeth are embedded in the denture base, just like the partial denture.

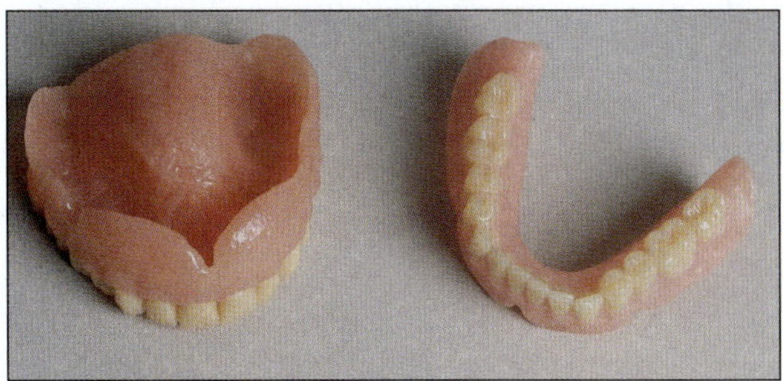

FIGURE 36-14

Full maxillary and mandibular denture: denture base, artificial teeth, tissue side of denture on the left and occlusal view on the right.

Denture Teeth. The denture teeth used in the construction of the denture are made of porcelain or acrylic resin. The porcelain teeth are more resistant to stain and wear but are more brittle than the resins. They may wear away the opposing natural tooth structure, so they are used more often when the opposing teeth are also porcelain. Porcelain teeth sometimes cause a "clicking" sound when the patient is eating or talking.

Acrylic resin (plastic) teeth have the advantage of greater resistance to breakage. They are quieter and bond more efficiently to the denture base. The adjustments require less time, because the acrylic teeth can be polished in the office, whereas porcelain teeth must go to the laboratory to be refinished. The acrylic resin teeth are used when the patient has natural opposing teeth and in patients with poor ridges.

Porcelain teeth are secured in the denture base by mechanical means of pins on the anterior teeth and diatoric (a recess in the denture base for attachment) holes on the posterior (Figure 36-15A). The plastic teeth adequately bond to the denture base material and do not require mechanical retention.

Posterior denture teeth are either **anatomical** or **nonanatomical**. The anatomical teeth resemble natural teeth, with cusps and developmental grooves. The nonanatomical teeth do not have detailed anatomy on the occlusal surface but are concave and somewhat flat. Nonanatomical occlusals are designed for additional strength for patients with too little alveolar ridge to retain dentures.

Denture teeth come in sets for the anterior and for the posterior. The anterior set includes six teeth: two cuspids, two laterals, and two central incisors. The posterior set includes eight teeth: four bicuspids and four molars. (Third molars are not placed in dentures.) These sets have matching shades and molds (shapes) (Figure 36-15B).

Immediate Dentures. The sequence of appointments for the complete denture depends on whether the patient is edentulous or has remaining teeth. When the patient is edentulous

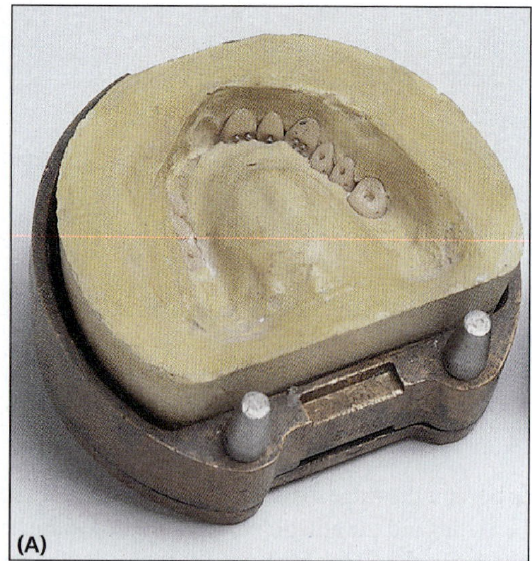

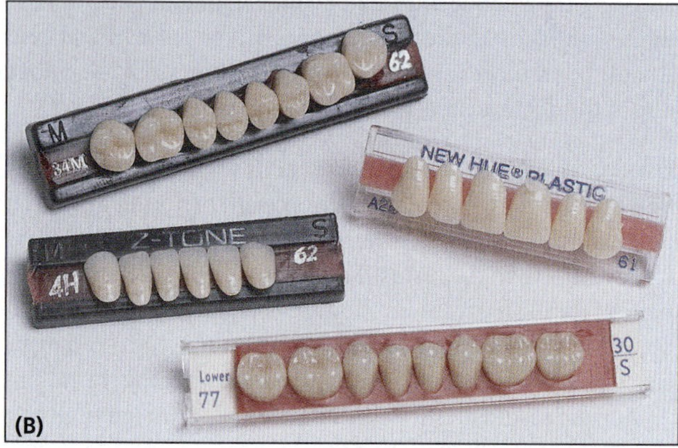

FIGURE 36-15

(A) Porcelain teeth showing pins and diatoric holes. (Note: These teeth are in a model in a flask ready for acrylic base material to be placed over them.) (B) Sets of denture teeth showing shade and mold.

he or she may already have a complete denture. This denture may have to be replaced with a new denture for better fit and retention, or the denture may have broken or been lost.

When the patient has remaining teeth, he or she will need to have the teeth extracted before receiving the denture. In this situation, there are two treatment sequences:

1. In the first treatment sequence, the patient can have all remaining teeth extracted and the alveolar bone shaped and contoured (**alveoplasty**). The patient waits for 4 to 6 months for the tissues and the alveolar bone to heal before the denture construction begins. The *advantage* of this sequence is that the tissues have healed and the alveolar ridge has resorbed to a stable position before impressions for the denture are started and the denture is fabricated. The *disadvantage* is that the patient is without teeth for the healing period. Esthetics and diet restrictions are concerns for the patient.
2. In the second treatment sequence (the immediate denture sequence), the patient has only the posterior teeth extracted—the anterior teeth remain. Another option is for the patient to have all their mandibular teeth and the maxillary posterior teeth extracted leaving the maxillary anterior teeth to be removed just before the immediate denture is seated. This works for patients who do not show much of their mandibular teeth, the patients still have their maxillary anterior teeth left for appearance.
3. Construction of the denture begins as soon as the hard and soft tissues of the posterior areas have healed completely. The patient is scheduled for several appointments to take impressions and then for try-ins of the waxed up denture without the anterior teeth. The jaw relations are determined and final adjustments are made. The articulated base plates and bite rims are sent back to the lab.
4. When the dentures are completed, the patient is scheduled to have the anterior teeth extracted, an alveolectomy is performed, and the denture is inserted. This is called an **immediate denture** (Figure 36-16).

After the surgery the patient is given postsurgical and home care instructions including: patient should wear the denture continuously for 24 hours, except when removed to be cleaned. An appointment is made for a postoperative checkup in 24 hours. During the examination the dentist removes the denture, irrigates, and checks the tissues and sutures. The dentist can relieve the denture if there are pressure sensitive areas. Once the sutures are removed and tissues are healing the patient is scheduled for a reline appointment in several months.

The advantages of the immediate denture are that the patient is never without teeth, the dentist and the laboratory have the patient's remaining teeth to reproduce his or her original appearance, there are no extreme diet restrictions,

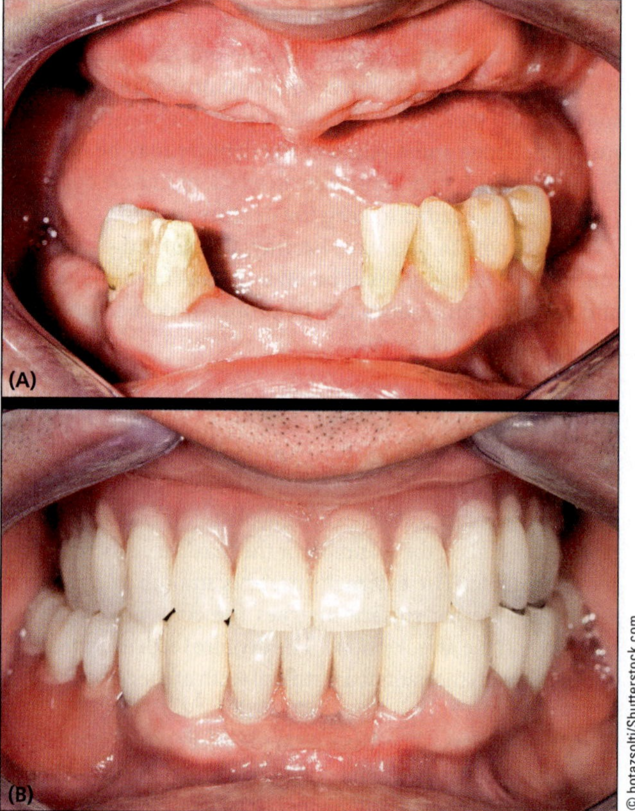

FIGURE 36-16

Immediate Denture. (A) Patient ready for surgery to remove remaining teeth. (B) Immediately after surgery patient with immediate denture in place.

and the immediate denture acts as a compress and bandage to protect the extraction sites.

The disadvantages include lack of an anterior try-in to evaluate the fit; the alveolar ridge changes after the extractions and alveoplasty; the denture needs to be relined in 4 to 6 months; and, because of the reline and the two appointments with the oral surgeon, this process is more costly to the patient.

The following sequence of appointments takes into consideration surgery appointments. Most patients elect to have the immediate denture sequence, and such additional appointments are noted in the procedure descriptions. For a brief overview of the appointments for a complete denture, see Table 36-2.

Examination and Diagnosis Appointments for Complete Denture

The examination appointment for complete dentures is similar to that of the examination for the partial denture. The dentist completes a detailed examination of the condition of the tissues, the shapes and sizes of the ridges, the retromolar and tuberosity areas, the frenum attachments, and the undercut areas. Radiographs and preliminary impressions are taken. Current photographs are made and the patient is asked to bring in other photographs for reference to create a natural appearance for the patient.

Preparation of the diagnosis, treatment plans, and the financial estimate are similar to those of the partial denture prosthesis preparation.

Consultation and Oral Surgery Appointments

The dental assistant has the study models, photographs, x-rays, visual aids, and the patient file ready for the consultation appointment. The dentist presents the information to the patient, explaining what needs to be completed, and discusses with the patient any options he or she may have, such as having all of his or her remaining teeth extracted and being without teeth while the tissues heal, or having an immediate denture. It is also explained to the patient what they can expect including type of anesthetic, discomfort/pain management, the time frame, number of appointments, and the cost.

Oral surgery appointments are scheduled if necessary and then the prostheses appointments are made according to the healing time the patient needs.

Final Impressions Appointment

Once the tissues have healed after the extractions, the patient is scheduled for final impressions. Using the study model impressions, custom trays are fabricated and detailed for the patient. Final impression material is prepared and placed in the custom trays to get an exact impression of the patient's mouth (Procedure 36-4). Once the final impressions are taken and meet the dentist's criteria, they are prepared to be sent to the laboratory. A lab prescription form is filled out and the impressions are ready to be sent to the lab. The impressions will be used to make the baseplates and the bite rims (Figure 36-17).

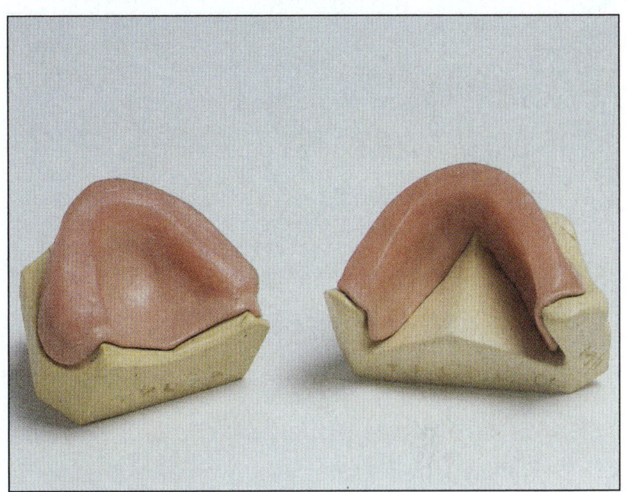

FIGURE 36-17

Baseplates and bite rims made in dental laboratory from final impressions.

TABLE 36-2 Appointments for Complete Denture (Brief Overview)

Appointment	Procedure
Examination	An oral exam is completed. Preliminary impressions and radiographs are taken. The patient is asked to bring photos for the next appointment.
Consultation	Treatment is explained to the patient. Discussion of the treatment includes the dentist's and the patient's responsibilities.
Oral surgery	During the appointment, the posterior teeth are removed and the alveolar bone is contoured.
Final impressions	When the posterior extractions have healed completely, the patient returns to the dental office and final impressions are taken.
Jaw relationship	The jaw relationship is determined with baseplates and bite rims.
Try-in appointment	Completed wax try-in dentures are returned to the dental office for final adjustments.
Denture delivery	The patient is scheduled for surgery to have the anterior teeth extracted and the immediate denture seated.
First follow-up (scheduled several days after the patient receives the denture)	With the immediate denture, the patient is seen the next day in the dental office.
Adjustments	As needed, adjustments are made.

Procedure 36-4
Final Impression Appointment

This procedure is performed by the dentist. Materials are prepared and transferred to the dentist by the dental assistant.

Equipment and Supplies (*Figure 36-18*)

- Basic setup: mouth mirror, explorer, and cotton pliers
- HVE and tip air–water syringe tip
- Cotton rolls and gauze
- Mouthwash for patient to rinse with prior to impressions being taken
- Custom tray (see Chapter 39, Laboratory Materials and Techniques)
- Compound wax and Bunsen burner for border molding the rims of the trays
- Laboratory knife to trim border molding
- Impression materials—spatulas and mixing pads or dispensing gun and tips
- Laboratory prescription form
- Disinfectant and container for impressions and bite registration

Procedure Steps (*Follow aseptic procedures*)

1. The final impressions are taken after custom trays have been fabricated from the casts taken at the examination appointment. The custom trays are inserted into the patient's mouth and evaluated for fit.
2. The impression compound is heated and placed along the borders of the custom tray (Figure 36-19). The tray is cooled and then placed in the patient's mouth. With the tray in the patient's mouth, the lips, cheeks, and tongue are moved to establish accurate length for the periphery and adjacent tissues to be included in the final impression. This is called **border molding** or **muscle trimming**.
3. Final impression materials are prepared and placed in the custom trays. The maxillary impression must include the tuberosities, frenum attachments, and other landmarks of the arch. The mandibular impression must include retromolar pads, oblique ridge, mylohyoid ridge, and frenum attachments.
4. Once the material has set, it is removed from the patient's mouth. The mouth is then rinsed thoroughly.
5. This procedure is repeated with the opposing arch if a full denture is being fabricated for both arches.
6. The impressions are disinfected and sent to the dental laboratory with the prescription form.
7. After the impressions have been taken, the patient is dismissed.

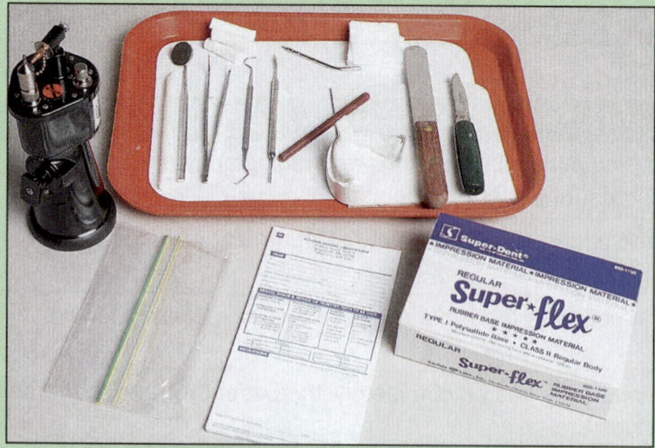

FIGURE 36-18

Tray setup for final impressions of complete denture with custom trays.

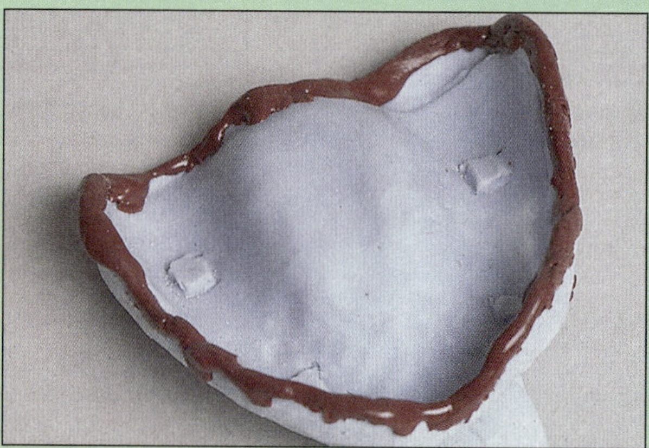

FIGURE 36-19

Custom tray that has been border molded to fit patient for the final impression.

Jaw Relationship Appointment

Once the completed baseplates and bite rims are articulated by the laboratory, they are sent back to the dental office to be used to determine the patient's jaw relationship (Procedure 36-5). The dentist and the laboratory technician need a detailed and accurate model of the patient's occlusion, along with the other measurements. A caliper-like device called a **facebow** is used to record the relationship of the maxillary dentition to the temporomandibular joints so that the maxillary cast can be mounted on the articulator in the correct anatomic position. The lab technician will use this information to orient the casts in this same relationship to the opening axis of the articulator. This allows the laboratory technician to have a model of the patient and how the patient bites when fabricating the complete denture.

A procedure called a **facebow transfer** (refer to Chapter 39, Laboratory Materials and Techniques) is used to take these measurements to be transferred to the articulator. In some states the dental assistant is allowed to perform this skill. To complete the other measurements, the dentist will insert the baseplates/bite rims in the patient's mouth and take measurements including the following:

- **Vertical dimension**—a vertical measurement of the face between two selected points, one located above the mouth and one located below, usually at the midline (Figure 36-20). The dentist places a sticker on the nose and the chin to establish the distance between the dots on the sticker. With the baseplates/bite rims in place the dentist determines an esthetic lip drape for the patient. If the bite rims are too large the patient will struggle to close their lips around them and if the bite rims are too small the patient's mouth will look too full and like they are "pouting."
- **Centric relation**—the position of the mandible when the condyles are positioned posterosuperiorly in an unstrained position in the glenoid fossae.

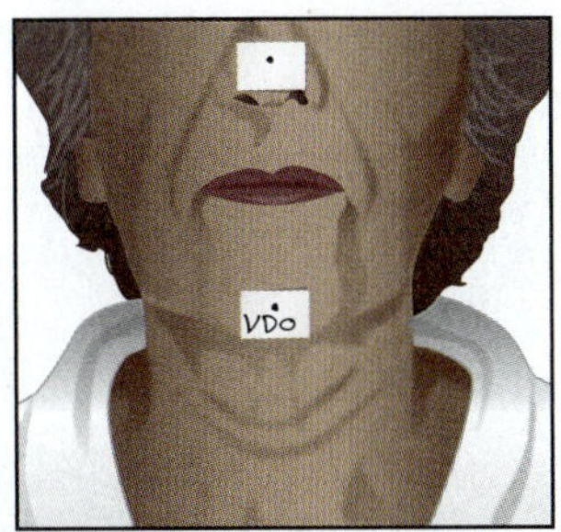

FIGURE 36-20
Patient with tape markings placed to determine vertical dimension occlusion (VDO).

- **Intercuspation**—the cusp-to-fossa relationship of the upper and lower posterior teeth to each other.
- **Centric occlusion**—the relation of opposing occlusal surfaces that provides the maximum planned contact and/or intercuspation. Centric occlusion should exist when the mandible is in centric relation to the maxilla.
- **Retrusion**—posterior movement: the patient moves the mandible as far back as possible.
- **Protrusion**—anterior movement: the patient moves the mandible as far forward as possible.
- **Lateral excursion**—the movement of the mandible from the centric position to a lateral or protrusive position.

Once the dentist has completed the measurements, the baseplates and bite rims are disinfected and sent back to the lab along with the facebow transfer information.

At the dental lab, the lab technician places the denture teeth in the bite rims and articulates the maxillary and mandibular teeth using the measurements the dentist prescribed. The wax try-in dentures are returned to the dental office for the patient's next appointment.

Procedure 36-5
Jaw Relationship Appointment

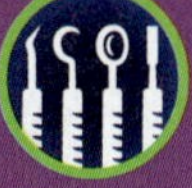

This procedure is performed by the dentist. During this appointment, the measurements, shape, and shade of the denture are determined. The dental assistant prepares equipment and materials and assists the dentist throughout the procedure.

Equipment and Supplies (*Figure 36-21*)

- Basic setup: mouth mirror, explorer, and cotton pliers
- HVE tip and air–water syringe tip
- Hand mirror
- Laboratory knife, #7 wax spatula, and Bunsen burner
- Shade guide
- Millimeter ruler and Boley gauge
- Baseplates and bite rims
- Face bow
- Photographs of the patient, showing the shapes and shades of the teeth
- Laboratory prescription form
- Disinfectant

(continues)

Procedure 36-5 (continued)

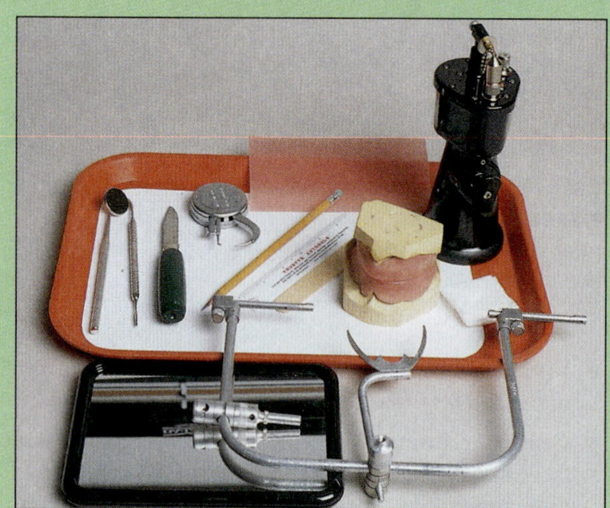

FIGURE 36-21
Tray setup for jaw relationship appointment.

Procedure Steps (*Follow aseptic procedures*)

1. Facebow transfer is taken with rigid bite registration materials and bite fork and transfer assembly, plane locator, plane marker, and ear bow. (Refer to Chapter 39, Laboratory Materials and Techniques.)
2. The baseplates and bite rims are inserted into the patient's mouth. The dentist determines and marks the midline of the maxillary and mandibular arches.
3. The bite rims represent the teeth and provide the vertical dimension. The dentist adjusts the wax bite rims with the laboratory knife and wax spatula until the patient has a natural lip drape and the correct amount of tooth and gingiva is visible when the patient is talking and smiling and the lips are in a resting position. The cuspid lines are determined to position cuspids at the corners of the mouth.
4. The centric occlusion is determined when the jaws are closed in a position that produces maximal contact between the occluding surfaces of the maxillary and mandibular arches. The jaw relationships are determined by evaluating how the mandible relates to the maxilla. The patient moves the mandible as far backward (retrusion) and forward (protrusion) as possible, and then as far as possible to the right and then the left (lateral excursion). Specially designed baseplates and materials assist in determining these measurements. Once determined, the information is used to articulate the casts to duplicate the normal motions of the patient. The laboratory technician constructs the complete denture in wax and with artificial teeth from these records.
5. After the jaw relationships are determined, the denture teeth are selected, and the appearance of the anterior teeth is discussed with the patient. The proper shade is determined using the shade guide and natural light. To achieve a natural look, the shade guide is compared with the patient's complexion and remaining natural teeth or photographs. Usually, the age of the patient indicates the shade range (the teeth stain and become darker with age). The shape (mold) of the teeth is determined by evaluating remaining natural teeth or from photographs. Sometimes, the shape of the patient's face also is used to guide the selection.
6. Because patients are concerned about the natural appearance of the teeth, some patients want to duplicate the arrangement of the teeth, including spaces, overlapping, and so on. Other patients want to correct the alignment of the natural teeth in the new denture. Spending a little more time at this point and having clear communication with the patient to determine what the expected outcome is often pays off when the patient receives the denture and is pleased with his or her appearance.

Denture Construction between Appointments

Between the consultation and the final impressions appointment, the alginate impressions are poured in plaster or stone. On these models, custom acrylic trays are constructed. In the case of an immediate denture, the custom trays are fabricated to allow space for the anterior teeth present in the mouth and the posterior edentulous areas.

Between the final impression appointment and the measurements appointment, at the dental laboratory the master cast is poured in stone from the final impressions. The master cast is used to construct a **baseplate**. A baseplate is a preformed, semi-rigid, acrylic resin material that temporarily represents the denture base.

On the baseplate, several layers of baseplate wax are attached (see Figure 36-17), called the **bite rim**. The bite rims represent the space provided by the teeth in normal occlusion. The bite rims, then, provide the vertical dimension for the denture and establish the position of the mandible to the maxilla. In the natural dentition, the length of the crowns of the teeth determines the distance between the upper and lower jaws. This distance is called the vertical dimension.

Immediate Denture

If the patient is receiving an immediate denture, the baseplate and bite rims are fabricated to fit over the posterior areas only. The patient's existing anterior teeth are used for jaw relationships and measurements.

Once the baseplate and bite rims are constructed, they are sent back to the dental office for the patient's next appointment.

Denture Construction between Appointments—Laboratory Procedures

Between appointments, the laboratory prepares a try-in denture. Denture teeth are mounted in the wax bite rim/base plate and are articulated (Figures 36-22A and B). The laboratory technician positions the teeth according to the dentist's directions and the position can be altered at the try-in appointment. The process of shaping the wax to include normal contours of the gingival tissues is known as *festooning*. With this step the denture takes on a natural look for the patient.

Try-In Appointment

The try-in appointment is the last time the dentist can make any adjustments before the denture is actually completed. The wax try-in dentures are completed by the dental laboratory and sent to the dental office prior to the try-in appointment (Procedure 36-6).

Denture Construction between Appointments—Final Laboratory Procedures

The denture is returned to the laboratory for final processing. This is a multistep process that converts the wax try-in denture to a denture with an acrylic resin base and plastic or porcelain teeth. A dental flask is utilized for this process

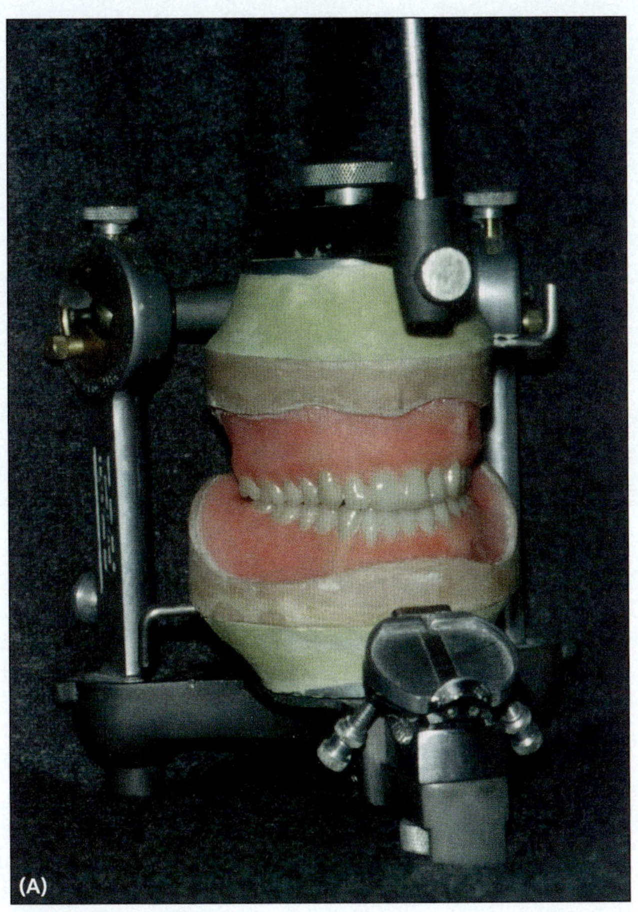

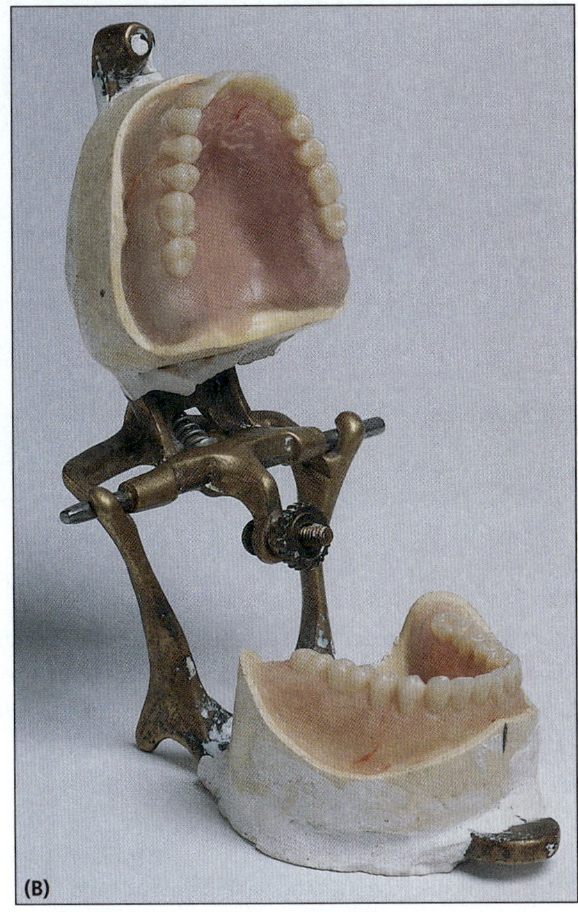

FIGURE 36-22

Wax bite rims with denture teeth on an articulator ready for try-in appointment. (A) Maxillary and mandibular dentures articulated in a closed position. (B) Maxillary and mandibular dentures articulated in an opened position.

Procedure 36-6
Try-In Appointment

This procedure is performed by the dentist. The dental assistant prepares the patient, instruments, and materials, and coordinates with the dental laboratory.

Equipment and Supplies

The dental assistant makes sure the denture is back from the laboratory and prepares the equipment and supplies for the try-in appointment (Figure 36-23).

- Basic setup: mouth mirror, explorer, and cotton pliers
- HVE tip and air–water syringe tip
- Hand mirror
- Laboratory knife, #7 wax spatula, and Bunsen burner
- "Try-in" denture mounted on the articulator from the laboratory
- Shade guide
- Articulating forceps and paper
- Laboratory prescription form
- Photographs of patient's teeth
- Disinfectant

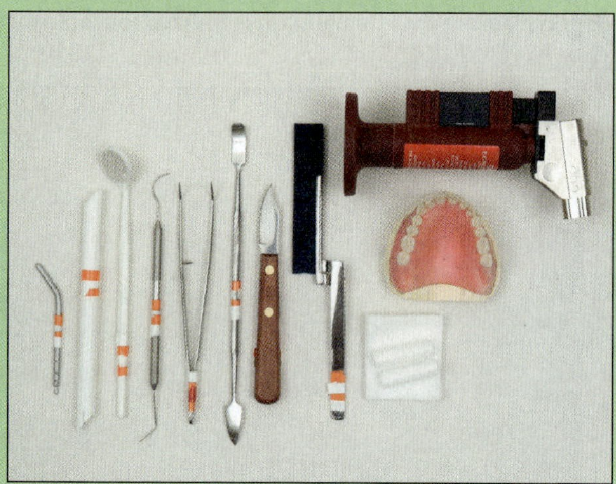

FIGURE 36-23
Tray setup for try-in appointment for full denture.

Procedure Steps (*Follow aseptic procedures*)

1. The "try-in" denture is disinfected before being placed in the patient's mouth.
2. The patient is seated and the denture is inserted into the patient's mouth. The dentist and/or the dental assistant spends a few minutes talking with the patient. This allows the patient time to adjust to the denture.
3. The denture is evaluated for esthetics, retention, and comfort. The occlusion is checked with articulating paper.
4. The dentist makes adjustments to the position of the teeth. The shade can be changed by the dental laboratory technician in the dental laboratory, if necessary.
5. Once the dentist and the patient are satisfied with the denture, it is disinfected and placed back on the articulator to be returned to the laboratory.

(Figure 36-24). The dental assistant should visit the dental laboratory and observe the steps involved in processing a denture to better understand and visualize the steps involved.

Denture Delivery Appointment

During the delivery appointment for the edentulous patient the denture is inserted into the patient's mouth and instructions are given for the insertion and removal techniques and how to maintain the denture. If the patient is receiving immediate dentures, the dentures may be sent to the oral surgeon's office so they can be placed immediately following the removal of the remaining teeth (Procedure 36-7).

Denture Adjustment Appointments

After receiving the immediate denture, the patient returns to the office the next day. The denture is removed and the tissues are examined. If any areas are uncomfortable to the patient at this time, the dentist performs minor adjustments. Because of the swelling and tenderness from the surgery, the dentist will

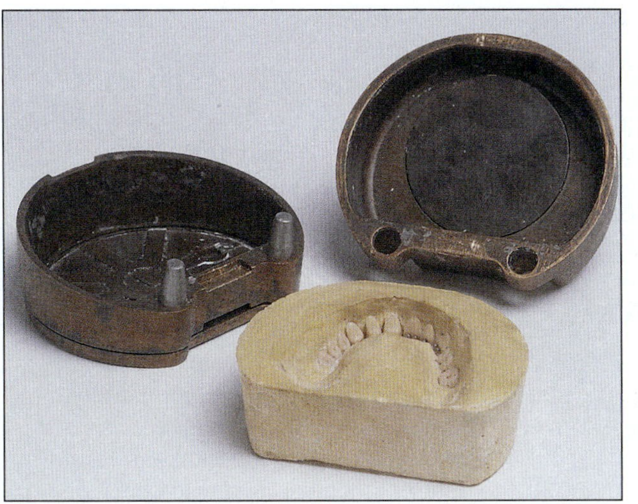

FIGURE 36-24

Dental flask and investment material used with denture teeth to fabricate the denture base.

not remove too much of the denture surface at this time. The patient is taught how to insert and remove the dentures and oral hygiene techniques. He or she is rescheduled in a couple of days for any adjustments.

The patient returns to the office after wearing the denture for several days. The dentist evaluates the tissues and may smooth rough areas, relieve pressure spots, and adjust the occlusion. The amount of adjustment varies with every patient, and this process may require several appointments over a period of time until the denture is comfortable.

The occlusion is adjusted with the burs, stones, and discs on the cusps of the denture teeth. Pressure spots are relieved on the tissue surface of the denture base. Pressure indicator paste is placed on the internal surface of the denture and then inserted into the patient's mouth. Pressure areas are marked and the dentist then uses acrylic burs and stones for adjustments.

Procedure 36-7
Delivery Appointment for Complete Denture

This procedure is performed by the dentist. The dental assistant prepares the patient and coordinates with the dental laboratory. The dentures come back from the laboratory in a container that keeps them moist.

Equipment and Supplies (*Figure 36-25*)

- Basic setup: mouth mirror, explorer, and cotton pliers
- HVE tip and air–water syringe tip
- Dentures from the laboratory
- Hand mirror
- Articulating forceps and paper
- High-speed handpiece and diamond and finishing burs
- Low-speed handpiece and assorted acrylic burs and discs
- Home care instructions pamphlet, denture brush, and container to place dentures in when they are not in the patient's mouth

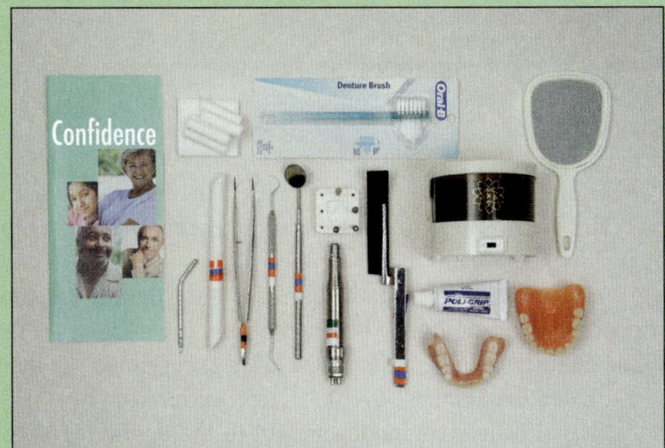

FIGURE 36-25

Tray setup for seating of complete denture.

Procedure Steps (*Follow aseptic procedures*)

1. The patient is seated and the appliances are removed and placed in a container to keep them moist.
2. If the patient is receiving an immediate denture, the denture is inserted after the extractions and alveoplasty. If there are more than simple extractions, the patient is scheduled with an oral maxillofacial surgeon. The dental laboratory sends the denture to the surgeon's office instead of to the dentist's office before the patient's surgery.
3. The new denture is inserted into the patient's mouth and the patient is given a few minutes to adjust. The dentist then begins the examination.

(continues)

Procedure 36-7 (continued)

4. The patient's occlusion is evaluated and, if adjustment is needed, burs and discs are used. The denture is removed from the patient's mouth and the dentist uses a low-speed handpiece and acrylic burs to reduce any high spots on the inside of the base (the part of the denture that is against the tissues) of the denture. Sometimes after the adjustments, the denture needs to be polished in the laboratory. If this process is necessary, the denture must be disinfected before replacing it in the patient's mouth.
5. The dentist evaluates the retention of the denture and the jaw relationships by having the patient demonstrate various facial expressions, swallowing, chewing actions, and speaking.
6. The patient learns to insert and remove the denture and is given oral hygiene and daily maintenance instructions on the care of their denture (see Table 36-3).
7. The patient is given instructions to call the office with any questions or problems and is scheduled for an adjustment appointment in a few days. The patient is then dismissed. As a courtesy, often the dentist or dental assistant calls the patient the following day to check on the patient's progress with the new denture.

TABLE 36-3 Home Care Instructions

- Keep the denture moist when not wearing it to prevent dimensional change.
- Place the dentures in an air-tight container with water or a denture soaking solution overnight. Follow the manufacturer's instructions on cleaning and soaking solutions.
- Do not use abrasive dentifrice on the acrylic, because it abrades easily.
- Do not clean acrylic dentures in hot water, because the acrylic can be deformed and distorted when exposed to high temperatures.
- Dentures have low thermal conductivity, so the patient will notice a decrease in thermal changes to the tissues under the acrylic denture base.
- Rinse thoroughly twice a day and after eating, if possible. If using a denture-soaking solution be sure to rinse the dentures thoroughly before putting them back in your mouth. These solutions may contain chemicals that can cause vomiting, pain, or may burn the tissues if swallowed.
- Use a soft denture brush and toothpaste designed for dentures (Figure 36-26).
- Remove the denture and rinse the oral cavity daily.
- Denture adhesives are not needed with a well-fitting denture. As the tissues change and the denture does not adapt as well, adhesives will fill in the spaces so that retention is increased.
- Commercial cleaners are available for overnight soaking. Use warm water with these products.
- The patient may wish to fill the sink with water or place a washcloth in the sink in case the denture is dropped (Figure 36-27).
- If the denture becomes loose, see the dentist as soon as possible. Loose dentures can cause sores and discomfort.
- The dentist will schedule regular dental checkups according to the patient's needs. They will examine the denture for wear and may professionally clean them. Your dentist will also examine the tissues in the oral cavity to make sure they are healthy and there are no irritations.

Denture Reline

The tissue side of the denture bases may need to be adjusted and/or **relined** to improve the fit of the denture and the comfort of the patient. After a period of time, the supporting tissues often shrink and change in size because of the pressure put on them by the complete or the partial denture. To evaluate how the denture fits over the tissues, a white silicone paste (Pressure Indicating Paste (PIP)) is placed over the tissue side of the denture and then seated in the patient's mouth. The material is allowed to set about 2 minutes and then the denture is removed. On the areas where the PIP is thin or displaced it is indicated that these areas on the denture need to be reduced to relieve the pressure on the tissues. The dentist will use an acrylic bur to make the minor adjustments on the denture outside the patient's mouth.

As changes occur with the tissues and the denture becomes loose or ill-fitting it may be time to have the denture relined. The denture relining adds a new layer of acrylic to the inside of the denture (Figure 36-28). This procedure can be done in the dental office (chairside) or sent to the dental laboratory (Procedure 36-8).

The chairside (soft) reline saves the patient time and makes it possible for the patient to never be without the denture. This reline process is a temporary solution, because the soft reline is not as durable and will not last as long as the laboratory reline.

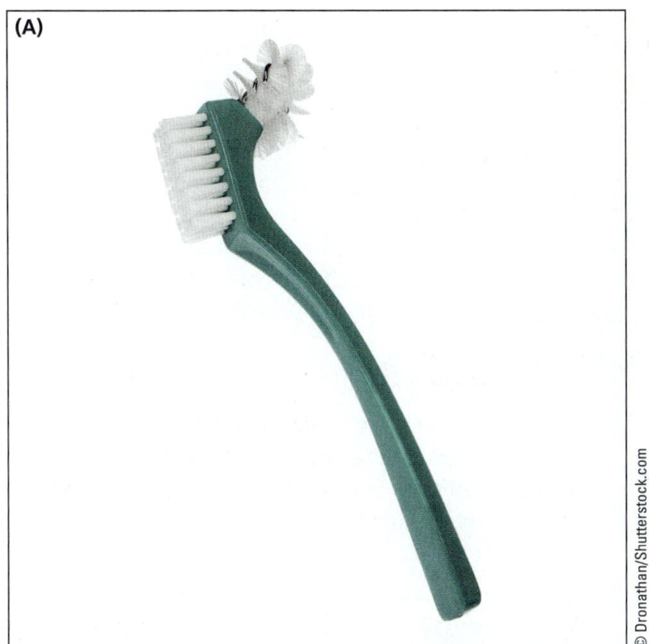

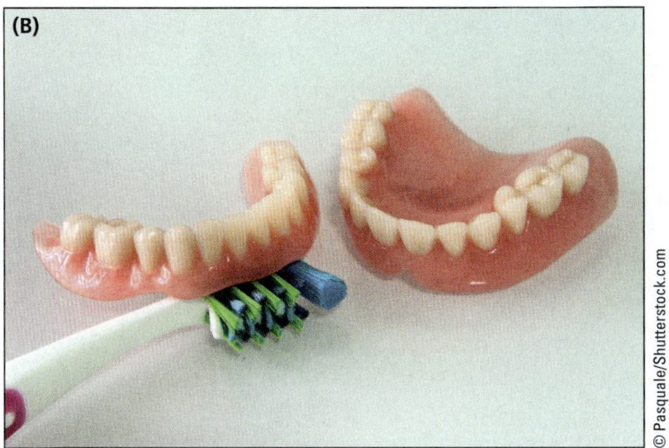

FIGURE 36-26
(A) Denture brush. (B) Brushing the tissue side of the denture.

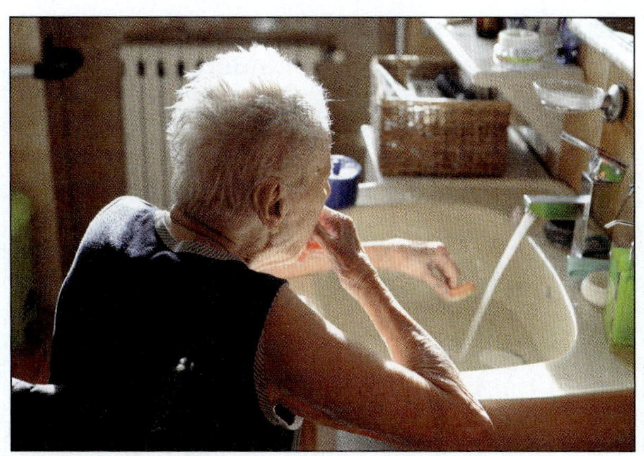

FIGURE 36-27
Elderly woman cleaning her denture over a sink of water.

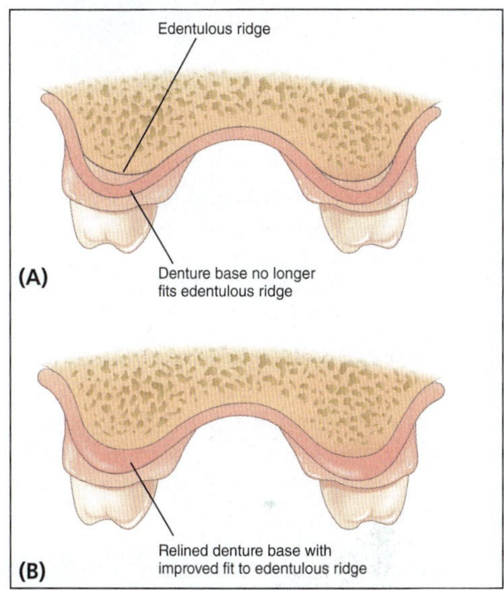

FIGURE 36-28
(A) An ill-fitting denture. (B) Denture fit after denture has been relined.

Procedure 36-8
Denture Relining

   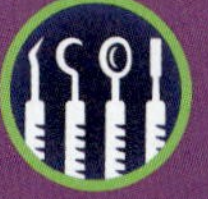

This procedure is performed by the dentist. The dental assistant prepares the patient and the materials. The reline materials are available in either hard or semi-soft materials. There is a variety to choose from, depending on the dentist's preference.

Equipment and Supplies (*Figure 36-29*)

- Basic setup: mouth mirror, explorer, and cotton pliers
- Low-speed handpiece with acrylic burs
- Chairside reline materials
- Mouth rinse
- Chairside relining

Procedure Steps (*Follow aseptic procedures*)

1. Clean the denture by placing it in an ultrasonic unit for a few minutes.
2. The dentist uses acrylic burs to roughen the tissue side of the denture.
3. The material is mixed according to manufacturer's directions and then placed in the clean denture, covering the entire tissue surface. The

(continues)

Procedure 36-8 (continued)

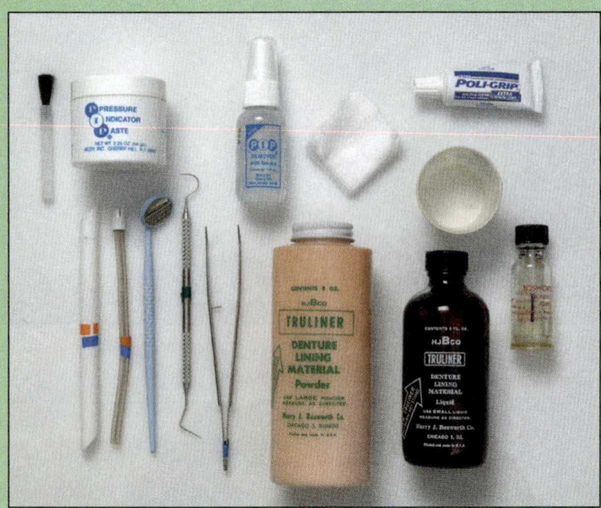

FIGURE 36-29

Tray setup for denture reline.

materials have low thermal reaction and cure directly in the patient's mouth.

4. The patient rinses with mouthwash to clean saliva and debris from the tissues.
5. The denture is inserted into the patient's mouth and the patient is asked to bite until the material reaches the initial set stage. Explain to the patient that sometimes the tissue will have a slight burning sensation from the acrylic material during the setting time.
6. The denture is removed to complete the setting process.
7. Excess material is trimmed away and the denture is polished. Follow routine disinfecting before the denture is inserted into the patient's mouth.

Laboratory Relining

The patient's denture is prepared in the same manner as it is for the chairside relining procedure. The following are the impression and laboratory steps. The tray setup is the same as that in the chairside relining, except for the types of materials used. Often, the denture or partial is used as the tray for the impression materials. A variety of impression materials, including polysulfides, polyethers, and silicone, are used to take the impression.

Procedure Steps (*Follow aseptic procedures*)

1. The impression material is mixed and placed in the denture (tray) according to the manufacturer's directions. The material should cover the entire tissue surface of the denture evenly and without excess.
2. The denture is inserted into the patient's mouth and positioned firmly. The patient should occlude and hold until the material is set.
3. After the material sets, the denture is removed from the patient's mouth, disinfected, and prepared to be sent to the dental laboratory. The laboratory prescription is completed and the patient is dismissed.
4. The dental laboratory processes the impression materials into an acrylic resin base that is fused to the denture.
5. The patient returns to the dental office as soon as the laboratory can process the denture. The turnaround time varies from hours to several days. The procedure is scheduled with the laboratory to minimize the time the patient is without the denture.
6. When the patient returns to the office, the denture is seated and adjustments are made as needed.
7. Postoperative instructions: The patient is given instructions to call the office with any questions or problems. Home care instructions for the prostheses are reviewed (see Table 36-3).

Tissue Conditioning

Sometimes the tissues are irritated and inflamed due to an ill-fitting denture. These tissues must be healed before a denture reline is completed. This process is called tissue conditioning. A temporary soft lining material is placed in the denture to relieve the pressure and allow the tissues to heal. The healing usually takes several weeks and then the denture can be relined.

The laboratory reline takes more time, and the patient may be without the dentures for a day. The laboratory reline replaces the tissue side of the denture.

Denture Repair

The denture may need repair from time to time. Sometimes a denture tooth becomes loose or is lost or the denture is dropped and fractured (Figure 36-30). When the patient brings the denture or partial to the office for repair, the dental assistant should disinfect it before the repair process begins. Some of the repairs can be completed in the dental office, but other, more complex repairs must be sent to the dental laboratory. The patient may need to be seen by the dentist if an impression is needed. In some cases, the dentures can be left at the office for repairs. The repairs often do not take long and the patient returns later in the same day or the next day to pick up the denture. Sometimes the patient is seen by the dentist for minor adjustments.

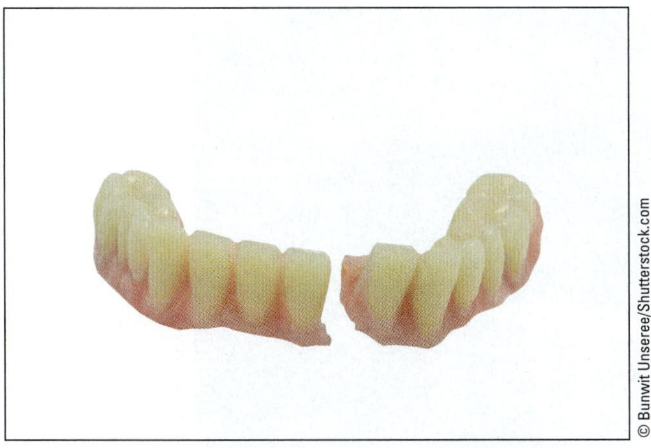

FIGURE 36-30

Mandibular denture in need of repair.

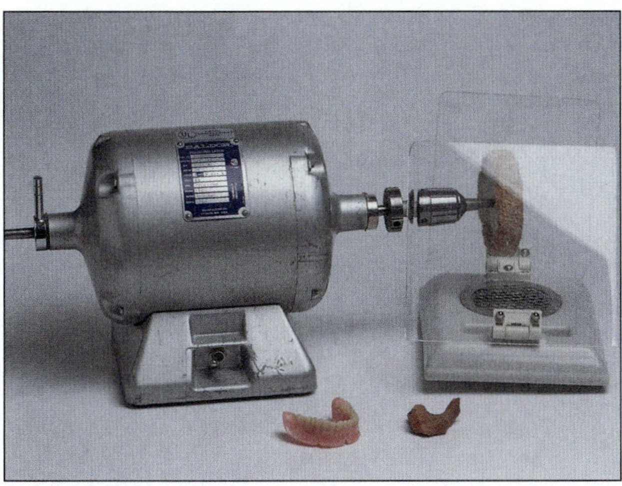

FIGURE 36-31

Dental lathe with rag wheel and Tripoli to polish prosthesis.

Polishing Removable Prostheses

After the dentist has adjusted the tissue surface of the removable prosthesis with acrylic burs, discs, and stones, it may need to be polished to smooth the surface. The polishing can be accomplished on a dental lathe with rag wheels, pumice slurry, and various other polishing agents, such as Tripoli or a paste of tin oxide and water (Figure 36-31). Care must be taken not to overheat the denture, because the denture base has a relatively low heat-transfer temperature. If the denture is overheated, it may be distorted, which affects the fit and the appearance of the denture. Also, the plastic teeth should be protected because they will abrade easily. Once the polish is complete, the prosthesis is washed in soap and water, disinfected, and stored in water until it is delivered to the patient. For each patient, separate burs, rag wheels, and pumice should be used to maintain infection control. Burs and rag wheels can be sterilized. The pumice is mixed with a disinfectant and green soap mixture and should be changed after each use.

Overdenture

Over time, the pressure applied during mastication on the mucosa and the supporting underlying alveolar bone causes the bone to shrink/absorb. The denture is not as stable, and retention becomes a problem for the patient. An **overdenture** can be fabricated to prevent or reduce this problem. The patient with overdentures has shown less alveolar bone loss.

To fabricate an overdenture, the dentist saves certain parts of the patient's remaining teeth or places dental implants in the dental arch on which the denture will attach. Instead of the denture base resting on the mucosa and the alveolar bone, the denture is supported by the retained prepared teeth (Figure 36-32) or the dental implants (Figures 36-33 A and B and 36-34 A and B).

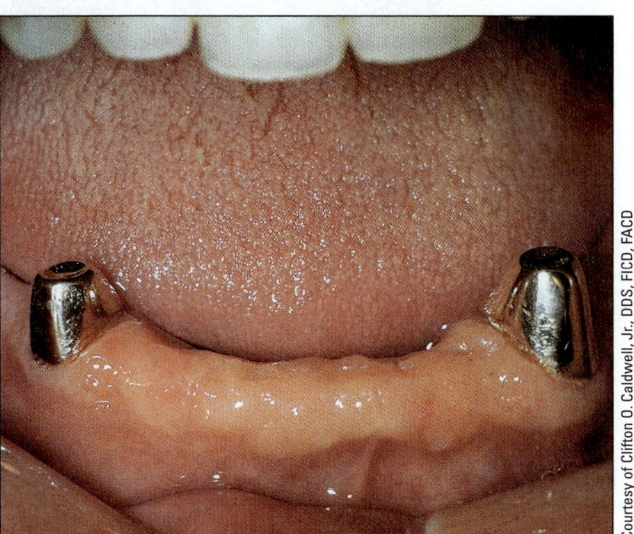
Courtesy of Clifton O. Caldwell, Jr., DDS, FICD, FACD

FIGURE 36-32

Overdenture supported with abutments (roots are restored with cast-gold post and dome-shaped core combination).

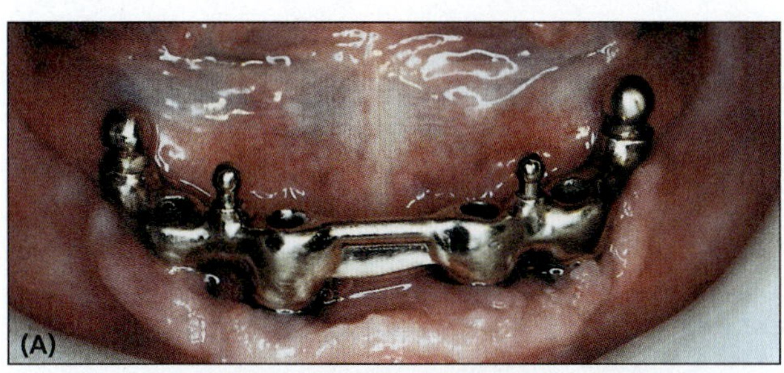

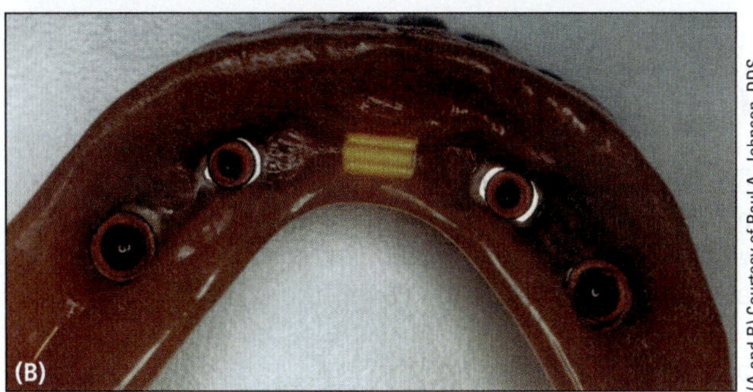
(A and B) Courtesy of Paul A. Johnson, DDS

FIGURE 36-33

(A) Dental implants for a denture. (B) Denture to fit over dental implants.

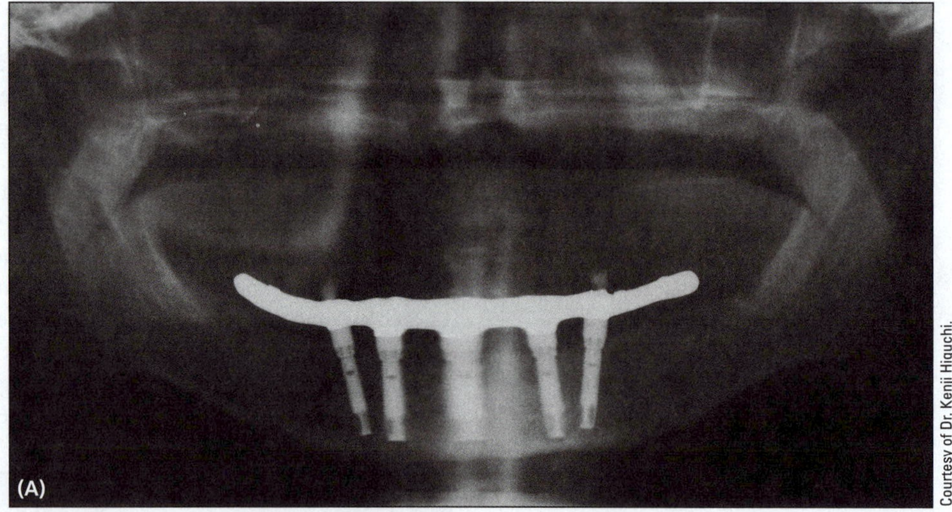
Courtesy of Dr. Kenji Higuchi.

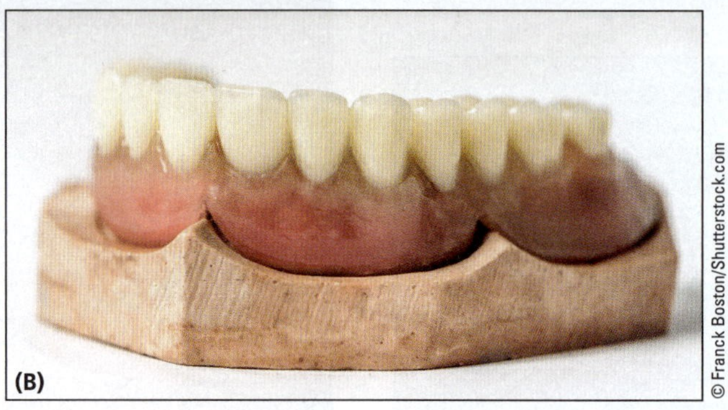
© Franck Boston/Shutterstock.com

FIGURE 36-34
(A) Panoramic radiograph showing dental implants to secure a denture. (B) Denture in place over the dental implants.

Endosseous Implant and Overdenture

The retained teeth are endodontically treated and prepared with posts and cores or with special prefabricated attachments. The tissue side of the denture is constructed with part of the attachment aligned with the implant or retained tooth. There are various types of attachments, including magnets and a "snap" design.

The advantages include retention and stability of the denture, especially if the patient does not have much alveolar ridge to retain a denture to begin with. The disadvantages include an increase in the cost and time involved because of the surgeries, endodontic treatment, and restorative procedures. Also, the patient must maintain the retained teeth and/or the dental implants. Plaque control is essential to prevent bone loss around the implants and the retained teeth and to inhibit root caries on the retained teeth. The patient must be diligent and motivated for the success of the overdenture.

Chapter Summary

Removable prosthodontics, like fixed prosthodontics, refers to the replacement of missing teeth and tissues with artificial structures, or prostheses. With removable prosthodontics, however, the prosthesis can be removed from the mouth of the patient. Most patients prefer to have fixed prostheses, but in some cases it may not be the treatment of choice due to existing conditions.

The dental assistant's main functions are to prepare materials, record measurements and details for the fabrication of the denture, provide patient education and support, and perform some laboratory procedures. The procedures in removable prosthodontics do not require many instrument exchanges, and the assistant does not continually maintain the oral cavity throughout the appointment with the air–water syringe and the HVE. The steps in removable prosthodontics involve as many extraoral as intraoral procedures. The dental assistant has all the items prepared so that the dentist can explain to the patient the diagnosis, the proposed treatment plan, and the prognosis.

Both full dentures and partial dentures are discussed including advantages, disadvantages, the components of both prostheses, and the appointment schedules. Steps of a denture reline and repairs are described, as well as how to polish a removable appliance. The overdenture procedure is explained along with the advantages and disadvantages relating to it.

CASE STUDY

Julie Davidson has been told by Dr. Jacobson that she needs a maxillary full denture. Mrs. Davidson has had problems with her teeth over the years because of advanced periodontal disease. She is an office manager for a group of physicians, and is very conscientious about her appearance and apprehensive about wearing dentures.

Case Study Review

1. What denture procedure would allow Julie to continue to function with her natural teeth while her maxillary denture is fabricated?
2. What types of patient information are available?
3. To prepare the patient for the denture procedure, what should the dental assistant consider?

Review Questions

Multiple Choice

1. Removable prosthodontics include all of the following procedures *except*
   a. partial denture.
   b. full denture.
   c. crown and bridge.
   d. immediate denture.
2. Parts of the partial denture that contact the teeth to provide vertical and horizontal support are
   a. connectors.
   b. rests.
   c. retainers.
   d. denture bases.
3. Denture teeth are made of
   a. porcelain.
   b. plastic.
   c. both porcelain and plastic.
   d. amalgam.
4. When the jaws are closed to produce the maximum contact, ________ can be determined.
   a. vertical dimension
   b. centric occlusion
   c. vertical occlusion
   d. horizontal dimension
5. All of the following are correct home care instructions for a patient just receiving a full denture *except:*
   a. Rinse the denture twice a day and after eating, if possible.
   b. Use a soft denture brush and toothpaste designated for dentures.
   c. Place water or a washcloth in the sink in case the denture is dropped while cleaning it.
   d. Use hot water when cleaning the denture to remove bacteria.
6. A ________ is the part of the removable partial denture that contacts the tooth to provide vertical and horizontal support.
   a. connector
   b. hinge
   c. rest
   d. retainer
7. The ________ retainer encircles and adapts to the contours of the abutment tooth.
   a. circumferential-type clasp
   b. bar-type clasp
   c. stress-breaker
   d. major connector
8. The part(s) of the partial denture that rest(s) upon the oral mucosa, providing coverage and stability, is (are) called the
   a. retainer.
   b. metallic framework.
   c. denture base.
   d. connectors.
9. All of the following statements are true about immediate dentures *except:*
   a. Patients are never without teeth with this technique.
   b. The patient has all teeth extracted, waits 4 to 6 months, and then the denture is fabricated.

c. The patient's remaining teeth assist the laboratory to reproduce the original appearance of his or her teeth in the denture.
d. This denture needs to be relined in 4 to 6 months.

10. The process of using impression compound to modify the custom tray is called
a. centric rotation.
b. vertical dimension.
c. the smile line.
d. border-molding/muscle trimming.

Critical Thinking

1. What types of materials can be used to take the final impression for a partial denture?
2. During which complete denture appointment must the baseplates and bite rims be ready for use?
3. What is an overdenture? When would a patient be a good candidate for an overdenture?

Web Activities

1. Find out how patients should care for their dentures. Go to *Public Resources*, Oral Health Topics, Dentures, and the questions patients frequently ask at http://www.ada.org.
2. Go to http://www.nadl.org and find out their mission statement and goals and public awareness programs.
3. Go to http://www.valplast.com to learn more about flexible partials.
4. Find out what the American College of Prosthodontists is and what information they have to assist patients and the public at http://www.prosthodontics.org.

Section VIII

Restorative and Laboratory Materials and Techniques

CHAPTER 37

Dental Cements, Bases, Liners, and Bonding Agents

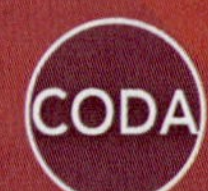

Specific Instructional Objectives

The student should strive to meet the following objectives and demonstrate an understanding of the facts and principles presented in this chapter:

1. Differentiate between dental cements, bases, liners, and bonding agents.
2. List the dental standards, and the organizations responsible for those standards.
3. Explain the role of the dental assistant in preparing materials.
4. List and explain the properties of dental materials.
5. Identify the types of dental cements. Explain the properties, composition, uses, and manipulation of zinc phosphate cement, zinc-oxide-eugenol (ZOE) cement, polycarboxylate cement, glass ionomer cement, resin-modified glass ionomer cement, calcium hydroxide, varnish, resin cement, and compomer cement.
6. Explain etchants and their function.
7. Describe bonding agents and their manipulation.
8. Discuss restorative dentistry and the various materials and techniques involved, including cavity detection and cavity cleaners, disinfectants, and desensitizers.
9. Identify cavity preparation terminology.
10. Describe the steps of cavity preparation.

Advanced Chairside Functions

11. Classify cavity preparations according to their relationships with the pulp.
12. Explain options for protecting the pulp with cavity liners, cavity varnish, and cement bases.
13. Describe the purpose of using cavity liners. List the types of materials that can be used and explain the placement procedure.
14. Describe the purpose of using cavity varnish and explain the placement procedure.
15. Describe the purpose of using cement bases. List the types of materials that can be used and explain the placement procedure.

Key Terms

adhesives (879)
axial wall (882)
base (865)
Bonding (864)
bonding agent (864)
bonding resins (879)
bruxism (862)
Calcium hydroxide (875)
cavity detection methods (881)
cavity liner (886)
cavity preparation (885)
cavity varnish (876)
cavosurface margin (883)
cement base (886)
chemical retention (863)
Compomer (878)
Composite resin cement (877)
copal varnish (876)
Corrosion (863)
desensitizer (882)
desiccating (881)
DIAGNOdent caries detection (881)
Dimensional change (863)
direct pulp capping (DPC) (886)
dual-cured material (864)
ductility (862)
elasticity (863)
etchant (877)
exothermic (865)

(continues)

Key Terms (continued)

flow (863)
force (862)
galvanism (863)
gingival wall (883)
glass ionomer (871)
high-strength base (886)
indirect pulp capping (886)
intermediate luting cement (865)
intermediate restorative material (IRM) (868)
light cured (864)
line angle (883)
liner (865)
low-strength base (886)
luting (865)
malleability (862)
mechanical retention (863)
microleakage (863)
palliative effect (865)
permanent luting cement (865)
point angles (883)
Polycarboxylate (868)
pulpal wall (882)
reinforced zinc-oxide-eugenol (865)
resin-modified (reinforced) glass ionomer (874)
retention (863)
sedative (865)
self-curing (864)
smear layer (881)
soluble (864)
strain (862)
stress (862)
tarnish (863)
temporary luting cement (865)
thermal conductivity (864)
thermal expansion (864)
universal varnish (876)
varnish (865)
viscosity (864)
wettability (864)
zinc-oxide-eugenol (868)
zinc phosphate (865)

Introduction

When the dentist fills (restores) a patient's tooth there are many dental materials that are used depending on how deep the cavity is, how much tooth structure is left, and the type of restorative material being used. In this chapter, dental cement, bases, liners, and bonding agents will be discussed explaining what they are; when they are used; and how each material is prepared, manipulated, and placed.

Dental cements are either permanent or temporary and are used to retain crowns, bridges, inlays, and onlays. Bases are used to protect the pulp when the cavity is deep and when the pulp may be sensitive. Liners are low-strength materials that are placed under the restoration. Some liners stimulate the formation of secondary dentin, some seal the dentin tubules, and some have fluoride in them. Bonding agents are used to improve the retention between the tooth and the restoration.

Before discussing each category of materials, the properties of dental materials will be covered. This will give the dental assistant a basic background on how the material works and the aspects that need to be considered when a material is selected.

The elements of cavity preparations are discussed before the expanded function section, which covers the placement of cements, bases, and liners. Dental assistants need to understand cavity preparation and know the correct terminology when assisting the dentist and when actually placing the materials.

Although some materials used in dentistry have been around for a long time, there are constant changes and new products that are always being introduced. The dental team should be updated by attending seminars and dental conferences, reading books and trade magazines, and through local sales representatives.

Generally, the materials are divided and categorized by function. Some materials have a broad spectrum of uses. After the tooth has been prepared and the decay removed, certain materials are utilized to restore the tooth. Dental materials are regulated and tested for function and safety before they become available for use. The ADA and the Food and Drug Administration (FDA) regulate dental materials. The ADA Council on Scientific Affairs is responsible for the testing of dental materials, and periodically publishes a listing of certified dental materials in the *Journal of the American Dental Association* and in *Clinical Products in Dentistry: A Desktop Reference.*

In addition, the following international organizations develop standards for materials, instruments, and equipment produced around the world: the Fédération Dentaire Internationale and the International Standards Organization (ISO). (See Chapter 1, Introduction to the Dental Profession.)

The ADA Seal of Acceptance

The ADA, in cooperation with the government, sponsored research on more than 50 types of dental materials. From this research, specifications and standards were established. These standards are updated continually, and are used to evaluate new materials. If a material meets specification requirements, the *ADA Seal of Certification* is awarded. This certifies that the material meets the criteria established by the ADA and the government, and that it is safe and effective.

For new types of dental materials, the ADA Council on Scientific Affairs conducts the program for evaluation and acceptance. Before these products are eligible to apply for the ADA Seal they must be cleared by the U.S. Food and Drug Administration to be marketed directly to the consumer. These products may be marketed for over-the-counter sales, or solely for oral health care professionals. The Council utilizes published technical standards, including ADA guidelines and specifications. There are guidelines to follow for companies and manufacturers that want to be in the acceptance program. Once the company or manufacturer has applied and been granted the Seal of Acceptance by the Council of Scientific Affairs, and after a license agreement has been signed, they can use the ADA Seal of Acceptance on their products. The *Seal of Acceptance of the ADA* indicates that the material has been proven to be safe and effective through biological, laboratory, and clinical evaluation. The following types of products may be included: therapeutic agents, drugs, chemicals, materials, instruments, and equipment used in the prevention of dental diseases. Cosmetic products may also be eligible for the seal. The ADA Seal of Acceptance is recognized by the public as a product endorsement by the dental profession, this assists them in making an informed decision when purchasing over-the-counter dental products.

The Role of the Dental Assistant

The dental assistant's role when working with dental restorative materials depends on the expanded functions of individual state practice acts, which regulate dentistry. The chairside dental assistant generally prepares and mixes the material, while the dentist places the material in the oral cavity. Some states allow the dental assistant to perform these basic responsibilities, as well as placing the materials in the oral cavity.

Knowledge of dental-material properties is necessary for the dental assistant to properly prepare and manipulate the materials, and is also beneficial for patient education and protection. Expanded-function dental assistants must understand and be competent with placing and finishing such materials.

Properties of Dental Materials

Replacing the natural tooth structure has presented a number of challenges. The oral cavity environment and functions create complex situations. Properties that are considered for dental materials include the following: acidity, adhesion, biting force, corrosion, dimensional change, elasticity, flow, galvanism, hardness, microleakage, retention, bonding, solubility, thermal conductivity, viscosity, and wettability.

Acidity

Acidity is viewed in terms of its effect on a given material and on the tissues in the mouth.

- The normal pH of the oral cavity is about neutral (pH 7.0). Some foods, such as citrus fruits, and some bacteria found in the plaque are acidic. Saliva aids in reducing the acidity of the mouth, but dental materials are subject to varying amounts of acid. How materials react to changing acidity levels in the mouth determines their use in the oral cavity.
- Another consideration is that the acidity of the materials may cause irritation to the gingival tissues or damage to the pulp. These materials can be used successfully in the mouth, but care is taken to prepare and/or place them following the manufacturer's directions.

pH Scale

The pH scale, which ranges from 0 to 14, measures the level of acidity or alkalinity of a substance. A pH of 7 is neutral, a pH less than 7 is acidic, and a pH greater than 7 is basic.

Adhesion

Adhesion is the force of attraction that holds unlike substances together. Adhesion involves physical or chemical forces. Chemical adhesion is quite strong and preferable, but physical adhesion is more common. Adhesion is a way to attach solid structures to each other. An example of physical adhesion is dental plaque adhering to a tooth. Certain dental cements function on the basis of a chemical reaction, which results in chemical adhesion.

Biting Forces

Dental materials are subject to various types of biting forces. Natural dentition can withstand much more force than prostheses, such as dentures and bridges. A **force** is defined as any push or pull on an object. The result of force on an object is resistance. **Stress** is defined as the force per unit area of a material. As force is applied the reaction of the object to resist the external force is **stress**. Forces can cause stress over a large area, such as a quadrant, or over a small area, such as the occlusal surface of a tooth. Enough stress can be placed on an object to cause a change. This change, or deformation, is known as **strain**.

- Types of stress and strain are described in the following (Figure 37-1): *Tensile*—pulls and stretches a material. Under tensile stress and strain, the structure tends to be elongated. An example of tensile stress and strain are wires that are pulled in opposite directions, or elastic, rubber bands used in orthodontics. The ability of a material to withstand forces of tensile stress without failing is known as **ductility**.
- *Compressive*—pushes, or compresses, a material. An example of compressive stress and strain is chewing or biting. The ability of a material to withstand compressive stresses without fracturing is known as **malleability**.
- *Shearing*—slides one part of a material parallel to another part in a back-and-forth motion. An example of shearing stress and strain is **bruxism**, or grinding of the teeth.

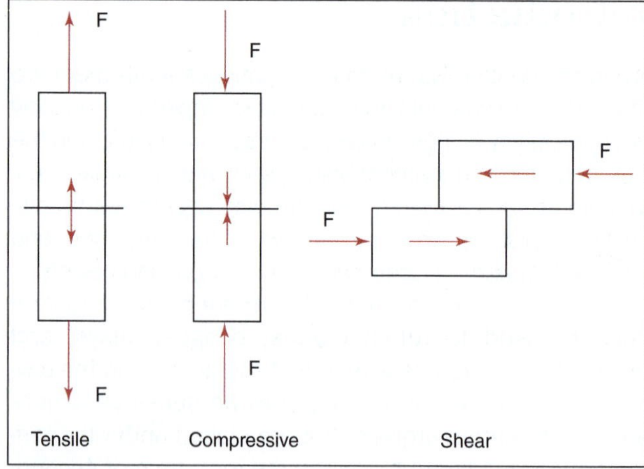

FIGURE 37-1
Tensile, compressive, and shearing stress and strain.

Biting Force

The average biting force for a person with natural dentition varies from 130 to 170 pounds on the molars, and progresses downward to about 40 pounds on the incisors. When force is applied on an individual tooth, this represents about 25,000 pounds per square inch (psi) on a single cusp or a molar.

Corrosion

Corrosion is the result of chemical or electrochemical attacks by the oral environment on pure metal, such as gold, or on an alloy, such as amalgam. Components of food or saliva react with the metals and cause deep pitting and roughness. Sometimes the metals become dull and discolored. This effect is referred to as **tarnish** (Figure 37-2).

Dimensional Change

Dimensional change in a material can occur from a variety of causes, such as the setting process of a material, or exposure to heat or cold. The change in a material is usually measured as a percentage of the original length or volume. If an impression material goes through dimensional change, the permanent restoration may not fit on the tooth, because the impression material does not represent the exact dimensions of the prepared tooth.

Elasticity

Some materials have the property of **elasticity**, which is the ability of a material to return to its original shape, after being distorted or deformed by an applied force, once that force is removed. Rubber bands exhibit this property; but if they are stretched for too long or too far, they reach their *elastic limit* and will not return to their original shape.

The *elastic modulus*, or modulus of elasticity, is a measure of the stiffness of a material below the elastic limit. This is a measure of how a material can resist deformation or change.

Flow

A **flow**, or creep and slump, is a continuing deformation of a solid. Under a constant force, certain materials change and deform. Examples of materials in which flow is a factor are dental waxes and certain impression materials. Amalgam is also subject to flow under constant compressive forces.

Galvanism

When two different metals are present in the mouth, there is a potential for the creation of small electrical shocks. This is known as **galvanism**. The oral fluids act as a carrier between the two metals to cause an electrical shock. This can occur when a gold restoration in one arch contacts an amalgam restoration in an opposing tooth on the opposite arch. The same shock happens if an individual bites a piece of tin foil and it contacts a tooth with a restoration.

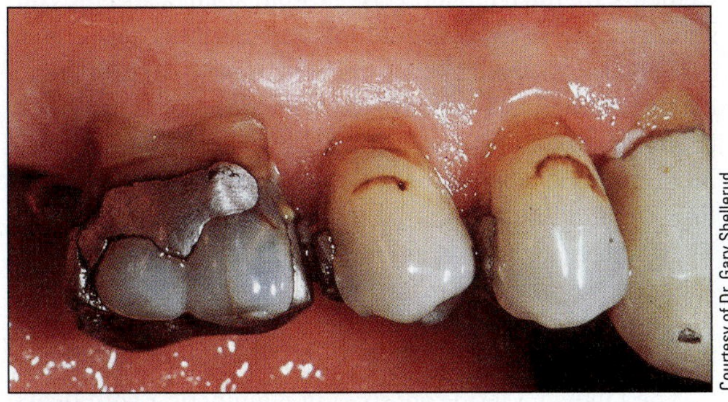
Courtesy of Dr. Gary Shellerud

FIGURE 37-2
An amalgam restoration showing corrosion and tarnish.

Hardness

The resistance of a material to scratching or indentation is known as the material's hardness. There are various ways to measure the hardness of a material. Dental materials that can be dented or scratched will show wear.

Microleakage

When saliva and debris from the oral cavity seep between the tooth structure and restorative materials, this is known as **microleakage**. The dentist prepares the cavity and places materials to prevent microleakage, but some microleakage still occurs. Recurrent decay and tooth sensitivity are some of the problems resulting from microleakage (Figure 37-3).

Retention

In dentistry, **retention** is the means by which materials are held in place. Different types of retention methods are used with the various types of restorative materials. Materials placed directly into the cavity preparation (direct restorative materials), such as amalgam and composites, are retained in place by mechanical means. A **mechanical retention** includes preparing the walls of the cavity preparation to be convergent (slanted in), roughening the tooth surface with etchant, or placing retentive grooves into the cavity walls.

Retention for indirect restorations, such as gold inlays or crowns, is accomplished with bonding agents and cements. Cements and bonding agents may be retained to the tooth surface by mechanical or chemical means. A **chemical retention** involves a chemical reaction between the tooth surface and the material.

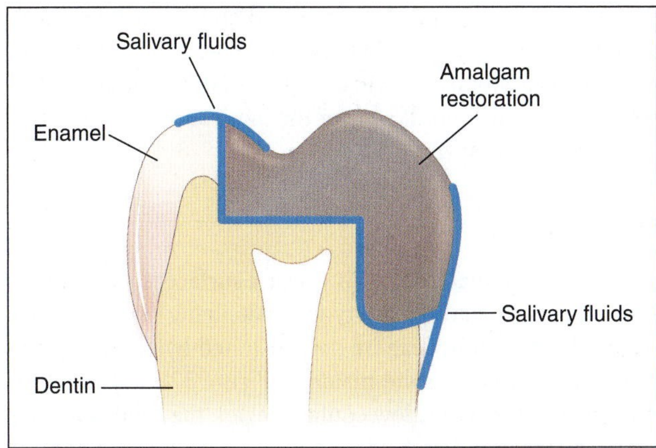

FIGURE 37-3
Microleakage can occur around the margins of an amalgam restoration.

Bonding

Bonding is the process by which materials adhere firmly or hold together. In dentistry, a **bonding agent** is used to bond the dentin and enamel with restorative materials. These materials are discussed later in this chapter.

Solubility

When a material is **soluble**, it dissolves in fluid. The solubility of a dental material is one factor used to determine its success in the oral cavity. A material that is soluble may be useful as a base or liner where it is not exposed to oral fluids. However, if the material is exposed to saliva, it dissolves and exposes the tooth structure.

Thermal Properties

Thermal conductivity is the ability of a material to transmit heat. With some materials heat transmits rapidly, while with others the process is very slow. The thermal conductivity of a material is a consideration when it is placed near the dental pulp, because a material that has a low rate of thermal conductivity offers more protection. Materials are placed in layers over the pulp to protect it from thermal changes. For example, the patient with a denture can drink hotter coffee because the denture base material has low thermal conductivity; thus, it protects the tissues under the denture.

Thermal expansion is another consideration for dental materials. With temperature changes, materials expand and contract. When materials are used in the oral cavity, they must expand and contract at a rate close to that of the tooth structure. Dimensional changes that occur from thermal expansion and contraction can lead to microleakage and sensitive teeth (Figure 37-3).

Viscosity

The **viscosity** of a material is related to its ability to flow. The thicker the material, the less it flows; therefore, it is said to be more viscous than a thin material that flows easily. Honey that is cool is thick and viscous, but when heated, it becomes thinner and less viscous. Materials that are more viscous do not spread easily over a surface. For example, if cement is too viscous, it will not flow over the tooth surface to produce adequate retention.

Wettability

The ability of a material to flow over a surface is **wettability**. This is an important property when applying certain dental materials. Wettability can be demonstrated by observing the shape of a drop on a solid material (Figure 37-4). If the drop spreads out (forming a low contact angle), the solid is readily wetted by the liquid. If the drop beads (forming a high contact angle), there is poor wetting of the solid. For instance, pit and fissure sealants should have good wettability in order to cover the grooves of the occlusal surface.

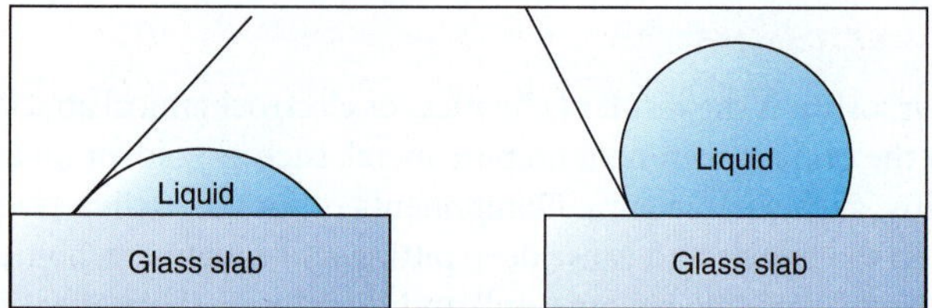

FIGURE 37-4
Examples of two materials' wettability.

Types of Restorative Dental Materials

The ADA and the International Standards Organization (ISO) have classified restorative materials into three types according to their use and properties:

- Type I materials include cements or *luting* agents. They may be permanent or temporary materials. These cements may be used as an adhesive for indirect restorations, as a temporary adhesive for provisional restorations, or as an adhesive for orthodontic appliances.
- Type II materials include amalgam, composite, and glass ionomer, which may be permanent restorative materials (see Chapter 38, Restorative Materials, Matrix, and Wedge) or temporary restorative materials, such as intermediate restorative materials (IRM). Dental Sealants are also included in this type (see Chapter 30, Dental Sealants).
- Type III materials include liners, bases, and bonding agents, which are placed in the cavity preparation.

These materials are mixed at chairside by the dental assistant as indicated by the dentist, following the manufacturer's instructions and the dentist's preferences. It is the dental assistant's responsibility to maintain the materials and the mixing equipment.

Dental Cements

Dental cements usually come in a powder/liquid form, two-paste system, capsule, or in a dispensing syringe. Most of these materials are mixed manually, but a few of the powder/liquid cements come in capsules that are mixed mechanically. Cements are mixed in a precise ratio to attain a specific consistency, ranging from a liquid solution to a putty consistency.

Dental cements can be set, or cured, by **self-curing** (chemical reaction between two materials), by means of a curing light (**light cured**), or by dual curing. Light-cured materials are becoming very popular because the operator has more time to place and manipulate the materials before curing them. These materials are sensitive to overhead lights, however, and must be protected from light if dispensed ahead of time. A **dual-cured material** combines self-curing properties with light-curing techniques.

The following terms are used in conjunction with dental materials. Knowing these terms assists in understanding their material uses and functions:

- **Luting**—bonding or cementing together. Dental cements may be used as luting agents to bond inlays, bridges, and so on to teeth.
- **Permanent luting cement**—a long-term cementing agent.
- **Temporary luting cement**—a short-term cementing agent.
- **Intermediate luting cement**—a material that lasts six months to a year.
- **Liner**—A material placed in a thin layer on the walls and floor of the cavity preparation. The liner protects the pulp from bacteria and irritants.
- **Base**—applied in a putty or thick layer between the tooth and the restoration in order to protect the pulp from chemical irritation, temperature changes, electrical shock, and mechanical injury. Bases are strong enough to be placed under restorative materials and to support the materials from occlusal stresses.
- **Sedative** or **palliative effect**—a soothing effect that a material may have on a tooth. The sedative or palliative material may relieve pain, but does not cure the problem.
- **Varnish**—a thin layer of material that is placed to seal the walls and floor of the cavity preparation.

Uses of Dental Cements

There are many types of dental cements, and each type of cement can have several uses (see Table 37-1 for the types of cements and their uses). Some cements are combined with other materials to modify or expand their functions. Examples are **reinforced zinc-oxide-eugenol** cements and glass ionomers.

Dental Cements

Dental cements are usually mixed on a paper pad. Although the paper pads are easy to use and clean up, they present a disinfection problem. After mixing, the top sheet of the paper pad is discarded and the rest of the pad is placed on the tray. Once in the sterilizing area, the paper pad is wiped with a disinfectant around the edges where the assistant may have held the pad. While this method works, after a while the edges of the paper pad begin to curl and the pad becomes difficult to use. An alternative to using paper pads is a Teflon slab or, for smaller mixes, the plastic that comes in x-ray packages. Be creative!

Zinc Phosphate Cement

Zinc phosphate cement is one of the oldest cements, and while it does have some disadvantages, it is still a reliable choice for a permanent luting (Type I) cement and a base (Type II) cement. It comes in a powder/liquid form, and several brands are available.

Composition. The zinc phosphate powder is primarily zinc oxide with a small amount of magnesium oxide and pigments. The powder is available in shades of white, yellow, and gray. The liquid is a solution of phosphoric acid in water buffered by agents to slow down the setting reaction. Because the liquid is acidic and irritating to the pulp, the tooth must be protected with a base, sealer, desensitizer, or liner before the cement is placed.

When the powder and liquid are mixed together, a chemical reaction occurs and heat is released. This reaction is called **exothermic**. As heat is produced, the reaction speeds up even more. There are specific guidelines to follow when mixing zinc

TABLE 37-1 The Functions of Dental Cements, Bases, Liners, and Varnish

Type of Cement	Uses or Functions
Zinc Phosphate	Permanent cementation of crowns, inlays, onlays, bridges, and orthodontic bands and brackets—an insulating base.
Zinc-Oxide-Eugenol	Temporary cementation of crowns, inlays, onlays, and bridges; and a temporary restoration and a low-strength base (palliative base). Is also a periodontal dressing after periodontal surgery and a root canal sealer.
Reinforced Zinc-Oxide-Eugenol	Permanent cementation of crowns, bridges, inlays, and onlays—an insulating base and temporary restoration.
Polycarboxylate	Permanent cementation of crowns, bridges, inlays, onlays, and orthodontic bands and brackets—a high-strength base and a temporary restoration.
Glass Ionomer	Permanent cementation of crowns, bridges, inlays, onlays, and orthodontic bands and brackets. A high-strength base and a low-strength liner. A permanent bonding liner for composites. Also a root canal sealer, restorative material, and core buildup material.
Calcium Hydroxide	Low-strength liner
Varnish	Thin liner
Resin Cement (Composite or Composite Resin)	Permanent cementation of cast crowns, bridges, inlays, onlays, and endodontic posts. Cementation of ceramic or composite inlays and onlays, resin-bonded bridges, and orthodontic bands.
Resin-Modified Glass Ionomer	Used to cement metallic restorations or porcelain-fused-to-metal restorations to the tooth structure—a core buildup material and high-strength liner.
Compomers	Referred to as polyacid-modified resins. They are used to cement all types of dental restorations.

phosphate cement in order to minimize the temperature rise and slow down the reaction process. This provides reasonable working time and allows for maximum incorporation of the powder.

Properties. When mixed, the zinc phosphate cement is high in strength and reaches two-thirds of this strength in less than an hour. Zinc phosphate sets (hardens) in 5 to 9 minutes, and has a long mixing time of up to 2 minutes. Viscosity is affected by mixing time and temperature. Zinc phosphate bonds to the tooth by means of mechanical interlocking.

Manipulation Considerations. When the zinc phosphate powder is mixed with the liquid, an exothermic reaction occurs. The cement is mixed on a cool glass slab in order to *dissipate* (spread) the heat of the mix. The slab is cooled in cold water and then dried completely. Any moisture left on the slab affects the properties of the cement. The glass slab should be clean and free of scratches and dried cement. A stainless steel cement spatula is used to mix the powder into the liquid. The spatula should also be cool.

The powder and liquid should be the same brand and type of cement. The powder and liquid may come in dispensing bottles; or a scoop for the powder and a dropper for the liquid may be required. The bottle of powder is fluffed/lightly shaken. The powder is placed on one side of the slab, and then proportioned for mixing. Then the liquid is dispensed on the slab (Figure 37-5). The powder is usually divided into differently sized sections for easier mixing. Follow the manufacturer's instructions.

As mentioned previously, one objective in mixing the cement is to dissipate the heat from the exothermic reaction. If the heat is dissipated, the setting reaction is slowed and more powder can be incorporated to make the cement stronger. To accomplish this goal, several mixing techniques are used:

- The glass slab is cooled.

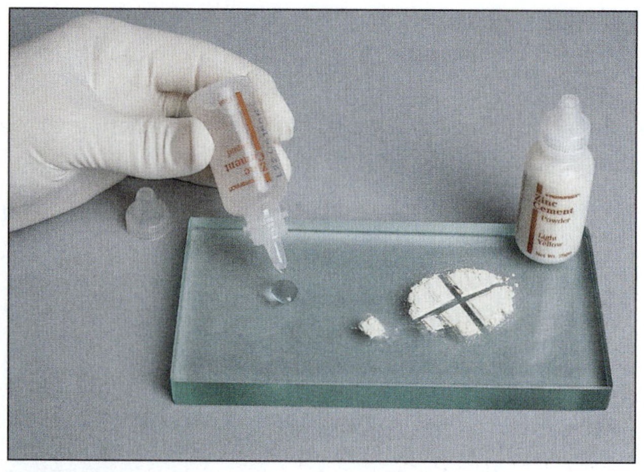

FIGURE 37-5

Zinc phosphate powder dispensed and divided into portions, with liquid being dispensed.

- The first increment of powder is mixed into the liquid for 10 to 15 seconds before more powder is brought into the mix.
- Spatulate the mix slowly when incorporating the powder into the liquid.
- Mix slowly over a large area of the slab, wiping both sides of the spatula.

Of all the cements, mixing zinc phosphate is the most critical, and each procedural step must be followed (see Procedure 37-1). When zinc phosphate cement is mixed into a luting consistency, the cement is creamy and follows the spatula about 1 inch above the mixing slab. When zinc phosphate cement is mixed into a base consistency, the cement resembles thick putty.

Procedure 37-1
Mixing Zinc Phosphate Cement

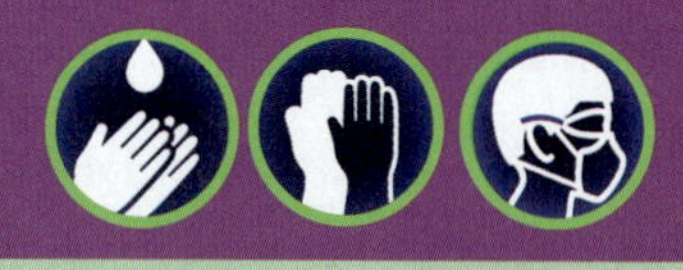

The dental assistant prepares the material and passes it to the dentist. Sometimes the dental assistant places the cement in the cast restoration while the dentist places material on the prepared tooth.

Equipment and Supplies (*Figure 37-6*)

- Zinc phosphate powder and liquid (dispensers, if needed)
- Cooled glass slab
- Flexible stainless steel cement spatula
- 2 × 2 inch gauze sponge
- Timer
- Plastic filling instrument

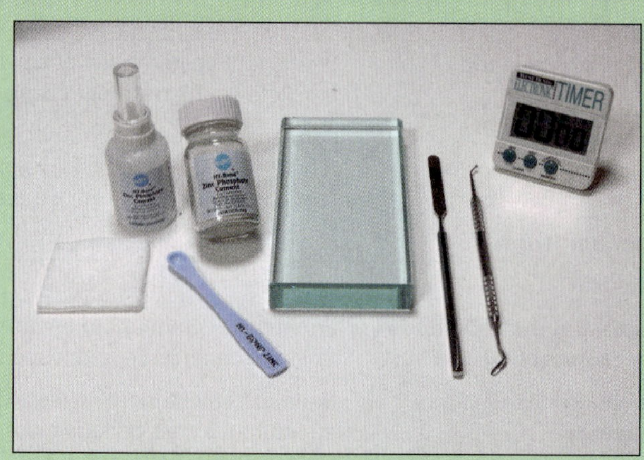

FIGURE 37-6

Zinc phosphate tray setup.

(continues)

Procedure 37-1 (continued)

Procedure Steps (*Follow Aseptic Procedures*)

1. Shake the powder before removing the cap.
2. Place an appropriate amount of powder on one end of the slab. The amount of powder to be used is determined by the powder-liquid ratio, and the amount of cement required for the procedure.
3. Level the powder with the flat side of the spatula blade into a layer of about 1 mm thick.
4. Divide the powder into small increments according to the manufacturer's directions.
5. Gently shake the liquid. Dispense the liquid from a dropper bottle onto the opposite side of the glass slab. Hold the liquid vertical (perpendicular to the slab) while dispensing in order to produce uniform drops.
6. Incorporate a small portion of powder into the liquid, following the specific manufacturer's directions on mixing times.
7. Using a *wide sweeping motion*, spatulate the powder and liquid over a *large area of the glass slab* (Figure 37-7).
8. Adding small amounts of powder will help neutralize the acid, control the setting time, and achieve a smooth consistency of the mix. Incorporate each increment of powder thoroughly into the mix before adding more powder.
9. The mix will appear watery at first, and then, as more powder is incorporated, the mix will become creamy.
10. Continue to add additional increments to the mix within the prescribed time until the desired consistency is reached.
11. The consistency for luting (cementing) will be creamy. It will follow the spatula for about 1 inch as it is lifted off the glass slab (Figure 37-8A).
12. The consistency for a base should be putty-like, and you should be able to roll the base into a ball or cylinder with the flat side of the spatula (Figure 38-8B).
13. Once the cement has been mixed to the desired consistency, wipe off the spatula with 2 × 2 inch gauze. Hold the glass slab under the patient's chin, and pass the plastic filling instrument to the dentist.
14. When the dentist has finished with the mixed cement, wipe the spatula and glass slab with a moistened 2 × 2 inch gauze.

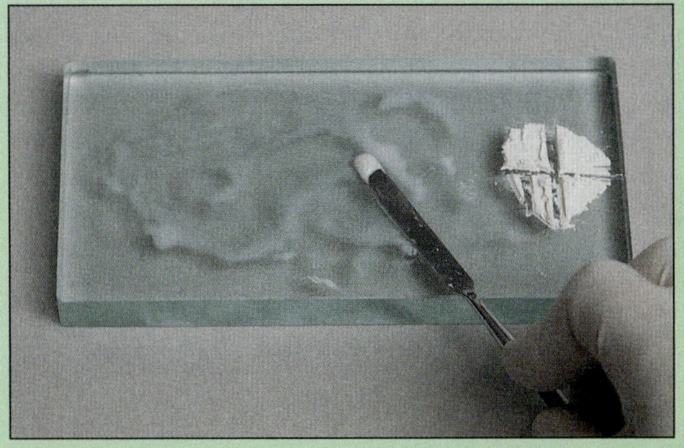

FIGURE 37-7
Mixing zinc phosphate powder and liquid. As the powder is incorporated, a larger area of the glass slab is used.

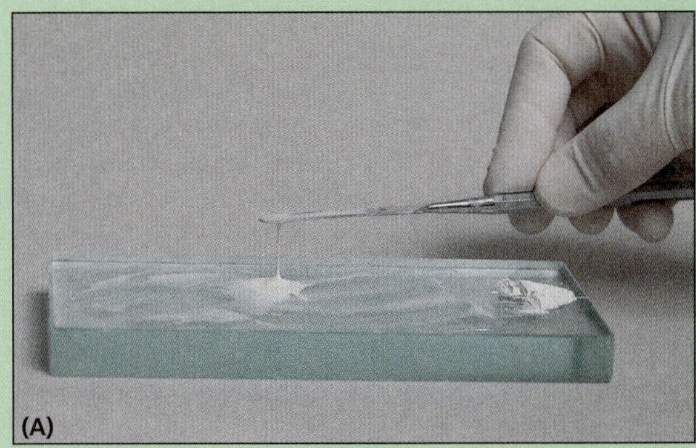

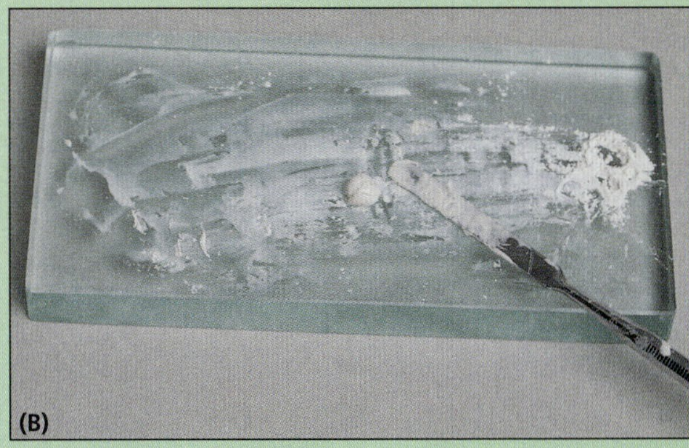

FIGURE 37-8
(A) Demonstration of luting consistency—the cement is creamy and the spatula lifts the cement 1 inch from the glass slab.
(B) Base consistency—thick putty. *Note:* Most of the glass slab was used, and there is excess powder with which to pick up and manipulate the base.

15. To clean the glass slab and spatula, soak them in water or a solution of soda bicarbonate to loosen the hardened cement, and then sterilize/disinfect.

Zinc-Oxide-Eugenol Cement

Zinc-oxide-eugenol cement, often referred to as "ZOE," is another cement that has been used for many years. It is noted for its sedative or soothing effect on the dental pulp (refer to Table 37-1 for the various uses of zinc-oxide-eugenol). The functions of this cement are diverse because of additives that enhance its properties. There are two types of this cement: *type I* is not as strong and is used for temporary restorations and cementation; *type II* has been reinforced and is stronger, and can be used for permanent cementation.

One type II zinc-oxide-eugenol cement is different from the rest in function. It is called an **intermediate restorative material (IRM)**. This material is placed in the patient's mouth and lasts up to 1 year. This material comes both in a powder/liquid form and in capsules (Figure 37-9). It is used when a tooth cannot be restored immediately, such as during illness, when the patient is moving, or because of economic reasons.

Eugenol

Although eugenol has long been known for its sedative effect on the pulp, it can also be irritating to the gingival tissues and the pulp when applied directly to these tissues. Sometimes, when a product containing eugenol contacts the oral mucosa, the patient feels a burning sensation, and the tissues become red and irritated. The tissues will sometimes slough off and are tender to the touch, thereby making eating and brushing uncomfortable. Several days may be necessary for the tissues to heal and become less sensitive. Eugenol also has a strong odor, which may be offensive to some patients.

Manufacturers of eugenol containing products, such as zinc-oxide-eugenol cements and periodontal dressing, now offer products containing a eugenol substitute, called non-eugenold products.

Composition.

ZOE is available in several forms, including powder/liquid, two-paste systems, capsules, and syringes. The powder for the conventional (type I) ZOE cement consists of zinc oxide, resin, zinc acetate, and an accelerator. The liquid is eugenol, which is sometimes mixed with other oils, such as clove oil. The reinforced (type II) ZOE cement includes the addition of alumina and polymers (resins) to the powder, and the addition of ethoxybenzoic acid to the eugenol. Non-eugenol zinc oxide cements are available for patients who are sensitive to eugenol. The non-eugenol cements (type I) are formulated with other oils.

Properties.

ZOE has several properties that affect the selection of this material. ZOE is very soluble in the mouth and dissolves quickly. Reinforced ZOE has the strength required for permanent cementation and retention, but it is not as strong as zinc phosphate. The pH of zinc-oxide-eugenol cements is neutral. With their sedative effect on the tooth, these materials do not require a protective base or liner.

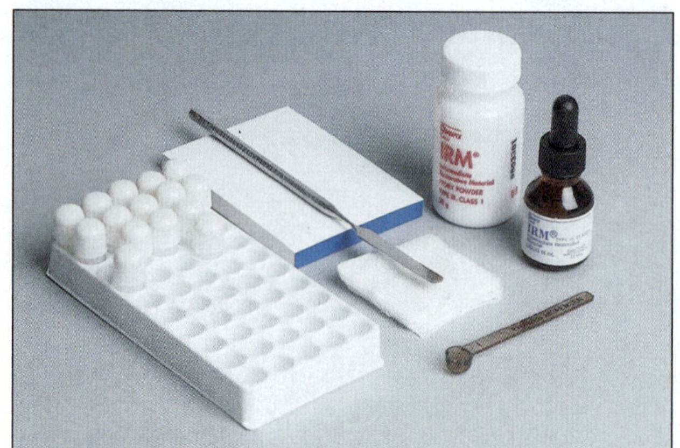

FIGURE 37-9

IRM-Type II (ZOE) comes in powder/liquid form and in premeasured capsules.

ZON materials are not used under composites or acrylic restorations, because the eugenol is not compatible with these materials, as the eugenol retards the setting process.

Manipulation Considerations.

Most ZOE materials are mixed on a paper pad with a stainless steel cement spatula (see Procedures 37-2 and 37-3). A glass slab may be used to control the setting time. Gently shake the powder before dispensing and swirl the liquid. Usually these materials have specific powder dispensers and liquid droppers. Care should be taken not to allow the eugenol into the rubber bulb of the dropper. The eugenol breaks down the rubber, thereby contaminating the liquid.

The type of material being mixed determines whether the powder is incorporated into the liquid in increments or brought in all at once. Usually, the mixing time is 30 to 60 seconds. All of the powder is mixed into the liquid to produce a uniform, smooth, creamy mix. ZOE cements set quickly in the mouth because of the moisture and the warmth.

Some ZOE cements are two-paste systems comprised of an accelerator and a base. They are dispensed in equal lengths on a paper pad. The two pastes have different colors and are mixed until a uniform color is achieved, which takes about 10 to 15 seconds.

The setting time ranges from 3 to 5 minutes in the oral cavity for most ZOE materials. They are mixed to either a luting or base consistency depending on their use and the specific material.

Polycarboxylate Cement

Polycarboxylate cement, also known as zinc polycarboxylate, is used for permanent cementation and as an insulating base. This cement is said to be kind to the pulp, and was the first

Procedure 37-2
Mixing Zinc-Oxide-Eugenol Cement—Powder/Liquid Form

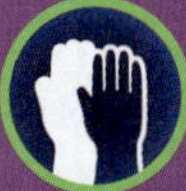

This procedure is completed by the dental assistant when the dentist signals. The equipment and materials are prepared and the material is mixed and passed to the dentist. The dental assistant follows the manufacturer's directions for specific information on proportions, incorporation technique, and mixing and setting times.

Equipment and Supplies (*Figure 37-10*)

- Zinc-oxide-eugenol cement
- Dispensers for specific material
- Paper pad or glass slab
- Cement spatula
- Timer
- Plastic filling instrument
- 2 × 2 inch gauze sponges
- Alcohol or orange solvent

Procedure Steps (*Follow aseptic procedures*)

1. Fluff the powder before removing the cap.
2. Place the powder on the mixing pad according to the manufacturer's directions. Replace the cap to avoid spilling and contamination.
3. After swirling, place the liquid on the paper pad. Hold the dispensing dropper perpendicular to the mixing pad and dispense the drops. Dispense near the powder but not touching it.
4. Incorporate the powder into the liquid in divided increments or all at once, according to the manufacturer's directions.
5. Spatulate with the flat part of the blade and with an even pressure to wet all particles of the powder. With some cements, a firm pressure is required to accomplish this.
6. Gather up the powder and liquid from the edges of the mix.
7. Gather up the entire mass into one unit on the slab to test its consistency.
8. The consistency for temporary luting will be creamy, like frosting (Figure 37-11).
9. The consistency for an insulating base or IRM will be putty-like, and can be rolled into a ball or cylinder.
10. Once the material has been mixed to the desired consistency, wipe the spatula with a 2 × 2 inch gauze. Hold the pad under the patient's chin, and pass the cement on the plastic filling instrument to the dentist.
11. Receive the plastic filling instrument and wipe it off. The top page of the paper pad is removed and folded to prevent accidental contact with the cement.
12. To clean material that has hardened on the spatula or glass slab, wipe it with alcohol or orange solvent as seen in Figure 37-10.

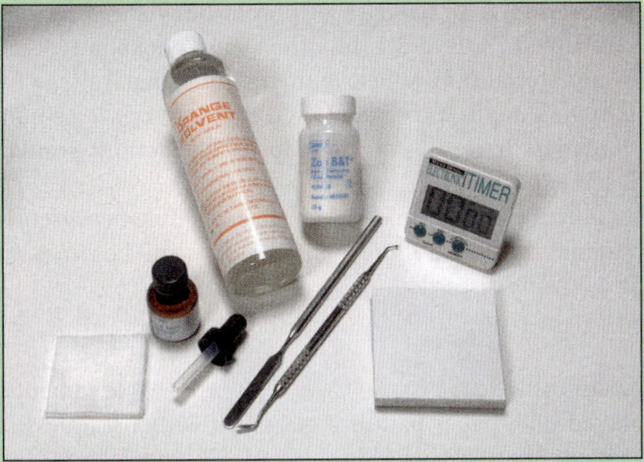

FIGURE 37-10
Tray setup for zinc-oxide-eugenol cement in powder/liquid form.

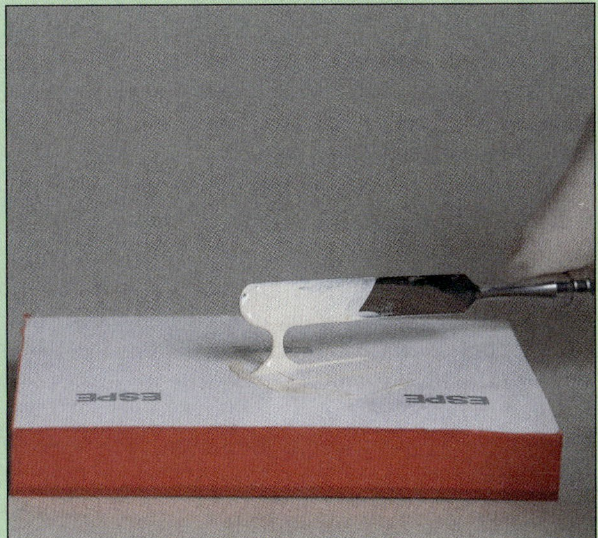

FIGURE 37-11
Consistency of ZOE temporary luting cement.

Procedure 37-3
Mixing Zinc-Oxide-Eugenol Cement—Two-Paste System

This material is often used for temporary luting of provisional coverage. The dental assistant dispenses and mixes the material according to the manufacturer's directions. The dental assistant assists the dentist during the placement of the temporary provisionals. Because sometimes the dental assistant places the cement for the provisional coverage of the tooth, this procedure is included in the expanded-function regulations.

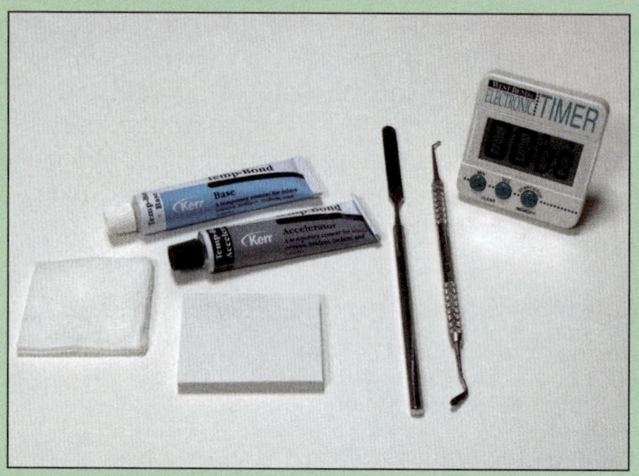

FIGURE 37-12
Tray setup for the zinc-oxide-eugenol cement two-paste system.

Equipment and Supplies (*Figure 37-12*)

- Two-paste zinc-oxide-eugenol (accelerator and base)
- Paper pad
- Cement spatula
- 2 × 2 inch gauze sponge (moistened)
- Plastic filling instrument

Procedure Steps (*Follow aseptic procedures*)

1. Dispense the amount of material required for the procedure. Equal lengths of the accelerator and the base are usually placed parallel to each other on the paper pad.
2. Gather the materials and mix into a homogeneous mass. Spread over a small area, and then gather. Repeat the process. The material should be a creamy mix that follows the spatula up for an inch (luting consistency).
3. Wipe both sides of the spatula, and then gather all the material into one area.
4. Wipe off the cement spatula with the moist 2 × 2 inch gauze sponge.

cement that had the ability to chemically bond to the tooth structure. There are several brands of polycarboxylate cement, and this cement comes both in a powder/liquid form and in capsules.

Composition. The powder of the polycarboxylate cement is similar to the zinc phosphate powder, with zinc oxide as the main component and a small amount of magnesium oxide. Some stannous fluoride is added to most polycarboxylates to improve its strength and reduce film thickness, not necessarily for anticarious effect. The liquid is what makes this cement different; it is a viscous solution of polyacrylic acid copolymer in water. The powder comes in a bottle with a specific dispenser, and the liquid comes in a squeeze bottle or a calibrated syringe. Polycarboxylate cement also comes in a capsule delivery system (Figures 37-13A and B).

Properties. Polycarboxylate cement sets in 3 to 5 minutes and does not exhibit exothermic heat. This material bonds chemically to the tooth structure and mechanically to the restoration. The strength of polycarboxylate is similar to reinforced ZOE and is less than zinc phosphate cement. The material may appear quite viscous, but it flows readily when applied to a surface. Polycarboxylate cement is much less irritating to the pulp, with reactions similar to 3 cement.

Polycarboxylate materials have a shelf life because of the water in the liquid. If the liquid discolors and becomes thick, it should be discarded.

Manipulation Properties. Polycarboxylate cements are mixed on a paper pad or a glass slab with a stainless steel cement spatula (Procedure 37-4). The powder is fluffed

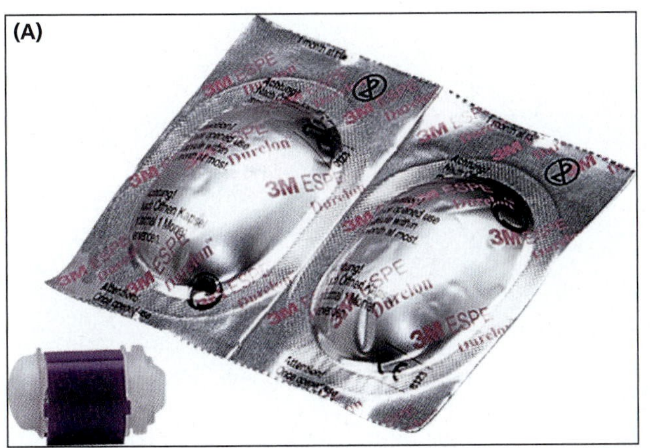

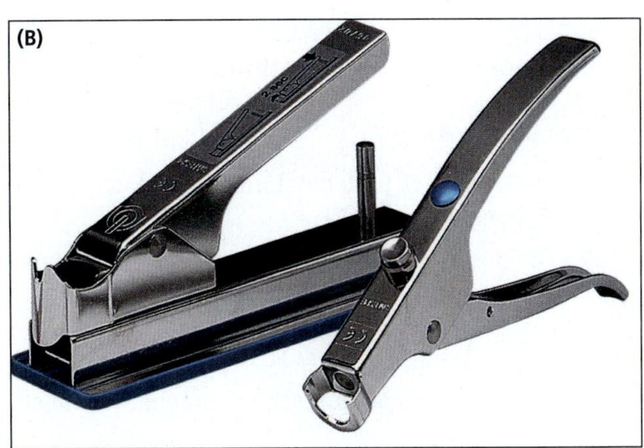

(A and B) Courtesy of 3M ESPE

FIGURE 37-13

(A) Polycarboxylate capsule and (B) activator/applier set.

before the dispenser is used. The viscous liquid is dispensed from a squeeze bottle or a calibrated syringe. The liquid bottle is held perpendicular to the pad or slab, and is squeezed until a drop begins to fall. The size of the drop varies because of this dispensing technique and the viscosity of the liquid. Using a syringe improves the accuracy of dispensing the liquid.

Polycarboxylate cements are mixed in 30 to 60 seconds and have a working time of about 3 minutes. The material loses its shine and becomes stringy, or forms cobwebs. At this point, the cement should not be used.

Glass Ionomer Cement

Glass ionomer cement is one of the most popular systems. The glass ionomer cements are a combination of the silicate and polycarboxylate cements. Their applications are very diverse and have been modified for many uses. Thus, there is

Procedure 37-4
Mixing Polycarboxylate Cement

The dental assistant prepares and mixes the polycarboxylate materials to the desired consistency. The amount of materials dispensed depends on the restoration size and the number of units involved.

Equipment and Supplies (*Figure 37-14*)

- Polycarboxylate powder and dispenser for powder
- Polycarboxylate liquid (in squeeze bottle or calibrated syringe)
- Paper pad or glass slab
- Flexible stainless steel spatula
- 2 × 2 inch gauze sponge (moistened)
- Timer
- Plastic filling instrument

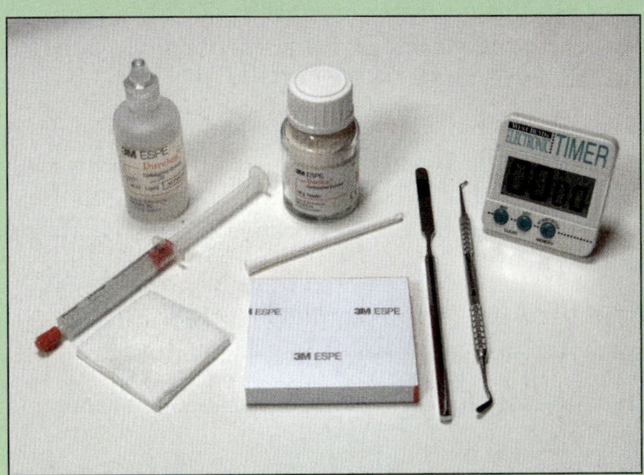

FIGURE 37-14

Mixing polycarboxylate cement tray setup (*Note:* liquid is shown in both dispenser bottle and calibrated syringe forms).

(continues)

Procedure 37-4 (continued)

Procedure Steps (*Follow aseptic procedures*)

1. The powder is fluffed before dispensing with the dispensing scoop.
2. The powder is measured and dispensed on one side of a paper pad or a glass slab.
3. Uniform drops of liquid are placed toward the opposite side of the powder. Follow the manufacturer's directions for the appropriate number of drops per scoop of powder.
4. Incorporate from three-fourths to all of the powder into the liquid, and use a folding motion while applying some pressure to wet all the powder. Mix the powder and liquid together quickly until all the powder is incorporated. Because the liquid is thick, it is harder to incorporate it into the powder.
5. The mix will be glossy and slightly more viscous than zinc phosphate cement. Gather all the cement, wiping both sides of the spatula.
6. For luting consistency, the mix should follow the spatula up 1 inch.
7. For a base consistency, the same amount of powder is used, but the liquid ratio is decreased. The mix for the base should be glossy, but the consistency is tacky and stiff.

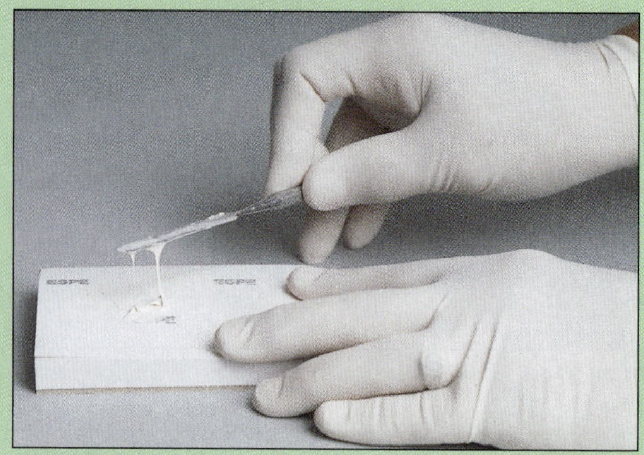

FIGURE 37-15
When cement is mixed for too long, the mix becomes thick and cobwebs form.

8. The mix must be used immediately before it becomes dull and stringy, and forms cobwebs (Figure 37-15).
9. The cleanup is done immediately by wiping the spatula with a wet 2 × 2 inch gauze, or by soaking the spatula with the dried cement in a 10 percent sodium hydroxide solution. The paper pad sheet is removed, folded, and disposed of. Fold the paper pad to prevent touching the cement and spreading it onto instruments and the patient's face.

more than one type of glass ionomer material. Some of which are listed as follows:

- Type I—a fine-grain glass ionomer is used for the cementation of crowns and bridges because it chemically bonds to the tooth structure.
- Type II—a coarser-grain glass ionomer available in various shades for use in selected restorations, such as Class III and V, and pediatric restorations (discussed in Chapter 38, Restorative Materials, Matrix and Wedge).
- Type III—a liner and dentin bonding agent.
- Type IV—pit and fissure sealants.
- Type V—used for the bonding of orthodontic bands and brackets.
- Type VI—silver or amalgam fillings are combined with glass ionomer material and are used for crown and core buildups.
- Type IX—designed to be used for some posterior restorations, especially for children.

Glass ionomer cements are available in powder/liquid, paste systems, syringes, and premeasured capsule forms. The glass ionomers come in self-curing, light-curing, and dual-curing materials (Figure 37-16).

Composition. Glass ionomer powder is a silicate glass powder containing calcium, aluminum, and fluoride (calcium-fluoroaluminosilicate glass). The liquid is an aqueous solution

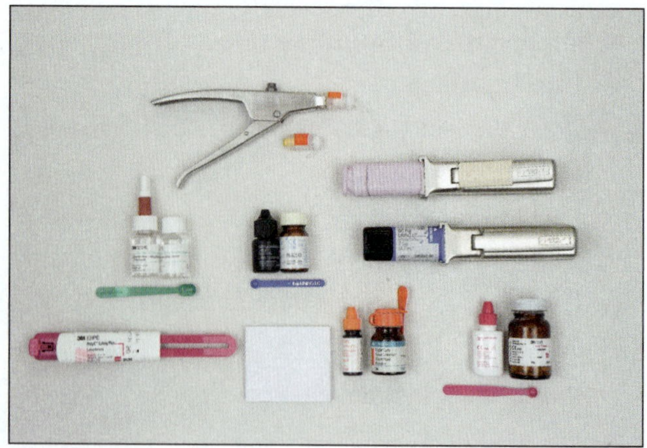

FIGURE 37-16
Various brands of glass ionomer cements.

(i.e., the solution contains water) of polyacrylic acid. The water is important for the setting of the cement, therefore do not dispense it until just before mixing.

Properties. Glass ionomer material is strong enough to act as a supportive base and is similar to zinc phosphate cement in strength. It mechanically and chemically bonds to the enamel, dentin, and metallic materials, and releases fluoride ions, which prevent secondary decay by strengthening the tooth structure. Glass ionomer cement has low solubility in the mouth. Glass ionomers have nonirritating qualities similar to polycarboxylate cements. They, therefore, will be tolerated by the pulp and are free from phosphoric acid. The complete setting reaction of glass ionomers takes up to 24 hours. After it is set, the cement has reached its maximum strength and resistance to the oral cavity environment.

Manipulation Considerations. It is important to read the manufacturer's instructions. Mixing and setting times will vary by manufacturer, and the type of glass ionomer. Glass ionomer cements are mixed on a paper pad or a cool glass slab (Procedure 37-5). The paper pads are preferred for easy cleanup, but glass slabs may be used to retard the setting action. Because of the water content, the materials should be mixed quickly, following the manufacturer's directions. Water evaporation affects the properties of the cement.

Although many properties of the glass ionomers are the same as those of the polycarboxylate cements, the liquid of the glass ionomers is not as viscous (thin film thickness), and is, therefore, easier to dispense and mix. The powder is dispensed first, using the scoop and the amount indicated in the manufacturer's instructions, and the liquid is dispensed just prior to manipulation. Mixing time is usually 30 to 60 seconds, and working time for the material is about 2 minutes.

The tooth is isolated, cleaned, and dried before the cement is placed. The tooth does not have to be completely dry because this cement sticks to a slightly moist tooth surface. The glass ionomer cement sets in the mouth in about 5 minutes. The excess cement is allowed to stay on the margins until the cement is set. Then an explorer or excavator is used to remove the excess cement. This is different than polycarboxylate cement, which is removed before it is set.

Procedure 37-5
Mixing Glass Ionomer Cement

This procedure is completed by the dental assistant. The equipment and materials are prepared and mixed when the dentist indicates. The material must be used immediately after it is mixed. This material requires that the tooth be clean of debris and dry, so the dental assistant should rinse and evacuate, and then isolate the area before beginning to mix the cement.

Equipment and Supplies (*Figure 37-17*)

- Glass ionomer materials and appropriate dispensers
- Paper pad or cool glass slab
- Flexible stainless steel spatula
- 2 × 2 inch gauze sponges (moistened)
- Timer
- Plastic filling instrument

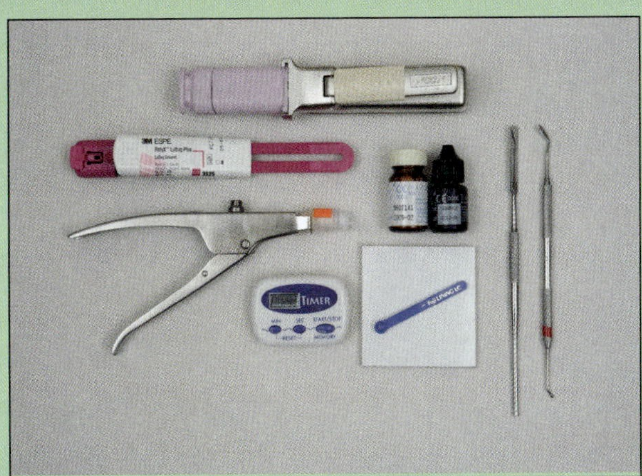

FIGURE 37-17
Tray setup for mixing the glass ionomer cement.

Procedure Steps (*Follow aseptic procedures*)

1. Fluff the powder and, using the recommended scoops, place the appropriate number of scoops on the paper pad or glass slab.
2. Swirl the liquid and then place the specified number of drops on the pad near the powder. Replace the cap on the liquid immediately to prevent evaporation (Figures 37-18A and B).
3. Divide the powder into halves or thirds, and then draw the sections into the liquid one at a time.

(continues)

Procedure 37-5 (continued)

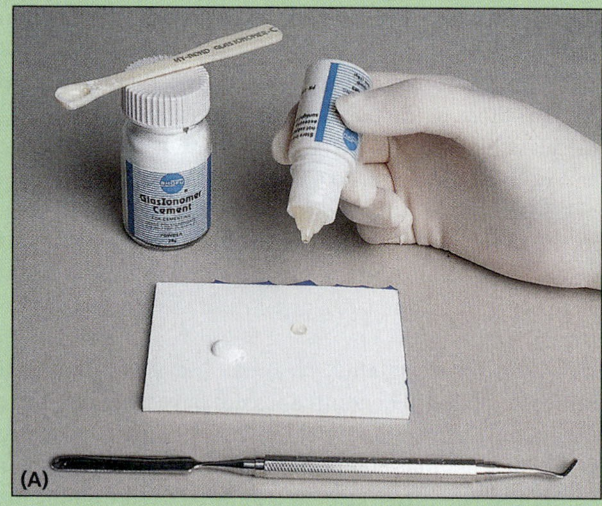

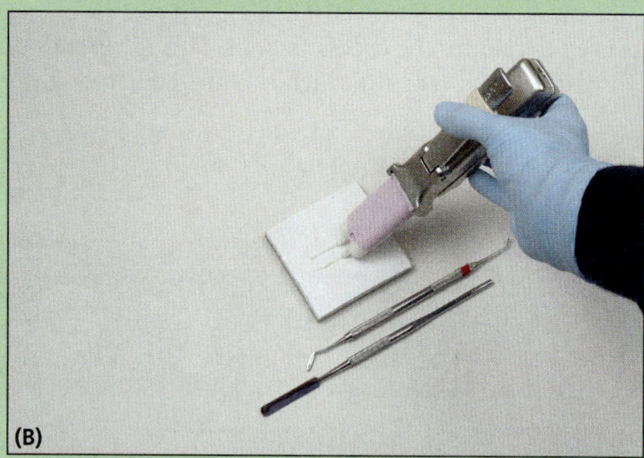

FIGURE 37-18

(A) Dispensed glass ionomer powder and liquid. (B) Dispensed glass ionomer using the syringe material.

4. Mix over a small area until all the powder is incorporated. The cement should be creamy and glossy for the luting consistency, and tacky and stiff for the base consistency.
5. Once the cement has obtained the final consistency, wipe off the spatula with a 2 × 2 inch gauze. Hold the paper or glass slab under the patient's chin and pass the plastic filling instrument to the dentist.
6. To clean up, remove the top paper, fold it, and dispose of it. The instruments are wiped after use for easier cleanup.
7. Glass ionomer capsules are also available. They are activated by placement in an activator or dispenser to break the seal between the powder and liquid in the capsule.
8. The capsules are then placed in an amalgamator to be mixed (triturated) for a specific amount of time, usually 10 seconds. Follow the manufacturer's directions.
9. Insert the capsule in the appropriate dispenser and pass it to the dentist for dispensing the material needed.
10. To clean up, the capsule is discarded, and the activator and dispenser are disinfected.

Resin-Modified Glass Ionomer Cement

The composition of the **resin-modified (reinforced) glass ionomer** cement is modified to include a light-curing resin component in addition to the traditional glass ionomer setting reactions. The material is supplied in protective containers because both components are light sensitive. Resin-modified glass ionomer cements are stronger, more water insoluble, and more adhesive to tooth structures than conventional glass ionomer cement (Figure 37-19). Resin-modified glass ionomer cement comes in a variety of forms including powder/liquid form and capsules. Like glass ionomer cement, the resin-modified glass ionomer cement releases fluoride to protect the enamel against decalcification and demineralization.

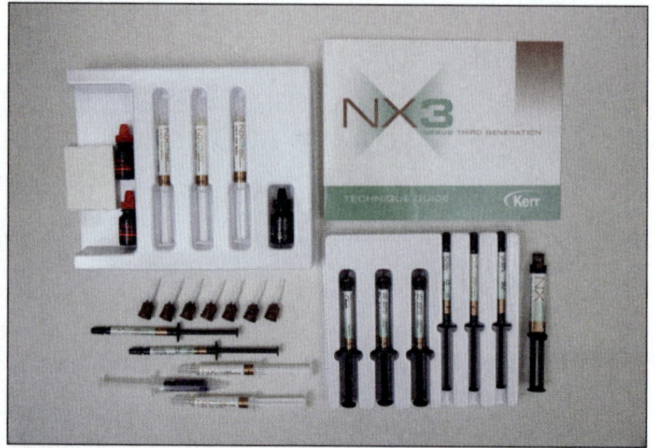

FIGURE 37-19

Resin-modified glass ionomer materials.

Calcium Hydroxide Material

Calcium hydroxide cement is used as a low-strength base or liner under any restoration, such as in indirect or direct pulp capping procedures (near or direct pulp exposures). This material has a therapeutic effect on the pulp; the area is sealed so that secondary dentin may form. Calcium hydroxide is not necessary to form secondary dentin, but its slightly irritating effect provides the mild irritant that encourages secondary dentin to form. Also, calcium hydroxide has antibacterial properties that keep bacteria from actively spreading.

Calcium hydroxide comes in a powder/liquid form, a two-paste system, or a one-paste system. The form many offices use is the two-paste system: catalyst and base. Calcium hydroxide comes in a self-curing and a light-curing formula (Figure 37-20).

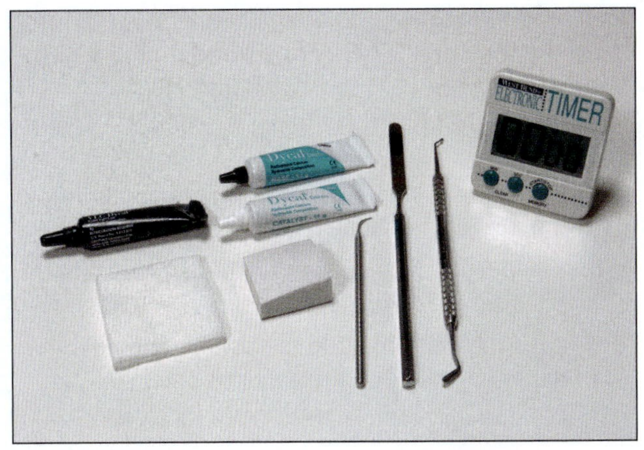

FIGURE 37-20

Various forms of calcium hydroxide, including the light-cured material (in the dark tube), and the two-paste materials.

Composition. Calcium hydroxide has a complicated formula, with several ingredients in addition to calcium hydroxide. The light-cured calcium hydroxide formula also contains a polymer resin.

Properties. Calcium hydroxide is low in strength and is placed in a thin layer near or over the pulp. It is easy to mix and place. The cement has low thermal conductivity, but is usually not used in a thick enough layer to provide thermal protection. An insulating base is often placed over the thin layer of calcium hydroxide.

Manipulation Considerations. The two-paste system is mixed on a small paper pad with a metal spatula, an explorer, or a small ball-ended instrument (Procedure 37-6). The base and the catalyst of the two-paste system come as a set and cannot be interchanged with those of other calcium hydroxide paste systems.

This material is dispensed in equal portions and mixed for about 10 to 15 seconds. Setting times vary from 2 to 7 minutes.

Procedure 37-6

Mixing Calcium Hydroxide Cement—Two-Paste System

This material is dispensed and mixed by the dental assistant. It is often the first step in restoring (filling) the cavity preparation.

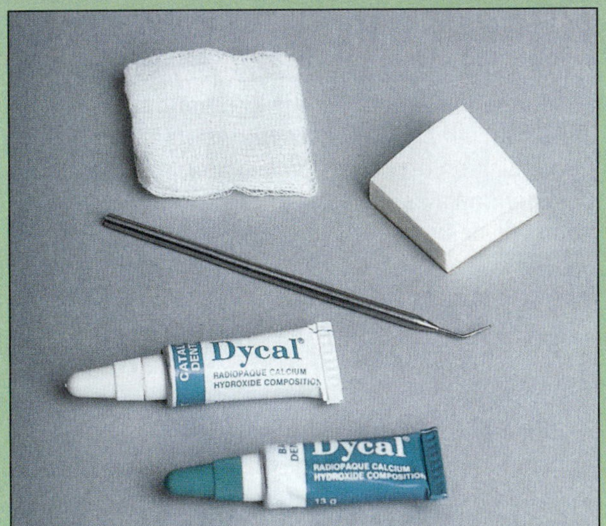

FIGURE 37-21

A two-paste calcium hydroxide tray setup.

Equipment and Supplies (*Figure 37-21*)

- Calcium hydroxide two-paste system
- Small paper pad
- Small ball-ended instrument or explorer
- 2 × 2 inch gauze sponge

Procedure Steps (*Follow aseptic procedures*)

1. Dispense small and equal amounts of both the catalyst and the base onto the paper pad.
2. Wipe off the ends of the tubes and replace the caps.

(continues)

Procedure 37-6 (continued)

3. Mix the two materials together using a circular motion.
4. Mix until the materials are a uniform color within the 10- to 15-second mixing time.
5. Use a 2 × 2 inch gauze to remove excess material from the mixing instrument.
6. Pass the instrument to the dentist and hold the paper pad close to the patient's chin.
7. Between applications, wipe off the instrument with gauze for the dentist.
8. Receive the instrument and wipe it off, and then tear and fold the top page of the paper pad and dispose of it.

Cavity Varnish

A **cavity varnish** is a material used to seal the dentin tubules that are exposed during an amalgam cavity preparation. This thin liquid is placed on the surface of the dentin only. There are various types of varnish, and some come with solvents.

Composition. Cavity varnishes are resin solutions of different compositions. The **copal varnish** contains organic solvents (ether, acetone, or chloroform) and is used only under metal restorations because the solvent material in the varnish may interfere with the setting action of composite and resins. A **universal varnish** does not have organic solvents and may be used under all restorations.

Properties

Varnishes are placed in a thin layer over the dentin tubules. The varnishes do not exhibit any strength and do not provide any thermal insulation. Cavity varnishes are insoluble in oral fluids, and reduce leakage around the margins of restorations, thereby preventing microleakage. Varnish also prevents the penetration of acids from some cements into the dentin. These materials are nonacidic and nonirritating.

Manipulation Properties. Cavity varnishes are often placed in two layers for greater protection, and to prevent voids. Recap the varnish immediately to minimize its evaporation. The cavity varnish comes with a separate bottle of solvent. If the varnish becomes too thick, solvent can be added. The solvent can also be used to clean the applicator and to remove any varnish on the external tooth surfaces.

Cavity varnish is not mixed; it is placed over the liner, or it is placed directly on the tooth with various types of applicators, such as small cotton pellets or brushes (Procedure 37-7).

Fluoride Varnish

Fluoride varnish is used to prevent dental decay. It is also a cavity varnish and desensitizer. This natural resin contains fluoride, which is slowly released once applied to the tooth surface. It

Procedure 37-7
Preparing a Cavity Varnish

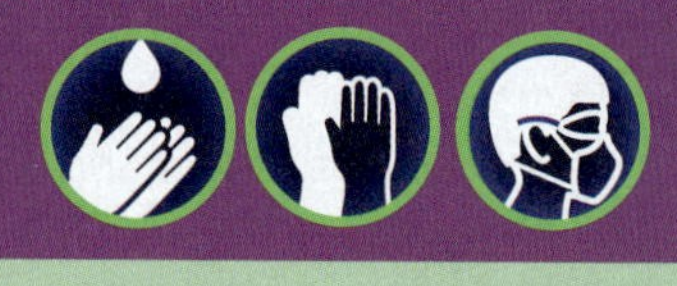

The materials needed for the application of a cavity varnish are prepared by the dental assistant. Depending on expanded-function laws, the dental assistant applies the varnish or assists the dentist during placement.

Equipment and Supplies (*Figure 37-22*)

- Cavity varnish and solvent
- Two cotton pliers
- Small brushes or cotton-tipped applicators. Some dentists may use cotton pellets or pieces of cotton rolled into small, football-shaped balls.
- Cotton roll

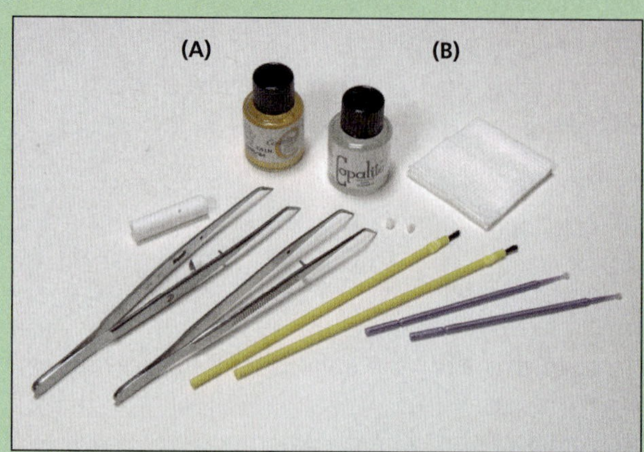

FIGURE 37-22

(A) Varnish and (B) solvent with materials needed for placement. Cotton pellets and cotton pliers, as well as microbrushes and applicator tips, are used for placement.

(continues)

Procedure 37-7 (continued)

Procedure Steps (*Follow aseptic procedures*)

1. Clean and dry the cavity preparation.
2. Prepare small brushes, cotton-tipped applicators, or cotton pellets for the application of two layers of varnish. The pellets must be small in order to apply the varnish on the dentin surface.
3. Remove the cap from the varnish bottle. Place the small brushes or applicators in the varnish, or, while holding two cotton pellets in a pair of pliers, dip them into the varnish until they are moistened. Then replace the cap on the varnish.
4. Place the brushes, applicators, or cotton pellets on a 2 × 2 inch gauze and dab off the excess varnish.
5. Using one brush, applicator or pellet, apply the varnish to the cavity preparation. Coat the surface of the preparation.
6. Allow the first coat to dry, and then apply a second coat in the same manner with the second brush, applicator, or cotton pellet. Prepare the cotton pellets one at a time—two separate cotton pliers must be used to avoid contamination.
7. Dispose of the brushes, applicators, or cotton pellets and, if used, clean the cotton pliers with solvent before sterilizing them.

is painted on the teeth and then sets on contact with the salvia (Figure 37-23). The patient can feel the varnish on the teeth for a while but it slowly seeps into the tooth structure and wears away. Refer to Chapter 4, Oral Health and Preventive Techniques, and Chapter 8, Pediatric Dentistry, for more information.

Composite Resin Cement

Composite resin cement has multiple uses for a wide variety of procedures, including permanent cementation of cast metal–based restorations, porcelain/resin restorations and veneers, orthodontic bands and brackets, and endodontic posts. Resin cements may be supplied in a two-paste system, powder/liquid set, or syringe. The manufacturer may supply **etchant** gel or liquid (refer to "Etchants" later in the chapter) with the material. Some of these materials may be shaded to complement the translucency of the crown or inlay.

There are three types of resin cements: self-curing (chemical), light cured, and dual cured. Dual-cured materials contain chemicals for a self-curing as well as a light-curing reaction. The self-cured materials are used with metal or metal combination materials and endodontic posts; the light-curing materials are used with porcelain/resin restorations, veneers, and orthodontic brackets.

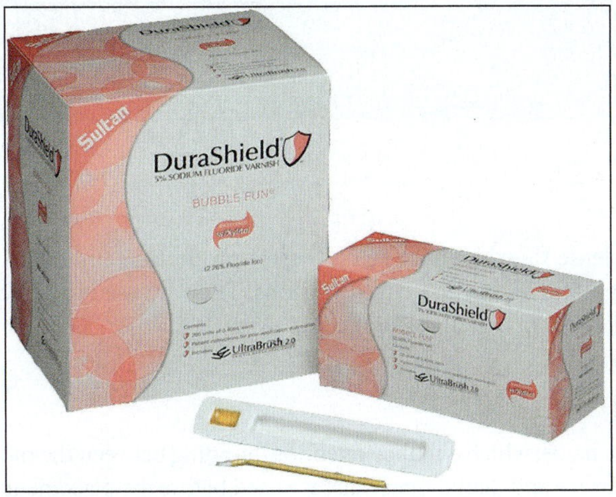

Courtesy of Sultan Healthcare

FIGURE 37-23
Fluoride varnish with disposable brush.

Composition. The resin cements are similar to composites in composition. Variation comes with individual products adjusted for different functions. The resin matrices are BIS-GMA (bisphenol A-glycidyl methacrylate) or dimethacrylate resin diluted with low-viscosity monomers. The resin cements are more fluid than direct filling composites because the amount of filler particles is reduced to create low viscosities for cementation purposes.

Properties. Most resin cements are radiopaque, and exhibit adequate strength and wear resistance for luting. These materials are insoluble in oral fluids but are irritating to the pulp; thus, protective cement is required. Some of the products contain fluoride.

Manipulation Considerations. With resin cements, the tooth must be cleaned to be free of plaque and debris before the cementing process can begin. Resin cements do not adhere directly to metal or ceramic materials. These materials must be roughened with etchants to produce mechanical bonding; or, alternatively, the tissue surfaces of the ceramics are treated with a silane-coupling agent to produce a chemical bond with the resin cements. Sometimes, a wire mesh or undercuts may be added to the tissue side of the prosthesis to aid in retention.

Self-cured materials come with an initiator and an activator. These are mixed on a paper pad for 20 to 30 seconds. Excess cement must be removed before the material is set completely to prevent any marginal leakage. Light-cured materials come in syringes and must be cured for at least 40 seconds. Dual-cured materials come in two component systems that are mixed together for 20 to 30 seconds. Once mixed,

Procedure 37-8
Placing Composite Resin Cement—Dual-Curing Technique

This procedure is performed by the dental assistant for the dentist. The equipment and materials are prepared, and the material is mixed and passed to the dentist. Because this material is dual curing, a curing light and eye protection are needed.

Equipment and Supplies (*Figures 37-24A and B*)

- Resin cement system
- Paper pad
- Stainless steel spatula
- Plastic filling instrument
- Curing light and protective shield or glasses
- 2 × 2 inch gauze sponges

Procedure Steps (*Follow aseptic procedures*)

1. Clean and dry the tooth and isolate the area with cotton rolls.
2. Pass the etchant to the dentist.
3. Wait the required time for the etchant and rinse the tooth thoroughly.
4. Lightly air dry the tooth and apply the adhesive.
5. Dispense and mix the two components together into a homogeneous, creamy mixture.
6. Hold the pad close to the patient and pass the placement instrument. The dentist places the material on the tooth and restoration.
7. Hold 2 × 2 inch gauze to remove any excess materials.
8. Receive the placement instrument and prepare the curing light.
9. Either the dental assistant or the dentist holds the curing light and uses the protective shield when the light is activated.
10. Clean up immediately. Wipe any excess cement off the instruments and discard disposable items.

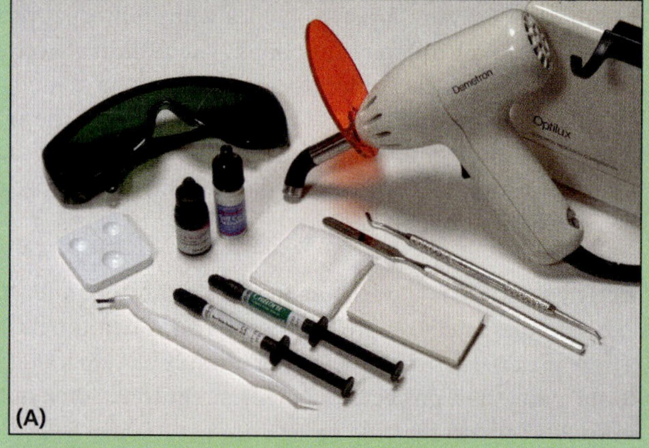

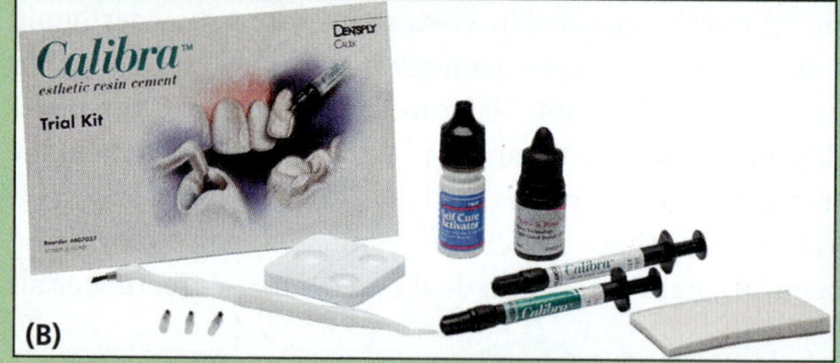

FIGURE 37-24
(A) Resin cement tray setup. (B) Resin cement system.

these materials begin to set slowly, allowing for the placement of the cement on the prosthesis, and the prosthesis to be seated into the oral cavity. Once in position, the visible light unit is activated to harden the cement (Procedure 37-8).

Compomer Cement

Compomer cements are basically polyacid-modified composites. They are like composites and do not contain water, and have properties similar to resin cements. The compomers release fluoride, have self-adhesive properties, and come in light-cured and self-cured versions. They are used to cement all types of dental restorations.

Etchants

Etchants, which enhance retention/bonding between the tooth surface and dental materials, are used before the placement of bonding agents, restorative materials, dental cements, and pit and fissure sealants. Etching products are typically comprised

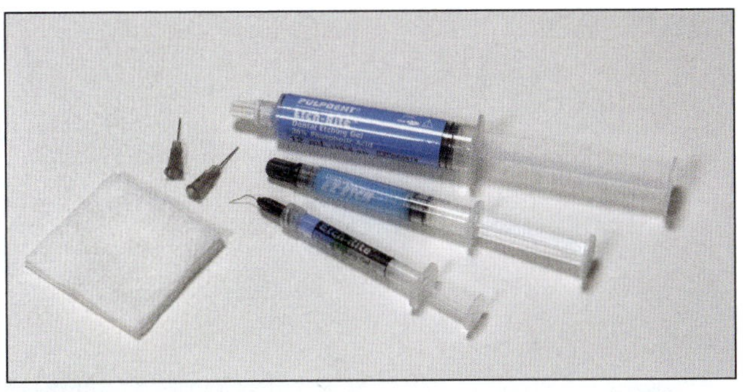

FIGURE 37-25
Various types of etchant materials.

of a 30 to 40 percent phosphoric acid solution. The etchant comes in liquid or gel form and is packaged in bottles or syringes. Liquids are placed with microbrushes or small cotton pellets. Gel etchants placed with a syringe tip are the most common. Gels are packaged with a number of disposable tips (Figure 37-25).

Etchants are used both on enamel and dentin tooth surfaces and are tinted for more accurate placement. The etchant is usually left on for 30 to 60 seconds and rinsed thoroughly (Procedure 37-9). For more information on etchants refer to Chapter 30, Dental Sealants.

Procedure 37-9
Placing the Etchant

The dental assistant prepares the materials and isolates the area. The dentist places the etchant. When the allotted time has passed, the dental assistant thoroughly rinses the tooth.

Equipment and Supplies (*Figure 37-26*)

- Acid etchant, usually a 30 to 40 percent phosphoric acid solution
- Isolation materials (rubber dam or cotton rolls)
- Applicator (syringe, cotton pellets, or small applicator tips)
- Dappen dish
- Air–water syringe
- Timer

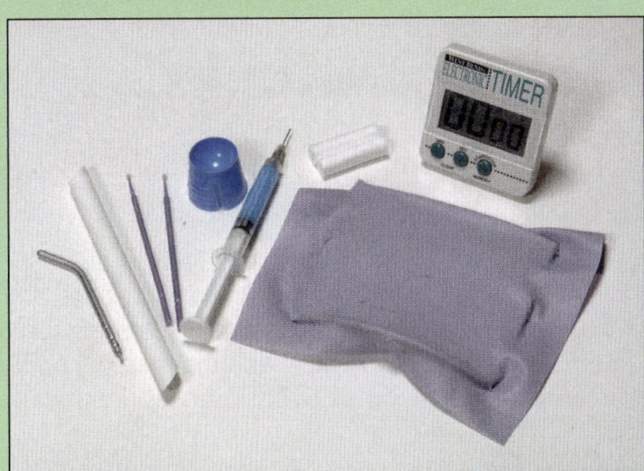

FIGURE 37-26
Tray setup for placing the etchant materials.

Procedure Steps (*Follow aseptic procedures*)

1. Isolate the area.
2. Clean the surface thoroughly.
3. Prepare the etchant applicator or syringe.
4. Place the etchant on the surface for 15 to 30 seconds, depending on the manufacturer's directions.
5. Rinse the tooth after the designated time for 15 to 20 seconds with the air–water syringe, and evacuate thoroughly for 10 to 20 seconds.

NOTE: The etched surface will have a frosty appearance. This surface needs to be isolated until the cementation is complete. If saliva or other fluids contact the surface, the etching process must be repeated.

Bonding Agents

Bonding agents are also known as **adhesives** or **bonding resins**. These materials are used to improve the retention between the tooth structure (enamel and dentin) and the restoration. These materials come in many forms and are often complete systems (Figure 37-27). These materials bond enamel and dentin to porcelain, resins, precious and nonprecious metals, composites, and amalgam.

Bonding materials are low-viscosity resins that may or may not contain fillers. Some of the bonding agents contain additives with adhesive enhancers, and some contain fluoride. These materials are mainly light cured or dual cured. Procedure 37-10 outlines the steps for placing a bonding agent.

Enamel Bonding

Adhesion of dental materials to enamel is accomplished by etching with phosphoric acid. This solution alters the surface of the enamel and creates microscopic undercuts between the enamel rods (Figure 37-28). Low-viscosity, unfilled resin bonding agents then penetrate into these undercuts and mechanically lock into them.

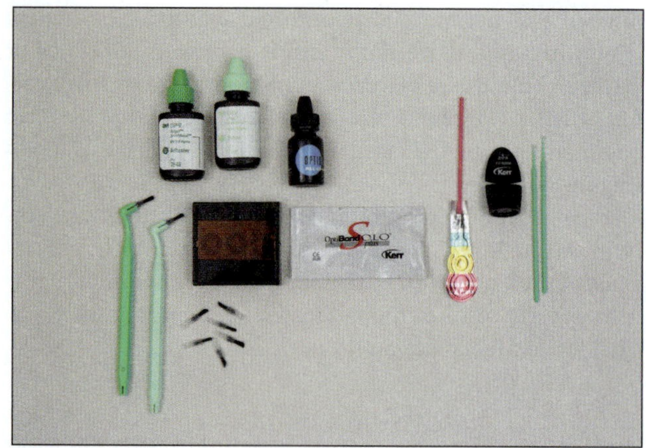

FIGURE 37-27
Bonding agents and systems.

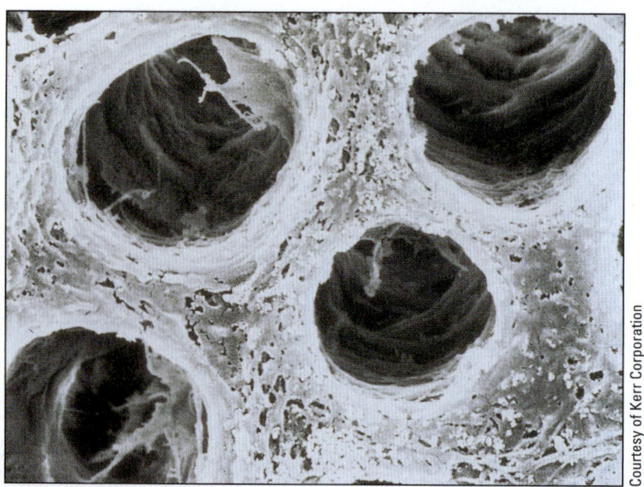

Courtesy of Kerr Corporation

FIGURE 37-28
Microscopic view of etched dentin.

Procedure 37-10
Placing the Bonding Agent

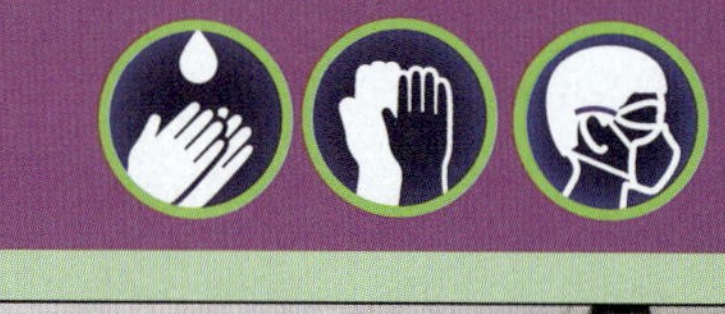

Steps in the application of bonding agents vary by manufacturer, so follow the directions that come with the product. The dental assistant prepares the materials for each step and keeps the area dry and free of debris (sometimes cavity cleaners are used).

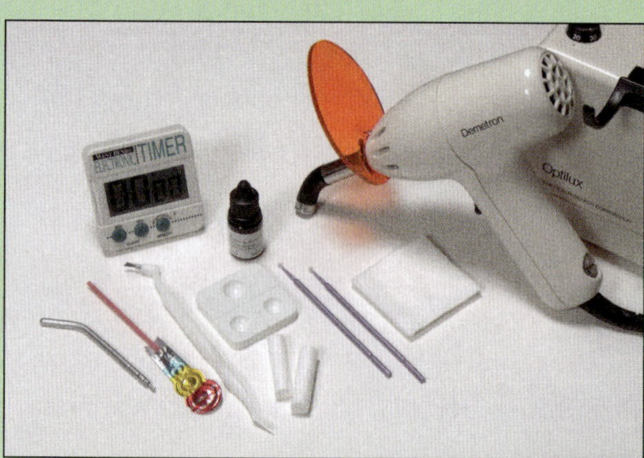

FIGURE 37-29
Tray setup and materials for placing bonding agents.

Equipment and Supplies (*Figure 37-29*)

- Bonding system that contains acid etchant, primer or conditioner, and adhesive material
- Applicators (disposable tips or brushes)
- Dappen dish
- Isolation means
- Air–water syringe
- Curing light and shield
- Timer

Procedure Steps (*Follow aseptic procedures*)

1. If the cavity preparation is near the pulp, place calcium hydroxide or glass ionomer lining cement over the area.
2. The etchant is placed on the enamel and the dentin for the specified amount of time, usually 15 to 20 seconds. Usually, the etchant is placed on the enamel first, and then the dentin, because the dentin is more sensitive to the etchant.
3. Rinse the tooth as soon as the time is up. Continue to rinse for at least 5 to 10 seconds. Move quickly to prevent bacterial contamination of the dentin.
4. If the bonding involves both the enamel and the dentin, a primer step is included. The primer or conditioner is placed with a brush or an applicator. This material wets the dentin and penetrates the dentin tubules.
5. The bonding resin is then applied, and the curing light is used to harden the material.
6. Cleanup involves the disposal of the applicator tips or brushes.

The restorative material then bonds to this layer and becomes a solid unit. Bonding to enamel is required before placement of composite restorations, pit and fissure sealants, veneers, resin-cemented crowns and bridges, and orthodontic brackets.

Dentin Bonding

Dentin bonding is more challenging than enamel bonding. Some of the obstacles are listed as follows:

- Dentin has a high water content, which can interfere with the bonding to the tooth.
- The composition of the dentin is more organic than inorganic.
- However, the dentin must maintain a small amount of moisture to prevent **desiccating**, or drying out the tooth. If this happens the structure of the tooth could be damaged.
- Dentin is directly above the pulp, so the operator must take care not to injure the pulp.
- When the dentin is cut with a bur during cavity preparation, it forms a **smear layer**. This layer of debris lies on the cavity floor and walls and prevents contact between the intact dentin and the bonding agent or adhesive.

Current dentin bonding materials use an etchant to remove the smear layer, because the smear layer is not attached firmly and is unreliable. When the smear layer is removed, the adhesives achieve a mechanical bond with the dentin. Many of the bonding agents are suitable for both enamel and dentin surfaces because of the etchant application.

Restorative Dentistry

Restorative dentistry, also known as operative dentistry, involves various materials and techniques. There are many reasons a tooth needs to be restored, including decay, fracture, abrasion, esthetics, and attrition. Restorative materials such as amalgam and composites are used to restore the tooth. These materials are called direct restorative materials because they are mixed and then placed directly in the cavity preparation in a single appointment.

Reasons for restoring teeth include the following:

- Arresting the loss of the tooth structure. Stopping the decay process early allows the preparation to be conservative, and small restorations to be stronger.
- Preventing the recurrence of decay by placing margins that can be reached easily for cleaning. This is known as *extension for prevention.*
- Restoring the contour of the tooth (shape and design of crown). The proper contour prevents food impaction and gingival irritation.
- Restoring the function of the tooth, and establishing occlusion with opposing teeth for the mastication of food.
- Restoring or improving the appearance of the teeth.

Classification

Dental caries are classified to simplify examination, charting, diagnosis, and patient communication. There are several ways to classify cavities and restorations (see Chapter 14, Dental Charting). One method used is Black's, which identifies areas of decay according to the surfaces they are located on, such as Class I for occlusal caries on the posterior teeth, and Class III for dental caries on the mesial or distal sides of the anterior teeth, where the incisal edge is not involved. Another classification is based on the number of surfaces involved, such as simple, compound, and complex. A third method of classifying dental caries is based on whether the caries are pit and fissure areas, or smooth surface areas.

Cavity Detection

The dentist is able to diagnose tooth decay through a variety of **cavity detection methods**. Cavities can be detected with radiographs, by probing with an explorer, or with the use of a special dye. This dye detects caries by distinguishing between good, sound, hard dentin and dentin that is infected with bacteria and softened. The dye is placed in the preparation early in the procedure to avoid removing too much tooth structure. The dye is applied for about 10 seconds and then rinsed off. Burs and spoon excavators usually remove all the stained dentin. This process is repeated until no caries remain. This material can also be used to identify cracks and root canals.

Caries are also detected via manual probing with an explorer and through radiographs. Another noninvasive diagnostic tool, called the **DIAGNOdent caries detection**, is a Class II laser that measures fluorescence levels in the tooth structure to quantify caries progression. The DIAGNOdent comes in a battery-operated, microprocessor-controlled display unit with handpiece and tips, or a handheld pen unit for easier handling and greater mobility. Several tips are packaged with the units, and the tips can be sterilized (Figures 37-30A and B). Altered tooth structures and bacteria fluoresce (give off light) when exposed to specific wavelengths of light. A clean, healthy tooth structure exhibits little or no fluorescence, while a tooth with decay fluoresces according to the extent of the caries. Thus, healthy teeth register a low reading, while teeth with decay register higher readings. Laser units may also emit audio signals, which allow the dentist to hear as well as see display changes.

Benefits of using a laser caries detection unit include the following:

- Accurate diagnosis of tooth decay
- Simple, fast, and painless
- Quantification of caries over time
- Early detection of caries
- Can be used by hygienist to detect suspicious areas requiring further examination
- Provides accurate visual and audio representation of the measured tooth structure

Cavity Cleaners/Disinfectants

Cavity cleaners/disinfectants can be used in the cavity preparation. As with any body wound, the cavity should be cleaned and disinfected to reduce the growth of bacteria under restorations, which can lead to sensitivity. This step is completed before the tooth is etched.

(A)

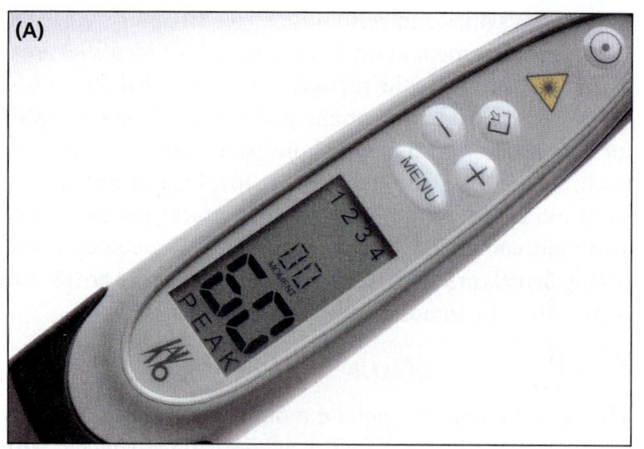

(B)

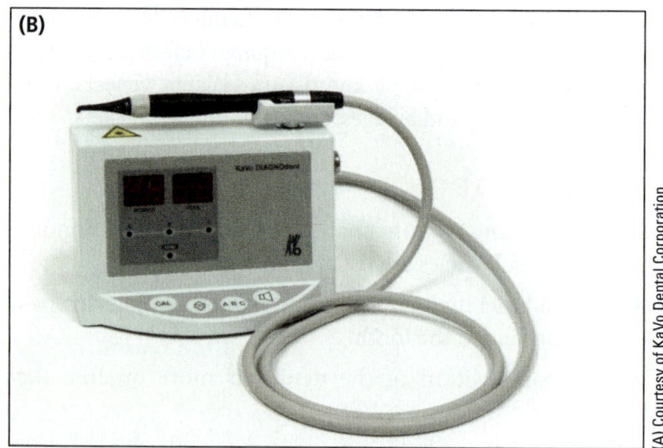

(A) Courtesy of KaVo Dental Corporation

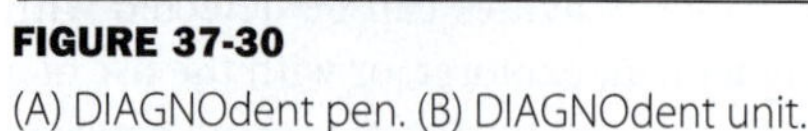

FIGURE 37-30
(A) DIAGNOdent pen. (B) DIAGNOdent unit.

How to Use the KaVo DIAGNOdent pen

1. Clean tooth surfaces, preferably with an air-polishing device (e.g., PROPHYflex), to remove plaque, stains, and calculus from fissure areas.
2. Dry the tooth.
3. Perform a clinical examination (scanning of tooth surface).
4. Diagnose and evaluate the quantitative measurements from the DIAGNOdent pen. Possible courses of action include the following:
    - Chart readings and monitor over time.
    - Initiate prophylactic treatment (fluoridation, etc.) and monitor the success/results.
    - Restore and check for residual caries.

Therapy Information According to the KaVo DIAGNOdent Pen

Display value	Therapy
0–14	No special measures
15–20	Usual prophylactic measures
21–30	More intensive prophylaxis or restoration, indication is dependent on: • Caries activity • Caries risk • Recall interval, and so on
≥30	Restoration and more intensive prophylaxis

Desensitizers

A **desensitizer** is used to treat or prevent hypersensitivity in the teeth. They are sometimes called *primers*. Hypersensitivity can be caused by cold, heat, or contact. In some procedures, etchants are used to increase bonding/retention of the tooth surface and restorative materials. The etchant opens and exposes dentin tubules, which sometimes cause hypersensitivity. In addition, patients who use certain whitening agents need to be treated with a desensitizer to reduce tooth sensitivity. Desensitizers can be used under all types of restorations, bonding agents, temporary fillings, and permanent cement. Some can also be used to desensitize an exposed root surface.

Desensitizers contain hydroxyethyl methacrylate (HEMA) and glutaraldehyde; because of this, soft tissues should be protected, as well as the skin. Use these materials sparingly with an appropriately sized applicator. Many types of desensitizers are available, some of which contain fluoride, while others contain antimicrobial additives that remove residual bacteria from the tooth surface.

Desensitizers are available in liquid or gel form, or in a dispensing syringe, and are placed with an applicator brush or syringe tip (Figure 37-31). A few of the materials are tinted to show where they have been placed, and that they have been completely rinsed off after application and drying. Some are single-dose, or, cartridges. These materials may be self-curing or light curing (Procedure 37-11). Some desensitizers require isolation before placement, usually cotton rolls or dental dam materials are used.

Cavity Preparation and Identification

Once the tooth is prepared, there are terms used to describe the inside of the cavity preparation. Knowledge of these terms helps the dental assistant to communicate better with the dentist, and also understand the details of the cavity preparation.

The preparation of the tooth forms walls, lines, and angles. A wall is the side or floor of the cavity preparation. The wall is named according to the surface of the tooth it is nearest to, such as the buccal wall or distal wall. The internal wall that runs parallel to the long axis of the tooth is the **axial wall**. The wall that overlies the pulp is the **pulpal wall** or floor. The wall

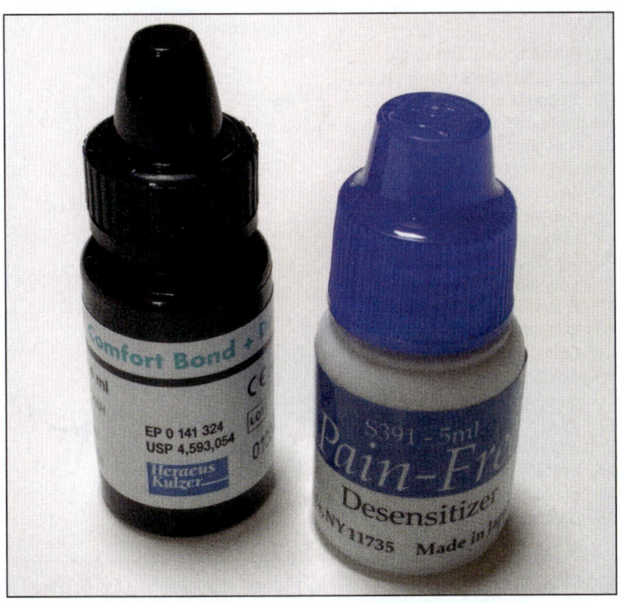

FIGURE 37-31

Desensitizers.

nearest the gingiva that is perpendicular to the long axis of the tooth is the **gingival wall**.

Lines are formed when two surfaces meet and form a **line angle**. The line angles are named according to the two surfaces, such as the distopulpal line angle or the axiogingival line angle (Figure 37-32). Note that the names of the two surfaces are usually joined with an "o" between the words. At the corners of the cavity preparation, three lines (surfaces) come together to form **point angles**. The point angles are named by joining the names of the walls, such as the mesiolinguopulpal point angle or the distobuccopulpal point angle (Figure 37-33).

The **cavosurface margin** is the angle that is formed by the junction of the wall of the preparation and the untouched surface of the tooth (Figure 37-34). The sealing of this margin is critical to prevent marginal leakage. Sometimes, this margin is beveled (slanted) during the preparation.

Elements of Cavity Preparations

The cavity preparation is a systematic cutting of the tooth structure that depends on the location of the decay, the extent of the decay, the amount of lost tooth structure, and the type of restorative material to be used. When the dentist prepares the cavity, some basic considerations are followed. Understanding these steps helps the dental assistant to know what is coming next so that he or she can be prepared to change burs, rinse and evacuate the oral cavity, mix materials, and so on. It also keeps the focus on the preparation, and the dental assistant more involved in the procedure.

Procedure 37-11
Placing a Desensitizing Agent

This procedure is performed by the dentist or expanded-function dental assistant. Preparation of the cavity has been completed, and this procedure is part of the cavity preparation before the restoration is placed. Steps in the application of desensitizing agents vary by manufacturer, so follow the directions that come with the product.

Equipment and Supplies

- Mouth mirror, explorer, and cotton pliers
- Desensitizing agent (Gluma Desensitizer PowerGel)
- Syringe or applicator
- Cotton rolls, gauze, or dental dam set up
- Air–water syringe
- HVE and salvia ejector

Procedure Steps (*Follow aseptic procedures*)

1. Examine the cavity preparation. Determine where the desensitizer is to be placed.
2. Remove any debris from the cavity preparation. Gently rinse and dry the cavity preparation. Be careful not to over dry the dentin.
3. Isolate the cavity preparation or area with cotton rolls or a dental dam.
4. Prepare the desensitizer to be used. Dispense according to the directions. Some materials are prepared by placing an application tip on the syringe material, or by preparing an applicator to use with liquids or gels.

Note: Usually light-cured materials do not have to be mixed, but are placed directly in the preparation.

5. Place the desensitizer on the dentin tubules in the cavity preparation for 30 to 60 seconds, using an applicator or syringe tip, and carefully place the desensitizing material. Be careful not to touch the tissues.
6. Using the air syringe, dry the area for 30 seconds to 2 minutes (depends on the material), and light-cure the material if necessary.
7. Rinse the area carefully. Have the dentist evaluate and finish the restoration.

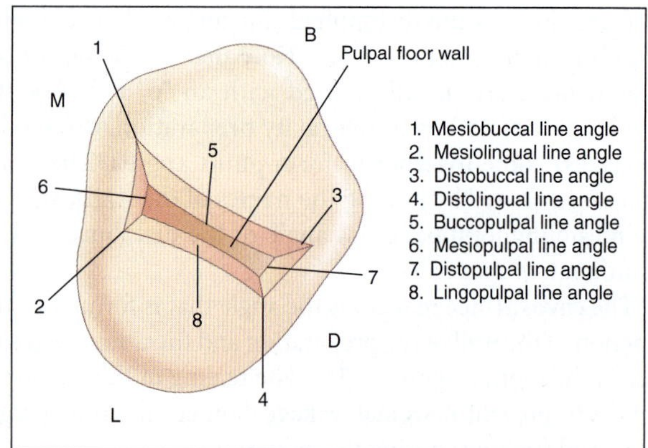

FIGURE 37-32

Cavity preparation line angles (looking down on an occlusal view).

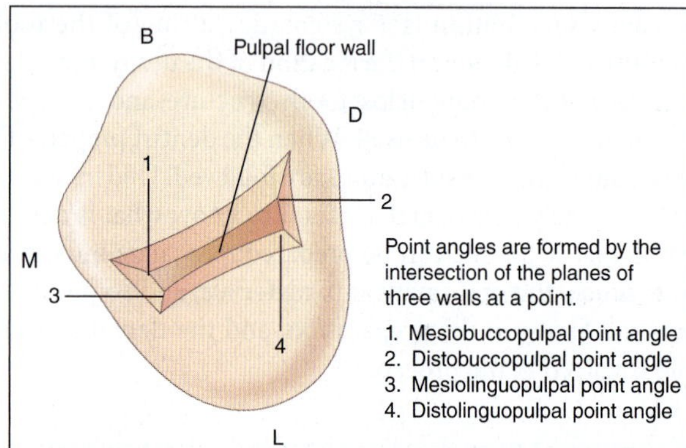

FIGURE 37-33

Cavity preparation point angles.

1. Buccogingival line angle
2. Linguogingival line angle
3. Buccoaxial line angle
4. Linguoaxial line angle
5. Axiogingival line angle
6. Gingivobuccoaxial point angle
7. Gingivolinguoaxial point angle
8. Buccodistal line angle
9. Linguodistal line angle
10. Distopulpal line angle
11. Linguopulpal line angle
12. Buccopulpal line angle
13. Distobuccopulpal point angle
14. Distolinguopulpal point angle
15. Additional line angle, the pulpoaxial line angle is formed by the intersection of the pulpal and axial walls
16. Pulpolinguoaxial point angle
17. Pulpobuccoaxial point angle
18. Cavosurface margin

Pulpal floor D 15 18 B L 16 17 4 3 7 6 2 1 Axial wall 5 M Gingival floor

B D 8 13 12 10 M 9 14 11 L

FIGURE 37-34

Cavity preparation line angles, point angles, and cavosurface margins. (The top figure is a mesial view; the bottom figure is an occlusal view.)

Cavity Preparations. Cavity preparations include the following considerations (Figure 37-35):

- **Outline form**—designates overall shape of the cavity preparation. This form is determined by the extent of the decay, the type of restorative material, and the retention of this material.
- **Resistance form**—the internal shape of the cavity that protects the tooth and restoration from the stresses of mastication.
- **Retention form**—the internal shape of the cavity walls that retains the restoration. In an amalgam preparation, the walls of the preparation are often slightly undercut for mechanical locking of the amalgam and the cavity preparation.
- **Convenience form**—an alteration to the cavity preparation that is necessary for instrumentation during the preparation and insertion of restorative materials. This is usually beyond the outline form and opens the tooth for the dentist to have enough space to prepare the cavity properly.
- **Finishing** or **refinement of the cavity preparation**—the final planning of the cavity walls before the placement of the restoration.
- **Cleansing** or **debridement of the cavity preparation**—spraying and rinsing of the cavity preparation to remove debris. The dental assistant uses the spray from the air-water syringe and the HVE to cleanse the area.

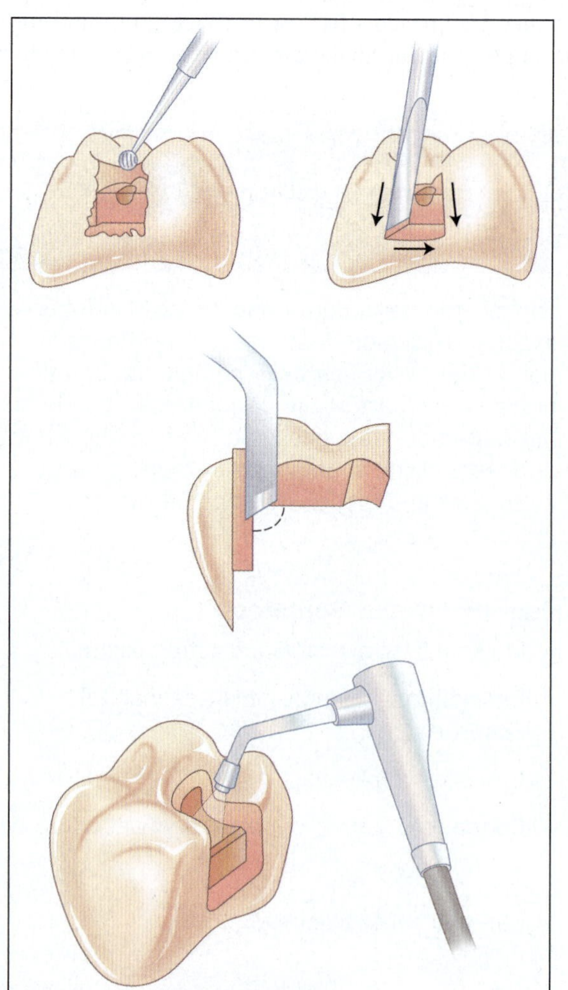

FIGURE 37-35

The steps of cavity preparation: opening the cavity with a bur, outlining the cavity, refining, and then finishing the cavity preparation.

Advanced Chairside Functions

Placing Cements, Bases, and Liners

The dental assistant should be familiar with and knowledgeable about the properties and preparation of cavity liners, varnishes, and cement bases. Cavity preparation and terminology should also be familiar so that the dental assistant can plan ahead and be ready to prepare and place the materials the dentist asks for. Some states allow dental assistants to place bases, liners, and cavity varnish; in others, the dental assistant assists the dentist during this step of the restorative procedure.

Cavity Preparation/Pulpal Involvement

The **cavity preparation** for a restoration depends on the amount of decay, the location of the decay, and the type of materials used to restore the tooth. If the dental assistant is placing the liners, base, or varnish, he or she should examine the cavity preparation to assess pulpal involvement (Table 37-2).

Treatment of Cavity Preparations

Treatment of cavity preparations varies with the amount of enamel and dentin removed, and how near the prep is to the pulp. Using the categories from Table 37-2, possible treatments are summarized as follows:

1. Treatment for an ideal cavity preparation:
   - A base is not required because only a minimal amount of enamel and dentin has been removed. Some dentists place only the restoration, while others prefer to place a fluoride-releasing liner. If an amalgam restoration is going to be placed, two thin layers of cavity varnish are often placed over the dentin.

TABLE 37-2 Depth of Cavity Preparations and Pulpal Relation

Pulpal Involvement	Illustration
1. Ideal level This preparation does not involve the pulp but is through the enamel and just into the dentin. It is large enough to retain a restoration.	
2. Beyond ideal More enamel and dentin are removed, but the preparation is not close to the pulp.	
3. Near exposure This cavity preparation involves a large amount of enamel and dentin being removed, but the pulp is not exposed. The floor of the preparation may be slightly pink due to proximity to the pulp.	
4. Pulp exposure Enough enamel and dentin have been removed to expose a portion of the pulp. There will be blood in the cavity preparation.	

Advanced Chairside Functions (Continued)

If a composite restoration is going to be used, calcium hydroxide or a glass ionomer liner is placed over the exposed dentin.

2. Treatment for a beyond-ideal cavity preparation:
   - With a beyond-ideal preparation, the level of the dentin is restored with a cement base.
   - With an amalgam restoration, there are several options. One option is to place two thin layers of varnish to seal the dentin tubules, and then place a layer of a cement base, such as zinc phosphate.
   - Another option is a reinforced ZOE base, which has a soothing effect on the pulp. Varnish is not used with this material.
   - Other options include a polycarboxylate or glass ionomer base, which also do not require a varnish.
   - Under composite restorative materials, use a glass ionomer base or calcium hydroxide.
3. Treatment for a near-exposure cavity preparation:
   - The closer the cavity preparation comes to the pulp, the more precautions are needed. There are also several options for treatment of the near-exposure preparation.
   - With preparations that are going to be restored with amalgam, a liner of calcium hydroxide, glass ionomer, or ZOE is first placed over the deepest portion of the prep in the dentin. Once this layer is placed, two thin layers of varnish may be inserted over the exposed dentin. Then, a layer of cement base is applied. Zinc phosphate, polycarboxylate, or glass ionomer cements can be used for this layer.
   - Another option for amalgam restorations is to place a liner over the deepest portion of the preparation, then a layer of reinforced ZOE, polycarboxylate, or glass ionomer cement. This is then sealed with a cavity varnish.
   - With some preparations, the dentist may choose not to place a cavity varnish.
   - When composite materials are going to be used to restore the tooth, a liner is placed first, then a layer of either polycarboxylate or glass ionomer cement. Varnish is not placed and a ZOE base liner is not used because they inhibit the setting of the composite.
   - When a cavity liner is placed on a near exposure, the procedure is often referred to as an **indirect pulp capping**.
4. Treatment for an exposed-pulp cavity preparation:
   - With an exposed pulp, the dentist must decide whether endodontic treatment is indicated, or if an attempt should be made to save the vitality of the tooth. If the treatment of choice is to save the pulp, a procedure called a **direct pulp capping (DPC)** is performed.
   - One treatment involves the placement of calcium hydroxide or a glass ionomer liner, which is then reinforced by ZOE as a temporary restoration. This gives the dentist time to see whether the pulp is going to heal.
   - Another treatment involves the placement of a liner, followed by a layer of ZOE cement, two thin layers of varnish, and a cement base.
   - Some dentists prefer to place a liner, and then a layer of polycarboxylate or glass ionomer cement base.

Cavity Liners

A **cavity liner** is placed in the deepest portion of the cavity preparation on the axial walls or pulpal walls (Procedure 37-11). After the liners harden, they form a cement layer with minimum strength. They are placed on the dentin or on an exposed pulp, and protect the pulp from chemical irritations as well as provide a therapeutic effect to the tooth. Examples of cavity liners are calcium hydroxide, ZOE, and glass ionomer. A liner is often called a **low-strength base**.

Cavity Varnish

A cavity varnish is used to seal the dentin tubules to prevent acids, saliva, and debris from reaching the pulp (Procedure 37-12). Cavity varnish is used under amalgam restorations to prevent microleakage, and under zinc phosphate cements to prevent penetration of acids to the pulp. If cavity liners or medicated bases are used, varnish is placed after or on top of these materials.

Cement Bases

A **cement base** is mixed to a thick putty consistency and placed in the cavity preparation to protect the pulp and provide mechanical support for the restoration. These cement bases are placed on the floor of the cavity preparation to raise the level of the floor of the preparation to the ideal height (Procedure 37-14). There are several different types of cements that can be used for bases. These include glass ionomers, hybrid ionomers, reinforced ZOE, zinc phosphate, and polycarboxylate. The preparation, sensitivity of the pulp, and type of restoration indicates which cement to use. These materials are often referred to as a **high-strength base**.

Advanced Chairside Functions

Procedure 37-12
Placing Cavity Liners—Glass Ionomer

This procedure is performed by the dentist or expanded-function dental assistant. Preparation of the cavity has been completed, and this procedure begins the restorative process.

Equipment and Supplies (*Figure 37-36*)

- Cavity liner—glass ionomer
- Application instrument—small, ball-shaped instrument or explorer
- Gauze sponges and cotton rolls
- Mixing pad and spatula, if material is mixed
- Curing light (if material is light cured)

Procedure Steps (*Follow aseptic procedures*)

1. Examine the cavity preparation. Determine the deepest portion of the cavity preparation, and access that area.
2. Clean and dry the cavity preparation. Remove any debris from the cavity preparation. Wash and dry the area with the air–water syringe.
3. Prepare the liner to be used. Dispense and mix according to directions.

Note: Usually, light-cured materials do not have to be mixed but are placed directly in the preparation.

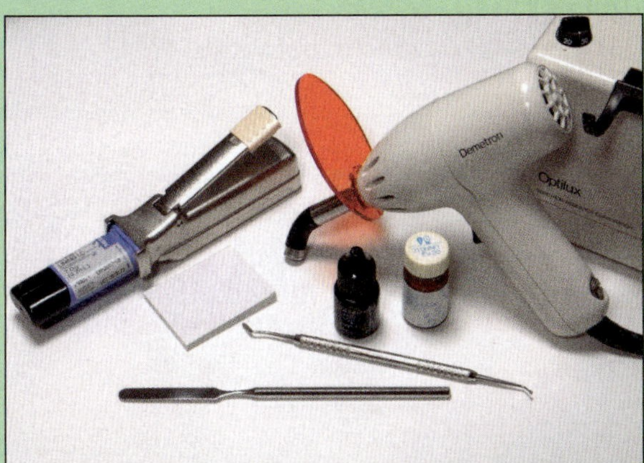

FIGURE 37-36
Glass ionomer tray setup—placing cavity liners.

4. Place the liner in the cavity preparation. Using a small, ball-ended instrument, place the material in the deepest portion of the cavity preparation in a thin layer. Be careful not to touch the instrument to the sides of the preparation. The material will flow into the area and can be spread by pushing the liner in the direction desired with the small ball of the instrument.
5. Complete the placement. Remove the instrument, wipe it clean with gauze, and repeat this procedure until the liner covers the deepest portion of the cavity preparation (Figure 37-37).
6. If the liner is self-curing, the mix must be allowed to harden. If the liner is light cured, the light is held over the tooth and activated to cure the material for the appropriate time (usually 10 to 20 seconds).
7. Examine the cavity preparation. After the liner has cured, examine the preparation. If any material is on the enamel walls, remove it with an explorer.

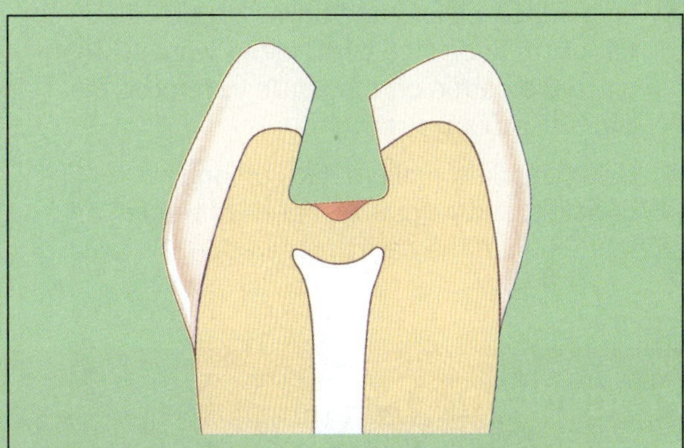

FIGURE 37-37
Placement of cavity liner in preparation.

Advanced Chairside Functions (Continued)

Procedure 37-13
Placing a Cavity Varnish

This procedure is performed by the dentist or expanded-function dental assistant. Preparation of the cavity has been completed, and this procedure is part of preparing the tooth for the restoration.

Equipment and Supplies

- Cavity varnish (varnish and solvent)
- Cotton pliers
- Application instruments (cotton balls, cotton pellets, sponge applicators, or brush applicators)
- Gauze sponges

Procedure Steps (*Follow aseptic procedures*)

1. Shape two very small cotton balls or pellets about 2 mm in size to look like small footballs.
2. Evaluate the cavity preparation to determine access, visibility, and placement of the liners or bases.
3. If the tooth has not been washed and dried, do so at this time with the air–water syringe.
4. To prevent contamination of the varnish, pick up both cotton pellets and balls with the sterile cotton pliers and place them in the varnish. Then, place the cotton on the gauze to remove the excess varnish.
5. Using the cotton pliers, pick up one cotton ball or pellet, and paint a thin layer of varnish on the dentin in the cavity preparation. A sterile disposable brush or sponge may also be used (Figure 37-38).
6. Allow the cavity to dry for 30 seconds. Place a second coat of varnish. Using the cotton pliers, pick up the second cotton pellet or ball from the gauze and apply a second layer of varnish (this prevents any voids). To prevent contamination, never place an applicator that has been used in the mouth back in the bottle of varnish.
7. Clean up after the procedure. If any excess varnish was placed on the enamel surface, remove it with varnish solvent and a small applicator.

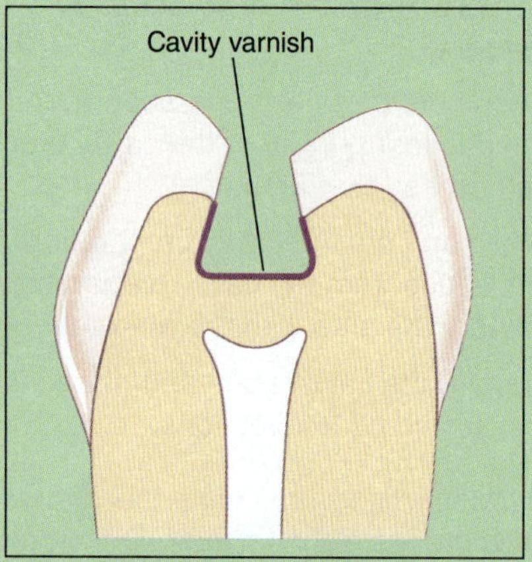

FIGURE 37-38
Placement of cavity varnish in preparation.

Procedure 37-14
Placement of Cement Bases

This procedure is performed by the dentist or expanded-function dental assistant. Preparation of the cavity has been completed, and this procedure is part of preparing the tooth for the restoration.

Equipment and Supplies (*Figures 37-39A and B*)

- Cement base materials, usually powder/liquid
- Mixing pad
- Cement spatula
- Gauze sponges
- Plastic filling instrument
- Explorer or spoon excavator

(continues)

Advanced Chairside Functions

Procedure 37-14 (continued)

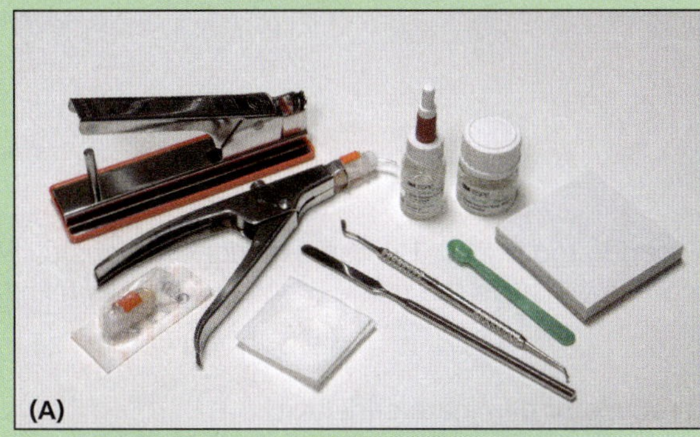

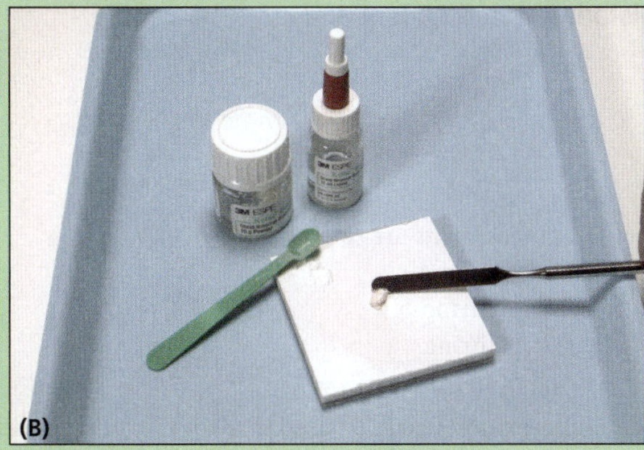

FIGURE 37-39

Placement of the cement base. (A) Cement base tray setup. (B) Cement base consistency.

Procedure Steps (*Follow aseptic procedures*)

1. Determine where to place the base and the size of the area. Evaluate access and visibility.
2. Prepare the preparation area. Remove any debris with the air–water syringe and HVE.
3. Prepare the cement base materials according to the manufacturer's instructions. Mix the cement base into a thick putty consistency and gather it into a small ball.
4. Collect the base on the blade of the plastic filling instrument. Place the base in the cavity preparation.
5. Using the small condensing end of the plastic filling instrument, condense the base into place on the floor of the cavity prep (Figure 37-40). If the material is sticky, place a small amount of the cement powder on the mixing pad and dip the end of the condenser as needed. Continue until a sufficient base layer is placed.
6. Evaluate the placement. The base should cover the floor of the cavity preparation, leave enough room for the restorative materials, and should not be on pins or in retentive grooves.
7. Remove any excess materials with a spoon excavator or an explorer.
8. Clean up the mixing materials. Remove cement from the spatula as soon as possible, and remove the paper from the pad.

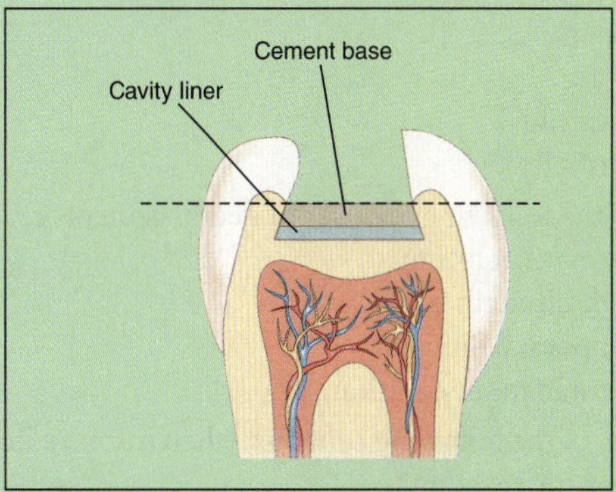

FIGURE 37-40

Placement of the cement base in a cavity preparation.

Chapter Summary

The general chairside assistant prepares and mixes the material, while the dentist places the material in the oral cavity. Some states allow the assistant to also place some of the materials in the oral cavity. Knowledge of dental cements, bases, liners, and bonding agent properties is necessary for the dental assistant to properly prepare and manipulate the materials. The assistant's knowledge of these dental materials is beneficial for patient education and protection. Expanded-function dental assistants must understand and be competent in the placement and finishing of materials.

CASE STUDY

Garrett Greenwood is having a large filling placed in tooth #30. He has experienced sensitivity in the past after restorations, and is concerned he will have the same problem with this filling.

Case Study Review

1. Discuss the steps that can be taken to reduce or eliminate sensitivity.
2. What information could the dental assistant give the patient about his concerns?

Review Questions

Multiple Choice

1. ________ is defined as the force per unit area of a material
   a. Strain
   b. Stress
   c. Shearing
   d. Elasticity
2. All of the following are uses of dental cements *except*
   a. permanent luting.
   b. high-strength base.
   c. temporary filling.
   d. permanent restoration.
3. Which of the following cements, when mixed, exhibits an exothermic reaction?
   a. Calcium hydroxide
   b. Zinc-oxide-eugenol
   c. Zinc phosphate
   d. Glass ionomer
4. Luting cement that has reached the correct consistency
   a. is granular.
   b. is of a putty consistency.
   c. follows the spatula up an inch off the mixing pad.
   d. forms a ball.
5. The two types of retention are
   a. mechanical and chemical.
   b. mechanical and surgical.
   c. chemical and surgical.
   d. none of the above.
6. Dental cements are set by
   a. self-curing.
   b. light curing.
   c. dual curing.
   d. all of the above.
7. Zinc-oxide-eugenol is used in all of the following *except*
   a. permanent cement.
   b. temporary cement.
   c. intermediate cement.
   d. temporary restoration.
8. ________ cement has many uses, it can be used for permanent cement, a pit and fissure sealant, as restorative material, and as a liner and bonding agent.
   a. Zinc phosphate
   b. Polycarboxylate
   c. Zinc-oxide-eugenol
   d. Glass ionomer
9. ________ is used as a low-strength base or liner, and is slightly irritating, which stimulates secondary dentin to form.
   a. Glass ionomer
   b. Zinc-oxide-eugenol
   c. Calcium hydroxide
   d. Cavity varnish
10. Which of the following materials is used to improve retention between the tooth structure and the restoration?
   a. Compomer cement
   b. Bonding agents
   c. Zinc phosphate cement
   d. Desensitizing materials

Critical Thinking

1. Give two examples of thermal conductivity relating to dentistry.
2. Explain how the correct amount of powder and liquid to be dispensed is determined.
3. Would cavity varnish be placed under or over calcium hydroxide? Explain.

Web Activities

1. Go to http://www.kavo.com and download and watch the video presentation on the DIAGNOdent pen.
2. To find out the latest information about cement and bonding materials, go to http://www.kerrdental.com.
3. To learn more about the specifications for dental materials go to http://www.ada.org.

CHAPTER 38

Restorative Materials and Matrix and Wedge

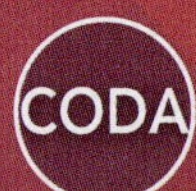

Specific Instructional Objectives

The student should strive to meet the following objectives and demonstrate an understanding of the facts and principles presented in this chapter:

1. Explain the properties, composition, and manipulation of dental amalgam.
2. Identify the armamentarium and the steps of an amalgam procedure.
3. Explain the composition of composite resins.
4. Explain the properties and manipulation of various composite restorations.
5. Identify the armamentarium and the steps of a composite restoration.
6. Explain the use of glass ionomer, resin, resin-reinforced glass ionomer, and compomer restorative materials.

Advanced Chairside Functions

7. Define matrix and wedge and list the uses and types of matrices.
8. Describe the functions, parts, placement, and removal of the Tofflemire matrix.
9. Discuss the function and placement of the wedge.
10. Describe the AutoMatrix and the sectional matrix, and where they are used in restorative procedures.
11. Explain and demonstrate the placement and removal of the strip matrix.

Key Terms

alloy (893)
amalgam (893)
amalgamation (895)
amalgamator (896)
AutoMatrix (907)
band (907)
burnish (913)
capsule (895)
circumference (908)
composite (901)
compules (900)
condensable composite (902)
contra-angle (908)
creep (895)
crown matrix form (914)
Direct restorative material (893)
flowable composite (901)
hybrid composite (901)
inorganic filler particles (901)
macrofilled composite (901)
matrix (907)
mercury (893)
microfill composite (901)
organic polymer matrix (901)
organic silane-coupling agent (901)
packable composite (902)
pestle (895)
plastic strip matrix (907)
primer (905)
retainer (907)
sectional matrix system (907)
shell matrix (907)
Tofflemire matrix (907)
trituration (895)
triturator (896)
wedge (907)

Introduction

This chapter discusses direct restorative materials, the dental dam, and the matrix and wedge. **Direct restorative materials** include dental amalgam, composite resin materials, and glass ionomers. Dental amalgam has been used successfully for filling posterior teeth for many years. Composition, types, and safety concerns are discussed, as well as proper handling and mixing techniques. There are some concerns about the mercury in the dental amalgam, and the dental assistant should keep up to date on current information to stay informed. Tooth-colored materials are the most popular and most widely used, because patients want a more natural appearance for their teeth. There are several types and categories of materials used to fill both the anterior and posterior teeth. The various composites and combinations are discussed, as well as the placement techniques for them.

Toward the end of the chapter, we discuss the dental dam, and the matrix and wedge materials, as well as placement techniques. Placing the dental dam, matrix, and wedge are considered expanded or advanced functions. Each state has regulations delegating whether the dental assistant can actually place the dental dam, matrix, and wedge, or if the assistant can only assist during their placement and removal.

The dental assistant can stay current on restorative materials and the dental dam, matrix, and wedge procedures by attending seminars and dental conferences, reading books and trade magazines, and through local sales representatives. The American Dental Association Council on Dental Materials, Instruments, and Equipment is responsible for information on, and the testing of, dental materials, and periodically publishes a listing in the *Journal of the American Dental Association and in Clinical Products in Dentistry: A Desktop Reference*.

Amalgam Restorative Materials

After the cavity has been prepared and the liners and bases have been placed, the tooth is ready to be restored. One of the most common restorative materials is dental **amalgam**, which has been used for many years (Figure 38-1). Dental amalgam is an effective, long-lasting, and comparatively inexpensive restorative material. Amalgam is a combination of an alloy with mercury. An **alloy** is the combination of two or more metals.

Dental amalgam is pliable when first mixed, so it is easily placed in the cavity preparation. It is carved before hardening to resemble the tooth structure. This material is used only on the posterior teeth because of its strength and because it is not esthetically pleasing.

The indications for placing amalgam fillings include the following:

- A long success record
- Working well in areas that are difficult to keep dry (moisture control)

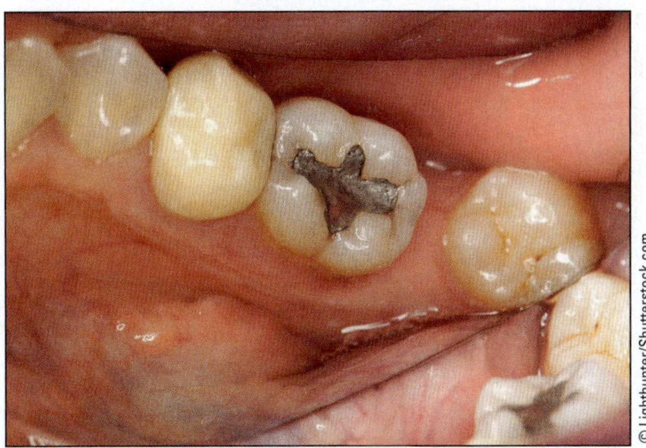

FIGURE 38-1
Occlusal amalgam restoration on a mandibular molar.

- Can be used on both primary and permanent teeth
- Less technique sensitive
- Patient's oral hygiene is poor
- Less expensive restorative material

The contraindications include the following:

- Poor esthetics, as amalgam is a silver material
- There is some controversy about the mercury content and allergies
- Used only on the posterior teeth
- Sometimes there is discoloration around the margins of the restoration

Composition

Dental amalgam is composed of silver, tin, copper, and zinc (optional) to form an alloy. This alloy is mixed with mercury to form the amalgam. The ADA has specifications that regulate the composition of dental amalgam (see Table 38-1 for the characteristics of each of the alloy components).

Types of Dental Amalgam

Dental amalgam consists of a low- and a high-copper alloy. Metals for the alloys are prepared in several ways to produce the lathe cut (comminuted particles) and spherically shaped particles. The way these metals are prepared affects their properties. Low-copper alloys are available with comminuted and spherical particles. High-copper alloys are supplied as *comminuted*, *spherical*, or *combination particles* (admix).

Spherical alloys have smoother surfaces that require less mercury when mixed. These alloys are also easier to condense, and have improved carving and polishing properties. Combination alloys adapt better to the cavity preparation and produce better contacts with the adjacent teeth.

Mercury Used in Dental Amalgam

Dental **mercury** is a very toxic chemical and must meet the specifications listed by the ADA. Dental professionals are aware of the hazards and safety measures when working with dental mercury to prevent problems from occurring.

TABLE 38-1 Dental Alloy Composition

Silver	**40 to 70 percent**	**High-copper amalgam**
	68 to 72 percent	**Low-copper mix**
	• Used to form a metallic compound with mercury (Hg), which determines the dimensional changes that occur during hardening • Increases restoration strength • Increases expansion • Is slow to amalgamate • Hardens rapidly • Tarnishes easily • Decreases setting time	
Tin	**22 to 30 percent**	**High-copper amalgam**
	26 to 37 percent	**Low-copper amalgam**
	• Aids in amalgamation (chemical combining) of alloy with Hg because of its strong Hg affinity • Reduces expansion during setting • Reduces strength • Setting time is slower • Is more susceptible to corrosion (conventional alloy) • Tends to weaken amalgam	
Copper	**12 to 30 percent**	**High-copper amalgam**
	4 to 5 percent	**Low-copper amalgam**
	• Increases strength and hardness • Increases expansion of amalgam during hardening • Reduces the flow of finished restoration • Resists corrosion (high copper) • Reduces marginal failure (high copper)	
Zinc	**0 to 1 percent**	**For high- and low-copper amalgams**
	• Minimizes the oxidation of other metals in the alloy during manufacturing. Zinc is a scavenger and reacts with oxygen, preventing it from combining with silver, tin, or copper. Note: Should moisture contamination occur during the manipulation or condensation of the amalgam, delayed expansion might occur. Zinc-containing dental amalgams are particularly sensitive to moisture. Zinc reacts with water to form zinc oxide and hydrogen gas, which may cause the unwanted and excessive expansion of the set amalgam restoration.	

Mercury is the only metal that is in a liquid state and vaporizes (particles of mercury scatter and float freely in the air) at a relatively low room temperature. Mercury is absorbed through the pores of the skin and through inhalation. Some potential sources of mercury contamination in the dental office are as follows:

- Mercury leaking out of a capsule during trituration
- Mercury vapor may occur during triturating and dispensing
- Polishing an amalgam restoration
- Removal of a hardened amalgam restoration
- Contact with the amalgam during the procedure
- Carpeting in the treatment rooms could retain amalgam particles and vacuuming these surfaces disperses the mercury through the air
- Scraps of amalgam left in an open container

Studies have revealed that in most dental offices, the level of mercury vapor is well below the maximum safe environmental concentration levels. Another study testing the blood mercury level in dentists displayed a reading well below the level at which symptoms begin to show.

There has been some concern about the level of mercury in patients with numerous amalgam restorations. Recent studies have shown that these patients ingest a very low amount of mercury from the amalgam fillings, well below what they would ingest from food, water, and the atmosphere. A very small number of people have a possible risk for an allergic reaction to mercury. The response manifests as a skin reaction that appears after the placement of an amalgam restoration. Including questions on the medical history is a prevention step. Because of these concerns, the dentist and dental assistant should stay current with research and ADA recommendations.

The ADA recommends that a program of mercury hygiene be established at every dental practice. Potential office hazards involving mercury can be eliminated by practicing appropriate mercury hygiene. Guidelines should include the following:

- Wear disposable gloves, a facemask, and glasses when working with the amalgam.
- Educate all personnel regarding the potential hazards of mercury, as well as good mercury hygiene practices.

- A no-touch technique should be used when handling mercury. If the skin is exposed, wash with soap and water, and rinse under running water.
- Use capsules containing a measured amount of mercury and alloy.
- Use an amalgamator with a protective cover both to reduce the chance of any mercury vapor being released, and to confine any mercury that might be sprayed from an ill-fitting capsule.
- Store mercury and amalgam scraps in capped, wide-mouthed, unbreakable jars containing used x-ray fixer, finely divided sulfur, glycerin, or mineral oil.
- Carpeting in dental treatment rooms is not recommended. Carpeting retains mercury, which is difficult to retrieve.
- Use water spray and high-volume evacuation when cutting old amalgams or polishing new restorations. Wear a mask during these procedures.
- Avoid working with mercury or amalgam near a heat source, such as the autoclave.
- Handle mercury only over impervious surfaces. The area should have a continuous lip to retain any spillage.
- The office should have proper ventilation to reduce the possibility of mercury vapor inhalation. Change the air filter frequently.
- Change the chairside traps by placing the disposable traps into a container that is marked "Contact Amalgam Waste for Recycling". For the reusable traps, remove the trap from the dental unit and empty contents in the marked container.
- Office personnel should have periodic urinalyses to check for any mercury in the body.
- Monitor the dental office to determine mercury levels.
- Keep a mercury spill kit if the office uses large quantities of mercury. Clean up any mercury scraps or spills immediately, following OSHA recommendations (Figure 38-2).

For more information on handling amalgam wastes go to the ADA website and look for the brochure on *Best Management Practices for Amalgam Wastes* and a *Practical Guide to Integrating BMP's Into Your Practice.*

Forms of Dental Alloy

Dental alloy is purchased in a disposable **capsule** form. The capsule contains a premeasured amount of alloy and mercury, and sometimes a **pestle**. The pestle, a small pellet, is made of metal or plastic and aids in the mixing of the alloy and mercury. In the capsule, a thin membrane separates the alloy and the mercury until they are mixed. Some capsules come with activators to break the membrane, while others are twisted or compressed before being mixed. The capsules are most often plastic and come with screw-type or friction-fit caps. Disposable capsules are color coded to distinguish single, double, and triple mixes (Figure 38-3).

Amalgam Properties

The strength of the amalgam is not adequate to withstand occlusal forces alone. The preparation is designed so that the remaining tooth structure sustains the forces to the amalgam.

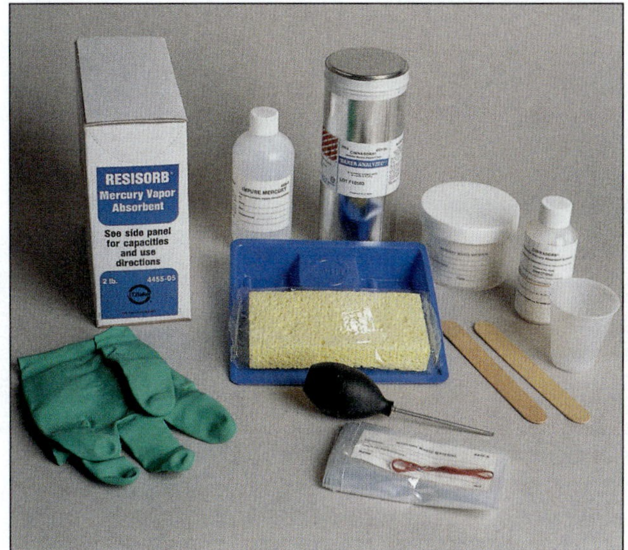

FIGURE 38-2
Mercury spill kit.

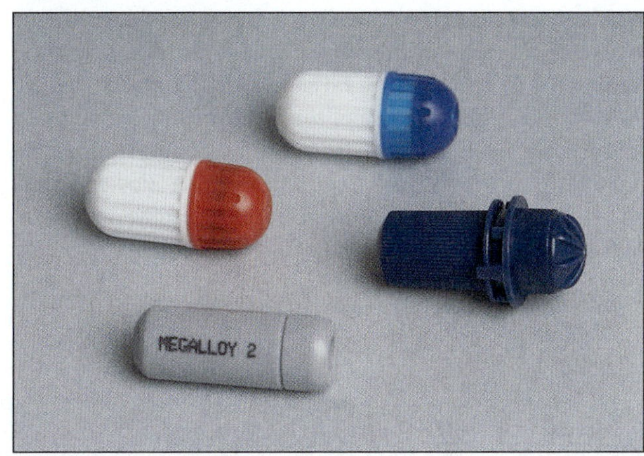

FIGURE 38-3
Samples of amalgam capsules.

Proper manipulation of the amalgam is important in the overall strength and success of the restoration.

Amalgam is subject to dimensional change, such as expansion and contraction. The amount of expansion and contraction is controlled by the composition of the alloy, and manipulation techniques.

Another property of amalgam is the ability of the material to **creep**. Creeping is a change in the material when under a constant load.

Amalgam restorations are subject to corrosion and tarnish in the oral cavity. Tarnish is the discoloration of the surface, and corrosion is the deterioration of the surface (Figure 38-4). The combination (admixed) and the spherical high-copper amalgams are less susceptible to corrosion. Careful finishing and polishing of the amalgams reduces tarnish and corrosion.

Amalgam Manipulation

The process of **trituration** is the combining (mixing) of the dental alloy and mercury mechanically. The process of **amalgamation** is the actual chemical reaction that occurs between

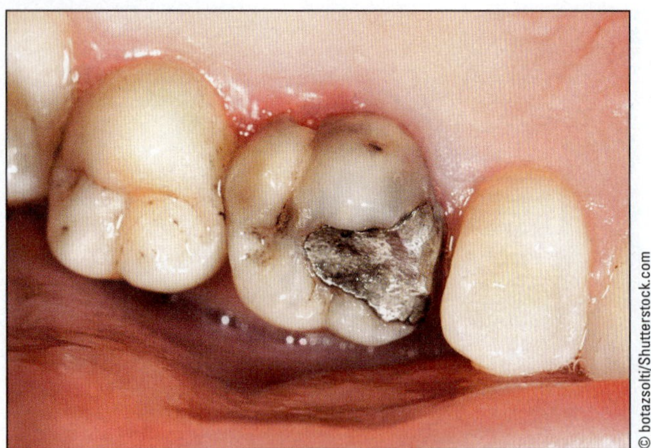

© botazsolti/Shutterstock.com

FIGURE 38-4

Tarnished and corroded amalgam restoration and decay are present.

the alloy and the mercury that forms the silver amalgam. A specially designed machine is used to triturate (amalgamate) the alloy and mercury; it's called a dental **amalgamator** or **triturator**. These machines have cradles to hold the capsules, cradle covers, timers, and variable speed controls (Figure 38-5). General steps for use of the amalgamator are outlined in Procedure 38-1. Each amalgamator must be set for the type of dental alloy used. Usually, trituration of the alloy and mercury is 10 to 15 seconds. This produces a homogeneous and uniform mix. Follow the manufacturer's directions and alloy specifications.

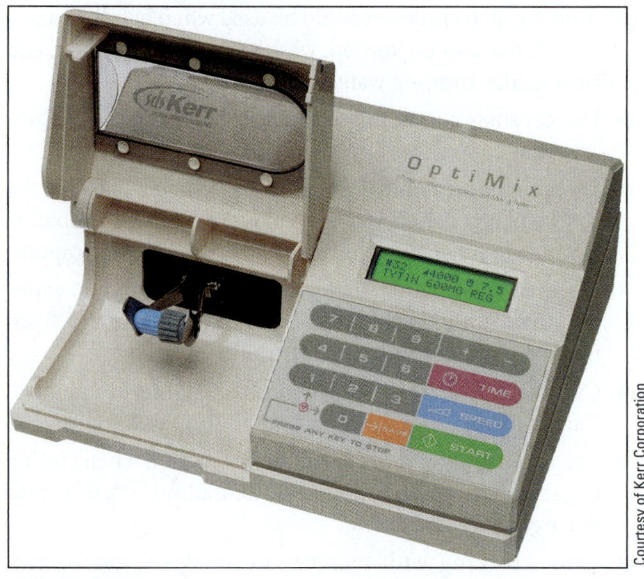

Courtesy of Kerr Corporation

FIGURE 38-5

A dental amalgamator.

Trituration of the amalgam is an important step for restoration success. The quality of the mix is determined by the mixing time, speed of the amalgamator, and the force being applied during the trituration. Varying conditions in the trituration process can cause certain problems. If the amalgam is mixed too long (over triturated), it will be soupy before hardening and difficult to remove from the capsule. If the amalgam is undermixed (under triturated), it will be crumbly and dull in appearance, and the strength of the amalgam will be reduced.

Procedure 38-1
Using the Dental Amalgamator

This procedure is completed by the dental assistant. The materials and equipment are prepared before the procedure begins. The types of amalgamator and capsules vary.

Equipment and Supplies *(Figure 38-6)*

- Amalgamator
- Premeasured capsule of dental alloy and mercury
- Amalgam well, dappen dish, or squeeze cloth
- Amalgam carrier/condenser
- Scrap container for excess amalgam

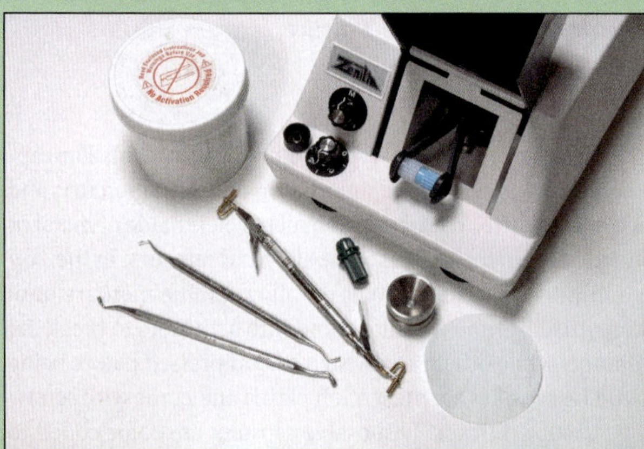

FIGURE 38-6

Items needed to mix and place an amalgam restoration, including two condensers, a container for amalgam scraps, an amalgam carrier, an amalgamator, an amalgam capsule, an amalgam well, and squeeze cloth.

Procedure Steps *(Follow aseptic procedures)*

1. Assemble the materials for the procedure. Select the trituration time and speed for the type of alloy and amalgamator.

(continues)

Procedure 38-1 (continued)

2. Prepare the capsule by twisting the cap, squeezing the capsule, or using an activator.
3. Insert the capsule into the cradle (prongs) of the amalgamator. Place one end first, and then slide the other end down into place. Practice placing the capsules into the cradle with one hand (Figure 38-7A).
4. Close the cover of the amalgamator.
5. Activate the amalgamator for the prescribed time and speed (Figure 38-7B). The timer will automatically switch off after the prescribed trituration time.
6. Lift the cover and remove the capsule.
7. Open the capsule and empty the amalgam into an amalgam well. Avoid touching the amalgam with gloved hands. Use cotton pliers, if necessary. A well-mixed amalgam will have a glossy appearance with a smooth, velvety consistency.
8. Reassemble the capsule and place it to the side.
9. Hold the carrier and load the amalgam (Figure 38-8).
10. Pack the carrier, applying pressure so that the cylinder is packed tightly. Wipe excess material from the end of the carrier onto the sides of the amalgam well.
11. Pass the amalgam carrier to the dentist and prepare to exchange a condenser for the carrier. When practicing, dispense the amalgam from the carrier into a dappen dish and evaluate the mix. The cylinders of amalgam should be smooth and shiny.
12. Repeat the loading and dispensing of all the material. Toward the end of the manipulation, the amalgam becomes harder to load into the carrier because it begins to set. This is the stage that takes practice in order to become proficient.
13. To clean up, expel any excess amalgam into the appropriate container. The instruments are then cleaned and sterilized (Figure 38-9).

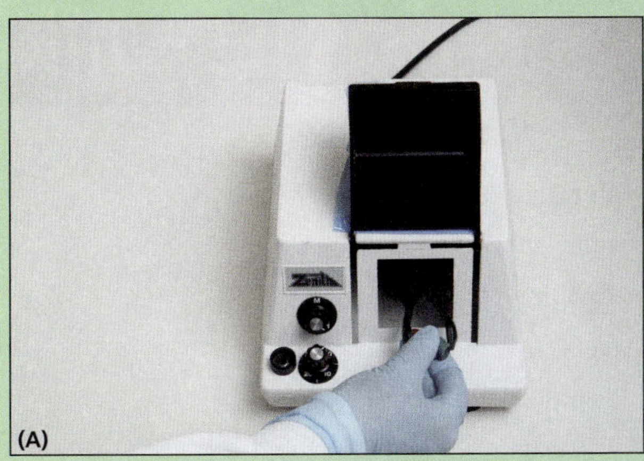

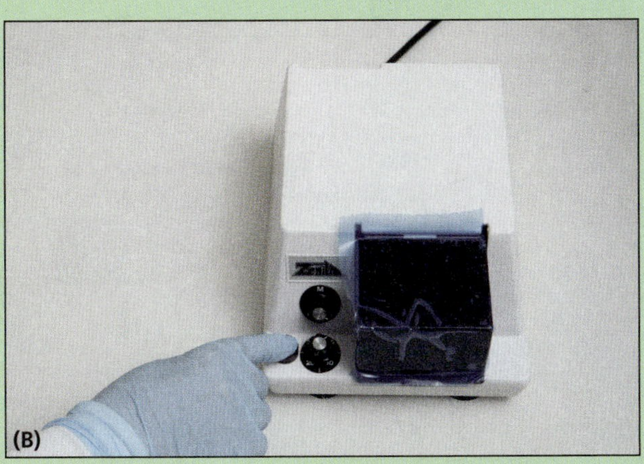

FIGURE 38-7
(A) Placing a capsule in an amalgamator. (B) Activating the amalgamator timer.

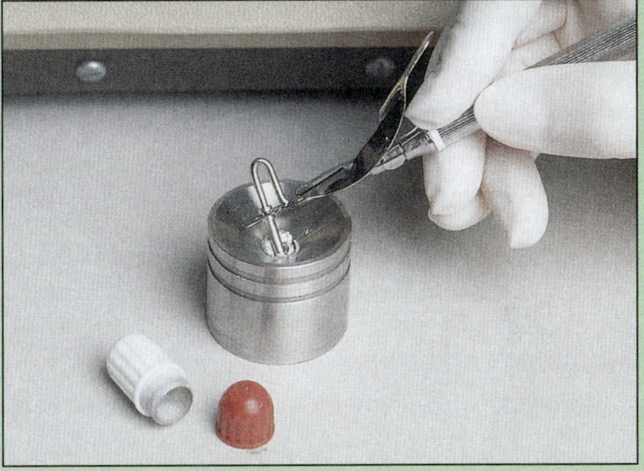

FIGURE 38-8
Loading the amalgam carrier.

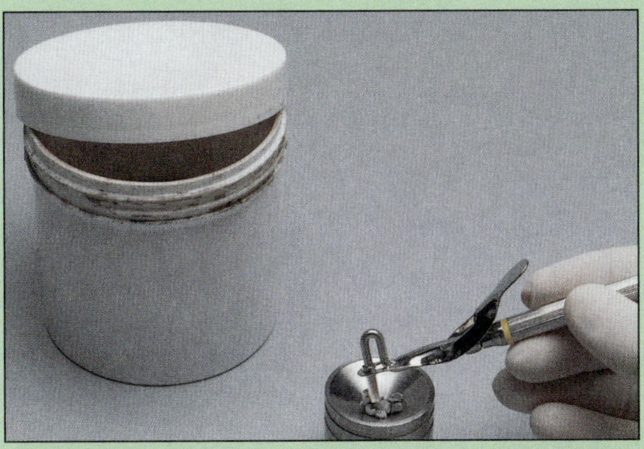

FIGURE 38-9
Placing amalgam scraps into a sealed container.

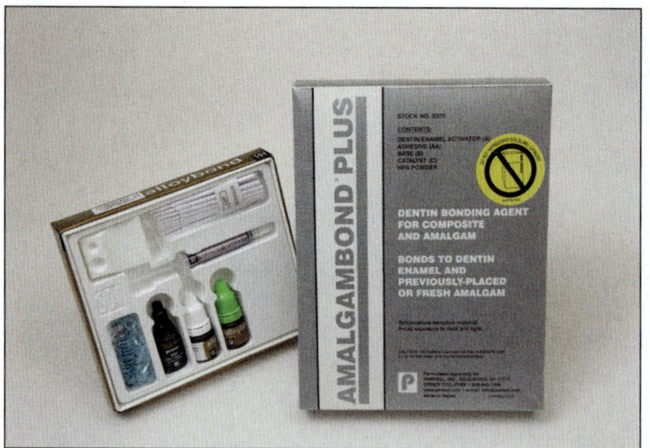

FIGURE 38-10
Amalgam bonding materials.

Amalgam Bonding

Amalgam bonding agents are available and used in many restorations to bond the amalgam to the tooth surface (Figure 38-10). Amalgam bonding increases the retention of the restoration and decreases marginal leakage. The bonding agent is a low-viscosity resin, similar to those discussed in Chapter 37, Dental Cements, Bases, Liners, and Bonding Agents. The procedure 37-10 in Chapter 37 describes the application of bonding agents. The placement of the amalgam follows immediately, before the bonding agent sets.

NOTE: Other retention methods, including the placement of retention pins and core buildups, have been discussed in Chapter 33, Fixed Prosthodontics and Gingival Retraction.

A Complete Amalgam Procedure

The sequence for the following procedure is for a complete amalgam restoration. The steps include administering an anesthetic; placing the rubber dam; placing liners, bases, and bonding agents; assembling the matrix and wedge; and mixing, placing, condensing, and finishing the amalgam restoration. Procedure 38-2 gives the dental assistant an overall view of assisting during an amalgam procedure. Many of these steps, such as placing the rubber dam, are discussed in detail later in this chapter because they can be performed by an expanded-function dental assistant.

Procedure 38-2
Amalgam Restoration—Class II

   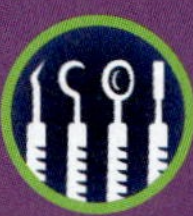

This procedure is completed by the dentist and dental assistant. The tooth is prepared with the dental handpiece and assorted burs. Once the tooth is prepared, it is restored with dental amalgam.

Equipment and Supplies (*Figure 38-11*)

- Basic setup: mouth mirror, explorer, and cotton pliers
- Air–water syringe tip, HVE tip, and saliva ejector
- Cotton rolls, gauze sponges, pellets, cotton-tip applicators, and floss
- Topical and local anesthetic setup
- Rubber dam setup
- High- and low-speed handpieces
- Assortment of dental burs
- Spoon excavator
- Hand-cutting instruments (hatchets, chisels, hoes, and gingival margin trimmers)
- Base, liner, varnish, and/or bonding agent
- Paper pad, cement spatula, and placement instrument
- Matrix retainer, matrix bands, and wedges
- Locking pliers or hemostat
- Amalgam capsules
- Amalgam well
- Amalgam carrier and condensers
- Amalgamator
- Carving instruments
- Articulating paper and forceps

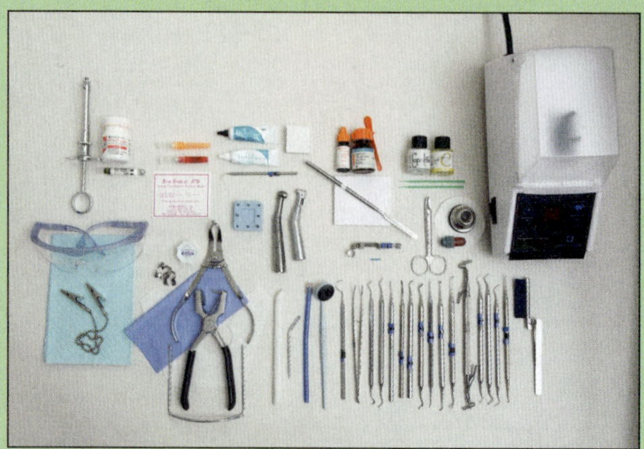

FIGURE 38-11
Amalgam procedure tray setup.

(continues)

Procedure 38-2 (continued)

Procedure Steps (*Follow aseptic procedures*)

1. Greet and prepare the patient for the procedure. Review his or her medical history.
2. Prepare for the administration of the topical and local anesthetic. Dry the injection site and apply topical anesthetic (expanded function—EF). Prepare the syringe and summon the dentist. Transfer the mirror and explorer to the dentist to examine the tooth before beginning the procedure. When the dentist is ready, transfer a 2 × 2 inch gauze in one hand and the syringe in the other. The dentist replaces the needle cap and places the syringe on the tray. After the injection, rinse and evacuate the patient's mouth.
3. Prepare the rubber dam materials and equipment to assist the dentist in the placement (EF).
4. Transfer the mouth mirror and the high-speed handpiece with a bur. Position the HVE tip and maintain visibility throughout the procedure by retracting the cheek and tongue, keeping the mirror clear with the air–water syringe, and evacuating the site (Figure 38-12). Transfer and receive instruments at the dentist's signals. Instruments used at this point may include the explorer, the excavator, hatchets, hoes, angle formers, gingival margin trimmers, and chisels.
5. When the preparation is finished, transfer a cotton pellet with a cavity cleaning preparation to clean the inside of the tooth (EF). The area is then rinsed and dried. At the dentist's direction, mix the cavity liner (calcium hydroxide or glass ionomer); prepare the varnish (if used), the base (glass ionomer, polycarboxylate, zinc phosphate, or modified zinc oxide-eugenol (ZOE), and the bonding agent (if used), and transfer them to the dentist for placement. If the materials are light cured, hold the light tip near the material to be cured and, with the protective shield in place, activate the light to cure the material.
6. Assemble the matrix retainer and the band into the correct position according to the tooth being restored, and transfer it to the dentist (EF). After the matrix is placed, transfer the wedge in cotton pliers (locking is best) or in a hemostat. The dentist places the wedge.
7. When the dentist is ready, prepare the amalgam capsule by twisting the cap, squeezing the capsule together, or placing it in an activator, and then placing the capsule in the amalgamator. The amalgamator is set for the specific type of amalgam material, and for the size of the mix. When the amalgam material has been mixed, remove the capsule from the amalgamator and place it in the amalgam well or a dappen dish. The amalgam is loaded into the amalgam carrier. If the carrier is double ended, both ends are filled and the loaded carrier is passed to the dentist (Figure 38-13). The carrier and the condenser are used alternately until the restorative material fills the cavity. In some offices, the dental assistant loads the carrier and, at the dentist's direction, places the amalgam in the cavity preparation, eliminating the exchanging of instruments and allowing the dentist to focus on the condensing of the amalgam. After the last exchange, transfer an explorer to the dentist to loosen the amalgam from the matrix band. While

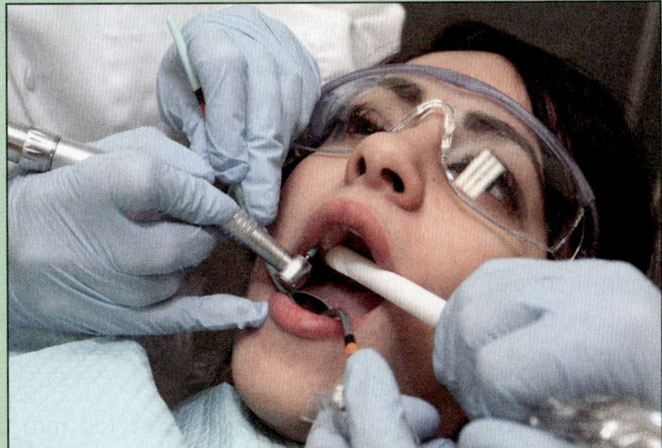

FIGURE 38-12
Cavity being prepared by the dentist with a dental assistant evacuating, and keeping the mirror dry and clean.

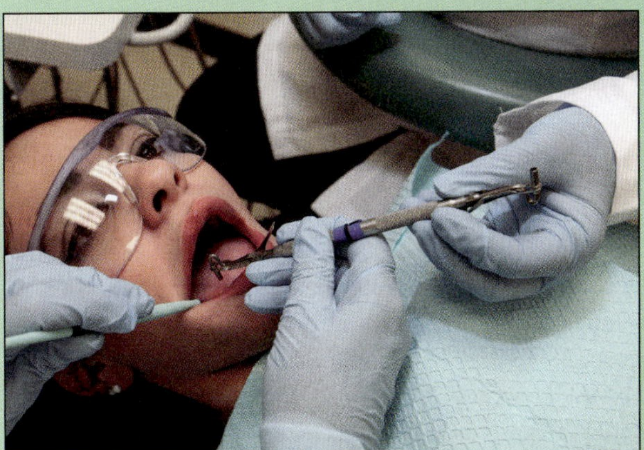

FIGURE 38-13
A loaded amalgam carrier ready for use.

(continues)

Procedure 38-2 (continued)

the dentist is using the explorer, clean up any amalgam scraps from the carrier and the well, and place them in a sealed container.

8. Receive the explorer, transfer carving, and finishing instruments at the dentist's signals. Operate the HVE tip near the site to evacuate any amalgam particles. After the dentist completes the preliminary carving, pass the cotton pliers to remove the wedge, and then receive the wedge, pliers, and matrix retainer. The cotton pliers may be used again to remove the matrix band. Receive the cotton pliers and band, and then transfer the carver of the dentist's choice for finishing the carving of the anatomy in the restoration.
9. The rubber dam is carefully removed at this time (EF). Transfer the clamp forceps, receive the forceps with the clamp, and then transfer the scissors to cut the interseptal dam. Receive the scissors, frame, napkin, and dam material. Rinse and evacuate the patient's mouth.
10. Dry the area and transfer the articulating paper positioned on the forceps to the dentist. The assistant may be instructed by the dentist to place the articulating paper over the restoration. The patient is instructed to gently tap the teeth together (Figure 38-14). Additional carving and checking of the occlusion are continued until the dentist is satisfied and the patient is comfortable.
11. The restoration is wiped off with a wet cotton roll to remove blue marks left by the articulating paper. Rinse and evacuate the patient's mouth thoroughly and clean any debris from the patient's face. The patient is cautioned not to chew on the side of the restoration for a few hours and is then dismissed (Figure 38-15).

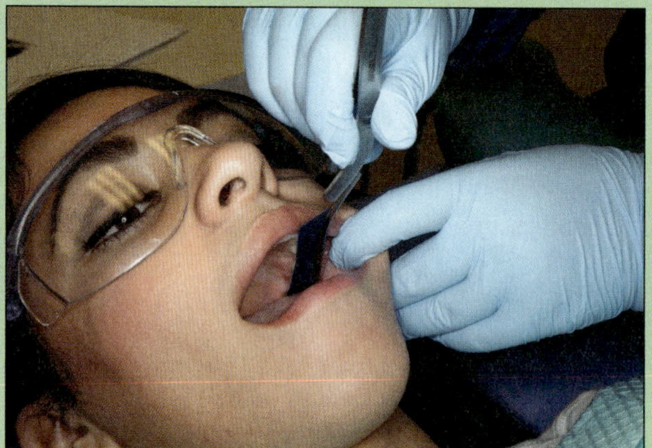

FIGURE 38-14
Articulating paper positioned for the patient to gently close on to check the occlusion.

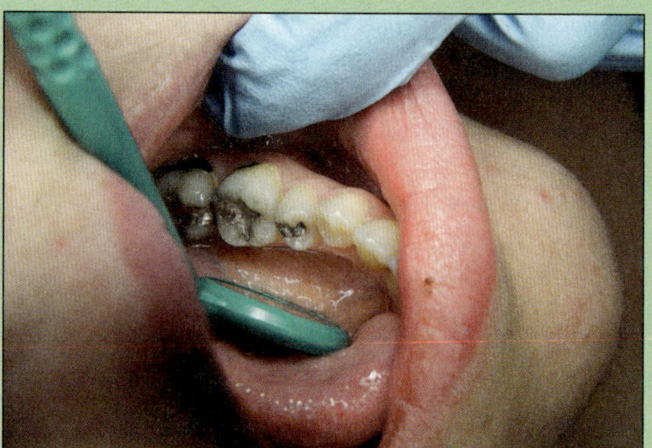

FIGURE 38-15
A finished amalgam restoration.

Composite Restorative Materials

Composite restorative materials dominate the field of esthetic restorations. These materials have a natural appearance, and were used primarily for anterior restorations but have now developed as esthetic restorations for the posterior teeth (Figures 38-16 and 38-17). Composite restorative materials can be used for Class I, II, III, IV, V, and VI caries. Composite materials are also used for veneers on anterior teeth that have been stained or that have some erosion. They are also used to close a diastema or to esthetically re-contour teeth. These procedures are discussed in Chapter 33, Fixed Prosthodontics and Gingival Retraction.

Technology is expanding the types of materials available as alternatives to dental amalgam. With concerns over the mercury in amalgams and the desire for the natural appearance of teeth, there is ongoing research and development with composite restorative materials. Composites, glass ionomers, resins, and porcelain materials, as well as combinations of these materials, are used for esthetic restorations.

These direct restorative materials are inserted into the cavity preparation and then self-cured, light cured, or dual cured. They come in syringes or single-application cartridges (**compules**), and have a variety of shades or shade modifiers. The location and the size of the cavity determine which material the dentist chooses.

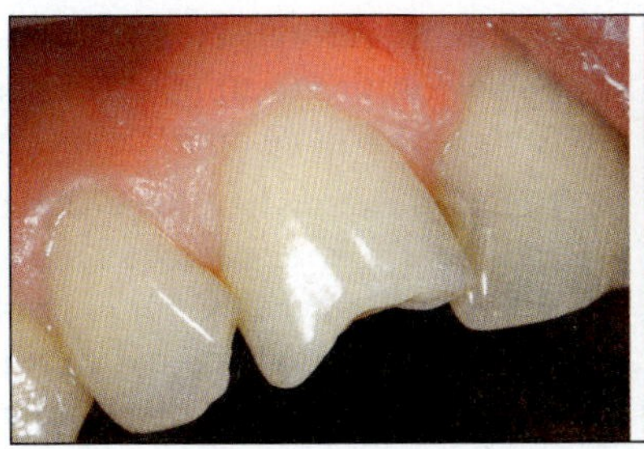
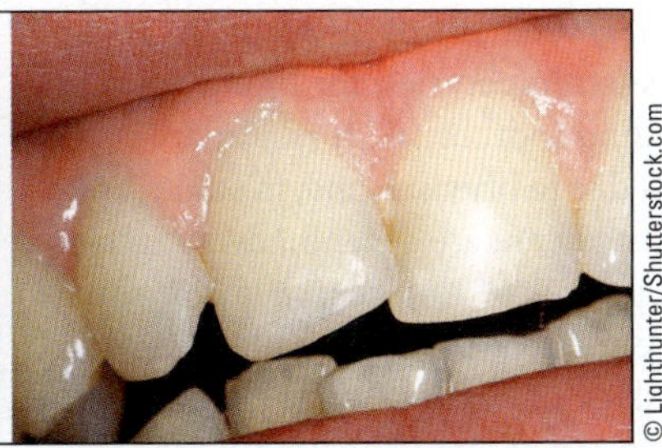

FIGURE 38-16

Before and after photos of a fractured anterior tooth (#8) that was restored with composite material.

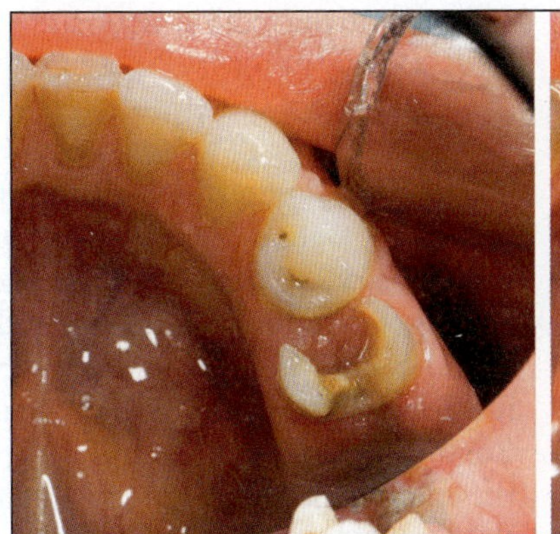
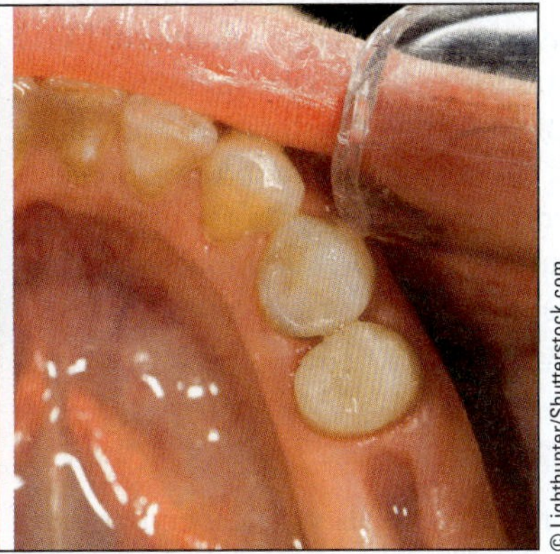

FIGURE 38-17

Before and after photos of a posterior tooth (#29MOD) that was restored with composite restorative material.

Composition

A **composite** restorative material is composed of the following components:

- An **organic polymer matrix**, such as dimethacrylate, identified as BIS-GMA or urethane dimethacrylates.
- Some **inorganic filler particles**, such as quartz, silica, and lithium aluminum silicate.
- An **organic silane-coupling agent**. The inorganic filler particles are treated with an organic silane-coupling agent to provide a bond between the inorganic fillers and the resin matrix.

Barium, strontium, zinc, or zirconium may be added to make the composite material more radiopaque.

The composites are classified according to the type, amount, and size of the filler particles, but all are referred to as composite resins. Composite particles come in fine, microfill, or combinations of the fine and microfill filler particles, which are called *hybrids*. The filler particles can make up as much as 84 percent of the composite material by volume.

- The **macrofilled composite** contains filler particles that range in size from 1 to 3 microns. These materials are used for Class IV restorations because they are strong enough to resist fracture and are esthetically pleasing. They do not polish to the same high finish as the microfill and the hybrids.
- The **microfill composite** contains fillers that range in size from 0.01 to 0.1 microns. They are used as a cosmetic filling material for Class III and V restorations. Microfills are also used for direct veneers and diastema closures. Some microfills are reinforced for Class IV restorations, and the occlusal portion of Class I and II restorations. Microfill composites are esthetic restorations that resist wear due to abrasion, and they polish well, leaving a high-luster finish.
- The **hybrid composite** is a combination of both macrofillers and microfillers. They contain more than one type of filler particles, usually glass and silica. The glass particles are in the 1- to 3-micron range, and the silica is around 0.04 microns. These composites are stronger and less likely to fracture in high-stress areas than the microfill composites. The hybrids combine the strength and esthetics of the other composites to make a restoration that is strong and polishable. They are used in both the anterior and the posterior areas of the mouth.

Flowable Composites. A **flowable composite** is similar to the microfill and hybrid composites in filler content and particle size. It has a low viscosity that allows for an easy flow, direct application into cavity preparations by small syringe tips. Flowable composites can adapt to the irregularities of cavity walls and flow into narrow preparations of conservative dentistry. It has many uses, such as linings for large cavity preparations; as additives to temporaries; for filling voids in non-carious areas, including toothbrush abrasion areas, or areas of occlusal tooth loss due to bruxism; and, in some cases, as a pit and fissure sealant. There are several advantages of flowable composites: they are easy to place, they can reach small areas, and they are esthetic with many shades available. Disadvantages include a lack of strength, they shrink more than hybrid composites, and they cannot be used alone to fill large preparations (Figure 38-18).

Packable Composites. The **packable composite** is sometimes called a **condensable composite**. They are more putty-like and stiffer in consistency than other composites, and they are highly viscous and contain large amounts of fillers. They are used in posterior areas for core buildups, and in places requiring a resistant, stronger restoration. Packable composites can be pressed into the restoration in layers. Sometimes, various types of composite are layered for optimum results. Packable composites are not subject to as much shrinkage when polymerized as certain other composites because they contain less resin and more filler.

Composite Properties

Properties of composite resin materials vary depending on the type and size of the filler. These aspects of the composites are constantly being improved for a strong, esthetic, long-lasting restoration. Overall, composites exhibit the following properties:

- Resistance to fracturing.
- Occlusal wear resistance is improving.
- Good esthetics for matching the tooth structure .
- Some composites are radiopaque, making them more visible on radiographic film.
- Composites bond efficiently to dentin and enamel in the cavity preparation, unlike amalgam where the cavity preparation is designed to hold or retain the amalgam in place.
- Composites are often placed in layers to reduce the effect of polymerization (setting) shrinkage. See Chapter 30, Dental Sealants, for more information on polymerization.
- Composite resins have adequate strength for specific applications. The strength requirement varies for various classifications of cavities. For example, the anterior Class III and V cavities do not require great strength but do require color stability. The posterior Class I and II must exhibit enough strength to withstand occlusal stresses, but appearance is not as critical. All composite restorations require a smooth finish to reduce the potential for plaque and debris accumulation, and for staining.
- Expansion and contraction rates of composite materials are similar to the tooth structure.

Manipulation Considerations

To bond the composite material and tooth structure, the cavity preparation is acid etched for 30 to 60 seconds. The etchant is rinsed completely and the surface is dried. After etching, the tooth has a chalky, dull appearance. Adhesion of the composite to the etched surface is rated high, but it can be further improved by the use of a bonding agent. Bonding agents are applied as described previously to both the enamel and the dentin. The composite then adheres to the bonding agent.

Shrinkage of composites can be minimized by placing the composite in small layers in the cavity preparation. After each layer is placed, it is light cured into a hardened form. Layering of the composite is also a method to modify the restoration shade. The layers can be composed of various types of composites with diverse properties to enhance the qualities of the material.

Composites are mainly packaged as one-paste systems that are light cured. The paste may come in a syringe for multiple applications or in single-dose cartridges that are used with a syringe (Figure 38-19). The pastes also come in a variety of shades. A specific shade guide comes with composite systems

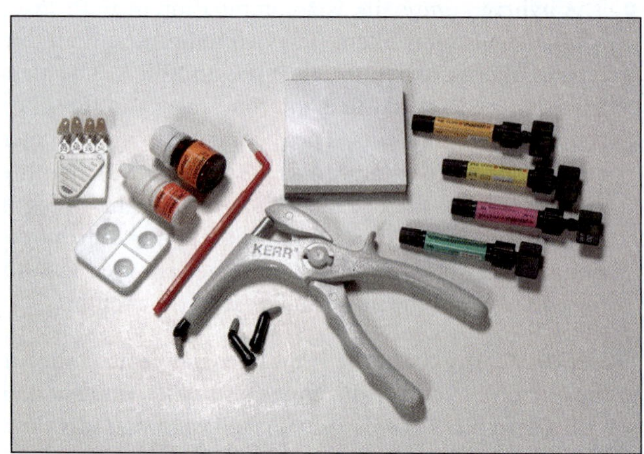

FIGURE 38-18

A flowable composite system.

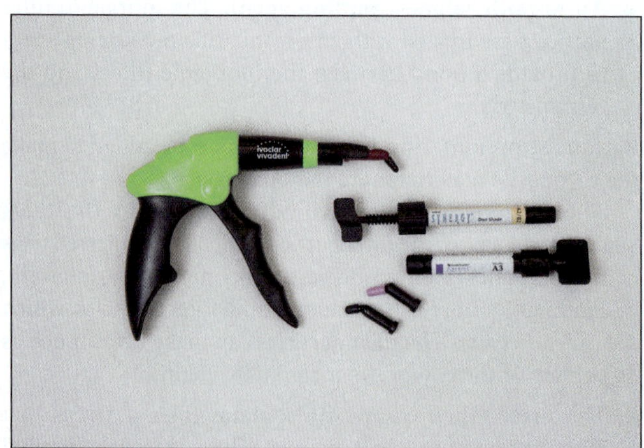

FIGURE 38-19

Composite material dispensing units including syringes and tips and individual cartridges and a dual-clicker dispenser.

to assist in the selection of a shade that matches the patient's natural dentition.

The pulp can be protected with a cavity liner before the etching, bonding, and composite placement steps.

Often, a plastic or Teflon-tipped filling instrument is used to place and shape the composite. These instruments come in various sizes and shapes, which aid in adapting the composite material to the cavity preparation.

A shade guide is always used when selecting the composite material. Determine the shade with the patient in natural light (Figures 38-20A and B). Use the designated shade guide for the material being placed, or use the VITA Shade Guide, which is a universally accepted shade guide.

Modifications

Procedure 38-3 is for a Class III restoration. Some modifications to the procedure may be required for Classes I, II, IV, and V. Most of the procedures are similar, but there are a few changes or considerations.

Classes I and II. Classes I and II are posterior restorations. Shade selection is not as critical with these restorations as it is with the anterior classes. The Class I restoration does not require a matrix, because only the occlusal surface is involved. For Class II restorations, some operators prefer the clear matrix band, which is used with a retainer and wedges, which facilitate the light-curing process.

Some anatomy may be carved into the composite before the final curing. Discs may be difficult to use in some areas, but diamonds, finishing burs, and polishing points are used to smooth and finish the restoration.

Class IV. Class IV anterior restorations involve the proximal surface and incisal edge. In some cases, retention pins are required because of the amount of lost tooth structure. The pins are positioned once the tooth is prepared, and before the placement of the composite material.

A matrix strip or preformed celluloid crown can be used to mold the composite (Figure 38-21). If the celluloid crown form is used, the dentist places the composite into the cavity preparation in layers, curing after each step. A crown form is partially filled and placed over the cured resin in the preparation to form the incisal angle of the restoration. The crown form is prepared with a small hole placed into the incisal edge to prevent air from being trapped. Excess material is removed, and the curing light is used to harden the composite.

After the material is cured, the crown form is removed and the final shaping and finishing are completed with finishing burs, polishing discs, and strips.

Class V. A Class V, gingival, one-third restoration may not require a matrix strip. A pre-contoured matrix may be used, or a matrix may not be used at all. The restorative materials can be placed in the cavity preparation, shaped with a plastic or composite filling instrument, and then light cured. Finishing should be minimal with these restorations.

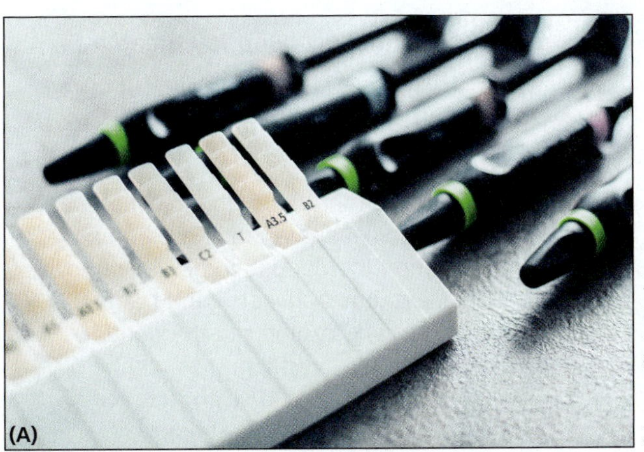

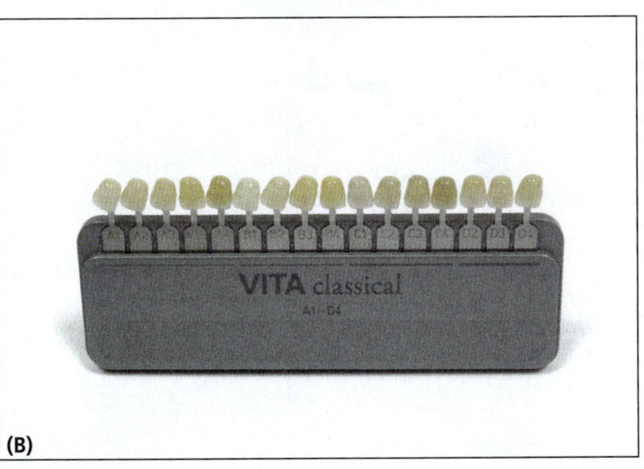

FIGURE 38-20

(A) A shade guide that came with the composite material. (B) The VITA Shade Guide.

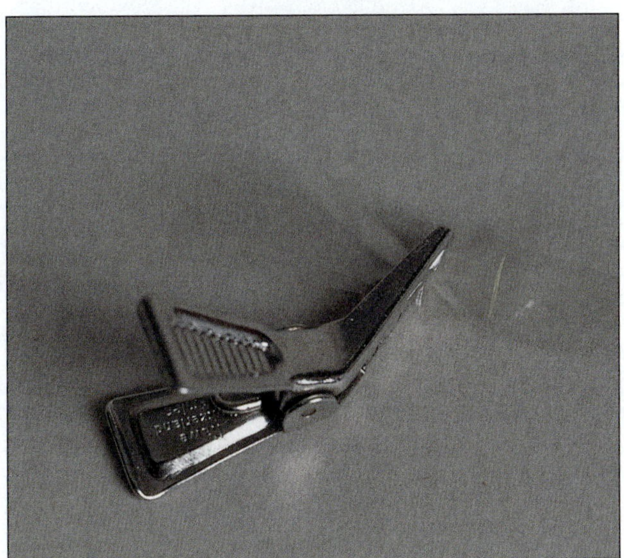

FIGURE 38-21

A celluloid matrix strip with metal clip.

Procedure 38-3
Composite Restoration—Class III

   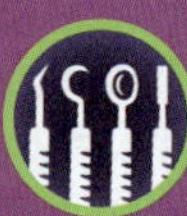

This procedure is completed by the dentist and dental assistant. The tooth is prepared with the dental handpiece and assorted burs. Once the tooth is prepared, it is restored with composite.

Equipment and Supplies (*Figure 38-22*)

- Basic setup: mouth mirror, explorer, and cotton pliers
- Air–water syringe tip, HVE tip, and saliva ejector
- Cotton rolls, gauze sponges, cotton pellets, cotton-tip applicators, and dental floss
- Topical and local anesthetic setup
- Rubber dam setup
- High- and low-speed handpieces
- Assortment of dental burs (including diamond and cutting burs)
- Spoon excavator
- Hand-cutting instruments (dentist's choice may include binangle chisel and Wedelstaedt chisel)
- Base and liner with mixing materials and placement instruments
- Bonding materials
- Etchant and applicator, if necessary (usually comes with the composite system)
- Primer (usually comes with the composite system)
- Composite materials, including a shade guide
- Composite placement instrument (plastic filling instrument)
- Curing light with protective shield
- Celluloid matrix strip and wedges
- Locking pliers or hemostat
- Finishing burs or diamonds
- #12 scalpel (optional)
- Abrasive strips
- Polishing discs
- Lubricant
- Articulating paper and forceps

Procedure Steps (*Follow aseptic procedures*)

1. The patient is seated and prepared for the procedure. Confirm the procedure and review the medical history.
2. Rinse the patient's mouth, dry the injection site, and place the topical anesthetic (EF). Prepare the syringe. When the dentist comes in, remove the topical anesthetic applicator and transfer the mouth mirror and explorer to the dentist.

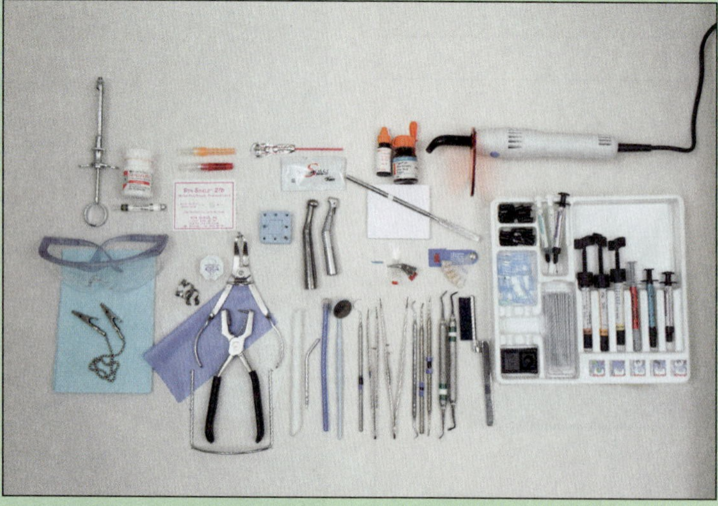

FIGURE 38-22

A composite procedure tray setup.

(continues)

Procedure 38-3 (continued)

After receiving the mirror and explorer, transfer a 2 × 2 inch gauze to the dentist and then transfer the anesthetic syringe. While following the administration of the local anesthetic, rinse the patient's mouth.

3. The shade is determined for the composite material before the placement of the rubber dam (Figure 38-23). Under natural light, the dentist compares a shade guide to the patient's teeth. A shade, or a combination of shades, is selected to match the patient's teeth as closely as possible. The shade is recorded on the patient's chart for future reference.
4. The dental dam is placed by the dental assistant, or with the dental assistant helping the dentist.
5. Transfer a mirror, high-speed handpiece, and bur to the dentist. Maintain visibility throughout the procedure by cleaning the mirror, retracting the tissues, and evacuating the area. During the cavity preparation, transfer instruments and change burs as indicated by the dentist.
6. When the cavity preparation is complete, rinse and dry the preparation. Proximity of the pulp to the cavity preparation determines the type of base or liner needed for protection. Mix the appropriate materials, usually a calcium hydroxide or glass ionomer liner, and hold the mixing pad, applicator, and 2 × 2 inch gauze near the patient's chin. After each application, wipe the instrument. If the materials need the curing light to cure, it is prepared and positioned.

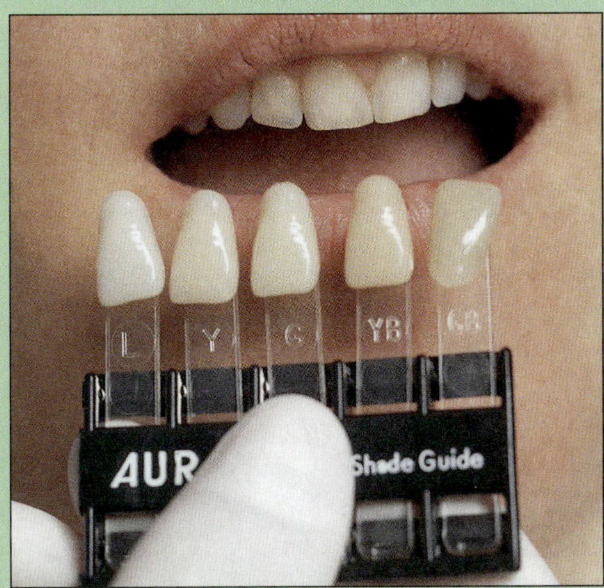

FIGURE 38-23
Determining a shade before the procedure begins.

7. Transfer a syringe, brush, or applicator tip containing the acid etching materials to the dentist, who applies it to the cavity preparation. The etchant is rinsed thoroughly after the recommended time.
8. The celluloid matrix strip is placed by the dentist. If required, a plastic wedge is also placed. The plastic wedges permit light curing of the bonding agent and the composite.
9. The bonding material is placed according to the manufacturer's instructions. With some bonding resins, a **primer** or conditioner is placed before the bonding material.
10. Most composites are applied with a single-application syringe, which can be used to place the material directly into the cavity preparation. Sometimes, a composite placement instrument is used for the placement. The matrix is held around the tooth to restore contour. If the material is light cured, it is placed in incremental layers, and then light cured after each layer is placed. The self-curing composites are mixed and placed in the cavity preparation. Within a few minutes, the material begins to chemically set.
11. Transfer cotton pliers to remove the wedge and the matrix strip. After receiving these items, an explorer is transferred to check the restoration.
12. Transfer the low-speed handpiece with finishing bur to the dentist. When the dentist is using the handpiece, use the air syringe. Finishing burs, diamonds, and abrasive discs may be used to finish the composite restoration. Abrasive strips may be used to smooth the interproximal areas. Composite polishing points, discs, and cups are then used to smooth the restoration (Figure 38-24).
13. The dental dam is carefully removed and the oral cavity is rinsed.
14. Transfer the mirror and explorer to the dentist for examination, dry the tooth, receive the mirror and explorer, and pass the articulating paper. The occlusion is checked and any high marks are removed. The patient's mouth is rinsed and the patient is given postoperative instructions (Figure 38-25).

(continues)

Procedure 38-3 (continued)

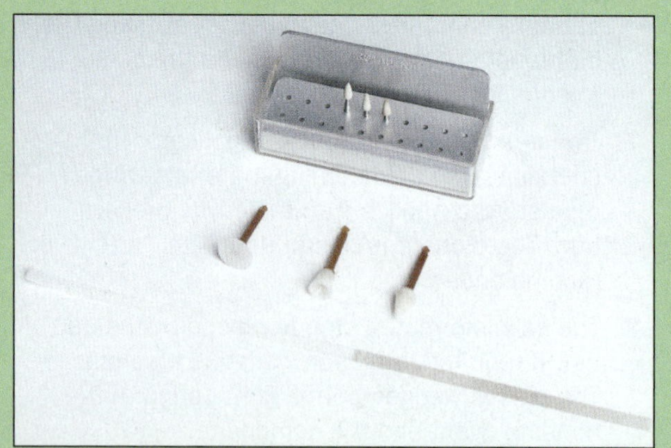

FIGURE 38-24

Polishing burs and an abrasive strip for composites.

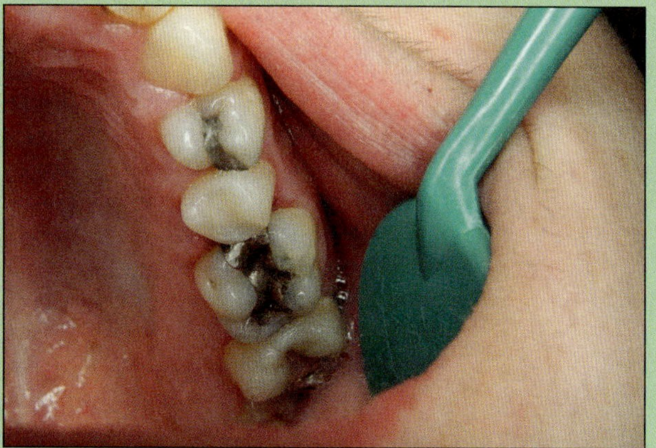

FIGURE 38-25

A completed composite restoration on maxillary second bicuspid.

Glass Ionomer Restorations

Glass ionomer materials are used as an esthetic restoration most often in non-stress-bearing restorations (Figure 38-26). Examples include Class I, (both stress and non-stress-bearing areas), II (non-stress-bearing areas), and V (non-stress-bearing areas). Class V includes restoring the gingival one-third, and root surface cavities. These materials are often used in pediatric and geriatric restorations, sealants, long-term temporaries, and core buildups. Glass ionomers bond well by adhering chemically to the tooth structure. Upon setting these materials, release fluoride on the finished preparation, to resist recurrent decay. The materials have low solubility; therefore the tooth does not have to be totally dry. They are available in multi-shades, are radiopaque, and come in powder/liquid and capsules.

Hybrid (or Resin-Modified) Glass Ionomers

The combination of composite resins and glass ionomers has improved the quality of glass ionomer restorations. They are used for Class III and V restorations. They come in various shades and are light-cured materials.

The technique for placement is similar to that for composites, with the following exceptions: The tooth is conservatively prepared with no need for mechanical retention or bevels. A retraction cord may be placed with the Class V preparations to expose the entire margin of the cavity preparation. The preparation is cleaned with a chlorhexidine soap solution. Follow the manufacturer's directions on the finishing and polishing of the restoration. Some need

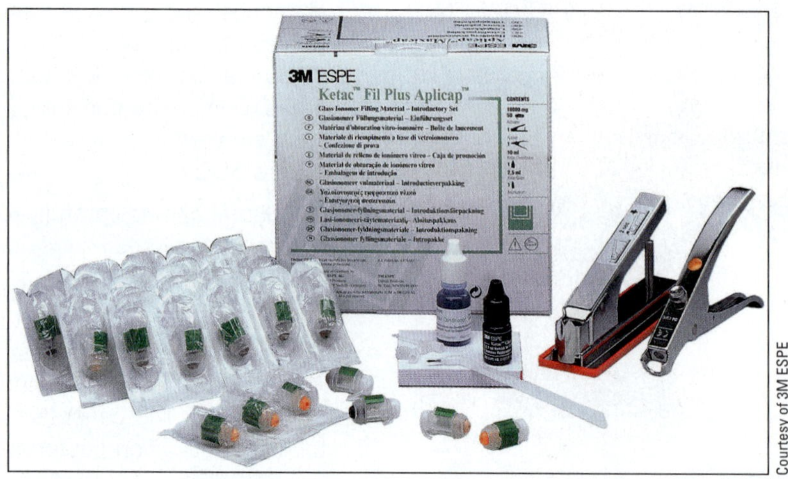

Courtesy of 3M ESPE

FIGURE 38-26

A glass ionomer restorative material kit.

to be kept moist or have lubricants placed when polishing. A layer of light-cured enamel bonding agent is applied over the finished restoration.

Compomers

Compomers are a cross between composites and glass ionomers in characteristics and properties. They are single-paste, light-cured systems that release fluoride, and are bonded to the walls of the cavity with dentin or enamel adhesives. Compomers are mostly used on all types of restorations for primary teeth, and on Class III and V restorations for permanent teeth. They adhere to dentin without etching the tooth, but a primer or adhesive must be used (Figure 38-27).

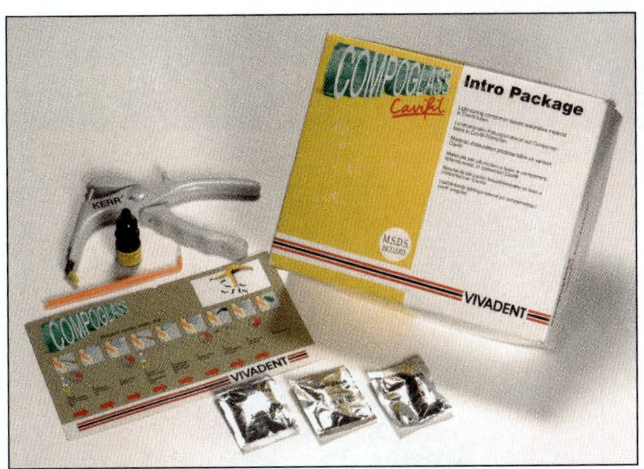

FIGURE 38-27

A compomer restorative material kit.

Advanced Chairside Functions

Matrix and Wedge

During the preparation of a tooth for an amalgam or a composite restoration, often, one or more axial surfaces are removed. Once these surfaces are removed, the only way to restore the tooth is to have an artificial wall in place of the missing wall or surface. This wall holds the restorative materials in the preparation during the filling of the cavity. A matrix replaces the surface and acts as the artificial wall.

The **matrix** is a collective term used to refer to the matrix **band** and the **retainer**. The matrix band forms the missing surface or wall, and reestablishes the normal contour of the prepared tooth while the tooth is being filled with the restorative material. The matrix band is inserted into the retainer and then placed on the tooth. The retainer is the device that holds the band. It is tightened on the tooth and secures the band in place.

In addition to replacing the missing tooth surface of the cavity preparation, the matrix restores the natural contours of the tooth and the proximal contact with the adjacent tooth. A matrix also contains the restorative material within the walls, thereby preventing any excess material from getting near the gingiva. In addition, the matrix must be stable enough to withstand the pressure of the restorative material being placed in the cavity preparation.

Matrices

Several different matrices are available, and the type of matrix selected depends on the type of restorative materials being used. For amalgam restorations, the **Tofflemire matrix** or the **AutoMatrix** is used. With composite material, a **plastic strip matrix**, **shell matrix**, or a **sectional matrix system** is used.

Wedges

Once the matrix is in place, a wedge (a small, triangular piece of wood or plastic) is inserted interproximally against the matrix band or strip near the gingival margin of the preparation. This **wedge** holds the band securely in place and also prevents excess filling material from escaping between the tooth and the matrix band. This excess is called an *overhang*. An overhang can be damaging to the gingival tissues if left in place, so the correct positioning of the wedge is important in order to prevent this from occurring. The wedge also slightly separates the teeth to compensate for the thickness of the band. This ensures good contact with the adjacent tooth after the band has been removed.

Wedge Types. Wedges come in different sizes and are either natural wood, clear, or colored. The clear or transparent wedges are used with light-curing restorative materials. These wedges deflect light into the restoration to ensure a thoroughly cured material without marginal gaps. They usually come in an assortment kit with various sizes, with colors marking the different sizes (Figure 38-28). Some wedges can be altered in shape with a knife, if needed. Once the procedure is complete, the wedges are discarded.

Wedge Placement. Wedges are only used when the preparation includes a proximal surface(s). For example, if the tooth had a mesio-occlusal (MO) cavity preparation, only one wedge would be needed on the mesial. On the posterior teeth, either the wooden or plastic wedges can be used. On the anterior teeth, when light-cured materials are used, the plastic wedges are the best.

The wedges are usually placed from the lingual side on the posterior teeth. This makes placement easier and prevents interference with the retainer. Cotton pliers or a hemostat is used to place and remove the wedges. When placing the wedge, the smallest of the three sides is placed toward the gingiva. The wedge should fill the space and fit snugly (Figure 38-29A).

Tofflemire Matrix

The Tofflemire matrix is the most common matrix used for amalgam restorations. It has two parts: the retainer and the band (Figure 38-29B). The retainer can be sterilized and

Advanced Chairside Functions (Continued)

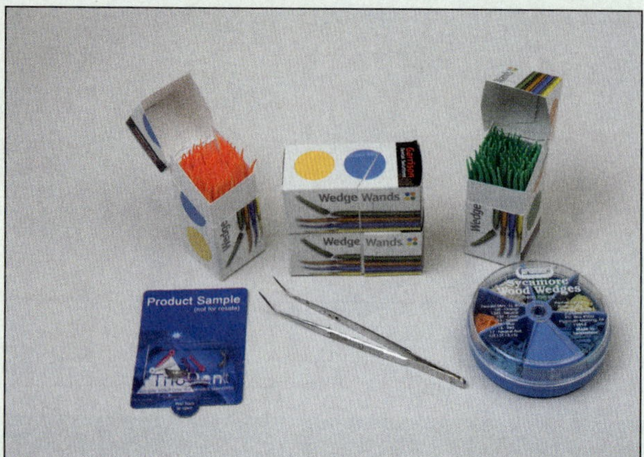

FIGURE 38-28
Assortment of wedges showing different sizes and types.

reused, but the bands are disposed of in the sharps container after the procedure.

Parts of the Tofflemire Matrix Retainer. Table 38-2 identifies the parts and functions of the Tofflemire matrix retainer. This retainer has a top (occlusal) side and a bottom (gingival) side. The occlusal side is directed toward the occlusal surface and is the smooth side of the guide channels and the vise. The gingival side is directed toward the gingival tissues and has the diagonal slot on the vise and the open ends of the guide channels. Assembly of the matrix is outlined in Procedures 38-7 and 38-8.

Tofflemire Retainer Styles. The Tofflemire retainer is available in several styles so that it can be positioned from either the lingual or the facial surfaces. The straight Tofflemire retainer is the most commonly used, and it is placed on the buccal or facial side, while the **contra-angle** Tofflemire retainer is placed on the lingual surface. It is angled slightly to accommodate the clearance of the anterior teeth (Figure 38-30).

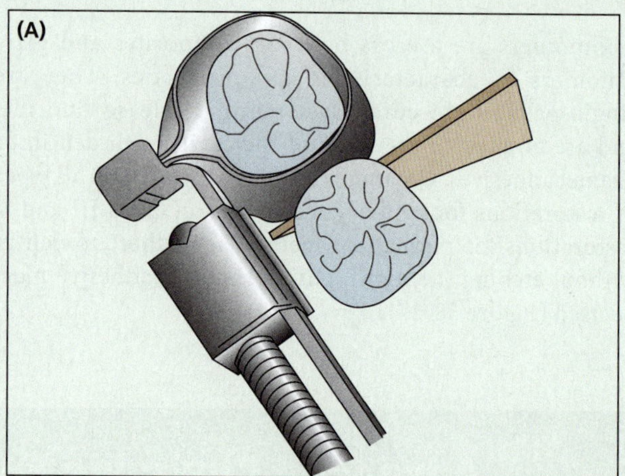

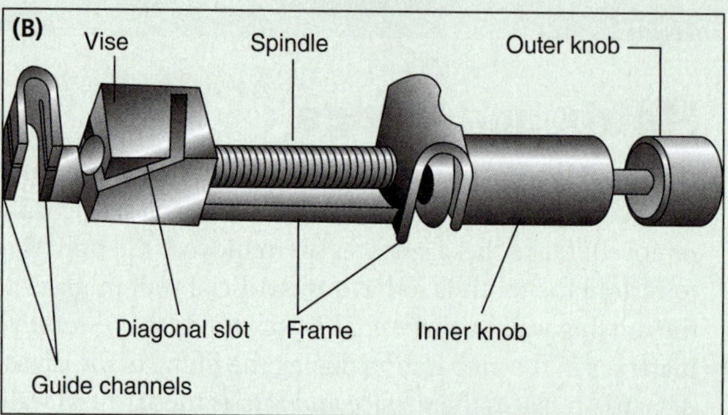

FIGURE 38-29
(A) Occlusal aspect of the Tofflemire matrix with a wedge in place. (B) Parts of a straight Tofflemire retainer: guide channels, vise, diagonal slot, spindle, inner knob, outer knob, and frame.

Matrix Bands

Matrix bands are made of stainless steel and are approximately all the same length. They differ in the shape of one edge and their widths (Figure 38-31). The size and shape of the cavity prep indicate which band is used. The more the prep extends toward the gingiva, the wider the matrix band needs to be. The matrix band is slightly curved, and when it is looped over so that both ends meet, the small **circumference** edge faces toward the gingiva, and the larger circumference edge faces toward the occlusal surface.

TABLE 38-2 Components of the Tofflemire Matrix Retainer

Part	Function
Frame	Main body of retainer.
Guide channels	Slots on the end of the retainer that hold the matrix band. The slots direct the band to the right or left of the retainer.
Vise (locking)	Holds the ends of the matrix band in place, in the diagonal slot.
Spindle	A screw-like rod used to secure the band in the vise.
Inner knob (adjusting knob)	Adjusts the size of the matrix band loop by moving the vise along the retainer frame.
Outer knob (locking knob)	Tightens and loosens the spindle against the band in the vise.

Advanced Chairside Functions

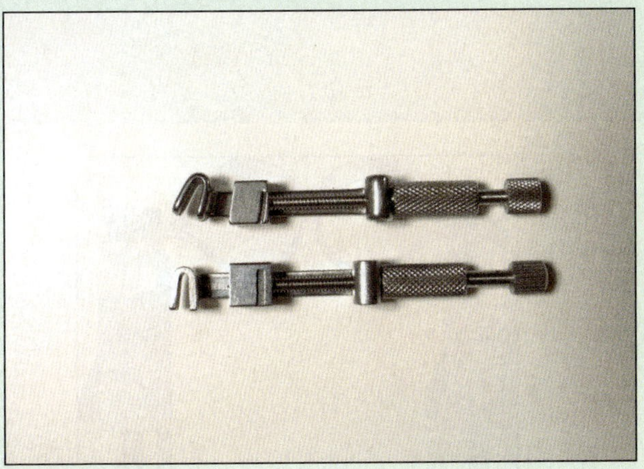

FIGURE 38-30

Top: Contra-angle Tofflemire retainer (note the angle of the guide channel section). Bottom: Straight Tofflemire retainer.

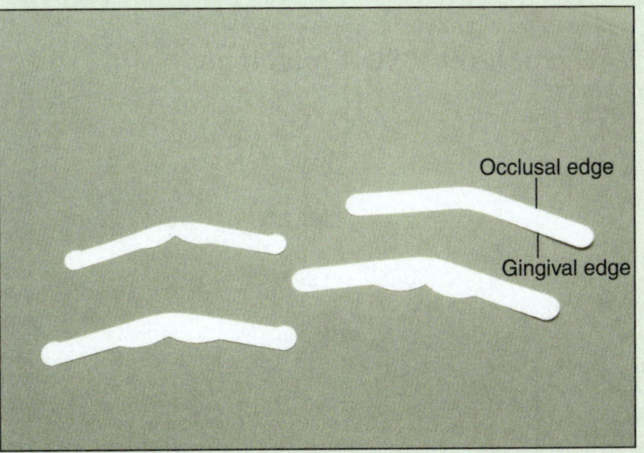

FIGURE 38-31

Examples of various matrix bands. The extension of cavity preparation determines the width of the band selection. The gingival and occlusal edge on the matrix band is shown.

- Hold the retainer with the guide channels and diagonal slot on the vise facing the operator.
- Keep the guide channels and the vise within 1/4 inch of each other.
- The looped matrix band correlates to the shape of the tooth, with the smaller circumference at the gingiva and the larger circumference at the occlusal.

Procedure 38-4
Assembly of the Tofflemire Matrix

This procedure is performed by the dentist or dental assistant. The assembly is completed before the procedure begins.

Equipment and Supplies

- Tofflemire retainer
- Assortment of matrix bands

Procedure Steps (*Follow aseptic procedures*)

1. Hold the retainer so that the guide channels and the diagonal slot on the vise are facing the operator.
2. Holding the frame of the retainer, rotate the inner knob (adjustment knob) until the vise is within ¼ inch of the guide channels.
3. Turn the outer knob (locking knob) until the pointed end of the spindle is clear (below) of the slot in the vise.
4. Prepare the matrix band for placement in the retainer by holding the band to look like a smile, with the gingival edge on the top and the occlusal edge on the bottom.
5. Bring the ends together to form a teardrop-shaped loop (Figure 38-32). Be careful not to crease the band at any time. The larger circumference of the

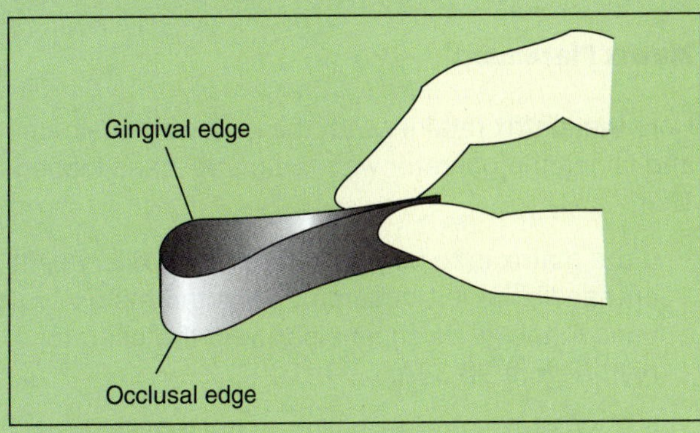

FIGURE 38-32

Hold the matrix band in a smile and loop the ends of the band together. The smaller circumference, the gingival edge, will be on the top, and the larger circumference, the occlusal edge, will be on the bottom.

(continues)

Advanced Chairside Functions (Continued)

Procedure 38-4 (continued)

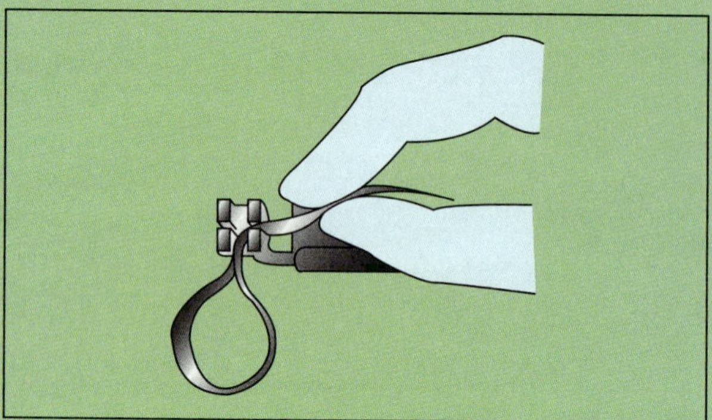

FIGURE 38-33
Hold the Tofflemire retainer with the guide channels and slot facing up, and insert the matrix band into the vise slot and guide channels.

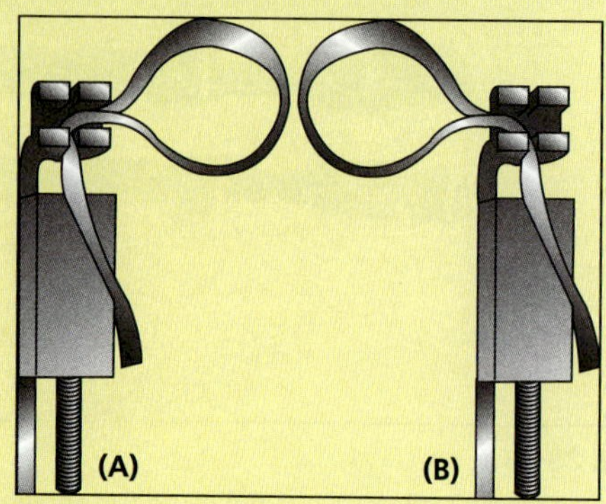

FIGURE 38-34
Two matrix bands are positioned in guide channels for the quadrants. (A) Maxillary right/mandibular left. (B) Maxillary left/mandibular right.

band, the occlusal edge will be on the bottom, and the smaller the circumference, the gingival edge, will be on the top.

6. With the gingival edge still on the top, place the occlusal edge of the band in the diagonal slot of the vise. The loop is extended toward the guide channels.
7. Place the matrix band in the appropriate guide channels. The direction of the matrix band depends on the tooth being restored (Figure 38-33).
8. Once the band is placed in the vise slot with the guide channels, turn the outer knob until the tip of the spindle is tight against the band in the vise slot (Figure 38-35A).
9. Move the inner knob to increase or decrease the size of the loop to match the diameter of the tooth (Figure 38-35B).
10. If the band becomes creased or bent during the assembly, it can be smoothed out by inserting the handle of the mouth mirror into the loop and running it around the inside of the loop (similar to curling ribbon when wrapping a gift).

Matrix Placement

Hold the matrix retainer with the guide channels up and facing the operator with the matrix band looped. Then:

- If the matrix is to be applied to the maxillary right or mandibular left quadrant, place the matrix band in the guide channels toward the operator's right (Figure 38-34A).
- If the matrix is to be applied to the maxillary left or mandibular right quadrant, place the matrix band in the guide channels toward the operator's left (Figure 38-34B).

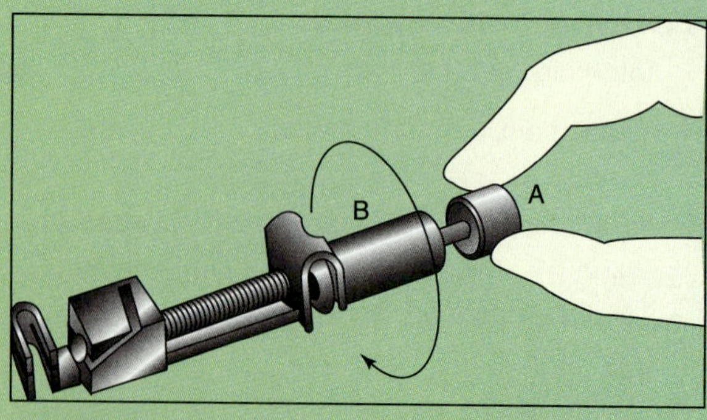

FIGURE 38-35
(A) By turning the outer knob of the Tofflemire retainer, the band will be secured. (B) By turning the inner knob of the Tofflemire retainer, the matrix band loop increases and decreases in size.

Advanced Chairside Functions

Procedure 38-5
Placement of the Tofflemire Matrix

This procedure is performed by the dentist or dental assistant. After the Tofflemire matrix is assembled, it is ready for positioning on the prepared tooth.

Equipment and Supplies (*Figure 38-36*)

- Assembled Tofflemire retainer and matrix band
- Cotton pliers or hemostat
- Ball burnisher
- 2 × 2 inch gauze sponges
- Assortment of wedges

Procedure Steps (*Follow aseptic procedures*)

1. Place the matrix band over the prepared tooth with the smaller edge of the band toward the gingiva. The slot on the vise is directed toward the gingiva. Keep the retainer parallel to the buccal surface as the loop is placed around the tooth.
2. Move the loop through the interproximal surface. Place one finger over the loop to stabilize the loop and the retainer.
3. Once the matrix band is around the tooth, adjust the guide channel to center the retainer on the buccal surface of the tooth (Figure 38-37).
4. Turn the inner knob to tighten the band around the tooth. The band should be securely around the tooth, and the retainer should be snug to the tooth. If the band is too tight or too loose, the contour of the restoration may change the contours of the tooth and the proximal contact.
5. Check the margins of the matrix band. The band should extend no more than 1 to 1.5 mm beyond the gingival margin of the cavity preparation on the gingival edge; and the occlusal edge should extend no more than 2 mm above the highest cusp (Figure 38-38).
6. To ensure contact with the adjacent teeth, the band needs to be contoured. To accomplish this, use a ball burnisher. Place the burnisher on the inner surface of the band and apply pressure until the band becomes slightly concave at the contact area.
7. Once the matrix band has been placed on the tooth, a wedge(s) is (are) placed to stabilize the band at the gingival margin of the preparation. (Refer to the Wedges section of this chapter for placement suggestions.)
8. Check the seal at the gingival margin of the preparation with an explorer. There should be no gap between the band and the preparation.

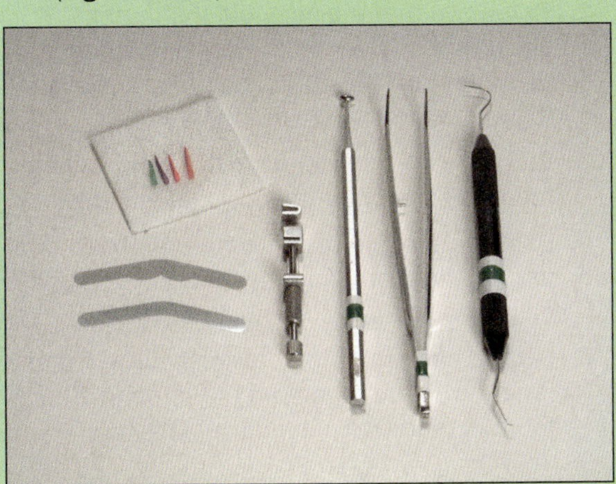

FIGURE 38-36

The materials needed for the placement of the Tofflemire matrix.

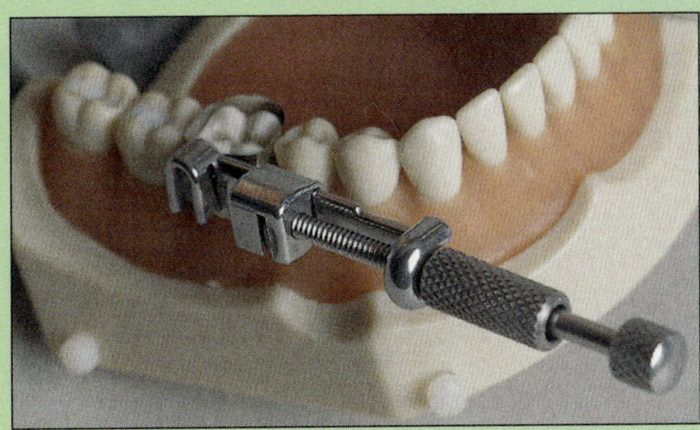

FIGURE 38-37

Placing the Tofflemire retainer with a matrix band on a tooth, and centering the retainer on the buccal surface of the tooth.

(continues)

Advanced Chairside Functions (Continued)

Procedure 38-5 (continued)

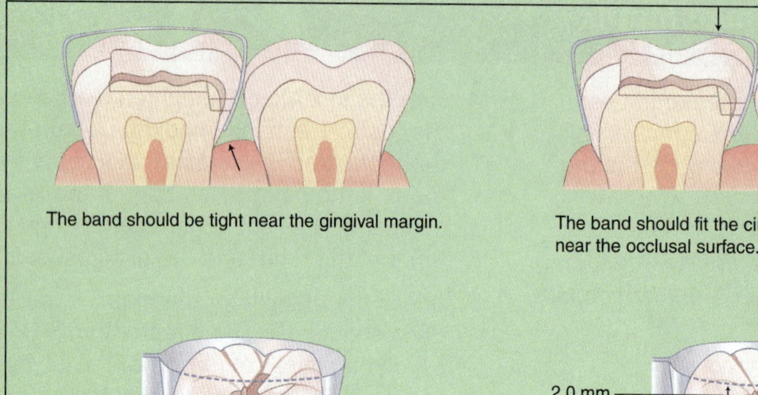

The band should be tight near the gingival margin.

The band should fit the circumference of the tooth near the occlusal surface.

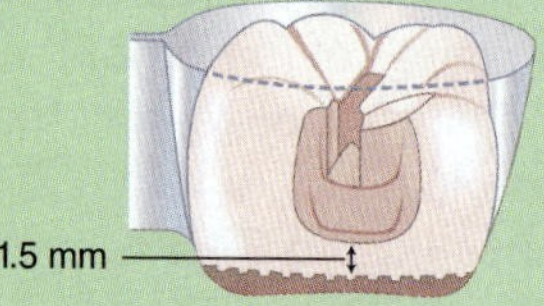

The band should extend 1.0 to 1.5 mm beyond the cavity preparation near the gingiva.

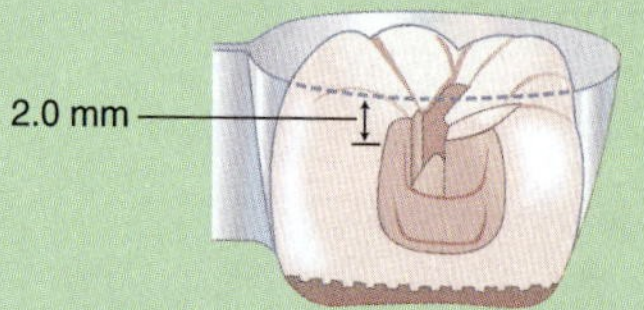

The band should extend no more than 2 mm above the cusp of the tooth and occlusal ridge.

FIGURE 38-38

Criteria for correctly placing a matrix band.

Procedure 38-6
Removal of the Wedge and Tofflemire Matrix

This procedure is performed by the dentist with assistance by the dental assistant. Once the tooth has been filled with restorative material, the matrix and wedge are removed to finish carving the anatomy of the tooth.

Equipment and Supplies

- Cotton pliers or hemostat
- 2 × 2 inch gauze

Procedure Steps (*Follow aseptic procedures*)

1. To remove the wedge, use cotton pliers or a hemostat. Grasp the wedge at the base and pull in the opposite direction of the insertion.
2. To remove the retainer, hold the matrix in place with a finger on the occlusal surface, and then turn the outer knob of the retainer to loosen the spindle in the vise.
3. Separate the retainer from the band by lifting the retainer toward the occlusal surface.
4. Using cotton pliers, gently free the band from around the tooth, and then lift one end of the band in a lingual-occlusal direction.
5. Lift the band from the proximal surface and repeat with the other end of the band. The tooth is ready for the final carving.

Advanced Chairside Functions

AutoMatrix

The AutoMatrix is a matrix without a retainer. The stainless steel bands are conical shaped and come in four sizes. The conical shape makes the band easy to **burnish** (smooth) for better contact in proximal areas. The bands are circles with autolock loops that lock the matrices on the teeth. The tightening coil on the outside of the band is where the matrix is adapted to the tooth. There is no retainer to obstruct the operator's access or vision. The AutoMatrix comes in a kit that contains clipping pliers, a tightening device, and bands in assorted sizes (Figure 38-39).

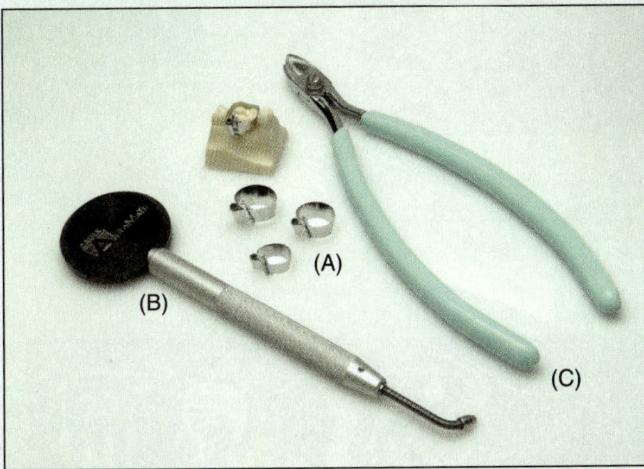

FIGURE 38-39
AutoMatrix kit including (A) matrix with coil, (B) tightening device, (C) removal pliers.

To place the AutoMatrix, position the matrix on the tooth following the same criteria as with the Tofflemire. Place the tightening device in the coil and rotate the handle to tighten the band around the tooth. Once the matrix is securely on the tooth, place the wedges as needed. To remove the AutoMatrix, remove the wedges and then, using the removal pliers, clip the end of the autolock loop. The pliers have a plastic cover to catch the ends of the loop as they fall after being cut. Open the matrix and slide it toward the buccal or lingual sides while pulling it occlusally.

Plastic Strip Matrix

The thin, transparent, strip matrix is used with composite, glass ionomer, or compomer restorative materials on the anterior teeth (see Procedures 38-10 and 38-11). The strip can be made of nylon, acetate, celluloid, or resin, and is approximately three inches long and three-eighths inch wide. The functions of the strip matrix are as follows:

- Provides an anatomical contour and proximal contact relation
- Prevents excess material at the gingival margin
- Confines the restorative material under pressure while the material is being cured
- Protects the restorative material from losing or gaining moisture during the setting time
- Allows the polymerizing light to reach the composite restorative material

Procedure 38-7
Placement of the Strip Matrix

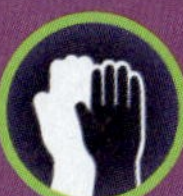

This procedure is performed by the dentist or dental assistant. After the tooth has been prepared, the strip matrix is placed.

Equipment and Supplies

- Strip matrix
- Cotton pliers
- Mouth mirror
- Assortment of clear wedges

Procedure Steps (*Follow aseptic procedures*)

1. Contour the strip by drawing the strip over the rounded edge of the handle of the mouth mirror. The procedure is the same here as it is with the Tofflemire matrix band.
2. Place the strip matrix between the teeth. Hold the strip tightly and slide toward the gingiva.
3. Adjust the position of the strip so that the entire preparation is covered by the strip.
4. Seat the wedge to secure the strip in place.
5. Restorative materials are placed and the strip matrix is pulled tightly around the tooth to adapt the material to the convex surface of the tooth.
6. The strip matrix is held in place by hand or with a clip retainer until the material has been cured (Figure 38-40).

(continues)

Advanced Chairside Functions (Continued)

Procedure 38-7 (continued)

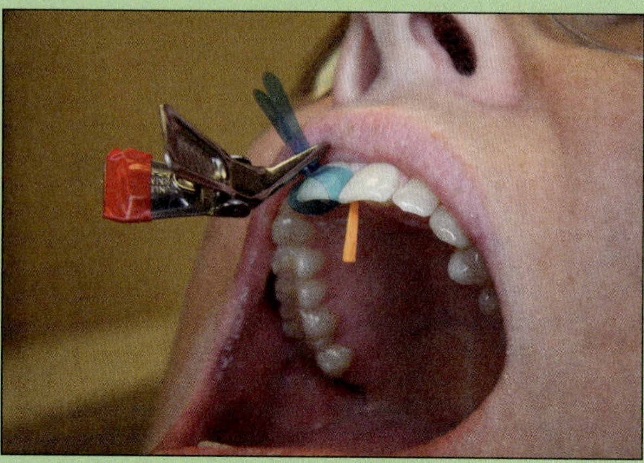

FIGURE 38-40
A strip matrix and wedges on a tooth.

Procedure 38-8
Removal of Strip Matrix

This procedure is performed by the dentist once the restorative material is placed and cured.

Equipment and Supplies

- Cotton pliers or hemostat
- 2 × 2 inch gauze sponges

Procedure Steps (*Follow aseptic procedures*)

1. Once the material has been cured and is completely hardened, remove the clip retainer if one was used. Then, remove the wedges with cotton pliers.
2. The strip matrix is gently pulled away from the restorative material.
3. Remove the matrix strip by pulling it in a lingual-incisal or facial-incisal direction.

Crown Matrix Form. The **crown matrix form** is a thin, plastic form that is shaped like the crown of a tooth. On anterior teeth, when the incisal edge is involved (Class IV restorations), a crown form is often used to restore the tooth. The crown forms come preformed in various designs and sizes. The restorative material is placed both in the cavity preparation and in the crown form. The crown form is then placed on the tooth. These crown forms are clear and can be used with light-cured materials. Once the restorative material is set, the crown form is removed and the tooth is ready for final contouring and finishing.

Sectional Matrix Systems

A sectional matrix system is most often used on Class II restorations to restore anatomical contacts. The matrix is stable and produces a tight contact with no overhangs. The system consists of oval matrix bands, rings to hold the matrix bands, and forceps to place the rings. The oval-shaped matrix bands are contoured and come in different sizes. They are slightly thicker than the Tofflemire bands. The rings are used to hold the matrix bands in place and usually come in two different sizes. The forceps are designed to open the rings for placement

Advanced Chairside Functions

and removal. They are like dental dam forceps except the ends are shorter, broader, and angled slightly for better retention.

A separate matrix band/ring is used for each surface, so on a mesio-occluso-distal (MOD) two-matrix bands/rings would be used. Placing the sectional matrix takes some practice, but once the procedure is learned it can be done quickly to produce a functional matrix. Wedges are used with this matrix system. They are usually placed after the band is placed and before the ring is positioned. The main function of the wedge with this system is to prevent gingival overhangs (Figure 38-41).

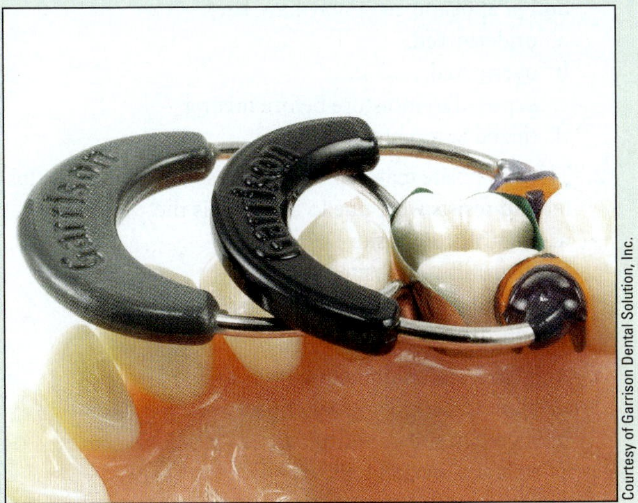

Courtesy of Garrison Dental Solution, Inc.

FIGURE 38-41
A sectional matrix system in place for a MOD restoration placement.

Chapter Summary

The general chairside assistant prepares restorative materials for the dentist to place in the prepared cavity. In some states dental assistants and/or hygienists are allowed to place restorative materials. The restorative dental assistant or restorative dental hygienist completes specific education including didactic and clinical training to become licensed to perform these skills.

Knowledge of the properties of restorative materials is necessary for the dental assistant to properly prepare and manipulate the materials, and also allows the dental assistant to be a step ahead of the dentist.

One expanded function included in this chapter is the placement and removal of a matrix when restoring a tooth. Several types of matrices are discussed including the Tofflemire, the AutoMatrix system, sectional matrix systems, and the plastic strip matrix. Matrices are used to contour, and hold the restorative materials in place. The dental assistant assembles and readies the matrix for placement, except in states that allow the dental assistant to place and remove the various matrices. The dental assistant gains knowledge of sequence and techniques in this chapter.

CASE STUDY

Charlotte Larson needs to replace several restorations in her maxillary molars. Over the years, she has had numerous amalgam restorations placed throughout her mouth. Although Charlotte has never had any trouble, she is concerned after reading articles about restorations containing mercury. She is also interested in more natural-looking restorations.

Case Study Review

1. List some of the concerns Charlotte may have read regarding restorations containing mercury.
2. What information could the dental assistant give to Charlotte in response to her concerns? What resources are available for information?
3. Are there any alternative restorative materials available for Charlotte?

Review Questions

Multiple Choice

1. If, after the amalgam has been triturated, it is crumbly and dull in appearance, it may have been
   a. undermixed.
   b. overmixed.
   c. exposed to moisture before mixing.
   d. mixed at too high a speed.
2. The composite material that finishes with the highest luster and resists wear due to abrasion is the
   a. fine-fill composite.
   b. microfill composite.
   c. hybrid composite.
   d. extra-course composite.
3. Amalgam is a combination of
   a. alloy and copper restorations.
   b. mercury and dental alloy.
   c. dental alloy and high-copper alloy.
   d. mercury and copper.
4. All of the following statements are true about the properties of amalgam except:
   a. Amalgam can withstand occlusal forces alone.
   b. Proper manipulation is important to overall strength.
   c. Amalgam is subject to dimensional change.
   d. Amalgam has the ability to creep.
5. The process of mixing amalgam is called
   a. trituration.
   b. amalgamation.
   c. polymerizing.
   d. both a and b.
6. ________ dominate the field of esthetic restorations.
   a. Composite restorations
   b. Dental amalgam restorations
   c. Glass ionomer restorations
   d. Resin-modified glass ionomer restorations
7. This type of composite contains a combination of fillers and are stronger.
   a. Macrofilled composites
   b. Hybrid composites
   c. Microfill composites
   d. None of the above
8. When is the shade taken when placing esthetic restorations?
   a. Before the procedure begins
   b. After the tooth has been prepared
   c. Before the bases and liners have been placed
   d. After the etchant and bonding agent have been placed
9. Once the matrix is placed, a(n) ________ is placed near the gingival margin of the preparation.
   a. overhang
   b. dental dam clamp
   c. AutoMatrix
   d. wedge
10. All of the following statements are true about the Tofflemire matrix *except:*
    a. This matrix consists of two parts, the retainer and the band.
    b. Adjustment is not possible.
    c. Bands are made of stainless steel.
    d. The retainer has guide channels in which to place the band.

Critical Thinking

1. Discuss the pros and cons of using amalgam as a restorative material.
2. How can pulp be protected when using a composite restorative material?
3. Discuss alternatives to composite restorations.
4. In your own words, describe how to assemble the band in the Tofflemire retainer.

Web Activities

1. To study the latest information about dental amalgam fillings, go to http://www.ada.org, *Public Resources*, Oral Health Topics.
2. Go to http://www.kerrdental.com to compare the types of composites.
3. Go to http://www.garrisondental.com to learn about matrix systems and composite instruments, and view product videos.

CHAPTER 39

Laboratory Materials and Techniques

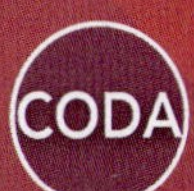

Specific Instructional Objectives

The student should strive to meet the following objectives and demonstrate an understanding of the facts and principles presented in this chapter:

1. Identify materials used in the dental laboratory and perform associated procedures.
2. Demonstrate the knowledge and skills needed to prepare, take, and remove alginate impressions and wax bites.
3. Demonstrate the knowledge and skills necessary to prepare reversible hydrocolloid impression material for the dentist.
4. Demonstrate the knowledge and skills necessary to prepare elastomeric impression materials such as polysulfide, silicone (polysiloxane and polyvinyl siloxanes), and polyether for the dentist.
5. Explain the process for debriding and disinfecting impressions, bite registrations, wax bites, and facebow registrations.
6. Demonstrate the knowledge and skills necessary to use gypsum products such as Type I, impression plaster; Type II, laboratory or model plaster; Type III, laboratory stone; Type IV, die stone; and Type V, high-strength die stone.
7. Demonstrate the knowledge and skills necessary to pour and trim a patient's alginate impression (diagnostic cast).
8. Identify use of a dental articulator and facebow for dental casts or study models.
9. Demonstrate taking a facebow transfer and mounting models on an articulator.
10. Identify various classifications and uses of waxes used in dentistry.
11. Demonstrate the knowledge and skills necessary to fabricate acrylic tray resin self-curing and light-curing custom trays, vacuum-formed trays, and thermoplastic custom trays.
12. Demonstrate the knowledge and skills necessary to contour prefabricated temporary crowns and to fabricate and fit custom temporary restorations.

Key Terms

accelerates (929)
articulator (945)
beading (921)
calcination (934)
catalyst (929)
centric relationship (948)
distortion (929)
exothermic reaction (935)
facebow (945)
gel (918)
gelatin time (918)
gypsum (934)
homogeneous (951)
imbibition (918)
irreversible hydrocolloid (918)
matrix (957)
monomer (950)
polymer (950)
polymerization (929)
polysulfide (929)
potassium alginate (918)
potassium titanium fluoride (918)
reversible hydrocolloid (928)
silicone (931)
sol (918)
study models (926)
syneresis (918)
thermoplastic (953)
undercuts (918)

Introduction

A number of materials that are used by dental assistants specifically in the dental laboratory are not used in the dental treatment room. Other materials are used initially in the treatment room and then taken by the dental assistant to the laboratory, where a second procedure is completed. Many models are taken to an in-office dental laboratory, where the laboratory technician completes the procedures, or the models are sent out to a commercial dental laboratory for additional procedures. It is always important to ensure that cross-contamination does not occur when working with laboratory materials. The dental assistant must pay special attention when taking materials from the treatment room to the dental laboratory.

Any dental assistant who has skills in performing laboratory duties is an asset to his or her employer. The better cross-trained the dental team members are, the better the dental office functions. A number of basic functions in the dental laboratory are routinely performed by the dental assistant, such as pouring and trimming study models, fabricating custom trays, and fabricating provisional temporaries. To accomplish these procedures, the dental assistant must understand the materials that are used, the properties of each material, and the steps in each procedure.

Hydrocolloid Impression Materials

Impressions are taken to produce an accurate three-dimensional duplicate of an individual's teeth and surrounding tissues. The impression makes a negative reproduction in which gypsum material can be poured and therefore creates a completed positive model. Varying degrees of accuracy can be obtained depending on the type of impression material and gypsum used. The operator gives directions to the dental assistant on the type of model that is desired. Models can be used for many purposes. One of the most common models that the dental assistant will make is the study cast or primary model. Normally, the impression material used is irreversible hydrocolloid, which is commonly called alginate.

Alginate (Irreversible Hydrocolloid) Impression Material

Alginate is a generic name used for a group of **irreversible hydrocolloid** impression materials. Alginate is used when less accuracy is needed. One of the most common areas in which alginate is used is in making diagnostic casts or study models. Alginate impression material is used routinely in making opposing models for fixed and removable prosthetics, orthodontic appliances, mouth guards, bleach trays, provisional restorations, and custom trays.

Alginate material's primary ingredient is **potassium alginate**, therefore giving the material its generic name. Potassium alginate is extracted from seaweed and kelp, which is a marine growth found primarily off the coastline of Japan. This material readily dissolves in water to form a viscous **sol** (liquid). Added to this potassium alginate is a calcium sulfate which, through a chemical reaction, forms a **gel** (solid). To control the setting time and allow for the material to be placed in a tray and into the patient's mouth, tri-sodium phosphate is added. Without this retarder, the material would be set before it could be inserted into the patient's mouth. A retarder slows the setting of the material. To increase the strength and stiffness and make up the bulk of the material, fillers are used. Some of the fillers that may be in alginate are diatomaceous earth, zinc oxide, color, and flavoring. The fillers constitute from one-half to three-quarters of the total composition of the material. A small amount of **potassium titanium fluoride** is added to the material to counteract a specific action of the alginate whereby it tends to soften the surface of the gypsum products and not allow it to fully set on the surface. Due to the particularly chalky taste, alginate may come in assorted flavors or liquid flavoring drops may be added during mixing.

Advantages and Disadvantages of Alginate. Alginate has a number of advantages that explain its extensive use in the dental office:

- Ease of manipulation
- Minimal equipment required
- Economical
- Meets the requirements for accuracy for a number of applications
- Rapid setting
- Comfort for the patient
- Can be used for both teeth and tissue impressions
- Withdraws over **undercuts** (recessed areas that are wider on the bottom than on the top) because of its elastic properties

The disadvantages of alginates primarily come from the loss of accuracy due to atmospheric conditions. If the impression is stored prior to pouring, it is susceptible to dimensional change due to loss or gain of water. If the impression loses water content due to heat, dryness, or exposure to air, it causes shrinkage. This condition is known as **syneresis** (sin-er-**EE**-sis). If the reverse happens and the impression takes on additional water and causes swelling, the impression will have a dimensional enlargement, known as **imbibition** (im-bah-**BIH**-shun). The material also can cause some tissue distortion or displacement due to its thickened consistency. Another disadvantage is that it is not as precise or accurate as some of the other materials on the market.

Setting Time for Alginate. The time from which the alginate powder material is mixed with water until it is completely set is called the **gelatin time**. The gelatin time is different depending on the type of material used. Most of the materials come in two types: Type I is a fast-set alginate and Type II is a regular-set alginate. The gelatin time for both is broken into two different increments. The first is the working time, where the dental assistant mixes the material to the desired consistency, loads it into the tray, and inserts and positions the tray into the patient's mouth. The working time for the regular set is approximately 1 minute and even less than that for the fast set. The second phase is the setting time, where the material remains in the patient's mouth and sets until the chemical reaction is completed, the gel is formed completely, and the tray is removed from the patient's mouth. The Type I gelatin time including both the working and setting times ranges from 1 to 2 minutes. The Type II gelatin time normally ranges from 2 to 4½ minutes including both working and setting times. The setting times can be altered. The most convenient way to control the setting time is to adjust the temperature of the water. The suggested temperature of water to be used is room temperature (70°F or 21°C). If the temperature of the water is higher, working and setting times are shorter. If the water is cooled, the working and setting times are longer. Warm weather causes the alginate to set more rapidly as well. Some offices refrigerate the water during hot humid times.

The choice of whether to use Type I or Type II is made according to the preference of the operator and the conditions of the patient needing the impression. The outcome of both materials is the same. Cases in which the slower Type II material is beneficial would be where the operator is working alone or the tray is going to be difficult to insert into the oral cavity in the correct position in the patient's mouth. The faster set, Type I, is beneficial where the patient is a child or where the patient has a problem with gagging and the tray needs to be removed as rapidly as possible for patient comfort.

Some alginates contain chromatic agents that cause the alginate to change color throughout the mixing and setting of the material. Once the powder is incorporated into the water, the alginate will be a bright pink or purple. The color will begin to fade to a lighter pink signaling the amount of time left to load the tray and seat it in the patient's mouth. Once seated, the alginate will fade completely white, indicating the complete set-time and removal from the patient's mouth.

Alginate Packaging, Storage, and Shelf Life. Normally, alginate is purchased in airtight plastic canisters the size of coffee cans (Figure 39-1). The powder may be inside, in a foil or plastic bag, to be placed in the mixing container when ready for use. Along with the powder are the measuring devices for the powder and the water. Some of the canisters have built-in areas on the outside for the water-measuring devices. This makes it convenient for the dental assistant. Alginate can be bought in premeasured sealed bags, but this is much more costly and normally unnecessary because measuring the powder is not a difficult procedure. Most dental offices currently use powder/water alginate.

It is important that alginate not be stored in an area that can have temperatures over 120°F because it causes loss of strength and lower resistance to deformation. If kept in an area where moisture can contaminate it, the material will demonstrate erratic setting times. Optimum storage is in a cool, dry place. Keeping the lid screwed tightly in place while not in use aids in prevention of unintentional moisture contamination. The normal shelf life for alginate materials is not more than 1 year.

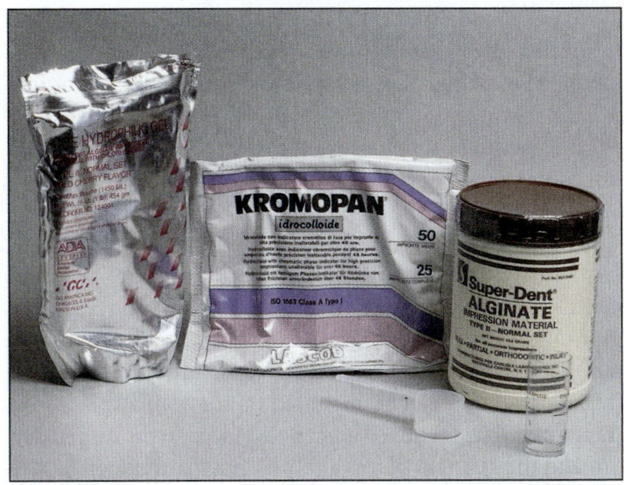

FIGURE 39-1
Foil bags and plastic canister of alginate with measuring devices.

Alginate Powder/Water Ratio. All the alginate materials come with their own specific measuring devices for both the powder and the water. First, read the manufacturer's directions for dispensing the material. The dispensing of each material may be slightly different. For instance, some of the materials direct that the powder be fluffed with the lid on prior to putting it into the powder scoop, while others may indicate that the powder should be packed into the scoop. This makes a definite difference regarding the amount of powder that is used. The water measure is normally a plastic cylinder with lines on it to indicate the amount of water for each scoop of powder. Normally, it takes two scoops of powder to two increments of water for each mandibular impression. Three of each are normally needed for the maxillary impression. (These amounts can change depending on the size of the patient's arches.)

It is important that the correct amounts of both powder and water are used. If a lower water-to-powder ratio transpires, a stiffer, thicker mix is produced. Along with being more difficult to use, the material has decreased detail, decreased ability to pull from undercuts, decreased flexibility, increased tissue displacement, rapid setting time, increased strength, and a mix that is not as uniform in consistency. If a higher water-to-powder ratio is used, the impression has a decreased resistance to deformation, decreased strength, and increased setting time. Both increases and decreases in spatulation affect the setting time and decrease the strength of the material.

Bowls and Spatulas Used for Alginate Impressions. The operator can either use a flexible rubber bowl and a flexible spatula to mix the alginate or use a disposable bowl with built-in water measuring lines. The flexible rubber bowl allows easy mixing of the alginate but must be sterilized or disinfected after use. The disposable bowl comes with a disposable spatula that can be used for mixing alginate at one end and mixing plaster at the other end. The disposable bowl and spatula can be thrown away and they eliminate the aseptic procedures required after contamination of the rubber bowl and spatula (Figure 39-2).

Alginate Substitute. Alginate substitutes are silicone-based impression materials intended as an alternative to traditional alginate materials. One popular brand is available in a premixed package with a dispensing unit (Figure 39-3). This alginate unit can be mounted on the wall or placed on the counter. The premixed alginate is placed in the dispensing unit and the assistant places a dispensing tip on the unit. The material is then dispensed directly into the tray (Figure 39-4). This unit is similar to, or the same as, the unit for dispensing some polysiloxane or polyether materials (final impression materials). It can also come in a cartridge with a mixing tip and a gun for dispensing. This extruder operation for mixing eliminates hand mixing. The mixing unit must be wiped down with surface disinfectant thoroughly after each use to prevent cross-contamination.

Trays Used for Alginate Impressions. Several trays are available for alginate impressions (Figure 39-5). Most commonly used are the perforated trays that come in metal and plastic. The trays have holes in them for the material to ooze through and lock the impression material in the tray. If not using the perforated trays, the material may stay in the patient's mouth as the tray is removed. The impression then has to be retaken due to loss of accuracy from the flexible material coming loose from the rigid tray. Some operators use a rim lock tray in place of the perforated tray. The rim lock tray has a border around the top of it to aid in holding the material in place. This tray has no perforations in it. Alginate

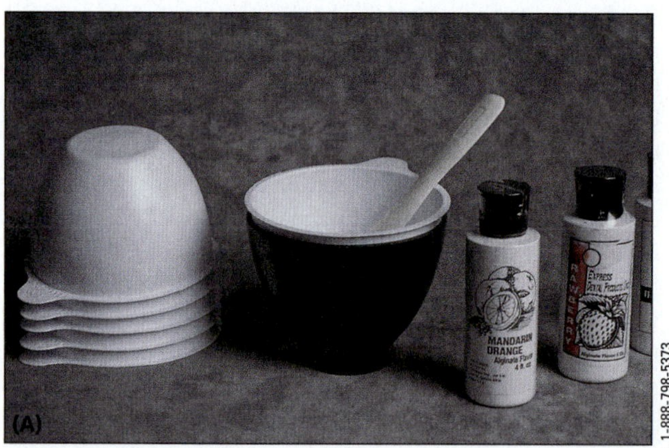

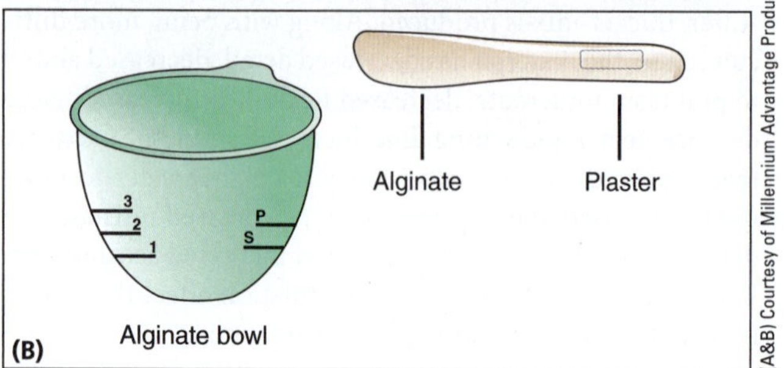

(A&B) Courtesy of Millennium Advantage Products, 1-888-798-5373

FIGURE 39-2

(A) Bowl-Away and Spat-Away disposable bowl and spatula used for mixing alginate and plaster. (B) Bowl-Away and Spat-Away show water measuring lines in mixing bowl. The disposable spatula shows ends, one for alginate and one for plaster.

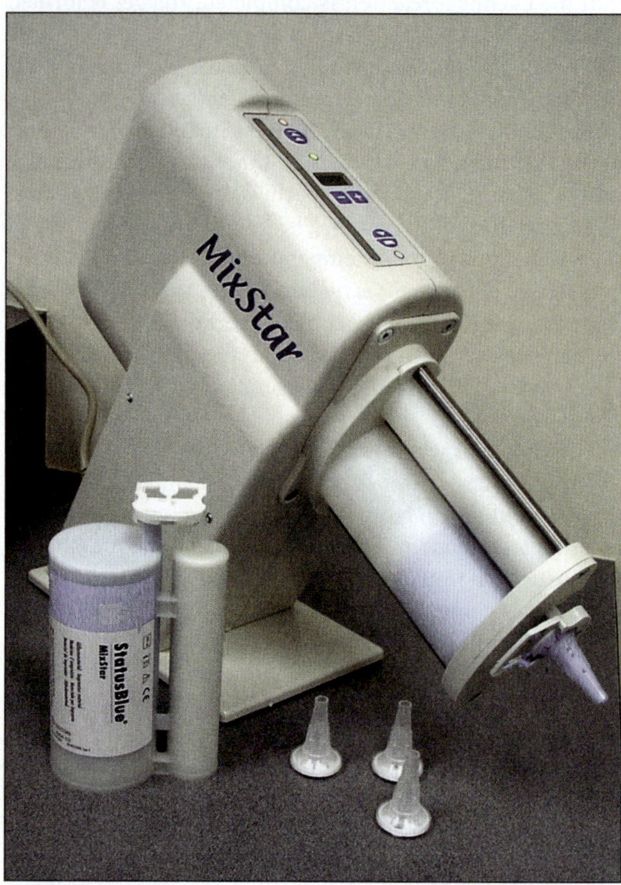

FIGURE 39-3

Unit for dispensing premixed alginate substitute.

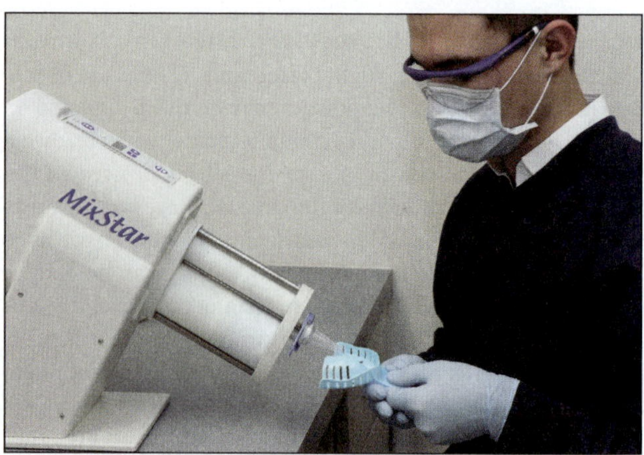

FIGURE 39-4

Dispense material directly in tray.

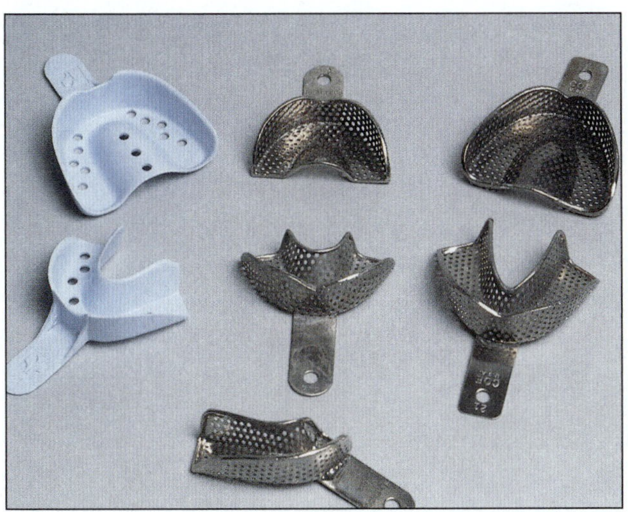

FIGURE 39-5

Assortment of alginate trays.

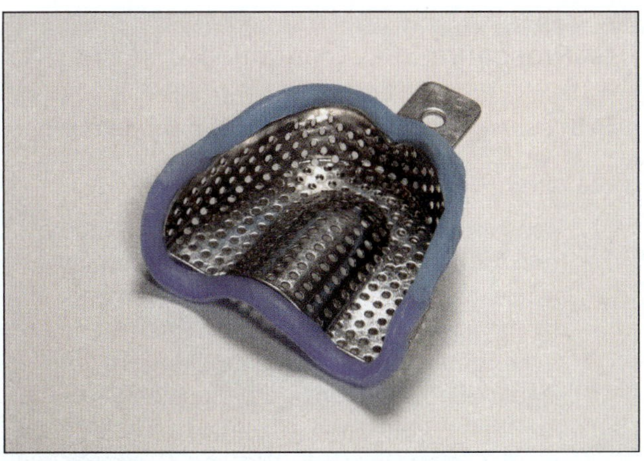

FIGURE 39-6

Alginate tray with beading wax on the periphery. The wax aids in tray extension and patient comfort.

adhesive may also be applied to the impression tray to prevent the impression from lifting out of the tray upon removal from the mouth. Both the perforated tray and the rim lock tray come in plastic and metal. The metal trays can be cleaned and reused after sterilization. In order to achieve complete sterilization of reusable metal trays, it is important to remove all debris from the trays prior to heat sterilization.

Whichever tray is used, the operator must make sure that the tray fits correctly in the patient's mouth. Selecting the correct tray is essential to obtaining an accurate impression. The trays come in several sizes. The operator first examines the patient's mouth and identifies a sterilized or disposable tray that he or she thinks will fit. The trays should be tried in the patient's mouth to ensure a correct fit and comfort for the patient. The tray should extend 2 or 3 mm beyond the last molar area and below both the lingual and facial tooth surfaces. Keep in mind that there should be enough room for 2 mm of the alginate material between the tray and all surfaces of the teeth and tissue. If the size of the tray seems appropriate but the tray does not extend over the last molar area, utility wax strips can be used. The wax is placed in layers until the desired length is achieved. The wax also can be placed around the border of the tray to lengthen it on the lingual and facial areas and to provide more comfort for the patient (Figure 39-6). The process of placing the wax around the border of the tray is called **beading**.

Taking Alginate Impressions for Diagnostic Casts (Study Models)

In some states, dental assistants are allowed to take the alginate impressions, while in other states, the dental assistant can select the tray, mix the material, load the material into the tray, and pass the tray for the dentist to place in the patient's mouth.

The alginate material can be mixed using the Alginator II® method (Procedure 39-1) or the manual method (Procedure 39-2). The material can also be mixed in a plastic bag: place powder in the bag, add water, and knead. The "bag procedure" is very effective in ensuring aseptic technique because the bag can easily be disposed of, but mixing in this manner incorporates more air bubbles if not done properly.

The Alginator II device makes mixing easier, as well as increasing the likelihood of a bubble-free mixture. Rather than the operator rotating the bowl, the device spins the bowl about 300 times a minute.

Procedure 39-1
Mixing Alginate with an Alginator II Mixing Device

This procedure is performed by the dental assistant in the states where allowed. The materials are prepared and the Alginator II mixing device is prepared and ready.

Equipment and Supplies

- Flexible spatula/broad blade or disposable spatula
- Flexible rubber bowl(s) or Alginator II flexible bowl only
- Alginate material with water and powder measuring devices
- Water
- Alginate flavoring (optional)

(continues)

Procedure 39-1 (continued)

Procedure Steps (*Follow aseptic procedures*)

Material Preparation

1. Measure the impression water (room temperature) for the mandibular impression, normally two calibrations of the water measurement device supplied by the manufacturer. Place water in the rubber bowl attached to the Alginator II (Figure 39-7). Some operators use an additional bowl in the Alginator II so that it can be cleaned easily. Leaving the bowl attached allows for more control; attach it by rotating slightly to the side and fitting into the grooves on the bottom of the bowl.
2. Fluff the powder before opening the powder canister, if indicated by the manufacturer's directions.
3. Fill the measure with powder by overfilling and then leveling off with the spatula (use the flat blade, not the edge blade of the spatula). Dispense two corresponding scoops into the water in the rubber bowl. Add drops of flavoring to the water, if using.
4. Incorporate the mixture slightly.
5. Hold the spatula to the side of the bowl with the mixture and use slight pressure. Turn on the Alginator II; the material is mixed as the bowl rotates (300 times a minute). Use the side of the spatula blade during this process.
6. When the material is completely mixed, it can be easily collected by using the edge of the spatula starting from the deepest area in the bowl.
7. Upon completion, the material should be homogeneous and smooth without bubbles.
8. Remove excess material from bowls with paper towels, and then clean thoroughly and disinfect.

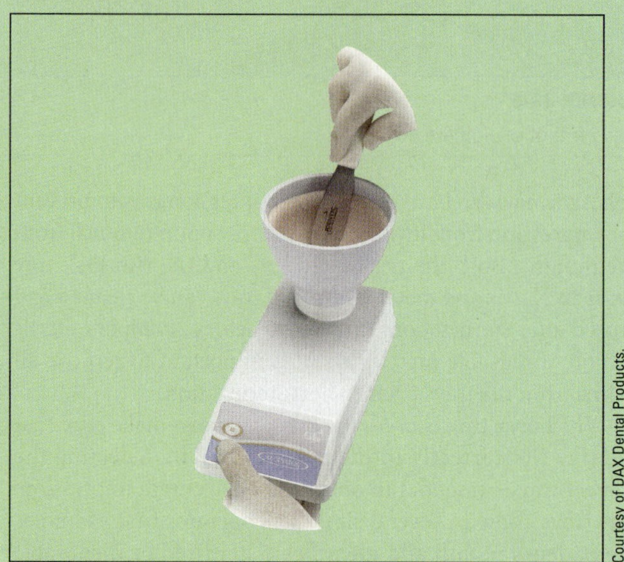

Courtesy of DAX Dental Products.

FIGURE 39-7
Alginator II used for mixing alginate.

Procedure 39-2
Preparing for Alginate Impression

This procedure is performed by the dental assistant in states where allowed. The materials are prepared and the alginate impression is taken on the maxillary and mandibular arches.

Equipment and Supplies

- Flexible spatula/broad blade or disposable spatula
- Flexible rubber bowl(s) or disposable bowl
- Alginate material with water and powder measuring devices
- Water
- Alginate flavoring if used
- Impression tray(s)
- Beading wax (if necessary)

(continues)

Procedure 39-2 (continued)

Procedure Steps (*Follow aseptic procedures*)

Patient Preparation

1. Health history is reviewed.
2. Patient is seated in an upright position with a patient napkin in place.
3. Patient's mouth is rinsed with water or mouth rinse to remove any food debris and to aid with removing thick saliva.
4. The procedure is explained to the patient.
5. Impression trays are tried in the oral cavity to determine the correct size.

Material Preparation

1. Wax is placed around the borders of the impression trays, if necessary, to extend the borders of the trays or to provide additional patient comfort (Figure 39-6).
2. The impression water (room temperature) is measured for the mandibular model, normally two calibrations of the water measurement device supplied by the manufacturer. The water is placed in the flexible mixing bowl. Flavoring is added if being used.

Order of Taking Impressions

Taking the mandibular model first allows the patient to build confidence and feel more secure before the maxillary impression, which often causes more gagging.

NOTE: Place the water in the bowl first to ensure that all the powder is incorporated into the mixture.

3. Fluff the powder prior to opening the powder canister, if indicated by the manufacturer's directions.
4. Fill the measure of powder by overfilling and then leveling off with the spatula (use the flat blade, not the edge blade of the spatula) to get an accurate measure. Dispense two corresponding scoops into a second flexible rubber bowl.
5. When ready, place the powder in water.
6. Mix the water and powder first with a stirring motion. Then mix by holding the bowl in one hand, rotating the bowl occasionally, and using the flat side of the spatula to incorporate the material through pressure against the side of the bowl (Figure 39-8). The mixing time for Type I fast set is 30 to 45 seconds, and for Type II regular set, 1 minute.
7. Upon completion, the mixture should be homogeneous and creamy. When the material is mixed correctly, load it into the impression tray. On the mandibular tray, the material should be loaded from both lingual sides (Figure 39-9). Use the flat side of the blade to condense the material firmly into the tray. If necessary to further smooth the surface, take a gloved hand, moisten, and smooth the top.

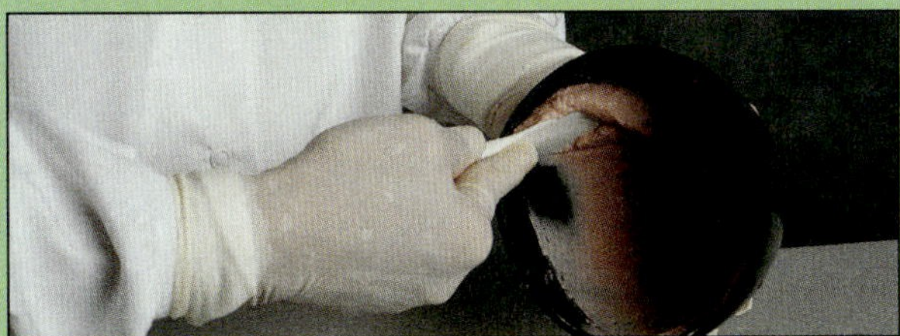

FIGURE 39-8
Mixing alginate material in a flexible rubber bowl, while pushing on sides of bowl to eliminate air bubbles.

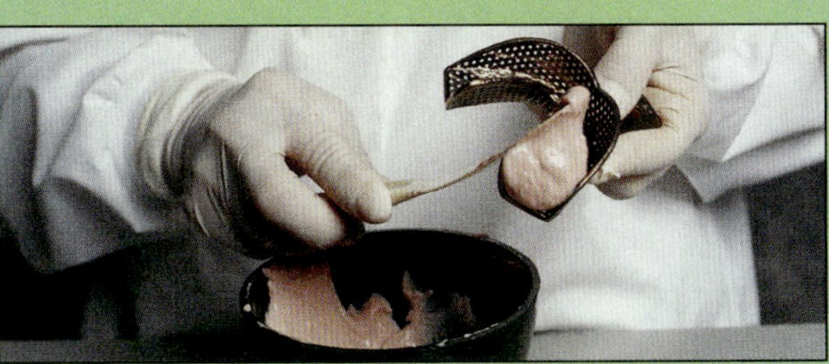

FIGURE 39-9
Loading mandibular alginate tray from lingual side to eliminate air spaces.

Procedure 39-3
Taking an Alginate Impression

Refer to Procedure 39-2, Preparing for an Alginate Impression, to identify PPE, equipment, and supplies.

Procedure Steps *(Follow aseptic procedures)*

1. When taking the mandibular impression, face the patient, and retract the right cheek slightly.
2. Use the excess alginate material to rub onto the occlusal surfaces of the teeth in order to obtain more accurate anatomy.
3. Invert the impression tray so that the material is toward the teeth.
4. Turn the tray so that it passes through the lip opening with one side of the tray entering first, using the other hand to retract the opposite corner of the mouth.
5. When the tray is completely in the patient's mouth, center it above the teeth.
6. Lower the tray onto the teeth, placing the posterior area down first, leaving the impression tray slightly anterior.
7. Have the patient raise the tongue and move it side to side to ensure that the lingual aspect of the alveolar process is defined in the impression.
8. Pull out the lip from the center with the other hand.
9. Finish placing the impression tray down and, as this is being done, push slightly toward the posterior area with the tray. This pushes the impression material down into the patient's anterior vestibule area, therefore producing a good esthetic model. One area that often lacks detail in the impression is the anterior segment. By leaving the tray slightly anterior and pushing the tray toward the posterior while making sure the lip is out of the way, this problem can be overcome.
10. Allow the lip to cover the tray. It should be close to the handle portion of the tray.
11. Hold it in the patient's mouth with two fingers on the back of the tray, one on the right side, one on the left side, until set (Figure 39-10). Check the excess material around the edges of the impression tray, or in the bowl, to determine if the material is set. The material should feel firm and not change shape when pushed.
12. The maxillary alginate impression is loaded from the posterior, making sure that the material completely fills the tray without voids (Figure 39-11A). Smooth the material (Figure 39-11B). Take a small amount of alginate out from the palate area to prevent the impression material from going down the patient's throat after insertion (Figure 39-11C). Place some alginate on the occlusal surfaces of the maxillary teeth.
13. Stand behind or to the side of the patient, place the maxillary tray in the patient's mouth by turning the tray so that it passes through the lip opening with one side of the tray entering first, using the other hand to retract the opposite corner of the mouth (Figure 39-11D). Raise the tray to the maxillary arch and hold out the lip before seating the tray in place. Hold it in position until the material is set in the bowl (Figure 39-11E).

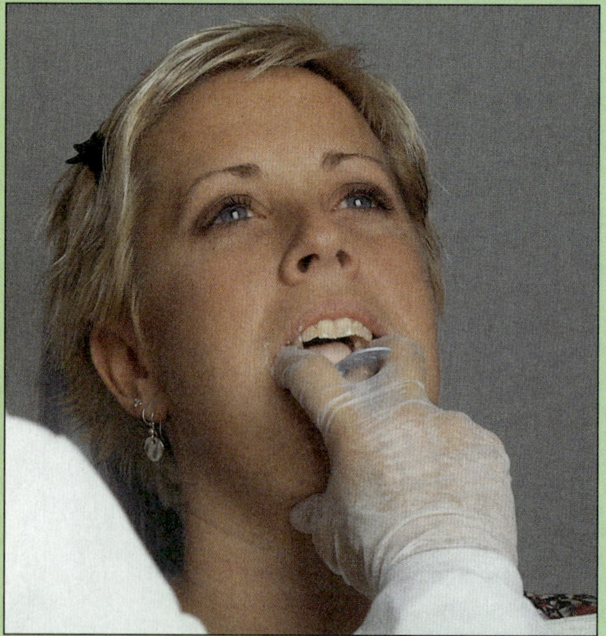

FIGURE 39-10
Holding mandibular alginate tray in patient's mouth, maintaining a stable force while material is setting.

(continues)

Procedure 39-3 (continued)

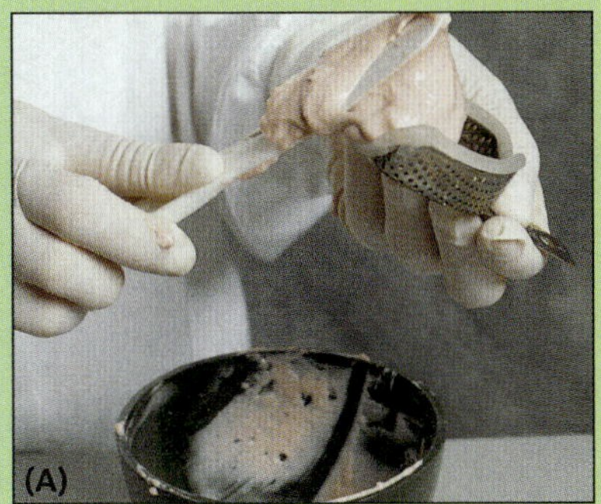
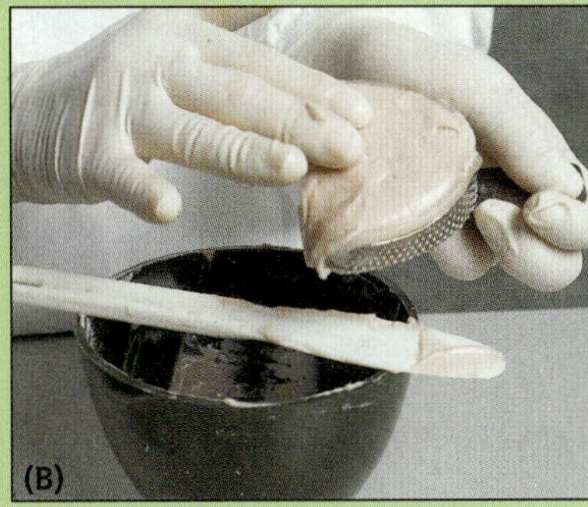
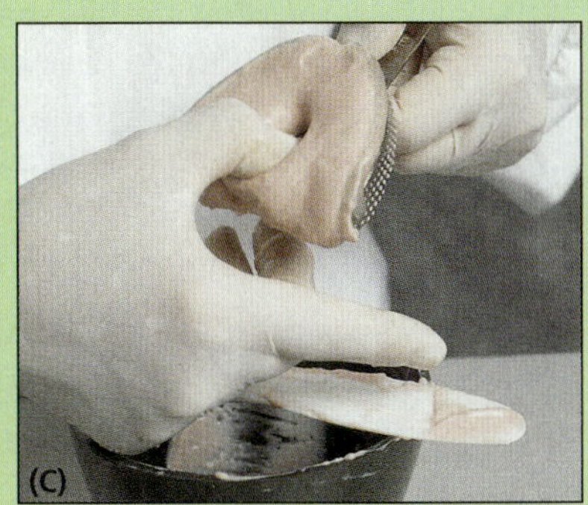
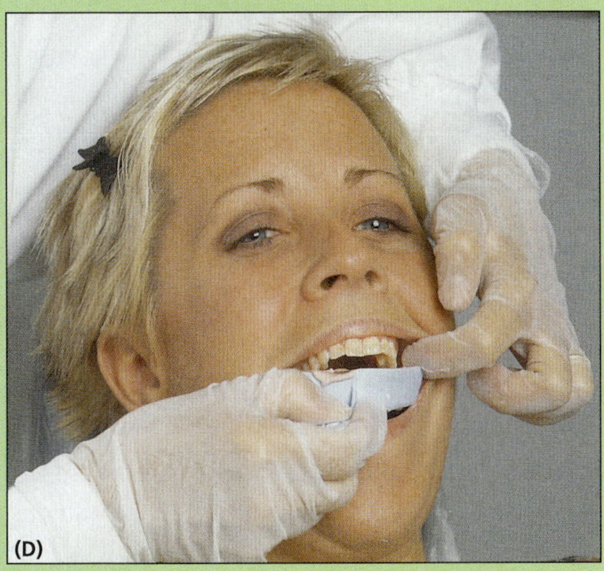
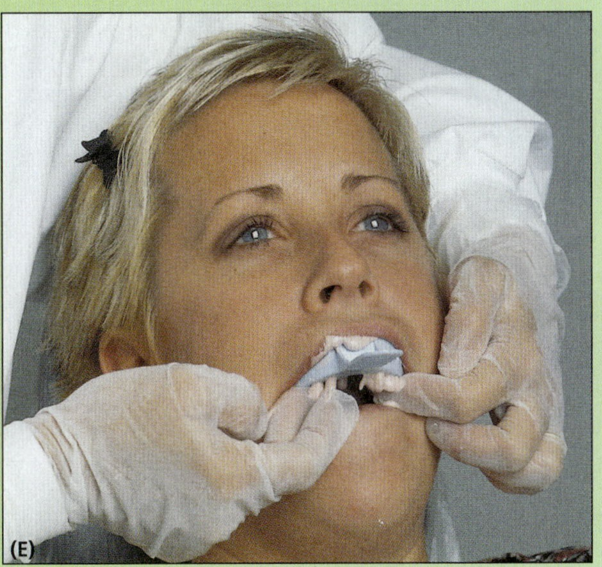

FIGURE 39-11

(A) Load maxillary alginate tray from posterior area of tray. (B) Smooth the material. (C) Before seating tray in patient's mouth, remove a small amount of alginate from palate area. Doing so prevents material from descending into the patient's throat. (D) Insert tray into patient's mouth one side first, and then rotate the entire tray into the patient's mouth. (E) Hold the tray in place until the material sets.

Procedure 39-4
Removing the Alginate Impression

Refer to Procedure 39-2, Preparing for an Alginate Impression, to identify PPE, equipment, and supplies.

Procedure Steps (*Follow aseptic procedures*)

1. When the material is completely set, remove it from the mouth by first loosening the tissue of the lips and cheek around the periphery with fingers to break the suction-like seal.
2. Place fingers of the opposing hand on the opposite arch to protect the adjacent arch as the tray is being removed.
3. Remove the tray in an upward or downward motion (depending on the arch) with a quick snap. Turn it to the side to allow it to be removed from the oral cavity.

(continues)

Procedure 39-4 (continued)

4. Remove any excess alginate material from the patient's mouth with the evacuator and have the patient rinse. Check the patient's face for any excess alginate material. If present, give the patient a tissue and mirror to remove the material.
5. Check the impression for accuracy (Figure 39-12).
6. Rinse the impression gently with water to remove saliva, blood, or debris.
7. Spray with approved surface disinfectant.
8. If there is a time lapse (maximum of 20 minutes) before pouring, wrap the alginate impression in an airtight container or a moist towel and place it in a plastic bag labeled with the patient's name. If the impression is placed in a wet towel for an extended period of time, imbibition (taking up extra moisture) may occur.

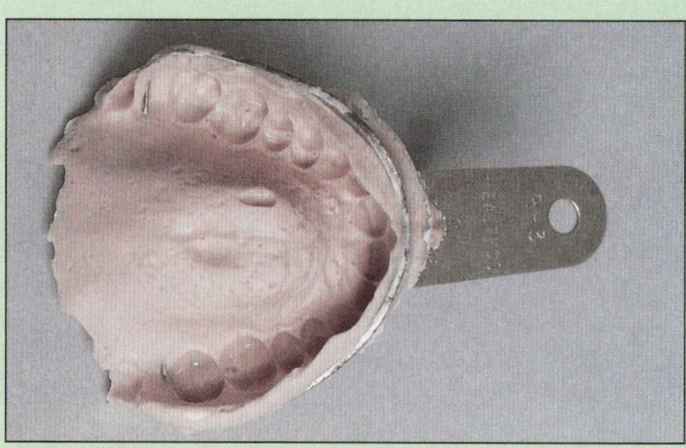

FIGURE 39-12

The alginate impression is checked for accuracy after removal from the patient's mouth.

Procedure 39-5

Disinfecting Alginate Impressions

This procedure is performed by the dental assistant immediately after removing the alginate impressions from the patient's mouth and caring for the patient.

Equipment and Supplies

- Approved disinfectant
- Covered container or sealable plastic bag

Procedure Steps (*Follow aseptic procedures*)

1. Rinse the impressions gently under tap water to remove any debris, blood, or saliva.
2. Spray the impressions with an approved disinfectant (see Chapter 11, Infection Control).
3. If not pouring immediately, place the impressions in a covered container.
4. Label the container with the patient's name.

Accuracy of Alginate Impression

- Tray covers all necessary areas.
- Tray is centered on central incisors.
- Tray is not pushed down or up too far, allowing teeth to penetrate through material to tray.
- Impression is not torn.
- Impression is free of bubbles and voids.
- Impression shows sharp anatomic detail of all teeth and tissues.
- Impression has a good "peripheral roll" and includes all vestibule areas.
- Mandibular impression shows good detail in retromolar area and shows lingual frenum and mylohyoid ridge area.
- Maxillary impression shows good detail in tuberosities and palate areas.

Wax Bite Registration

A wax bite registration is taken to establish the relationship between the maxillary and mandibular teeth (see Procedure 39-6). It can be used to verify the occlusal relationship when trimming the diagnostic casts (**study models**). Normally, wax that is formed in a horseshoe shape is used, but the flat sheets of utility wax can be used as well.

Other materials are also used in taking a bite registration. Polysiloxane impression material, specifically designed for occlusal registration, can be dispensed using a dispensing gun and cartridge tip. It is dispensed directly onto the occlusal surface, and the patient is asked to close in the normal biting position and remain closed until the material sets, normally within 2 minutes. The set material is removed, disinfected, stored, and used to establish the patient's occlusal relationship.

Procedure 39-6

Taking a Bite Registration

This procedure is performed by the dental assistant under direction of the dentist or by the dentist with the dental assistant assisting.

Equipment and Supplies

- Bite registration wax or wax horseshoe or polysiloxane and extruder gun and disposable tips
- Laboratory knife
- Warm water or torch

Procedure Steps (*Follow aseptic procedures*)

1. The patient remains seated in an upright position with a patient napkin in place after the impressions are taken.
2. Explain the procedure.
3. The bite registration wax is tried to determine correct length. If correction is needed, the laboratory knife is used to trim off the excess.
4. Instruct the patient to practice biting to establish occlusion. You may have to instruct the patient in biting in occlusion.
5. Bite registration wax is heated in warm water or with a torch to soften it.
6. Place wax on the mandibular occlusal surface of the patient. If using polysiloxane, the bite registration material is extruded from the disposable tip directly onto the occlusal surface of the mandibular teeth (Figure 39-13A).
7. Instruct the patient to bite together gently in the correct occlusion. You need to make sure the patient is in proper occlusion.
8. The wax will cool in 1 to 2 minutes while the patient keeps the teeth together in occlusion. If using polysiloxane, the patient gently occludes until the material sets (Figure 39-13B).
9. Gently remove wax or polysiloxane bite without distortion.
10. The wax or polysiloxane bite registration is rinsed, disinfected, with appropriate surface disinfectant, labeled, and stored for use during trimming of the diagnostic casts (Figure 39-13C).

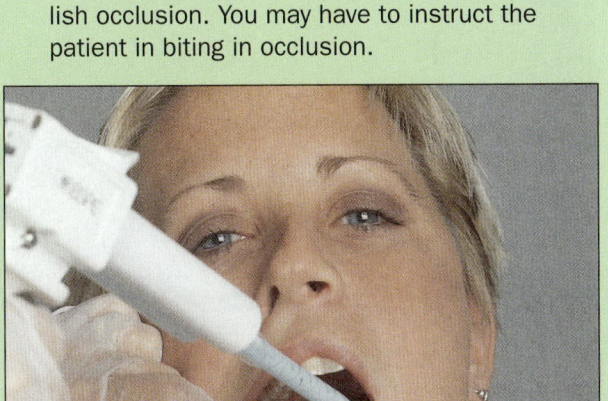

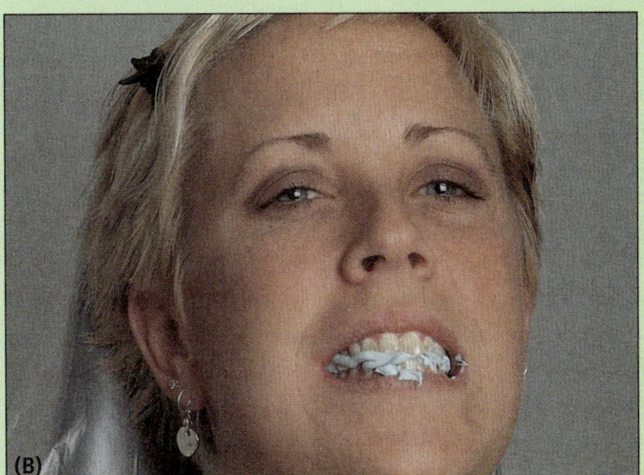

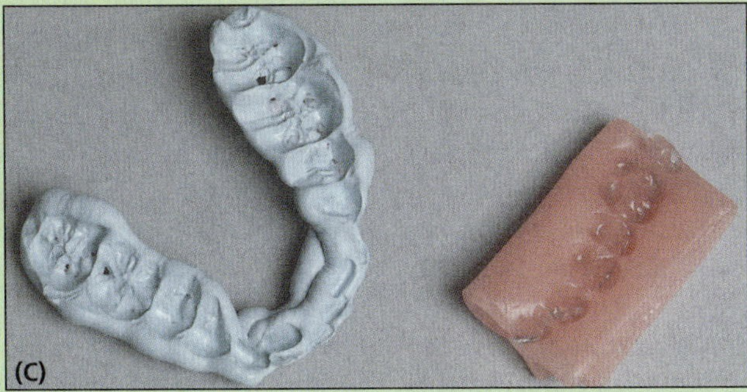

FIGURE 39-13

(A) Bite registration material is extruded from the tip directly onto the occlusal surface of the mandibular teeth. (B) Patient occludes gently until the material sets. (C) Polysiloxane or wax bite taken on a patient for use in establishing patient's occlusion.

Reversible Hydrocolloid Impression Material (Agar-Agar)

One of the oldest impression materials that has good detail and is used for final impressions is **reversible hydrocolloid** impression material, sometimes referred to as agar-agar. The composition for this material is somewhat similar to alginate in that the main component is derived from seaweed and kelp. It also has fillers, additives, coloring, and flavoring. The unique difference between reversible and irreversible hydrocolloid material is the setting reaction. The setting of the irreversible hydrocolloid (alginate) is accomplished by a chemical reaction. Reversible hydrocolloid changes from a gel to a sol and back again due to thermal reaction. The material begins in a gel (solid) state and, after boiling in a hydrocolloid conditioner unit for 10 minutes, it becomes liquid and remains in that state for hours if placed in a water storage bath of 150°F or 66°C until the operator is ready to use it. Five minutes before taking the impression, the tray material is moved into a water bath of 110°F or 45°C. It is further cooled in the mouth as cool water flows through the water trays, connected to hoses at the dental unit. Most units have two water connectors where the hoses can be attached. Due to the equipment needed and sensitivity of the technique for tempering the alginate, many dental offices do not use or have discontinued the use of reversible hydrocolloid.

Advantages and Disadvantages of Reversible Hydrocolloid. The primary advantage of using reversible hydrocolloid is the accuracy of the impression. Accuracy is more precise and more detailed than that for alginate (irreversible hydrocolloid), and reversible hydrocolloid can be used for impressions for crown and bridge construction. This material can be used for impressions for both teeth and tissue. After the initial equipment has been purchased, it is more economical than many materials on the market for final impressions.

The main disadvantage is the additional equipment needed to prepare the material. In addition, reversible hydrocolloid can lose accuracy due to atmospheric conditions. Also, the preparation and setting time is increased to 10 minutes. This material was used widely in earlier years and now has somewhat declined due to the emergence of a number of elastomeric impression materials available with similar accuracy.

Reversible Hydrocolloid Packaging and Equipment. The tray material is supplied in collapsible plastic tubes (Figure 39-14). The syringe material is supplied in either cylinders in a jar or syringe carpules. Both materials come in several colors and strengths. Special water-cooled trays and attachment hoses to circulate the water must be used with this material.

A hydrocolloid conditioner unit is used to prepare the material for use. This electric unit has three compartments (Figure 39-15). As with all equipment and material, read the manufacturer's directions and specific times for the material to be placed in each compartment. Normally, a timer is built into the conditioner. Each compartment in the conditioning unit is filled with clean water. The first compartment on the left (facing the unit) is for boiling the material. The tubes are placed, with the lids tight and upside down, in the unit. The syringe material is placed in a holding case for the cartridges or inside the boiling syringes if cylinders are used. The material must stay in the syringes or tubes or it will disperse throughout the water and be unusable. There, the material is boiled for 10 minutes. Digital machines can be set to start the timer for 10 minutes as soon as the boiling temperature is reached. If not using a digital machine, the dental assistant has to monitor the boiling temperature and time carefully. After the boiling process is complete, the temperature drops to the preset storage temperature.

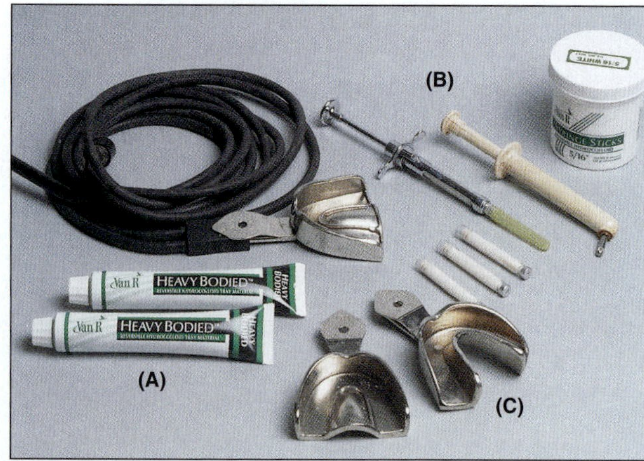

FIGURE 39-14

Hydrocolloid. (A) Tubes. (B) Syringes and cartridges. (C) Trays used with hydrocolloid conditioning unit to obtain final impressions.

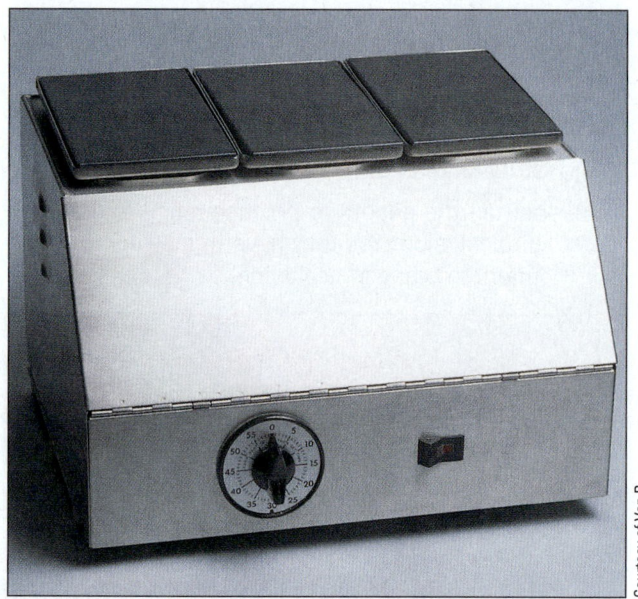

Courtesy of Van R.

FIGURE 39-15

Hydrocolloid conditioning unit with boiling bath, storage bath, and conditioning bath.

After the tubes and syringe material is boiled, it is moved to the middle compartment for storage. In this compartment, the temperature is set to maintain the material in a liquid state. The material can stay in this compartment for hours or days before use.

The third compartment on the right, facing the unit, is for tray material only. The material is placed in a water-cooled tray and then in the compartment to be tempered for 5 minutes. This cools the material so that it does not burn the patient's mouth upon insertion. The syringe material remains in the fluid state to get into the crevices around the prepared tooth and obtain the necessary anatomy on the adjacent teeth. Because of the small opening in the syringe, the amount coming from the syringe cools rapidly as it is used.

The hydrocolloid conditioner unit requires very little maintenance. The compartments should be emptied and rinsed out on a regular basis and then wiped with a soft cloth and refilled with clean water. A condition cleaner can be placed in the compartments and left for 1 hour to remove any buildup. The cleaner is then rinsed out prior to placing clean water in the compartments.

Elastomeric Impression Materials

Elastomeric impression materials have rubber-like qualities and are used for areas that require precise duplication. Materials in this classification are not as affected by atmospheric changes as are hydrocolloids. They are more elastic and rubber-like when set, and thus allow removal from the mouth to take place without tearing and distortion. A **distortion** is a dimensional change in shape. There are three primary groups of materials in this classification: polysulfide, silicone (polysiloxane and polyvinyl siloxanes), and polyether. Each group has slightly different properties and characteristics, even though all have elastic qualities. All the materials have a catalyst and base that are mixed together to start the chemical self-curing process. The **catalyst** is the ingredient that **accelerates** or starts the process of setting the material. The process by which the catalyst and accelerator begin to cure and the material changes from a paste to an elastic, rubber-like material is called **polymerization**. The accelerator is dispensed as a paste from a small tube or in liquid form from a bottle with a dropper. The base that makes up the volume of the material is normally dispensed in a paste. Often, the tube openings of base and catalyst are different sizes, with the catalyst tube opening being smaller. Many of the materials are now dispensed in an "extruder gun" with a mixing tip. The mixing tip brings together the correct amount of the base and the catalyst material and dispenses it, premixed (Figure 39-16). If this technique is used, there is no need for a mixing pad and a spatula. A new tip is required for each application and the material must be purchased in special cartridges. Additionally, a fine tip may be added to the mixing tip for the light body elastomeric material to dispense around prepared teeth to ensure all details are captured in the impression. Dental offices that use a large volume of elastomeric impression material may use an automatic mixing unit which holds a bulk amount of base and catalyst that is mixed and then dispensed on to an impression tray (Figure 39-17). The benefits of the mixing unit are that there is minimal waste of material, and clean-up and cross-contamination are minimized. Light, medium, or heavy body material can be mixed in the unit. As with the extruder gun technique, a new mixing tip must be used each time. The mixing unit must be wiped with a surface disinfectant after each use to prevent cross-contamination.

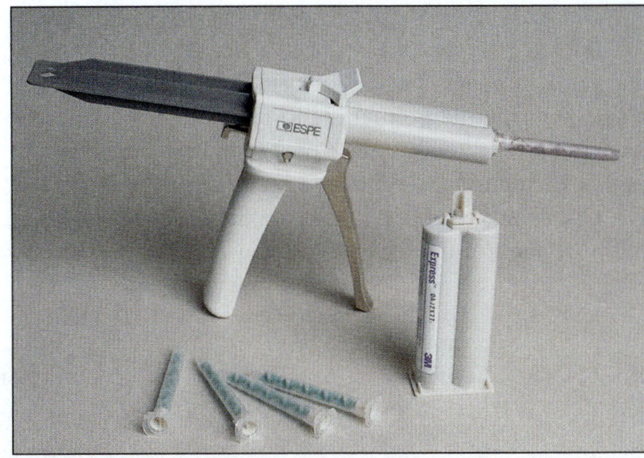

FIGURE 39-16
Extruder gun cartridge and tips used to mix and dispense the material.

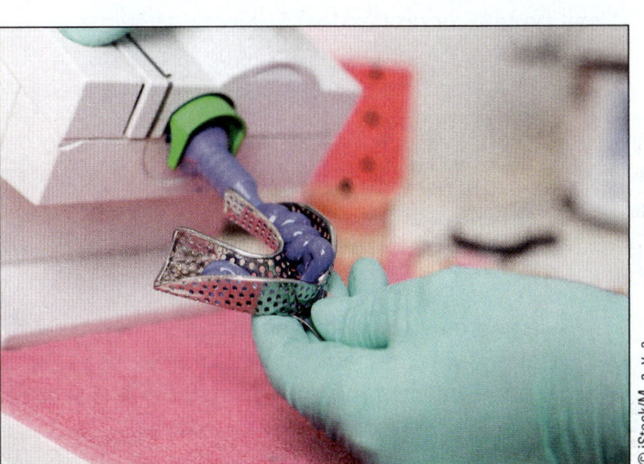

FIGURE 39-17
Dispensing using a large volume mixing unit.

Polysulfide

The **polysulfide** impression materials have been around for a long time, and may be called mercaptan or rubber-base materials. They are supplied in two pastes: a base and a catalyst. The base is the larger tube and the whiter color of the two. It is made from liquid polysulfide polymer (thiokol polysulfide rubber) with filler added. The dark brown accelerator is made from lead peroxide. These pastes can be purchased as light (syringe material), regular, heavy, and extra heavy (tray material).

Advantages of the polysulfide material include relative stability after the final set has been achieved, good accuracy, sharpness of detail, and a relatively long shelf life (several years). Pouring the polysulfide impression within an hour is advisable, but impressions have been known to be left for days before pouring with no noticeable change in dimension. The disadvantages of polysulfide are the odor (it smells like sulfur because of the base), taste, staining (it permanently stains clothes because of the accelerator), and the relatively long setting time (10 minutes is required from the start of the mix to the setting of the material prior to removal from the patient's mouth). The setting time can be accelerated slightly by increasing temperature, moisture, and amount of accelerator. Polysulfide is not used very much anymore due to the taste, staining, and long setting time. Procedure 39-7 outlines how to take an impression with polysulfide.

Procedure 39-7
Taking a Polysulfide Impression

This procedure is performed by the dentist with assistance by the dental assistant. This procedure can be four- or six-handed. Everyone should wear protective overclothing. Polysulfide is a material used in taking final impressions for which extreme accuracy is required.

Equipment and Supplies

- Two rigid laboratory spatulas
- Paper pad, provided by the manufacturer
- Two pastes each (two syringe pastes and two tray pastes) from the same manufacturer (a base and an accelerator of the syringe material and a base and an accelerator of the tray material)
- Impression syringe with tip in place and plunger out of the cylinder
- Custom tray that has been painted with corresponding adhesive and permitted to dry

Procedure Steps (*Follow aseptic procedures*)

1. Health history is reviewed.
2. The patient is seated in an upright position with a patient napkin in place and a large drape over the clothes.
3. The procedure is explained to the patient.
4. The patient's mouth is rinsed with water or a mouth rinse to remove any food debris and aid with removing thick saliva.
5. The materials are mixed concurrently by two individuals. The syringe material is mixed slightly ahead of the tray material.
6. Dispense the accelerator onto the pad in a long, even line about 4 inches long. If more material is needed, additional lines can be placed together on the paper pad.

NOTE: Be sure to wipe the end of the tube before placing the lid back on to prevent mess and sticking of the top.

7. Dispense the base onto the pad in a long, even line the same length as the accelerator (Figure 39-18). Additional lines can be dispensed, but they should not touch the accelerator until the operator wants the process of polymerization to begin.
8. When ready, the individual with the syringe material begins mixing by first gathering up the accelerator with the spatula and placing it in the base material. Spatulate the pastes together with broad sweeps. After a minute has lapsed, the individual mixing the tray material begins the same process.
9. When the mix is homogeneous and lacks brown or white streaks, it is completely mixed. This process takes from 45 seconds to 1 minute.

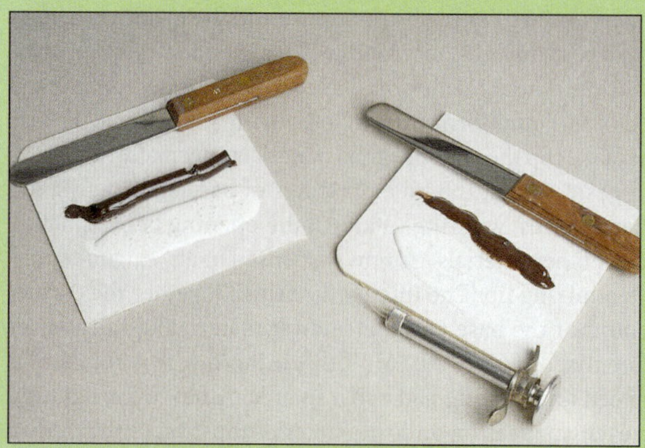

FIGURE 39-18
Polysulfide material is dispensed and ready to mix. The lines are equally long, but the amount of material differs.

(continues)

Procedure 39-7 (continued)

10. The syringe material is then loaded into an impression syringe using the back portion or the working end nozzle of the barrel and pushing the syringe over the material repeatedly to force the material into the chamber (Figure 39-19). When the material is in the syringe chamber, wipe the edges quickly and place the plunger in the syringe. Extrude the material slightly to make sure it is working and pass it to the dentist.

11. The tray material is mixed to the same consistency and within the same time frame. The bulk of the tray material is picked up by the spatula and loaded into the impression tray and spread evenly. The tray is then transferred to the dentist after the syringe has been used. The mixing and loading (working time) must be completed within 4 minutes.

12. The impression must remain in the patient's mouth, held by the operator or the dental assistant, for 6 minutes in order to achieve a final set.

13. Cleanup is accomplished after the material has reached the rubber stage. The material peels off the spatula. The paper pad normally has a corner for the spatula to fit under to aid in removing the soiled top sheet (Figure 39-20). The disposable impression syringe and paper sheet can be disposed of and the spatula sterilized.

14. The removal of the tray is done in much the same manner as was the alginate. Remove the impression after releasing the seal, taking care to protect the opposing teeth from the quick snap.

15. The impression is rinsed with water to remove saliva, blood, and debris and then sprayed with a surface disinfectant.

16. The impression is placed in a sealed container or bag that is labeled.

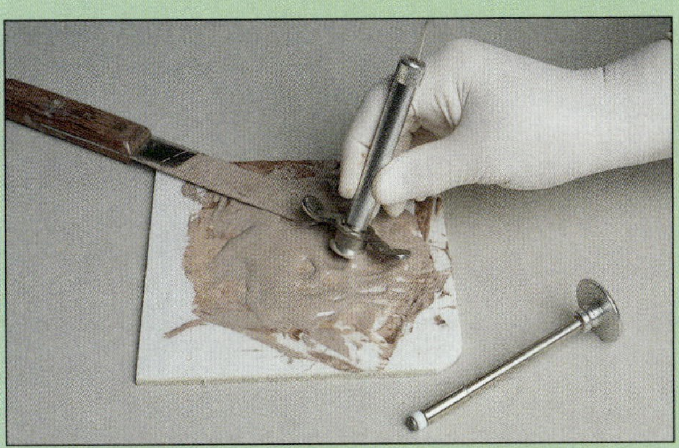

FIGURE 39-19
Loading mixed polysulfide syringe material into syringe for placement directly around prepared tooth.

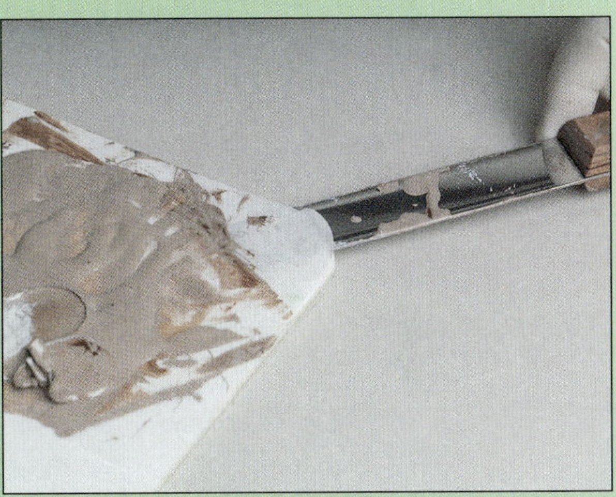

FIGURE 39-20
Polysulfide material cleans easily after it sets. The paper pad has a precut corner to allow the easy insertion of the spatula for cleanup and disposal.

Silicone (Polysiloxane and Polyvinyl Siloxanes)

A number of new silicone materials have been introduced in recent years. A **silicone** has the advantages of polysulfide without the disadvantages. It is more expensive than the polysulfide, however. Advantages of the material include high accuracy, no shrinkage, dimensional stability, high tear resistance, no taste, and no odor.

The material comes in a number of forms, including putty for making a custom tray, in tubes of base and accelerator (catalyst) for injection, and regular and heavy type for impressions. It is also available in cartridge form to be used with the mixing tip and extruding gun (automix cartridge system), and in bulk containers to be used in an automatic mixing unit.

The putty material comes in two colors. Each container of putty has a colored scoop that is used for either the base or the catalyst (Figure 39-21). Do not mix up the scoops because doing so will contaminate the material and cause the polymerization process to start, making the material hard and useless. The material is dispensed with an equal volume of base and catalyst putties. Knead and mix the putty quickly until a homogeneous color is achieved. This mixing

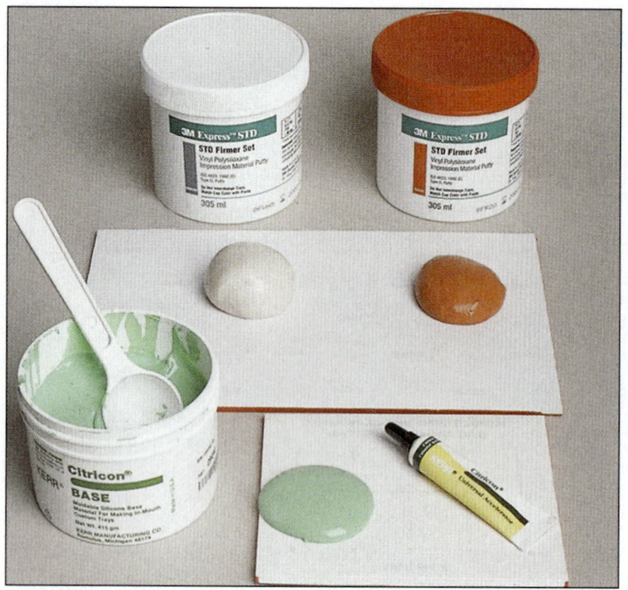

FIGURE 39-21

Two scoops of putty, or putty and a tube of accelerator, are dispensed for easy incorporation.

takes about 30 seconds. Mixing putty with latex gloves will adversely affect the set of some materials—read the directions. The silicone is placed in the tray, covered with a thin plastic sheet, and placed in the patient's mouth or over the model. It takes about 3 minutes for the material to harden. Remove the plastic, and a custom tray is ready for the impression material. The putty material is not suitable for detailed impressions.

When ready for the impression, the tray is loaded by the operator squeezing the dispenser handle of the extruding gun and engaging the plunger. The plunger enters the cartridge and extrudes the material through the mixing tip and into the putty material in the impression tray. The syringe material can also be injected from the mixing tip into the impression syringe for use around the sulcus of the tooth. When ready, the tray is placed in the patient's mouth and immobilized until set (3½ minutes for a fast set and 5 minutes for a regular set). The impression is removed after the seal is loosened and the opposing teeth are protected. The impression is run under cold water and sprayed with disinfectant. The impression is very stable and can be poured weeks later. The total time from mixing to the final set is from 4 to 6 minutes (see Procedure 39-8).

Procedure 39-8

Taking a Silicone (Polysiloxane) Two-Step Impression

This procedure is performed by the dentist with assistance by the dental assistant. Silicone (polysiloxane) is a material used in taking final impressions for which extreme accuracy is required.

Equipment and Supplies

- Spatula
- Paper mixing pad
- Vinyl overgloves
- Two containers of putty (one base and one catalyst) with color-coordinated scoops or one putty base and liquid dropper of catalyst (Figure 39-20)
- Stock tray with adhesive painted on interior
- Plastic sheet for use as a spacer
- Extruder gun, mixing tip with intraoral delivery tip or injection syringe (Figure 39-22)
- Cartridges of impression material (light-body or wash material)

Procedure Steps *(Follow aseptic procedures)*

Patient Preparation

1. Health history is reviewed.
2. The patient is seated in an upright position with a bib in place.
3. Retraction cord is placed around prepared tooth.
4. The procedure is explained.

Preliminary Putty Impression

1. Don vinyl gloves.
2. Equal scoops of the putty are mixed together, or the putty base and drops of catalyst are mixed together. The putty must be kneaded until a homogeneous mixture is obtained within the manufacturer's recommended timeframe (normally 30 seconds). The mixture must be a single color with no streaks.
3. After the material is mixed, pat it into a patty and load it into the prepared tray. With a finger, make a slight indentation where the teeth are located.

(continues)

Procedure 39-8 (continued)

4. Place the plastic spacer sheet over the material and insert it into the patient's mouth. The objective is to create 2 mm of space for the final syringeable viscous impression material.
5. The setting of the putty takes about 3 minutes. The tray is then removed from the patient's mouth, the spacer is removed, and the putty is checked for accuracy and left to set further.

Final Impression

1. After the tooth has been prepared, the area is cleaned and dried, the retraction cord is placed, and the doctor indicates that he or she is ready for the final impression, prepare the material.
2. The tray with the preliminary impression is ready with the spacer removed. The extruder gun is prepared and loaded with the light-body or wash material.
3. The syringe (light-body) material is extruded through the mixing tip and placed in the preliminary impression (Figure 39-23).
4. The tip is wiped off and an intraoral delivery tip is placed on for direct injection around the prepared tooth after the retraction cord has been removed. The extruder gun is transferred to the dentist. Instead of using the intraoral delivery tip, some dentists prefer to use an injection syringe, which can be loaded with the mixing tip.
5. The tray is seated by the dentist immediately into place and held steady for 3 to 5 minutes, depending on the material used.
6. After the material has set, the impression tray is removed after releasing the seal and taking care to protect the opposing teeth from the quick snap.
7. Immediately rinse the impression under water and lightly air blow dry. Disinfect according to the manufacturer's directions.
8. Impressions should be poured immediately, but can be poured up to weeks later and still remain dimensionally stable.

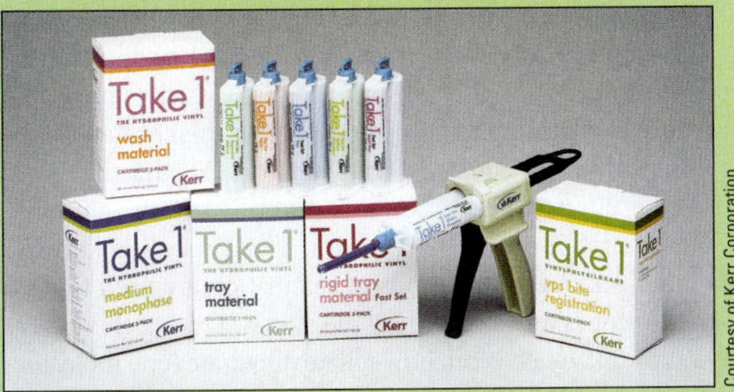

Courtesy of Kerr Corporation

FIGURE 39-22
Extruder gun, mixing tips, and cartridges of impression material.

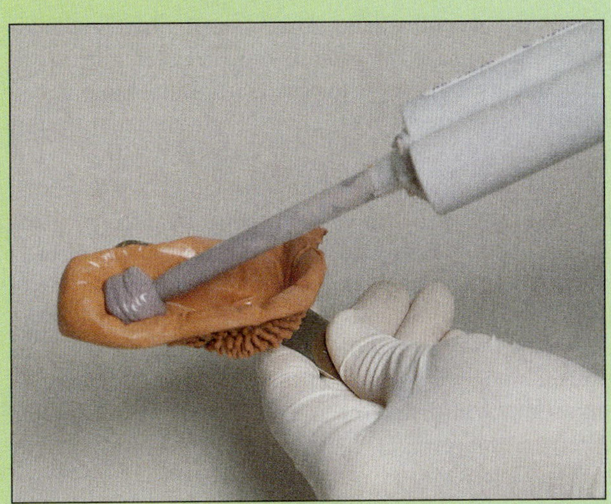

FIGURE 39-23
Syringe material extrudes from extruding gun into prepared tray.

Light-cured impression materials are also available. The advantage of this material is that the setting time is controlled by the operator. The disadvantage is that it is sometimes difficult to move the curing light over the complete surface of the material. A clear-plastic impression tray must be used. The light must hit all areas in order to bring about the curing. The light acts as a catalyst to set up the material.

Polyether

Polyether, an impression material used for crowns and bridges, has excellent accuracy and dimensional stability. It is supplied in tubes as pastes, the larger tube for the base and the smaller one for the catalyst. The material comes only in regular body and is stiffer than many other materials. It can be used for both the custom tray and the syringe. If used for a custom tray, a tray is chosen that is the correct size, painted with adhesive, and allowed to dry for 1 minute. The material is dispensed on a paper pad, supplied by the manufacturer, 1 inch per tooth involved in the impression. Equal lengths of material are placed on the pad, not equal amounts (Figure 39-24). This material is then mixed by placing the catalyst in the base in a figure-eight motion and obtaining a homogeneous mixture free of streaks. The mixing should not take longer than 30 seconds. When mixing is complete, the material is loaded onto the spatula and into the tray. The tray is seated by the

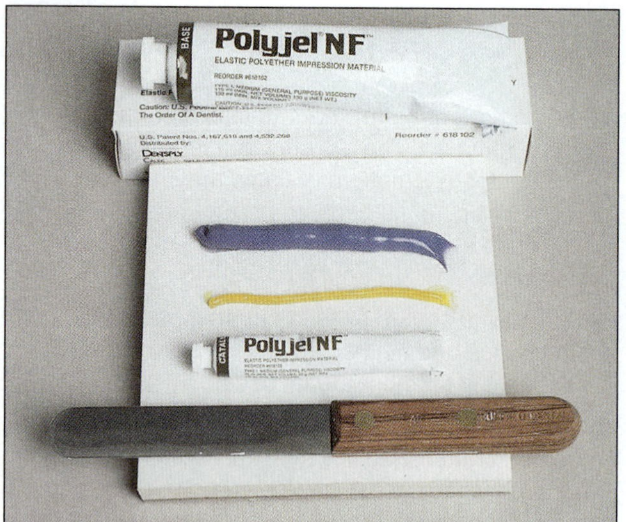

FIGURE 39-24
Polyether impression materials are dispensed on paper pad, ready to be mixed. Material swaths are equally long, but of unequal length.

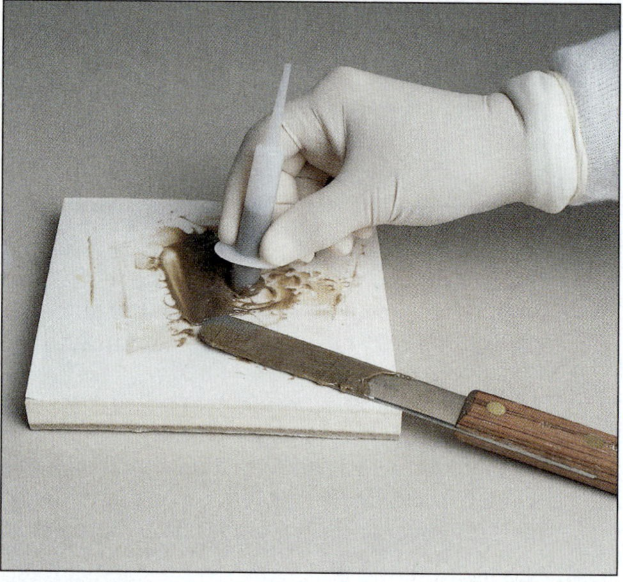

FIGURE 39-25
Mixed polyether is loaded into a syringe.

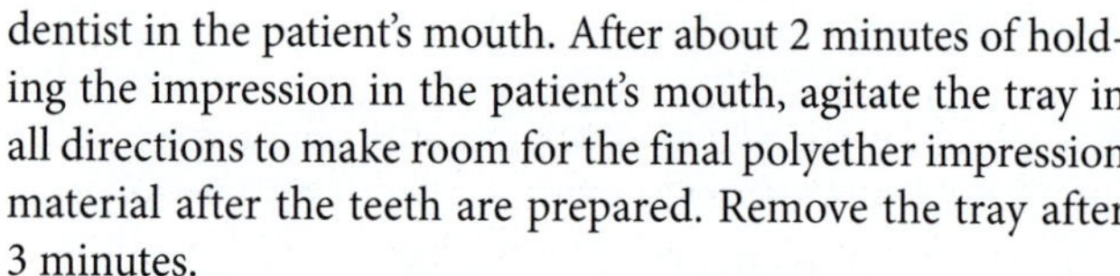

dentist in the patient's mouth. After about 2 minutes of holding the impression in the patient's mouth, agitate the tray in all directions to make room for the final polyether impression material after the teeth are prepared. Remove the tray after 3 minutes.

To take the final impression with polyether after the teeth are prepared, dispense the material in a similar manner. Less material is needed because of the volume already in the preliminary tray. If a less viscous impression material is desired by the dentist, a thinner (or body modifier) can be added to the mixture. The catalyst and the modifier are mixed into the base material. The material is loaded into an injection syringe, and the excess material is placed in the preliminary impression (Figure 39-25). The impression tray is then reinserted into the patient's mouth and held for 4 minutes to obtain an accurate impression. This technique can be accomplished in a one-step technique as well, eliminating the preliminary tray.

After the tray is loosened from the mouth and removed with a quick snapping motion, protecting the opposing arch, it is rinsed with cold water and then completely air dried. The impression can be disinfected with a 2 percent solution of glutaraldehyde for 10 minutes.

Gypsum Materials

Several different **gypsum** materials are used when pouring an impression to make a model. It is important to identify the application for the material before determining the type of gypsum product to use. Gypsum materials vary in strength, dimensional accuracy, resistance, reproduction detail, water/powder ratio, and setting times.

Primary types of gypsum used in dentistry are as follows:

- Type I: Impression plaster
- Type II: Model or laboratory plaster
- Orthodontic stone/combination of Type II: Model or laboratory plaster, and Type III: Laboratory stone
- Type III: Laboratory stone
- Type IV: Die stone
- Type V: High-strength, high-expansion die stone

During the process of manufacturing the various types of plasters and stones, the gypsum product (which is mined as a hard rock) is ground to a fine powder. It is then heated in large, cylindrical kettles equipped with agitators. The heating is controlled accurately and is continued until a specific amount of water is driven out of the gypsum. This process is known as **calcination**. Several methods of calcination are used to derive various stones and investment die stones. During this process, the gypsum, which is calcium sulfate dihydrate (one molecule of calcium sulfate to two molecules of water), is changed to hemihydrate powder (one water molecule to every two molecules of calcium sulfate). Because both plaster and stone are white in color, yellow, blue, and pink pigments are added to the stone to make it easier to distinguish which material is being used.

Strengths of the gypsum products are determined by the calcination process and the water/powder ratio needed to incorporate the mixture. Plaster (beta hemihydrate) comprises gypsum particles that are larger and more irregular than the particles of stone (alpha hemihydrate), which have undergone further processing and were transformed into denser particles. It is important to follow the manufacturer's directions when mixing gypsum products. One of the chief obstacles to overcome when mixing these products is incorporating air and wetting each particle. Plaster particles are more irregular and require more water to wet each surface of each particle. The ratio of water to powder for plaster is 50 mL of water to 100 grams of powder; stone requires only 30 mL of water to 100 grams of powder. Die stones require even less water because the particles are smaller, less irregular, and more dense.

Incorporating the water is an important step in mixing gypsum products. Using a flexible rubber bowl and a stiff spatula allows the operator to stir the viscous material and press against the sides of the bowl to eliminate air bubbles. Avoid whipping the powder and the water together, because doing so adds air to the mixture. It should be mixed to a creamy, putty-like consistency. A grainy mixture will not pour into the impression. The incorporating and spatulating procedure should take about 1 minute. Overspatulating causes a breakdown of crystals and soft spots in the model.

Gypsum sets when the plaster or stone transforms back to the dihydrate through a chemical reaction. This process gives off heat, called an **exothermic reaction**. The temperature of the water increases or decreases the setting time. The hotter the water, the more rapidly the material sets. There are retarders such as borax and sodium citrate that can be added to the material to slow down the set. Potassium sulfate accelerates the setting time. The manufacturers add small concentrations of the retarders or accelerators to cause a decrease or an increase in the setting rate of the gypsum.

The gypsum powder is measured by weight and the water is calibrated by volume. It is important to have the correct water-to-powder ratio. If less water is incorporated, the model can have greater setting expansion. It will have increased strength and hardness but may result in a thick mixture that becomes a dry, crumbly mass that cannot flow into the impression. At this stage, more water cannot be added to the mixture. It will need to be disposed of and a new mixture made. If too much water is incorporated into the mixture, the model will be weak, slow setting, and filled with air spaces. A plaster model will set in 10 to 20 minutes and can be determined by feel. If the heat has dissipated, the model is set. It goes through a cycle and heats up and seems to perspire; then, the heat diminishes and the model is cool and dry. The final set occurs after 24 hours when the model reaches the optimum hardness.

All gypsum products are packaged in some type of plastic bag or container to ensure that they do not become contaminated with moisture. If contaminated, the properties and the setting reaction may be altered. These plastic bags are normally further packaged in a cardboard box for easier handling.

Plaster

Plaster (plaster of Paris) is a white gypsum referred to as beta-hemihydrate. It was one of the first gypsum products available to dentistry. It is the weakest and least expensive of gypsum products. It is calcinated in an open kettle method, and the result is particles that are rough, irregular, and porous. The final product is a powder that, when mixed with water, reverts to a gypsum product or dihydrate. Plaster takes more water to incorporate the powder. After the model dries and the water evaporates, the areas where the water was become air bubbles. This is the primary reason that plaster is weaker than stone. Stone is more compact and requires less water, therefore making a stronger model. Plaster is used in areas where detail and strength are not as important. Plaster is used to pour up study models, for opposing models, in mounting study models and casts, and for repairing casts (See Procedures 39-9 through 39-12).

Type I: Impression Plaster

Impression plaster (modified Type II: Laboratory or model plaster) was used to take impressions before the newer, easy-to-manipulate impression materials now on the market. This plaster (Type I), mixed with a water-to-powder ratio of 60 mL of water to 100 grams of powder, is placed in the mouth carefully on the area to be duplicated, and then the operator must wait for the plaster to set. After the set (usually 4 to 5 minutes), the material is broken apart and reassembled in the laboratory. Because the material is so rigid, it fractures and breaks easily. Today, this material is rarely used for impressions; it is used primarily to mount casts on an articulator because of its quick setting time.

Type II: Laboratory or Model Plaster

Model plaster is used routinely in the dental office by the dental assistant to pour diagnostic casts or study models. It is normally white in color, and is slightly stronger than the Type I: impression plaster, because it requires a water-to-powder ratio of 50 mL of water to 100 grams of powder, making the material less porous.

Type III: Laboratory Stone

Type III: Laboratory stone is stronger than plaster and is used where more strength is needed. It requires 30 mL of water to 100 grams of powder, making it denser, harder, and stronger. It is normally yellow in color due to the manufacturer's added pigments, more expensive than plaster, and referred to as alpha-hemihydrate. It is used for study models (diagnostic casts) that require greater strength, working casts, and models for partial and full dentures.

Orthodontic Stone

Orthodontic stone is a mixture of laboratory or model plaster and laboratory stone. This white stone allows for a stronger model to be used for the diagnosis and treatment of orthodontic cases.

Type IV: Die Stone

Type IV: Die stone is calcinated by autoclaving in the presence of calcium chloride. This modified alpha-hemihydrate is referred to as "die stone." A die is a positive replica of the prepared tooth made from stone. It requires much less water (less than 24 mL to 100 grams of powder) to incorporate its small, uniform particles. More stone with less water and air makes the model strong and resistant to abrasion. It is used most often for dies or where a very strong model or cast is needed.

Type V: High-Strength, High-Expansion Die Stone

Recently, the ADA added a new material to its list of gypsum products. Type V: Die stone requires from 18 to 22 mL of water to 100 grams of powder, making it the strongest accepted gypsum product available for use in the dental office.

Water-to-Powder Ratio Recommendations

Type I: Impression plaster	100 grams powder	to	60 mL water
Type II: Laboratory or model plaster	100 grams powder	to	50 mL water
Type III: Laboratory stone	100 grams powder	to	30 mL water
Type IV: Die stone	100 grams powder	to	24 mL water
Type V: Die stone	100 grams powder	to	18–22 mL water

Procedure 39-9
Pouring an Alginate Impression with Plaster

This procedure is performed by the dental assistant in the dental laboratory.

Equipment and Supplies (*Figure 39-26*)

- Spatula, metal with rounded end and stiff, straight sides
- Two flexible rubber mixing bowls
- Scale
- Plaster (100 grams)
- Gram measuring device
- Water measuring device (calibrated syringe or vial)
- Vibrator with paper or plastic cover on platform
- Room-temperature water
- Alginate impression (disinfected)

Procedure Steps (*Follow aseptic procedures*)

Mixing the Plaster

1. Measure 50 mL of room-temperature water into one of the flexible mixing bowls (Figure 39-27).
2. Place the second flexible mixing bowl on the scale and set the dial to zero. This allows the plaster powder to be weighed (Figure 39-28).
3. Weigh out 100 grams of plaster in the second rubber bowl.
4. Add the powder from the second bowl to the water of the first bowl. Placing the water in first allows for all the powder to become incorporated into the mixture. Allow several seconds for the powder to dissolve into the water.

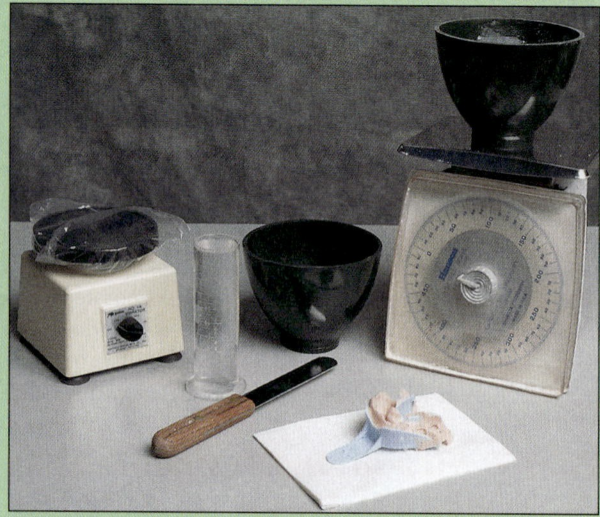

FIGURE 39-26
Equipment for pouring plaster.

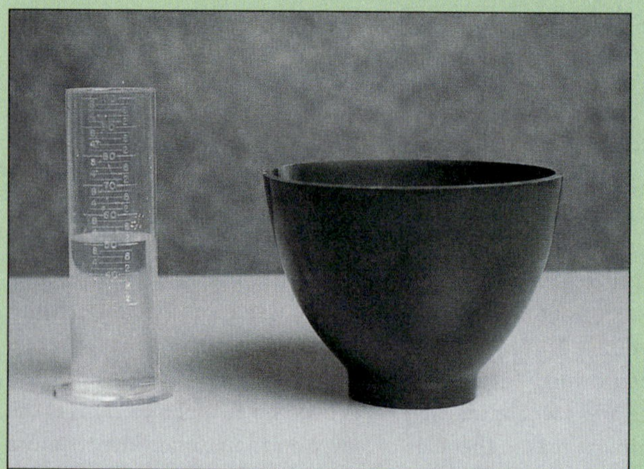

FIGURE 39-27
Measure 50 mL of water into a flexible mixing bowl.

(continues)

Procedure 39-9 (continued)

5. Use the spatula to slowly mix the particles together. The initial mixing should be completed in 20 seconds. The total mixing procedure should take about 1 minute.
6. Turn on the vibrator to medium or low speed.
7. Place the rubber bowl on the vibrator platform, pressing lightly.
8. Rotate the bowl on the vibrator to allow the air bubbles to rise to the top surface (Figure 39-29). The mixing and vibrating should be completed within a couple of minutes. The mixture is ready if the spatula can cut through it and it stays to the sides without changing positions. It will appear like whipped cream with a smooth, creamy texture (Figure 39-30). Another way to check whether the powder/water is in correct ratio is to place a spoonful on the spatula and turn it upside down. If the material remains in place, the mixture is ready.

Note: When the spatula is held sideways, mixture will fall from it.

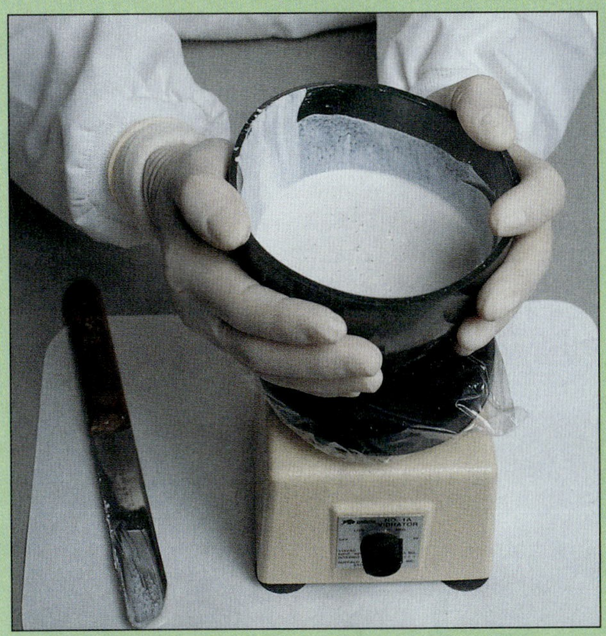

FIGURE 39-29

Vibrator brings air bubbles to surface of plaster mixture.

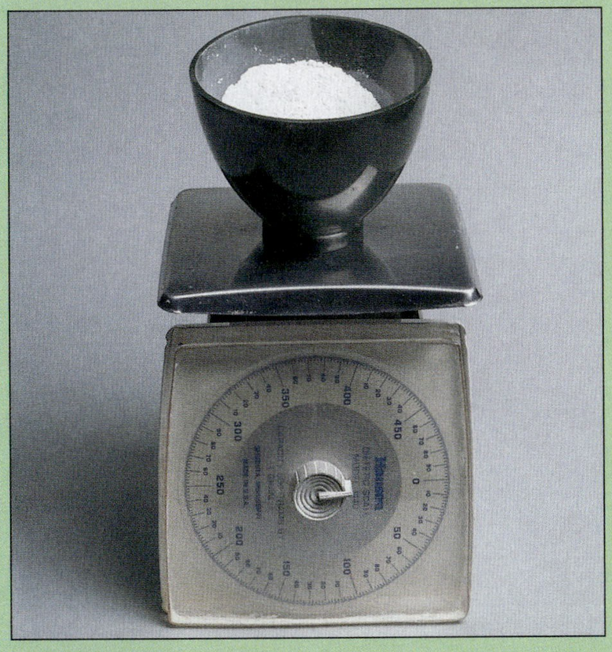

FIGURE 39-28

Measure 100 g of plaster into a bowl for pouring alginate impression.

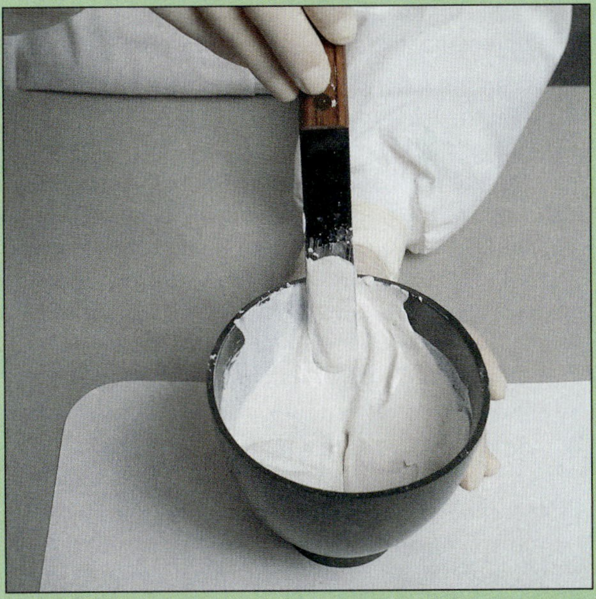

FIGURE 39-30

Plaster's consistency should allow it to retain position as spatula slides through it.

Procedure 39-10
Pouring Alginate Impression for Study Model

This procedure is performed by the dental assistant in the dental laboratory immediately after mixing the plaster. The impression is ready to pour, the excess moisture is removed, and a laboratory knife has been used to eliminate any excess impression material that will hamper the pouring of the model.

Equipment and Supplies

- Metal spatula (stiff blade with rounded end) or disposable spatula
- Mixed plaster from Procedure 39-9, Pouring an Alginate Impression with Plaster
- Vibrator with paper towel or plastic cover on platform

Procedure Steps (*Follow aseptic procedures*)

1. Use the vibrator at low or medium speed.
2. Hold the impression by the handle with the tray portion on the platform of the vibrator. Allow a small amount of plaster to touch the most distal surface of one side of the arch in the impression (Figure 39-31).
3. When the plaster touches the impression that is on the vibrating platform, it flows down the back of the impression and into the anatomy of the teeth. Continue to add small increments of the plaster in the same area as the plaster flows around toward the anterior teeth and to the other side of the arch. (Using this technique allows the air to push ahead of the plaster material, and eliminates bubbles. This produces a model that has detailed anatomic qualities.)
4. Add the plaster in this manner until it flows out the other side of the impression and fills the anatomic portion of the model. Rotating the impression around on the platform of the vibrator aids in allowing the material to travel around the arch.
5. After the anatomy portion is filled with plaster, use larger increments to fill the entire impression (while off the vibrator). When filled, place lightly on the vibrator to coalesce (combine). Overvibration can cause bubbles to form.
6. If a two-pour method is to be used, small blobs should be left on the top of the plaster so that it can attach to the art portion of the model. (A flat surface may break apart at a later date.)

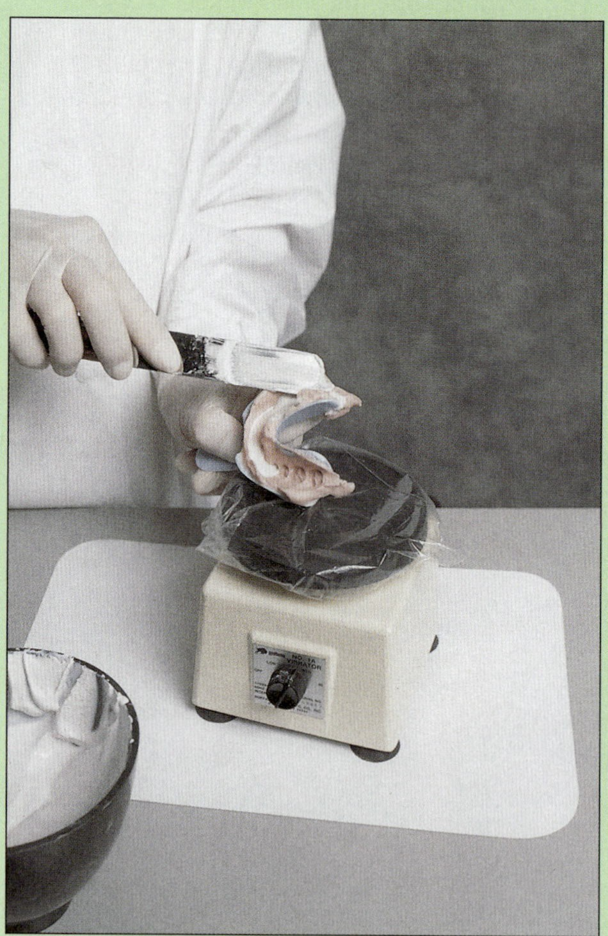

FIGURE 39-31
Mixed plaster is vibrated into alginate impression, starting at the posterior area of arch and continuing to fill from that area while material rotates around to the opposite side of arch.

Procedure 39-11
Pouring Art Portion of Plaster Study Model Using Two-Pour Method

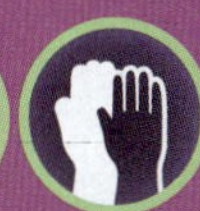

This procedure is performed by the dental assistant in the dental laboratory after the anatomic portion of the study model has set.

Equipment and Supplies

- Metal spatula (stiff blade with rounded end) or disposable spatula
- Flexible rubber bowl or disposable bowl
- Vibrator with a paper towel or plastic cover on platform
- Paper towels
- Plaster
- Calibration measurement device
- Room-temperature water
- Water measuring device

Procedure Steps (*Follow aseptic procedures*)

1. After pouring the anatomical portion of the impression, allow it to set for 5 to 10 minutes.
2. Wipe the rubber bowl and spatula with a paper towel and dispose of the material. Wash, clean, and ready the rubber bowl and spatula for a second pour of plaster.
3. The ratio of powder to water can be altered to create a thicker mix, which is desirable for bases. If pouring the bases or art portion of both the maxillary and the mandibular casts, use 100 grams of powder to 40 mL of water. If pouring only one model, mix half the amount of powder and water.
4. Mix the plaster in the same manner as before. It will appear much thicker. This part of the model is not as crucial as the anatomical portion. Areas that have bubbles can be repaired easily.
5. Gather the plaster on the spatula and place it on a glass slab or a paper towel (Figure 39-32). It is important to allow the material to mass upward and not to spread out like a pancake.
6. After all the material is on the paper towel, invert the poured anatomy portion onto the base material.
7. Hold the tray steady and situate the handle so that it is parallel to the paper surface or glass slab. It is important to get a base that is even and uniform in thickness. This makes it easier to trim the model later.
8. Carefully drag the excess plaster up over the edges of the cast, filling in any voided areas (Figure 39-33). Try not to cover any margins of the impression tray while doing this. This locks the plaster onto the tray and may cause the cast to fracture when removing the impression material and the tray.

NOTE: If using a one- or single-pour method, the base is poured immediately after the anatomical portion is poured. The two-pour method allows the material to initially set in the anatomical portion prior to inverting it and ensures that the plaster does not flow from any crucial areas.

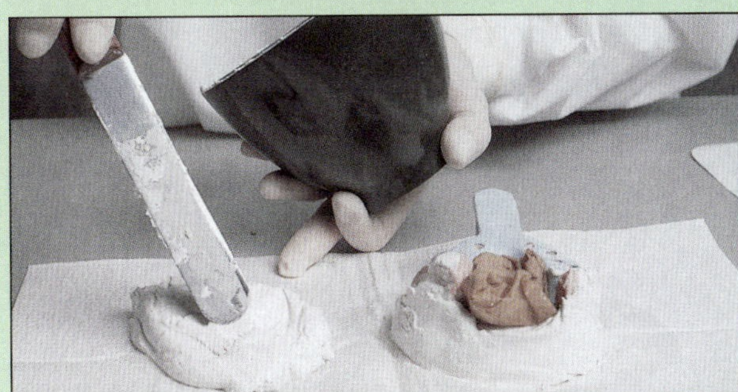

FIGURE 39-32
Plaster is gathered to make a base. The plaster must have enough body so that it does not flatten.

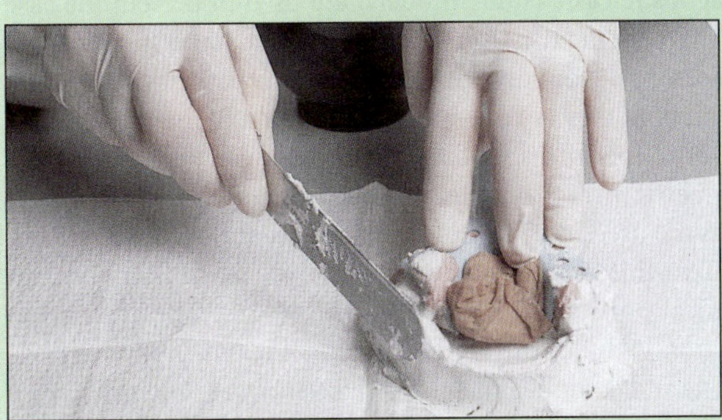

FIGURE 39-33
Operator must smooth plaster sides of base after inversion of filled impression.

Procedure 39-12
Removing Plaster Model from Alginate Impression

This procedure is performed by the dental assistant in the dental laboratory after the study model has set.

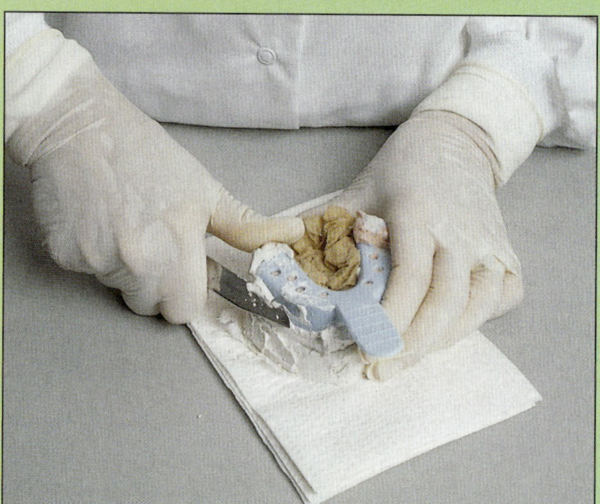

FIGURE 39-34
Before removing the impression from the model, use knife to remove remaining plaster from the impression.

Equipment and Supplies

- Laboratory knife
- Maxillary and mandibular plaster models, set in alginate impressions

Procedure Steps (*Follow aseptic procedures*)

1. Allow the plaster to set for 40 to 60 minutes before removing the impression material and the tray. The exothermic heat should be gone from the plaster material to indicate it is set.
2. Using a laboratory knife, gently remove any plaster on the margin of the tray (Figure 39-34).
3. Holding the handle of the impression tray, lift the tray straight upward.
4. If the tray does not come off, identify the area that is holding it back. Remove the necessary plaster in that area to release the tray and the impression material. Be sure to lift in an upward motion to remove the tray. Wiggling side to side or lifting sideways may fracture the teeth and anatomical portion of the cast.

Trimming and Finishing Diagnostic Casts

Diagnostic casts (study models) are used to present the case to the patient. It is important that they have an attractive appearance. Not only are they part of the patient's permanent record, but they are also a direct reflection of the type of work the office performs for the patient. They can be trimmed in a geometric form that is pleasing in appearance. Standard guidelines are used in trimming the casts (see Procedure 39-13).

Two-thirds of the trimmed model are made from the anatomical portion of the cast (Figure 39-35). The anatomical portion includes the teeth, the mucosa, and frenum attachments and is about 1 inch high. This area was duplicated from the oral cavity. The remaining one-third is the base or art portion of the cast. This portion is trimmed in a geometric form with specific angles and is about 1 inch high. When maxillary and mandibular models are trimmed and in occlusion, they should have an overall height of 3 inches.

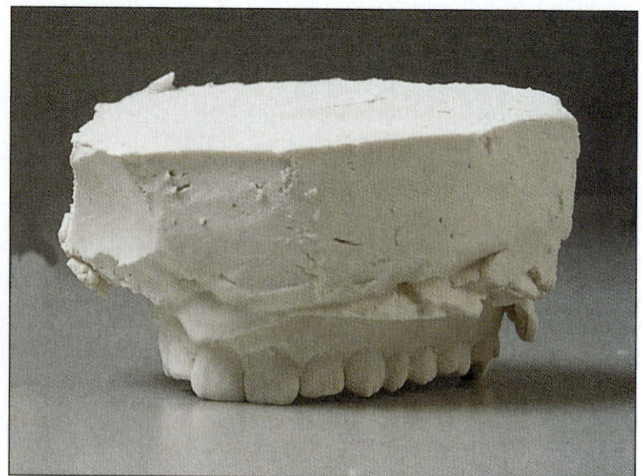

FIGURE 39-35
After trimming, the anatomical portion of the cast will make up two-thirds of the model.

Procedure 39-13
Trimming Diagnostic Casts/Study Models

This procedure is performed by the dental assistant in the dental laboratory after the study model has set, been separated from the alginate impression, and prepared for trimming.

Equipment and Supplies

- Safety glasses
- Maxillary and mandibular models
- Two flexible rubber mixing bowls
- Laboratory knife
- Pencil
- Measuring straight edge

Procedure Steps (*Follow aseptic procedures*)

1. If the maxillary and mandibular plaster models are dry, soak the bases of the models in rubber mixing bowls for 5 minutes prior to trimming. The trimming wheel on the model trimmer is more effective if the models are wet prior to trimming.
2. Don safety glasses and mask and adjust the model trimmer so that the water runs freely over the grinding wheel when the trimmer is on.
3. Invert the models so that the teeth are resting on the counter. Evaluate whether the base is parallel to the counter (Figure 39-36). Keep in mind that the art portion is ½ inch high when completed.
4. Turn on the model trimmer and trim the base so that it is parallel to the occlusal plane. The model trimmer works best if light even pressure is used when applying the models to the grinding wheel. Hold the model as level as possible during this procedure (Figure 39-37).
5. Rest hands on the table of the model trimmer and keep fingers away from the grinding wheel.
6. The model may have to be returned to the counter for re-evaluation and then again to the model trimmer to achieve a parallel surface. Trim both models to this stage.

NOTE: Move the models back and forth once across the grinding surface as the model comes off the grinding wheel. This eliminates the circular grinding marks made as the wheel rotates.

7. Place the models together in occlusion (a wax bite may be necessary) and again evaluate whether the objective of obtaining parallel models has been achieved. If not, grind to get the models to this stage. All other cuts will be off if this stage is not properly achieved, because this flat surface is laid on the model trimming table guide to grind the other areas.

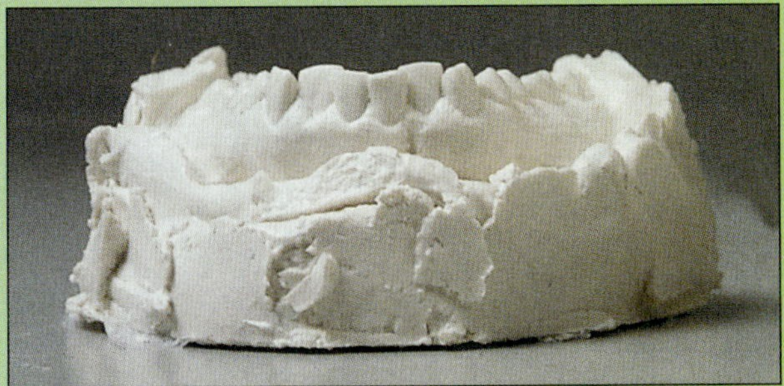

FIGURE 39-36
Before proceeding to trim study model, model base should be parallel to counter.

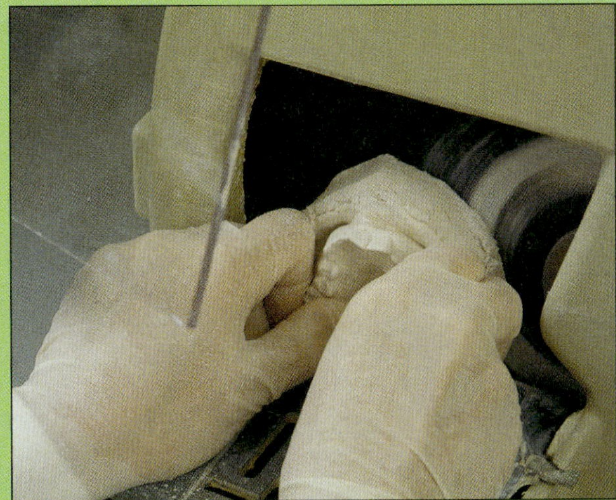

FIGURE 39-37
Study model base is trimmed as the operator maintains even pressure on the trimming wheel.

(continues)

Procedure 39-13 (continued)

8. When the cut maxillary and mandibular models are parallel as a pair, keep them in occlusion and evaluate which posterior teeth are the most distal: maxillary or mandibular. When that has been determined, take that model and draw with a pencil a line behind the retromolar area indicating where to trim (Figure 39-38).
9. Place the base surface of that model on the model trimmer table guide and cut the posterior area at a right angle with the base up to the indicated lines (Figure 39-39).
10. Put the two models back into occlusion and place the cut model (whether maxillary or mandibular) on the top. Place the opposite base on the model trimmer table guide while holding the models together and trim the posterior at a right angle to the base (Figure 39-40). The trimmed model acts as a guide to follow while trimming. When small particles of plaster are trimmed off the first base, it indicates that they are trimmed to the same plane. To evaluate this, the models are taken off the grinding wheel and placed on their backs (Figure 39-41). The occlusal plane is at a right angle to the counter. If the models stay in occlusion, the objective has been met. If they fall apart and out of occlusion, then place them back onto the grinding wheel until they stay in the correct position.

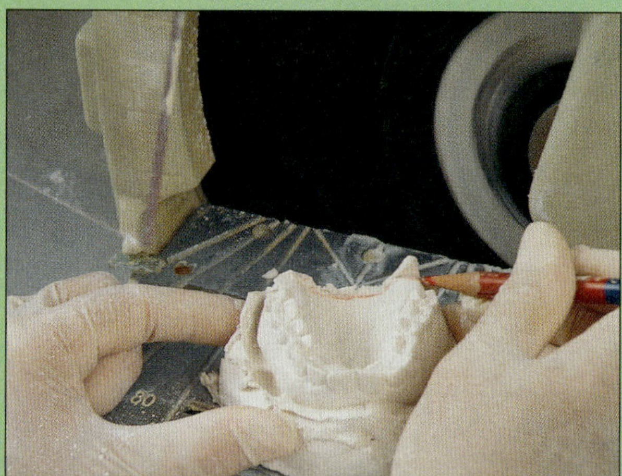

FIGURE 39-38
Pencil line is drawn from 2 mm distal from the last molar to 2 mm distal from the molar on the opposite side of the arch. This establishes a cutting line for back cut.

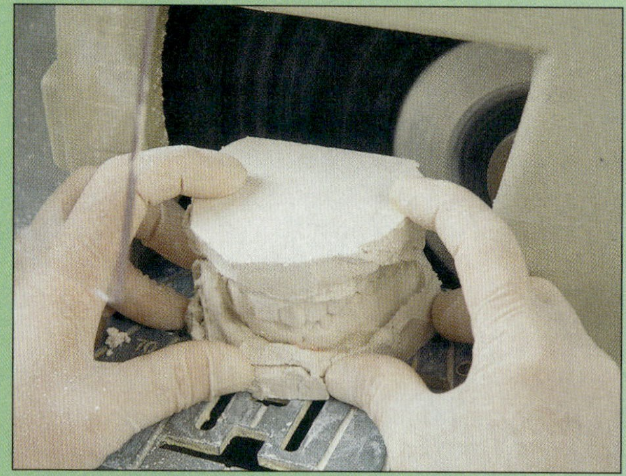

FIGURE 39-40
Models are placed together to trim back cut.

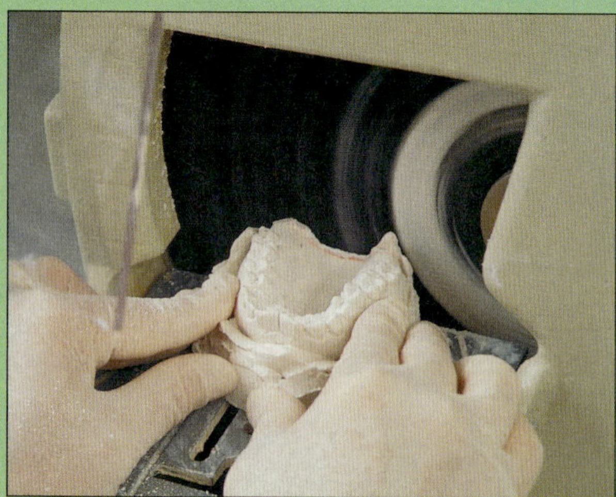

FIGURE 39-39
Posterior of model base is cut at right angle to base.

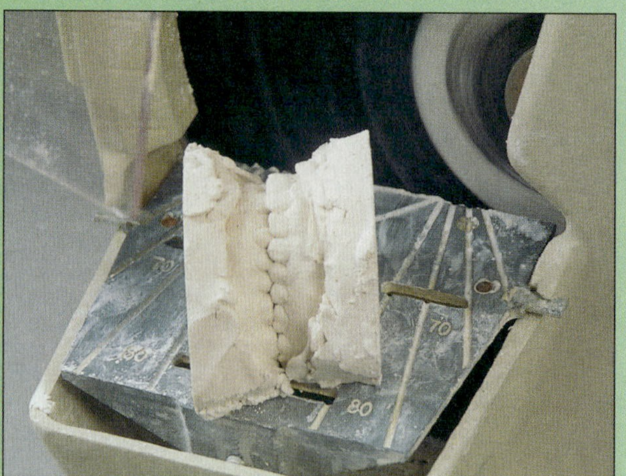

FIGURE 39-41
Models are placed on their backs on a hard, flat surface in occlusion to verify whether back cuts are correct.

(continues)

Procedure 39-13 (continued)

11. The top, bottom, and back now are trimmed. Left to trim are the heel, side, and anterior cuts. The first to be cut are the side angles. Take the pencil and mark the following areas: outward from the middle of the mandibular premolars to the edge of the model and the maxillary cuspids in the same manner. Draw a line running parallel to the teeth at the greatest depth of the buccal vestibule, from the molars to the premolars. This line will be about 5 mm from the buccal surface of the teeth. Mark both sides of the maxillary and the mandibular models in this manner.
12. Place the model base back on the model trimmer table guide and trim the model to the pencil lines on both sides (Figure 39-42). Repeat this procedure with both models.
13. Using the straight edge of the measuring device, draw a line from the dot to the canine/cuspid line on each quadrant (Figure 39-43). Make both anterior cuts, forming a pointed area at the midline and center of both cuspids. If the teeth are highly irregular, adjustments may have to be done. After the lines are drawn, make sure that the cuts will not trim away the protruding teeth. If it appears that this may happen, move the lines out on each side to accommodate this. The model should appear symmetrical (Figure 39-44).
14. A pencil line can be drawn at the depth of the anterior vestibule as a guide for trimming (Figure 39-45).

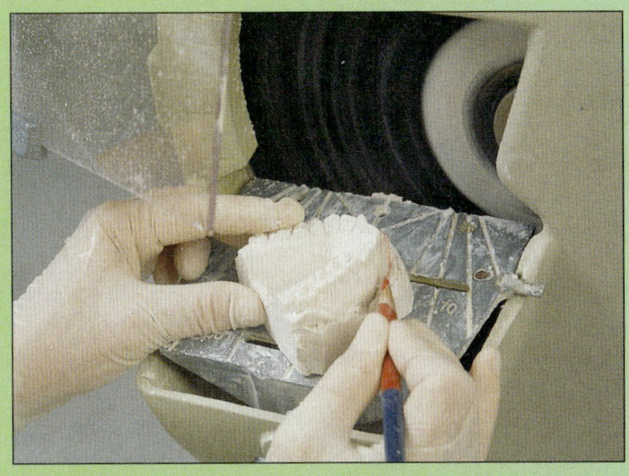

FIGURE 39-43
Line is drawn from midline of central incisors to middle of cuspid to establish a cut line for anterior.

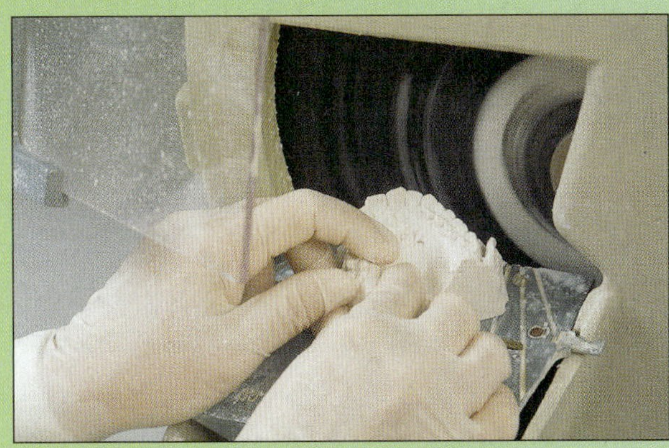

FIGURE 39-44
Maxillary anterior area is cut to a point, bringing both cuspid cuts to midline between maxillary central incisors.

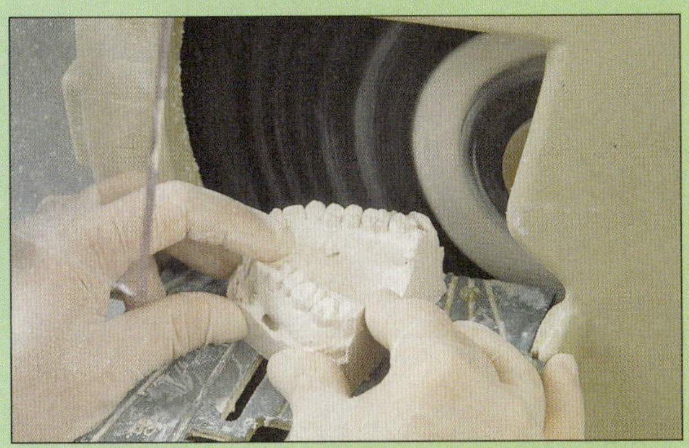

FIGURE 39-42
Vestibule or side area is cut at deepest area. A line can be drawn to establish a proper cut line.

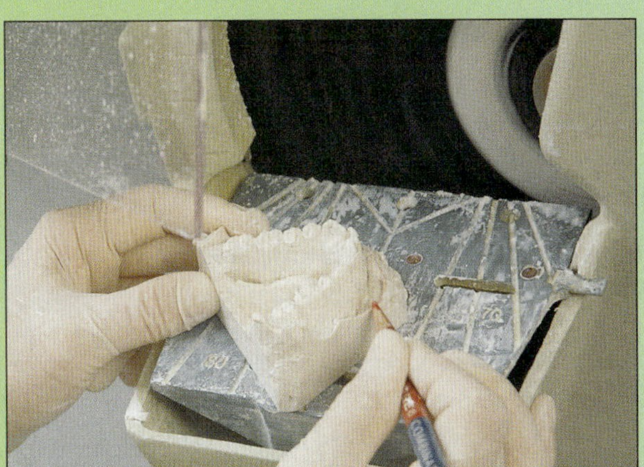

FIGURE 39-45
A rounded line is drawn on mandibular from cuspid to cuspid to indicate where the cut should be made.

(continues)

Procedure 39-13 (continued)

15. The heel cuts on both the maxillary and mandibular models are ⅜ to ⅝ inches wide and should appear symmetric in length. They can be drawn on the model by turning the base upward and placing an imaginary diagonal line from the cuspid (maxillary) premolar (mandibular) to where the side and back cuts meet. Draw a 90 degree angle across the base, opposite the anterior area. The heel cuts are small cuts on both the maxillary and the mandibular models that finish the trimming of the models (Figure 39-46).
16. After the models are trimmed symmetrically, a laboratory knife is used to trim the tongue area flat and smooth other areas on the art portion. Take care not to destroy the anatomy of the diagnostic casts. Any air bubbles can be filled with plaster. Use dry plaster on the finger, and push it into the wet model to fill small air bubbles. To complete the smoothing of the flat surfaces, a fine wet/dry sandpaper can be used under water. Any small beads of plaster can be removed carefully from the surfaces of the teeth.
17. Place the models in a model gloss for 10 minutes or spray with gloss to provide a professional appearance and add strength. The models need to be polished with a dry cloth to buff the surface in order to achieve the desired high gloss.
18. Label both models with the patient's name and the date the models were taken. In an orthodontic office, the patient's age may also be identified on the models.

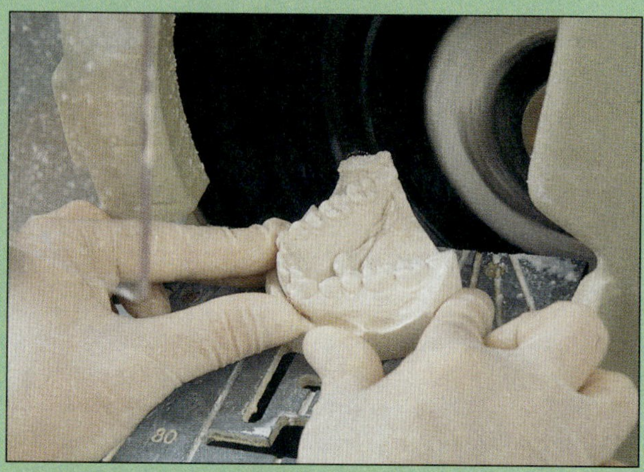

FIGURE 39-46
Heel cuts are established on models and cut.

Note: The grinding stone on the model trimmer can be cleaned with a brush and the water increased to run over the surface. Shut off the machine and clean the guide table and the reservoir beneath where the plaster accumulates. If this is allowed to build up, the water will back up and cause water to splash out while trimming.

Trimmed Diagnostic Casts (Study Models) Evaluation

- Both maxillary and mandibular models are trimmed symmetrically following specific cut angles indicated.
- All anatomic portions of the model are accurate.
- Trimmed models sit on end and maintain occlusion.
- Each model exhibits a ½-inch base and a 1-inch anatomic portion.
- Final finishing is accomplished and the models present a professional appearance (Figure 39-47).

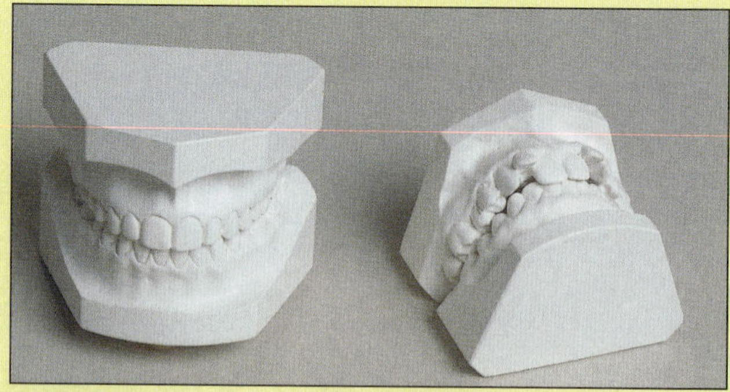

FIGURE 39-47
Trimmed study models.

Articulating Casts or Study Models

An articulator is used to duplicate the patient's occlusion on models (Figure 39-48). An **articulator** is a frame that holds models of the patient's teeth in order to maintain the patient's occlusion and represent his or her jaws. Articulators can be simple, such as hinges that only duplicate the up-and-down motions, or they can be complex, where they are adjustable and can duplicate the side-to-side motions as well as the up-and-down motions.

Articulators can be used to study malocclusion, to wax and carve teeth for crowns and bridges, and to demonstrate to the patient the action that is of concern. They also have a number of other desired uses. The dental assistant may perform the task of mounting models or assist the dentist in this task.

Facebows and Articulators

Dental offices will use a **facebow** and an articulator to duplicate the function of the tempormandibular joint. The facebow allows the operator to obtain the records about the placement of the maxillary arch and its location to the joint. From this the mandibular arch can be mounted and the biting function can be duplicated. This provides the dentist the information for diagnosis or for constructing dental appliances such as crowns, bridges, veneers, partials, and dentures.

Facebow Transfer

Dental assistants will need to prepare the patient and the parts of the facebow (Figure 39-49) for the facebow transfer. This skill is allowed for dental assistants to complete under general supervision in some states. Following all aseptic techniques and informing the patient, the operator will use the reference plane marker and locator to mark the anterior reference point on the patient's right side according to the manufacturer's directions. (See Procedure 39-14, Completing a Facebow Transfer.) The bite registration material or baseplate wax is then placed on the top side of the bitefork, which is then inserted into the patient's mouth where they close on it to secure it in place while the material sets. The facebow is secured to the bitefork and the earbow assembly is attached. The finger screws are tightened to obtain the needed records and then the release screws are loosened and the patient opens and the entire facebow and bitefork is removed from the patient. It is disinfected and either sent to the laboratory or the dentist or auxiliary will mount it to an articulator (see Procedure 39-15).

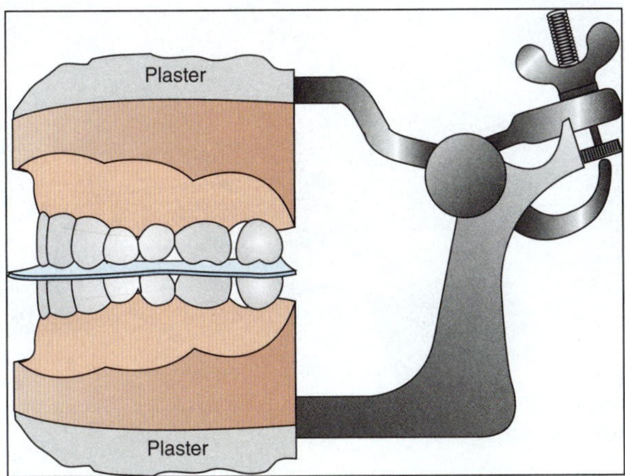

FIGURE 39-48
Articulator.

Articulator

An articulator (Figure 39-50) is used to replicate the up-and-down motion and lateral movement of the joint. Many articulators are on the market and used for specific

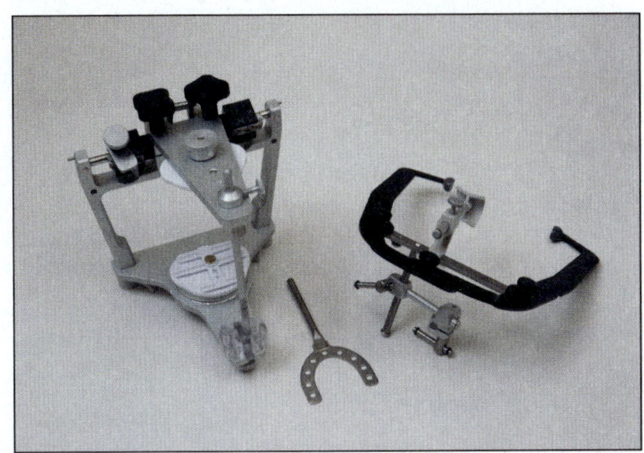

FIGURE 39-49
Facebow parts.

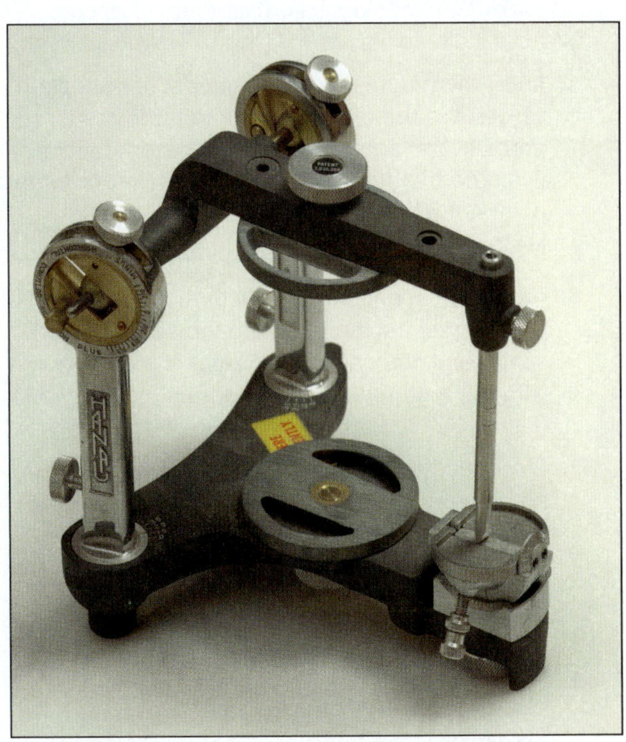

FIGURE 39-50
Articulator that can duplicate an individual's bite and mastication.

Procedure 39-14
Taking the Records and Performing a Facebow Transfer

This procedure is performed by the dental assistant under the general supervision of the dentist in some states, or by the dentist with the auxiliary assisting. The patient is seated and prepared for dental treatment. The operator has washed hands and donned gloves, eyewear, and mask.

Equipment and Supplies

- Earbow
- Bitefork and transfer jig assembly
- Reference plane marker
- Reference plane locator
- Firm cotton roll
- Bite registration material or baseplate wax

Procedure Steps (*Follow aseptic procedures and wear PPE*)

1. Assemble equipment and supplies.
2. Explain the procedure to the patient.
3. Use the reference plane marker and locater and mark the anterior reference point on the patient's right side according to the manufacturer's directions.
4. Apply the bite registration material or baseplate wax on the top of the bitefork in three areas, normally the anterior and both posterior sides. Evaluate the arch to ensure that there are three points of reference.
5. Insert the bitefork into the mouth.
6. Align the patient's midline with the index notch; ensure that it is parallel with the patient's horizontal and coronal planes. Move the bitefork with the material into place on the maxillary arch (Figure 39-51).
7. Place a cotton roll or two under the bitefork to stabilize as the patient bites and this will avoid movement as the material sets.
8. Attach the vertical shaft to the measuring facebow with the clamp and tighten the screw. This should hold the facebow onto the shaft.
9. Loosen the side finger screws as well as the center wheel so that the earbow assembly on the facebow will open.
10. Have the patient place the bow earpieces in the ears (Figure 39-52). Have them slide the earpieces forward to ensure they are in the ears snugly.
11. Tighten the finger side screws.
12. Raise or lower the bow so that the pointer aligns precisely with the anterior reference point. When it is aligned, tighten the clamps. If necessary adjustments are made, retighten the side finger screws to accommodate changes (Figure 39-53). Make sure not to alter the bow when tightening all of the screws.

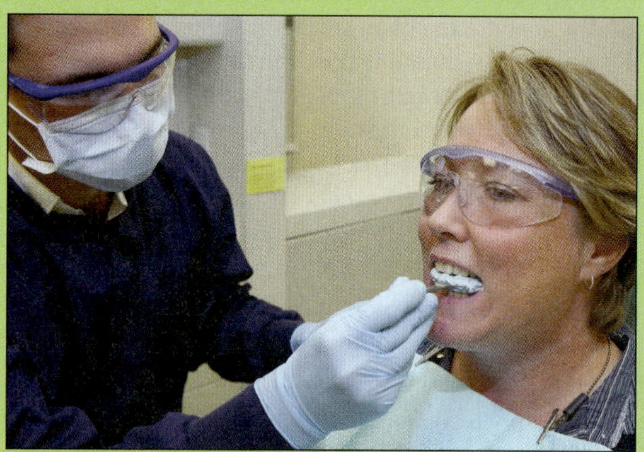

FIGURE 39-51
Move the bitefork with the material into place on the maxillary arch.

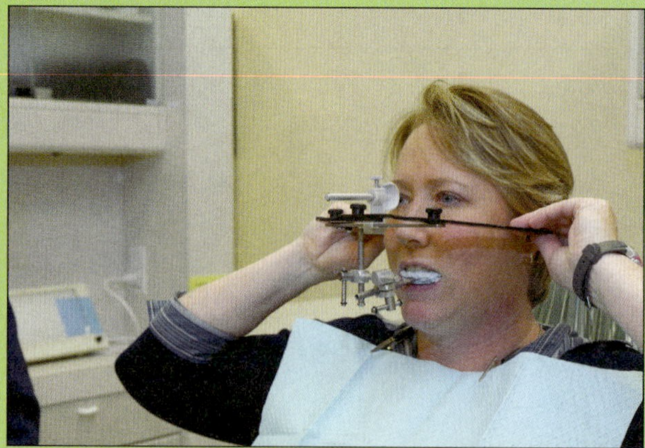

FIGURE 39-52
Have the patient place the bow earpiece into the ears.

(continues)

Procedure 39-14 (continued)

13. Loosen the anterior finger grip and screw on the measuring bow, move the measuring bow away from the patient's face, and instruct the patient to open while holding the bow and removing it and the bitefork from the patient's mouth (Figure 39-54).

14. The bitefork is to be disinfected prior to sending to the laboratory or mounting it to the articulator.

15. Dismiss the patient, document the procedure on the patient's chart, and give postoperative instructions.

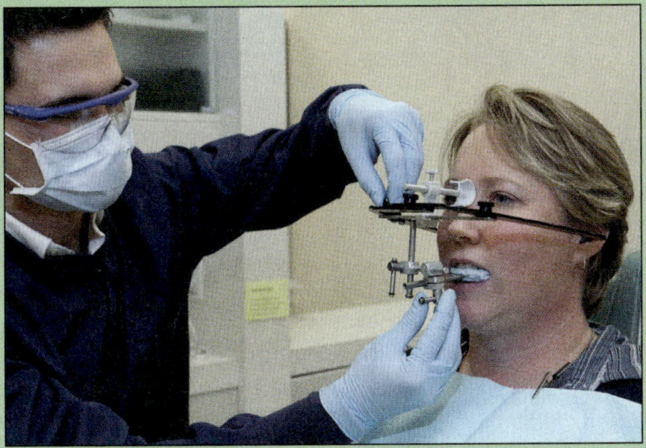

FIGURE 39-53
Retighten side finger screws to accommodate changes.

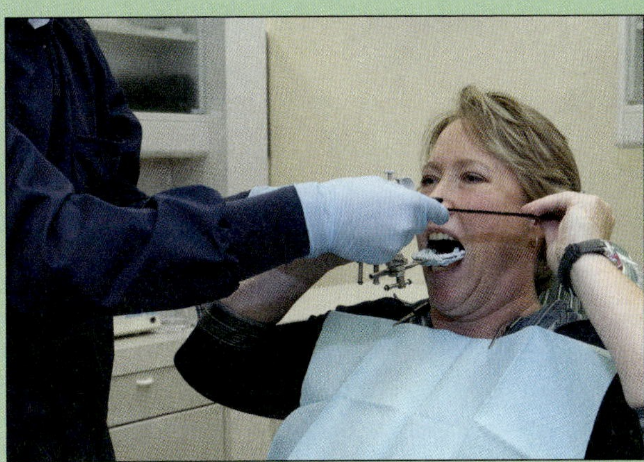

FIGURE 39-54
Removing the bitefork from the patient's mouth.

Procedure 39-15
Mounting Models on an Articulator After Facebow Records Have Been Completed

This procedure is performed by the dental assistant under the general supervision of the dentist in some states or by the dentist with the auxiliary assisting. It is done in the office dental laboratory or at a commercial dental laboratory. The facebow is disinfected and ready to be mounted.

Equipment and Supplies

- Facebow and bitefork assembled
- Articulator
- Two mounting rings
- Trimmed models
- Type I plaster and water
- Mixing bowl and spatula

Procedure Steps (*Follow aseptic procedures and wear PPE*)

1. Assemble equipment and supplies.
2. Trim models so that they fit within the two bows easily.
3. Score the models with a knife.
4. Attach the facebow to the articulator according to the manufacturer's directions.
5. Place the maxillary model into the bite registration material or baseplate wax that was used on the patient. Make sure that it is seated into the impression that was established.
6. Lift the articulator arm up to expose the scored area on the maxillary model.

(continues)

Procedure 39-15 (continued)

7. Mix Type I Plaster to a thick consistency and place it on the model. Fill the entire space between the model and the top of the articulator, then bring the top arm with the articulator ring down onto the plaster (Figure 39-55). Make sure some of the plaster goes through the open areas of the ring. Remove excess plaster and smooth the plaster around the ring and the model.
8. After the maxillary model is set, remove the facebow and bite stick. The maxillary model is now attached to the articulator. Use the bite registrations that were obtained during the appointment to mount the mandibular model. Hold the models together in correct bite and mix additional plaster. Mound the plaster on the lower articulator ring until the space is filled and then allow the area of the mandibular scored model to be placed into the plaster (Figure 39-56).
9. After the initial set, clean any excess plaster up and smooth the plaster that has been added. After the plaster has set, the models remain in the articulator and then can be opened and closed as if biting. They also allow for side to side excursions to be accomplished so that the dental appliance can be made properly.
10. The pin is added to the articulator and now the centric relationship has been established for the models. The **centric relationship** is where the teeth are positioned when the joints are aligned. Patients often rest in this centric relationship.
11. After this is accomplished the dentist can diagnosis or work with the dental laboratory to fabricate crowns, veneers, or partials.

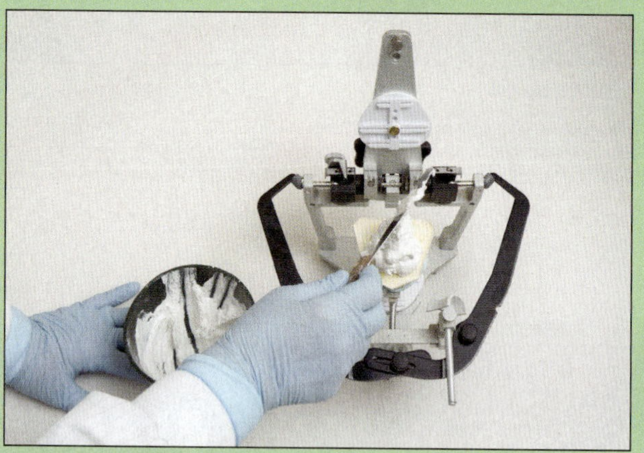

FIGURE 39-55

Fill the entire space between the model and the top of the articulator, and then bring the top arm with the articulator ring down onto the plaster.

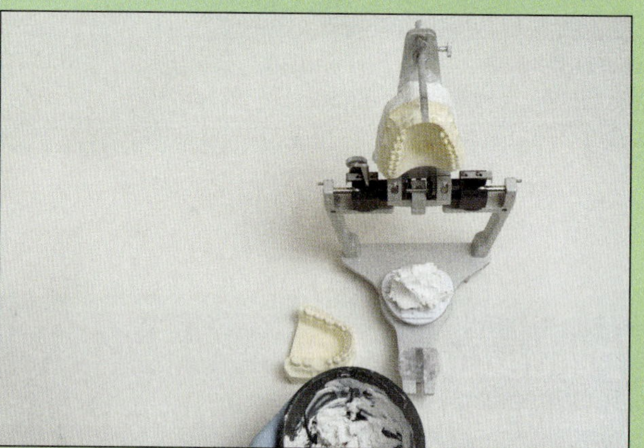

FIGURE 39-56

Mound the plaster on the lower articulating ring until the space is filled.

reasons with enhanced functions. They have two support bows: one to stabilize the maxillary and one to stabilize the mandibular.

The hinge represents the temporomandibular joints. The first step in using this articulator is to trim the models so that they fit within the two bows easily. The top portion of the bases can then be scored. To score a model is to make cut marks in the smooth surface so that the added gypsum can adhere. The models are placed within the bows in the correct bite. Normally, the wax bite is used to establish the correct occlusion. The models are then attached to the bows using impression plaster, which flows into the scored area and around the bow. After the plaster has set, the models remain fastened to the articulator and can be opened and the wax bite removed.

Dental Waxes

Waxes are among the oldest materials used in dentistry. Over 200 years ago, impressions were taken of specific areas in the mouth with wax. The waxes are derived from a number of sources, including bees, plants, and minerals. Beeswax has to be refined and bleached to obtain uniformity of color and character. Differences in color and texture may take place if the bee has been feeding on something unusual, for example, plants all yellow in color. Certain plants in South America and Brazil bring to dentistry a hard wax that is gathered from the fronds of a tree. This wax also is used for polishing automobiles to a high gloss shine. From minerals come petroleum products, such as paraffin wax. In dentistry, only the highest grade of wax is used. It must be uniform and provide consistent results when used.

Wax Groups

Waxes are classified into three broad groups: pattern, processing, and impression. Pattern waxes are hard waxes used in crown and bridge casting (inlay wax) and the construction of the baseplate tray (baseplate wax). Processing and impression waxes have many uses in dentistry.

Pattern Wax. Pattern, or inlay, wax normally is supplied in dark-colored sticks (Figure 39-57A). It is used on a die, a positive replica of the prepared tooth made from stone. The wax is melted and applied to the die, making a wax pattern that is used to create the metal and/or porcelain restoration. The composition varies from manufacturer to manufacturer, but most waxes have a certain degree of hardness, toughness, resistance to flaking, and ability to achieve a smooth surface. Desirable properties of inlay wax are that it flows at a temperature slightly above the mouth temperature, it achieves complete burnout at temperatures above 900°F, and it carves away easily without chipping or cracking. These properties are essential in using the *lost wax* technique of casting. The lost wax technique refers to the wax pattern after the wax is enclosed in investment stone and heated to high temperatures. The high temperatures cause the wax to vaporize, leaving behind a void or an empty space (lost wax) where the melted metal can be invested using centrifugal force.

The baseplate wax is a hard wax that can be heated to make the initial base on which to form a denture (Figure 39-57B). It comes in Types I, II, and III. Type III is the hardest, and Type II is most often used in the fabrication of baseplates.

Processing Wax. Several waxes used in dentistry are in the processing wax classification (Figure 39-58). Boxing wax is a soft, pliable wax that is used to form a wax box around an impression prior to pouring it with gypsum. It comes in wax strips 1 and 1½ inches wide and can be reused for the purpose of making a ring around the impression to hold the runny gypsum in place until it sets.

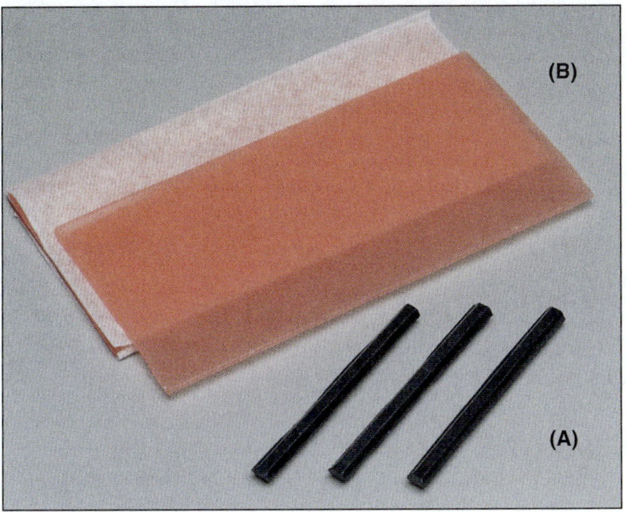

FIGURE 39-57

Pattern waxes. (A) Inlay wax. (B) Baseplate wax.

Sticky wax is another type of processing wax. It is very brittle at room temperature but when melted with a flame source becomes soft and sticky. It adheres to a number of surfaces, such as metal, gypsum, and porcelain. It is used to hold two fractured pieces together until they can be repaired.

Utility wax, also called periphery or bending wax, is a soft wax that is adhesive and pliable. It does not require additional heat and can be molded to most surfaces. This is the wax used to bead around trays to extend them and assist in patient comfort. This wax is also used for orthodontic patients to cover the brackets and uncomfortable areas until the cheeks and lips can adjust. It is supplied in long ropes or strips and in a number of colors.

Impression or Bite Registration Waxes. Normally containing copper or aluminum particles, impression waxes are used to take bite registrations. They are supplied in horseshoe shapes for obtaining the maxillary and mandibular biting surfaces.

Additional Waxes. Other waxes used in dentistry that are not in the three primary classifications are the study wax and the undercut wax. The study wax is hard wax supplied in blocks used for carving teeth and anatomy (Figure 39-59). Undercut wax is a putty-type wax used to fill in the undercuts prior to the impression being taken.

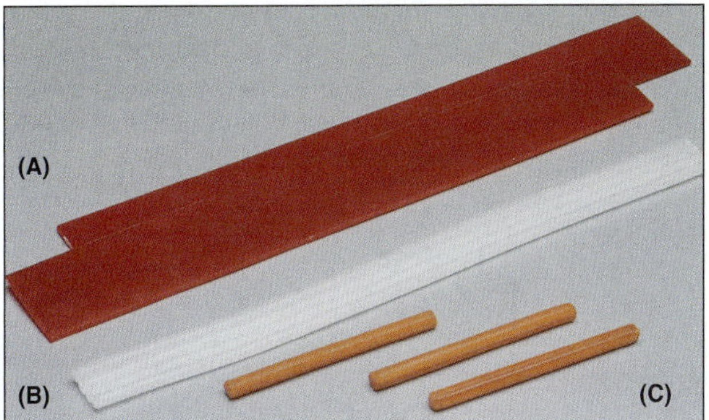

FIGURE 39-58

Processing waxes. (A) Boxing wax. (B) Utility wax. (C) Sticky wax.

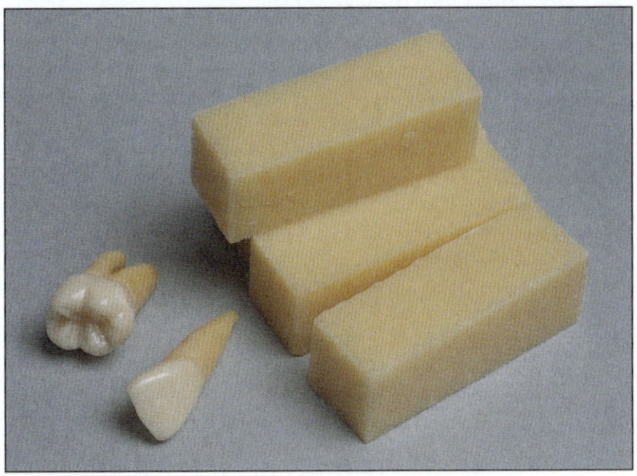

FIGURE 39-59

Study wax blocks.

Custom Trays

The dentist may ask for a custom tray for the patient in order to obtain an accurate impression. This may be because a regular stock tray does not fit. The stock tray will not allow a minimum amount of space for the material to flow around the prepared area, or it may require that an overabundance of impression material be used to obtain the impression, therefore risking an inferior outcome. In any case, a custom tray can be fabricated to meet the need. Several materials are available to make a custom tray. It can be constructed from self- or light-curing acrylic resin, a vacuum resin, or a thermoplastic material. All materials must be rigid enough to provide subsistence for the material as it is inserted into and removed from the mouth. It is important that the material adapts well during the construction so that the final tray meets the required criteria.

Required Criteria for a Custom Tray

- Stable enough to hold the material rigid during placement and removal.
- Can be smoothed and contoured to the arch.
- Can be adapted to an edentulous, a partially edentulous, and a full dentition.
- Can be adapted to allow uniform thickness of impression material in all areas of the arch.
- Can be altered and contoured to any irregular area.
- Can be designed so that stops are in the spacer, therefore holding the material in a stable, specifically determined area, providing a more accurate impression.

Self-Curing Acrylic Tray Resin Custom Trays

The most common material used to make custom trays is the self-curing acrylic tray resin (Procedure 39-16). It consists of a liquid catalyst (**monomer**) that mixes with a powder (**polymer**) to start the process of curing (polymerization). Polymerization occurs when material changes from a plastic pliable state to a rigid state. Once this process starts, it continues until the material is set completely. The material goes through several stages as it is cured. The first stage is after the liquid and the powder are mixed together. This initial set is when the material appears sticky and, if pulled apart, appears to have spider-web strands from particle to particle. The second stage is where the material can be gathered into a ball, kneaded, and contoured to the model. The third stage is where the material goes through an exothermic reaction, giving off a great deal of heat while setting. When the heat has diminished and the material can no longer be shaped, the final set stage is completed. A custom tray should be allowed to set for 24 hours prior to use due to the fact that it is still dimensionally unstable.

Light-Cured Acrylic Tray Resin Custom Trays

Acrylic tray resin is supplied in light-cured custom trays. The primary difference between this material and the self-curing material is that the setting time is operator controlled. The material stays pliable and workable until a light source initiates polymerization. The polymerization process happens quickly.

Procedure 39-16

Procedure Constructing a Self-Curing Acrylic Resin Custom Tray

This procedure is performed by the dental assistant in the dental laboratory on a working cast.

Equipment and Supplies

- Maxillary and/or mandibular casts
- Laboratory knife
- Pencil (plain or red and blue)
- Wax spatula
- Baseplate wax and heating source (warm water or laboratory torch)
- Tray resin with measuring devices
- Separating medium with brush
- Wooden tongue blade and wax-lined paper cup
- Petroleum jelly
- Tray adhesive

Procedure Steps (*Follow aseptic procedures*)

Preparing the Cast

1. Outline the area of the cast for the spacer to be placed (see Figure 39-71). This is 2 to 3 mm below the margin of the prepared tooth or 2 to 3 mm above the lowest point in the vestibule if the arch is edentulous.

(continues)

Procedure 39-16 (continued)

2. Fill any undercuts in the cast or cover with the spacer material. Heat the spacer material and contour to the pencil line.
3. Using a laboratory knife, trim the wax or spacer to the line using an angled cut instead of a blunt cut (Figure 39-60).
4. Cut the appropriate stops in the spacer (Figure 39-61).
5. Cover the spacer with aluminum foil or paint it with separating medium.

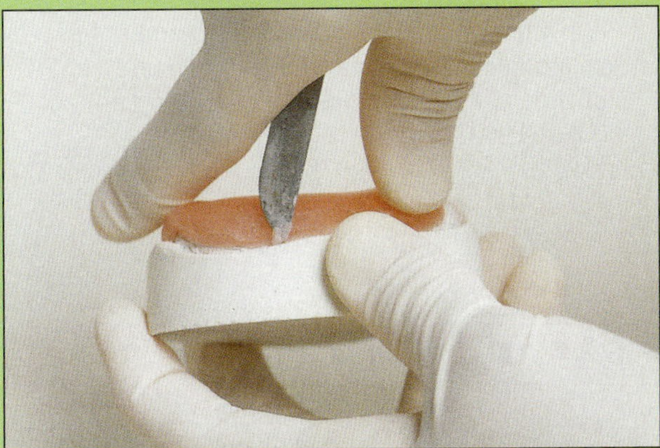

FIGURE 39-60
Wax spacer is trimmed to line on working cast.

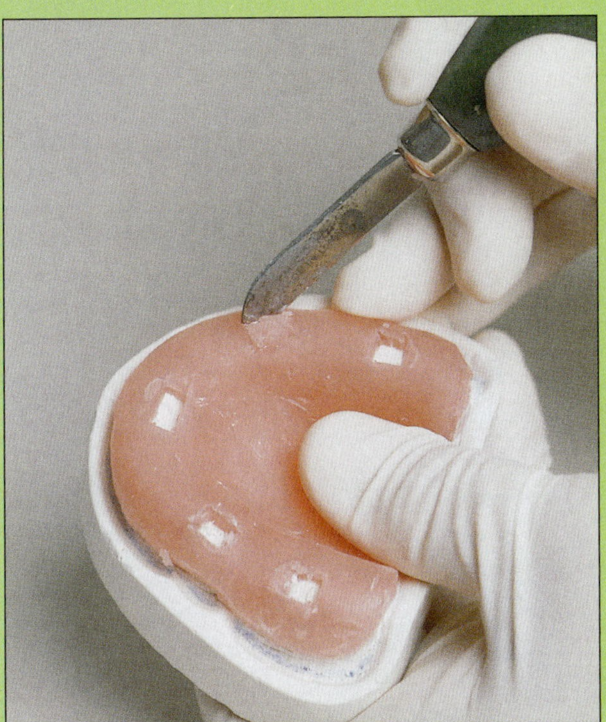

FIGURE 39-61
Stops cut into wax spacer allow room for impression material.

Mixing Custom Tray Acrylic Self-Curing Resin

1. Measure the powder and the liquid to the correct calibrations on the measuring devices according to the manufacturer's directions.
2. Mix the powder and liquid together in the wax-lined paper cup with the wooden tongue blade until the mixture is **homogeneous** (uniformly mixed).
3. Allow the mixture to go through initial polymerization for 2 to 3 minutes. Some manufacturers indicate that a cover be placed over the material during the polymerization.
4. During this time, place petroleum jelly over the cast and on the palms of your hands.

Contouring Custom Tray Acrylic Self-Curing Resin

1. The material is ready to conform to the tray after the initial set when the material is no longer sticky and can be gathered into a ball. Knead the material to further mix the material and set a small amount aside for the handle (Figure 39-62). This doughy stage allows the material to be formed into a patty for the maxillary arch or a roll for the mandibular arch.
2. Place the dough-like patty for the maxillary cast, covering the wax spacer. Contour and adapt it to extend 1 to 2 mm over the wax spacer (Figure 39-63A). Try to complete the adaptation with a rolled edge at the designated area. If unable to accomplish this, a laboratory knife can be used to trim the material back. (Doing this causes rough edges that need to be smoothed back later.)

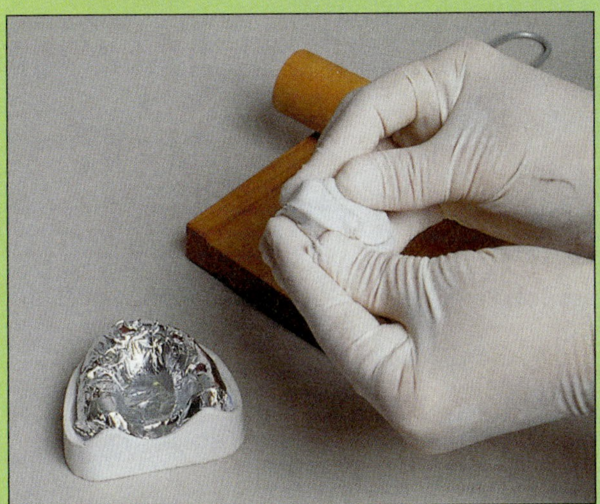

FIGURE 39-62
Custom tray material is kneaded for use.

(continues)

Procedure 39-16 (continued)

3. The material set aside for the handle is shaped and a drop of the monomer liquid placed on the tray where the handle is to be adapted and then on the handle where it will be placed on the custom tray. This allows the materials to join together for a better outcome.
4. Place the handle in the midline area of the arch (Figure 39-63B). If making an edentulous custom tray, the handle should come up from the ridge and then outward. A custom tray handle that is made for an area that has teeth can come directly outward.
5. Place the handle and hold it in the proper position until the material becomes firm.

Finishing Custom Tray Acrylic Self-Curing Resin

1. The setting takes about 8 to 10 minutes. Remove the custom tray from the cast and take out the spacer material.
2. If foil has been used, the cleaning will not take a great deal of time. If only wax was used, melt it. A wax spatula is used to remove it, along with hot water and an old toothbrush.
3. After the final set (30 minutes minimum), use an acrylic bur (Figure 39-64) or an arbor band to trim the edges of the custom tray. Do not trim the inside of the tray.
4. Clean and disinfect the custom tray according to the manufacturer's directions. Write the patient's name on the tray.
5. Apply the adhesive provided by the manufacturer of the impression material to the inside of the custom tray and along the margins (Figure 39-65).

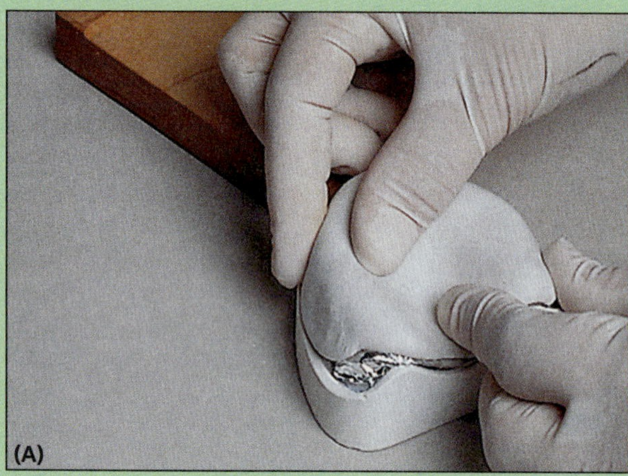

(A)

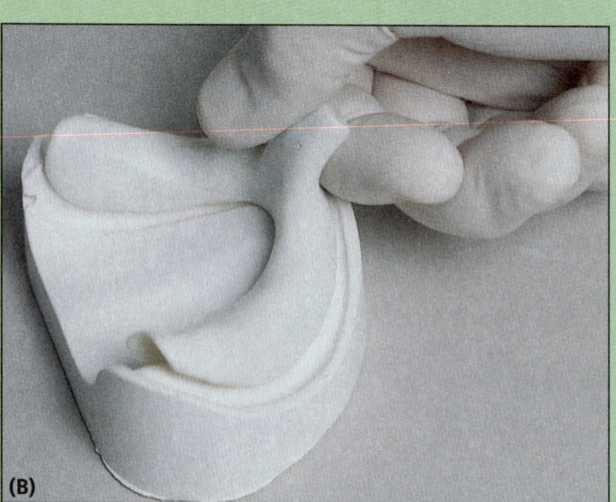

(B)

FIGURE 39-63

(A) Custom tray material is adapted to model over wax spacer. (B) Handle is attached to adapted custom tray.

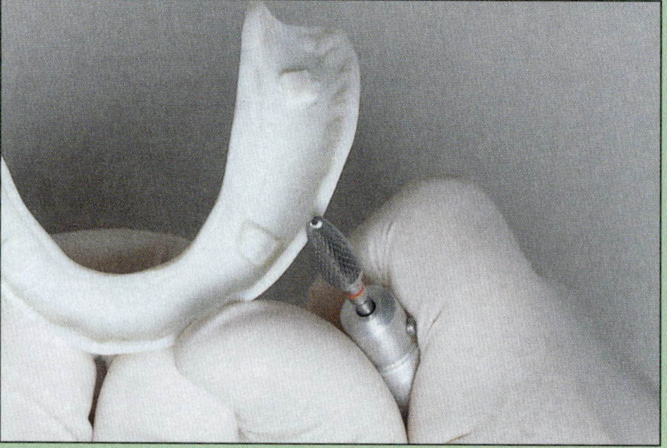

FIGURE 39-64

Custom tray is trimmed with an acrylic bur.

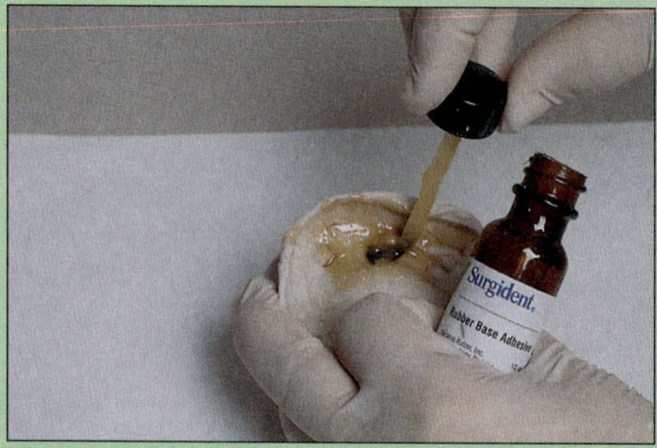

FIGURE 39-65

Adhesive is applied to custom tray in a thin coat and allowed to dry.

This technique requires special equipment: an oven-like appliance with a special curing light in it (Figure 39-66). The custom tray is designed and placed in the oven for a quick setting and then is ready for use.

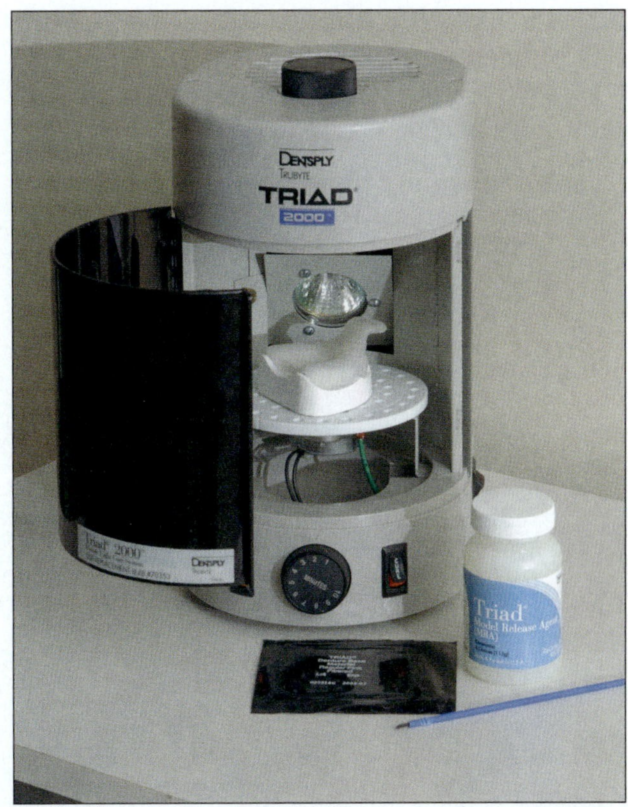

FIGURE 39-66

Triad® Visible Light Cure unit.

Vacuum-Formed Custom Trays

Like the acrylic tray resin that is light cured, the vacuum-formed custom trays require additional equipment (Procedure 39-17). This unit has a frame that holds the sheets directly under a heating element and, when they are softened, the frame drops the sheet onto the cast as vacuum pressure draws the material to the model. The vacuum-forming unit has other applications in dentistry. Acrylic resin sheets are supplied in several gauges for different applications. The custom tray requires the use of a rigid, heavy, plastic resin.

Thermoplastic Tray Material Custom Trays

Other materials used for making custom trays are the **thermoplastic** beads and buttons. When these small, round beads or buttons are placed in warm water, the thermoplastic reaction takes place. Thermoplastic means that the material becomes soft and pliable when exposed to heat. Once the material is soft, it can be conformed to the model in the desired shape. As the heat dissipates, the material hardens. It is easy to identify when the material is soft enough because it appears clear and then becomes dense when it hardens.

Procedure 39-17
Constructing a Vacuum-Formed Acrylic Resin Custom Tray

This procedure is performed by the dental assistant in the dental laboratory on a working cast.

Equipment and Supplies

- Maxillary and/or mandibular casts
- Laboratory knife
- Laboratory scissors
- Vacuum former with heating element
- Acrylic sheets

Procedure Steps (*Follow aseptic procedures*)

Preparing the Cast

1. The cast is soaked in warm water for up to 30 minutes prior to forming a custom tray on it. This eliminates small air bubbles. (These air bubbles coming to the surface [percolating] will cause small spaces between the cast and the acrylic sheet. Then, the custom tray would not have the accuracy desired.)
2. Place the spacer, if indicated. (A wax spacer will melt under the heating element, if used.)
3. Mark the desired outer margin of the custom tray.
4. Place the cast on the platform of the vacuum-forming unit.

Contouring Acrylic Resin Sheets during Vacuum-Forming Process

1. Select the appropriate acrylic resin sheets to be used for the procedure.
2. Place the acrylic resin sheets between the heater frame and the gasket frame and tighten the anterior knob to secure the material in place. Place the cast on the platform (Figure 39-67).
3. Make sure the heating element is in the correct place above the acrylic resin sheet and turn it on.

(continues)

Procedure 39-17 (continued)

4. Watch the resin as it heats. It will begin to sag downward (Figure 39-68). Allow this to continue until the resin droops downward about 1 inch. (Overheating causes air bubbles to form on the surface of the acrylic resin.)
5. After the material is heated properly, take both handles on the frame and pull the frame downward, over the cast. Only touch the handles because the entire area is extremely hot.
6. Turn on the vacuum immediately after the resin sheet is entirely over the cast (Figure 39-69).
7. Turn off the heating unit.
8. Allow the vacuum to continue for 1 to 2 minutes in order to cool the resin so it becomes firm again.

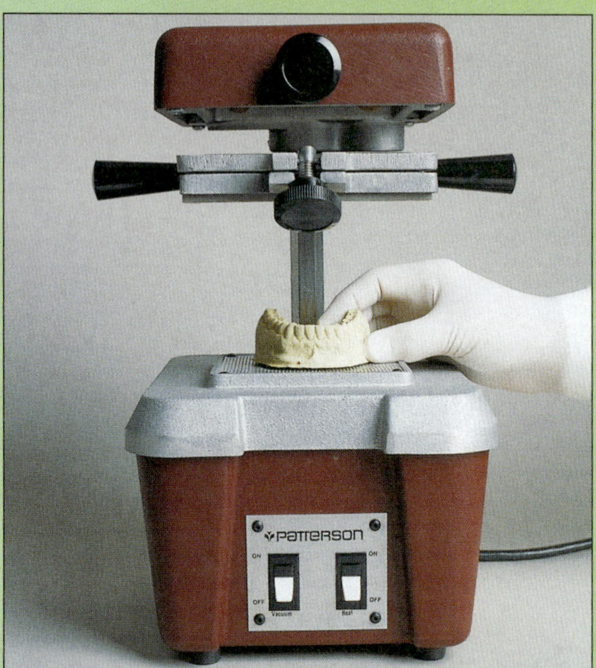

FIGURE 39-67

Resin sheets are secured in place, and the cast is placed on the platform of a vacuum-forming unit.

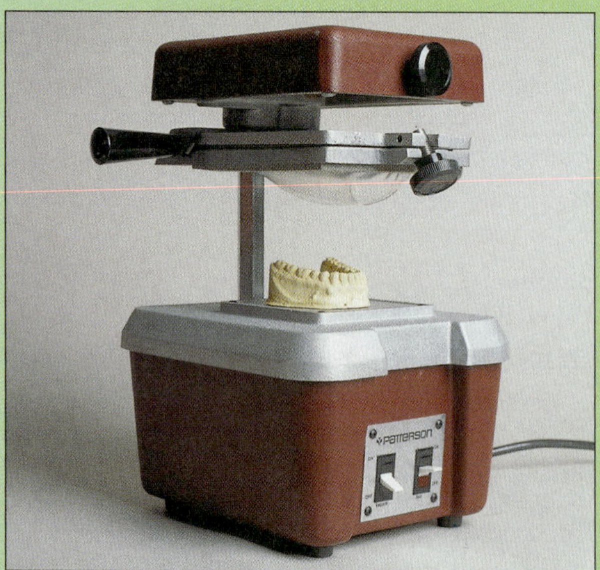

FIGURE 39-68

Resin sheet begins sagging as material is heated.

Finishing Vacuum-Formed Acrylic Resin Custom Tray

1. After the resin material is cooled, remove it from the vacuum-form frame.
2. Separate the resin-formed custom tray from the cast and, using laboratory scissors, trim to the desired form (Figure 39-70).
3. Use a torch to heat and apply a cutout handle section to the custom tray.
4. Clean and disinfect the custom tray according to the manufacturer's directions and write the patient's name on it.

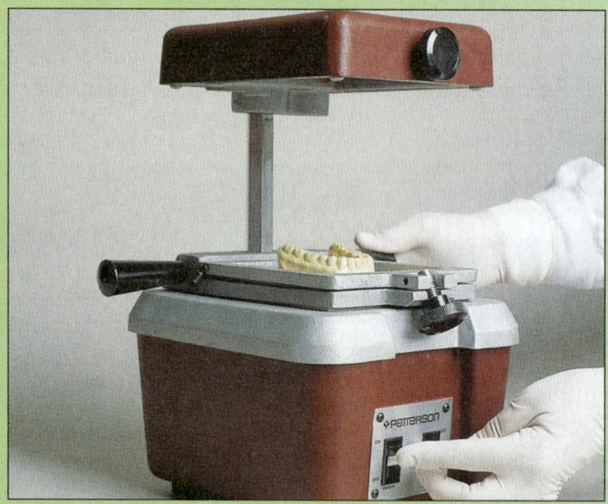

FIGURE 39-69

When resin material has sagged 1 inch below the holding ring, it is ready to be dropped into position over cast. The unit is held by handles to ensure that the operator is not burned.

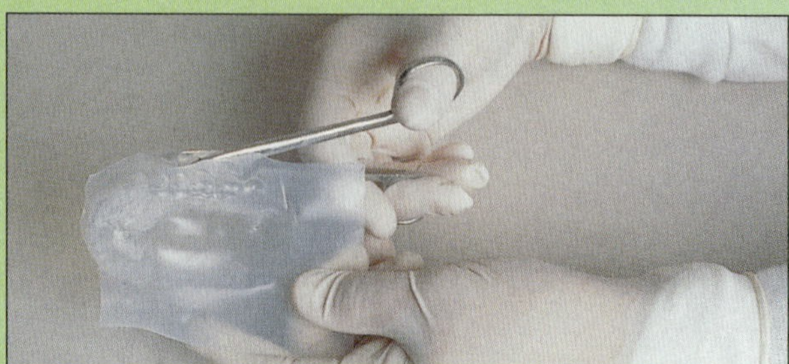

FIGURE 39-70

Vacuum form can be trimmed with scissors.

Constructing a Custom Tray

Regardless of the material type used, the custom tray model is prepared in the same manner.

Outlining Tray Margins

If a full custom tray is desired on an edentulous arch, draw a blue line at the bottom of the vestibule area around the facial surface, across the palate area on the maxillary model, around the posterior retromolar area, along the bottom of the vestibule area, and across the opposite posterior retromolar area on the mandibular model (Figure 39-71). From that first marking, make a red line 2 mm upward (toward the ridge). This gives a definite line to follow when adapting the spacer. A spacer is placed on the model to allow room in the tray for the impression material. This spacer normally is made of pink baseplate wax, but a commercial nonstick molding material may be used (especially when using the vacuum-formed custom tray because of the heating element) or a moist paper towel can be used. When the spacer is placed, the undercuts are filled in. Undercuts are recessed areas in the model that make it impossible to seat or remove the custom tray properly. Undercuts are caused by bubbles in the plaster, cavities, or the shape of the arch or dentition. If using baseplate wax for the spacer, it can be heated with warm water or butane torch (Figure 39-72) and conformed to the model. Cut it back to the red line in an angle-forming manner (see Procedure 39-16, Constructing Self-Curing Acrylic Resin Custom Tray). This provides a smoother tissue side to the custom tray and is more comfortable to the patients than a blunt-edge cut. After the spacer is in place, take a warm plastic instrument to lute (secure) the edges of the wax to the cast. After the securing is accomplished, cut into the crest of the wax with a laboratory knife, making small rectangular or round holes. These stops (holes on the spacer that allow bumps to be formed on the tissue side of the tray) allow the tray to be seated 2 to 3 mm from the teeth or tissue and to prevent it from seating too deeply. This allows an adequate amount of impression material to flow around the prepared teeth or the tissue. There should be a minimum of four stops on an edentulous model, two on each first molar and cuspid area. When making a custom tray for crowns and bridges, the stops should be placed one tooth distal and mesial from the prepared tooth.

The self-curing material is exothermic. It heats up and causes the wax to melt slightly. It is advisable to place a layer of aluminum foil over the wax spacer and into the stops. The foil makes it easier to remove the wax from the tissue side of the tray after the custom tray is made. If foil is not used, a toothbrush and hot water will aid in getting the wax out of the inside (tissue side) of the custom tray.

After the cast is prepared, the custom tray material is mixed according to the manufacturer's directions and formed to the cast. In the doughy stage, the maxillary material can be shaped into a patty and the mandibular can be rolled into a log shape prior to placing the materials on the cast. A handle can be made from the remaining material. It is placed on the anterior of the tray near the midline of the arch. It is secured by wiping the anterior area and the handle area that is to be attached with the resin liquid and then placing it on the custom tray. Because the handle is still soft when it is applied to the cast, it must be held in place until initially set up. Make sure the handle is large and strong enough to allow for leverage in placing and removing the custom tray from the mouth. Remember that the dentist will have his or her fingers and thumb on the handle while performing the procedure, so make sure it can be held easily. When working on edentulous custom trays, the handles

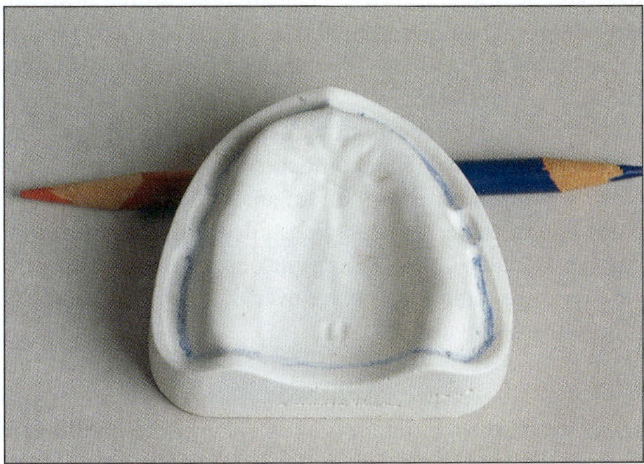

FIGURE 39-71

Tray margin is outlined on plaster or stone cast. The deepest area is marked in blue; 1 or 2 mm above this point, a red line indicating where the wax spacer is to be located can be drawn.

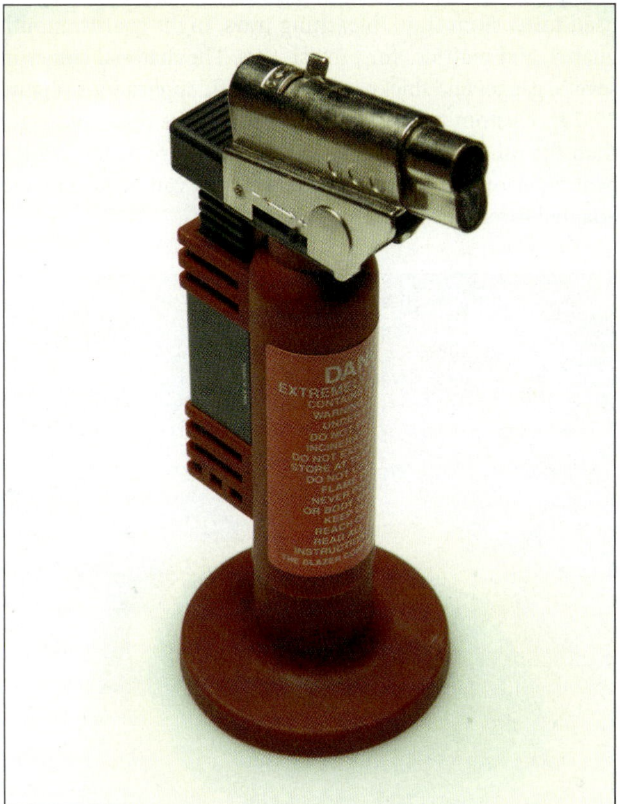

FIGURE 39-72

Butane torch.

should extend upward and outward from the model. If this is not done, the handle is placed so that it protrudes directly through the lip of the patient.

When the exothermic reaction has completed and the model has cooled (about 10 minutes), remove the spacer and evaluate the tray. The inside of the tray does not need to be smooth because the impression material covers this area. Any rough areas on the margins and on the outside of the tray can be smoothed for patient comfort. This can be accomplished by using an acrylic bur in a straight handpiece or with an arbor band on the laboratory lathe. Wear protective glasses when performing either of these trimming procedures. When completed, clean and disinfect the custom tray according to the manufacturer's directions and place it in a barrier ready for patient use.

An adhesive is painted on the tissue side of the tray prior to taking the impression. It is normally applied in two coats. The first is allowed to dry and the second is placed 10 minutes or so before the impression is taken. This secures the material to the custom tray. Some dentists may want holes placed in the custom tray to further lock the impression material into the tray. This can be accomplished by wearing protective glasses and using a straight handpiece with a round bur to penetrate the custom tray. Either or both techniques will secure the material into the custom tray.

Vacuum-Formed Tray

Trays that are vacuum formed can be used for a number of applications in the field of dentistry. Most often they are used for custom trays, bleaching trays, night guards, mouth guards, and matrices for provisionals. The material comes in several gauges and thicknesses for specific applications (Figure 39-73). Custom tray material is much more thick and rigid than the other applications. All use a vacuum former with a heating element, a cast, and material that can be heated and adapted through vacuum pressure.

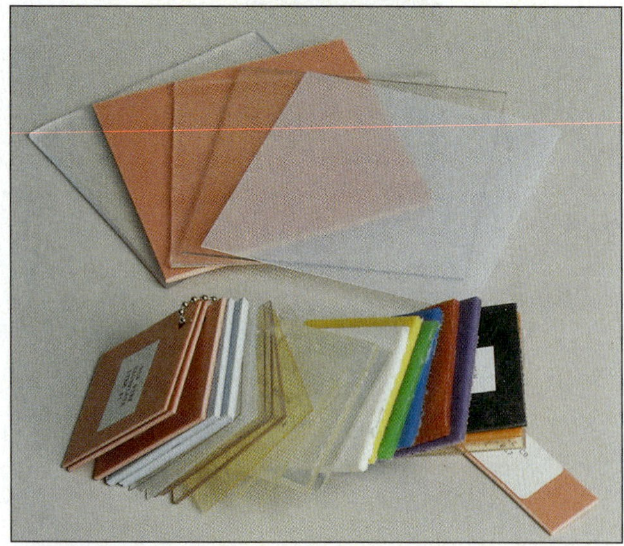

FIGURE 39-73
Various vacuum-formed materials.

Temporary (Provisional) Restorations

After a tooth has been prepared for a crown and prior to the seating of the crown, a temporary restoration must be adapted and temporarily cemented on the tooth to protect it in the interim. These temporary restorations stabilize and protect the tooth for the 2 days to 2 weeks it takes to make the crown(s) or bridge(s).

Temporary Restoration Criteria

- Comfortable and esthetically acceptable to patient.
- Remains stable, with proper mesial and distal contacts and occlusal alignment, until permanent crown is cemented.
- Easily removed, without damaging tooth, when the permanent restoration is ready for placement.
- Fits snugly and accurately along prepared margin of the tooth. There is less than 0.05 mm of space between the temporary restoration and finish line of the margin.
- Contoured in a similar fashion to original tooth, therefore protecting gingiva from irritation and interproximal areas from food impaction.

Types of Temporary Restorations

Temporary restorations, also known as provisional restorations, can be made of a number of materials, both custom and preformed. In many states, the function of fabricating and placing a temporary restoration is delegated to the dental assistant under the supervision of the dentist. Most offices use the preformed aluminum and acrylic crowns, along with the custom acrylic or composite crowns.

Preformed Aluminum Temporary Crowns. Preformed aluminum temporary crowns are supplied in different sizes and anatomic features. They are used on the posterior teeth because they lack esthetic value. Some are made without any anatomy and resemble thimbles with parallel straight sides and flat, occlusal surfaces. More contouring is necessary to adapt this model to the tooth. Others have anatomies similar to the natural teeth and are contoured much like stainless steel crowns. Both the crowns without anatomic features and the ones with anatomic features can be filled with acrylic or composite material to obtain a more custom fit prior to setting the temporary restorations in place over the prepared teeth (see Procedures 39-18 and 39-19).

Preformed Acrylic Temporary Crowns. Preformed acrylic or plastic temporary crowns are available in different sizes, shapes, and shades (Figure 39-74). The advantage of this type of crown is that it is more esthetically pleasing for anterior use. The plastic temporary crown is a form used to match the appropriate shape and contour of the tooth. It is filled with acrylic material and then removed. The preformed acrylic

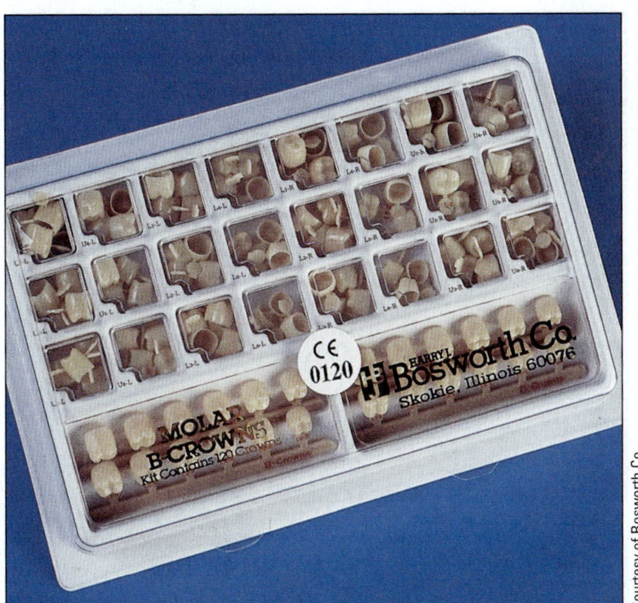

Courtesy of Bosworth Co.

FIGURE 39-74

Preformed acrylic temporary crowns.

crowns have tabs on the incisal edge for easy placement. These tabs are removed prior to cementation. The preformed acrylic crowns are used more easily because they require little adjustment and can be seated immediately. One disadvantage is that they are shorter in length, or more closely trimmed to the optimum margin length of the prepared tooth. If a patient has had periodontal disease and the crown must be lengthened to cover any areas of recession, the clear-plastic crowns adapt better. They are supplied with longer "necks" on the crown for this purpose. See Procedure 39-20.

Custom Acrylic or Composite Temporary Restorations. When making custom acrylic or composite temporary restorations, a matrix is used. The matrix can be direct or indirect. A **matrix** is a form shaped in the pattern of the tooth prior to preparing the tooth (Figure 39-75). The *Direct matrix technique* (making the matrix directly from the tooth) uses alginate, impression material, the freehand (block) technique, wax, thermo-forming beads, or a thermoplastic button in the matrix. The *indirect matrix technique* (making the matrix on a model or cast) utilizes wax, a vacuum-formed shell, and thermo-forming bead and button matrices.

The alginate and impression materials render more anatomically accurate temporaries. The other materials meet the criteria for a temporary restoration form adequately and may prove to be less costly and more easily made. The utility wax is heated in warm water and then formed over the tooth or model to obtain the shape of the tooth and then cooled. Thermo-forming beads and buttons are heated in hot water and formed on the tooth prior to preparation or on a cast when using the indirect matrix technique. The vacuum-formed shell is made on a vacuum unit using a cast covered with very thin sheets of acrylic resin. After it is heated, this sheet is cut to the desired size for use in making the temporary restoration.

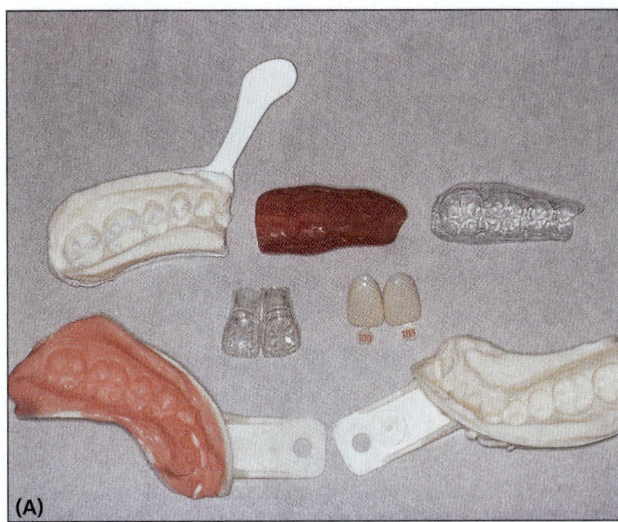
(A)

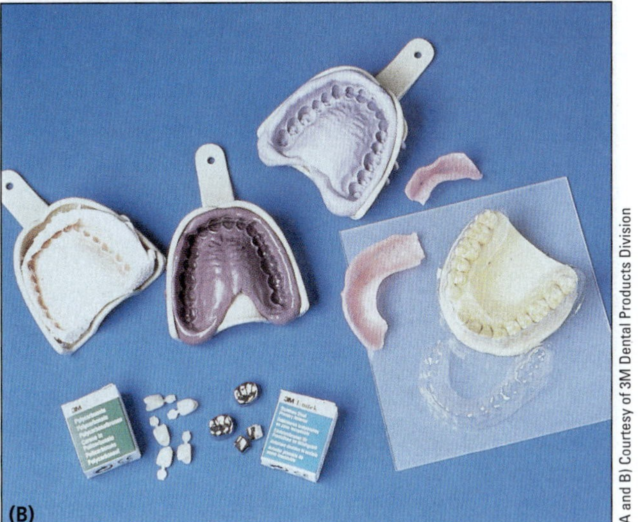
(B)

(A and B) Courtesy of 3M Dental Products Division

FIGURE 39-75

Figures A and B both show various types of temporary/provisional matrices.

Matrix Used for Direct Technique in Making Temporary Restorations

- Alginate impression
- Impression material
- Freehand (making a block of the material and covering the prepared tooth)
- Wax
- Thermo-forming beads or buttons

Matrix Used for Indirect Technique in Making Temporary Restorations

- Wax
- Thermo-forming beads or buttons
- Vacuum-formed shell

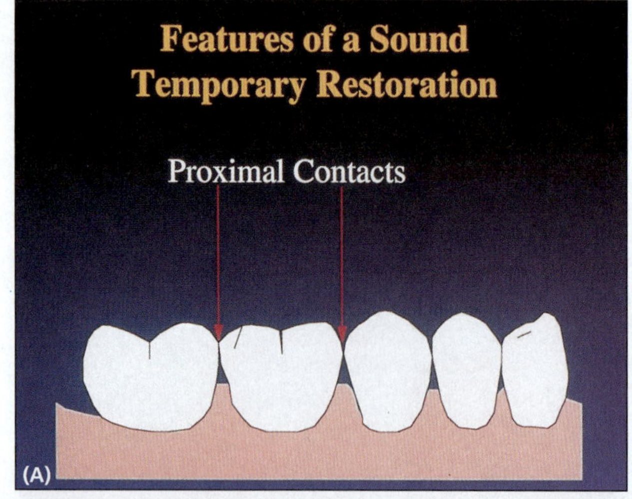

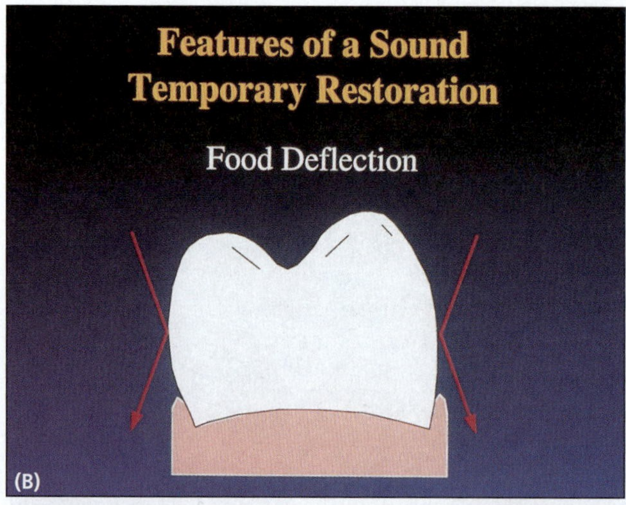

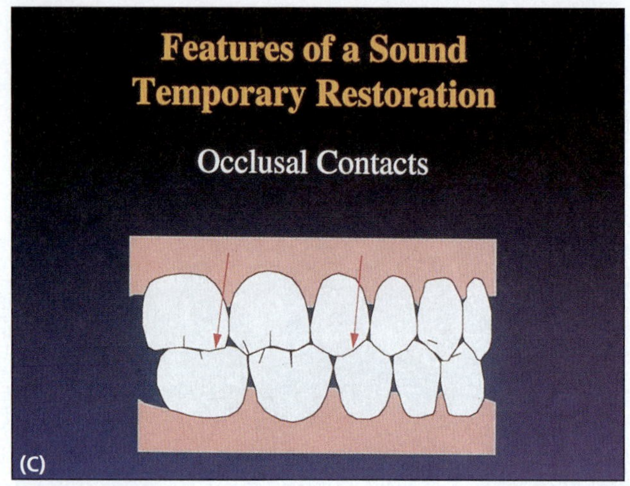

Features of a Sound
Temporary Restoration
Occlusal Contacts
(C)

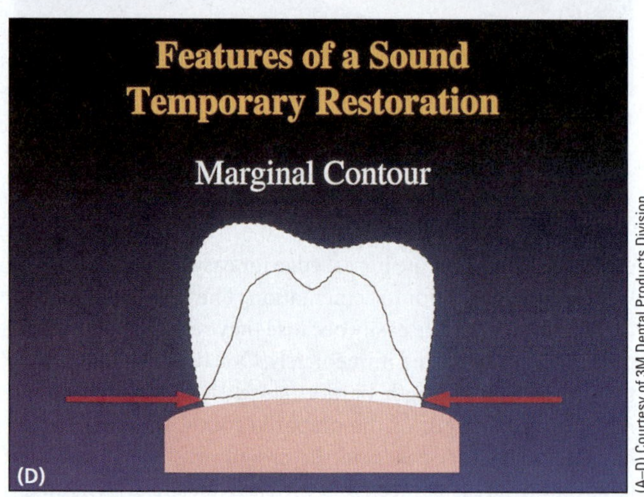

(A–D) Courtesy of 3M Dental Products Division

FIGURE 39-76

Criteria for custom acrylic or a composite temporary restoration. (A) Good proximal contacts. (B) Good occlusal contacts. (C) Good food deflection. (D) Good marginal contours.

A custom acrylic or composite temporary restoration (Procedure 39-21) must have good proximal contacts, good occlusal contacts, good food deflection, and good marginal contours (Figures 39-76A through D). Using the correct burs when making a temporary is essential. For making proper margins and contacts, use burs and discs (Figure 39-77) that have been developed specifically for this purpose, as the outcome of the temporary will be much more accurate.

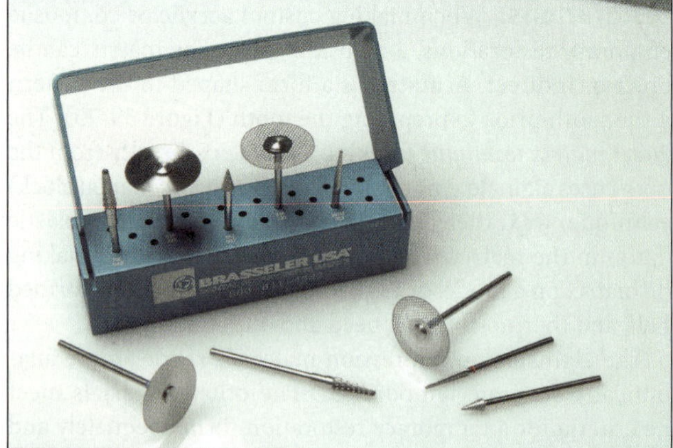

FIGURE 39-77

Provisional bur kit used when trimming temporary restorations.

Self-Curing Methyl Methacrylate. There are several categories of materials that achieve the desired outcome of a custom temporary restoration. Each material has advantages and disadvantages. One of the routinely used older materials is methyl methacrylate. The advantages of this material are that it has good physical properties, good esthetics, better color stability than the R9 methacrylates, and a lower cost. The disadvantages are the strong odor, high shrinkage, and high exothermic heat given off during the self-cure chemical setting.

Self-Curing R9 Methacrylate. The R9 (resin) methacrylates have one of the active ingredients, such as vinyl, ethyl, or isobutyl, in place of the methyl. In comparison to the methyl methacrylates, they have lower shrinkage and a lower level of exothermic heat given off during the self-cure chemical setting. They are similar in price per temporary, but they are the weakest of the methacrylates, they have poor color stability, and they have the same strong odor that the methyl methacrylates have.

Both the methyl and the R9 methacrylates come in powder and liquid forms that are mixed together to form a creamy mix. After mixing, they are allowed to condition for approximately 30 seconds and then are placed in the matrix. A dull surface appears on the top of the material, and it is placed in the mouth over the prepared tooth and held in place for the initial set. It has a rubber appearance at this time. Most manufacturers suggest that the material be taken off and on the prepared tooth during the time of 4 to 6 minutes. This is when the exothermic heat is the greatest. The excess can be trimmed off easily with scissors during this time. The final set is from 6 to 8 minutes, and the material becomes hard plastic. The range of setting time from start to finish is from 8 to 10 minutes for the materials in these two groups. Many of the newer materials are completed in half the time. The temporary restorations are removed from the matrix and trimmed with an acrylic bur to the desired shape and size.

After the temporary has been trimmed, it is polished with pumice and a rag wheel. Some of the materials in this category come with glazes. This glaze is applied after the polishing and allowed to dry for 5 minutes before the temporary is cemented.

Self-Curing Composite Material. Materials in the category of self-curing composite are double the price of the methacrylates. They are much stronger materials because they are made as composites and not plastics. They do not have the odor, the shrinkage, or the exothermic reaction during setting, and they have excellent color stability.

Materials in this category come in two pastes. They are supplied in either two tubes or in a cartridge that fits into extruding guns with auto mixing tips. Both the tubes and the cartridge tips must remain clean and flowing to obtain the correct dispensed amount of the material. If they become clogged with old material, use an explorer to clear the old material out. Dispense a small, pea-shaped amount on the pad before beginning, to ensure that everything is working properly.

The material is placed in the matrix and over the prepared tooth for up to 2 minutes. During the rubber stage (from 4 to 6 minutes), it is removed from the mouth to complete curing. The total time from start to finish for this material classification is up to 7 minutes. After the material is set, the surface has a greasy layer due to the oxygen in the air, which can be removed with alcohol or any other organic solvent. The trimming is done with a diamond bur and no polish is necessary. If additional material is required on the temporary, light-cured composite or flowable resin repair can be used and trimmed accordingly.

Multi-cured Temporary Materials. Several multi-cured temporary materials are on the market. They have extended working time in the rubbery stage and improved operator control because they can be light cured on demand. They have good strength and are higher in cost. Some of the materials in this group are methacrylates and some are composites having the characteristics of the self-curing materials. The biggest advantage of this group is light-curing control, which allows for a quicker set and unlimited setting time.

Procedure 39-18

Sizing, Adapting, and Seating Aluminum Temporary Crown

 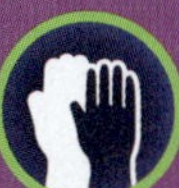  

This procedure is performed by the dentist or the dental assistant at the dental unit after tooth has been prepared for a crown.

Equipment and Supplies

- Maxillary and/or mandibular selection of aluminum temporary crowns (Figure 39-78)
- Millimeter ruler
- Basic setup: mouth mirror, cotton pliers, and explorer
- Crown and collar scissors
- Contouring pliers
- Acrylic or composite temporary material (optional)
- Sandpaper discs, rubber wheel, and mandrel
- Temporary cement, pad, and spatula
- Articulating paper
- Dental floss

Procedure Steps *(Follow aseptic procedures)*

1. Measure the available space for the temporary crown from the mesial to distal with the millimeter ruler. This aids in the selection of a preformed crown having the appropriate mesial and distal contact.
2. Determine the correct crown to try in. The aluminum crown is for the correct tooth in the dentition and the size is chosen according to the measurement taken with the millimeter ruler. (Prevent cross-contamination while taking the crown from the container. Do not use contaminated instruments.) Any crown tried that does not fit must be sterilized before replacing it in the selection tray.

(continues)

Procedure 39-18 (continued)

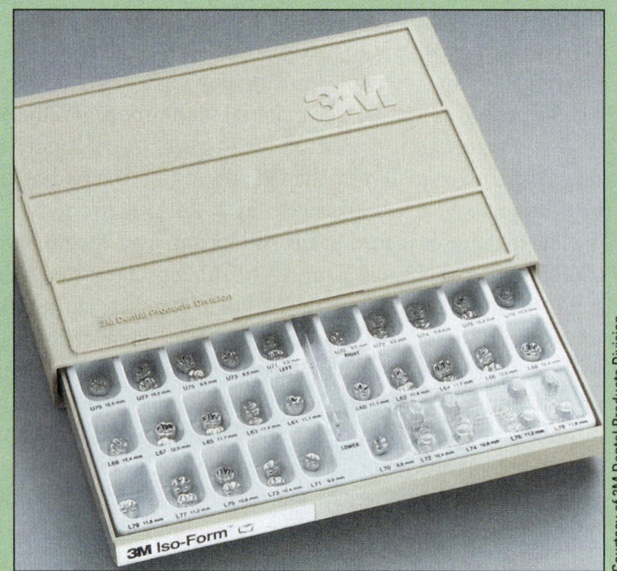

Courtesy of 3M Dental Products Division

FIGURE 39-78
Selection of Iso-Form temporary crowns.

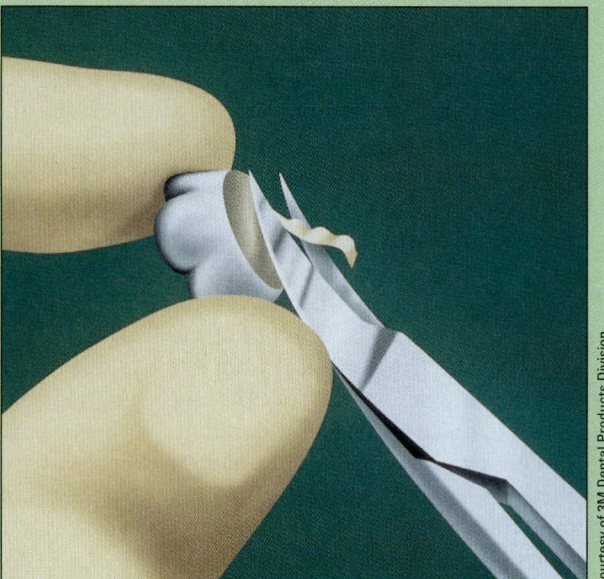

Courtesy of 3M Dental Products Division

FIGURE 39-80
Trimming aluminum crown with crown and collar scissors.

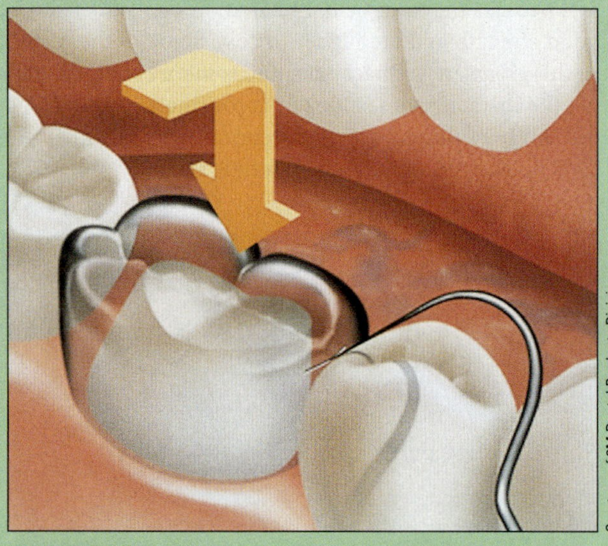

Courtesy of 3M Dental Products Division

FIGURE 39-79
Explorer used to establish height of temporary aluminum crown.

3. Try the selected crown on and check for mesial and distal width. The crown will be above the occlusal plane at this time.
4. The length of the crown is determined by placing the aluminum crown over the prepared tooth and using an explorer to mark the height (Figure 39-79). Another way to accomplish this is to scribe the tooth at the occlusal surface with an instrument where it aligns with the other teeth on the arch and then take that same amount off the gingival area. Either method shows that the margin of the gingival needs to be trimmed in order to fit.
5. Using a crown and collar scissors (with curved blades), trim the gingival margin. Crowns are never straight across the surface but are longer on the buccal and lingual margins. Use the rounded edges of the scissors to trim.

NOTE: Trimming a small amount at first allows refitting to further check the desired result (Figure 39-80). Taking too much off renders the crown useless. Making several trims to get the desired effect is a better method. Using the scissors in a continuous cutting action gives a much smoother surface. Avoid sharp, uneven edges that cause the patient discomfort around the gingival surface.

6. After the desired length is achieved, use the contouring pliers to invert the gingival edge in an inward manner. This crimping aids in the adaptation of the circumference edge of the aluminum crown to the finish line of the preparation.
7. Smoothing of the rough and jagged edges is accomplished through use of sandpaper discs and a rubber wheel. Check that all edges are smooth and polished (Figure 39-81).
8. Place the aluminum crown on the prepared tooth and check the occlusion with the articulating paper and the contacts with dental floss.

NOTE: If the contacts are weak, use a burnisher on the inside to extend the crown outward to get a better contact.

(continues)

Procedure 39-18 (continued)

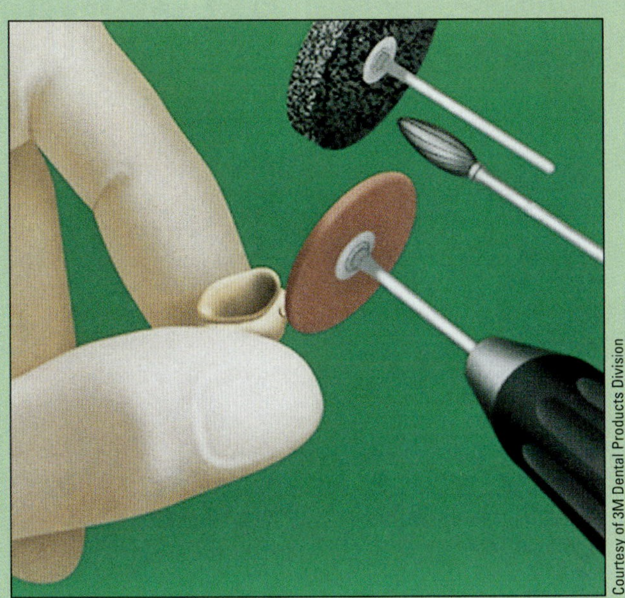

Courtesy of 3M Dental Products Division

FIGURE 39-81
Smooth rough and jagged edges of temporary with rubber wheel.

9. If an acrylic or a composite lining is used, the crown is filled with the material and placed on the prepared tooth. The patient is asked to bite into normal occlusion.

NOTE: The tooth may require light lubrication with petroleum jelly to avoid retention of the material.

The material sets according to the manufacturer's directions and is then removed. Any excess material is polished away.

NOTE: Some operators prefer to do this step earlier in the procedure.

10. A final check for marginal fit, contour, and occlusion is done before cementation takes place.

Procedure 39-19
Cementing the Aluminum Crown

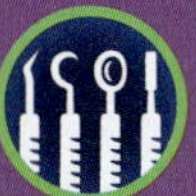

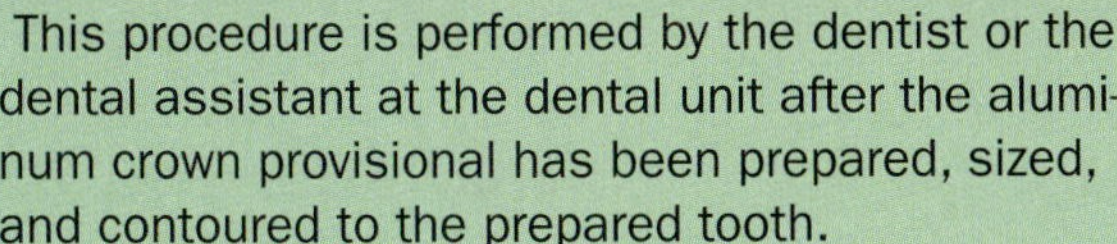

This procedure is performed by the dentist or the dental assistant at the dental unit after the aluminum crown provisional has been prepared, sized, and contoured to the prepared tooth.

Equipment and Supplies

- Fitted aluminum temporary
- Cotton rolls
- Temporary cementation material
- Mixing pad
- Plastic filling instrument
- Basic setup: mouth mirror, explorer, and cotton pliers

Procedure Steps (*Follow aseptic procedures*)

1. The prepared tooth is rinsed and dried with cotton rolls in place.
2. The temporary cementation material, such as zinc oxide eugenol, is mixed with a spatula and placed in the aluminum crown.
3. The aluminum crown is placed in position over the prepared tooth and the patient is asked to bite in occlusion until the cement is set.

NOTE: Some operators like the patient to bite on a cotton roll over the aluminum crown while the cement sets.

4. After the cement is set, the excess is removed with an explorer.
5. The contacts are checked with floss and the margins are inspected to determine whether all excess cement has been removed and the crown fits correctly.
6. A final check for occlusion is done with articulating paper.
7. Instructions are given to the patient for care of the temporary aluminum crown.

Procedure 39-20

Sizing, Adapting, and Seating a Preformed Acrylic Crown

This procedure is performed by the dentist or the dental assistant at the dental unit after the preformed acrylic provisional has been prepared, sized, and contoured to the prepared tooth.

Equipment and Supplies

- Maxillary and/or mandibular selection of acrylic temporary crowns
- Mirror, explorer, and cotton pliers
- Acrylic or composite temporary material (optional)
- Acrylic bur
- Temporary cement, pad, and spatula
- Articulating paper
- Dental floss

Procedure Steps (*Follow aseptic procedures*)

Preparing a Preformed Acrylic Temporary Restoration

1. After the tooth has been prepared for a crown, a preformed acrylic temporary restoration is selected and adapted. Choose a crown that has enough width to contact on the adjacent teeth, is long enough to be in proper occlusion, and is the correct shade.
2. Retrieve this crown without cross-contaminating the other acrylic crowns. The tab at the incisal edge allows the operator to try the crown over the prepared tooth (Figure 39-82).
3. If necessary, adjustments are made with an acrylic bur. Polish with a rag wheel and pumice.
4. Take off the tag, place the crown, and check the occlusion with articulating paper.
5. Make adjustments, if necessary, and again polish the adjustment areas for a smooth surface for patient comfort.

Cementing Acrylic Provisional Crown

1. The prepared tooth is rinsed and dried with cotton rolls in place.

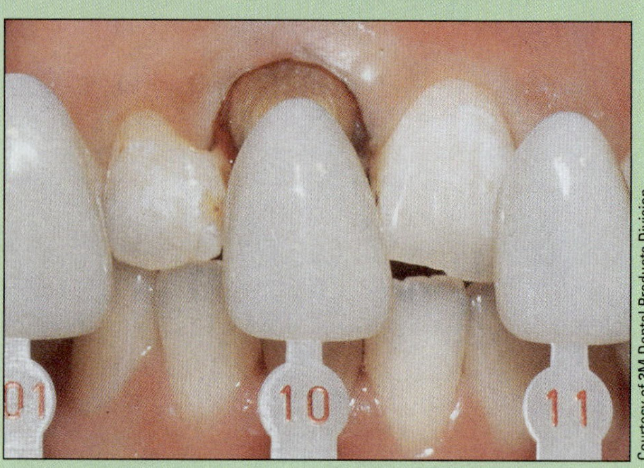

Courtesy of 3M Dental Products Division

FIGURE 39-82
Acrylic crown is tried over prepared tooth, holding onto incisal tab.

2. The temporary cementation material, such as zinc oxide eugenol, is mixed with a spatula and placed in the preformed acrylic crown.
3. The preformed acrylic crown is placed in position over the prepared tooth and the patient is asked to bite in occlusion or the operator holds the crown in place until the cement is set.

NOTE: Some operators like the patient to bite on a cotton roll over the preformed acrylic crown while the cement sets.

4. After the cement is set, the excess is removed with an explorer.
5. The contacts are checked with floss and the margins are inspected to determine whether all excess cement has been removed and whether the crown fits correctly.
6. A final check for occlusion is done with articulating paper.
7. Instructions are given to the patient for care of the temporary preformed acrylic crown.

Procedure 39-21

Develop or Place a Pontic in a Model for a Three-Unit Bridge on a Dental Model; Adapt a Matrix; Make, Trim, and Place the Three-Unit Provisional Temporary

This procedure is performed by the dentist or the dental assistant at the dental unit after tooth has been prepared for a crown.

Equipment and Supplies

- Basic setup: mouth mirror, explorer, and cotton pliers
- Thermoplastic buttons/hot water (one possible option for use in making a matrix)
- Composite temporary material
- Diamond bur and disc
- Temporary cement, pad, and spatula
- Articulating paper
- Dental floss
- Dental model with missing tooth

Procedure Steps (*Follow aseptic procedures*)

Developing or Placing a Pontic on the Model Where the Tooth Is Missing

1. To develop a pontic, block-out putty can be manipulated to fit into the space. Ensure that the material is not wider than the other teeth in the arch (Figure 39-83).
2. There are also pontics that are available by using a multi-cure provisional material; they can be placed into the space and light cured in place prior to making a matrix.

Making Thermo-Forming Matrix before Tooth Preparation

1. Place the thermo-forming matrix buttons in hot water (one button per prepared tooth).
2. Allow the white color of the button to become clear. When that takes place, the material is pliable and able to be adapted.
3. Adapt the material over the teeth and tightly conform it to the teeth area and slightly below the gingival. Insure that the matrix covers all teeth that will be in the bridge. They should cover about one half of an extra tooth on each side of the matrix.
4. When the material cools (air can be used to make this more rapid), the matrix appears white and firm. Remove the matrix from the area and set it aside (Figure 39-84).

Preparing Custom Bridge Temporary Restoration

1. After the teeth have been prepared for a bridge, coat the teeth on the model with a light application of petroleum jelly (Figure 39-85).
2. If using the composite self-curing temporary material in two tubes, dispense on the paper pad by holding tubes at a 45 degree angle.
3. Rotate the end-dispensing handle of the base until a click is heard. (The base is the larger of the two tubes. The smaller of the two holds the catalyst and has two dispensing ends.) Rotate the

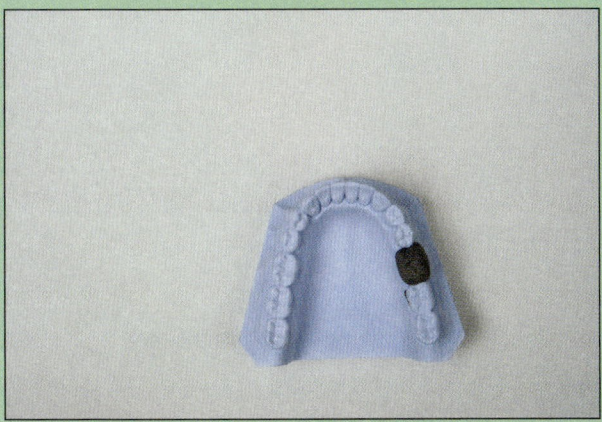

FIGURE 39-83
Develop a pontic out of block-out.

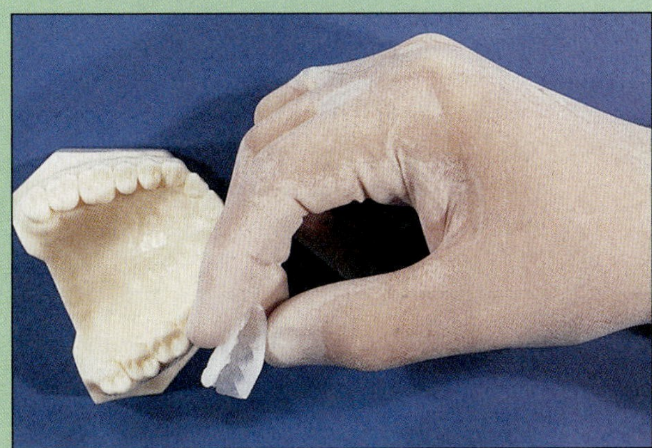

FIGURE 39-84
Matrix is removed.

(continues)

Procedure 39-21 (continued)

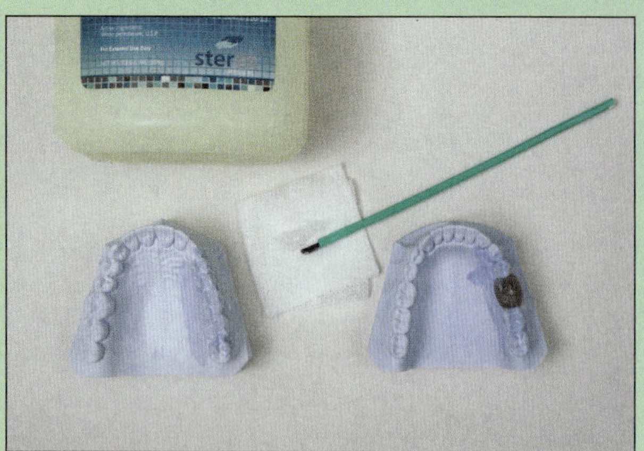

FIGURE 39-85

Place the lubricant on the model so the material will not stick to the gypsum.

end-dispensing handle of the catalyst. Two small amounts are expelled. Each click of the dispensing handle is enough material for one temporary.

4. If a shade is being used, mix it with the base. If a mottled effect is desired, mix the shade after the base and catalyst are mixed together.
5. Mix the material together to obtain a creamy substance (about 30 seconds).
6. Place the material in the matrix.
7. Place the matrix over the prepared tooth (manipulation time is about 1½ minutes).
8. Hold it in place in the mouth for 2 minutes.
9. Remove it from the mouth and set it aside for 2 minutes.
10. Remove the crown or bridge from the matrix (Figure 39-86). The additional curing time takes 1 minute. There are 7 minutes total time from start to finish of the set.
11. Remove the greasy layer with alcohol or any other organic solvent.
12. Mark the contact areas (Figure 39-87).
13. Trim with scissors, a diamond, or an acrylic bur.
14. Trim and smooth all areas (Figure 39-88), make sure that the area that was marked as the contact point is not trimmed away. Use a disc (Figure 39-89) to cut the embrasure area. Always use a fulcrum when trimming provisional restorations.
15. If too much material was trimmed away, use a flowable temporary (provisional) material that can be placed on the restoration with a tip and dispenser (Figure 39-90) and then light cure it (Figure 39-91). The material can then be trimmed again to get the desired finished products.

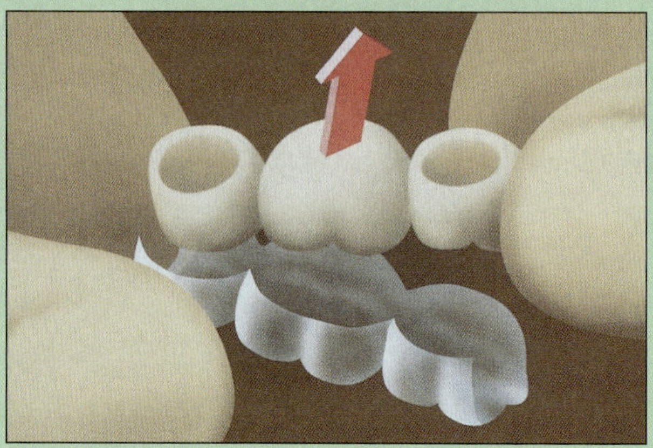

FIGURE 39-86

Remove acrylic bridge from matrix.

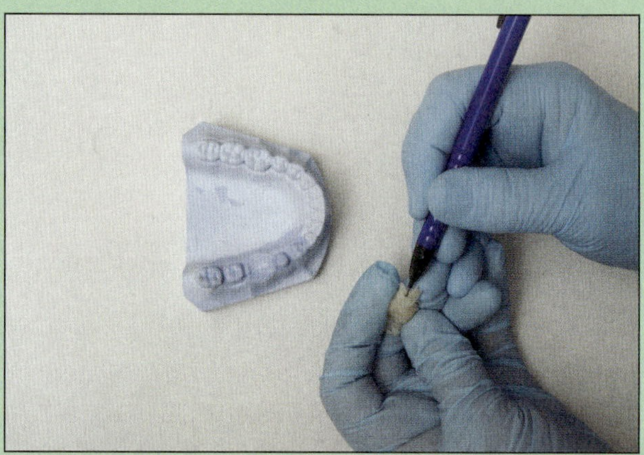

FIGURE 39-87

Mark the contact areas.

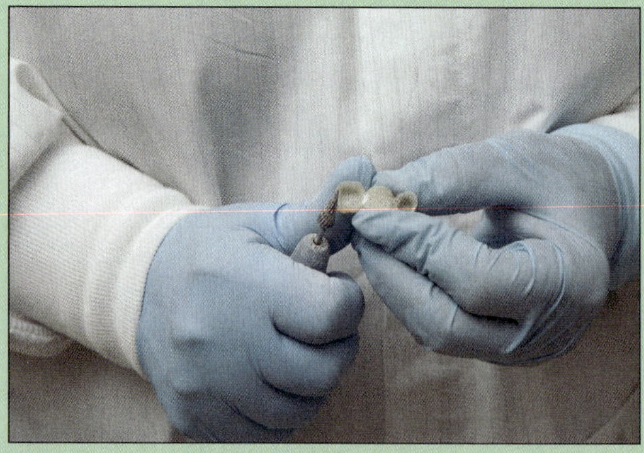

FIGURE 39-88

Trim and smooth entire provisional bridge.

16. Check the contacts (Figure 39-92) and occlusion.
17. If desired, place a glaze on the provisional (Figure 39-93) and light cure it to give it a smoother surface.

(continues)

Procedure 39-21 (continued)

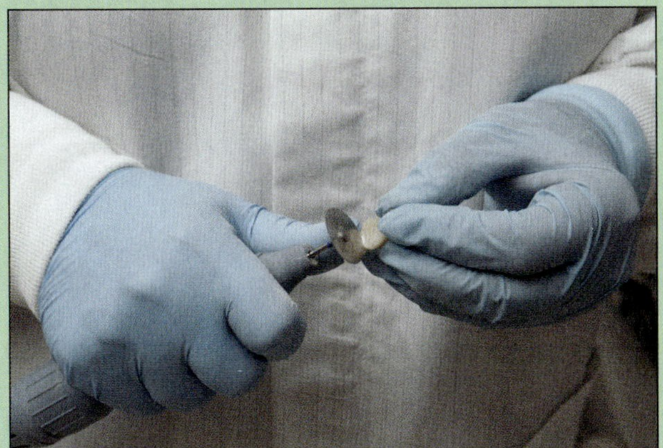
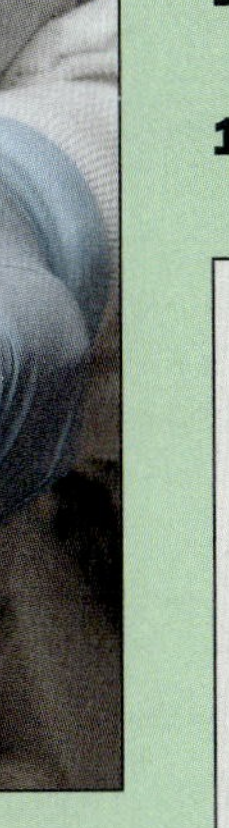

FIGURE 39-89
Use a disc to cut the embrasure area.

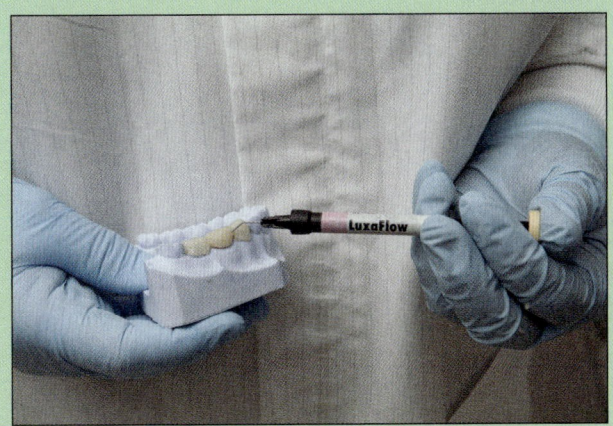

FIGURE 39-90
Place flowable temporary material on areas in need.

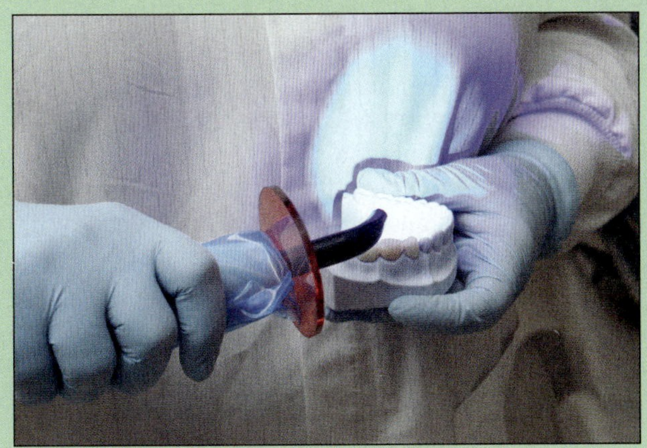

FIGURE 39-91
Light cure flowable provisional material.

18. Check occlusion by having patient bite on articulating paper.

19. Check margins with explorer and mirror.

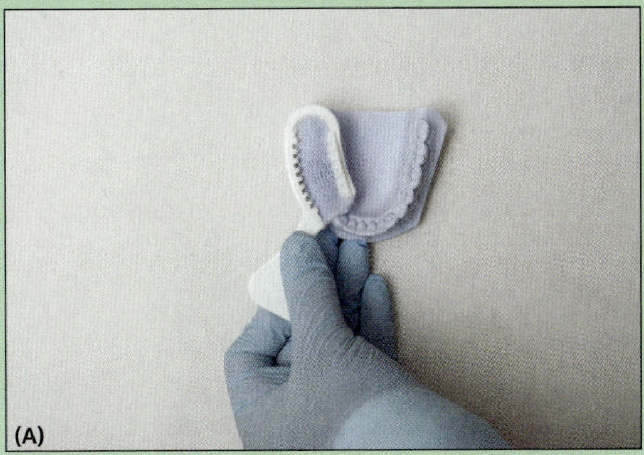
(A)

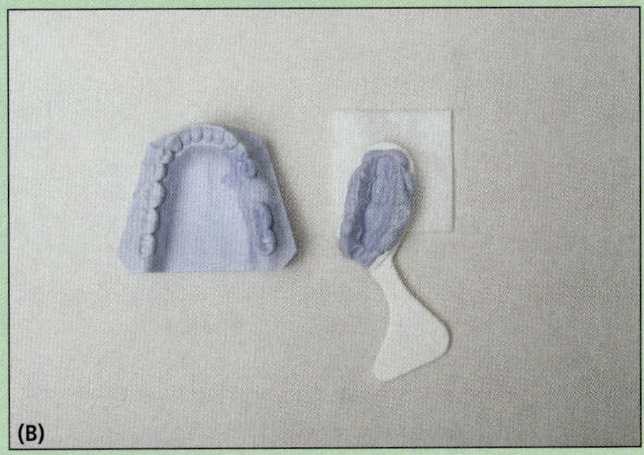
(B)

FIGURE 39-92
Check the contacts and occlusion.

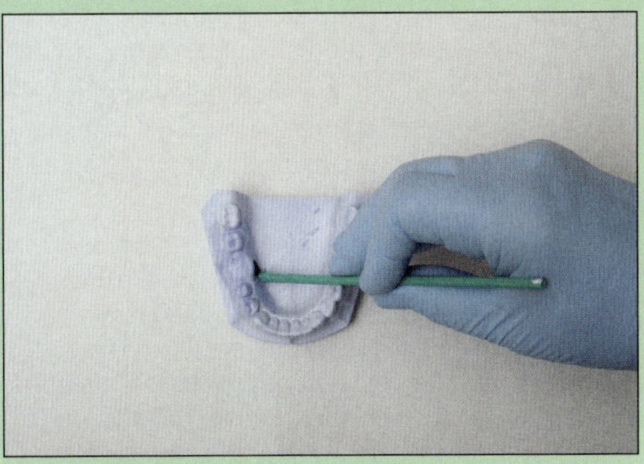

FIGURE 39-93
Place a glaze on the provisional if desired.

Procedure 39-22

Preparing a Full Crown Provisional on a Lower Left Molar on a Patient

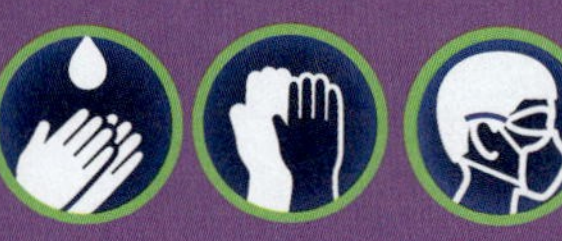

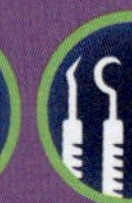
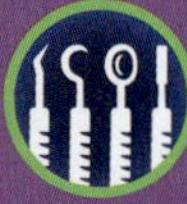

This procedure is performed by the dental assistant under the general supervision of the dentist most often. It can also be done by the dentist with the auxiliary assisting.

Equipment and Supplies

- Basic setup: mouth mirror, explorer, and cotton pliers
- Impression material for matrix
- Triple tray for matrix
- Composite temporary (provision) material
- Diamond bur
- Articulating paper
- Dental floss

Procedure Steps (*Follow aseptic procedures and wear PPE*)

1. Assemble equipment and supplies.
2. Inform the patient that the doctor is going to prepare the tooth for a crown and you are taking an impression for the temporary. Evaluate the tooth that is to receive the temporary and later the crown.
3. Use the impression material and triple tray to make a matrix for the provisional prior to the tooth being prepared. Place the material in the mouth and have the patient close lightly or hold it in place until the material sets.
4. When the dentist arrives, turn off the operatory light and obtain a shade for the crown.
5. After the procedure is completed and the tooth is prepared, fill the impression matrix that you prepared earlier two-thirds full with composite temporary material (Figure 39-94).
6. Make sure it is in the same position that it was when the matrix was obtained. Follow the manufacturer's directions as the material sets. It may have to be removed and replaced several times until set. Composite or multi-cured provisional materials will take 1 to 3 minutes to set up. The multi-cured material will set with a curing light immediately.
7. When the temporary is set, remove it from the patient's mouth or the matrix, wherever it is when the matrix is removed from the patient's mouth.

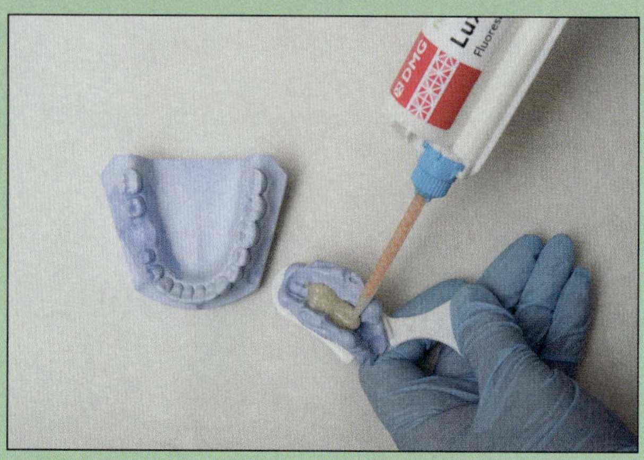

FIGURE 39-94

Filling the dental matrix with composite temporary/provisional material.

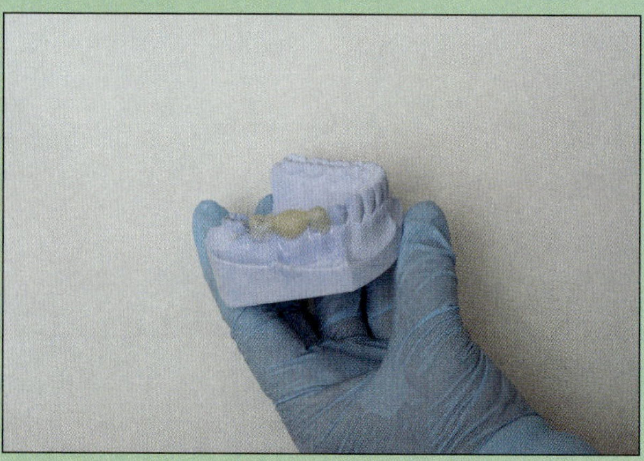

FIGURE 39-95

Evaluate the initial temporary/provisional.

8. Evaluate the temporary (Figure 39-95). This temporary needs to have the additional flash around the edges cut off and some trimming done. It also appears thin on the occlusal surface. If this is due to not enough clearance, the dentist will need to be informed for further evaluation.
9. Remove the greasy layer with alcohol or any other organic solvent.
10. Mark the contact point with a pencil if you are just learning to do temporaries. This will indicate that this area should not be removed. Often assistants start trimming and the contact area quickly gets overlooked and is trimmed away.
11. Trim this full crown with a diamond bur (Figure 39-96).

(continues)

Procedure 39-22 (continued)

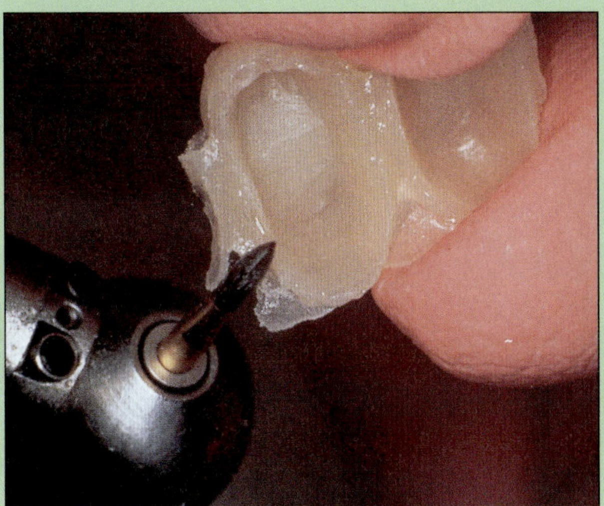

FIGURE 39-96

Trim temporary restoration.

12. If too much material was trimmed away, use a flowable temporary (provisional) material that can be placed on the restoration with a tip and dispenser and then light cure it. The material can then be trimmed again to get the desired finished product.
13. Check the contacts and occlusion. Evaluate the provisional. This completed provisional appears to have the correct occlusion on the mesial side because it is the same height as the crown in front of it. It also appears to have a good contact. It appears to be covering the entire prepped area and smooth. Most temporaries do not have the same occlusion as the final crown. It is trimmed in a fluted figure eight pattern as the mandibular molar should have. It appears to be a good temporary.
14. If desired, place a glaze on the provisional and light cure it to give it a smoother surface.

Procedure 39-23

Cementing Custom Self-Curing Composite Temporary Crown

This procedure is performed by the dentist or the dental assistant at the dental unit after the temporary restoration has been prepared and is ready to be cemented in place over the prepared tooth.

Equipment and Supplies

- Basic setup: mouth mirror, explorer, and cotton pliers
- Cotton rolls
- Temporary luting cement
- Paper pad
- Mixing spatula
- Plastic filling instrument
- Dental floss

Procedure Steps (*Follow aseptic procedures*)

1. The prepared tooth is rinsed and dried with cotton rolls in place.
2. The temporary cement material is mixed with a spatula and placed in the custom composite temporary crown.
3. The temporary crown is placed in position over the prepared tooth and the patient is asked to bite in occlusion or the operator will hold the crown in place until the cement is set.

NOTE: Some operators like the patient to bite on a cotton roll over the preformed acrylic crown while the cement sets.

4. After the cement is set, the excess is removed with an explorer (Figure 39-97). Make sure that a fulcrum is used so that if the explorer slips, it does not go into the sulcus and cause tissue trauma. If feeling unsure with this skill, position the explorer so that the point is facing away from the tissue during removal of the cement.
5. The contacts are checked with floss and the margins are inspected to determine whether all excess cement has been removed and whether the crown fits correctly.

(continues)

Procedure 39-23 (continued)

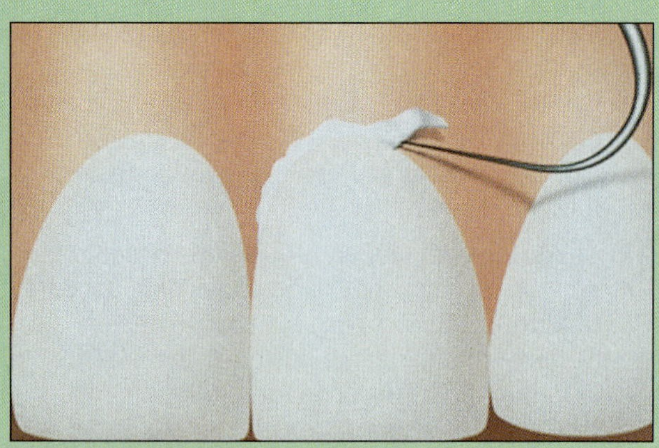

FIGURE 39-97
Temporary is placed and excess cement is removed.

6. A final check for occlusion is performed with the articulating paper.
7. Instructions are given to the patient for care of the temporary preformed acrylic crown.

Chapter Summary

A number of basic functions in the dental laboratory are routinely performed by the dental assistant, such as pouring and trimming study models, fabricating custom trays, and fabricating provisional temporaries. Many newer technologies are completed by dental assistants today such as mounting models on the articulator, taking digital impressions, and designing and fabricating crowns through computer-aided manufacturing. To accomplish these procedures, the dental assistant must understand the materials that are used, the properties of each material, the steps in each procedure, and seek ongoing education and training on new technologies introduced in the field. Any dental assistant who has skills in performing laboratory duties will be an asset to his or her employer. The better crossed-trained the dental team members are, the better the dental office functions.

CASE STUDY

Patrick Norman came into the dental office and wanted to talk to the doctor about a space in the anterior region of his maxillary teeth. After Dr. Smith completed a clinical examination, he asked the dental assistant to make diagnostic casts for further study. After talking to Patrick, the dental assistant found that Patrick has difficulty when anything is placed in his mouth and that gagging is a problem.

Case Study Review

1. What can the dental assistant do to help Patrick with the gagging problem while taking impressions for the diagnostic casts?
2. What material is used routinely for obtaining preliminary impressions?
3. Would the fast or regular set be more beneficial in this case?
4. Which arch would be taken first? Why?

Review Questions

Multiple Choice

1. If an impression loses water content due to heat, dryness, or exposure to air, the condition is known as
   a. imbibition.
   b. syneresis.
   c. distortion.
   d. acceleration.
2. The broad group title that encompasses the hard waxes used in crown and bridge casting (inlay wax) is
   a. pattern.
   b. processing.
   c. impression.
   d. study wax.
3. The liquid catalyst for the self-curing acrylic tray resin is a
   a. polymer.
   b. thermoplastic.
   c. monomer.
   d. spacer.
4. The strongest temporary (provisional) restoration is the
   a. aluminum shell temporary.
   b. self-curing methyl methacrylate temporary.
   c. self-curing R9 (resin) methacrylate temporary.
   d. self-curing composite temporary.
5. Which processing wax is used around trays to extend them and assist in patient comfort?
   a. Study wax
   b. Beading wax
   c. Sticky wax
   d. Boxing wax
6. Trays used for irreversible hydrocolloid are
   a. water cooled.
   b. perforated.
   c. rim locked.
   d. both b and c.
7. The final impression material that smells like sulfur is
   a. polysulfide.
   b. polyether.
   c. polysiloxane.
   d. silicone.
8. The highest-strength type of gypsum material is
   a. Type I.
   b. Type II.
   c. Type III.
   d. Type IV.
9. The ________ allows the operator to obtain the records about the placement of the maxillary arch and its location to the joint.
   a. facebow
   b. articulator
   c. amalgamator
   d. study model
10. What is used to present a case to the patient?
    a. Wax bite registrations
    b. Study models
    c. Articulator
    d. Elastomeric impressions

Critical Thinking

1. Name several types of final impression materials and identify factors that affect usage with each.
2. What are the effects of a lower water-to-powder ratio in a mixture of irreversible hydrocolloid?
3. What are some of the advantages of polyether impression material?

Web Activities

1. Go to http://www.dentsply.com and review the product catalog for new products. Be prepared to discuss new products in class.
2. Go to http://www?bosworth.com, access techniques, and find the technique for Ultra Trim. Is this technique different from the one discussed in this book under temporary restorations? Compare and contrast information about each.

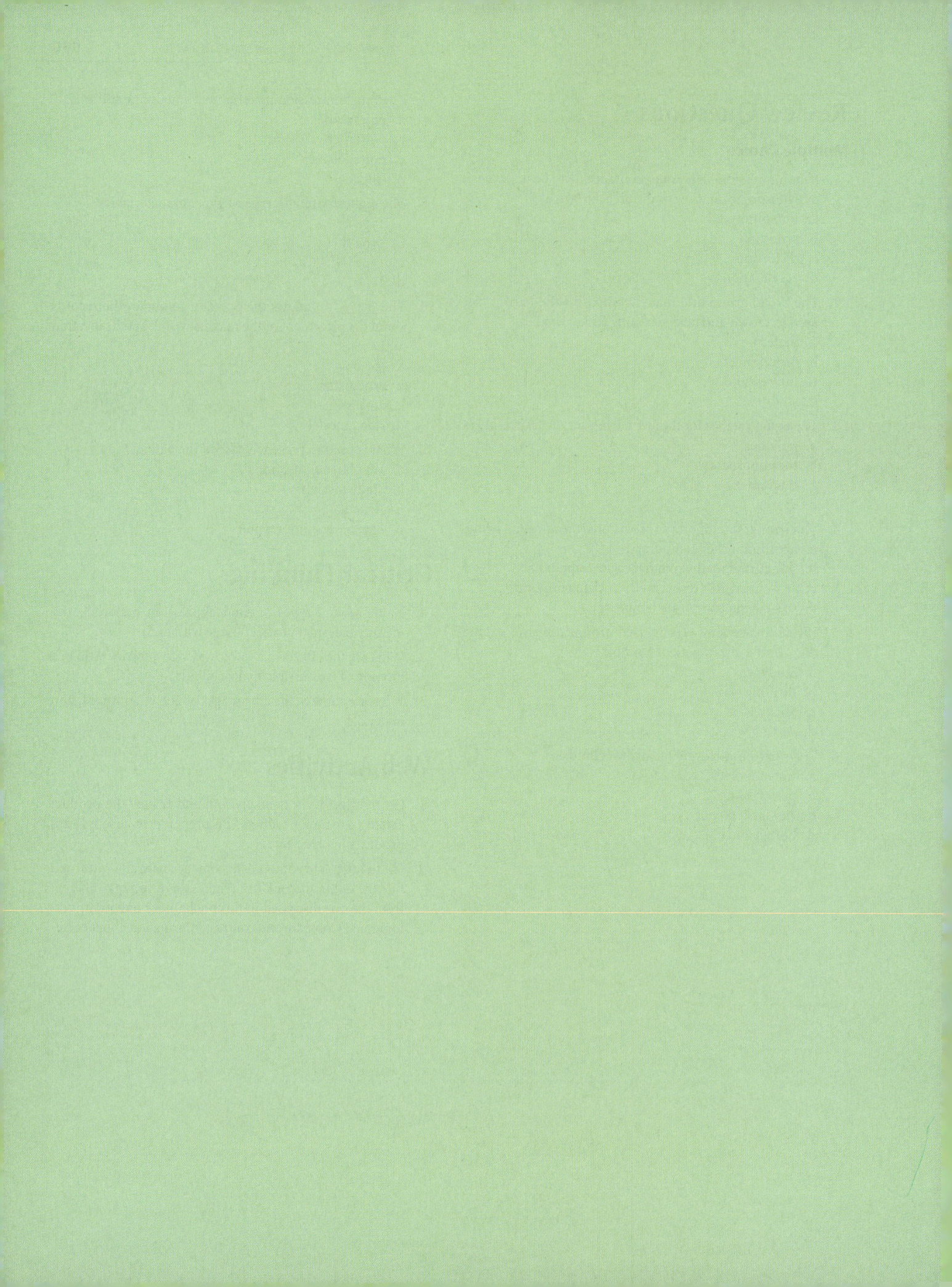

Section IX

Dental Practice Management

CHAPTER 40

Dental Office Management

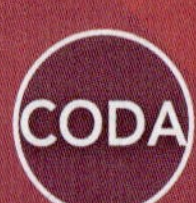

Specific Instructional Objectives

The student should strive to meet the following objectives and demonstrate an understanding of the facts and principles presented in this chapter:

1. Identify the dental office staff and their areas of responsibility.
2. Identify marketing ideas for dentistry.
3. Outline the proper procedure for answering an incoming call.
4. Describe the information every message should contain.
5. Describe telephone and business office technology and its uses.
6. Give examples of the ways in which computers are used in the dental office.
7. Explain how database management concepts can be used in the dental office.
8. Explain why ergonomics is important at a computer workstation.
9. Explain ways in which effective patient scheduling can be accomplished in the dental office.
10. Identify the equipment needed for record management.
11. Define key terms related to accounts receivable.
12. Identify computerized and manual systems for the management of patient accounts.
13. Identify the accounts payable expenses that the dental practice is responsible for.

Key Terms

accounts payable (974)
accounts receivable (974)
Americans with Disabilities Act (973)
certified mail (975)
check register (1002)
computerized system (979)
coordination of benefits (COB) (997)
double booking (983)
downtime (985)
ergonomics (982)
etiquette (976)
expendable (1000)
Fair Debt Collection Practices Act (998)
gross income (1000)
hardware (979)
net income (1000)
nonexpendable (1000)
overhead (1000)
overlap of time (985)
overtime (985)
petty cash (1002)
professional courtesy (990)
software (979)
tickler file (987)
Truth in Lending Act (TILA) (994)
usual, customary, and reasonable fee (990)

Introduction

The dental reception area needs to be an environment in which all patients feel welcome and can relax. Dentists have worked long and hard to overcome the negative image of dentistry prevalent in the past. Today, dentistry can be a positive experience, and dental treatment can be comfortable. In fact, many patients look forward to their dental visits. Some dentists have hired interior design consultants and space-planning advisors to aid the practice in developing an area that is inviting and pleasant for their patients. Offices may have themes, while others are designed to have warm, friendly, home-like atmospheres. The creation of this area not only requires appealing colors, but also a staff that greets patients with smiles, and makes them feel welcome.

Reception Area

The reception area is a place where patients are greeted. (Figure 40-1). Calling it a waiting room gives it a negative connotation: patients are busy, their time is important, and they do not want to wait. The colors, design, and artwork should be relaxing and comfortable, and seating should be available so that each patient can have his or her own space. Keep in mind that individuals from different cultures have varying personal space requirements. The seating should be arranged in a way that allows people to cluster together or remain distant from others.

The reception area should be kept neat and clean. This may require frequent attention throughout the day. Patients looking around the reception area and seeing dust, dirty glass, or discarded trash will wonder if this is a reflection of the overall cleanliness of the practice. Special attention should be taken to keep children's toys or puzzles clean. Patients are also acutely aware of dental office smells so efforts should be made to eliminate them as much as possible.

Provide magazines containing short stories so that patients can read them if they are waiting. The magazines should be current. An office that has out-of-date magazines shows indifference to the patient, and it reflects negatively on overall care. Many dentists have brochures and pamphlets related to the procedures performed in the office. This is also an area in which to display marketing materials. Some offices have photos of staff members. Patients like to feel that they can get to know the staff members who are taking care of them. Dental offices may have areas where patients can relax with a beverage (coffee and juice), or areas with toys and games for children and teens. Providing internet access for patients in the reception area is a growing trend.

Reception areas must be comfortable for everyone regardless of ability. In 1990, Congress originally passed the **Americans with Disabilities Act** (ADA), since then it has been amended several times. It mandates that individuals with disabilities have access to health care facilities including dental offices. Patients with sight or hearing impairments must be provided with assistance to enable them to complete forms and fully understand treatment plans. To accommodate physically disabled patients, all doors and hallways should be wide enough for wheelchair access, and a ramp should be available in areas where stairs are present and no elevator is available. Restrooms must be accessible and ADA compliant.

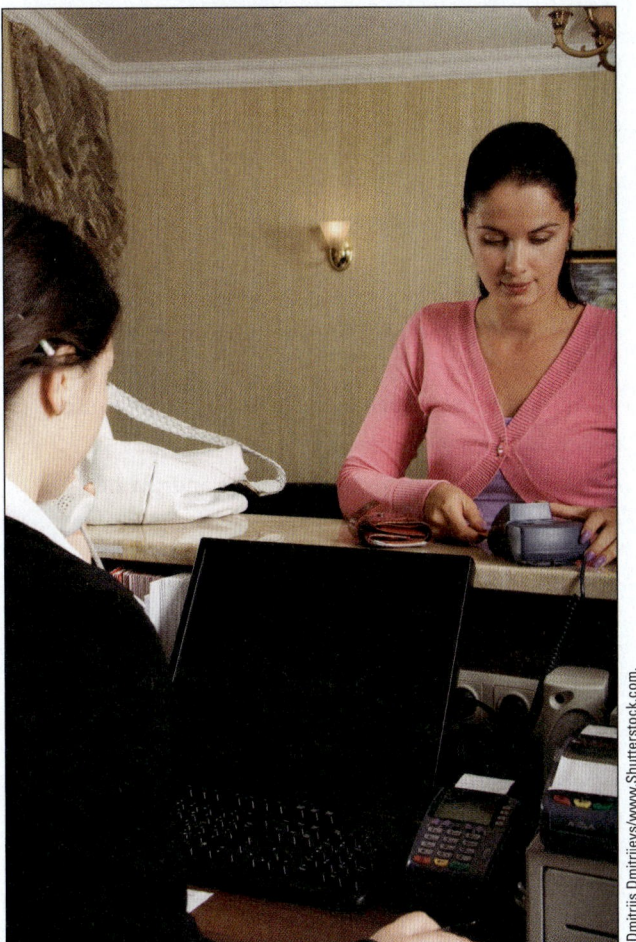

FIGURE 40-1
The reception area, where the patient first encounters the dental office, should be a welcoming environment.

The overall appearance and initial impression of the reception area should give the patients a feeling of well-being and confidence. The patients may not consciously realize the message that is being received, but the dental office should present an atmosphere that relieves feelings of anxiety.

Business Office Staff

The front office staff has changed dramatically in recent years. One person used to greet patients and perform all the paperwork for the office. This is no longer the case due to the increased demand for skills that front office personnel are required to perform.

Front Office Assistant

The front office assistant in a dental office needs to be able to organize time efficiently and handle multiple tasks concurrently. Despite constantly being interrupted, the front office assistant must be able to complete tasks on time, paying close attention to details. The front office assistant must be able to communicate effectively, listen to and observe patients, and serve as a liaison between the patient and clinical staff. This individual must be able to respond to patients who may be upset in a calm, tactful, and appropriate manner.

The front office assistant is normally responsible for, but not limited to, the following tasks:

- Greeting patients
- Assisting patients in filling out initial paperwork required for treatment
- Answering the telephone and taking messages as necessary
- Scheduling appointments
- Maintaining the patient chart system and records
- Accepting and recording patient payments

Dental Office Manager

The dental office manager might be the same person as the front office assistant, or another individual, depending on the size of the office. This person must pay close attention to detail. All office finances are handled by this person, including **accounts receivable**, the money owed to the practice; and **accounts payable**, the money the office owes to others. These finances are normally handled in two separate bookkeeping systems. This individual may handle patient dental insurance and make financial arrangements with the patients for payment of the dental service. The inventory and supply system may also be handled by this individual with the help of the clinical staff. This person must be organized, have knowledge of dental treatments, and exhibit good communication and problem-solving skills. These tasks may be shared with other individuals, such as the front office assistant, depending on the size of the practice. All individuals in the front office need to be knowledgeable in using business machines such as computers, scanners, faxes, copy machines, and high-tech phone systems.

Marketing a Dental Practice

Even though the first priority of the office team is to care for patients' dental needs, this cannot be accomplished when the patient numbers are inadequate. A dental office is a business as well as a health care facility. Marketing is a means of attracting and retaining patients who are satisfied with the practice. All members of the dental team need to be involved in marketing the practice. It can be rewarding for dental assistants to attract patients to the practice, whether through external or internal methods.

Even during off hours, a dental assistant is still associated with the dentist practice where he or she is employed. When people ask what your occupation is, it provides an opportunity to do external marketing for the practice. Other planned external activities can be done, such as dental health education in the community at schools and senior centers. Professionalism and enthusiasm enhance any marketing attempts.

Internal marketing can be accomplished in a number of ways. One person or the whole staff can participate. The ideas are limitless, but the following are suggestions:

- Monthly newsletters with tips for dental health
- Referral contests for patients allowing them the chance to win prizes for recommending the office to friends and family
- Flowers sent to patients as a referral thank you
- Birthday greetings or cards for special occasions, such as a new baby, an anniversary, or a graduation
- Special dental services coupons, such as discounts on services like whitening
- Refrigerator magnets noting the dental office and phone number

Online Marketing

Marketing using the internet is increasingly popular with dental offices. It allows them to reach large numbers of existing and potential patients for a relatively small cost.

Website. An office website is an example of both internal and external marketing. It serves as a way for existing patients to contact the practice or learn about new dental techniques being offered by the practice. Some offices set up secured websites that allow patients to make or check appointments, review their accounts, and make payments online. Websites also attract new patients to the practice by providing information about the dentist and staff, practice philosophy, location details, and the hours that the practice sees patients. The office website provides a way for the office to introduce the dentist and staff. Each individual can have a photo accompanied by an overview of his or her professional qualifications, and, often, a brief personal fact that patients can relate to, such as favorite hobbies or pets.

A dental practice can set up a website using one of the many templates available, but offices can also use a professional website developer to assist them in the design to create a more unique appearance (Figure 40-2). Once the website is online it must be maintained. Someone in the office needs to check to make sure that the links work so that patients and future patients can obtain information. New and updated material needs to be added to keep the website current. Finding fun facts and news can involve everyone in the practice.

Remember that the practice's online presence must be HIPAA compliant (See Chapter 3, Ethics, Jurisprudence, and the Health Information Portability and Accountability Act.) Having a photo release form ready for patients to sign will save time. Even if your practice is posting smile transformation photos that don't show the patients' entire face, ask and receive their written permission.

Social Media. Social media, such as Facebook, Twitter, and Instagram, can also be used to attract patients and stay in contact with existing patients. This type of marketing seems simple, but it takes time and must be monitored closely. The practice should

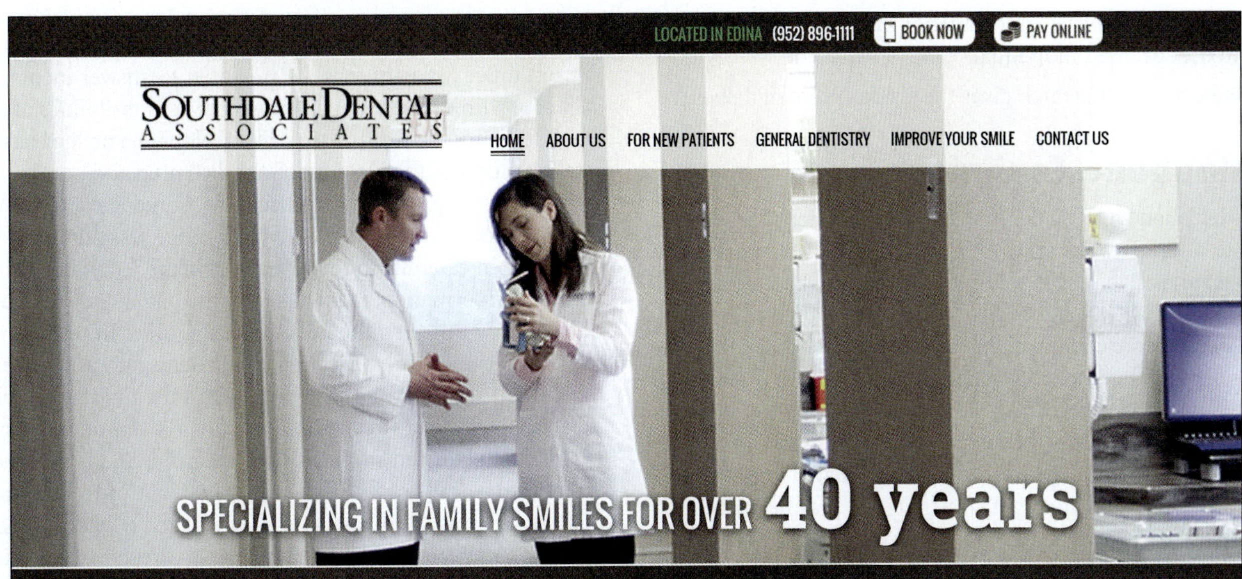

FIGURE 40-2

The office website should be visually appealing and functional.

Source: www.sdadental.com

have a plan for the types of things the practice would like to post and follow. Remember that posts on social media create a personality for the practice! Think about how the patients see a post as compared to how the office staff may see it. For example, Dr. Smith gets a new boat and tweets out photos. Some patients may see it as a sign they are paying too much for their dental care, rather than Dr. Smith's reward for working hard. However, Dr. Smith tweets out photos of his new baby and patients feel like part of the family. You want to update frequently enough to keep patients engaged, but not overwhelm them with content.

Reviews. Positive reviews can be extremely helpful in building a dental practice, but if you have negative reviews patients and prospective patients see those too. There is nothing wrong with asking patients who have had a good experience in your office to write a review.

While it is always disappointing to receive a poor review, it may be good for your practice. Sometimes the person is right, and by letting you know, they have given the practice an opportunity to correct the problem. We can always wish the patient had talked to us personally, and not on a public forum, but patients may take comfort in anonymity. The practice may also receive a poor review that is unjustified. If this happens it is best not to argue about the validity online since it draws attention to the comment.

The goal of marketing is to attract new patients to the practice and retain current patients. Go that *extra mile* to make patients comfortable. Treat them with dignity every time they are in the office.

U.S. Postal Service

The U.S. Postal Service (USPS) has numerous ideas and plans for small businesses. Check their website www.usps.com under business solutions to find services that may help your dental office. Several additional private vendors are available with new ideas and services available for mail and shipping as well. If your practice has a need for a confirmation of delivery, use certified mail. The mailperson has the individual receiving the mail sign for it, and then a copy of the signature is given to the sender for the sender's records. **Certified mail** is used when the practice must prove that a patient has received a letter. If no proof is required, but the dental practice wants to track the package or letter, a tracking number can be obtained and used to track it online. USPS can be used to send greeting cards and postcards, which are especially good for marketing. Many services from the post office can be purchased online, for example, stamps and priority mailing for packages. The front office assistant or office manager may want to check the services that the USPS offers to track mailing expenses and expand marketing.

USPS Services

As noted, there are many USPS services that a small business, such as a dental office, can use, including the following:

- Certificate of mailing, which is a receipt showing that an item was mailed.
- Certified mail, which gives the sender a mailing receipt at the time of mailing and online access to the date and time of delivery. It also provides the recipient's signature at the delivery time.
- Collect on delivery (COD), which is when the mailer wants to collect payment when the merchandise is delivered.
- Delivery confirmation, which is an online service that verifies the delivery date, location, and time.
- Insured mail, which is like an insurance coverage that is purchased when the mailer sends the items.
- Registered mail, the most secure type of mail, which ensures the protection of important mail.

- Restricted delivery, which is when the mail is delivered only to the specified individual.
- Return receipt, which gives the sender proof of delivery.

Telephone Technique

The telephone may be the first contact the patient has with the office, and it sets the stage for the kind of care the person can expect to receive. The first impression tends to be a lasting one. Make sure that the tone of voice and message substance are informational and welcoming to the caller. Handle the call in the same manner as when meeting the patient face to face. Posture and the way the body is carried, along with attitude through facial expressions, are carried through the telephone line to the patient. If the telephone is answered by an individual who is slumped over, leaving the diaphragm constricted, it may be interpreted on the other end as being tired or frustrated. Correct posture allows an individual to sound alert and more professional. Attitude is heard by the patients over the phone. Never forget that the patients who are calling are not interrupting work but, rather, are the reason that the job exists. Some reception areas have mirrors placed in front of the phone so that anyone answering can look at the expression on his or her face, and be reminded of the importance of communicating a good attitude to the caller.

Answer the telephone in a manner that depicts pleasure that the individual called the office. Speak clearly and distinctly, identify the dental practice and yourself, and ask, "How can I help you?" Then, listen carefully. Personality and attitude can sparkle through the telephone, or come out flat and drab.

Basic Telephone Techniques

- No food or drink while on the telephone
- Answer within two or three telephone rings.
- Smile, because the patient can "hear your smile."
- Speak directly into the mouthpiece; keep it no more than one and one-half inches away.
- Use the same volume you would use if speaking to the person directly.
- Enunciate, speak clearly, and articulate carefully.
- Speak at a normal rate of speed.
- Pronounce words correctly.
- Always use telephone **etiquette** (good manners).
- Get the caller's name and use it during the conversation.
- Listen carefully.
- Have a pen and paper close by.
- Use caution not to repeat personal details where they can be overheard by other patients.
- Allow the caller to end the call.

Call Types

Several types of calls come into the dental office. They all should be handled in a professional manner. Some of the calls are more critical for patient care than others.

Answering Calls

A front office assistant must be prepared to answer incoming calls at any time, while juggling the other responsibilities of the front desk. It is crucial that the caller feel that he or she has the total attention of the assistant. Good listening and communication skills help portray an image of an organized, efficient, and courteous dental office. The front office assistant must be able to listen carefully to the caller, and make judgments, after gathering information, that will aid in the patient's care. It may be necessary to *screen* the calls to get the caller in touch with the right person to solve the problem. Patients may ask to speak to the dentist. The front office assistant must first try to help, identify the patient's concern, and take a telephone number where the doctor can call back. Give the caller an idea of when to expect the call from the dentist. The front office assistant must ensure that the dentist's time is managed efficiently. Most dentists prefer not to be interrupted at chairside while caring for another patient. With infection control concerns, the chance of being inconsiderate to the current patient, and the delay in patient treatment during the day's schedule, it is important not to disrupt the dentist with a telephone call. Some dentists will take calls from another dentist, the dental laboratory technician needing an answer to further a case, and/or family members. Know your doctor's policies in regard to taking incoming phone calls. Handle the calls with tact by saying something such as, "The doctor is with a patient. Can I help you?"

Placing Callers on Hold

If it becomes necessary to place the caller on hold and handle emergent situations or answer another phone line, ask the patient if he or she would mind holding for a minute, and then listen to the answer. One of the rudest ways to handle patients on the telephone is by asking, "Can you hold, please?" and then, without waiting for an answer, pushing the hold button and cutting the patient off.

The caller should never have to wait any longer than 1 minute on hold. If necessary, check in and ask whether the caller would like to continue to hold, or whether it would be more convenient to receive a call back. Handle on-hold calls in this manner and the patients will know that their time is being respected, and that their needs will be facilitated as soon as possible. Some offices have 1-minute timers by the telephone to remind the front office assistant of the person waiting, and how long he or she has been on the other line. Do what is necessary to get back to the person on hold or that patient may be lost to the practice.

Taking Messages

When taking messages, be thorough. It is advisable to use standard telephone message pads with carbon so that the office can retain copies of all messages. Record the date and time and ask the caller the following information:

- Name and telephone number of the caller
- Who the message is for
- Message and urgency of the telephone call

- What action is required
- A good time to return the call

After the message is written, repeat it to the caller to verify that it was written correctly. Also, enter your initials or name in case the person receiving the messages has questions. Give the caller an approximate time when to expect the return call to be placed.

Outgoing Calls

When telephone calls are made from the office, the same professional, positive approach should be followed. Be prepared and know the information that needs to be conveyed or sought. Most offices call the next day's patients to confirm their appointments. Performing this tedious task requires attention. More than one front office assistant has called a patient to confirm the appointment, and totally forgotten which individual was dialed. Use some type of indication system to keep track of which patients have been called. If calling an insurance company, have all the information handy, including the patient's chart and forms, so that any questions that come up can be answered readily.

If calling and leaving a message, take care with any information recorded on the answering machine. Remember that all health care issues are confidential and should be discussed only with the patient. Try not to leave the information with small children, because the information can become confusing and get passed on to the adult inaccurately.

It is best if no personal telephone calls are made at the office. If the need arises, make them during your lunch hour, if possible. The telephone is for dental office business, and personal matters belong outside the office.

When phone calls need to be made to insurance companies and patients living or working in other parts of the country, keep in mind that there is a 3-hour time difference from one zone on the Pacific coast to the other time zone on the Atlantic coast.

English as a Second Language

It is probable to encounter many patients whose primary language is not English in the dental office. The dentist is responsible for providing an interpreter, if necessary, for communication. Some patients bring family members who speak English to translate. It is important that communication on the telephone and in the office be handled in a manner that provides the patient with the pertinent information. There are several things to remember when speaking to patients whose first language is not English:

- Be patient.
- Speak at a normal volume. Raising the voice does not increase the other person's ability to understand the words.
- Speak more slowly, if necessary, and avoid complicated words, phrases, or slang terms.
- A patient who does not speak English may be able to understand English well. Do not assume that the patient does not comprehend what is being said.
- Ask the patient if clarification is needed.
- Repeat the information, if necessary, until understood.

Telephone and Communication Technology

Most offices have multifunctional telephones. Normally, the telephones have hold buttons and a minimum of three lines. It is important to understand the functions of the phone system so that if transfers are done, the patient is not lost. Spend time thoroughly learning the entire system. The cost of telephone systems has become a great expense to the dental office but they are designed to save time when used effectively. Once a phone system is installed in the practice there may be options available to update and expand functions to meet the dental practice's changing needs. Caller identification systems have become common as a part of the dental office phone system, and aid the front office assistant in helping patients more quickly by providing a visual display of the caller's name. Advances in telecommunications have a tremendous impact on dental office communication, so stay informed.

Answering Systems. Dental offices need to provide a way for patients to contact them when the office is closed. Answering systems, such as answering machines or as part of the telephone system, are commonplace today, and patients have grown to accept them. They are not replacements for a live person answering, but can be utilized to give patients emergency telephone numbers and information. Many offices use answering systems that are turned on each evening when the dentist and staff leave for the day, as well as during lunch hours or staff meetings. These systems are checked promptly for messages. They may be turned off during the day, or left on and used as a backup when a phone cannot be answered personally, such as when all the lines are busy. If the phone system is used to take messages during the work day, the front office assistant must remember to check for those messages. Generally, phone systems have something, such as a blinking light, to notify staff that a message has been received.

It is the responsibility of the front office assistant to record the message on the answering machine and check for messages. Often, offices have several messages recorded that they can choose from when leaving the office. They might have a lunch message, an evening message, a weekend message, or even a message that lets the caller know that the practice is open but you are currently assisting other patients and will return the call as quickly as possible. The front office assistant should call the number occasionally to check that the message being received by the patients is acceptable, and the system is functioning properly. The phone message reflects the dental office and, like all other aspects, it is important that the recording is clear and of good quality.

Answering with Headphones. The front office assistant completes numerous tasks where her or his hands are needed, so offices may use headphones (Figure 40-3) to answer calls. These allow the person taking the calls to be able to write

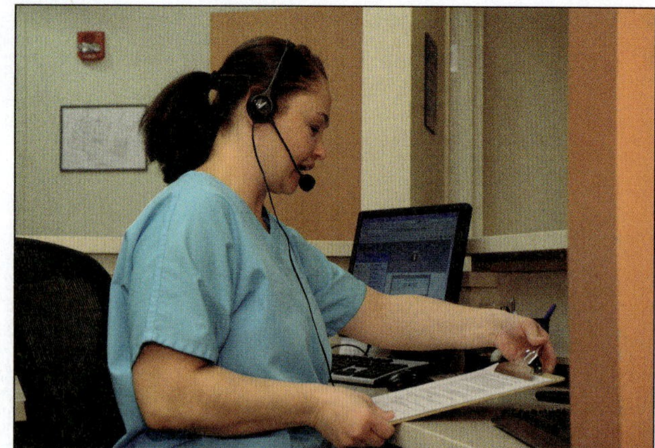

FIGURE 40-3
A dental office team member utilizing a headset to communicate with a patient.

things down much easier. They are also utilized to talk to other team members throughout the office. This interactive ongoing communication will help make the office run smoothly.

Answering Services. Some offices have opted for answering services that are staffed by live operators. Having a person at the other end of the line is more reassuring to patients and other callers. These services also can provide flexibility in screening and routing calls. Most of the fees for the answering services are by the month or by the number of calls received. This service is more expensive than that of an in-office answering system.

Voice Mail. If working at a large group practice, a voice mail or automated routing unit may be used. This system answers the call, and a recorded voice identifies choices for the caller to select by pressing a specific number on a touch-tone telephone. Some of the automated routing systems have mailboxes for the caller to leave a message for a specific person being called. All the messages are delivered by a recorded voice. Some patients can become frustrated by it, especially elderly patients who may have more difficulty hearing the directions.

Fax Machines. Fax machines are common in the dental office. A fax is a facsimile transmission used to send and receive written messages through the telephone lines. It can contain typed or written data, pictures, and line art. It is important that it be sent to the correct address, taking care that confidential information be handled conscientiously. The fax is used to relay information to and from patients and insurance companies, and to order dental supplies, among other things.

Email. Email (electronic mail) is another common form of communication used by dental practices. It can be very convenient and saves time and money over traditional mail. Email can be saved so that all the parties involved in the electronic conversation have a history of it. It is a great way to send messages to other members of the dental team. Multiple email addresses can be used to send the same message to a group of people, or a message can be forwarded to a third party for whom the message might be relevant.

Email can be used, with their consent, to contact patients. Patient privacy rules apply to this form of contact, so the use of personal health information (PHI) should not be included unless the patient has asked you in writing to do so. When sending an email, either to patients or co-workers, some guidelines should be followed:

- Use complete sentences.
- Grammar and spelling should be accurate.
- Be polite.
- Proofread your email before sending it.
- Never send an email when you are upset, mad, or frustrated.
- Capitalize appropriately. Using all CAPITAL letters is viewed as yelling.
- Keep your message brief and to the point.
- Use an appropriate salutation and closing.
- Using an electronic signature can be helpful in providing additional contact information.
- Use the subject line to summarize the message in a few words.
- Keep your correspondence professional—don't forward things you think are funny or cute.
- Do not send personal email from an office computer.
- Never include credit card or other personal/office financial information.

Cell Phones. Patients, dentists, and staff members may use cell phones routinely for communication. In fact, cell phones have become so common many families no longer have traditional land lines. When updating patient records, document what the best number to reach them is for confirmation of appointments and other communication.

Cell phones can also be used as an alternative to an after-hours answering service. The office cell phone belongs to the office, but staff members take it home at night and weekends to answer possible emergency calls. The dental team member talks to the patient and determines if he or she should contact the dentist, schedule an emergency visit, or if the call can be returned during business hours. Remember that emergencies can be anything from a true dental emergency to a problem that needs to be scheduled quickly but not immediately.

Cell phone etiquette:

- Turn your cell phone to vibrate when you are in the office.
- Leave your phone in your purse or locker during work hours.
- During lunch or break times, speak quietly or walk outside of the office.
- If you use your cell phone to take photos, keep in mind what or who is in the background. A patient or PHI that might be visible is a violation of HIPAA.

Text messaging using a cell phone has become a very popular means of communication. The same rules of etiquette apply to texting and verbal cell phone communication. When you are working with patients they deserve 100 percent of your attention. The chime of a phone receiving texts messages is distracting to both you, your patient, and other staff members.

Business Office Systems

Historically, business office systems were manual, but today most offices use a **computerized system** made up of hardware and software (Figure 40-4). The dental practice may use the computer for everything and be completely paperless, or use some manual systems in conjunction with their computer system. In today's fast-paced dental office, time and efficiency are important. Computers reduce the time involved in many routine office procedures. Once the dental assistant becomes familiar with the computer software and applications, he or she will find more and more uses for the computer. When choosing the **hardware** (the computer's physical equipment) and **software** (a computer program or set of instructions), the dentist may rely heavily on the dental office manager and business office staff. Determine how the system will be used in the practice and evaluate each system based on the needs of the practice. Talk to other practices using the systems being considered, and evaluate the pros and cons of each one. Work with a trusted and knowledgeable vendor who understands the needs of the practice before making such a significant purchase.

After the research is completed, bring it to the staff members for their input. It is important that all the staff members be familiar with the system. It takes a great deal of time to convert all the information to the new system, and staff training will be necessary, so it is best if everyone is involved in the process. Make sure the system that is purchased meets not only current needs, but allows for future growth within the practice (Figure 40-5).

Dental Office Software

A large variety of dental office software programs are available for use in the dental office. Choose the software that best meets the office's needs. It should have general-purpose functions that includes database management, word processing, graphics, spreadsheets, bookkeeping, insurance, and online communication. It is possible to purchase software that has many clinical functions too.

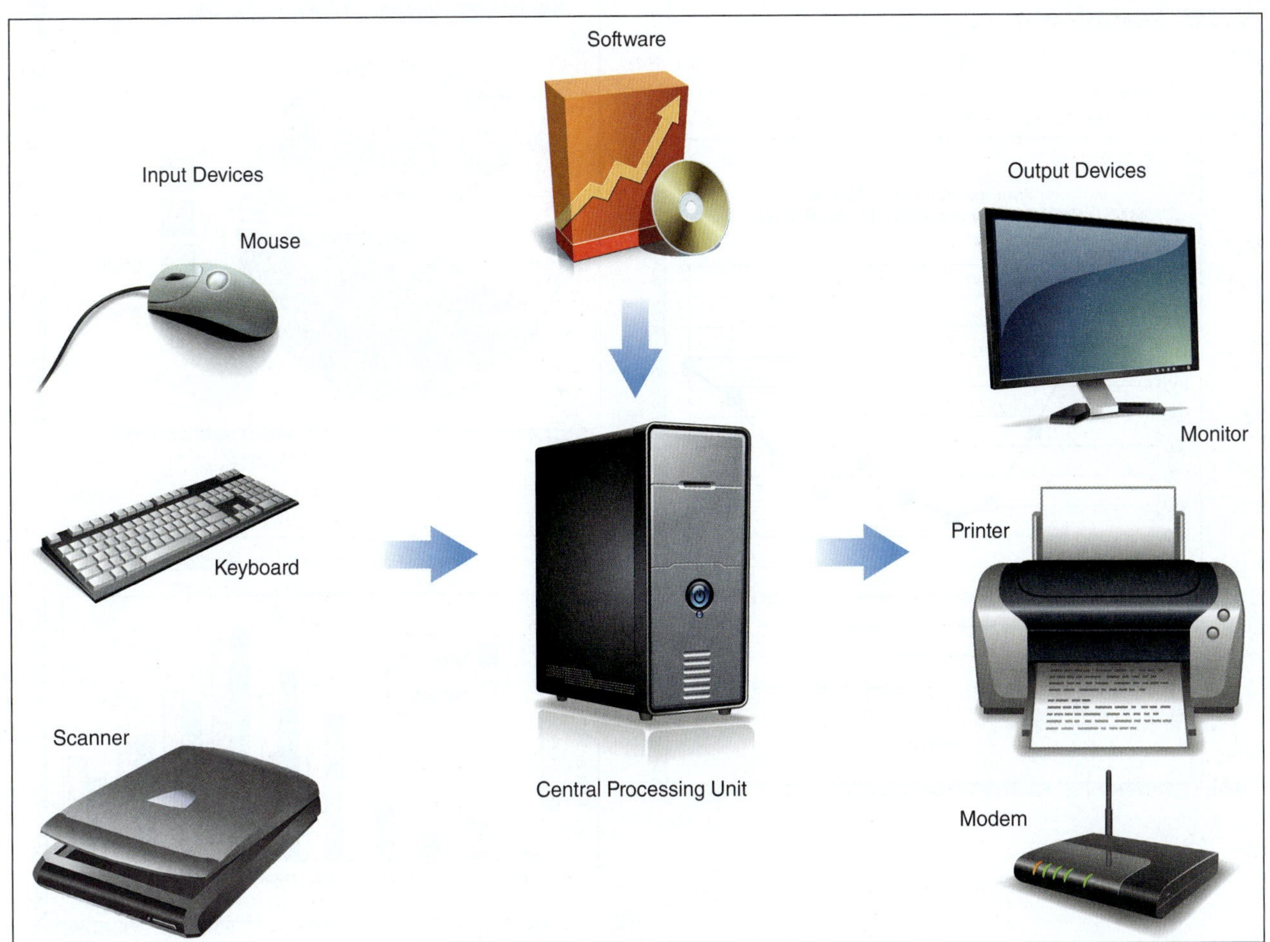

FIGURE 40-4
Components of a computer system in the dental office.

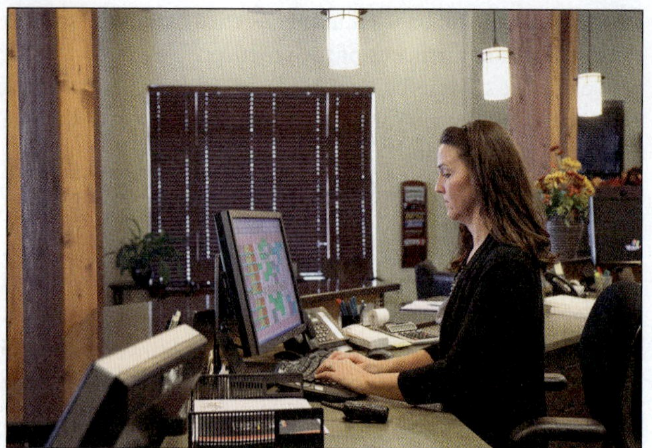

FIGURE 40-5

Front office personnel with computer system components.

There are lots of software programs available. Two software programs that are commonly used within dental offices are the Dentrix system available from Henry Schein Inc. and Eaglesoft available from Patterson Dental. Both software programs have a wide range of applications and training. This training may be provided by the manufacturers of the software, or by alternate training sites. Both programs are updated often to provide the newest services available to the dental team.

Word Processing. Word processing has largely replaced typewriters. It allows the dental team member to use a computer keyboard to type memos, letters, and reports, and to make corrections easily. Word processing software allows for spelling checks, deletions, cutting and pasting information, and much more. The documents can be stored and retrieved at a later time, and then changed slightly and used again without having to create a whole new document. Typing a letter has been made much easier via computer and word processing software. Dental management software often contains prewritten letters as part of its word processing function. They can be used as is, customized, or even integrated with a patient database to send personally addressed letters to a large number of patients.

Graphics. With the use of graphic software, numeric information can be transformed into graphs, pie charts, and bar graphs (Figure 40-6). This allows information to be summarized in a graphic format for easy visualization. Dental software uses a practice's data to allow the practice to create graphs that track trends and evaluate possible changes.

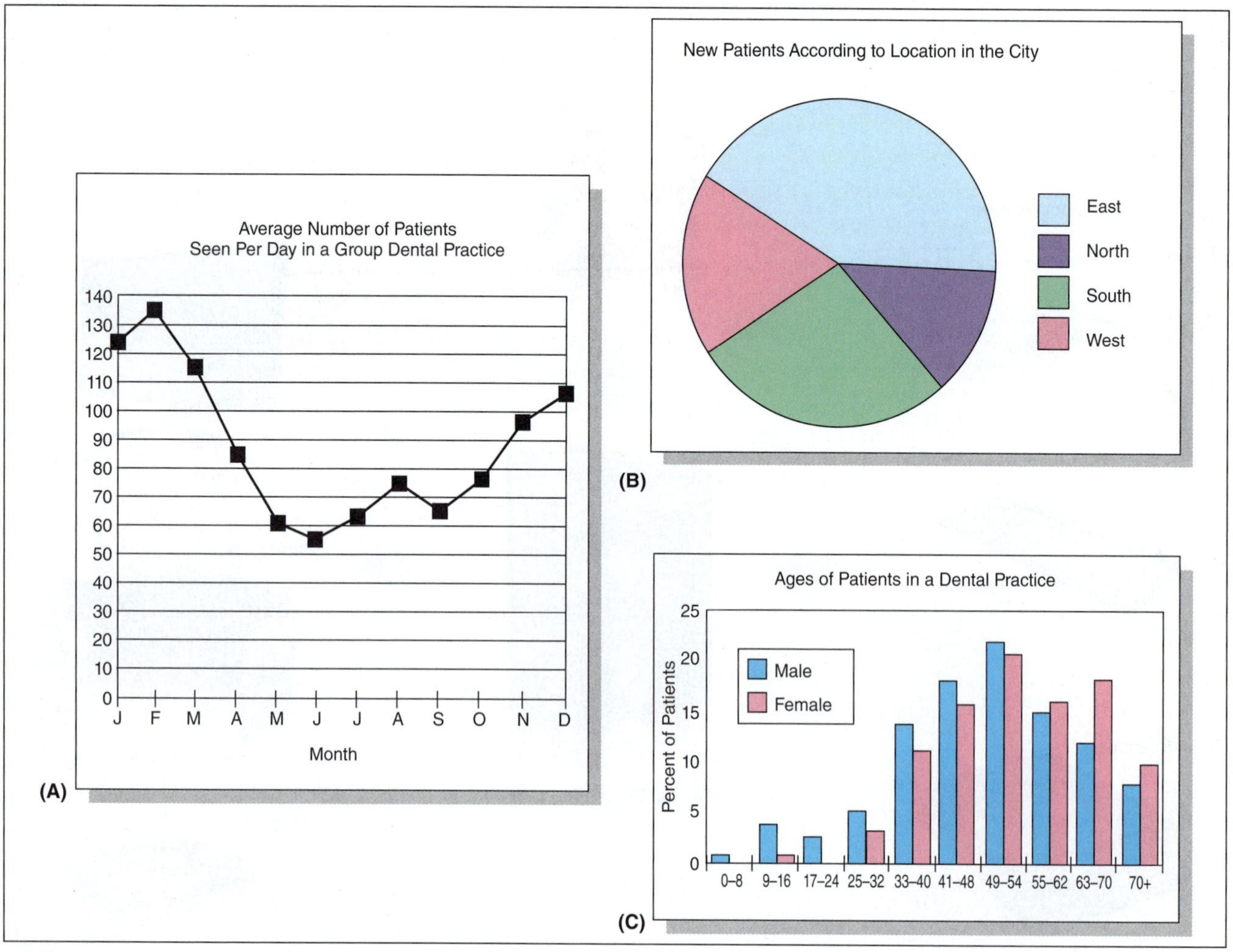

FIGURE 40-6

Graphs and charts make information easier to interpret. (A) Line graph. (B) Pie chart. (C) Bar graph.

Spreadsheets. Spreadsheets are a computerized worksheet that allows for programmed calculations. Spreadsheets electronically calculate the numerical data to be analyzed. This calculation and recalculation, which used to take hours, is completed in seconds with spreadsheet software. Spreadsheets are used in the dental office to prepare monthly and yearly financial statements and accounts payable, along with other uses. The data from a spreadsheet can be converted into a graph or chart, presenting information that can be interpreted at a glance.

The software used in dentistry can track the practice's success in many ways. The office can view office totals according to specified criteria, and through any time frame. It can also be viewed in a graphic display (Figure 40-7). Many patient groups can be identified, and a report generated. For instance, if the office wanted to see how many patients had porcelain crowns in the past year, it can be easily found. This would allow the office to assess whether there is a need to purchase a machine (CAD/CAM) for designing and manufacturing crowns. All types of information are available and can be readily accessed.

Database Management

To organize large quantities of related data into useful forms, computer database management software is used. The patient database allows staff to quickly access information and would include basic information such as the

- patient's name,
- patient's date of birth,
- spouse's name and/or other family members,
- patient's address,
- patient's home phone number,
- patient's work phone number, and
- patient's insurance.

Many office database systems have additional information about the patient, such as his or her preferred name, place of employment, Social Security number, preferred provider, privacy requests, medical alerts, or even a photo of the patient. The patient's continuing care schedule can be placed in the computer with the other information. Once the information is in the computer database, it can be used with the word processor, graphs, or spreadsheets. This information can be grouped in a number of ways. For example, an office could identify all the patients who have birthdays in the current month and send birthday cards to them, or all the new patients could be identified so that welcome letters could go out to them. A variety of database applications are beneficial to the dental practice, both for marketing and in collecting data.

Computer Safety

Use computer virus software to protect the office system if there is any chance that the office may download information from the internet or accept files from other computer systems. Everything could be lost if unprotected. Most offices backup their files daily to make sure that a copy of the information is available if the system crashes due to an internet virus, fire, or water damage. Even if the possibility of losing the data is remote, it takes a great deal of time to reconstruct the system if this happens. Always have a backup of critical information.

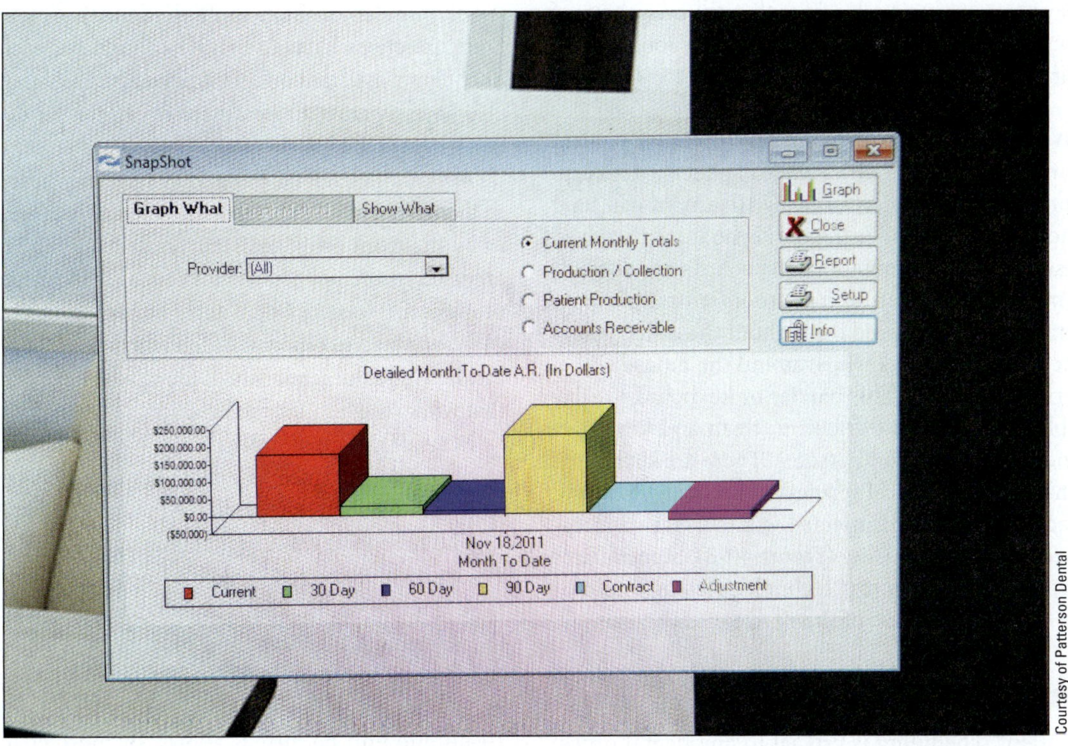

FIGURE 40-7
Computer software graph showing dental office production.

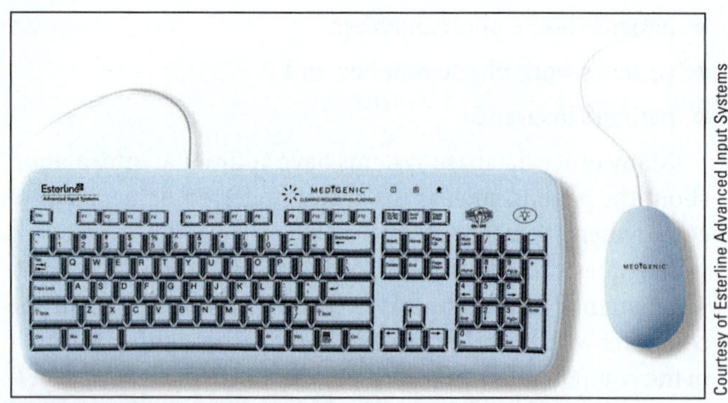
Courtesy of Esterline Advanced Input Systems

FIGURE 40-8

Flat keyboard design and mouse allow for easy disinfection, with timed alert for users to become aware that disinfection has not occurred.

Computer Ergonomics and Eye Care. For those individuals who spend a great deal of time on the computer, it is important to practice recommended computer **ergonomics** (human factors that affect the design and operation of tools and the work environment). For instance, posture is critical for preventing injury. Choose a comfortable cushioned chair with back support and four to five casters forming a stable base. The height of the chair should allow the feet to be on the floor with the desk surface slightly lower than elbow level. Keep items used frequently close at hand.

Other recommended aids include an ergonomic keyboard, which allows the wrists to remain in a flat position. A wrist rest for the mouse is used to keep the wrist in a level position. Screen glare protectors can be used to deflect and reduce monitor glare. Eye care professionals advise that, for every hour of computer use, the user should relax the eyes by looking at a distance for 10 minutes to reduce eye fatigue.

Infection Control for Keyboards. Infection control for keyboards in the dental office has long been a concern. Aerosol spray from handpieces during treatment can land on computer keyboards; and using the keyboard with gloved hands causes cross-contamination. Keyboards are difficult or nearly impossible to clean, and microorganisms multiply and are spread and transferred throughout the office. Many dental offices are covering keyboards and the mouse with a barrier during treatment. This barrier or keyboard overlay is acceptable, but it is still difficult to clean and keying in patient procedure data is cumbersome. There are keyboards available that act like a typical spring-key keyboard, but have a flat surface that can be disinfected with surface disinfectant or placed in the dishwasher (Figure 40-8). Some offices have incorporated voice to text technology using a microphone and eliminating some of the need for keyboards.

Patient Scheduling

Effective patient scheduling is crucial to any dental office, and the appointment book is the heart of a dental practice. Basics of scheduling remain the same regardless of whether the appointment book is on a computer or in a traditional paper format. Maintaining a smooth patient flow throughout the day determines the success and profitability of the dentist and the practice. Scheduling may seem to be a mundane task, but in reality it takes an organized person with good interpersonal and communication skills to schedule in a way that maximizes production, while also reducing stress. If the task is done well, this job can be very challenging and satisfying. When scheduling, the front office assistant acts as a coordinator to help all team members work together, keep their timing perfect, and reach goals. One of the first steps in the process is to acquire the proper materials for scheduling effectively. Analyze the needs of the practice and plan accordingly. Understand that the needs may change and adjustments will have to be made.

Appointment Books

Appointment books are available in several forms. To choose the correct one for the office situation, evaluate the qualities of each. Manual appointment books come in ringed or bound copies. The ringed appointment book allows for the addition or deletion of additional pages. It lays open and flat on the counter during use. A bound appointment book needs to be replaced when the current one is filled. This leaves a time frame during which two books are utilized, making it more difficult for the scheduling to be completed.

Another consideration is the number of appointment columns required. This is dependent on the unique needs of the physical facilities and staff. Solo practitioners have two or three columns for scheduling patients. Larger practices need six or more columns if multiple dentists practice together. Some practices have a separate column for each expanded-duty dental assistant or dental hygienist. Dental practices may also have separate appointment books for the dental hygienist's patient schedule.

Appointment book pages may have day headings printed in them. Alternatively, pages with blank headings can be filled in by the front office assistant so that only the days worked are used in the appointment book and a minimum number of pages are wasted. Some appointment books have the days of the week across the top of the schedule and the correct day can be circled or underlined. Identify the appointment book that works the best for the practice.

Many of the appointment books are set up so that the pages show a week at a glance. The days not worked can be crossed out, while still allowing the user to see the entire week at one time.

The time intervals in an appointment book are normally 10- or 15-minute intervals and are described as units of time (Figure 40-9). There are six units in an hour if using the 10-minute intervals, and four units in an hour if using the 15-minute intervals. The 15-minute unit is routinely utilized in some offices. However, most dental offices use the 10-minute unit because it allows for more effective patient scheduling. The treatment procedures are broken down into units. For example, the doctor may request five units for a

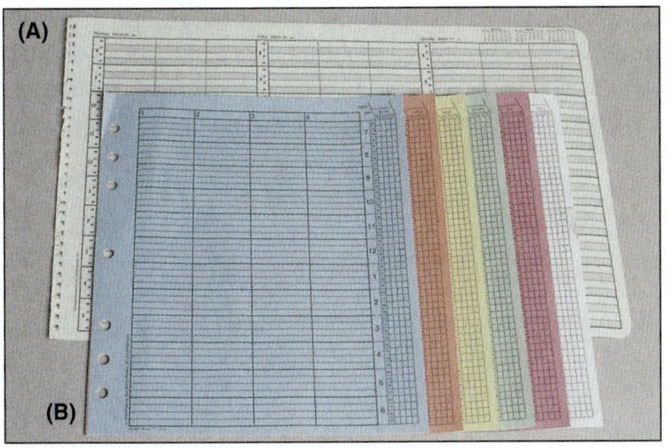

FIGURE 40-9

(A) Appointment book pages showing 15-minute units for patient scheduling. (B) Color-coded appointment book for efficient use of dentist's and dental assistant's time. Both allow for a week at a glance.

crown preparation. This equals 50 minutes of time in the appointment book.

Front office assistants who are advanced and production conscious can color code the scheduling of appointments. The appointment book indicates whether the dentist or expanded-duty dental assistant is performing treatment for the patient. For example, if using the crown preparation appointment, the schedule would reflect that the first 5 minutes of the 50-minute allotted time are for the dental assistant to set up and take the preliminary impressions; the next 30 minutes are for the dentist to anesthetize the patient, prepare the tooth for the crown preparation, and take the final impression; and the final 15 minutes are for the dental assistant to make the temporary (provisional) restoration and dismiss the patient. Therefore, the dentist's time can be scheduled for other patient's care after the initial 35 minutes with the crown preparation patient. This method is utilized in a practice in which patients can be attended to by other staff members. This approach, called **double booking**, uses the dentist's time in the most productive manner. If patients are waiting for the staff or the dentist to attend to them, then the double-booking approach is not working effectively. Double booking can be done in a manual appointment book or on the computer.

Appointment Book Matrix. After the appointment book is selected with the appropriate days, columns, and units, the front office assistant can begin establishing the appointment book matrix. This is where the whole year (if possible) can be mapped out to avoid scheduling patients when the dentist has other commitments or when the office is closed. It is advisable to use pencil in a manual appointment book, because even the best laid out plans may change. First, mark an "X" through the days when the office is closed. Identify all the continuing education seminars and meetings that the dentist and staff will be attending, along with the holidays when the office is closed.

In many offices, specific periods of time are set aside for emergencies. This time is referred to as buffer time. Each dental office identifies which time is best for buffer time. The most common buffer time is late morning, right before lunch, and late afternoon, right before closing. Buffer time is not previously scheduled but is reserved for emergency patients only.

Lunch time is marked out in the appointment book with an "X" or a diagonal line. The columns are identified for treatment rooms or for specific dental team members, such as the dental hygienist. Color coding can be used in defining the appointment book matrix.

When scheduling the dental appointments or developing the treatment plan for patients, it is important to know the specific time intervals needed between appointments. For instance, after a crown is prepared and a provisional is placed, the dental laboratory needs time to process the case and return the finished product to the dental office before the next appointment. This interim time may be from 2 to 7 days. Each dental laboratory varies in the amount of time needed to process the case. Whatever the time required by the laboratory, allow a couple of additional days to ensure that the case is complete prior to the patient's appointment. At times, multiple appointments are required in a series. The front office assistant may have to consider healing time, as well as laboratory production time when scheduling the advance appointments.

Special Patient Appointment Times. All practices have patients who require special scheduling of appointment times due to health concerns, age, or just nervousness. If young children are to be scheduled for dental appointments, it is best to care for them in the morning or after nap times. Treating a child prior to nap time when he or she is cranky and unhappy may make it difficult for everyone. Children of school age normally require appointments after school or during vacation days. Obtain the calendar for local schools to become aware of the academic calendar year so that the appointment book can be scheduled according to children's needs.

Elderly patients should be scheduled at a time when they are not fatigued. They may have concerns about transportation, bus routes, and the weather. Arrange times for their appointments that are convenient for them. Morning appointments often work well.

It is well documented that patients who are extremely anxious about dentistry have a greater cancellation rate for their appointments. If a patient expresses fear, the assistant can reassure him or her and make a notation for the front office assistant. This alerts the front office assistant that a short, easy appointment should be scheduled the first time to build the patient's confidence and lessen the risk of cancellation. Calls may be made prior to the appointment to confirm the time, and follow-up calls may be made after the appointment to ensure that everything went well for the patient.

Health concerns impact patient appointment scheduling. If a patient has diabetes or hypoglycemia, schedule the patient after a mealtime. Confirm that the patient has eaten and verify that the diabetic patient has taken the needed medication. A patient with heart problems may require shorter appointments so that the patient does not become over fatigued.

Other Scheduling Concerns. Discuss the appointment book scheduling with the dentist and the staff. The dentist may have the highest energy level in the morning. Scheduling a difficult, tedious treatment at the end of the day may be overtaxing. Also, scheduling the same procedure repeatedly may make it difficult on the dental team members. Staggering the types of treatment allows the dental team to be prepared for the procedures and makes the day go smoother and faster. Also, scheduling the same procedure several times in a row may make it difficult to accomplish the sterilization procedures when only a limited number of specific instruments are available for the specific procedure. During staff meetings, talk over appointment scheduling that works well, and define the best policy approach.

Computer Scheduling

Dental offices today most often use computer scheduling (Figure 40-10). Many software packages, offering a variety of services, are available. The office can determine the type of software needed for the practice. The same information is needed for computer scheduling as with a manual appointment book. Computer scheduling is, however, completed more rapidly and quickly for the patient, and the front office assistant.

When using computer scheduling, the program searches through the database for open appointment time frames based on the treatment plan. After finding a time and date that are convenient for the patient, the data is keyed into the computer schedule and the appointment is automatically scheduled. Dental management software is available to develop any matrix that the practice desires for scheduling appointments. The schedule can be designed to highlight open appointment times with very few directions.

Appointment Book Entries

When making appointment book entries using the manual system, it is important to write in pencil. Of course, entering appointments with a computer is much easier. First, establish an appointment time with the patient, noting any special considerations, such as laboratory work, that might affect the appointment. Record the entry in the schedule. The entry should include the patient's name and phone number, the procedure to be completed (abbreviated), the length of the procedure (identified by an arrow), and the age if the patient is a child (these things can be done automatically in a computerized system). Write out the information on an appointment card for the patient, including the day, date, and time (Figure 40-11). Clearly repeat the information to the patient as the card is given to him or her, to verify it once again.

The front office assistant must know the time units for each procedure in order to schedule patient appointments. The more productive treatment procedures are

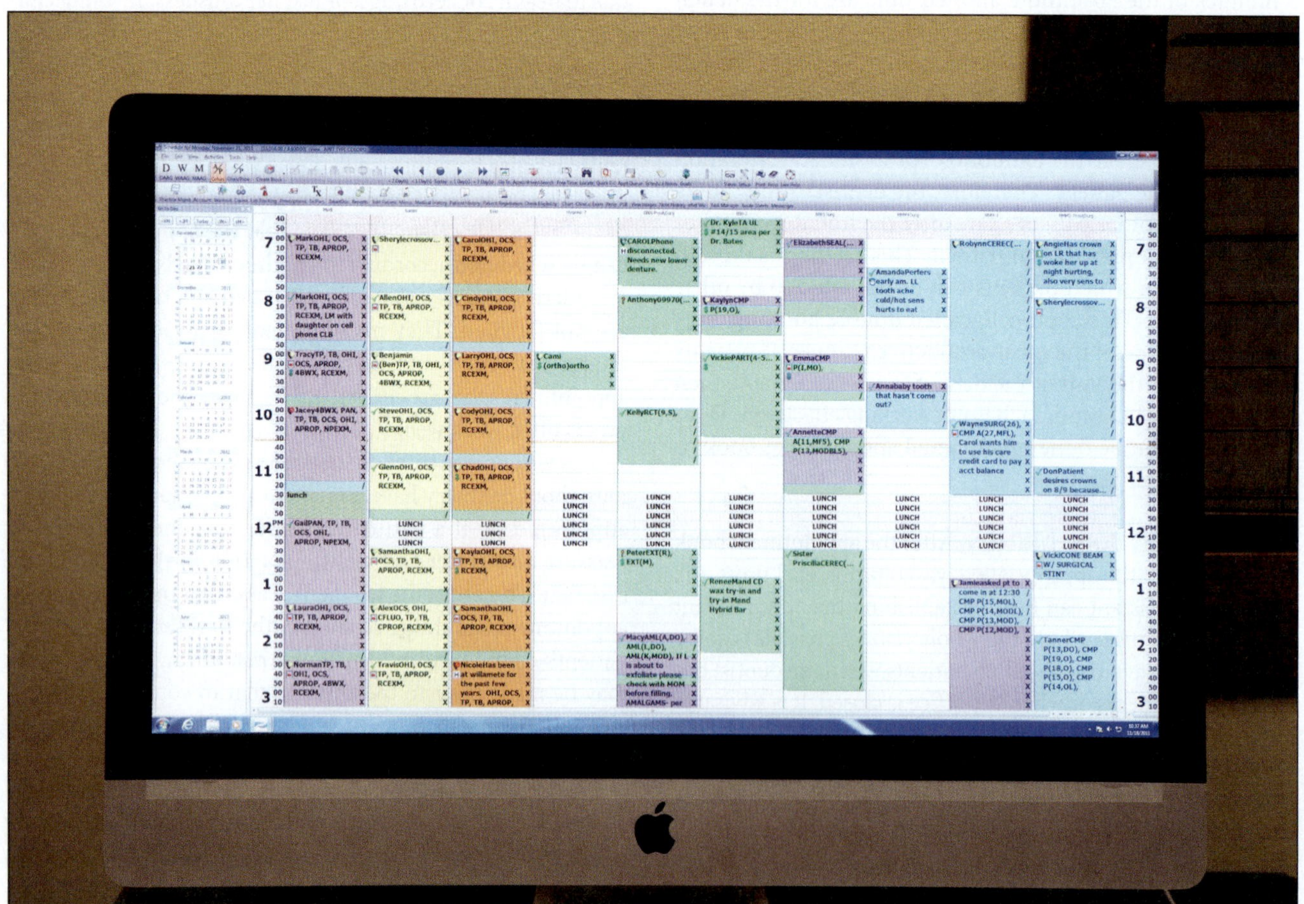

Courtesy of Patterson Dental

FIGURE 40-10

Computer software system showing patient scheduling.

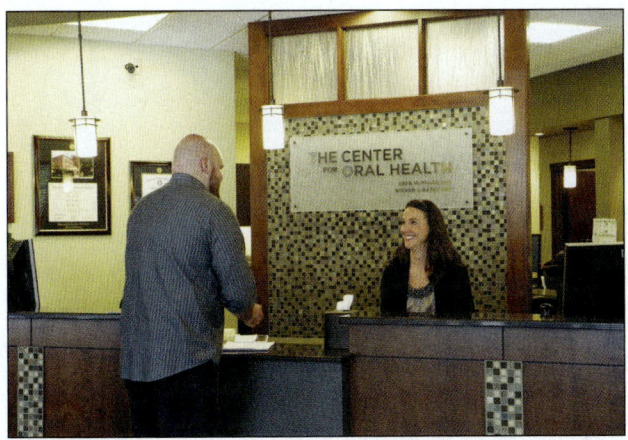

FIGURE 40-11

Patients are given appointment cards with their next appointment, and preoperative instructions printed neatly.

called primary procedures. They tend to be the longer appointments dealing with crown and bridge preparations, amalgam and composite fillings, surgery, and endodontic treatment. With the increased time spent placing and removing barriers and sterilization, it is much more productive to take care of several teeth at the same appointment. Around the primary procedures, the front office assistant can schedule a dovetail or conjunctive procedure that does not require the same concentrated attention by the dentist. These conjunctive procedures include routine examinations, consultations, or adjustments.

The front office assistant's goal is to fill the appointment book with patient care so that the scheduling problems such as downtime, overtime, and overlap time are nonexistent for the dentist and dental assistants.

- **Downtime**—is time in the appointment book that is not scheduled. If an appointment time using 10-minute units is open from 2:00 to 2:30, it is referred to as three units of downtime. Downtime can be costly for the practice since many of the expenses for the practice remain the same, but there is no production during that time.
- **Overtime**—is where the patient treatment time went beyond the estimated time frame. This can affect the entire schedule. It can cause other patients to wait for their appointments, therefore making them unhappy.
- **Overlap of time**—occurs when the dentist or dental assistant is required to be in two places at the same time, or when two patients need to be seated in the same treatment room at the same time.

All three scheduling problems occur, and care should be taken to eliminate them whenever possible. Careful estimation of accurate time units reduces or eliminates some of these problems. If this is an ongoing concern, scheduling adjustments should be made accordingly. The office team should meet and discuss ideas to eliminate scheduling problems.

Office policies for handling patients with special needs, repeated appointment delays, and repeated missed appointments must be developed. The computer can note these and, after several missed appointments, it may be office policy to avoid rescheduling the patient. All these topics should be discussed so that the front office assistant knows how to handle these situations.

Recall Patients

Established dental offices consider the recall system the backbone of the dental practice. A recall system ensures that patients return for continued care and maintenance of their dental needs. These appointments are called recall or recare appointments. Bringing patients back into the office at regular intervals allows the dentist to assess their teeth and tissues, and keep them in optimum condition. This preventive measure prevents serious discomfort for the patient. During the recall (recare) appointment, the dental team reinforces oral hygiene techniques and educates the patient concerning any new products or other dental aids on the market that will help the patient with overall oral care. Questions may arise about whitening techniques, types of toothbrushes, and mouth rinses. It also allows the dentist to assess pathology concerns at an early stage.

Computer Recall. Recalling patients for their ongoing care can be accomplished with a number of methods. With increased computer use in dental offices, most current recall is done from a computer-generated printout. Information is placed in the computer after the regular appointment is completed. The program allows a date for the recall or recare appointment to be indicated. At the end of the month, an alphabetical list of patients needing recall for the following month, along with their addresses and phone numbers, can be generated. This list can be used to contact the patients by telephone or through the mail. The patients who schedule appointments can be removed from the list, while the others stay on the printout automatically.

Advance Appointment Scheduling

The appointment book allows for advance scheduling of recall appointments immediately after regular dental care is complete. This allows an appointment to be scheduled for the patient 3 to 6 months in advance. The appointment book in this system is used as the primary listing. The patients need to reaffirm their appointments 2 weeks in advance as well as the day prior. The advantage to this system is that the task is completed immediately for the patient as well as the dental office. The disadvantage of this system is obvious: The patient does not always know what will be happening in his or her life that far in advance, and may need to cancel or reschedule the appointment.

Chronological Card File. A minimum amount of time is invested in the chronological card file system. In this system, the patient fills out a postcard so that the next recall date will be mailed directly to his or her address. The cards are filed according to the month the patient is to be recalled. The card is mailed to the patient 2 weeks before the given recall date. If this system is used alone, the card is sent to the patient, and then all references for the patient recall are lost, unless someone goes through all the charts and makes a list of patients needing recall appointments. It is better to make a list and note the patients who do not schedule appointments, and follow up with telephone calls to schedule the appointment.

Color-Tagged Card File. Another type of recall system is the color-tagged card file. In this system, every patient has an index card with his or her name, address, telephone number, and any other special notations printed on it. The cards are filed alphabetically, and a colored tag is clipped to each card indicating in which month the patient requires a recall appointment. For example, a yellow tag is clipped to a card if the patient needs a recall appointment in January. The tagged file cards are reviewed each month, and calls are made to schedule the patients needing continued care. If they do not schedule, they can be moved up to the next month or later, if requested. After the patient is scheduled, the card is attached to the chart and updated at the time of the patient's appointment. A new color-coded tag is then attached to the card and filed in the index system. The advantage of this system is that the cards are available with information on them about prior appointments. Disadvantages are the time it takes to complete a card for each patient and the possibility of the tag falling off.

Regardless of which system is used, the goal is to make sure that every patient in the dental office is either under regular treatment or on a recall system.

Dental Records Management

Accurate dental records management is essential for quality patient care at any dental office. It is also necessary because of the legal issues that every dental office must face today. The records must be filled out completely, reflecting all pertinent information.

Equipment and Supplies for Record Management

The dentist decides on the type of file folder to use in the office, normally after consulting with the front office and clinical staff. File folders are designed in many different ways to meet office needs. They should provide easy accessibility and yet enclose the information and protect it during storage. A patient folder may be like an envelope or have a book-type opening. The envelope folder may have preprinted data on the outside and all the information sheets, x-rays, and so on placed inside. The book type normally keeps the patient information in constant order. The book type is normally more costly because it requires added pockets and fasteners to hold the information sheets secure.

File cabinets are also available in several primary types, such as vertical, open-shelf lateral, and movable. The vertical file cabinet is widely used in home filing (Figure 40-12A). The files are retrieved by lifting the appropriate file upward and outward. Open-shelf file cabinets seem to

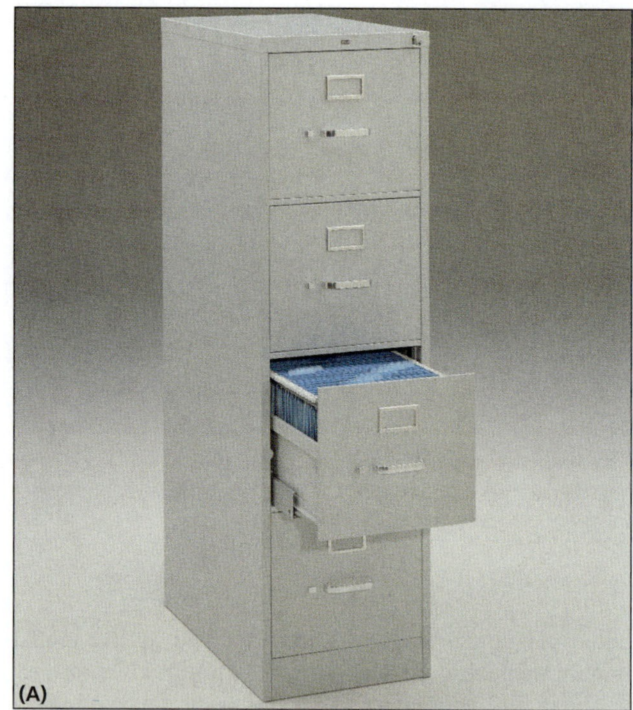

(A)

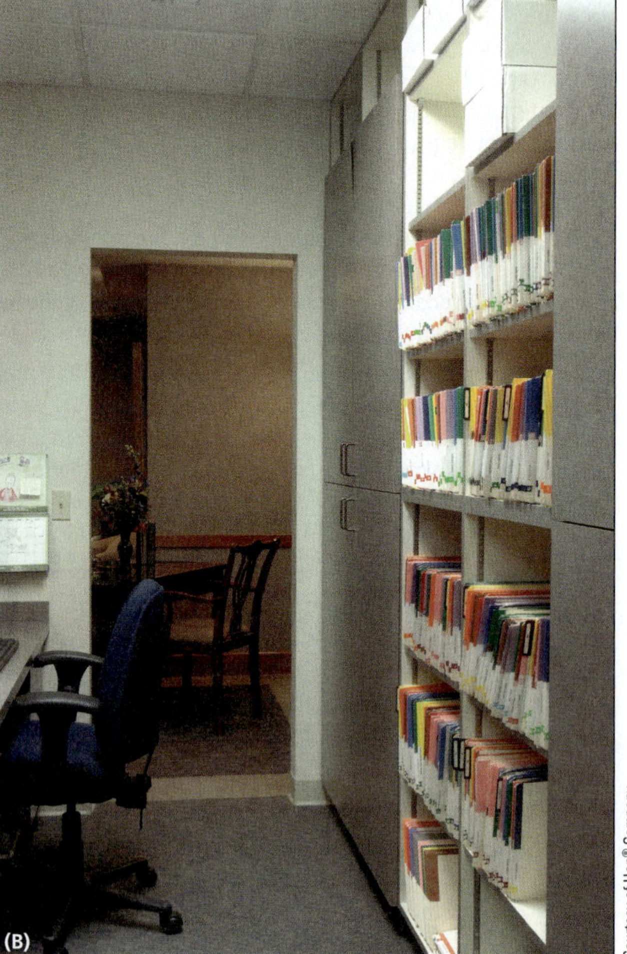

(B)

Courtesy of Hon® Company

FIGURE 40-12
(A) Vertical file cabinet. (B) Open-shelf lateral file cabinet.

FIGURE 40-13

Color-coded patient files. Yellow file selected for "Carl"; "F" side tab selected for "Friend."

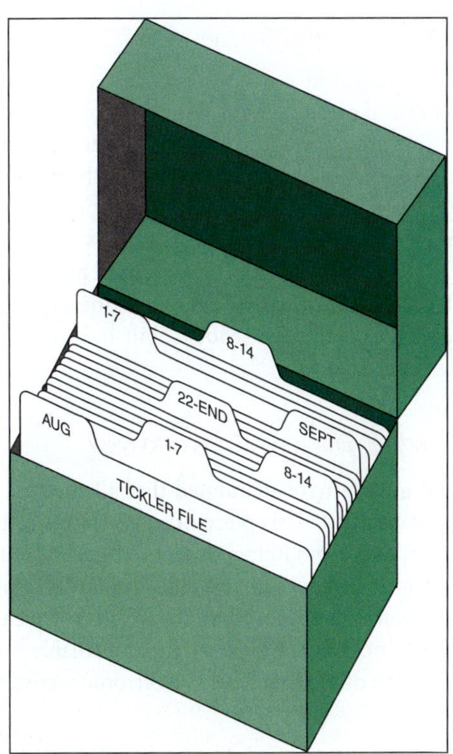

FIGURE 40-14

Tickler file for daily review and follow-up actions in patient management.

be the most widely used in the dental office, normally with a color-coding system that allows for easy chart identification (Figure 40-12B). The records from the open-shelf lateral files are retrieved by pulling them out laterally from the shelf. Some large offices may have movable file units that are powered electrically or physically by easy handles. Patient names are typed on the labels and attached to the file for quick identification.

Patient Chart Filing

Most filing systems used are organized alphabetically. These systems index the individual names. The patient name is divided into three units: the last name, first name, and middle name or initial. File all the charts according to the last name; if two patients have the same last name, such as Smith, then file by the first names. For example, if the office has a John Smith and a Jim Smith, Jim is filed before John in the file cabinet. Occasionally, two patients with the same first and last name become patients. Use their middle names or initials to file properly. Alphabetical filing requires accuracy during the removal and replacement of the chart. These tasks must be done correctly, or a lot of time can be wasted trying to find a chart.

Most dental offices use some form of color coding in regards to their patient filing (Figure 40-13). The file folder may be color coded so that all the patients with a last name beginning in A or S have yellow charts, and all the patients with B or T have blue charts. Other charts may have colored tabs that are placed on either plain or colored charts to make the filing and retrieval of files more efficient. The larger the practice, the more tabs are required to break down the charts into smaller groupings. This makes filing easier and reduces the number of errors and lost charts that may occur, because any visible color differences are quickly identified. Color coding by adding date stickers helps clinical assistants and front office assistants track active and inactive accounts.

Tickler File. A well-organized office has a **tickler file** that serves as a reminder of any action that needs to be taken in the future. Most offices use sticky notes (reminder notes that have adhesive strips on one side) to remind office personnel of things that need to be taken care of immediately. A tickler file normally uses index cards in an index box marked with approximate dates in which certain tasks should be completed (Figure 40-14). Many computer software programs have tickler files available so that information can be stored and retrieved when necessary.

Record Confidentiality

The patient has the right to confidential treatment and records (see Chapter 3, Ethics, Jurisprudence, and the Health Information Portability and Accountability Act). The patient chart contains private information that must be kept confidential. With the usage of computers and fax machines, great care must be used when placing anything where others can see it. Place computer monitors out of the view of other patients. When sending a fax, attach a cover sheet that advises the receiver of the confidential nature of the material, and make sure that the fax machine that is receiving the material is located in an area where only the appropriate individuals can access it.

Archival Storage

Dentists are required to keep records for the entirety of their careers and often beyond. This can create storage concerns for the practice when there are older paper charts. The contents of older paper charts can be scanned and stored electronically in an archive file. Computer systems allow a practice to archive charts of patients that move from the area or die. Even though the patient's chart is archived, the electronic record is still available quickly and easily within inactive or archive records, but it is not cluttering the active records.

Electronic Record Keeping

The federal government mandated that all medical records be electronic by 2014. This piece of legislation is called "The American Recovery and Reinvestment Act of 2009," or ARRA. While this legislation does not specifically require dental practices to have electronic records, dental practices have used this date as a goal. Incentives have been made available to ease the financial burden of moving toward electronic record keeping.

Paperless Dental Practice

With current dental software, it is possible for a dental practice to be paperless. This is the goal of the electronic records mandate: to eliminate physical patient charts that must be stored and retrieved. The advantages are that patient information can be accessed by the dentist from multiple locations, and dental office staff never has to search for a chart, saving time and improving efficiency. The disadvantage is that if there is a computer problem it affects everything.

A paperless (computerized) patient chart should contain a health history completed online or scanned into the computer, all the patient's information including insurance information, a clinical chart with radiographs, treatment notes, and dental charting. Any letters or additional information can be scanned and linked from the treatment or administrative notes. Things like insurance claim forms are already part of the patient computer ledger and can be viewed without printing. Basically, everything is available with a few clicks on a keyboard from anywhere.

The process of converting from paper to paperless charts can seem overwhelming at first, but the convenience of accessible legible patient records soon outweighs the problems.

Daily Schedule

The daily schedule is developed directly from the information in the appointment book for that day (Figure 40-15). It shows the time that each patient is scheduled and the treatment that is to be provided. Normally, several daily schedules are generated so that one can be placed in each treatment room and one in the sterilization area. These schedules must be placed out of patient view. The schedule allows the clinical staff to plan ahead and set up for the upcoming patients. Any changes throughout the day are changed on each printed copy of the schedule. If computer monitors are used in the treatment area, the daily schedule can be viewed or changed from there as well as the front desk.

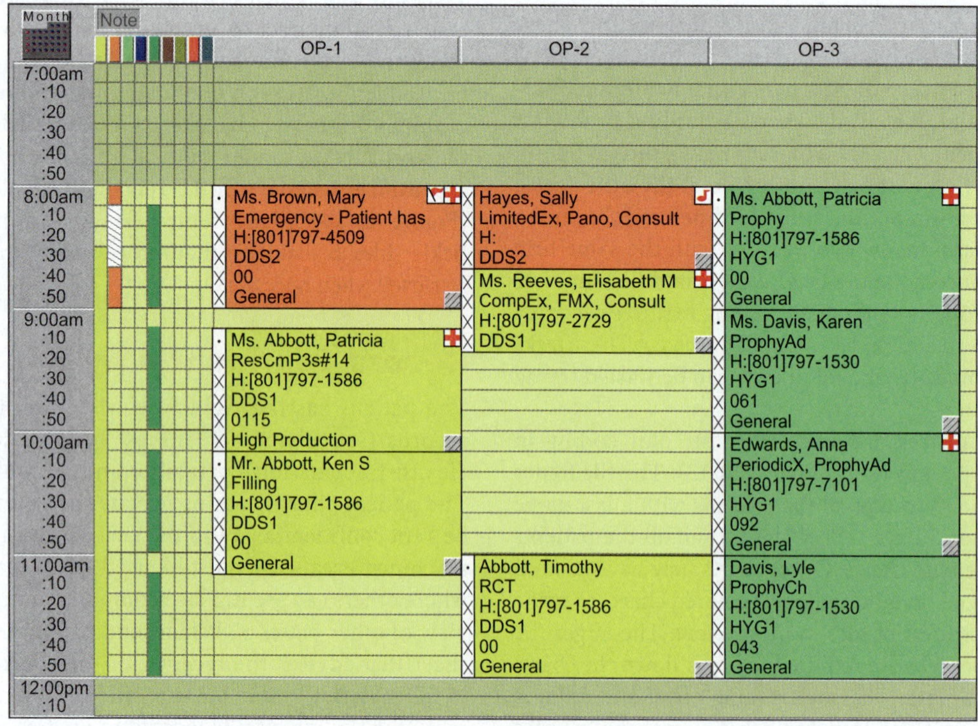

FIGURE 40-15

A computer-generated daily patient schedule.

Procedure 40-1
Preparing for the Day's Appointments

Preparing for the upcoming day is important to ensure that optimal care is provided to patients in a calm efficient environment.

Equipment and Supplies

- Patient charts
- Phone or automated confirmation system
- Word processor—if schedule is in an appointment book
- Computer and printer—if the schedule is computerized

Procedure Steps

Day Before Appointment:

1. Patient charts are pulled, if necessary.
2. Laboratory work is checked to ensure it is ready.
3. Records are reviewed for any special concerns.
4. Patient account balances are reviewed.
5. Any health concerns are identified.
6. Daily schedule is created.
7. Patient appointments are confirmed.
8. Schedules are given to the dental team.

Day of the Appointment:

1. Office staff meets in the morning to review the daily schedule. This brief meeting allows staff to discuss any patient concerns and create a plan to make the day run smoothly.
2. The clinical team is provided with patient information or a chart.
3. Patients are greeted and seated in the treatment rooms.
4. After treatment is completed the patient is escorted back to the front desk.

Patient Account Management

Patient accounts can be managed through either a computerized bookkeeping system or a manual system, such as the pegboard system. Most dental offices have converted from a manual bookkeeping system to a computerized system because it offers great versatility and the ability to quickly analyze the finances of the practice.

Pegboard System of Account Management

Since so few offices use a pegboard system anymore the focus of the chapter will be on computerized account management. Because the pegboard systems were an important part of dental practices in the past, and a few offices may still use them, a brief description seems appropriate.

The pegboard system is designed as a "write it once" system that uses no-carbon-required paper, permitting the user to enter the data only once. The system consists of day sheets, charge slips, ledger cards, and receipt forms. The forms are designed to work together and are aligned on a pegboard with matching columns. The system is relatively inexpensive. Each patient has a ledger card with this system, and the charges to that ledger are duplicated onto the day sheet. At the end of the day, the day sheet is balanced. When the accounts are balanced for the day the ledger cards are placed in a fireproof safe as a "back up" system. At the end of the month, ledger cards with balances are copied and sent out as statements. Changing from the manual pegboard system is initially time consuming until all the data are entered into the computer.

Computerized Account Management Systems

Most dental offices use computerized account management systems. They are much quicker and allow offices to gather information more rapidly. Computerized patient ledgers contain information about each patient, including name, address, telephone number, insurance coverage, and the person responsible for the account (Figure 40-16). This ledger also lists office visits, the services provided, and procedure codes. Dental software is very user friendly and, with some practice, managing financial accounts is easy. Many software programs use icons (small pictures) to direct the user to the exact function needed.

Accounts Receivable

The primary concern of the dental office is patient care, but without sound financial management, the office will not thrive and the patients will ultimately suffer. With the high cost of materials and equipment, profit management is critical. The accounts receivable of the dental office encompasses the money owed to the practice. The bookkeeping in this area must be accurate, and carries with it a great responsibility. This position may be occupied by the front office assistant or the dental

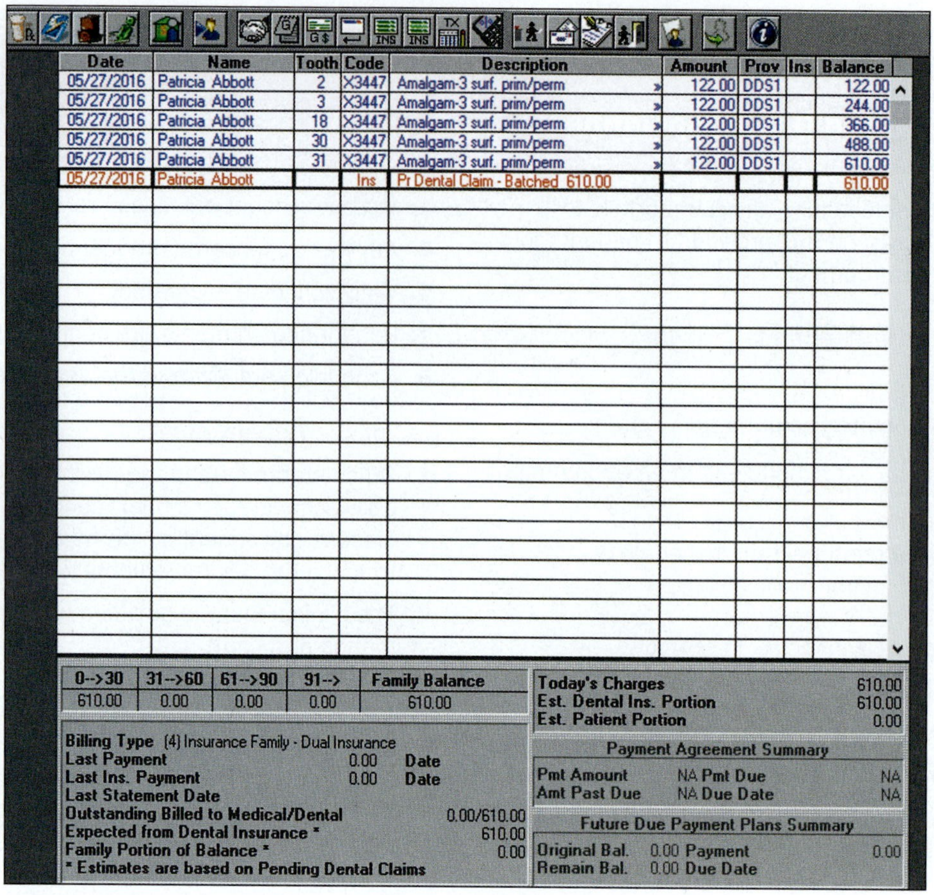

Date	Name	Tooth	Code	Description	Amount	Prov	Ins	Balance
05/27/2016	Patricia Abbott	2	X3447	Amalgam-3 surf. prim/perm	122.00	DDS1		122.00
05/27/2016	Patricia Abbott	3	X3447	Amalgam-3 surf. prim/perm	122.00	DDS1		244.00
05/27/2016	Patricia Abbott	18	X3447	Amalgam-3 surf. prim/perm	122.00	DDS1		366.00
05/27/2016	Patricia Abbott	30	X3447	Amalgam-3 surf. prim/perm	122.00	DDS1		488.00
05/27/2016	Patricia Abbott	31	X3447	Amalgam-3 surf. prim/perm	122.00	DDS1		610.00
05/27/2016	Patricia Abbott		Ins	Pr Dental Claim - Batched 610.00				610.00

0-->30	31-->60	61-->90	91-->	Family Balance
610.00	0.00	0.00	0.00	610.00

Billing Type (4) Insurance Family - Dual Insurance
Last Payment 0.00 Date
Last Ins. Payment 0.00 Date
Last Statement Date
Outstanding Billed to Medical/Dental 0.00/610.00
Expected from Dental Insurance * 610.00
Family Portion of Balance * 0.00
* Estimates are based on Pending Dental Claims

Today's Charges 610.00
Est. Dental Ins. Portion 610.00
Est. Patient Portion 0.00

Payment Agreement Summary
Pmt Amount NA Pmt Due NA
Amt Past Due NA Due Date NA

Future Due Payment Plans Summary
Original Bal. 0.00 Payment 0.00
Remain Bal. 0.00 Due Date

FIGURE 40-16

Computer patient ledgers provide a summary of all fees, payments, and insurance.

office manager. Like the information on the patient's records, the financial information must remain confidential. All transactions, payments, adjustments, and charges must be handled in a safe and professional manner. Any employee engaging in unlawful activities may be prosecuted under the law and required to repay the employer for any theft. Insurance fraud also brings with it prosecution and possible imprisonment.

Patient Fees

In the dental office, a fee schedule is used to define what patients are charged for each service. It is referred to as the **usual, customary, and reasonable (UCR) fee**. The usual fee refers to the fee that is typically charged by the dentist for a specific procedure. The customary fee is the average fee up to the 90th percentile that the dentists in the area charge for the same procedure. The reasonable fee is the midrange of fees charged for the same procedure. If a procedure is a difficult case, then the usual fee may be raised to reflect the difficulty of the case. However, if a dentist feels that he or she would like to charge a greater amount for a service, insurance companies will not pay above the usual, customary, and reasonable fee schedule. Therefore, the patient will be billed for the overage unless the dentist is contracted with the insurance company and has agreed to accept their payment as payment in full. Patients may question the additional charge and become upset with the practice if this has not been discussed previously in the treatment plan or at the consultation appointment. Most dentists stay within the fee range. The UCR fee schedule is reviewed annually and adjusted as necessary.

Dentists have the right to adjust fees by means of a **professional courtesy**. This professional courtesy, a discounted amount, may be offered to other dentists for dental work or to employees, family, and friends. The dentist has the discretion to make any adjustments desired. Another area in which dentists may make adjustments is with insurance. Dentists who accept assignments in specific programs agree to accept a payment in full by the insurance company. For instance, if a patient is covered on a program, and the dentist does a restoration for this patient at a fee of $75, but the insurance company only pays $55 for this particular service, the dentist has to adjust, or "waive," the remaining $20 of the fee; and the patient will not be responsible for it. This can only be done if the insurance company pays a flat fee. If the insurance company pays a percentage of a fee and a discount is given, it must be given to the insurance company too. For example, if an insurance company pays 80 percent for a restoration, the dentist should not take the 80 percent and then adjust, or "write-off" the 20 percent balance. Dental team members must be aware that the practice cannot survive if constant adjustments to the fees are made. Production must be balanced by other cases that meet the regular fee schedule to maintain a viable practice.

Posting Patient Fees

Each time the patient is in the office, information about the treatment received by the patient is entered into the computer system using CDT (current dental terminology) codes. Most computer programs have the UCR fees for the practice preprogrammed into the system. Once the CDT code is entered, the fee automatically appears. Of course, the system can be overridden and a custom fee added if necessary. This auto-fee generation eliminates errors and having to look up fees. The computer automatically updates the ledger, posts the charges, and calculates the patient's balance and the practice's accounts receivable balance. As the treatment fee is being posted, it can be assigned to any provider in a multi-provider practice. Discounts the patient might receive can also be given, and notes can be added regarding the treatment.

After the fee is posted and added to the ledger, the computer can automatically create an insurance claim form for patients with insurance. The claim form contains the patient and insurance information, and uses the CDT code so that the insurance company recognizes the procedure.

Posting Patient Payments

Ideally, every patient should pay for the dental treatment that he or she receives the day of service, either in full or the estimated portion that is their responsibility after insurance. Every time a patient makes a payment, or an insurance company makes a payment on behalf of a patient, it must be entered into the ledger. This is done by adding a payment. Once you access the payment screen, either by selecting it by name or by its icon, it is as simple as filling in the blanks. It is important to designate how the payment was made so at the end of the day you can balance your accounts. If a patient makes a payment with a credit card then this option is selected. If the payment was by check, then the assistant enters the check number as well as the amount. Cash payments are designated as cash. If payment is from an insurance company, it will be either by check, or by an electronic transfer of funds, and the option of payment by an insurance company must be specified.

Cash Payments. Few patients pay for their dental treatment in cash. However, it is important to keep enough cash in the office to make change if the need arises. Some dental offices offer a discount to patients who pay cash in advance (checks included) for the entire treatment the patient is to receive. If a patient pays in cash, it is important to give a written receipt showing the payment on the account. This can be done easily by printing a walkout statement.

Check Payments. The majority of patients pay for their dental services with personal checks. Some offices require that the patient use a driver's license number on the check and/or another form of identification for the check. Some regular patients may take offense to this requirement, so be sure to identify how the dentist would like to handle this.

Other checks that may be received in the dental office are cashier's checks. A cashier's check is guaranteed by the bank for the amount in which it is written. It is actually the bank's own check that the patient has paid for. Traveler's checks may be used by out-of-town patients. They are safer than cash for the user. They are written in specific denominations ($20, $50, and so on) and require a signature from the user that matches the one on the check at the time of use. A certified check could be used by a patient as well. A certified check is one that the bank has verified as good for the amount indicated.

Credit Cards. Patients may use credit cards to pay for services. The office takes the card and uses a card reader to enter the amount, and swipes the card or inserts a chipped card. The patient signs electronically or on a print out of the transaction. The payment is entered into the computer as a credit card payment and the patient is given a receipt.

With practice, the front office assistant can accomplish these tasks quickly and accurately. After posting a fee that the patient owes or a payment that the patient has made, the patient account can be viewed on the computer monitor or printed out if the patient desires a copy. This copy is often called a walkout statement (Figure 40-17).

Bank Deposits

Patient and insurance payments are deposited into the bank daily. The cash is noted separately and all the checks are endorsed with the office endorsement stamp, which indicates the specific bank that is utilized. Most offices have restrictive endorsement stamps that state "for deposit only." This protects the office if the check is stolen or lost. A deposit slip with the date, practice name, account number, listed currency and checks, and the total amount of the deposit identified on it is written for each deposit. Most computer software can automatically generate a deposit slip based on the day's entries. The front office assistant must make sure the deposit slip is generated and the cash, checks, and credit card receipts match before making the deposit.

Monthly Billing

Sending monthly billing statements is expensive and time consuming, so, ideally, patients pay at the time of services in order to avoid having to print and mail statements; but sometimes, statements do need to be sent.

The computer generates monthly statements from the ledger in the database with an age analysis of the balance. Many offices include return envelopes to aid the patient in sending a payment. Reviewing the statements before sending them is a good idea so that statements for very small amounts are not sent. If your cost of sending a statement is $3, sending out a statement asking for a payment of $1 would be inefficient. Keep in mind, the patient did receive a walkout statement when he or she left the office. If a patient has insurance, often those accounts are not sent statements until the insurance has paid and any remaining balance is actually owed by the patient. A good rule is to send out statements only when necessary and not for informational purposes.

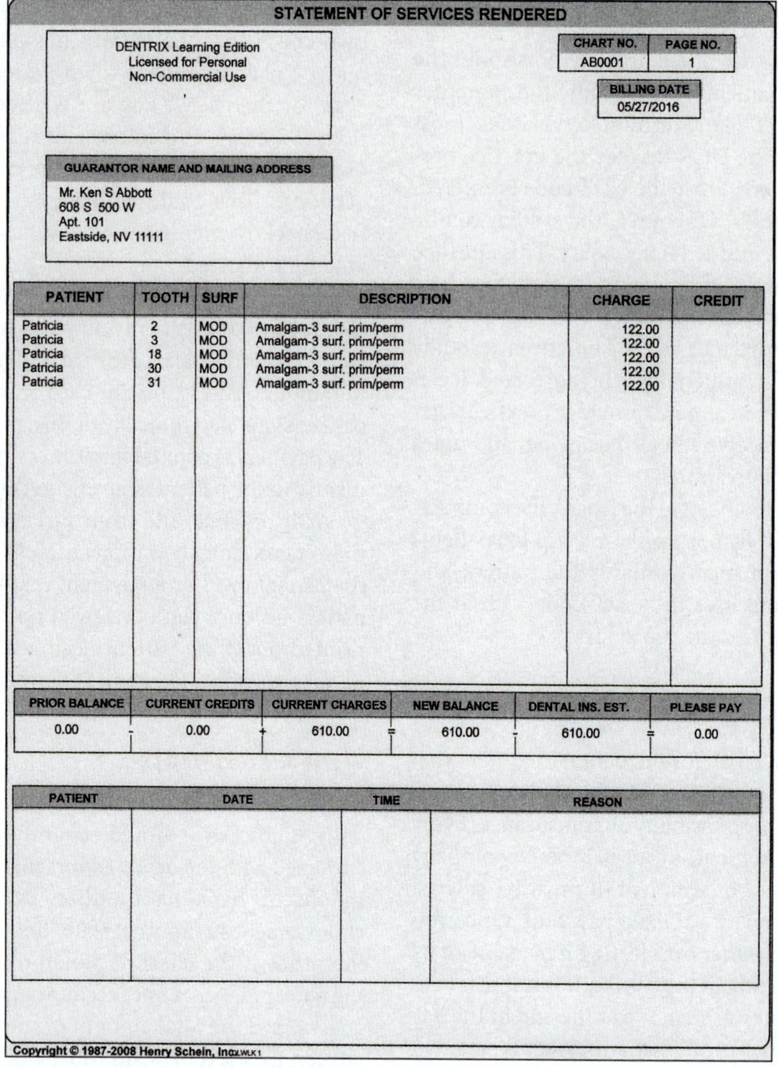
STATEMENT OF SERVICES RENDERED

DENTRIX Learning Edition
Licensed for Personal
Non-Commercial Use

CHART NO.	PAGE NO.
AB0001	1

BILLING DATE
05/27/2016

GUARANTOR NAME AND MAILING ADDRESS

Mr. Ken S Abbott
608 S 500 W
Apt. 101
Eastside, NV 11111

PATIENT	TOOTH	SURF	DESCRIPTION	CHARGE	CREDIT
Patricia	2	MOD	Amalgam-3 surf. prim/perm	122.00	
Patricia	3	MOD	Amalgam-3 surf. prim/perm	122.00	
Patricia	18	MOD	Amalgam-3 surf. prim/perm	122.00	
Patricia	30	MOD	Amalgam-3 surf. prim/perm	122.00	
Patricia	31	MOD	Amalgam-3 surf. prim/perm	122.00	

PRIOR BALANCE	CURRENT CREDITS	CURRENT CHARGES	NEW BALANCE	DENTAL INS. EST.	PLEASE PAY
0.00	- 0.00	+ 610.00	= 610.00	- 610.00	= 0.00

PATIENT	DATE	TIME	REASON

FIGURE 40-17
Patients should receive a walkout statement when they leave the office.

Procedure 40-2
Posting Patient Charges

The front office assistant performs this task during or at the end of the day.

Equipment and Supplies

- Access to the computer
- Confirmation of treatment done
- Current dental terminology (CDT) codes
- Financial agreement, if one was made
- Printer
- Appointment cards

Procedure Steps

1. The treatment fee is posted in the computer using CDT codes.
2. If there are discounts that the patient will be receiving, these can be deducted according to its category such as courtesy, or professional discounts. If multiple dentists are in the practice, make sure the production is credited to the correct dentist.
3. Using the financial agreement, the patient is asked to pay all or part of the treatment fee. Some practices collect this before treatment is started to avoid any surprises.

(continues)

Procedure 40-2 (continued)

4. Any new treatment plan is discussed.
5. Any new financial arrangements, if necessary, are agreed upon.
6. The next appointment is scheduled.
7. If the next appointment is a periodic recall, it is scheduled or added to a file so it isn't forgotten. Every patient should leave knowing when they should return and why!
8. The patient is given a walkout statement that includes charges, payments, insurance information, any outstanding balance, and when their next appointment is scheduled.
9. The patient is given an appointment slip or card.

Procedure 40-3
Balancing Day Sheets

The front office assistant balances the day sheets at the end of each day.

Equipment and Supplies

- Access to the computer
- Printer
- The day's schedule

Procedure Steps

End of Day

1. Choose "end of day" on the computer and the information you want to include on your day sheet. Computer software will allow you to view the information chronologically, alphabetically, or by provider.
2. Print out an end of day sheet following your software instructions. *Hint: Some dental office managers in practices that take in lots of payments, do a test close earlier in the day so that mistakes are discovered before they are ready to leave for the day.*
3. Total the payments you collected and make sure they equal the amount on the day sheet.
4. Prepare a deposit slip. *Directions are in Procedure 40-4.*
5. When your accounts balance, close the day and back up the computer. Once the day is closed, the next work date will automatically appear and you will no longer be able to make changes on the day you just closed.

Procedure 40-4
Preparing a Deposit Slip

The front office assistant creates the deposit slip, and either the front office assistant takes it to the bank or the dentist takes it to the bank to be deposited. Deposits are normally made in person or placed in a night deposit box.

Equipment and Supplies

- Deposit slip (Figure 40-18)
- Copy of the day's schedule
- Cash and checks received for that day
- Office stamp for endorsing the check
- Envelope in which to place the deposit slip, checks, and cash
- Access to a computer and printer

Procedure Steps

1. Place the date on the bank's deposit slip, or use the computer to print a deposit slip.
2. Separate the currency (coin and paper money) from the checks.

(continues)

Procedure 40-4 (continued)

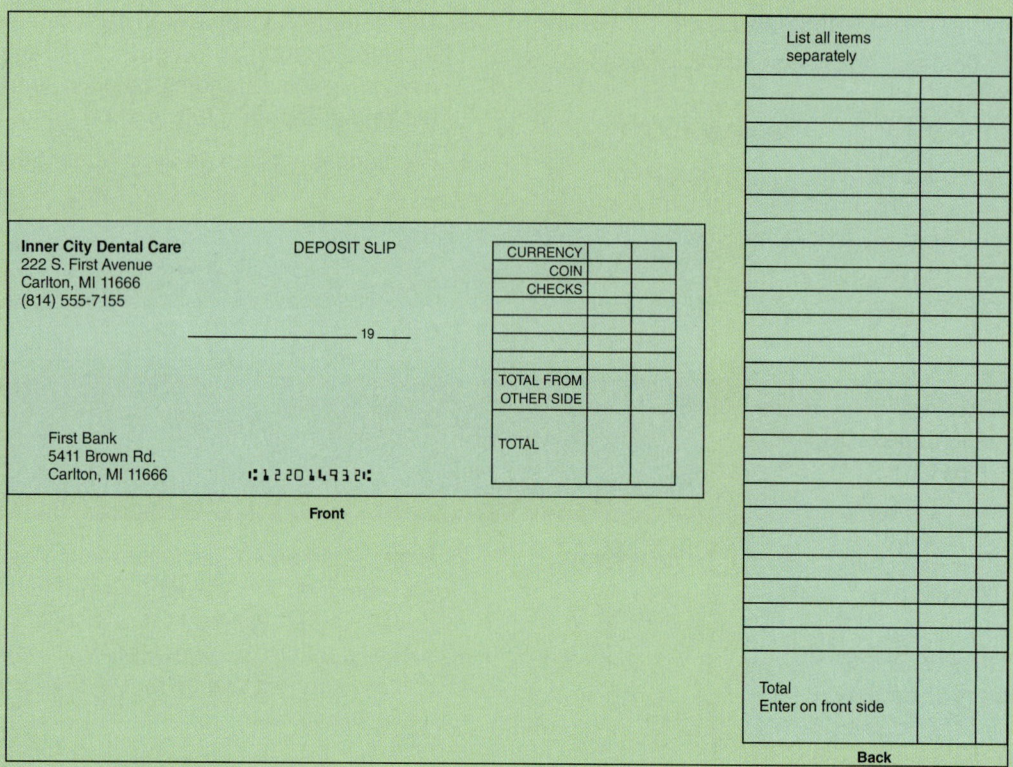

FIGURE 40-18
Sample deposit slip.

3. Tally the coins and place or confirm the total sum in the designated space on the deposit slip.
4. Tally the paper money and place or confirm the total sum in the designated space on the deposit slip.
5. On the back of the deposit slip, list each check separately, listing the patient's last name and the amount of the check in the space provided in the right-hand column. With a computerized system, if you have entered the information correctly throughout the day, the checks will be listed for you. Double-check for errors using the day's schedule.
6. Total the list amounts from the checks on the back of the deposit slip and place this sum in the area on the front of the deposit slip in the space identified as checks.
7. Total the currency (both coins and paper money) and the check amount, and place this sum at the bottom of the deposit slip under "Total." This amount should match the total identified on the payments column on the day sheet. One way to check that the total is accurate is to add up the coins, paper money, and each check. This verifies that the sum is correct.

Payment Plans. For more expensive dental treatment, offering several payment options after the treatment plan is discussed helps the practice remain healthy and productive. When treatment is diagnosed, the front desk assistant or dental office manager may set up financial arrangements. Often, an initial down payment is requested when treatment is done. The balance is then divided and this fixed amount is paid over an arranged time frame. For instance, a patient may have $1,000 worth of dentistry to complete. The office may request 20 percent as a down payment, with the additional $800 dollars being paid in $200 increments over the next 4 months. The patient signs the payment plan along with the dental office manager or dentist. If payments extend over 4 months, and finance charges are added to the unpaid balance, the patient must be notified in advance under the federal **Truth in Lending Act (TILA)**. This law, which is designed to protect consumers in credit transactions, requires that clear disclosure of contract terms and any associated costs be given to the consumer. The dental office should use a truth-in-lending form, which can be custom designed from a computer-generated template, to notify the consumer of financial arrangements The patient is given one copy of the payment plan and the original is kept in the patient's record. This information may also be noted on the ledger to remind the patient of the arrangements when the statement is sent out.

Loans. An additional payment option is a loan. These dental/medical loans are becoming very popular and often have no interest payments for 12–18 months if paid in full during that time period. Many dental offices provide this information to patients and assist them in completing the paperwork. Some patients may have their own loan sources and use a bank they work with already. To receive loans, patients must complete the appropriate paperwork. Some loan agencies can quickly verify that patients meet requirements; others need a day or two. In this system, the patient may pay additional loan fees, but payments can be established through loan agencies over an extended period of time.

Credit Reports. It may be necessary to obtain credit reports for patients who have large financial responsibilities for dental treatment. Essentially, the dental practice is loaning the patient the money to pay for this treatment. There are lab fees and overhead that must be paid, and the patient is requesting to be trusted to pay this at a later date. Consumer credit reporting agencies provide financial profiles on individuals, and verify whether they meet their obligations or are slow to meet their obligations through a rating system. The patient must be informed prior to requesting a credit report. The patient's Social Security number and birth date may be necessary to obtain the pertinent information. Any bankruptcies and lawsuits are identified on the credit report. After the report is received, the dentist or business assistant can determine whether the patient can pay in installments for dental treatment.

Financial Information

When a patient calls for an appointment, it is beneficial to gather all the information in regard to dental insurance. When the patient comes in, be sure to get a copy of his or her insurance card and have the patient complete and sign a consent to allow the office to release information to the insurance company and assign the benefit to your office. With this information, the front office assistant can gather information concerning the patient's dental coverage. Insurance coverage can have yearly limits and may have restrictions for specific services. By having knowledge about the most commonly used insurance plans, the business assistant can help patients with making decisions concerning dental treatment.

Dental Insurance

Dental insurance represents a large portion of accounts receivable in most dental practices. While the computer system automatically creates the claim form, the accuracy of the claim depends on the information entered into the computer system (Figure 40-19). Dental insurance seldom covers the entire fee, and the patient is responsible for the balance.

Dental Insurance Terms

Assignment of benefits—the patient assigns benefits to be paid directly to the dentist or the provider.

Beneficiary—the patient who is entitled to dental insurance benefits.

Benefit-less-benefit—refers to nonduplication of benefits pertinent to subscribers of more than one plan. Such plans allow reimbursement to be limited to the higher level allowed of the two plans.

Birthday rule—refers to cases when both parents have coverage for a child patient: the primary carrier is held by the parent whose birthday month and day (not year) comes earliest in the calendar year.

Carrier—usually the dental insurance company.

Coordination of benefits (COB)—refers to provisions made by two carriers to coordinate (share) benefits between them, which are not to exceed 100 percent of the dental charges for an eligible subscriber.

Coverage—benefits available to the person covered by dental insurance.

CDT codes—codes that are published in the Current Dental Terminology under the ADA's jurisdiction.

Deductible—the amount paid before benefits take effect.

Dependents—children covered under dental insurance.

Dual coverage—two dental coverages; the primary is in first position and the balance is normally paid by the secondary insurance.

Eligibility—determining if a patient is eligible for dental benefits.

Exclusions—items that dental insurance does not cover.

Explanation of benefits (EOB)—a detailed description showing the payment or denial of an insurance claim.

Fee for service—a payment to providers on a service-by-service, rather than a salaried or capitated, basis.

Group plan—a plan in which several individuals are covered.

Individual plan—a plan in which an individual has a plan without a group of individuals.

Patient—a person receiving treatment.

Predetermination of benefits—submitting the treatment plan to the carrier to determine what the insurance will pay on the dental services; this is often called the pretreatment estimate (estimate completed before treatment).

Premium—the amount the carrier charges the subscriber.

Primary insurance—the insurance of the subscriber.

Provider—the dentist who performs the dental service.

Reimbursement—a payment made by the carrier to the patient, or the dentist on behalf of the beneficiary, toward the dental fee incurred.

Secondary insurance—the insurance of the subscriber's spouse.

Subscriber—an individual with dental insurance.

Dental Claim Form © American Dental Association, 2006

HEADER INFORMATION

1. Type of Transaction (Mark all applicable boxes)

[X] Statement of Actual Services [ ] Request for Predetermination/Preauthorization

[ ] EPSDT/Title XIX

2. Predetermination/Preauthorization Number

INSURANCE COMPANY/DENTAL BENEFIT PLAN INFORMATION

3. Company/Plan Name, Address, City, State, Zip Code

Aetna
PO Box 706
Windsor CT 06095-2222

OTHER COVERAGE

4. Other Dental or Medical Coverage? [ ] No (Skip 5-11) [X] Yes (Complete 5-11)

5. Name of Policyholder/Subscriber in #4 (Last, First, Middle Initial, Suffix)
Abbott, Ken S

6. Date of Birth (MM/DD/CCYY) 03/02/1973 | 7. Gender [X] M [ ] F | 8. Policyholder/Subscriber ID (SSN or ID#) 000-00-0001

9. Plan/Group Number 21440 | 10. Patient's Relationship to Person Named in #5 [ ] Self [X] Spouse [ ] Dependent [ ] Other

11. Other Insurance Company/Dental Benefit Plan Name, Address, City, State, Zip Code

Blue Cross Blue Shield
5575 Tech Center Drive, Suite 320
Colorado Springs CO 809195555

POLICYHOLDER/SUBSCRIBER INFORMATION (For Insurance Company Named in #3)

12. Policyholder/Subscriber Name (Last, First, Middle Initial, Suffix), Address, City, State, Zip Code

Abbott, Patricia
608 S 500 W
Apt. 101
Eastside NV 11111

13. Date of Birth (MM/DD/CCYY) 09/28/1974 | 14. Gender [ ] M [X] F | 15. Policyholder/Subscriber ID (SSN or ID#) 000-00-0002

16. Plan/Group Number 01278 | 17. Employer Name JC Penny - Active

PATIENT INFORMATION

18. Relationship to Policyholder/Subscriber in #12 Above [X] Self [ ] Spouse [ ] Dependent Child [ ] Other | 19. Student Status [ ] FTS [ ] PTS

20. Name (Last, First, Middle Initial, Suffix), Address, City, State, Zip Code

21. Date of Birth (MM/DD/CCYY) | 22. Gender [ ] M [ ] F | 23. Patient ID/Account # (Assigned by Dentist)

RECORD OF SERVICES PROVIDED

	24. Procedure Date (MM/DD/CCYY)	25. Area of Oral Cavity	26. Tooth System	27. Tooth Number(s) or Letter(s)	28. Tooth Surface	29. Procedure Code	30. Description	31. Fee
1	05/27/2016		JP	2	MOD	X3447	Amalgam-3 surf. prim/perm	122 00
2	05/27/2016		JP	3	MOD	X3447	Amalgam-3 surf. prim/perm	122 00
3	05/27/2016		JP	18	MOD	X3447	Amalgam-3 surf. prim/perm	122 00
4	05/27/2016		JP	30	MOD	X3447	Amalgam-3 surf. prim/perm	122 00
5	05/27/2016		JP	31	MOD	X3447	Amalgam-3 surf. prim/perm	122 00
6								
7								
8								
9								
10								

MISSING TEETH INFORMATION

34. (Place an 'X' on each missing tooth)

Permanent: 1 2 3 4 5 6 7 8 9 10 11 12 13 14 15 16 / 32 31 30 29 28 27 26 25 24 23 22 21 20 19 18 17

Primary: A B C D E F G H I J / T S R Q P O N M L K

32. Other Fee(s)

33. Total Fee 610 00

35. Remarks

AUTHORIZATIONS

36. I have been informed of the treatment plan and associated fees. I agree to be responsible for all charges for dental services and materials not paid by my dental benefit plan, unless prohibited by law, or the treating dentist or dental practice has a contractual agreement with my plan prohibiting all or a portion of such charges. To the extent permitted by law, I consent to your use and disclosure of my protected health information to carry out payment activities in connection with this claim.

X SIGNATURE ON FILE 05/27/2016
Patient/Guardian signature Date

37. I hereby authorize and direct payment of the dental benefits otherwise payable to me, directly to the below named dentist or dental entity.

X SIGNATURE ON FILE 05/27/2016
Subscriber signature Date

ANCILLARY CLAIM/TREATMENT INFORMATION

38. Place of Treatment [X] Provider's Office [ ] Hospital [ ] ECF [ ] Other

39. Number of Enclosures (00 to 99) Radiograph(s) 00 Oral Image(s) 00 Model(s) 00

40. Is Treatment for Orthodontics? [X] No (Skip 41-42) [ ] Yes (Complete 41-42)

41. Date Appliance Placed (MM/DD/CCYY)

42. Months of Treatment Remaining | 43. Replacement of Prosthesis? [X] No [ ] Yes (Complete 44) | 44. Date Prior Placement (MM/DD/CCYY)

45. Treatment Resulting from [ ] Occupational illness/injury [ ] Auto accident [ ] Other accident

46. Date of Accident (MM/DD/CCYY) | 47. Auto Accident State

BILLING DENTIST OR DENTAL ENTITY (Leave blank if dentist or dental entity is not submitting claim on behalf of the patient or insured/subscriber)

48. Name, Address, City, State, Zip Code

Dennis Smith D.D.S.
DDS1_727 E Utah Valley Drive
Suite #500
American Fork UT 84003

49. NPI DDS1_NPI | 50. License Number DDS1_StateID | 51. SSN or TIN DDS1_TIN

52. Phone Number (801) 555 – 4121 | 52A. Additional Provider ID DDS1_Provider

TREATING DENTIST AND TREATMENT LOCATION INFORMATION

53. I hearby certify that the procedures as indicated by date are in progress (for procedures that require multiple visits) or have been completed.

X 05/27/2016
Signed (Treating Dentist) Date

54. NPI DDS1_NPI | 55. License Number DDS1_StateID

56. Address, City, State, Zip Code | 56A. Provider Specialty Code 122300000X

DDS1_727 E Utah Valley Drive , Suite #500
American Fork UT 84003

57. Phone Number (801) 555– 4121 | 58. Additional Provider ID DDS1_Provider

FIGURE 40-19

Dental insurance assists patients in paying for their treatment.

The individual who has dental insurance through employment or an individual plan is referred to as the subscriber. The patient who is entitled to benefits under any dental plan is referred to as the beneficiary. Some patients have dental insurance through their employment for themselves, and have other coverage through their spouses. They would then be the subscribers for their primary insurance and the beneficiaries for the other dental insurance, or secondary insurance. This person is said to have dual coverage and may not have to pay for any additional expenses for dental treatment. If two coverages are used, the primary pays the normal fees and the secondary covers up to the amount owed. Together they pay the entire bill.

The **coordination of benefits (COB)** applies to patients eligible for benefits under two carriers, in which the primary carrier pays part of the allowed amount and the secondary carrier pays the balance. For instance, if allowed dental charges were \$500 and the primary paid \$350 of the fee, the secondary would only pay \$150, regardless of allowed benefits for the services rendered under the secondary policy. Together the two carriers pay 100 percent of the dental fee.

Other plans may specify nonduplication of benefits, known as benefit-less-benefit. This provision applies to subscribers eligible for benefits under more than one plan. Reimbursement is limited to the highest level allowed by either plan, not a combined total or limit of 100 percent of the dental charge. For instance, assume that the dental fee is \$500, the primary carrier allows \$200, and the secondary carrier allows \$300. In this instance, the secondary carrier would reimburse the dentist for \$300, and the patient would be responsible for \$200.

A person could also obtain insurance through an individual plan instead of a plan through an employer. A plan through an employer is normally a group plan, in which several individuals are covered. The larger the group in the plan, the better the benefit coverage and the more reasonable the premium or monthly costs. Individual plans are normally much more costly and often offer lesser benefits.

Children covered under dental insurance are referred to as dependents by the dental insurance carrier. Health care reform includes many new rules for medical insurance that may not apply separately to dental coverage. Dental is classified as an "excepted benefit" under the provisions of the Public Health Service Act, so the rules of exactly who is a dependent may vary. Many carriers have adjusted the benefit age for dependents to 26 to correspond with medical coverage. The carrier is the dental insurance company that pays the agreed benefits for the patient treatment. Patients who have benefits are normally provided information that states the coverage that the patients are eligible for. Exclusions, items the dental coverage does not cover, are noted in this information. The coverage is normally negotiated by the employer for their employees. Limitations for benefits may be noted in the information along with the coverage. For children who are eligible under both parents' insurance, benefit payout may be determined by the birthday rule. Under this rule, the carrier for the parent subscriber whose birthday (day and month) comes first in the calendar year is the primary. Many insurance plans have an identified deductible amount. This means that a specified amount is deducted from the benefit amount before any benefits are paid. For example, if the policy has a \$100 deductible each year, the individual must pay this amount before becoming eligible for payment of any benefits.

Some insurance plans have maximum amounts that can be paid out for the year. This means that no matter what the dental treatment is, the plan will not pay over a specified amount. So, if an insurance plan pays a maximum annual amount of \$2,000 per year and a patient has four crowns costing \$800 each (total cost = \$3,200), the insurance will only pay \$2,000 of the bill. The patient would be responsible for the remaining \$1,200 balance. So, for this patient, it would be beneficial to have two crowns completed each year for 2 years in order to utilize maximum benefits from the dental insurance.

If the dental coverage, or benefits available, is difficult to determine, send the planned treatment to the insurance company to get a predetermination of benefits. This predetermination is often referred to as a pretreatment estimate. The insurance carrier may request dental radiographs before the predetermination can be made. After receiving the predetermination, both the dentist and the patient will know the exact amount of benefits available toward the cost of the entire dental treatment.

Capitation Program

In a capitation program, the dentist or dentists contract with the program's administrator to provide subscribers all the services covered in the program for a payment on a per capita basis. The dentist receives a fixed fee for each patient in the program and is not paid for the services that are provided. The subscriber has a limited number of dentists from which to choose (only those contracted). This type of plan is used for health maintenance organizations (HMOs).

Contract Fee Schedule Plan

A contract fee schedule plan is a dental benefit plan in which participating dentists agree to accept the fees listed under the plan for the total fees. The government program, Medicaid, is a contract fee schedule plan. Dentists who accept Medicaid agree to accept the amounts paid by the carriers, and do not bill for the remaining amounts. Most contract fee schedule plans offer reduced payments.

Direct Reimbursement Plans

With a direct reimbursement plan, the patient pays the dental treatment fee and is reimbursed the agreed upon amount by the employer. An insurance carrier is uninvolved in this plan.

Preferred Provider Organizations

Under a preferred provider organization (PPO), the insurance company negotiates discounted rates for dental services with selected dentists. Many subscribers with a PPO use providers outside of the PPO, although financial incentives encourage patients to use preferred providers. Providers in the PPO benefit through increased patient volume and prompt payment. In return, providers agree to a fee schedule and, if requested, to have the practice reviewed.

Submitting Dental Insurance Claims

As a courtesy to patients, most dental offices submit insurance claims. The entire claim must be filled out. The computer software will use the information in the patient database, and the information the front office assistant has entered regarding insurance coverage to generate the claim form. The American

Dental Association developed a *Code on Dental Procedures and Nomenclature* to simplify the reporting of confidential information regarding the patient's dental treatment.

The current dental terminology (CDT) codes are published in the *Current Dental Terminology* under the ADA's jurisdiction. The codes are updated every 2 years—new codes are added and obsolete codes are deleted. CDT codes follow a five-digit system for identifying dental procedures and services. The first digit of the code is the letter D for dental, which distinguishes the codes from medical ones. The second digit designates the category of service (e.g., preventative is 1). The third digit designates the class of service in the category, the fourth the subclass of service, and the fifth is open for expansion. An example of a CDT code is D1110 for adult prophylaxis. The CDT code for a child's prophylaxis is D1120. Most computer applications have the codes programmed. The dental assistant identifies the service, and the code appears. As CDT codes change, software is updated. (See Chapter 3, Ethics, Jurisprudence, and the Health Information Portability and Accountability Act, for more information and a list of the CDT codes.)

The insurance claims are completed using an ADA claim form. The name and address of the carrier are noted on the form as well as the patient's name, address, date of birth, ID number (this is different than the patient's Social Security number), sex, and phone numbers. In addition, the employer, the relationship to the subscriber, the subscriber ID, and the group number are also noted on the form. Secondary insurance is also included on the form when applicable. The claim form also has two boxes for patients to sign. One of the boxes is for *release of information*. The release of information allows the dentist to release the patient's dental treatment information to the carrier (insurance company). Without this consent, the dentist cannot release this confidential information. The other box for the patient to sign is the assignment of benefits. Assignment of benefits authorizes the carrier to pay the dentist directly. If this box is unsigned, the check goes directly to the patient. When this box is unsigned, the office should arrange for payment of the entire dental treatment, because the office is not guaranteed to receive the insurance money. To facilitate electronic filing, dental offices use *signature on file*. This form is completed during patient registration and covers both the release of information and the assignment of benefits, if the patient has signed for both. When an office uses signature on file it is critical that the form is signed and is part of the patient's chart.

After the patient treatment is complete, the insurance is sent in for payment. The codes for service and their descriptions are completed, along with the fee and the date the service was performed. The form is submitted to the carrier via electronic claims processing. Dental software applications allow for the transmission of insurance claims online through the modem. The claims are transmitted either directly to the carrier, or to a national clearinghouse and then to the carrier.

The front office assistant is responsible for tracking insurance claims and making certain that payment is received. A copy of each submitted insurance claim is essential for tracking. It is essential to follow up on claims that are not paid promptly in order to identify the problem so that it can be corrected.

The benefit checks received from the carrier are accompanied by an explanation of benefits (EOB). The benefit check is posted to the bookkeeping system on the patient ledger with information explaining the services covered. The check is then deposited along with other checks and cash in the daily deposit.

Insurance Schedule of Benefits. Insurance companies may list their schedules of benefits, also known as the schedule or table of allowances. This is a list of specified amounts that the carrier will pay for the service. This schedule is not in any way related to the dentist's actual fees. The schedule of benefits also identifies the services that are covered under the plan. Some dental insurance policies will not pay for orthodontic benefits. They may provide reimbursement (the payment made by the carrier to the patient or the dentist on behalf of the patient) toward the dental fee incurred. This amount might only cover two surface restorations at an $80 fee, or a percentage of this established fee. The patient is responsible for the balance of uncovered fees. Medicaid, a government program, requires that the dentist accept the reduced amount as payment in full without being able to bill the patient for the balance. Participation in any managed care program is always the dentist's choice.

Collection Management

Collection on some accounts is necessary no matter how effective the billing process. The best front office assistant still has to collect from individuals who have past due accounts. There are individuals who have financial difficulties. Work with these patients so that they can continue paying small amounts on the accounts until they are in better financial states. There are also patients who are negligent in meeting their financial obligations. The longer the dental office puts off contacting these people, the less chance there is in receiving the delinquent amounts.

The dentist will give guidelines for patient collections. They must be handled carefully and tactfully. The best way to address this issue with a patient is in a manner that aids the patient in finding a way to pay the account balance. The **Fair Debt Collection Practices Act** makes it illegal to telephone a debtor at inconvenient hours. It also prevents collection calls from being made to the debtor's employer, except to verify employment. It prevents anyone seeking collection from obtaining information through false pretense or by threatening violence.

The telephone is the most effective way to contact the debtor. First, identify that the person is the individual who is responsible for the account, and then discuss the methods for resolving the problem. Always set a date when the payment can be expected. If it does not arrive as promised, then contact the responsible party immediately to let them know that the dental office is not letting the debt slide.

Collection Letters. If unable to reach the debtor by telephone, a collection letter is necessary. The letters are sent to encourage responsible parties to pay their overdue balances. Collection letters can be sent through regular mail (Figure 40-20). A final collection letter notifying the responsible party that the account will be turned over to a collection

Procedure 40-5
Filing Insurance Claims

The front office assistant will prepare, complete and send insurance claims for patients at the end of each appointment or at the completion of their treatment.

Equipment and Supplies

- Access to a computer
- Access to the internet
- Completed insurance claim forms

Procedure Steps

1. If you have made errors in charges, or failed to update patient and insurance information, update the information before sending insurance claims. Errors on claims delay payments.
2. Create insurance claims according to your software instructions. Commonly, this is done through the patient ledger and is done daily.
3. Before sending them electronically, they are batched into a group so that they all go together at the end of the day.
4. The last step is to send them electronically. Follow the specific directions for the software being used. You do not have to send each claim to each insurance company individually. The computer software allows you to send them as a group.
5. Confirmation that the claim was sent is automatically added to the patient ledger.
6. If, at a later date, you want to print the claim you can do so by selecting it from the ledger and clicking on print.

Tamara Riegel, D.D.S.
909 Central
Rockford, LA 20011

December 1, 20XX

Mr. John Cooper
41 Sandiford Drive
Locust, LA 22011

Dear Mr. Cooper:

Your account with our office is three months past due, and you have not responded to our previous requests for payment. Please pay your balance of $152 at this time, or contact us with an explanation of why you cannot pay.

Please call me at 555-7823 if you have a question about your account. Otherwise, we expect your payment immediately.

Sincerely,

Natalie Short
Accounts Manager

Tamara Riegel, D.D.S.
909 Central
Rockford, LA 20011

December 29, 20XX

Mr. John Cooper
41 Sandiford Drive
Locust, LA 22011

Dear Mr. Cooper:

Your son, Royce, had a seriously infected tooth in March when he came to Dr. Riegel for treatment. Dr. Riegel was pleased to use her experience and education to treat Royce, and it was in this same spirit of cooperation that we expected you to pay your account within a reasonable amount of time.

Four months have passed and you have still not remitted the $152 outstanding balance on your account. We cannot continue to keep your unpaid account on our books. If you are experiencing financial difficulties, please call the office so we can arrange a payment schedule that is agreeable to both of us.

Sincerely,

Natalie Short
Accounts Manager

Tamara Riegel, D.D.S.
909 Central
Rockford, LA 20011

February 1, 20XX

Mr. John Cooper
41 Sandiford Drive
Locust, LA 22011

Dear Mr. Cooper:

You have not replied to our previous notices regarding your unpaid balance of $152. Unless we hear from you personally within 14 days, your account will be given to the Rockford Medical and Dental Collection Service.

Do not wait any longer to contact me at 555-7823 if you wish to maintain your previous good credit record with Dr. Riegel. As previously suggested, we will cooperate in arranging a suitable payment schedule, if needed.

Sincerely,

Natalie Short
Accounts Manager

FIGURE 40-20

Collection letters sent to patients with delinquent accounts, drafted to encourage patients to pay their bills.

agency is often sent by certified mail. Any letters received via certified mail are signed by the people receiving them. This receipt is sent back to the sender to verify that the letter was received. The receipt should be kept in the patient's chart, along with a copy of the letter.

Occasionally, dental offices have to turn highly delinquent accounts over to an outside collection agency. The agency will normally charge one-third to one-half of the balance collected as its fee. All accounts that reach collection are reported to the credit bureau. After the money is collected, the fees are subtracted and the balance is sent to the office.

Special Collection Situations

- If the patient has declared bankruptcy, the dental office is notified. The dental office is no longer able to send statements or attempt to collect the amount owed. The patient's debt is written off as a loss for the dental office.
- If the patient has died, and his or her finances are tied up, a person is designated to execute the deceased individual's estate and oversee payment of outstanding bills. The statements should be addressed to the "Estate of" from that time forward until paid.
- Some patients may "skip" town and leave no forwarding addresses. The statement will be returned with "no forwarding address" on the unopened envelope. Verify that the address was correct. If it is, the office needs to decide whether to pursue the unpaid debt or turn it over to a collection agency.

Accounts Payable

The accounts payable are the amounts that the practice owes others, such as necessary expenses. The expenses that are required to run the dental practice are called **overhead**. The total accounts receivable is calculated as the **gross income**. Subtract the accounts payable from the gross income to identify the net income. The **net income** is the true profit the practice makes. The practice cannot remain vital if there is no net income for the dentist. It is not advisable to operate a business in an unprofitable manner for long.

Some of the expenses are *fixed* (remain the same) each month. These include the mortgage, full-time salaries, and some utilities. Other expenses are *variable*, meaning that they fluctuate and are dependent on the needs for the month. Variable overhead expenses include dental supplies, dental laboratory costs, and equipment repairs. The front office assistant, along with the dentist, can document the monthly overhead and evaluate whether costs can be cut without decreasing patient service. One of the highest monthly variable overhead costs is in the area of dental supplies.

Inventory Supply Systems

There are different types of supplies utilized in the dental office. Some of these supplies are disposable and used up quickly. They are referred to as **expendable**. Examples of expendable supplies are cotton rolls and stationery. Other supplies are retained in the office for long periods of time and are referred to as **nonexpendable** supplies, such as the autoclave and light-curing unit.

A number of things must be taken into account when developing an efficient inventory supply system. Products need to be looked at according to the following factors:

- Shelf life—length of time the product can be stored until it begins to deteriorate.
- Item price—cost of one item.
- Unit price—cost of a commonly grouped package of an item (for example, a dozen toothbrushes).
- Bulk price—reduced price for a minimum of units (for example, 12 dozen units of toothbrushes).
- Price break—the minimum quantity of a supply at which the per unit or per item cost is reduced.
- Lead time—the time between when an order is placed and the time it is received.
- Rate of use—how much of a product is used in a specific period (for example, 20 toothbrushes per week are given out to patients).
- Reorder point—the point refers to a point of time that items should be reordered to ensure that an adequate supply is available, taking into consideration the lead time and the rate of use for the product.

There are several inventory records systems that can be utilized in the dental office to keep track of supplies. The goal of any system is for supplies to be available when they are needed. Maintenance of an adequate supply of materials and supplies is essential. Placing the supplies in a central location makes it easier to manage and restock. In most offices, one person is assigned to oversee the inventory system. The system should be simple, easy to use, and accurate. The computer has made an inventory list system easier to maintain. The system can be further designed to meet the needs of the practice. Another system that is routinely used in dental offices is the tag system. The tag system makes use of a reorder tag that is attached to an item in the inventory and represents the reorder point for that particular supply. Tags can be attached with rubber bands. The information on the tag may include only the name of the item. Some dental supply companies come into dental offices and set up this system by placing the initial tags on the inventory.

When supplies get down to the tagged item, the tagged item is placed in an area to be ordered from the dental supply representative or mail-order supply company.

Mail-order supply companies require slight increases in lead time.

Another supply inventory system that has become more popular is the bar code system. This system allows dental assistants to use a bar code wand, which reads the bar code information and electronically transmits this data to the dental supplier to be ordered (Figure 40-21). This system cuts down on the time spent on ordering supplies for the dental assistant.

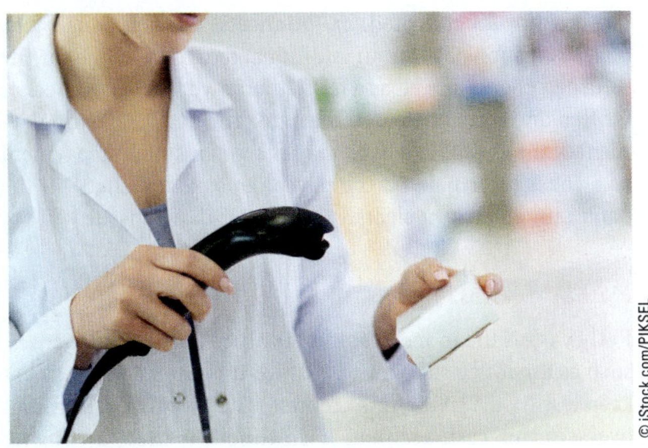

FIGURE 40-21
An electronic bar code ordering system.

Receiving Supplies. When the supplies are delivered, check them for damage. If there is damage, immediately notify the manufacturer or distributor. A packing slip listing everything that was shipped is enclosed with the supplies. Check the items received against the packing slip list; if there are any discrepancies, contact the manufacturer.

The packing slip does not have price information. This is sent separately on the *statement*, a monthly summary with all the supply charges listed.

If any items are returned for any reason to a supplier, a *credit slip* is issued. The credit slip assures the office that they will not be charged for the returned item. If the supplier cannot supply an item on the order, a *back order slip* is issued. This slip lists the items the supplier could not ship immediately, and gives an estimated date when the items will be available.

Storing Supplies. After supplies are received and checked, the dental assistant places them in the storage area. The supplies should be rotated so that the older supply items are used before the more recently purchased items. The older supplies are placed directly in the front, ready for use. Some of the supplies require special storage. For example, some of the dental medications and restorative materials require refrigeration, while others require dry, dark areas. Read the manufacturer's instructions for special storage concerns.

Procedure 40-6
Reordering Supplies

The front office assistant may be assigned specifically to order supplies, or this task may be shared by several dental assistants.

Equipment and Supplies

Red Flag Reorder Tag System

- Red flag reorder tags that have surfaced for reordering
- Telephone
- Index card with order information

Electronic Bar Code System

- Bar code wand
- Telephone
- Access to the computer

Procedure Steps

Red Flag Reorder Tag System

1. Gather the red flags indicating the items that require reordering.
2. Check the index card to obtain the ordering information for each item.
3. Place an indicator in the upper-right corner to indicate that this item is to be ordered immediately.
4. After the item is ordered, place the indicator in the upper-left corner until the product arrives.
5. When the item arrives, remove the indicator from the tag, place the most recently received items to the back of the supply (using the older materials first), and place the red flag ordering tag on the minimum quantity needed in stock before reordering must be accomplished again.

Electronic Bar Code System

1. Identify the items that require reordering. This system is used for commonly ordered items.
2. Obtain the book that has the product information and bar codes identified.
3. Use the bar code wand to input the items needed. Run the wand over the bar codes of the items needing to be ordered. Indicate on the transmitter the number of items needed. The order is then transmitted directly to the dental supply company for ordering.
4. Place a date on the listed items, and indicate the number that have been ordered on the forms provided with the electronic bar code system.

Account Payment

The accounts payable for a dental office are paid monthly or bimonthly by the dentist. The dentist reviews the accounts payable and approves payment, and then the front office assistant or dental office manager prepares the checks for the dentist to sign. All statements are checked for accuracy prior to being paid.

The checks, which are orders for the identified banks to pay the specific amounts indicated to the payee, should be dated. The name of the payee must be clearly indicated following the preprinted "Pay to the Order of." The amount of the payment must be entered in both figures and in words. It is advisable to complete the check stub information needed for tax purposes. The **check register** is a record of all the deposits and checks made from the account. It provides a running balance of the funds within the account.

Each month, the bank sends a statement showing any transactions that took place within the account during the month. It lists all checks that have cleared the bank, any deposits received by the bank, and any service charges that were deducted from the account. It should be reconciled against the entries made in the dental office check register (Procedure 40-7).

Nonsufficient Funds. If any check is written in excess of the amount in the account, it is returned to the payee and marked "NSF" for nonsufficient funds. The bank charges the account for returned, or "bounced," checks. Usually the payer is responsible for an additional fee to the office for the returned check, as well as a fee to their own bank. If a check is written and has not cleared the bank, the payer can stop payment of the check. The bank may charge for stopping payment of a check. Normally, if the payee deposits the check in the bank immediately, it clears within 1 to 3 days of issue.

Petty Cash

Petty cash is the money kept in the office for minor expenses, such as for coffee supplies or postage-due letters. Most offices keep less than $100 in this account. The front office assistant oversees this cash account. Each time it is used, a voucher or receipt is placed in the cash box until the money gets low. Then, the fund is replenished by writing another check to the cash fund, bringing it up to the original amount. The check is noted as petty cash and the receipts total the amount replenished to the account.

Payroll

The front office assistant or dental office manager may complete the employee payroll. Each employee fills out a W-4 form, or the Employee's Withholding Allowance Certificate, when he or she begins employment, which includes

Procedure 40-7
Reconciling a Bank Statement

The front office assistant or dental office manager reconciles the bank statement each month. This can be done manually or with the help of a computer, but, regardless of the method, the process remains the same.

Equipment and Supplies

- Bank statement (Figure 40-22)
- Checkbook
- Calculator
- Access to a computer

Procedure Steps

1. Make sure that all checks and deposits have been added to or subtracted from the checkbook.
2. Subtract any bank service charge from the last balance listed in the checkbook.
3. Check off each listed check in the bank statement against the checkbook and verify the amount listed.
4. Check off each deposit listed in the bank statement against the checkbook and verify the amount listed.
5. On the back of the bank statement, place the ending balance from the front of the statement in the ending balance space on the worksheet.
6. List all checks from the checkbook that have not cleared the bank in the section provided on the back worksheet.
7. List all deposits from the checkbook that have not been received by the bank on the space provided on the worksheet on the back of the statement.
8. Total the checks not cleared and the deposits not received. Subtract the checks not received from the ending balance on the bank statement, and add the deposits not received to the ending balance on the bank statement. This balance should agree with the checkbook balance. If there are any bank charges on the statement, make the corresponding adjustments to the checkbook balance.

(continues)

Procedure 40-7 (continued)

Summary of Account Balance — Closing Date 1/15/XX

Account # 1257-164013 — Ending Balance $8,347.62

Beginning Balance	$ 7,152.18
Total Deposits and Additions	$ 8,643.86
Total Withdrawals	$ 7,433.21
Service Charge	$ 15.24

Number	Date	Amount	Number	Date	Amount
201	12/18/XX	173.82	234	1/4/XX	96.31
223*	12/18/XX	44.12	235	1/4/XX	73.48
224	12/20/XX	586.00	236	1/6/XX	325.40
225	12/21/XX	24.15	237	1/7/XX	40.00
226	12/22/XX	33.90	238	1/8/XX	66.77
228*	12/23/XX	1250.00	241*	1/9/XX	15.55
229	12/24/XX	11.75	242	1/10/XX	12.45
230	12/24/XX	19.02	243	1/10/XX	4441.64
231	1/2/XX	43.80	244	1/10/XX	64.55
232	1/3/XX	39.00			
233	1/4/XX	71.50			

*Denotes gap in check sequence

Date	Deposit Amount	Date	Deposit Amount
18-Dec	361.75	4-Jan	825.00
19-Dec	586.00	5-Jan	1286.71
20-Dec	918.21	7-Jan	608.00
21-Dec	201.00	8-Jan	811.15
2-Jan	475.00	9-Jan	1092.68
3-Dec	1478.36		

(A) Front

1. Enter ending balance from the front of this statement
$ 8,347.62

2. Enter deposits not shown on this statement.
$ 3,162.50

3. Subtotal (add 1 and 2)
$ 11,510.12

4. List outstanding checks or other withdrawals here

Check #	Amount
222	37.89
227	161.15
239	11.50
240	92.12
245	835.17
246	21.75
247	586.00

5. Total outstanding checks.
$ 1,745.58

Balance (subtract 5 from 3)
$ 9,764.54
This should equal your checkbook balance

(B) Back

FIGURE 40-22
A sample bank statement.

Procedure 40-8
Writing a Business Check

The front office assistant or dental office manager writes out the office accounts payable for the dentist to review and sign.

Equipment and Supplies

- Checkbook with check and stub (Figure 40-23)
- Calculator
- Access to a computer and printer, if checks are written electronically

Procedure Steps

1. Write or type in the date. Make sure the date is current.
2. Write or type in the name of the payee. Verify that this is the correct payee.
3. Write in the correct numbers for the correct amount and write out the amount in the designated area. Check that the numerical and written amounts agree and are correct.
4. Fill out the memo, indicating what the check is for.
5. Fill out the date, payee, memo information, and amount on the check stub.
6. Verify that everything is accurate, including spelling.
7. Have the dentist sign on the signature line after reviewing the account payable.

(continues)

Procedure 40-8 (continued)

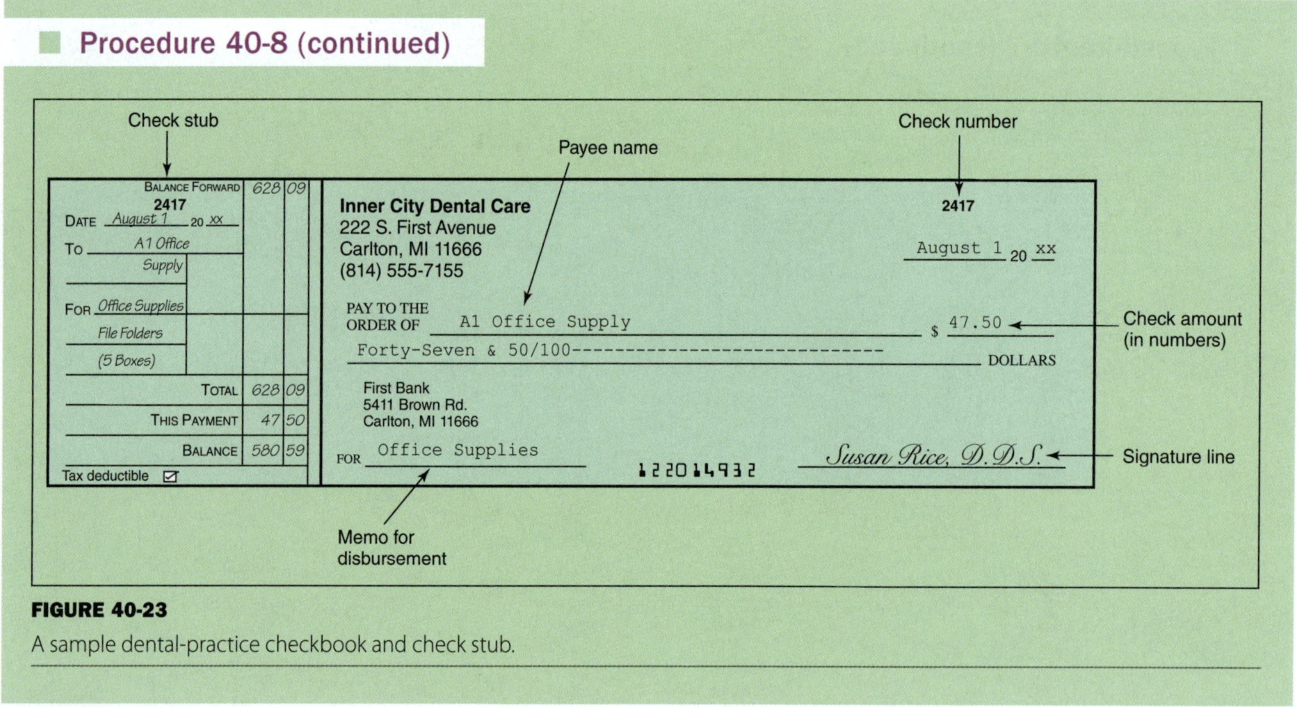

FIGURE 40-23

A sample dental-practice checkbook and check stub.

his or her name, address, Social Security number, and the total number of allowances (exemptions) to be claimed. With this information, payroll is calculated using the charts provided by the Internal Revenue Service. Federal taxes are based on the amount earned, marital status, number and type of allowances claimed, and length of pay period. Most state and local taxes are calculated on the total gross earnings of the employee. A required deduction under the Federal Insurance Contributions Act (FICA), commonly called Social Security, is calculated on the basis of gross pay. The employer is required to match this deducted amount and send both contributions to the federal government quarterly. Other deductions that may be taken from the employee's paycheck are health and life insurance payments, along with retirement or savings contributions that are put in another account.

At the end of the year, the employer is required to give each employee a W-2 wage and tax statement (Figure 40-24). This statement is used by the employee to submit his or her federal income tax. The statement includes total wages earned and the tax deductions made for the year by that employee.

Staying Current

Keeping up with all the new trends in the dental office comes from attending seminars, researching the internet, reviewing information from numerous companies, reading dental magazines, and attending local, regional, national, and international meetings. Much of this information can be accessed via the internet, allowing the dentist to stay up to date on available information. However, it is also helpful to go to booths at meetings and conferences where vendors will allow dental team members to learn from using the instruments, seeing and hearing about equipment, and so forth.

Connecting with the Office Through Mobile Devices

Dentists can now stay current with their practices by utilizing mobile dental software. This software allows the dentist to access practice information through smart phone technology via an application (or "app" for short). If a patient has an after-hours dental emergency, the patient is able to call the dentist, and the dentist is able to review the patient file over the telephone. The dentist can see if the patient has been prescribed medications, when medications and treatments were provided, and quickly scan for an available emergency appointment. The dentist can also review financial records and stay up to date on how the practice is doing.

Web Conferencing

In a busy office, taking time to attend a conference is difficult. Many practices are seeking webinars (Web-based seminars) for training and information. Offices can view a seminar, lecture, workshop, or presentation that is broadcast over the Web to the dental team members watching online. Some of the workshops are interactive and allow the participants to respond to the speaker. Brainstorming sessions can also be done through interactive webinars.

Distance Learning

Online education for health care professionals is an easy, convenient, and cost effective way to learn. Many courses are accepted for all or part of continuing education requirements. Colleges, universities, private companies, DANB, ADA, and ADAA all have a wide variety of courses available. These courses can be taken using a computer from any location, and at any time that is convenient for the dental assistant.

a Control number 3203	22222	Void ☐	For Official Use Only OMB No. 1545-0008

b Employer's identification number 317 600 23	1 Wages, tips, other compensation 18,500.00	2 Federal income tax withheld 2,950.00
c Employer's name, address, and ZIP code Lewis & King, D.D.S. 2501 Center Street, Suite 23 Northborough, OH 12345	3 Social security wages 18,500.00	4 Social security taxes withheld 1200.00
	5 Medicare wages and tips 18,500.00	6 Medicare tax withheld 220.00
	7 Social security tips	8 Allocated tips
d Employee's social security number 263-58-5296	9 Advance EIC payment	10 Dependent care benefits
e Employee's name (first, middle initial, last) Ellen L. Armstrong	11 Nonqualified plans	12 Benefits included in box 1
498 Menaul Road Northborough, OH 12345	13 See Instrs. for box 13	14 Other 360.00 Dental Care
f Employee's address and ZIP code	19 Statutory employee ☐ Deceased ☐ Pension plan ☐ Legal rep. ☐ Hshld. emp. ☐ Subtotal ☐ Deferred compensation ☐	

16 State	Employer's state I.D. No.	17 State wages, tips, etc.	18 State income tax	19 Locality name	20 Local wages, tips, etc.	21 Local income tax
OH	24	18,500.00	750.00	OH	18,500.00	63.50

Cat. No. 10134D Department of Treasury—Internal Revenue Service

Form **W-2** Wage and Tax Statement **20--**

For Paperwork Reduction Act Notice, see separate instructions

Copy A For Social Security Administration

FIGURE 40-24

W-2 form, summarizing all earnings and deductions for the year. The employer prepares a yearly W-2 form for each employee by January 31.

Chapter Summary

The dental reception area must be an environment in which all patients feel welcome and comfortable. Today, dentistry can be a positive experience, and dental treatment can be pain free. This positive image is developed when the patient first steps into the reception area. Patients may not consciously realize the message that is being received, but the dental office should present an atmosphere that relieves anxiety.

Front office staff has changed dramatically in recent years. All individuals in the front office require knowledge of business machines such as computers, fax machines, and copy machines. These individuals must be organized, have knowledge of dental treatments, and have good communication and problem-solving skills.

Marketing is also an important part of the dental practice. A dental office is a business as well as a health care facility. Dental assistants, along with all members of the dental team, need to be involved in marketing the practice.

This chapter will discuss business operations and the application of computerization in the dental office. Accurate information on dental record management is essential to every dental office. There is discussion on handling patient charts, record confidentiality, appointment scheduling, new patient's information, and patient recall. Financial management of the dental office is also covered including monthly billing, dental insurance, collection management, account receivable/payable, and supplies and inventory.

CASE STUDY

Melissa Jones is a new graduate of an accredited dental assisting program and has received her dental assisting national certification. She will be the front office assistant in the office of Dr. Ward. Dr. Ward is using practice management software and would like to expand on marketing ideas.

Case Study Review

1. Which types of effective marketing and practice management functions can be done from a computer-based practice management system?
2. What types of reports can be generated by a computer-based practice management system?
3. Identify the background knowledge Melissa received in her dental assisting program that will aid her in this task.

Review Questions

Multiple Choice

1. Basic telephone techniques include
   a. speaking loudly so the person can hear you.
   b. not asking the patient's name for privacy reasons.
   c. answering within three to four rings.
   d. allowing the caller to end the call.
2. A check guaranteed by the bank is called a
   a. certified check.
   b. cashier's check.
   c. voucher check.
   d. money order.
3. One of the primary reasons that dental patients do not pay their dental bills is that
   a. patients consider the cost of dental care to be too high.
   b. patients think that the insurance company should pay the entire dental bill.
   c. patients become unable to pay their dental bills because of financial hardship.
   d. the treatment plan was not discussed, and sound financial arrangements were not made at the time of the dental services.
4. An example of a fixed cost is
   a. the cost of supplies.
   b. the cost of treating dental patients.
   c. salaries.
   d. the cost of dental materials.
5. The Employee's Withholding Allowance Certificate, which is completed by all employees, is the
   a. W-2.
   b. W-4.
   c. accounts payable.
   d. accounts receivable.
6. In what year was the Americans with Disabilities Act passed by Congress?
   a. 1980
   b. 1990
   c. 2000
   d. 2005
7. Eye professionals advise that for every hour of computer use the user should relax the eyes by looking at a distant spot for how long?
   a. 5 minutes
   b. 10 minutes
   c. 20 minutes
   d. 30 minutes
8. Appointment books are normally set up in ________ minute units.
   a. 10
   b. 15
   c. 30
   d. both a and b
9. The insurance birthday rule pertains to the
   a. primary carrier.
   b. dependent child of two parents who have dental coverage.
   c. stepchildren who have dental coverage.
   d. secondary carrier.
10. Assume that a patient had dental work totaling $600, and is eligible for benefits under two insurance carriers that have a benefit-less-benefit provision. One carrier allows $400 for this service and the other allows $450. The second carrier would pay $450 and the other would pay
    a. $0.
    b. $100.
    c. $450.
    d. $50.

Critical Thinking

1. Why is billing patients promptly and accurately critical to the success of the dental office?
2. List the five sections of the pegboard day sheet and describe the functions of each.
3. Explain why a color-coding system is used for filing charts.

Web Activities

1. Practice management is an important part of being successful in dentistry. Visit http://www.dentaleconomics.com and review an article in the magazine under Front Office Review.
2. Do an internet search for "dental practice management software." Compare and contrast several programs on the market.
3. Do an internet search for "professional grade dental office keyboards." Research five keyboards and be prepared to share your findings and to discuss how this would help with infection control. In what other areas of the dental office would this be useful?
4. You need CEUs and would like to find an online course focusing on Office Management. Go to http://www.ineedce.com and search for courses available. Note the topic, hours, and cost for three courses you think sound interesting. Be prepared to share your results.
5. Dentistry IQ is a comprehensive resource for dental professionals. It collects articles from several publications. Go to http://www.dentistryiq.com and choose Office Managers, and find an article relating to insurance or CDT coding to review.

CHAPTER

41

Employment Strategies

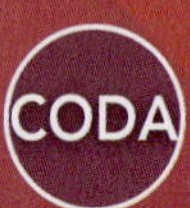

Specific Instructional Objectives

The student should strive to meet the following objectives and demonstrate an understanding of the facts and principles presented in this chapter:

1. Identify three pathways to obtain DANB certification.
2. Explain how to obtain employment and identify types of practices.
3. Set goals and identify sources to obtain employment in the dental field.
4. Identify the steps in preparing a cover letter and a résumé.
5. Explain how to prepare for the interview.
6. Describe the interview process, and identify the skills and preparation techniques that will aid in obtaining a job.
7. Identify the skills that a successful dental assistant possesses.
8. Explain how to terminate employment.

Key Terms

American Dental Assistants Association (ADAA) (1009)

American Dental Association (ADA) (1009)

Dental Assisting National Board, Inc. (DANB) (1009)

dental associate (1010)

partnership (1010)

Introduction

As the required formal training necessary to become a dental assistant nears completion, the student must switch his or her goals toward becoming an employed dental assistant. The first step in this process is obtaining national certification, and state registration or licensure. Then, the employment search begins.

When conducting the search for suitable employment, it is necessary to be well prepared and goal oriented. Being knowledgeable about how to write a cover letter and prepare a résumé is very important. Effective cover letters and résumés lead to job interviews. Understanding the interview process, and possessing the skills necessary to interview successfully lead to job offers.

Obtaining National Certification

National certification for dental assistants is not mandatory in every state. Once obtained, however, the patients and the dentist can be assured that the assistant has the basic knowledge and background necessary to perform as a professional on the dental team. The **Dental Assisting National Board, Inc. (DANB)** assumes the responsibility for credentialing dental assistants. This board is independent of the **American Dental Association (ADA)** and the **American Dental Assistants Association (ADAA)**. Upon completing and passing the chairside dental assisting examination of the DANB, the dental assistant can display the certificate that verifies successful completion of the DANB test (Figure 41-1). The assistant can also wear the official certified dental assistant (CDA) pin acknowledging that he or she is a CDA, and can use that title. The DANB examination is divided into three major categories: radiology, infection control, and general chairside. An assistant must pass all three sections in order to become a CDA. Maintenance of the CDA credential is through yearly continuing education hours and a renewal fee.

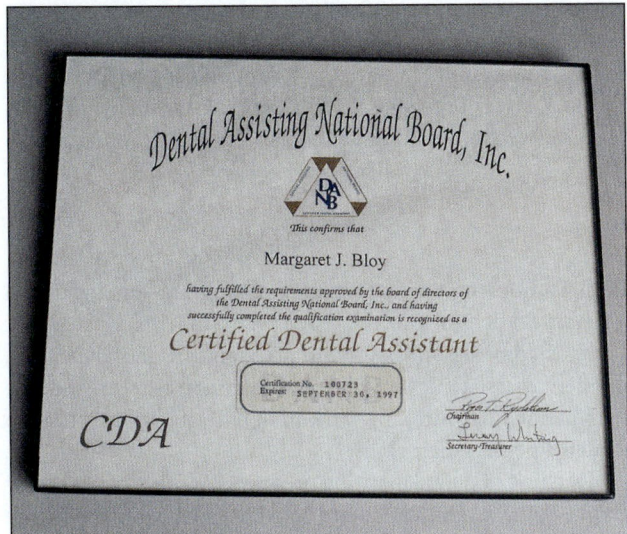

FIGURE 41-1
Dental Assisting National Board (DANB) certificate.

A dental assistant is eligible to take the dental assisting examination, and can obtain national certification by DANB through three pathways:

DANB Pathways

Pathway I

- Graduation (or anticipated graduation) from a Commission on Dental Accreditation (CODA) accredited dental assisting or dental hygiene program, or current registered dental hygienist (RDH).
- Current cardiopulmonary resuscitation (CPR), basic life support (BLS), or advanced cardiac life support (ACLS)

Pathway II

- Minimum of 3,500 hours work experience as a dental assistant, accrued over a period of at least two years to a maximum of four years; employment must be verified by a licensed dentist
- High school graduation or equivalent
- Current cardiopulmonary resuscitation (CPR), basic life support (BLS), or advanced cardiac life support (ACLS)

Pathway III

- Former DANB CDA certificant or graduation from a D.D.S. or D.M.D. program
- Current cardiopulmonary resuscitation (CPR), basic life support (BLS), or advanced cardiac life support (ACLS)

Reprinted with permission of the Dental Assisting National Board, Inc., (DANB).

Every dental assistant should obtain national certification to ensure that his or her patients receive the best care possible, as well as to build self-esteem.

State Requirements

Many states have requirements, job titles, and specific allowable functions for various levels of dental assisting. Many states have some type of registration that allows dental assistants to take radiographs after some education and skill proficiency are met. This may be part of the dental assisting program. Some states have a variety of requirements for various levels of dental assisting skills. There may be an entry level *registration*, where the dental assistant fills out a form, pays a fee, and receives a registration card. There is no examination, but the registration requires the dental assistant to know and follow the laws and rule changes of the state. In other states the registration is for dental assistants who have successfully completed a dental assisting program and have met certain criteria to perform dental assisting skills. States may also require a *license* (or registration, terms vary with each state) in order for dental assistants to perform certain expanded functions/duties. Licensed dental assistants must pass a written exam and, in some states, a clinical exam on specific skills. The Dental Assistant National Board (DANB) provides written examinations that states can use for the different levels of dental assisting skills. Go to the DANB website to find information on your state's requirements.

Note: There are publications that offer state-by-state information about dental assisting regulations and allowable duties called *DANB's State Career Ladder Templates for Dental Assistants and DANB's State Fact Booklet.*

Employment

Whether graduating from an accredited program or just trying to obtain a position in a dental office, there are several important tasks that must be accomplished first. Planning future employment is very important. It may be necessary to obtain dental assisting national certification for the state in which employment is sought. If this is the case, reflect on the pathways available and seek the one that best suits your needs.

After obtaining the necessary credentials, the next goal is to prepare for obtaining successful employment. Research should be done to identify the type of practice that will be the most interesting, stimulating, and enjoyable. When choosing an employer, find one who has a good reputation and whose philosophy is similar to your own. A dental assistant needs to feel that he or she is working with the dentist and other team members to care for patients in the best manner possible. Prior to obtaining the position, do research and talk to employees who work for the dentist to make sure that this practice would be a good employment match for you. Another aspect of employment is working well with other employees. Are they team players? Will compatibility be possible?

It is important to find employment that best suits the individual's needs and allows for the best possible situation for the dental assistant, the employer, and the patients. Before taking the first position offered, consider the following:

- What qualities are desired in an employer?
- What areas of growth are available in this situation?
- From an employee's position, what strengths can be brought to this position?
- What individual areas can be improved upon?
- Overall, what type of dentistry is interesting?

Solo or Partnership Practice

The majority of dentists practice in solo practices in which there is only a single dentist. A dentist may hire another dentist under a contractual agreement; this hired dentist is a **dental associate**. An associate relationship may turn into a **partnership**, in which each dentist has equal rights and duties. A partnership is developed through a legal agreement, which makes both dentists responsible for any accounts payable. However, a partner is not held responsible for malpractice suits against the other partner.

Partnerships in dental practices are increasing. This is due to the tremendous startup cost that a dentist faces upon graduation from dental school. Therefore, a newly graduated dentist may work in an established practice as a dental associate for some time, and then, after an allotted period of time, become a partner. Another way that dentists are dealing with the costs of their practices is to share a building and/or front office employees while still maintaining solo practices.

Group Practice

Another type of dental office is the group practice. In a group practice, any number of dentists (both general and specialty) can share a building and still remain independent. Positive aspects of this type of practice are the opportunities to talk over cases with each other, reduced overhead, and increased patient coverage on weekends and holidays. In addition, the total number of employees in the group practice may lend itself to offering more complete and extensive benefit packages. The more employees under the same insurance plan, the better the rates for the employer.

Dental Specialty Practice

If a dental assistant likes to assist primarily in oral surgery, endodontics, periodontics, orthodontics, prosthodontics, pathology, pediatric dentistry, or dental public health, specialty offices are available. Fewer employment opportunities are available in the areas of pathology and dental public health. Dental specialists work with general dentists to care for specific cases. The general dentist refers the patient to a specialty office to obtain a special service, and then the patient returns to the general dental office for routine care.

Public Health and Government Programs

Public health programs often include oral health care. Dental assistants can gain employment in these public health/government clinics to provide oral health information, collect data, and provide dental treatment. These programs care for patients who are eligible to receive dental care for free or at a reduced rate. They are local, state, and/or federally funded. Often, federal or state grants set up programs to meet the specific needs of people who cannot afford dental care. These programs may also collect data on specific diseases this group of people may have. Usually, the guidelines of the programs change or have to be renewed annually. A dental assistant is an employee hired by the overseer of the grant. This dental assistant may receive great satisfaction treating patients in this type of program.

Teaching, School Clinics, and Laboratories

Dental schools and dental assisting schools also employ dental assistants who work in the clinic with students, or teach or serve as administrators for the program. In dental schools, the dental assistants work with student dentists to simulate four-handed dentistry, or work in dental laboratories to help students perfect their skills.

Teaching in dental assisting programs or schools is a career choice some dental assistants consider after working in the field for a while. Teaching often requires additional education that varies with each state. Some require a bachelor's degree, and a certificate, registration, and/or license from the state.

If the school is ADA accredited, a bachelor's degree for the program director and faculty is now required. This is a challenging and rewarding career path for dental assistants that find teaching an area they are interested in, but still want to stay in dental assisting.

Veterans' Hospitals

Veterans' hospitals hire dental assistants to assist the dentists on staff in the clinics. Employment in this area must be obtained through the civil service office. Points are given to individuals who have worked in the service, or have been employed in veterans' programs before. A list of qualifications can be obtained from the civil service office that advertises the employment position.

Dental Supply Companies

Dental supply companies hire dental assistants as sales representatives for goods and supplies. Normally, a dental assistant in this position does not utilize his or her chairside skills, but becomes knowledgeable about products, traveling from dental office to dental office providing product information and ordering supplies.

Insurance Companies

Dental assistants are also hired by insurance companies to process dental insurance claims. Having knowledge of and a background in dental terminology and procedures is an asset for understanding situations and processing dental insurance claims.

Employment Search

After a decision is made about the desired type of dental practice, locating open positions is the next step. Many dentists advertise in *daily newspapers* in the classified section, and on online job search websites. Other areas where employment opportunities are posted include *local dental and dental assistant societies/associations*. Most local societies have newsletters or other services that list job openings. If graduating from a dental assisting program, *career placement services* may be available at the school. Some *employment agencies* have listings for dental assistant jobs, and most *dental supply houses* know of dentists who are hiring. Leaving a cover letter and résumé with some of these agencies may be a consideration.

An additional resource for an employment search is the *Internet*, start with a search for "employment in dental professions." This is especially helpful when planning to relocate.

Preparing a Cover Letter and Résumé

The next step in the employment search is to prepare a cover letter and a résumé. These documents introduce the prospective employee, and present the individual's educational background, training, and previous employment experience. The cover letter states why the individual is right for the position, and when he or she is available for employment.

The cover letter and the résumé should be printed on quality paper (normally white, light gray, or off-white), and follow a professional format. It is crucial that the cover letter and résumé be printed on a laser printer or high-quality dot matrix printer, and that they demonstrate correct spelling, punctuation, and grammar. Every cover letter and résumé must be proofread several times before being submitted to a prospective employer.

Cover Letter

A cover letter is an introduction to a prospective employer (Figure 41-2). It communicates to the employer or hiring personnel the individual's potential value, and any specific personal attributes that should be called attention to. A cover letter should accompany every résumé (Procedure 41-1). A standard format can be used to develop a cover letter.

- **Return address**—include a street address, city, state, and zip code.
- **Date**—month, day, and year.
- **Inside address**—the addressee's name and title, company name (if different), street address, city, state, and zip code.
- **Salutation**—make every effort to use the correct name. If unknown, and as a last resort, use "To Whom It May Concern:" At the end of every salutation, a colon (:) is used.
- **First paragraph**—tell why the letter is being written and indicate where the information about the employment opportunity was obtained, and which position is desired.
- **Second paragraph**—identify the reasons for the interest in the position, such as the dental office having a good reputation for providing quality dental care. List the qualifications that would be assets to the employer and dental team members, for example, being a graduate of an accredited dental assisting program (with an explanation on how this academic background makes for a qualified dental assistant). Mention any relevant work experience. Refer the employer to the résumé, which lists individual qualifications, education, training, and experience.
- **Third paragraph**—ask for a personal interview, indicate flexible available times to be reached, and list a phone number with area code, if applicable, and an email address. Close with a statement that encourages a speedy response: "I am available for an interview at your convenience and will be calling within the next five days to confirm an interview time with you," or "I am looking forward to meeting with you and your dental team in the near future."
- **Closing**—Close the letter with "Sincerely" and a comma. Then, type four returns and your name. The four spaces provide room for a signature, written in black ink. Using other colors may detract from the professionalism that has been established in the cover letter.
- **Enclosures**—After the typed name, type two returns and then type the words "Enclosure: Résumé." Any other enclosures can be listed beneath the word "Résumé," such as letters of recommendation.

625 "B" Street
Spokane, WA 99228

January 12, 20XX

Dr. Conrad Jones
312 33rd
Spokane, WA 99205

Dear Dr. Jones:

I am writing in response to your advertisement in the April edition of the *Spokesman Review* for an expanded-function dental assistant.

I believe that I am the "gentle, caring, enthusiastic" dental assistant that you are looking for. You will find me to be flexible and capable of working individually or as a team member. A recent graduate of the Spokane Community College Dental Assisting program, I am currently awaiting the results of my Dental Assisting National Board examination. With the combination of my training, my desire to work, and my love of helping people, I will be a valuable asset to your office.

Looking at my enclosed résumé, you will see that I have worked in several offices during my training. I have also assisted several dentists in the volunteer clinic, provided dental education in the area schools, and worked with patients in my other health-related employment. Computer proficiency was obtained during my other employment opportunities.

Please contact me for a personal interview to further discuss the position and to answer any questions you may have. My schedule is flexible so feel free to call me at (509) 555-1857 as soon as is convenient so an appointment can be arranged.

Looking forward to meeting you and your staff and to getting the opportunity to demonstrate my abilities as a valuable member of your office team.

Sincerely yours,

Jean Lucas
Dental Assistant

Enclosure: résumé

FIGURE 41-2

Cover letter for employment as a dental assistant in a dental office.

Résumé

A résumé should fit on one page (Figure 41-3), and it should be attractive and professional. Present specific information, and stress achievements and skills related to employment. Include personal data, career objective, education, employment history (including qualifications, skills, and abilities), and references (Procedure 41-2).

- **Personal data**—include personal name, address, phone number or numbers, and email address, if available, where you can be reached. Marital status and birth date are no longer appropriate for a résumé.
- **Career objective**—identify the desired goal, for example, "To gain a position in a dental office as a dental assistant where I will utilize skills and abilities obtained in dental assisting school."
- **Education**—list certificates, registration, degrees, and continuing education courses that have been completed. Do not include grade point average unless it is in some way pertinent to the position. Also, list any academic awards received, such as scholarships. List the most recent education first with corresponding dates. High school graduation information is not necessary.

625 "B" Street
Spokane, WA 99228

Phone: 509-555-1857
Fax: 599-555-3038
E-mail:
Jlucas@spokane.wa.us.com

Jean Lucas

Career Objective — To obtain a dental assisting position in which my education and skills can be utilized, in an office that uses the team approach to providing quality dental care.

Education — 2014–2016 Spokane Community College Spokane, WA

AAS Degree, Dental Assisting

- Vice President's Honor Roll for academic achievement

Employment History — 2014–Present Community Clinic Palouse, WA

Chairside Dental Assistant

- Assisted in a variety of dental procedures
- Developed and taught a program in oral hygiene to elementary children
- Provided patient care and service
- Maintained inventory and supplies
- Volunteered in community clinic care programs

2012–2014 Ice Cream Delight Seattle, WA

Senior Assistant Manager

- Supervised employees while providing customer service
- Created and decorated cakes
- Managed telephones
- Maintained accounts payable and receivable
- Organized employee work schedule

References: Available on request

FIGURE 41-3
Résumé for employment as a dental assistant in a dental office.

- **Employment history**—employment history should be listed with an idea of what was accomplished in each position. Use action words to explain what was done. For instance, instead of writing, "I worked as a cashier," it would be better to write, "I was responsible for maintaining cash payables while resolving daily problems, projecting a positive attitude, and developing good customer relations." Present the abilities in the best manner, but always be honest about the job description.
- **References**—it is appropriate to use the sentence, "References are available upon request." In many areas of the country, it is beneficial to list three references using name, title, and phone number. It is likely that a dentist will call a fellow dentist to inquire about an individual's skills and abilities. Make sure that the references listed have been checked first to ensure that they will give positive references, and that they are aware that they have been listed as references. It is important to have references who relate specifically to the desired characteristics, and pertain to the employment that is sought. Some characteristics include integrity, reliability, work ethic, good communication skills and a team spirit.

Procedure 41-1
Preparing a Cover Letter

The dental assistant prepares a cover letter as an introduction to a future employer when applying for employment.

Equipment and Supplies

- Quality paper
- Information to be included in the cover letter
- Computer
- Printer

Procedure Steps

1. Have correct names and addresses.
2. Select a format for the cover letter.
3. Select the font and font size (usually 12-point size).
4. Outline the information to include in the cover letter.
5. Create the cover letter including a return address, date, inside address, salutation, first paragraph, second paragraph, third paragraph, a closing, and enclosures.
6. Ensure that the cover letter is neat and free of errors.

Procedure 41-2
Preparing a Professional Résumé

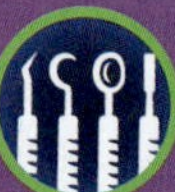

The dental assistant prepares a résumé for a future employer when applying for employment.

Equipment and Supplies

- Quality paper
- Information to be included in the résumé
- Computer
- Printer

Procedure Steps

1. Have correct names, addresses, and dates (Figure 41-4).
2. Select a format for the résumé.
3. Select the font and font size (usually 12-point size).
4. Outline the information to be included in the résumé.

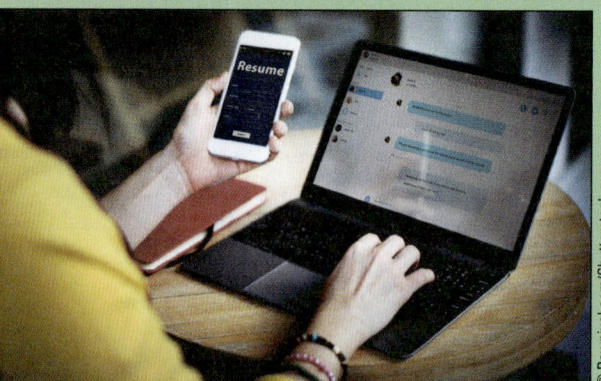

FIGURE 41-4
Using technology for reference while preparing a résumé.

5. Create the résumé including personal data, career objective, education, employment history, and references.
6. Ensure that the résumé is neat and free of errors.

Setting Up an Interview

Follow through on what was said in the cover letter. For example, if the letter mentions making a follow-up call in 5 days, be sure to call back on that fifth day. When making a follow-up call, make sure that background noises are not distracting. If you are nervous about using the telephone to set up the interview, visit the dental office in person to set it up. It may be beneficial to develop a script that is comfortable to use prior to making contact. Try it out on a friend or two, and obtain their feedback first. When setting up an interview, you should make sure that your schedule can accommodate the appointment time. It is also important to make sure that it is scheduled at a convenient time for the dentist and staff.

Interview Process

When preparing for the interview, there are several things to consider. It is important to be at least 5 minutes early for the interview, so allow additional time to get there. It is important that some research has been done regarding the dental office. The additional interest in the dental office will have a positive effect on the prospective employer. Know yourself and know your strengths and abilities in order to be prepared for the question that is most often asked: "Why should we hire you for this position?"

Develop questions that can be asked of the dentist and staff. Salary questions should not be the only thing that is brought up in the interview. Ask questions related to teamwork, prevention programs, or continuing education.

Prepare a portfolio with letters of recommendation, copies of certificates, radiographs you have taken, or any additional items that attest to your abilities and skills (Figure 41-5). Place them in a folder to present to the dentist and staff.

Practice the interview before actually going to one. Ask a friend or family member to do a mock interview and to give feedback on any areas that can be improved. A firm handshake, eye contact, and a smile are still important in the interview process. Sit up straight and speak distinctly. Try to relax and enjoy it. Identify possible situations that might come up and plan ahead. For example, how is the situation going to be handled if the office staff asks if you would like a cup of coffee?

Appearance is crucial. Wear something that feels comfortable, but the rule of thumb is to dress like an individual who cares about being hired (Figure 41-6). Many individuals feel comfortable in jeans, but jeans are not appropriate attire for an interview. Dress appropriately and demonstrate good hygiene. Make sure that clothes are clean and pressed. Do not wear clothes that appear to be flamboyant or dowdy; instead, err on the side of conservatism. Think about the small details, such as where your car keys or purse are going to be placed during the interview. Is a pen available if asked to fill out an application? If necessary, are references with addresses and phone numbers available? If asked to write a paragraph about yourself, can you do this while correctly spelling the words needed to express yourself properly? Will it be legible? Are your questions readily

Common Interview Questions

- How well do you handle stress at work?
- How would you describe yourself?
- Where do you see yourself in 5 years? 10 years?
- Why did you quit your last job?
- Who was your best employer and why?
- What did you dislike about your previous job?
- What have you learned from your mistakes?
- What are you passionate about?
- What motivates you?
- What is your greatest weakness/strength?
- When was the last time you were angry? What happened?
- Give some examples of teamwork and how you participated in it.
- Tell me about yourself.
- Describe what success means for you personally.
- If you know your employer is 100 percent wrong about something, how do you handle it?
- Why should this office hire you?
- What are your career goals?
- Tell me about your abilities and how they would work out in this office.
- Why do you want to work here?
- Do you see dentistry as your lifelong career?
- What type of challenges are you looking for in this position?
- Tell me about your dental assisting skills.
- Tell me about your interpersonal skills.
- Describe your work style.

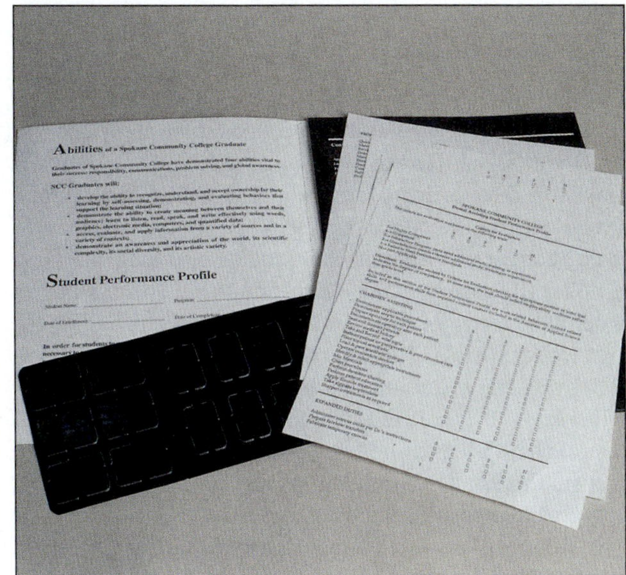

FIGURE 41-5

A personal portfolio is an effective way to share your certificates and letters of recommendation with the dental office.

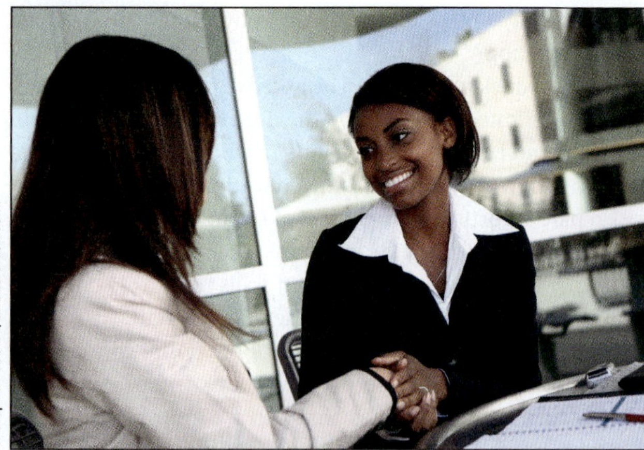

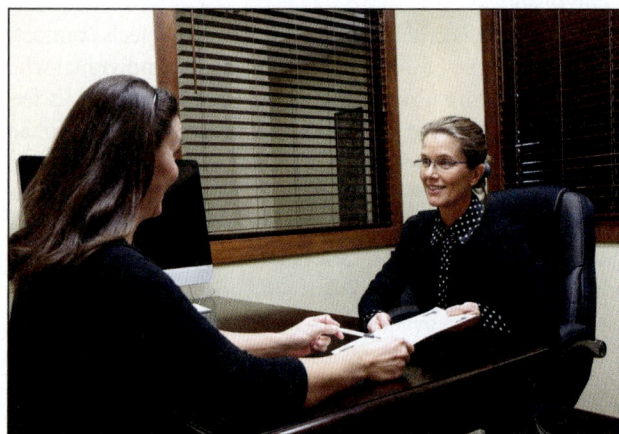

FIGURE 41-6
Appearance should be professional and neat.

FIGURE 41-7
During the interview be prepared, and listen carefully to the interviewer before answering questions.

available to ask the dental team members? Many of these items may not be necessary, but it is important to be prepared.

Be yourself and, if nervous, say so, and then continue on. Make sure that the dentist's name is pronounced correctly and always address the dentist as "Dr.__________" unless asked to do otherwise. The dentist may request a working interview. If this is the case, ask about time, uniform, and parking in order to be ready for the identified day. Stay calm and do the best work possible. The interviewer usually closes the session by asking if the interviewee has any further questions (Figure 41-7). This is the time to ask prepared questions. If all areas have been covered, say, "The specific questions I had prepared to ask have been answered. Can I clarify anything in regard to my background and experience?" If all questions have not been answered show them that you are prepared and have done your research. For example: "I have reviewed your Web page and found that you are very team oriented, do you have regular staff meetings?" See sample questions to ask employers in the following box.

Sample Questions to Ask Employers

- Normally there is time at the end of the interview for questions to be asked.
- Note that they may have scheduled a certain amount of time for the interview and that time has lapsed leaving very little time for you to ask questions. Only ask one or two questions if running out of time; otherwise ask up to five questions.
- Make sure you have done your research on the office—don't ask questions that are covered on the Web page.
- Ask questions that are intelligent and thoughtful.
- Do not ask about salary and benefits initially.
- Sometimes the questions were answered during the interview, and you can simply express that the interview was very thorough.
- Good questions are open ended.

Examples:

- Please tell me about the best dental assistant that you ever employed. What qualities did or does this person have that were beneficial to this office?
- Can you tell me when the interviews will be completed, and if you will be conducting working interviews with the top candidates?
- I noticed on your website that you have done presentations to other study clubs. What do your team members in this office do to help facilitate this? Do you anticipate that other seminars or presentations will occur, and how would you see a dental assistant supporting you in this endeavor?
- I had checked with the dental society in this area and found that you are an officer. That is exciting! It seems like you are interested in staying up on all the changes in dentistry. Do you also seek continued education opportunities? Is that a quality that you seek in a dental assistant as well?
- You have a copy of my cover letter and résumé, and you have covered many of my questions during the interview. I am excited about the possibility of employment here. Would you like me to check back with you at the end of the week to see if you need any further information, or would like to set up a working interview?

Leaving the Interview and Following Up

Be sure to thank the interviewers for their time and shake their hands. It is good to close by stating that you are interested in the position and look forward to hearing from them. If they have not stated it during the interview, ask when they anticipate making a decision on the open position. Dentists look for dental assistants who have positive attitudes, good interpersonal skills, good clinical skills, good dental educational foundations, flexibility, team player attitudes, and the willingness to learn.

If the interviewee decides after the interview that he or she would like to obtain a position in that dental office, he or she would then send a follow-up letter referring (Procedure 41-3)

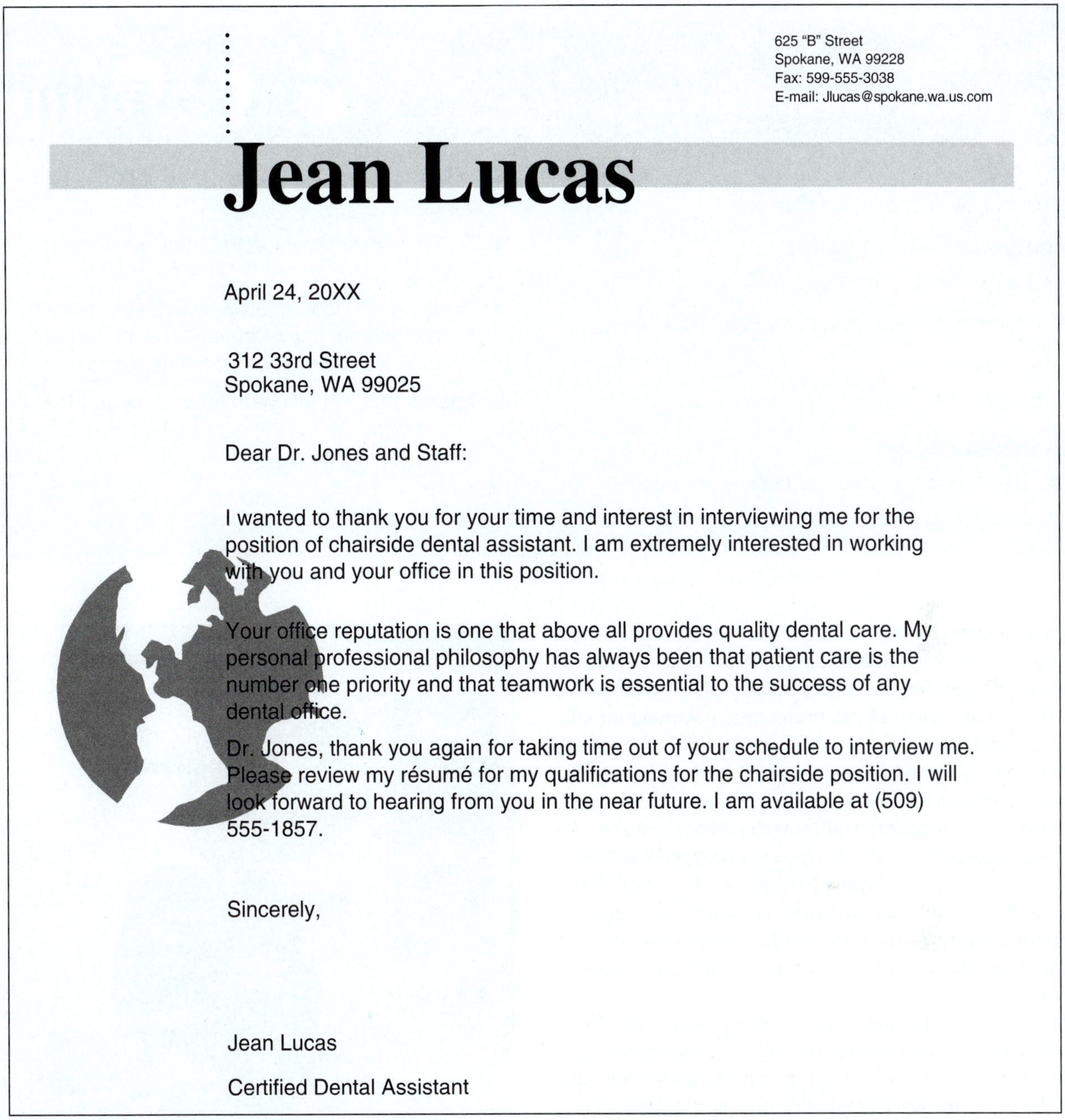

625 "B" Street
Spokane, WA 99228
Fax: 599-555-3038
E-mail: Jlucas@spokane.wa.us.com

Jean Lucas

April 24, 20XX

312 33rd Street
Spokane, WA 99025

Dear Dr. Jones and Staff:

I wanted to thank you for your time and interest in interviewing me for the position of chairside dental assistant. I am extremely interested in working with you and your office in this position.

Your office reputation is one that above all provides quality dental care. My personal professional philosophy has always been that patient care is the number one priority and that teamwork is essential to the success of any dental office.

Dr. Jones, thank you again for taking time out of your schedule to interview me. Please review my résumé for my qualifications for the chairside position. I will look forward to hearing from you in the near future. I am available at (509) 555-1857.

Sincerely,

Jean Lucas

Certified Dental Assistant

FIGURE 41-8

Sending a follow-up letter is advisable after an interview.

the office to the résumé, and restating an interest in becoming part of the dental team (Figure 41-8).

Receiving an Employment Offer

Before accepting an employment offer, it is important to ask a few more questions. If it was not mentioned during the interview, now is an appropriate time to discuss salary. Also, ask about benefits, such as medical insurance, dental care, and retirement plans. Check the office's policies on requirements for uniforms, payment of professional dues, opportunities for continued education, sick days, holidays, and vacation time. Know what the dental assistant's specific responsibilities are, and what the office hours will be. Find out when performance evaluations are conducted, and which performance objectives lead to a raise in pay.

Professional Conduct During Employment

Once the job is obtained, the dental assistant's goal becomes keeping the job. Basic requirements for keeping the job are to always be on time, be ready to accomplish the necessary skills, plan ahead, and prepare for success. Take care of all outside

Procedure 41-3
Preparing a Follow-Up Letter

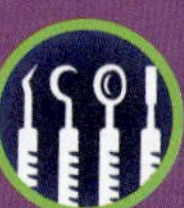

The dental assistant prepares a follow-up letter after an interview with a future employer.

Equipment and Supplies

- Quality paper
- Information to be included in the follow-up letter
- Computer
- Printer

Procedure Steps

1. Have correct names, addresses, and dates.
2. Select a format for the follow-up letter.
3. Select the font and font size (usually 12-point).
4. Outline the information to be included in the letter.
5. Create the follow-up letter including reference to the résumé, and restating an interest in becoming a member of the office team.
6. Ensure that the follow-up letter is neat and free of errors.

practical matters so that attention can be placed on fulfilling employment responsibilities. Make sure that childcare is arranged (if applicable), and that backup care is available in case the primary caregiver has an emergency. Arrange for reliable transportation.

Maintain high standards of personal hygiene (Figure 41-9). As an employee in a health profession, it is important to present good health standards. Uniforms should be clean and well pressed, and shoes should be clean and in good condition. Unfortunately, an employer's perception of an employee's abilities may be influenced by the employee's appearance. Therefore, dental assistants should always look and act like professionals, and be well prepared for the job every work day.

Make sure that the expectations of the job are identified, and then try to go above and beyond those expectations, especially if planning to advance. If expectations are unclear, talk with the office manager or employer to clarify areas of concern. A positive attitude is key to becoming an ideal employee. The dental office can be stressful, especially when a patient procedure changes and the schedule is off course, so tackling each challenge with a positive attitude and flexibility makes the office environment better for everyone. It is a well-known fact that the majority of patients who leave one dental office for another do so because of the poor attitude of one particular employee. Each dental assistant is responsible for maintaining a positive attitude at work.

Set goals to learn new skills, and stay current with the changes in technology and materials. One way to continue education is through the Dental Assistant Association, other professional courses, and seminars. Other courses offered by nearby community or 4-year colleges may be of benefit to an individual's professional growth. Seek them out. Occasionally, perform a self-evaluation. Be honest and look at overall

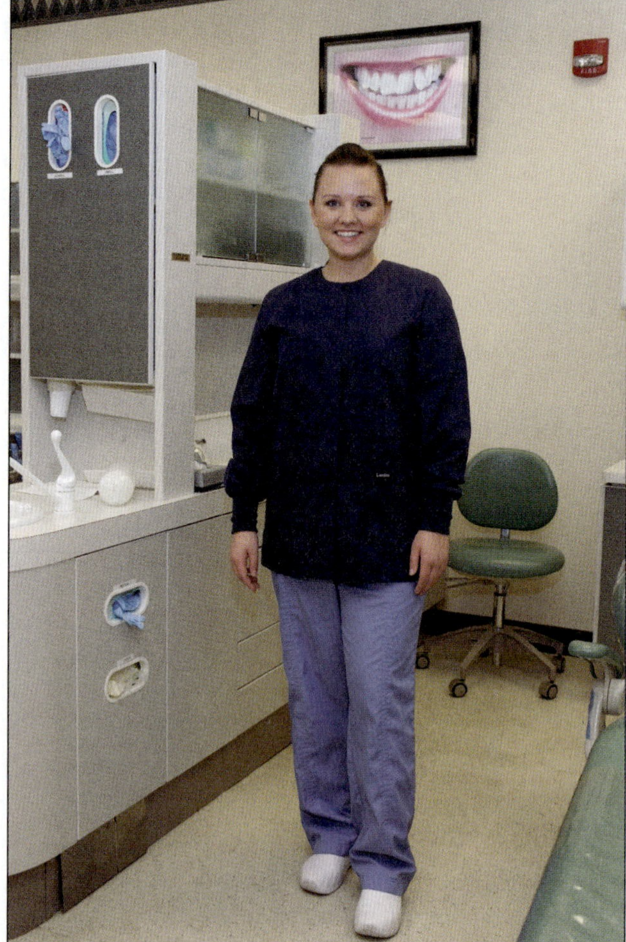

FIGURE 41-9
Maintaining a professional appearance on the job is important for the dental assistant.

individual attitude, skill, and professionalism. Try not to look at others to correct these behaviors, because the only person an individual can change is himself or herself.

Terminating Employment

If you begin to dread going to work each day, determine where employment could be obtained that would correct the problem. Evaluate your career goals, your qualifications pertaining to these goals, and the new path that is desired. If it is determined that employment in a different office is the required plan of action, submit a letter of termination, or verbally notify the employer, and allow him or her 2 weeks' notice so that a replacement can be found. Do everything possible to leave a position on good terms with the employer. Then, if the new career does not proceed as planned, returning to the prior job when an opening is available is a possibility.

Continued Success

The career of dental assisting is a very rewarding one, both professionally and personally. The work environment is a pleasant one that usually does not require evenings or night shifts. The goal of dental offices is to provide the best care possible for their patients. The patients are appreciative of the dental assistants who care for their needs. The dental assistant who provides a pleasant smile while providing care makes everything go better for the patient. Most days, dental assistants go home feeling good about the skills and knowledge they used to provide quality dental care to their patients. Continue to improve dental assisting skills and knowledge through continuing education, and stay challenged to stay knowledgeable about new techniques and materials. Be the best dental assistant possible. Good luck in your career!

Chapter Summary

It is important to find employment that will best suit individual needs and that allows for the best possible situation for the dental assistant, employer, and patients. Before taking the first position available, plan ahead. It may be essential to obtain dental assisting national certification for the state in which employment is sought. National certification for dental assistants is not mandatory in every state, but it assures patients and the dentist that the assistant has the basic knowledge and background to perform as a professional on the dental team. Make sure that the expectations of the job are identified, and then try to meet and exceed them if planning to advance. Learn how to prepare a cover letter and resume that reflects your experience and skills. The interview process is discussed including how to prepare for the interview and then how to complete the process with a follow-up letter. Each dental assistant is responsible for maintaining a positive attitude at work. Set goals to learn new skills and stay abreast of changes in technology and materials. A dental assisting career is very rewarding, both professionally and personally. Be the best dental assistant possible.

CASE STUDY

Dr. Bryan and Dr. Lucas are hiring a dental assistant to replace Phong Ho, a dental assistant who is leaving at the end of the month. Phong has been a chairside dental assistant for 7 years for Dr. Bryan and Dr. Lucas. Svetlana Maklavic has applied for the position, and will be the first dental assistant applicant to be interviewed.

Case Study Review

1. What paperwork should Svetlana bring to the interview?
2. How should Svetlana prepare for the interview?
3. What clothes should Svetlana wear for an interview with Dr. Bryan and Dr. Lucas?
4. Why should Svetlana arrive for the interview 5 minutes early?

Review Questions

Multiple Choice

1. A cover letter is a(n)
   a. listing of personal data for the employer.
   b. listing of education.
   c. introduction to your employer.
   d. career objective for the position being sought.
2. The interview
   a. does not require a follow-up.
   b. is a time for questions and answers about salary and benefits.
   c. requires very little preparation.
   d. requires that you prepare, listen carefully, and think before answering questions asked.
3. If an individual is a graduate of an accredited dental assisting program, what would not be required in order to be eligible to take the Dental Assisting National Board?
   a. Current cardiopulmonary resuscitation care certificate, health care provider level
   b. Verification of work experience by dentist employer
   c. Completed application
   d. Application fee
4. A ________ practice is one in which any number of dentists can share a building and still remain independent.
   a. group
   b. specialty
   c. general
   d. partnership
5. The key to becoming an ideal employee is/are:
   a. a high standard of personal hygiene.
   b. skill and knowledge.
   c. a positive attitude.
   d. all of the above.
6. The ________ provides national certification for dental assistants.
   a. American Dental Assisting Association
   b. Dental Assisting National Board, Inc.
   c. American Dental Association
   d. Commission on Dental Accreditation
7. To apply for the certification examination, Pathway I, the applicant must
   a. have graduated from a dental assisting or dental hygiene program accredited by the ADA Commission on Dental Accreditation.
   b. have a current CPR card.
   c. pay a fee to take the examination.
   d. accomplish all of the above.
8. A dentist may hire another dentist under a contractual agreement; the hired dentist is
   a. a partner.
   b. a dental associate.
   c. both a and b.
   d. neither a nor b.
9. The document that introduces the prospective employee and presents the individual's educational background, training, and previous employment experiences is a
   a. cover letter.
   b. résumé
   c. follow-up letter.
   d. interview
10. Which of the following is one of the most frequently asked questions in the interview process?
    a. Do you have childcare for your child?
    b. Do you have transportation to and from home?
    c. Do you have a background in dentistry?
    d. Why should we hire you for this position?

Critical Thinking

1. Discuss methods for researching a prospective employer.
2. Identify the differences between a solo, partnership, group, and specialty dental practice.
3. Identify the areas in which a dental assistant can obtain employment.

Web Activities

1. Identify possible employment opportunities by performing a Web search on dental assistant employment in your area.
2. Find the site http://www.danb.org and download an application. While on this site, also read the results of the salary survey "Show Me the Money."
3. Go to your state dental practice act and look up the requirements and list of skills for the various levels of dental assisting.

APPENDIX

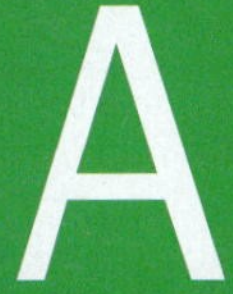

Dental and Dental-Related Organizations and Publications Resource List

United States Organizations

American Dental Association (ADA)
211 E. Chicago Avenue
Chicago, IL 60611
312-440-2500
online: *www.ada.org*

American Dental Assistants Association (ADAA)
140 N. Bloomingdale Road
Bloomingdale, IL 60108-1017
630-994-4247
877-874-3785
online: *www.adaausa.org*

Dental Assisting National Board, Inc. (DANB)
444 N. Michigan Avenue, Suite 900
Chicago, IL 60611
312-642-3368
800-347-3262
Email: danbmail@danb.org
online: *www.danb.org*

Centers for Disease Control and Prevention (CDC)
1600 Clifton Rd.
Atlanta, GA 30329-4027
800-232-4636
online: *www.cdc.gov*

American Dental Education Association
655 K Street, NW, Suite 800
Suite 1100
Washington, DC 20001
202-289-7201
online: *www.adea.org*

American Dental Hygienists' Association
444 N. Michigan Avenue, Suite 3400
Chicago, IL 60611
312-440-8900
online: *www.adha.org*

American National Standards Institute
1899 L Street NW
11th Floor
Washington, DC 20036
202-293-8020
online: *www.ansi.org*

ASTM International Standards Worldwide
100 Barr Harbor Drive
P.O. Box C700
West Conshohocken, PA 19428
610-832-9585
online: *www.astm.org*

Environmental Protection Agency (EPA)
1200 Pennsylvania Avenue, NW
Washington, DC 20460
Toxic Substances Control Act Hotline: (202) 554-1404
202-272-0167
online: *www.epa.gov*

Food and Drug Administration (FDA)
10903 New Hampshire Avenue
Silver Spring, MD 20993
888-463-6332
Devices and Radiological Health (800) 638-2041
Drug Evaluation Research (301) 796-3400
online: *www.fda.gov*

United States Occupational Safety and Health Administration (OSHA) Department of Labor
200 Constitution Avenue NW
Washington, DC 20210
800-321-6742
online: *www.osha.gov*

American Latex Allergy Association
63334 Lohman LN
Eastman, WI 54626
608-972-5378
1-888-972-5378
online: *www.latexallergyresources.org*

National Association of Dental Laboratories
325 John Knox Road # L103
Tallahassee, FL 32303
800-950-1150
online: *www.nadl.org*

Organization for Safety, Asepsis, and Prevention (OSAP)
3525 Piedmont Rd
Building 5, Suite 300
Atlanta, GA 30305
800-298-6727
online: *www.osap.org*

Canadian Organizations

Canadian Dental Assistants' Association
1150 – 45 O'Connor Street
Ottawa, ON K1P 1A4
Canada
Phone 1-613-521-5495
Toll-Free 1-800-345-5137
Email: info@cdaa.ca
online: *www.cdaa.ca*

Canadian Dental Association
1815 Alta Vista Drive
Ottawa, ON K1G 3Y6
Canada
Phone 1-613-523-1770
Email: reception@ada-adc.ca
online: *www.cda-adc.ca*

College of Alberta Dental Assistants (CADA)
166-14315 118 Avenue, NW
Edmonton AB T5L 4S6
Canada
780-486-2526
Email: contact@abrda.ca
online: *www.abrda.ca*

Certified Dental Assistants of British Columbia
102-221 Columbia Street
Vancouver, BC V6A 2R5
Canada
604-714-1766
Email: info@cdabc.org
online: *www.cdabc.org*

Saskatchewan Dental Assistants' Association
P.O. Box 294
Kenaston, SK S0G 2N0
Canada
306-252-2769
online: *www.sdaa.sk.ca*

Ontario Dental Assistants Association
869 Dundas Street
London, ON N5W 2Z8
Canada
519-679-2566
Email: info@odaa.org
online: *www.odaa.org*

Nova Scotia Dental Assistants Association
P.O. Box 9142
Station "A"
Halifax, NS B3K 5M8
Canada
902-405-1122
Email: nsdaa@eastlink.ca
online: *www.nsdaa.ca*

Product Guides

Reality
(Guide to dental products and techniques)
Reality Publishing Company
11757 Katy Freeway, Suite 210
Houston, TX 77079
281-558-9101
Email: info@realirtesthetics.com
online: *www.realityesthetics.com*

The Dental Advisor
(Product and equipment guide and evaluation)
Dental Consultants, Inc.
3110 West Liberty
Ann Arbor, MI 48103
734-665-2020
Email: info@dentaladvisor.com
online: *www.dentaladvisor.com*

Dental Products Report
(Product equipment guide and techniques)
641 Lexington Avenue, 8th Floor
New York, NY 10022
212-951-6600
Email: info@dentalproductsreport.com
online: *www.dentalproductsreport.com*

Dental Office
(Innovative ideas for dentists and assistants)
Penn Well Publications
1421 S. Sheridan Road
Tulsa, OK 74112
(800) 331-4463
online: *www.dentistryiq.com*

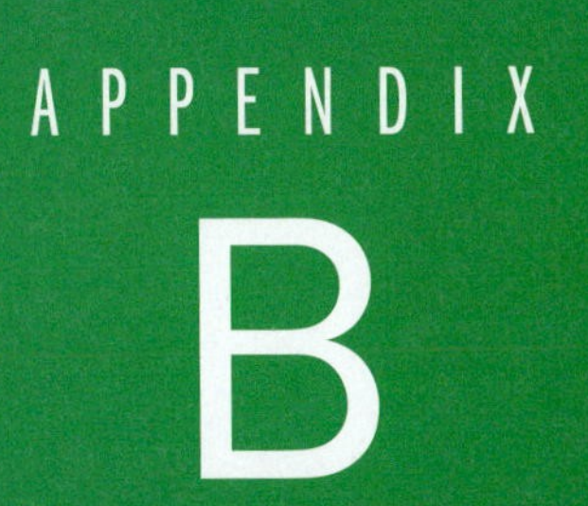

Stages of Tooth Eruption

Development of Human Dentition

Prenatal	Infancy	Early Childhood
4 months in utero	Birth	18–30 months
6 months in utero	4–8 months	2–3 years
Primary Dentition Permanent Dentition	8–12 months	3–4 years
	9–15 months	4–5 years
	15–21 months	5–6 years

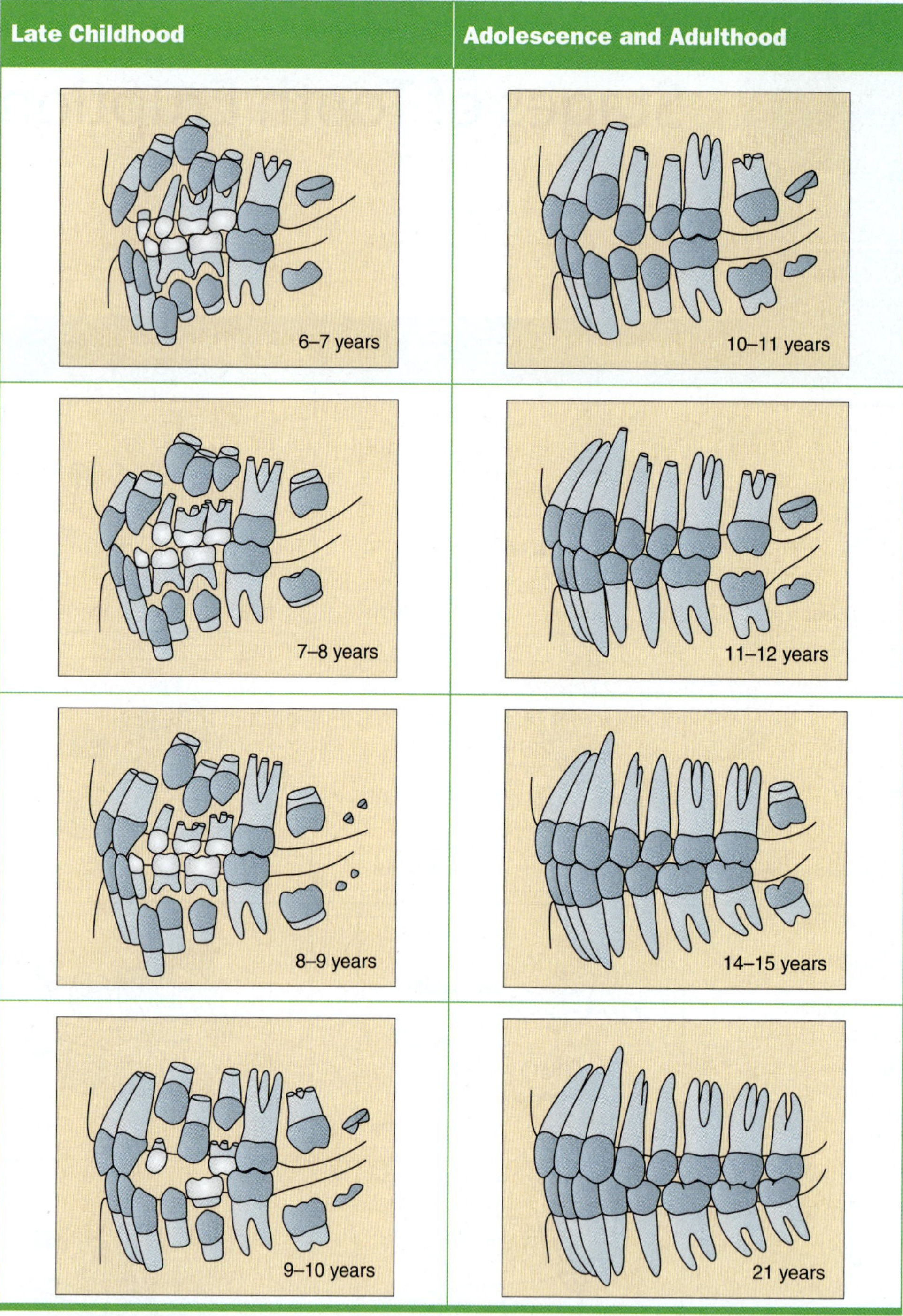
Late Childhood
Adolescence and Adulthood
6–7 years
10–11 years
7–8 years
11–12 years
8–9 years
14–15 years
9–10 years
21 years

GLOSSARY

A

3D dental imaging 3 dimensional imaging technology that shows a 3-D dental image scan of a patient's mouth, face, and jaw areas including the condyles and surrounding structures (Ch. 23)

3D Radiographic imaging an imaging technique that shows immediate three-dimensional reconstruction of a patient's mouth, face, and jaw areas including condyles and surrounding structures; tooth positions are visualized to show impactions in alveolar bone, location of adjacent teeth, and proximity to vital structures such as the mandibular nerve canal and sinus walls (Ch. 23)

abandonment desertion; refusal to treat a patient without notice (Ch. 3)

abrasive materials that cut or grind a surface leaving grooves and a rough surface; in powder or paste form (Ch. 32)

abrasive polishing strip used for small stains and only on enamel surfaces; also called finishing strips (Ch. 32)

Abrasive rotary instrument a non-bladed instrument used to finish and polish restorations and appliances (Ch. 18)

abscess local area of pus and infection (Chs. 14, 24, and 27)

abscessed tooth an infected tooth that causes the patient pain (Ch. 16)

abutment a tooth, a root, or an implant for retaining a fixed or removable prosthesis; the teeth adjacent to a pontic in a bridge (Chs. 14 and 33)

abutment post a post that is screwed into the implant after the healing cap is removed (Ch. 26)

accelerates speeds the process of (Ch. 39)

accounts payable amount a business or an office owes for goods or services (Ch. 40)

accounts receivable amount a business or an office is owed for goods or services (Ch. 40)

acetic acid chemical used in development of radiographs to stop the developing action and provide the required acidity for the sodium thiosulfate to work (Ch. 22)

acidulated phosphate fluoride APF solutions and gels are the preferred method of topical fluoride treatment because of patient acceptability and greater uptake of the fluoride by the surface enamel of the tooth (Ch. 4)

acquired immunity protection developed as a result of exposure to a pathogen (Ch. 10)

acrylic bur tool used to adjust acrylic materials, such as partials, dentures, and custom trays; also referred to as a laboratory bur (Ch. 18)

actinomycosis an infection caused by bacteria, characterized by painful swelling followed by discharge of pus and yellow granules (Ch. 27)

activator orthopedic appliance that widens the maxillary arch (Ch. 28)

activity zones four zones of an area around the patient: operating, assisting, static, and transfer (Ch. 17)

acute fluoride poisoning this occurs when large amounts of fluoride are ingested, inhaled, or absorbed into the body at one time (Ch. 4)

acute inflammation when the body's response to injury is minor and doesn't last long. Tissues heal quickly (Ch. 27)

ADA seal of acceptance products are subjected to a rigorous scientific review by the ADA Council on Scientific Affairs (CSA) to determine if they meet ADA criteria for safety and effectiveness; products that meet these criteria are awarded the ADA Seal of Acceptance, which will appear on product packaging and labeling (Ch. 4)

addiction physical or psychological dependency (Ch. 15)

adhesives materials that improve retention between two objects; also known as bonding agents (Ch. 37)

administrative area where the office manager or business assistant manages the business part of the dental practice. This area is close to the front of the office and has a desk, computer system, copier, phone system, and the business files (Ch. 17)

aerobic bacteria require oxygen to grow and live (Ch. 10)

aerosol a spray of particle-containing air (Ch. 11)

agenesis occurs when the tooth buds do not form (Ch. 9)

agent 1. a person whose discussions and actions are a reflection and representation of the person he or she is working for (Ch. 3); 2. an entity that is capable of causing a disease (Chs. 3 and 33)

air abrasion a technique used for specific dental procedures to remove micro amounts of tooth structure in the cavity preparation (Ch. 18)

air compressor tool that provides compressed air for handpieces and air–water syringes (Ch. 17)

airborne transmission mode of disease transmission through contaminated droplets or dust particles that are suspended in the air (Ch. 11)

air–water syringe a device the dentist uses that provides air or water or a combination spray of air and water (Chs. 17 and 19)

alcohol-based hand antiseptic a substance containing either isopropanol, ethanol, n-propanolol, or a combination of two of these products used for antimicrobial properties to cleanse the hands (Ch. 11)

alkalosis an increase in blood alkalinity (Ch. 16)

allergens substances that produce allergic reactions (Ch. 10)

allergic reactions the overreactions of the body to particular allergens; itching, redness of the skin, and hives are symptoms (Ch. 16)

alloy combination of two or more metals (Ch. 38)

aluminum filter a solid metal filter, usually made of aluminum that is put in the path of x-rays to eliminate the soft x-rays (Ch. 21)

alveolar crest where two cortical bone plates come together between each tooth (Ch. 8)

alveolar mucosa thin, loosely attached mucosa covering the alveolar bone; alveolar process forms the bone that supports the maxillary and mandibular teeth (Ch. 8)

alveolar process the bone that supports the teeth in both arches (Ch. 8)

alveoli part of the alveolar sacs in the lungs where gas exchange occurs (Ch. 6)

alveolitis complication following tooth extraction involving the loss of the blood clot, leaving a "dry socket" that can be very painful (Chs. 16 and 25)

alveolodental ligament fiber groups six groups of fibers in the alveolodental tissues; alveolar crest, horizontal, oblique, apical, interradicular, and interdental fiber groups (Ch. 8)

alveolus the bone that surrounds the root of the tooth, the socket (Ch. 8)

alveoplasty surgical contouring of the alveolar bone (Ch. 25)

amalgam an effective, long-lasting, and comparatively inexpensive material (an alloy with mercury) used for tooth restoration (Ch. 38)

amalgam carrier an instrument designed to carry and dispense amalgam or composite into the cavity preparation (Ch. 18)

amalgam condenser an instrument used to pack amalgam into the cavity preparation (Ch. 18)

amalgam gun an instrument used to carry and place composites, glass ionomers, and amalgam alloys (Ch. 18)

amalgam tattoo blue-to-gray gingival tissue in an area where amalgam particles have become trapped in the tissue (Ch. 27)

amalgamation the actual chemical reaction that occurs between the alloy and the mercury to form the silver amalgam (Ch. 38)

amalgamator a small machine that mixes dental amalgam and other dental materials (Chs. 17 and 34)

ameloblasts enamel-forming cells (Chs. 4 and 8)

amelogenesis imperfecta genetic condition where tooth enamel is either discolored, partially missing, or extremely thin (Ch. 27)

amenorrhea absence of monthly menstrual periods (Ch. 5)

American Academy of Cosmetic Dentistry (AACD) largest international organization dedicated to the art and science of cosmetic dentistry (Ch. 35)

American Dental Assistants Association (ADAA) the national professional organization for dental assistants; local and state branches exist with a national office in Chicago (Chs. 1 and 41)

American Dental Association (ADA) the national professional organization for dentists (Chs. 1 and 41)

American Dental Hygienists' Association (ADHA) Association (ADHA) the national professional organization for dental hygienists (Ch. 1)

American Dental Laboratory Technician Association (ADLTA) national organization that represents dental laboratory technicians (Ch. 1)

Americans with Disabilities Act legislation passed by Congress in 1990 to end discrimination against people with disabilities (Chs. 3 and 40)

American National Standards Institute (ANSI) is the organization that classifies dental x-ray film (Ch. 21)

anaerobic bacteria can only survive without the presence of oxygen and are destroyed by oxygen (Ch. 10)

analgesic a drug that relieves pain (e.g., aspirin or morphine) (Ch. 15)

Analgesia the absence of pain (Ch.20)

analog image an image depicted as a continuous spectrum of gray shades between black and white (Ch. 23)

anaphylactic shock an immediate, severe, sometimes fatal reaction to allergens (Ch. 10)

anatomical term for posterior denture teeth; resemble natural teeth with cusps and developmental grooves (Ch. 36)

anatomical crown portion of the tooth covered with enamel (Ch. 9)

anatomical root the portion of the tooth covered with cementum (Ch. 9)

anatomy the study of the body structure (Ch. 6)

anchor tooth tooth on which the dental dam clamp is placed; usually one or two teeth distal to the tooth or teeth being restored (Ch. 19)

anesthesia drugs that cause a loss of pain but not a loss of all sensation; usually used before surgeries (Chs. 15 and 20)

angina pectoris pain in the chest that may radiate into the jaw, neck, or arm (Ch. 16)

angioedema large urticaria (hives) brought on by an allergic reaction (Ch. 16)

angle former a tool used in a downward pushing motion to form and define point angles and to sharpen line angles (Ch. 18)

Angle's classification system used to classify malocclusion (Ch. 28)

Angulation in reference to dental radiology, is the alignment of the central x-ray beam in vertical and horizontal planes (Ch. 22)

angular cheilitis inflammation of the corners of the mouth (Ch. 27)

ankyloglossia a condition in which the lingual frenum is attached near the tip of the tongue thus limiting movement of the tongue (Ch. 27)

ankylosis a condition in which the tooth, cementum, or dentin fuses with the alveolar bone, restricting movement of the tooth (Ch. 27)

anode the positive terminal of an electrolytic cell (Ch. 21)

anodontia the congenital absence of teeth (Ch. 27)

anorexia nervosa an eating disorder characterized by severe weight loss, an extreme aversion to food, and a fear of being fat (Ch. 5)

antagonistic pair sets of muscles where when one set contracts, the corresponding set relaxes; the body moves and functions through these coordinated efforts (Ch. 6)

antecubital space the indented area inside of the elbow as the arm is stretched straight (Ch. 13)

antibacterial effect the condition that inhibits the growth of acids responsible for decay (Ch. 4)

Antibody produce immunity against any foreign substance or pathogen. The body utilizes antibodies as its final defense (Ch.10)

antigenic capable of causing the production of an antibody (Ch. 27)

antigens pathogens that stimulate the production of antibodies (Ch. 10)

antihistamine drugs that counteract the body's production of histamine (Ch. 16)

antimicrobial a microorganism growth inhibitor (e.g., antimicrobial soap) (Ch. 11)

antipyretic an agent that reduces fever (Ch. 13)

antisepsis the inhibition of the growth of causative microorganisms (Ch. 11)

antitoxin an antibody produced in response to and capable of neutralizing a biologic toxin (Ch. 10)

aorta largest artery that receives blood directly from the heart (Ch. 6)

apex at or near the end of the root (Ch. 9)

apex finder a unit that measures the distance to the apex of a tooth and displays the information on a digital readout (Ch. 24)

apexification the treatment of the apex of the root canal in a tooth that is necrotic (Ch. 24)

apexogenesis pulpotomy of permanent tooth whereby pulp vitality is maintained, allowing time for the root end to develop and close (Chs. 24 and 29)

aphthous ulcers painful ulcers that appear in the oral cavity; a circular lesion appears with a yellow center and red "halo" surrounding the lesion; sometimes called a canker sore (Chs. 10 and 27)

apical curettage removal of diseased tissues by scraping with a curette after the apex of the tooth has been removed (Ch.24)

apical elevator similar to elevators but with a larger handle and smaller working ends; used to loosen and remove roots or bone fragments (Ch. 25)

apical foramen an opening in the end of the tooth through which nerve and blood vessels enter (Ch. 9)

apical periodontitis pulpal inflammation that extends into the periapical tissues (Ch. 24)

apical third the root of the tooth is divided into imaginary thirds with the area nearest the apex as the apical third (Ch. 9)

apicoectomy removal of the apex of the root and infection surrounding the area (Ch. 24)

aponeurosis a specialized connective tissue extension, broad and flattened, attaches muscle to bone and binds muscle to muscle (Ch. 6)

appendicular skeleton one of the two main divisions of the skeleton, composed of the bones from the upper and lower extremities including arms, hands, legs, feet, shoulders, and hips (Ch. 6)

apposition in the life cycle of a tooth when the calcium salts and other minerals are deposited and when the tissues or enamel, dentin, and cementum are formed in layers (Ch. 8)

arch wire wires used to apply force to move or hold teeth in desired positions (Ch. 28)

argon laser a curing light technology, light amplification by stimulated emission of radiation; produces a relatively high-intensity light that does not generate noticeable heat; some disadvantages include lack of compatibility with some dental materials and the expense (Ch. 17)

armamentarium all materials and instruments needed to complete a dental procedure (Ch. 25)

arrhythmia irregular pattern of the heartbeat (Ch. 13)

arteriole smallest arteries (Ch. 6)

arteriosclerosis hardening of the arteries (Ch. 16)

artery carries oxygenated blood from the heart to the capillaries of the tissues (Ch. 6)

arthrocentesis the irrigation of the joint, a minimally invasive procedure used to treat TMJ disease (Ch. 25)

arthroplasty surgery to relieve pain and restore range of motion by realigning or reconstructing a joint; includes several types of surgeries for the TMJ (Ch. 25)

arthroscopy involves the surgeon inserting a tiny instrument through a small incision to remove adhesions and place anti-inflammatory agents (Ch. 25)

articular disc also known as meniscus, it is a dense, fibrous connective tissue that is thicker at the ends attached to the condyle (Ch. 7)

articular eminence recontouring shortening and smoothing of the articular eminence to prevent or reduce the excessive forces, and improve the range of motion and lessen the pain (Ch. 25)

articulation joint where two or more bones meet or form a junction (Ch. 6)

articulator a frame representing the jaw that holds models of the patient's teeth to maintain the patient's occlusion; a mechanical device that represents the temporomandibular joints to which upper and lower casts of the dental arches may be attached to simulate mouth functions (Ch. 39)

artificial acquired immunity protection from a pathogen for an individual who has been vaccinated with a specific antigen (Ch. 10)

artificial teeth a component of the removable denture that is made of either acrylic resin or porcelain and secured to the denture base by pins or holes on the undersides of the teeth (Ch. 36)

as low as reasonably achievable (ALARA) the principle of keeping radiation exposure "as low as reasonably achievable"; it involves combining radiation protection procedures with commonsense practices (Ch. 21)

asepsis the creation of an environment free of pathogens (Ch. 11)

aseptic technique steps necessary to ensure an environment free from pathogens; handwashing, for example (Ch. 11)

Aspirates process of drawing back, such as when the operator retracts the thumb ring on the syringe once the needle is in the tissues and a negative pressure is created (Ch. 20)

aspirating syringe most common type of syringe designed to allow the operator to check the position of the needle before depositing the anesthetic solution (Ch. 20)

assault threat of touching a person without consent (Ch. 3)

assessment a judgment about the patient's health based on an understanding of the situation and upcoming treatment that is completed by the auxiliary and the findings reported to the dentist (Ch. 13)

assistant's cart a mobile cart that is usually set up with the air–water syringe, saliva ejector, and HVE (Ch. 17)

assisted whitening combination of dental office and home bleaching process (Ch. 35)

assisting zone the area in which the dental assistant is positioned to easily assist the dentist and have access to instruments, the evacuator, and the dental unit or cart without interference (Ch. 17)

asymmetric unequal shapes, sizes, and relative positions of body parts on opposite sides (Ch. 13)

asymptomatic having no symptoms (Ch. 11)

Atom makes up all matter, composed of a nucleus, inner core that is positively charged and negatively charged particles (electrons) that orbit the nucleus (Ch. 21)

attached gingiva extends from the mucogingival junction to the gingival groove; it is stippled and attached tightly to the alveolar bone (Ch. 8)

attrition the wearing away of the incisal or occlusal surfaces of the tooth during normal function; the final stage of the life cycle of the tooth (Ch. 8)

atypical unusual, not the normal finding (Ch. 27)

automatic processing processing of dental x-rays using automated equipment (Ch. 22)

autoMatrix a matrix without a retainer (Ch. 38)

autonomic nervous system (ANS) collection of nerves, ganglia, and plexuses through which visceral organs, heart, blood vessels, glands, and smooth muscles receive their innervation (Ch. 6)

auxiliary polishing aid aids used during coronal polishing procedures, including bridge threaders, abrasive polishing strips, soft wooden points, and small interproximal brushes (Ch. 32)

avulsed tooth a tooth that has been removed from the mouth; avulsed teeth should be replanted immediately (if possible) or transported to the dentist in milk, saliva, saline, or water (Chs. 16 and 29)

axial plane plane around which computed tomography is achieved (Ch. 23)

axial skeleton one of the two main divisions of the skeleton includes bones of the cranium, face, spinal column, ribs, and sternum (Ch. 6)

axial wall walls parallel to the long axis of the tooth (Ch. 37)

axons nerve fibers that conduct impulses away from the cell body (Ch. 6)

B

baby boomer generation set of individuals who were born in the United States between the years 1946 to 1964, and is often thought of as those born after World War II (Ch. 2)

bacilli a type of bacteria that produces spores (Ch. 10)

bacteria tiny, simple, single-celled plants that contain no chlorophyll (Ch. 10)

bacterial plaque a local irritant that is a common cause of the inflammation of the gingival tissues (Ch. 31)

band part of the matrix that forms the missing surface or wall of a tooth (Ch. 38)

barbed broach endodontic instruments used to remove soft tissue from the pulp canal (Ch. 24)

barriers coverings used wherever possible in all aspects of the dental office. Inside the operatory, barriers cover the patient dental chair, light (handles and operating switch), handpieces, air–water syringe, high-volume evacuator, saliva ejector, tubing, writing utensils, and surfaces (Ch. 11)

bar-type clasp a retainer design that extends from a gingival direction toward the occlusal (Ch. 36)

basal cell carcinoma most common form of skin cancer (Ch. 27)

basal cells some of the deepest cells in the dermis (Ch. 21)

basal metabolic rate (BMR) the energy that is used when a person is at rest (Ch. 5)

base material applied in a putty or thick layer between the tooth and restoration to protect the pulp from chemical, electrical, mechanical, or thermal irritation (Ch. 37)

baseline vital signs the initial reading of basic signs of life, including body temperature, pulse, blood pressure, and respiration rate (Ch. 13)

baseplate preformed, semirigid acrylic resin material that represents the denture base temporarily (Ch. 36)

battery according to the law, the actual touching of another individual without consent (Ch. 3)

beading process used with utility wax to curb impressions before boxing and pouring (Ch. 39)

behavior management plan to modify or maintain the desired behavior of a person or group of persons (Ch. 29)

bell stage the stage where cell specialization or histodifferentiation takes place (Ch. 8)

Bell's palsy the temporary paralysis of the muscles on one side of the face (Ch. 27)

bevel slanted edge or side on the working end of an instrument (Chs. 18 and 33)

bi-beveled beveled (slanted) on both sides of the blade (Ch. 18)

bicanineate a larger single buccal cusp and a lingual cusp (Ch. 9)

bicuspids another term used for premolars—they have two cusps (Ch. 9)

bifid tongue the failure of the lateral halves of the anterior two-thirds of the tongue to fuse completely (Ch. 27)

bifurcated one tooth with two roots (Ch. 9)

bile substance produced by the liver, emulsifies fat (Ch. 6)

binangle dental instrument on which the shank has two angles (Ch. 18)

binging overeating that is a response to stress or depression (Ch. 5)

bioburden the number of microorganisms, such as blood, saliva, and other body fluids contaminating an object, that has not been sterilized (Ch. 11)

biofilms microscopic communities that allow bacteria, fungi, and viruses to multiply (Ch. 11)

biological monitor most accurate way to assess whether sterilization has occurred, often commercially prepared (Ch. 11)

bionator appliance an acrylic appliance that fits on the upper and lower teeth, and positions the lower jaw forward; it is used to encourage lower jaw growth (Ch. 28)

biopsy surgical removal of a small amount of tissue (Chs. 25 and 27)

biotin a vitamin found in both plant and animal foods; helps in energy metabolism (Ch. 5)

bisecting technique x-ray technique that applies the geometric principle in which the central ray bisects the angle formed by the dental film and the long axis of the tooth (Ch. 22)

bite registration an occlusal record of the relationship between the upper and lower teeth (Ch. 33)

bite rim several layers of baseplate wax that are attached to the baseplate to represent the space provided by teeth in normal occlusion, registering the vertical dimension for the denture and establishing the occlusal relationship of the mandibular and maxillary arches (Ch. 36)

bitewing radiograph an x-ray of the crowns of the teeth, interproximal spaces, and the crest area of the alveolar bone of both the maxillary and the mandibular teeth. Used to detect caries, faulty restorations, and calculus (Ch. 22)

black line stain formation of a thin black to dark brown line slightly above the gingiva and following the contour of the gingival margin; found primarily in women and often in cases of excellent oral hygiene (Ch. 32)

black's formula formula developed by G. V. Black to stan-dardize the exact size and angulation of an instrument (Ch. 18)

blade flat working end on a dental instrument (Ch. 18)

bleaching/whitening procedure for lightening teeth. Esthetically improving the shade of a person's teeth (Ch. 35)

Bleeding Index part of the periodontal examination that involves recording the amount of blood/fluid present during probing (Ch. 31)

blister a raised, fluid-filled area, usually oval or circular (Ch. 27)

blood main functions include transportation of nutrients, gases, waste products, and hormones; regulation of the amount of body fluids, pH balance, and body temperature; and protection against pathogens and blood loss after injury through clotting mechanism (Ch. 6)

blood pressure indicator of the health of a patient's cardiovascular system. Measured by systolic blood pressure and diastolic blood pressure using a sphygmomanometer and stethoscope

bloodborne pathogens disease-spreading organisms found in the blood, can be passed on by contact with the blood of an infected individual (Ch. 10)

Bloodborne Pathogens Standard effective in 1992, a federal standard instituted in the hope of reducing the occupational-related cases of HIV and hepatitis B infection among health care workers (Ch. 11)

blurred image images on x-ray film that are out of focus (Ch. 22)

body cavity space or area in the body where various structures and organs are found (Ch. 6)

body mass index (BMI) energy that is used when a person is at rest (Ch. 5)

body substance isolation (BSI) a system of techniques requiring personal protective equipment to be worn to protect against contact with all body fluids, whether or not blood is visible (Ch. 11)

Bonding the process by which materials adhere firmly or hold together (Chs. 30 and 37)

bonding agent materials, usually low-viscosity resins, used to improve retention between two objects (in dentistry, between the tooth structure [enamel and dentin] and the restoration); also known as adhesives, bonding resins; mainly light or dull cured (Ch. 39)

bonding resins materials used to improve the retention between the tooth structure (enamel and dentin) and the restoration; also called bonding agents and adhesives (Ch. 37)

bone grafting moving tissue from one area to another; adding bone or a bone substitute to fill areas (Ch. 31)

bones of the cranium eight bones that make up the cranium, including frontal, parietal, temporal, occipital, ethmoid, and sphenoid (Ch. 7)

bones of the face fourteen bones that make up the face, including nasal, vomer, inferior conchae, lacrimal, maxillae, zygomatic, palatine, and mandible (Ch. 7)

border molding when receiving a final impression, the impression compound is heated and placed along the borders of the custom tray; the tray is cooled and placed in the patient's mouth; and the lips, cheeks, and tongue are moved to establish accurate length for the periphery and adjacent tissues to be included in the final impression (Ch. 36)

brachial artery main artery of the arm (Ch. 13)

brackets devices attached to the teeth to hold the arch wire in place and transmit the force of the arch wire to move the tooth (Ch. 28)

bradycardia abnormally slow heart rate (Ch. 13)

bradypnea abnormally slow respiratory rate at rest (Ch. 13)

brand name manufacturer assigns name to the drug they created. Often referred to as trade names, are always capitalized and have registered trademarks (Ch. 15)

breach of contract breaking of a contract (Ch. 3)

Bremsstrahlung radiation is the primary type of radiation in the x-ray beam going out from the tubehead (Ch. 21)

bridge a fixed prosthetic device placed in the mouth to replace missing teeth (Ch. 14)

bridge threader used to pull the dental tape and floss under fixed appliances, around orthodontic appliances, and around splints so that all proximal surfaces can be cleaned and polished (Ch. 32)

broad spectrum refers to drugs, specifically antibiotics, that are effective against a wide range of bacteria, not just one specific bacteria (Ch. 15)

broad spectrum activity to kill a wide range of microbes. Phenolics, or synthetic phenolics are used for intermediate-level disinfectants and have this ability (Ch. 11)

bronchi two branches that form at the end of the trachea and enter the lungs (Ch. 6)

bronchioles small branches of the bronchiole tubes that divide into alveolar sacs (Chs. 6 and 16)

brown stain staining of the teeth generally associated with plaque and most commonly found on the buccal surface of the maxillary molars and lingual surface of the mandibular incisors (Ch. 32)

bruxism teeth grinding (Chs. 31 and 37)

buccal the surface of the posterior tooth that is toward the cheeks (Ch. 9)

buccal groove a linear depression forming a groove that extends from the middle of the buccal surface to the occlusal surface of the tooth (Ch. 9)

buccal tubes small cylinders of metal welded to the molar bands providing a means of attachment for the arch wire to the band in the posterior area (Ch. 28)

buccoversion a tooth that is tipped toward the lip or cheek (Ch. 27)

bud stage the first stage of odontogenesis, initiation of the tooth begins (Ch. 8)

bulimia a psychological disorder that is characterized by secretive bouts of gross overeating followed by methods of weight control such as purging, laxative abuse, excessive exercise, and over usage of diuretics (Ch. 5)

bulla a large, fluid-filled blister; greater than 1/2 inch in diameter (Ch. 27)

bur device used to store rotary instruments (Ch. 18)

bur block device used to store rotary instruments (Ch. 18)

burnish to smooth (Ch. 38)

burnisher instrument used to smooth rough margins of the restoration and to shape metal matrix bands (Ch. 18)

business associates indirect providers of health care services and supplies such as accounting firms, consultants, legal firms, management companies, data/record copying, storage and destruction companies, and suppliers (Ch. 3)

C

CAD/CAM restorative systems a restoration system that allows metal-free, tooth-colored restorations to be fabricated in one appointment (Ch. 34)

calcification the process of depositing calcium salts and other materials in the formed tooth, it takes place in the apposition stage of tooth development (Ch. 8)

calcination the process of driving a specific amount of water out of gypsum to create specific plasters, stones, or investment die stones (Ch. 39)

calcium a major mineral found in bones and teeth and functions in muscle contraction, the nervous system, and the blood (Ch. 5)

Calcium hydroxide type of cementation used as a low-strength base under any restoration (Ch. 37)

calculus hard, calcified deposit of mineralized plaque that forms on teeth, restorations, and dental appliances; also known as tartar (Ch. 31)

Calorie units of heat; the large Calorie (which is always capitalized) is the amount of heat needed to change the temperature of l gram of water from 14.5° C to 15.5° C; one thousand kilo calories make up l calorie (Ch. 5)

cancellous bone sponge-like tissue (Ch. 6)

candida albicans yeast-like fungus (Ch. 26)

canine cuspid; third tooth from the midline; bulkier and aids in tearing food (Ch. 9)

canine eminence a bony ridge covering the labial portion of the roots (Ch. 9)

canker sores painful ulcers that appear in the oral cavity; circular lesions appear with yellow centers and red "halos" surrounding the lesion; sometimes called aphthous ulcers (Ch. 27)

cannula small hollow tube (Ch. 30)

cantilever bridge prosthetic device in mouth attached at only one side; useful in an area with little stress such as a missing lateral (Chs. 14 and 33)

cap stage the bud of the tooth grows and changes shape (Ch. 8)

capillary the connection between the arteries and the veins where the exchange is made between the blood and body cells (Ch. 6)

capnograph a medical device that is used to measure the carbon dioxide (CO_2) concentration in an air sample (Ch. 16)

capnometry the measurement and numerical display of maximum inhalation and expiratory CO_2 concentrations during a respiratory cycle (Ch. 16)

capsule cylindrical device that contains a premeasured amount of alloy and mercury (Ch. 38)

carbamide peroxide a material used for teeth whitening and is used in a 10–20 percent solution; a thickening agent is added to increase adhesion (Ch. 35)

carbohydrates one of the six broad categories of nutrients primarily found in fruits, grains, legumes, and some vegetable roots (Ch. 5)

carborundum disc thin, brittle discs: double-sided and are used primarily in the dental laboratory to cut and finish gold restorations, but they can be used intraorally as well (Ch. 18)

Cardiac muscle found only in the heart, receives an impulse, responds and relaxes at a rapid pace that keeps the heart beating in an even rhythm (Ch. 6)

cardiopulmonary rescue breathing and chest compressions performed on a patient experiencing cardiac arrest (Ch. 16)

caries dental cavities; tooth decay (Chs. 4 and 14)

cariogenic foods that break down into simple sugars in the mouth and can be used by the bacteria to cause dental caries (Ch. 5)

carotene vitamin A that comes from plants (Ch. 5)

carotid pulse pulse found in the carotid artery located in the neck (Ch. 13)

carpules glass containers of anesthetic solution (Ch. 20)

cartilage a tough nonvascular, resilient, specialized connective tissue (Ch. 6)

cartridges glass containers of anesthetic solution (Ch. 20)

carver instrument used to remove excess restorative material and to carve tooth anatomy in the restoration before the material hardens (Ch. 18)

cassette a container for extraoral radiographic film containing intensifying screens; available in hard or soft lightproof containers (Ch. 23)

cast restoration prosthetic device that is cemented and bonded in place to restore tooth function (Ch. 30)

catalyst an ingredient that starts or accelerates a process (Ch. 35)

cathode the negative terminal of an x-ray tube (Ch. 21)

cavitation a process where bubbles are formed (Ch. 11)

cavity detection methods use of radiographs, by probing with an explorer, with use of a special dye or with a Class II laser that measures fluorescence levels in the tooth structure to quantify (37)

cavity liner low-strength bases placed in the deepest portion of the cavity preparation, on the dentin or exposed pulp, which harden to form a cement layer to protect the pulp from chemical irritations and provide a therapeutic effect on the tooth (Ch. 33)

cavity preparation preparation for a restoration; technique depends on the amount and location of decay, degree of pulpal involvement, and type of materials used to restore the tooth (Ch. 33)

cavity varnish used to seal the dentin tubules to prevent acids, saliva, and debris from reaching the pulp; when used with cavity liner or medicated base, it is placed on top of these materials (Ch. 33)

cavosurface margin angle that is formed by the junction of the wall of a cavity preparation and the untouched surface of the tooth; sealing of this margin is critical to prevent marginal leakage (Ch. 33)

cell the smallest functioning unit of the body; contains cell membrane, nucleus, cytoplasm, and chromosomes (Ch. 6)

cellulitis swelling and discomfort of facial tissues caused by an abscess (Chs. 24 and 27)

celsius the centigrade measure of temperature; the freezing point is 0 degrees and the boiling point is 100 degrees (Ch. 13)

cement base high-strength bases of thick, putty-like consistency placed on the floor of a cavity preparation to protect the pulp and provide mechanical support for the restoration; preparation, pulp sensitivity, and type of restoration indicate which cement to use (Ch. 37)

cement spatula instrument used to mix dental materials (Ch. 18)

cemental spur found near the cementoenamel junction (CEJ), it appears similar to calculus (Ch. 8)

cementoblasts cementum-forming cells (Ch. 8)

cementoclasts cells that resorb cementum (Ch. 8)

cementum the tooth structure that is located around the root covering the dentin on the root portion of the tooth (Ch. 8)

central beam the primary ray emitting from the x-ray tube head (Ch. 21)

central groove most prominent developmental groove on the occlusal surface of the posterior teeth (Ch. 9)

central incisor the first tooth starting from the midline; used to cut or bite the food that is ingested (Ch. 9)

central nervous system (CNS) the brain and the spinal cord (Ch. 6)

central ray x-rays at the center of the x-ray beam (Ch. 22)

central vacuum system system that provides suction for saliva ejectors and oral evacuators (Ch. 17)

centric occlusion closing of the jaws in a position that maximizes contact between the occluding surfaces of the maxillary and the mandibular arch (Ch. 36)

centric relation position of the mandible when the condyles are positioned posterosuperiorly in an unstrained position in the glenoid fossae (Ch. 36)

centric relationship where the teeth are positioned when the joints are aligned. Patients often rest in this centric relationship (Ch. 39)

cephalometric extraoral radiographs showing patient profiles, including bones and tissues (Ch. 23)

cephalostat head holding device used to position the patient's head when taking a cephalometric x-ray (Ch. 23)

CERAC CAD/CAM retraction systems a restoration system that allows metal-free, tooth-colored restorations to be fabricated in one appointment (Ch. 34)

ceramometal restoration used in conditions of heavy occlusal stress and for multiple-unit fixed prostheses (Ch. 35)

cerebral embolism a blood clot that blocks the normal flow of blood to the brain (Ch. 16)

cerebral hemorrhage rupture of a blood vessel in the brain (Ch. 16)

cerebral infarction an interruption of the flow of blood to the brain (Ch. 16)

certified dental assistant(CDA) a dental assistant who has obtained national certification through the Dental Assisting National Board (Ch. 1)

certified mail mail sent that provides the sender confirmation of delivery (Ch. 40)

cervical clamps double-bowed clamps used for Class V restorations on anterior teeth; help with gingival retraction; often must be stabilized with stick impression compound after the teeth have been exposed (Ch. 19)

cervical line where the anatomical crown and root join (Ch. 9)

cervical third the area on the crown of the tooth that is nearest the cervical (or nearest the gingival) (Ch. 9)

chain of asepsis aseptic procedures ensuring that no cross-contamination occurs (Ch. 11)

chain of infection the elements of an infectious process. It is an interactive process that involves the agent, host, and environment (Ch. 11)

chalk a mild abrasive used in some prophylactic pastes; also known as whiting (Ch. 32)

chamfer a type of crown preparation that provides adequate bulk and extends easily into the gingival sulcus (Ch. 33)

Chapin A. Harris started the first dental college in the world, the Baltimore College of Dental Surgery in 1840 (Ch. 1)

Charge-coupled device (CCD) an image receptor; converts x-rays to electrons (Ch. 23)

check register record of all checking account transactions; includes deposits to and checks made from the account (Ch. 40)

cheek retractor instrument used to keep the cheek out of the way during dental procedures (Ch. 25)

cheilosis a condition due to Vitamin B deficiency where lips become red and fissures develop in the corners of the mouth (Ch. 5)

chelating a process by which an agent encloses or grasps a toxic substance and makes it nontoxic (Ch. 24)

chemical retention a chemical reaction occurs between the tooth surface and a material that allows the material to be held in place (Ch. 37)

chemical vapor sterilizer uses a pressurized gaseous vapor of formaldehyde and alcohol for sterilization. Heat unit to 132°C (270°F) for 20 minutes in order to sterilize either loose or wrapped instruments (Ch. 11)

Chemically cured type of sealant material that is hardened by use of a catalyst and a base; also known as self-cure or autopolymerization (Ch. 30)

chisel used to shape and plane (make surface flat or level) enamel and dentin walls of the cavity preparation. The blade of the chisel is straight and has a cutting edge with a one-sided bevel (Ch. 18)

chisel scaler a periodontal instrument used most often in the anterior of the mouth (Ch. 31)

chlorine a mineral which maintains the correct pH balance in blood (Ch. 5)

chroma the intensity or quality of the hue (Ch. 35)

chromium a trace mineral involved in the process of metabolism (Ch. 5)

chronic a disease or disorder that is present throughout one's life (Ch. 13)

chronic fluoride poisoning this occurs over a period of time with ingestion of high fluoride levels in the water or by a combination of several fluoride sources (Ch. 4)

Chronic inflammation occurs when the tissues do not heal quickly and the inflammation process continues (Ch. 27)

chronological order dates in order of occurrence (Ch. 13)

chuck a small metal cylinder in the head of the handpiece that holds rotary instruments (Ch. 18)

chyme mixture of food and gastric juices (Ch. 6)

cingulum a convex area on the lingual surface of the anterior teeth near the gingiva (Ch. 9)

circumference the distance around (Ch. 38)

circumferential-type clasp a retainer design that encircles and adapts to the contours of the abutment tooth (Ch. 36)

cirrhosis liver deterioration (Ch. 15)

civil law law related to actions and circumstances between individuals; civil law can be broken into contract law and tort law (Ch. 3)

classifications of motion the five classifications that show the amount of motion with which the dental team is involved (Ch. 17)

clear film a film that was not exposed to radiation (Ch. 22)

cleft lip cleft in or separation of the upper lip; also known as harelip; failure of the maxillary processes to fuse with the medial nasal process (Ch. 8)

cleft palate a fissure in the roof of the mouth that forms a passage between the nasal cavities and the mouth; failure of the palatal shelves to fuse with the primary palate or with each other (Ch. 8)

cleft uvula the uvula is separated slightly (Ch. 8)

clinical contact surface surfaces of concern by OSAP including areas that are directly touched and contaminated during dental treatment procedures, the surfaces not directly touched, but are areas or items that are indirectly contaminated, surfaces that dental personnel do not actually contact, but still may be contaminated (Ch. 11)

clinical crown exposed coronal portion of the crowns (Ch. 9)

clinical root the portion of the root seen in the oral cavity (Ch. 9)

closing prescription closing; area on the prescription where dentists sign their names and authorize whether prescriptions can be refilled and how many times; also notes whether a generic brand of the medication can be dispensed in place of that written (Ch. 15)

coagulation blood clotting (Ch. 15)

coalesced fused (Ch. 30)

cobalt a trace mineral that helps in the functioning of red blood cells (Ch. 5)

cocci round or bead-shaped bacteria (Ch. 10)

cold sore a blister (Ch. 10)

collimator a device used to eliminate peripheral radiation (Ch. 21)

color-changing sealants sealants with a photoactive color additive that change to opaque after being light cured (Ch. 30)

commissures corners of the mouth where the upper lip meets the lower lip (Ch. 13)

common carotid artery supplying blood to most of the head and the neck, divided into internal and external branches (Ch. 7)

communication exchange of information and ideas (Ch. 2)

compact bone the strong and hard section of a bone is dense and forms the main shaft of long bones and the outer layer of other bones (Ch. 6)

complementary metal oxide semiconductor (CMOS) type of a sensor with technology that coverts x-rays into an electronic signal, which is sent to the computer (Ch. 23)

Compomer polyacid-modified resin used to cement all types of dental restorations and to restore teeth in non-stress-bearing areas (Ch. 37)

composite direct, tooth-colored restorative material (Ch. 38)

Composite resin material used to restore a tooth (Ch. 30)

Comprehensive Drug Abuse Prevention and Control Act of 1970 law that identifies drugs according to five schedules of potential abuse (Ch. 15)

compromised host an individual whose normal defense mechanisms are impaired (Ch. 11)

compules single-application cartridges (Ch. 38)

computed tomography (CT scanning) computer-produced image (Ch. 23)

computer surface A computerized system used to create a 3D record of the geometry of a preparation used in the creation and design of crowns, bridges, and veneers (Ch. 35)

computer-aided design (CAD) a computerized system used to create impressions for ceramic crowns, bridges, and veneers (Ch. 34)

computer-aided manufacturing (CAM) a computerized system used to construct ceramic crowns, bridges, and veneers (Ch. 34)

computer-controlled local used to administer all traditional infiltration and block injections; delivers a pressure and volume of anesthetic solution at a controlled rate (Ch. 20)

computerized units of computer parts that function together to perform tasks (Ch. 36)

concave recessed or indented (Ch. 9)

condensable composite also called packable composites, are putty-like and stiff in consistency; used in posterior areas (Ch. 38)

condensation build-up of particles, moisture, and algae in the compressor, to prevent filters should be changed routinely (Ch. 17)

cone cutting partial image created when the central beam misses the x-ray film (Ch. 22)

cone socket handle an instrument in which the working ends can be replaced (Ch. 18)

conflict disagreement or power struggle between individuals or groups (Ch. 2)

congenital present at birth (Ch. 27)

congestive heart failure a condition that occurs as the heart weakens, rendering it unable to achieve the level of cardiac output that meets the body's needs (Ch. 16)

conjunctivitis also called pink eye, is an inflammation of the eye caused by infection or the herpes simplex virus type 1 (Ch. 10)

connector elements that unite the parts of the partial into one unit; hold working parts in proper positions (Ch. 36)

conscious sedation a very safe means for patients to be free of pain and discomfort during dental procedures; patient can communicate during this process (Ch. 20)

consent form form signed by the patient indicating the patient's agreement to a particular procedure (Ch. 13)

consultation room/area private area away from the main flow of the office where the dentist can sit down with the patient and discuss the treatment plan and financial arrangement (Ch. 17)

contact area the proximal sides of where two teeth come together and touch; normally the medial of one tooth and the distal of another tooth (Ch. 9)

contact dermatitis disorder of the skin due to an irritant (Ch. 11)

contact transmission the physical transfer of an agent from an infected person to an uninfected person through direct contact with the infected person (Ch. 11)

continuous simple suture series of stitches that look like hem stitching; placed in areas of multiple extractions and tied with a surgeon's knot at either end (Ch. 25)

continuous sling suture series of sling stitches placed in areas with a large flap involving several teeth (Ch. 25)

contour lines of Owen contour lines in dentin that demonstrate a disturbance in the body metabolism (Ch. 8)

contra-angle attachment head for the low-speed handpiece; contra-angles hold burs, discs, stones, rubber cups, and brushes for intraoral and extraoral procedures; type of Tofflemire retainer, placed on the lingual side, angled slightly to clear the anterior teeth (Chs. 18 and 38)

contract a binding agreement between two or more persons (Ch. 3)

contrast difference between shades or colors (Ch. 21)

control panel device on a radiography machine where settings can be adjusted and changed and from which the operation of the machine takes place (Ch. 21)

Controlled Substances Act gives the power of enforcement of this act to the DEA, which is part of the U.S. Department of Justice (Ch. 15)

convex to bulge or curve outward (Ch. 9)

convulsion seizure (Ch. 16)

coordination of benefits (COB) when two insurance carriers coordinate the benefits not to exceed the total cost of the actual dental expense (Ch. 40)

copal varnish a cavity varnish containing organic solvents (ether, acetone, or chloroform) and is used only under metal restorations because the solvent material in the varnish may interfere with the setting action of composite and resins (Ch. 37)

copper a trace mineral involved in the process of metabolism (Ch. 5)

core buildup treatment performed for vital teeth and nonvital teeth that have very little crown structure; for this procedure, the dentist removes any decay and defective restoration and then builds a core that supports and provides more retention for the cast restoration (Ch. 33)

corneal ulcer an inflammatory condition of the cornea that results in the loss of the outer layer; can be caused by trauma, burns, infections, or the herpes simplex virus type 1 (Ch. 10)

coronal polish procedure whereby coronal surfaces of the teeth are polished with rubber cups, brushes, an abrasive, polishers, and dental tape (also known as prophylaxis) (Chs. 31 and 32)

corrective orthodontics the improvement of orthodontic problems (Ch. 28)

Corrosion the result of chemical or electrochemical attacks (Ch. 37)

cortical bone compact bone plates on the facial and lingual surfaces (Ch. 8)

cotton plier instrument used to pass cotton or other materials to the dentist (Ch. 18)

Council on Dental Therapeutics part of the ADA, a body that gathers and releases to dentists information about drugs being used in dentistry (Ch. 15)

covered entities providers of health care services and supplies such as hospitals, clinics, nursing homes, assisted-living facilities, home health agencies, physicians, dentists, and alternative medicine (Ch. 3)

creep a change in a material when under a constant load (Ch. 38)

crepitus crackling sound (Ch. 25)

criminal law law related to wrongs committed against the welfare and safety of society as a whole (Ch. 3)

cross-contamination pathways formed when pathogens travel from patients to dentists, dental assistants, dental hygienists, dental laboratory technicians, and other patients (Ch. 11)

cross-section technique used to expose occlusal radiographs (Ch. 22)

crown top or highest part of a tooth; often called a cap (Chs. 9 and 14)

crown and collar (bridge) scissors instrument used to trim crowns (Ch. 18)

crown lengthening procedure in which the gingival tissue is removed to allow more of the crown of the teeth to show; eliminates a gummy smile (Ch. 35)

crown matrix form a thin, plastic form that is shaped like a crown used on anterior teeth when the incisal edge is involved (Ch. 38)

culture the shared beliefs and values of a group (Ch. 2)

curette hand instruments for removing subgingival calculus, smoothing the root surface, and removing the soft tissue lining of the periodontal pocket (Ch. 31)

curing light a high-intensity light that hardens or sets many dental materials (Ch. 17)

Current Dental Terminology (CDT) CDT represents the collaboration of dental vendors, payers, providers, clearinghouses, and the government for a standard code set; initially developed in 1969, it is now revised every 2 years (Ch. 3)

curve of Spee a slight anatomical curve of the occlusal alignment of the teeth, beginning with the mandibular cuspids/canines and following the buccal cusps of the premolars/bicuspids and molar (Ch. 22)

cusp pointed or rounded mounds on the crown of the tooth (Ch. 9)

cusp of Carabelli a fifth cusp on the mesial lingual surface of most maxillary first molars (Ch. 9)

cuticle nail bed (Ch. 6)

cutting edge on a dental instrument, the sharpened edge used for refining the cavity preparation (Ch. 18)

cutting instrument instruments designed to cut and shape walls of the cavity preparation. The blade ends in a sharp, beveled end. Examples include chisels and hatchets (Ch. 18)

cyst fluid-filled or semisolid fluid-filled sac (Ch. 27)

cytodifferentiation the development of different cells during the embryonic stage of pregnancy (Ch. 8)

D

darkroom a small room near the treatment rooms where x-ray processing is done (Ch. 17)

debride to remove debris (dead tissue) (Ch. 25)

debridement removal of diseased and necrotic tissues from the canal (Ch. 24)
deciduous primary (Ch. 9)
defamation of character causing injury to another's reputation, name, or character; can be verbal or written (Ch. 3)
defendant the individual a charge is brought against (Ch. 3)
defibrillation mechanical application of an electrical charge to restart the heart (Ch. 16)
deglutition also known as swallowing, provides the movement for the food to move from the mouth to the stomach (Ch. 6)
demineralization case in which calcium and phosphorus are lost from the enamel surface (Ch. 4)
demographic identifying factors of groups of people such as age, gender, ethnicity, location, etc. (Ch. 13)
dendrites nerve fibers that conduct impulses toward the cell body (Ch. 6)
density degree of darkness on an x-ray (Ch. 21)
Dental Assisting National Board, Inc. (DANB) independent organization that administers the credentialing examinations for dental assistants (Chs. 1 and 41)
dental associate a dentist who works under contract, usually for a dentist with a solo practice (Ch. 41)
dental casting alloy combination of metals (gold, iron, tin, and zinc) used in crowns (Ch. 33)
dental composite resins (BIS-GMA) BIS-GMA material commonly used as a sealant for occlusal pits and fissures (Ch. 30)
dental dam clamps tools that stabilize and secure the dental dam material in place; they come in numerous designs and sizes to fit around the teeth (Ch. 19)
dental dam forceps forceps with two beaks that fit in the holes of the jaws of the clamp; used to place and remove the dental dam clamp (Ch. 19)
dental dam frame holder designed to stretch and secure the dam in place across the patient's face; keeps the operating area open (Ch. 19)
dental dam napkin soft, precut, disposable, absorbent fabric pieces used for patient comfort and for absorbing saliva, water, and perspiration (Ch. 19)
dental dam punch a tool similar in action to a paper punch, although much differently designed, with a sharp projection to punch through the dental dam to create holes for the teeth (Ch. 19)
dental dam scissors any small pair of scissors the operator uses to cut the interseptal dental dam during removal of the dam from the patient's mouth (Ch. 19)
dental floss placed interproximally, wrapped around the tooth, and moved in an up-and-down motion (Ch. 32)
dental fluorosis a condition caused by an excess intake of fluorides during tooth development; enamel surface appears mottled and stained but is caries free (Ch. 32)
dental history questions regarding the patient's past dental treatment, information regarding any concerns the patient has regarding his or her current dental health (Ch. 13)
dental implant fixed prostheses, attached to bone, used to replace missing teeth (Ch. 26)
dental jurisprudence the law(s) governing dentistry (Ch. 3)
dental lamina a growth from the oral epithelium that gives rise to the tooth buds (Ch. 8)
dental phobia patients who have a fear of dentistry and of receiving dental care (Ch. 2)
dental Practice Act state regulations that describe legal restrictions and controls on the dentist, the hygienist, and other dental assistants (Ch. 3)
dental public health the specialty in dentistry that is concerned with dental disease; works with the community to promote dental health (Ch. 1)
dental sac an enclosed area formed by the mesenchyme tissue that matures into the dentin, cementum, and the pulp of the tooth (Ch. 8)
dental tape used on the interproximal surfaces of the teeth with an abrasive agent (Ch. 32)
dental unit positioned according to the dentist, unit that consists of handpieces, an air–water syringe, a saliva ejector, an oral evacuator (HVE), an ultrasonic scaling unit, and numerous other options (Ch. 17)
dentifrice toothpaste used with brushing and flossing for patient oral hygiene self-care (Ch. 4)
dentin makes up the bulk of the tooth structures located around the pulp cavity and under the enamel within the anatomical crown, and under the cementum within the root (Ch. 8)
dentinal fluid tissue fluid surrounding the cell membrane of the odontoblast (Ch. 8)
dentinal hypersensitivity pain that may occur if dentin is exposed (Ch. 8)
dentinal tubule tubules that pass through the entire surface of the dentin and contain dentinal fluid (Ch. 8)
dentinogenesis imperfecta a hereditary condition in which the enamel appears to be opalescent and chips away from the dentin soon after tooth eruption (Ch. 27)
dentition natural teeth in position (Ch. 9)
denture a prosthesis that replaces missing teeth in the same arch; a full denture is used when all the natural teeth are missing, a partial denture when some natural teeth are missing (Chs. 14 and 36)
denture base sometimes called the saddle, holds denture teeth (Ch. 36)
dependent children covered under dental insurance (normally up to age 18) (Ch. 15)
deposition the process in which new cells are created and deposited to hold restorations in place (Ch. 28)
depressant substance that slows body functions (Ch. 15)
desensitizer materials that are used to treat or prevent hypersensitivity in the tooth (Ch. 37)
desiccating to dry out the tooth (Ch. 37)
developer solution the first chemical solution used to process radiographs (Ch. 22)
developmental groove groove formed by the uniting of lobes during development of the crown of the tooth (Ch. 9)
diabetic acidosis a serious consequence of hyperglycemia when the patient has too much sugar and not enough insulin; the body produces acids and the pH level is lowered, often resulting in a coma and death if left untreated (Ch. 16)
DIAGNOdent caries detection Class II laser that measures fluorescence levels in the tooth structure to quantify caries progression. Is battery-operated microprocessor unit with handpiece and tips (Ch. 37)
diagnosis the decisions made regarding a disease process based upon assessment of signs and symptoms (Ch. 13)
diastema space between the maxillary central incisors in humans; can also be used to denote a space between two adjacent teeth in the same dental arch (Chs. 9 and 14)
diastolic blood created as the arteries return to their original state when the heart relaxes between contractions (Ch. 13)
die mold (Ch. 33)
diet food an individual eats (Ch. 5)
diffuses after the local anesthetic is injected into the tissue it spreads into the nerve fibers (Ch. 20)
digestion the process by which food is broken down into small nutrient molecules that the cells can use (Ch. 6)

digital image an image made up of many small pieces to make a whole picture (Ch. 23)

digital impression computerized image captured on a computer screen with a CAD system. A specially designed scanner and software is used to capture a digital impression of the prepared tooth, the adjacent teeth, and the opposing arch (Ch. 34)

digital radiology a computerized system that allows the dentist to take an intraoral or extraoral radiograph and display the image on a computer screen without exposing and processing dental film (Ch. 23)

digital subtraction allows images that were taken at different times to be compared (Ch. 23)

digitization (CSD) A computerized system used to create a 3D record of the geometry of a preparation used in the creation and design of crowns, bridges, and veneers (Ch. 34)

dimensional change change in length or volume of a material, usually from exposure to heat or cold (Ch. 37)

diplococcic pairs of bacteria (Ch. 10)

direct contact something an individual has with a lesion or microorganism while performing intraoral dental procedures; touching or first-hand contact (Ch. 11)

direct digital imaging the image is produced on a surface sensor, digitized, and then transmitted to a computer monitor (Ch. 23)

direct providers the HIPAA provisions apply to direct providers of health care services and supplies including hospitals, clinics, nursing homes, assisted-living facilities, home health agencies, physicians, dentists, and alternative medicine (Ch. 3)

direct pulp capping (DPC) technique used to treat permanent tooth when pulp has been exposed due to mechanical or traumatic means but chance exists that the pulp will heal; involves placing of medicament directly over exposed pulp, followed by tooth restoration (Chs. 29 and 37)

direct resin veneer made in dental office directly on patient's tooth (Ch. 33)

direct restorative material materials that are placed directly in the mouth after the tooth has been prepared. **Including dental amalgam, composite resin materials, and glass ionomers** (Ch. 38)

direct supervision the dentist must be physically in the treatment facility to authorize this function and he or she must be available within an immediate distance to respond to the patient needs and must evaluate the performance of the procedure (Ch. 3)

disc repositioning one type of arthroplasty surgery, where the displaced disk is moved back into its original position (Ch. 25)

discectomy the surgical removal of the disk; when it has become deteriorated and damaged, and the disk is out of place or popping back and forth, then as a last resort, this surgery is performed (Ch. 25)

disease outbreak when disease happens and it infects a greater number of individuals than expected (Ch. 10)

disinfection occurs when some microorganisms are destroyed; cleaning and sanitizing (Ch. 11)

distal the surface of the tooth that is away from the midline (Ch. 9)

distortion change in shape (Ch. 39)

distoversion a deviation in tooth positioning; the tooth is distal to normal position (Ch. 28)

distribution when a drug attaches to the protein in the blood and circulates throughout the body, affecting the destination area (Ch. 15)

diuretic substances that cause the body to lose water (Ch. 5)

doctrine of respondeat superior simply put, the dentist is responsible for the actions of the dental assistant, as well as any assistant; when there is a complaint or an act of negligence on the assistant's part, the dentist is liable for the act (Ch. 3)

documentation the writing down of all tasks completed; record keeping (Ch. 35)

domestic violence behaviors used by one person in a relationship to control the other person in the relationship are defined as emotional abuse (Ch. 3)

dosage correct amount of a drug formulated for dispensing (Ch. 15)

dosage indicator method of sterilization monitoring that works in much the same manner as a process indicator (Ch. 11)

dosimeter is a badge that monitors an individual's radiation exposure and accumulated dosage in the office. Also known as the radiation monitoring device (Ch. 21)

double booking booking additional patients at down times with the initial patient's procedures (Ch. 40)

double exposure a technique error in which film was exposed twice (Ch. 22)

downtime time in the appointment book that is not used for appointments (Ch. 40)

Dr. C. Edmund Kells hired a female to replace a male assistant in 1885. He wanted this "lady assistant" to be "quick, quiet, gentle, and attentive" (Ch. 1)

Dr. Greene Vardiman Black he invented numerous machines for testing alloys and instruments to refine cavity preparations. Referred to as the "grand old man of dentistry" (Ch. 1)

Dr. Samuel D. Harris instrumental in founding the Dr. Samuel Harris National Museum of Dental History (Ch. 1)

drifting a tooth moving into the space created by a missing tooth (Ch. 14)

drug any substance that changes the body's life chemical processes (Ch. 15)

drug abuse the use of a substance in a manner that is excessive or not the approved intended use (Ch. 15)

Drug Enforcement Agency (DEA) number number assigned by the agency that regulates controlled substances; part of the U.S. Department of Justice (Ch. 15)

drug interaction the effect one drug can have on another when taken at the same time; intended results may be increased or decreased (Ch. 15)

dry angle triangular pads that absorb the flow of saliva and protect the cheek (Ch. 19)

dry heat sterilizer sterilizing unit where dry instruments do not experience corrosion or rust. Good for delicate or instruments that have a movable joint or sharp edges. Heat to 171°C (340°F) for 1 hour to sterilize (Ch. 11)

dry socket common complication after an extraction where the blood clot has not formed or is lost; also called alveolitis (Ch. 25)

dual-cured material materials containing chemicals for self-curing as well as materials set by light curing (Ch. 37)

ductility the ability of a material to withstand forces of tensile stress without failing (Ch. 37)

due care the care that any reasonable and prudent dental care personnel would do in the same circumstances (Ch. 3)

duplication technique a technique whereby dental radiographs are reproduced on specialized film (Ch. 22)

duration the time during which something continues or exists (Ch. 20)

Dycal instrument/small-balled instrument usually a smaller instrument in size than the plastic filling instrument and has a small ball tip on the working end. Used to place dental liners in the cavity preparation (Ch. 18)

dysplastic cells abnormal cell features such as size, shape, and rate of multiplication (Ch. 27)

E

ecchymosis the bruising of tissue (Ch. 27)

echo generation is another name for Generation Y, the children of the baby boomers (Ch. 2)

edema excessive amounts of fluid in body tissue; swelling (Ch. 16)

effectiveness (rbe) unit used to compare the biological effects of different tissues irradiated by different forms of radiation (Ch. 21)

elasticity the ability to be distorted or deformed by an applied force and then return to its original shape once the force is removed (Ch. 37)

elastics rubber bands or elastic threads, often used between the upper and lower arches to provide force for movement (Ch. 28)

elder abuse abuse of persons 65 and older (Ch. 3)

electric handpiece an alternative to the air-driven handpieces; units can be calibrated to be used with existing air pressure and rheostats; may be low or high speed (Ch. 18)

electrocardiography the ability to use a mechanical device to read and record the electrical activity of the heart (Ch. 16)

electrolytes minerals that have positive or negative charges (Ch. 5)

electromagnetic energy a form of energy that is the result of electric and magnetic disturbances in space (Ch. 21)

electronic dental anesthesia used with patients who are allergic to local anesthetics or who are extremely fearful of the injection. It is also used with nitrous oxide inhalation sedation in many dental procedures (Ch. 20)

electronic pulp tester tool, usually battery operated, that creates an electrical stimulus to the tooth indicating whether pulp is vital or nonvital (Ch. 24)

electrons negatively charged particles that orbit the nucleus (Ch. 21)

electrosurgery procedure that uses tiny electrical currents to incise gingival tissue and coagulate blood; setup consists of control box, foot-operated on-off controls, a terminal plate that is placed behind patient's back or shoulders, and a terminal probe with various cutting tips (Ch. 31)

elevator instruments that loosen and remove teeth, retained roots, and root fragments (Ch. 25)

elon a chemical reducer used in development of radiographs to blacken the exposed silver halide crystals (Ch. 22)

elongation a technique error that elongates the image of the teeth (Ch. 22)

emaciation extreme thinness (Ch. 5)

embrasure the triangular space in the gingival direction that is made when two adjoining teeth are contacting (Ch. 9)

embryo the study of prenatal growth and the developing process of an individual (Ch. 8)

embryology the study of prenatal growth and the developing process of an individual (Ch. 8)

embryonic layers three primary layers formed early in the embryo phase include ectoderm, mesoderm, and endoderm layers (Ch. 8)

embryonic phase in this prenatal phase of pregnancy cells are differentiating (developing individual characteristics) and integrating to form cell layers that develop into a human being (Ch. 8)

emollient a substance that help reduce drying of the skin (Ch. 11)

emotional abuse behaviors used by one person in a relationship to control the other person in the relationship (Ch. 3)

emulsion part of the dental film, which is made of a homogeneous mixture of silver halide crystals suspended in a gelatin (Ch. 21)

enamel tooth structure that covers the outside of the crown of the tooth; the hardest living tissue in the body (Ch. 8)

enamel dysplasia a developmental disturbance during the apposition stage, perhaps from a nutritional loss, resulting in the surface of teeth becoming grooved and pitted (Ch. 8)

enamel hypocalcification soft and undercalcified tooth enamel (Ch. 4)

enamel hypoplasia incomplete development of tooth enamel (Ch. 4)

enamel lamellae narrow and long enamel tufts that extend from the dentinoenamel junction to the enamel surface (Ch. 8)

enamel matrix produced by the ameloblast cells (Ch. 8)

enamel spindles short, dentinal tubules that seem to have crossed over into the enamel and were trapped there during the process of enamel mineralization (Ch. 8)

enamel tufts similar to enamel spindles but with bases near the dentinoenamel junction that appear as small, dark brushes (Ch. 8)

encoding the use of specific signs, symbols, interpersonal communication, or language used in communicating a message (Ch. 2)

endocardium thin lining on the inside of the heart (Ch. 6)

endodontic bender device designed to carefully bend endodontic reamers, files, posts, pluggers, and spreaders to conform to the shape of the root canal (Ch. 24)

endodontic handpiece an attachment to a low-speed handpiece that supplies quarter-turn motion consistently and evenly (Ch. 24)

endodontic microscope a device with a variety of high levels of magnification, with levels ranging from 2x to 20x; there is also the high-intensity illumination that adds brightness in a concentrated area and is designed to be shadow free (Ch. 24)

endodontic obturation system this system is provided by a cordless unit that warms the filling material (either brand name materials or traditional gutta percha) and then allows the dentist to place the material into the canal for vertical and backfill obturation (Ch. 24)

Endodontics the branch of dentistry that deals with the diagnosis and treatment of diseases of the pulp and the periapical tissues (Chs. 1 and 24)

endogenous originating from within the tooth (Ch. 32)

endospores a dormant, nonreproductive structure produced by a small number of bacteria, with the primary function to ensure survival through periods of environmental stress (Ch. 10)

endosteal implants implants placed into the bone surgically; used to replace single teeth and for patients who are partially edentulous (Ch. 26)

enteric-coated a coating found on some medications that resists breakdown by gastric juices and dissolves in the intestines (Ch. 15)

epidemic an infectious disease spreads quickly to a large number of individuals (Ch. 10)

epiglottis a leaf-shaped organ at the end of the larynx whose function is to close off the larynx during swallowing (Ch. 6)

epilepsy a recurrent disorder of cerebral function, due to excessive neuronal discharge (Ch. 16)

epinephrine the most common vasoconstrictor used in dentistry (Ch. 20)

epithelial attachment the gingiva in the floor of the gingival sulcus that attaches to the enamel surface of the teeth just above the CEJ of the tooth (Ch. 8)

equipment (PPE) items that should be worn to protect against contact with all body fluids (e.g., protective eyewear) (Ch. 11)

ergonomics study of work and space, including factors that affect worker's health, productivity, and mental well-being (Chs. 17 and 40)

erosion wearing away (Ch. 27)

eruption when the tooth emerges from the gum tissue (Ch. 8)

erythema redness or inflammation of the skin (Ch. 16)

erythroplakia any red patch of tissue in the oral cavity that cannot be associated with inflammation (Ch. 27)

esophagus extends from the pharynx to the stomach; includes muscles that help food move toward the stomach (Ch. 6)

essential amino acid ten are needed; part of the protein molecule that the body cannot synthesize or produce; must be obtained through diet (Ch. 5)

etchant substance used to roughen a surface before bonding; increases strength of the bond (Ch. 37)

etched conditioned tooth surface with phosphoric acid. Tooth becomes more porous and frosted in appearance. Used to prepare the tooth for sealants and some bonding agents (Ch. 30)

ethics although different from person to person, ethics are what is morally right or wrong (Ch. 3)

ethnicity a group that shares cultural characteristics (Ch. 2)

ethylene oxide sterilizer instrument sterilizer that comes in two different types: a heated unit and a unit that can be used at room temperature. Both units are reliable for sterilization (Ch. 11)

etiologic agent causative agent of a disease (Ch. 10)

etiology cause of a disease (Ch. 27)

etiquette treating people/customers with respect; manners, politeness (Ch. 40)

evanesce dissolve (Ch. 8)

excavator also known as spoon excavators, are used to remove carious material and debris from the teeth (Ch. 18)

excisional biopsy complete removal of a lesion along with a small border of the normal tissue surrounding it (Ch. 25)

excitability when muscle tissue responds to stimuli (Ch. 6)

excretion process by which excess drugs are eliminated through the liver or kidneys (Ch. 15)

exfoliated shed from the oral cavity (Ch. 9)

exfoliative cytology or "smear biopsy" involves removal of a layer of cells from the surface of the lesion. This is a nonsurgical procedure in which the gathered cells are spread on a glass slab (Ch. 25)

exhalation phase of respiration when muscles relax and the air is moved out of the lungs; breathing out (Chs. 6 and 13)

exogenous originating from outside the tooth (Ch. 32)

exophthalmos bulging of the eyeballs (Ch. 15)

exostosis an enlargement of nodular outgrowth of dense lamella bone that appears on the facial surfaces of the mandibular and the maxillary palate (Ch. 27)

exothermic a chemical reaction that releases heat (Ch. 37)

exothermic reaction a chemical reaction that releases heat (Ch. 39)

expanded Function Dental Assistant dental assistant who completes additional education and training to perform advanced functions and skills. Some states require registration and or licensure (Ch. 1)

expanded functions skills and functions beyond those normally associated with dental assisting that require increased skill and responsibility; delegated by dentists according to the Dental Practice Acts in their states (Chs. 3 and 19)

expendable supplies that are used up or disposed of after use (e.g., cotton balls and envelopes) (Ch. 40)

explorer are single- or double-ended instruments; the working end is a thin, sharp point of flexible steel (Ch. 18)

expressed contract a contract, written or verbal, that describes what each party in the contract will do (Ch. 3)

extensibility the ability of the muscle to stretch or spread in order to perform tasks (Ch. 6)

extirpate to remove pulpal contents (Ch. 24)

extraction forceps instruments used to remove teeth from the alveolar bone (Ch. 25)

extraoral film film used outside the oral cavity (Ch. 23)

extraoral imaging radiographs taken outside the patient's mouth. Include panoramic, cephalometric, lateral jaw, and temporomandibular joint radiographs (Ch. 23)

extrinsic on the outside (Ch. 32)

exudate pus (Ch. 24)

F

facebow a device that allows the operator to obtain the records about the placement of the maxillary arch and its location to the joint (Chs. 36 and 39)

facebow transfer transfer measurements from the facebow to an articulator (Ch. 36)

facial either the labial surface of the anterior teeth or the buccal surface of the posterior teeth (Ch. 9)

facial nerve one of the four cranial nerves that innervates the face (Ch. 7)

facultative anaerobic bacteria grow with or without oxygen (Ch. 10)

Fahrenheit system used to measure temperature; the freezing point is 32 degrees and the boiling point is 212 degrees (Ch. 13)

Fair Debt Collection Practice Act legislation making it illegal to phone a debtor at inconvenient hours or to phone the debtor's employers (Ch. 40)

fascia a fibrous sheet of connective tissue that covers, supports, and separates each group of muscle cells, or fibers (Ch. 6)

fats derived from solids, fat provides a source of energy in addition to carbohydrates; fat insulates the body from heat loss, protects vital organs, and aids in the transportation of fat-soluble vitamins (Ch. 5)

Fédération Dentaire Internationale (FDI) system for numbering international system used for coding teeth and the oral cavity in charting (Ch. 14)

fetal phase ninth week pregnancy term until birth (Ch. 8)

fever elevation of the body's temperature above the normal range (Ch. 13)

fiber-optic light sources available with high-speed handpieces, fiber-optic systems greatly improve visibility of the treatment area for the operator (Ch. 18)

fibroblast cells that form connective tissue (Ch. 8)

fibroma a benign tumor of connective tissue cells; a reactive hyperplasia rather than a true neoplasm (Ch. 27)

field block anesthesia injection method that places the anesthetic solution near larger terminal nerve branches (Ch. 20)

files endodontic instruments used to enlarge and smooth the canal (Chs. 18 and 24)

film artifact marks on x-ray film that are caused by errors or other substances on the patient such as surgical staples, earrings, etc. (Ch. 22)

finishing knife used to trim excess filling material. The working ends of the finishing knives have sharp, knife-like blades and variety of shapes and angles to access restoration margins (Ch. 18)

fissure a developmental groove that has an imperfect union where the lobes join (Ch. 9)

fissured tongue a wrinkled, deeply grooved surface on the tongue (Ch. 27)

fistula a tube-like passage from an abscess to the external surface; used to drain the abscess (Chs. 16 and 24)

fixed appliance appliances attached to the teeth that cannot be removed by the patient (e.g., braces) (Ch. 28)

fixer solution the second chemical solution used in processing radiographs (Ch. 22)

flagella long, thread-like appendage on protozoa that assist with movement (Ch. 10)

flange part of the denture base that covers the alveolar ridge and gingival tissues (Ch. 36)

flex files endodontic files made of stainless steel or nickel- titanium and used for curved and narrow canals that require flexibility to negotiate (Ch. 24)

floor of the mouth area that includes the sublingual caruncles, sublingual folds, and sublingual sulcus and the base of the tongue (Ch. 7)

floss holder a Y-shaped device with a handle that makes flossing easier for individuals with arthritis, poor manual dexterity, or large hands (Ch. 4)

floss threader a device used to remove plaque and debris from under fixed bridges, orthodontic wires, and retainers (Ch. 4)

flour of pumice a relatively coarse (abrasive) material used to remove stains from enamel; should be followed by a fine polishing agent (Ch. 32)

flow continuing deformation of a solid; also called creep and slump (Ch. 37)

flowable composite similar to microfilled and hybrid composites in content and particle size; can be applied directly into cavity preparations by small syringe tips (Ch. 38)

fluorescence a glow that results when a fluorescent substance is struck by cathode rays, light, or x-rays) was occurring on the other side of the room (Ch. 21)

fluoridation the process of adding fluoride to the water supply (Ch. 4)

fluoride a natural mineral nutrient, derived from fluorine, which comes from fluorspar, the thirteenth most abundant chemical element in the earth's crust; fluoride is essential to the formation of healthy bones and teeth (Ch. 4)

fluoride application fluoride applied to the teeth in the dental office (Ch. 29)

fluoride prophylaxis commercially prepared pastes with the addition of fluoride (Ch. 29)

fluoride prophylaxis pastes commercially prepared pastes with the addition of fluoride (Ch. 29)

fluoride varnish paint on method to apply topical fluoride to the teeth for longer exposure (Ch. 29)

fluorine a trace mineral that helps strengthen teeth and may help prevent osteoporosis (Ch. 5)

fluoroapatite crystal tooth structure formed when fluoride replaces the hydroxyl ion of the enamel (Ch. 4)

fluorosis mottled enamel; results from excessive fluoride during tooth development; tooth enamel appears pitted and multicolored (Ch. 4)

focal spot area on the anode that electrons hit during x-ray production (Ch. 21)

focal trough a three-dimensional curved zone in a panoramic radiographic machine in which the dental arches are positioned to achieve the sharpest image; also called the image layer or sharpness (Ch. 23)

focusing cup area on the anode that directs the electrons to the focal spot during x-ray production (Ch. 21)

fogged film an x-ray film that appears dark and dense related to old or overused chemicals (Ch. 22)

folic acid also known as folacin, is a water-soluble vitamin found in plants such as spinach, asparagus, broccoli, and kidney beans; its primary function is the synthesis of red blood cells (Ch. 5)

fomite objects contaminated with infectious agents such as instruments or dressings (Ch. 11)

Food and Drug Administration (FDA) federal regulation agency (Ch. 15)

force the push or pull of an object (Ch. 37)

Fordyce's spots sebaceous oil glands near the surface of the epithelium that appear in the oral cavity as round, yellow spots (Ch. 27)

foreign body airway obstruction (FBAO) obstruction of normal breathing; dental instruments, crowns, amalgams, composite, cotton rolls, and gauze are items that may obstruct the airway (Ch. 16)

forensic dentistry area of dentistry that deals with identification of an individual through tooth restorations and morphology using dental records (Ch. 1)

forensics area of investigation in which identity of the patient is established though scientific methods by the use of the charting and radiographs (Ch. 13)

foreshortening a technique error whereby the image of the teeth is shortened (Ch. 22)

Formocresol a solution of formaldehyde, cresol, glycerin, and water; it is used in vital pulpotomy and as a temporary intracanal medicament used during root canal therapy (Ch. 29)

fossa a shallow, rounded, or angular depression (Ch. 9)

four-handed system in which the dentist and dental assistant work together at the dental chair (Chs. 17 and 18)

framework the skeleton of the removable partial to which rests, connectors, and retainers are attached (Ch. 36)

Frankel appliance device that assists the mandible to advance and move forward while stopping the maxilla from growing; the front teeth are pulled back, which results in flattening the open bite (Ch. 28)

Frankfort plane the imaginary horizontal plane from the bottom of the eye socket to the top of the ear canal (Ch. 23)

fraud a deliberate deception that is practiced to secure unfair or unlawful gain (Ch. 3)

free gingiva or marginal surrounds the teeth and is attached only at the gingival groove, appears lighter in color (if healthy) and is about 1 mm in width (Ch. 8)

frenectomy complete surgical removal of the frenum, including the attachment to the underlying bone (Ch. 31)

friction grip shank short, small, and smooth portion of a bur or tool that attaches to a handpiece (Ch. 18)

frictional heat heat produced when a moving surface contacts another (Ch. 18)

front delivery system one of three types of dental unit with the equipment designed to be pulled over the patient's chest and located between the dentist and the assistant (Ch. 17)

fulcrum the support or point on which a level turns (e.g., position of finger rest for support when working in a patient's mouth) (Ch. 19)

full-cast crown full covering over a tooth that has extensive decay or damage (Ch. 33)

fungi mold (Ch. 10)

fungicidal a biological organism or biological chemical compound used to kill or inhibit fungi or fungal spores (Ch. 11)

furcation the dividing point of a multirooted tooth; division of the roots (Ch. 14)

fusion a condition in which the enamel and dentin of two or more individual teeth join together (Ch. 27)

G

gallbladder muscular sac that stores bile from the liver (Ch. 6)

galvanism creation of electrical shock caused by two different metals coming together (Ch. 37)

galvanometer instrument for detecting and measuring electric current (Ch. 16)

gauge the diameter of needles used in dentistry. Usual sizes are 25, 27, and 30 gauge. The smaller the gauge, the larger the diameter of the needle (Ch. 20)

gel a solid (Ch. 39)

gelatin time the time from which the alginate powder material is mixed with water until it is completely set and considered alginate (Ch. 39)

general anesthesia when the patient goes into an unconscious state, by temporarily altering the central nervous system so that sensation or feeling is lost (Ch. 20)

general supervision the dentist is to diagnosis and authorize the work to be performed on the patient by the dental auxiliary but he or she is not required to be on the premises while the treatment is being completed (Ch. 3)

generalized hypoxia is a pathological condition in which either the whole body (Ch. 16)

generation X also called the MTV generation, is thought to be those born during the 1960s and 1970s, and some consider it to include the 1980s (Ch. 2)

generation Y those born between 1977 and 1994, known as the generation following Generation X (Ch. 2)

generation Z was born in the mid-1990s to early 2000s. In American culture specifically this group is a more diverse mix of ethnicities than the generations before them (Ch. 2)

generic name drug names unprotected by trademark; are less expensive than brand names and may be used by any business (Ch. 15)

genetic effects one of the classifications of the effects of radiations, that may not involve the primary individual exposed to the radiation. Genetic effects cannot be repaired and are passed to future generations (Ch. 21)

germination when one tooth bud appears to divide, leaving an indentation on the incisal or occlusal surface (Ch. 27)

gestational period the period of carrying an offspring in the womb during pregnancy; the fetus can grow to a length of 19–21 inches (or 48–52 cm) (Ch. 8)

ghost image a radiopaque artifact seen on panoramic film caused by metal or dense objects being exposed twice by the x-ray beam (Ch. 23)

gingiva composed of a mucosa that surrounds the necks of the teeth, and covers the alveolar processes (Ch. 8)

gingival dense, fibrous tissue located between the alveolar mucosa and the teeth and covered with mucous membrane (Ch. 7)

gingival cleft a fissure or elongated opening that extends toward the root of the tooth; the margin of the gingival tissue forms a "V" instead of a smooth rounded border, exposing the cementum covering the root (Ch. 31)

gingival fiber groups found in the lamina propria, they support the marginal gingival tissues in relationship to the tooth, and lie above the alveolar bone crest and below the epithelium (Ch. 8)

gingival grafting procedure in which tissue is taken from one site and placed on another (Ch. 31)

gingival groove line of demarcation between attached gingiva and the marginal gingival; also called the free gingival groove (Ch. 8)

gingival hyperplasia an overgrowth of gingival tissue (Ch. 27)

gingival margin trimmer (GMT) is similar to the hatchet regarding the position of the blade to the handle, but there are two distinct differences: First, the blade on the GMT is curved, not flat like the hatchet; second, the cutting edge is at an angle, not straight across like the hatchet (Ch. 18)

gingival recession loss of gingival tissue, exposing the underlying cementum/dentin, usually seen on the facial surface (Ch. 14)

gingival retraction chemical, mechanical, surgical, or combination process used to ensure an impression with clear margins can be obtained when preparing a tooth for a crown (Ch. 33)

gingival sulcus the space between the attached gingiva and the tooth (Ch. 8)

gingival wall the side or floor of the cavity preparation nearest the gingival that is perpendicular to the long axis of the tooth (Ch. 37)

gingivectomy surgical removal of diseased gingival tissue (Ch. 31)

gingivitis (NUG) also called Vincent's disease or trench mouth, a common disease found in teenagers and young adults; causes include stress, smoking, poor diet, and poor oral hygiene (Ch. 31)

gingivitis inflammation of the gingival tissues, marked by red, swollen, and/or bleeding gums; caused by buildup of plaque and calculus, poorly fitting appliances, or malocclusion; may occur with certain systemic diseases, hormonal changes, or prolonged drug therapy (Ch. 31)

gingivoplasty reshaping of the gingival tissue to remove such deformities as clefts, craters, and enlargements; performed only to recontour the gingiva (Ch. 31)

glass ionomer permanent cementation with diverse types and applications: Type I is a finer grain that bonds chemically to teeth; Type II is coarser grain and is used in selected restorations; Type III is used as a liner and dentin bonding agent; Type IV is admixtures of glass ionomers used for buildups (Chs. 30, 37)

Glick #1 endodontic instrument used to remove excess gutta percha (Ch. 24)

Globally Harmonized System of Classification and Labeling of Chemicals (GHS) part of the 2012 revision of the Hazardous Communication Standard. Chemicals and materials are classified and labeled the same way internationally, regardless of where the chemicals are manufactured, sold, or used (Ch. 12)

glossitis a condition due to Vitamin B deficiency causing inflammation of the tongue and Pellagra, where mucous membranes atrophy and ulcers develop (Chs. 5 and 27)

glossopharyngeal one of the four cranial nerves innervate the oral cavity (Ch. 7)

gold foil restoration created when several layers of pure gold are placed in the cavity preparation (Ch. 14)

good Samaritan Law protection for people who provide medical assistance to those in emergency situations who are not seeking payment for it; those providing the assistance are given immunity (Ch. 3)

Gracey curette a set of several instruments that are designed and angled to be used in specific areas (Ch. 31)

gram negative a cell wall's lack of dye color under a microscope (Ch. 10)

gram positive a cell wall's retention of dye color under a microscope (Ch. 10)

Gram stain a procedure to differentiate cells into two specific groups using special dyes (Ch. 10)

gram variable classification of bacteria that are not consistently stained (Ch. 10)

grand mal seizure seizure marked by person becoming unconscious and the body jerking, twitching, and stiffening; usually lasts 2 to 5 minutes (Ch. 16)

granuloma a neoplasm or tumor filled with granulation tissue (Ch. 27)

gray (GY) the Systeme Internationale unit of absorbed dose of ionizing radiation (Ch. 21)

gray scale the contrast found in an image related to the degrees of gray found in the image (Ch. 23)

green stain discoloration most often found in children; found on the facial surface of the maxillary anterior teeth at the cervical third, containing chromogenic bacteria and fungi; varies from light to dark green or yellowish-green (Ch. 32)

gross income total accounts receivable (Ch. 40)

guided tissue regeneration a technique that uses barrier membranes to maintain a space between the gingival flap and the root surface of the tooth in order for tissues to regenerate in a periodontal defect (Ch. 40)

gumma a localized lesion that occurs in the third stage of syphilis (Ch. 27)
gutta percha filling material; usually thermoplastic (Ch. 24)
guy de Chauliac from France, a surgeon who became one of the fourteenth century's most influential authors on surgery and she wrote "Hygienic Rules for Oral Hygiene" (Ch. 1)
gypsum calcium sulfate dihydrate; used when pouring an impression to make a model; water–powder ratio dictates strength, accuracy, resistance, reproduction detail, and setting times (Ch. 39)

H

habit forming leading to psychological or physical drug dependency (Ch. 15)
hairy leukoplakia a white, patterned lesion normally found on the borders of the tongue in patients infected with HIV (Ch. 27)
hairy tongue a condition in which the filiform papillae of the tongue become elongated and appear like hairs (Ch. 27)
halide crystals component of film's emulsion suspended in a gelatin; stores the energy from which they have been exposed and reacts with the chemicals in the processing tank to form a black region on the film (Ch. 21)
halitosis bad breath (Ch. 4)
hallucinate to cause the drug user to see images and hear sounds that do not exist (Ch. 15)
handheld intraoral radiography low-radiation dose, battery-operated machine to take dental x-rays. Used in a variety of dental clinics, military bases, teaching facilities, and nursing homes (Ch. 23)
hand-over-mouth (HOM) technique act by which a medical or dental professional places the hand over the patient's mouth and calmly explains behavior expectations; requires informed consent (Ch. 29)
handpieces instruments used with rotary burs, discs, and stones; connected to power, air, and water sources (Chs. 17 and 18)
hands-free a communications device consisting of a headset and speakers that allow reception to communicate with the rest of the staff without tying up hands and to improve office efficiencies (Ch. 17)
hard deposits hard, calcified deposits (mineralized plaque) firmly attached to teeth, restorations, and dental appliances; also called calculus or tartar (Ch. 32)
hard radiation short wavelengths with high frequency, high energy, and high penetrating power (Ch. 21)
hard tissue impaction occurs if the teeth are impacted in bone and not through the gingival tissues (Ch. 25)
hardware physical computer equipment that processes data (Ch. 40)
hatchet sometimes called enamel hatchets, are similar to hatchets used to cut wood; there is an angle in the shank of a hatchet and the blade is flat; used in a downward motion to refine the cavity walls and to obtain retention in the cavity preparation (Ch. 18)
Hawley retainer custom-made appliance fitted to patient's arch to retain the teeth in position after orthodontic treatment (Ch. 28)
headgear orthodontic appliance composed of a strap that goes behind the patient's head or neck and a facebow that attaches to buccal tubes on molar bands; applies force to move teeth, restrain or alter facial bone growth, and reinforce the stability of intraoral appliances (Ch. 28)
heading portion of the prescription that includes the doctor's name and degrees, the DEA number, the office address, and the phone number (Ch. 15)
healing cap a metal cap/screw that fits on the dental implant and keeps tissue and debris from getting into the implant (Ch. 26)
health information (HI) information provided to a health care institution related to a specific person's care as well as personal information (Ch. 3)
Health Insurance Portability the Health Insurance Portability and Accountability Act of 1996 (HIPAA), also known as the Kennedy-Kassebaum Act, was enacted to establish safeguards for health care transactions transmitted electronically (Ch. 3)
Health Insurance Portability and Accountability Act of 1996 (HIPAA) the Health Insurance Portability and Accountability Act of 1996 (HIPAA), also known as the Kennedy-Kassebaum Act, was enacted to establish safeguards for health care transactions transmitted electronically (Ch. 3)
heart a hollow muscular organ that acts as a pump, which circulates blood throughout the body (Ch. 6)
heart valves four valves in the heart regulate the flow of blood in one direction (Ch. 6)
heating unit recent technology that has many applications such as providing heat for vitality testing, warming the gutta percha for obturation, and providing heat for bleaching procedures (Ch. 24)
hedström file endodontic files that are very sharp and cut aggressively; used in a push-and-pull motion (Ch. 24)
heimlich maneuver the procedure performed when a person is in distress and unable to breathe due to a foreign body airway obstruction (Ch. 16)
hematoma appearing as a bruised area, a lesion caused by bleeding from a ruptured blood vessel (Chs. 20 and 27)
hemiplegia weakness, numbness, or paralysis on one side of the body (Ch. 16)
hemisection surgical removal of one root and the overlying crown (Ch. 24)
hemostasis process by which the body controls bleeding (Ch. 6)
hemostat forceps instruments used during surgery to retract tissue, remove small root tips, clamp off blood vessels, and grasp objects (Ch. 25)
Herbst appliance a fixed appliance that improves the overbite by encouraging lower jaw growth (Ch. 28)
herpes labialis form of herpes simplex type I; also known as fever blisters (Ch. 27)
herpes zoster unilateral, painful lesions that can last up to 5 weeks; also known as shingles (Ch. 27)
herpetic gingivostomatitis inflammation of the gingiva caused by a virus (Ch. 27)
herpetic whitlow exposure to the herpes virus that manifests itself as a crusting ulceration on the fingers or hands; may be very painful (Chs. 10 and 27)
herringbone pattern a cross pattern that appears on film that has been placed backward in the mouth; caused by the pattern on the lead foil (Ch. 22)
high-speed handpieces handpieces used to rapidly cut tooth structure and finish restorations; rotates between 10,000 and 800,000 rpm (Ch. 18)
high-strength base cement bases including glass ionomers, hybrid ionomers, reinforced zinc oxide eugenol, zinc phosphate, and polycarboxylate (Ch. 37)
high-volume evacuator (HVE) increased evacuation system to remove fluids from the patient's mouth. Uses stainless steel or plastic tips (Chs. 17 and 19)
hinge a metal device—similar to a hinge—that may be built into the partial denture that relieves pressure on the abutment teeth; also called a stress-breaker (Ch. 36)
Hippocrates known as the father of medicine; the Oath of Hippocrates serves as the code of ethics for the medical and dental professions (Ch. 1)
histamines some chemicals released by specialized cells in an area. They are thought to bring about inflammation

by increasing blood flow to the involved area and causing redness and heat (Ch. 27)

histodifferentiation the development of different tissues during the embryonic stage of pregnancy (Ch. 8)

histology the study of the microscopic structure and function of tissues (Ch. 8)

hoe an instrument that is used in a pulling motion to smooth and shape the floor of the cavity preparation (Ch. 18)

hoe scaler instrument with sharp, beveled, 90-degree angled blade that, when placed in the periodontal pocket to the base and pulled toward the crown of the tooth with even pressure, planes and smooths the root surface (Ch. 31)

homeostasis cells, tissues, organs, and systems all functioning together to maintain harmony in the body (Ch. 6)

homogeneous uniformly mixed (Ch. 39)

Horace H. Hayden (1769–1844) established the Baltimore College of Dental Surgery with Chapin Harris; it was the first dental college in the world (Ch. 1)

horizontal angulation adjustment of angulation from left to right; improper angulation shows overlapping teeth (Ch. 22)

horizontal bone a result of periodontal disease when there is equal crestal bone loss on the mesial and distal surfaces of the proximal teeth (Ch. 29)

horizontal mattress suture used when suturing a flap, goes in and out of the tissue on the same surface; identified by a horizontal stitch or "bite"; tied with one surgeon's knot on the surface where suture procedure began (Ch. 25)

hormone secretions released from the endocrine glands into the bloodstream (Ch. 6)

host a simple or complex organism that can be affected by an agent (Ch. 11)

housekeeping surfaces CDC environmental surfaces of concern, including the floors, walls, sinks, windows, and in the general overall patient care areas (Ch. 11)

hue color; the hue of mature teeth varies due to intrinsic and extrinsic stains from smoking, foods, and restorative materials (Ch. 35)

human immunodeficiency virus (HIV) the AIDS virus; ultimately destroys immune system cells (Chs. 10 and 27)

humectant material or substance that retains moisture (Ch. 32)

Hutchinson's incisors the appearance of indentations on the incisal edges of the anterior dentition; this is characteristic of the teeth of children born to mothers with syphilis (Ch. 27)

hybrid composite includes more than one type of filler particle, usually glass and silica; stronger and less likely to fracture in high-stress areas (Ch. 38)

hydrogen peroxide material used for whitening teeth that causes temporary sensitivity of the pulp, irritates tissue, and discolors clothing (Ch. 35)

hydroquinone a chemical used in development of radiographs; a reducing agent used to blacken exposed silver halide crystals (Ch. 22)

hydroxyl ion located on the surface of the apatite crystal in the enamel (Ch. 4)

hyoid bone a horseshoe-shaped bone lying at the base of the tongue; all the muscles of the tongue and the floor of the mouth attach to this bone for support (Ch. 7)

hypercementosis a thickening of cementum around the apex that is caused by trauma to the tooth (Ch. 8)

hyperglycemia too much glucose in the blood (Ch. 16)

hyperkeratinized epithelium tissue that has built a layer of keratin as a protective coating (Ch. 27)

hyperplasia excess tissue; in dentistry, resulting from ill-fitting dentures that initially cause small ulcers that, after continued irritation, become folds of excess tissue (Chs. 16 and 27)

hypersensitive repeated contact with an allergen that causes the body to overreact (Ch. 16)

hypertension higher-than-normal blood pressure (Ch. 13)

hyperventilation abnormally rapid and deep breathing resulting in decreased carbon dioxide levels (Ch. 16)

hypoglossal nerve supplies motor fibers to all of the muscles of the tongue, except the palatoglossus muscle (Ch. 7)

hypotension lower-than-normal blood pressure (Ch. 13)

hypothermic having a body temperature below normal (Ch. 13)

hypoxia low oxygen levels in the blood (Ch. 16)

I

idiopathic a disease or disorder that has no known cause (Ch. 27)

illusion the art of making something appear different than it actually is (Ch. 35)

imbibition enlargement due to swelling or the absorption of fluid (Ch. 39)

imbrication lines small, curved lines running parallel to the CEJ near the gingival area of the labial of the crown of a tooth (Chs. 8 and 9)

imbrication lines of Von Ebner stained growth rings or incremental lines in dentin (Ch. 8)

immediate denture the dentures are completed, the anterior teeth are extracted, an alveolectomy is performed, and the denture is inserted (Ch. 36)

immunization a process that increases an individual's resistance to a particular disease (Ch. 10)

implied consent consent for a procedure given by the patient's act (e.g., patients who roll up their sleeves for blood pressure readings or to receive injections (Ch. 3)

implied contract a contract implemented by actions, not words (Ch. 3)

incipient beginning tooth decay that has not broken through the enamel into the dentin (Ch. 14)

incisal edge cutting or tearing edge of the anterior teeth (Ch. 9)

incisal third the area on the crown of the tooth that is nearest the incisal edge on the anterior tooth (Ch. 9)

incisional biopsy removal of a small section of a lesion along with a small border of normal tissue (Ch. 25)

indirect contact contact with a microorganism through such means as contaminated instruments, supplies, and equipment (Ch. 11)

indirect digital imaging converts traditional x-rays to digital images (Ch. 23)

indirect providers the HIPAA provisions apply to indirect providers of health care services and supplies such as laboratories, pharmacies, surgical centers, and any others that would deal with any patient information (Ch. 3)

indirect pulp capping when there is a near pulp exposure a cavity liner is placed to protect the pulp before the restoration is placed (Ch. 37)

indirect pulp treatment (IPT) technique used when treating permanent teeth with potentially infectious tissue (due to caries or traumatic injury), when pulp is not exposed but when pulp may be exposed during tissue removal; also known as indirect pulp capping (Ch. 29)

indirect resin veneer requires two dental appointments; first an impression is made, and then the fabricated veneer is bonded in place (Ch. 33)

indirect restoration impressions are taken and then these "fixed prostheses" are fabricated in a dental laboratory (Ch. 33)

infection control methods to eliminate or reduce the transmission of infectious microorganisms (Ch. 11)

inflammation body's defense against infection or trauma; redness, pain, and swelling may occur (Ch. 27)

informed consent agreement by the patient to the procedure that is about to be performed after being told of the procedure, risks involved, expected outcomes, and alternative treatments; patients acknowledge their understanding and acceptance by signing (Ch. 3)
infraversion tooth is positioned below the normal line of occlusion (Ch. 28)
inhalation breathing in; in the administration of drugs, the patient breathes in gas or aerosol; an individual contacts a microorganism by "breathing it in" (Chs. 11, 13, and 15)
inhalation sedation a general anesthesia used when IV sedation would be difficult to administer; the inhalation causes sleepiness and the patient doesn't remember much of the procedure (Ch. 20)
inherent filter This aluminum filter, known as the inherent filter, is placed in the path of the x-rays to eliminate the soft x-rays (those with low penetrating power) (Ch. 21)
initiation when the tooth begins formation from the dental lamina (Ch. 8)
inlay restoration replacements for missing tooth structure in teeth; covers the area between the cusps in the middle of the tooth and the proximal surfaces (Ch. 33)
innocuous causing no harm (Ch. 27)
inorganic filler quartz, silica, and lithium aluminum silicate (Ch. 34)
inorganic filler particles quartz, silica, and lithium aluminum silicate (Ch. 38)
inscription name of the drug prescribed and the dosage; appears in the prescription (Ch. 15)
insertion point part of a muscle where the bone is moveable (Ch. 6)
integrating indicators A method of monitoring all critical parameters covering a sterilization cycle (Ch. 11)
intensifying screen screens in cassettes used with extraoral films (Ch. 23)
Intensity (combination of the number of photons (product of the quantity or milliamperage), and the energy of the photons (product of the quality or kilovoltage) affected by time and distance (Ch. 21)
intercellular substances substances between the cells (Ch. 8)
interceptive prevention and treatment of orthodontic problems (Ch. 28)
intercuspation the cusps to fossa relationship of the upper and lower posterior teeth to each other (Ch. 36)
interdental gingiva an extension of unattached gingiva between adjacent teeth; it is also called interdental papilla (Ch. 8)
interdental knives periodontal knives used to remove soft tissue interproximally; spear shaped with long, narrow, double-edged blades (Ch. 31)
interdental septum a bony projection that separates each socket of the interradicular septum (Ch. 8)
intermediate luting cement material that lasts 6 months to a year (Ch. 37)
intermediate restorative a type II zinc oxide eugenol cement that is placed in the patient's mouth and lasts up to one year; used when a tooth cannot be restored immediately (Ch. 33)
intermediate restorative material (IRM) a type II zinc oxide eugenol cement that is placed in the patient's mouth and lasts up to 1 year; used when a tooth cannot be restored immediately (Ch. 37)
interprismatic substance the hardest substance surrounding the core of each enamel rod (Ch. 8)
interproximal radiographs; also known as bitewing radiographs (Ch. 22)
interproximal brush small, soft-bristled brush attached to a metal or plastic handle for cleaning open contact areas, around orthodontic braces and wires, around exposed bifurcation or trifurcation of the roots, or on abutment teeth of a hygienic bridge (Chs. 4 and 32)
interradicular septum the bone that separates multiple roots in a tooth (Ch. 8)
Intersecting lines lines that cross each other at some point (Ch. 22)
interseptal dental dam material that goes between adjacent teeth (Ch. 19)
intracanal instruments instruments used in endodontics with precise diameters and lengths; made of stainless steel and nickel titanium alloy wire (Ch. 24)
intradermal administering drugs by injection under the epidermis (Ch. 15)
intramuscular administering drugs by injection into muscle tissue (Ch. 15)
intraoral film used inside the oral cavity (Ch. 21)
intraoral camera a small camera attached to the intraoral wand that transmits images to a television monitor (Ch. 17)
intraosseous anesthesia an injection of a local anesthetic directly into the cancellous bone (spongy bone) (Ch. 20)
intrapulpal injection a technique that deposits the anesthetic directly into the pulp chamber or root canal of the involved tooth (Ch. 20)
intravenous administering drugs by injecting directly into the vein (Ch. 15)
intravenous conscious sedation a very common way to keep patients relaxed, comfortable, and pain-free during dental procedures; sedative drugs are administered through an IV and directly into the patient's blood stream (Ch. 20)
intrinsic discolorations, usually permanent, inside the tooth structure (Ch. 32)
inverting tucking of the dental dam material around the teeth to prevent moisture leakage (Ch. 19)
iodine a trace mineral, found in the thyroid gland, regulates metabolism (Ch. 5)
ionization process by which atoms change into negatively or positively charged ions during radiation (Ch. 21)
iron a trace mineral whose primary function is to carry oxygen through the blood to the cells (Ch. 5)
irreversible hydrocolloid commonly called alginate, material used in the formation of dental impressions; setting of the material is accomplished by chemical reaction (Ch. 39)
irreversible pulpitis inflammation of the pulpal tissue to the point where it cannot recover; treatment includes root canal or extraction (Ch. 24)
irritability when muscle tissue responds to stimuli (Ch. 6)
ischemia shrinking of tissues (Ch. 33)
Isolite system system that provides isolation, retraction, evacuation, and a light source in one piece of equipment (Ch. 19)

J

James B. Morrison manufactured and patented the first dental engine with a functioning handpiece, motor, and foot-treadle (Ch. 1)
Jo-dandy disc thin, brittle discs that are double-sided and are used primarily in the dental laboratory to cut and finish gold restorations, but they can be used intraorally as well (Ch. 18)
John Greenwood the favored dentist of George Washington; proponent for pediatric dentistry; constructed dentures (Ch. 1)
Josiah Flagg (Late 1700s) notable dental surgeon; developed the first dental chair (Ch. 1)
Juliette Southard founded the American Dental Assistants' Association in 1924 (Ch. 1)

K

Kaposi's sarcoma malignant neoplasm, normally flat, reddish purple to dark blue; most commonly occurring in AIDS patients and men over 60 (Ch. 27)
key hole punch the largest hole punched in the dental dam; slides over the clamp and onto the anchor tooth; point from which next holes are punched (Ch. 19)
kilovoltage (kV) unit of electrical potential equal to 1,000 volts; dental kilovoltage is responsible for the quality of radiographs or penetrating power (Ch. 21)

kinetic energy energy of motion created during the x-ray process. Approximately 1 percent of kinetic energy is converted into useful x-rays (Ch. 21)
korotkoff sounds sounds heard through a stethoscope when taking a blood pressure (Ch. 13)
K-type file standard files used to scrape and widen the walls of the canal and to remove necrotic tissue (Ch. 24)

L

labial the "inside" surface, which is toward the lips (Ch. 9)
labioversion also called buccoversion, when a tooth is tipped toward the lip or cheek (Ch. 28)
laboratory area of the dental office where non-patient work is performed; may be used for finishing crowns, bridges, and so on (Ch. 17)
laboratory spatula tool used to mix dental materials (Ch. 18)
lamina dura radiopaque line that represents the thin compact alveolus bone lining the socket (Ch. 8)
lamina propria the connective tissue of the marginal gingiva and the location of the gingival fiber groups (Ch. 8)
landmarks of the face structures or tissues to recognize on the face include ala of the nose, nasolabial groove, philtrum, vermilion border, vermilion zone, the tubercle of the lip, labial commissures, and the labio-mental grooves (Ch. 7)
landmarks of the oral cavity structures or tissues to recognize in the oral cavity include vestibule, vestibule fornix, labial mucosa, buccal mucosa, parotid papilla, Stensen's duct, linea alba, Fordyce's spots, alveolar mucosa, gingiva, labial and buccal frenum (Ch. 7)
lanugo baby-like hair on the body (Chs. 5 and 8)
large intestine extending from the small intestine to the rectum, stores and excretes the waste products of digestion (Ch. 6)
laryngopharynx the lower section of the pharynx (Ch. 6)
larynx also known as voice box, connects the pharynx and the trachea, is made up of cartilage and supported by muscles (Ch. 6)
laser a medical device that generates a precise beam of concentrated light energy (Ch. 31)
laser handpiece used to cut and remove both hard and soft tissue, control bleeding (cauterize), and biopsy tissue. It is attached to a unit with a fiber-optic cable and has water and air to cool the tooth and tissues (Ch. 18)
latch-type shank contains a notch that fits into the contra-angle/right-angle handpiece and latches securely in place (Ch. 18)
latent suppressed or dormant for a period of time (Ch. 10)
latent image During radiation exposure, the silver halide crystals store the energy to which they have been exposed, and react with the chemicals in the processing tank to form a black region on the film. This energy, or latent image, does not become visible until the film has been exposed to chemicals for a given time at a given temperature (Ch. 21)
latent period time elapsed between exposure and response (e.g., time between exposure to the sun and sunburn) (Ch. 21)
lateral excursion the movement of the mandible from the centric position to a lateral or protrusive position (Ch. 36)
lateral incisor the second tooth from the midline used for cutting (Ch. 9)
lateral jaw radiograph takes an image depicting a large area of the jaw and is used in dental offices lacking a panoramic x-ray machine (Ch. 23)
latex allergies commonly presented in three primary types of reactions; the first one is contact dermatitis and involves only irritation to the top layers of the skin; the second one is Type IV and it is the most common; Type IV allergic reaction is primarily limited to the areas that contacted the latex (Ch. 11)
lead apron a common panoramic radiography error resulting from a patient wearing a lead apron with a thyroid collar (Ch. 21)
lead apron artifact a common panoramic radiography error resulting from a patient wearing a lead apron with a thyroid collar (Ch. 23)
leakage radiation the radiation comes out in all directions from the tube or tube head due to a malfunction or leakage (Ch. 21)
legal form documents that can be used in a court proceeding (Ch. 35)
lesions tissue damage; in dentistry, all abnormal structures in the oral cavity (Ch. 27)
leukemia a malignant, progressive disease of the blood-forming organs that is marked by unrestrained growth of abnormal leukocytes (Ch. 27)
leukoplakia a condition in the oral cavity with a white, leathery patch that cannot be identified as any other white lesion (Ch. 27)
libel false and malicious written comments (Ch. 3)
lichen planus a condition first appearing on the lower leg or ankle and then appearing in the oral cavity as small, white papules that group and form interlacing white lines (Ch. 27)
ligament fiber groups circles and tightens the gingival margin around the neck of the tooth; located in the lamina propria of the marginal gingival (Ch. 8)
ligaments composed of bands or sheets of fibrous tissue that act to connect or support two or more bones (Ch. 6)
ligature a piece of floss or a cord that stabilizes the dental dam in different applications; used in fixed bridge isolation, bleaching procedures, and tooth isolation (Ch. 19)
ligature wire a thin, flexible wire that holds the arch wire to the brackets (Ch. 28)
light cured type of sealant that is hardened by use of a single-component system activated by a curing light (Chs. 30 and 37)
light emitting diode (LED) A type of curing light that is durable, portable, produces minimal heat, does not require bulbs, and is quiet (Ch. 17)
line angle when two surfaces of a tooth meet (Ch. 37)
Liner material in a thin layer on the walls and floor of the cavity preparation (Ch. 37)
lines of Retzius incremental lines or bands around the layers of the enamel matrix (Ch. 8)
lingual surface of the tooth that is toward the tongue (Ch. 9)
linguoversion a deviation in tooth positioning; the tooth is lingual to normal position (Ch. 28)
lip retractor used to hold the patient's cheeks away from the operating site (Ch. 25)
lipids fat or similar compound found in cells (Ch. 5)
litigation the act or process of seeking or contesting a lawsuit (Ch. 13)
liver largest of the glandular organs, main function is the production of bile as well as aiding in the digestive process (Ch. 6)
load amount of pressure or strain put on a dental implant once placed in the bone (Ch. 26)
lobes divisions that join to form a tooth; often in molars, lobes become cusps (Ch. 9)
local anesthesia anesthesia that produces a deadened or pain-free area (Ch. 20)
local drugs Drugs that are applied in a specific area (Ch. 15)
local infiltration anesthesia an injection method that places anesthetic solution into the tissues near the small terminal nerve branches for absorption (Ch. 20)

Long axis of the tooth a line that divides a tooth into equal halves starting from the incisal/occlusal surface and ending at the apex of the tooth (Ch. 22)
long wavelengths in dental radiographs, wavelengths that have low energy, low frequency, and are unsuitable for exposing dental radiographs (Ch. 21)
low-speed handpieces handpieces used to polish teeth and restorations, remove soft carious material, and define cavity margins and walls; achieve between 6,000 and 25,000 rpm (Ch. 18)
low-strength base also called cavity liners, materials placed on dentin or on exposed pulp to protect the pulp from chemical irritation and provide therapeutic effect to the tooth; include calcium hydroxide, zinc oxide eugenol, and glass ionomer (Ch. 37)
Lucy Beaman Hobbs Taylor the first woman to graduate from a recognized dental college, earned her dental degree in 1866 (Ch. 1)
lumbar lower region of the back (Ch. 17)
lumen the internal opening of the needle where the anesthetic solution flows through (Ch. 20)
Lungs two cone-shaped organs inside the rib cage (Ch. 6)
Luting bonding or cementing together (Ch. 37)
luxates to move or dislocate (e.g., the dentist uses forceps to luxate a loose tooth from the socket) (Ch. 25)
lymph also called tissue fluid, is a clear liquid formed in tissue spaces; it enters the lymphatic capillary system and drains away excess fluid and carries proteins back to the blood stream (Ch. 6)
lymph nodes found in groups along the lymphatic vessels, their purpose is to filter the lymph as it moves back to the blood stream and to manufacture antibodies and other active materials of the immunity process (Ch. 6)

M

macrodontia abnormally large teeth (Ch. 27)
macrofilled materials used for Class IV restorations because they are strong enough to resist fracture and are esthetically pleasing (Ch. 34)
macule spot on the skin of abnormal texture or color (Ch. 27)
magnesium a mineral involved in energy metabolism and stabilizing the components of the bones and teeth once they are formed (Ch. 5)
magnetic resonance imaging (MRI) technique used mainly in the diagnosis of TMJ disease; allows the dentist to look at soft tissues of TMJ with little patient risk (Ch. 23)
Malaligned teeth that are out of line or order (Ch. 19)
malignant cancerous (Ch. 27)
malleability ability of a material to withstand compressive stresses without fracturing (Ch. 37)
malnutrition disorder resulting from lack of correct nutrients for the body (Ch. 5)
malocclusion any deviation from normal occlusion; may be a missing tooth, a group of teeth, or an entire arch (Ch. 28)
malpractice incorrect or negligent treatment given to a patient by a doctor, dentist, or health care provider (Ch. 3)
mamelons three bulges on the incisal edge of a newly erupted central incisor (Ch. 9)
mandible the only movable bone of the face (Ch. 7)
mandibular arch lower arch in the dentition (Ch. 9)
mandibular occlusal view patient is positioned in the supine position parallel to the floor with head tilted back; one assistant places the retractors and another positions the mirror (Ch. 35)
mandrel rods of various lengths used in low-speed handpieces; mandrels are available in three shanks: latch, friction grip, or straight (Ch. 18)
manganese a trace mineral involved in the process of metabolism (Ch. 5)
manual processing processing dental x-rays using a manual tank with developer, running water, and fixer (Ch. 22)
manual toothbrush a handheld toothbrush that only moves by the individual using it (Ch. 4)
manufacturer's number number found on the handle of the instrument; used for ordering and identifying the instrument placement in a set (Ch. 18)
marginal groove developmental groove that provides a spillway for food to escape during chewing (Ch. 9)
marginal ridges elevated areas of enamel that form the mesial and distal borders of the lingual surface on the anterior teeth and the mesial and distal borders of the occlusal surface of the posterior teeth (Ch. 9)
Maryland bridge a resin-retained, fixed bridge that replaces one tooth (Chs. 14 and 33)
Maslow's hierarchy of needs ranking of human needs developed by Maslow in which physiological needs are on the lowest level and self-esteem and self-actualization are on the highest (Ch. 2)
master cone the primary cone, normally gutta percha, used in a root canal (Ch. 24)
mastication process of chewing (Ch. 7)
matrix an essential artificial wall used to replace the missing or removed surfaces of a tooth during the filling of a cavity; composed of a band and a retainer (Chs. 38 and 39)
maturation growth to and learning on a certain level (Ch. 27)
maxilla the largest of the facial bones extending from the floor of each orbit and the floor and exterior walls of the nasal cavity to form the roof of the mouth (Ch. 7)
maxillary arch upper arch in the dentition (Ch. 9)
maxillary occlusal view patient is positioned in a semi-upright position with the mouth open; one assistant holds the lip and cheek retractors in the patient's mouth while another assistant positions the mirror (Ch. 35)
maximum permissible dose (MPD) the maximum dose of radiation that, in light of present knowledge, would not be expected to produce negative effects in a life (Ch. 21)
mechanical bond bonding of sealant accomplished as sealant flows into the irregularities of the treated enamel and locks into place (Ch. 30)
mechanical monitoring some sterilizers have gauges that monitor sterilization, and provide ongoing reports. Information covered is normally the temperature, of the cycle, the pressure, and exposure time (Ch. 11)
mechanical retention the attachment of materials to surfaces by means of grooves in the cavity preparation (Ch. 37)
mechanical toothbrush a handheld toothbrush, powered by electricity or batteries that move the brush (Ch. 4)
medical history contains questions about past surgeries, systemic diseases, injuries, and allergies (Ch. 13)
medicine drugs used to treat diseases (Ch. 15)
mercury a toxic chemical element that is the main ingredient of dental amalgams (Ch. 38)
mesenchyme tissue the primary embryonic mesoderm layer that develops during the morphodifferentiation period (Ch. 8)
mesial surface of the tooth toward the midline (Ch. 9)
mesioversion when a tooth is mesial to normal position (Ch. 28)
metabolic rate the physical and chemical changes that take place in relationship to the usage of energy (Ch. 5)
metabolism sum of chemical and physical changes occurring in tissue (Chs. 5 and 15)

metallic stain discolorations of the teeth due to metals and metallic salts inhaled (in industrial settings), taken orally in certain drugs, or as part of the materials used in tooth restoration; copper dust, amalgam, iron dust, and iron drugs can cause permanent stains (Ch. 32)

metastasize the spreading of a carcinoma (Ch. 27)

microbiology the study of microorganisms (Ch. 10)

microdontia abnormally small teeth; commonly seen in people with Down syndrome or people with congenital heart disease (Ch. 27)

microetcher a smaller version of the air abrasion units; they are used for intraoral sandblasting and dentin bonding (Ch. 18)

microfilled composite materials used as a cosmetic filling material for Class III and V restorations; used for direct veneers and diastema closures (Ch. 38)

microleakage the seepage of saliva and debris from the oral cavity between the tooth structure and restorative materials (Ch. 37)

middle third the root of the tooth is divided into imaginary thirds with the area between the incisal third and the cervical third is called the middle third (Ch. 9)

midsagittal plane sagittal plane divided into equal left and right sides of the body (Ch. 23)

milliamperage (mA) a measurement unit for electrical current (Ch. 21)

milliamperage seconds (mAs) determines the amount of radiation exposure the patient receives (Ch. 21)

milliroentgen (mr) one one-thousandth (1/1,000) of a roentgen (Ch. 21)

mini dental implant (MDI) type of dental implant that is smaller in diameter (less than 3 mm) and narrower than other dental implants. It can be placed directly through the mucosal tissue and into the bone (Ch. 26)

mitosis cell division in the sex cells in which the number of chromosomes in each is reduced by one-half (Ch. 21)

mixed dentition the period when primary teeth and permanent teeth are in the dentition lasting from approximately 6 to 12 years of age (Ch. 9)

mobile cart movable cart that contains dental equipment (Ch. 17)

mobility tooth movement in the socket; may be due to periodontal disease or trauma (Ch. 14)

mode of transmission the process that bridges the gap between the portal of exit and the infectious agent from the reservoir and the portal of entry of the susceptible host (Ch. 11)

modeling technique technique that aims to modify a patient's undesirable behavior by pairing the patient with another who demonstrates more desirable behavior (Ch. 29)

modified pen grasp grasping an instrument as one would with a pen, except the pad of the middle finger is placed on the top of the instrument with the index finger (Ch. 19)

molars molars are used to chew food, found in the posterior in maxillary and mandibular arches (Ch. 9)

molybdenum a trace mineral involved in the process of metabolism (Ch. 5)

monangle a dental instrument with a shank that has one angle (Ch. 18)

monomer self-curing acrylic tray resin (liquid catalyst) (Ch. 39)

morphodifferentiation the development of different forms during the embryonic stage of pregnancy (Ch. 8)

mottled enamel another name for dental fluorosis (Ch. 4)

mouth guard protective device that prevents premature loss or fracture of teeth (Ch. 29)

mouth mirror tool used for better visualization in the oral cavity (Ch. 18)

MTV Generation Generation X, born during the 1960s and 1970s (Ch. 2)

mucocele trauma to a minor salivary gland resulting in a bubble on the inside of the lip (Ch. 27)

mucogingival junction the line of demarcation between the attached gingiva and the alveolar mucosa (Ch. 8)

mucogingival surgery reconstructive surgery on the gingiva and/or mucosa tissues; involves covering exposed roots, increasing the width of gingival tissue, and reducing frenum or muscle attachments (Ch. 31)

mucoperiosteum mucosa and periosteum surfaces that combine to form a membrane (Ch. 25)

mulberry molars the appearance of a more rounded occlusal surface on the permanent molars; this is characteristic of the teeth of children born to mothers with syphilis (Ch. 27)

multi-parameter indicators react to two or more parameters, such as time and temperature. These indicators reference the exposure of dental instruments to the desired parameters during a sterilization cycle. Only available for steam sterilizers (i.e., autoclaves) (Ch. 11)

muscle trimming molding the borders of the custom tray to achieve margin adaption of the tray before final edentulous impression (Ch. 36)

muscles of facial expression allow for a wide variety of facial expressions, including smiling and whistling (Ch. 7)

muscles of mastication provide movement for the mandible as they protrude, retract, elevate, and lateral movement (Ch. 7)

muscles of the floor of the mouth four muscles between the mandible and the hyoid bone that assist in opening the mouth, depressing the mandible, and elevating the tongue (Ch. 7)

muscles of the neck draw down the mandible, the corners of the mouth, and the lower lip. Moves the head backward and laterally and elevates the chin (Ch. 7)

muscles of the soft palate raise the soft palate during the swallowing process (deglutition) (Ch. 7)

muscles of the tongue are responsible for shaping the tongue during speech, mastication, and swallowing (Ch. 7)

myelin sheath the protective and insulating covering of some nerves (Ch. 6)

N

napkin bib (Ch. 17)

nasmyth's membrane a covering over the enamel of newly erupted primary teeth left over from the epithelium and the ameloblasts (Ch. 8)

nasolacrimal groove extends from the medial corner of the eye to the nasal cavity along the maxillary process to the medial nasal process (Ch. 8)

nasopharynx first section of the pharynx; located behind the nasal cavity (Ch. 6)

National Fire Protection Association's color and number method labeling system for hazardous chemicals using data from MSDS (Ch. 12)

National Institute of Occupational Safety and Health (NIOSH) the federal agency responsible for conducting research and making recommendations for work-related sickness and health issues; it is part of the Centers for Disease Control (CDC) (Ch. 20)

natural acquired protection when an individual has had a disease, the body manufactured antibodies to the disease, and the individual recovered (Ch. 10)

natural immunity the innate ability for our bodies to experience local inflammation and the existence of blood phagocytes to fight pathogens (Ch. 10)

natural light multidirectional light that casts shadows and shows texture (Ch. 35)

necrosis tissue death (Ch. 27)

necrotizing ulcerative gingivitis (NUG) also called Vincent's disease or trench mouth, a common disease found in teenagers and young adults; causes include stress, smoking, poor diet, and poor oral hygiene (Ch. 31)

necrotizing ulcerative periodontitis (NUP) disease found in patients with HIV infection and in patients with severe malnutrition and suppressed immune systems; symptoms include pain, bleeding, and extensive tissue and bone destruction (Ch. 31)

needle holder hemostat-like instruments with grooved beaks to hold the suture needles (Ch. 25)

Needlestick Safety and Prevention Act passed by the U.S. Congress and became effective in April 2001; directs OSHA to revise the bloodborne pathogens standard (Ch. 12)

negligence the failure to exercise the standard of care that a reasonable person would exercise in similar circumstances (Ch. 3)

neonatal line an accentuated incremental line on the enamel matrix layer of a tooth that indicates the trauma of birth; found in all the primary teeth and several of the permanent teeth (Ch. 8)

neonatal teeth teeth present at birth or within the first month after birth (Ch. 27)

neoplasm an abnormal growth that can be malignant (cancerous) or benign (noncancerous); a tumor (Ch. 27)

nerve block injection of anesthesia near a main nerve trunk (Ch. 20)

net income the accounts payable subtracted from the gross income (Ch. 40)

neuromuscular dentistry the science of occlusion that objectively measures the physiological functions affected by occlusion to achieve an optimal relationship between the skull and the mandible (Ch. 35)

neuron basic structural unit of the nervous system comprised of a nucleus surrounded by a cell membrane with thread-like projections called nerve fibers (Ch. 6)

neutrons are part of the nucleus that is not charged (Ch. 21)

niacin one of the B Complex vitamins found in animal products; helps prevent gastrointestinal and nervous system disturbances (Ch. 5)

nib blunt end of an instrument that is serrated or smooth (Ch. 18)

nicotine stomatitis the heat and the irritating effect of chemicals in tobacco causing irritation to tissue that over time presents as whitened and red hyperkeratinized nodules (Ch. 27)

nitrous oxide odor-free gas derived from nitrogen and oxygen; used as a sedative before anesthesia; relieves anxiety and fear (Ch. 20)

nodule small lump of tissue, hard or soft, usually more than 1/4 inch in diameter (Ch. 27)

nonanatomical term for describing posterior denture teeth; nonanatomical teeth lack detailed anatomy on the occlusal, usually a concave and flat surface (anatomical teeth have cusps and developmental grooves) (Ch. 36)

noncompliant unwilling to follow treatment plans or directions from the dentist or another party (Ch. 3)

noncutting classification of operative hand instruments that are not used to shape or plane the cavity preparation (Ch. 18)

non-cutting instrument not used for cutting tooth structure (e.g., mouth mirrors and cotton pliers) (Ch. 18)

nonexpendable supplies that are not used up or disposed of after use (e.g., the dental chair or an autoclave) (Ch. 40)

nonspecific immunity the body's defense against any harmful agents (Ch. 6)

nonsuccedaneous pertain to the teeth that do not replace primary teeth (Ch. 9)

Nonverbal communication communication that takes place without verbal communication (Ch. 2)

nonvital pulp the pulp of the tooth that does not respond to sensory stimuli (Ch. 24)

normal flora bacteria in the human body that perform tasks that are essential to human survival (Ch. 10)

normal occlusion term that describes the contact relationship of the mandibular arch with the maxillary arch (Ch. 28)

nursing bottle syndrome (NBS) tooth decay develops in infants who have erupted teeth and are given bottles of milk, fruit juice, or sweet substances over a long period of time (Ch. 5)

nutrient chemical substances in food that provide the body tissues and structures with the elements needed for growth, maintenance, and repair (Ch. 5)

nutrition the manner in which foods are used to meet the body's needs (Ch. 5)

O

objective fears fears based on a person's experiences (Ch. 29)

oblique ridge elevated area of enamel that extends obliquely across the occlusal of the tooth (Ch. 9)

obturating process of filling the root canal (Ch. 24)

occlude to cause to become closed; obstruct (Ch. 14)

occlusal chewing surface of the molars and premolar teeth (Ch. 9)

occlusal equilibration process of alleviating areas with an excessive force (Ch. 31)

occlusal radiograph radiographs that expose the maxillary or mandibular occlusal surface of the dental arch (Ch. 22)

occlusal third the area on the crown of the tooth that is nearest the occlusal surface of the posterior tooth (Ch. 9)

occupational exposure any reasonably anticipated exposure to secretions of the eye, mucosa, skin, parenteral (cut, needlestick, puncture, abrasions, etc.), or any contact with blood or saliva that may be a result of employment tasks (Ch. 11)

odontoblast dentin-forming cells (Ch. 8)

odontogenesis origin of the tooth (Ch. 8)

one-stage implant technique the implant is inserted into the bone, but the extruding end is not covered with gingival tissue and a healing cap is placed (Ch. 26)

onlay replacements for missing tooth structure in the tooth (Ch. 33)

opacity not allowing any light to pass through (Ch. 35)

operating light adjustable light used by the dentist during examinations and procedures (Ch. 17)

operating zone the area where the operator (dentist) is positioned to access the oral cavity and have the best visibility (Ch. 17)

operator's cart a mobile cart that is usually set up for two or three dental handpieces plus an air–water syringe (Ch. 17)

operatory dental treatment room (Ch. 17)

opportunistic infections infections resulting from a weakened immune system (Ch. 27)

oral by mouth; with medications usually in tablet, capsule, pill, or liquid form (Ch. 15)

oral and maxillofacial pathology dental specialty concerned with the diagnosis and nature of the diseases that affect the oral cavity (Ch. 1)

oral and maxillofacial radiology dental specialty that covers radiology of the oral and maxillofacial area (Ch. 1)

oral and maxillofacial surgery dental specialty concerned with the diagnosis and surgical treatment of the oral and maxillofacial region (Chs. 1 and 25)

oral brush biopsy type of biopsy in which the surface of the lesion is wiped or scraped to remove a layer of the lesion (Ch. 25)

oral cavity the mouth, a part of the digestive system (Ch. 6)

oral pathology the study of oral diseases, their causes (if known), and their effects on the body (Ch. 27)

oral prophylaxis two-fold procedure involving removal of hard deposits and polishing of the teeth with a rubber cup (Ch. 32)

oral sedation a commonly prescribed drug is taken by the patient the night before their dental appointment (Ch. 20)

organic a product that is grown without the use of herbicides, chemical pesticides, or fertilizers; the seeds must not have been prepared with the use of hormones or any other enhancement (Ch. 5)

organic polymer matrix dimethacrylate, identified as BIS-GMA or urethane dimethacrylates (Ch. 38)

organic silane coupling agent barium, strontium, zinc, or zirconium may be added to make the composite material more radiopaque (Ch. 38)

organs tissues grouping together (Ch. 6)

orifices openings of the salivary glands (Ch. 27)

origin the part of a muscle that attaches to the more stationary bone (Ch. 6)

oropharynx middle section of the pharynx behind the mouth (Ch. 6)

orthodontic bands stainless steel bands fitted around teeth to hold and control tooth movement (Ch. 28)

orthodontics and dentofacial orthopedics dental specialty concerned with the diagnosis, supervision, guidance, and correction of the malocclusion in the dental facial structures (Ch. 1)

orthognathic surgery surgery involving the face, maxilla, and mandible (Ch. 25)

osseointegration compatible interface between the bone and the dental implant (Ch. 26)

osseous surgery restoration of bone by removal of defects and deformities caused by periodontal disease and related conditions; can be either additive (augmentive) or subtractive (Ch. 31)

osseous tissue the connective tissue of bones; is hard due to deposits of mineral salts (Ch. 6)

ostby frame a plastic dental dam frame that is oval-shaped and designed to follow the shape of the lower face; the frame is radiotransparent and autoclavable (Ch. 19)

ostectomy form of osseous surgery in which deformed bone is removed (Ch. 31)

osteoblasts bone-forming cells (Ch. 6 and 28)

osteomyelitis an advanced stage of periapical infection that spreads into and through the bone (Ch. 24)

osteoplasty form of osseous surgery in which deformed bone is reshaped (Ch. 31)

other potentially infectious materials (OPIM) any materials or bodily fluids other than blood; precautions should be taken to avoid contact (Ch. 11)

overbite projection of the upper teeth over the lower (Ch. 28)

overdenture retained roots providing support to a complete or partial denture (Ch. 36)

overgloves also known as food handler's gloves, are big, loose gloves that do not have the tactile touch that latex and vinyl gloves have, but quickly fit over the gloves to obtain something in a sterile area (Ch. 11)

overhang excess restorative material projecting over the cavity margin (Ch. 14)

overhead expenses required to run the practice (Ch. 40)

overlap of time when a doctor/dentist is required to be in two different places at once, or when two patients are scheduled for treatment at once (Ch. 40)

overlapping x-ray technique error resulting from improper horizontal angulation (Ch. 22)

over-the-counter (OTC) drug drugs that can be purchased without prescriptions (Ch. 15)

overtime treatment time beyond that scheduled (Ch. 40)

oxidation a process where solutions combine with oxygen and then the solutions lose strength and volume (Ch. 22)

P

packable composite more putty-like and stiff in consistency than other composites; used in posterior areas that need a stronger restoration (Ch. 38)

palatal expanding appliance composed of an acrylic palatal portion that is split along the midline; the acrylic palatal portion is attached to bands, and the bands are cemented to the posterior teeth for stability; in the middle of the acrylic is a screw-like device that can be adjusted to expand the arch called the rapid palatal Expander (RPE); the function of the palatal separating appliance is to spread the mid-palatal suture (Ch. 28)

palate roof of the mouth (Ch. 7)

palatine bone joined at the midline; are often referred to as the median palatine suture (Ch. 7)

palliative effect soothing effect a material may have on a tooth; also called sedative effect (Ch. 37)

palm grasp holding an instrument in the palm of the hand (Ch. 19)

Palmer System for numbering system of teeth identification that numbers permanent teeth 1 through 8, divided into quadrants; the deciduous teeth are labeled A through E, also by quadrant (Ch. 14)

palm-thumb grasp the grasping of an instrument that has the handle in the palm of the hand, four fingers wrapped around the handle, and the thumb extended upward from the palm (Ch. 19)

palpate to examine the body with the hands or fingers for detection of abnormalities, checking pulse rate, and so on (Chs. 13 and 27)

palpation pressure is applied to the mucosal tissue to test a suspicious root area (Ch. 24)

pancreas produces pancreatic juices that are emptied into the duodenum to aid digestion and produce insulin (Ch. 6)

pandemic wide spread epidemic of infectious disease. It may be spread worldwide or just across a large region (Ch. 10)

panoramic radiography type of extraoral radiograph that shows the entire maxilla and mandible on one film (Ch. 23)

pantothenic acid a vitamin found in both animal and plant foods; helps in energy metabolism (Ch. 5)

papilla small, raised projection covering the dorsal side of the tongue (Ch. 7)

papilloma a benign lesion of squamous epithelium tissue resembling a cauliflower in appearance (Ch. 27)

papoose board gentle restraint of the arms and legs to reduce or eliminate movement. This is for the safety of the patient and the operator and used with the informed consent of the parent/guardian (Ch. 29)

papule a small, solid, raised area of skin less than 1/2 inch in diameter (Ch. 26)

paradigm how individual views life due to life patterns (Ch. 2)

Parallel lines lines that are always the same distance apart, never intersecting (Ch. 22)

paralleling technique x-ray technique, also known as the right-angle technique, whereby the film and tooth and PID are parallel (Ch. 22)

parenteral piercing of the mucous membranes of the skin through such events as needlesticks, cuts, and abrasions (Chs. 11 and 12)

paresthesia sensation of being numb (Chs. 20 and 25)

partial crown covers only part of the tooth, not the entire crown of the tooth (Ch. 33)

partial denture prosthetic devices containing artificial teeth supported on metal frameworks and attached by clasps to natural teeth (Chs. 14 and 36)

partial image an x-ray film processing error due to the film placement in the processing tank when the solution levels are low (Ch. 22)

partnership legal agreement that makes doctors and dentists responsible for accounts payable; partners are not responsible for malpractice suits against the other (Ch. 41)

passive acquired immunity protection from a specific disease provided by an injection of antibodies from another animal or person (Ch. 10)

patch area of the skin that differs in color or texture (Ch. 27)

patent medicine over-the-counter drugs (Ch. 15)

pathogens disease-producing microorganisms (Chs. 10 and 11)

Paul Revere (1735–1818) a silversmith who was known to practice dentistry; his greatest contribution was making artificial teeth and surgical instruments (Ch. 1)

Pediatric dentistry dental specialty concerned with prevention of oral disease, diagnosis, and treatment of oral care in children from birth to adolescence (Ch. 1)

pedodontics dental care for children (Ch. 29)

peg lateral a diminutive, peg-shaped crown with a smooth surface lacking contact on the mesial and distal surfaces (Ch. 9)

pellicle thin, clear film of insoluble proteins, fats, and other materials from saliva that forms within minutes of removal; may protect enamel or provide breeding ground for plaque and calculus (Ch. 32)

pen grasp the grasping of an instrument in the same manner as one would grasp a pen or pencil (Ch. 19)

percussion examination of a tooth by tapping on the occlusal or incisal surface with fingers or instruments (Ch. 24)

Perforation going beyond the length of the root canal (Ch. 24)

periapical abscess localized destruction of tissue and accumulation of exudate in the periapical region (Ch. 24)

periapical cyst common cyst of the jaw, result of infection of the tooth. The cyst is caused by pulpal necrosis that is secondary to dental caries or trauma. Also called a "periradicular cyst" (Ch. 24)

periapical radiograph this radiograph pictures the entire tooth and surrounding area (Ch. 22)

pericardium double-wall sac that forms the outer layer of the heart (Ch. 6)

perikymata small grooves on some teeth (Ch. 8)

periodontal dressing bandage-like material applied to protect a surgical site as it heals (Ch. 31)

periodontal flap surgery surgical separation of the gingiva from the underlying tissue (Ch. 31)

periodontal knive instruments used to remove gingival tissue during periodontal surgery; also known as gingivectomy knives (Ch. 31)

periodontal ligament connective tissue that is formed by the fibroblast cells and secures the tooth into the socket by a number of organized fiber groups; contains two types of nerves (Ch. 8)

periodontal pocket space in the gingival sulcus (beyond the normal 1–3 mm) created by periodontal disease (Chs. 14 and 31)

periodontal probe calibrated instrument used to measure the depths of periodontal pockets, areas of recession, bleeding, or exudate; primary instrument in periodontal examinations (Chs. 18 and 31)

periodontal probing measuring of the depth of the periodontal pocket with a periodontal probe (Ch. 31)

periodontal scissors used during periodontal surgery mainly to remove tags of tissue and to trim margins (Ch. 31)

periodontal screening and recording (PSR) screening system for monitoring and documenting the periodontal health of a patient (Ch. 31)

periodontics dental specialty concerned with the diagnosis and treatment of the diseases of the supporting and surrounding tissues of the tooth (Ch. 1)

periodontitis the formation of periodontal pockets, occurring when margins of the gingiva and periodontal fibers recede and the supporting bone becomes inflamed and destroyed (Chs. 24 and 31)

periodontium a collective term for the periodontal tissues (Chs. 8 and 31)

periosteal elevator tool used to reflect soft tissue from the bone; usually double-ended with one long, tapered end and one round, bladed end (Chs. 25 and 31)

periotomes instrument used to sever the periodontal ligament (PDL) prior to a traumatic extraction as well as to prepare the tissue for dental implants. Come in a variety of shapes and can be used on anterior and posterior teeth (Ch. 31)

peripheral nervous system (PNS) all of the nerves outside of the central nervous system (Ch. 6)

periradicular cyst another name for a periapical cyst (Ch. 24)

peristalsis the process of involuntary wave-like successive muscular contractions by which food is moved through the digestive tract (Ch. 6)

permanent luting cement long-term cementing agent (Ch. 37)

permanent teeth second set of teeth humans grow (Ch. 9)

permeates spreads or covers throughout the nerve fibers to block the normal action until the bloodstream carries the anesthetic away and the sensations return (Ch. 20)

Perpendicular lines when one line is exactly vertical, and is intersected with a horizontal line to form a right angle (Ch. 22)

personal protective items that should be worn to protect against contact with all body fluids (e.g., protective eyewear) (Ch. 11)

pestle a small pellet made of metal or plastic that aids in the mixing of the alloy and mercury (Ch. 38)

petechiae small red or purple spots that appear on the skin or Mucosal tissue (Ch. 27)

petri dish a cylindrical shallow dish or plate with a cover used to grow bacteria under sterile conditions (Ch. 10)

petty cash small amount of money kept in the office for minor expenses, such as for coffee supplies or postage due letters, etc. (Ch. 40)

pharmacokinetics the study of the stages of drug action in the body (Ch. 15)

pharmacology the study of all drugs (Ch. 15)

pharynx connects the oral cavity to the esophagus; where food is swallowed (Ch. 6)

phosphorus a mineral found in bones and teeth and involved in energy metabolism and maintenance of proper pH balance in the blood (Ch. 5)

photopolymerized sealants contain a photoactive color additive; they are tinted (usually pink or green) on the initial application, and then change to opaque white after being light cured (Ch. 30)

photostimulable phosphor (PSP) a sensor plate technology, that is a wireless system that uses specially coated imaging plates instead of sensors to record the image. It is also called "storage phosphor imaging" (Ch. 23)

Physician's Desk Reference (PDR) published annually, comprehensive listing of drugs and drug information; lists drugs by trade or product name, generic and chemical name, and category (Ch. 15)

physiology the study of how the body functions (Ch. 6)

pictogram a picture on the label of materials that may present a health and physical hazard. Part of the 2012 revision to the HCS (Ch. 12)

Pierre Fauchard (1678–1761) founder of modern dentistry, organized all known information about dentistry and compiled it into a textbook (Ch. 1)

pit area on the occlusal surface of the teeth where the grooves come together or the fissures cross (Ch. 9)

pit and fissure hard resin materials that are applied to the occlusal surface of caries-free posterior teeth to prevent decay; also known as enamel sealants (Ch. 28)

pixels picture element; a small dot in a digital image (Ch. 23)

plaintiff the individual who brings charges against another individual (Ch. 3)

plane using a chisel cutting instrument make enamel and dentin walls of the cavity preparation flat or level (Ch. 18)

planes imaginary lines used to define areas of the body and parts within those areas (Ch. 6)

plaque any raised or flat patch in the oral mucosa; common cause of inflammation of gingival tissues; a sticky mass that contains bacteria and grows in colonies on the teeth (Chs. 4, 27, and 31)

plasma liquid portion of blood is 91 percent water and carries nutrients, hormones, and wastes (Ch. 6)

plasma arc (PAC) a type of light curing that is very fast and powerful; disadvantages include the expense and some are not portable (Ch. 17)

plastic filling used to place and condense pliable restorative materials and to place cement bases in the cavity preparation (Ch. 18)

plastic rings also called elastic ties, are small bands that are used to hold the arch wire to the brackets (Ch. 28)

plastic spatula tool used to mix dental materials (Ch. 18)

plastic stint clear denture base material, molded to the same shape and size as the denture (Ch. 25)

plastic strip matrix a thin, transparent, strip matrix used with composite, glass ionomer, or compomer restorative materials on anterior teeth (Ch. 38)

plugger used in amalgam fillings and root canal filling to pack amalgam into the tooth; the working end is short and comes in a variety of shapes and sizes; endodontic versions have long working ends with blunt ends; also known as condensers (Ch. 24)

pocket marking plier instruments with two beaks that, when pinched together, leave small pinpoint perforations on the gingival tissue; used to transfer measurement of a pocket to the outside of the tissue so the operator can see the depth of the pocket (Ch. 31)

point angles in the corners of a cavity preparation, the place where three lines (surfaces) come together (Ch. 37)

polishing process of using fine abrasives to produce a smooth, glossy surface (Ch. 32)

polycarboxylate type of permanent cementation for crowns, bridges, inlays, onlays, and orthodontic bands and brackets; sets in 3 to 5 minutes, does not exhibit exothermic heat (Ch. 37)

polymer self-curing acrylic tray resin (powder) (Ch. 39)

polymerization process by which a material changes from a plastic, pliable state to a rigid state (Chs. 30 and 39)

polysulfide material used in taking final impressions; composed of a base and lead peroxide accelerator, resulting in good stability, accuracy, sharpness of detail, and a relatively long shelf life (Ch. 39)

pontic portion of a bridge that replaces the missing tooth (Chs. 14 and 33)

porcelain restoration made of porcelain material for esthetic restorations, such as full crowns/coverage or as partial veneers/coverage (Ch. 35)

porcelain veneer requires two dental appointments; natural in appearance and are durable (Ch. 33)

porcelain-fused-to-metal crowns crowns with veneers (veneers are used to cover badly stained teeth and to reshape the anatomy of teeth) (Ch. 30)

portal of entry the route by which an infectious agent enters the host (Ch. 11)

portal of exit the route by which an infectious agent leaves the reservoir to be transferred to a susceptible host (Ch. 11)

position indicator device (PID) the open-ended tube in a dental x-ray unit, commonly called the cone (Ch. 21)

posteruption stage immediately after the tooth has erupted into the oral cavity, the absorption rate of fluoride is the highest (Ch. 4)

post-retained core metal posts fitted into the pulp canal of endodontically treated teeth for crown retention (Ch. 33)

potassium a mineral that helps release energy and synthesize protein; works together with sodium to regulate the electrolyte balance (Ch. 5)

potassium alginate an ingredient extracted from seaweed and kelp that is used for alginate impression material (Ch. 39)

Potassium alum a chemical used in development of radiographs that shrinks and hardens the emulsion gelatin (Ch. 22)

potassium bromide a chemical used in development of radiographs to slow the developing process to a practical speed and prevent film fog (Ch. 22)

potassium titanium fluoride an ingredient added to alginate impression material to counteract a specific action of the alginate where it tends to soften the surface of the gypsum products, not allowing it to fully set on the surface (Ch. 39)

power whitening process involving the reapplication of a bleach mix every 10 to 15 minutes (Ch. 35)

preemption related to HIPAA, when state laws conflict with federal laws (Ch. 3)

preeruption stage before the tooth has erupted into the oral cavity (Ch. 4)

premolars often called bicuspids, used to pulverize the food. Two premolars are in each arch and are posterior to the canines (Ch. 9)

prescription an authorization written by a doctor, dentist, or other that makes drugs available to patients (Ch. 15)

preservatives chemicals added to food to keep the contents fresh for a longer period (Ch. 5)

preset tray system instruments and auxiliary items are placed on a tray in the order of their use during the procedure; then the tray is covered and carried to the treatment room when the patient is seated (Ch. 18)

preventive orthodontic treatment to eliminate problems that may disrupt normal development of the teeth and facial structures (Ch. 28)

primary palate also known as primitive palate, appears as a triangular mass and contains the four maxillary incisor teeth; primary function is to separate the developing oral and nasal cavities (Ch. 8)

primary radiation central beam of the x-ray tube head (Ch. 21)

primary teeth first set of teeth humans grow. They are replaced with permanent teeth between ages 6 to 21 (Ch. 9)

primer conditioner used before a bonding material is placed (Ch. 38)

privacy officer the person in the dental office responsible for keeping all office personnel updated on HIPAA (Ch. 3)

process indicators normally heat-sensitive tapes or inks printed either on sterilization packaging materials, or on sterilization tape that can be placed on any packaging (Ch. 11)

professional courtesy discount the provider gives the patient (Ch. 40)

proliferation the cap stage in the life cycle of a tooth where the primary embryonic ectoderm layer matures into the enamel of the developing tooth (Ch. 8)

prophy brush used for the coronal polish procedure; only used on the enamel surface and should never contact the gingival tissues (Ch. 32)

prophylactic antibiotics that are prescribed as a measure to prevent infection (Ch. 15)

prophylaxis procedure whereby soft and hard deposits are removed from teeth; includes scaling and polishing (Ch. 31)

prostheses replacements for missing body parts; in dentistry, missing teeth and tissues are replaced with artificial structures (Ch. 33)

Prosthodontics dental specialty concerned with the diagnosis and restoration and maintenance of oral function with replacement of missing teeth and supporting structures through artificial means (Ch. 1)

prosthodontist dentist that has completed additional education on fixed and removable prosthodontic procedures (Ch. 33)

protected health information (PHI) PHI, an integral part of HIPAA, covers any information that identifies the individual or reveals information identifying the individual; this includes information such as name, telephone number, email address, and birth date (Ch. 3)

prothrombin substance produced by Vitamin K that is responsible for blood clotting and coagulation (Ch. 5)

protons are the positive charged part of the nucleus (Ch. 21)

Protozoa organisms just below visibility of the naked eye (about 100 microns in size) (Ch. 10)

protrusion anterior movement—patient moves the mandible as far forward as possible (Ch. 36)

Psychologically dependent person taking the drug has developed a strong emotional need to take that drug. It is similar to a craving (Ch. 15)

psychology profession and science concerned with the behavior of humans and animals (Ch. 2)

pulmonary circulation the pathway of blood circulation through the heart to the lungs and back to the heart (Ch. 6)

pulp vascular and nerve network of fleshy connective tissue that fills the center of the tooth in the cavity formed by the dentin (Ch. 8)

pulp canal is in the root of the tooth (Ch. 8)

pulp chamber a large portion of the pulp which is in the crown of the tooth (Ch. 8)

pulp horns pointed elongations of the pulp that extend toward the incisal or occlusal portion of the tooth (Ch. 8)

pulp stones calcified masses of dentin that can be attached or unattached to the pulpal wall (Ch. 8)

pulpal necrosis death of pulpal cells; often results from irreversible pulpitis (Ch. 24)

pulpal wall the side or floor of a cavity preparation that overlies the pulp (Ch. 37)

pulpectomy nonvital pulp therapy involving the complete removal of the dental pulp (Chs. 24 and 29)

pulpitis inflamed tissues due to injury (Chs. 24 and 8)

pulpotomy removal of pulp exclusively in the coronal portion of the tooth (Chs. 24 and 29)

pulse rate number of beats per minute of the heart (Ch. 13)

pulse rhythm expansion and contraction of an artery (Ch. 13)

pulse volume the strength of the pulse (Ch. 13)

punch table/punch part of the working end of a dental dam punch that includes four or five differently sized holes and rotates to facilitate punching holes for the various teeth (Ch. 34)

Pure Food and Drug Act law passed in 1906 by the U.S. government; controlled and regulated the composition, sale, and distribution of drugs (Ch. 15)

purging self-induced vomiting (Ch. 5)

purpura small purplish or reddish-brown areas or spots caused by bleeding in underlying tissues (Ch. 27)

purulence pus containing (Ch. 10)

pustule small, pus-containing blister (Ch. 27)

pyogenic membrane the membrane that builds a wall to contain the infection and does not allow it to spread to other parts of the body (Ch. 10)

Q

quadrants two sections formed by the imaginary line dividing the dental arches in two halves; actually there are four quadrants each containing eight permanent teeth (Ch. 9)

quality assurance (QA) routine procedures that have been developed to ensure the highest quality x-ray with minimal risk to the patients due to radiation exposure (Ch. 22)

quality control tests tests of equipment, solutions, and procedures to ensure that consistent high quality is maintained (Ch. 22)

quickdam an alternative to the full dental dam placement; an oval piece of dental dam with a border of flexible plastic that lies in the vestibular area of the patient's mouth (Ch. 19)

R

race grouping of people based upon biological resemblance (Ch. 2)

radial pulse site of palpating a pulse on the wrist (Ch. 13)

radiation absorbed dose (rad) amount of ionizing radiation absorbed in a substance (Ch. 21)

radiation monitoring device Any dental assistant producing radiographs should wear a radiation monitoring device or dosimeter badge. This badge monitors an individual's radiation exposure and accumulated dosage in the office (Ch. 21)

radiographs x-rays taken and processed to be used as a diagnostic tool (Chs. 21 and 23)

radiology The science or study of radiation as it is used in medicine (Ch. 21)

radiolucency the dark region of the images on radiographs. The dentist relies on the variations in the gray scale to determine the presence of disease (Ch. 23)

radiolucent black region on the x-ray indicating where radiation passed through the tissue (Ch. 21)

radiometer (light meter) a meter that measures the intensity of a light bulb (Ch. 17)

radiopacity the light region of the images on a radiograph. The dentist relies on the variations in the gray scale to determine the presence of disease (Ch. 23)

radiosensitive condition of being sensitized and affected by radiant energy (Ch. 21)

radiotransparent allows radiation to pass through it so that it does not interfere with images on an x-ray. Ostby dental dam frame is radiotransparent (Ch. 19)

rare earth phosphors phosphor substance that emits green light when struck by x-rays. These phosphors react fast, thus, the patient receives fewer x-rays during exposure (Ch. 23)

reamer endodontic instrument with a tapered metal shaft used to clean and enlarge a root canal (Ch. 24)

rear delivery system one of three types of dental unit with the equipment located behind the patient's head (Ch. 17)

reception room area the patient initially enters in the dental office (Ch. 17)

recession movement of gingival tissue away from the tooth (Ch. 31)

reciprocity one who has passed the medical/dental requirements for one state that applies for the same "rights" in another state, without taking another written or clinical examination (Ch. 3)

rectal administration of drugs through the anus; enemas and suppositories may be used (Ch. 15)

referral when a patient is sent to another dentist, usually a dental specialist, for a consult or treatment (Ch. 13)

reflex arc occurs when a stimuli is sent through the sensory neurons into the spinal cord and a response is automatically processed and sent back through motor neurons for an action (Ch. 6)

reflux when the water button is released, the normal action on the three-way syringe tip causes "suck back" to occur. This action allows contaminated fluids to retract back into the tip due to negative water pressure (Ch. 19)

registration form information on personal history of the patient, including the following: full name, address, phone numbers, Social Security number, insurance, emergency contacts, and financial information (Ch. 13)

regurgitation vomiting (Ch. 5)

reinforced zinc oxide eugenol dental material used for permanently cementation of crowns, bridges, inlays, and onlays; an insulating base and temporary restoration (Ch. 37)

relative biological effectiveness (RBE) measurement unit used to compare the biological effects of different tissues irradiated by different forms of radiation (Ch. 21)

relined resurfacing of the under surface or tissue surface of a full or partial denture to improve the fit (Ch. 36)

remineralization the minerals are replaced in the tooth (Ch. 4)

removable appliance devices inserted into the mouth and removed by the patient (e.g., retainers) (Ch. 28)

replenish to refill or fill with new solutions (Ch. 22)

res gestae meaning "part of the action"; any statements made during the time of an alleged act can be made admissible in a court of law (Ch. 3)

res ipsa loquitur when an act speaks for itself (Ch. 3)

reservoir a place where the agent can survive (Ch. 11)

residual activity where the effect of ideal surface disinfectants continue long after initial application (Ch. 11)

resin-modified (reinforced) glass ionomer a dental material used to cement metallic restorations or porcelain-fused-to-metal restorations to tooth structure (Ch. 37)

resolution the act of finding an answer or a solution to a problem (Ch. 2)

resorption the body's process of removing bone (Chs. 28 and 31)

respiration the process of breathing and exchanging oxygen and carbon dioxide between the body and its environment (Ch. 6)

respiration depth the amount of air that is inhaled and exhaled, which is recorded as shallow and deep (Ch. 13)

respiration rate number of breaths per minute (Ch. 13)

respiration rhythm the pattern of breaths (Ch. 13)

rest the part of the removable partial denture that contacts a tooth to provide vertical and horizontal support (Ch. 36)

restoration process of replacing missing tooth structure; results in "fillings" (Ch. 14)

resuscitation (CPR) rescue breathing and chest compressions performed on a patient experiencing cardiac arrest (Ch. 16)

retainer tool used to tighten and support the matrix band on the tooth while the tooth is being restored; part of a partial denture that contacts the abutment teeth and prevents the partial from moving (Chs. 36 and 38)

retention the means by which materials are held in place (Ch. 37)

retention core core buildup made of amalgam, composite, or a silver alloy/glass ionomer combination (Ch. 33)

retention pin small metal pins placed for restoration retention (Ch. 33)

reticulation processing error that shows on the dental film when the film emulsion is exposed to extreme temperature variations; normally shows as pitting or wrinkling of the emulsion (Ch. 22)

retinol Vitamin A that comes from an animal source (Ch. 5)

retractor oral surgery instruments that clear tissue from the surgical site (Ch. 25)

retrograde filling filling material placed in the apex of a tooth during an apicoectomy (Ch. 24)

retrusion posterior movement—patient moves the mandible as far back as possible (Ch. 36)

reuse life the time period that a disinfectant remains effective (Ch. 11)

reverse palm-thumb grasp grasp with the evacuator tip held in the palm of the hand, thumb directed toward the assistant instead of toward the patient (Ch. 19)

reversible hydrocolloid sometimes called agar-agar; used in the formation of dental impressions that can be converted from a gel to a sol back to a gel due to thermal reaction; produces accurate impressions (Ch. 39)

reversible pulpitis inflammation of the pulp caused by an irritant; when irritant is removed, the pulp heals (Ch. 24)

revolutions per minute (rpm) speeds of dental handpieces (Ch. 18)

Rh factor blood variable that is either positive or negative and an important consideration for blood transfusions (Ch. 6)

rheostat foot pedal on a dental handpiece that controls handpiece speed (Chs. 17 and 18)

riboflavin also known as Vitamin B2, found in milk, green vegetables, cereals, and enriched bread; it aids in growth, release of energy from food, and helps produce proteins (Ch. 5)

rickettsiae a parasitic form of bacteria. Lice, fleas, ticks, and mites are often hosts to rickettsiae. They multiply only by invading the cells of another life form. The hosts then transmit the disease to humans (Ch. 10)

ridge a linear elevation of enamel found on the tooth (Ch. 9)

right angle is formed when two perpendicular lines form a 90 degree angle (Ch. 22)

Robert Woofendale one of the first dentists from England to establish a practice in the United States (Ch. 1)

rod core the inner portion of an enamel rod (Ch. 8)

roentgen (R) the amount of radiation that ionizes one cubic centimeter of air (Ch. 21)

roentgen equivalent man (rem) also called sievert (Sv), is a radiation unit of measurement (Ch. 21)

rongeurs forceps with sharp cutting edges used to trim and shape the alveolar bone following tooth extraction (Ch. 25)

root divided into anatomical and clinical portions; the anatomical root is covered with cementum and the clinical root is the root seen in the oral cavity (Ch. 9)

root amputation surgical procedure to remove one or more roots of a multi-rooted tooth (Ch. 24)

root canal where the pulp is removed and replaced with a filling material (Ch. 14)

root canal sealer cement used with gutta percha to seal the pulp canal (Ch. 24)

root planing process of smoothing the root surface with curettes and other periodontal instruments to leave a smooth root surface (Ch. 31)

root tip pick delicate instrument used to tweeze the root tips or fragments from the bone socket (Ch. 25)

rotary instruments instruments that are mechanically driven (Ch. 18)

rotational centers the part of the panoramic x-ray machine where the rotation of the tubehead and the cassette that rotate around the patient is synchronized (Ch. 23)

rubber dental stimulator a device placed into the interproximal area that is angled toward the occlusal surface and rotated in a circular pattern (Ch. 4)

rubber stop pieces of rubber placed on files and reamers to mark the length of the root canal (Ch. 24)

S

saliva clear fluid secreted from the salivary glands and mucous glands throughout the mouth (Ch. 7)

saliva ejector a low-volume suction device that removes saliva and fluids from the patient's mouth (Chs. 17 and 19)

salivary gland produces saliva to dissolve food, facilitates the process of chewing, and coats food for ease in swallowing; three types include parotid, submandibular, and sublingual (Ch. 7)

sanitization process much like cleaning, area has been decontaminated, but it does not mean that all microorganisms in the area have been destroyed (Ch. 11)

sarcoma type of cancer cell that occurs in connective tissue cells. These tissues support the body and include cartilage, tendons, bones, muscles, and the fibrous tissue in organs (Ch. 27)

scaler sharp hand instruments used to remove hard deposits, such as supragingival and subgingival calculus, from the teeth (Ch. 31)

scaling technique to remove plaque, calculus, and stains from the surfaces of the teeth (Ch. 31)

scatter radiation radiation that is deflected from its path as it strikes matter (Ch. 21)

scored when a drug capsule is cut superficially to allow it to separate or break apart more easily (Ch. 15)

sealants enamel sealant is a resin material used to seal pits and fissures to prevent future decay (Chs. 14 and 30)

secondary palate the separation between the oral and nasal cavities evolves to form the remaining two-thirds of the hard palate and contains remaining teeth (beyond the four maxillary incisor teeth), forming the soft palate and uvula (Ch. 8)

secondary radiation formed when the primary x-rays strike the patient or come in contact with any matter or substance (Ch. 21)

sectional matrix system used to restore anatomical contacts during the filling process; consists of an oval matrix band, rings to hold the matrix band, and forceps to place the ring (Ch. 34)

security rule the ability to control access and protect information from accidental or intentional disclosure to unauthorized persons and from alteration, destruction, or loss (Ch. 3)

sedative a soothing effect a material may have (Ch. 37)

selective anesthesia one area of a patient's mouth is selected for an injection to identify which tooth or arch is problematic (Ch. 24)

selenium a trace mineral involved in the process of metabolism (Ch. 5)

self-curing materials set by means of a chemical reaction (Ch. 37)

self-ligating bracket does not require ligature ties; instead, the bracket has a slot that opens for placement and removal of the arch wire (Ch. 28)

sensor used in place of the dental film to caption a digital image (Ch. 21)

separating disc thin, brittle discs that are double-sided and are used primarily in the dental laboratory to cut and finish gold restorations, but they can be used intraorally as well (Ch. 18)

separators devices placed in the contact areas between teeth, forcing teeth to spread apart to accommodate the orthodontic bands; the separators are placed a few days before the patient is to have bands placed (Ch. 28)

septum amount of dental dam that slides between the teeth (Ch. 19)

seroconversion the process after exposure to a disease in which the blood changes from a negative to a positive serum marker for that disease (Ch. 10)

serrated lines or ridges on the working ends of dental instruments (Ch. 18)

sextants dividing the dental arches into sixths (Ch. 9)

shade guide samples of tooth shades used for tooth-colored restorations and denture teeth (Ch. 33)

shaft the handle of an instrument (Ch. 18)

shank the section of the instrument that connects the handle to the working end (Ch. 18)

Sharpey's fibers collagen fibers from the periodontal ligament, found within the outer part of the cementum (Ch. 8)

shelf life indefinite period of time materials as long as the packaging material remains intact and uncontaminated (Ch. 11)

shell matrix a type of matrix used with composite material (Ch. 38)

short wavelengths radiation wavelengths that have high frequency, high energy, and high penetrating power; also known as hard radiation (Ch. 21)

shoulder a type of crown preparation that provides a ledge that is sometimes beveled (Ch. 33)

side delivery one of three types of dental unit with the equipment located on the dentist's side and mounted to a moveable arm or mobile cart (Ch. 17)

side effect unintended result of drug use (Ch. 15)

sievert (Sv) also called roentgen equivalent man (rem), is a radiation unit of measurement (Ch. 21)

signature in the closing of the prescription the dentist signs his or her name, authorizes whether the prescription can be refilled and how many times (Ch. 15)

Silane coupling material that provides a secure bond between otherwise nonbonding or incompatible materials (Ch. 30)

silicone materials available in various forms that are used in taking final impressions; benefits include high rate of accuracy, no shrinkage, dimensional stability, high tear resistance, no taste, and no odor (Ch. 39)

simple suture most versatile, widely used stitch; suture goes into the facial surface and emerges from the lingual surface, and is tied with a surgeon's knot (Ch. 25)

single-parameter indicators are on paper, or paper-plastic sterilizing pouches or bags, and respond to time or temperature (Ch. 11)

six-handed system in which the dentist and two dental assistants work together at the dental chair (Ch. 17)

skin composed of several layers including the epidermis, dermis, and subcutaneous layers (Ch. 6)

slander false and malicious spoken words (Ch. 3)

sling suture used for interproximal suturing, stitch wraps around tooth to act like a sling; especially useful when a flap is necessary (Ch. 25)

small intestine connects the stomach to the large intestine; includes the duodenum, where digestive breakdown continues, and villi, where digested food is absorbed into the blood stream (Ch. 6)

small-balled instrument/ Dycal instrument instrument that has a small ball tip on the working end. It is used to place dental liners in the cavity preparation (Ch. 18)

smear layer layer of debris (created when the dentin is cut with a bur during cavity preparation) that lays on the cavity floor and walls and prevents contact between the intact dentin and the bonding agent/adhesive (Ch. 37)

smile line position of the lips when the patient smiles (Ch. 13)

Smooth muscle involuntary muscle that is under the autonomic nervous system's control; they are found in internal organs, blood vessels, skin, and ducts from glands (Ch. 6)

sodium a mineral that maintains fluid balance in the blood; works with potassium to regulate the electrolyte balance (Ch. 5)

Sodium carbonate a chemical used in radiographs as an alkaline medium in developer (Ch. 22)

sodium fluoride mouth rinses purchased at pharmacies generally contain 0.05 percent sodium fluoride and are fine for daily use; prescribed mouth rinses generally contain 0.2 percent sodium fluoride; sodium fluoride is used in the community water supply (Ch. 4)

sodium hypochlorite the most common biomechanical cleaner; also known as household bleach (Ch. 24)

sodium perborate a material used for teeth whitening that is a non-hydrogen peroxide system that contains sodium chloride, oxygen, and fluoride; used in household bleaching agents (Ch. 35)

sodium sulfite a chemical used in radiographs to prevent oxidation and to increase the life span of the developer solution (Ch. 22)

sodium thiosulfate a chemical used in development of radiographs for removal of unexposed and undeveloped crystals from the film (Ch. 22)

soft deposit acquired dental pellicle, materia alba, food debris, and plaque, removed during coronal polish (Ch. 32)

soft radiation long wavelengths with low energy, low frequency, and low penetrating power; also called Grenz rays (Ch. 21)

soft tissue impaction when third molars are partially erupted through the bone and into the soft tissues (Ch. 25)

soft tissue rongeur also called nippers; hinged pliers used to shape the soft tissue (Ch. 31)

soft wood points sometimes used with polishing agents to polish occlusal grooves and pits, proximal surfaces of sensitive teeth, and areas other polishing instruments cannot reach (Ch. 32)

software computer program (set of instructions) that tells the hardware what to do (Ch. 40)

sol a liquid (Ch. 39)

soluble ability of a material to dissolve in a fluid (Ch. 37)

somatic effects one of the classifications of the biological effects of radiation that leaves the individual in poor health and with cataracts, cancer, or leukemia (Ch. 21)

space maintainer device (fixed or removable) designed to hold a space (left from the premature loss of a primary tooth) until the permanent tooth erupts (Chs. 28 and 29)

specific immunity the body's defense against selected agents (Ch. 6)

sphygmomanometer instrument used to measure blood pressure (Ch. 13)

spinal canal also known as vertebral canal, is the space in vertebrae through which the spinal cord passes (Ch. 6)

spirilla/spirochetes S-shaped bacteria (Ch. 10)

splash, splatter, and droplet surfaces are areas that dental personnel do not actually contact, but still may be contaminated, such as counter tops or front of the dental light (Ch. 11)

spleen largest lymphoid organ, functions include the removal of bacteria and other foreign materials, filtering out of old red blood cells, production of red blood cells before birth, and acts as a storage for blood in case of hemorrhage (Ch. 6)

spore dormant stage of bacteria (Ch. 10)

sporicidal high-level disinfection that is extremely strong and can kill all the bacterial spores (Ch. 11)

sporulating a means of survival for bacteria where spores become enclosed in several protein coats that resist drying, heat, and most chemicals (Ch. 10)

spot-welded matrix band custom-made bands constructed with the use of a spot-welding unit and used in class II restorations; does not require a retainer (Ch. 29)

spray-wipe-spray technique universally accepted technique for cleaning and disinfecting surfaces. Surface is sprayed, then wiped to eliminate debris, then a second spray, is left on the item or surfaces for the specific time (Ch. 11)

spreader endodontic instrument used when sealing the root canal (Ch. 24)

springs specially bent or shaped wires attached to the main arch wire; used to exert pressure on the teeth (Ch. 28)

squamous cell a cancer of the squamous epithelium usually found in adults 40 years or older; lesions appear under the tongue, on the sides or borders of the tongue, and on the soft palate tonsil area (Ch. 26)

stainless steel crown used in the restoration of badly decayed teeth; usually used as a space maintainer in primary tooth replacement, or as temporary crown to be replaced by cast gold or porcelain (Ch. 29)

stamp used with an ink pad to indicate where the holes for the teeth should be punched on a dental dam (Ch. 19)

standard precaution universal precautions plus body substance isolation techniques. These are practiced prior to, during, and after each procedure in the dental office (Ch. 11)

stannous fluoride a stannous fluoride mouth rinse prescribed by a dentist can be used for decreasing the sensitivity of the tooth to hot and/or cold dental hypersensitivity (Ch. 4)

staphylococci diseases such as staph infection, gangrene, toxic shock syndrome, venereal diseases, and some forms of pneumonia caused by bacteria groups that grow in clusters (Ch. 10)

static zone the activity zone where rear delivery systems are located along with dental instruments and equipment used at the dental chair (Ch. 17)

statutory law law written and enacted by a legislative body (Ch. 3)

steam under pressure sterilization sterilizer that uses distilled water, can be used with wrapped or unwrapped packs, or handpieces. It has four preselected cycles that can be chosen (Ch. 11)

step wedge used to monitor the quality of the processing solutions. There are commercial step wedges or they can be made by placing several lead foil pieces from the x-ray film packet together in a stair-step manner and solder them (Ch. 22)

sterilization process by which all forms of life are completely destroyed in a controlled area (Ch. 11)

sterilization assistant dental assistant to do all the disinfecting/sterilizing of treatment rooms and instruments. This individual is responsible for monitoring all sterilizers, water lines, ultrasonic, cold chemical solutions, and biohazard materials (Ch. 1)

sterilization indicator a device used to determine if instrumentation has been properly sterilized once autoclaved (Ch. 11)

sterilizing area area of the dental office where all sterilization procedures are performed (Ch. 17)

stethoscope instrument used to listen to body sounds; for example, heartbeat and breathing (Ch. 13)

stimulant a drug that speeds up the body's activities (Ch. 15)

stippled healthy gingival tissue's appearance that is similar to the texture of an orange (Ch. 8)

stomach an organ, extending from the esophagus to the small intestine, that acts as a storage area and a churn to mix food with gastric juices (Ch. 6)

stomodeum in the primitive mouth it appears between the maxillary and mandibular processes. It initially appears as a shallow depression in the embryonic surface (Ch. 8)

storage phosphor imaging a type of indirect digital imaging; a wireless system that uses specially coated plates instead of sensors to record the image (Ch. 23)

straight shank functions with the straight, low-speed handpiece (Ch. 18)

strain change or deformation of an object brought about by the object's resistance to a stress (Ch. 37)

streptococci a species of streptococcus that has been implicated in dental caries and endocarditis; requires prompt use of antibiotics (Ch. 10)

stress reaction of an object to resist an external force (Chs. 2 and 33)

Striated muscle also known as skeletal muscles, its function is to provide for external body movement; these are the only muscles under conscious control (Ch. 6)

study models diagnostic casts (Ch. 39)

stylet a thin wire used to clear blood and tissue from the surgical tips (Ch. 15)

subcutaneous beneath the skin (Ch. 15)

subgingival below the gingival margin (Ch. 31)

subjective fears fears based on feelings, attitudes, and concerns that have developed from suggestions by others (Ch. 29)

sublingual in the administration of drugs, this method places the medication under the tongue and lets it dissolve (Ch. 15)

subperiosteal implant implanted beneath the periosteum, placed on top of the bone (Ch. 26)

subpoena court order mandating an individual to appear at a particular time and date with a specific reason to testify (Ch. 3)

subscription part of the prescription, it is the area where the doctor writes the name and strength of the drug being prescribed, the dosage, and the form in which the drug is to be dispensed (Ch. 15)

substance abuse use of a drug for other than medicinal purposes (Ch. 15)

subsupine position the patient is in a reclined position with the head lower than the feet (Ch. 17)

succedaneous permanent teeth that replace primary teeth (Ch. 9)

sulfur a mineral found in protein and involved in energy metabolism (Ch. 5)

supernumerary teeth extra teeth, usually dwarfed in size or shape (Ch. 27)

superscription part of the prescription directly below the heading that is used for filling in patient information; includes blank lines where the dentist can fill in the name and address of the patient, space for when the prescription was written, patient's phone number, age, gender, etc. (Ch. 15)

supine position the patient is in a reclined position with the nose and knees on the same plane (Ch. 17)

supplemental groove shallow linear grooves that radiate from the developmental groove (Ch. 9)

supragingival above the gingival margin (Ch. 31)

supraversion when a tooth extends above the normal line of occlusion (Ch. 28)

surgical aspirating tips tools used to aspirate blood and debris from the surgical site (Ch. 25)

surgical bone file instruments used to trim and smooth the edges of the alveolar bone following tooth extraction (Ch. 25)

surgical chisel instruments used to remove or shape the bone (Ch. 25)

surgical curette instruments used for debridement of the tooth socket or diseased tissue (Ch. 25)

surgical mallet instrument used to remove bone; shaped like a small hammer and used with a chisel (Ch. 25)

surgical rotary instruments include low- and high-speed surgical handpieces and a variety of burs and discs (Ch. 25)

surgical scissors instruments made of stainless steel and available in various sizes; used to cut sutures and trim soft tissues (Ch. 25)

surgical stent made of clear acrylic and placed over the tissues during surgery to guide the dentist in the placement of the implant; sometimes called a template (Ch. 26)

susceptible host an individual who lacks resistance to an agent and is vulnerable to disease (Ch. 11)

symmetric shape, size, and relative position of body parts on opposite sides are equal (Ch. 13)

synapse the conduit through which nerve fibers move impulses from one to another (Ch. 6)

syneresis shrinkage from a loss of water content due to heat, dryness, or exposure to air (Ch. 39)

syphilis a chronic sexually transmitted infection caused by the spirochete bacterium. The primary route of transmission is through sexual contact (Ch. 27)

system a grouping of tissues and organs (Chs. 17, 38 and 40)

systemic circulation carries the blood from the aorta to the smallest blood vessels and back to the heart (Ch. 6)

systemic drugs drugs that are taken internally (Ch. 15)

systemic fluoride one of the two ways that fluoride is used for dental health care needs; the sources for systemic fluoride include fluoridated water, foods with fluoride, fluoride tablets, and drops (Ch. 4)

systemic toxicity the anesthetic affecting a particular body system or the entire body (Ch. 20)

systems formed by tissues and organs forming together (Ch. 6)

systolic blood pressure created when the heart contracts and forces blood through the arteries (Ch. 13)

T

tachycardia abnormally rapid heart rate (Ch. 13)

tachypnea abnormally rapid respiratory rate at rest (Ch. 13)

tactile the feeling sensed by touch (Ch. 19)

tarnish dulling and discoloration of metal resulting from chemical or electrochemical attacks of the oral cavity (Ch. 37)

taste buds oval structures located on the dorsal surface of the tongue that provide our sense of taste (Ch. 7)

T-band matrix restorative band made of brass strips that are crossed at one end; secured on primary teeth; adjustable, do not require a retainer (Ch. 29)

tell, show, and do technique for easing a patient's fears by introducing the patient to the instrument to be used, demonstrating the instrument's use, and then performing the technique (Ch. 28)

temperature measurement of body temperature is an essential component of every patient's health evaluation. Body temperature is compared to the normal body temperature range and, if higher or lower, it should be further investigated (Ch. 13)

template guide showing the adult or pediatric arches indicating where the holes for the teeth should be punched (Ch. 19)

temporal pulse site of palpating a pulse at the temple of the head (Ch. 13)

temporary luting cement short-term cementing agent (Ch. 37)

temporomandibular joint (TMJ) structure made of muscles, bones, and the joints of the jaw; work together closely to make it possible to chew, speak, and swallow without discomfort (Ch. 7)
tendon skeletal muscle attached through specialized connective tissue extending beyond the muscle in the form of a cord (Ch. 6)
tetracycline stain discoloration of the teeth resulting from high concentrations of tetracycline antibiotics taken while the tooth was developing; vary in color from light green or yellow to dark gray-brown (Ch. 32)
The Federal Food, Drug, and Cosmetic Act law to control the sale of narcotic drugs. It was passed in 1938 and allowed Food and Drug Administration (FDA) to have control of all food, cosmetics, and drugs sold (Ch. 15)
thermal conductivity the ability for a material to transmit heat (Ch. 37)
thermal disinfector a device that uses heat to kill most vegetative microorganisms (Ch. 11)
thermal expansion the ability for a material to expand and contract with temperature changes (Ch. 37)
thermionic emission the process of heating the current to an extremely high temperature to allow electrons to be given off (during radiation production) (Ch. 21)
thermometer device used to measure body temperature (Ch. 13)
thermoplastic properties of becoming softer when heated and harder when cooled (Ch. 39)
thiamin a B-complex vitamin that provides energy as well as helps to prevent cardiovascular changes (Ch. 5)
three-quarter crown a fixed prosthesis that covers a tooth so that the mesial, distal, and lingual surfaces are reduced but the facial surface is left intact (Ch. 33)
thrush fungal infection of candidiasis in children, appearing as a thick, white covering over the oral mucous membrane (Ch. 27)
thumb-to-nose grasp the reverse palm-thumb grasp is sometimes called the thumb-to-nose grasp: with this grasp, the evacuator tip is held in the palm of the hand with the thumb directed toward the assistant instead of toward the patient, as with the palm-thumb grasp (Ch. 19)
thymus located under the sternum, it is large and active before birth and through puberty but gradually shrinks; important to the development of the immune system (Ch. 6)
tickler file system that serves as a reminder that events are to occur on specific dates (Ch. 40)
tidal volume normal volume of air inhaled and exhaled with each breath. Many offices begin with the flow of oxygen for a minute before the nitrous oxide to determine the patient's tidal volume (Ch. 20)
tin oxide very fine polishing agent used on enamel and metallic restorations (Ch. 32)
tinnitus ringing or tinkling sound (Ch. 25)
tissue forceps instruments used to hold and retract tissue during dental procedures (Chs. 25 and 31)
tissue retractor either a forceps (hinged) or cotton-plier style; the working end of both types has small teeth to assist in grasping the tissue securely (Ch. 25)
tissues specialized group of cell (Ch. 6)
TMJ replacement the joint is badly damaged and cannot be repaired, it is removed and replaced (Ch. 25)
tobacco stain light brown to black discolorations of the teeth caused by coal tar combustion in cigarettes, and pigments from chewing tobacco, penetrating the pits and fissures on the enamel and dentin surfaces (Ch. 32)
tofflemire matrix most common matrix used for amalgam restorations; the retainer can be sterilized and reused but the bands are disposable (Ch. 38)
tolerance when a person requires larger amounts of a drug in order to produce the same effect (Ch. 15)
Tome's process a secretory surface of the ameloblast that is responsible for laying down and guiding the enamel matrix into place (Ch. 8)
tomography the fundamental principle governing panoramic radiography that shows the imaging of one layer or section of the body while blurring images from the other areas (Ch. 23)
tongue moves food from the anterior teeth to the posterior teeth and gathers the food before it is swallowed (Chs. 25 and 7)
tongue retractor retractors that are spoon shaped or with long blades used to retract the tongue or cheeks from the operating site (Ch. 25)
tongue thrusting habit whereby a person's (usually a child's) tongue pushes against the anterior teeth during swallowing, causing an anterior open bite (Ch. 29)
tonsils forms a protective circle around the inside of the oral cavity that guards against bacteria entering the body through the digestive and respiratory systems (Ch. 6)
tooth mobility movement of the tooth within the socket (Ch. 31)
tooth morphology the study of the structure and form of teeth (Ch. 9)
tooth positioner a flexible or soft-plastic appliance that surrounds the crowns of all teeth, in both arches, when positioned in the patient's mouth (Ch. 28)
topical administration of drugs to the skin's surface, usually in ointment, lotion, gel, or cream form; in dentistry, topical drugs are sometimes used as anesthesia prior to surgery (Ch. 15)
topical anesthetic anesthesia that numbs the area about to be injected with local anesthesia; the patient will not feel the pain of the needle (Ch. 20)
topical fluoride one of the two ways that fluoride is used for dental health care needs; the direct application of fluoride only penetrates the outer layer of the tooth enamel; it is available as a gel, rinse, foam, and liquid (Ch. 4)
topographic technique technique used to expose occlusal radiographs (Ch. 22)
tori boney outgrowths of tissue in the oral cavity that are benign (Ch. 27)
torsoversion when a tooth is rotted or turned (Ch. 28)
tort a wrongful act that results in injury to one person by another (Ch. 3)
torus excess bone that is occasionally in the middle of the palate (Ch. 7)
touch surface surface that is directly touched and contaminated during dental treatment procedures, such as light handles, unit controls, material containers, dental trays, pens, and drawer handles (Ch. 11)
toxic reaction symptoms that appear due to overdose or excessive administration of the anesthetic solution (Ch. 20)
trabeculae sponge-like appearance of the cancellous bone as seen on dental x-rays (Ch. 6)
trachea also known as the windpipe, consists of C-shaped cartilage that allows for expansion of the esophagus during the process of swallowing (Ch. 6)
tragus of the ear projection on the anterior portion of the ear that helps position the arches when exposing x-rays using the bisecting technique (Ch. 23)
transcranial temporomandibular joint radiograph radiograph taken with the patient holding a cassette against the side of the head (Ch. 23)
transdermal a method of delivery of medication using a patch applied to the skin (Ch. 15)
transfer surface surface is not directly touched, but are areas or items that are indirectly contaminated, such as

air–water syringe holders, dental trays, and handpiece holders (Ch. 11)

transfer zone the area below the patient's nose where instruments and materials are passed and received (Chs. 17 and 19)

transformers part of the tubehead where the voltage is adjusted up and down (Ch. 21)

transillumination test reflection of fiber-optic light through the crown of a tooth to indicate vertical fractures (Ch. 24)

transitional line angles surround the tooth and mark the boundaries of the face of the tooth (Ch. 35)

translucency allows light to pass through (Ch. 35)

transosteal implant is used in an edentulous area of the mandible and is also known as staple or transosseous implants. They consist of screws, nuts, and a pressure plate (Ch. 26)

transposition when a tooth is in the wrong order in the arch (Ch. 28)

transverse ridge the union of two triangular ridges produces a single ridge of elevation across the occlusal surface of a posterior tooth (Ch. 9)

transversion when a tooth is in the wrong order in the arch (Ch. 28)

traumatic intrusion occurs when the teeth are forcibly driven into the alveolus (Ch. 29)

treatment plan the outline of what will be done to address the needs of a patient and remedy a condition (Ch. 13)

treatment room areas of the dental office where the patient is examined (Ch. 17)

triangular ridge ridge or elevation that descends from the cusp and widens as it runs downward to the middle area of the occlusal surface (Ch. 9)

tricanineate three-cusp type of tooth (Ch. 9)

trifurcated when there are three roots coming from the main trunk of the tooth (Ch. 9)

trigeminal nerve the largest cranial nerve and most important to dental auxiliaries because it innervates the maxilla and the mandible dividing the semi-lunar ganglion into three branches (Ch. 7)

triglycerides neutral fats from plant and animal food found in a normal diet (Ch. 5)

trismus limited opening of the mouth (Chs. 23 and 25)

triturates mechanically combines dental materials (Ch. 17)

trituration mixing (Ch. 38)

triturator specially designed machine used to triturate (mix) the alloy and mercury; also called amalgamators (Ch. 38)

Truth in Lending Act (TILA) a U.S federal law that is designed to protect consumers in any credit transactions (Ch. 40)

tubehead where the x-ray tube and step-up and step-down transformers are located (Ch. 21)

tuberculocidal high-level disinfection that kills most, but not all, bacterial spores (Ch. 11)

tungsten halogen the traditional curing light that is durable, less expensive, cures quickly, and is fairly effective; disadvantages include emitted heat, requires a filter, and lack of portability (Ch. 17)

tungsten target an area located on the anode, where electrons directed from the cathode hit. The anode tungsten target is attached to a copper stem that is located in the glass envelope in the tube head (Ch. 21)

twinning a condition where two separate teeth are made from one tooth bud (Ch. 27)

two-stage implant technique technique where the implant is placed into the bone and gingival tissue is sutured into place to cover the implant. After 3 to 4 months of healing time a second surgery is scheduled to uncovered and a cap or abutment is placed (Ch. 26)

tympanic membrane the eardrum (Ch. 13)

tympanic thermometer a device used to measure the temperature by inserting it into the ear (Ch. 13)

type I allergic reaction a very serious adverse reaction to a substance can occur minutes after exposure and can result in death if the patient has an anaphylaxis reaction (Ch. 11)

type IV allergic reaction a mild adverse reaction to a substance (Ch. 11)

U

U-frame a plastic dental dam frame that is easy to apply, comfortable for the patient, radiolucent, and autoclavable (Ch. 19)

ulcer an open sore, usually inflamed and painful, that forms on tissue (Chs. 15 and 27)

ultrasonic cleaner metal or plastic containers for cleaning instruments before being sterilized (Ch. 11)

ultrasonic handpiece handpiece that is attached to ultrasonic scaler unit. The unit converts electrical energy into ultrasonic vibrations that are transmitted to the handpiece. Mainly used for scaling procedures and root canal therapy (Ch. 18)

ultrasonic instruments instruments used to remove hard deposits, stains, and debris through the high-power vibrations of scaling, curettage, and root planing procedures (Ch. 31)

ultrasonic scaler through a vibrating action, removes hard deposits (e.g., calculus) from the teeth (Ch. 17)

ultrasonic unit used for troughing (making a groove or channel) around a post and opening calcified canals, breaking away cement or calculus, and vibrating a post out of a canal or vibrating a crown or bridge off (Ch. 24)

undercuts recessed areas that are wider on the bottom than on the top (Ch. 39)

underexposed when the film appears light and has a thin image (Ch. 22)

undernourished lacking proper nutrients (Ch. 5)

units represent each tooth in a bridge. For example, a three-unit bridge involves three teeth (Ch. 33)

universal curette a hand instrument used for removing subgingival calculus, smoothing the root surface, and removing the soft tissue lining of the periodontal pocket (Ch. 31)

universal forceps forceps that can be used on any of the four quadrants (Ch. 25)

Universal/National System for numbering system adopted in 1968 by the ADA to identify the teeth; permanent teeth are numbered 1 to 32 (maxillary right to left; mandibular left to right); primary teeth are labeled A to T (Ch. 14)

universal precautions guidelines established by the CDC to help protect health care workers and patients from the transmission of infectious diseases (Ch. 11)

universal varnish a cavity varnish that does not have the organic solvent and may be used under all restorations (Ch. 37)

upright position the back of the dental chair is in a 90-degree angle to provide comfort and support for the patient (Ch. 17)

usual, customary, and reasonable fee is a fee schedule used to define what patients are charged for each service. The usual fee is typically charged by the dentist for a specific procedure. The customary fee is the average fee charge in the area for the same procedure. The reasonable fee is the midrange of fees charged (Ch. 40)

utility gloves thicker gloves used during disinfection and cleanup procedures (Ch. 11)

V

value corresponds to brightness, which is very important when matching shades (Ch. 35)

varix weakening and extension of blood vessels in the oral cavity beneath the tongue, primarily seen in the elderly (Ch. 27)

Varnish thin layer of material that is placed to seal the walls and floor of a cavity preparation (Ch. 37)

vasoconstrictor drugs added to anesthetic solutions that constrict blood vessels around the injection site, reducing the blood flow in the area (Ch. 20)

vectorborne transmission mode of transmission of infectious agents through animate means such as mosquitos, ticks, lice, and other animals (Ch. 11)

vehicle transmission mode of transmission of infectious agents through contamination of inanimate objects such as water, food, meat, drugs, and blood (Ch. 11)

vein carries blood that has drained from the capillaries back to the heart (Ch. 6)

VELscope a screening system used to detect diseased tissues in the oral cavity (Ch. 25)

vena cava the large vessel where blood enters the heart (Ch. 6)

veneer items used to cover badly stained teeth and to reshape the anatomy of teeth; thin layers of tooth-colored material that cover much of the facial surface (Ch. 33)

verbal communication using words and voice to communicate (Ch. 2)

vermilion border line around the lips (Ch. 13)

vertical angulation adjustment of angulation from top to bottom; improper vertical angulation shows teeth elongated or foreshortened (Ch. 22)

vertical bone resorption receding of the alveolar bone vertically on individual teeth and the interproximal surface (Ch. 31)

vertical dimension space provided by the teeth in normal occlusion, or, with the teeth in occlusion, a measurement of the face at the midline (Ch. 36)

vertical mattress suture used when suturing a flap, goes in and out of the tissue on the same surface; identified by vertical stitch or "bite"; tied with one surgeon's knot on surface where suture procedure began (Ch. 25)

vesicle small, fluid-filled blisters (Ch. 27)

vibrios curved like a comma (Ch. 10)

viewbox a lighted box with a white, frosted surface, used to mount dental radiographs (Ch. 22)

virucidal an agent that neutralizes or destroys viruses (Ch. 11)

viruses smallest microorganisms known to date that reproduce inside host cells and are difficult to grow in a culture (Ch. 11)

viscosity the ability of liquid to flow (Ch. 37)

vital pulp term used to describe healthy pulp (Ch. 24)

vital signs the basic signs of life; for example, body temperature, pulse, blood pressure, and respiration rate (Ch. 13)

vitality scanner an electronic pulp testing unit that measures whether a tooth is vital or nonvital (Ch. 24)

Vitamin B12 a water-soluble vitamin found in animal products; functions include the synthesis of red blood cells and maintenance of myelin sheaths (Ch. 5)

Vitamin B6 essential in the synthesis and metabolism of protein, carbohydrates, and fat; if taken in large quantity, it could be toxic (Ch. 5)

vitamins a class of nutrients that do not provide the body with energy but perform other necessary functions (Ch. 5)

ViziLite a screening system used to detect diseased tissues in the oral cavity (Ch. 25)

vocal cords cords that stretch across the width of the larynx to produce sound (Ch. 6)

vulcanite bur used to adjust acrylic materials, such as partials, dentures, and custom trays; they are also used on plaster, stone, and metal materials (Ch. 18)

W

walking whitening technique teeth whitening techniques in which a bleach mixture is temporarily sealed in place; it allows the patient to leave the office and return for evaluation at a later date (Ch. 35)

water irrigation device used to clean away debris from orthodontic brackets and other prosthetic devices (Ch. 4)

water reservoir bottle on the dental unit that supplies water to the water syringe and the dental handpieces (Ch.17)

waterline shock initial tablet in waterline treatment (Ch. 11)

wedge small, triangular piece of wood or plastic (Ch. 38)

Wells, Horace (1815–1848) Connecticut dentist who was the first to use nitrous oxide as an anesthetic during dental surgery (Ch. 20)

wettability ability of a material to flow over a surface (Ch. 37)

white light teeth whitening systems home lightening system that uses a light transmitter to activate the whitening gel (Ch. 35)

Wickham's striae interlacing white lines formed by a grouping of white papules; usually on the buccal mucosa (Ch. 27)

Wilhelm Conrad Roentgen (1845–1923) discovered x-rays in 1895 (Ch. 1)

winged clamps clamps with extra projections (wings) that are angled toward the gingiva for better retraction and holding of the dental dam (Ch. 19)

wingless clamps clamps with no projections (wings) and with the letter "W" in front of the numbers of the clamps (Ch. 19)

withdrawal symptoms that occur when a person addicted to a drug stops taking that drug; nervousness, stomach cramps, diarrhea, shaking, and depression may be symptoms (Ch. 15)

wooden dental stimulator elongated, soft-wood wedges placed into the interproximal area, angling them toward the biting surface and rotating them in a circular pattern; the action stimulates the soft tissues and removes plaque in the area (Ch. 4)

working end part of the instrument that performs the instrument's function (Ch. 18)

X

xerostomia dryness of the mouth caused by saliva reduction (Ch. 4)

x-ray tube part of the dental x-ray unit that houses the coolidge, vacuum tube, filters, Collimator, and cone (Ch. 21)

x-rays invisible, odorless electromagnetic radiation (Ch. 21)

XTS composite instrument aluminum-titanum nitride instruments are non-adhering, hard, and scratch resistant. These composite instruments are ergonomically designed handles and black working ends for contrast with the tooth surface (Ch. 18)

Y

yellow stain discolorations of the teeth usually associated with poor oral hygiene and plaque; dull yellow to light brownish (Ch. 32)

young frame metal U-shaped dental dam frame that is made of stainless steel, easy to apply, and comfortable for the patient (Ch. 19)

Z

zinc a trace mineral that aids in tissue growth and maintenance of the immune system (Ch. 5)

zinc oxide eugenol type of temporary cementation of crowns, inlays, onlays, and bridges (Ch. 37)

zinc phosphate permanent cement for crowns, inlays, onlays, bridges, and orthodontic bands and brackets (Ch. 37)

zirconium silicate material used for stain removal and polishing on gold restoration, exposed dentin, tooth-colored restoration, and enamel (Ch. 32)

zygote state during which cells proliferate (Ch. 8)

REFERENCES

Abrahams, P.H., Marks, S.C. Jr., Hutchins, R.T. (2014). *McMinn and Abrahams' Clinical Atlas of Human Anatomy*, 7th ed. St. Louis, MO: Mosby.

American Dental Assistants Association. (1999). *Introduction to Basic Concepts in Dental Radiography*. Chicago, IL: ADAA.

American Dental Association. (2016). *ADA Principles of Ethics and Code of Professional Conduct*. Chicago, IL: The Association. www.ada.org

American Dental Association. *The ADA Practical Guide to HIPAA Compliance*. Chicago, IL: The Association.

American Dental Association. (2012). *The ADA Practice Guide to Dental Procedure Codes*. Chicago, IL: The Association.

American Dental Association. *OSHA: Training for Dental Professionals*. Chicago, IL: The Association.

American Heart Association. (2015). *The American Heart Association Guidelines for Cardiopulmonary Resuscitation and Emergency Cardiovascular Care*. www.heart.org

Anderson, Pauline C., Pendleton, Alice E. (2001). *The Dental Assistant*, 7th ed. Clifton Park, NY: Delmar Cengage Learning.

Anusavice, K.J. (2012) *Phillips Science of Dental Materials*, 12th ed. St. Louis, MO: Elsevier.

Appleton & Lange's Health Professionals Drug Guide. (2000). Stamford, CT: Appleton & Lange.

Aschheim, K.W., Dale, B.G. (2014). *Esthetic Dentistry: A Clinical Approach to Techniques and Materials*, 3rd ed. St. Louis, MO: Mosby, Inc.

Ash, M., Nelson, S. (2015). *Wheeler's Dental Anatomy, Physiology, and Occlusion*, 10th ed. St. Louis, MO: Elsevier.

Ash, M.M. 10th ed. (2015). *Wheeler's Atlas of Tooth Form*, 5th ed. Philadelphia, PA: W.B. Saunders.

Beirle, J.W. (1993). "Dental Operatory Water Lines." *Canadian Dental Association Journal*, 211(2), 13–15.

Berkovitz, B.K.B., Holland, G.R., Moxham, B.J. (2009). *Oral Anatomy, Histology, and Embryology*, 4th ed. St. Louis, MO: Mosby.

Brand, R.W., Isselhard, D.E. (2014). *Anatomy of Orofacial Structures*, 7th ed. St. Louis, MO: Mosby.

Burt, B.A., Eklund, S.A. (2005). *Dentistry, Dental Practice, and the Community*, 6th ed. Philadelphia, PA: W.B. Saunders.

Burton, G., Engelkirk, P. (2014). *Microbiology for the Health Sciences*, 10th ed. Philadelphia, PA: J.B. Lippincott Co.

Carranza, F., Newman, M. (2014) *Carranza's Clinical Periodontology*, 12th ed. St. Louis, MO: W.B. Saunders.

Chapman, S. (1998). *Medical & Dental Associates, P.C.: Insurance Forms Preparation*, 3rd ed. Clifton Park, NY: Delmar Cengage Learning.

Chernega, J.B. (2013). *Emergency Guide for Dental Auxiliaries*, 4th ed. Clifton Park, NY: Delmar Cengage Learning.

Christensen, G.J. (2002). *A Consumer's Guide to Dentistry*, 2nd ed. St. Louis, MO: Mosby.

Cohen, B.J., Hull, Kerry (2015). *Memmler's the Human Body in Health and Disease*, 13th ed. Philadelphia, PA: Lippincott-Raven.

Craig, R.G., Powers, J. (2002). *Restorative Dentistry Materials*, 13th ed. St. Louis, MO: Mosby.

Darby, M., Walsh, M. (2014). *Dental Hygiene Theory and Practice*, 4th ed. Philadelphia, PA: W.B. Saunders.

Dean, J. (2015). *Dentistry for the Child and Adolescent*, 10th ed. St. Louis, MO: Mosby.

Dietz, E. (2000). *Dental Office Management*. Clifton Park, NY: Delmar Cengage Learning.

Dietz, E., Badavinac, R. (2002). *Safety Standards and Infection Control for Dental Hygienists*, Clifton Park, NY: Delmar Cengage Learning.

Dofka. C. (2013). *Dental Terminology*, 3rd ed. Clifton Park, NY: Delmar Cengage Learning.

Dorland's Pocket Medical Dictionary, 29th ed. (2012). Philadelphia, PA: W.B. Saunders.

Drafke, M.W. (2002). *Working in Health Care: What You Need to Know to Succeed*, 2nd ed. Philadelphia, PA: F.A. Davis.

Ehrlich, A., Schraeder, C. (2017). *Medical Terminology for Health Professions*, 8th ed. Clifton Park, NY: Delmar Cengage Learning.

Fehrenbach, M., Herring, S. (2016). *Illustrated Anatomy of the Head and Neck*, 5th ed. Philadelphia, PA: W.B. Saunders.

Fehrenbach, M.J., Popowics, T. (2016). *Illustrated Dental Embryology, Histology, and Anatomy*, 4th ed. Maryland Heights, MO: Elsevier.

Ferracane, J.L. (2001). *Materials in Dentistry*, 2nd ed. Philadelphia, PA: J.B. Lippincott Co.

Finkbeiner, B.L., Finkbeiner, C.A. (2015). *Practice Management for the Dental Team*, 8th ed. St. Louis, MO: Mosby.

Fordney, M.T. (2016). *Insurance Handbook for the Medical Office*, 14th ed. Philadelphia, PA: W.B. Saunders.

Frommer, H.H. (2010). *Radiology for the Dental Professional*, 9th ed. St. Louis, MO: Mosby.

Genco, R.J., Goldman, H.M., Cohen, D.W. (1990). *Contemporary Periodontics*. St. Louis, MO: Mosby.

Gladwin, M., Bagby, M. (2012) *Clinical Aspects of Dental Materials: Theory, Practice, and Cases*, 4th ed. Baltimore, MD: Lippincott Williams & Wilkins.

Gluck, G., Morganstein, W. (2003). *Jong's Community Dental Health*, 5th ed. St. Louis, MO: Mosby.

Graber, T.M., Vanarsdall R.L. (2017). *Orthodontics: Current Principles and Techniques*, 6th ed. St. Louis, MO: Mosby.

Grembowski, D. (1992). "How Fluoridation Affects Adult Dental Caries." *Journal of the American Dental Association*, 1123, 49–54.

Guerini, V. (1909). *A History of Dentistry from the Most Ancient Times Until the End of the 18th Century*. Philadelphia, PA: Lea & Febiger.

Haring, J.I., Howerton, L.J., (2016). *Dental Radiography: Principles and Techniques*, 5rd ed. Philadelphia, PA: W.B. Saunders.

Harris, N., Garcia-Godoy, F., Nielsen Nathe, C. (2013). *Primary Preventive Dentistry*, 8th ed. Upper Saddle River, N.J.: Pearson Education.

Hatrick, C., Eakle, W., Bird, W., (2010). *Dental Materials: Clinical Applications for Dental Assistants and Dental Hygienists.* 2nd ed. St. Louis, MO: Elsevier Saunders.

Haveles, E. (2002). *Delmar's Dental Drug Reference.* Clifton Park, NY: Delmar Cengage Learning.

Haveles, E.B. (2015). *Applied Pharmacology for the Dental Hygienist*, 7th ed. St. Louis, MO: Mosby Elsevier.

Helgeson, B. (1974). "American Dental Assistants Commemorate 50th Anniversary." *Journal of the American Dental Association*, 89, 539–544.

History of the American Dental Assistants Association. (1970). Chicago, IL: American Dental Assistants Association.

Iannucci, J.M., Howerton, L.J. (2016). *Dental Radiography: Principles and Techniques*, 5th ed. St. Louis, MO: Elsevier Saunders.

Ibsen, O.A., Phelan, J. (2013). *Oral Pathology for the Dental Hygienist*, 6th ed. Philadelphia, PA: W.B. Saunders.

Ingle, J.I., Bakland, L.K. (2016). *Ingle's Endodontics*, 7th ed. Hamilton, Ontario: BC Decker Inc.

Jaroski-Graf, J. (2000). *Dental Charting: A Standard Approach*, Clifton Park, NY: Delmar Cengage Learning.

Johnson, O.N. (2011). *Essentials of Dental Radiography*, 9th ed. Stamford, CT: Pearson.

Kimbrough, Vickie J., Lautar, C.J. (2012) *Ethics, Jurisprudence, & Practice Management in Dental Hygiene*, 3rd ed. Upper Saddle River, NJ: Pearson–Prentice Hall.

Kumar, V., Cotran, R.S., Robbins, S.F. (2012). *Basic Pathology*, 9th ed. Philadelphia, PA: W.B. Saunders.

Landgland, O., Langlais, R., Preece, J. (2002). *Principles of Dental Imaging*, 2nd ed. Baltimore, MD: Lippincott Williams & Wilkins.

Langlais, R., Miller, C.S. Nield-Gehrig, J.S. (2016). *Color Atlas of Common Oral Diseases*, 5th ed. Philadelphia, PA: Lea & Febiger.

Lindh, W.Q., Pooler, M.S., Tamparo, C.D., Cerrato, J.U. (2018). *Delmar's Comprehensive Medical Assisting*, 6th ed. Clifton Park, NY: Delmar Cengage Learning.

Little, J., Falace, D., Miller, C., Rhodus, N. (2012). *Dental Management of the Medically Compromised Patient*, 8th ed. St. Louis, MO: Mosby.

Logan, B., Reynolds, P. (2016). *Color Atlas of Head and Neck Anatomy*, 5th ed. St. Louis, MO: Mosby-Wolfe.

Mahan, L.K., Raymond, J. (2016). *Krause's Food, Nutrition, and Diet Therapy*, 14th ed. Philadelphia, PA: W.B. Saunders.

Malamed, S.F. (2007). *Handbook of Medical Emergencies in the Dental Office*, 6th ed. St. Louis, MO: Mosby.

Malamed, S.F. (2012). *Handbook of Local Anesthesia*, 6th ed. St. Louis, MO: Mosby.

Malamed, S.F. (2014). *Medical Emergencies in the Dental Office*, 7th ed. St. Louis, MO: Mosby.

Miller, B., Keanne, B. (2005). *Encyclopedia and Dictionary of Medicine, Nursing, and Allied Health*, 7th ed. Philadelphia, PA: W.B. Saunders.

Miller, C.H. (2017). *Infection Control and Management of Hazardous Material for the Dental Team*, 6th ed. St. Louis, MO: Mosby.

Mosby's Dental Dictionary, 3rd ed. (2013). St. Louis, MO: Mosby Elsevier.

Mosby's Dental Drug Reference, 11th ed. (2013). St. Louis, MO: Mosby Elsevier.

Mosby's Dictionary of Medicine, Nursing & Health Professions, 10th ed. (2017). St Louis, MO: Mosby Elsevier.

Nield-Gehrig, J.S., Houseman, G.A. (2004). *Fundamentals of Periodontal Instrumentation*, 5th ed. Baltimore, MD: Williams & Wilkins.

Nielsen Nathe, C. (2017). *Dental Public Health & Research*, 4th ed. Boston, MA: Pearson Education.

Pickett, F.A., Terezhalmy, G.T. (2009). *Dental Drug Reference with Clinical Implications*, 2nd ed. Baltimore, MD: Lippincott Williams & Wilkins.

Powers, J, Wataha, J. (2016). *Dental Materials: Foundations and Applications*, 11th ed. St. Louis, MO: Mosby.

Proffit, W.R. (2012). *Contemporary Orthodontics*, 5th ed. St. Louis, MO: Mosby.

Purtilo, R. (2015). *Ethical Dimensions in the Health Professions*, 6th ed. Philadelphia, PA: Elsevier Saunders.

Regezi, J., Sciubba, J.J. (2016). *Oral Pathology: Clinical Pathologic Correlations*, 7th ed. Philadelphia, PA: W.B. Saunders.

Rizzo, D. (2016). *Delmar's Fundamentals of Anatomy & Physiology*, 4th ed. Clifton Park, NY: Delmar Cengage Learning.

Roberson, T.M., Heymann, H., Swift, E. (2012). *Sturdevant's Art and Science of Operative Dentistry*, 6th ed. St. Louis, MO: Mosby.

Robinson, D., Bird, D. (2016). *Essentials of Dental Assisting*, 6th ed. Philadelphia, PA: W.B. Saunders.

Rose, L.R. DDS, Mealey, B.L. DDS. (2004). *Periodontics Medicine, Surgery, and Implants.* St. Louis, MO: Mosby.

Rosenstiel, S.T., Land, M.F., Fujimoto, J. (2015). *Contemporary Fixed Prosthodontics*, 5th ed. St. Louis, MO: Mosby.

Sapp, P.J., Eversole, L.R., Wysocki, G.P. (2004). *Contemporary Oral and Maxillofacial Pathology*, 2nd ed. St. Louis, MO: Mosby.

Short, M.J. (2012). *Head and Neck Dental Anatomy*, 4th ed. Clifton Park, NY: Delmar Cengage Learning.

Soloman, E.P. (2015). *Introduction to Human Anatomy and Physiology*, 4th ed. Philadelphia, PA: W.B. Saunders.

Sroda, R. (2010). *Nutrition for Dental Health*, Baltimore, MD: Wolters Kluwer, Lippincott Williams & Wilkins.

Stedman's Concise Medical Dictionary for the Health Professions, 4th ed. (2003). Baltimore, MD: Williams & Wilkins.

Taber's Cyclopedic Medical Dictionary, 22nd ed. (2013). Philadelphia, PA: F.A. Davis Company.

Tamparo, C.D., Lewis, M.A. (2016). *Diseases of the Human Body*, 6th ed. Philadelphia, PA: F.A. Davis.

Ten Cate, A.R. (2012). *Oral Histology: Development, Structure, and Function*, 8th ed. St. Louis, MO: C.V. Mosby Co.

Thibodeau, G.A., Patton, K.T. (2006). *Anatomy and Physiology*, 6th ed. St. Louis, MO: Mosby.

Thibodeau, G.A., Patton, K.T. (2014). *The Human Body in Health and Disease*, 6th ed. St. Louis, MO: Mosby.

Topazin, R.G., Goldberg, M.H., Hupp, J. (2011). *Oral and Maxillofacial Infections*, 4th ed. Philadelphia, PA: W.B. Saunders.

Tyler, L., (2009). *Pearson's Comprehensive Dental Assisting.* Upper Saddle River, NJ: Pearson Education Inc.

Vernino, A., Gray, J., Hughes, E. (2007). *The Periodontic Syllabus*, 5th ed. Baltimore, MD: Williams & Wilkins.

Walton, R.E., Torabinejad, M. (2014). *Principles and Practice of Endodontics*, 5th ed. Philadelphia, PA: W.B. Saunders.

Williams, S.R. (2016). *Basic Nutrition and Diet Therapy*, 15th ed. St. Louis, MO: Mosby.

Woelfel, J.B., Scheid, R.C. (2016). *Dental Anatomy*, 9th ed. Philadelphia, PA: Lippincott Williams & Wilkins.

INDEX

Note: Page numbers followed by "f" indicate figures; page numbers followed by "t" indicate tables; page numbers followed by "b" indicate boxes; page numbers followedby "n" indicate notes.

B

C

D

F

G

H

J

K

L

N

O

P

Q

R

S

T

U

V

W

X

Y

Z